QUICK-REFERENCE INDEX

Nursing Care of Children

Nursing Care of Children

PRINCIPLES AND PRACTICE

Jean Weiler Ashwill, MSN, RN, CPNP
Director of Continuing Nursing Education
University of Texas at Arlington School of Nursing
Arlington, Texas

Formerly, Associate Professor of Nursing and
Coordinator of Maternal-Child Health
Nursing Department
Tarrant County Junior College
Fort Worth, Texas

Susan Colvert Droske, MSN, RN, CPN
Associate Professor of Nursing
Texarkana College
Texarkana, Texas

Formerly, Assistant Professor of Nursing
University of Texas at Arlington School of Nursing
Arlington, Texas

W.B. SAUNDERS COMPANY
A Division of Harcourt Brace & Company
Philadelphia London Toronto Montreal Sydney Tokyo

W.B. SAUNDERS COMPANY
A Division of Harcourt Brace & Company

The Curtis Center
Independence Square West
Philadelphia, Pennsylvania 19106

Library of Congress Cataloging-in-Publication Data

Nursing care of children : principles and practice / edited by Jean Weiler Ashwill, Susan Colvert Droske. — 1st ed.
p. cm.
ISBN 0–7216–6488–1
1. Pediatric nursing. I. Ashwill, Jean Weiler. II. Droske, Susan Colvert.
[DNLM: 1. Pediatric Nursing. WY 159 N97388 1997]
RJ245.N856 1997
610.73′62—dc20
DNLM/DLC 96–16728

Pediatric nursing is an ever-changing field. Standard safety precautions must be followed, but as new research and clinical experience broaden our knowledge, changes in treatment and drug therapy become necessary or appropriate. Readers are advised to check the product information currently provided by the manufacturer of each drug to be administered to verify the recommended dose, the method and duration of administration, and contraindications. It is the responsibility of the treating physician relying on experience and knowledge of the patient to determine dosages and the best treatment for the patient. Neither the Publisher nor the editor assumes any responsibility for any injury and/or damage to persons or property.

THE PUBLISHER

NURSING CARE OF CHILDREN: PRINCIPLES AND PRACTICE ISBN 0–7216–6488–1

Printed in the United States of America.

Last digit is the print number: 9 8 7 6 5 4 3 2 1

To my husband, Vince, who gives me love, support, and joy.

To my children, Vin, Amy, and Heidi, who taught me growth and development and whom I cherish.

To my granddaughter, Avery, who has brought awe, laughter, and pure joy into my life.

To my mother, Leona, who provided me with the gifts of trust and love.

—Jean Weiler Ashwill

With love and thanks to my husband, Terry,

and to our children, Mike, Katie, and David, who fill our home with laughter, music, and love.

With loving memories of my parents, Dr. and Mrs. J. R. Colvert, who showed me greatness.

And to my finest friend, Jesus Christ, who always sees me through.

—Susan Colvert Droske

CONTRIBUTORS

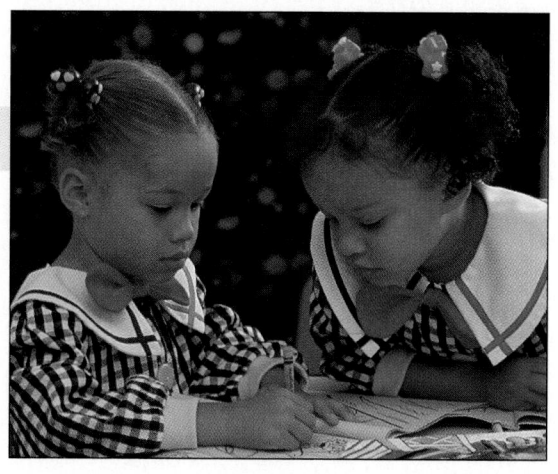

Jane A. Ahlrichs, BSN, MEd, RN
Director, Nursing Services
Pediatric Rehabilitation/Transitional Care
Children's Hospital Medical Center
Cincinnati, Ohio
Chapter 10, Communicating With Children

Susan Allen, RN, MSN
Clinical Director/Clinical Nurse Specialist
Emergency Department
Blank Children's Hospital
Des Moines, Iowa
Chapter 27, The Child With Genitourinary Alterations

Jean Weiler Ashwill, MSN, RN, CPNP
Director of Continuing Nursing Education
University of Texas at Arlington School of Nursing
Arlington, Texas
Chapter 1, Introduction to Pediatric Nursing
Chapter 9, The Child and Play
Chapter 12, Nutrition
Chapter 15, The Ill Child in the Hospital and Other Care Settings
Chapter 20, The Child in Pain
Chapter 28, The Child With an Acute Respiratory Disorder

Ann Aurigemma, RN, BS, MA
Head Nurse, Pediatrics
New York University Medical Center
New York, New York
Chapter 40, The Child With Neurologic Alterations

Karen Bernardy, RN, MSN
Child Health Consultant
Conyers, Georgia
Chapter 25, The Child With Upper Gastrointestinal Alterations
Chapter 26, The Child With Lower Gastrointestinal Alterations

Marilyn Cox Borgersen, MSN, RN
Endocrine Clinical Nurse Specialist
Children's Medical Center
Dallas, Texas
Chapter 39, The Child With Diabetes Mellitus

Susan Burkett, RN, MSN, CPNP, CPN
Administrator
T. C. Thompson Children's Hospital
Chattanooga, Tennessee
Chapter 32, The Child With Hematologic Alterations
Chapter 33, The Child With Cancer

Nancy H. Busen, PhD, RN, C-FNP
Associate Professor of Nursing
Coordinator, Graduate Pediatric Nurse Practitioner Program
University of Texas Houston Health Science Center
School of Nursing
Houston, Texas
Chapter 8, The Adolescent

Dolores W. Clark, RN, BSN, MSN, FNP
Specialist
University of Texas at Arlington School of Nursing
Arlington, Texas
Advanced Pediatric Nurse
Community Oriented Primary Care Clinic
Parkland Memorial Hospital
Dallas, Texas
Chapter 11, Physical Assessment

Joan Marie Cutrone, BSN, MA, RN
Head Nurse, Neonatal ICU
New York University Medical Center
New York, New York
Chapter 40, The Child With Neurologic Alterations

Bernadette Daborn, RN, MA
Head Nurse, Pediatrics
New York University Medical Center
New York, New York
Chapter 40, The Child With Neurologic Alterations

Kimberly L. Davies, BS, RN, CEN
Pediatric Trauma Coordinator
Children's Medical Center of Dallas
Dallas, Texas
Chapter 13, Safety

Susan Colvert Droske, MSN, RN, CPN
Associate Professor of Nursing
Texarkana College
Texarkana, Texas
Chapter 1, Introduction to Pediatric Nursing
Chapter 5, The Toddler
Chapter 6, The Preschool Child
Chapter 7, The School-Age Child
Chapter 29, The Child With Chronic Respiratory Alterations
Chapter 34, The Child With Integumentary Alterations

Dallas Estey, RNC, MSN
Neonatal Nurse Practitioner
Woman's Hospital
Baton Rouge, Louisiana
Chapter 21, The High-Risk Neonate

Joan Holter Gildea, MA, RNC
Clinical Assistant Director of Nursing
New York University Medical Center
New York, New York
Chapter 40, The Child With Neurologic Alterations

Judith W. Gross, PhD, RN
Assistant Professor
College of Nursing
Medical University of South Carolina
Charleston, South Carolina
Chapter 36, The Child With Musculoskeletal Alterations
Chapter 37, The Child With Structural Disorders of the Bones and Joints

Julie F. Gwin, BSN, RN, MN
Assistant Professor
Department of Nursing
Tarrant County Junior College
Staff Nurse
Cook Children's Medical Center
Fort Worth, Texas
Chapter 22, The Child With an Infectious Disease

Deborah Parkman Henderson, PhD, RN
Lecturer
UCLA School of Medicine
University of California Los Angeles
Harbor–UCLA Medical Center
Torrance, California
Chapter 14, Emergency Care of the Child and Family

Jill Howie-Stites, RN, MN
Nurse Practitioner
Children's Hospital of Orange County
Orange, California
Chapter 38, The Child With Endocrine Alterations

Sylvia H. Imhoff, RN, MSN, JD
Attorney
Slack & Davis
Austin, Texas
Chapter 1, Introduction to Pediatric Nursing

Stephen Jones, MS, RNC, PNP, ET
Assistant Professor
Clinical Nursing Education
Albany Medical College
Albany, New York
Adjunct Clinical Instructor
Russell Sage College
Troy, New York
Chapter 24, The Child With Fluid and Electrolyte Alterations

Kathleen A. Koszarek, RNC, MSN
Neonatal Nurse Practitioner
Ochsner Foundation Hospital
New Orleans, Louisiana
Chapter 21, The High-Risk Neonate

Melva Kravitz, PhD, RN
Director, Research & Education
Division of Nursing
Yale–New Haven Hospital
Associate Professor
Yale School of Nursing
New Haven, Connecticut
Chapter 35, The Child With Burns

Gwendolyn T. Martin, RN, BSN, MSN, CNS, CPN
Pediatric Coordinator
Community Hospice of Texas
Fort Worth, Texas
Chapter 17, The Child With a Chronic or Terminal Illness

Sharon M. McLeod, MS, CCLS, CTRS
Director, Child Life Department
Children's Hospital Medical Center
Cincinnati, Ohio
Chapter 10, Communicating With Children

Michele Michael, PhD, CRNP
Assistant Professor
School of Nursing
University of Maryland
Baltimore, Maryland
Chapter 36, The Child With Musculoskeletal Alterations

Maribeth Moran, MSN, RN, CPN
Assistant Professor
College of Nursing
University of Oklahoma
Oklahoma City, Oklahoma
Chapter 2, Growth and Development
Chapter 4, The Infant

Donna Nash Parnell, RN, BSN, MNSc
Trauma Coordinator
Arkansas Children's Hospital
Little Rock, Arkansas
Chapter 18, Application of Nursing Principles to Pediatrics

Therese L. Polacek, RN, MSN, CPNP
Assistant Professor
College of St. Scholastica
Duluth, Minnesota
Chapter 31, The Child With Cardiovascular Alterations

Mary C. Rathlev, RN, MSN
Program Manager
Project CHAMP (Children's HIV/AIDS Model Program)
Children's National Medical Center
Washington, District of Columbia
Chapter 23, The Child With Immunologic Alterations

Leslie M. Reed, RN, MSN
Renal Transplant Nurse Specialist
Children's Mercy Hospital
Kansas City, Missouri
Chapter 27, The Child With Genitourinary Alterations

Janice G. Sample, BSN, MNSc, CNRN
Certified Neuroscience Registered Nurse
American Association of Neuroscience Nurses
Assistant Professor
Texarkana College
Texarkana, Texas
Chapter 40, The Child With Neurologic Alterations

Anne Scott, PhD, RN
Per Diem Staff Nurse-Pediatrics
Bulloch Memorial Hospital
Director of Nursing Research
Associate Professor
Georgia Southern University
Statesboro, Georgia
Chapter 16, Family-Centered Nursing Care

Mary Ellen Sheldon, RNC, MA, CCRN
Pediatric Staff Development Instructor
New York University Medical Center
New York, New York
Chapter 40, The Child With Neurologic Alterations

Nedra Skale, MS, MJ, RN, CNA
Nurse Associate
Midwest Orthopaedics
Chicago, Illinois
Chapter 40, The Child With Neurologic Alterations

Dotty Volz, RN, MSN
Clinical Nurse Specialist
T. C. Thompson Children's Hospital
Chattanooga, Tennessee
CEO, Dotty Volz & Associates
Hixson, Tennessee
Chapter 15, The Ill Child in the Hospital and Other Care Settings

Brenda J. Wagner, RN, BSN, MSN, PhD
Clinical Psychologist
Scottish Rite Children's Medical Center
Atlanta, Georgia
Chapter 41, The Child With a Psychosocial Disorder
Chapter 42, The Child With a Cognitive Deficit

Anne Weir, RNP, C, MSN
Clinical Instructor
Arkansas Children's Hospital
Little Rock, Arkansas
Chapter 3, The Newborn
Chapter 19, Medicating Infants and Children
Chapter 43, The Child With Sensory Alterations

Sharon Whalen, RN, MS
Clinical Nurse Specialist
Huntington Beach, California
Chapter 14, Emergency Care of the Child and Family

Vicki L. Zeigler, RN, MSN
Pediatric Arrhythmia Case Manager
Cardiology Department
Cook Children's Medical Center
Forth Worth, Texas
Chapter 30, The Child With Congenital Cardiac Defects

REVIEWERS

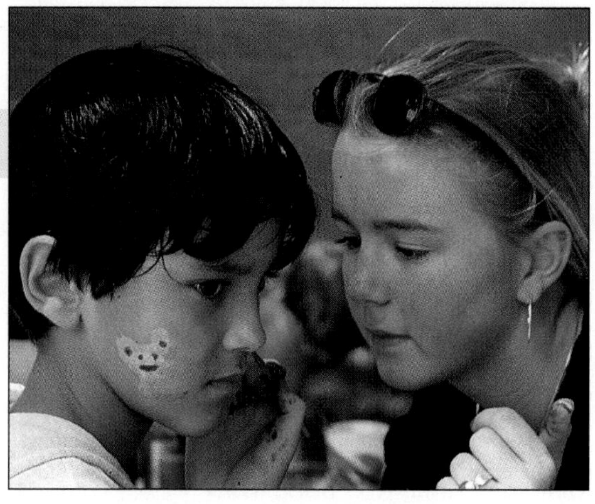

Stephanie S. Allen, MS, RN, CNS
Baylor University School of Nursing
Children's Medical Center of Dallas
Southwestern Medical School
Dallas, Texas

Lisa Anderson-Shaw, RN, C, MSN, MA
University of Illinois at Chicago Medical Center
University of Illinois at Chicago College of Nursing
Chicago, Illinois

Betty L. Ashe, MSN, RN, C
School of Nursing
Mississippi Gulf Coast Community College
Gulfport, Mississippi

Pamela A. Bachmeyer, PhD, CPNP, RN
School of Nursing
Chicago State University
Chicago, Illinois

Sherry D. Baker, BSN, RNC, CPN
Nursing Department
Hillcrest Baptist Medical Center
Waco, Texas

Corazon B. Barbon, MSN, RN, C, CCRN
Department of Education and Standards
Columbia Presbyterian Medical Center
New York, New York

Lynn C. Barnhart, RN, MSN
School of Nursing
Cameron University
Lawton, Oklahoma

Louise S. Barton, BA, BSN, RN
Nursing Department, Pediatrics
Rose Medical Center
Denver, Colorado

Mary M. Bartos, RN, BSN, MSN
Nursing Department
St. Luke's Medical Center
Cleveland, Ohio

Celine M. Belling, RN, BSN, CNOR
Nursing Department
The Children's Hospital of Buffalo
Buffalo, New York

Lisa Marie Bernardo, RN, PhD, CEN
Children's Hospital of Pittsburgh
School of Nursing
University of Pittsburgh
Pittsburgh, Pennsylvania

Patricia Bielecki, RNC, MS
Nursing Department
Resurrection Medical Center
Chicago, Illinois

Kathy R. Birt, RNC
Nursing Department
Mother Frances Hospital
Tyler, Texas

Shawn Renee Brekke, RN, RNCPN, BSN, FNP, MSN
Nursing Department
Hoag Memorial Hospital Presbyterian
Newport Beach, California

Sandra L. Brisendine, MSN, ARNP, CNS, FNP, RN
School of Nursing
Seward County Community College
Liberal, Kansas

Bonita E. Broyles, RN, BSN, EdD
School of Nursing
Piedmont Community College
Roxboro, North Carolina

Maureen Cahill, RN, BSN, MSN
Nursing Department
Rush Medical Center
Chicago, Illinois

Judith R. Campsey, BSN, MEd, MNEd, RNC
Nursing Department
The Washington Hospital
Washington, Pennsylvania

Rebecca Coffey, RN, MSN
Nursing Department
Ohio State University Hospitals
Columbus, Ohio

Elizabeth Conklin, RN, BSN, MN
School of Nursing
Orangeburg-Calhoun Technical College
Orangeburg, South Carolina

Gretchen R. Cornell, RN, PhD
School of Nursing
Northeast Missouri State University
Kirksville, Missouri

Genean Crosby, RN
JPS Health Network
Fort Worth, Texas

Diane L. Davis, BSN, MSN
Department of Health & Human Services
Washington, DC

Elizabeth Ann Deaton, RN, MSN
School of Nursing
Cape Fear Community College
Wilmington, North Carolina

Caryn E. Decker, MSN, RN, CPNP, CDE
Nursing Department
James Whitcomb Riley Hospital for Children
Indianapolis, Indiana

Deborah M. Dee, RN, CPNP
Mercy Hospital of Buffalo
School of Nursing
University of Buffalo
Buffalo, New York

Lisa L. Depperman, BSN, RN, C
Nursing Department
A.O. Fox Memorial Hospital
Oneonta, New York

Anne M. Desmond, RN, MN, CPN
Nursing Department
Medical College of Georgia
Athens, Georgia

Kathleen Doering, RN, MN, ET
School of Nursing
Hawaii Community College
School of Nursing
University of Hawaii
Kealakekua, Hawaii

Carol L. Doubblestein, RN, MSN
School of Nursing
Grand Rapids Community College
Grand Rapids, Michigan

Beth S. Dullanty, RN, C, BSN
Nursing Department
Sacred Heart Medical Center
Spokane, Washington

Carol E. Elmer, RN, MSN
School of Nursing
Henderson Community College, Henderson, Kentucky
University of Kentucky, Lexington, Kentucky

Denise D. Estridge, RN, BSN, MPH
School of Nursing
Guilford Technical Community College
Jamestown, North Carolina

Salva Failla, RN, BSN, MN, DNS
School of Nursing
Louisiana State University Medical Center
New Orleans, Louisiana

Linda R. Franck, MS, RN, C
Nursing Department
Upper Valley Medical Centers
Troy, Ohio

Diane E. Fritsch, RN, MSN, CCRN, CS
Nursing Department
MetroHealth Medical Center
Cleveland, Ohio

Barbara Gerwatosky, RN, C
Nursing Department
Martin Luther Hospital
Anaheim, California

Linda Howard Glenn, RN, C, MN
Nursing Department
Friendly Hills Healthcare Network
La Habra, California

Sharon K. Grider, RN, BS, MSN
Nursing Department
St. Elizabeth's Hospital
Belleville, Illinois

Lynn Rice Grommet, RNC, MNSc
School of Nursing
East Arkansas Community College
Forrest City, Arkansas

Cynthia L. Grubbs, MNSc, RN, CS, FNP/PNP
Nursing Department
Family Health Center
Battle Creek, Michigan

C. Magee Grundmann, RN, BSN
Cook Children's Medical Center
Fort Worth, Texas

Lisa R. Guerrieri, RN, C, BSN, MBA
Nursing Department
Hospital of St. Raphael
New Haven, Connecticut

Mary Gustafsson, RN, AS
Nursing Department
Community Hospital of Monterey Peninsula
Monterey, California

Mary Hagedorn, RN, PhD, CS
The Children's Hospital
School of Nursing
University of Colorado
Denver, Colorado

Betty W. Hamlisch, RN, BSN, MS
School of Nursing
Tompkins-Cortland Community College
Dryden, New York

Kirsten Sueppel Hanrahan, RN, MA, CPNP
Nursing Department
University of Iowa Hospitals and Clinics
Iowa City, Iowa

Mary Katherine Bourgeois Harris, RN, MSN, CFNP
Nursing Department
Kaiser Permanente
Huntington Beach, California

Margaret J. Harvey, RN, MSN
School of Nursing
Ravenswood Hospital Medical Center
Chicago, Illinois

Amy Zlomek Hedden, RN, MS, CNS, NP
School of Nursing
California State University Bakersfield
Bakersfield Family Medical Center
Bakersfield, California

Jule Anne D. Henstenburg, MS, RD
Department of Medical Affairs
Wyeth-Ayerst Laboratories
St. Davids, Pennsylvania

Sandra Herliczek-Lebow, MS, RN
Nursing Department
Berkshire Medical Center
Pittsfield, Massachusetts

Sally Higgins, RN, PhD, FAAN
School of Nursing
University of San Francisco
Nursing Department
Children's Hospital of Oakland
Oakland, California

Nancy G. Hinzman, RNC, BSN, MSN
School of Nursing
Northern Kentucky University
Highland Heights, Kentucky

Judy L. Hollingsworth, MSN, RN
School of Nursing
Indiana University
Nursing Department
Riley Hospital for Children
Indianapolis, Indiana

Mary Ellen Howell, RNC, MN
School of Nursing
Florence Darlington Technical College
Florence, South Carolina

Mary L. Jackson, RN
Cook Children's Medical Center
Fort Worth, Texas

Nancy Kadavy-Clark, BSN, RNC, NNP
Nursing Department
Foster G. McGraw Hospital
School of Nursing
Loyola University at Chicago Medical Center
Maywood, Illinois

Kelly A. Keefe, MSN, RN, CS
Nursing Department
Maimonides Medical Center
Brooklyn, New York

Jeanene Kelly, RNC, MS, CNS
Nursing Department
Hillcrest Baptist Medical Center
Waco, Texas

Patti M. Kendall, RN
School of Nursing
Decatur Memorial Hospital
Nursing Department
Sarah Bush Lincoln Health Center
Mattoon, Illinois

Mary T. Kenney, BSN, RN
Nursing Department
Cleveland Clinic Foundation
Cleveland, Ohio

Joan Marie Ketchur, RN, BSN, MSN
School of Nursing
Cape Fear Community College
Wilmington, North Carolina

Susan Kitchell, RNC, MS, PNP
Nursing Department
Kaiser Permanente Medical Center
San Francisco, California

Debra L. Klein, RN, BSN
Nursing Department
Hahnemann University Hospital
Philadelphia, Pennsylvania

Suzan C. Knoblauch, RN, MS
School of Nursing
St. Francis College of Nursing
Peoria, Illinois

Linda S. Kocent, RN, MSN, CCRN
Nursing Department
Thomas Jefferson University Hospital
Philadelphia, Pennsylvania

Patricia Koren-Robinson, BSN, MSN, RN
School of Nursing
Mercy Hospital
Pittsburgh, Pennsylvania

Martha D. Krull, BS, MS, CCLS
Nursing Department
Cook Children's Medical Center
Fort Worth, Texas

Janet Kuhn, EdD, RN
School of Nursing
Villanova University
Haverford, Pennsylvania

Audrey J. LaPenta, BSN, MA, RN, C
Charles E. Gregory School of Nursing
Raritan Bay Medical Center
Perth Amboy, New Jersey

Maureen Lancellot, MBA, MSN, RN
Nursing Department
Broward General Medical Center
Fort Lauderdale, Florida

Margo E. Layman, RN, MSN, RNC, CNA
Nursing Department
Clinton County Hospital
Frankfort, Indiana

Glenda Le Maitre, RN, C, MSN
School of Nursing
University of the District of Columbia
Washington, DC

Mary F. Lepley, RN, MSN, CNP
Nursing Department
St. Elizabeth Hospital
Chicago, Illinois
School of Nursing
Triton College
River Grove, Florida

Rose Mary Leppert, RN, BSN
Nursing Department
Memorial Hospital of Bedford County
Everett, Pennsylvania

Mira L. Lessick, PhD, RN
Rush University College of Nursing
Chicago, Illinois

Ann M. Lupica, RN, C
Nursing Department
Morton Hospital and Medical Center
Taunton, Massachusetts

Janetta R. McFarland, RN, BSN, MSN, CPNP
Citizens General Hospital School of Nursing
New Kensington, Pennsylvania

Sharon A. Mandell, RN, BSN
School of Nursing
Springfield Technical Community College
Springfield, Massachusetts

Theresa Marvelli, RN, C, BSN, MA
Nursing Department
Maimonides Medical Center
Brooklyn, New York

Georgiann Massa, RN, MSN
Nursing Department
Cleveland Clinic Foundation
Cleveland, Ohio

Sandra S. Mattox, RN, BSN, OCN
School of Nursing
University of Arkansas for Medical Sciences
Little Rock, Arkansas

Cindy Matyus, RN, BSN, BA
Nursing Department
Easton Hospital
Easton, Pennsylvania

Linda M. Mayer, RN, MSN
School of Nursing
Umpqua Community College
Roseburg, Oregon

Ann F. Mead, RN, MN, GPN
School of Nursing
Mississippi Gulf Coast Community College
Gulfport, Mississippi

Ellen Meeropol, RN, MS
Nursing Department
Shriners Hospital
Springfield, Massachusetts

Carmella Mikol, RNC, MN, CPNP
School of Nursing
College of Lake County
Grayslake, Illinois

Patricia Dillon Montpas, RN, BSN, MSN, EdD
School of Nursing
Mott Community College
Flint, Michigan

Martha J. Morrow, RN, MSN, PhDC
School of Nursing
Shenandoah University
Winchester, Virginia

Carole T. Murtha, RN, BSN, MA
School of Nursing
Gloucester County College
Sewell, New Jersey

Tracey R. Neff, BSN, RN, PHN
Nursing Department
Kaweah Delta District Hospital
Visalia, California

Roseanne Ellen Nolan, RN, BSN
Nursing Department
Parkland Memorial Hospital
Dallas, TX

Ruth Novitt-Schumacher, RN, MSN
School of Nursing
University of Illinois at Chicago
Chicago, Illinois

Jane O'Donnell, RN, BSN, MSN
School of Nursing
Ocean County College
Toms River, New Jersey

Nancy O'Donnell, RN, BSN, MSN
J. Sergeant Reynolds Community College
School of Nursing
Medical College of Virginia Hospital
Richmond, Virginia

Maureen T. O'Hara, RN, MS, CNS
School of Nursing
University Hospital–State University of New York
Syracuse, New York

Netha O'Meara, RN, MSN
School of Nursing
Wharton County Junior College
Wharton, Texas

Mary O'Pray, RN, C, PhD
School of Nursing
Santa Fe Community College
Gainesville, Florida

Bobbie J. Williams Ogg, BSN, RN
School of Nursing
Houston Baptist University
Houston, Texas

Susan Rearden, RN
Cook Children's Medical Center
Fort Worth, Texas

Nancy E. Rooker, RNC, MS
School of Nursing
Elgin Community College
Elgin, Illinois

Maureen T. Rorke, RN, MSN, CCRN
Schneider Children's Hospital
Nursing Department
Long Island Jewish Medical Center
New Hyde Park, New York

Patricia A. Rowland, RN, BSN
Consultant
Boardman, Ohio

Rose A. Runnels, BSN, RN
Nursing Department
Wilford Hall Medical Center
San Antonio, Texas

Teresa A. Savage, PhD (C), MS, BSN, RN
Rush University College of Nursing
Chicago, Illinois

Amy Sintros, BSN, MS, RNC
The Cheshire Medical Center
Keene, New Hampshire
Nursing Department
Monadnock Community Hospital
Peterborough, New Hampshire

Patricia Soran, RN, MS
School of Nursing
Boise State University
Boise, Idaho

Beth A. Speckhart, RN, MS, OCN, CPON
Nursing Department
St. Jude Midwest Affiliate, Children's Hospital of Illinois
Peoria, Illinois

Geralyn R. Spollett, MSN, C-ANP, CDE
Yale University School of Medicine
Yale-New Haven Hospital, Nursing Department
New Haven, Connecticut

Nikki Spriggs, RN
Nursing Department
Arkansas Children's Hospital
Little Rock, Arkansas

Jodie Stabinski, RN, BS, CCRN
Nursing Department
Penn State University Children's Hospital
Hershey, Pennsylvania

LuAnn Starzynski, BSN, RNC
Nursing Department
Mercy Hospital of Buffalo
Buffalo, New York

Patricia A. Sullivan, RN, CPN, BSN, MS
Nursing Department
Holy Name Hospital
Teaneck, New Jersey

Patricia R. Teasley, MSN, RN, CS
School of Nursing
Columbus College
Columbus, Georgia

Nancy Thornton, RN, MSN
Nursing Department
British Columbia's Children's Hospital
Vancouver, British Columbia CANADA

Roselena Thorpe, RN, PhD
School of Nursing
Community College of Allegheny County
Pittsburgh, Pennsylvania

Joyce R. Tiede, BSN, RN
Nursing Department
The William W. Backus Hospital
Norwich, Connecticut

Beverley Tipsord-Klinkhammer, RN, MS, CEN
Nursing Department
MacNeal Hospital
Berwyn, Illinois

Paula Dunn Tropello, MN, RN, C, CNS, ACCE
Elizabeth General School of Nursing Cooperative Program with Union County College
Elizabeth, New Jersey

Donna G. Truesdell, MS, RNC
Nursing Department
Franklin Medical Center
Greenfield, Massachusetts

Susan Valentin-Cubing, RNC, MS, CNS
Nursing Department
California Pacific Medical Center
San Francisco, California

Janice I. Vanderlaan, RN, MSN
School of Nursing
Stephen F. Austin State University
Nacogdoches, Texas

Carole J. Petrosky Vozel, RN, C, PhD
Western Pennsylvania Hospital School of Nursing
Pittsburgh, Pennsylvania

Frances S. Wall, RN, MN
Providence General Medical Center
Everett, Washington

Geraldine Walsh, RNC, MA, CNS, PNP
Beth Israel Medical Center
New York, New York

Kathy Washburn, RNC, MSN
Nursing Department
Mount Sinai Medical Center
Miami Beach, Florida

Linda Waters, MSN, RN, C
Nursing Department
Columbia-Presbyterian Medical Center
New York, New York

Nancy Ruth West, MN, BSN, RN
School of Nursing
Johnson County Community College
Overland Park, Kansas

Shannon E. West-Buxton, RN, MS, CNS
Nursing Department
Baystate Medical Center Children's Hospital
Springfield, Massachusetts

Julia C. Whelan, RN, BSN, MN
School of Nursing
Ocean County College
Toms River, New Jersey

Susan Karm Wieczorek, RN, MSN
Health Education Consulting Institute
Fortson, Georgia

Catherine L. Witt, RNC, MS, NNP
University of Colorado Health Sciences Center, School of Nursing
Presbyterian St. Luke's Medical Center, Nursing Department
Denver, Colorado

Jodi Young, MSN, NNP, PNP
Nursing Department
St. Peters Medical Center
New Brunswick, New Jersey
School of Nursing
Columbia University
New York, New York

Susan C. Zappa, RN, CPN, CPON
Nursing Department
Cook Children's Medical Center
Fort Worth, Texas

PREFACE

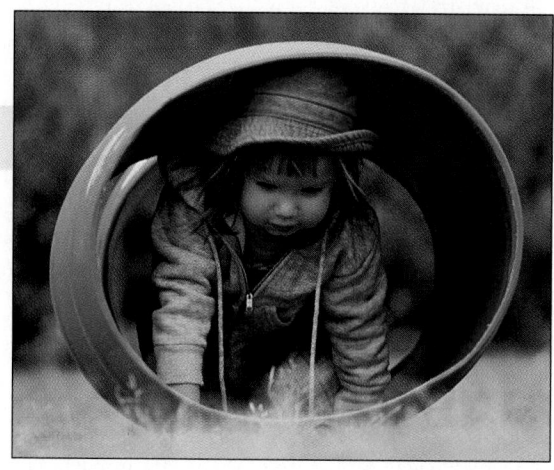

There is nothing more precious than a child, and nothing more rewarding than caring for the health of children and their families. Holding a child, talking softly, singing with a child, playing with a child—all are a part of pediatric nursing. Hugging a parent, explaining a procedure or a disease, sitting quietly with a parent, or providing reassurance through quiet, competent care can literally change the way a parent acts or reacts to his or her child's illness.

High-quality pediatric nursing care combines compassion with the most up-to-date clinical knowledge grounded in the basic principles of pediatric nursing care. In our years of teaching, we have found that nursing students are often overwhelmed by the amount of information they are expected to absorb while studying pediatric nursing. As technology and scientific research add to the amount of information available, students find it difficult to sort out that which is most important. As pediatric nursing instructors we have looked for tools to help students focus on commonalities, underlying principles, main points, and the most essential information—both for today's clinical experience and as preparation for a lifetime of professional practice. ***Nursing Care of Children: Principles and Practice*** was written to fulfill this need.

This text was also written to address contemporary changes in health care, in order to meet the needs of the pediatric nursing student preparing to practice into the next century. Because health care costs have led to shorter hospital stays and a shift to health care provided in the community and the home, ***Nursing Care of Children*** provides a strong focus on the growing and changing roles of nurses caring for children in varied settings. The text's emphasis on health and wellness is revealed in a comprehensive unit covering growth and development, with anticipatory guidance for families. Teaching guidelines provided throughout the text assist students to teach parents and children about home care, self-care, preventive care, and follow-up care.

PRINCIPLES OF PEDIATRIC NURSING

The foundation principles of pediatric nursing we identify for students in this text are as follows:

- *Growth and development,* with a strong emphasis on anticipatory guidance provided at each developmental stage. Individual chapters discuss a concept (play, pain, illness, etc.), and help a student apply it to each age group. Each of the growth and development chapters provides a review of physical and psychosocial changes unique to that age group, with an emphasis on the nurse's role. Health promotion in each chapter prepares students for parent teaching, ambulatory care, and home care.
- *Family*—The nurse must care for the child within the context of the family. In this text, emphasis is placed on the importance of focusing on the family in caring for children of all ages and in many different settings. Changing family structure and diversity in types of families are considered. Parent teaching boxes and home care are directed toward the child's family. Special sections are devoted to the needs of siblings.
- *Health promotion*—Concepts of health promotion provide the theoretical base that students need about important aspects of the health of children: nutrition, safety, parenting, assessment, self-esteem, communication, immunizations, and play.
- *Child advocacy*—Legal and ethical responsibilities of nurses are identified and explained in such areas as violence, abuse, neglect, drug abuse, and access to health care.
- *Communication*—Tips and techniques are offered to enhance therapeutic communication with children and families and to facilitate client teaching. An entire chapter is devoted to communicating with children. Throughout the book communication cues assist the student in applying principles of communication.

- *Concepts and skills*—These are the chapters in Unit II that guide students as they discover what is different, what is special about caring for infants and children. Within these chapters students study nutrition, play, pain, emergency care, medicating the pediatric patient, assessment, procedures, and other concepts and skills pertaining to pediatric nursing.

Organization of the Text

The text uses an objective-oriented approach that makes it easy for students to understand and retain important material. Nursing care is organized by the nursing process because of the ability to teach easily using a problem-solving method.

The text is presented in four units:

Unit I, Introduction to Pediatric Nursing, offers an insightful overview of contemporary pediatric nursing.

Unit II, Growth and Development: The Child and the Family, contains seven comprehensive chapters which cover child growth and development, from the neonatal period through adolescence. Chapter 2, an overview, discusses the stages and principles of growth and development, as well as theories, influencing factors, assessment methods, and the nurse's role in promoting optimal growth and development. Six subsequent chapters cover normal growth and development and anticipatory guidance for the family, in relation to both developmental milestones and health promotion. *Summary of Growth and Development* tables and *Health Screening, Health Maintenance and Anticipatory Guidance* tables in Chapters 4 through 8 consolidate the information for quick reference and review. These chapters reflect contemporary issues affecting children, such as violence, stress, and poverty.

In **Unit III, Special Considerations in Caring for Children** are presented in twelve chapters that provide students with a solid foundation for understanding children's needs. These chapters feature in-depth coverage, with complete chapters on important topics such as play, communication, nutrition, safety, emergency care, administration of medications, and pain management. Separate comprehensive chapters also discuss physical assessment, care of the hospitalized child, adapting nursing procedures to children, and care of the child with a chronic condition.

Unit IV, Caring for Children With Health Problems, is an extensive unit of twenty-three thorough chapters covering the care of children with alterations in health.

Presentation of material has been designed to promote learning. For example, Unit IV contains colored Clinical Reference Pages to visually separate reference material from narrative text. The Clinical Reference Pages serve two purposes—they make review material, medication tables, and laboratory test tables easy to locate, and they make the narrative pages easier to read by separating out reference material.

The greatest amount of discussion is devoted to the major and the most common disorders of childhood and adolescence. We have chosen these carefully, consulting with many clinicians and educators, to reflect what students will encounter most often, what is statistically most prevalent, and what presents the best opportunities for teaching nursing care. Major disorders include full text discussion and detailed, two-column Nursing Care Plans focusing on helping students understand the thought process involved in planning and evaluating. NANDA-approved diagnoses, expected outcomes, interventions with rationales, and evaluation statements are included, as are Teaching Guidelines for hospital and home care as appropriate.

Narrative coverage of other important childhood disorders is consistently organized in a nursing process format, again with NANDA diagnoses, expected outcomes, and evaluation questions. Less common disorders are grouped and discussed in tables in each body system chapter.

PEDAGOGICAL FEATURES

- The most important points for students to remember are highlighted throughout the text in red boxes.
- Guidance on effective communication with parents and with children at various ages is highlighted in tan *Communication Boxes* throughout the text.
- *Clinical Reference Pages* throughout Unit IV provide easy-to-locate reference and review sections. Anatomy and physiology, pediatric differences, related laboratory and diagnostic tests, and commonly prescribed medications are highlighted in the Clinical Reference Pages.
- *Pathophysiology Boxes* explain changes in physiology occurring in a variety of diseases and disorders in children. This concise presentation of altered function provides the specific disease-related foundation that the student needs to care for sick children and adolescents.
- Photo stories are used effectively to capture student interest and to provide exposure to a variety of nursing settings and roles.
- *Teaching Guidelines* boxes guide the student in teaching the parent and child about self-care, preventive care, and follow-up care.
- Organizational aids are used liberally in each chapter. A Chapter Overview in outline format with page num-

bers identifies key content, along with specific tables and boxes, at the beginning of each chapter. Learning Objectives tie in with the Key Concept summary at the end of the chapter. Key Terms with definitions begin each chapter, and a comprehensive glossary is provided for the entire book.

Original full-color artwork and photography illustrate the text generously. Each illustration has been chosen to provide maximum information in minimum space. Illustrations reinforce knowledge of growth and development, explain pathophysiology, make learning procedures easier, show manifestations of diseases and disorders, and provide models of interactions with patients and families.

ANCILLARIES

Complements to the text include the *Clinical Companion to Accompany Nursing Care of Children,* a compact source of essential information featuring an alphabetical listing of disorders and essential lab values, medications, and other clinical reference material in an easy-to carry, pocket-sized format.

The *Study Guide to Accompany Nursing Care of Children,* provides an overview of anticipated learning, helpful hints of topics learned from other courses, learning exercises and activities, critical thinking exercises with case studies, and multiple choice review questions.

Ancillaries available to educators include the *Instructor's Manual to Accompany Nursing Care of Children,* which provides convenient outlines to assist in lecture preparation, ideas for clinical and classroom learning activities, and audiovisual resources. A printed Test Bank and a computerized version, ExaMaster, which provide the educator with a variety of testing options, are available to qualified adopters, as is a package of 40 full-color acetate transparencies to enhance classroom presentation.

In summary, ***Nursing Care of Children: Principles and Practice*** offers a fresh, contemporary approach to the teaching of pediatric nursing. By careful choice of content and expert contributors, we believe this text balances the need for comprehensive coverage with the need for focused learning. The student is guided through pediatric nursing by building on previous knowledge, reviewing key information and concepts, and focusing on underlying principles. We believe that, in practice, the nurse who has an understanding of the principles of care can more readily think critically and apply those principles in any clinical situation.

As educators we owe our students guidance, nurturing, and support as they experience the challenge of pediatric nursing. One way we can do this is by providing learning materials that support and strengthen their ability and desire to read and learn; we hope we can share with you the enthusiasm and pleasure of teaching through ***Nursing Care of Children: Principles and Practice.***

Jean Weiler Ashwill, MSN, RN, CPNP
Susan Colvert Droske, MSN, RN, CPN

ACKNOWLEDGMENTS

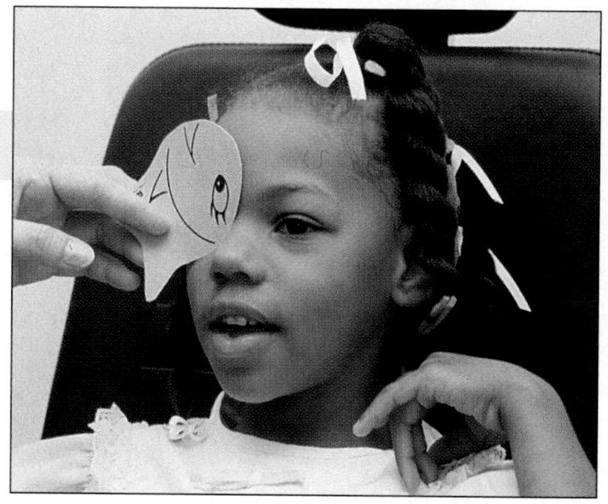

Writing ***Pediatric Nursing: Principles and Practice*** was a group effort. We would like to thank our families and friends who supported us by understanding when we were unavailable and encouraging us when we were overwhelmed.

We express our sincere appreciation to the clinicians, experts in their fields, who contributed to the book. They provided the up-to-date clinical information needed in a teaching text. We appreciate their many hours of research, writing, and rewriting. Friendships have developed from working with these professionals (their names are listed on pages vii–ix).

Educators and clinicians reviewed our manuscripts and provided valuable input and insight into each chapter (their names are listed on pages xi–xvii). Bonita Broyles, RN, BSN, EdD, reviewed the book and also provided many helpful comments while writing the Clinical Companion which accompanies the text. We also would like to express warm appreciation to J. R. Colvert, Jr., MD, Terry Droske, DDS, and Littleton Fowler, OD, for their manuscript review, helpful comments, and encouragement.

A special thank you to Emily McKinney, MSN, CRN, who put many miles on her car, spent hours looking at file pictures generously provided by William Benge, and, together with Wayne Eppstein, photographer, provided photographs from the Dallas–Fort Worth area. We would also like to thank Cook Children's Medical Center in Fort Worth, Texas, and Parkland Memorial Hospital in Dallas, Texas, who very generously allowed us access to their photo files and allowed us to take photographs on their premises. Dottie Volz, RNC, MSN, CPNP, and Jim Dove, photographer, collaborated to provide additional photographs, with the cooperation of T. C. Thomson Children's Hospital and Siskin Hospital for Physical Rehabilitation, both in Chattanooga, Tennessee. Judith W. Gross, PhD, RN, provided the spica cast photo story, with the cooperation of Nicole and her family and the Medical University of South Carolina in Charleston, South Carolina. The staff at each of the above-mentioned facilities went out of their way to assist us in obtaining the specific pictures we needed. We also thank Mark Patterson and Randall Brown, RN, for the photographs they provided.

Sandra Sevigny, medical illustrator, worked with the contributors and us to create the most realistic illustrations. Her ability to bring life to an illustration is evident in the children portrayed in her work.

A special thanks to the many children, parents, and nurses who posed for the pictures. Dolores Clark, who contributed the physical assessment chapter, coordinated many of the physical assessment and growth and development pictures taken at The University of Texas at Arlington, Arlington, Texas. She also provided children and grandchildren for the long day of picture taking. Gwen Martin, MSN, RN, who contributed Chapter 17, also provided some photographs via *Children's Promise*/Cook Children's Medical Center, as well as some children's drawings that appear in the book.

Ilze Rader, Senior Nursing Editor at W. B. Saunders, nurtured the idea of a more student-friendly text and guided us as we developed the plan for such a text. She assisted us in defining the core of the book and inspired us to be creative as the project took hold.

Rosanne Hallowell joined the project as Developmental Editor and used her quiet, calm manner to guide us through the critical process of putting it all together. She was always just a phone call away when any question or concern arose.

Marie Thomas and Rachel Hubbs, Editorial Assistants at W. B. Saunders Company, spent many persuasive hours on the phone arranging for educators and clinicians to review chapters. Joan Sinclair, Production Manager at W. B. Saunders, along with P. M. Gordon Associates, handled the many details involved in copy-editing and typesetting the text, and merging words and pictures into a cohesive whole.

Finally, a thank you to all of our students and all the children and their families who have taught us what pediatric nursing is really about.

CONTENTS

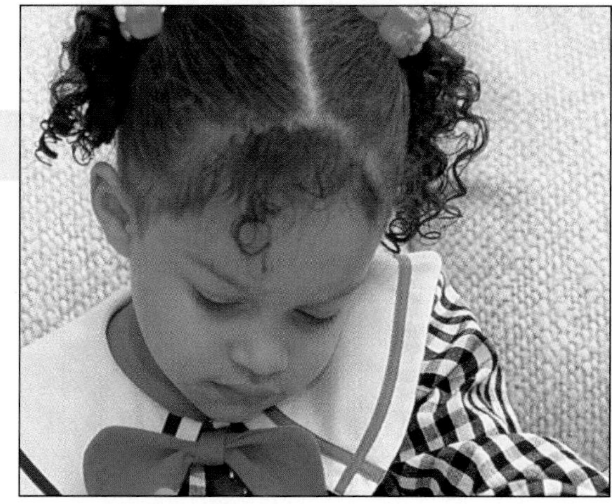

Note: Detailed Nursing Care Plans within chapters are indicated by boldface entries in the contents.

28 The Child With an Acute Respiratory Disorder 810

29 The Child With Chronic Respiratory Alterations 860

30 The Child With Congenital Cardiac Defects 906

31 The Child With Cardiovascular Alterations 938

32 The Child With Hematologic Alterations 960

33 The Child With Cancer 990

34 The Child With Integumentary Alterations 1028

UNIT I

INTRODUCTION TO PEDIATRIC NURSING

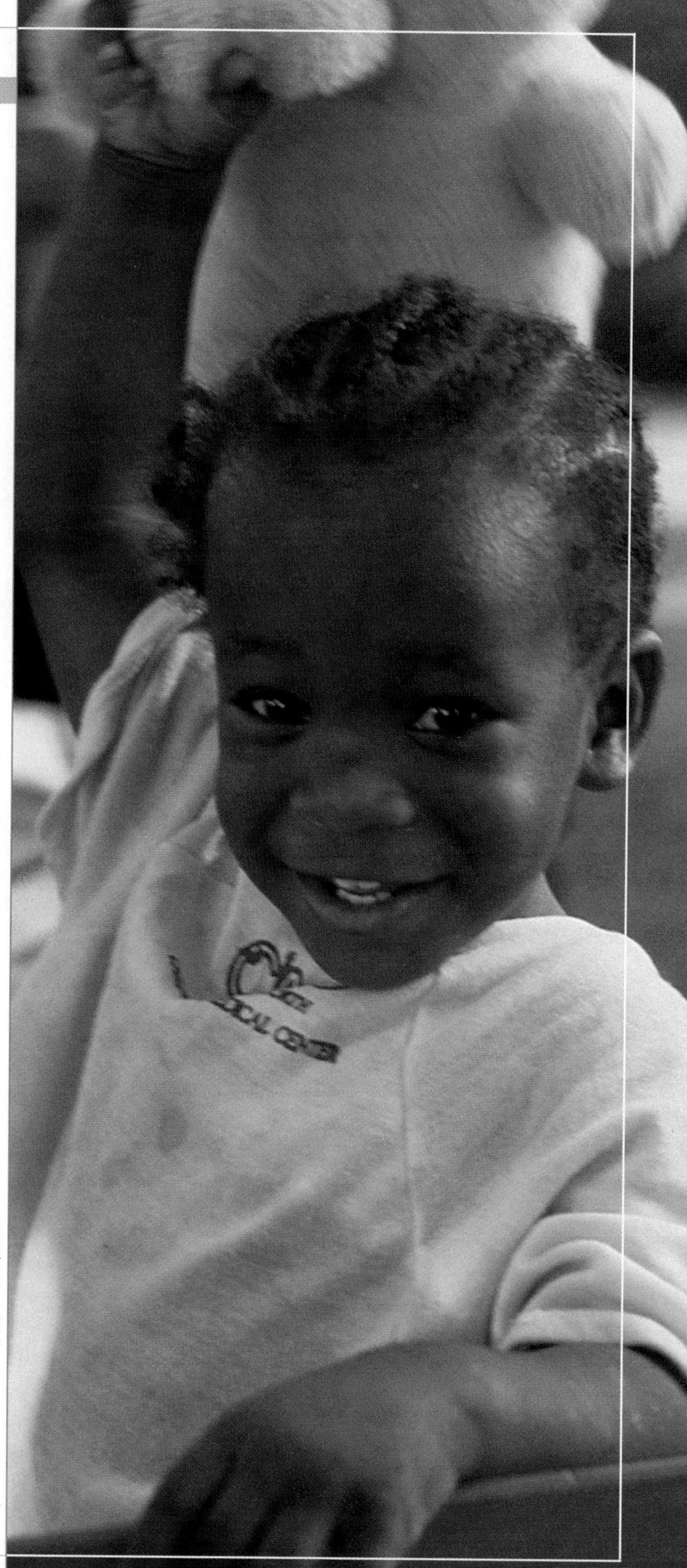

Courtesy of Cook Children's Medical Center, Fort Worth, Texas

1

Introduction to Pediatric Nursing

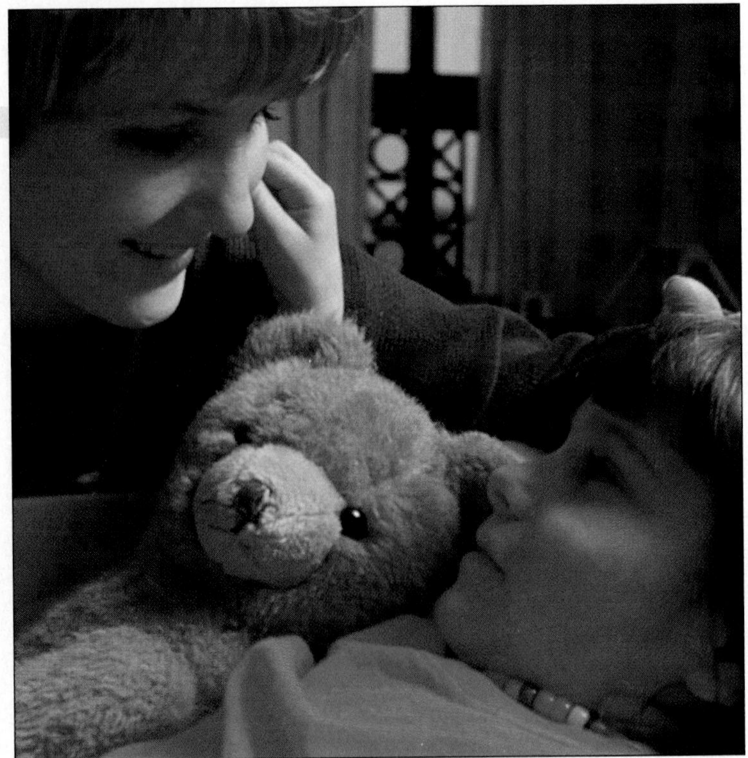

Courtesy of Cook Children's Medical Center, Fort Worth, Texas

CHAPTER OVERVIEW

LEARNING OBJECTIVES

After studying this chapter, you should be able to:

- List the major principles of pediatric nursing that form the basis of this text.
- Describe how the principles of pediatric nursing apply to nursing practice.
- Discuss society's treatment of children throughout history, and how this relates to the health care of children.
- Discuss current trends in the health care system in relation to the care of children and their families.
- Identify some of the effects of poverty and violence on the well-being of children and families.
- Describe how cultural background can affect a child's health care.
- List and describe five roles of the pediatric nurse.
- Describe the various settings in which pediatric nurses practice.
- Give examples of legal concerns specific to pediatric nurses.
- Name some factors that affect infant mortality in the United States.
- Explain why each step of the nursing process in pediatric nursing must incorporate the child's family.
- Describe how clinical pathways might be used in the pediatric setting.

KEY TERMS

advocacy: speaking or arguing in support of a policy or a person's rights

case management: a practice model that uses a systematic approach to identify specific patient needs and to manage patient care to ensure optimal outcomes

culture: shared values, beliefs, and practices of a particular group of people

Medicaid: a state-operated program providing medical care to certain eligible persons

morbidity: ratio of sick to well persons in a defined population

mortality: ratio of the number of deaths to the total number of persons in a given population

neonatal mortality: infant deaths that occur during the first 27 days of life

nursing diagnosis: a clinical judgment about individual, family, or community responses to actual or potential health problems/life processes. Nursing diagnoses provide the basis for selection of nursing interventions to achieve outcomes for which the nurse is accountable (NANDA, 1990)

postneonatal mortality: infant deaths occurring between the ages of 28 days and 1 year

WIC: the special supplemental food program for women, infants, and children which provides nutritious food and nutrition education to low-income pregnant and postpartum women and their children

Whether it be in the area of health promotion or caring for an ill child, there is no greater challenge or satisfaction than pediatric nursing. Often, pediatric nurses are asked, "How can you care for sick children?" The pediatric nurse has the unique opportunity to make a difference in a child's life. Whether it be to prevent an accident, to lessen pain, to facilitate communication between an adolescent and a parent, or simply to comfort a child, pediatric nursing is special.

This chapter provides a foundation for the student by defining the principles and the practice of pediatric nursing. It also provides a historical background for the specialty. Using the principles of pediatric nursing as a base of knowledge, the student can begin to understand what makes pediatric nursing unique. The student can also begin to learn the application of these principles in the practice of pediatric nursing.

PRINCIPLES AND PRACTICE OF PEDIATRIC NURSING

When you, the student, enter the specialty area of pediatrics, you may experience emotions ranging from curiosity to fear, to excitement, anticipation, and uncertainty. All these are normal emotions because, although you build on previous learning, pediatric nursing is a unique area with its own principles. This book guides the novice nurse through pediatrics by building on previous knowledge, reviewing key information and concepts, and focusing on underlying principles. It is neither necessary nor possible to study every pediatric disease. In this book, you are introduced to those diseases that are common, those that are most often encountered by pediatric nurses, and those that best illustrate the special care needs of children. The nurse who gains an understanding of the principles of care will be prepared to think critically and apply those principles in any clinical practice situation.

The principles upon which pediatric nursing care is founded, as identified in the text, are outlined as follows:

GROWTH AND DEVELOPMENT Nurses who care for children must apply knowledge of growth and development in order to meet the child's physical and emotional needs. An understanding of normal physiologic processes that occur during the child's maturation must guide all nursing care of children. Physiologic immaturity affects the child's immunity, fluid balance, function of organ systems, and response to illness. All aspects of care must be carefully tailored to each child's chronological and developmental age. For example, preparing a child for a procedure, administering medications and fluids, communicating, teaching, providing anticipatory guidance, and gauging a child's expected responses to illness all have growth and development principles at their core. For these reasons, this text devotes separate chapters to growth and development so that the nursing student is well versed in this area.

HEALTH PROMOTION The promotion of health in the pediatric setting is attained through education and counseling. The goal is to guide the child and the family toward independence and to help them to take responsibility for their health. In some families, this may never be completely accomplished; however, the goal remains the same, even if the methods must change.

Parents need to be educated about growth and development to form a foundation of knowledge with its natural flow to anticipatory guidance. Inherent in health promotion are nutrition, well-child care, exercise, parenting, and safety.

Through education and health promotion, there has been an increase in the number of children being immunized, a decline in the mortality rate, a dramatic decrease in accidental poisonings, and a decrease in the rate of children injured in motor vehicle accidents.

FOCUS ON THE FAMILY Family-centered care is at the core of pediatric nursing. The child's health and development are profoundly influenced by the values, beliefs, attitudes, and health practices of the family. The child's need for support, love, and security, which are essential to normal growth and development, is suddenly increased during illness.

The focus of pediatric nursing is not only to care for the ill child, but to care for the ill child and his family. It is important that families be treated as partners in the child's care, not passive recipients. Parents should be provided with accurate information in order to enable them to participate in decision making regarding their child's care. The family's needs should be assessed and necessary resources made available through collaboration with other health care providers. Throughout the text, there is frequent reference to the family and how the family is involved in the care of their child. In addition, Chapter 16 is devoted entirely to the family and to the multiple aspects of family-centered care.

CHILD ADVOCACY Legally and ethically, the nurse must assume the role of advocate for the child. All nurses have legal and ethical responsibilities. Pediatric nurses have specific responsibilities as child advocates in the areas of health promotion, violence, abuse, neglect, drug abuse, infant morbidity and mortality, and access to care. The nurse may be the only voice for a child seen in the emergency room for suspected neglect or abuse. The nurse is a "mandated reporter" for suspected child abuse. The nurse should exercise this responsibility cautiously, but must be aware of the accountability.

CONCEPTS APPLIED ACROSS AGE GROUPS Central concepts fundamental to the care of children extend across many disorders and through all age groups. During any given health care encounter, the child may have needs related to play and activity, pain, chronicity, nutrition, illness, and family. Each of these concepts requires a knowledge base that extends across age groups and settings of care. By integrating these concepts with a knowledge of developmental levels, family, and pathophysiology, the nurse is able to meet the challenge of caring for children.

COMMUNICATION Most students enter pediatric nursing with a knowledge of therapeutic communication. In order to care for infants and children, that knowledge must be expanded to include children and their families. Communicating with children can be intimidating, especially if the student has had limited experience with or exposure to children. Chapter 10 guides the student through an approach to communication that is very clear and easy to apply to the clinical situation. Communication cues are interspersed throughout the text to guide the student in the practical application of communication techniques in caring for children and their families.

FOCUS ON COMMON PEDIATRIC DISORDERS The incidence, care, and treatment of pediatric disorders change over time as research discoveries are made. No text can cover every disorder, nor should it. By focusing on common, recurring disorders, principles are established that will guide the student throughout his nursing career.

Knowledge Base for Practice. The practice of pediatric nursing requires access to specific information about normal growth and development parameters, appropriate preventive care, guidance for specific age groups, medications, laboratory values, vital signs in children of different ages, and immunization schedules. The nurse also needs to understand the importance of adapting procedures for children. For instance, in a hospital setting, how does one: Transport children of different ages? Protect children? Provide for activity? Administer medications? Assess children's nonverbal behaviors? Plan and carry out care for a child? Teach home care to the child and family?

This text includes a number of features that facilitate access to this vital information. Critical Elements (red-shaded boxes) throughout the text focus on key information. Nursing care plans, pediatric procedures, immunization schedules, and numerous other tables, boxes, and illustrations provide specific, practical information on caring for children. Screened ( ) Clinical Reference Pages review anatomy and physiology and highlight anatomic differences between children and adults. This enables the student to critically analyze why infants and children can become so acutely ill in such a short time, and illustrates why there is a smaller "margin of safety" when administering fluids or medications. The Clinical Reference Pages provide quick access to commonly used medications and diagnostic tests for specific groups of disorders. Pathophysiology is highlighted in special boxes, and illustrations throughout Unit IV help to promote an understanding of why a particular change may take place. This information can then be applied to similar disorders. Teaching Guidelines and the Home Care sections help prepare the student to teach families and children self-care.

HISTORICAL PERSPECTIVES

As Vaughn (1992) observed:

> *The caring qualities of any society may best be measured by the concerns it manifests for its aged, its disadvantaged, . . . and its young. The young are often among the most vulnerable and disadvantaged in society.*

Children have not always enjoyed the valued position that they hold in most families today. Historically, in times of economic or social instability, children have been viewed as expendable. In societies in which the struggle for survival is the central issue and only the strongest survive, the needs of children are secondary. The well-being of children in the past has depended on the economic and cultural conditions of the society. Children have at times been viewed as property by their parents, and have been bought and sold, beaten, or, in some cultures, sacrificed in religious ceremonies. At times, infanticide has been a routine practice. Conversely, children have been highly valued and their birth considered a blessing.

In Greek and Roman civilizations, attention was given to the education of children, and although their physical needs were provided for, there was no regard shown to weak, handicapped, or, in some instances, female infants, who were routinely exposed to the elements, abandoned, or killed. In the history of Europe, attitudes toward children have varied. For example, after the weakening of the Roman empire in the fourth century AD, war, famine, disease, and poverty were widespread. Children were often sold into slavery in payment of their parents' debts, and infanticide was practiced. One teaching of the Christian church included limiting the cruel treatment of children, but just as punishment of adults was cruel by today's standards, abuse of children continued as common practice.

By the 15th century, foundling homes for abandoned children had been established. It is estimated that as many as 95 percent of the infants in these homes died as a result of difficulties with artificial feeding. Nearly 65% of all children died before the age of 5 years (Forsyth, cited in Brodie, 1986). Viewed by society as miniature adults, children received the same remedies as adults and, during illness, were cared for at home by family members, just like adults.

17th and 18th Centuries. On the North American continent, as European settlements expanded during the 17th and 18th centuries, children were valued as assets to the community because of the desire to increase the population and to share the work to be done. Expansion of settlements depended upon survival and growth of families (Brodie, 1986). Public schools were established, and the courts began to view children as minors and to protect them accordingly. Devastating epidemics of smallpox, diphtheria, scarlet fever, and measles took their toll on children in the 18th century. Children often died of these virulent diseases within 1 day. Medical care was provided by families, neighbors, midwives, ministers, and doctors.

The high mortality rate of children led some physicians to examine common child care practices. In 1748, William Cadogan's "Essay on Nursing" discouraged unhealthy child care practices, such as swaddling infants in three or four layers of clothing and feeding them thin gruel within hours after birth. Instead, Cadogan urged mothers to breastfeed their infants and identified certain practices that were thought to contribute to childhood illness. Unfortunately, despite the efforts of Cadogan and others, child care practices were slow to change. Later in the 18th century, the health of children improved with the development of certain advances, such as innoculation against smallpox.

19th Century. In the 19th century, with the flood of immigrants to eastern American cities, infectious diseases flourished as a result of crowded living conditions, inadequate and unsanitary food, and harsh working conditions for men, women, and children. Twelve- and 14-hour work days were common for children working in factories, whose earnings were essential to the survival of the family. The most serious child health problems during the 19th century were caused by poverty and overcrowding. Infants were fed contaminated milk, sometimes from tuberculosis-infected cows; milk was carried to the cities and purchased by mothers with no means to refrigerate it. Infectious diarrhea was a common cause of infant death.

During the late 19th century, conditions began to improve for children and families. Lillian Wald initiated public health nursing at Henry Street Settlement House in New York City, where nurses taught mothers in their homes. In 1889, a milk distribution center opened in New York City to provide uncontaminated milk to sick infants.

Hygiene and Hospitalization. Knowledge of the discoveries of scientists, such as Pasteur, Lister, and Koch, who proved that many diseases were caused by bacteria, became widespread. The use of hygienic practices in hospitals and foundling homes gradually increased. Hospitals began to require personnel to wear uniforms and to limit contact between children in the wards. In an effort to prevent infection, hospital wards were closed to visitors. Because parental visits were noted to cause distress, particularly when parents had to leave, parental visitation was considered to be emotionally stressful to hospitalized children. In an effort to prevent such emotional distress, and the spread of infection, parents were prohibited from visiting hospitalized children. As hospital care focused on preventing disease transmission and curing physical diseases, the emotional health of hospitalized children received little attention.

20th Century. During the 20th century, dramatic changes in child health began to occur owing to increased knowledge about nutrition, sanitation, bacteriology, pharmacology, medication, and psychology. In the 1940s and 1950s, the introduction of penicillin, corticosteroids, and vaccines against many communicable diseases saved tens of thousands of children. Technologic advances in the 1970s and 1980s led to increasing survival rates among infants and children with previously fatal conditions, resulting in increased numbers of children with chronic disabilities. An increase in societal concern for children brought about the development of federally supported programs, such as school lunch programs, The Supplemental Food Program for Women, Infants, and Children (WIC), Medicare, and **Medicaid,** under which the Early Periodic Screening, Diagnosis, and Treatment (EPSDT) program, WIC, and Project Head Start were implemented.

In recent decades, increasing attention has been focused on the psychological and emotional effects of hospitalization during childhood. In response to increasing knowledge about the emotional effects of illness and hospitalization, hospital policies and health care services for children have changed. Twenty-four hour parental visitation, sibling visitation policies, and home care services have become increasingly commonplace. The Association for the Care of Children's Health (ACCH) has been a major force in promoting humanized, family-centered pediatric care. Psychological preparation of children for hospitalization and surgery has become standard nursing practice. In many hospitals, child life programs have been established to help children and their families cope with the stress of illness. Shorter hospital stays, home care, and day surgery have also helped to minimize the emotional impact of hospitalization and illness on children.

History reveals that progress in the area of child health has been slow and, at times, tentative. As the 21st century approaches, pediatric nurses face unprecedented challenges as they work to provide care and to promote health among today's children. Health care in the future will be affected by economic realities, technologic innovations, consumer expectations, and changes in the system of care delivery. Pediatric nurses are among the most knowledgeable and caring of those providing input for new health care policies. Continuing their tradition of caring, nurses can significantly affect the future of America's children.

CURRENT TRENDS AND ISSUES

Health care in the 1990s is in transition, and health care providers in all settings are being affected. The year 2000 looms uncomfortably near as we look at the goals set by the United States Department of Health and Human Services in *Healthy People 2000.* Can the United States reduce infant mortality to no more than 7 deaths per 1000 births, increase childhood immunization levels to at least 90% of 2-year-olds, and eliminate measles by the year 2000 (U.S. Department of Health and Human Services, 1990)? These questions, and many more affecting the care of infants and children, are being asked in light of major changes in the way health care is delivered and proposed funding cuts by the government.

Ten trends for pediatric care are developing:

- a decreasing patient base in the acute care setting
- sicker children in the hospital
- inadequate Medicaid coverage
- increasing numbers of uninsured Americans
- the development of managed care
- increasing costs accompanied by decreasing profits

- consolidation of community pediatric units
- growth of children's hospitals, particularly children's hospitals within other hospitals
- a shift to ambulatory care
- an increasing youth market (Society of Pediatric Nurses, 1995)

Health Care Reform

The health care reform and universal health coverage package proposed in 1994 was not passed by the United States government. It is expected that the federal government will continue to work on health care reform during the second half of the 1990s by focusing on specific areas of health care rather than developing a comprehensive plan. Most experts agree that insurance reform, malpractice reform, Medicare and Medicaid reform, and medical costs will be areas targeted for change.

Nurses will continue to be involved in the health care reform debate. Many believe that Medicaid restructuring will mean less money for children's health. Special interest groups are expected to vie for the moneys that are available. Because each individual state is assuming greater control of the money for health care, there may be wide variances from state to state in how children's health needs are met. Nurses cannot remain silent, but rather must speak out as child advocates.

Managed Care

Even while health care reform was being debated, changes were occurring. One of the biggest changes has been the tremendous growth of managed care, whereby care is provided through health maintenance organizations (HMOs), point of service plans (POSs), and preferred provider organizations (PPOs). Managed care providers emphasize coordination of care, utilization review, and preventive and primary care. The basic goals are to maintain quality care, prevent unnecessary care, and contain costs. The challenge is to make sure that cost containment does not override the other goals of care. An outcry against early discharge of maternity patients led to the passage of a law guaranteeing availability of at least 48 hours of stay in the birth center after a normal vaginal delivery.

Nurse practitioners and certified nurse midwives, are increasingly being employed by managed care agencies. These nurses with advanced education are being utilized to deliver both primary and preventive care at less cost to the managing agency. As advanced practice nurses provide care in community and rural areas and school-based clinics, it is hoped that access to care for children will improve. It is believed by many that the opportunities for nurse practitioners will increase as this trend continues.

Home Care

Children with complex, chronic health problems who at one time would have died are now living. Many of these children require complex care which, through the use of specialized equipment, can often be provided at home. First and foremost, caring for a child at home maintains the integrity of the family, and it also decreases health care costs. Pediatric home care is expected to continue to grow. For a further discussion of home care, see Chapter 15.

Health Insurance

In the 1990s, the percentage of children covered by Medicaid increased significantly, whereas the percentage of children with employer-based or private health insurance decreased significantly. At the same time, the number of children in the United States who were uninsured decreased slightly (American Academy of Pediatrics, 1995). The increase in Medicaid coverage was related to the federal government's expansion of eligibility.

More than two-thirds of uninsured children live in families with incomes below the poverty level. Nearly 80% of uninsured children are dependents of working parents who do not have insurance for a variety of reasons:

- Increasing numbers of children now live with single mothers who work in low-paying service jobs without medical insurance.
- Employer health care benefits have declined over the past decade.
- If family coverage is offered, the employee may decline it because of the high cost of the premiums (Carnegie Corporation of New York, 1994).

Besides the obvious implication of not having health insurance—the inability to pay for health care during illness—there is another very important effect on children who are not insured. They are less likely to receive preventive care. This places them at increased risk for preventable illnesses and, because preventive health care is a learned behavior, adults who are less healthy.

Health Care Assistance Programs

There are many programs, funded both privately and by the government, which assist in the care of infants and children. Some programs have been more successful than others.

The supplemental food program known as WIC, which was established in 1972, is the largest federal health program in the United States. WIC provides supplemental food supplies to low-income women who are pregnant or breastfeeding and to their children up to the age of 5 years. The WIC program has long been heralded as a cost-effective program that not only provides nutritional support but also links families with other services, such as prenatal care and immunizations.

Medicaid's EPSDT program was developed to provide comprehensive health care with the aim of preventing health problems, before they become severe, in Medicaid recipients from birth to 21 years of age. This program pays for well-child examinations and for treatment of any medical problems diagnosed during such checkups. However, a study conducted by Richardson, et al., (1994), which evaluated the results obtained by EPSDT in 76 children in a poor rural area, revealed that health care providers frequently failed to document—and possibly may have failed to perform—the required components of the EPSDT well-child checkup. Programs such as this will need to adhere strictly to the standards set by both medicine and nursing in order to survive in an increasing quality-and cost-conscious society.

Public Law 99-457 is part of the Individuals with Disabilities Act, which provides financial incentives to states to establish comprehensive early intervention services for infants and toddlers with, or at risk for, developmental disabilities. Services include screening, identification, referral, and treatment.

The Healthy Start initiative, begun in 1991, has as its goal a 50% reduction in infant mortality. In order to reach this goal, 15 key communities with high infant mortality rates were selected for demonstration projects. A few of the needs that are being addressed in these projects include outreach to high-risk women, child care, housing, public awareness, and new solutions for delivering health care (Struk, 1994).

Poverty

The number of American children under the age of 6 years living in poverty has increased over the last decade. Childhood poverty has been linked to a drop in parental earnings, particularly of male family members, which has brought many working families into poverty; family breakdown associated with an increase in teen pregnancies, family dissolution, and abandonment of children by their fathers; and inadequate governmental policy (Children's Defense Fund, 1991).

In the United States, 3.9 million children grow up in "severely distressed neighborhoods"—communities with four or more of the following characteristics: poverty, female-headed households, high-school dropouts, unemployment, and reliance on welfare. Nearly half of these children live in California, Illinois, Michigan, New York, Ohio, and Texas (Fig. 1–1). More than 80% are African-American or Latino (Larson, 1995). Compared to families making $35,000 or more a year, families with incomes of less than $10,000 are more than twice as likely to report that illnesses limit their children's activities, and six times more likely to report that their children are in poor or fair health. Poor children and adolescents have also been found to have a higher incidence of vision and hearing

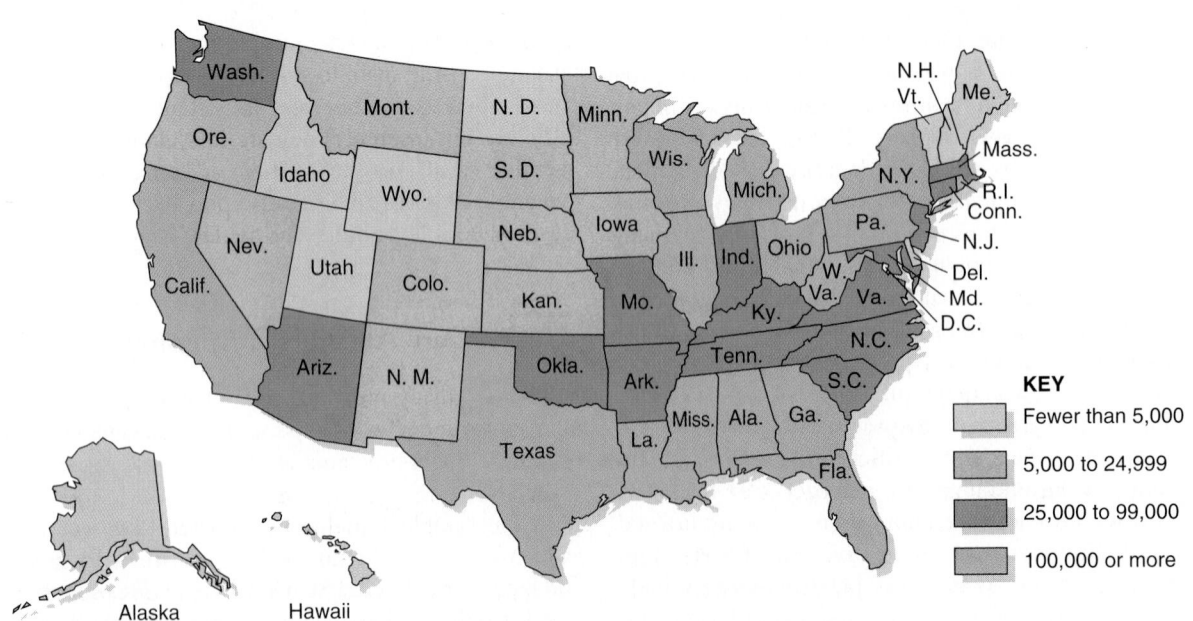

Figure 1–1
Number of children living in severely distressed neighborhoods, by state. (From the 1994 KIDS COUNT Data Book from the Annie E. Casey Foundation, Baltimore, MD, and 1990 U.S. Census figures.)

TABLE 1–1 *Preventable U.S. Childhood Diseases*

Yesterday's neglected immunizations become today's childhood diseases. This comparison shows federally reported vaccine-preventable disease rates in the United States from January to September for 1993 and 1994. Data for 1994 are provisional.

	1993		1994	
	TOTAL CASES (JAN.–SEPT.)	CASES AMONG CHILDREN YOUNGER THAN AGE 5	TOTAL CASES (JAN.–SEPT.)	CASES AMONG CHILDREN YOUNGER THAN AGE 5
Congenital rubella syndrome (CRS)	5	4 (80%)	3	2 (66.7%)
Diphtheria	0	0 (0%)	1	1 (100%)
Haemophilus influenzae*	958	292 (30.5%)	874	234 (26.8%)
Measles	269	102 (37.9%)	844	194 (23%)
Mumps	1244	209 (16.8%)	1068	170 (15.9%)
Pertussis	4366	2598 (59.5%)	2553	1457 (57.1%)
Poliomyelitis, paralytic	3	1 (33.3%)	1	1 (100%)
Rubella	165	25 (15.2%)	210	21 (10%)
Tetanus	33	0 (0%)	26	0 (0%)

*Invasive *H. influenzae* disease serotype is not routinely reported to the National Notifiable Diseases Surveillance System.

From Office of the Director, National Immunization Program. (1994, December). *Immunization action news.* Hyattsville, MD: U.S. Centers for Disease Control and Prevention.

problems, oral health problems, nonacne skin lesions, and elevated blood lead levels than their wealthier counterparts (Newacheck et al., 1994).

The number of uninsured American children has also increased owing to a decline in private, employer-paid coverage. This has had a tremendous impact on the low-income worker who does not have employer-paid coverage and is unable to afford individually purchased insurance. Although Medicaid has expanded its coverage, there are millions of children who live in households with incomes just above the Medicaid eligibility level whose families cannot afford to purchase private insurance.

The infant mortality rate is increased in infants born to mothers living in poverty. A high percentage of postnatal (28–364 days) deaths in this population are linked to infections and injuries (Centers for Disease Control, 1995a). Studies in the early 1980s determined that a large number of infants who were at risk for death during the postnatal period received little or no care during that same period of time. In response to this information, a program was developed in West Virginia that has resulted in a significant decline in the infant mortality rate in that state. Much of their success has been attributed to identifying high-risk infants and linking them to a medical home where both preventive and acute care needs are met and outcomes are tracked (Jakubeck, 1995). The success in West Virginia underscores the importance of early identification of risk factors and case management.

Nurses can play a role in meeting the health care needs of all children by recognizing the effect of poverty on child health and identifying poverty as a practice concern. The United States Public Health Service's Objectives for the Nation for 2000 outlines goals for improving the health care of all children (Malloy, 1992). The targeted objectives from *Healthy People 2000* include the following:

- Reduce the *infant mortality rate* to no more than 7 per 1000 live births, and mortality among black infants to no more than 11 per 1000 live births. The current rates are 7.9 per 1000 live births and 16.8 per 1000 black live births.
- Reduce the incidence of low birth weight no more than 5% of live births and no more than 9% of black infants. The current rates are 6.0% and 13.3%, respectively.
- Ninety percent of all pregnant women will receive prenatal care in the first trimester of pregnancy. The current rate is 79%.
- At least 90% of children younger than 2 years of age will complete the basic immunization series. At the present time, 89.6% receive the measles vaccine; 25.5% receive the hepatitis B vaccine, 87% are immunized against diphtheria, tetanus, and pertussis (DTP), 76% receive the polio vaccine, and 70.6% are immunized against *Haemophilus influenzae* type b (Hib).
- Vaccine-preventable disease will be reduced as follows: (1) measles and rubella to zero cases; (2) mumps to no more than 500 cases per year; and (3) pertussis to no more than 1000 cases per year. Table 1–1 shows current data on preventable childhood diseases.*

There has been an increase in the national vaccination levels for Hib and hepatitis B. Vaccination levels are near the highest ever for three doses of DTP, three doses of polio vaccine, and one dose of the measles vaccine and for the combined series. However, an estimated 2 million children ages 19 to 35 months still need one or more doses of DTP, polio, or measles, mumps, and rubella (MMR) vaccine to be completely vaccinated (Centers for Disease Control, 1995b).

*Current data reflect available statistics in 1996.

Violence

In today's society, children are the victims and the perpetrators of violence. Violence is not only a social problem, it is a health problem. Acts of violence can include child abuse, domestic abuse, and murder. Children who live in an environment of violence feel helpless and ineffective. These children have difficulty sleeping and show increased anxiety and fearfulness. Repeated exposure to violence is a threat to the healthy physical, intellectual, and emotional development of children (Carnegie Corporation of New York, 1994).

Violence in schools continues to rise, and for many children, it is a daily stressor (see box). Many see this as a result of the social problems that plague the country. Experts in the field of education have cited socioeconomic disparity, language barriers, diverse cultural upbringing, lack of supervision and behavioral feedback, domestic violence, and changes within the family as possible causes for the increased violence. Traditional approaches to aggressive behavior in the school, such as suspension, detention, and being sent to the principal's office, have been ineffective in changing behavior, and serve only to exclude the student from education, leading to an increased drop-out rate. One program, Project Achieve, a school-based reform curriculum, teaches at-risk youth behavioral alternatives to aggression. Schools using Project Achieve have seen 50% to 75% student compliance with school procedures and significantly reduced physical aggression (Larson, 1995). An antiviolence curriculum called Second Step is based on stopping aggressive behavior before it becomes a part of a violent personality. The Second Step curriculum offers an anti-violence curriculum for preschool through eighth grade, a truancy-reduction program, a peer court, youth activities, and Second Chance, a program for delinquent youth (Larson, 1995). Nurses must educate themselves on the issue of violence and, in turn, work with schools and parents to combat the problem. In addition, they should not ignore the child who is afraid to go to school or is having other school-related problems.

There is also increased concern over media violence. Children and adolescents are being exposed to violence via television, movies, video games, and youth-oriented music. Nurses should make this issue a part of anticipatory guidance. Parents should be encouraged to monitor their children's media exposure and limit their children's television viewing to two hours or less per day.

There is an increasing awareness of the problem of violence and much dialogue is taking place. The American Academy of Pediatrics encourages clinicians to be concerned about adolescents who display aggressive or acting-out behaviors, such as lying, stealing, temper outbursts, vandalism, excessive fighting, and destructiveness. They further recommend that health care providers promote the responsibility of every family to create a gun-safe home environment, including asking about the presence of guns in the home and counseling patients, parents, and relatives on the importance of firearm safety and the dangers of having a gun, especially a handgun.

Nurses working with children should ask them about violence in their school, home, or neighborhood, and if they have had any personal experiences with violent behavior. In some cases, it may be necessary to contact parents, human resource departments, police, or other authorities in order to protect children and adolescents who are either in violent situations or at risk for violence.

Violence in U.S. Schools

A 1993 U.S. Centers for Disease Control and Prevention survey of 16,000 U.S. high school students revealed that:

- 4.4% had skipped at least 1 day of school in the month preceding the survey because they felt unsafe.
- 7.3% had been threatened or injured with weapons on school property within the past year.
- 11.8% carried a weapon on school property within the past 30 days.
- 16.2% had been in a physical fight on school property within the past year.
- 32.7% had property stolen or damaged on school grounds within the past year.

Cultural Diversity

Nursing has long recognized the impact that **culture** has on the care of patients. It is difficult to imagine any health care setting where nurses will not have contact with more than one cultural background. Some of the major factors to consider when assessing culture in children and their families are religion, diet, health beliefs and practices, family values, parenting practices, and language and communication.

Although an awareness of specific cultural beliefs and nursing care practices is essential to provide holistic care, the nurse must always remember that each child and family has its own unique set of needs and beliefs. Beliefs may vary widely within the same ethnic and cultural background. The nurse is cautioned to avoid generalizing about a specific group. Culturally sensitive care focuses on diversity while maintaining the individuality of each child and family (Ahmann, 1994). The cultural aspects of families are addressed in Chapter 16, and cultural implications are interwoven throughout the chapters of this text.

ROLE OF THE PEDIATRIC NURSE

The professional nurse has a responsibility to provide the highest quality care to every child. Nurses are accountable for the care they provide for children and families. Standards of practice describe the level of performance expected of a professional nurse as determined by an authority in the practice. The American Nurses' Association (ANA) and the Society of Pediatric Nurses (SPN) recently formed a task force to develop *Standards of Care* and *Standards of Professional Performance* for pediatric nurses (see box). These standards can be used by nurses caring for children in all clinical settings as a guide for their practice. Other standards of practice for specific clinical areas are available from nursing specialty groups, such as pediatric oncology nursing or emergency nursing. The American Nurses Association (ANA) Code for Nurses provides guidelines for ethical and professional behavior (see box). The Code for Nurses emphasizes the nurses' accountability to the patient, the community, and to the profession. The nurse should understand the implications of this code and strive to practice accordingly. Professional nurses have a legal obligation to know and understand the standard of care imposed on them. It is critical that nurses maintain competence and a current knowledge base in their areas of practice.

Pediatric nurses function in a variety of roles, including those of care provider, teacher, collaborator, researcher, and advocate.

ANA-SPN Standards of Care and Standards of Professional Performance for Pediatric Nurses

STANDARDS OF CARE*

Comprehensive pediatric nursing care focuses on helping children and their families and communities achieve their optimum health potentials. This is best achieved within the framework of family-centered care and the pediatric nursing process, including primary, secondary, and tertiary care coordinated across health care and community settings.

Standard I. Assessment
The pediatric nurse collects health data.

Standard II. Diagnosis
The pediatric nurse analyzes the assessment data in determining diagnoses.

Standard III. Outcome Identification
The pediatric nurse identifies expected outcomes individualized to the client.

Standard IV. Planning
The pediatric nurse develops a plan of care that prescribes interventions to attain expected outcomes.

Standard V. Implementation
The pediatric nurse implements the interventions identified in the plan of care.

Standard VI. Evaluation
The pediatric nurse evaluates the child's and family's progress toward attainment of outcomes.

From the American Nurses' Association and the Society of Pediatric Nurses. (1996). *Statement on the scope and standards of pediatric clinical practice* (pp. 25–35). Washington, DC: American Nurses Publishing.

STANDARDS OF PROFESSIONAL PERFORMANCE*

Standard I. Quality of Care
The pediatric nurse systematically evaluates the quality and effectiveness of pediatric nursing practice.

Standard II. Performance Appraisal
The pediatric nurse evaluates his or her own nursing practice in relation to professional practice standards and relevant statutes and regulations.

Standard III. Education
The pediatric nurse acquires and maintains current knowledge in pediatric nursing practice.

Standard IV. Collegiality
The pediatric nurse contributes to the professional development of peers, colleagues, and others.

Standard V. Ethics
The pediatric nurse's decisions and actions on behalf of children and their families are determined in an ethical manner.

Standard VI. Collaboration
The pediatric nurse collaborates with the child, family, and health care providers in providing client care.

Standard VII. Research
The pediatric nurse uses research findings in practice.

Standard VIII. Resource Utilization
The pediatric nurse considers factors related to safety, effectiveness, and cost in planning and delivering care.

*See the original source for measurement criteria.

ANA Code for Nurses

1. The nurse provides services with respect for human dignity and the uniqueness of the client unrestricted by considerations of social or economic status, personal attributes, or the nature of health problems.
2. The nurse safeguards the client's right to privacy by judiciously protecting information of a confidential nature.
3. The nurse acts to safeguard the client and the public when health care and safety are affected by the incompetent, unethical, or illegal practice of any person.
4. The nurse assumes responsibility and accountability for individual nursing judgments and actions.
5. The nurse maintains competence in nursing.
6. The nurse exercises informed judgment and uses individual competence and qualifications as criteria in seeking consultation, accepting responsibilities, and delegating nursing activities to others.
7. The nurse participates in activities that contribute to the ongoing development of the profession's body of knowledge.
8. The nurse participates in the profession's efforts to implement and improve standards of nursing.
9. The nurse participates in the profession's efforts to establish and maintain conditions of employment conducive to high-quality nursing care.
10. The nurse participates in the profession's effort to protect the public from misinformation and misrepresentation and to maintain the integrity of nursing.
11. The nurse collaborates with members of the health professions and other citizens in promoting community and national efforts to meet the health needs of the public.

From *Code for nurses with interpretive statements* (1985). American Nurses' Association, 600 Maryland Avenue, SW, Suite 100W, Washington, DC 20024–2521.

Care Provider. The pediatric nurse provides direct nursing care to children and their families in times of illness, injury, and recovery. Care of children and families is based on the nursing process. The nurse caring for pediatric clients will obtain health histories, assess client needs, monitor growth and development, perform health screening procedures, develop comprehensive plans of care, provide treatment and care, make referrals, and evaluate care. Care is based on an understanding of the child's developmental stage, and is aimed at meeting the child's physical and emotional needs. Developing a therapeutic relationship and providing support to children and their families are essential components of nursing care. Pediatric nurses practice family-centered care, embracing diversity in family structures and cultural backgrounds. These nurses strive to empower families, encouraging them to participate in their child's care and to provide care and comfort whenever possible.

Teacher. Education is one of the most important roles of the pediatric nurse. In the acute care setting, nurses prepare children for procedures, hospitalization, or surgery, using a knowledge of growth and development to teach children at various levels of understanding. The nurse explains procedures and treatments, ensuring that the child and family have adequate information to consider their options and to make decisions about the child's care. The nurse answers questions and helps families understand their child's condition as fully as possible. Families need information as well as emotional support so that they can cope with the anxiety and uncertainty of illness in their child. Nurses teach parents to provide care, watch for important signs, and increase the child's comfort. They also work with parents so they are prepared to assume responsibility for the child's care at home after discharge from the hospital.

Education is essential for promotion of health. Teaching facilitates positive changes in attitudes toward health in children and families. The nurse applies principles of teaching and learning to change behavior of family members. Nurses motivate children and families to take charge of and make responsible decisions about their own health. In order for teaching to be effective, it is essential to incorporate the family's values and health beliefs.

Pediatric nurses play an important role in the prevention of illness and injury through education and anticipatory guidance. Teaching about immunizations, safety, dental care, socialization, and discipline are essential components of care. Nurses offer guidance to parents with regard to childrearing practices and preventing potential problems. They also answer questions about growth and development and assist families in understanding their children. Teaching often involves providing emotional support and counseling to children and families.

Collaborator. Pediatric nurses collaborate with other members of the health care team, often coordinating and managing the child's care. Care is improved by an interdisciplinary approach as nurses work together with dieticians, social workers, physicians, home care nurses, and others.

Managing a child's transition from hospital or any other acute care setting to home or another facility involves discharge planning and collaboration with other health care professionals. The trend toward home care makes collaboration increasingly important. The nurse must be knowledgeable about community resources, home care agencies qualified to care for children, and financial resources. Collaboration is the keystone to family-centered care, as nurses work with families in providing care for their children. Cooperation and communication are essential as parents are encouraged to participate in their child's care. In order to provide the highest quality of care, pediatric nurses must build collaborative relationships with parents and other health professionals.

Researcher. Nurses contribute to their profession's knowledge base by systematically investigating theoretical or practice issues in child nursing. Nursing does not merely "borrow" scientific knowledge from medicine and basic sciences. Nursing is demonstrating the ability to generate and answer its own questions based on research of its own unique subject matter. The responsibility of research within nursing is not limited to nurses with graduate degrees. It is important that all nurses apply research findings to their practice, rather than basing care decisions merely on intuition or tradition. Nurses can contribute to the body of professional knowledge by demonstrating an awareness of the value of nursing research and assisting in problem identification and data collection. Nurses should keep their knowledge current by "networking" and sharing research findings at conferences and by reading research journal articles.

Child and Family Advocate. An advocate is one who speaks on behalf of another. As the health care environment becomes increasingly complex, care can become impersonal. The wishes and needs of children and families are sometimes discounted or ignored in the effort to treat and to cure. The nurse, as the health professional who is closest to the patient, is in an ideal position to "humanize" care and to intercede on the child's behalf. As an advocate, the nurse considers the family's wishes in planning and implementing care. The nurse informs families of treatments and procedures, ensuring that they are involved directly in decisions and activities related to the child's care. The nurse must be sensitive to the values, beliefs, and customs of families. The nurse makes families aware of resources available in the hospital and community and assists them in accessing the services required by the child.

Pediatric nurses must be advocates for health promotion for all children. Nurses can promote the rights of children and/or families through participation in groups dedicated to the welfare of children, such as professional nursing societies, parent support groups, religious organizations, and voluntary organizations. Through involvement with health care planning on a political or legislative level, and by working as a consumer advocate, nurses can initiate changes for better quality health care. Nurses are on the "front line" of health care. Because of their interactions with parents, health care professionals, and the public, nurses have the potential not only to influence but to shape important health policies for children (Velsor-Freidrich & Frager, 1990). Nurses possess unique knowledge and skills and can make valuable contributions in developing health care strategies to ensure that every child receives optimal care.

Settings of Care

Pediatric nurses are involved in all aspects of child health care and practice in many different settings. Social and political forces have resulted in a changing, cost-conscious health care environment with a great diversity of care settings. Pediatric nurses perform their roles virtually everywhere there are children, including:

- acute care settings: general pediatric hospital units, intensive care units, surgery, postanesthesia units, emergency care facilities, and on board air-life helicopters and emergency transport craft
- clinics, physicians' offices, and health maintenance organizations (providing direct care, telephone triage, teaching regarding health promotion, growth and development, safety, and nutrition)
- home health agencies (providing home care to children with acute and chronic conditions)
- schools (performing screening, health teaching, and monitoring of health status)
- rehabilitation centers or long-term care hospitals (providing inpatient care to children in order to restore their level of function to an optimal state)
- summer camps and day care centers
- administrative positions to provide quality assurance and control of infectious diseases
- hospice programs, respite care programs
- psychiatric centers

Expanded Roles

Expanded roles exist for pediatric nurses with master's degrees and doctorates in nursing. These include positions for nurse practitioners, clinical specialists, nurse administrators, nurse educators, and nurse researchers. *Pediatric nurse practitioners* (PNPs) use advanced skills in the assessment and treatment of ill children using established protocols. PNPs also provide well-child care and perform developmental screening. The PNP role emphasizes health promotion, illness prevention, and wellness maintenance. The *clinical nurse specialist* (CNS) in child health care is an example of another expanded role in which nurses provide specialized care for families and children. Clinical specialists have been educated beyond the basic preparational stage in areas of child health, and function in expanded roles in a variety of settings.

LEGAL CONCERNS

Nursing practice must comply to the standard of care determined by various state nursing practice acts, state and federal laws, state courts, and U.S. Supreme Court decisions. Deviation from the standard of care may result in nursing malpractice or negligence, which can lead to conviction and/or revocation of a nursing license.

Malpractice and Negligence

In the past, a nurse was rarely drawn into a lawsuit involving medical negligence. Instead, the physician and hospital were the typical parties sued by the injured patient, the plaintiff. Today, the nurse is frequently named as one of the defendants in a lawsuit because recent legislation mandates that all negligent parties be named in the suit, in order for the plaintiff to seek full or complete recovery.

The number of medical malpractice lawsuits is increasing, largely because of the public's awareness of legal remedies for medical negligence, advanced technology requiring complex and specialized care, and increasingly sophisticated means of early assessment and diagnostic testing for various health problems. For example, in nursing a child with meningitis, a misdiagnosis or a delayed nursing diagnosis can cause permanent neurologic sequelae or even death.

Accountability

Accountability in pediatric nursing requires special consideration because the nurse must be accountable to the child, as well as to the family. Accountability involves a knowledge of current laws. For example, the National Childhood Vaccine Injury Act mandates that explanations about the risks of communicable diseases and the risks and benefits associated with immunizations should be given to all parents to enable them to make informed decisions about their child's health care. Parents need to know the common side effects and what to do in an emergency if any occur. The law stipulates that children injured by the vaccine must go through the administrative compensation system (funds from an excise tax levied on the vaccines) and reject an award before attempting to sue in a civil suit either the manufacturer or the person who gave the vaccine. Furthermore, the law mandates certain record keeping and reporting requirements for nurses.

In 1984, the subject of handicapped infants was addressed by the Child Abuse Amendments and delegated to state child protective agencies to investigate allegations of necessary medical care being denied. These regulations come into play when caring for children with symptoms of acquired immunodeficiency syndrome (AIDS).

Both federal and state legislative bodies have addressed the issue of child abuse. Considerable variation exists among state laws in the investigative authority and procedures granted to child protective workers. When child abuse is suspected, issues often arise as to whether a health care provider may investigate the home situation and obtain relevant records.

A recent issue pertaining to nursing accountability is inadequate hospital staffing owing to budget cuts. A nurse has a duty to immediately communicate concerns about staffing levels through established channels. A nurse will not be excused from responsibility (e.g., late medication administration or injury resulting from inadequate supervision of a child), just as a hospital will not be excused for insufficient staffing because of budget cuts.

Accountability also involves competency. If a nurse is not competent to perform a particular nursing task (e.g., to administer a new chemotherapeutic drug), or if a patient's status worsens to a point at which her care needs are beyond the nurse's competency level (e.g., a patient requiring hemodynamic monitoring), the nurse must immediately communicate this to the nursing supervisor and/or physician. The fact that a patient's transfer to the intensive care unit (ICU) was requested but denied because the ICU was at full capacity is an insufficient defense in a charge of nursing negligence. Additionally, the fact that a call was placed to a physician but there was no return call is no excuse for harm caused to a child because of delayed treatment.

Documentation: Nursing Notes

Nursing documentation in the care of a child, differs in several respects from that required in caring for an adult. The child may not be able to communicate the source of pain or discomfort. For example, a child's inconsolable crying may be an indication of increased intracranial pressure, an infiltrated IV line, or sepsis.

Documentation of a child's behavior and state of alertness is important in assessing changes in the child's neurologic status. The child's health status can change rapidly without any verbal warnings from the child. A compliant, sleepy, or lethargic child may actually be experiencing a worsening condition (e.g., sudden intracranial bleed).

Practical nursing guidelines to follow when charting include charting total body assessment of each body system and charting all communications with doctors and parents.

A minimum of a one-sentence summary should be included at the onset and end of a shift and at any time when the child's condition changes. The following information should be included in the summary: behavior status; fluid and food intake, and last urine and stool output; location of restraints; location and condition of IV sites (past and present); IV fluid content, flow rate, manual drip or machine, and IV medications piggybacked; status of neurological, respiratory, cardiovascular, gastrointestinal, and integument systems; and whether parents or other caregivers are at bedside. It is advisable to chart every two hours during the shift.

Legal Rights of the Child and Family

Terminating Life Support. Decisions to terminate life support systems continue to present gut-wrenching situations to the pediatric nurse, especially when an infant or child is involved. Contrary to the common belief that such decisions should be determined by what is termed "quality of life," the legal system plays a major role in this area of health care.

A recent Georgia court decision, *In re Jan Doe* [418 S.E.2d 3 (GA. 1992)] involved a 13-year-old child who had an unknown degenerative neurologic disease. She had limited cognitive skills and was dependent on a ventilator and a gastrostomy tube. A dispute arose between her parents as to the appropriateness of a "do not resuscitate" (DNR) order requested by the mother. A hospital ethics committee agreed with the mother's wishes.

However, the guardian appointed for the child argued that such an order was not necessary because death was not imminent. The court disagreed and held that the decision was one of personal autonomy. If the parents could not decide, it was inappropriate to ask the legal system to determine what was in the best interests of the child. Furthermore, it was determined that, if the parents can decide mutually on a course of action, the legal system should not undo their decision.

Frequently, parents become attached to a primary care nurse and request that the nurse participate in the decision as to whether or not to terminate life support for their child. A pediatric nurse might be faced with such a situation in the neonatal ICU with a teenage parent of a premature infant with a congenital defect, or in a chronic care oncology unit with a terminally ill child.

In such instances, a team conference should be arranged with the parents, primary nurse, physician, and a hospital staff attorney who is knowledgeable about applicable laws in that particular state. Problems may arise when there is a discrepancy between what families, physicians, and nurses think is best.

The issue of when to first discuss with adolescents the idea of cardiopulmonary resuscitation, mechanical ventilation, and DNR orders is always sensitive. Adolescent patients who have reached majority age must give consent if they are of sound mind. In most states, minority status ends at the age of 18 years.

Informed Consent. As in other areas of nursing, the pediatric nurse must obtain properly executed informed consent to treat or not treat a particular child. Without proper informed consent, assault and battery charges can result. Consent must be obtained from the child's parent or legal guardian (differentiated from caregiver, relative, etc.). Minors are not allowed to give consent; however, children should have procedures explained to them in terms appropriate for their age.

The law mandates what procedures require informed consent. The same laws govern both adults and children. The law mandates what to inform about as "risks" specific to each procedure. Nurses must be familiar with those procedures requiring consent.

Most states allow some exceptions for parental consent in cases involving emancipated minors. An emancipated minor is a minor child who has the legal competency of an adult because of circumstances involving marriage, divorce, parenting of a child, living independently without parents, or enlistment in the armed services. Legal counsel may be consulted to verify the status of the emancipated minor for consent purposes.

Most states allow minors to obtain treatment for drug or alcohol abuse, or sexually transmitted diseases, and to have access to birth control without parental consent. At present, laws governing adolescent abortion vary widely from state to state.

When parents refuse to give consent for what is deemed necessary treatment of a child, the state may be petitioned to intervene. The child may temporarily be placed by the court in the custody of the government or a private agency. The nurse may be asked to witness such a transaction when physicians act in cases of emergencies.

Closed, Open, and Semi-open Adoption. Nurses may care for infants involved in "open," or "semi-open," or "closed" adoptions. The nurse may need to consult with the birth parents, adoptive parents, social workers, obstetrician, or pediatrician to determine the various rights of the child, birth parents, and adoptive parents (e.g., in matters concerning visitation rights, informed consent, or discharge planning).

In open adoptions, the birth mother may opt to room in with the baby during hospitalization. The birth mother and adopted parents typically have had contact prior to the delivery and have an informal agreement regarding shared responsibility for the baby. The birth parent may even participate in discharge planning because she may have extended rights to visit the child after adoption.

Issues may develop as to the state of mind of the birth mother at the time of relinguishing parental rights (which cannot occur until after birth, unlike the relinguishment of the birth father's rights). State laws vary as to the legal time period necessary (1 day to several weeks) before a birth mother can lawfully relinguish her rights to the child after the birth of the child.

Some state laws allow the birth mother to relinguish her rights immediately after birth. In such cases, the nurse has the responsibility of protecting the birth mother and child to ensure that the birth mother is not coerced into making a decision while under the effects of anesthesia. Factual documentation of such circumstances may be requested if the birth mother later asserts her rights to the child, claiming "undue influence" or "coercion."

Although birth fathers rarely participate in the care of the baby during hospitalization, they have the same rights as the birth mother. Unless the birth father relinguishes his legal rights to the child, the adoptive parents are taking a risk when taking custody of the child at the time of discharge from the hospital. The birth father may later assert his rights to the child after bonding has occurred with the adoptive parents.

MORTALITY AND MORBIDITY

Mortality

Mortality statistics describe the number of individuals in a given population who have died over a specified period. They are usually presented as rates per 100,000, although the infant mortality rate is presented as the number of deaths per 1000 live births.

Infant Mortality. Infant mortality rates are deaths that occur among infants younger than 1 year of age from a specified period (monthly, year-to-date, or 12-month period). The infant mortality rate for the year ending in December of 1994 was 7.9 per 1000 live births, 4% lower than the preceding 12-month period. This is the lowest rate ever recorded in the United States (Fig. 1–2). The rate for infants younger than 28 days (**neonatal morality** rate) was 5.0 deaths per 1000 live births, which was 8% lower than the 1993 rate. The change in mortality rate for infants ages 28 days to 11 months (**postneonatal mortality**) was not statistically significant. There was a decrease in infant mortality related to respiratory distress syndrome and sudden infant death syndrome between 1993 and 1995. However, the infant mortality rate from accidents increased by 35% (Guyer et al., 1995).

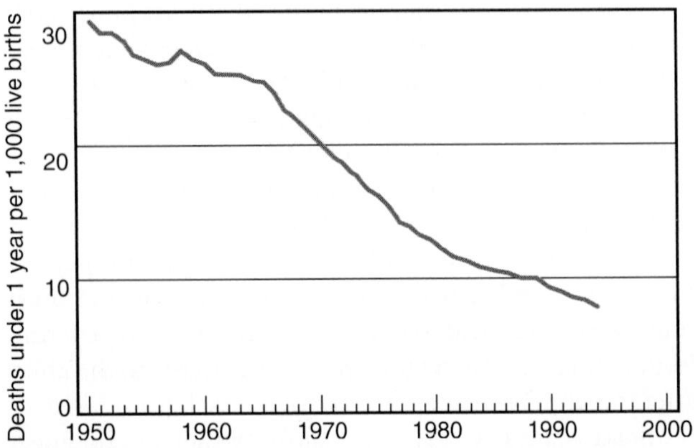

Figure 1–2
Infant mortality rates in the United States, 1950–1994. (From *Monthly Vital Statistics Report.* [1995, October 23], *43*[13], 9.)

There has been declining mortality from pneumonia and influenza, respiratory distress syndrome, prematurity and low birth weight, and congenital anomalies. However, race, socioeconomic background, and education are strong variables within the population (Singh & Yu, 1995). For example, declines in neonatal mortality rates have been more rapid for the white population than for other racial groups (Centers for Disease Control, 1994; Fig. 1–3). The Hispanic infant mortality rate is similar to that of white infants. However, this number may be underestimated because deaths and live births of unknown origin are not distributed among the specified Hispanic and non-Hispanic groups (Singh and Yu, 1995).

The race disparity, in terms of mortality, between blacks and whites is not expected to decrease in the near future. The risk for mortality is currently 2.2 times higher for black infants than for white infants. This ratio is expected to prevail during the first decade of the 21st century.

Japan, Sweden, Finland, Switzerland, Singapore, and Canada have the lowest infant mortality rates in the world. Although the infant mortality rate has dropped in the United States, it has also dropped in other countries. In 1992, published rates for 1990 showed the United States to have a higher mortality rate than that of 20 other countries (Population and Vital Statistics Report, 1992). Comparisons between the 1994 infant morality rate for the United States and other countries are currently not available. Those statistics will have implications for changes in health care delivery and further research because some of the countries with low infant mortality rates (e.g., Sweden, Switzerland, Canada), provide free prenatal care for all women and have lower rates of adolescent pregnancy (Gorrie et al., 1994).

Childhood Mortality. Mortality rates for children older than 1 year of age are lower than for infants. School-age children have the lowest rate of deaths, with adolescent rates rising significantly. Seventy-two percent of all deaths among school-age youths and young adults are from four causes: motor vehicle crashes (30%), other unintentional injuries (12%), homicide (19%), and suicide (11%). Table 1–2 shows the leading causes of death in children.

Morbidity

Morbidity is the ratio of sick to well persons in a community. This ratio is presented as rates per 1000 population because of the increased frequency of occurrence. This term is used in reference to acute and chronic illness, as well as disability. Because morbidity statistics are col-

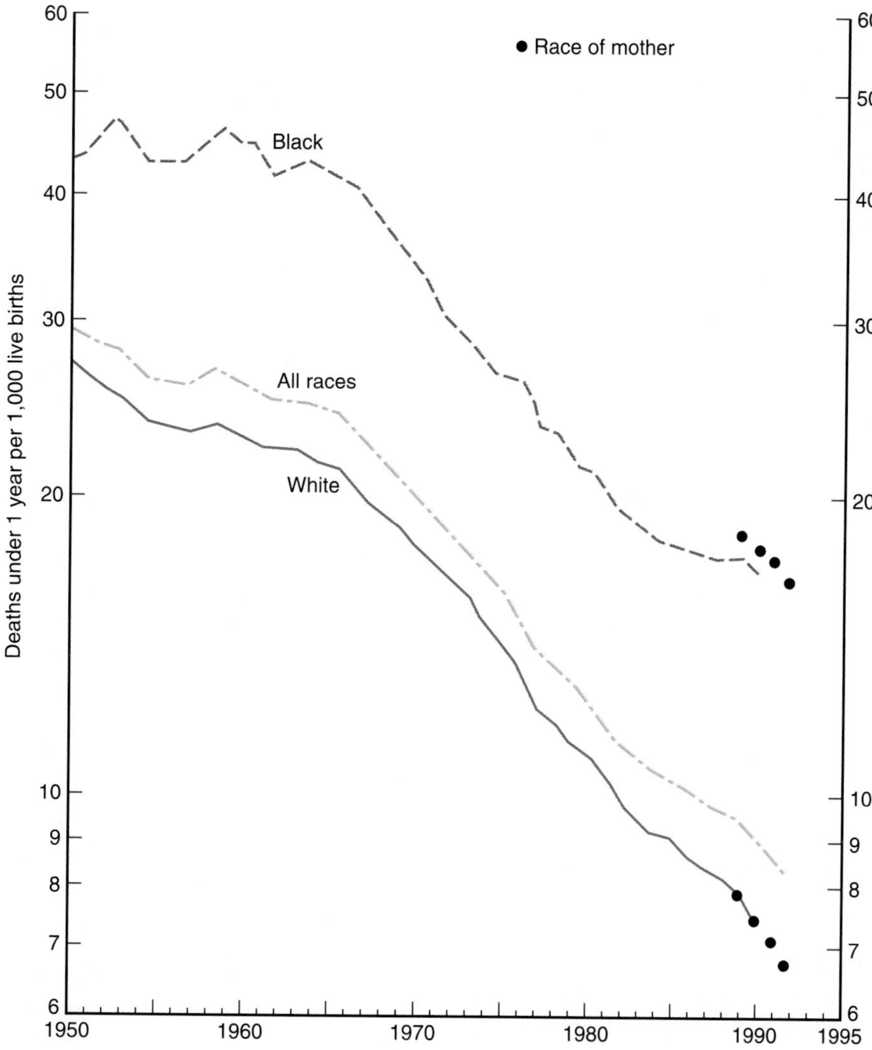

Figure 1–3

Infant mortality rates by race in the United States, 1950–1992. (From *Monthly Vital Statistics Report.* [1994, December 8], *43*[6S], 11.)

lected and updated less frequently than mortality statistics, it is difficult to present current data in all areas of pediatrics. Statistics regarding morbidity related to particular disorders are available throughout the text as the information is presented.

The Youth Risk Behavior Surveillance System has identified six categories of health risk behaviors among youth that contribute to increased morbidity: tobacco, alcohol, and other drug use; risky sexual behaviors; poor dietary behaviors; and lack of physical activity. Behaviors that lead to problems include rarely or never using a safety belt, riding with a driver who has been drinking alcohol, carrying a weapon, using drugs, and attempting suicide. Morbidity and other problems also result from unplanned pregnancies and sexually transmitted diseases, including infection with the human immunodeficiency virus (HIV) (Centers for Disease Control, 1995c).

THE NURSING PROCESS

The nursing process is a systematic method for providing patient care. It provides a framework for independent nursing action. *Key to the use of the nursing process in the care of children is the involvement of the family.* Nursing students in pediatric courses typically are taught the use of the nursing process prior to beginning pediatrics. Therefore, this section will serve as a quick review of the nursing process and its application to pediatrics.

TABLE 1–2 *Death Rates per 100,000 Population for the 15 Leading Causes of Death: Birth Through 24 Years**

CAUSE OF DEATH†	YEAR	ALL AGES, INCLUDING ADULTS‡	YOUNGER THAN 1 YEAR§	1–14 YEARS	15–24 YEARS
Chronic obstructive pulmonary diseases and allied conditions	1994	39.1	*	0.3	0.5
	1993	39.2	*	0.2	0.3
Accidents and adverse effects	1994	34.6	25.3	11.7	39.0
	1993	34.4	18.9	11.9	37.2
Motor vehicle accidents	1994	16.2	7.2	5.7	29.4
	1993	15.9	3.3	5.3	27.5
All other accidents and adverse effects	1994	18.4	18.1	6.0	9.5
	1993	18.5	15.3	6.6	9.7
Pneumonia and influenza	1994	31.5	11.6	0.4	0.8
	1993	31.7	11.7	0.6	0.7
Diabetes mellitus	1994	21.2	*	*	0.4
	1993	21.4	*	*	0.4
Human immunodeficiency virus infection	1994	16.1	0.8 (younger than 1 year and 1–14 years combined)		1.8
	1993	14.9	0.7 (younger than 1 year and 1–14 years combined)		1.8
Suicide	1994	12.4	. . .	0.7	14.9
	1993	12.1	. . .	0.6	13.8
Chronic liver disease and cirrhosis	1994	9.9	*	*	*
	1993	9.6	*	*	*
Homicide and legal intervention	1994	9.1	8.0	1.7	21.6
	1993	9.9	7.4	2.2	22.5
Nephritis, nephrotic syndrome, and nephrosis	1994	9.1	3.9	*	*
	1993	9.1	3.6	*	*
Septicemia	1994	7.6	4.7	0.2	*
	1993	7.9	4.8	0.3	*
Atherosclerosis	1994	6.9	*	*	*
	1993	6.6	*	*	*
Certain conditions originating in the perinatal period	1994	5.4	359.9	0.3	*
	1993	6.1	399.0	0.3	*

*Excerpted from a larger table that includes death rates through age 85 and older. Data are provisional, estimated from a 10% sample of deaths. Rates are per 100,000 population in a specified group. For further details, see original source.

†Ninth revision, International Classification of Diseases, 1975.

‡Figures for all ages include adults ages 25 to 85 years and older. See original source for adult figures. Figures for ages not stated (*) are included in "all ages" but are not distributed among age groups.

§Death rates for those of ages "younger than 1 year" (based on population estimates) differ from infant mortality rates (based on live births).

Adapted from National Center for Health Statistics, Department of Health and Human Services, *Monthly Vital Statistics Report.* (1995, October 23). *43*(13), 25.

Steps of the Nursing Process

- **Assessment:** The systematic collection of relevant data to determine a child's and family's current health status, coping patterns, needs, and problems
- **Diagnosis:** Analysis leading to the identification of a nursing diagnosis
- **Planning:** The process of prioritizing nursing diagnoses, writing goals and expected outcomes, and prescribing nursing interventions
- **Implementation:** The actual initiation and completion of nursing interventions essential to meet the stated goals. This step concludes when the nursing interventions are completed and have been documented.
- **Evaluation:** The examination of the results of nursing interventions in relation to the stated expected outcomes, which may include a review of the entire care plan

Assessment

During the assessment phase, three things take place: data collection, grouping of findings, and writing of the nursing diagnoses. Data can be collected through interview, physical examination, observation, review of records, and diagnostic reports, as well as through collaboration with other health care workers and the family.

There are several frameworks that may be used to guide the nurse in data collection. Two of the most common models are Gordon's Functional Health Patterns and the North American Nursing Diagnosis Association's (NANDA) Human Response Patterns. Chapters 10, (Communication), 11, (Physical Assessment), and 15 (The Ill Child) will assist in the assessment process by giving direction in interviewing, obtaining histories, using communication techniques, and performing the actual physical assessment.

Once the data are collected, they are grouped or organized into clusters that are made up of similar categories or cues. The process of clustering results in the formulation of a nursing diagnosis.

Nursing Diagnosis

A **nursing diagnosis** is a clinical judgment about the response of an individual, family, or community to actual and potential health problems/life processes. Nursing diagnoses provide the basis for selecting nursing interventions to achieve outcomes for which the nurse is accountable (North American Nursing Diagnosis Association, 1992). There are three types of nursing diagnoses. An actual nursing diagnosis describes a human response to a health condition/life process affecting an individual, family, or community. It is supported by defining characteristics (manifestations/signs and symptoms) that can be clustered in patterns of related cues or inferences. *Risk nursing diagnoses* describe human responses to health conditions/life processes that may develop in a vulnerable individual, family, or community. They are supported by risk factors that contribute to increased vulnerability. *Wellness nursing diagnoses* describe human responses to levels of wellness in an individual, family, or community that have a potential for enhancement to a higher state.

Each nursing diagnosis is a concise term or phrase that represents a pattern of related cues or signs and symptoms. The nursing diagnosis guides the nurse in planning care. One problem that nurses often encounter is writing nursing diagnoses that nursing actions cannot address. For example, a medical diagnosis, such as pyloric stenosis, cannot be treated by a nurse. However, it is appropriate to say that there are nursing actions that can decrease the fluid volume deficit associated with pyloric stenosis.

A nursing diagnosis consists of two sections joined by the phrase "related to." The statement begins with the child's response to the current problem and then describes the causative factor or factors. For example: *Altered Family Processes* related to *the diagnosis of a child with cancer.* The causative factors can be physiologic, psychological, sociocultural, environmental, or spiritual. They assist the nurse in identifying nursing interventions as planning takes place.

See Appendix J for a listing of the current NANDA-approved nursing diagnoses.

Planning

During the planning stage, the nursing diagnoses are prioritized, expected outcomes or goals are identified, and nursing interventions are prescribed. The diagnoses of highest priority are focused on the child's and family's most urgent needs. Actual nursing diagnoses do not necessarily have priority over high-risk nursing diagnoses.

Expected outcomes should be measurable child- or family-focused goals, and should be derived from the nursing diagnosis. Outcomes can be short- or long-term. Each expected outcome is stated in measurable terms. There should be a realistic time frame within which to achieve the outcome. Outcome criteria give direction to planning, implementation, and evaluation.

Nursing interventions may also be called *nursing orders* or *nursing actions;* they provide specific directions for nursing care. Through nursing interventions, the care of the child and family becomes individualized. There are three types of nursing interventions: independent, dependent, and interdependent.

- Independent—actions that can be performed by a nurse without another practitioner's direction or supervision
- Dependent—actions that require written or oral directions from another practitioner, but involve the nurse taking the action
- Interdependendent—actions involving collaboration between professionals, with possible establishment of standing orders or protocols

All three types of nursing interventions involve a nursing action to determine whether the intervention is appropriate for that child and family at that moment. This is part of ongoing assessment and utilizes the nurses' critical thinking skills.

Implementation

Implementation is the action phase of the nursing process. It begins with the initiation of nursing interventions and ends when the nurse documents the actions and the responses of the child and family. During this phase, the nurse is constantly reassessing to determine that the interventions remain appropriate. As the child's condition changes, so does the plan of care.

Evaluation

The effectiveness of the nursing care plan is appraised during the evaluation phase. The nurse determines whether the child and family have made progress according to the stated outcomes. In a way, it is also a time of assessing, as the nurse not only evaluates the plan of care but also seeks to identify new problems. Finally, the nurse determines whether the plan of care needs to be revised, and if so, which part of the plan presents a problem. Perhaps one or more of the nursing diagnoses were not appropriate. Nursing interventions may have been incomplete or not relevant to that child or family.

All steps of the nursing process are ongoing as long as the infant or child is receiving nursing care.

Documentation

Documentation establishes a mechanism for communication among members of the health care team, facilitates the delivery of quality client care, assures a mechanism for the evaluation of individual client care, and creates a permanent legal record of the care provided to the client (Iyer et al., 1991). Although documentation is not listed as a step in the nursing process, it is an integral part of the process.

Closure is brought to the nursing process when the care given is documented. Within the framework of documentation, the patient's records should show assessment data, nursing diagnoses, nursing care given, and the evaluation of that care. Documentation should be all-inclusive of the care given, including teaching and care of the family.

CASE MANAGEMENT

Case management is a practice model that uses a systematic approach to identify specific patients and to manage patient care to ensure optimal outcomes (Ignatavicius & Hausman, 1995). Within this model, services required by the patient and family are coordinated by a case manager or case coordinator, who focuses on both quality and cost outcomes. Inherent to case management is the coordination of care by all members of the health care team.

The guidelines established in 1995 by the Joint Commission on the Accreditation of Health Care Organizations (JCAHO) require an interdisciplinary, collaborative approach to patient care. This concept is at the core of case management.

Some of the identified strengths of case management include the following:

- Patients have a direction, are more aware of their progress, and have more insight into their care, thus increasing participation.
- Nursing practice becomes more outcome-oriented.
- The length of hospital stay is controlled.
- Staff nurses experience a greater sense of control and satisfaction about their care of patients.
- Increased collaboration is promoted among everyone involved with the patient, including patients and their families (Bower, 1988).

One question that continues to be asked is, "Who should the case manager be?" Many agencies employ baccalaureate- or masters-prepared nurses, but others may employ other health care providers, such as social workers. The use of the case manager also varies from institution to institution. The case manager may provide total patient care, may coordinate care provided by other health care givers, or may function in a consultant role. The role of the nurse in case management will continue to evolve as the delivery of health care continues to change.

Clinical Pathways

Clinical pathways provide for the case manager a tool for measuring outcomes. Clinical pathways are interdisciplinary plans of care that outline the optimal sequencing and timing of interventions for patients with a particular diagnosis, procedure, or symptom (Ignatavicius & Hausman, 1995). Clinical pathways are also referred to as clinical paths, critical paths or pathways, care maps, collaborative plans of care, multidisciplinary action plans (MAPS), care paths, and anticipated recovery paths. Although the concept of clinical pathways is not new, it has only recently been widely accepted as the use of case management has become more widespread in various health care settings. The purpose, as in managed care and case management, is to provide quality care while controlling cost.

Clinical pathways identify patient outcomes, specify timelines, promote collaboration, and involve a comprehensive approach to care. They are characterized by the following:

- Expected patient outcomes by the time of discharge are listed.
- Specific timelines for sequencing interventions are outlined.
- Jointly developed by multiple health care professionals, including physicians, clinical pathways reflect interdisciplinary interventions.
- The approach to care is comprehensive and includes nutrition, diagnostic tests, treatments, medications, mobility and activity, patient teaching, and discharge planning (Ignatavicius & Hausman, 1995).

Clinical pathways (Fig. 1–4) can be used in settings other than the hospital. Home health agencies are developing clinical pathways, and in some settings, these are developed in collaboration with hospital staff. (See Appendix K for additional samples of clinical pathways used in pediatrics.)

ASTHMA (Uncomplicated-without multi-system problems)
ICD-9 Codes 493, 493.01, 493.11, 493.91

Expected LOS-3 Days
D#.# = Key interventions for this study.

Examples of appropriate Co-morbidities
Acute Pharyngitis
Acute Sinusitis NOS
Cellulitis
Other Specific Viral Infection
Otitis Media NOS

Examples of Co-morbidities that are not appropriate
Bronchiolitis
Bronchopneumonia
Bronchopulmonary Dysplasia
Cardiac Conditions that extend the LOS
Cerebral Palsy
Cystic Fibrosis
Esophageal Reflux
HIV
Pneumonia
Pulmonary Collapse
Respiratory Failure
Sickle Cell Anemia

Refer to Tracking Sheet for Recording

Clinical Pathway	**Admission Day (Includes first 30 hrs)**	**Day 2**	**Day 3**
Aspect of Care	Date____ Unit____ ED	Date____ Unit	Date____ Unit
DAILY OUTCOME		↓ O2/Off O2 ↓ NEBS Off IV meds	↓ O2/Off O2 Discharge (D4.7 If not d/c by Day 3. record on tracking sheet)
TESTS	*D1.1 Waters view* Chest x-ray (if indicated)	*D2.5 Potassium level*	
CONSULTS	*D1.2 Discharge Planner* Asthma Education *Specialist (if high risk)*		Specialist (if not clearing)
FLUID/ELECTROLYTE MANAGEMENT	IV (pump & site check) I & O Q2-4 hr	Hep lock Routine I & O	Routine I & O
TREATMENTS/ PROCEDURES	*D1.3 NEBS Q2-4 hr* O2 (if indicated) Pulse oximeter	Nebs Q 3-8 hr Wean 02 to RA D/C oximeter when on room air	Neb Q 4-8 hr
MEDICATIONS	*D1.4 Steroid use* Zantac (consider) Antibiotics (if indicated)	Wean to po meds	*D3.6-Anti-Inflammatory Rx @ Discharge Y or N* (Record Y or N on tracking sheet) p.o. meds
CLINICAL SUPPORT	Anticipated LOS Basic Asthma Education tape Bed rest Extra patient checks Diet as tolerated Emotional support for patient/family	Nebulizer teaching (if indicated) Reinforce Asthma Education Up ad lib Routine safety Regular diet Emotional support for patient/family	Discharge meds & activity Up ad lib Routine safety Regular diet Emotional support for patient/family

Original Date 5/11/95 Revision Dates: 7/28/95 8/3/1995 1/1/96

This pathway is not a permanent part of the patient's medical record.

ANTI-INFLAMMATORY AGENTS

Corticosteroids, Inhaled
- Beclomethasone: Beclovent, Vanceril
- Dexamethasone: Decadron Respihaler
- Triamcinolone: Azmacort
- Flunisolide: AeroBid, AeroBid-M

Miscellaneous Agents, Inhaled
- Cromolyn: Intal
- Nedocromil: Tilade

Corticosteroids, Oral (multiple generics available)
- Prednisone: Liquid Prednisone
- Prednisolone: Prelone
- Triamcinolone: Kenacort, Aristocort
- Methylprednisolone: Medrol
- Dexamethasone: Decadron
- Betamethasone: Celestone

Disclaimer: This clinical pathway document is provided as a general guideline for use by physicians and staff in planning the care and treatment of patients and their families. It is not intended to be and does not establish a standard of care. Each patient's care is individualized according to their specific needs.

Cook Children's Medical Center
N:\WPFILES\COMM-MS\CCAR\ASTHMACP.FRM

Privileged and cofidential committee Document
TEX.REV.CIV.STAT.ANN art. 4995b §5.06

Figure 1–4
A clinical pathway for a child with uncomplicated asthma. (Courtesy of Cook Children's Medical Center, Fort Worth, Texas)

KEY CONCEPTS

- The major principles of pediatric nursing on which this textbook is based are (1) growth and development, (2) family-centered care, (3) health promotion, (4) child advocacy, (5) concepts applied across age groups, (6) focus on common pediatric disorders, and (7) communication.
- Current trends that affect the roles of nurses who care for children and their families include: changes in the health insurance system; the increasing number of children living in poverty; the increase in violence in U.S. society; the growth of children's hospitals and pediatric units; a shift to home-and community-based care; and the increasing cultural diversity of the population.
- Culture affects health care in the areas of nutrition, family values and parenting styles, language and communication, and individual family health beliefs and practices.
- Five roles of the pediatric nurse are care provider, teacher, collaborator, researcher, and advocate.
- The care settings in which pediatric nurses may practice include acute care settings, clinics, physicians' offices, HMOs, home health agencies, schools, rehabilitation centers, summer camps, day care centers, and hospice programs.
- Legal issues of particular concern to nurses caring for children include informed consent of the family for treatment, documentation of nonverbal behaviors, child advocacy (including reporting of suspected child abuse), issues related to adoption, and issues of confidentiality in dealing with adolescent health problems.
- Race, socioeconomic background, and education are variables that affect infant mortality in the United States.
- Health risk behaviors of youth include tobacco, drug, and alcohol use; risky sexual behaviors; poor diet; lack of physical activity; nonuse of safety belts or protective gear; and carrying of a weapon.

REFERENCES

Ahmann, E. (1994). "Chunky stew": Appreciating cultural diversity while providing health care for children. *Pediatric Nursing, 20*(3), 320–321.

American Academy of Pediatrics. (1995). The health insurance status of children: 1989–1992. *AAP News, 11*(2), 10–11.

Bower, K. (1988). Managed care: Controlling costs, guaranteeing outcomes. *Definition, 7*(3), 1–3.

Brodie, B. (1986). Yesterday, today, and tomorrow's pediatric world. *Children's Health Care, 14,* 168–173.

Carnegie Corporation of New York. New York. (1994). *Starting points: Meeting the needs of our youngest children.* New York: Author.

Centers for Disease Control. (1995a, March 24). *Morbidity and Mortality Weekly Report, 44,* No. SS1.

Centers for Disease Control. (1995b, May 26). Vaccination coverage levels among children aged 19–35 months—United States, April–June, 1994. *Morbidity and Mortality Weekly Report, 44*(20), 396–398.

Centers for Disease Control. (1995c). Poverty and infant mortality—United States, 1988. *Morbidity and Mortality Weekly Report. 44*(49), 922–926.

Centers for Disease Control. (1995d, March 22). Advance report of final monthly statistics, 1992. *Monthly Vital Statistics, 43*(6), Suppl.

Children's Defense Fund. (1991). *The state of America's children.* Washington, DC: Author.

Gorrie, T. M., McKinney, E. S., & Murray, S. S. (1994). *Foundations of maternal newborn nursing.* Philadelphia: W. B. Saunders.

Guyer, B., Strobino, D. M., Ventura, S. J., & Singh, G. K. (1995). Annual summary of vital statistics. *Pediatrics, 96*(6), 1029–1039.

Ignatavicius, D., & Hausman, K. (1995). *Clinical pathways for collaborative practice.* Philadelphia: W. B. Saunders.

Iyer, P., Taptich, B., & Bernocchi-Losey, D. (1991). *Nurisng process and nursing diagnosis.* Philadelphia: W. B. Saunders.

Jakubec, P. (1995). West Virginia effort reduces infant mortality rate. *AAP News, 11*(12), 18.

Larson, L. (1995). Violence casts fear over schools. *AAP News, 11*(9), 1–7.

Malloy, C. (1992). Children and poverty: America's future at risk. *Pediatric Nursing, 18*(6), 553–557.

Newacheck, P., Jameson, W., & Halfon, N. (1994). Health status and income: The impact of poverty on child health. *Journal of School Health, 64*(6), 229–233.

North American Nursing Diagnosis Association (1992). *NANDA Nursing Diagnosis: Definitions and Classifications: 1992.* St. Louis: Author.

Population and Vital Statistics Report. (1990). Series A, 44(1). New York: United Nations.

Richardson, L. A., Selby-Harrington, M. L., Krowchuk, H. V., Cross, A. W., & Williams, D. (1994). Health promotion and injury prevention. *Journal of Pediatric Health Care, 8,* 212–220.

Singh, G. K., & Yu, S. M. (1995). Infant mortality in the United States: Trends, differentials, and projections, 1950 through 2010. *American Journal of Public Health, 85*(7), 957–964.

Society of Pediatric Nurses. (1995). Changing practice, changing roles, and changing environments: *Report of the Fifth Annual SPN Conference, 4*(2), 4–5.

Struk, C. (1994). Women and children: Infant mortality, urban programs, and home care. *Nursing Clinics of North America, 29*(3), 395–407.

U.S. Department of Health and Human Services. (1990). *Healthy People 2000.* Washington, DC: Author.

Vaughn, V. C. (1992). The field of pediatrics. In R. E. Behrman & V. C. Vaughn (Eds.), *Nelson's textbook of pediatrics* (14th ed., p. 1). Philadelphia: W. B. Saunders.

Velsor-Friedrich, B., & Frager, B. (1990). The federal government and child health. *Journal of Pediatric Nursing, 5*(1), 56–58.

BIBLIOGRAPHY

Alfaro-LeFevere, R. (1995). *Critical thinking in nursing.* Philadelphia: W. B. Saunders.

Allen, J. M., & Hollowell, E. E. (1990). Nurses and child abuse/neglect reporting: Duties, responsibilities, and issues. *Journal of Practical Nursing, 40*(2), 56–59.

American Academy of Pediatrics Committee on Communications. (1995). *Media violence.* Elk Grove Village, IL: American Academy of Pediatrics.

Ballard, D. (1993). The legal side. *American Journal of Nursing, 93*(12), 21.

Blendon, R., Altman, D., Benson, J., Brodie, M., James, M., & Chervinsky, G. (1995). The public and the welfare reform debate. *Archives of Pediatric and Adolescent Medicine, 149,* 1065–1069.

Bocchino, C. (1993). Legislative update: Immunizing America's children. *Pediatric Nursing, 19*(3), 281–282.

Broome, M. E., & Stieglitz, K. A. (1992). The consent process and children. *Research in Nursing and Health, 15,* 147–152.

Carpenito, L. (1995). *Nursing diagnosis: Application to clinical practice.* Philadelphia: J. B. Lippincott.

Centers for Disease Control. (1996). Monthly immunization table. *Morbidity and Mortality Weekly Report, 45*(1), 10.

Clayton, E. W., & Hickson, G. B. (1990). Compensation under the National Childhood Vaccine Injury Act. *Journal of Pediatrics, 116*(4), 508–513.

Davia, A. J. (1980). When parents disagree on treatment. *American Journal of Nursing, 80*(11), 2082.

Demos, J. (1970). *A little commonwealth: Family life in a Plymouth colony.* New York: Oxford University.

Doenges, M., Moorhouse, M., Burley, J. (1995). *Application of nursing process and nursing diagnosis: An interactive text for diagnostic reasoning.* Philadelphia: F. A. Davis.

Dolan J., Fitzpatrick M., & Hermann, E. (1983). *Nursing in society: A historical perspective* (15th ed.). Philadelphia: W. B. Saunders.

English, A. (1990). Treating adolescents: Legal and ethical considerations. *Pediatric Clinics of North America, 74,* 1097.

Fiesta, J. (1991). Mother vs. child—A legal controversy. *Nursing Management, 22*(10), 14–17.

Frenkel, L. D. (1990). Pediatric vaccinations: Update 1990. Routine immunizations for American children in the 1990s. *Pediatric Clinics of North America, 37*(3), 531–548.

Hogue, E. E. (1988). Informed consent: Implications for critical care nurses. *Pediatric Nursing, 14*(4), 315–316.

King, J. (1986). Nature of the duty owed—The standard of care. In *The Law of Medical Malpractice in a Nutshell* (2nd ed.). St. Paul: West Publishing Co.

Lannon, C., Brack, V., Stuart, J., Caplow, M., McNeill, A., Bordley, W. C., & Margolis, P. (1995). What mothers say about why poor children fall behind on immunizations. *Archives of Pediatric and Adolescent Medicine,* 149, 1070–1075.

Mandell, M. (1992). Practical ways to survive a lawsuit. *Nursing '92, 22*(8), 56–57.

Melina, L. R., & Roszia, S. K. (1993). The open adoption experience. New York: Harper Perennial.

Moore, G. M. (1993). Surviving a malpractice lawsuit: One nurse's story. *Nursing '93, 23*(10), 55–58.

National Center for Children in Poverty. (1990). *Five million children: A statistical profile of our poorest young citizens.* New York: Columbia University School of Public Health.

National Center for Family-Centered Care. (1990). *What is family-centered care?* Bethesda, MD: Association for the Care of Children's Health.

Olson, V. T., & Hooke, M. M. (1988). The complexities of do not resuscitate orders. *MCN, 13*(3), 157–162.

Pieranunzi, V. R., & Freitas, L. G. (1992). Informed consent with children and adolescents. *JCPN, 5*(2), 21–26.

Plotnick, J., & Presler, B. (1996). Rugged individualism and compassion: The foundation of public policy. *Maternal and Child Nursing, 21,* 20–33.

President's Commission for the Study of Ethical Problems in Medicine and Biomedical and Behavioral Research. (1982). *Making health care decisions* (Vol. 1). Washington, DC: U.S. Government Printing Office.

Rachuba, L., Stanton, B., & Howard, D. (1995). Violent crime in the United States. *Archives of Pediatric and Adolescent Medicine, 149,* 953–960.

Rhodes, A. M. (1991). Major legal initiatives in MCH (1975–1990). *Maternal and Child Nursing, 16*(1), 45.

Rushton, C. H., et al. (1993). End of life care for infants with AIDS: Ethical and legal issues. *Pediatric Nursing, 19*(1), 79–83.

Silber, K., & Dorner, P. M. (1990). *Children of open adoption.* San Antonio, TX: Corona Publishing Company.

Sklan, M. L. (1994, Winter). Medicine and law: Recent developments. *Tort & Insurance Law Journal, 22*(2), 347–348.

Smith, J. B. (1989). Ethical issues raised by new treatment options. *Maternal and Child Nursing, 14*(3), 183–187.

Solar, J. M. (1994). Analysis of legal issues, pharmaceutical cases. Part II: Over-the-counter medications and drug samples. In *Medical Device and Pharmaceutical Litigation.* Houston, TX: University of Houston Law Foundation.

Sparks, S., & Taylor, C. (1993). *Nursing diagnosis reference manual.* Springhouse, PA: Springhouse Corporation.

Spence, A. (1995). Family instability leaves children vulnerable. *AAP News, 11*(8), 10–12.

Steinbock, B. (1984). Baby Jane Doe in court. *The Hastings Report, 40*(1), 13–19.

Torres, J. L., & Blair, T. M. (1992). Administering emergency medical care to minors. *Topics in Emergency Medicine, 14*(4), 20–23.

Weese, C. B., Drauss, M. R. (1995). A "barrier-free" health care system does not ensure adequate vaccination of 2-year-old children. *Archives of Pediatric and Adolescent Medicine, 149,* 1130–1135.

White, C. C. (1995). Migrant farmworker children suffer inferior health care. *AAP News, 11*(10), 8–25.

Yoos, H. L., Kitzman, H., Olds, D. L., & Overacker, I. (1995). Community: Implications for culturally competent pediatric care. *Journal of Pediatric Nursing, 10*(6), 343–353.

UNIT II

GROWTH AND DEVELOPMENT: THE CHILD AND THE FAMILY

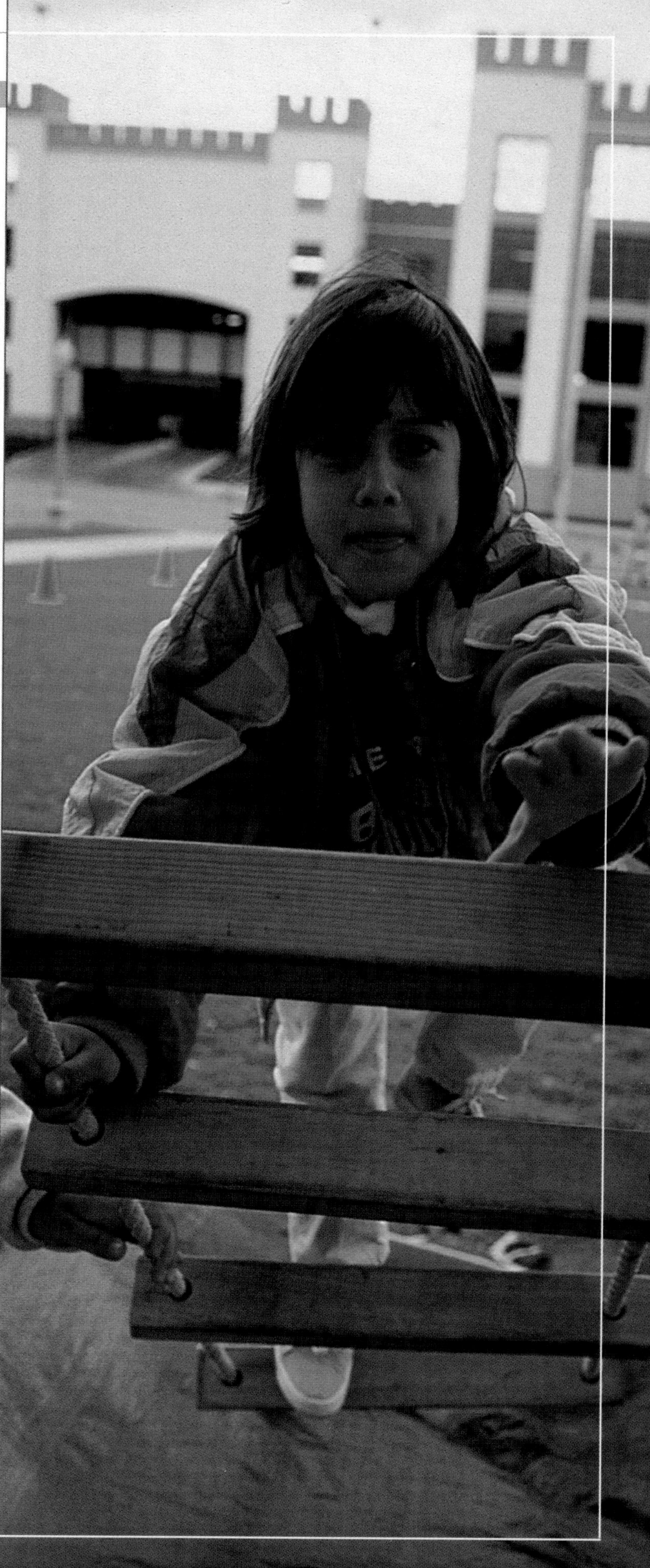

Courtesy of Cook Children's Medical Center, Fort Worth, Texas

2

Growth and Development

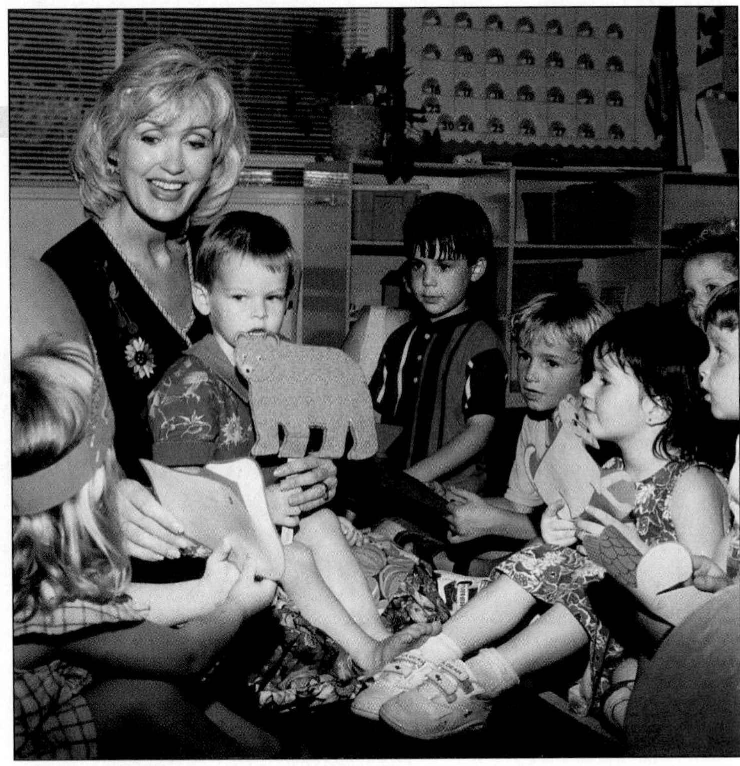

CHAPTER OVERVIEW

LEARNING OBJECTIVES

After studying this chapter, you should be able to:

- Define terms related to growth and development.
- Discuss principles of growth and development.
- Describe various factors, including genetics, that affect growth and development.
- Discuss the following theorists' ideas about growth and development: Piaget, Freud, Erikson, Kohlberg.
- Discuss theories of language development.
- Identify methods used to assess growth and development.
- Use knowledge of growth and development to formulate a developmentally appropriate nursing care plan.

KEY TERMS

cephalocaudal: growth and development that proceeds from head to toe

chromosomes: packages of genetic material that occur in pairs within the nucleus of cells; contain genes

chronological age: age in years

developmental age: age based on functional behavior and ability to adapt to the environment; does not necessarily correspond to chronological age

genes: units of heredity that control formation and function of proteins throughout the body and transmit inherited information

genetics: the study of heredity

growth spurts: brief periods of rapid increase in growth rate

heredity: the transmission of genetic characteristics from parent to offspring

learning: behavior changes that occur as a result of both maturation and experience with the environment

regression: use of behavior that is more appropriate to an earlier stage of development; often used to cope with stress or anxiety

Humans grow and change dramatically during childhood and adolescence. Parents watch with wonder as their tiny, helpless newborns grow and develop into self-sufficient, independent individuals. Changes occur so rapidly and completely that parents may have trouble remembering what their children were like at earlier stages of development.

Normal growth and development proceed in an orderly, predictable pattern that provides the basis for assessing an individual's abilities and potential. Nurses provide health care teaching and anticipatory guidance about the growth and development of children in many settings, such as newborn nurseries, emergency departments, clinics, and pediatric inpatient units.

Because nurses are often the most approachable members of the health care team, they must be prepared to deal with questions asked by parents. Parents are often concerned that their children are not progressing normally. Nurses can reassure parents about normal variations in development and also identify problems early so that developmental delays can be addressed as soon as possible.

Nurses who work with ill children must have a clear understanding of how children differ from adults and from each other at various stages. This awareness is essential to allow nurses to create developmentally appropriate plans of care to meet the needs of their young patients.

This chapter provides an introduction to growth and development and an overview of theories on intellectual, psychosocial, language, and moral development. It discusses principles of growth and development as well as factors that influence how children progress. In addition, various methods of assessing growth and development are described. The theories presented provide a basis for the application of the nursing process to the care of children. More in-depth discussion of growth and development follows in chapters devoted to each age group.

OVERVIEW OF GROWTH AND DEVELOPMENT

Definition of Terms

Although the terms "growth" and "development" are often used together and interchangeably, they have distinct definitions and meanings. Growth is generally referred to as an increase in the physical size of a whole or any of its parts, or an increase in the number and size of cells.

Growth can be measured easily and accurately. For example, any observer can see that an infant grows rapidly during the first year of life. This growth can be measured readily by determining changes in weight and length. The difference in size between a newborn and a 12-month-old is an obvious sign of the remarkable growth that occurs during the first year of life.

Development is a more complex and subtle concept. Development is generally considered a continuous, orderly series of conditions that lead to activities, new motives for activities, and eventual patterns of behavior.

Another definition of development is an increase in function and complexity that occurs through growth, maturation, and learning; in other words, an increase in capabilities. Development is illustrated by the process of language acquisition. The use of language becomes increasingly complex as the child matures. At 10 to 12 months of age, a child uses single words to communicate simple desires and needs. By age 4 to 5 years, she uses complete and complex sentences to relate elaborate tales. Language development can be measured by determining vocabulary, articulation skill, and word use.

Maturity and learning also affect development. Maturation is the physical change in the complexity of body structures that enables a child to function at increasingly higher levels. Maturity is programmed genetically and may occur as a result of several changes. For example, maturation of the central nervous system is dependent on changes that occur throughout the body, such as an increase in the number of neurons, myelinization of nerve fibers, lengthening of muscles, and overall weight gain.

Learning involves changes in behavior that occur as a result of both maturation and experience with the environment. Predictable patterns are observed in learning, and these patterns are sequential, orderly, and progressive. For example, when learning to walk, a baby first learns to control his head, then to roll over, next to sit, then to crawl, and finally to walk. The child's muscle mass and nervous system must grow and mature as well.

These examples show how complex and interrelated the processes of growth, development, maturation, and learning are. Children must be monitored carefully to ensure that these complicated events and activities unfold normally. Wide variations occur as children grow and develop. Each child has a unique rate and pattern of development, although parameters are used to identify abnormalities. Nurses must be familiar with normal parameters so that delays can be detected early. The earlier that delays are discovered and treated, the less dramatic their effect will be.

Stages of Growth and Development

The following stages and age groupings are used throughout this book in referring to stages of childhood growth and development.

Newborn	Birth–1 month
Infancy	1 month–1 year
Toddlerhood	1–3 years
Preschool age	3–6 years
School age	6–11 or 12 years
Adolescence	11 or 12–21 years

Stages of Growth and Development

To simplify analysis and discussion of the complex processes and theories related to growth and development, researchers and theorists have identified stages or age groupings (see box). These stages serve as reference points in describing various features of growth and development. Chapters 3 through 8 discuss the physical growth and cognitive, emotional, language, and motor development specific to each stage.

Parameters of Growth

Statistical data derived from research studies of large groups of children provide health care professionals with information about how children normally grow. Throughout infancy, childhood, and adolescence, growth occurs in bursts separated by periods when no growth occurs (Lampl, 1995). Although heredity determines each individual's growth rate, the normal pace of growth of all children falls into four distinct patterns: (1) a rapid pace from birth to 2 years; (2) a slower pace from 2 years to puberty; (3) a rapid pace from puberty to approximately 15 years of age; and (4) a sharp decline from 16 years to approximately 24 years, when full adult size is reached.

Weight, height, and head circumference are parameters that are used to monitor growth. They should be measured at regular intervals during childhood. The weight of the average term newborn is approximately 7 to 8 pounds, (3.2–3.6 kg). Male infants are usually slightly heavier than female infants. Usually, the birth weight doubles by 6 months of age and triples by 1 year of age. Between 2 and 3 years of age, the weight quadruples. Slow, steady weight gain during childhood is followed by a growth spurt during adolescence.

The average newborn is approximately 20 inches (50 cm) long, with an average increase of approximately 1 inch (2.54 cm) per month for the first 6 months, followed by an increase of approximately ½ inch per month for the remainder of the first year. The child gains 3 inches (7.6 cm) per year from age 1 through 7 years, then 2 inches (5 cm) per year from age 8 through 15 years. Boys generally add more height during adolescence than do girls. Body proportion changes are shown in Figure 2–1.

Head circumference indicates brain growth. The normal occipital–frontal circumference of the term newborn head is 13 to 14 inches (33–35 cm). Average head growth occurs according to the following pattern: 4 inches (10 cm) during the first year; 1 inch (2.5 cm) during the second year; ½ inch (1.2 cm) per year from 3 to 5 years; and ½ inch per 5 years until puberty. The average adult head circumference is approximately 21 inches (53 cm).

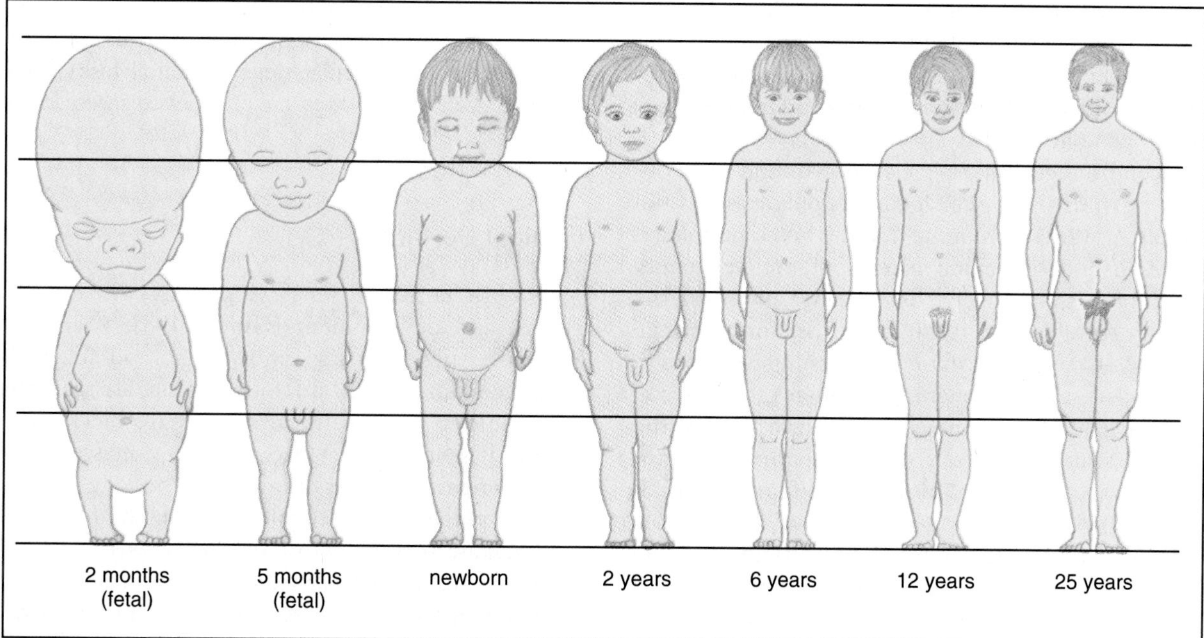

Figure 2–1
Changes in body proportions with growth.

Dentition, the eruption of teeth, also follows a sequential pattern. Primary dentition usually begins at approximately 6 to 8 months. Most children have 20 teeth by $2\frac{1}{2}$ years. Permanent teeth, 32 in all, erupt beginning at approximately age 6 years, accompanied by the loss of primary teeth (see Chapter 11). Although some parents place importance on eruption of the teeth as a sign of maturation, dentition is not related to the level or rate of development.

PRINCIPLES OF GROWTH AND DEVELOPMENT

Patterns of Growth and Development

Growth and development are directional and follow predictable patterns (see box). The first direction of growth is **cephalocaudal,** which means that growth and development proceed from head to tail (or toe). Structures and functions originating in the head develop before those in the lower parts of the body. At birth, the head is large, a full one-fourth of the entire body length, the trunk is long, and the arms are longer than the legs. As the child matures, his body proportions gradually change, and by adulthood, the legs have increased in size from approximately 38% to 50% of the total body length (see Figure 2–1).

Directional growth and development is illustrated further by the myelinization of nerves, which begins in the

Directional Patterns of Growth and Development

CEPHALOCAUDAL PATTERN (HEAD TO TOE)

Examples:

- Head initially grows fastest (fetus), then trunk (infant), then legs (child).
- Infant can raise his head before sitting and can sit before standing.

Cephalocaudal (head to toe)

Proximal distal (from the center outward)

PROXIMODISTAL PATTERN (FROM THE CENTER OUTWARD)

Examples:

- In the respiratory system, the trachea develops first in the embryo, followed by branching and growth outward in the bronchi, bronchioles, and alveoli in the fetus and infant.
- Motor control of the arms comes before control of the hands, and hand control comes before finger control.

brain and spreads downward as the child matures. Growth of the myelin sheath and other nerve structures contributes to cephalocaudal development, which is illustrated by the infant's ability to raise his head before he sits and to sit before he stands.

A second directional aspect of growth and development is proximodistal, which means progression from the center outward, or from the midline to the periphery. The growth and branching pattern of the respiratory tract illustrates this concept. The trachea, which is the central structure of the respiratory tree, forms in the embryo by 24 days of gestation. Branching and growth outward occur in the bronchi, bronchioles, and alveoli throughout fetal life and infancy. Alveoli, which are the most distal structures of the system, continue to grow and develop in number and function until middle childhood.

Growth and development follow patterns, one of which is general to specific. As a child matures, her activities become less generalized and more focused. For example, a newborn's response to pain is usually a whole-body response, with flailing of the arms and legs even if the pain is in the abdomen. As the child matures, the pain response becomes more localized to the stimulus. An older child with abdominal pain guards his abdomen. Another example is palmar grasp (using the whole hand to grasp an object) at 4 to 5 months of age. At approximately 9 months of age, the palmar grasp is gradually replaced by the pincer grasp (using the thumb and forefinger). The pincer grasp requires the use of more specific fine motor muscle control than does the palmar grasp.

Another pattern is the progression of functions from simple to complex. This pattern is easily observed in language development. A toddler's first sentences are formed simply, using only a noun and a verb. By age 5 years, she constructs detailed stories using many complex modifiers.

The rate of growth is not constant as the child matures. **Growth spurts,** alternating with periods of slow or stagnant growth, are observed throughout childhood. Spurts are frequently seen as the child prepares to master a significant developmental task, such as walking. An increase in growth around a child's first birthday may promote the neuromuscular maturation needed for him to take his first steps.

All facets of development (cognitive, motor, emotional, language) normally proceed according to these patterns. Knowledge of these concepts is useful when determining how a child's development is progressing and when comparing a child's development with normal patterns.

Mastery of developmental tasks is not static or permanent, and developmental stages do not always correlate with chronological age. Children progress through developmental stages at varying rates within normal limits and may master developmental tasks only to regress to earlier levels when ill or stressed. Also, people can struggle repeatedly with particular developmental tasks throughout life, even though they have achieved more advanced levels of development.

Critical Periods

After birth, critical or sensitive periods exist for optimal growth and development (Hinde, 1983; Crain, 1992). Similar to times during embryologic and fetal life in which certain organs are formed and are particularly vulnerable to injury, critical periods are blocks of time during which children are ready to master specific developmental tasks. During these periods, which are not tied precisely to chronological age, children seem to demonstrate a readiness to learn (Thomas, 1992). Children can master tasks outside of these critical periods, but some tasks are learned more easily during particular periods.

Many factors affect a child's sensitive learning periods, such as injury, illness, and malnutrition. For example, the sensitive period for learning to walk seems to be during the latter part of the first year and the beginning of the second year. Children seem to be driven by an irresistible urge to practice walking and display great pride as they succeed. If a child is immobilized, for instance for the treatment of an orthopedic condition from age 10 months to 18 months, he may have difficulty learning to walk. He can learn to walk, but the task may be more difficult for him than for others.

Factors Influencing Growth and Development

Genetics. One of the factors with the greatest influence on a child's growth and development is genetics. Genetic potential is affected by many factors. Environment influences how and to what extent particular genetic traits are manifested. A more complete discussion of genetics is included later in this chapter (see Hereditary Influence on Growth and Development).

Environment. The environment is a significant determinant of growth and developmental outcome, both before and after birth. Prenatal environmental factors include maternal smoking, alcohol intake, and disease, such as diabetes. Socioeconomic status, interpersonal relationships, and environmental hazards are only a few of the factors affecting children both before and after birth. For a discussion of environmental factors that affect children, see Chapters 13 and 16.

Culture. Culture is the way of life of a people, including their habits, beliefs, language, and values. It is a significant factor influencing children as they grow toward adulthood.

For example, Victora et al. (1990) found that preschool British children performed better on tests of fine motor and practical reasoning skills than did their counterparts from Brazil. On the other hand, the Brazilian preschoolers were more advanced in their gross motor skills and speech than the British children.

These differences may be attributed to cultural features of the two countries. Brazilian culture stresses vigorous activities, such as running, jumping, and playing in groups outdoors, perhaps because of the warm climate and the relatively large family size. British children may spend more time indoors, perhaps because of the cool weather and industrialized economy. These children may develop fine motor and problem-solving skills through drawing, solving puzzles, and assembling structure-building toys.

When gathering data, nurses must recognize how the common family structures and traditional values of various groups affect children's performance on assessment tests. For example, Seideman et al. (1994) found that Native American mothers were likely to use nonverbal parenting techniques and unlikely to structure and intervene in their children's activities. This preference for nonverbal teaching and visual learning affects the child's verbal development and performance on assessment tests. The child's progress in schools that emphasize verbal skills may also be affected.

Nurses should consider the patient's cultural and ethnic background while assessing growth and development. Standard growth curves and developmental tests do not necessarily reflect the normal growth and development of children of various cultural groups. Growth curves for children of various racial and cultural backgrounds are increasingly available. Studies are conducted by nurse researchers and others to determine the effectiveness of measurement tools for culturally diverse populations. In addition, culturally sensitive instruments are being developed to gather data to determine appropriate nursing interventions. To provide quality care to all patients, nurses must consider the effect of culture on children and families.

Nutrition. Because children are growing constantly and need a continuous supply of nutrients, nutrition plays an important role throughout childhood. Adequate nourishment is necessary for brain growth, prenatally and especially during the first year of life (Pipes, 1993). Good nutritional status is also needed for normal function of hormones, especially growth factor and sex hormones. The effect of nutrition on growth and development is discussed in Chapter 12.

Health Status. Overall health status plays an important part in the growth and development of children. At the cellular level, inherited or acquired disease can affect the delivery of nutrients, hormones, or oxygen to organs and also organ growth and function. Disease states that affect growth and development include digestive or malabsorption disorders, heart defects, and metabolic diseases.

Play. Play is the work of children. To adult observers, children's play may appear unorganized, meaningless, and even chaotic. However, anyone who watches carefully quickly discovers that play is a rich activity, intricately woven with meaning and purpose. Play is most frequent during periods of rapid growth and development, and play may be related directly to expanding intellectual, motor, language, and social development (Garvey, 1990). In adulthood, work is any activity during which one uses time and energy to create a product or achieve a goal. Play in childhood is similar to adult work in that it is undertaken by the child to accomplish developmental tasks and master the environment. Play is described in Chapter 9.

Family. A child is an inseparable part of a family. Family relationships and influences are major determinants of how children grow and progress. Because of the special bond and influence of the family on the child, there can be no separation of child from family in the health care setting. For example, to diminish anxiety in a child, nurses sometimes attempt to reduce parental anxiety, which may then reduce the stress on the child. Nursing care of children involves nursing care of the whole family and requires skill in dealing with both adults and children. The family is discussed in Chapter 16.

COMMUNICATION CUE Nurses might reduce parental anxiety about an ill child by saying the following: "Your child is in the best place possible here at the hospital. You brought him in at just the right time so that we can help him."

Family structures are in a constant state of change, and these dynamic states influence how children develop. Within the family, relationships change because of marriage, birth, divorce, death, and new roles and responsibilities. Societal forces outside the family, such as economics, population shifts, and migration, change how children are raised. Perhaps one of the most dramatic changes in the American family over the last 30 years has been an increase in the number of single-parent families. Nearly 50% of children born today will spend an extended period in a family headed by only one adult (Lewis & Volkmar, 1990). These forces cause changes in family structures and the outcomes of child rearing that must be considered when planning nursing care for children.

Parental Attitudes. Parental attitudes affect growth and development. Growth and development continue throughout life, and parents have stage-related needs and tasks that affect their children. Superimposed on these developmental issues are other factors influencing parental attitudes: educational level, childhood experiences, financial pressures, marital status, and available support systems. Parental attitudes are also affected by the child's temperament, the child's unique way of relating to the world. Temperament is discussed in Chapter 16, which describes the easy child, the slow-to-warm child, and the difficult child. These different temperaments affect parenting practices and whether a child's unique personality traits develop into assets or problems.

Child-Rearing Philosophies. Child-rearing philosophies, shaped by a myriad of life events, have an effect on how children grow and develop. For example, well-educated, well-read parents often provide their children with extra stimulation and opportunities for learning, beginning at a young age. This enrichment includes extra parental attention and interaction, not necessarily expensive toys. Generally, development progresses best when enriched opportunities for learning are provided.

Other parents may not recognize the need to provide a rich learning environment at home, may not have time, or may not value this type of parenting. Children of these parents may not progress at the same rate as those raised in a more enriched atmosphere.

A significant point for parents to remember is that children must be ready to learn. If motor and neurologic structures are not mature, no amount of added stimulation will produce new behavior. The result of an overzealous approach toward accomplishing a specific task is frustration for both child and parent. For example, a child who is 6 months old will not be able to walk alone, no matter how much time and effort the parent expends. However, at 12 to 14 months, a child usually is ready to begin walking and will do so with ease if given opportunities to practice.

THEORIES OF GROWTH AND DEVELOPMENT

Many theorists have attempted to organize and classify the complex phenomena of growth and development. No single theory can adequately explain the wondrous journey from infancy to adulthood. However, each theorist contributes a piece of the puzzle. Theories are not facts, but merely attempts to explain human behavior. Table 2–1 compares and contrasts theories discussed in the text. The chapters on each age group provide further discussion of these theories.

Piaget's Theory of Cognitive Development

Jean Piaget (1896–1980), a Swiss theorist, made major contributions to the study of how children learn. His complex theory provides a framework for understanding how thinking during childhood progresses and differs from adult thinking. Like other developmental theorists, he postulates that as children develop intellectually, they pass through progressive stages. The ages assigned to these periods are only averages.

During the sensorimotor period of development, infant thinking seems to involve the entire body. Reflexive behavior is gradually replaced by more complex activities. The world becomes increasingly solid through the development of the concept of object permanence, which is the awareness that objects continue to exist even when they disappear from sight. By the end of this stage, the infant shows some evidence of reasoning.

During the period of preoperational thought, language becomes increasingly useful. Judgments are dominated by perception and are illogical, and thinking is characterized, especially during the early part of this stage, by egocentrism. In other words, the child is unable to think about another person's viewpoint and believes that everyone perceives situations as she does. Magical thinking, or the belief that events occur because of wishing, and animism, or the perception that all objects have life and feeling, characterize this period.

At the end of the preoperational stage, the child shifts from egocentric thinking and begins to look at the world from another's view. This shifting enables the child to move into the period of concrete operations, during which he is no longer bound by perceptions and can distinguish fact from fantasy. The concept of time becomes increasingly clear during this stage, although far past and far future events remain obscure. Although reasoning powers increase rapidly during this stage, the child cannot deal with abstractions or socialized thinking.

Normally, adolescents progress to the period of formal operations. In this period, the child can create new ideas by combining previous thoughts. He can analyze situations and think abstractly through the use of concepts. All of these stages of cognitive development are discussed in the chapters on each age group (Dixon & Stein, 1992; Flavell, 1963; Lewis & Volkmar, 1990).

Nursing Implications of Piaget's Theory. Piaget's theory is especially significant to nurses as they develop teaching plans of care for children. Piaget believed that learning should be geared to the child's level of understanding and that the child should be an active participant in the learning process. For health teaching to be effective, nurses must understand the different cognitive abilities of children at various ages. Nurses also must know how to engage children in the learning process with developmentally appropriate activities.

Because hospitalization is often frightening to children, especially toddlers and preschoolers, nurses must understand the cognitive basis of fears related to treatment and be able to intervene appropriately (see Chapter 15).

Freud's Theory of Psychosexual Development

Sigmund Freud (1856–1939) developed theories to explain psychosexual development. His theories were in vogue for many years and provided a basis for other theories. Freud postulated that early childhood experiences provide unconscious motivation for actions later in life. According to Freudian theory, certain parts of the body assume psychologic significance as foci of sexual energy. These areas shift from one part of the body to another as the child moves through different stages of development. Recently, experts have been critical of Freud's psychoanalytic theories, citing that they are too narrow and simple to explain such complex behavior (Lewis & Volkmar, 1990; Crain, 1992). However, Freud's work may help to explain normal behavior that parents may confuse with abnormal behavior, and it also may provide a good foundation for sex education.

Freud believed that during infancy, sexual behavior seems to focus around the mouth, the most erogenous area of the infant body (oral stage). The infant derives pleasure from sucking and exploring objects by placing them in his mouth. During toddlerhood, when toilet training becomes a major developmental task, sensations seem to shift away from the mouth and toward the anus (anal stage). Psychoanalysts see this period as a time of holding on and letting go. A sense of control or autonomy develops as the child masters bodily functions.

During the preschool years, interest in the genitalia arises (phallic stage). Children are curious about anatomic differences, childbirth, and sexuality. Children at this age often ask many questions, freely exhibit their own sexual organs, and want to peek at those of others. Children often masturbate, sometimes causing great concern in parents. Although it is not universal, a phenomenon described by Freud as the Oedipal conflict in boys and the Electra complex in girls is seen in preschool children. This possessiveness of the child for the opposite-sex parent, marked by aggressiveness toward the same-sex parent, is considered normal behavior, as is a heightened interest in sex. To resolve these disturbing sexual feelings, the preschooler identifies with or becomes more like the same-sex parent. The superego (an inner voice that reprimands and evokes guilt) also develops. The superego is similar to a conscience (Freud, 1923).

The school-age period is described by Freud as the latency stage, when sexuality plays a less prominent role in the everyday life of the child. Best friends and same-sex peer groups are influential in the school-age child's life. Younger school-age children often refuse to play with children of the opposite sex, whereas prepubertal children begin to desire the companionship of opposite-sex friends.

During adolescence, interest in sex again flourishes as the child searches for his identity (genital stage). Under the influence of fluctuating hormone levels, dramatic physical changes, and shifting social relationships, the adolescent develops a more adult view of sexuality. However, their cognitive skills are not fully developed, and adolescents often make questionable judgments about sexual matters and may have questions and concerns about their behavior and feelings (Freud, 1974; Lewis & Volkmar, 1990; Litt & Martin, 1992).

Nursing Implications of Freud's Theory. Both children and parents may have questions and concerns about normal sexual development and sex education. Nurses must understand normal sexual growth and development to help parents and children form healthy attitudes about sex.

Erikson's Psychosocial Theory

Born in 1902, Erik H. Erikson, inspired by the work of Sigmund Freud, created a popular theory about child development. He viewed development as a lifelong series of conflicts affected by social and cultural factors. Each conflict must be resolved for the child and adult to progress emotionally. There is wide variation in how individuals address the conflicts. However, according to Erikson, unsuccessful resolution leaves the individual emotionally handicapped.

Each stage of development has a specific central conflict or developmental task. These eight tasks, divided into stages of development, are described in terms of a positive or negative resolution. The actual resolution of a specific conflict lies somewhere along a continuum between a perfect positive and a perfect negative.

The first developmental task is the establishment of trust. The basic quality of trust provides a foundation for the personality. If an infant's physical and emotional needs are met in a timely manner through warm and nurturing interactions with a consistent caregiver, the infant begins to sense that her world is trustworthy. She begins to trust, not only her caregivers, but herself as a being worthy of love. Through successful achievement of a sense of trust, the infant can move on to subsequent developmental stages.

According to Erikson, unsuccessful resolution of this first developmental task results in a sense of mistrust. If needs are consistently unmet, acute tension begins to appear in children. During infancy, signs of unmet needs include restlessness, fretfulness, whining, crying, clinging, physical tenseness, and physical dysfunctions such as vomiting, diarrhea, and sleep disturbances. All children exhibit these signs at times. However, if these behaviors become personality characteristics, unsuccessful resolution of this stage is suspected. Prolonged deprivation leads to personality dysfunction that is reflected in clinging, dependent behavior, eating disorders, or chronic envy (Lewis & Volkmar, 1990). Negative resolution of any developmental task leads to decreased ability to handle

TABLE 2–1 *Comparison of Theories of Growth and Development*

	PIAGET'S PERIODS OF COGNITIVE DEVELOPMENT	FREUD'S STAGES OF PSYCHOSEXUAL DEVELOPMENT	ERIKSON'S STAGES OF PSYCHOSOCIAL DEVELOPMENT	KOHLBERG'S STAGES OF MORAL DEVELOPMENT
Infancy	***Period 1 (Birth–2 Years): Sensorimotor Period*** Reflexive behavior is used to adapt to the environment; egocentric view of the world; development of object permanence.	***Oral Stage*** Mouth is a sensory organ; infant takes in and explores during oral passive substage (first half of infancy); infant strikes out with teeth during oral aggressive substage (latter half of infancy).	***Trust versus Mistrust*** Development of a sense that the self is good and the world is good when consistent, predictable, reliable care is received; characterized by hope.	***Stage 0 (0–2 Years): Naivete and Egocentrism*** No moral sensitivity; decisions are made on the basis of what pleases the child; infants like or love what helps them and dislike what hurts them; no awareness of the effect of his actions on others. "Good is what I like and want."
Toddlerhood	***Period 2 (2–7 Years): Preoperational Thought*** Thinking remains egocentric, becomes magical, and is dominated by perception.	***Anal Stage*** Major focus of sexual interest is anus; control of bodily functions is major feature.	***Autonomy versus Shame and Doubt*** Development of a sense of control over the self and bodily functions; exerts self; characterized by will.	***Stage 1 (2–3 Years): Punishment–Obedience Orientation*** Right or wrong is determined by physical consequences: "If I get caught and punished for doing it, it is wrong. If I am not caught or punished, then it must be right."
Preschool Age	↓	***Phallic or Oedipal/ Electra Stage*** Genitals become focus of sexual curiosity; superego (conscience) develops; feelings of guilt emerge.	***Initiative versus Guilt*** Development of a can-do attitude about the self; behavior becomes goal-directed, competitive, and imaginative; initiation into sex role; characterized by purpose.	***Premorality or Preconventional Morality Stage 2 (4–7 Years): Instrumental Hedonism and Concrete Reciprocity*** Child conforms to rules out of self-interest: "I'll do this for you if you do this for me"; behavior is guided by an "eye for an eye" orientation. "If you do something bad to me, then it's OK if I do something bad to you."
School Age	***Period 3 (7–11 Years): Concrete Operations*** Thinking becomes more systematic and logical, but concrete objects and activities are needed.	***Latency Stage*** Sexual feelings are firmly repressed by the superego; period of relative calm.	***Industry versus Inferiority*** Mastering of useful skills and tools of the culture; learning how to play and work with peers; characterized by competence.	***Morality of Conventional Role Conformity Stage 3 (7–10 Years): Good-Boy/ Girl Orientation*** Morality is based on avoiding disapproval or disturbing the conscience; child is becoming socially sensitive. ***Stage 4 (Begins about 10–12 Years): Law and Order Orientation*** Right takes on a religious or metaphysical quality. Child wants to do her duty, show respect for authority, and maintain social order; obeys rules for their own sake.

TABLE 2–1 *Comparison of Theories of Growth and Development (continued)*

	PIAGET'S PERIODS OF COGNITIVE DEVELOPMENT	FREUD'S STAGES OF PSYCHOSEXUAL DEVELOPMENT	ERIKSON'S STAGES OF PSYCHOSOCIAL DEVELOPMENT	KOHLBERG'S STAGES OF MORAL DEVELOPMENT
Adolescence	*Period 4 (11 Years–Adulthood): Formal Operations* New ideas can be created; situations can be analyzed; use of abstract thinking. ↓	*Puberty or Genital Stage* Stimulated by increasing hormone levels; sexual energy wells up in full force, resulting in personal and family turmoil.	*Identity versus Role Confusion* Begins to develop a sense of "I"; this process is lifelong; peers become of paramount importance; child gains independence from parents; characterized by faith in self.	*Morality of Self-Accepted Moral Principles* *Stage 5: Social Contract Orientation* Right is determined by what is best for the majority; exceptions to rules can be made if a person's welfare is violated; the end no longer justifies the means; laws are for mutual good and mutual cooperation. ↓
Adulthood			*Intimacy versus Isolation* Development of the ability to lose the self in genuine mutuality with another; characterized by love.	
			Generativity versus Stagnation Production of ideas and materials through work; creation of children; characterized by care.	*Stage 6: Personal Principle Orientation* Achieved only by the morally mature individual; few people reach this level; this person does what he thinks is right, regardless of others' opinions, legal sanctions, or personal sacrifice; actions are guided by internal standards; integrity is of utmost importance; may be willing to die for his beliefs.
			Ego Integrity versus Despair Realization that there is order and purpose to life; characterized by wisdom.	*Stage 7: Universal Principle Orientation* This stage is achieved by only a rare few; Mother Teresa, Ghandi, Socrates are examples; the individual transcends the teachings of organized religion and perceives herself as part of the cosmic order; understands the reason for her existence and lives for her beliefs.

problems, whereas a positive resolution builds a stronger personality or ego (Crain, 1992).

The toddler's developmental task is to acquire a sense of autonomy rather than a sense of shame and doubt. A positive resolution of this task is accomplished by his ability to control his body and bodily functions, especially elimination. Success at this stage does not mean that the toddler, even as an adult, will exhibit autonomous behavior in all life situations. In certain circumstances, feelings of shame and self-doubt are normal and may be adaptive.

Erikson's theory describes each developmental stage, with crises related to individual stages emerging at specific times and in a particular order. Likewise, each stage is built on the resolution of previous developmental tasks.

However, during each conflict, the child spends some energy and time resolving earlier conflicts (Erikson, 1963; Crain, 1992; Thomas, 1992; Freiberg, 1992). These concepts are illustrated by the adolescent who grapples with establishing a sense of identity rather than identity confusion. As she looks to her peers to help craft an image of herself, she must deal with her ability to trust her friends. Even if she successfully established a sense of trust and autonomy during her earlier life, these issues surface again, although to a lesser degree, as she struggles with the independence of adolescence.

Nursing Implications of Erikson's Theory. In stressful situations, such as hospitalization, children, even those with healthy personalities, evoke defense mechanisms that protect them against undue anxiety. **Regression,** a behavior used frequently by children, is a reactivation of behavior more appropriate to an earlier stage of development (Freiberg, 1992). This defense mechanism is illustrated by a 6-year-old boy who reverts to sucking his thumb and wetting his pants under increased stress, such as illness or the birth of a sibling. Nurses can educate parents about regression and encourage them to offer their children support, not ridicule. They can provide constructive suggestions for stress management and reassure parents that regression normally subsides as anxiety decreases. This phenomenon is discussed in Chapter 15.

Erikson's main contribution to the study of human development lies in his outline of a universal sequence of phases of psychosocial development. His work is especially relevant to nursing because it provides a theoretical basis for much of the emotional care that is given to children. The stages are discussed in the chapters on each age group.

Kohlberg's Theory of Moral Development

Lawrence Kohlberg (1927–1987), a psychologist and philosopher, described a stage theory of moral development, closely paralleling Piaget's stages of cognitive development. He discussed moral development as a complicated process involving the acceptance of the values and rules of society in a way that shapes behavior. Morality is influenced by many external and internal factors. External factors include family structure, punishment and rewards, and contact with parents and peers. Internal factors include intelligence, capacity for empathy with others, and the ability to control impulses and to judge behavior (Lewis & Volkmar, 1990).

Guilt, an internal expression of self-criticism and feeling of remorse, is an emotion closely tied to moral reasoning. Most children 12 years or older react to misbehavior with guilt. Guilt helps them to realize when their moral judgment fails.

Building on Piaget's work, Kohlberg studied boys and girls from middle- and lower-class families in the United States and other countries. He interviewed them by presenting scenarios with moral dilemmas and asking them to make a judgment. His focus was not on the answer, but on the reasoning behind the judgment (Kohlberg, 1964). He then classified the responses into a series of levels and stages as follows:

Level 1—Premorality (Preconventional Morality). The child demonstrates acceptable behavior because he fears punishment from a superior force, such as a parent. At this stage of cognitive and moral development, children cannot reason as mature members of society. They view the world in a selfish, egocentric way, with no real understanding of right or wrong. They view morality as external to themselves, and their behavior reflects what others tell them to do, rather than an internal drive to do what is right. In other words, they have an external locus of control. Premorality is illustrated by a child who thinks, "I will not steal money from my sister because my mother will spank me."

Within this level are three stages:

- Stage 0 (0–2 years): The infant has no awareness of right or wrong and does not consider the effect of his actions on others.
- Stage 1 (2–3 years): The child obeys rules to avoid punishment, and she acts to avoid displeasing those who are in power.
- Stage 2 (4–7 years): The child conforms to rules to obtain rewards or have favors returned. This type of behavior coincides with Piaget's preconceptual stage of cognition in which thinking is dominated by perception and egocentrism.

Level 2—Morality of Conventional Role Conformity (Conventional Morality). The child conforms to rules to please others. The child still has an external locus of control, but a concern for social order begins to emerge and replace the more egocentric thinking of the earlier stage. The child has an increased awareness of others' feelings. In the child's view, good behavior is that which those in authority will approve. If behavior is not acceptable, the child feels guilty.

Within this level are Stage 3 (7–10 years), in which conformity occurs to avoid disapproval or dislike by others, and Stage 4 (10–12 years), in which the child has more concern with society as a whole. In these stages, emphasis is on obeying laws to maintain social order. This level of moral reasoning develops as the child shifts the focus of living from the family to peer groups and society as a whole. As the child's cognitive capacities increase, an internal sense of right and wrong emerges and the individual is said to have developed an internal locus of control. Along with this internal locus of control comes the ability to consider circumstances when judging behavior.

Level 3—Morality of Self-Accepted Moral Principles (Postconventional Morality). The person focuses on individual rights and principles of conscience during this stage. There is an internal locus of control. Concern about what is best for all is uppermost, and the person steps back from her own viewpoint to consider what rights and values must be upheld for the good of all. Because abstract thinking abilities are necessary for this type of reasoning, this level is not attained until adolescence. Some individuals never reach this point. Within this level is Stage 5, in which conformity occurs because individuals have basic rights and society needs to be improved. The adolescent in this stage gives as well as takes, and does not expect to get something without paying for it. In Stage 6, conformity is based on universal principles of justice and occurs to avoid self-condemnation (Colby, Kohlberg, & Kauffman, 1987; Crain, 1992; Kohlberg, 1964; Lewis & Volkmar, 1990). Stage 6 is achieved by only a few morally mature individuals. These people, committed to a moral idea, live and die for their principles.

Kohlberg believes that children proceed from one stage to the next in a sequence that does not vary, although some people may never reach the highest levels. Even though children are raised in different cultures and with different experiences, he believes that all children progress according to his description.

Nursing Implications of Kohlberg's Theory. Nurses must be aware of how moral development progresses to provide anticipatory guidance to parents about expectations and discipline of their children. Parents are often distraught because their young children apparently do not understand right and wrong. For example, a 6-year-old girl who takes money from her mother's purse does not show remorse or seem to recognize that stealing is wrong. In fact, she is more concerned about her punishment than about her misdeed. With an understanding of normal moral development, the nurse can reassure the concerned parents that the child is showing age-appropriate behavior. As she matures, she will show more interest in the well-being of others and a more internal sense of right and wrong than she displays at this age.

Theories of Language Development

Human language has a number of characteristics that are not shared with other species of animals who communicate with each other. Human language has meaning, provides a mechanism for thought, and permits tremendous creativity.

Because language is such a complex process and involves such a vast number of neuromuscular structures, brain growth and differentiation must reach a certain level of maturity before a child can speak. Language development closely parallels cognitive development and is discussed by most cognitive theorists as they explain the maturation of thinking abilities. However, the process of how language develops remains a mystery.

Passive or receptive language is the ability to understand the spoken word. Expressive language is the ability to produce meaningful vocalizations. In most people, the areas in the brain responsible for expressive language are close to motor centers in the left cerebral area that control muscle movement of the mouth, tongue, and hands. Humans use a variety of facial and hand movements as well as words to convey ideas. Infants also use gestures as they acquire language skills (Oller, 1980; Freiberg, 1992).

Crying is the infant's first method of communication. These vocalizations quickly become distinct and individual and accurately convey such states as hunger, diaper discomfort, pain, loneliness, and boredom. Vowel sounds appear first, as early as 2 weeks of age, followed by consonants at approximately 5 months of age.

By age 2 years, children have a vocabulary of roughly 300 words and can construct simple sentences. By age 4 years, children have gained a sense of correct grammar and articulation, but several consonants, including "l" and "r" remain difficult to pronounce. For example, the sentence "The red and blue bird flew up to the tree" might be pronounced by the preschooler as "The wed and boo bud fwew up to the twee!"

The language of school-age children is less concrete and much more articulate than that of the preschooler. Between the ages of 5 and 10 years, children begin to understand the structure of language. By adolescence, as cognitive skills develop, language becomes a mechanism for abstract thinking (Nelson, 1977; Lewis & Volkmar, 1990).

Infants learn much of their language from their parents. Children who are raised in homes where verbalization is encouraged and modeled tend to display advanced language skills. Also, in infancy, receptive ability (the understanding of language) is more developed than expressive skill (the actual articulation of words). This tendency persists throughout life and is important to realize when caring for children.

> In clinical situations, nurses must communicate what is happening to their young patients, using simple, age-appropriate words, even though the child may not verbalize understanding.

Language development is discussed in more depth in chapters on each age group.

HEREDITARY INFLUENCE ON GROWTH AND DEVELOPMENT

Heredity is the transmission of genetic characteristics from parent to offspring and is one of the most significant determinants of growth and development. Because all humans are products of the biologic composition of their parents, heredity must be considered when assessing a child's growth and patterns and when caring for children with inherited diseases. Nurses need a working knowledge of how common genetic disorders are transmitted, how common chromosomal abnormalities occur, and what effects these diseases have on children and families.

Nurses play many roles in the health care of children and families with genetic problems. Early assessment and identification can be provided by alert and skilled nurses in hospital, clinic, and home settings. Nurses should be knowledgeable about appropriate referral sources so that prompt genetic evaluation and counseling can be provided. After genetic counseling sessions, nurses can interpret, clarify, and reinforce information that is provided to families.

A significant role of nurses is offering families support in coping with genetic abnormalities. Nurses can act as patient and family advocates, helping them to maneuver through the complexities of the health care system. Finally, nurses are in an excellent position to educate families and communities about the causes of birth defects and the prevention of environmentally induced disorders (Thomson, 1988).

Genetics is the study of how inherited traits are transmitted and how genetic material, deoxyribonucleic acid (DNA), affects the physiology of cells. The transmission of traits from parents to offspring is a complex process involving basic structures called chromosomes and genes.

Chromosomes, which lie within the nucleus of all body cells, consist of long strands of DNA. These packages of genetic material contain genes and normally occur in pairs. The normal number of chromosomes in human cells is 46, including 22 pairs of autosomes and 1 pair of sex chromosomes. Autosome pairs are numbered 1 through 22; sex chromosomes are labeled pair 23. If the 23rd pair consists of two large X chromosomes, the individual is female. If the pair consists of an X and a smaller Y chromosome, the individual is male.

Chromosomes contain **genes,** the functional units of heredity. Genes, which also occur in pairs, control the formation and function of proteins throughout the body and are responsible for the transmission of inherited information. Most cells of the body contain approximately 50,000 to 100,000 genes (Heim, 1988).

Structurally, genes are much smaller than chromosomes. If a chromosome could be compared to a high-rise apartment building, a gene could be compared to a closet in one of the apartments. With the aid of high-resolution chromosome analysis, cytogeneticists can examine specific chromosomes and detect small abnormalities. No techniques exist to directly visualize genes, although specific genes have been identified and located on specific chromosomes.

Chromosome Abnormalities. Chromosome abnormalities occur in approximately 1 in 150 live births and are most likely the cause of 50% of first-trimester spontaneous abortions (Ward, 1988). An increased incidence of abnormalities is often observed in the children of mothers who are older than 40 years. One type of chromosome defect is an abnormal number of chromosomes, as seen in Down syndrome, the most common chromosomal defect in humans. Down syndrome is usually caused by faulty cell division that results in three number 21 chromosomes (trisomy 21) instead of the normal pair. Dramatic mental and physical abnormalities occur because a large amount of genetic material is affected. Down syndrome is discussed in Chapter 42.

Gene Abnormalities. Approximately 4000 genetic conditions resulting from single-gene abnormalities have been identified, resulting in an incidence of 2 to 3 per 100 live newborns (Heim & Scott, 1988). Effects vary widely, from barely perceptible to lethal.

Like chromosomes, genes are paired, with one gene from each parent. Abnormal genes are generally either dominant or recessive and can be located on autosomal or sex chromosomes. There are four basic patterns of inheritance: autosomal dominant, autosomal recessive, X (sex)-linked dominant, and X-linked recessive patterns (Fig. 2–2). Because X-linked dominant disorders are rare, they are not discussed here.

Three principles aid in understanding these patterns of inheritance: (1) genes are paired; (2) one gene comes from the mother, and one comes from the father; (3) only one gene of each pair from the parents is passed on to the child (Heim & Scott, 1988).

Autosomal dominant disorders occur when an abnormal dominant gene is carried on one of the autosomal chromosomes with a normal gene. Because the affected gene is dominant, abnormalities occur even when only one gene of the pair is defective. A parent with an autosomal dominant gene has a 50% chance of passing the defect on to a child, as seen in the disfiguring disease neurofibromatosis.

Autosomal recessive disorders occur only when both genes of the pair are abnormal. Therefore, both parents must pass on a defective gene to the child. The child then has a pair of defective genes or is homozygous and exhibits the disease. A person who has one defective gene and one normal gene is said to be a carrier or heterozygous and does not exhibit the abnormality. Parents with an autosomal recessive disorder (carrier state) have a 25% chance of passing the defect on to each child, a 50% chance of passing on the carrier state, and a 25% chance of passing on normal genes. Sickle cell disease and cystic fibrosis demonstrate an autosomal recessive pattern of inheritance.

An X-linked recessive disorder is carried on the sex or X chromosome of women. Because normal women have two X chromosomes, a recessive gene on one X chromosome is compensated for by the other normal X chromosome. Thus, the woman would not have the disease.

Autosomal Dominant Inheritance Pattern

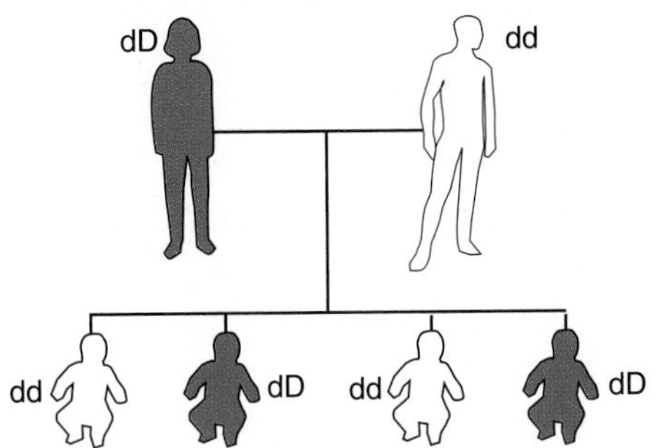

Each child has:
- 50% chance of having the disease
- 50% chance of being normal

No carrier state

No relationship to sex of the child

Example : Neurofibromatosis

Key: d = normal gene; D = abnormal, *dominant* gene

Autosomal Recessive Inheritance Pattern

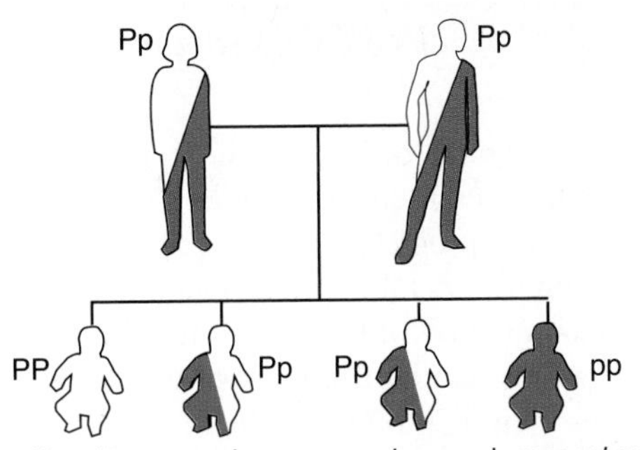

Each child has:
- 25% chance of having the disease
- 50% chance of being a carrier
- 25% chance of being normal

No relationship to sex of the child

Examples : Sickle cell disease, cystic fibrosis

Key: P = normal gene; p = abnormal, *recessive* gene

X-Linked Recessive Inheritance Pattern

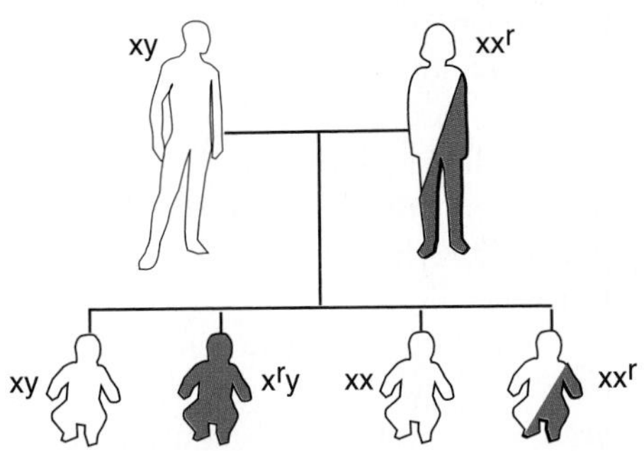

Each *female* child has:
- 50% chance of being a carrier
- 50% chance of being normal

Each *male* child has:
- 50% chance of having the disease
- 50% chance of being normal

Females do not usually have X-linked recessive disorders

Males are not usually carriers

Example : Hemophilia

Key: xy = normal *male* sex chromosome pattern;
xx = normal *female* sex chromosome pattern;
r= sex-linked *recessive* gene

Figure 2–2

Inheritance patterns.

However, a man, with only one X chromosome, would be affected because there are no genes on his Y chromosome to compensate for the abnormal gene. Women with the genetic defect on one X chromosome are known as carriers. Hemophilia A is a classic example of this type of inheritance pattern.

Many other genetic abnormalities occur as a result of the combined effect of more than one gene and the environment. The term multifactorial inheritance refers to this interactional process. Common congenital defects, such as neural tube defects, and many other medical problems, such as schizophrenia and allergies, demonstrate this type of inheritance pattern.

Prenatal Diagnosis of Genetic Disorders. Many chromosomal and genetic disorders can be diagnosed prenatally. A variety of prenatal diagnostic tools are available to aid in the prediction of the pregnancy outcome of at-risk couples. Among these are chorionic villi sampling, ultrasonography, and fetal blood sampling. The most widely used technique is genetic amniocentesis with the guidance of ultrasound. Chromosomes and biochemical substances, such as alpha-fetoprotein obtained from fetal cells in the amniotic fluid after 15 to 16 weeks of gestation, can be analyzed. Although there is a slight degree of risk during amniocentesis, this technique is frequently used to diagnose numerous chromosomal and genetic abnormalities, including neural tube defects. The sex of the fetus can also be determined by amniocentesis.

> Genetic disorders occur frequently and have a significant effect on the growth and development of children. Because genetic diseases are complex, permanent, and chronic, children, families, and entire communities are affected.

ASSESSMENT OF GROWTH

Because growth is an excellent indicator of physical well-being, accurate assessments must be obtained at regular intervals so that patterns of growth can be determined. Growth measurement should be performed by trained individuals using calibrated equipment and proper techniques. Methods of obtaining accurate measurements of children are described in Chapter 11. To minimize the chance of error, data should be collected on children under consistent conditions on a routine basis, and values should be recorded and plotted on growth charts immediately.

Standardized growth charts are tools that are used to compare an individual child's growth with statistical norms. The most commonly used growth charts are those developed by the National Center for Health Statistics. Separate charts are available for boys and girls. One set of charts is used for children from birth to 3 years, and another set is used for children 2 years to 18 years (see Appendix).

Because height and weight are the best indicators of growth, these parameters are measured, plotted on growth charts, and monitored over time. Brain growth can also be monitored by measuring infant frontal–occipital circumference (FOC) at intervals and plotting the values on growth charts. It is important to relate head size to weight because larger babies have bigger heads. These measurements are routinely performed during the first 2 years of life. Chapter 11 describes appropriate techniques for obtaining growth measurements.

Growth rate is measured in percentiles. The area between any two percentiles is referred to as a growth channel (see Growth Charts in Appendix). Childhood growth normally progresses according to a pattern along a particular growth channel. Deviations from normal growth patterns may suggest problems. Any change of more than two growth channels indicates a need for more in-depth assessment.

> Recognition of abnormal growth patterns is an important role of the nurse. The earlier the detection, diagnosis, and treatment of growth disorders, the better the long-term prognosis.

For example, if a growth hormone deficiency is discovered and growth hormone replacement is begun early in childhood, the child may be able to achieve his genetically determined height. On the other hand, if the abnormality is not detected until late in childhood, the child's growth would be diminished.

ASSESSMENT OF DEVELOPMENT

Assessment of development is a more complex process than assessment of growth. To accurately assess developmental progress, nurses must gather data from many sources, including observation and interview, physical examination, interaction with the child and parents, and various standardized assessment tools.

Observation is a valuable method most often used to obtain information about a child's **developmental age** (level of functioning). By watching a child during daily activities, such as eating, playing, toileting, and dressing, nurses gather a great deal of assessment data. Observation of the child's problem-solving abilities, communication patterns, interaction skills, and emotional responses can yield valuable information about his level of development. Similarly, interviews and physical examinations can provide much needed information about how the child functions.

In addition to these sources of data, many standardized assessment tools are available for nurses and other health care professionals to use for developmental screening. Screening should be included in newborn assessment and as part of every well-child examination for several reasons. One reason is that parents want to know how their child compares with others and whether her development is normal, especially if they experienced a difficult pregnancy or if they have developmentally delayed children. Screening tends to allay fears. Another reason to screen children is that abnormal development must be discovered early to obtain optimal outcomes through early intervention.

Newborn Assessment

The most commonly used newborn screening tools are the Brazelton Neonatal Behavior Assessment Scale and the Dubowitz system for estimation of gestational age. These tools are described in Chapters 3 and 21.

Denver II Developmental Screening Test

The most widely used screening tool for infants and young children is the Denver II Developmental Screening Test (DDST-II; see Appendix D). First developed as the Denver Developmental Screening Test (DDST) in 1967, the Denver II, a renormed and revised version, helps to provide the health care worker with "an organized clinical impression of a child's overall development and to alert the user to potential developmental difficulties" (Frankenburg & Dodds, 1990).

The Denver II, designed to be used with children between birth and 6 years of age, assesses development based on performance of a series of age-appropriate tasks. There are 125 tasks or items arranged in four functional areas:

1. **Personal–social** (getting along with others, caring for personal needs)
2. **Fine motor** (eye–hand coordination, problem-solving skills)
3. **Language** (hearing, using and understanding language)
4. **Gross motor** (sitting, jumping)

Items for rating the child's behavior are also included at the end of the test (Frankenburg & Dodds, 1990).

The test form is arranged with age scales across the top and bottom. (see Appendix for a sample test form). After calculating the child's **chronological age** (age in years), the test administrator draws an age line on the form. Each of the 125 tasks or items is arranged on a shaded bar depicting at which ages 25%, 50%, 75%, and 90% of the children in the research sample completed that particular item. The child is presented with the items clustered around her age line. The directions must be followed exactly during administration of the test. A score for performance on each item is recorded according to the following scale: pass (P), fail (F), no opportunity (NO), and refusal (R). Test behavior ratings (located at the bottom left of the form) are scored by the screener at the completion of the test.

Interpretation of the test is based first on individual items, then on the test as a whole. Individual items are considered as "advanced, normal, caution, delayed, or no opportunity." The Denver II as a whole is interpreted as follows:

Normal: no delays and a maximum of 1 caution
Abnormal: 2 or more delays
Questionable: 1 delay or 2 or more cautions
Untestable: 2 or more refusals

Recommendations based on the interpretation of the test are as follows (Frankenburg & Dodds, 1990):

Normal: routine rescreening at next well-child check
Abnormal: refer for diagnostic evaluation
Questionable: provide teaching for parents on how to practice delayed skills or tasks; rescreen in 3 months
Untestable: rescreen in 2 to 3 weeks

Results of the test can be used to identify a child's developmental age and to determine how a child compares with others of the same chronological age. This information can be used to alert health care providers to potential problems. To ensure that the results are accurate, testing should be performed only by individuals who are trained to administer the test in a standardized manner. Training is obtained through study of the testing manual, review of the accompanying videotape, and supervised practice with children of various ages.

Although the Denver II is used widely, it is a screening test only, not an intelligence quotient (IQ) test. It is not a definitive predictor of future abilities, and it should not be used to determine diagnostic labels. However, it is a useful tool for noting problems, validating hunches, monitoring development, and providing referrals.

Principles Guiding Screening With the DDST-II

Preterm Delivery. Allowance must be made for prematurity in calculating the age line. For example, a 9-month-old child who was born 2 months prematurely should be compared with a normal 7-month-old infant.

Optimum Performance. A child's performance must be judged as the best of which he is capable. Results obtained when a child is tired, hungry, bored, frightened, ill, or under the influence of drugs cannot be considered reliable or valid.

Parental Input. Parents provide important, useful information about their child's normal behavior and should be present during the screening. Their input also helps to determine whether the child's development is steady, accelerating, or slowing.

Gross Motor Development Versus Fine Motor Development. Assessment of large muscle development is less significant for overall evaluation than assessment of fine motor development. For example, developmentally delayed infants often sit and walk at appropriate ages; however, their use of their hands, especially the pincer grasp, is a much more reliable indicator of overall development.

Interactive Features. Even though alertness, responsiveness, imitation, and quality of vocalization cannot be scored, these features provide valuable data to the experienced screener and should be considered in the overall assessment (Illingworth, 1988).

Administering the Denver Developmental Screening Test II

INTRODUCTION

TeVonte ("T") is visiting the clinic for preventive health care shortly after his third birthday. The nurse will administer a Denver II Developmental Screening Test (DDST-II) to evaluate his development in each of four areas: personal-social, fine-motor-adaptive, language, and gross motor.

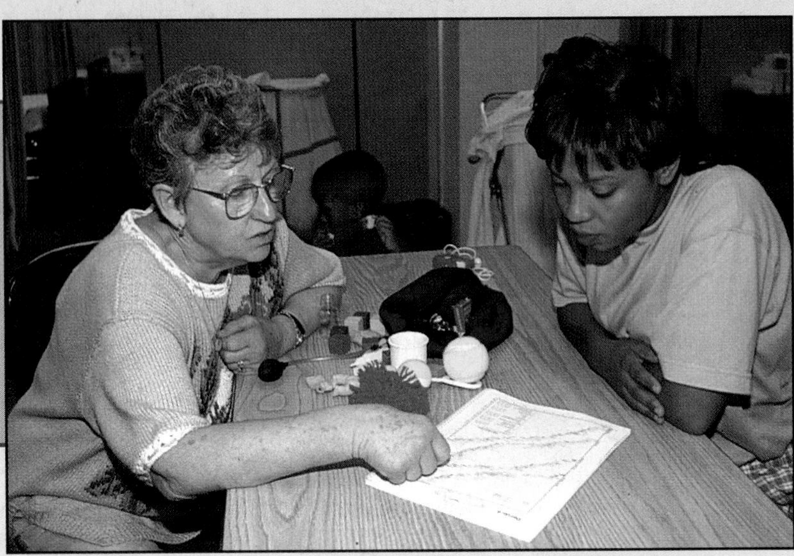

Before beginning T's DDST-II screening test, the nurse explains its purpose to his mother, Monifa Lee. The test assesses the child's performance of various age-appropriate tasks. The nurse emphasizes to the mother that the DDST-II is not an IQ test, but rather compares her child's development to that of other children of the same age.

After verifying T's age, the nurse begins the test with personal-social items. After helping him remove his shirt, the nurse asks T to put it back on. T pulls the shirt over his head, then slips each arm into the sleeves.

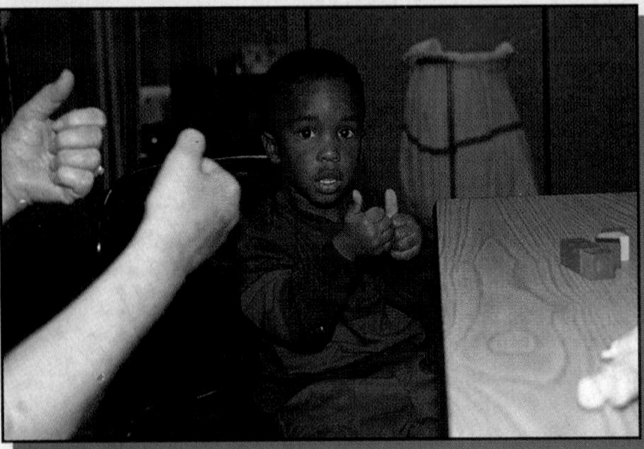

The nurse shows T how to wiggle his thumbs. T passes this part of the test because he keeps his fists closed and wiggles only his thumbs.

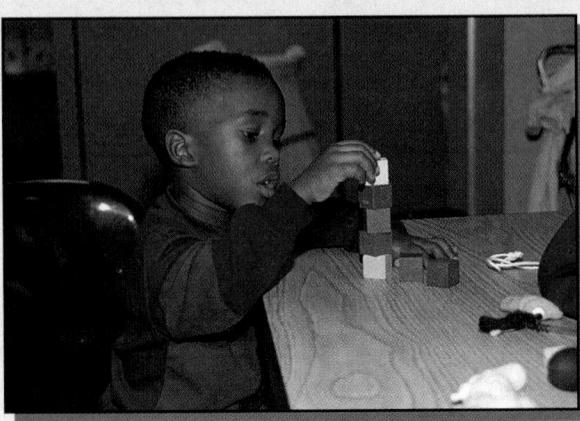

Colored cubes are used to evaluate T's ability to name colors and to build a tower. T is building a tower of 8 blocks, which allows the tester to evaluate his fine-motor-adaptive development.

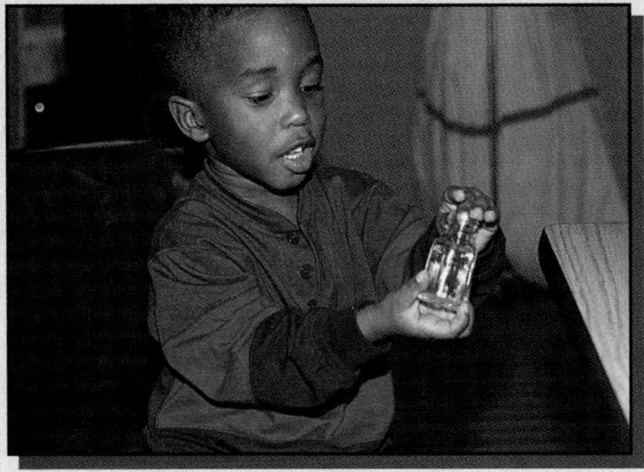

T plays with a raisin in a jar as part of the fine motor screening. The nurse observes to see whether T will pick up the raisin using his thumb and forefinger. T is really more interested in eating the raisin!

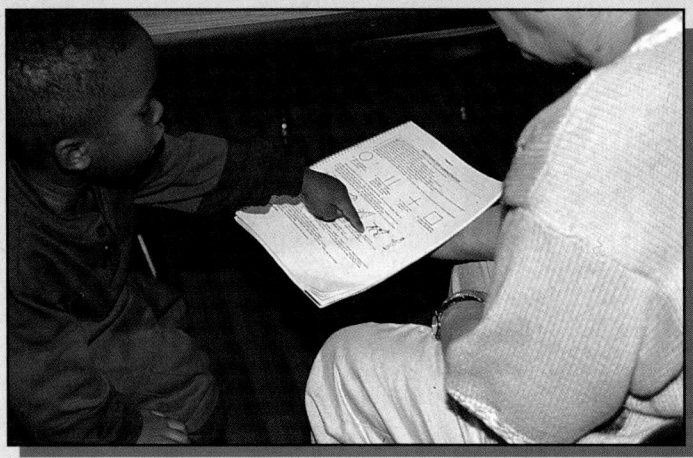

As she administers the DDST-II, the nurse evaluates T's speech, which is completely understandable, as it should be at his age. An additional part of the language section of the test is to identify at least four of the pictures printed in the test manual. T correctly names the dog as well as the other objects.

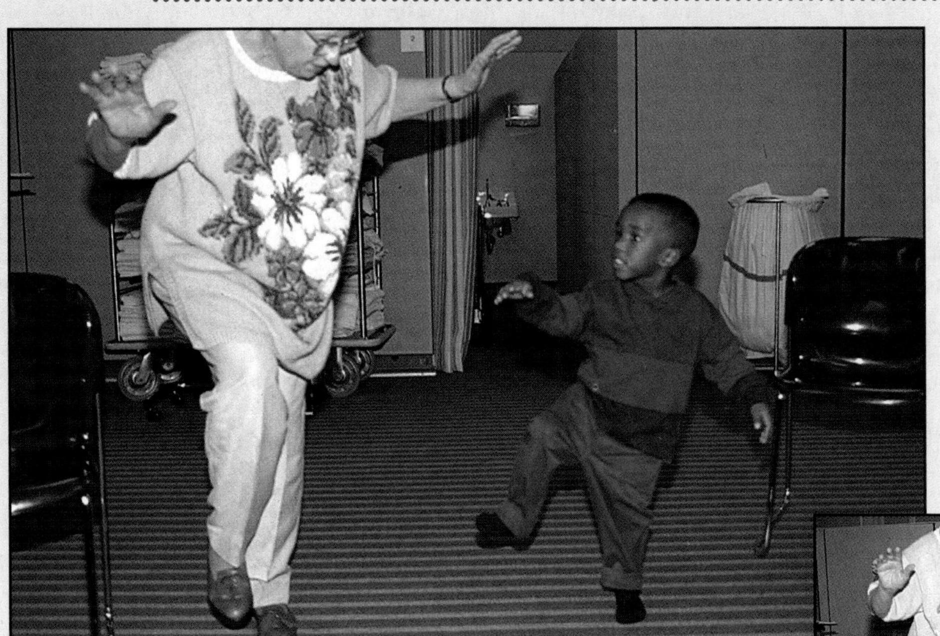

As the nurse shows T how to hop, he hops quickly in response. T's expression shows that he enjoys the gross motor part of the DDST-II.

Tevonte shows the nurse that he can balance on each foot for 3 seconds. Note that he is effectively using his arms to help maintain his balance.

CONCLUSION

After completing the DDST-II, the nurse shares the results with T's mother. The screening indicates that T's development is appropriate for his age. The nurse recommends that TeVonte continue to have well-child screenings each year, including a DDST-II up to the age of 6 years.

Photos courtesy of the University of Texas at Arlington School of Nursing.

Implications for Nurses

To ensure the child's best performance, nurses must first establish rapport and create a comfortable screening environment. The test should be administered in a comfortably warm room with the child dressed, but with restrictive clothing and shoes removed. Test materials should be located where the child can easily reach them. Only materials that are being used immediately for testing should be available to the child. All other materials should be out of sight. Young children may be held, but they should be able to rest their elbows on the testing table to manipulate objects. Other techniques for establishing rapport with children are discussed in Chapters 10 and 18.

Nurses should avoid making prejudgments about how a child will perform on the tests based on the child's or the parents' physical appearance. It is important to avoid being misled by a child's charm, facial features, small or large size, handicap, or oddly shaped head. Children should be given every opportunity to perform to the best of their ability.

As the testing progresses, it is important to avoid causing unnecessary worry in parents. Doubts should not be expressed until the screener is certain that the child should be seen for further evaluation. The slightest suggestion of concern, which may be communicated by even a casual facial expression, can create unnecessary concern and diminished trust. Words such as spastic, retarded, hydrocephalic, developmentally behind, and cerebral palsy should be avoided during the screening process (Illingsworth, 1988).

Again, the role of the nurse is to gather valid assessment data, determine deviations from normal, make appropriate referrals, and provide support. Diagnosis of developmental delay is the role of other health care professionals.

THE NURSE'S ROLE IN PROMOTING OPTIMAL GROWTH AND DEVELOPMENT

Nurses are particularly concerned with preventing disease and promoting health. One aspect of preventive care is providing anticipatory guidance or basic information for parents about normal growth and development as their child reaches different age levels.

Brazelton (1992) described "touchpoints" as predictable times during which health care professionals can reach into a family system and, through supportive help, diminish or prevent problems. These points generally occur just before a growth or developmental spurt in which the child's behavior changes and the parents' normal modes of handling behavior do not work. During these periods, the child becomes difficult to understand. These predictable periods can be anticipated by the nurse, and they provide a window of opportunity to offer information about normal growth and development as well as practical interventions to prevent problems characteristic of that age. Age-appropriate topics for anticipatory guidance are discussed further in the chapters on specific age groups.

THE DEVELOPMENTAL NURSING CARE PLAN

Nursing care for children is not complete without addressing the developmental issues that are unique to each child. Because children are rapidly growing and changing, the nurse must use knowledge of theories of growth and development to create plans of care for both healthy and ill children. Assessment data are collected from a variety of sources, categorized, and analyzed with a theoretical knowledge base and clinical experience. A list of strengths and problems related to growth and development is generated. Nursing diagnoses are formulated with individualized goals, interventions, and evaluation to address specific problems that are related to, but differ from, physiologic and psychosocial needs.

The following case study illustrates the nursing process used to address for the growth and developmental needs of an ill child.

> Shannon, a 4-year-old white girl, is admitted to the hospital with a diagnosis of acute lymphocytic leukemia. Her parents are with her. She has a 6-year-old brother and an 18-month-old sister. She was healthy until about 3 months ago, when she began to have numerous upper and lower respiratory infections. She lost 6 pounds over the last 2 months, and her mother stated that Shannon has been tired and irritable. She has never been hospitalized and appears to be frightened and cautious of the staff and equipment. Diagnostic studies for leukemia will continue in the morning, and a treatment regimen will be developed based on the results of her studies.

Assessment

In an initial interview with Shannon and her parents, the nurse would ask questions about her cognitive, language, motor, and emotional level of development. The parents' emotional state, level of education, and culture must be considered when information is gathered. In speaking with Shannon's parents, the nurse might use the following questions and statements, among others, to gather information about Shannon's cognitive, motor, and language development.

What does Shannon like to do at home?
Can she recite the alphabet, poems, songs?
Tell me about a typical day for Shannon.
Does Shannon attend preschool?
Can she throw a ball, ride a tricycle, climb?
Can she print her name, draw pictures, color them?
How effective is her use of language?
How did her development progress during infancy and toddlerhood?

The nurse also obtains input from Shannon about how she thinks through situations and communicates verbally. As Shannon interacts with different hospital personnel, the nurse can observe her cognitive abilities. The number, type, length, appropriateness, and correct use of words and sentences she uses must be noted. Careful observation of the child in a variety of situations, including play, provides valuable information about her cognitive development.

Shannon's stage of emotional development can be assessed in a number of ways. Based on Erikson's theory, it is expected that Shannon's major conflict would be developing a sense of initiative rather than a sense of guilt. However, she might exhibit regressive behaviors if the anxiety of hospitalization is overwhelming. Questions directed to the parents, such as the ones that follow, could help to validate inferences about Shannon's psychosocial development.

What types of play activities does Shannon like best?
How does she get along with other children? With adults?
How does Shannon usually handle stressful situations?
What do you do to help her cope with problems?
How does her ability to cope compare with your other children?
Is the behavior she displays now usual for her?

The nurse can also obtain valuable information from careful observation of Shannon as she experiences her illness and hospitalization. The nurse should note how she deals with pain, intrusive procedures, and separation from her parents.

Nursing Diagnoses

- Ineffective Individual Coping related to painful procedures, separation from family, and unfamiliar, frightening experiences.
- Altered Growth and Development of motor skills in a preschooler related to confinement, isolation from friends and siblings, and pain.

Planning, Implementation, and Evaluation

NURSING DIAGNOSIS

- Ineffective Individual Coping related to painful procedures, separation from family, and unfamiliar, frightening experiences.

Expected Outcome:

- Shannon will develop a healthy sense of initiative rather than feelings of guilt and responsibility.
- Shannon's coping skills will be more effective as evidenced by an ability to tolerate painful procedures, endure short separations from family members, and deal with unfamiliar, frightening experiences in the hospital.

Intervention	Rationale
1. Establish a relationship with Shannon and her family. Introduce yourself, and state how long you will be caring for Shannon. Answer all questions truthfully and accurately. If you do not know the correct answer to a question, tell the family that you will find out, and do so. Follow through on all commitments.	To intervene effectively, the nurse must develop a relationship with the child and family. During the initial phase of development, the nurse creates a sense of trust and caring. This phase is important because the feelings established here provide the foundation for all interventions.
2. Provide comments and praise such as "It's OK to cry when it hurts," and "You really did a fine job of holding still while I gave you your medicine."	Comments such as these help the preschool child, who is struggling with initiative versus guilt, to develop a sense of competence and control in stressful situations.
3. Provide play opportunities during which she can have hands-on experiences with equipment such as syringes, cotton, and alcohol. Offer her dolls, puppets, and dress-up clothes.	Children can cope with pain and stress through play. Allowing them to play with the medical equipment that is used helps to diminish anxiety and fear.

Intervention	Rationale
4. Allow acceptable acting out behavior.	Children need an outlet for their fears and anxiety. A certain amount of crying, whining, and demanding attention is to be expected because children have limited capacity to cope with threat. These regressive behaviors, although not desirable, can be used to deal with anxiety and pain.
5. Discourage self-deprecating comments or self-destructive behavior.	These methods of coping are never acceptable. Because preschool children are especially likely to feel guilty about life situations or to blame themselves for being ill, they need extra positive support.
6. Explain to Shannon and her parents what will happen to her during each procedure and experience. Gear explanations to her level by using simple words and concepts that she will understand. Draw pictures and use models to explain.	Preparing children for frightening and painful procedures is one of the most effective means nurses have to help children cope. However, it is important to assess the child's cognitive developmental level and to gear explanations to that level. Preschoolers do not understand much about how body parts look and function. However, their ability to understand probably is greater than their ability to communicate understanding.
7. Enlist her participation in procedures as much as possible. Praise her efforts. Suggest developmentally appropriate coping mechanisms, such as blowing out imaginary candles.	Active participation can help the child to feel more in control and can reduce anxiety.
8. Provide books depicting hospital situations or other stories that might help her to work through some of her anxiety. Provide art materials.	Both of these play activities can help her to work through anxiety and guilt.
9. Allow parents to support the child during painful procedures if possible.	Parental presence can be of great comfort to the child during stressful situations. It is important to remember that the role of the parent is that of support only. Parents should not be asked to restrain the child or otherwise assist medical personnel.

Evaluation: Because growth and development are continuous processes and personality unfolds over a long period, it is more difficult to evaluate specific developmental interventions than to evaluate other types of nursing interventions. If the child exhibits signs that development is progressing normally and can use healthy coping mechanisms to deal with stress, the nurse can be fairly confident that the developmental care plan is appropriate. If behavior becomes abnormal, alternative interventions must be used. If these attempts fail, referral to a psychologist or social worker may be necessary.

NURSING DIAGNOSIS

- Altered Growth and Development of motor skills in a preschooler related to confinement, isolation from friends and siblings, and pain.

Expected Outcome:

- Shannon will demonstrate motor development appropriate for her age.

Intervention	Rationale
1. Offer play activities appropriate for her activity level, such as a Nerf ball, dancing, or exercises.	These activities promote gross and fine motor development and can be performed in the restricted environment of the hospital.
2. Provide opportunities for her to practice fine motor skills, such as drawing, coloring, or sewing.	See Chapter 6 for more specific gross and fine motor play activities.
3. Encourage her to play with age-mates in the hospital.	Playing with other children is an important way in which children develop and learn. Because hospitalized children are isolated from their peers, nurses should provide opportunities for interaction.
4. Offer pain medication as needed. Be sure that she has adequate time for rest.	For play to be effective as a learning tool, the child must be able to concentrate on and enjoy the activity. Rest and medication might be necessary to ensure that the child is comfortable.
5. Restrict the amount of TV watching time.	TV watching is an acceptable activity as long as it is not overused. Interactive and active play promotes motor development much more than does passive TV viewing.

Evaluation: Again, because motor development is a continuous process, the results of developmental interventions will not be evident immediately. Motor development can be monitored by observing Shannon's play activities and comparing them with norms for her age.

KEY CONCEPTS

- Growth, development, maturation, and learning are complex, interrelated processes that produce complicated series of changes in individuals from conception to death.
- Growth and development proceed from simple to complex, proximal to distal, and from the head downward (cephalocaudal).
- As children grow and develop, wide variations within normal limits occur.
- Weight, height, and head circumference, common parameters used to monitor growth, should be measured and evaluated at regular intervals.
- The earlier that delays and deviations from normal are treated, the less severe the effect will be on growth and developmental outcomes.
- Numerous factors, including genetics, environment, culture, nutrition, health status, and family structure, affect how children grow and develop.
- Piaget's theory of cognitive development describes how children learn to deal with their environment through thinking and reasoning. Progress in learning through various periods is based on the child's ability to create patterns of understanding and behavior.
- Freud's psychosexual theory attempts to explain how humans struggle in both conscious and unconscious ways to become individual beings. During each stage of sexual development in children, a different area of the body is the focus of attention and pleasure.
- Erikson's theory of psychosocial development describes a series of conflicts that are built on one another. These stages occur throughout life, and each must be resolved to progress emotionally.
- Kohlberg discusses moral development as a complex process involving progressive acceptance of the values and rules of society in a way that determines behavior. As an individual matures, he is less concerned with avoiding punishment and more interested in human rights and universal justice.
- Language development, a complex process involving extensive neuromuscular maturation, begins as undifferentiated crying at birth and proceeds throughout life to provide a vehicle for communication, thought, and creativity.
- Genetics is the study of how traits are transmitted from parents to children in a complicated process involving chromosomes and genes. Chromosome and genetic

abnormalities are common in humans and result in a wide range of disorders.

- A variety of screening tools, such as the Denver II, are used by nurses to provide an overall picture of a child's developmental progress and to alert the nurse to potential developmental delays.
- Preventive care for children is easier, more efficient, and more cost-effective than curative care.
- To provide high-quality, developmentally appropriate care to children and parents, nurses must be aware of normal patterns of growth and development.

REFERENCES

Brazelton, T. B. (1992). *Touchpoints.* Menlo Park, CA: Addison-Wesley.

Colby, A., Kohlberg, L., & Kauffman, K. (1987). Theoretical introduction to the measurement of moral judgement. In A. Colby & L. Kohlberg. *The measurement of moral judgement:* Vol. 1. Cambridge, England: Cambridge University Press.

Crain, W. C. (1992). *Theories of development: Concepts and applications.* Englewood Cliffs, NJ: Prentice-Hall.

Dixon, S. D., & Stein, M. T. (1992). *Encounters with children* (2nd ed.). St. Louis: Mosby–Year Book.

Erikson, E. H. (1963). *Childhood and society* (2nd ed.). New York: Norton.

Flavell, J. (1963). *The developmental psychology of Jean Piaget.* Princeton, NJ: Van Nostrand.

Frankenburg, W. K., & Dodds, J. B. (1990). *Denver II screening manual.* Denver, CO: Developmental Materials.

Freiberg, K. L. (1992). *Human development.* Boston: Jones and Bartlett.

Freud, A. (1974). *Introduction to psychoanalysis.* New York: International Universities Press.

Freud, S. (1923). *The ego and the id.* (J. Riviere, Trans.). New York: Norton 1960.

Garvey, C. (1990). *Play.* Cambridge, MA: Harvard University Press.

Heim, W. G. (1988). Genetics principles: Genes. In *Genetics applications: A health perspective.* Lawrence, KS: University of Colorado Health Sciences Center, Learner Managed Designs.

Heim, W. G., & Scott, J. A. (1988). Gene abnormalities. In *Genetics applications: A health perspective.* Lawrence, KS: University of Colorado Health Sciences Center, Learner Managed Designs.

Illingworth, R. S. (1988). *Basic developmental screening: 0–4 years.* Boston: Blackwell.

Kohlberg, L. (1964). Development of moral character. In M. Hoffman & L. Hoffman (Eds.), *Review of Child Development Research:* Vol. 1. New York: Russell Sage Foundation.

Lampl, M. (1995). Leaps and bounds: How children grow. *Pediatric Basics, 72,* 10–16.

Lewis, M., & Volkmar, F. (1990). *Clinical aspects of child and adolescent development* (3rd ed.). Philadelphia: Lea and Febiger.

Litt, I. F., & Martin, J. A. (1992). Development of sexuality and its problems. In M. D. Levin, W. B. Carey, & A. C. Crocker (Eds.), *Developmental-behavioral pediatrics* (2nd ed.). Philadelphia: W. B. Saunders.

Nelson, K. (1977). Aspects of language acquisition and use from 2 to 20. *Journal of the American Academy of Child Psychiatry, 16,* 584–607.

Oller, D. (1980). Patterns of infant vocalization. In A. Reilly (Ed.), *The communication game: Pediatric round table series.* Vol. 4. Skillman, NJ: Johnson & Johnson.

Pipes, P. L. (1993). *Nutrition in infancy and childhood.* St. Louis: Mosby–Year Book.

Seideman, R. Y., Williams, R., Burns, P., Jacobson, S., Weatherby, F., & Primeaux, M. (1994). Culture sensitivity in assessing urban Native American parenting. *Public Health Nursing, 2*(2), 98–103.

Thomas, R. M. (1992). *Comparing theories of child development* (3rd ed.). Belmont, CA: Wadsworth.

Thomson, E. (1988). Professional roles and responsibilities. In *Genetics applications: A health perspective.* Lawrence, KS: University of Colorado Health Sciences Center, Learner Managed Designs.

Victora, M.D., Victora, C. G., & Barros, F. C. (1990). Cross-cultural differences in developmental rates: A comparison between British and Brazilian children. *Child: Care, Health, and Development, 16,* 151–164.

Ward, B. E. (1988). Genetic principles: Chromosomes. In *Genetics applications: A health perspective.* Lawrence, KS: University of Colorado Health Sciences Center, Learner Managed Designs.

BIBLIOGRAPHY

Baldwin, A. L. (1967). *Theories of child development.* New York: Wiley.

Colby, A., Kohlberg, L., & Kauffman, K. (1987). Theoretical introduction to the measurement of moral judgement. In A. Colby & L. Kohlberg. *The measurement of moral judgement,* Vol. 1. Cambridge, England: Cambridge University Press.

Dixon, S. D., & Stein, M. T. (1992). *Encounters with children* (2nd ed.). St. Louis: Mosby–Year Book.

Dudek, S. (1993). *Nutrition handbook for nursing practice* (2nd ed.). Philadelphia: J. B. Lippincott.

Field, T. (1990). *Infancy.* Cambridge, MA: Harvard University Press.

Garcia Coll, C. T. (1990). Developmental outcome of minority infants: A process-oriented look into our beginnings. *Child Development, 61,* 270–289.

Giordano, B. P. (1992). The impact of genetic syndromes on children's growth. *Journal of Pediatric Health Care, 6*(5), Part 2, 309–315.

Henry, J. J. (1992). Routine growth monitoring and assessment of growth disorders. *Journal of Pediatric Health Care, 6*(5), Part 2, 291–300.

Hinde, R. A. (1983). Ethology and child development. In M. M. Haith & J. J. Campos (Eds.), *Handbook of child psychology: Vol. 2. Infancy and Developmental Psychology* (pp. 27–93). New York: Wiley.

Kohlberg, L. (1984). *The psychology of moral development.* San Francisco: Harper & Row.

Levine, M. D., Carey, W. B., & Crocker, A. C. (Eds.). (1992). *Developmental-behavioral pediatrics* (2nd ed.). Philadelphia: W. B. Saunders.

Pineyard, B. J. (1992). Assessment of infant growth. *Journal of Pediatric Health Care, 6*(5), Part 2, 302–307.

Rasbridge, L. A., & Kuliz, J.C. (1995). Infant feeding among Cambodian refugees. *MCN, The American Journal of Maternal/Child Nursing, 20*(4), 213–218.

Teung, A. G. (1982). *Growth and development: A self mastery approach.* Norwalk, CT: Appleton-Century-Crofts.

University of Colorado Health Sciences Center. (1988). *Genetics applications: A health perspective.* Lawrence, KS: Learner Managed Designs.

3

The Newborn

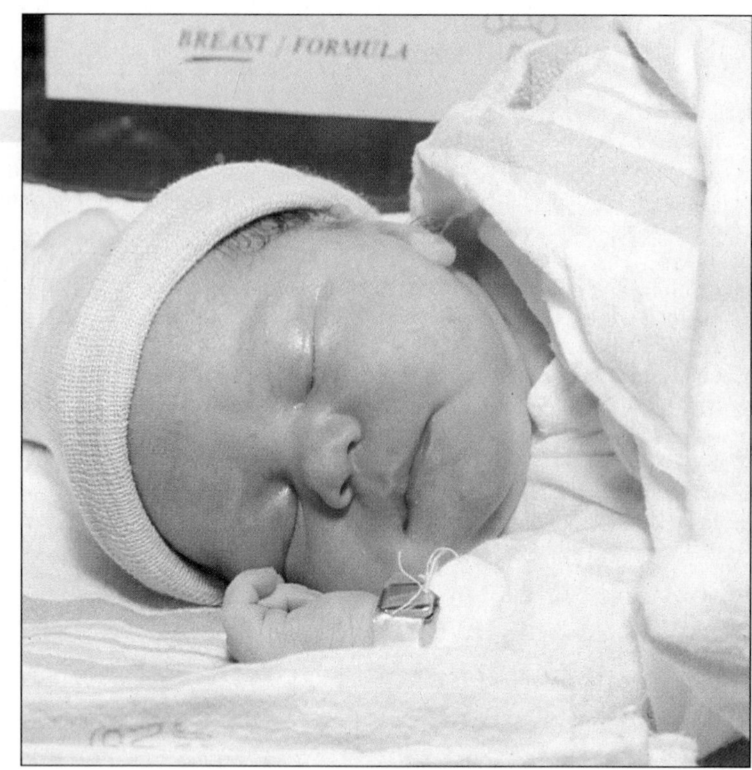

CHAPTER OVERVIEW

LEARNING OBJECTIVES

After studying this chapter, you should be able to:

- Describe the major physiologic changes that the infant undergoes at birth.
- Discuss the major responsibilities of the nurse regarding the newborn's adaptation to extrauterine life.
- Describe the factors that predispose the infant to rapid heat loss.
- Describe the initial assessment of the newborn.
- Identify the factors included in the assessment of neurologic functioning in the infant.
- Discuss which factors have become vitally important as newborns and their mothers are being discharged sooner from the hospital.

KEY TERMS

Apgar: scoring system that looks at the newborn's heart rate, respiratory rate, muscle tone, irritability, and color and is indicative of adaptation to extrauterine life

caput succedaneum: edema of the soft tissues of the scalp and head caused by squeezing during the delivery process; usually disappears in 2 to 3 days

cephalhematoma: unilateral swelling caused by bleeding below the periosteum of the cranium; swelling does not cross suture lines

Dubowitz: scale developed in 1970 to assess gestational age according to 10 neurologic and 11 physical criteria

gestation: length of pregnancy

gestational age: age of a fetus or newborn stated in terms of the number of weeks dating from the first day of the mother's menstrual period

LGA: large for gestational age infant; most often associated with maternal diabetes, but may also be caused by genetics

postmature infant: infant born after 42 weeks of gestation

preterm infant: infant born before 38 weeks of gestation

SGA: small for gestational age infant; may be of two types: (1) symmetrical, in which the whole body, including the head, is involved; and (2) asymmetrical (most common), in which the body is starved in appearance, but the head is of normal size.

term newborn: infant born between 38 and 42 weeks of gestation

vernix caseosa: cheesy, white substance composed of epitrichium (outer layer of embryonic skin) cells and secretions from the sebaceous glands; appears at about 20 weeks of fetal life and is present until about 42 weeks of gestational age

At birth, the newborn faces the enormous tasks of homeostasis and adaptation to extrauterine life. These include the change from fetal to extrauterine circulation, temperature regulation, elimination, and the establishment of respiration. The infant must also establish a relationship with his caregivers and learn to adapt and interact with the world surrounding him. The infant's family is adapting too: first-time parents are assuming new roles and tasks, while already established families are adapting their roles and patterns to the new member.

The nurse's role includes physical assessment of the newborn, both in the transitional phase immediately after birth, and later after physiologic adaptation. The nurse must be alert for any physical or behavioral indicators of abnormalities (see Chapter 21, The High Risk Neonate). The nurse also plays a role in promoting parent-infant bonding and must be alert for any problems in attachment. Finally, the nurse prepares the family for discharge by demonstrating physical care of the newborn and by providing information and anticipatory guidance.

IMMEDIATE PHYSIOLOGIC CHANGES AFTER BIRTH

The most profound changes noted at birth are found in the cardiovascular and respiratory systems of the neonate. Respiration is stimulated by birth. This stimulus is probably initiated by the hypoxia that results from clamping of the umbilical cord and cessation of placental blood flow. This hypoxia causes chemical changes in medullary, aortic, and carotid receptor sites, which stimulate respiration.

The first breath expands collapsed alveoli. A large negative intrathoracic pressure is required for this first breath. Pulmonary resistance is high because of the smaller size of the bronchi and alveoli. Of this first volume inspired, about half remains in the lungs as residual volume.

With the infant's first breath, pulmonary vascular resistance to blood flow decreases. There is also a resultant drop in pulmonary artery pressure. The pressure changes within the heart result from clamping of the umbilical cord, increasing PaO_2 levels, and a decrease in pulmonary vascular resistance. Right atrial pressure declines. Pulmonary blood flow to the left side of the heart increases, causing an increase in left atrial pressure. A higher systemic vascular resistance also results in a rise in pressure in the left side of the heart. This rise results in a shifting from fetal to postnatal circulation. This shift allows blood to be circulated to the lungs, PaO_2 levels to increase, and pH to decrease. The changes that occur in the prenatal vessels are shown in Table 3–1.

Most heart murmurs noted during the newborn period are benign and are the result of the infant's adaptation to extrauterine life. However, they should be reported for

TABLE 3–1 *Changes That Occur in the Prenatal Vessels*

	PRENATAL STATUS/FUNCTION	POSTNATAL STATUS/FUNCTION
Foramen ovale	Opening that allows oxygenated blood from the placenta to flow in a right to left direction from the right to left atrium, decreasing pulmonary blood flow	Functionally closes at birth and anatomically closes in several weeks to 1 year. Increase in pressure in the right side of the heart (crying) may cause shunt to reopen in the newborn period.
Ductus venosus	Connects the umbilical vein with the inferior vena cava	Becomes the ligamentum venosus.
Ductus arteriosus	Shunts deoxygenated blood from the pulmonary artery to the descending aorta	Functionally closes as PaO_2 levels rise after birth. Anatomically closes in 1–3 months and becomes the ligamentum arteriosum.
Umbilical vein	Carries oxygenated blood from the placenta to the liver and ductus venosus	Closes with clamping of the umbilical cord and becomes the ligamentum teres hepatis.
Umbilical arteries	Carry deoxygenated blood from hypogastric arteries to the placenta	Closes with the clamping of the umbilical cord. Proximal portions become superior vesicle arteries, and distal portions become lateral vesicoumbilical ligaments.

further evaluation, especially if other signs and symptoms of cardiac defect, such as decreased or absent pulses in the lower extremities, bounding pulses, or respiratory distress, are noted.

INITIAL ASSESSMENT AND STABILIZATION

One of the earliest indicators of successful adaptation is the **Apgar** score. Developed by Virginia Apgar in the 1950s, this test is performed immediately at birth, 1 minute after birth, and 5 minutes after birth. It uses five criteria to measure the infant's adaptation: heart rate, respiratory effort, muscle tone, irritability (reflexes), and color. Scoring ranges from 0 to 10. A score of 8 to 10 is predictive of an infant who is adjusting well to extrauterine life. A score of 5 to 7 often indicates an infant who requires some resuscitative intervention. Scores of less than 5 indicate infants who are having difficulty adjusting to extrauterine life and will require vigorous resuscitation. Low Apgar scores may be the result of maternal sedation, prematurity, or neuromuscular disorders (American Academy of Pediatrics and American College of Obstetricians and Gynecologists, 1988). Table 3–2 illustrates the Apgar scoring system.

Stabilization and facilitation of the infant's adaptation to extrauterine life are critical responsibilities of the nurse caring for the infant in the delivery room. Immediately after delivery, the delivery room nurse dries and stimulates the infant. A radiant heat source and dry, warmed blankets should be available to provide warmth for the infant. The newborn's respiratory system should be assessed for airway patency and respiratory status. Starting with the mouth, the nurse uses a bulb syringe or suction catheter to clear the airway of secretions (Fig. 3–1). The airway should be suctioned carefully so as not to induce apnea, which may result from vigorous suctioning and/or stimulation of the posterior pharynx (Bloom, 1991, p. 309).

If meconium-stained amniotic fluid was noted before delivery, the airway must be protected, and prevention of

TABLE 3–2 *The Apgar Scoring System*

	POINTS		
	0	1	2
Heart rate	Absent	Slow (<100)	>100
Respiratory effort	Absent	Slow or irregular, weak cry	Good, crying lustily
Muscle tone	Limp, hypotonic	Some extremity flexion	Active, moving, well flexed
Irritability (measured by bulb suctioning)	No response	Grimace	Cough, sneeze, vigorous cry
Color	Cyanotic or pale	Acrocyanotic, cyanosis of extremities	Pink

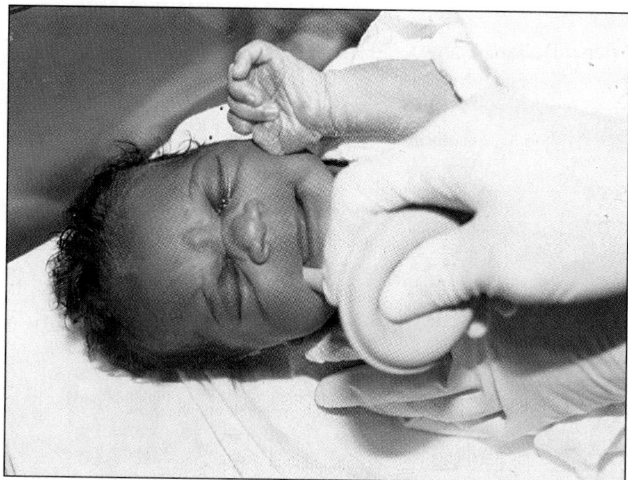

Figure 3–1
Suctioning secretions to clear the newborn's airway. A bulb suction can be used to clear most of the newborn's excess secretions. The mouth is suctioned before the nose. If the nose is suctioned first, any secretions in the mouth can be aspirated as the infant gasps. The nurse first compresses the bulb, then inserts the tip into one side of the infant's mouth. The bulb is released, creating the suction that removes secretions. The same procedure is used for the nares, if needed. The bulb syringe should always be kept with the infant, and the parents should be taught how to use it. (Courtesy of Parkland Memorial Hospital, Dallas, Texas)

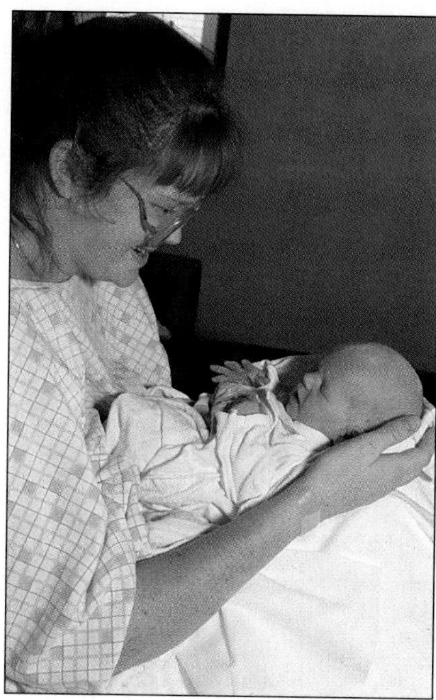

Figure 3–2
The mother demonstrates the en face position as she becomes acquainted with her newborn. She positions her infant so that their faces are aligned, aiding the eye contact that is important in the bonding process.

aspiration is essential. The infant should be intubated and the airway cleared after the head is delivered and before the rest of the body is delivered. If this intubation is not possible, the infant should not be stimulated until the airway is cleared of any aspirated meconium. The airway is cleared by visualizing the infant's hypopharynx with a laryngoscope and removing any meconium by suctioning. The trachea is then intubated, and deep suctioning into the lower airway is performed. If the meconium is thick, suction may be applied directly to the end of the endotracheal tube. It may be necessary to repeat the procedure, each time with a clean endotracheal tube, before the airway is cleared of meconium. Warming and drying should take place only after the airway is cleared of meconium (Chameides, 1994).

The nurse should perform an initial physical assessment in the delivery room, including assessing the infant's ability to maintain a patent airway. The infant's respiratory rate and rhythm should be noted and the lungs auscultated for the presence of crackles, which indicate fluid in the alveoli. Any passage of urine or meconium should be documented. The umbilical cord is examined for the presence of two arteries and one vein and any meconium staining. The neurologic system is assessed by testing for the presence of the Moro reflex. The anterior fontanel is checked for bulging or depression, and approximated, split, or overriding suture lines are noted. Finally, any gross structural abnormalities are documented.

A rapid assessment of maturity is usually performed in the delivery room. This evaluation includes skin color, presence of desquamation or vernix, length of fingernails, visibility of veins, and development of creases on the soles of the feet. The presence of breast tissue and development of the genitalia are also noted.

The infant may be weighed and measured in the delivery room. Footprints are obtained, and identification bands are placed on both the infant and the mother. The baby is then wrapped in warmed, dry blankets, and a stocking cap is placed on his head. If no problems are noted and the mother is able, the infant may be left with his parents for bonding and quiet time (Fig. 3–2).

NURSERY ASSESSMENT AND CARE

Physical Measurements

If the infant was not weighed and measured in the delivery room, these measurements are obtained on admission to the newborn nursery. The admitting nurse plots the infant's physical measurements (height, weight, and head circumference) on a growth chart. Most infants fall between the fifth and 95th percentiles.

Average weight varies from 2500 to 4000 g (5 lb, 8 oz to 9 lb, 13 oz). Birth weight greater than 4000 g indi-

MATURATIONAL ASSESSMENT OF GESTATIONAL AGE (New Ballard Score)

NAME ____ DATE/TIME OF BIRTH ____ SEX ____

HOSPITAL NO. ____ DATE/TIME OF EXAM ____ BIRTH WEIGHT ____

RACE ____ AGE WHEN EXAMINED ____ LENGTH ____

APGAR SCORE: 1 MINUTE ____ 5 MINUTES ____ 10 MINUTES ____ HEAD CIRC. ____

EXAMINER ____

NEUROMUSCULAR MATURITY

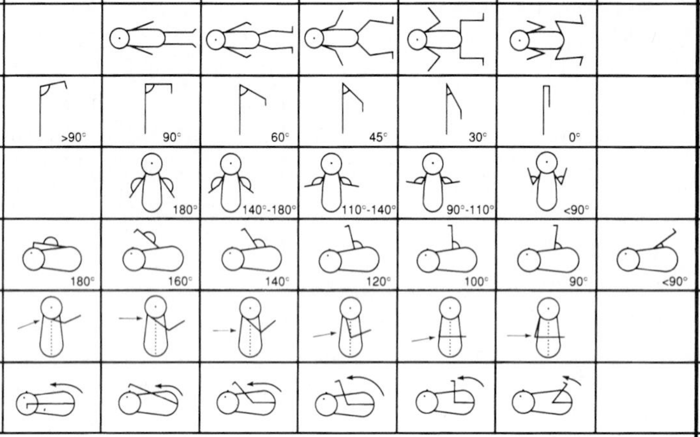

NEUROMUSCULAR MATURITY SIGN	SCORE -1	0	1	2	3	4	5	RECORD SCORE HERE
POSTURE								
SQUARE WINDOW (Wrist)	>90°	90°	60°	45°	30°	0°		
ARM RECOIL		180°	140°-180°	110°-140°	90°-110°	<90°		
POPLITEAL ANGLE	180°	160°	140°	120°	100°	90°	<90°	
SCARF SIGN								
HEEL TO EAR								

TOTAL NEUROMUSCULAR MATURITY SCORE ____

PHYSICAL MATURITY

PHYSICAL MATURITY SIGN	SCORE -1	0	1	2	3	4	5	RECORD SCORE HERE
SKIN	sticky friable transparent	gelatinous red translucent	smooth pink visible veins	superficial peeling &/or rash, few veins	cracking pale areas rare veins	parchment deep cracking no vessels	leathery cracked wrinkled	
LANUGO	none	sparse	abundant	thinning	bald areas	mostly bald		
PLANTAR SURFACE	heel-toe 40-50 mm:-1 <40 mm:-2	>50 mm no crease	faint red marks	anterior transverse crease only	creases ant. 2/3	creases over entire sole		
BREAST	imperceptible	barely perceptible	flat areola no bud	stippled areola 1-2 mm bud	raised areola 3-4 mm bud	full areola 5-10 mm bud		
EYE/EAR	lids fused loosely: -1 tightly: -2	lids open pinna flat stays folded	sl. curved pinna; soft; slow recoil	well-curved pinna; soft but ready recoil	formed & firm instant recoil	thick cartilage ear stiff		
GENITALS (Male)	scrotum flat, smooth	scrotum empty faint rugae	testes in upper canal rare rugae	testes descending few rugae	testes down good rugae	testes pendulous deep rugae		
GENITALS (Female)	clitoris prominent & labia flat	prominent clitoris & small labia minora	prominent clitoris & enlarging minora	majora & minora equally prominent	majora large minora small	majora cover clitoris & minora		

TOTAL PHYSICAL MATURITY SCORE ____

SCORE

Neuromuscular ____

Physical ____

Total ____

MATURITY RATING

score	weeks
-10	20
-5	22
0	24
5	26
10	28
15	30
20	32
25	34
30	36
35	38
40	40
45	42
50	44

GESTATIONAL AGE (weeks)

By dates ____

By ultrasound ____

By exam ____

Figure 3–3

The new Ballard gestational age assessment scoring system. (From Ballard, J. L., Khoury, J. C., Wedig, K., Wang, L., Ellers-Waisman, B. L., & Lipp, R. [1991]. New Ballard score, expanded to include extremely premature infants. *Journal of Pediatrics, 119*[3], 418.)

cates a large for gestational age **(LGA)** infant and may be associated with maternal diabetes or heredity. A birth weight less then 2500 g may be associated with prematurity, an infant that is small for gestational age **(SGA)**, or an infant that has intrauterine growth retardation (IUGR). Low birth weight may be associated with placental insufficiency, maternal malnutrition, pregnancy-induced hypertension (PIH), or maternal use of nicotine, drugs, on alcohol. The frequency of low birth weight is also higher in lower socioeconomic classes, minorities, and teenage mothers.

Head size is measured by placing the measuring tape in a "hat band" position just above the eyebrows. Normal head circumference varies from 32 to 38 cm, with the average being 34 cm. A larger than normal circumference for gestational age that is associated with a bulging fontanel may indicate hydrocephalus, whereas a smaller than normal circumference may indicate microcephaly or a growth-retarded infant. Chest circumference is measured at the nipple line. Average chest size ranges from 30 to 37.5 cm. The chest should be approximately 2 cm smaller than the head. Length is measured from crown to heel. Average length varies from 45 to 52.2 cm.

Gestational Age

Gestational age is assessed according to the new Ballard gestational age assessment scoring system (Ballard, 1991). The scale assesses six neurologic and six physical signs. A numeric score ranging from −1 to 5 is assigned to each sign. The total score corresponds to a gestational age. Figure 3–3 illustrates the Ballard scale.

Vital Signs

Vital signs are measured when the infant is still and quiet. Respiratory and heart rates and blood pressure fluctuate with stress, crying, movement, and sleep–wake cycles. Heart and respiratory rates should be counted for 1 full minute to detect any irregularities. Heart rate commonly increases with respiration. Although the heart rate is measured apically, brachial and femoral pulses should be assessed for equality and strength.

> Weak or absent femoral pulses and systolic blood pressures in the lower extremities that are 10 mm less than those in the upper extremities are associated with coarctation of the aorta and should be reported immediately.

Blood pressure should be measured in all four extremities on admission. The blood pressure cuff size should be 75% of the width of the upper arm. When measuring blood pressure electronically, the nurse should follow the manufacturer's directions for cuff size.

Normal Ranges for Newborn Vital Signs

Respiratory rate	30–60 breaths/minute
Heart rate	120–150 beats/minute
Blood pressure	Systolic = 96–64 mmHg Diastolic = 62–30 mmHg
Temperature	36.5–37.6°C rectal 36.5–37.9°C axillary

The infant's temperature is measured soon after birth. The infant is placed in a radiant warmer and a skin probe is attached to the abdomen. The probe allows the warmer to measure and display the infant's temperature continuously. It is set to regulate the amount of heat produced by the warmer according to the infant's skin temperature. The temperature should be noted and recorded every 15 minutes during the first hour and hourly during the next few hours. The temperature can be measured every 8 hours thereafter if it remains stable.

In some agencies the first temperature is taken rectally, although recent research reveals risks of this practice. Rectal temperature provides information about the infant's temperature as well as patency of the anus. The thermometer should be inserted no farther than 0.5 inch into the anus. The colon turns at a sharp right angle approximately 1 inch from the anal sphincter. Inserting the thermometer farther might cause potentially fatal perforation of the intestinal wall. The thermometer should never be forced into the rectum because there may be an imperforate anus (Gorrie et al., 1994).

Axillary temperature measurement is safer than taking rectal temperature. Axillary measurement provides a reading very close to rectal temperature. Skin temperature is slightly lower than core temperature, so axillary temperature is usually slightly lower. Normal ranges for vital signs are listed in the accompanying box.

PHYSICAL ASSESSMENT OF THE NEWBORN

The nurse must remember certain key points when preparing to assess the newborn. The first is the preparation of the environment. The room should be warm to prevent hypothermia. To accurately assess skin color, walls should be white or off-white. Noise levels should be low to prevent stressing the infant.

The infant should be assessed during a quiet alert state. Assessments should not be performed when the

Basic Principles of Physical Assessment of the Newborn

According to Tappero and Honeyfield (1993), the following are essential elements of any newborn examination:

- Review the perinatal history for clues to potential abnormalities
- Assess the infant's color for clues to potential abnormalities
- Auscultate only in a quiet environment
- Keep the infant warm during examination
- Have the necessary tools at hand
- Calm the infant before beginning the examination
- Handle the infant gently

Adapted from Tappero, E. P., & Honeyfield, M.E. (1993). *Physical assessment of the newborn* (p. 4). Petaluma, CA: NICUINK Publications.

infant is hungry or has just been fed, when stressed, or immediately after delivery (Judd, 1985).

The examination should be organized, orderly, and methodical (head-to-toe) (see *Basic Principles of Physical Assessment of the Newborn* box). The nurse should perform the examination as quickly as possible and start with the least threatening parts of the examination, such as auscultation. These assessments usually require the infant to be calm and quiet.

General Appearance. The newborn has a posture of flexion. Preterm and neurologically impaired infants have deviations from this posture. They are often limp and hypotonic. Other variations in posture may result from intrauterine positioning, such as breech position (Fig. 3–4).

Integumentary System. The skin structure of the infant is similar to that of the older child or adult. It contains the same three layers: epidermis, dermis, and subcutaneous. The skin maintains temperature and provides sensory per-

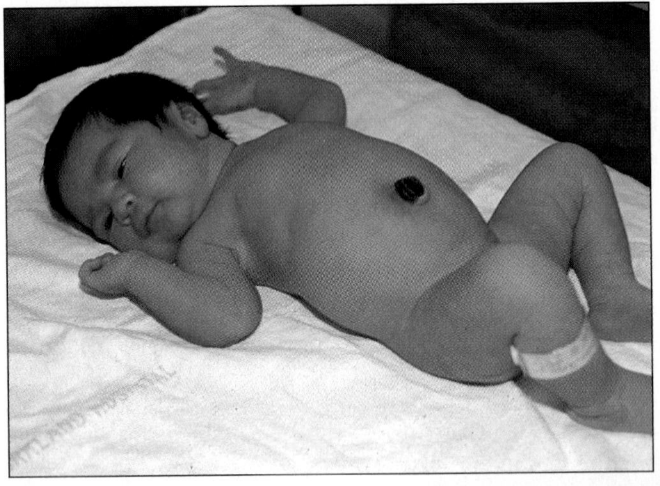

◄ Flexed position of the full-term newborn infant, similar to the position in utero. Flexion limits heat loss because it reduces the amount of body surface that is exposed. Note: This infant would be positioned on her side if a nurse were not beside her.

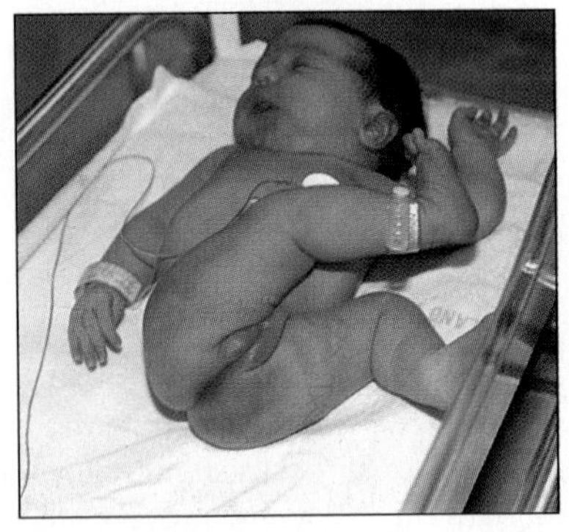

◄ After vaginal birth in the breech presentation, this newborn's legs remain in a position of extension. Bruising of her buttocks and labia occurred because of pressure on these parts as they passed through the mother's pelvis. The small gold disc on her upper abdomen is a temperature probe that regulates the heat output of the radiant warmer over her crib.

Figure 3–4
Newborn posture. (Courtesy of Parkland Memorial Hospital, Dallas, Texas)

ception and protection from infection. The more immature the infant, the more immature the skin and the less likely it is to be able to protect the infant from heat loss and infection. Finally, the infant's skin is thin, and the epidermis and dermis are loosely attached. Therefore, the infant is at a higher risk of separation of these layers, which may result in blistering.

By the time the infant reaches 36 weeks of gestation, the skin is generally soft and pink, with few visible vessels. Skin color, however, is dependent on several factors, such as activity level, temperature, hematocrit levels and race. The skin of infants of darker races will appear light at birth, but will darken as time passes. An infant with a high hematocrit level (high red blood cell count relative to blood volume) will appear plethoric. Plethora is a ruddy (red) appearance of the skin. A plethoric infant should have his hematocrit and hemoglobin values checked by heelstick. If the hematocrit level is greater than 65%, a central hematocrit value should be checked. A central hematocrit value greater than 65% indicates polycythemia.

> A polycythemic infant should be monitored closely for signs and symptoms of cyanosis, respiratory distress, hypoglycemia, and jaundice (Blanchette and Zipursky, 1987).

When an infant cries, her skin becomes bright red. Because the capillary system is immature, acrocyanosis (cyanosis or blue color of hands and feet) is common. The infant may also have a mottled appearance (called cutis marmorata) when stressed, cold, or overstimulated. It should disappear as the infant is warmed. A Harlequin sign may also be noted, especially in the low–birth-weight infant (Margileth, 1987), and is seen in both normal and ill newborns. When the infant is turned on his side, his body has a sharp line of demarcation dividing a bright red dependent half and a pale superior half. This condition is attributed to an immature autonomic regulatory system and usually disappears within 30 minutes if the infant is turned to his back or abdomen.

> Persistent cutis marmorata may be associated with trisomy 21, trisomy 18, or Cornelia de Lange syndrome (Jones, 1988).

Sebaceous glands are active and are responsible for producing the vernix caseosa. **Vernix caseosa,** a cheesy white substance composed of sebum and skin cells, is present on the back, head, and in body creases (Fig. 3–5). If it is not washed off, it dries and disappears within 48 hours. Lanugo, a fine, downy hair, is noted on the cheeks, forehead, shoulders, and back. Milia, small white papules, are often present on the nose and chin and are caused by a blockage of the sebaceous glands.

The eccrine sweat glands are active at birth, but require a higher temperature than those of an adult to produce sweat. The aprocrine sweat glands do not function until adolescence. Miliaria is caused by obstructed sweat glands. The most common type, miliaria crystallina, is characterized by clear vesicles noted over the forehead, scalp, groin, and in creases.

Finally, any birthmarks are noted and documented. Common findings include erythema toxicum neonatorum (small red patches on the cheeks or trunk) and Mongolian spots (dark, bluish-black areas noted on the buttocks of Asian and black infants). Other findings may include forceps marks (bruising on the face), stork bites, port wine stains, and café au lait spots (see Fig. 3–5). Documentation of birthmarks should include the type of marking, size, location, and any distinguishing characteristics.

The Head and Facies. The head should be inspected and palpated for shape and symmetry. The circumference should be measured. If the measurement is abnormally large or small, the infant's head should be examined for variations caused by the birthing process. If the abnormal measurement is caused by the birthing process, the measurements should be within normal limits several days after delivery (Tappero and Honeyfield, 1993). Microcephaly (head circumference less than the 10th percentile) is associated with inadequate brain growth and may be associated with a genetic syndrome or a congenital infection. Macrocephaly (head circumference greater than the 90th percentile) may be associated with hydrocephalus, congenital dwarfism, or osteogenesis imperfecta.

The anterior and posterior fontanels and suture lines should be palpated while the infant is quiet. Fontanel size is measured diagonally from bone to bone. The anterior fontanel is diamond-shaped and located on the top of the head. It should be soft and flat and may range in size from almost nonexistent to 4 to 5 cm across. In a normal infant, it is soft and flat. It normally closes by 18 to 24 months of age. The posterior fontanel is located in the midline in the occipital region of the skull. It is small (1–2 cm) and normally closes by 2 to 3 months of age.

> A bulging or tense fontanel may result from crying or may be a sign of increased intracranial pressure. A large anterior fontanel is often associated with hypothyroidism (Jones, 1988).

Normal suture lines may be approximated or overriding. They are also mobile. A split in the sutures of as much as 1 cm is considered normal (Tappero and Honeyfield, 1993). Overriding suture lines are most often caused by the birthing process and resolve spontaneously.

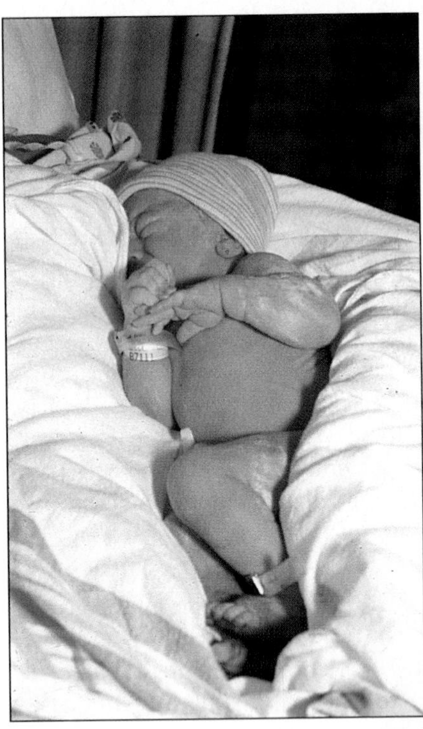

◀ Vernix caseosa, the white cheesy substance that protects the skin before birth. Newborns have varying amounts of vernix, but preterm infants usually have little, if any. Note: The stockinette cap slows heat loss from the large surface area of the newborn's head, reducing the risk of cold stress.

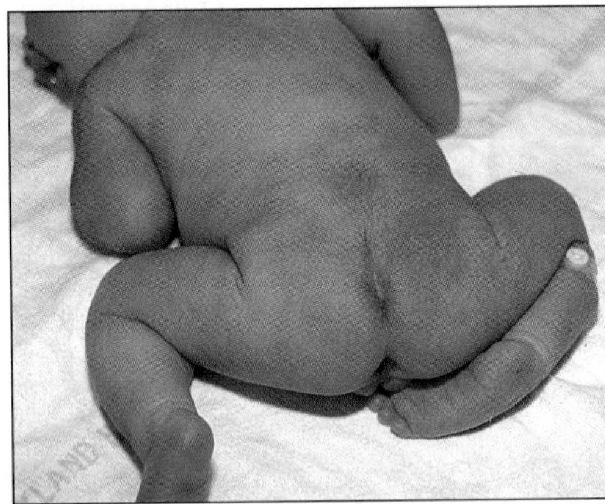

◀ Mongolian spots are normal bluish areas of the skin that are sometimes mistaken for bruises. Most common in dark-skinned infants, Mongolian spots usually fade within the first few years. This Hispanic infant has abundant dark body hair, which is common in this ethnic group. (Courtesy of Parkland Memorial Hospital, Dallas, Texas)

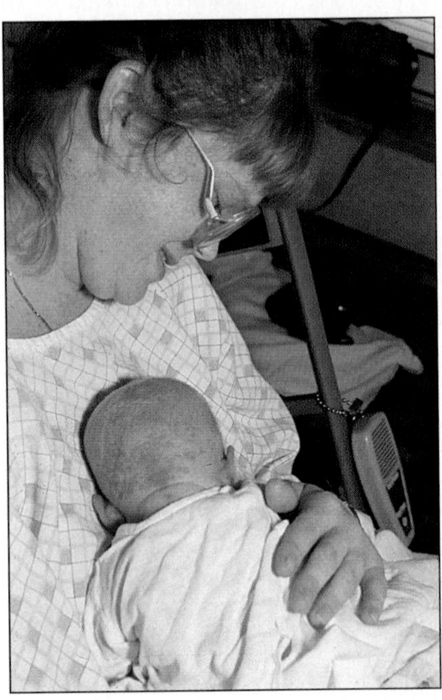

◀ Telangiectatic nevi (stork bites) are flat, pink areas usually seen on the back of the neck, on the eyelids, or on the bridge of the nose. They are more common in fair-skinned newborns, and they gradually fade.

Figure 3–5
Common neonatal skin features.

A suture split of greater than 1 cm may indicate increased intracranial pressure. A hard, ridged, or immobile suture line may be associated with premature closure or craniosynostosis and should be investigated further.

The shape of the head may be indicative of ethnic origin. Other variations in head shape occur as a result of the birthing process. Molding is often present in babies born vaginally (Fig. 3–6). Molding is caused by the movement of flexible suture lines to allow passage of the infant's head through the birth canal. A **caput succedaneum** (swelling of the soft tissues of the head and scalp) or **cephalhematoma** (edema resulting from bleeding below the periosteum of the cranium) may also be noted (Fig. 3–6).

Molding

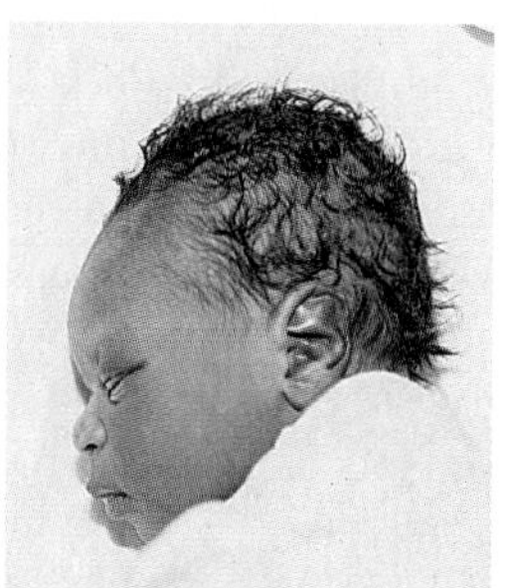

- Adjustment of skull bones to fit birth canal
- Disappears in a few days

Caput succedaneum

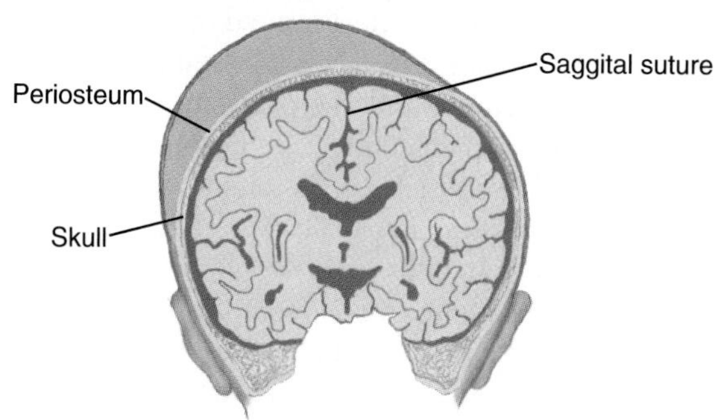

- Swelling of soft tissues of scalp
- May extend across suture lines
- Most pronounced after a long labor
- Evident within 24 hours after birth
- Resolves within a few days

Cephalhematoma

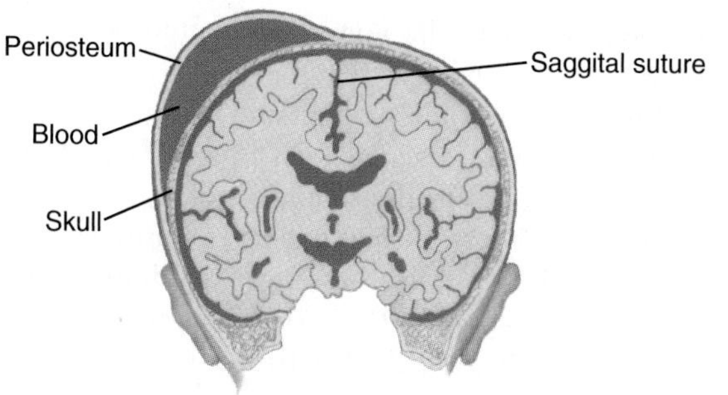

- Blood between skull bone and periosteum
- Does not cross suture lines
- Due to ruptured blood vessels from head trauma during birth
- Develops 24-48 hours after birth
- May take 2 to 3 weeks to resolve

Figure 3–6
Variations in head shape. (Photo courtesy of Parkland Memorial Hospital)

> A caput is differentiated from a cephalhematoma in that the edema of a cephalhematoma is unilateral and does not cross suture lines.

The scalp and hair should be examined for hair growth patterns and any trauma or abnormalities. Infants may have punctures or lacerations from scalp electrodes, blood sampling, or delivery trauma. Other abnormalities, such as scalp defects, may be associated with certain congenital anomalies. Brittle or excessive hair or a low hairline may also be associated with congenital abnormalities.

The facies should be examined for symmetry, positioning of the facial features, and movement and expression. Intrauterine positioning may lead to asymmetry of the facial features. This asymmetry is usually transient and normally disappears within a few weeks or months. Unusual asymmetry, irregularities of the facies during crying, or other deficits should be reported.

Eyes. Eyes may be edematous from the administration of ointment to prevent gonococcal conjunctivitis. Examination of the eyes is easier if they are opened by the infant rather than the examiner. The infant may open her eyes if the lights are dimmed and she is given an auditory stimulus. The outer canthus of the eye should fall into a horizontal line with the external ear. The lids should completely cover the eyes when closed. There should be no slanting of the epicanthal folds in non-Asian children. The infant may normally exhibit nystagmus (rhythmic back-and-forth lateral or vertical movement of the eyes), strabismus (crossed eyes), or pseudostrabismus (the illusion of crossed eyes).

> A slant of the epicanthal fold in a non-Asian child may indicate Down syndrome.

The color of the iris of light-skinned newborns is usually dark blue, whereas dark-skinned infants usually have brown eyes. Tears are seldom formed until the infant is about 2 to 3 months old (Tappero and Honeyfield, 1993). The sclera should be white or bluish-white. Yellow sclera indicates jaundice, and blue sclera may indicate osteogenesis imperfecta. Subconjunctival hemorrhages may result from the pressure exhibited during labor and delivery, but should disappear by 2 to 3 weeks of age.

> Purulent drainage is abnormal and may be indicative of bacterial or chlamydial conjunctivitis.

Pupils should have an equal reaction to light. Absence of this reflex may indicate blindness. The nurse should be able to elicit a red reflex to light in both eyes. Absence of the red reflex may indicate retinal hemorrhage, cataract, glaucoma or retinoblastoma. The corneas should be clear. A cloudy or milky appearance may indicate congenital cataracts. The infant can see clearly and in color for a distance of about 8 inches (approximately the distance from breast to face in an adult).

Nose. The nose should be positioned in the midline, and the nares should be of equal size and shape. The bridge is lower than in an older child or adult, but a very low bridge may be associated with congenital malformations, such as Down syndrome. Sneezing is normal in the newborn, but a severely stuffy or runny nose is abnormal and may indicate a condition such as congenital syphilis.

> Nasal flaring is abnormal and is indicative of respiratory distress.

Patency of the nares may be assessed with a feeding tube or suction catheter. A lack of patency in one or both nares may indicate choanal atresia. If the infant has had vigorous nasal suctioning with a bulb syringe, stuffiness may result. In this situation, attempts to pass a feeding tube will only increase the edema and should not be attempted. Newborn infants are preferential nose breathers. This condition usually lasts 3 to 4 months. Because mouth breathing must be learned, the infant responds to a blockage of the nose with anoxia. The anoxia then causes the infant to cry or open his mouth and take a single gasp.

Mouth. The mouth should be located in the midline. The lips and gums should be intact, pink, and moist. Although it is easiest to examine the mouth while the infant is crying, if necessary, the mouth may be opened by gently applying pressure to the chin. A tongue depressor should not be used because it usually stimulates a protrusion reflex of the tongue.

The nurse examines the hard and soft palates by placing a gloved finger in the infant's mouth. The arch should be intact. An extremely high or narrow palate or any cleft should be reported. The gag and suck reflexes may also be assessed at this time.

Epstein's pearls may be noted when examining the inside of the mouth. These are small, shiny, yellow-white nodules located at the junctions of the hard and soft palates. Occasionally, the examiner notes a tooth that has erupted prematurely. These teeth have no roots, are attached loosely to the gums, and should be removed to decrease the risk of aspiration.

The tongue should be pink and completely contained within the mouth. Macroglossia, a protruding tongue that appears too large for the infant's mouth, is indicative of endocrine disorders, such as hypothyroidism, or congenital or genetic disorders, such as Down syndrome. Excessive salivation is abnormal in the newborn and may indicate a tracheoesophageal fistula. If a fistula is suspected, an orogastric tube may be passed.

> Inability to pass an orogastric tube or an orogastric tube that curls back out of the mouth is indicative of a tracheoesophageal fistula and should be reported immediately.

Ears. The ear is assessed for form and the presence of cartilage. By 36 weeks, the pinna has curved and the ear recoils if folded. By 39 weeks, the ear is well defined and holds its shape away from the head. Vernix and amniotic fluid may make observation of the tympanic membrane impossible. The ear should sit nearly vertically on the head and intersect an imaginary line drawn from the outer canthus of the eye (see Fig. 11–7 in Chapter 11).

> Low set or oddly placed ears are associated with a variety of congenital defects and should be reported immediately.

Hearing acuity may be assessed by evaluating the infant's blink or startle reflex. Several conditions, such as congenital infections, family history, low birth weight, and asphyxia are associated with hearing loss. Most hospitals screen for hearing loss risk factors. If these are present, audiology testing is usually recommended.

Neck. The newborn's neck is short. Any noted asymmetry is usually caused by positioning in utero. The neck should be soft and free of masses. The thyroid is difficult to palpate, except in instances of hypothyroidism. The most common neck mass noted in the newborn is a cystic hygroma (a mass of lymphatic channels that form a large cystic mass). These masses range in size from a few centimeters to large enough to impede the airway).

While palpating the neck, the nurse should note any webbing (extra or redundant skin). A webbed neck is often associated with such genetic syndromes as Down syndrome or Turner syndrome. Finally, the clavicles should be palpated to assess for a fracture that may have occurred during delivery. If a fracture is present, the bone ends may seem to move freely or the broken edges of the bone feel gritty or sandy.

Chest. The chest is barrel-shaped. The anteroposterior and lateral diameters are approximately equal. The chest circumference usually ranges from 30 to 36 cm and is approximately 2 cm smaller than a normal head circumference. The sternum should lie in the center of the chest and should not be protruding (pectus carinatum or pigeon chest) or sunken (pectus excavatum or funnel chest). A deviation in the shape of the sternum may be associated with congenital anomalies such as Marfan syndrome. A marked barrel chest (a chest with an increased anteroposterior diameter) may be seen in the infant with an aspiration syndrome. The xiphoid process is visible at the end of the sternum.

The size and shape of the breasts should be noted. Breast enlargement caused by maternal hormones is common in both sexes. A white, milky substance known as witch's milk may be secreted by the breasts of infants of both sexes for 1 to 2 weeks. The distance between the infant's nipples should equal about 25% of the total chest circumference. Widely spaced nipples are often seen in genetic syndromes such as Turner syndrome. Supernumerary nipples are extra nipples that most often are found between 5 and 6 cm below the true nipple. They may, however, occur anywhere in the midclavicular line. Supernumerary nipples are often associated with congenital anomalies in white infants (Seidel et al., 1991).

Lungs. Newborns are diaphragmatic breathers, and accessory muscles, in particular the diaphragm, are used for respiration. The infant may also have paradoxical breathing (the thorax pulls inward and the abdomen bulges outward).

The infant may have slight nasal flaring and grunting immediately after delivery. These should resolve soon after birth, however. Periods of apnea or periodic breathing lasting less than 15 seconds may also occur during the newborn period.

> A lapse of breathing for longer than 15 to 20 seconds is considered apnea and may indicate a serious problem, such as sepsis, seizures, hypoglycemia, or maternal sedation.

Auscultation should be performed while the infant is quiet and still. All fields should be auscultated. Breath sounds should be equal and essentially clear. Abnormal breath sounds, such as crackles or wheezing, should be noted and reported.

Heart. An assessment of the cardiovascular system begins with an assessment of color. The infant should be centrally pink, including the mucous membranes and the scrotum in boys. The chest should be palpated for the point of maximum intensity (PMI). The heart rate, rhythm, and quality of heart sounds should be auscultated.

> Although most murmurs noted in the neonatal period are functional murmurs and result from anatomic changes that occur as the infant shifts from a fetal to a postnatal circulatory pattern, they should be reported, especially if they are accompanied by other signs of congenital heart disease, such as cyanosis, paleness, or sweating when feeding.

The infant's peripheral pulses should be assessed for rate, character, and equality. Pulses should be strong and equal, both side to side and upper and lower. In other words, the brachial pulses should feel equal when compared with each other and with the femoral pulses. Bounding pulses are often associated with a patent ductus arteriosus or aortic lesions. Weakened or absent femoral pulses may be associated with lesions that impede aortic outflow, such as coarctation of the aorta. Finally, weak or absent pulses may be the result of low cardiac output.

Abdomen. Infants normally have a potbellied appearance. A congenital absence of the abdominal muscles is known as prune-belly syndrome. It is more common in boys and is associated with anomalies of the renal and urinary systems (Tappero and Honeyfield, 1993). Visible peristalsis (pyloric stenosis) or a scaphoid appearance (diaphragmatic hernia) is abnormal and should be reported immediately.

The umbilicus should be located in the midline. Any umbilical hernias should be reported. Three vessels (two arteries and one vein) should be visible. The cord yellows as it dries. Absence of one of the umbilical arteries may be associated with cardiovascular or renal anomalies and should be reported. If an antibacterial agent has been applied, the color of the cord may be that of the agent (such as deep blue with triple dye).

> There should be no odor, redness, induration, or discharge from the umbilical cord. The presence of one of these abnormalities indicates an umbilical infection, which can lead quickly to sepsis and should be reported.

Bowel sounds are audible in the first 15 minutes after birth (Cohen & Koffler, 1987). They should be auscultated before palpation. On palpation, the liver should be noted 1 to 2 cm below the right costal margin. The spleen may be felt 1 to 2 cm below the left costal margin. The lower portion of the kidney is usually found 1 to 2 cm above the umbilicus on deep palpation.

Genitourinary System. At birth, the female genitalia are edematous, especially in cases of breech delivery. In full-term infants, the labia major are enlarged so that the clitoris is nearly covered. Vernix may be noted in the folds. The urethra lies directly behind the clitoris. Hymenal tags are common. A white mucoid discharge is also common for approximately 1 week. A blood-tinged discharge may also be noted as a result of the withdrawal of maternal hormones.

The foreskin often completely covers the glans penis. The urinary meatus normally appears as a slit in the middle of the glans. Abnormal positions include hypospadias (the meatus is on the ventral side of the penis) and epispadias (the meatus is on the dorsal side of the penis). The prepuce is commonly tight in the newborn and does not indicate phimosis (an abnormal condition in which the foreskin adheres to the glans and cannot be retracted). It should not be forcibly retracted.

The scrotum may appear edematous. In full-term male infants the scrotum is pendulous and completely covered by rugae. Testes are present in the lower portion of the scrotum. The inguinal canal remains open in the newborn, and the testes can easily migrate back into the canal when the infant is exposed to cold. The testicles may be palpated by blocking the inguinal canal with the forefinger and thumb of one hand and following the scrotum down with other hand until the testicle is felt. Undescended testicles (cryptorchidism) are not uncommon. This condition is more common on the right side (Tappero and Honeyfield, 1993). One-half of undescended testicles descend into the scrotum by the age of 6 weeks (Danish, 1992). If the testicles have not descended by 18 months of age, surgical intervention is necessary.

The bladder is palpable 1 to 4 cm above the symphysis. It is not uncommon to note a full, distended bladder immediately after birth, before the first void, or after feeding (Tappero and Honeyfield, 1993).

> All infants should void within the first 24 hours of life. Failure to do so may indicate a urinary blockage or a renal abnormality.

Normally, the anus is located approximately 1 finger width below the vagina in girls. The anus should have a tightly closed sphincter. An anal wink (a tightening or winking of the sphincter with stimulation) may be elicited by gently stroking the area near the anus. This area should be inspected for tags, imperforation, or membranes.

> Meconium should be passed within the first 24 hours. If it is not or if there is suspicion of an imperforation, the anus should be inspected with a well-lubricated, gloved little finger.

Musculoskeletal System. The back should be examined with the infant prone. The back is gently rounded. The curves typical of older children are not found. The skin along the spine should be intact. Any openings may indicate a neural tube defect or spina bifida. A dimple in the sacral area is called a pilonidal sinus and should be reported. It may be covered with a tuft of hair and is often associated with spina bifida occulta.

Because passive range of motion is easy in the newborn, examination of the extremities is easy. Full range of motion should be easy in the newborn. When the infant's arms or legs are extended fully, they should return to a flexed position.

The hands and feet should be examined for the presence of extra digits (polydactyly) or the absence of a digit (syndactyly). The palms should be examined for webbing of the fingers or the presence of a simian crease (a single long crease that crosses the entire palm), which may indicate Down syndrome. The fingers and toes should be straight. Macrodactyly (an enlarged finger or toe) could be indicative of neurofibromatosis, and an overlapping of the second and third fingers is often seen in infants with trisomy 18.

Infant Reflexes

Rooting: If the infant's cheek is stroked or her mouth is touched, she should respond by searching for and attempting to suck the examiner's finger.

Sucking: If a nipple or finger is placed in the infant's mouth so that it touches his hard palate, he should suck vigorously. This reflex is also indicative of functional gag and swallowing reflexes.

Ciliary: If the infant's eyelashes are stroked, she should close one or both of her eyes.

Doll's eyes: If the infant is placed in a supine position and his head is turned from side to side, his eyes should move to the opposite side.

Moro: If the infant is held in a supine position and her body is quickly displaced a few centimeters lower, she should extend, then abduct her extremities, with fingers spread in a symmetrical fashion. She may also cry.

Tonic neck: The infant is placed in a supine position and his head is turned to one side with the ipsilateral arm and leg extended and the contralateral arm and leg flexed. If the head is turned to the other direction, the positioning of the extremities is reversed. This reflex may or may not be present at birth, and its absence is not considered abnormal.

Palmar: If a finger is placed in the infant's palm, she should respond by grasping the examiner's finger. The grasp should be symmetrical. If pressure is put on the balls of her feet, she should grasp with her toes.

Step: If the infant is held upright with his feet touching a flat surface, he should make stepping motions.

Babinski: If the infant's foot is stroked on the outside (little toe) edge, she should fan her toes up and outward.

The thighs and gluteal folds should be examined for symmetry. The hips should be flexed and the thighs abducted to an angle of about 160°. Any clicks or slipping of the hip joints should be reported immediately.

Feet should be examined for deformities. Intrauterine positioning may cause the feet to turn inward (varus), but this positioning is usually transitory. Any evidence of clubfoot should be reported immediately.

Neurologic System. Neurologic assessment is a crucial part of the physical assessment. It is based on the presence of expected reflexive actions (see box). All infants are born with a series of reflexive actions that are indicative of neurologic well-being.

Neurologic functioning is displayed as a series of primitive reflexive actions. Myelinization is incomplete. It occurs in the same pattern that growth and development is noted (cephalocaudal and proximodistal). The achievement of neurologic milestones is closely related to this myelinization. Cranial nerves, except for the optic and olfactory nerves, are myelinated. The infant's senses of smell, taste, and hearing are well developed at birth, as is the sensation of pain.

Type and level of the baby's activity should be noted. Her posture should be one of flexion. Unless she has physical needs (hunger, wet diaper), she should appear quiet and contented. Jitteriness (shaking) may indicate hypoglycemia or infection. Crying is inevitable, but the pitch and any irritability should be noted. A high-pitched, irritable cry may indicate a neurologic deficit or disease and should be referred. The newborn sleeps about 16 hours per day, and this sleep is organized as a series of naps that last from 30 minutes to 4 hours.

STATUS OF OTHER BODY SYSTEMS

Gastrointestinal System. The gastrointestinal system has an adequate ability to meet the infant's needs for digestion, absorption, and metabolism. Because pancreatic enzymes are not available in the same amounts as in older infants, the ability to digest fat is decreased. Glycogen stores are low in the newborn, leaving him at greater risk for hypoglycemia.

The stomach holds approximately 90 ml at birth. Gastric emptying is unpredictable, and peristalsis is increased in the infant. An immature cardiac sphincter often leads to regurgitation or spitting up. The small intestine is immature and does not reabsorb water from the stool effectively. The large intestine absorbs more water from the stool, but because motility is rapid, the result is soft, liquid, and frequent stools.

Stools are composed of meconium for the first 2 days or so. Meconium is a sticky, dark greenish-black substance made up of bile, epithelial cells, digestive secretions, and amniotic fluid. Stools then enter a transition stage (a combination of meconium and regular stool) before becoming soft and yellow-brown. The stools of breastfed infants are looser and more yellow than those of formula-fed infants.

Renal System. Daily urine output is usually about 250 ml. This amount varies with fluid intake. The infant's bladder capacity is about 15 ml, and it empties spontaneously on reaching this amount.

Signs and Symptoms of Infection

- Hypothermia
- Poor feeding
- Vomiting or diarrhea
- Jitteriness
- Jaundice
- Apnea
- Hypotension
- Tachycardia
- Dyspnea
- Lethargy
- Cyanosis

Because the renal system is immature, urine is not concentrated. Reabsorption and filtration are limited, and the infant excretes a large amount of water. The urine is colorless or clear yellow, odorless, and has a specific gravity of approximately 1.020.

Immune System. Neonates have several protective mechanisms against infection. Infants are born with passive immunity. The infant receives immunity from the mother in the form of immunoglobulin G (IgG) near the end of gestation. Passive immunity and immunity received from breast milk provide protection against major childhood illnesses. This immunity lasts 3 to 6 months. Because this passive immunity is not permanent, infants must receive immunizations against childhood diseases as recommended by the Centers for Disease Control and the American Academy of Pediatrics. Breastfed infants also receive cellular and humoral protection (especially large amounts of IgA) from breast milk. These offer additional protection from infectious diseases, such as influenza, mumps, and chickenpox.

Infants begin to produce antibodies at 3 months after delivery. Because the immune system is immature, infants are susceptible to pathogens that normally do not affect older children, such as *Staphylococcus epidermidis* and *Escherichia coli.*

Leukocytosis (high white blood cell count) is normal at birth. Neonates, however, do not respond to sepsis with an increase in the white blood cell count. A decrease in the white blood cell counts is the typical response to sepsis.

Thermoregulation. The neonate has a limited ability to regulate heat production and loss. Hypothermia poses a serious, life-threatening problem for the newborn. The infant's ability to produce heat is immature and ineffective. The metabolic rate is higher in infants than in adults, and the body surface area is relatively larger. Therefore, in the infant, heat production is less than in an adult, and heat losses are greater.

The infant cannot shiver to generate heat. Infants metabolize brown fat stores to generate heat. Brown fat is a rich, well-vascularized fat store located between the scapulae; in the neck and axilla; behind the sternum; around the kidneys, trachea, and esophagus; and around major blood vessels and the adrenal glands (Poissonet et al., 1988). When the infant is cold stressed, he begins to metabolize this rich fat source, increasing oxygen consumption and ultimately heat production.

Heat loss occurs in four ways. The first is convection. This principle is illustrated by heat loss from a warm body to the cooler ambient air (drafts). Radiant heat loss occurs when the body loses heat to solid items that are not in contact with the body, but are in close proximity. This principle is illustrated by the infant losing heat to walls and windows in a cool nursery. Heat loss by evaporation is of major concern. This loss occurs when the infant's body cools as moisture that is present on the skin evaporates, such as after birth in the delivery room. Conduction is the fourth way that the body loses heat. The body loses heat to a cooler solid surface with which it is in direct contact (scales, examining tables).

Because cold stress can cause serious metabolic and physiologic problems for the neonate, attention must be paid to heat loss. At birth, the infant is dried thoroughly and placed under a radiant heat source until her temperature stabilizes (> 36.5° C). The first bath should take place under the radiant heat source.

Hemopoietic System. Blood volume ranges from 80 to 110 ml/kg of body weight, with an average volume of 200 ml in the neonate. The volume is often dependent on how much placental transfer of blood occurred in the delivery room.

The lifespan of the infant's red blood cells is considerably shorter than that of an older child or adult. The average lifespan of the infant's red blood cells is 50 to 90 days (Stockman, 1988). In the older child and adult, red blood cells usually have a lifespan of about 120 days. One theory about this difference is the decreased deformability of the newborn's red blood cells. This decrease impedes splenic filtering, thus leading to cell destruction (Shaw, 1993).

Hepatic System. Most infants have some physiologic jaundice after the first day of life characterized by a yellow-gold color of the skin. This jaundice is caused by the increased number of erythrocytes (red blood cells) in circulation, the shorter lifespan of the erythrocytes, and the inability of the immature neonatal liver to conjugate (indirect) bilirubin out of the bloodstream. Because unconjugated bilirubin is bound to albumin, any medications that can interfere with these albumin binding sites (such as phenobarbital) may also interfere with the excretion of bilirubin.

Indirect bilirubin levels usually peak at about 4 days of age. Their maximum level is usually 6 to 7 mg/dl. After this point, levels should continue to fall.

> Jaundice that appears in the first 24 hours is usually caused by hemolytic disease (Rh incompatibility). Jaundice that appears after the third day of life may be associated with illness, such as sepsis.

Two types of jaundice have been identified in breastfed babies. The first type is early-onset jaundice, which is seen in 10% to 25% of infants. As with formula-fed infants, this type of jaundice occurs 2 to 4 days after birth and usually resolves within 1 week. Early and frequent breast feedings appear to decrease the incidence (Osborn, 1986). The second type of jaundice is termed breast milk jaundice and appears in 2% to 3% of breastfed infants. This type of jaundice appears at 4 to 5 days of age and may last 3 to 12 weeks. This type of jaundice may be related to certain factors in the breast milk that break bilirubin down into a lipid-soluble form. This bilirubin is then reabsorbed by the gut (Lascari, 1986).

Decreased ability of the liver to form plasma proteins leads to edema after birth. Decreased levels of prothrombin and other coagulation factors cause an increased risk of bleeding. Low glycogen stores in the liver predispose the newborn to hypoglycemia. For these reasons, early feeding and protection from infection and injury are important.

A summary of the physical assessment of newborns is shown in Table 3–3.

BEHAVIORAL CHARACTERISTICS

Infants are born with distinctive temperaments or behavior styles. Temperament affects the child's interaction with the environment, his consolability, and his adaptation to change in routine.

Several researchers have studied the relationship of the newborn's temperament to later personality. Three basic types of infant temperament have been identified. A newborn who is quiet and alert is easygoing and adaptable to changes in routine. He responds to stimuli appropriately. The overresponsive infant does not adapt well to changes in routine, is fussy, and responds to new or different stimuli by crying. The third type, the unresponsive infant, is often difficult to arouse and may initially respond to stimuli negatively (Als and Brazelton, 1981).

In 1973, T. Berry Brazelton developed the Brazelton Neonatal Behavioral Assessment Scale (BNBAS) (Brazelton, 1984). This scale focuses on the behavior of infants. It measures both behavioral and elicited responses to stimuli. This scale is useful to help parents and caregivers learn to read infant cues and react appropriately.

BNBAS scores are based on the infant's best performance for each response (instead of an average of all responses). Performance is directly related to the sleep–wake state of the infant. Brazelton identified these states as follows:

1. *Deep sleep*: Regular respiratory rate, no rapid eye movements, little spontaneous movement
2. *Light sleep*: Irregular respirations, rapid eye movements, occasional movement
3. *Drowsy*: Semi-asleep, variable activity level
4. *Quiet alert*: Bright-eyed, alert, attentive, calm, quiet
5. *Active alert*: Increased activity, fussy, less attentive
6. *Crying*: Loud crying, large amounts of motor activity, inattentive to stimuli

Infants are most reactive to stimuli and most interactive with others during the quiet alert state. It is helpful to parents and others who will interact with the infant to learn to recognize these states, note when the infant is becoming overstimulated, and adjust stimuli accordingly.

Infants are fascinated with adults. From about 3 days of age, they can identify their mother by the sound of her voice (DeCasper and Fifer, 1980). The infant may also identify other members of his family from the sounds he has heard frequently in utero. An infant also responds physically to the rhythm of speech.

Studies have shown that infants prefer moving objects (Kessen et al., 1970). Neonates prefer large objects to small ones and respond well to black and white contrasts. Greenberg (1971) found that infants prefer patterns that offer increasing visual complexity. They prefer faces to inanimate objects (Bushnell, 1982). Scanning the face occurs primarily in the young infant. The older infant focuses on specific parts of the face (Hainline and Lemerise, 1982).

The infant prefers sweet to salty tastes and will turn toward her mother's milk (MacFarlane, 1975). Sucking responses are also patterned according to the taste. An infant will suck less when a liquid is salty or unsweetened and more when it is sweet.

New babies imitate the behavior of adults. Meltzoff and Moore (1977) showed that infants as young as 12 days would imitate an adult sticking out his tongue. Infants learn through operant conditioning. Response to stimuli is noted in differing ways, depending on the temperament of the infant.

Play dominates the infant's waking hours. Play is body-focused and consists of being talked to, held, rocked, and tickled. Piaget found that infants will repeat behaviors simply for the pleasure of performing the act.

TABLE 3-3 *Summary of Physical Assessment*

USUAL FINDINGS	USUAL VARIATIONS FROM NORMAL	ABNORMALITIES
General Appearance		
Flexion, with extremities pulled in close to the chest and abdomen.	Breech (frank): legs extended and rotated externally.	Limp, hypotonia, or stiffened posture.
Integument		
Smooth, reddened, and slightly edematous at birth. Pale pink to tan, drier, and slightly flaky by the second to third day. Vernix caseosa and lanugo in varying amounts. Edema may be noted in the face, extremities, and genitalia. Color changes with stress: reddening with crying, acrocyanosis, and cutis mamorata (mottling when exposed to cold).	Bruising from birth trauma or forceps. Milia: small white papules located on the nose and chin caused by maternal hormones. Miliaria: tiny vesicles on the face resulting from blockage of the sweat glands. Jaundice after 24 hours. Erythema toxicum: "newborn rash" or red papular rash with yellow or white vesicles located in the center. Mongolian spots: dark blue-black pigments on the sacral and gluteal region of black, Hispanic, and Asian infants. Telangiectatic nevi or stork bite: reddened area at the nape of the neck. Strawberry nevi: deep red, raised areas located primarily on the head and face.	Jaundice appearing before 24 hours. Pallor. Cyanosis. Plethora: extreme redness caused by a high hematocrit value. Petechiae. Rashes or papules other than newborn rash. Café au lait spots: sharply demarcated, hyperpigmented macules that may be associated with neurofibromatosis. Port wine stains.
Head and Facies		
Both anterior and posterior fontanels are open, soft, and flat. Facies are symmetrical. Some edema may be present, especially around the eyes.	Unilateral edema from forceps. Forceps marks. Molding. Caput succedaneum: edema of the soft tissue on the back of the scalp; crosses suture lines. Cephalhematoma: hematoma formed between the periosteum and bone of the skull; unilateral and does not cross suture lines.	Asymmetrical features. Fused sutures (craniosynostosis). Widened sutures or fontanels. Bulging or tense fontanel when quiet. Craniotabes: snapping or popping of bones along lambdoid suture; resembles indentations on a table tennis ball.
Eyes		
Edema. Dark blue, gray, or brown. No tears. Pupils react to light. Blink response to bright light. Fixation on objects of interest (black and white objects, human faces).	Epicanthal folds in infants of Asian descent. Nystagmus. Strabismus. Subconjunctival hemorrhages from delivery.	Epicanthal folds in non-Asian infants. Cloudy or hazy lens. Fixed constricted or dilated pupil. Absence of pupillary reflex (blindness). Absence of red reflex. Blue sclera (osteogenesis imperfecta). Yellow sclera (jaundice).
Nose		
Patent. Located in the midline. Two nares.	Flattened. Edematous. Milia.	Nonpatent nares. Thick, copious discharge. Nasal flaring.
Mouth		
High, arched palate. Uvula in the midline. Frenulum noted on the tongue and upper lip. Sucking reflex. Rooting reflex. Gag reflex. Extrusion reflex. Little or no salivation.	Epstein pearls. Natal teeth.	Cleft lip or palate. Large, protruding tongue. Excessive salivation or drooling: tracheoesophageal fistula. Posteriorly placed tongue or small chin (Pierre Robin syndrome).
Ears		
Top of the pinna is level with the outer canthus of the eye. Near vertical placement. Reacts to loud noise with startle reflex.	Inability to visualize the tympanic membrane. Pinna is soft and flexible, flat to the head. Small pits or skin tags directly in front of the ear.	Low-set ears. Failure to elicit startle reflex. Abnormalities of shape and size.

TABLE 3–3 *Summary of Physical Assessment (continued)*

USUAL FINDINGS	USUAL VARIATIONS FROM NORMAL	ABNORMALITIES
Chest		
Rounded, barrel-shaped appearance. Xyphoid process is visible at the end of the sternum. Mild intercostal retractions.	Supernumerary nipples. "Witch's milk" excreted from the breast.	Funnel chest (pectus excavatum). Pigeon chest (pectus carnatum). Broad, shield-like shape, with widely spaced nipples. Moderate retractions. Asymmetrical shape.
Lungs		
Diaphragmatic breathing. Bilateral breath sounds are equal, essentially clear.	Fine crackles immediately after birth. Irregular rate and rhythm of breathing. Periodic apnea (<15 seconds).	Grunting. Stridor. Persistent moderate to coarse crackles. Wheezing. Grunting. Decreased breath sounds. Long periods of apnea (>15 seconds). Seesaw respirations. Bowel sounds.
Heart		
PMI at fourth to fifth intercostal space. Rate increases with crying, excitement.	Functional murmurs. Sinus tachycardia.	Murmurs, especially if associated with cyanosis, pallor, or sweating with feeding. Thrills.
Abdomen		
Potbellied shape. Liver 1–2 cm below the right costal margin. Spleen 1–2 cm below the left costal margin. Kidneys 1–2 cm above the umbilicus. Umbilical cord contains two arteries and one vein. Bowel sounds present.	Umbilical hernia.	Distension. Masses. Visible peristalsis. Absent bowel sounds. Small, hard, pea-shaped mass (pyloric stenosis). Umbilicus with only one artery. Scaphoid appearance.
Genitalia		
Edema. Vernix in folds. Female urethra located behind the clitoris. Male urethra located at the tip of the glans penis. Testes in the scrotum. Urine within 24 hours.	Blood-tinged or milky discharge from female. Hymenal tags. Prepuce tightly adherent to the glans penis. Testes retracting into the inguinal canal when exposed to cold.	Urinary meatus located at the tip of the clitoris. Fused labia. Absence of vaginal opening. Fecal material draining from the vagina. Hypospadias. Epispadias. No urine in 24 hours.
Anus		
Anal wink reflex. Patent anus. Sphincter tightly closed. Meconium stool within 24–36 hours.		Anal fissures. Fistulas. Imperforate anus. No wink reflex (spina bifida). Failure to pass meconium.
Back		
Spine intact and rounded.		Spina bifida. Hair tufts or sinuses along the sacrum.
Extremities		
Ten fingers. Ten toes. Muscle tone equal bilaterally. Flexed against the chest and abdomen. Acrocyanosis.	Partial syndactyly between second and third toes. Wide space between great and second toes.	Polydactyly. Syndactyly. Simian crease. Decreased range of motion. Absence of any part of an extremity. Dislocation of the hips. Fractures.
Neurologic System		
Flexion. Presence of primitive reflexes.	Slight quivering or tremors, especially when crying.	High-pitched cry. Hypo- or hypertonia. Opisthotonos (hypertonia with arching of the back: common with meningeal irritation). Paralysis. Seizures (tremors do not stop when the extremity is held by the examiner).

NURSING CARE OF THE NEWBORN

Because of the relative immaturity of their body systems, newborns require a great deal of physical care. Promotion of parental attachment and assimilation of the infant into the family is also of vital importance.

Actual physical care includes the promotion of growth through appropriate nutrition, thermoregulation, airway maintenance, and protection from illness and injury.

Nutrition: Breast and Bottle Feeding

The method of feeding is a major decision to be made by parents. Both breastfeeding and commercial cow's milk formulas offer advantages and disadvantages. Many factors affect the family's choice of feeding method.

Culture greatly affects the family's food choices. Beliefs about breastfeeding and bottle feeding, the introduction of solid foods, and ethnic food preferences also affect the nutritional choices made by the family.

> Infants need about 108 kcal/kg/day. Infant formulas and breast milk both provide 20 kcal/ounce.

Ethnicity, education, and socioeconomic factors are all related to the choice of feeding method. In the United States, white, middle- and upper-income, college-educated, married women are the most likely to breastfeed (Dix, 1991). Factors associated with choosing not to breastfeed are poor health, delivery of a preterm infant, and not attending childbirth classes. Old wives' tales and taboos about breastfeeding may also influence the decision. For example, some women believe that the breasts will become pendulous after breastfeeding.

The food of choice for the newborn is milk, either human or prepared formulas. A comparison of the two shows that both contain fat, protein, and sugar (see Chapter 12). The protein in breast milk is a more complete protein, is more easily digested, and results in a more rapid gastric emptying time than the protein in cow's milk. Therefore infants fed breast milk require more frequent feedings. Human milk is higher in lactose, which is converted into the monosaccharide galactose. Galactose is essential for central nervous system development and growth. The fat in breast milk is higher in monosaturated fat, which is more easily digested and absorbed than the fat in cow's milk. Finally, with the exception of vitamin D and fluoride, breast milk provides everything that the newborn needs, including added antibodies against disease.

Breastfed babies are rarely overfed because there is less tendency to finish the rest of a bottle. Breastfeeding also facilitates a bond between the infant and her mother. Breastfeeding should be initiated within the first hour after delivery, if possible. The infant is in a quiet alert state during this time, has a vigorous suck, and will often nurse well. Studies show that the longer after a birth an infant waits to be put to the breast, the more difficult it is for him to suckle well (Panetta, 1993).

For breastfeeding to be successful, the mother should use a comfortable position that allows the infant to latch onto the nipple well. The mother and infant should be "tummy to tummy." A pillow may be needed to bring the infant's mouth to the level of the breast (Winthrop, 1995).

For mothers who have difficulty, a lactation specialist or breastfeeding support group may be helpful. Nipple confusion may occur if the infant is switched often between the bottle and breast. Tsang and Nichols (1988) stated that bottle feeding may be introduced as an alternative to breastfeeding once lactation has been well established, usually 2 weeks postpartum. Mothers can also pump and store their breast milk.

Bottle feeding is the method chosen more frequently in the United States. This method is often easier for the mother who must return to work soon after the delivery of her infant, and it has the advantage of allowing other members of the family to participate in the feeding of the infant. The ability of others to provide nutrition for the infant also allows the mother to rotate the responsibility of some late-night feedings. If bottle feedings are used, the formula should be an iron-fortified formula. Cow's milk formulas without added iron do not provide enough iron to meet the infant's daily requirements. If bottle feeding is the choice made by the mother, she should be supported in her decision by the nurse. Mothers should never be made to feel guilty for not breastfeeding.

It should never be assumed that parents know how to bottle feed an infant. They should be taught how often and how much to feed the infant, how to hold and cuddle him while feeding, when and how to burp, and how to prepare formula. While in the hospital, they should be provided with a new, sterile nipple for each feeding. Mothers should be discouraged from reusing the nipples sent with bottles of formula because there is no way to properly clean and sterilize them.

Teaching Guidelines for breast and bottle feeding appear in Chapter 12.

Infants are born with an extrusion reflex (tongue thrust) that helps them learn to effectively suck, swallow, and breathe. This reflex also prevents infants from effectively taking solid foods from a spoon until about the age of 6 months.

Newborn infants usually consume 2 to 3 ounces per feeding in six to eight feedings per day. The amount of formula consumed at each feeding increases with a growth spurt at about 2 weeks to 3 to 5 ounces per feeding in five to six feedings per day (Heslin, 1988).

Protection From Illness and Injury

Because the infant has an immature immune system, special attention should be paid to avoid exposure to pathogens. The nurse should use good infection control practices. These include washing hands on entering the nursery and between caring for infants and isolating potentially infectious infants (including infants colonized, although not sick with such pathogens as methicillin-resistant *Staphylococcus aureus*). Some nurseries also use cover gowns worn over street clothes. As with all patients, standard precautions should be used in the nursery.

Vitamin K (Aquamephyton) is administered to all infants shortly after birth to prevent bleeding. Vitamin K is synthesized in the intestinal tract by intestinal flora. Because a newborn's intestinal tract is sterile, supplementary vitamin K is necessary to produce prothrombin in the liver until the body begins to synthesize vitamin K (about 3–4 days after delivery).

Eye care should be performed after delivery to prevent ophthalmia neonatorum. The most frequently used preparations are 0.5% erythromycin ointment or drops and 1% tetracycline ointment or drops. Silver nitrate is not often used because it is not effective against *Chlamydia trachomatis*. Application of the ointment or drops may be delayed for 1 hour after delivery to facilitate the bonding between the infant and parents.

Bathing is frequently done after the infant is admitted to the nursery and has warmed to an axillary temperature of 36.6°C. The bath should be done with warm water and a mild soap. The primary reason for the bath is to remove blood from the infant. Although vernix is removed, there is some indication that the vernix provides lubrication and protection for the skin. The bath is performed from head to toe. The infant should be placed under a radiant heat source for the first bath. The female genitalia should be cleansed in a front-to-back manner to prevent urinary tract infection. In boys, any smegma noted around the glans penis should be wiped away, but the foreskin should not be forcefully retracted.

The umbilicus requires special attention. It provides an excellent medium for infection and should be cleaned with alcohol after each diaper change. Many institutions use triple dye (a brilliant blue antibiotic preparation) to facilitate drying and prevent infection. Triple dye stains the cord a bright blue.

> There should be no odor, redness, induration, or discharge from the umbilical cord. Any of these would indicate an umbilical infection, which can lead quickly to sepsis.

Circumcision

Circumcision is a frequently performed surgical procedure that removes the foreskin of the penis. In 1992 the American Academy of Pediatrics stated that there is no medical indication for circumcision, and the procedure remains a source of great debate (Podnar, 1992). Circumcision may be performed with a scalpel, Gomco clamp, or Hollister Plastibell.

If a scalpel or Gomco clamp is used to remove the foreskin, the glans will appear dark red and have some bleeding. The end of the penis is generally covered with a petroleum jelly gauze to prevent its adherence to the diaper. The diaper is applied loosely to decrease friction against the penis. The infant must be closely observed for voiding after circumcision.

A yellowish exudate appears on the glans at about the second day after removal of the foreskin. This exudate is part of the normal healing process. If a Plastibell is used, it is applied like a tourniquet and the excess foreskin trimmed. The bell automatically falls off in about 5 to 8 days.

Promotion of Parent–Infant Attachment

Facilitating the parent–infant bond is important. Many parents are overwhelmed at the prospect of a newborn infant who is completely dependent on them for care. It is important to allow parents time to get to know their infant. Nurses can facilitate the bonding process by anticipating knowledge deficits and providing anticipatory guidance. Many parents are too embarrassed to ask questions. The nurse should anticipate and identify these questions and foster a nonthreatening environment. Fostering positive interactions between the infant and his family supports the infant's sense of trust and increases the parents' confidence in their abilities.

Ways to facilitate infant–parent attachment include teaching parents to recognize their infant's response to stimuli, recognizing the threshold at which the infant becomes overstimulated, and noting behavioral cues. Most infants block out noxious or overwhelming stimuli through a process called habituation. Habituation means that the infant gradually decreases his response to noxious stimuli until the response disappears. Infants who do not have the ability to habituate will be irritable and fussy, and show signs of overstimulation. They exhibit feeding difficulties because they cannot shut out environmental stimuli (Tappero and Honeyfield, 1993). Parents should be taught to read the infant's cues and respond in ways that decrease the overstimulation.

Infants provide their caregivers with specific cues to have their demands met. A reciprocal relationship develops between the infant and caregiver when appropriate responses are given to cues. Appropriate responses also reinforce the infant's behavioral organization (Creger,

1992; D'Apolito, 1991). Signs that the infant is ready for interaction include a quiet alert state with a focused stare, regular breathing patterns, sucking, and hand-to-mouth behaviors (Creger, 1992). The infant who is ready to terminate interaction will avert his gaze, sneeze, frown, or hiccup (Creger, 1992).

PREPARATION FOR DISCHARGE (ANTICIPATORY GUIDANCE)

Unless the health of the infant or mother is a concern, most infants remain in the hospital nursery less than 72 hours. Discharge planning is crucial, particularly if the infant is a firstborn. Much of discharge planning focuses on anticipatory guidance and should include hygiene, signs and symptoms of illness, nutrition and growth, elimination, thermoregulation, and safety.

Hygiene. Because thermoregulation may be a problem and because the newborn's skin is sensitive, tub baths with soap are not given for the first few days of life. Sponge baths will suffice until the cord stump has dried and fallen off. Few infants require a daily bath. If soap is used, it should be unscented and mild. As in the hospital, the bath should proceed from head to toe, with special attention paid to folds of skin. To maintain temperature, the infant should be completely dried after each bath. If dry skin is noted, baths should be given less frequently and a lotion that can be absorbed by the skin applied. Baby oil should not be used to lubricate the skin because it is not completely absorbed and can promote the growth of bacteria.

Seborrheic dermatitis or cradle cap is seen in some infants. It appears as thick, yellow, scaly patches that are found on the scalp (most often over the anterior fontanel), but may also appear on the eyebrows or eyelids. The scales may be removed by warming a small amount of baby oil, applying it to the patches, and allowing it to penetrate the crusts. The crusts may then be washed away with baby shampoo. It is important to reassure parents that the condition is usually temporary and disappears by 12 months.

Cord care should be performed after each bath and diaper change. The umbilical stump and the area where it attaches to the abdomen are cleaned with rubbing or isopropyl alcohol. The umbilical cord usually falls off about 10 days after birth. Some slight bleeding may be noted. Parents should be taught to recognize the signs and symptoms of umbilical infection.

The diaper area, including the gluteal folds, should be cleaned and thoroughly dried with each diaper change. Either warm water or baby wipes can be used. Parents should be cautioned not to use commercial baby wipes if any diaper rash is noted. It is important to teach parents to wipe girls from front to back and to clean under the scrotum of boys.

If parents decide to have their male infant circumcised, informed consent must be obtained before the procedure. Parents should be taught to recognize the normal appearance of the glans after circumcision. If a plastic bell is applied to protect the glans, it will stay in place until the penis heals. The physician should be notified if the bell does not fall off.

If parents decide not to have their infant circumcised, they must be taught how to retract the foreskin and clean the glans. It is also important to teach parents that the foreskin may not be completely retractable until the child reaches preschool age.

Elimination. Infants frequently have a stool with each feeding and may void as many as 20 times per day. Parents should be taught that their infant should have at least one stool and eight wet diapers per day.

Growth and Development. Newborn infants usually lose between 5% and 10% of their birth weight in the first few days. They then stabilize, begin to gain weight, and return to their birth weight within 2 weeks. Parents can expect the infant to gain about 5 to 7 ounces (150–210 g) per week for the first 6 months of life. They can also expect him to grow about 1 inch per month in length. Head circumference increases by 0.5 inches per month. Infants have periodic growth spurts when they increase their food intake. The first of these spurts occurs at about 2 weeks, and another occurs at about 6 weeks. Parents should know that the infant will want to feed more often if she is breastfed (about every 2 hours) to increase the mother's milk supply or will take a larger volume if she is fed formula.

Nurses should teach parents growth and developmental milestones. Parents often have many questions about when to expect a child to perform certain tasks. It is important to stress that growth and development follow certain predictable patterns and that milestones are reached within a range of ages, but not necessarily at a specific age.

Thermoregulation and Clothing. Parents should be taught to protect their newborn from drafts and extremes of temperature. Infants should be dressed as other family members are dressed. Baths should take place in a warm area, and infants should be dried thoroughly to protect the infant from evaporative heat loss.

Safety. All states now have child restraint laws that require infants and young children to be restrained in an approved car seat. An infant held on a parent's lap is 14 times more likely to be killed in an accident than one who is restrained in an approved safety seat (Arnott and Wright, 1992). The distance traveled makes no difference; children should be restrained for any trip in a car. Car seats should have a label that states that the seat "meets or exceeds Federal Motor Vehicle Safety Standard #213" (Loomis, 1992). A car seat manufactured before 1981 does not meet these standards and should not be used.

Infants should be placed in a bucket-type car seat that faces backward in the backseat until they weigh 18 to 20 lb. The infant should never face forward or ride in the front seat. Parents should be taught to secure the seat in the car and place the child in the seat properly. Bottles should never be propped.

Studies in Europe and the Netherlands show as much as a 50% decrease in the incidence of sudden infant death syndrome (SIDS) when infants were put to bed in a supine rather than a prone position (Spiers and Guntheroth, 1994; Willinger et al., 1994). This recommendation was adopted by the National Institutes of Health (NIH) and the American Academy of Pediatrics in 1994. Parents, therefore, should be taught to put infants to bed on their backs.

Cribs should be finished with unleaded paint. Crib bars should be no more than 2 inches apart, and the mattress should be no more than 1 fingerwidth smaller than the crib.

Disease Prevention. It is important to teach the family about infection control. Newborn infants should not be taken out into crowded areas where they may be exposed to disease. The infant should not have visitors who have colds or other infectious diseases. New parents need not be housebound, however. Newborns may be taken out, but parents should remember that if the weather is too extreme for them, it is too extreme for their newborn.

Well-Baby Visits

Well-baby physical examination: 2–4 weeks; 2, 4, 6, 9, and 12 months
Measurements, including height, weight, and head circumference: 2–4 weeks; 2, 4, 6, 9, and 12 months
Sensory screening: 2–4 weeks; 2, 4, 6, 9, and 12 months
Developmental and behavioral assessment: 2–4 weeks; 2, 4, 6, 9, and 12 months
Metabolic/genetic screening: By 1 month
Tuberculin skin test: 12 months
Hematocrit or hemoglobin: 9 months
Urinalysis: 6 months
Anticipatory guidance/parent teaching: 2–4 weeks; 2, 4, 6, 9, and 12 months
Immunization: See immunization schedule, Appendix A

Signs and symptoms of illness should also be discussed with the parents. This discussion should include a definition of fever (usually a temperature of >100.8° F), distinguishing vomiting from spitting up, and diarrhea. Parents should also be taught how to recognize dehydration in an infant.

Finally, the importance of follow-up visits should be emphasized. These visits provide time for assessing the infant's growth and development. The importance of well-baby care, such as immunizations, should be stressed (see box). The infant should receive the first dose of hepatitis B vaccine before discharge from the newborn nursery. Parents should be taught the importance of follow-up visits and of keeping the infant's immunizations up-to-date.

KEY CONCEPTS

- The infant undergoes major physiologic changes at birth that include the change from fetal to postnatal circulation, temperature regulation, elimination, and the establishment of respiration.
- Stabilization and facilitation of the newborn's adaptation to extrauterine life are major responsibilities of the nurse.
- A large surface area, little subcutaneous fat, and inability to produce heat predispose the infant to rapid heat loss.
- Initial assessment of the newborn includes gestational age assessment, measurements and weight, and physical assessment.
- Assessment of neurologic functioning in the infant is based on a series of reflexive actions as well as an evaluation of general well-being.
- Because newborns and their mothers are being discharged from the hospital quickly, discharge planning and anticipatory guidance are vitally important.

REFERENCES

Als, H., & Brazelton, T. B. (1981). A new model of assessing the behavioral organization in preterm and full term infants. *Journal of the American Academy of Child Psychiatry, 20,* 239.

American Academy of Pediatrics and American College of Obstetricians and Gynecologists. (1988). *Guidelines for perinatal care* (2nd ed.). Elk Grove Village, IL: Author.

Arnott, N., & Wright, J. (1992). How to choose and use a car seat. *American Baby, 54*(5), B5–B8.

Ballard, J. L., Khoury, J. C., Wedig, K., Wang, L., Ellers-Waisman, B. L., & Lipp, R. (1991). New Ballard score, expanded to include extremely premature infants. *Journal of Pediatrics, 119*(3), 418.

Ballard, J. L., Novak, K. K., & Driver, M. (1979). A simplified score for assessment of fetal maturation of newly born infants. *Journal of Pediatrics, 95*(5), 769–774.

Blanchette, V., & Zipursky, A. (1987). Neonatal hematology. In G. B. Avery (Ed.), *Neonatology: Pathophysiology and management of the newborn* (3rd ed., pp. 638–690). Philadelphia: J. B. Lippincott.

Bloom, R. S. (1991). Delivery room resuscitation of the newborn. In A. A. Farnaroff & R. J. Martin (Eds.), *Neonatal-perinatal medicine.* St. Louis: Mosby–Year Book.

Brazelton, T. B. (Ed.). (1984). *Neonatal behavioral assessment scale* (2nd ed.). Philadelphia: J. B. Lippincott.

Britton, J. R., Britton H. L., & Beebe, S. A. (1994). Early discharge of the term newborn: A continued dilemma. *Pediatrics, 94,* 291–295.

Bushnell, I. W. R. (1982). Discrimination of faces by young infants. *Journal of Experimental Child Psychology, 33,* 298–308.

Chameides, L. (Ed.). (1994). *Pediatric advanced life support.* Dallas, TX: American Heart Association.

Cohen, R. W., & Koffler, H. (1987). *Primary care of the newborn* (pp. 20–28). Boston: Little, Brown.

Creger, P. (1992). Developmental support in the NICU. In P. Beadry & J. Deacon (Eds.), *Core curriculum for neonatal intensive care nursing.* Philadelphia: W. B. Saunders.

Danish, R. K. (1992). Abnormalities of sexual differentiation. In A. A. Fanaroff & R. J. Martin (Eds.), *Neonatal-perinatal medicine: Diseases of the fetus and infant.* (5th ed., pp. 1273–1275). St. Louis: C. V. Mosby.

D'Apolito, K. (1991). What is an organized infant? *Neonatal Network, 10*(1), 23–29.

DeCasper, A., & Fifer, W. P. (1980). Of human bonding: Newborns prefer their mothers' voices. *Science, 208,* 1174–1176.

Dix, D. N. (1991). Why women decide not to breastfeed. *Birth, 18*(4), 222–225.

Gorrie, T. M., McKinney, E. S., & Murray, S. S. (1994). *Foundations of maternal newborn nursing.* Philadelphia: W. B. Saunders.

Greenberg, D. J. (1971). Accelerating visual complexity in the human infant. *Child Development, 42*(3), 905–918.

Hainline, L., & Lemerise, E. (1982). Infants' scanning of geometric forms varying in size. *Journal of Experimental Child Psychology. 33,* 235–256.

Heslin, J. A. (1988). *No-nonsense nutrition for your baby's first year.* Englewood Cliffs, NJ: Prentice-Hall.

Heslin, J. (1992). If you bottlefeed . . . *American Baby, 54*(5), B10–B14.

Jones, K. L. (1988). *Smith's recognizable patterns of human malformation* (4th ed.). Philadelphia: W. B. Saunders.

Judd, J. M. (1985). Assessing the newborn from head to toe. *Nursing 85, 15*(12), 34–41.

Kessen, W., Haith, M. M., & Salapatek, P. H. (1970). Human infants: A bibliography and guide. In P. H. Mussen (Ed.), *Carmichael's manual of child psychology.* New York: Wiley.

Lascari, A. D. (1986). Early breast feeding jaundice: Clinical significance. *Journal of Pediatrics, 108*(1), 156–158.

Loomis, C. (1992). Buying guide: Car seats. *Parents Magazine, 67*(8), 101–103.

Margileth, A. (1987). Neonatal hematology. In G. B. Avery (Ed.), *Neonatology: Pathophysiology and management of the newborn* (3rd ed., pp. 1230–1273). Philadelphia: J. B. Lippincott.

MacFarlane, A. (1975). Olfaction in the development of social preferences in the human neonate. *CIBA Foundation Symposium, 33,* 1975.

Meltzoff, A. N., & Moore, M. K. (1977). Imitation of facial and manual gestures by human neonates. *Science, 198*(4312), 74–78.

Osborn, L. M. (1986). Management of neonatal jaundice. *Nurse Practitioner, 11*(14), 41–52.

Podnar, N. C. (1992). Circumcision. *American Baby, 54*(11), 72–76.

Poissonnet, C., LaVelle, M., & Burdi, A. (1988). Growth and development of adipose tissue. *Journal of Pediatrics, 113*(1), 1–9.

Seidel, H. M., Ball, J. W., Dains, J. E., & Benedict, G. W. (1991). *Mosby's guide to physical examination* (2nd ed.). St. Louis: Mosby–Year Book.

Shaw, N. (1993). Assessment and management of hematologic dysfunction. In C. Kenner, A. Brueggemeyer, & L. P. Gunderson (Eds.), *Comprehensive neonatal nursing.* Philadelphia: W. B. Saunders.

Spiers, P. S., & Guntheroth, W. G. (1994). Recommendations to avoid the prone sleeping position and recent statistics for sudden infant death syndrome in the United States. *Archives of Pediatric and Adolescent Medicine, 148,* 141–146.

Stockman, J. (1988). Physiology of the neonate as it relates to transfusion therapy. In D. Kasprisin, & N. Luban, (Eds.), *Pediatric transfusion medicine* (pp. 1–22). Boca Raton, FL: CRC Press.

Tappero, E. P., & Honeyfield, M. E. (1993). *Physical assessment of the newborn.* Petaluma, CA: NICUINK Publications.

Tsang, R. C., & Nichols, B. L. (Eds.). (1988). *Nutrition during infancy.* St. Louis: C. V. Mosby.

Willinger, M., Hoffman H. J., & Hartford R. B. (1994). Infant sleep position and risk for sudden infant death syndrome: Report of a meeting held January 13–14, 1994. *Pediatrics, 93,* 814–819.

Winthrop, A. (1995, July). Breastfeeding for beginners. *American Baby,* 68–71.

BIBLIOGRAPHY

Baker, K., Kuhlmann, T., & Magliaro, B. L. (1989). Homeward bound: Discharge teaching for parents of newborns with special needs. *Nursing Clinics of North America, 24*(3), 655–64.

Bindler, R. M., & Howry, L. B. (1991). *Pediatric drugs and nursing implications.* Norwalk, CT: Appleton & Lange.

Brans, Y. W. (1987). *Neonatology in obstetrical practice.* Philadelphia: J. B. Lippincott.

Bull, M. J., Stroup, K. B., & Gerhart, S. (1988). Misuse of car safety seats. *Pediatrics, 81*(1), 98–101.

Danner, S. (1991). How do we influence the breastfeeding decision? *Birth, 18*(4), 227–228.

Fanaroff, A., & Martin, R. (1992). *Neonatal-perinatal medicine: Diseases of the fetus and infant* (Vol. II, 5th ed.). St. Louis: Mosby–Year Book.

Frantz, K. (1991). Keep breastfeeding simple, keep it easy, keep it fun. *Birth, 18*(4), 228–229.

Greene, M. G. (Ed.). (1991). *The Harriet Lane Handbook* (12th ed.). Chicago: Year Book.

Grimes, J., & Burns, E. (1992). *Health assessment in nursing practice* (3rd ed.). Boston: Jones and Bartlett.

Johnson, P. A., & Gaines, S. K. (1988). Helping families to help themselves. *MCN: The American Journal of Maternal Child Nursing, 13*(5), 336–339.

Karlsrud, K. (1991). Can you spoil a baby? *Parents, 66*(1), 107.

Karlsrud, K., & Schultz, D. (1991). Weaning from the breast. *Parents, 66*(10), 158.

Kiernan, B. S., Scoloveno, M. A. (1986). Assessment of the neonate. *Topics in Clinical Nursing, 8*(1), 1–10.

Lawrence, R. A. (1991). When will it become American to breastfeed? *Birth, 18*(4), 226–227.

Maccagno-Smith, R., & Young, M. (1993). Breastfeeding the sleepy infant. *Canadian Nurse, 89*(2), 20–22.

Moore, K. L. (1982). *The developing human* (3rd ed.). Philadelphia: W. B. Saunders.

Panetta, I. (1993). Breastfeeding, A to Z. *Canadian Nurse, 89*(2), 17–19.

Rengucci, L. M. (1992). Neonatal nursing assessment by functional health patterns. *Critical Care Nursing Clinics of North America. 4*(3), 471–480.

Rivara, F. P., Kamisuka, M.D., & Quan, L. (1988). Injuries to children younger than 1 year of age. *Pediatrics, 81*(1), 93–97.

Sears, W. (1993, December–January). A family is born. *Parenting,* 96–101.

Smith, L. F. (1986). New-parent teaching in the ambulatory care setting. *MCN: The American Journal of Maternal Child Nursing, 11*(4), 256–258.

Tortora, G. J., & Anagnostakos, N.P. (1987). *Principles of anatomy and physiology* (5th ed.). New York: Harper & Row.

Wright, J., Arnott, N. (1992). Your baby head to toe. *American Baby, 54*(1), 56–59.

Ziai, M., Clarke, T. A., & Merritt, T.A. (Eds.). (1984). *Assessment of the newborn: A guide for the practitioner.* Boston: Little, Brown.

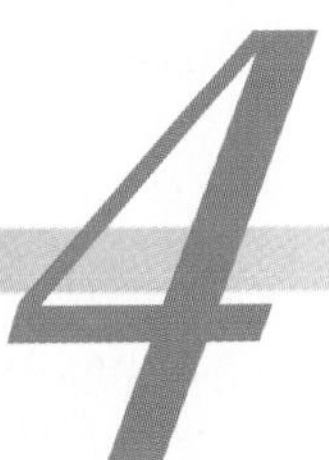

The Infant

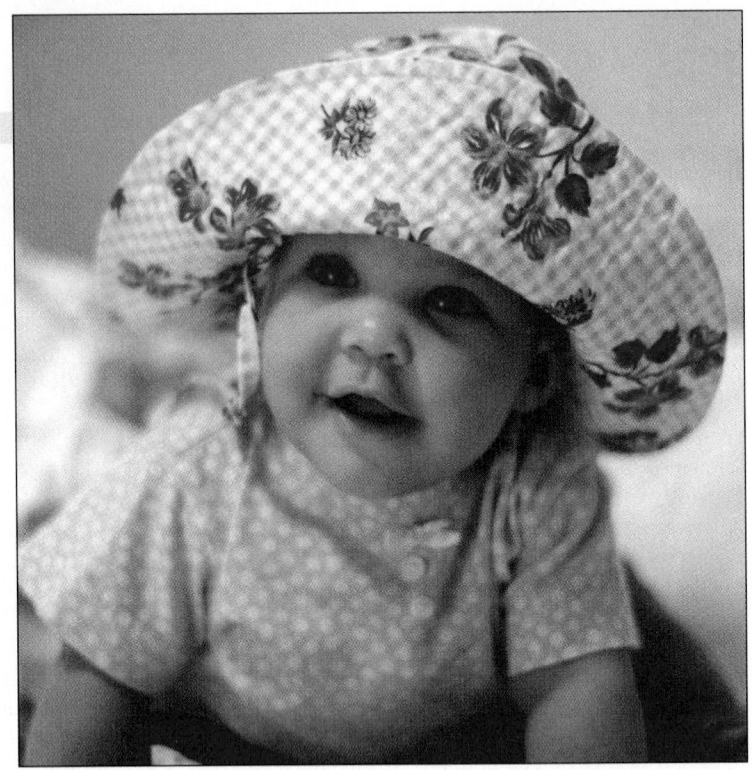

CHAPTER OVERVIEW

LEARNING OBJECTIVES

After studying this chapter, you should be able to:

- Describe the physiologic changes that occur during infancy
- Describe the motor, psychosocial, language, and cognitive development of the infant.
- Discuss common problems of infancy, such as separation anxiety, sleep, and irritability.
- Discuss the importance of immunizations, recommended immunization schedules, contraindications, and nursing care for the child receiving immunizations.
- Provide parents with anticipatory guidance for common concerns during infancy, such as sleep problems, introduction of foods, accident prevention, and dental care.

KEY TERMS

egocentrism: complete absorption with self; an inability to understand that others have a different point of view

mistrust: the negative resolution of the first developmental task according to Erikson's theory resulting in acute emotional tension and behavioral signs of unmet needs.

object permanence: the realization that objects continue to exist even though they are out of sight

parent/infant attachment: a sense of belonging to or connection with a parent and infant

pincer grasp: use of index finger and thumb to grip objects

sensorimotor stage: Piaget's first stage of cognitive development in which the infant and young toddler use mainly senses and movement to begin to understand and control their environment

stranger anxiety: the ability of an infant to distinguish between caregivers and others, to prefer parents over other caregivers, and to become distressed when separation occurs

trust: the basic emotion established during infancy as a result of satisfying interactions between child and caregiver that provides the foundation upon which a healthy personality is built

During no other time after birth does a human being grow and change as dramatically as during infancy. Between the ages of 1 month and 1 year, the infancy period, a child grows and develops from a tiny bundle of physiologic needs to a dynamo capable of locomotion and language, and ready to embark on the adventures of the toddler years.

Even though historically adults considered infants unable to do much more than eat and sleep, it is now well documented that even young infants can organize their experiences in meaningful ways and adapt to changes in the environment. There is evidence that they form strong bonds with their caregivers, communicate their needs and wants, and interact socially. By the end of the first year of life, infants can move about on their own, elicit responses from adults, communicate through the use of rudimentary language, and solve simple problems.

Infancy is characterized by the need to establish harmony between the self and the world. To achieve this harmony, the infant needs food, warmth, comfort, oral satisfaction, environmental stimulation, and opportunities for self-exploration and expression. Competent caregivers satisfy the needs of the helpless infant, providing a warm, nurturing relationship so that the infant experiences a sense of trust in the world and in herself. These challenges make infancy an exciting, yet demanding, period for both child and parents.

Nurses play an important role in the health promotion and maintenance of infants. Providing parents with information about immunization, feeding, sleep, and other common concerns is an important nursing responsibility. Nurses are in a good position to offer anticipatory guidance about injury prevention based on the infant's development and are instrumental in teaching parents how to make the infant's environment safe. Nurses can help parents to understand their infant's needs. By helping parents to identify their infant's personality or temperament characteristics and find the best ways to interact with them, nurses can help to strengthen the bond between parents and infants.

GROWTH AND DEVELOPMENT OF THE INFANT

Table 4–1 summarizes the growth and development of the infant.

Physical Growth and Development

Growth is an excellent indicator of overall health during infancy. Although growth rates are variable, infants usually double their birth weight by 6 months and triple it by 1 year of age. During the first 6 months, the average weight gain is 2.2 lb (1 kg) per month. Throughout the next 6 months, weight increase is approximately 1 lb (0.45 kg) per month. Weight gain in formula-fed infants is slightly greater than in breastfed infants.

During the first 6 months, infants increase their birth length approximately 1 inch (2.54 cm) per month, slowing to 0.5 inches (1.27 cm) per month over the next 6 months. By 1 year of age, most infants have increased their birth length by 50%.

The head circumference growth rate during the first year is slightly less than 0.5 inches per month. Usually, the

TABLE 4–1 *Summary of Growth and Development: The Infant*

PHYSICAL	MOTOR	PSYCHOSOCIAL	SENSORY/COGNITIVE	LANGUAGE/COMMUNICATION
1–3 Months Fast growth; upper limbs and head grow faster; posterior fontanelle closes; obligate nose breather. Primitive reflexes fading (3 months)	Gross: Can get hand to mouth. Can lift head off bed from prone position. Head lag present when pulled to sitting position. Fine: (1 month) Immediately drops object placed in hand. Fists usually clenched (grasp reflex). (2 months) Holds objects momentarily. Hands often open (grasp reflex fading). (3 months) Holds objects placed in hands. Hands open (grasp reflex absent).	Erikson's stage of trust versus mistrust. Learns that the world is good and "I am good." This stage is the foundation for other stages. Child is entirely dependent on mother and other caregivers. Needs should be met in a timely fashion. Touch is important.	Piaget's sensorimotor stage. Follows small moving objects. Shows active interest in face. Vision 20/100. Behavior is dominated by reflexes. Expects feedings at specific routine times.	Smiles. Sets up a reciprocal interactive cycle. Crying becomes differentiated. Cooing begins at 3 months. Responds to voice.
4–5 Months Can breathe when nose is obstructed; growth rate declines. Drooling begins. Moro, tonic neck, and rooting reflexes have disappeared.	Gross: Plays with feet. Puts foot in mouth. Bears weight when held in a standing position. Turns from abdomen to back. Fine: Begins reaching and grasping with palm. Hits at object, misses.	Mouth is a sensory organ used to explore the environment. Attachment is an ongoing process throughout infancy. Has increased interest in mother; shows trust; knows mother. Shows emotions of fear and anger (psychosocial, 4–5 months).	Vision 20/80. Begins to play with objects. Recognizes familiar faces. Turns head to locate sounds. Shows anticipation and excitement. Memory span is 5–7 minutes. Plays with favorite toys.	Crying becomes differentiated. Babbling is common. Begins consonant sounds: H, N, G, K, G, P, B (4 months). Makes vowel sounds: ee, ah, ooh (5 months).
6–7 Months Birth weight doubles; tooth eruption begins; chewing and biting occur; maternal iron stores are depleted.	Gross: Sits, leaning forward on both hands; when supine, lifts head off table. Turns from back to abdomen. Fine: Transfers objects from one hand to another. Picks up object well. Holds bottle well. Reaches with one arm.	Smiles at self in mirror. Plays peek-a-boo. Begins to show stranger anxiety.	Can fixate on small objects. Adjusts posture to see. Responds to name. Beginning sense of object permanence. Recognizes mother in other clothes, places. Is alert for $1\frac{1}{2}$–2 hours.	Produces vowel sounds and chained syllables. Begins to imitate sounds. Belly laughs. Babbles (one syllable) with pleasure. Calls for help. "Talks" to toys and image in mirror.

8–9 Months Continues to gain weight, length. Patterns of bladder and bowel elimination begin to become regular.	Gross: Sits steadily unsupported. Can crawl and pull up. Fine: Pincer grasp develops. Reaches for toys. Rakes for objects. Releases objects.	Stranger anxiety is at its height. Separation anxiety is increasing. Follows mother around the house.	Beginning development of depth perception. Object permanence continues to develop. Uses hands to learn concepts of in and out.	Stringing of vowels and consonants together begins. First few words begin to have meaning (Mama, Daddy, bye-bye, baby). Begins to understand and obey simple commands, such as "Wave bye-bye." Responds to "No!" Shouts for attention.
10–12 Months Triples birth weight; birth length increases by 50% (12 months). Head and chest circumference equal. Babinski reflex disappears.	Gross: Can walk with one hand held, but crawls to get places quickly. Fine: Releases hold on cup. Finger feeds self (10 months). Feeds self with spoon (12 months). Holds crayon to mark on paper. Pincer grasp is complete (12 months).	Has mood changes. Quiets self. Is quieted by music. Tenderly cuddles toy.	Vision 20/40. Searches for hidden toy. Explores boxes, inserts objects in container. Symbol recognition is developing (enjoys books).	Can say two or more words. Says "Mama or Dada" specifically. Waves bye-bye. Begins to differentiate between words. Enjoys jabbering. Vocalization decreases when walking. Knows own name.

posterior fontanelle closes by 6 to 8 weeks of age, whereas the larger anterior fontanelle can remain open until 18 months. Head circumference and fontanelle measurements indicate brain growth and are obtained, along with height and weight, at each well-baby visit. Chapter 11 discusses growth rate monitoring throughout infancy.

Maturation of Body Systems

In addition to height and weight, organ systems grow and mature rapidly in the infant. Even though body systems are developing rapidly, the infant's organs are different from those of older children and adults in both structure and function. These differences place the infant at risk for problems that might not be expected in older individuals. Knowledge of these differences provides the nurse with important rationale on which to base anticipatory guidance and specific nursing interventions.

Neurologic System. Brain growth and differentiation occurs rapidly during the first year of life and is dependent on nutrition and function of the other organ systems. At birth, the brain accounts for approximately 10% to 12% of body weight. By 1 year of age, the brain has doubled its weight, with two major growth spurts occurring between 15 and 20 weeks of age and another between 30 weeks and 1 year of age (Sinclair, 1989; Porth, 1994). Increases in the number of synapses and expanded myelination of nerves contribute to maturation of the neurologic system during infancy. Primitive reflexes disappear as the cerebral cortex thickens and motor areas of the brain continue to develop, proceeding in a cephalocaudal pattern, arms first, then legs.

Respiratory System. In the first year of life, the lungs increase to three times their weight and six times their volume at birth. In the newborn, alveoli number approximately 20 million, increasing to the adult number of 300 million by age 8 years. During infancy, the trachea remains small, supported only by soft cartilage.

> The diameter and length of the trachea, bronchi, and bronchiolus increase with age; however, these tiny, collapsible air passages leave infants vulnerable to respiratory difficulties caused by infection or foreign bodies (Burgess & Chernick, 1982).

The eustachian tube is short and relatively horizontal, placing the infant at risk for middle-ear infections.

Cardiovascular System. The cardiovascular system undergoes dramatic changes in the transition from fetal to extrauterine circulation. Fetal shunts close, and pulmonary circulation increases drastically (see Chapter 3). During infancy, the heart doubles in size and weight, the heart rate gradually slows, and blood pressure increases (Porth, 1994).

Immune System. Transplacental transfer of maternal antibodies supplements the infant's weak response to infection until approximately 3 to 4 months of age. Although the infant begins to produce immunoglobulins (Ig) soon after birth, by 1 year of age, the infant has only approximately 60% of the adult IgG level, 75% of the adult IgM level, and 20% of the adult IgA level. Breast milk transmits additional IgA protection. The activity of T lymphocytes also increases after birth.

> Even though the immune system matures during infancy, maximum protection against infection is not offered until early childhood. This immaturity places the infant at risk for infection (Korones, 1986).

Gastrointestinal System. The stomach capacity of a newborn is only approximately 30 ml, but with feedings, the capacity increases rapidly to approximately 200 ml at 1 year of age. In the gastrointestinal system, enzymes needed for the digestion and absorption of proteins, fats, and carbohydrates mature and increase in concentration. Although the newborn's gastrointestinal system is capable of digesting protein and lactase, the ability to digest and absorb fat does not reach adult levels until approximately 6 to 9 months of age. The infant usually is not ready to digest complex carbohydrates, such as those found in cereal, until at least age 3 to 4 months (Pipes & Trahms, 1993).

Renal System. Kidney mass increases threefold during the first year of life. Although the glomeruli enlarge considerably during the first few months of life, the glomerular filtration rate remains low. Thus, the kidney is not effective as a filtration organ nor is it efficient in concentrating urine until after the first year of life.

> Because of the functional immaturity of the renal system, the infant is at great risk for fluid and electrolyte imbalance.

Motor Development

During the first few months after birth, muscle growth and weight gain allow for increased control of reflexes and more purposeful movement (see Chapter 3). At 1 month, movement occurs in a random fashion, with the fists tightly clenched. Because the neck musculature is weak and the head is large, the infant can lift her head only briefly. By 2 to 3 months, the infant can lift her head 90° from a prone position and can hold it steadily erect in a sitting position. During this time, active grasping gradually replaces reflexive grasping and increases in frequency as eye–hand coordination improves. (See pages 80–83.)

The Moro, tonic neck, and rooting reflexes disappear at approximately 3 to 4 months. These primitive reflexes, which are controlled by the midbrain, probably disappear because they are suppressed by growing cortical layers. Head control steadily increases during the third month. By the fourth month, the infant's head remains in a straight line with the body when he is pulled to a sitting position. Most infants play with their feet by 4–5 months, drawing them up to suck on their toes.

During the fifth and sixth months, motor development accelerates rapidly. Infants of this age readily reach for and grasp objects. They can bear weight when held in a standing position and can turn from abdomen to back. By 5 months, some infants rock back and forth as a precursor to crawling.

Six-month-old infants can sit alone, leaning forward on their hands. This ability provides them with a wider view of the world and creates new ways to play. An infant of this age can roll from back to abdomen and can raise his head from the table when supine. He transfers objects from one hand to another. In addition, he can grab objects, even small ones, and insert them in his mouth with lightning speed.

At 6 to 9 months, the infant begins to explore the world by crawling. By 9 months, most infants have enough muscle strength and coordination to pull themselves up and cruise around furniture. These new methods of mobility enable the infant to follow her mother or caregiver around the house.

By 6 to 7 months, the infant can transfer objects from one hand to another and becomes increasingly adept at pointing to make her demands known. The 6-month-old grasps objects with all of her fingers in a raking motion, but the 9-month-old uses his thumb and forefinger in a fine motor skill called the **pincer grasp.** This grasp provides the infant with a useful, yet potentially dangerous ability to grab, hold, and insert tiny objects into her mouth.

The 9-month-old infant can wave bye-bye or clap his hands together. He can pick up an object, but has difficulty releasing it on request. By 1 year of age, he can extend an object and release it into an offered hand. Most 1-year-old children can balance well enough to walk when holding another person's hand. However, they often resort to crawling as a more rapid and efficient way to move about.

An increased ability to move about, reach objects, and explore their world places infants at great risk for accidents and injury.

Nurses should provide information to parents about how quickly infant motor skills develop. Specific suggestions, such as covering electric sockets with protective devices, using gates to restrict infant movement from room to room, and storing poisonous household products in high cupboards, can be offered to make the home environment safer. Nurses should also remind parents that mobile infants need vigilant supervision to prevent falls and other injuries.

> Parents need anticipatory guidance about ways to prevent accidents by "baby-proofing" their homes before each motor development milestone is reached: "It is best to begin 'baby-proofing' your home even before your infant begins to crawl. If you wait, she may fall or get burned or even drink something poisonous before you are able to make your home safe for her."

Cognitive Development

Many factors contribute to the way in which infants learn about their world. Besides innate intellectual aptitude and motivation, the infant's sensory capabilities, neuromuscular control, and perceptual skills all affect how his cognitive processes unfold during infancy and throughout life. In addition, variables such as the quality and quantity of parental interaction and environmental stimulation contribute to cognitive development.

Cognitive development during the first 2 years of life begins with a profound state of egocentrism. **Egocentrism** is the child's complete absorption with herself and the inability to view the world from anyone else's vantage point. As an infant's cognitive capacities expand, she becomes increasingly aware of the outside world and her separateness from it. Gradually, with maturation and experience, she becomes capable of differentiating herself from others and her surroundings.

According to Piaget's theory, cognitive development occurs in stages or periods (see Chapter 2). Infancy is included in the **sensorimotor stage** (birth to 2 years), during which the infant experiences the world through his senses and his attempts to control the environment. Learning activities progress from simple reflex behavior to trial-and-error experiments.

During the first month of life, infants are in the first substage, reflex activity, of the sensorimotor period. In this substage, behavior such as grasping, sucking, or looking is dominated by reflexes. Piaget believed that infants organize their activity, survive, and adapt to their world with the use of reflexes.

Primary circular reactions is the second substage, occurring from age 1 to 4 months. During this substage, reflexes become more organized and new schema are acquired, usually centering around the infant's body. Sensual activities, such as sucking and kicking, become less reflexive and more controlled, and are repeated because of the stimulation they provide. The baby also begins to recognize objects, especially those that bring pleasure, such as the breast or bottle.

During the third substage, secondary circular reactions, the infant performs actions that are more oriented toward the world outside his own body. The 4- to 8-month-old infant in this substage begins to play with objects in the external environment, such as a rattle or stuffed toy. The infant's actions are labeled as secondary because they are intentional (repeated because of the

Text continued on page 84

The First Year: Growth and Development Milestones

INTRODUCTION

During the first year after birth, the infant's development is dramatic as he grows toward independence. Knowledge of developmental milestones helps caregivers determine whether the baby is growing and maturing as expected. One should remember that these markers are averages, and that healthy infants often vary. Some infants reach each milestone earlier than average, while other normal infants reach each milestone later than most. Knowledge of normal growth and development helps the nurse promote the safety of children. Parents should be taught to prepare for their child's safety before she reaches each milestone.

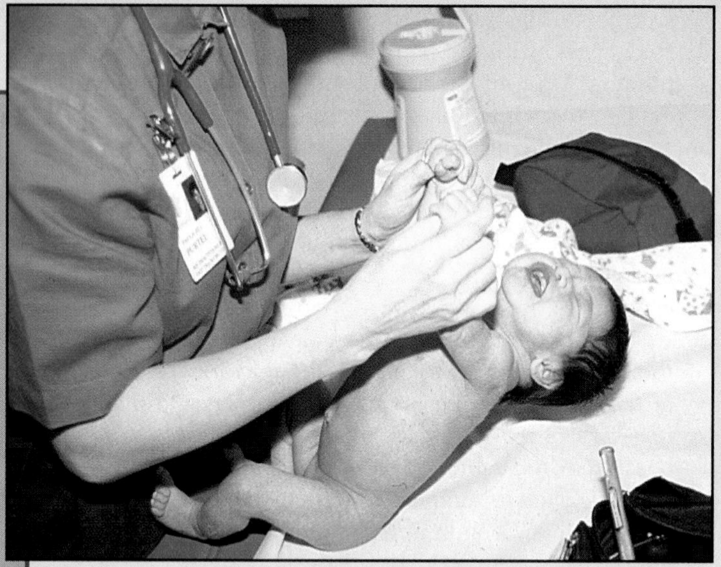

This 18-day-old infant demonstrates substantial head lag as the nurse lifts her trunk from the examining table. Weak neck muscles, combined with a large head, limit her ability to keep her head aligned with her spine as she is pulled toward a sitting position.

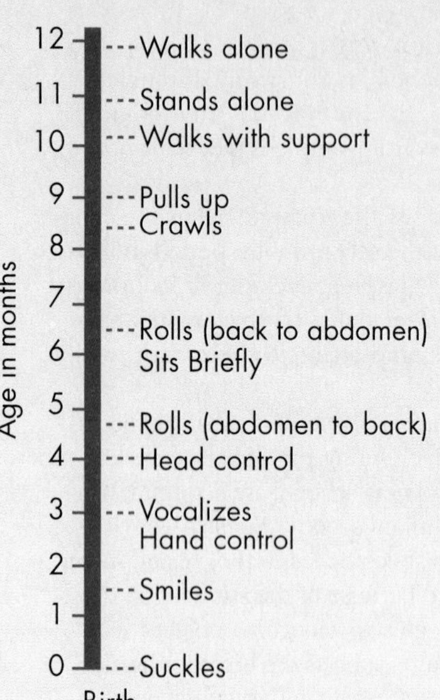

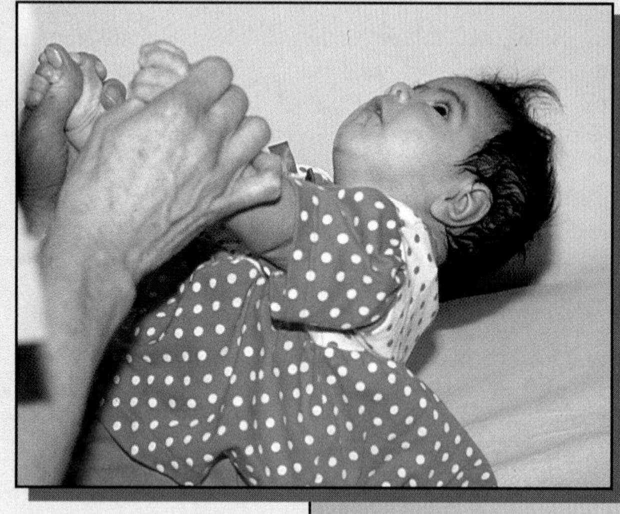

By 2 months, the infant has much less head lag as her neck muscles become stronger and better able to support her head.

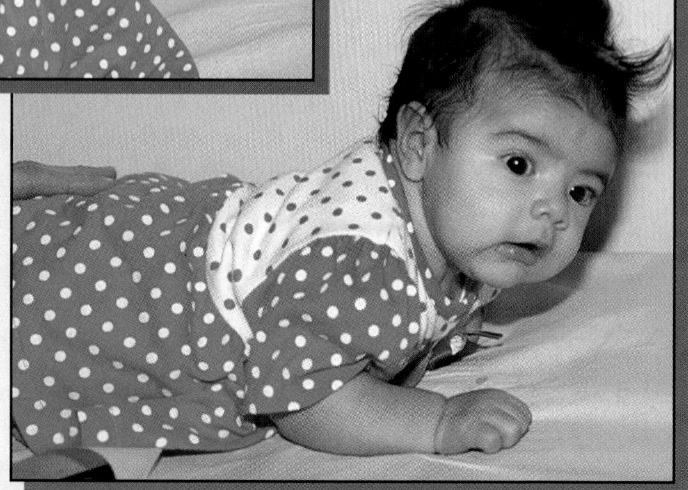

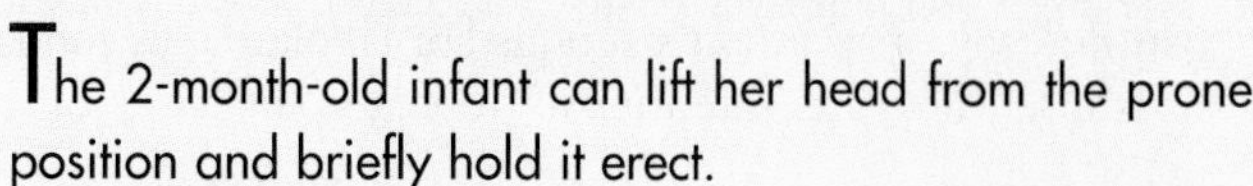

The 2-month-old infant can lift her head from the prone position and briefly hold it erect.

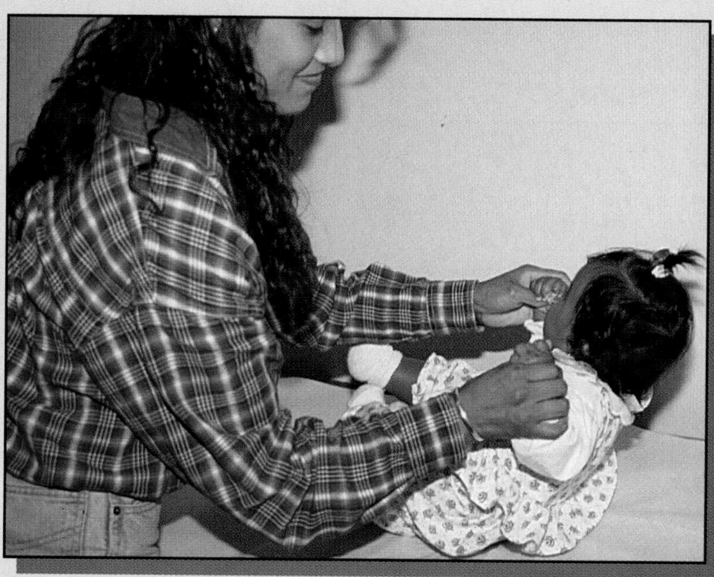

Head control steadily increases so that by 4 months, this infant keeps her head in a straight line as her mother pulls her to a sitting position.

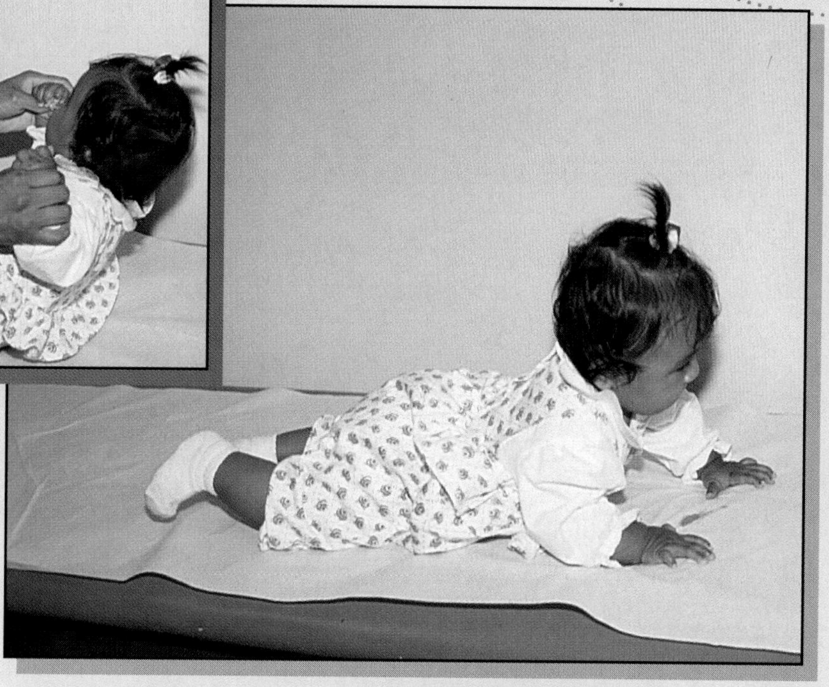

The 4-month-old infant can easily lift her head from a prone position and hold it steadily erect.

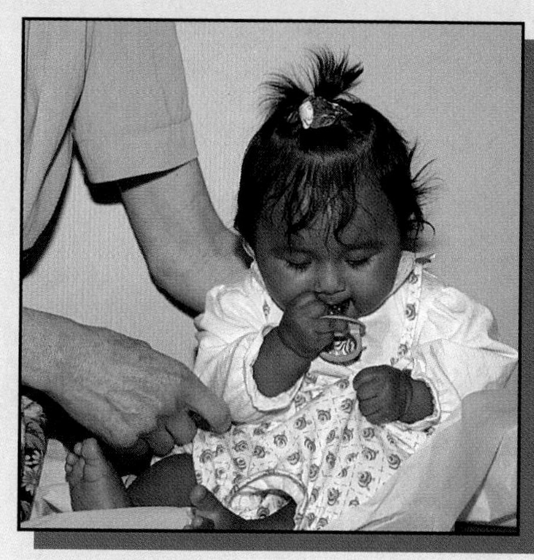

By 4 months, the infant can purposefully grasp objects with the palms of her hands.

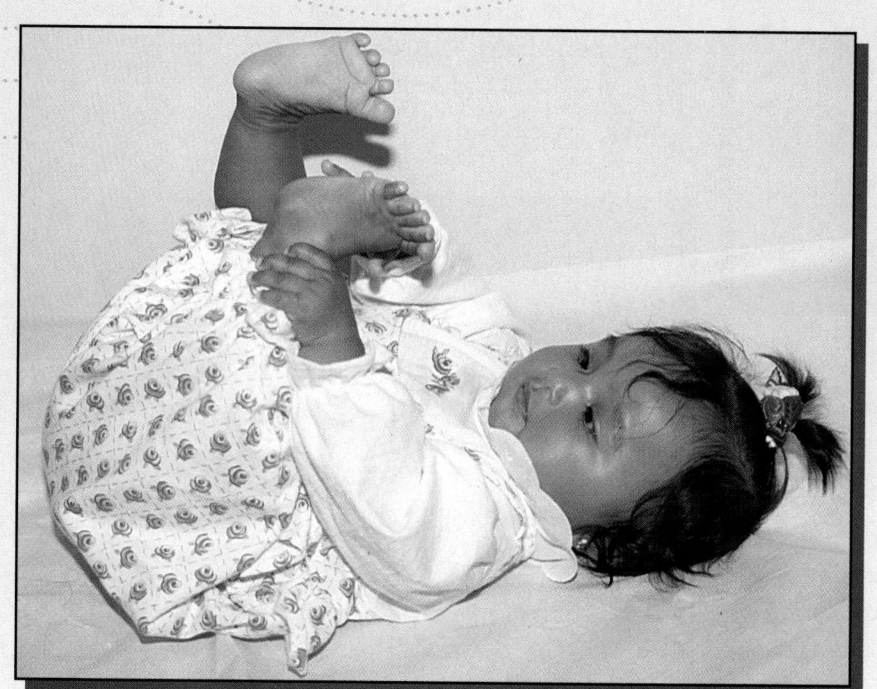

The 4-month-old infant takes pleasure in exploring her own body. She begins playing with her feet, and often puts her toes in her mouth.

CONTINUED

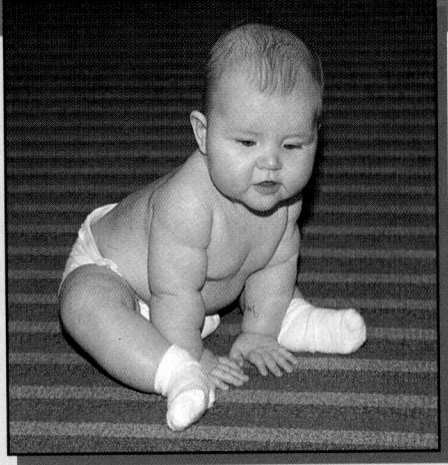

At 6 months, the infant can sit briefly if she leans forward on both hands for support.

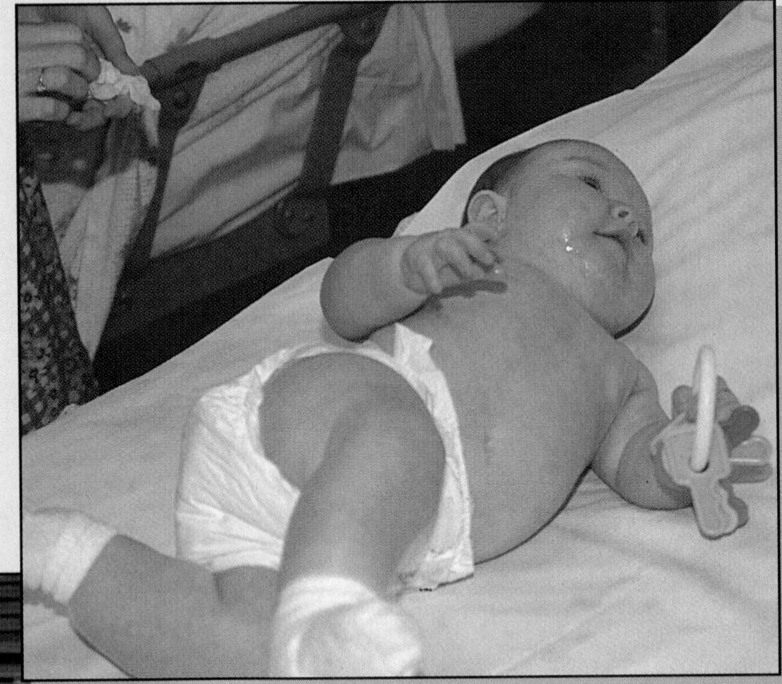

This 6-month-old infant can easily turn from her abdomen onto her back. An adult must be near if the infant of this age is on an elevated surface, such as an examining table or diaper-changing table. The nurse should teach parents about safety measures *before* their child reaches each developmental milestone to reduce the risk of accidents.

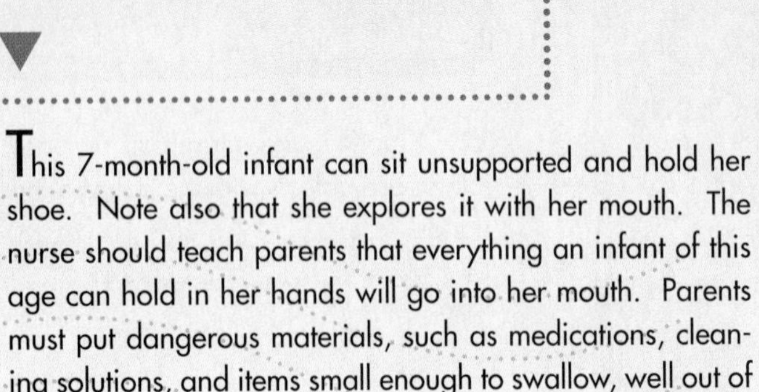

This 7-month-old infant can sit unsupported and hold her shoe. Note also that she explores it with her mouth. The nurse should teach parents that everything an infant of this age can hold in her hands will go into her mouth. Parents must put dangerous materials, such as medications, cleaning solutions, and items small enough to swallow, well out of reach.

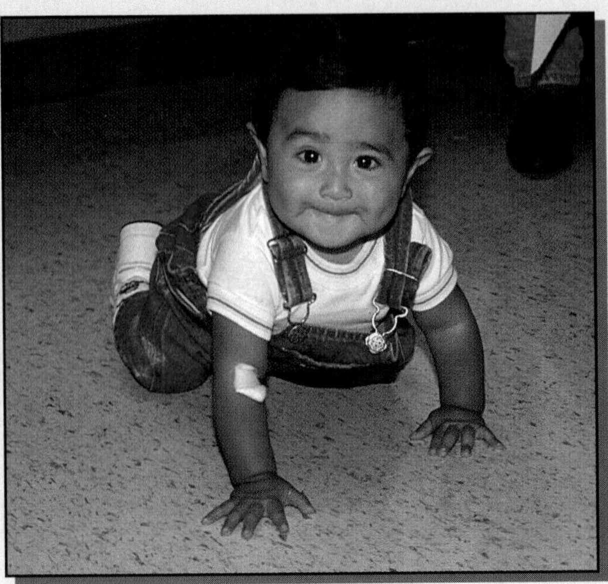

The 9-month-old infant crawls quickly, keeping his belly off the floor.

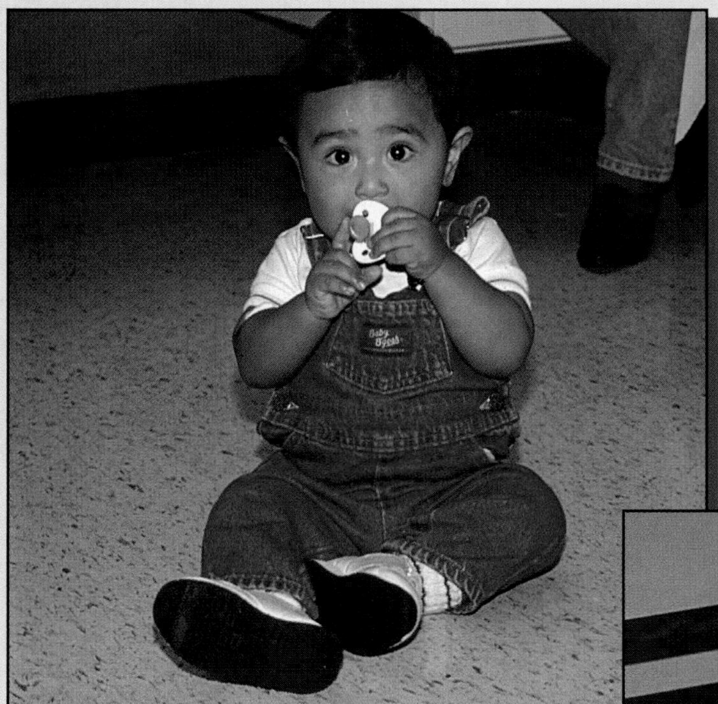

At 9 months, the infant can move easily from a crawling to a sitting position and can sit steadily with no support. He also begins grasping objects with the finer pincer grasp rather than the palmar grasp. If a parent tries to hide something, such as this pacifier, he will not forget the object and will search for it.

At 1 year, the infant can pull to a standing position. On a slick, hard floor such as this, an adult should be near to catch him if he slips backward while trying to pull up.

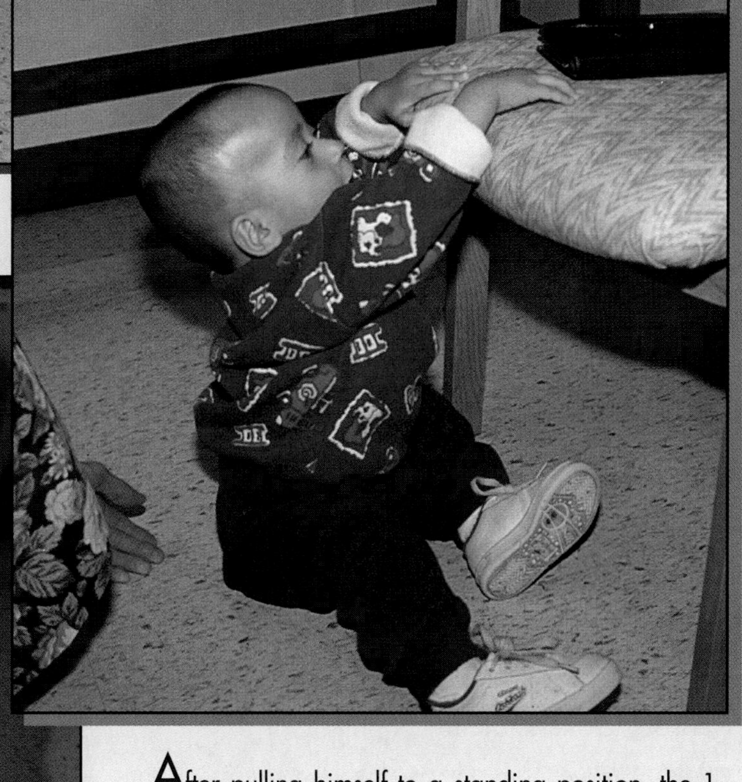

After pulling himself to a standing position, the 1-year-old can stand alone.

CONCLUSION

After the first year, motor development is less dramatic. Nevertheless, nurses must prepare parents for new milestones to promote the child's safety and normal development.

Photos courtesy of Dallas County Hospital District Community Oriented Primary Care Clinic and University of Texas at Arlington School of Nursing.

response that is elicited). For example, a baby in this substage intentionally shakes a rattle to hear the sound.

By age 8 to 12 months, infants in the fourth substage, coordination of secondary schemata, begin to relate to objects as if they realize that the objects exist even when they are out of sight. This awareness is referred to as **object permanence** and is illustrated by a 9-month-old infant seeking a toy after it is hidden under a pillow. In contrast, a 6-month-old can follow the path of a toy that is dropped in front of him; however, he will not look for the dropped toy nor protest its disappearance until he is older and has developed the concept of object permanence.

Infants in this substage solve problems differently than in earlier substages. Rather than randomly selecting approaches to problems, they choose actions that were successful in the past. This tendency suggests that they remember and can perform some mental processing. They seem to be able to identify simple causal relationships, and they show definite intentionality. For example, when an 11-month-old child sees a toy that is beyond reach, he uses the blanket that it is resting on to pull it toward him (Piaget, 1952; Flavell, 1964).

Cognitive development in the infant parallels motor development. It appears that motor activity is necessary for cognitive development and that cognitive development is based on interaction with the environment, not simply maturation. Infancy is when the child lays the foundation for later cognitive functioning. Nurses can promote the cognitive development of infants by encouraging parents to interact with their infants and provide them with novel, interesting stimuli. At the same time, parents should maintain familiar, routine experiences through which the infant can develop a sense of security about the world. Within this type of environment, infants will thrive and learn.

Sensory Development

Vision. The size of the eye at birth is approximately one-half to three-quarters of the adult size. Growth of the eye, including the internal structures, is rapid during the first year. As the infant grows and becomes more interested in the environment, his eyes remain open for longer periods. He shows a preference for familiar faces and is increasingly able to fixate on objects. Visual acuity is estimated at approximately 20/100 at birth, but improves rapidly during infancy and toddlerhood to 20/40 to 20/30 between 2 and 3 years of age. Infants show a preference for high-contrast colors, such as black and white and primary colors. Pastel colors are not easily distinguished until about 6 months of age.

Young infants may lack coordination of eye movements and extraocular muscle alignment, but should achieve proper coordination by age 4 to 6 months.

> Persistent lack of eye muscle control beyond the age of 4 to 6 months needs further evaluation.

Depth perception appears to begin at approximately 7 to 9 months and contributes to the infant's new ability to move about independently.

Hearing. Hearing seems to be relatively acute, even at birth, as evidenced by reflexive generalized reactions to noise. With myelination of the auditory nerve tracts during the first year, responses to sound become increasingly more specialized. By 4 months, the infant should turn her eyes and head toward a sound coming from behind, and by 10 months, the infant should respond to the sound of her name.

Language Development

The acquisition of language has its roots in infancy as the child becomes increasingly intrigued with sound, begins to realize that words have meaning, and eventually uses simple sounds to communicate. Although young infants probably understand tones and inflections of voice rather than words themselves, it is not long before repetition and practice of sounds enables them to understand and communicate with words. Infants can understand more than they can express.

The social smile develops early in the infant, usually by 3 to 5 weeks of age (Fig. 4–1). This powerful communication tool helps to foster attachment and demonstrates that the infant can differentiate between persons and objects within the environment.

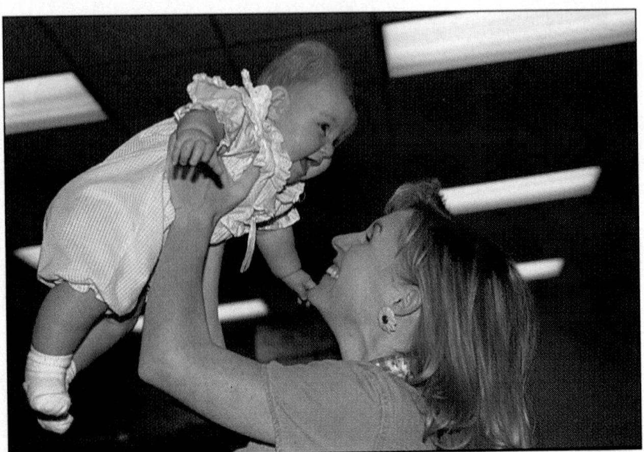

Figure 4–1
The 6-month-old infant delightedly responds to her mother with a true social smile. Such interactive responses between parent and child promote communication and emotional development.

The infant who does not display a social smile by the age of 8 to 12 weeks needs further evaluation and close follow-up because of the possibility of developmental delay.

During infancy, connections form within the central nervous system, providing fine motor control of the numerous muscles required for speech. Maturation of the mouth, jaw, and larynx; bone growth; and development of the face help to prepare the infant to speak (Netsell, 1980).

Vocalization does not appear to be reflexive, but rather a relatively high-level activity similar to conversation. Parents usually elicit vocalization in infants better than other adults can. Infants vocalize in response to adult voices (Oller, 1980).

Although there is great variability, most children begin to make nonmeaningful sounds, such as "ma," "da," or "ah," by 4 to 6 months. The sounds become more meaningful and specific by 9 to 15 months, and by age 1 year, the child usually has a vocabulary of several words, such as "mama," "dada," and "bye-bye" (Castiglia, 1987). Infants who have older siblings or are raised in verbally rich environments sometimes meet these developmental milestones earlier than other infants. On the other hand, infants with family members who discourage infant verbalization sometimes exhibit delayed speech patterns.

See the accompanying box for a summary of developmental milestones in infant language and communication.

Language and Communication: Developmental Milestones in Infancy

1–3 MONTHS

Reflexive smile at first, then smile becomes more voluntary; sets up a reciprocal smiling cycle with parent. Cooing.

3–4 MONTHS

Crying becomes more differentiated. Babbling is common.

4–6 MONTHS

Plays with sound, repeating sounds to self. Can identify mother's voice. May squeal in excitement.

6–8 MONTHS

Single consonant babbling occurs. Increasing interest in sound.

8–9 MONTHS

Stringing of vowels and consonants together begins. First few words begin to have meaning (Mama, Daddy, bye-bye, baby). Begins to understand and obey simple commands such as "Wave bye-bye."

9–12 MONTHS

Some children begin to use simple words on their own, such as "Mama, Dada, go." Gestures are used to communicate.

Psychosocial Development

Most experts agree that infancy is a crucial period during which the child develops the foundation of his personality and sense of self. According to Erik Erikson's theory of psychosocial development (1963), the infant struggles to establish a sense of basic **trust** rather than a sense of basic **mistrust** in his world, his caregivers, and himself. If provided with consistent, satisfying experiences delivered in a timely manner, the infant comes to rely on the fact that his needs will be met and that, in turn, he will be able to tolerate some degree of frustration and discomfort until his needs are met. This sense of confidence is an early form of trust and provides the foundation for a healthy personality.

On the other hand, if the child's needs are ignored or met in a consistently haphazard, inadequate manner, the infant has no reason to believe that his needs will be met or that his environment is a safe, secure place. According to Erikson, without consistent satisfaction of needs, the individual develops a basic sense of suspicion or mistrust.

Parallel to this viewpoint is Freudian theory, which regards infancy as the oral stage. The mouth is the major focus of this stage. Observation of an infant for a few minutes shows that most of her behavior centers around her mouth. Sensory stimulation and pleasure as well as nourishment are experienced through the infant's mouth. Sucking is an adaptive behavior that provides comfort and satisfaction while enabling the infant to experience and explore his world. Later in infancy, as teething progresses, the mouth becomes an effective tool for aggressive behavior (see Chapter 2).

Parent–Infant Attachment. One of the most important aspects of infant psychosocial development is parent–infant attachment. Attachment is a sense of belonging to or a connection with each other. This significant bond between infant and parent is critical to normal development and even survival. Initiated immediately after birth, attachment is strengthened by many mutually satisfying interactions between the parents and the infant throughout the first months of life.

For example, noisy distress in the infant signals a need, such as hunger. The parent responds by providing food. In turn, the infant responds by quieting and accepting nourishment. Pleasure is derived by the infant, who has his hunger satiated, and by the parent, who is able to successfully care for the child. A basic reciprocal cycle is set in motion in which parents learn to regulate infant feeding, sleep, and activity through a series of interactions. These interactions include rocking, touching, talking, smiling, and singing. The infant responds by quieting, eating, watching, smiling, or sleeping.

Conversely, parents who chronically are unable or unwilling to meet the dependency needs of their infant foster insecurity and dissatisfaction in their infants. A cycle of dissatisfaction is established in which parents become frustrated as caregivers and have further difficulty providing for the infant's needs.

It is well documented that the child, even as a newborn, is an active participant in interactions with parents and the process of attachment (Thomas & Chess, 1977). From birth, temperament influences the way the child interacts with parents and in turn the way parents interact with the child (see Chapter 16).

If a parent can adapt to the infant, meet his needs, and provide nurturance, attachment is secure. Psychosocial development can proceed based on a strong foundation of attachment. On the other hand, if a parent's personality and ability to cope with infant care do not match the infant's needs, the relationship is considered at risk.

Although the establishment of trust depends heavily on the quality of the maternal interaction, the infant also needs consistent, satisfying social interactions within a family structure. Family routines can help to provide this consistency. Touch is an important tool that can be used by all family members to convey a sense of caring.

Stranger Anxiety. Another important aspect of psychosocial development is stranger anxiety or separation anxiety. By 6 to 7 months, expanding cognitive capacities and strong feelings of attachment enable the infant to differentiate between caregivers and strangers and to act wary of the latter. The infant displays an obvious preference for parents over other caregivers and other unfamiliar people. Anxiety, demonstrated by crying, clinging, and turning away from the stranger, is manifested when separation occurs. This behavior peaks at approximately 7 to 9 months and again during toddlerhood, when separation may be difficult (see Chapter 4).

Although stressful for parents, stranger anxiety is a normal sign of healthy attachment and occurs because of cognitive development (**object permanence**). Nurses can reassure parents that although the infant seems distressed, no harm is done by leaving him for short periods. Separations should be accomplished swiftly, yet with care, love, and emphasis on the parent's return.

HEALTH PROMOTION FOR THE INFANT AND FAMILY

Parents, particularly new parents, often need guidance in caring for their infant. Nurses can provide valuable information about health promotion of the infant. Specific guidance about everyday concerns, such as sleep, crying, and feeding, can be offered as well as anticipatory guidance about injury prevention. An important nursing responsibility is to provide parents with information about immunizations and dental care. Nurses can offer support to new parents by identifying strategies for coping with the first few months with an infant. Table 4–2 at the end of this chapter presents an overview of health screening, health maintenance, and anticipatory guidance activities for infants.

Sleep, Rest, and Crying

Newborns may sleep as much as 17 to 20 hours per day. Sleep patterns vary widely, with some infants sleeping only 2 to 3 hours at a time. At approximately 3 to 4 months of age, most infants begin to sleep for longer periods during the night, although some children do not sleep through the night consistently until the second year.

Often one of the most difficult tasks for new parents is the regulation of their infant's sleep–wake cycles. Parents need anticipatory guidance about what to expect regarding sleep, rest, and crying. Nurses can suggest that parents console their infant when he cries by holding him, talking softly, or humming. Also gently stroking his head, back, and arms may be soothing. Infant massage techniques and simply "centering" are easily accomplished by positioning the infant's arms and legs toward the midline of the body. Swaddling a new infant is a consoling technique that assists the infant in centering. Some infants respond readily to attempts to comfort them, sleep a great deal, and fit easily into their family's lifestyle.

On the other hand, some infants cry more readily and for longer periods and spend more time in a fretful, restless state than others. These infants often experience more colic symptoms and sleep problems. This irritability may be caused by health problems such as feeding difficulties, infection, or allergies, but often, no clear cause emerges.

The Family's Need for Support. During the first few months after the addition of a new baby, demanding work schedules, lack of recovery time from childbirth, the needs of other family members, physical exhaustion, and sleep deprivation can combine with a fretful infant to create stressful situations for the entire family. Sometimes infant temperament and parental coping styles are not compatible. These families require an extended adjustment period and extra support and help from others.

New parents often feel anxious and guilty about not being able to console their infant. They may also worry about the child's health and feel resentful or frustrated about the disruption of the family. Infants sense anxiety and frustration in their parents and respond by becoming more upset and irritable. A cycle of negative emotional responses between infant and parents can occur and set the stage for later parenting difficulties.

Nurses can intervene by meeting the parents' needs for support and understanding, helping to restore their emotional reserve, and providing strategies for coping with the first few months of infancy. Keefe and Froese-Fretz (1991) found that parents, especially mothers, need empathy, validation, support, and reassurance. As an empathetic listener, the nurse can help the mother to feel supported while gathering data to determine whether the problem requires medical follow-up. In validating the mother's feelings, the nurse recognizes that the infant's irritability is real, not imagined, and that the infant is a challenge to handle. The nurse can reassure the mother that the infant is healthy, normal, and gaining weight, and that the mother is competent in her nurturing role.

> *Nurse (to new mother):* "It's not easy being a new parent. Sometimes your baby cries and it's hard to know what he needs since he can't tell you with words. But he looks so strong and healthy. You're doing a good job as a new mother."

The emotional reserve of the parents can be restored through rest and pleasurable activities. Parents may need brief periods of relief from infant care responsibilities. Grandparents or other family members may be able to provide the parents with an evening out or a night of uninterrupted sleep. This direct support can help to restore the parents' energy to cope with daily activities. In the study by Keefe and Froese-Fretz (1991), mothers who received support from significant family members or friends seemed less overwhelmed and stressed by the demands of infant care. Nurses intervene by helping parents to mobilize support systems.

Strategies for Soothing Infants. Specific strategies to diminish infant irritability include activities such as taking the baby for a car ride, carrying the infant in a front pack close to the parent's chest, or swinging the baby in an infant swing. Vertical positioning and constant motion, such as that obtained when walking with the baby carried over the shoulder, are sometimes helpful. The football carry position, with gentle patting on the back, can also be tried. Constant low-level noise, such as that provided by a hair dryer or clothes dryer, sometimes quiets fussy infants. Sometimes irritable infants need to be left alone to cry. If parents choose this strategy, they must be cautioned to limit the crying time to 15 to 20 minutes and to check the baby frequently.

Few interventions are consistently successful because infant responses may be variable. However, providing parents with strategies helps to decrease their anxiety and increase their feelings of control and competence. When parents' needs are met, they are increasingly calm and better able to deal with the demands of their irritable infants. As infants grow and develop, they are better able to regulate their sleep–wake cycles. Generally, during the third or fourth month of life, sleep problems and irritability improve.

Feeding and Nutrition

Because infancy is a period of rapid growth, nutritional needs are of special significance. During infancy, eating progresses from a principally reflex activity to relatively sophisticated, yet messy, attempts at self-feeding. Because the infant's gastrointestinal system continues to mature throughout the first year, changes in diet, introduction of new foods, and even upsets in routines can result in feeding problems. Parents often have many questions and concerns about nutrition. They are influenced by a variety of sources, including relatives and friends, who may not be aware of current scientific practices regarding infant feeding. The nurse must have a clear understanding of gastrointestinal maturation and knowledge about various infant formulas and foods to provide anticipatory guidance.

Families and cultures vary widely in food preferences and infant feeding practices. The nurse must remain cognizant of these differences when providing anticipatory guidance related to infant nutrition. Parents must be told that breast milk, formulas, and various combinations of semisolid and table foods provide adequate nourishment for their infants during the first year of life.

> It is generally recommended that breast milk or commercially prepared formulas provide the foundation of nutrition throughout infancy.

Whole milk can be introduced after 1 year of age, when the digestive tract is ready to process it and the chances of allergic responses are decreased. Generally, an infant should be permitted to establish his own feeding schedule and should be fed until he is satisfied. Normal growth patterns show that the child is ingesting adequate amounts of food.

Weaning. Weaning from the breast or bottle to a cup is a gradual process that is usually accomplished by 12 to 14 months of age, although some children continue to need a bottle at bedtime. The cup can be introduced gradually during meals while bottles are eliminated one by one during the day. Infants vary regarding their need for nonnutritive sucking. Pacifiers can be offered to babies who require increased opportunities to meet their sucking needs. If parents are concerned about their infant becoming attached to the pacifier, they should be instructed to begin weaning from the pacifier at 4 months of age because the sucking reflex naturally diminishes at this age.

Solid Foods. Introduction of solid foods should be delayed until age 4 to 6 months, when the gastrointestinal system has matured sufficiently to handle complex nutrients. Infants' suck reflex and tongue thrust reflex diminishes at around 4 months of age. Therefore, the introduction of solid foods should be delayed until that time. Usually, rice cereal is the first solid food offered because it rarely induces allergic reactions and it is a rich source of iron. Next, pureed fruits, vegetables, and meats can be introduced one at a time. When an infant can reach out, grasp food items, and place them in her mouth, finger foods may be offered (Pipes & Trahms, 1993). Other adult foods can be gradually introduced as tolerated.

Because of narrow air passages and occasional uncoordinated swallowing, infants are at risk for choking on food. The nurse should counsel parents to feed infants in an upright position and to avoid offering them foods that are easy to aspirate, such as raisins, nuts, hard candy, hot dogs, and popcorn. Parents should be instructed in the appropriate action to take if the infant chokes. (See Chapter 14 for a discussion of emergency procedures.)

For further discussion of infant nutrition, see Chapter 12.

Safety

It seems that the rapidly growing infant becomes mobile overnight. With newfound mobility comes the potential for accidents. As the infant's musculature strengthens and coordination improves, the infant has an insatiable desire to explore. Without the cognitive skills needed to differentiate danger from safety, the rolling, crawling, toddling infant is at great risk for accidents.

The most common causes of accidents in infancy are falls, aspiration, poisoning, burns, and motor vehicle accidents.

The nurse should counsel parents to protect the child against falls, never to leave the infant alone on a changing table or in an infant seat, and to anticipate increased mobility. They should keep all small objects that could be placed in the mouth, swallowed, or aspirated away from the baby, including toys and household items. This point is especially important for parents who have older children with toys that could be dangerous for infants. Baby-proofing the home before the infant begins to crawl is a must. Necessary steps include locking poisons in high cabinets, covering electric outlets, and removing poisonous plants. Hot water tanks should be set to deliver water that is no hotter than 120°F to help prevent scalds. Parents must also be reminded that infants must ride in federally approved car seats (see Chapter 13).

Immunization

The importance of childhood immunization against disease cannot be overemphasized. Infants are especially vulnerable to infectious disease because their immune systems are immature. Term newborns are protected from certain infections by transplacental passive immunity from their mothers. Breastfed infants receive additional immunoglobulins against many types of viruses and bacteria. However, transplacental immunity is effective only for approximately 3 months, and for a variety of reasons, many mothers choose not to breastfeed. In any case, this passive immunity does not cover all diseases, and infection in the infant can be devastating. Immunization offers protection that all infants need.

According to the United States Department of Health and Human Services, one of the national health objectives is that by the year 2000, at least 90% of all children will be immunized before their second birthday against diphtheria, pertussis, tetanus, poliomyelitis, measles, mumps, rubella, *Haemophilus influenzae* type b, and hepatitis B (American Public Health Association, 1990). Although there are many barriers to receiving immunizations and many misconceptions about their administration and safety, health professional groups continue to work toward meeting this objective. The American Academy of Pediatrics and the Centers for Disease Control and Prevention have made recommendations about the most effective way to administer immunizations (see Chapter 22).

Nurses play an important role in health promotion and disease prevention related to immunization. Nursing responsibilities include assessing current immunization status and recognizing contraindications to the receipt of vaccines. By working to remove barriers to the receipt of immunizations, providing effective tracking systems, and providing parent education about immunization, nurses can help to reduce the morbidity rate of American children while maintaining cost-effective health care (Havens and Bodenhorn, 1992).

Dental Care

Eruption of the infant's first teeth is a developmental milestone that has great significance for many parents. Deciduous or "baby" teeth usually erupt between 5 and 9 months of age. The first to appear are the lower central incisors, followed by the upper central, then the upper lateral incisors. The next teeth to erupt are usually the lower lateral incisors, first primary molars, canines, and the second primary molars. The average child has six to eight teeth by his first birthday (see Chapter 11, Fig. 11–9).

Teething. Although sometimes asymptomatic, teething is often signaled by behavior such as night wakening, daytime restlessness, an increase in nonnutritive sucking, excess drooling, and temporary loss of appetite. Some degree of discomfort is normal, but elevated temperature, irritability, ear tugging, or diarrhea should be investigated further by a health care professional.

To help parents to cope with teething, nurses can suggest that they provide cool liquids and hard foods (dry toast, popsicles, frozen bagels) for chewing. Hard, cold teethers and ice wrapped in cloth may also provide comfort for inflamed gums. Nurses should explain to parents that over-the-counter topical medications for gum pain relief should be used only as directed. Home remedies, such as rubbing the gums with whiskey or aspirin, should be discouraged, but acetaminophen administered as directed for the child's age can be used to relieve discomfort. Although these interventions can be helpful, parents should understand that absolute relief comes only with tooth eruption.

Cleaning Teeth. Because the primary teeth are used for chewing until the permanent teeth erupt and decay of the primary teeth often results in decay of the permanent teeth, dental care must begin in infancy. Cotton swabs or a soft washcloth can be used to clean the teeth with the child positioned in the parent's lap or on a changing table. Toothpaste is not recommended because infants tend to swallow it, possibly ingesting excessive amounts of fluoride. Too much fluoride can cause fluorosis, which results in staining of the teeth (Nowak, 1993).

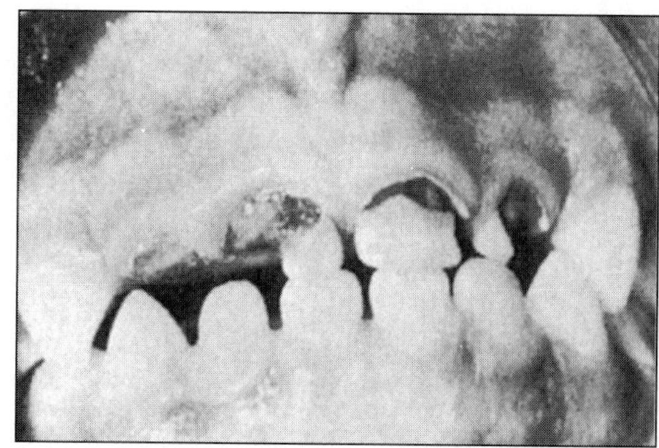

Figure 4–2
Bottle mouth caries. To avoid this decay pattern, discourage parents from giving milk or juice bedtime bottles to their infants and toddlers. A plain water bottle is an acceptable substitute. (From Caldwell, R. C., & Stallard, R. E. [1977]. *Textbook of preventive dentistry*. Philadelphia: W. B. Saunders.)

Appropriate amounts of fluoride, however, are necessary for the development of healthy teeth. Infants receive fluoride when formula and cereal are mixed with water from fluoridated water supplies. Supplements may be necessary, depending on the amount of fluoride in the local water system. See Chapter 5 for more information on fluoride and dental care for infants and older children.

Bottle Mouth Caries. Bottle mouth caries or nursing bottle syndrome is a well-described form of tooth decay that can develop in infants and children. The decay pattern usually involves the incisors initially, then spreads to other teeth (Fig. 4–2). Decay may be so serious that tooth loss occurs prematurely. Prolonged breastfeeding or bottle feeding, especially at night, puts infants at risk for the development of bottle mouth caries. When the infant is allowed to fall asleep with a bottle containing milk or juice, the carbohydrate-rich solution bathes the teeth for a long period and may cause dental caries (Barnes et al., 1992).

Nurses should discourage parents from giving bedtime bottles of milk or juice to infants. If a nighttime bottle is necessary, plain water is an acceptable substitute for carbohydrate-rich liquids (Von Burg, Sanders, Weddell, 1995). A pacifier is an acceptable alternative, although the practice of dipping the pacifier in Karo cornsyrup or honey to encourage acceptance poses the same problem. An additional danger of the use of honey in infancy is botulism (see Chapter 12).

TABLE 4–2 *Health Screening, Health Maintenance, and Anticipatory Guidance for Infants*

1–2 MONTHS	4 MONTHS	6 MONTHS	9 MONTHS	12 MONTHS
Immunizations DTP #1 OPV #1 HBV #1 Hib #1	DTP #2 OPV #2 HBV #2 Hib #2	DTP #3 OPV #3 HBV #3 Hib #3		DTP #4 at 12–15 months (may be given at 12 months if 6 months has elapsed since DTP #3). TB skin test. MMR #1 at 12–15 months. Varicella at 12–18 months.
Safety Use infant car seat throughout infancy. Be sure bath water is no hotter than 120°F. Never shake or vigorously jiggle baby's head. Do not hold infant while drinking hot liquids. Baby-proof home.	Guard infant on bed or changing table. Be sure safety straps are used for infant seat.	Remove chemicals, poisons, and plants from infant's reach. Cover electrical outlets. Do not leave unattended in bath.	Anticipate increased mobility. Protect from falls. Use gates to protect infant from stairs. Remove hazardous objects from low places. Cover electrical outlets. Keep syrup of ipecac and poison control number on hand. Be sure toys have no small pieces.	Prevent burns and scalding. Guard against falls. Supervise child in or near water. Keep older siblings toys with small pieces away from infant. Lock poisons away.
Nutrition Breast milk or formula is main food throughout infancy; no homogenized cow's milk. Vitamin, iron, and fluoride supplements should be used for breast-fed infants. Formula powder should be mixed with fluoridated tap water if fluoride levels are adequate. If not, give fluoride supplements to bottle-fed infants.	May offer rice cereal mixed with breast milk or formula.	Introduce strained vegetables, fruits, and meats one at a time. Begin use of cup for juice and water. Give only water if bottle taken to bed.	Table foods can be given when infant is sitting at family table. Self-feeding can begin. Avoid foods that might cause choking (e.g., popcorn, peanuts, hard candy, hot dogs, raw vegetables, raisins.	Self-feeding with help of table foods is appropriate. Liquids can be given with a cup. Weaning may be started. Bottle should be gradually eliminated.

Vision and Hearing				
Check for response to sound of bell. Assess ability to follow light past midline.	Assess for strabismus.		Assess for ability to look for objects.	Assess for ability to respond to name and other sounds. Assess ability to see and grasp.
Dental Care				
		Discuss teething and associated problems. When teeth erupt, they may be cleaned by using cotton swabs or soft cloth.	Discuss teething and associated problems. Compare growth to norms.	Continue to discuss teething and associated problems. Do not allow bottle in bed.
Screening				
Height, weight, and head circumference should be compared to norms at each well-child visit.	Height, weight, and head circumference should be monitored and compared to normals. Encourage parents to talk to infant.	Height, weight, and head circumference should be monitored and compared to normals. Hemoglobin and hematocrit screening for anemia (6–9 months). Urinalysis (1–12 months).	Compare height, weight, and head circumference to norms. Monitor deviations. Hemoglobin and hematocrit screening is done (6–9 months).	Monitor weight, height, and head circumference and compare to norms.
Teaching and Counseling				
Discuss irregular sleep patterns. Reinforce parents desire to cuddle and play with infant. Discuss importance of development of trust. Discuss needs and behavior of siblings.	Encourage parents to play with infant and provide safe, age-appropriate toys. Reassure parents that holding infant will not result in a "spoiled" child.	Discuss sleep problems and interventions. Encourage playing and talking to infant. Discuss stranger anxiety. Reassure that thumb-sucking is normal.	Discuss play and social games. Educate about normal behavior and expectations of growing infant. Discuss stranger anxiety. Encourage vocalization by talking to infant.	Discuss increasing mobility and growing need for autonomy. Encourage regular bedtime. Encourage vocalization and social play.

Abbreviations: DTP, diptheria and tetanus toxoids and pertussis vaccine; Hib, "Hemophilus influenzae" type B conjugate vaccine; HbV, hepatitis B virus vaccine; OPV, oral poliovirus vaccine.

Data from American Academy of Pediatrics, Committee on the Psychosocial Aspects of Child and Family Health. (1988). *Guidelines for health supervision.* Elk Grove Village, IL: American Academy of Pediatrics.

KEY CONCEPTS

- During the first year of life the infant's organs grow and mature at a rapid rate, yet organ systems of infants remain very different from those of older children and adults.
- Weight gain and muscle growth during infancy allow the infant to have increased control of reflexes and increasingly coordinated movement.
- Sensory capabilities, neuromuscular control, and perceptual skills as well as quality and quantity of parental interaction and environmental stimulation all impact cognitive development during infancy.
- Infants develop language by first listening to sounds of caregivers, then by realizing that certain sounds have special meaning, and eventually by using simple words to communicate.
- Infancy is the period during which a child develops the foundation of his personality, struggling to establish a sense of basic trust rather than mistrust.
- One of the most important features of psychosocial development during infancy is parent-infant attachment, or the sense of belonging with another.
- Common problems during infancy such as separation anxiety, sleep disorders, and fretfulness cause parents concern and distress. Nurses should be available with information and support to provide anticipatory guidance.
- Because infancy is a period of very rapid growth and development, nutritional needs are of special significance. Parents frequently have many questions and concerns about nutrition.
- Breast milk or commercially prepared formulas provide the foundation of nutrition throughout infancy.
- Introduction of solid foods should be delayed until age 4–6 months when the gastrointestinal system has matured sufficiently to handle complex nutrients.
- Improved motor development coupled with a keen desire to explore the environment places the infant at great risk for accidents and injury.
- Nurses play an important role in health promotion and disease prevention related to immunizations. Nursing responsibilities related to immunizations in infancy include educating parents about the necessity of immunizations, assessing current immunization status, and storing, administering, and documenting immunizations.
- Teething usually begins between 5 and 9 months of age. Some degree of discomfort is normal, and parents often need suggestions for coping with teething.
- Bottle mouth caries or nursing bottle syndrome is a form of tooth decay that can develop in infants and children as a result of prolonged breast feeding or bottle feeding, especially at night.

REFERENCES

American Public Health Association. (1990). *Healthy people 2000*. Washington, DC: U.S. Government Printing Office.

Barnes, G. P. (1992). Ethnicity, location, age and fluoridation factors in baby bottle tooth decay and caries prevalence of Head Start children. *Public Health Reports, 107*(2), 167–173.

Burgess, W. R., & Chernick, V. (1982). *Respiratory therapy in newborn infants and children*. New York: Thieme-Stratton.

Castiglia, P. T. (1987). Speech and language development. *Journal of Pediatric Health Care, 1*(3), 165–167.

Erikson, E. H. (1963). *Childhood and society* (2nd ed.). New York: Norton.

Flavell, J. H. (1964). *The developmental psychology of Jean Piaget*. New York: Van Nostrand.

Havens, D. H., & Bodenhorn, K. (1992). Standards for immunization practice. *Journal of Pediatric Health Care*, 275–278.

Keefe, M. R., & Froese-Fretz, A. (1991). Living with an irritable infant: Maternal perspectives. *MCN: The American Journal of Maternal Child Nursing, 16*(5), 255–259.

Korones, S. B. (1986). *High-risk newborn infants*. St. Louis: C. V. Mosby.

Netsell, R. (1980). Speech motor control development. In A. P. Reilly (Ed.), *Pediatric round table series: The communication game* (pp. 33–38). Baltimore: Johnson & Johnson.

Nowak, A. J. (1993). The pediatrician and pediatric dentist: partners in prevention. *Pediatric Basics, 64*, 6–12.

Oller, D. K. (1980). Patterns of infant vocalization. In A. P. Reilly (Ed.), *Pediatric round table series: The communication game* (pp. 43–48). Baltimore: Johnson & Johnson.

Piaget, J. (1952). *The origins of intelligence in children*. New York: International Universities Press.

Pipes, P. L., & Trahms, C. M. (1993). *Nutrition in infancy and childhood*. St. Louis: C. V. Mosby.

Porth, C. M. (1994). *Pathophysiology*. Philadelphia: Lippincott.

Sinclair, D. (1989). *Human growth after birth*. New York: Oxford University Press.

Thomas, A., & Chess, S. (1977). *Temperament and development*. New York: Brunner/Mazel.

Von Burg, M. M., Sanders, B. J., Weddell, J. A. (1995). Baby bottle tooth decay: A concern for all mothers. *Pediatric Nursing, 21*(6), 515–519.

BIBLIOGRAPHY

American Academy of Pediatrics. (1991). *Report of the Committee on Infectious Diseases* (22nd ed.). Elk Grove Village, IL: Author.

Bawden, J. W. (Ed.). (1992). Changing patterns of fluoride intake. *Journal of Dental Research, 71,* 1215–1265.

Behrman, R. E., Kliegman, R., & Nelson, W. E. (1992). *Textbook of Pediatrics.* Philadelphia: W. B. Saunders.

Bellanti, J. A. (1990). Basic immunologic principles underlying vaccination procedures. *Pediatric Clinics of North America, 37*(3), 513–530.

Castiglia, P. T. (1992). Teething. *Journal of Pediatric Health Care, 6*(3), 153–154.

Dixon, M., Keeling, A. W., & Kennel, S. (1994). What pediatric hospital nurses should know about immunizations. *MCN: The American Journal of Maternal Child Nursing, 19*(2), 74–78.

Field, T. (1993). Sucking for stress reduction, growth and development during infancy. *Pediatric Basics, 64,* 13–16.

Freud, A. (1974). *Introduction to Psychoanalysis.* New York: International University Press.

Gray, P. (1988). Cry-sis: Support group for parents of crying sleepless babies. *Midwife Health Visitor and Community Nurse, 26*(6), 211.

Greenspan, S. I. (1991). Clinical assessment of emotional milestones in infancy and early childhood. *Pediatric Clinics of North America, 38*(6), 1371–1385.

Henry, J. T. (1992). Routine growth monitoring and assessment of growth disorders. *Journal of Pediatric Health Care, 6,* 291–301.

Howard, B. J. (1990). Growing together: Parents and child from 3 months to 1 year. *Contemporary Pediatrics,* 81–98.

Immunization Practices Advisory Committee (ACIP). (1991a). Haemophilus b conjugate vaccines for prevention of *Haemophilus influenzae* type b disease among infants and children two months of age and older. *Morbidity and Mortality Weekly Reports, 40*(RR-1), 1–7.

Immunization Practices Advisory Committee (ACIP). (1991b). Diphtheria, tetanus, pertussis: Recommendations for vaccine use and other preventive measures. *Morbidity and Mortality Weekly Reports, 40*(RR-10), 1–28.

Immunization Practices Advisory Committee (ACIP). (1989). General recommendations on immunizations. *Morbidity and Mortality Weekly Reports, 38*(13), 205–227.

Jaques, S. (1992, April). Baby teeth. *American Baby,* B9–B120.

Kefalas, M. J. (1993). American children and immunizations: Part 1, How bad is it? *Journal of Pediatric Nursing, 8*(5), 345–347.

Lerner, H. (1993). Sleep position in infants: Applying research to practice. *MCN: The American Journal of Maternal Child Nursing, 18*(5), 275–277.

Lewis, M., & Volkmar, F. R. (1990). *Clinical aspects of child and adolescent development.* Philadelphia: Lea and Febiger.

Maikler, V. E. (1991). Effects of skin refrigerant/anesthetic and age on the pain responses of infants receiving immunizations. *Research in Nursing & Health, 14*(6), 397–403.

O'Laughlin, E. D. & Ridley-Johnson, R. (1995). Maternal presence during children's routine immunizations: The effect of mother in reducing child distress. *Children's Health Care, 24*(3), 175–191.

Peter, G. (1992). Childhood immunizations. *New England Journal of Medicine, 327*(25), 1794–1800.

Phillips, C. F. (1993). Vaccine update, 1993. *Contemporary Pediatrics, 10*(2), 75–77, 81–88, 92–96.

Pinyerd, B. J. (1992). Assessment of infant growth. *Journal of Pediatric Health Care, 6*(5), 302–307.

Sharts-Hopko, N. (1992). Preventing hepatitis B in infants. *MCN: The American Journal of Maternal Child Nursing, 17*(6), 336.

Sharts-Hopko, N. C. (1994). Current immunization guidelines. *MCN: The American Journal of Maternal Child Nursing, 19,* 82–84.

Stern, D. (1985). *The interpersonal world of the infant.* New York: Basic Books.

Wilson, C. B. (1986). Immunologic basis for increased susceptibility of the neonate to infection. *Journal of Pediatrics, 108*(1), 1–12.

White, B. L. (1975). *The first three years of life.* Englewood Cliffs, NJ: Prentice-Hall.

5

The Toddler

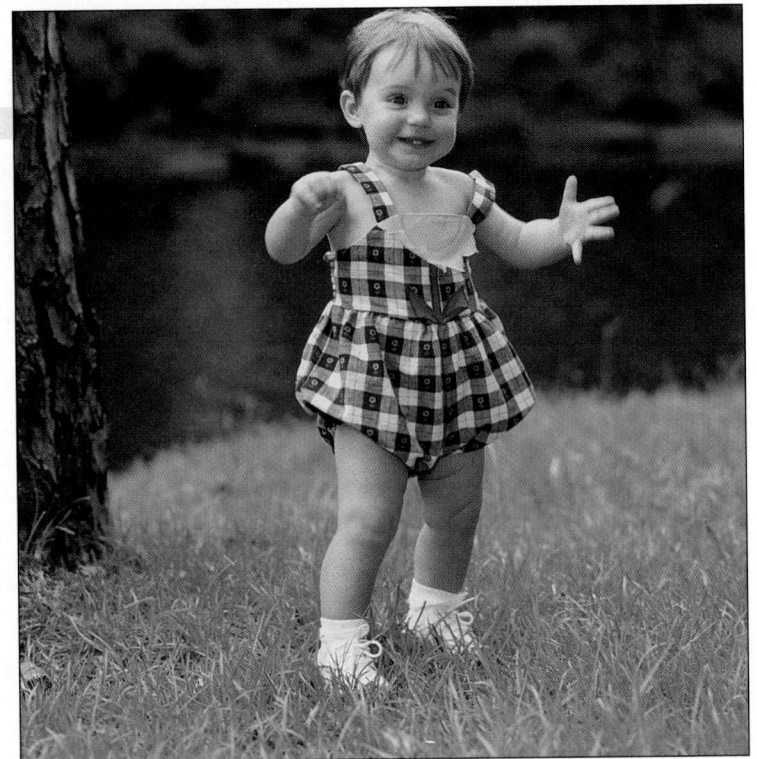

Courtesy of Mark Patterson

CHAPTER OVERVIEW

LEARNING OBJECTIVES

After studying this chapter, you should be able to:

- Describe the physiologic changes and motor, cognitive, language, and psychosocial development of the toddler.
- Discuss the cause of, and identify interventions to cope with, common toddler behaviors: temper tantrums, negativism, and ritualism.
- Discuss strategies for disciplining a toddler.
- Describe signs of a toddler's readiness for toilet training and offer guidelines to parents.
- Discuss ways to prepare a toddler for the birth of a sibling.
- Discuss anticipatory guidance for preventive dental care of the toddler.

KEY TERMS

animism: attributing lifelike characteristics to inanimate objects

autonomy: ability to function independently without the control of others

caries: tooth decay

negativism: attitude of opposing or resisting the directions of others

parallel play: playing alongside, but not with, other children

physiologic anorexia: decreased appetite because of relatively decreased caloric need

regression: return to a behavior characteristic of an earlier stage

ritualism: the need to maintain sameness and reliability

toddler: child between the ages of 12 and 36 months

The developmental changes that mark the transition from infancy to early childhood are dramatic. Between the ages of 12 and 30 months, the child begins to strike out independently from a secure base of trust established during the first year. As the toddler learns to walk, increased mobility provides new perspectives and access to new territory. Boundless energy and insatiable curiosity drive the child to explore the environment and master new skills. The combination of increased motor skills, immaturity, and lack of experience place the toddler at risk for accidental injury. One of the most important roles of the nurse is to provide anticipatory guidance to parents, teaching them strategies for protecting the toddler and setting appropriate limits while promoting autonomy and curiosity (see Chapter 13).

The toddler years (the period from 12–36 months of age) are characterized by the struggle for autonomy as the child develops a sense of herself as separate from the parent. Toddlers' egocentric and demanding behavior, often marked by temper tantrums and negativism, have given this age the label "the terrible twos." However, toddlers are also irresistibly charming. The toddler is enchanted with a world filled with discovery. Many parents find the toddler years a rewarding time as they watch their child learn and grow. Dramatic growth of language and cognitive skills during the second year enable the toddler to think and solve problems for the first time. The toddler years are some of the most exciting and magical of childhood.

GROWTH AND DEVELOPMENT OF THE TODDLER

Growth and development of the toddler are summarized in Table 5–1.

Physical Growth and Development

Physical growth slows during the toddler years. Average weight gain is 2.25 kg (5 lb) per year. Birth weight is quadrupled by 2 to 3 years of age. The rate of increase in height also slows, with the average toddler growing approximately 7.5 cm (3 inches) per year. Adult height may be estimated by doubling the child's height at 2 years of age.

The brain grows at a slower rate during toddlerhood than during infancy. Head circumference reflects this growth, increasing approximately 3.5 cm (1.8 inches) during the toddler years compared with the growth of 12 cm (4.7 inches) in the first 12 months. By the age of 2 years, the brain has attained 90% of adult size.

Because of their slower growth rate, toddlers require relatively fewer calories than infants. The child's appetite tends to drop off at this time, resulting in **physiologic anorexia.** The toddler needs an average of 1300 calories per day (see Chapter 12). The toddler's appetite tends to be erratic, often causing parents to be concerned that their child is not eating enough. The nurse should reassure parents that toddlers often go on "food jags" or assert their independence by refusing to eat meals offered by the parents. When providing anticipatory guidance for parents, the nurse should suggest that they offer small portions and recognize the ritualistic needs of the toddler (e.g., same dishes, utensils, chair). Nutritious foods, such as yogurt, fruit juice, peanut butter, and vegetables, should be offered throughout the day because toddlers usually eat "on the go." The child should never be forced to eat, as the child will ultimately win food-related battles. Toddlers who drink large quantities of milk often do not eat sufficient iron-rich foods and are prone to iron-deficiency

TABLE 5–1 *Summary of Growth and Development: The Toddler*

PHYSICAL	MOTOR	PSYCHOSOCIAL	SENSORY/COGNITIVE	LANGUAGE/COMMUNICATION
15 Months Gains 2.25 kg (5 lb) per year. Grows 7.5 cm (3 inches) per year. Twelve teeth erupt.	**Gross:** Walks alone. Climbs stairs; slides down backwards on abdomen. Enjoys throwing objects to the floor. May climb out of high chair, crib, or stroller. Constantly on the go. **Fine:** Builds a tower of two blocks. Drinks from a cup, holding the cup with both hands. Takes off socks and shoes. Puts a pellet in a bottle and pours it out. Wants to carry something in each hand.	Onset of negativism. Demands attention. Frequent mood swings. Begins to insist on doing things without help. Shows affection to parents. Recognizes herself in photographs, mirror. Imitates housework. Easily distracted and entertained. May indicate wet diaper. Likes to take off shoes and socks.	Places a round block in a round hole. Unable to transfer knowledge to a new situation. Pats picture in a book. Imitates simple actions. Binocular vision well developed. Looks at picture books with parent. Enjoys feeling different textures; dislikes substances that stick to fingers.	Vocabulary of four to six words. Uses gestures and expressive jargon (few real words can be recognized). May say "bye-bye." Asks for objects by pointing. Understands simple directions ("no," "show me," "look"). Points to and names one body part.
18 Months	**Gross:** Walks fast; seldom falls. Runs stiffly; falls. Pulls toys and large objects. Carries large toy while walking. Climbs. Walks up or down stairs with adult holding his hand. Squats fully and stands again without falling. Seats himself in a small chair. Jumps in place with both feet. **Fine:** Puts blocks in large holes, rings on peg. Scribbles; may attempt to draw horizontal lines. Can drink from a cup without much spilling. Feeds herself partially. Builds tower of four to five blocks. Turns knob of radio or TV. Shows hand preference.	Demands attention. Opposes parents with "No!" Less afraid of strangers. Little toleration for frustration. Temper tantrums may be triggered by fatigue, frustration, or anger. Unable to share. Imitates housework. Treats other toddlers as if they were objects. May indicate readiness for toilet training. Tries to brush teeth. Likes to undress. Is an entertaining show-off. Balances desire for independence with desire for closeness (e.g., explores across the room and then comes back to cuddle).	Imitates people and things in the environment. Explores environment extensively. Searches for desired object (toy) in more than one place. Follows simple, one-part directions. Infers causes from observing effects; beginning to figure out how things work. Short attention span. Remembers where objects belong. Has 20/40 vision.	Vocabulary of 30 or more words. "No" is chief word. Holographic speech (uses a single word with accompanying gestures to express whole ideas). Asks for some wants by naming (e.g., juice, cookie, outside). Gets coat and says "bye-bye." May not talk yet.

24 Months	**Gross:** Runs fairly well. Walks up and down stairs holding on to handrail (two feet on each step). Throws ball with both hands without falling. Kicks ball. **Fine:** Opens doorknob. Drinks from a small cup using only one hand. Uses a spoon, spilling little. Turns pages of a book one at a time. Unzips large zipper; unbuttons large buttons. Puts on coat without help. Builds tower of six to seven blocks. Lines blocks up, making a train.	Negativistic, stubborn. Wants to do things for herself. Likes to tell others what to do. Engages in pretend play. Still cannot share. May bite, slap, or hit. Wants his own way in everything. Affectionate. Has a positive self-concept. Likes to dress and take off clothes. Brushes teeth with help. May demonstrate readiness for toilet training by anticipating a need to defecate or urinate. May be afraid of the dark or of animals.	Places a square block into the appropriate hole. Magical thinking. Matches simple shapes and colors. Names three body parts on request. Beginning to understand time ("after lunch"), but does not understand clock or calendar time. Is learning to wait; understands "soon." Attention span of approximately 2 minutes.	Vocabulary of 300 or more words. Uses two- to three-word sentences ("Go bye-bye." "More milk."). Telegraphic speech ("Me do." "Daddy push."). Egocentric speech, monologues. Uses pronouns (I, me). Talks constantly. Refers to himself by his first name. Listens to and enjoys simple stories.
30 Months	**Gross:** Stands on one foot alone for 1 second. Jumps with both feet. Can throw a large ball about 5 feet. Catches a large ball with both arms and body. Can walk on tiptoe. **Fine:** Likes to fill containers with objects. Puts on simple clothes independently, snaps large snaps, and buttons large buttons. Twists lid off a jar. Places simple shapes in correct hole. Uses fork. May use toilet, but still needs help. Builds tower of eight blocks.	Plays in an organized, focused manner for 20 minutes or longer. Beginning to think about the consequences of her behavior. May sort blocks or dolls and pretend that they are members of a family (e.g., a big block is the head of the family).	Can think about the consequences of her behavior. Names six body parts on request. Beginning to understand "tomorrow" and "yesterday."	Vocabulary increases; can name almost everything at home or on walks. More conversation with others; less monologue. Sentences of three or more words. Knows her first and last name. Uses plurals.

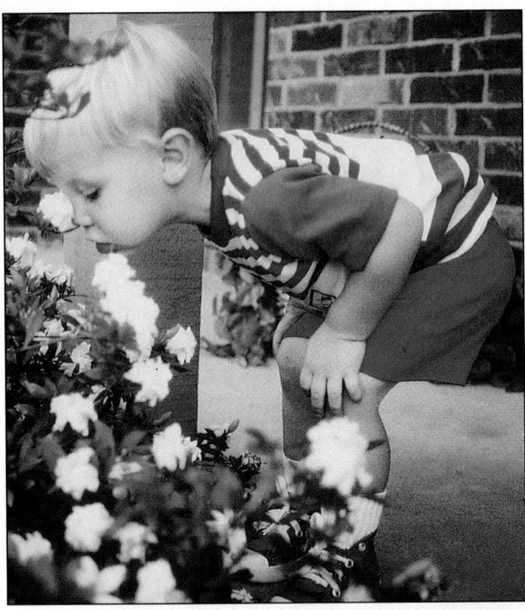

◄ The toddler is enchanted with a world filled with discovery. Curiosity provides resources for the tremendous cognitive growth that occurs during this period.

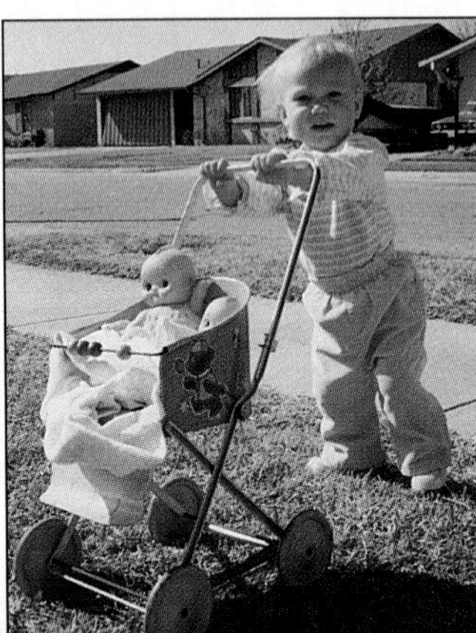

◄ Toddlers enjoy push-pull toys. Toys should be strong and sturdy; wheeled toys should not tip over easily.

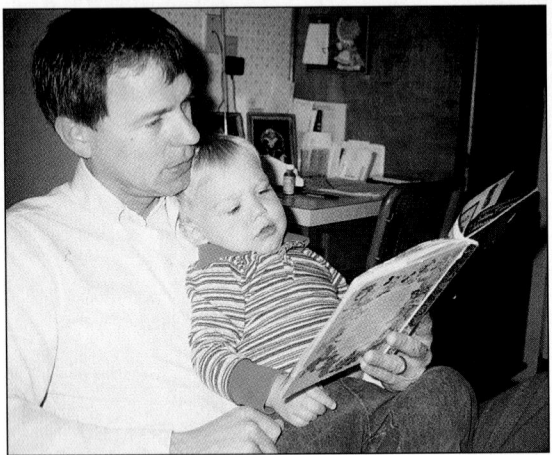

Reading simple stories provides quiet, enjoyable times for toddlers and parents and enhances speech and language development.

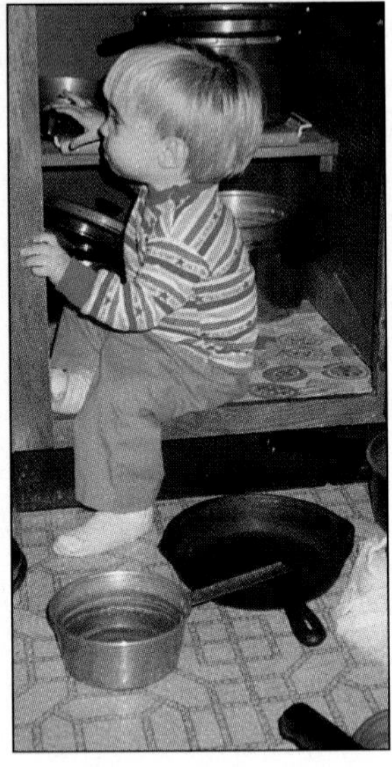

◄ Pots and pans are popular toys for inquisitive toddlers. However, exploring cupboards can be a dangerous activity for toddlers. Toxic cleaning substances and other dangerous objects must be kept behind locked doors or otherwise out of reach.

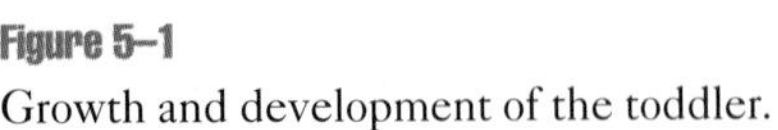

Figure 5–1
Growth and development of the toddler.

anemia. Milk intake should be limited to 24 to 32 ounces per day. A bottle should not be given as a substitute for solid foods, and solids should be offered before or with milk.

Immature abdominal musculature gives the toddler a potbellied appearance, with an exaggerated lumbar curve. The child's short legs may appear slightly bowed, and the feet seem flat because of a plantar fat pad that disappears around the age of 2 years. During the toddler years, muscle tissue gradually replaces much of the adipose tissue (baby fat) present during infancy. With increased ambulation and maturation of the musculoskeletal system, the child loses the cherubic appearance of the toddler and grows into a taller, leaner preschooler.

Motor Development

Learning to walk is the crowning achievement of the toddler period. Increased mobility opens up new vistas for the enthusiastic toddler. The toddler appears to spend every moment of his busy day perfecting motor skills, especially learning to walk. The child is in perpetual motion, seemingly compelled to pull himself up, take a few steps, fall, and repeat the process over and over, oblivious to bumps and bruises. The toddler will repeat this performance hundreds of times, until he has perfected the skill of walking. He is so absorbed in mastering the task that he will work at it from morning to night, until he is too exhausted to continue.

The age at which children learn to walk varies widely. Most children can walk alone by 15 months. By 18 months of age, toddlers walk well and try to run, but fall often. Nurses can help to prevent injuries by providing anticipatory guidance to parents about the selection of toys for toddlers. Toddlers enjoy push–pull toys and often carry large toys around as they walk. Toys should be strong and sturdy; wheeled toys should not tip over easily.

At approximately 15 months of age, many toddlers become avid climbers, scaling every available obstacle. Chairs, tables, and bookcases all present irresistible challenges. Parents may have difficulty keeping the toddler in a crib and may decide it is time to move her into a regular bed.

Toddlers are also engaged in perfecting fine motor skills. Hand–eye coordination improves with maturity and practice. Mealtimes are still messy. Although most 18-month-olds can hold a cup with both hands and drink from it without much spilling, eating with a spoon is difficult. Most of the food conveyed in a spoon is spilled. The child needs a great deal of practice with a spoon before he can feed himself without spilling. Most toddlers can feed themselves with a spoon by their second birthday if they have been allowed to practice.

At 18 months of age, the toddler enjoys removing clothing. By 24 months, the toddler can put on simple items of clothing, but cannot differentiate front from back. The child at this age also can zip large zippers, put on her shoes, and wash and dry her hands. Two-year-olds brush their teeth, but need help to adequately remove plaque.

The toddler's increasing motor skills allow him more independence in all areas of daily life. Feeding, dressing, and play provide opportunities for the child to develop his ever-increasing autonomy. Because the toddler's motor development is far ahead of his judgment and perceptions, he is at risk for accidental injury. Nurses must provide anticipatory guidance to parents on ways to keep the child safe from falls, burns, poisonous ingestions, and a myriad of other dangers.

> Essential teaching includes childproofing the home by keeping poisons and sharp objects locked up and out of reach, supervising children when near cars or traffic, using car safety seats, and being vigilant when children are near fireplaces, grills, or water.

See Chapter 13 for a more detailed discussion of safety issues for the toddler.

Cognitive and Sensory Development

Toddlers are consumed with curiosity. Their boundless energy and insatiable inquisitiveness provide them with resources for the tremendous cognitive growth that occurs during this period.

Toddlers between the ages of 12 and 18 months are in Piaget's sensorimotor period (see Chapter 2). Learning in this stage occurs mainly by trial and error. The toddler spends most of her busy day experimenting to see what will happen as she dumps, fills, empties, and explores every accessible area of her environment. Between 19 and 24 months, the child enters the final stage of the sensorimotor period. Object permanence is firmly established by this age. The child has a beginning ability to use symbols and words when referring to absent people or objects and begins to solve problems mentally rather than by repeating an action over and over. A toddler at this stage is often seen imitating the parent of the same sex performing household tasks (domestic mimicry). Late in this stage, the child displays deferred imitation (e.g., he imitates the parent putting on makeup or shaving hours after that parent has left for work). The 18-month-old has a beginning ability to wait, as evidenced by the toddler responding appropriately to a parent or caregiver who says, "just a minute." The child's concept of time is still immature, however, and "a minute" may seem like an hour to the toddler.

> Toddlers think in terms of the predictable routines of their daily schedule. When talking with the toddler, the nurse should use time orientation in relation to familiar activities. For example, a toddler would understand "Your mother will be here after your nap" better than "Your mother will be here at 2:00."

Many hours each day are spent putting objects into holes and smaller objects into each other as the child experiments with sizes, shapes, and space relations. Toddlers enjoy opening drawers and doors, exploring the contents of cabinets and closets, and generally wreaking havoc throughout the house. Their drive to explore is insatiable, placing them at risk for injury. The nurse should counsel parents to supervise the toddler at all times (see Chapter 3).

At around 24 months, the child enters the preconceptual phase of Piaget's preoperational period. This phase ends at age 4. The preoperational stage is characterized by an increased ability to think symbolically. The child begins to think and reason at a primitive level. The 2-year-old has a beginning ability to retain mental images. This ability allows him to internalize what he sees and experiences. Symbols in the form of words can be used to represent ideas. Increasing amounts of playtime are spent pretending. A box may become a spaceship or a hat; pebbles may be money or popcorn. The child's rapidly increasing

TABLE 5–2 *Characteristics of Preoperational Thinking*

CHARACTERISTIC	EXAMPLE
Egocentrism: Views everything in relation to himself, is unable to consider another's point of view.	Toddler takes a toy away from another child and cannot understand that the other child wants (or has a right to) the toy, too.
Animism: Believes that inert objects are alive and have wills of their own.	Toddler trips over a toy and scolds the toy for hurting her. She believes that the toy hurt her on purpose.
Irreversibility: Cannot see a process in reverse order. Cannot follow a line of reasoning back to its beginning. Cannot hold onto two or more sequential thoughts simultaneously.	If the child takes a toy apart, he cannot remember the sequence for putting it back together. If child is taken on a walk, he cannot retrace his steps and find his way home.
Magical thought: Believes that magical thought is the cause of events; that wishing something will make it so.	Toddlers often feel extremely powerful and believe that their thoughts cause events to happen. May believe that parents are all-powerful and can read minds or have magical powers.
Centration: Tends to focus on only one aspect of an experience, ignoring other possible alternatives. Focuses on the dominant characteristic of an object, excluding other characteristics.	May have difficulty putting together a puzzle, concentrating on only one detail of a piece (such as shape) and ignoring other qualities (such as color or detail). Cannot follow more than one direction at a time.

vocabulary enhances symbolic play. The toddler begins to think about alternate solutions to a problem and can even consider the consequences of an action without carrying it out (touching a hot stove, running too fast on a slippery sidewalk).

The toddler's thinking is immature, limited in its logic and bound to the present. Egocentrism, **animism** (attributing lifelike characteristics to inanimate objects), irreversibility, magical thought, and centration characterize the preoperational thought of the toddler (see Table 5–2).

Language Development

Acquisition of language is one of the most dramatic developments of early childhood. Although the age at which children begin to talk varies widely, most can communicate verbally by their second birthday. The rate of language development depends on physical maturity and the amount of reinforcement that the child has received. Language characteristics of toddlers at various ages are summarized in Table 5–1. Between 15 and 24 months of age, language ability develops rapidly. Toddlers understand many more words than they can say because receptive language (what the child understands) develops sooner and more quickly than speech. Sometime after 18 months, many children experience a sudden spurt in both speech and comprehension, resulting in a vocabulary of 300 or more words of 24 months. By 2 years of age, two-thirds of toddlers' speech should be understandable. Because children of 24 to 30 months are less egocentric and better able to consider another's point of view, they engage in more conversation with others and less monologue.

An important role of the nurse is to assess the language development of the toddler. Reports of parents can give the first clue to a child's hearing problems (Rapin, 1993). If language development is not progressing normally, parents should be advised to pursue follow-up care. Children of bilingual families, twins, and children other than firstborns may have slower language development.

Nurses should counsel parents about ways to promote language development. Parents should be encouraged to talk to the child and incorporate teaching into daily routines. Feeding, bathing, dressing, and outings to both new and familiar places offer opportunities for verbal interaction and practice of growing language skills. Children seem to talk sooner when parents encourage them to express their needs rather than anticipating what the child wants before he asks for it. Reading simple, entertaining stories with colorful pictures provides quiet, enjoyable times for toddlers and parents and enhances speech and language development.

Psychosocial Development

The toddler is developing a sense of **autonomy,** giving up the comfort of dependence she enjoyed during infancy. If a basic sense of trust was established during the first year, she can venture forward and leave her parents for short periods to explore and experience the world.

Important tasks of the toddler period include

- Recognition of himself as a separate person, with a will of his own.
- Toleration of separation from the parent.
- Control of impulses and acquisition of socially acceptable ways to communicate his wants and needs.
- Control of elimination.

According to Erikson, the toddler is struggling with the developmental task of acquiring a sense of autonomy while overcoming a sense of shame and doubt. The toddler discovers that he has a will of his own and that he can control others. However, asserting his will and insisting on his own way leads to conflict with those he loves, whereas submissive behavior is rewarded with affection and approval. Toddlers experience conflict because they want to assert their own will, but do not want to risk losing the approval of loved ones. The child doubts his abilities if he continues to practice dependent behavior. He may feel shame for his independent impulses, particularly if he is frequently punished for asserting his will.

As the toddler struggles to accomplish these tasks, he experiments with ways to control those around him. He learns which behaviors gain approval from those he loves and which result in censure and punishment. The 2-year-old does not have a conscience, but learns to control his behavior to avoid punishment. He determines right and wrong by the consequences of his actions.

At around 15 months, toddlers begin to demonstrate their developing autonomy with two almost universal behaviors: negativism and ritualism.

Negativism. **Negativism,** one of the most dramatic expressions of independence, is shown in a variety of ways. One child psychologist has described the toddler's negativism as "a preview of coming attractions of adolescence" (White, 1985). The toddler's favorite word seems to be "no," and any offer of help is met with an emphatic "Me do." When asked if she wants a cookie, the toddler may answer "No!" even though she wants it very much. Unable to distinguish between requests and directives, the toddler seems to feel that saying "yes" would mean giving up her free will. At this stage, the toddler is also possessive and seems to delight in testing her will against her parent's. Negativism may result in screaming, kicking, hitting, biting, or breath holding. Such displays make the terrible twos a trying time for parents. Parents often interpret the child's negative behavior as being bad or stubborn. Nurses can help parents to understand their toddler's behavior as an important sign of the child's progress from dependency to autonomy and independence. Parents should be given support and encouraged to deal with the toddler's trying behavior with patience and a sense of humor. Although general permissiveness is not recommended, too much pressure and forceful methods of control often lead to defiance, tantrums, and prolonged negative behavior.

Ritualism and the Importance of Routine. **Ritualism** helps the child to venture out and away from the safety of his parents by ensuring uniformity and security. Ritualism allows the toddler to have a sense of control. The child feels more confident with a secure home base. The toddler insists on sameness. Milk may need to be poured into the same cup, parents may need to sit in the same chairs at dinnertime, and a specified routine may need to be followed countless times throughout the day. The child may be unable to go to sleep unless a bedtime ritual is followed exactly (e.g., a drink of water, two stories, prayers, and a teddy bear). The child may experience distress if this routine is not followed exactly the next night. Failure to recognize the importance of such rituals may increase stress and insecurity.

Events such as hospitalization, where continuity of routine cannot be ensured, are difficult for the toddler. The nurse can decrease the stress of hospitalization by incorporating the child's usual rituals and routines from home into nursing care activities. Keeping routines as similar to home as possible and recognizing ritualistic needs gives the toddler some sense of control and security and decreases feelings of helplessness and fear. See Chapter 15 for further discussion of the hospitalized child.

Separation Anxiety. Separation anxiety peaks again in the toddler period. Although the concept of object permanence is fully developed in toddlerhood, the toddler cannot differentiate her own feelings from those of her parent. When the child experiences a strong desire to be independent and to leave her mother, she fears that her mother may also want to leave her. The child may strike out independently across the room, only to rush back in tears to her mother, as if the child were frightened and angry with the mother for leaving her. For a brief period, the parent may find it almost impossible to talk on the telephone without interruption or even to go into the bathroom without being followed. Leave-taking and brief separations are acceptable to the toddler if they are her idea, but her mother's departure may cause desperate clinging and crying. Games such as hide-and-seek help the child to master fears of separation. By repeating separation under conditions she can control, the toddler is helped to overcome the anxiety associated with separation. The child learns from experience that loved ones will return after separation.

The toddler is particularly vulnerable to separation. Being left with a stranger can be stressful. Toddlers should be told honestly and clearly about a separation shortly before it occurs. The child should also be reassured that the parent is coming back. When a parent returns, the toddler often shows his anger at being left by ignoring the parent or by pretending to be more interested in play than in going home. Parents of hospitalized toddlers are frequently distressed by such behavior when they visit their child. The nurse can offer support by explaining the behavior and telling the parents that plenty of affection and attention are needed to help the toddler to cope with the stress of separation.

Transition objects, such as a favorite blanket or toy, provide comfort to the toddler in stressful situations, such as separation, illness, or even bedtime. Such objects help children to make the transition from dependency to autonomy. The toddler may become so attached to his "lovey" that he can hardly bear to part with it, even for a quick run through the washing machine. Such objects provide extra security when the child must be separated from the parent, such as in daycare, while spending the night away from home, or during hospitalization. Tolerating brief separations from her parents is an important developmental task of toddlerhood. The nurse should counsel parents to leave a toddler only briefly initially and, if possible, to delay extended separations until the toddler can better handle them. The nurse who helps parents to understand normal toddler behavior in response to separation helps parents to cope with the frustrations of this transition.

Play. Toddlers spend most of their time at play. Play is serious business to the toddler—it is her work. Many hours are spent each day in play perfecting fine and gross motor skills, learning to control inner urges, and gaining self-esteem. Play during this period reflects the developmental level of the egocentric toddler (see Chapter 9). The toddler engages in **parallel play,** in which she plays alongside, but not with, other children. Little regard is given to the feelings of others. She frequently grabs toys away from other children or may hit or fight to obtain a wanted toy. Because the toddler is egocentric, she does not realize that she is hurting the other child and feels no shame for aggressive actions.

Imitation or acting out of scenes of everyday life are common as the toddler begins to try out roles and to identify with adults. Active, large-muscle play helps the toddler to vent frustrations and dissipate excess energy. The nurse can help parents to understand how play enhances the toddler's development. The nurse should encourage parents to play with their toddler and to provide opportunities for the toddler to play with other children. The nurse should teach parents that the house should be childproofed daily. Toys must be strong, safe, and too large to swallow or place in the ear or nose. Toddlers need supervision at all times. A variety of play materials, which need not be expensive, and a safe play environment enhance the toddler's development.

Psychosexual Development. At around 18 months, toddlers enter Freud's anal stage. Freud theorized that as the child focuses on mastery of bowel and bladder functions, his attention is also directed to the genital area. Even before the age of 2, children are aware of their own sex and begin to develop a sense of gender identity. By $2\frac{1}{2}$ or 3 years, toddlers can correctly identify anatomic pictures of boys and girls. It is not until the age of 5 years that gender identity is fully established and the child understands gender as permanent (e.g., that gender does not change with the addition of a wig or a dress) (Kohlberg, 1966).

Children begin to be aware of expected sex role behaviors at an early age. By age 3, most toddlers show an awareness of sex role stereotypes and tend to imitate the same-sex parent during play. Sex role identification continues throughout the toddler and preschool years as the child incorporates the attitudes, roles, and values of the same-sex parent. Although sex role stereotypes have relaxed somewhat in recent years, children behave according to adult expectations. Children learn behavior by reinforcement and punishment as well as by imitation. If a boy repeatedly hears that boys don't play with dolls, he will spurn such "girl's toys" and will play with toys that his parents consider masculine to gain their praise and approval. Nurses should be aware of their own biases about sex-typed behaviors and should support the parents in their choice of toys and activities for their child. The nurse can be most helpful by encouraging parents to make traditionally sex-typed toys available to both boys and girls if this approach is consistent with their own beliefs. Parents' expectations of appropriate sex role behavior differ according to their cultural backgrounds. In most cultures, boys and girls are treated differently and thus are taught "male" and "female" behaviors.

Parents are often concerned about their toddler's interest in and curiosity about sexual differences. Sex play and masturbation are common among toddlers. Nurses can reassure parents that self-exploration or exploration of another toddler's body is normal behavior during early childhood. Parents should respect the child's curiosity as normal without judging the child as "bad." The child should be told that touching private parts is something that is done only in private. When parents discover children involved in sex play, casually telling them to dress and directing them to another activity can limit sex play without producing feelings of shame or anxiety. The nurse should explain to parents that positive attitudes toward sexuality are learned from parents who are comfortable with their own sexuality. As young children learn about their bodies and explore anatomic differences, they frequently ask questions about where babies come from or why "Brian looks different from Emily." Honest, straightforward answers using the correct terminology satisfy the toddler's curiosity and lay the foundation for healthy sexual attitudes.

HEALTH PROMOTION FOR THE TODDLER AND FAMILY

Table 5–4 at the end of this chapter presents an overview of health screening, health maintenance, and anticipatory guidance activities for toddlers.

Sleep and Rest

During the second year, children require approximately 12 to 14 hours of sleep each day. Most 2-year-olds take an afternoon nap, and until their second birthday, some children also require a morning nap. Toddlers often resist going to bed, using dawdling or even temper tantrums to postpone separation from loved ones and the exciting events of the day. Firm, consistent limits are needed when toddlers try stalling tactics such as asking for one more drink of water.

Bedtime protests may be reduced by warning the child a few minutes before it is time for bed. Winding down with a quiet activity for 30 minutes before bedtime also helps toddlers to prepare for sleep. Bedtime offers an opportunity for some snuggle time, when the parent and toddler can read a story and share the events of the day. Children of this age often have trouble relaxing and falling asleep. A warm bath before bedtime promotes relaxation. Bedtime rituals are important and should be followed consistently. Transition objects, such as a favorite blanket or stuffed animal, are often an important part of the child's bedtime routine.

Toilet Training

Control of elimination is one of the major tasks of toddlerhood. Successful toilet training depends on the readiness of both the child and the parent. The parent must be willing to spend the necessary time and emotional energy to encourage the child on a daily basis.

> Toilet training is one of the most frustrating and time-consuming tasks that parents face. It can be so frustrating for some that researchers have linked toilet training accidents with many cases of child abuse. Parents who do not understand normal growth and development patterns often have unrealistic expectations and can become frustrated to the point of rage.

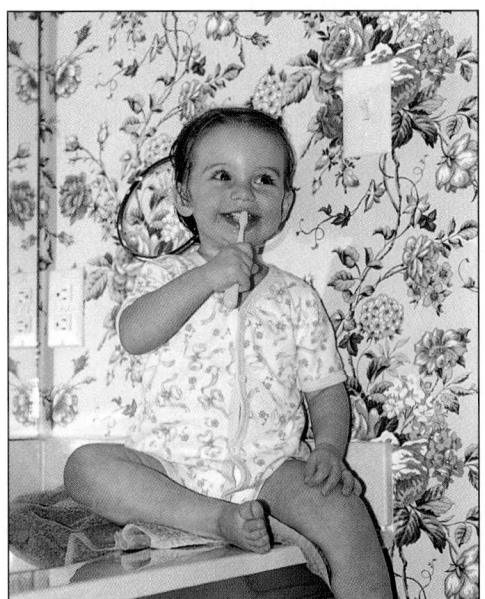

◀ Care of the deciduous teeth promotes healthy development of the permanent teeth. Because 2-year-olds lack the manual dexterity to adequately remove plaque, parents must assume responsibility for cleaning the toddler's teeth.

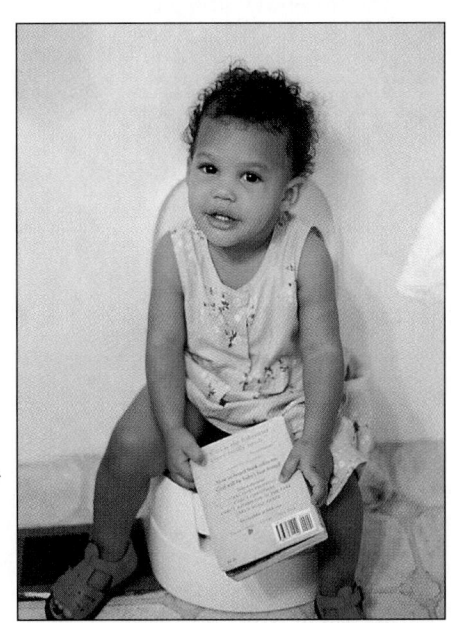

There are no set rules or timetables for toilet training. The nurse can help parents to understand that both physical and psychologic readiness are necessary for success. ▶

Figure 5–2

Health promotion for the toddler and family.

The nurse can assist parents by explaining developmental milestones and encouraging parents not to begin training until the child shows signs of readiness. Helping the parent recognize factors that interfere with toilet training, such as stress, can make the training easier. The parent may not have the necessary reserves of patience and energy for toilet training during stressful times, such as near the birth of another child or while moving to a new house. Training may be easier if it is postponed until routines return to normal.

The nurse can assist parents in toilet training the toddler by explaining the importance of maturation to successful toilet training. Parents need to know that both physical and psychologic readiness are necessary for toilet training to be successful. Myelinization of the spinal cord, which usually occurs between 12 and 18 months, must be complete before the child can voluntarily control bowel and bladder sphincters. The nurse can offer anticipatory guidance to parents by teaching them the signs that the toddler is ready for toilet training (see box, Signs of Readiness for Toilet Training). The average toddler is not ready for toilet training to begin until 18 to 24 months of age. Waiting until the child is 24 to 30 months old makes the task considerably easier because toddlers of this age are less negative and usually are more willing to control their sphincters to please their parents.

There are no set rules or timetables for toilet training. The age at which toilet training is usually begun varies from culture to culture. Bowel control is usually achieved before bladder control. Daytime bladder control occurs before nighttime bladder control. A relaxed, child-centered approach is most successful, with plenty of praise for each success. Punishment and coercive techniques cause feelings of shame and lead to power struggles. The child should never be forced to sit on the potty for long periods. Successful toilet training is a gradual process, and relapses must be expected. Accidents often occur when children are too busy playing to notice a full bladder until it is too late. Many children cannot remain completely dry until the age of 3 years. Parents should respond to accidents with tolerance instead of scolding or shaming the child.

Signs of Readiness for Toilet Training

PHYSICAL READINESS

Ability to remove clothing
Willingness to let go of a toy when asked
Ability to sit, squat, and walk well
Has been walking for 1 year

PSYCHOLOGIC READINESS

Ability to notice if his diaper is wet
May indicate that he wants to be changed by pulling on his diaper, squatting, or repeating a word or phrase
Ability to communicate a need to go to the bathroom or ability to get there on his own
Desire to please his parent by staying dry

Discipline

Toddlers need and want discipline to feel secure. They have little control over their behavior and need limits to learn how to behave and how to follow the rules and expectations of society. Toddlers' negativism, intense emotions, and curiosity place them at risk for injury. Because they are usually unaware of the consequences of their actions, vigilance and limits are needed for safety. Toddlers are frightened by a lack of limits and will deliberately test their parents until they are shown how far they can go. Firm discipline promotes the development of autonomy by giving the child a feeling of freedom within bounds.

The goal of discipline and limit setting is to teach self-control. Eventually the child internalizes controls established by parental limits and begins to develop a conscience. Toddlers often repeat parental prohibitions to themselves while engaging in a forbidden activity. For example, a toddler may walk over to an electric outlet, knowing that it is out of bounds, and mumble, "No, no, hurt!" as he plays with the outlet. Although the toddler remembers the prohibition, he lacks sufficient self-control to prevent the behavior.

Effective discipline techniques for children of this age include time-out (1 minute per year of age), diversion, and positive reinforcement. Physical punishment, such as spanking, is one of the least effective discipline techniques (see Chapter 16). Guidelines for disciplining toddlers are listed on the following page.

Temper Tantrums

Temper tantrums are a common toddler response to anger and frustration and often result from thwarted attempts at mastery and autonomy. Tantrums may also occur as an emotional release of tension after a long, tiring day. Unable to express anger in more productive ways because of limited language and reasoning abilities, toddlers may react by screaming, kicking, throwing things, or even biting themselves or banging their heads. Tantrums occur more often when toddlers are tired, hungry, bored, or excessively stimulated.

The nurse can help parents by identifying strategies to decrease the frequency of tantrums. Limiting situations

TEACHING GUIDELINES *for Disciplining a Toddler*

- Discipline must be consistent. Inconsistency is confusing and counterproductive. It is important to follow through every time.
- Discipline must be immediate. Consequences of behavior should occur as soon as possible after it occurs. Threats such as "Just wait until your father gets home!" are confusing and ineffective for a child of this age.
- Discipline must be realistic and age-appropriate. Toddlers should not be expected to act like "little ladies" or "little gentlemen."
- Discipline must be related to the incident. Consequences that are logical results of a behavior are most effective.
- Limits must be clearly explained to the child.
- Toddlers must be given time to respond to instructions.
- Withdrawal of love should never be used as punishment. Comforting the child after discipline promotes positive feelings. Love is the key to effective discipline.
- Arguments and extensive explanations should be avoided.
- Praise for good behavior should be used to build self-confidence and self-esteem.
- The toddler must be separated from the behavior ("I love you very much. Hitting your sister needs to stop.").

that are too much for the child to handle is helpful. Anticipating periods of fatigue, having a snack ready before the child gets too hungry, and offering the toddler choices when possible can minimize temper tantrums. Parental practices such as inconsistency, permissiveness, excessive strictness, and overprotectiveness increase the probability of tantrums.

Toddlers need appropriate and consistent limits. Letting the child know that temper tantrums will not be tolerated gives her a sense of security. The intensity of a toddler's outburst almost seems to be a plea for someone to stop her. Probably the most effective method for handling tantrums is to isolate and ignore the child. The child should learn that nothing is gained from a tantrum, not even attention. Giving in to the child's demands or scolding the child only increases the behavior. Toddlers stop using tantrums when they do not achieve their goals and as their verbal skills increase. Once the tantrum has subsided and the toddler has regained some self-control, the parent should comfort the child by letting her know that limits are necessary and that she is loved. Acknowledging the child's angry feelings and rewarding more mature ways of expressing them help the child to gain self-control.

Sibling Rivalry

Often toddlers have intense feelings of jealousy and envy toward a new infant sibling. Toddlers' egocentrism makes it difficult for them to understand that a parent can love more than one child at a time. Toddlers respond to a new sibling in various ways, depending on the child's personality, age, and interests (Murphy, 1993).

The nurse who helps parents to understand normal toddler behavior in response to separation can help parents to cope with the frustrations of this transition. Sharing parents' love and attention is difficult for most toddlers. Because the infant requires a great deal of time and attention, the toddler's routine is disrupted. Because a toddler has limited resources to cope with such stress, she may react by treating the baby roughly, damaging property, or harming pets. The toddler may seem to regress by asking for a bottle or pacifier, or by using baby talk. Recent research has explained such behavior as a form of imitation rather than **regression** (reversion to a younger level of maturity). Such behavior may be an attempt to find out what it feels like to be a baby and has been associated with more positive sibling relationships later on (Stewart, 1990).

The nurse may counsel parents about strategies to decrease sibling rivalry, such as including the toddler in preparations for the new baby. Explaining to the toddler what new babies are like, letting him feel the fetus move, and reading picture books about new siblings can ease the child's transition to the role of older sibling. Talking about changes that the newborn might create and acknowledging the older child's feelings about these changes also can improve the toddler's ability to cope. Referring to the baby as "ours" decreases the child's feelings of exclusion. Any changes, such as moving the toddler to a new bedroom or beginning daycare, should be made as far in advance as possible so that the toddler will not feel displaced by abrupt changes when the baby arrives. Sibling preparation classes, offered by many hospitals, decrease the signs of sibling rivalry. When the mother and infant come home from the hospital, the mother's first concern should be greeting the older sibling and letting him know how much she missed him. The father or another caregiver should carry the newborn, allowing the mother's arms to be free to hug the waiting toddler. A toddler's jealous feelings can become intense when visitors lavish gifts and praise on the baby. These feelings can be minimized by giving an inexpensive gift to the toddler each time the baby receives one. Visitors should be encouraged to pay attention to the older child as well as the baby. Parents should anticipate behavior changes, even if the toddler has been prepared for the arrival of a new baby.

The most important strategy for decreasing sibling rivalry is to affirm the older child's individuality and to let him know that he is loved as much as he was before. Planned, uninterrupted, private time is important to maintain feelings of closeness between parent and toddler. Even 10 or 15 minutes a day while the baby is sleeping is valuable. Allowing the toddler to choose an activity for this time with the parent makes it even more special. This special time should be given to the child each day, regardless of his behavior.

With the increased workload of a second child, fathers often become more involved in child care and household tasks (Murphy, 1993). Fathers play an important role in the toddler's adjustment to a new sibling. Research has shown that greater involvement by the father is associated with positive sibling–infant relationships (Kreppner, 1990).

It is important to help toddlers to recognize and identify negative feelings toward a new sibling. Firm limits must be set, however, if the toddler tries to harm the baby. The child may be told that it's okay to feel jealous, but it's not okay to hurt the baby. Praise should be given for affectionate, cooperative behavior.

Parents should give the older child plenty of attention and affection, letting him know that he is loved for who he is. Shaming, ridiculing, or punishing may reinforce angry and regressive behaviors.

With plenty of affection and understanding, the toddler gradually learns to share parental attention. A relationship between the toddler and the newborn develops gradually. Within the context of family interaction, the child learns caring, mutual respect, and effective ways of relating to others (Murphy, 1993).

Dental Care

Most toddlers have a complete set of 20 deciduous teeth by the time they are 30 months of age. Although the exact time of eruption of teeth varies, an approximate rule of thumb to assess the number of teeth is the age of the toddler in months minus 6. Usually, one tooth erupts for each month of age past 6 months up to 30 months of age.

Permanent teeth are calcifying during the toddler period, long before they are visible. Proper care of the deciduous teeth is crucial for the toddler's general health and for the health and alignment of the permanent teeth. Deciduous teeth play an important role in the growth and development of the jaws and face and in speech development. Premature loss of the deciduous teeth complicates eruption of the permanent teeth, often leading to malocclusion. It is the nurse's role to teach parents the importance of preventing tooth decay in toddlers. Many parents do not understand the value of preserving primary teeth. Dental **caries** (tooth decay) are preventable and should not occur if parents are given and follow appropriate guidelines.

Proper dental care includes adequate cleaning, removal of plaque, use of fluoride (Table 5–3), good nutrition, and regular dental checkups. Because toddlers do not have the manual dexterity to adequately remove plaque, parents must assume complete responsibility for cleaning their teeth. The child can be encouraged to brush her teeth after they have been thoroughly cleaned by a parent. Because toddlers like to imitate, watching parents brush their teeth can be motivating. A small, soft nylon-bristle brush works best. Optimum access and visibility are provided if the parent sits on the floor or bed with the child's head in the parent's lap and the child's body perpendicular to the parent's. This position also gives the parent some control of the child's head movement. Toothpaste is not recommended for young children because they often do not like the taste or, if they do, tend to swallow it. If the child receives fluoride from other sources, such as water or supplements, excess amounts of fluoride may be ingested if fluoride toothpaste is swallowed. Ingestion of excessive amounts of

TABLE 5–3 *Fluoride Supplementation Schedule for Infants and Children**

	FLUORIDE CONCENTRATION IN WATER SUPPLY (ppm)		
AGE	**<0.3**	**0.3–0.7**	**>0.7**
0–2 yr	0.25 mg/day	0 mg/day	0 mg/day
2–3 yr	0.50 mg/day	0.25 mg/day	0 mg/day
3–16 yr	1.00 mg/day	0.50 mg/day	0 mg/day

*Milligrams of fluoride supplement per day. Supplementation should begin in the first 2 weeks after birth.

From American Academy of Pediatrics, Committee on Nutrition. (1986). Fluoride supplementation. *Pediatrics, 77,* 758–761.

TABLE 5–4 *Health Screening, Health Maintenance, and Anticipatory Guidance for Toddlers*

15 MONTHS	18 MONTHS	30 MONTHS
Immunization		
OPV #3 (or #4), MMR #1. Routine TB skin test. DTP #4 is given 6–12 months after the third dose. Varicella vaccine (12–18 months). HbV #3 (6–18 months). Hib #4 (12–15 months).	DTP #4 if not given at 15 months.	
Safety		
Toddler car seat. Supervise child near water. Keep poisons and sharp objects locked up and out of child's reach. Do not leave child unattended in bathtub. Cover electric outlets. Supervise child near stove, fireplace.	Supervise child at playgrounds. Protect child from falling. Supervise child around pets: teach her not to approach strange dogs. Keep poison control center number and syrup of ipecac available in home.	Supervise child near outdoor hazard (street, swimming pools, garages, power tools, pesticides). Never leave child unattended in the car. Use sunscreen. Provide safe toys.
Nutrition		
Limit milk intake to 24–32 oz/day. Do not give bottle as a substitute for solid foods. Feeding: offer finger foods, cup.	Physiologic anorexia. Do not force child to eat. Recognize ritualistic needs. Toddlers often go on food jags.	Serve small portions. Child needs approximately 1300 calories per day. Avoid cariogenic foods.
Vision and Hearing		
Ask parents if child seems to hear and see well. Child should localize sounds. Child should accurately visualize small objects (i.e., raisins) Perform Hirschberg's light reflex test for overt strabismus.	Assess speech and language. Ear infections may affect hearing.	Assess speech and language. Two-thirds of child's speech should be intelligible. Perform audiometric hearing screening (with parental practice beforehand). Perform HOTV vision test (with parental practice beforehand). Perform Hirschberg's light reflex test for overt strabismus, cover test for latent strabismus.
Dental Care		
Brush and floss twice daily with help from parents. Use fluoridated water or supplements. Do not allow child to have a bottle in bed.	Limit concentrated sweets.	First visit to dentist should occur when all primary teeth have erupted.
Screening		
Monitor growth trajectory for deviations as indicated on growth chart. Evaluate hematocrit if not done at 9 months.	Screen for hypertension, iron deficiency anemia.	Screen for elevated cholesterol and triglyceride levels if family history of obesity, cardiovascular disease, or elevated cholesterol levels are present.
Teaching and Counseling		
Discuss limit-setting, discipline. Assess child's readiness for toilet training: suggest waiting if possible. Reassure parents that negativism will pass.	Assess readiness for toilet training. Discuss negativism and ways to handle it.	Toilet training: nighttime wetting and daytime accidents are common. Discuss possible night fears; warn parents that these may soon appear. Discuss discipline (consistency, positive techniques).

Abbreviations: HbV, hepatitis B virus vaccine; DTP, diphtheria and tetanus toxoids and pertussis vaccine; HiB, "Hemophilus influenzae" type B conjugate vaccine; OPV, oral poliovirus vaccine; MMR, measles, mumps, and rubella; TB, tuberculosis.

fluoride may lead to fluorosis, which produces white speckles or brown discoloration of the enamel. Toddlers should not be allowed to chew on toothpaste tubes because they may contain lead. Ideally, teeth should be brushed after every meal and especially at bedtime. Flossing between teeth helps remove plaque and should be done daily by the parent after the toddler's teeth are brushed.

Fluoride makes tooth enamel resistant to acid attack, preventing decay. Fluoride supplementation should begin early in infancy if drinking water is not fluoridated (see Chapter 4). The fluoride dosage should be adjusted at age 2 and again at age 3 (see Table 5–3).

A diet that is low in sweets and high in nutritious food promotes dental health. Sweets are most likely to cause caries if they are sticky or if they are eaten between meals rather than with meals. Nutritious snacks, such as fresh fruit, yogurt, or cheese, should be offered instead of candy, soda, or cookies.

The first dental visit should be made 6 months after the first primary tooth erupts and no later than 30 months of age. The first appointment should be made before any dental work needs to be done so that the visit is enjoyable and free from discomfort. This visit provides an opportunity for early assessment of the child's dental health as well as for teaching parents good preventive dental health practices.

> A toddler should never be allowed to fall asleep with a bottle because of the risk of bottle mouth caries (see Chapter 4). If a bottle is allowed in bed, it should contain only water.

KEY CONCEPTS

- Toddlerhood is characterized by the struggle for autonomy as the child develops a sense of herself as separate from the parent. The Eriksonian task for the toddler is autonomy versus shame and doubt.
- The combination of increased motor skills, immaturity, and lack of experience places the toddler at risk for accidental injury. Anticipatory guidance about childproofing the home is an essential nursing role.
- The slower physical growth rate of the toddler creates a relatively smaller demand for calories and decreased appetite (physiologic anorexia).
- Toddler behavior is characterized by negativism, ritualism, and egocentrism.
- Toddlers require approximately 12 to 14 hours of sleep.
- Nurses can help parents with toilet training by explaining the signs of physical and psychologic readiness. Readiness depends on myelinization of the nerve pathways that enable the child to control bowel and bladder sphincters.
- Firm, consistent discipline helps toddlers to learn self-control. Effective discipline techniques include time-out, diversion, and positive reinforcement.
- Sibling rivalry can be minimized with techniques such as including the toddler in preparations for the new baby, acknowledging the toddler's negative feelings while setting appropriate limits, and affirming the toddler as special and loved.
- Proper care of deciduous teeth is crucial for the child's general health and for the health and alignment of permanent teeth. Nurses should teach parents the importance of good oral hygiene, fluoride supplementation, good nutrition, and regular dental checkups.

REFERENCES

American Academy of Pediatric Dentistry. (1992). *Recommendations for preventive dental care.* Chicago: Author.

American Academy of Pediatrics, Committee on Nutrition. (1986). Fluoride supplementation. *Pediatrics, 77,* 758–761.

Bhatia, M. S., Dhar, P. K., & Singhal, V. R. (1990). Temper tantrums. *Clinical Pediatrics, 29*(6), 311–315.

Christopherson, E. R. (1992). Discipline. *Pediatric Clinics of North America, 39*(3), 395–411.

Christopherson, E. R. (1991). Oppositional behavior in children. *Pediatric Annals, 20*(5), 267–273.

Christopherson, E. R. (1991). Toileting problems in children. *Pediatric Annals, 20*(5), 240–244.

Forrester, D. J. (1978). Preventive aspects of dental care. In R. A. Hoekelman, et al. (Eds.), *Principles of pediatrics.* New York: McGraw-Hill.

Fortier, J. C., Carson, V. B., Will, S., & Shubkagel, B. L. (1991). Adjustment to a newborn: Sibling preparation makes a difference. *Journal of Gynecologic and Neonatal Nursing, 20*(1), 73–79.

Greenspan, S. I. (1991). Clinical assessment of emotional milestones in infancy and early childhood. *Pediatric Clinics of North America, 38*(6), 1371–1385.

Leung, A. K. C., & Fagan, J. E. (1991). Temper tantrums. *American Family Physician, 44*(2), 559–563.

Murphy, S. O. (1993). Siblings and the new baby: Changing perspectives. *Journal of Pediatric Nursing, 8*(5), 277–288.
Nelms, B. C. (1993). Discipline: What do you recommend? *Journal of Pediatric Health Care, 7*(1), 1–2.
Rapin, I. (1993). Hearing disorders. *Pediatrics in Review, 14*(2), 43–49.
Ripa, L. W. (1991, Winter). A critique of topical fluoride methods (dentifrices, mouth rinses, operator and self-applied gels) in an era of decreased caries and increased fluorosis prevalence. *Journal of Public Health Dentistry, 51,* 23–41.
Robson, W. L., & Leung, A. K. (1991). Advising parents on toilet training. *American Family Practice, 44*(4), 1263–1266.
Spadt, S. K., Martin, K. R., & Thomas, A. M. (1990). Experiential classes for siblings-to-be. *MCN: The American Journal of Maternal Child Nursing, 15,* 184–186.

BIBLIOGRAPHY

Advocacy for Head Start and children's dental health: Report of a workshop conducted by the National Dental Association. (1978). Washington, DC: U.S. Department of Health, Education and Welfare, Public Health Service, Health Services Administration, Bureau of Community Health Services.
Anderberg, G. J. (1988). Initial acquaintance and attachment behavior of siblings with the newborn. *Journal of Obstetric, Gynecologic, and Neonatal Nursing, 17*(1), 49–54.
Brazelton, T. B. (1974). *Toddlers and parents: A declaration of independence.* Lawrence, NY: Delacorte Press.
Calladine, C., & Calladine, A. (1979). *Raising siblings: A sane and sensible approach to raising brothers and sisters without raising the roof.* New York: Delacorte Press.
Castiglia, P. T. (1987). Speech-language development. *Journal of Pediatric Health Care, 1*(3), 165–167.
Decayed, Missing, and Filled Teeth Among Persons 1–74 Years: United States. (1981). Washington, DC: U.S. Department of Health and Human Services, Public Health Service, Office of Health Research, Statistics, and Technology, National Center for Health Statistics.
Demetras, M., Post, K., & Snow, C. (1986). Feedback to first language learners: The role of repetitions and clarification questions. *Journal of Child Language, 13,* 275–292.
Doleys, D., & Dolce, J. (1982). Toilet training and enuresis. *Pediatric Clinics of North America, 29,* 297–307.
Dunn, J., & Kendrick, C., (1982). *Siblings: Love, envy and understanding.* Cambridge, MA: Harvard University Press.
Ferber, R. (1987). Circadian and schedule disturbances. In C. Guilleminault (Ed.), *Sleep and its disorders in children.* New York: Raven Press.
Fraiberg, S. H. (1968). *The magic years: Understanding and handling the problems of early childhood.* London: Methuen.
Hakuta, K., & Garcia, E. (1989). Bilingualism and education. *American Psychologist, 44,* 374–379.
Horner, M., & McClellan, M. (1981). Toilet training: Ready or not? *Pediatric Nursing, 7,* 15–18.
Ingram, D. (1989). *First language acquisition: Method, description and explanation.* New York: Cambridge University Press.
Jacobbi, M. (1987). Ten ways to help your kids become friends. *McCalls, 145*(6), 57.
Kohlberg, L. (1966). A cognitive developmental analysis of children's sex-role concepts and attitudes. In E. E. Maccoby (Ed.), *The development of sex differences.* Stanford, CA: Stanford University Press.
Kreppner, K. (1990, April). *Father participation in family socialization during the first two years after a second child's arrival.* Paper presented at the Seventh International Conference on Infant Studies, Montreal, Canada.
McCormick, K. F. (1992). Attitudes of primary care physicians toward corporal punishment. *JAMA, 267,* 3161–3165.
McIntosh, B. (1989). Spoiled child syndrome. *Pediatrics, 83,* 108–121.
Reich, P. A. (1986). *Language development.* Englewood Cliffs, NJ: Prentice-Hall.
Rosemond, J. K. (1987). And baby makes four: Preparing your first child for the second. *Better Homes and Gardens, 65*(1), 38.
Rubin, N. (1986). Mom and dad always liked you better. *Parents, 61*(6), 86–92.
Sande, D. R., & Billingsley, C. S. (1985). Language development in infants and toddlers. *Nurse Practitioner, 10*(9), 39–47.
Snow, C. (1989). Understanding social interaction and language acquisition: Sentences are not enough. In M. Bornstein & J. Bruner (Eds.), *Interaction in human development.* Hillsdale, NJ: Erlbaum.
Stewart, R. B. (1990). *The second child: Family transition and adjustment.* Newbury Park, CA: Sage.
Sweet, P. T. (1979). Prenatal classes especially for children. *MCN: The American Journal of Maternal Child Nursing, 4,* 82.
Tomasello, M., & Farrar, M. (1986). Joint attention and early language. *Child Development, 57,* 1454–1463.
White, B. L. (1985). *The first three years of life.* New York: Prentice-Hall.
Whitehurst, G., & Valdez-Menchaca, M. (1988). What is the role of reinforcement in early language acquisition? *Child Development, 59,* 430–440.

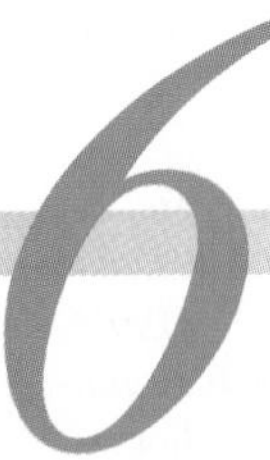

The Preschool Child

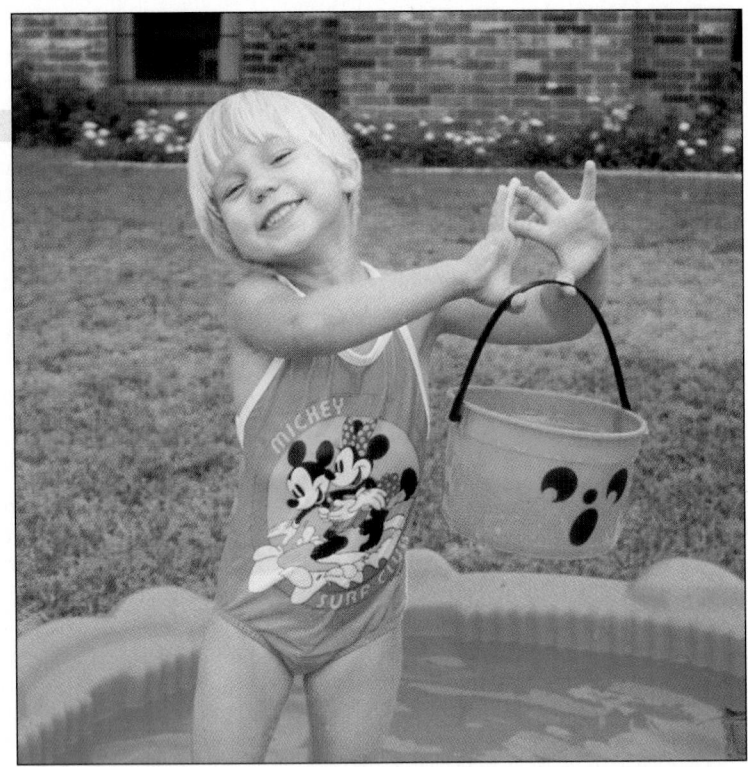

CHAPTER OVERVIEW

LEARNING OBJECTIVES

After studying this chapter, you should be able to:

- Identify normal physical, motor, psychosocial, moral, and cognitive development in preschool children.
- Describe the nursing assessment of the preschool child's development.
- Identify strategies for dealing with a preschool child's fears and sleep problems.
- Provide parents with anticipatory guidance for preventive dental care for the preschool child.
- Discuss guidelines for selecting daycare facilities.
- Offer parents suggestions for promoting school readiness in the preschool child.

KEY TERMS

animism: attributing lifelike characteristics to inanimate objects

centration: tendency to focus on only one aspect of an event or object rather than all aspects

irreversibility: inability to understand a process in reverse or to mentally undo an action that has been performed

symbolic thought: ability to allow a mental image (word or object) to represent something else that is not present

transductive reasoning: reasoning from the particular to the particular rather than from the general to the particular

The preschool period, from ages 3 through 5 years, is a time of relative tranquility after the tumultuous toddler period. The preschooler becomes increasingly independent, mastering many self-care and motor skills and developing greater social and emotional maturity. The preschooler is imaginative, creative, and curious. Many parents describe this period as their favorite age as they watch the dramatic transformation of a chubby toddler into an agile, articulate child who is ready to enter the world of peers and school.

The nurse's roles as health-care provider, family counselor, and child advocate continue during the preschool years. Well-child checkups provide the nurse with opportunities for anticipatory guidance related to safety and nutrition. The nurse can also address some of the common concerns of parents with preschoolers: limit setting, day care, and preparation for school.

GROWTH AND DEVELOPMENT OF THE PRESCHOOL CHILD

Growth and development of the preschooler is summarized in Table 6–1.

Physical Growth and Development

Growth of the preschool child is slow and steady. Height and weight gain is minimal during this period. Average weight gain is about 5 pounds per year, and height gain averages 2 to 3 inches per year. The child attains half of his adult height between the ages of 2 and 3 years. During this time, growth occurs more rapidly in the legs than in the trunk, accumulation of adipose tissue declines, and the child's appetite decreases. As a result, the preschooler loses the potbellied appearance of the toddler, becoming slimmer and more agile. Muscles grow faster than bones during the preschool period. Muscle strength is influenced by nutrition, genetic makeup, and opportunity to exercise and use the muscles. Knock-knees are common in 3-year-olds and are often associated with occasional stumbling and falling. Maturation of the knee and hip joints usually corrects this problem by age 4 or 5 years.

As lungs grow, vital capacity increases and respiratory rate slows. Respirations remain primarily diaphragmatic until age 5 or 6. Heart rate decreases and blood pressure increases as the heart increases in size (see the inside front cover for vital sign ranges). Cardiovascular maturation enables the preschooler to engage in more sustained and strenuous activity.

All 20 deciduous teeth are present by the age of 3. Deciduous teeth may begin to fall out at the end of the preschool period. The first permanent teeth to erupt, the back molars, usually appear in the early school-age years.

Motor Development

Coordination and muscle strength increase rapidly between the ages of 3 and 5. Increase in brain size and nerve myelinization enable the child to perfect fine and gross motor skills.

Motor abilities vary widely among children. Although motor skill is less influenced by environment than other areas of development, such as language, opportunities to practice may contribute to better motor skills. For example, a 4-year-old who often plays catch with a sibling or parent generally finds playing Little League baseball as a 7-year-old easier than a child without similar experience. Research shows that because of inadequate exercise, preschoolers today score lower on muscle strength, cardiovascular endurance, and body leanness than children 20 years ago (Gallahue, 1990, as cited in Poest et al., 1990).

Handedness begins to emerge at about 3 years of age and is usually clearly established by age 4. The nurse should encourage parents to provide left-handed children

TABLE 6–1 *Summary of Growth and Development: The Preschool Child*

PHYSICAL	MOTOR	PSYCHOSOCIAL	SENSORY/COGNITIVE	LANGUAGE/COMMUNICATION
3 Years Appears taller and thinner as body contours change. Growth occurs more in limbs than in trunk. Average growth 2–3 inches (6–8 cm) per year. Average weight gain 4–5 lb (1.8–2.3 kg) per year. Average weight 32 lb (14.6 kg). Average height 37.25 inches (95 cm). 20 teeth present.	**Gross:** Pedals tricycle. Goes up stairs (alternating feet) without holding on. Jumps from bottom step. Stands briefly on one foot. Walks well on uneven surfaces. Can walk a straight line. Walks backward. Throws ball with one hand. Catches large ball with both hands. **Fine:** Copies circle; copies cross. Draws a person with three parts (usually a circle with eyes). Can cut on a straight line with scissors. Strings large beads. Builds a tower of 10 cubes. Builds a bridge with three cubes.	Curious and energetic. Increasingly independent. Imitates role models. Wants to please. Thrives on routine. Bedtime rituals are important. Jealous of siblings. Play is parallel and associative. Understands turn-taking and is capable of sharing, but does not always want to share. Occasional feelings of guilt and shame. Fears of the dark, animals, shadows, and strangers. Feeds self well. Can go to the toilet without help; usually stays dry at night. Can wash and dry hands; brush teeth; dress self completely, except for back buttons. Puts shoes on. Can help with simple household tasks (dusting, picking up toys, setting the table). Sexual curiosity is common. May masturbate, knows sex differences and own sex.	Preconceptual phase. Egocentric in thought and actions (cannot appreciate another's viewpoint). Magical thinking; shifts between reality and imagination. Animism (believes anything that moves is alive). Lacks reversibility. Has an attention span of 10 minutes. Has a slight understanding of past and future, but tomorrow and yesterday are still confusing. Thinks illogically. Understands simple reasoning. Sense of humor. Follows simple directions.	Talks incessantly whether anyone is listening or not. Uses telegraphic speech. Constantly asks how and why questions. Speaks in sentences of three to four words. Vocabulary of 300–900 words. Uses pronouns (I, me, you). Talks to himself. Understands spatial relationships (in, on, under). Knows functions of common objects. Can count three objects. Can tell her full name, age, and sex.
4 Years Growth rate similar to previous year. Average weight 36.75 lb (16.7 kg). Average height 40.5 inches (103 cm). Birth length doubles.	**Gross:** Very active; constantly on the go. Runs well. Can catch and throw ball overhand. Jumps and climbs well. Swings. Goes up and down stairs without holding on. Hops on one foot. Heel-toe walks. **Fine:** Copies a square. Tries to print letters. Draws a person with two to four parts. Can cut on a curved line with scissors. Handedness is usually established.	Increasingly independent. Separates more easily from parent. Play is associative; cooperates with other children, but less likely to share than 3-year-old. May have an imaginary friend. Still jealous of siblings, but beginning to work through jealousy. Dresses and undresses himself. Can button front and side of clothes, but needs	Intuitive thought stage. Beginning to be less egocentric, but still unable to take another's point of view. Highly imaginative. Still believes that thoughts cause events. Lacks reversibility. Has an attention span of 20 minutes. Improved understanding of time (tomorrow, this afternoon, next week). Can name one or more colors.	Constantly asks questions. Vocabulary of 1500 words. Speaks in sentences of four to five words. Tells stories mixing reality and fantasy. Uses "I" frequently. Counts to 5. Understands same and different. Knows days of the week. Stuttering fairly common (normal language variation).

		help with zippers. Can lace shoes, but not tie them. Can brush teeth and bathe herself. Bossy, name-calling. Boasts, brags, and exaggerates. May use profanity to get attention. May "run away from home." Increased ability to think without acting out; anticipates events. Sexual curiosity and exploration is common. Identifies with opposite-sex parent.	Can complete an 8- to 10-piece puzzle. Has difficulty distinguishing reality from fantasy.	
5 Years Average weight 41.25 lb (18.7 kg). Average height 43.25 inches (110 cm). May begin to lose deciduous teeth. First permanent teeth (molars) may erupt.	**Gross:** Runs with more control and power. Throws and catches a ball well. Stands on one foot (10 seconds). Able to skip, roller skate, swing on a swing, and hit a ball with a bat. Can jump rope. Hops on either foot. **Fine:** Copies a triangle or diamond. Draws a person with a body and six parts. Prints first name and some letters. Cuts out simple shapes with scissors. Hits a nail on the head with a hammer.	Increasingly independent. Gets along well with parents. Industrious and proud of accomplishments. Play is associative; likes rules, but may cheat to win. More generous with toys. Less imaginative, more realistic. Daydreams. Less argumentative and rebellious. Responsible; values rules. Fewer fears. Protective of younger siblings. May show tension by biting nails, picking nose, or whining. Aware of cultural differences. Dresses without help. Can tie shoelaces. Can put toys away neatly. Pours from a small pitcher. Spreads butter with a knife; can cut own meat. Identifies with same-sex parent and enjoys doing things together.	Beginning to understand others' viewpoints. Has an attention span of 30 minutes. Lacks reversibility. Better understanding of time. Can name four or more colors. Can count 10 or more objects. May do simple addition, but cannot subtract. Can name a penny, nickel, and dime.	Asks questions and the meaning of words. Vocabulary of 2100 words. Speaks in sentences of more than five words. Uses all parts of speech. Can define simple words by describing their use or shape. May use fantasy in stories, but is aware of distortions made. Counts to 10. Understands basic number concepts. Recalls parts of a story. Follows three-part commands. Knows the days of the week, seasons. Knows his name and address.

◀ As the brain matures, the preschool child's motor development matures. Opportunities for practice contribute to the development of motor skills. (Courtesy of Cook Children's Medical Center, Fort Worth, Texas)

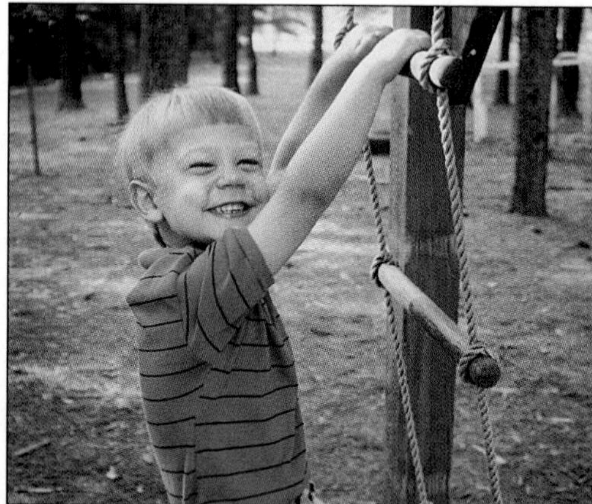

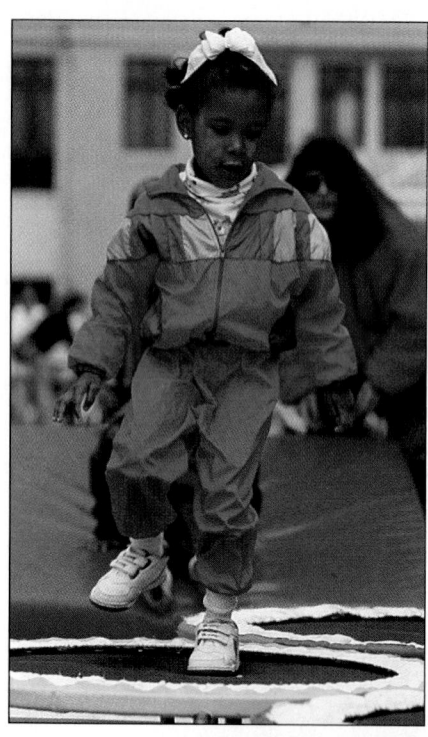

◀ The 4-year-old's motor development has increased to the point where he can jump and climb well. The 4-year-old can also throw a ball overhand and cut on a curved line with scissors.

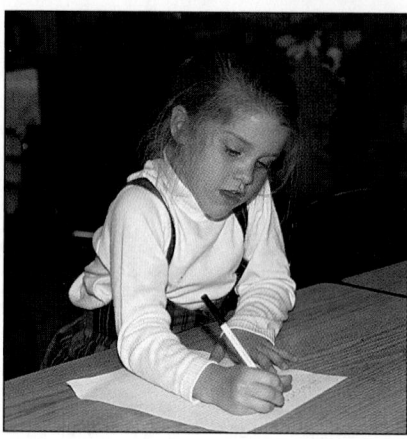

◀ This 5-year-old is printing her name in readable letters. Children of this age can usually skip and can both throw and catch a ball (Courtesy of University of Texas at Arlington School of Nursing, Arlington, Texas)

Figure 6–1
Growth and development of the preschooler.

with appropriate tools, particularly left-handed scissors. Left-handed children should not be forced to use their right hand because coordination is usually better when using the dominant side. Eye–hand coordination is usually good enough by age 5 for a child to hit a nail on the head with a hammer. Increased coordination allows the child to perform many self-care skills and to become more independent.

By age 4 or 5, the child is independent and can dress herself, eat, and go to the bathroom without help (see Table 6–1). Unlike the toddler, who must be restrained to avoid injury, the older preschooler can usually be trusted to heed verbal warnings of danger.

Cognitive and Sensory Development

By 3 years of age, the brain is two-thirds of its adult size. Maturation of the central nervous system contributes to the child's increasing cognitive abilities.

According to Piaget, the preschool child is in the preoperational stage of cognitive development. This stage is divided into two phases, the preconceptual phase (2–4 years) and the intuitive phase (4–7 years). During the preconceptual phase, the child is beginning to use **symbolic thought,** the ability to allow a mental image (words or ideas) to represent objects or ideas. Mental symbols allow the child to remember the past and to describe events that happened in the past. The 3-year-old can retain a mental image of a loved one and can periodically "refuel" by thinking about that person. A photograph can help some children to cope with separation by bridging the gap between physical presence and mental image. The preschooler's ability to remember the parent and to recognize that his needs can be met even though the parent is not present increases the child's ability to tolerate separation.

Because preschoolers still engage in **animism,** they often endow inanimate objects with lifelike qualities during play. A doll may become a crying baby, or a teddy bear may become a friend who listens sympathetically. Symbolic play is important for emotional development because it allows the child to work through distressing feelings. For this reason, it is therapeutic to allow a child to play with medical equipment after a painful procedure. A 4-year-old who has received an injection may be found working out her feelings by giving her doll "lots of shots."

During the preconceptual phase, reality may be distorted by **transductive reasoning.** The preschool child reasons from particular to particular, rather than from particular to general and vice versa, as adults do. The child cannot understand that relationships exist and cannot view the whole in relation to its parts. The preschool child has difficulty focusing on the important aspects of a situation. To a child, everything is important and interdependent. This type of thinking is called field dependency. For example, the preschooler may have difficulty falling asleep at night because the parent did not follow the usual bedtime routine. Objects, routine, and sameness are important to the preschool child. Rituals provide the preschool child with a feeling of control.

In a 3-year-old, logic is immature. This incomplete understanding is part of the reason for the preschooler's concern over body integrity. For example, a 3-year-old boy who sees a little girl undressed may believe that she has lost her penis and that the same thing may happen to him (Howard, 1990).

The intuitive phase is characterized by centration and lack of reversibility. **Centration** is the tendency to center or focus on one part of a situation and ignore the other parts. The child cannot understand logical relationships and is unable to focus on more than one aspect of a situation at a time. For example, the child may not be able to follow a sequence of directions, but will perform well if the directions are given one at a time.

The 4- or 5-year-old shows **irreversibility** in thought. The child cannot reverse a process or the order of events. He may be able to take a complex puzzle apart, but may have difficulty putting it back together. Likewise, the child might understand that two identical glasses contain the same amount of water. However, if the water in one of the glasses is poured into a third container of a different shape, the child will believe that the third container holds a different amount of water. The child will not realize that if the water is poured back into the original glass, the glass will contain the original amount. The 4- or 5-year old also lacks reversibility with mathematical concepts. She may be able to add 3 and 1 and get 4, but reversing the problem ($4 - 1 = 3$) would be too difficult.

The preschool years are a period of rapid learning. The preschool child is curious and wants to know how things work. Preschoolers' thinking is still magical and egocentric (self-centered). The child tends to understand events only as he is affected by them, believing that everyone else has had the same experience. The child may see his mother in distress and bring her a doll, assuming that it would comfort the mother as it does the child. Preschool children often think that their thoughts are powerful enough to cause things to happen. They may frighten themselves with some of their ideas, believing that they may become what they imagine they will be. A preschooler may feel overwhelmed with guilt when a sibling is hospitalized because he believes that his hostile feelings caused the sibling's illness. Likewise, a child of this age may say, "I got sick because I was bad."

Language Development

Acquisition of language is one of the most dramatic features of the preschool period. Increase in language skill allows greater self-control and increases the child's ability to direct and be directed by others. At 2 or 3, a child may be heard reminding herself of behavior she has been taught or verbally rehearsing an event in bed before falling asleep (Howard, 1990).

Vocabulary increases rapidly, from 200 words at age 2 to more than 2100 words at age 5. In less than 3 years, the child grows from a toddler who knows only a few words into a child who skillfully uses an extensive vocabulary to describe events, share feelings, and ask questions. Three-year-olds speak in short, telegraphic sentences. They may talk to themselves or to imaginary friends. A delightful characteristic of young preschoolers is the tendency to engage in lengthy monologues, regardless of whether anyone is listening or even present. Such self-talk provides the child with opportunities to practice speech and is often combined with symbolic play.

By age 4, children talk incessantly and tend to boast and exaggerate. They enjoy rhymes and silly ways to use similar words (Howard, 1990). The 4-year-old expects more detailed answers to his questions. He may use speech aggressively and may use profanity to gain attention. "Bad" language should be ignored, depriving the child of reinforcement of the behavior. When the child feels that he gains power over the parent by using bad language, these verbalizations will continue. Parents may also want to omit objectionable words from their own vocabulary (Howard, 1990).

Five-year-olds speak in sentences of adult length and use all parts of speech. They usually are proficient storytellers who produce elaborate tales for anyone who will listen. Their tendency to mix fantasy with reality may be perceived as lying by adults. The child of 5 usually can recite the days of the week and can name the seasons.

Nurses can teach parents strategies to promote their child's language development. It is important for parents to talk with the child and respond to the child's attempts at communication. Reading to the child and making reading materials available can help to build vocabulary and promote a lifelong love of reading. Watching educational TV programs, such as *Sesame Street,* with their child may augment parents' communication skills. Preschoolers spend a great deal of time asking how and why questions, often taxing parents' patience. Short, simple, honest answers encourage vocabulary building and boost self-esteem.

Stuttering occurs commonly in preschool children as ideas come faster than the words to express them (Howard, 1990). Stuttering usually disappears spontaneously if the child is not pressured by anxious parents. Interrupting the child or telling her to slow down tends to make stuttering worse. Nurses should teach parents to give the child prompt, full attention when she speaks and not to comment on the stuttering. If stuttering is accompanied by tics, grimacing, or abnormal language structure, or if stuttering persists for more than 6 months, referral to a speech pathologist should be considered (Howard, 1990).

Psychosocial Development

The preschool years are a critical period for the development of socialization. Children need opportunities to play with others to learn communication and social skills. They also need appropriate guidance to learn acceptable behavior.

According to Erikson, the developmental task of the preschooler is to achieve a sense of initiative. The preschooler is busy learning how to do things and takes great pride in his new accomplishments. If the child acts inappropriately or is repeatedly criticized or punished for his attempts to explore and learn, feelings of guilt, anxiety, and fear may result. Criticism may lead to the development of a sense of guilt and shame. For example, an adult's comment, "That's nice, but it would look better if you did it this way," may cause the child to feel that his effort was inferior. Such subtle criticism can make the child reluctant to try new activities. A feeling of inferiority may also develop if adults are always doing things for the child, rather than encouraging her to be independent. The child who does not achieve a sense of initiative will feel defeated, angry, and afraid of people and new situations. Nurses can promote the healthy psychosocial development of preschoolers and help them to gain a sense of initiative by teaching parents the importance of providing the child with opportunities to explore in a safe, stimulating environment. Adults should encourage the preschooler's imagination and creativity and should praise appropriate behavior.

Play. Learning to relate to age-mates is another developmental task that is significant during the preschool period. Preschoolers need experience playing with other children to learn how to relate to other people. The 3-year-old is capable of sharing and is more likely to do so than the toddler. The 4-year-old tends to be more argumentative and less generous with playmates. Although this behavior may appear to be a step backward to parents, it is actually a sign of growth because the 4-year-old feels more secure in a group and is testing his role and communication skills. The 5-year-old enjoys playing with other children and generally can play with another child for longer periods before arguments develop.

Children between the ages of 3 and 5 years enjoy parallel and associative play. Children learn to share and cooperate as they play in small groups. During play, preschoolers learn simple games and rules, language concepts, and social roles. Play is often imitative, dramatic, and creative. Various roles are explored through play as children imitate significant adults. Preschoolers enjoy dress-up clothes, housekeeping toys, dollhouses, and other toys that encourage pretending. Tricycles and climbing toys help to develop muscles and coordination. Preschoolers also enjoy materials for cutting, pasting, and painting. Such manipulative and creative materials stimulate imagination and fine motor development (see Chapter 9).

Imaginary friends are common around the age of 3. Boundaries between reality and fantasy are blurred at this age, and "pretend" can seem real, especially during play. Imaginary friends serve many purposes. They may take the blame when the child misbehaves, allowing the child to save face when he feels guilty about his behavior. Imaginary friends may be companions during lonely times. They may accomplish a task that the child is struggling with or allow the child to practice roles. For example, the child may scold an imaginary friend and administer punishment, just like a parent. Imaginary friends seem to be more common in highly imaginative and intelligent children.

Psychosexual Development

Sexual identity and body image are developing. Sexual curiosity and explorations are normal. Preschoolers are curious about anatomic differences and seek to investigate them. Preschoolers show interest in the differences between the sexes and often compare their bodies with those of others. "Playing doctor" and hiding with a friend to investigate anatomic differences are common activities during the preschool period. The nurse should reassure parents that the child is simply learning about his body and that this behavior is no indication of homosexuality or other problems. Parents should not shame the child, but merely direct him to another activity. Preschoolers are interested in where they came from and how babies are made. Parents should be encouraged to assess what the child already knows when she asks about these subjects and to determine why she is asking the question. Questions should be answered simply, honestly, and matter-of-factly. The child usually neither wants nor understands detailed explanations. Many books are available to help parents answer their child's questions about sexuality (Stein, 1984).

A warm, accepting, matter-of-fact attitude toward sexual matters promotes a positive healthy perspective in children. An atmosphere of acceptance can be created by parents in the early preschool years when the first questions arise. A parental attitude of "You can ask me anything" can set the stage for healthy interaction from early childhood on into adolescence, when parental guidance is so important.

Masturbation is common and may increase in frequency when the child is under stress. Parents are often concerned about such behavior. The nurse can help parents to handle these situations by explaining that such self-comforting behaviors are normal for this age. If the parent discovers the child masturbating, it is best to simply redirect the child's attention without punishing, shaming, or reprimanding. Children should be taught that touching their genitals is not appropriate in public.

At this age, a sense of rivalry with the same-sex parent develops. It is common for a preschool boy to compete with his father for the attention of his mother. A girl, likewise, may become "Daddy's girl," often cuddling and flirting with her father while excluding her mother from the relationship. Children often state their intention to marry the opposite-sex parent and become upset when their parents kiss or hug (Howard, 1990). Although this behavior is normal, limits may be necessary. Parents should tell the child that when he grows up he will have a spouse of his own. This rivalry is usually resolved early in the school-age period as the child identifies strongly with the same-sex parent and same-sex peers. According to Freudian theory, the oedipal stage is resolved when the child strongly identifies with the parent of the same sex. By the end of the preschool period, the child identifies with and imitates the same-sex parent. In single-parent homes, if the parent and child are not of the same sex it is important for the child to have a friendly, stable relationship with an adult relative or friend of the same sex who can serve as a role model. Divorced or separated parents should be careful not to speak badly of each other because this behavior can adversely influence the preschool child's developing gender identity and self-esteem (Howard, 1990). By age 3, children know sex differences. They imitate masculine and feminine behaviors in play, and gender identity is well established by age 6.

Spiritual and Moral Development

Learning the difference between right and wrong (the development of a conscience) is another important task of the preschool period. According to Kohlberg, children between the ages of 4 and 7 years are in the second stage of the preconventional level of moral development. In this stage, children obey rules out of self-interest. They tend to believe that if the consequences of an action are personally advantageous, the action is right. An "eye-for-an-eye" orientation guides their behavior.

The preschooler begins to use self-control to resist temptation and tries to "be good" to avoid feelings of guilt. Preschoolers determine right from wrong based on the consequences of disobeying their parents' rules. At this age, children have little understanding of the reason for a rule. For example, when asked why it is wrong to hit another child, the preschooler might reply, "Because my mother says so." Preschoolers adhere to parents' rules dogmatically and understand what is right and wrong as a result of reward and punishment. The preschooler decides whether to break a rule based on the punishment he thinks will follow. Preschoolers often have difficulty applying rules in different situations. Although the child may know that it is wrong to hit her brother at home, she may not understand that it is also wrong to hit another child at daycare. Because the preschooler is egocentric, he cannot understand another's viewpoint. The child begins to develop a conscience as a result of consistent rewards for good behavior and punishment for bad behavior. Guilty feelings result when a child breaks a rule.

The preschool child's concept of God is concrete. The family's religious beliefs and customs, such as bedtime prayers, mealtime grace, and Bible stories, are important to preschoolers. Such rituals, practiced in an atmosphere of love, can be deeply meaningful and comforting to children of this age.

HEALTH PROMOTION FOR THE PRESCHOOL CHILD AND FAMILY

Table 6–2 at the end of this chapter presents an overview of health screening, health maintenance, and anticipatory guidance activities for preschool children.

Sleep and Rest

Because preschoolers expend so much energy growing and learning, they need adequate rest. The preschooler requires an average of 10 to 12 hours of sleep in a 24-hour period. Some preschoolers do well without a nap during the day, but others still need a nap. Resistance to naps is common at this age. The child usually does not want to leave his family or playmates, toys, and exciting activities to go into a darkened room to lie down and rest. A quiet time spent listening to music or looking at a favorite book may help the child to relax and get some rest. Insufficient rest during the day may lead to irritability, decreased resistance to infection, and difficulty sleeping at night.

Sleep problems are more common during the preschool years than at any other period of childhood. Because of their active imaginations and immaturity, preschoolers often have nightmares and have trouble falling asleep at night. Because the boundaries between reality and fantasy are not well defined for children of this age, monsters and scary creatures that lurk in the preschooler's imagination become real to the child after the light is turned off. Patient reassurance from a caring parent may be needed again and again. Nightmares (frightening dreams that awaken the child from sleep) are common among preschoolers. As soon as the child recognizes his familiar environment and is comforted with a hug and verbal reassurance from a parent, he usually returns to sleep. Night terrors differ from nightmares. Night terrors occur during deep sleep. The child does not awaken, but moans, screams, or cries. He does not recognize his parents and may become agitated if they try to comfort him. The child does not remember the episode in the morning, even if he awakens during the night terror. Parents should be instructed not to attempt to comfort or awaken the child during a night terror, but to allow him to sleep.

The nurse should assess sleep patterns during well-child visits. Parental concerns should be addressed. The nurse can reassure parents that resistance to going to bed, fears, and nightmares are normal for children of this age. The nurse should assess the frequency of sleep problems and parents' reactions to them. If sleep problems occur often and are disruptive to the family, further investigation and intervention should be performed. Nurses can suggest strategies to decrease bedtime struggles. Techniques that are helpful in decreasing bedtime resistance include a consistent bedtime ritual (e.g., brush the child's teeth, read one story, make one trip to the bathroom, turn out the light, say prayers, and say goodnight). Avoiding high-carbohydrate snacks and excitement before bedtime promotes relaxation. The child should not be ridiculed for his fears, and the parent should not belittle the child's fear with a terse, "There's nothing to be afraid of. Now go back to sleep." Children should not be forced to face their fear alone by sleeping in a completely dark room or with the door shut. Supportive parents can search the child's room and under the bed for anything frightening, leave a nightlight on and the door open, and reassure the child that there is nothing that will harm him and that the parents are just down the hall if he needs them. Transition objects, such as a special blanket or teddy bear, are comforting to many preschoolers. Progressive head-to-toe relaxation is an effective technique for helping preschoolers to fall asleep. Parents should determine whether the child is actually tired at bedtime. A child who has slept for a long time at the babysitter's or at daycare may not be ready to sleep again. Communication with the child's daytime caretaker is important. A set bedtime promotes security and healthy sleep habits.

Discipline

Discipline is important for the child to learn how to get along with others and follow the rules of society. Discipline by the parents is the foundation of the child's self-discipline later in life. Preschoolers are struggling to gain control over their strong inner impulses. To achieve this control, they need limits set on their behavior. Setting limits increases a child's feelings of security and allows her to explore her environment and try out new roles in an atmosphere of freedom and safety. Appropriate limit setting helps the child to learn self-confidence, self-control, and moral values. The child must be consistently disciplined for acts that are destructive, socially unacceptable, or morally wrong. Limits must be clearly defined and consistently enforced to be effective. To prevent confusion and anxiety, the consequences of misbehavior should be spelled out in advance and carried out immediately after misbehavior occurs. When the child is disciplined for misbehavior, a simple, truthful explanation of why the behavior was unacceptable should be given. The focus should be on the behavior rather than on the child. For example, "I don't like to see you throwing toys" is a better response than "I don't want to be around you when you act like that" or "You're a bad girl for doing that."

Discipline techniques that are effective with preschoolers include:

1. Time-out (removing the child from a situation for a short period and offering an explanation for the punishment).
2. Time-in (frequent, brief, nonverbal, physical contact when the child is acting appropriately. For example, the mother periodically strokes the child's hair or rubs his back when he is quietly playing on the floor near his mother while she talks on the telephone. The child who receives this type of reinforcement is more likely to continue what he is doing and much less likely to interrupt the mother.).
3. Offering restricted choices (e.g., "You may drink your juice in the kitchen or you may go into the living room without your juice.").
4. Diversion (e.g., "You must stop marking on the wall with crayons. Here, mark on this paper instead.").

Consistent positive reinforcement for desired behavior is a powerful tool. The parent should "catch the child being good" and reward positive behavior to increase its frequency. For example, the mother wants Katie to keep her room neat. If the mother responds with a hug and a positive comment ("It makes me so happy that you remembered to pick up your toys.") each time the child straightens up her room without being told, the behavior will increase. Parents should model the behavior that they wish the child to display. A warm, consistent relationship with a parent is important for the development of a child's conscience. If the parent does not care or is too busy to consistently enforce rules, the child will not internalize rules and will not feel guilty about breaking them. The child will be unruly and will be unable to follow the rules set by society.

It is important for parents to spend enjoyable time with their children. Examples include playing outside with children or simply watching TV together and cuddling on the sofa. Many parents have schedules that are so hectic that they must rely on discipline to keep their chil-

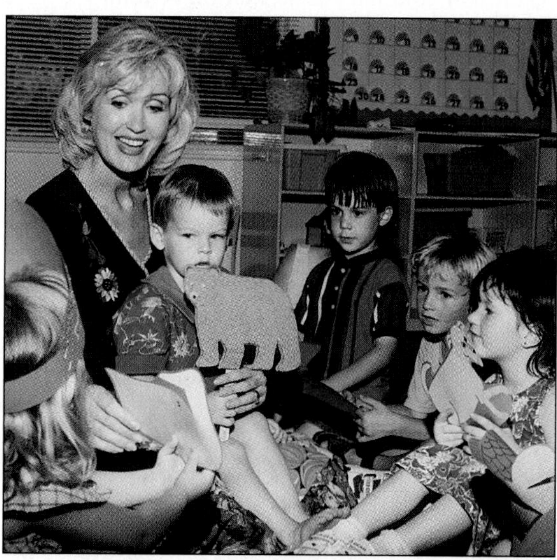

◄ Good daycare provides more than just safe custody of the child while the parent is away. Daycare helps the child learn how to interact with others and play with materials that may not be available at home.

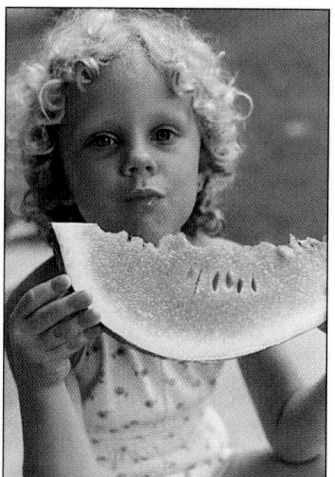

◄ The nurse should assess adequacy of the preschooler's diet. Fruit, instead of concentrated sweets, makes a nutritious snack.

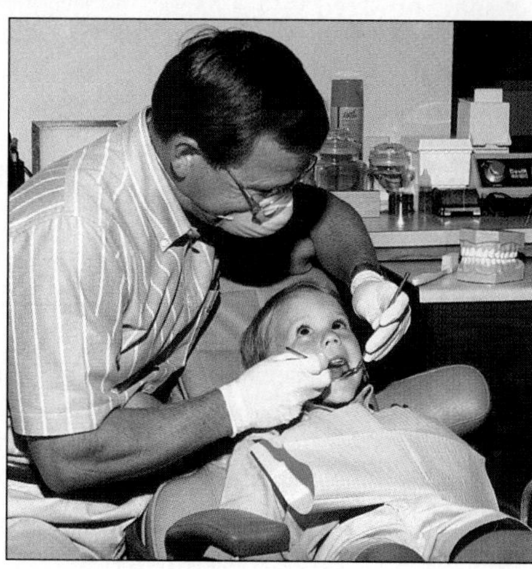

◄ The nurse plays an important role in teaching proper toothbrushing and encouraging visits to the dentist. The child's first visit to the dentist should occur during the toddler or preschool years, and it should be a pleasant experience.

Figure 6–2
Health promotion for the preschooler and family.

Factors to Consider When Evaluating Daycare Centers

- Attitude of the caregiver. Does the caregiver share the parents' value system about education, discipline, and nurturing? Are the staff members warm and attentive to the children?
- Daily program. Is there a routine that includes time for quiet play, group activities, active outdoor play, rest, and snacks? Is the schedule flexible? Do the children appear to be having fun?
- Teacher qualifications. Is the staff stable, qualified, and able to provide references? Have specific state certification and background check requirements been met?
- Student-to-staff ratio. Is the number of staff sufficient to provide adequate attention and care for children?
- Safety precautions. What are the policies for the safety and protection of children? Is the playground safe? Are toys age-appropriate? Are there fire drills? Who can pick up the child? How is child pickup monitored?
- Provision of meals. Are meals well balanced? Are nutritious snacks provided?
- Sanitary conditions. Are there adequate bathroom facilities? Does the staff practice handwashing, proper disposal of soiled diapers, and cleaning of surfaces after diaper changing? Are ill children cared for in a separate area or kept at home? Are children taught to wash their hands frequently, and are facilities accessible to them?
- Adequate indoor and outdoor play space. Is there appropriate play equipment for gross motor, dramatic, creative, and quiet play? Are children allowed freedom to explore? Is there space for the child's personal belongings? Is there adequate space for rest?
- Discipline of children. How are children disciplined? Are they allowed to take time-outs? Are problem-solving techniques taught and reinforced?
- Parent observation opportunities. Can parents drop in, or are appointments required?
- State license or voluntary accreditation system?
- Cost?
- Proximity to home and work. What are the hours of operation? What is the holiday observance schedule?

dren "in line" without ever developing a warm, caring relationship with them (Christopherson, 1991). Having good times with children increases their self-esteem and reinforces good behavior.

See Chapter 16 for further discussion of discipline.

Preschool and Daycare Programs

A quality daycare program provides an environment in which the child can expand social and play skills as well as manipulate play materials unavailable at home.

It is estimated that 57% to 70% of mothers of preschoolers in the United States work outside the home. (Cadden & Camerman, 1990; Garland, 1989) Working mothers often express guilt and concern about the effect of daycare on their child's emotional well-being and cognitive development. Some concerns about the effect of daycare on the child's development can be minimized by careful selection of a daycare facility. Factors to consider when choosing a daycare or preschool program are listed in the accompanying box.

The nurse is in an excellent position to advise parents about child care. Parents need specific advice about options that are affordable, but will not compromise the child's health and development. It is imperative that parents visit the daycare center to evaluate the quality of the program. Parents need to explore operating procedures, discuss costs, interview care providers, learn the child care and discipline practices of the center, and check references thoroughly (Busen, 1988).

The child needs preparation before beginning daycare. The parent should tell the child what to expect in simple, concrete terms. Emphasizing the exciting parts of the experience will help the child to view the experience positively. The parent should also explain the reason for separation. It is not uncommon for an imaginative preschooler to believe that she is being "sent away" because of some misdeed.

DISCUSSING SEPARATION When parents must take their child to a babysitter or daycare center, they should give the child an explanation for the separation. A statement such as "I have to work so I can buy food and clothes for the family and toys for you" is not adequate. In response to this explanation, one 3-year-old boy wailed, "But I have enough toys!"

It is important for the parent to reassure the child ("I'm really going to miss you today and I wish you could be with me.") and to let the child know that separation is painful for the parent as well, but necessary. At the end of the day, when the parent picks up the child, it is equally important to let the child know how happy he is to see the child. By responding to the child's feelings, parents can lessen the stress of separation.

Parents should accompany the child to the daycare facility and introduce him to the teacher. Staying on the first day until the child feels secure enough to let the parent go reduces separation anxiety. Transition objects may also help the child to adjust to the new environment. Providing the staff with information about the child's interests, home routine, special terms, and names of pets and siblings helps the new caregiver to make the child feel more comfortable. The parent should always tell the child that he will return to take him home.

Preparing the Child for School

Preparation for school begins long before the preschool period. The earliest interactions between parent and infant lay the foundation for school readiness. Research shows that the most important factor in the development of academic competency is the relationship between parent and child. Parents who are attuned to their child and who structure the environment to provide challenges as well as security facilitate the child's cognitive growth. An interesting environment, combined with parental encouragement and support, maximizes the child's potential. Responsive parenting is fundamental for learning. A parent who is sensitive and is able to synchronize communication and stimulation with the infant's cues promotes mastery of cognitive, language, and motor skills. However, if the infant finds that her actions do not affect her environment (or her parent's responses), she experiences a feeling of inadequacy called learned helplessness (Seligman, 1975). Helplessness results when a child feels that the situation is beyond her control and that there is nothing he can do to help herself. The child gives up and becomes listless, withdrawn, and apathetic. She seems to lose all motivation for learning and relating to other children (Elkind, 1987). Because the child feels unable to control or master her environment, she is overcome with anxiety, frustration, and fear, and performs inadequately, regardless of intelligence quotient (IQ). Learned helplessness results in the inability to learn how to learn. Such children exhibit motor, cognitive, and social delays. The helplessness syndrome can result from nonresponsive parenting or from stimulus deprivation.

Parents are the child's first and most important teachers. They structure the child's environment and offer opportunities for learning. Visiting a zoo, fire station, or museum and talking about the experience increases the child's general knowledge and vocabulary. Intellectual development is also fostered by cooking together, playing simple games, or putting together puzzles. Playing with clay, paint, and scissors promotes fine motor skills and provides opportunity for self-expression. Reading to the child is one of the most valuable activities for promoting school readiness. Listening to and discussing stories can promote reading readiness. Dramatic play encourages reading readiness by providing opportunities for symbolic thinking and problem solving. The skills necessary for academic success are promoted by parents who spend time with their children. However, the efforts of overly anxious or ambitious parents may be self-defeating. Too much parental pressure may lead to a dislike of schoolwork (Howard, 1990).

Preschool and daycare programs can supplement the developmental opportunities provided by parents at home. Opportunities to play with other children and to learn how to share the attention of an adult are benefits of a good preschool program. Head Start programs offer low-income children and their families opportunities for remedial and supportive activities. Kindergarten provides a transition between home and first grade through a structured learning environment. In kindergarten, children prepare for school by learning to cooperate with other children, developing listening skills, and forming a positive attitude toward school.

Nurses can provide parents with strategies designed to promote safety as part of preparation for school. Teaching children about street safety and dealing with strangers and ensuring that children know their telephone number and address are important aspects of preparation for school (see Table 6–3 and Chapter 13).

Checklist for School Readiness

- Physically healthy and strong enough to enjoy the challenge of going to school and to handle the increased stresses involved.
- Attends to own toileting needs and washes hands independently.
- Capable of separating from parent and spending several hours each day in an unfamiliar place with adults and children who are largely unknown at first.
- Long enough attention span to be able to sit for a fairly long period and to concentrate on one thing at a time, gradually learning to enjoy the practicing and problem-solving activity involved.
- Can listen to and follow two- or three-part instructions.
- Can restrict talking to appropriate times.
- Able to tolerate the frustration of not receiving immediate attention from the teacher or others; can wait for and take turns.
- Has some basic hand–eye skills necessary for learning to read and write.
- Can hold a pencil properly and turn pages one at a time.
- Knows the alphabet, including how to recognize letters.
- Counts to 10.
- Recognizes the colors of the rainbow.

TABLE 6–2 *Health Screening, Health Maintenance, and Anticipatory Guidance for Preschoolers*

3 YEARS	4 YEARS	5 YEARS
Immunization		
Review immunization record; administer appropriate immunizations if not up to date.	DTP #5, OPV #4 (or #5), MMR #2, (optional) between ages 4 and 6 years. Review reactions to previous immunizations.	Administer immunizations if not given at 4 years.
Safety		
Street supervision; car seat; booster seat and shoulder harness seat belt if child is > 40 lb (see Chapter 13). Teach child not to play with matches and how to escape from burning home. Supervise near fireplace or grill. Teach safety around pets and not to approach strange dogs. Avoid foods that may be aspirated.	Booster seat, safety belts; street safety (wait at the curb until told to cross, avoid riding cycles near street or driveways). Teach child to swim; supervise child near water. Teach child not to talk to strangers.	Booster seat, safety belts; playground safety; teach child not to talk to strangers. Child should know his name, address, and phone number, and how to seek help if lost.
Nutrition		
Review vitamin and fluoride dosage; discuss diet, feeding issues, and snacks.	Child needs approximately 1700 calories per day.	Assess adequacy of diet and snacks. Avoid concentrated sweets.
Vision and Hearing		
Parental perception. Assess readiness for objective screening. Speech should be 50%–75% intelligible. Address parental concerns. Stuttering is fairly common. Assess parents' reactions.	Parental perception. Assess readiness for objective screening. Assess speech intelligibility (most speech should be intelligible). Address parental concerns.	Vision and hearing screening. Assess parental concerns.
Dental Care		
First dental visit if not done previously. Does child brush his teeth with supervision?	Well-balanced diet. Limit sweets. Brush and floss twice daily. Dental visit every 6 months to 1 year.	Dental visit every 6 months to 1 year.
Screening		
Monitor height and weight for deviations as indicated on growth chart.	Review results of lead and TB screening if performed.	
Teaching and Counseling		
Discuss child's fears (the dark, monsters) and the results of active imagination. Discuss thumb sucking and masturbation. Assess parents' reactions. Discuss TV viewing, violence. Discuss elimination (bowel and bladder control). Encourage enrollment in nursery school.	Discuss imaginary friends, fantasies. Discuss sleep patterns and concerns (nightmares, fear of the dark, difficulty falling or staying asleep). Assess child's ability to separate from parents. Recommend TV restrictions. Prepare parents for child's increasing sexual curiosity.	Assess school readiness: child's reactions, parent's expectations, and child's ability to tolerate separation from parents and ability to do schoolwork.

Abbreviations: DTP, Diphtheria and tetanus toxoids with pertussis vaccine; OPV, oral poliovirus vaccine; MMR, measles, mumps, and rubella vaccine; TB, tuberculosis test.

Not every 5-year-old is ready for kindergarten. Both chronological age and developmental maturity should be considered when assessing a child's readiness for school. At this age, boys tend to lag behind girls developmentally by about 6 months. The accompanying Checklist for School Readiness lists areas of maturity needed by a child for school readiness.

Dental Care

Because the enamel on primary teeth is thinner than that on permanent teeth, preschoolers' teeth are prone to destruction from decay. The distance from the tooth surface to the pulp is shorter also, so tooth abscesses from caries can occur rapidly. Untreated caries can lead to pain, abscess formation, and poor digestion because of ineffective chewing. Many parents do not realize that the deciduous teeth are important to protect the dental arch. If deciduous teeth are lost early (e.g., because of decay) the remaining teeth may drift out of position, block proper eruption of the permanent teeth, and lead to malocclusion.

Nurses play an important role in the promotion of dental health by teaching proper tooth cleaning and the importance of adequate fluoride ingestion; a balanced diet, limited in sweets; and twice yearly visits to the dentist. Preschoolers can usually brush their own teeth and should be encouraged to do so at least once a day, especially at bedtime. Short back-and-forth or up-and-down strokes are easiest for the child to manage. Parents should monitor the child's toothbrushing and inspect the child's teeth to be sure that all plaque has been removed. Parents must help with flossing because it requires more manual dexterity than preschoolers have.

If the water supply does not contain fluoride in a concentration of at least 1 part per million (ppm), the child should be given a daily supplement of sodium fluoride (see Chapter 5, Table 5–3). Because excessive fluoride can cause mottling of enamel, parents should be cautioned not to exceed the prescribed dose. Topical fluoride also increases resistance to tooth decay and may be applied by the dentist. Fluoride rinses and toothpaste containing fluoride are also recommended.

If the child did not visit the dentist during toddlerhood, he should do so as soon as possible, preferably before any dental work needs to be done. The first dental visit should be a pleasant experience, and the parents should emphasize the concept of the dentist as a person who likes to help us stay healthy.

Nurses should teach parents the importance of a well-balanced diet that is low in sweets. Studies have shown that sweets are most likely to cause cavities when they are sticky or are eaten between meals rather than with meals (Wei, 1981). Nutritious snacks, such as raw vegetables and fruits, rather than sweets help to decrease tooth decay. If the child chews gum, it should be sugarless. Parents should be encouraged to monitor the types of snacks that their child receives at daycare or at a babysitter's.

KEY CONCEPTS

- Coordination and muscle strength increase rapidly between the ages of 3 and 5. Increases in brain size and nerve myelinization enable the child to perfect fine and gross motor skills. The preschool child has the skills needed to engage in activities such as running, riding a tricycle, cutting with scissors, and drawing.
- The preschool years are a critical period for the development of socialization. Children need opportunities to play with others to learn communication skills and ways to get along with others. Preschool children learn to share and cooperate as they play in small groups. Their play is often imitative, dramatic, and creative.
- According to Erikson, the developmental task of the preschooler is to gain a sense of initiative. The preschooler is busy learning how to do things and takes great pride in new accomplishments.
- Sexual identity and body image are developing in the preschool period. Sexual curiosity, anatomic explorations, and masturbation are common. The nurse should encourage parents to answer the preschooler's questions simply and honestly. Children should not be shamed or punished for self-comforting behaviors or for investigating sexual differences.
- Preschoolers' thinking is still magical and egocentric. The child tends to understand events only as he is affected by them, believing that everyone else has had the same experience. Preschool children may be overwhelmed with guilt if a loved one is injured or becomes ill because they think that their thoughts are powerful enough to cause events to happen.
- The preschooler requires an average of 10 to 12 hours of sleep in a 24-hour period. Because of the preschooler's active imagination and immaturity, sleep problems are common. Helpful techniques for decreas-

ing bedtime resistance include following a consistent bedtime ritual, avoiding high-carbohydrate snacks and excitement before bedtime, using a nightlight, maintaining a set bedtime, and using progressive relaxation.

- Preschool children need consistent discipline to learn acceptable behavior. Appropriate limit setting helps the child to learn self-confidence, self-control, and moral values. Discipline techniques that are effective at this age include time-out, time-in, the use of restricted choices, and diversion.
- All 20 deciduous teeth are present by the age of 3 years. If deciduous teeth are lost early (e.g., because of decay), the remaining teeth may drift out of position and block proper eruption of the permanent teeth, resulting in malocclusion. Nurses play an important role in promoting dental health by teaching proper methods for tooth cleaning and emphasizing the importance of adequate fluoride ingestion, a balanced diet with limited sweets, and visits to the dentist twice each year.
- The nurse can assist parents in selecting daycare for their children by suggesting that they evaluate the attitude and qualifications of the caregivers as well as operating procedures, costs, child care and discipline practices, meals, safety precautions, sanitary conditions, and the child–staff ratio.
- The nurse plays an important role in helping parents to prepare their children for school and in assessing children's readiness for school. Parents can help their child to succeed in school by providing a stimulating environment as well as encouragement and support.
- Health promotion of the preschool child includes adequate sleep, optimal nutrition, dental care, immunizations, and accident prevention.

REFERENCES

Busen, N. H. (1988). Societal values: A cause of stress in children. *Journal of Pediatric Health Care, 2*(6), 300–306.

Cadden, V., & Camerman, S. (1990, September). Where in the world is child care better? *Working Mother*, 62–68.

Christopherson, E. R. (1991). Oppositional behavior in children. *Pediatric Annals, 20*(5), 267–273.

Elkind, D. (1987). *The hurried child.* New York: Addison-Wesley.

Garland, S. B. (1989). America's child care crisis: The first tiny steps toward solutions. *Business Week, 3114,* 64–68.

Howard, B. J. (1990). Learning independence in the preschool years. *Contemporary Pediatrics,* 7, 11–26.

Poest, C. A., Williams, J. R., Witt, D. W., & Atwood, M. E. (1990). Challenge me to move: Large muscle development in young children. *Young Children, 45* (45), 4–10.

Seligman, M. E. P. (1975). *Helplessness: On depression, development, and death.* San Francisco: Freeman.

Stein, S. (1984). *Making babies.* New York: Walker.

Wei, S. (1981). Nutrition, diet, fluoride and dental health. *Pediatric Basics, 30,* 4–7.

BIBLIOGRAPHY

Betz C. L., Hunsberger, M., & Wright, S. (1994). *Family centered nursing care of children* (2nd ed.). Philadelphia: W. B. Saunders.

Boomer, H., & Deakin, A. (1991). Getting children to sleep. *Nursing Times, 87*(12), 40–43.

Christopherson, E. R. (1986). Anticipatory guidance on discipline. *Pediatric Clinics of North America, 33* (4), 789–798.

Crawford, W., Bennet, R., & Hewitt, K. (1989, March). Sleep problems in pre-school children. *Health Visitor, 62,* 79–81.

Davis, K. (1992). *How to live with your kids when you've already lost your mind.* Grand Rapids, MI: Zondervan.

Dobson, J. (1970). *Dare to discipline.* Wheaton, IL: Tyndale House.

Drabman, R. B., & Jarvie, G. (1987). Counseling parents of children with behavior problems: The use of extinction and time-out techniques. *Pediatrics, 59,* 78–85.

Edgil, A. E., Wood, K. R., & Smith, D. P. (1985). Sleep problems of older infants and preschool children. *Pediatric Nursing, 11* (2):87–89.

Feeg, V. D. (1987). Let's face it about day care. *Pediatric Nursing, 13*(3), 148–154.

Greenspan, S. I. (1991). Clinical assessment of emotional milestones of infancy and early childhood. *Pediatric Clinics of North America, 38* (6), 1371–1383.

Hauck, M. R. (1991). Cognitive abilities of preschool children: Implications for nurses working with young children. *Journal of Pediatric Nursing, 6*(4), 230–235.

Howard, B. J. (1991). Discipline in early childhood. *Pediatric Clinics of North America, 38,* 1351–1369.

Ogasawara, T., Watanabe, T., & Kasahara, H. (1992). Readiness for toothbrushing of young children. *Journal of Dentistry for Children, 59*(5), 353–359.

Schuster, C. S., & Ashburn, S. (1992). *The process of human development: A holistic life span approach.* New York: J. B. Lippincott.

Shelly, J. A. (1982). *The spiritual needs of children: A guide for nurses, parents and teachers.* Downers Grove, IL: InterVarsity Press.

Smardo, F. A., & Willis, T. B. (1983). Looking critically at dental health books for children. *Journal of School Health, 53*(10), 626–629.

Webster-Stratton, C. (1983). Intervention approaches to conduct disorders in young children. *Nurse Practitioner, 8*(5):23–4, 29, 33–4, 23–34.

Wong, D. L. (1986). Helping parents select day-care centers. *Pediatric Nursing, 12*(3),181–187.

7

The School-Age Child

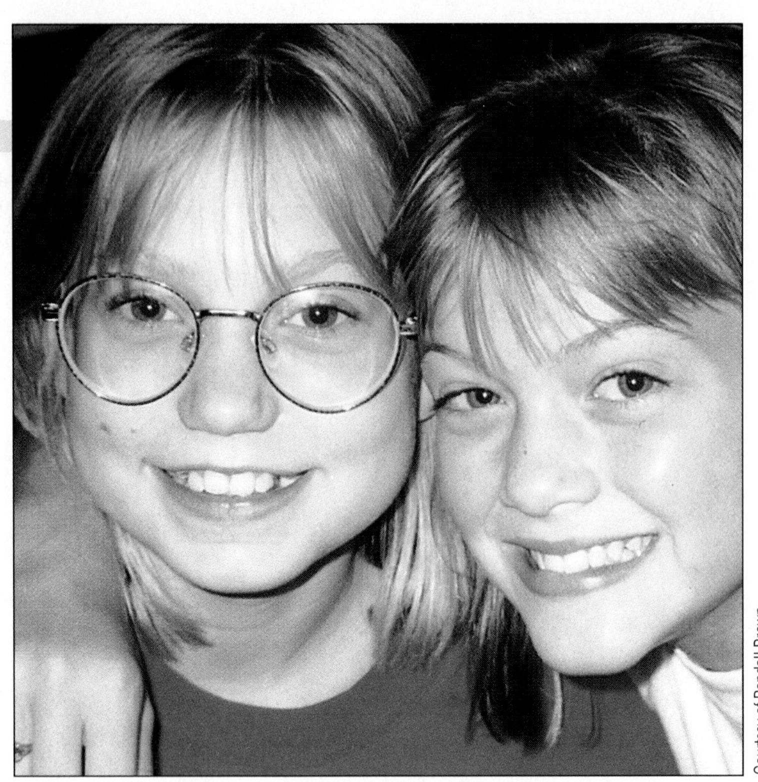

Courtesy of Randall Brown

CHAPTER OVERVIEW

LEARNING OBJECTIVES

After studying this chapter, you should be able to:

- Describe normal growth and development of the school-age child and assess the child for normal developmental milestones.
- Describe the maturational changes that take place during the school-age period and discuss implications for health care.
- Identify the stages of moral development of the school-age child and discuss implications for effective parenting strategies.
- Discuss the effect of schools on the development of the child and implications for teachers and parents.
- Discuss anticipatory guidance appropriate to offer to parents on discipline techniques for school-age children.
- Identify common causes of stress and their effects on school-age children. Describe anticipatory guidance that the nurse can offer to decrease children's stress.
- Discuss coping strategies that school-age children can implement to decrease the effects of stress.

KEY TERMS

caries: decay of the teeth

conservation: ability to understand that certain properties of objects do not change simply because their order, form, or appearance has changed

latchkey children: children who care for themselves at home after school

malocclusion: misalignment of the teeth or dental arches; teeth may be crowded, crooked, or out of alignment

menarche: onset of menstruation

The school-age years, from 6 to 12, are one of the healthiest periods of life. This time is characterized by slow, steady physical growth and rapid cognitive and social development. During these 6 years, the child's world expands from the tight circle of the family to include children and adults at school, at church, and in the community. The child becomes increasingly independent. Peers become important as the child starts school and gradually moves away from the security of home. This period is a time of best friends, sharing, and exploring.

The school-age child develops a sense of industry and learns the basic skills needed to function in society. The child develops an appreciation of rules and a conscience that bothers him if he disobeys. Cognitively, the child grows from the egocentrism of early childhood to more mature thinking. This maturity is characterized by the ability to solve problems and make independent judgments based on reason. The child is invested in the task of middle childhood: learning to do things and do them well. Competence and self-esteem increase with each academic, social, and athletic achievement. The relative stability and security of the school-age period prepare the child to enter the storm of adolescence.

GROWTH AND DEVELOPMENT OF THE SCHOOL-AGE CHILD

Growth and development of the school-age child is summarized in Table 7–1.

Physical Growth and Development

The school-age years are characterized by slow and steady growth. Physical changes that occur during this period are gradual and subtle. Although growth rates vary among children, average weight gain is 2.5 kg (5.5 pounds) per year, and the average increase in height is approximately 5.5 cm (2 inches) per year. During the early school-age period, boys are approximately 1 inch taller and 2 pounds heavier than girls. At around age 10 or 12 years, girls begin to catch up in size as they experience the preadolescent growth spurt. By age 12, girls are 1 inch taller than boys and 2 pounds heavier. This growth spurt, which signals the onset of puberty, occurs 2 years later in boys than in girls, usually between 12 and 14 years.

Body Systems. School-age children appear thinner and more graceful than preschoolers. Musculoskeletal growth leads to greater coordination and strength. The muscles are still immature, however, and can be injured from overuse. Growth of the facial bones changes facial proportions. As the facial bones grow, the eustachian tube assumes a more downward and inward position, resulting in fewer ear infections than in the preschool years. Lymphatic tissues continue to grow until about age 9. Enlarged tonsils and adenoids are common during these years and are not always an indication of illness. Frontal sinuses develop at age 7. The respiratory system also continues to mature. During the school-age years, the lungs and alveoli are fully developed, and fewer respiratory infections occur.

Dentition. During the school-age years, all 20 primary (deciduous) teeth are lost and are replaced by 28 of the 32 permanent teeth. All permanent teeth, except the second and third molars, erupt during the school-age period. The order of eruption and loss of primary teeth are shown in Figure 11–9. The first teeth to be lost are usually the lower central incisors at around age 6. Most first graders are characterized by a snaggle-tooth appearance, and visits from the "Tooth Fairy" are important signs of growing up.

Sexual Development

Puberty is a time of dramatic physical change. It includes the growth spurt, development of primary and secondary sexual characteristics, and maturation of the sexual organs

TABLE 7–1 *Summary of Growth and Development: The School-Age Child*

PHYSICAL	MOTOR	PSYCHOSOCIAL	SENSORY/COGNITIVE
6 Years Average weight gain: 2.5 kg (5.5 lb) per year. Average increase in height: 5.5 cm (2 inches) per year. Growth occurs in spurts; caloric needs increase during growth spurts. Growth of trunk, arms, and legs exceeds that of head. Posture becomes more erect. Dentition: Child loses the first primary teeth (usually lower central incisors). First molars erupt.	**Gross:** Full of energy; in constant motion. Needs activities that require use of large muscles. Can skip, jump rope; some can ride two-wheel bicycle. Balance and rhythm are good. Gross motor skills exceed fine motor coordination. **Fine:** Can tie shoelaces. Draws people with good detail. Prints; may reverse letters. Can cut with scissors; pastes. Can button and zip clothes; dresses without help. Draws a person with 12 parts.	Outgoing, boisterous, "know-it-all." Craves attention; insists on being first and will cheat to win. Loves new places, ideas, accomplishments. Has a good sense of humor. Loves parents; worries that something may happen to them. Argumentative. Uses tension outlets; wriggling, biting fingernails, twisting hair. Temper tantrums return.	Intuitive thought stage. Attends first grade. Learning to read. Knows right hand from left. Understands morning, afternoon, night. Understands numbers. Knows values of coins.
7 Years Boys are approximately 1 inch taller and 2 lb heavier on average than girls. Lymphatic tissue increases in size until age 9 years. Frontal sinuses develop. Dentition: Upper central incisors and lower lateral incisors erupt. Jaw begins to grow to accommodate permanent teeth; facial contours change. Brain attains 90% of adult size.	**Gross:** Quiter, more cautious than the 6-year-old. Jumps rope well. Plays "girls games" or "boy games" according to sex. **Fine:** Visual acuity fully developed; can read regular-size print. Draws a person with 16 parts.	Perfectionistic, self-critical. Becomes more sensitive, reflective, and quiet. Wants to be liked by peers. Likes to make things; often starts projects without finishing them. Aware of family roles and responsibility. Believes promises are important and should be kept. Strong sense of justice; may tattle.	Intuitive thought stage. Attends second grade. Understands clock time; can read time to the nearest quarter-hour. Can copy a diamond. Visual acuity fully developed (20/20 vision). Can read regular-size print.
8 Years Flexible and limber; bones grow faster than ligaments. Dentition: Upper lateral incisors and lower cuspids erupt. Eyes: Myopia may appear.	**Gross:** More coordinated and graceful, but rapid growth of arms and legs may cause frequent stumbling and spills at the table. Rides bicycle well. Enjoys sports. Plays and works hard.	Happy, cooperative with peers. Has a best friend. Prefers to play with same-sex peers. Dislikes being alone. Enjoys talking on the telephone. Enjoys dramatic play. Loves collections. Likes school. Enjoys running errands, helping.	Concrete operations stage. Attends third grade. Knows the date. Can name months in order. Understands conservation of mass, reversibility. Likes riddles and jokes. Can count backward from 20.

	Fine: Writes cursive.	May insist on changing the rules of games to win. Strong sense of humor. Modest.	
9–10 Years Brain growth complete by age 10 years. IgA and IgG reach adult levels.	**Gross:** High energy; always on the go. Coordination improves. Enjoys team sports. **Fine:** Eye–hand coordination well developed; enjoys crafts.	Clubs at a peak; likes secret codes and rituals. Peers' opinions are more important than parents'; child questions parental values. Fairly responsible, dependable. Increasingly polite with adults. Hero worship continues. Anger may flare, but child usually can control it. Ready for camp away from home.	Understands conservation of weight. Attends fourth and fifth grades. Reads more; enjoys books and comics. Understands fractions. Enjoys collections. Makes detailed drawings. Interested in how things work. Less easily distracted.
11–12 Years Rapid growth spurt and menarche occur in girls. Girls are 1 inch taller and 2 lb heavier on average than boys. Boys have greater physical strength, may become overweight. Eruption of permanent teeth complete except for third molars. About 90% of facial growth attained by age 12.	**Gross:** More awkward because of growth spurt. May drop out of team sports to avoid embarrassment. High energy level revealed in tapping pencils, drumming fingers, etc. **Fine:** Fine motor control begins to approximate that of adults.	Loyal to friends, team. Has a best friend. Boys tease opposite sex; girls flirt with boys. Girls may become "boy crazy." Modest, secretive. Needs privacy and time alone. Critical of own work. Wants more independence; may begin to rebel against parents. Begins to think about social problems, prejudices.	Formal operations stage. Attends sixth and seventh grades. Likes to talk on the telephone. Understands conservation of volume. Enjoys reading mysteries, romances, adventure stories; also reads for practical purposes.

Abbreviations: IgA, immunoglobulin A; IgG, immunoglobulin G.

(Jarvis, 1992). The age of onset of puberty varies widely, but the first physiologic signs—breast bud formation and enlargement of areolar diameter—usually begin to appear at about 9 years of age in girls. Puberty begins about $1\frac{1}{2}$ to 2 years later in boys. The average age of puberty is 12 for girls and 14 for boys. **Menarche,** the onset of menstruation, occurs about $2\frac{1}{2}$ years after the first physical changes of puberty. Wide variations in maturity at this age are a common cause of embarrassment because the school-age child does not want to appear different from her peers. Both early and late maturers may struggle with feelings of self-consciousness and inferiority. Puberty is occurring increasingly earlier, and many 10- and 11-year-old girls have already experienced menarche. Table 8-1 in Chapter 8 describes the usual sequence of appearance of secondary sex characteristics during the school-age and adolescent periods.

Because of earlier onset of puberty, sex education programs should be introduced in elementary and middle school. Nurses are in an excellent position to serve as resource persons for parents and teachers who are responsible for sex education. Children's questions about sexuality and related issues should be answered honestly and matter-of-factly. If sex education is presented within the context of learning about the human body, with its wonders and mysteries, children are less likely to feel embarrassment and anxiety. Regardless of whether sex education is a part of a formal school curriculum, children need accurate information. Basic anatomy and physiology, information about bodily functions, and the expected changes of puberty should be introduced to children by the age of 9. Older school-age children need information about menstruation, nocturnal emissions, and reproduction. Sex education programs must also include information about responsible sexuality and dangers, such as teenage pregnancy, acquired immune deficiency syndrome (AIDS), and sexually transmitted diseases.

Do not assume that children who use slang or street terms related to sex are knowledgeable about their meaning. Further questioning may uncover a child's confusion about a sexual issue.

Motor Development

The Importance of Active Play. School-age children spend much of their time in active play, practicing and refining motor skills. They seem to be constantly in motion. Children of this age enjoy active sports and games as well as crafts and fine motor activities. Activities requiring balance and strength, such as bicycle riding, tree climbing, and skating, are exciting and fun for the school-age child. Coordination and motor skills improve as the child is given an opportunity to practice.

Children should be encouraged to engage in physical activities. During the school-age years, children learn physical fitness skills that contribute to their health for the rest of their lives. Physical exercise promotes growth and ossification of bones and enhances academic learning (Bailey, 1978). Cardiovascular fitness, strength, and flexibility are improved by physical activity. Popular games, such as tag, jump rope, and hide-and-seek provide a release of emotional tension and enhance the development of leader and follower skills.

Team sports, such as soccer and baseball, provide opportunities not only for exercise and refinement of motor skills, but also for the development of the concepts of sportsmanship and teamwork. Nurses should advise parents on ways to prevent sports injuries. Sports activities should be well supervised, and protective gear (such as helmets for T-ball and shin guards for soccer) should be mandatory (see Chapter 13).

Unfortunately, the majority of United States children have a greater percentage of body fat than children had 20 years ago, and many are out of shape and unable to meet minimal standards on physical fitness examinations (Nelms, 1990). Time spent watching TV or playing computer games often diminishes a child's interest in active play outside. Nurses can help to reverse this trend by advising parents to limit their children's TV time to 2 hours per day or less and to encourage them to engage in more active play. Parents should provide adequate space for children to run, jump, and scuffle. The child should have enough free time to exercise and play. Nurses can play key roles, too, by encouraging parents to show an interest in their own fitness and by working as advocates for appropriate programs in the schools and community (Nelms, 1990).

Preventing Fatigue and Dehydration. Because children enjoy active play and are so full of energy, they often do not recognize fatigue. Six-year-olds, particularly, will not stop an activity to rest. Parents must learn to recognize signs of fatigue or irritability and enforce rest periods before the child becomes exhausted. Because the child's metabolic rate is higher than an adult's and sweating ability is limited, extremes in temperature while exercising can be dangerous. Dehydration and overheating can pose threats to the child's health. Frequent rest periods and adequate hydration are essential for the child during physical exercise.

Development of Fine Motor Skills. Increased myelinization of the central nervous system is shown by refinement of fine motor skills. Balance and eye–hand coordination improve with maturity and practice. School-age children take pride in activities that require dexterity and fine motor skill, such as model building, playing a musical instrument, or drawing.

Nursing Assessment of Motor Development. During physical examination, the nurse should assess the child's motor development, being alert for soft neurologic signs. These are findings that would be considered normal in a younger child, but if present in an older child, suggest neuromaturational immaturity. There may be a relationship between the presence of such soft signs and learning difficulties. Soft signs in school-age children include: dystonic posturing of the hands and arms while walking across the room on the heels, mirror movements of the opposite hand while performing rapid opposition movements of the thumbs and forefinger, and easily observed movements of the tongue while writing (Algranati, 1992; Dworkin, 1989).

Cognitive Development

Thought processes undergo dramatic changes as the child moves from the intuitive thinking of the preschool years to the logical operations of the school-age years. The school-age child gains new knowledge and develops more efficient problem-solving ability and greater flexibility of thinking. The 6- and 7-year-old remains in the intuitive thought stage (Piaget, 1962) characteristic of the older preschool child. By age 8, the child moves into the concrete operations stage, followed by formal operations at around age 12. See Chapter 8 for a discussion of formal operations; see Chapter 42 for a discussion of the child with cognitive defects, including mental retardation and developmental disabilities.

Intuitive Thought Stage

In the intuitive thought stage (6–7 years), thinking is based on immediate perceptions of the environment and the child's own viewpoint. Thinking is still characterized by egocentrism, animism, and centration (see Chapter 6). At 6 and 7 years old, children cannot understand another's viewpoint, form hypotheses, or deal with abstract concepts. The child in the intuitive thought stage has difficulty forming categories and often solves problems by random guessing. The game "Animal, Vegetable, or Mineral" is much more difficult for a 6-year-old than for a 10-year-old because of their differing abilities to organize objects and concepts according to categories (Schuster & Ashburn, 1992).

Concrete Operations Stage

By age 7 or 8, the child enters the stage of concrete operations. The child learns that his point of view is not the only one as he encounters different interpretations of reality and begins to differentiate his own viewpoint from those of peers and adults (Piaget, 1962). This newly developed freedom from egocentrism enables the child to think more flexibly and to learn about the environment more accurately. Problem solving becomes more efficient and reliable as the child learns how to form hypotheses. The use of symbolism becomes more sophisticated, and children now can manipulate symbols for things in the way that they once manipulated the things themselves. The child learns the alphabet and how to read. Attention span increases as the child grows older, facilitating classroom learning.

Reversibility. Children in the concrete operations stage grasp the concept of reversibility. They can mentally retrace a process, a skill necessary for understanding mathematic problems ($5 + 3 = 8$ and $8 - 3 = 5$). The child can now take a toy apart and put it back together or walk to school and find his way home the same way without getting lost. Reversibility also enables a child to anticipate the results of actions, a valuable tool for problem solving.

The understanding of time gradually develops during the early school-age years. Children can understand and use clock time at around age 8 years. Although calendar time is understood and dates are memorized by age 8 or 9, mastery of historical time does not occur until later.

Conservation. Gradually, the school-age child masters the concept of **conservation.** The child learns that certain properties of objects do not change simply because their order, form, or appearance has changed. For example, the child has mastered conservation of mass when he recognizes that a lump of clay that he has pounded flat is still the same amount of clay as when it was rolled into a ball. The child understands conservation of weight when he can correctly answer the classic nonsense question, "Which weighs more, a pound of feathers or a pound of rocks?" The concept of conservation does not develop all at once. The simpler conservations, such as number and mass, are understood first, and more complex conservations are mastered later. An understanding of conservation of weight develops at age 9 or 10, and volume at age 11 or 12.

Classification and Logic. Older school-age children are able to classify objects according to characteristics they share, to place things in a logical order, and to recall similarities and differences. This ability is reflected in the school-age child's interest in collections. Children love to collect and classify stamps, stickers, sports cards, shells, dolls, rocks, or anything imaginable. School-age children understand relationships such as larger and smaller, lighter and darker. They can comprehend class inclusion, the concept that objects can belong to more than one classification. For example, a man can be a brother, father, and son at the same time.

The school-age child moves away from magical thinking as he discovers that there are logical, physical explanations for most phenomena. The school-age child is a skeptic, no longer believing in Santa Claus or the

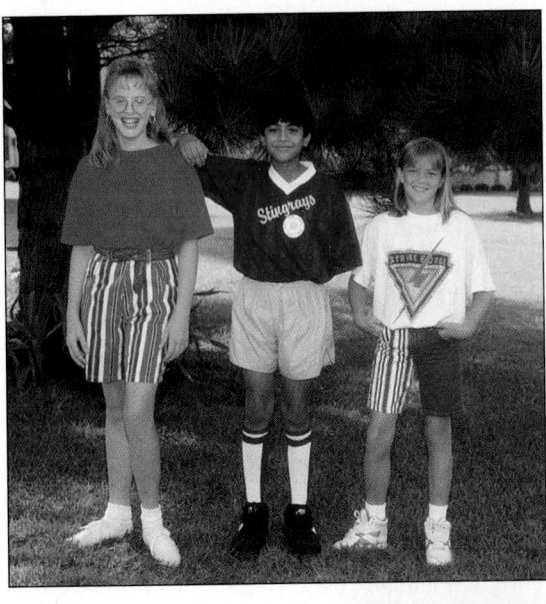

◀ Children of the same age can vary significantly in height and physical development.

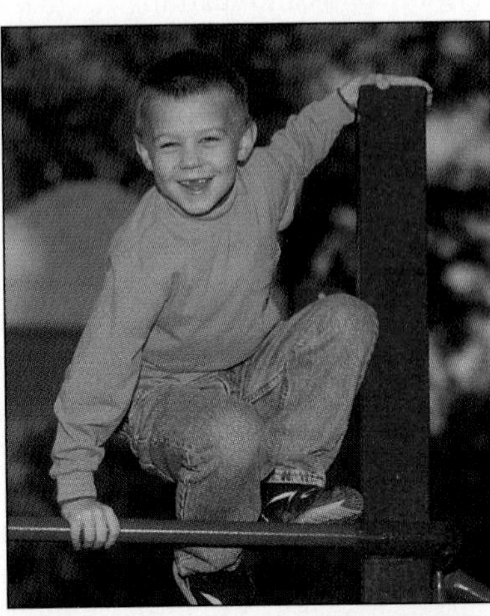

◀ School-age children often have a snaggle-tooth appearance while they are losing their primary teeth.

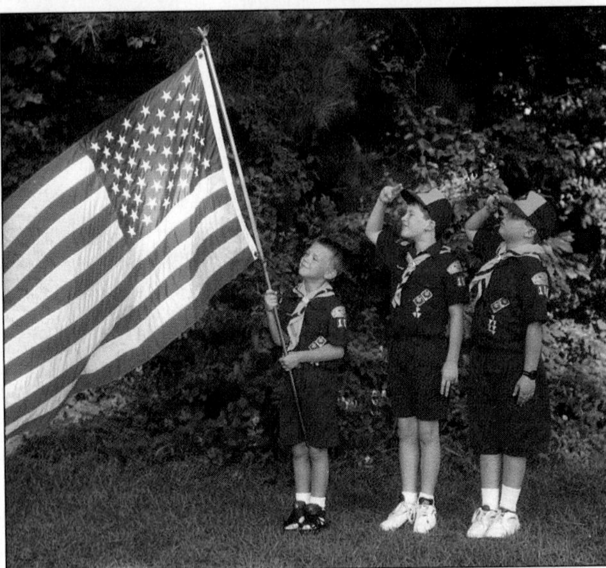

◀ Organizations such as Boy Scouts help to foster self-esteem and competence.

Figure 7–1
Growth and development of the school-age child.

Easter Bunny. As one 8-year-old laughingly answered, when asked if he believed in Santa, "I'm sure tryin', Mom!"

Humor. Children in the concrete operations stage have a delightful sense of humor. Around the age of 8, increased mastery of language and the beginning of logic enable children to appreciate a play on words. They laugh at incongruities and love silly jokes, riddles, and puns (e.g., "How do you keep a mad elephant from charging? You take away its credit cards!"). Riddle and joke books make ideal gifts for young school-age children.

Sensory Development

Vision. The eyes are fully developed by age 6. Visual acuity, ocular muscle control, peripheral vision, and color discrimination are fully developed by age 7. Just before puberty, some children's eyes experience a growth spurt, resulting in myopia. Children with poor visual acuity usually do not complain of vision problems because changes occur so gradually that they are difficult to notice. The young child may never have had 20/20 vision and has nothing with which to compare her imperfect vision. For these reasons, yearly vision screening is important for school-age children.

Hearing. With maturation and growth of the eustachian tube, middle-ear infections occur less frequently than in younger children. However, chronic middle-ear infections are a problem for a few children, resulting in hearing loss. Annual audiometric screening tests are important to detect hearing loss before unrecognized deficits lead to learning problems.

Language Development

Language development continues at a rapid pace during the school-age years. Vocabulary expands, and sentence structure becomes more complex. By age 6, the child's vocabulary is approximately 8000 to 14,000 words. There is an increase in the use of culturally specific words at this age. Bilingual children usually speak English at school and a different language at home.

Reading effectively improves language skills. Regular trips to the library, where the child can use her own library card to check out books of special interest, can promote a love of reading and enhance school performance. School-age children enjoy being read to as well as reading on their own.

School-age children often go through a period in which they experiment with profanity and dirty jokes. Parents who use four-letter words as part of their vocabulary are often imitated by their children.

Psychosocial Development

Development of a Sense of Industry. According to Erikson (1963), the central task of the school-age years is the development of a sense of industry. Ideally, the child is prepared for this task with a secure sense of himself as separate from loved ones in the family. The child should have learned to trust others and should have developed a sense of autonomy and initiative during the preceding years. The school-age child replaces fantasy play with "work" at school, crafts, chores, hobbies, and athletics. The child is rewarded by a sense of inner satisfaction in achieving a skill as well as by external rewards, such as good grades, trophies, or an allowance. School-age children enjoy undertaking new tasks and carrying them through to completion. Whether it is baking a cake, hitting a home run, or scoring 100 on a math test, purposeful activity leads to a sense of worth and competence. Successful resolution of the task of industry depends on learning to do things and do them well. School-age children learn skills that they will need later to compete in the adult world. A person's fundamental attitude toward work is established during the school-age years.

Fostering Self-Esteem. The negative component of this developmental stage is a sense of inferiority. If a child cannot separate psychologically from the parent or if expectations are set too high for the child to achieve, the child develops feelings of inferiority. If a child believes that she cannot succeed, she loses confidence and does not take pleasure in attempting new experiences. The child will then have a pervading feeling of inferiority and incompetence that will affect all aspects of her life. The child who lacks a sense of industry has a poor foundation for mastering the tasks of adolescence. The reality is that no one can master everything. Every child will feel deficient or inferior at something. The task of the caring parent or teacher is to identify areas in which a child is competent and to build on her successful experiences to foster feelings of mastery and success.

Nurses can suggest ways in which parents and teachers can promote a sense of self-esteem and competence in school-age children (see box).

Tips for Promoting Self-Esteem in Children

- Provide children with opportunities for assuming responsibility.
- Provide opportunities for making responsible choices and solving problems.
- Offer encouragement and positive feedback.
- Encourage self-discipline by providing guidelines and consequences.
- Help children feel okay about mistakes and failures.

Data from Brooks, R. B. (1992). Self-esteem during the school years: Its normal development and hazardous decline. *Pediatric Clinics of North America, 39*(3), 537–550.

Peer Relations. At this age, approval and esteem of those outside the family, especially peers, become important. Children learn that their parents are not infallible. As they begin to test parents' authority and knowledge, the influence of teachers and other adults is felt more and more. The peer group becomes the major socializing influence of the school-age child. Although parents' love, praise, and support are needed, even craved during stressful times, the child begins to prefer activities with friends to activities with the family. As the child becomes more independent, increasing amounts of time are spent with friends and away from the family.

The concept of friendship changes as the child matures. At 6 and 7 years old, children form friendships merely on the basis of who lives nearby or who has toys that they enjoy. By the time children are 9 or 10, friendships are based more on emotional bonds, warm feelings, and trust-building experiences. Children learn that friendship is more than just being together. Children at

11 and 12 years are loyal to their friends, often sharing problems and giving emotional support. School-age children tend to form friendships with peers of the same sex. Developing friendships and succeeding in social interactions lead to a sense of industry. Friendships are important for the emotional well-being of school-age children. Friends teach children skills they will use in future relationships.

Children learn a body of rules, sayings, and superstitions as they enter the culture of childhood. Rules are important to children because they provide predictability and offer security. Learning the sayings, jokes, and riddles are an important part of social interaction among peers. Sayings such as "Step on a crack and you'll break your mother's back" or "Finders, keepers; losers, weepers" have been a part of the lore of childhood for generations.

Children become sensitive to the norms and values of the peer group because pressure to conform is great. Children often find that it is painful to be different. Peer approval is a strong motivating force and allows the child to risk disapproval from parents.

The school-age years are a time of formal and informal clubs. Informal clubs among 6-, 7-, and 8-year-olds are loosely organized, with fluid membership. Membership changes frequently and is based on mutual interests, such as playing ball, riding bikes, or playing with dolls. Children learn interpersonal skills, such as sharing, cooperation, and tolerance, in these groups.

Clubs among older school-age children tend to be more structured, often characterized by secret codes, rituals, and rigid rules. A club may be formed for the purpose of exclusion, in which children snub another child for some reason.

Formal organizations, such as Boy Scouts, Girl Scouts, Campfire Boys and Girls, and 4H, organized by adults, also foster self-esteem and competence as children earn ranks and merit badges. Transmission of societal values, such as service to others, duty to God, and good citizenship, are important goals of these organizations.

Spiritual and Moral Development

The school-age years are pivotal in the development of a conscience and the internalization of values. Tremendous strides are made in moral development during these 6 years. Several theorists have described the dramatic growth that occurs during this stage.

Piaget. Piaget asserted that young school-age children obey rules because they are handed down by powerful, all-knowing adults. During this stage, children know the rules, but not the reasons behind them. Rules are interpreted in a literal way, and the child is unable to adjust rules to fit differing circumstances. The perception of guilt changes as the child matures. Piaget stated that up to about age 8, children judge degrees of guilt by the amount of damage done. No distinction is made between accidental and intentional wrongdoing. For example, the child believes that a child who broke five china cups by accident is more guilty than a child who broke one cup on purpose. By age 10, children are able to consider the intent of the action. Older school-age children are more flexible in their decisions and can take into account extenuating circumstances.

Kohlberg. Kohlberg described moral development in terms of three levels containing six stages (see Chapter 2). According to Kohlberg's theory, children who are 4 to 7 years of age are in stage 2 of the preconventional level, in which right and wrong are determined by physical consequences. The child obeys because of fear of punishment. If the child is not caught or punished for an act, the child does not consider the act wrong. At this stage, children conform to rules out of self-interest or in terms of what others can do in return ("I'll do this for you if you'll do that for me"). Behavior is guided by an "eye-for-an-eye" philosophy. Between the ages of 7 and 12, children are described by Kohlberg as being in stage 3 of the conventional level. A "good-boy" orientation characterizes this stage, in which the child conforms to rules to please others and avoid disapproval. This stage parallels the concrete operations stage of cognitive development. Around the age of 12, children enter stage 4 of the conventional level. There is an orientation toward respecting authority, obeying rules, and maintaining social order. Most religions place the age of accountability at approximately 12 years.

Influence of the Family. Moral development is profoundly influenced by parents and teachers. Parents can teach children the difference between right and wrong most effectively by living according to their values. A father who lectures his child about the importance of honesty gives a mixed message when he brags about fooling his boss or cheating on his income tax return. The moral atmosphere in the home is a critical factor in the personality development of the child. Children learn self-discipline and internalization of values through obedience to external rules. School-age children are legalistic, and they feel loved and secure when they know that firm limits are set on their behavior. They want and expect discipline for wrongdoings. For moral teaching to be effective, parents must be consistent in their expectations of their children as well as in administering rewards and punishment.

Spirituality and Religion. Spiritually, school-age children become acquainted with the basic content of their faith. Children reared within a religious tradition feel a part of their religion. They may believe in God with their whole being, and they affirm the reality of the divine in their life (Carlson, 1989). Although their thinking is still concrete, children begin to use abstract concepts to describe God and are able to comprehend God as a power greater than themselves or their parents. They have a great desire to learn about God and religion (Shelley, 1982). Because school-age children think literally, spiritual concepts take on materialistic and physical expression. They are fascinated by heaven and hell. Concern for rules and a maturing conscience may cause a nagging sense of guilt and fear of going to hell. Younger school-age children still tend to associate accidents and illness with punishment for real or imagined wrongdoing. One 6-year-old child hospitalized for an appendectomy said, "God saw all the bad things I did, and He punished me." Reassurance that God does not punish children by making them sick reduces anxiety.

At 8 and 9 years, children begin to relate to God through prayer, although their prayers are usually egocentric. They believe that if they have been "good" and ask God for something, He should give it to them. At ages 10 through 12, children tend to pray more spontaneously in response to their feelings, regarding prayer as a private conversation with God. Prayers gradually become more altruistic. By age 10 or 12, children begin to think about how faith relates to life, and they can discuss and explain what they believe. By age 12, some children begin to examine the validity of what they have been taught (Shelley, 1982). As children begin to realize that their parents are fallible, they welcome the assurance of someone or something greater. Adults who can communicate their faith without embarrassment can strengthen and comfort a child (Goldman, 1965).

HEALTH PROMOTION FOR THE SCHOOL-AGE CHILD AND FAMILY

Table 7–2 presents an overview of health screening, health maintenance, and anticipatory guidance activities for school-age children.

Sleep and Rest

The number of hours spent sleeping decreases as the child grows older. Children aged 6 and 7 years need about 12 hours of sleep per night. Some children also continue to need an afternoon quiet time or nap to restore energy levels. The 12-year-old needs about 9 to 10 hours of sleep at night (Coble et al., 1987). Increased amounts of sleep are needed when the child enters the preadolescent growth spurt. Adequate sleep is important for school performance and physical growth. Inadequate sleep can cause irritability, inability to concentrate, and poor school performance.

To promote rest and sleep, a period of quiet activity just before bedtime is helpful. A leisurely bedtime routine, with adequate time for the child to read, listen to the radio, or just daydream, promotes relaxation. When parents give in to bedtime struggles or allow late bedtimes followed by catch-up morning sleep on weekends and vacations, the child may have trouble waking up on time on school days (Ferber, 1987). A set bedtime and waking time, consistently enforced, promotes security and healthful sleep habits. Bedtime offers an ideal opportunity for parent and child to share important events of the day or give a kiss and a hug, unthinkable in front of peers earlier in the day.

Dental Care

Although the incidence of dental **caries** (tooth decay) has declined in recent years, tooth decay remains a significant health problem among school-age children. Unfortunately, many parents and school-age children consider dental hygiene to be of minor importance. Many parents erroneously believe that dental care, even brushing, is not important for primary teeth because they will all fall out anyway. However, premature loss of these deciduous teeth can complicate eruption of permanent teeth and lead to malocclusion. Statistics from the United States Government Public Health Service indicate that nearly half of the children in the nation have tooth decay or gum disease when entering school (United States Department of Health and Human Services, 1991). Gingivitis (inflammation of the gums) affects more than 60% of adolescents in the United States (Park et al., 1992).

Dental problems are more widespread among the poor. Low-income children have more than four times as many untreated decayed teeth as children from higher income families (United States Department of Health and Human Services, 1991). Unfortunately, children with the most decay are the least likely to receive dental treatment (Griffin & Goepferd, 1991). Dental caries are largely preventable with proper brushing, flossing, and fluoride supplementation.

School-age children are able to assume responsibility for their own dental hygiene. Good oral health habits tend to be carried into the adult years, reducing cavity formation for a lifetime. Thorough brushing with a fluoride toothpaste followed by flossing between the teeth should be done after meals and especially before bedtime. Proper brushing and flossing and a well-balanced diet promote healthy gums as well as prevent cavities (see Chapter 12). Sugary or sticky between-meal snacks should be limited. Candy that dissolves quickly, such as chocolate, is less cariogenic than sticky candy, which stays in contact with teeth longer.

Fluoride Supplements. The American Academy of Pediatrics recommends providing fluoride supplementation

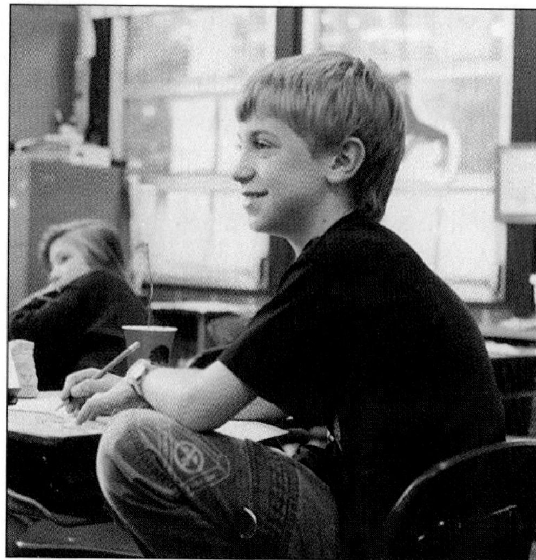

◀ Attention span increases during the school-age years, facilitating classroom learning.

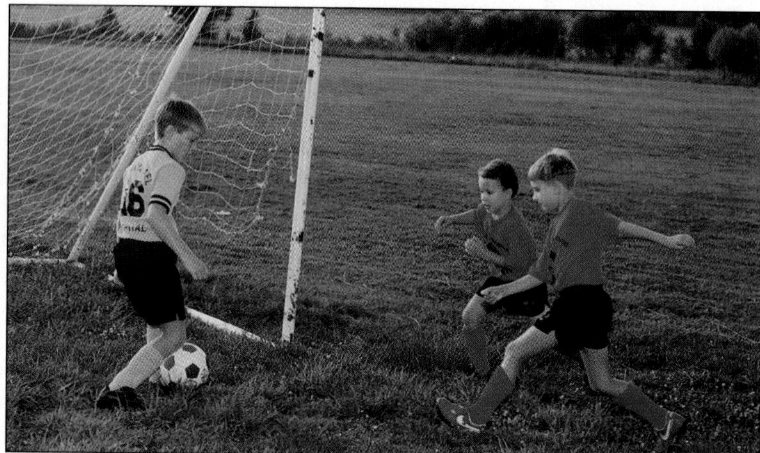

The nurse is in an excellent position to help parents and children identify factors that produce stress and to suggest ways to cope with its effects. Participation in competitive sports is stressful for some children, especially if parents push their child to play organized sports at an early age or overemphasize the importance of winning. Focusing on having fun and on the excitement of the game decreases competitive stress.

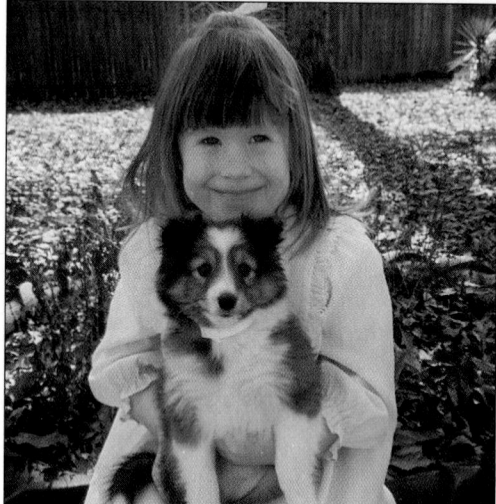

◀ Spending time playing with and caring for pets can be fun and relaxing. Children who are given time and encouragement to play are better able to deal with the stresses of life.

Figure 7–2
Health promotion for the school-age child and family.

from 2 weeks of age through at least 16 years of age to prevent dental caries. Community water fluoridation is the most efficient and cost-effective method of providing recommended levels of fluoride (Burt, 1989; American Academy of Pediatrics, 1986). Fluoride supplements are important for children who do not have access to fluoridated drinking water. Before fluoride supplements are recommended, however, assays of the drinking water should be obtained to decrease the risk of dental fluorosis (mottled enamel). This condition is caused by the ingestion of excessive fluoride during the years of tooth calcification (Leverett et al., 1988). Dosage of fluoride is dependent on the child's age and the water fluoride level (see Chapter 5, Table 5–3).

Dentist Visits and Application of Sealants. School-age children should visit the dentist at least twice yearly for a checkup, cleaning, and application of sealants and fluoride. Dental sealants are plastic coverings applied to the occlusal (chewing) surfaces of newly erupted permanent molars to prevent decay. These surfaces often decay because they contain pits and fissures (tiny grooves where plaque accumulates). Sealants have been shown to reduce decay by up to 45% (Griffin & Geopferd, 1991). According to the National Institute of Dental Research, two-thirds of decay is found on the chewing surfaces of teeth and could be eliminated with the combined use of fluoride and sealants (American Dental Association, 1993). First permanent molars erupt around age 6 and second molars at age 12. Children should be evaluated by their dentist at these ages to determine the need for dental sealants.

Malocclusion. Good occlusion of the teeth is important for tooth formation, speech development, and physical appearance. Many school-age children require braces to correct **malocclusion,** a condition in which the teeth are crowded, crooked, or out of alignment. Factors such as heredity, cleft palate, premature loss of primary teeth, and mouth breathing lead to malocclusion. Thumb sucking is not believed to cause malocclusion unless it persists past the age of 5 or 6. Malocclusion becomes particularly noticeable between the ages of 6 and 12, when the permanent teeth are erupting.

Children with braces are at increased risk for dental caries and must be scrupulous about their dental hygiene. School nurses can encourage children who wear braces to brush after every meal and snack, eat a nutritious diet, and visit the dentist at least once every 6 months. Use of a Water Pik appliance keeps gums healthy and helps to remove food particles from around wires and bands.

Braces cause many children to feel self-conscious and may be difficult for a school-age child to accept. However, for some children, orthodontic appliances may be a status symbol. Parental support and encouragement are important to help the child adjust to orthodontic treatment.

Preventing Dental Injuries. During the school-age years, injuries to the teeth can occur easily. Many injuries can be avoided by using mouth protectors. These resilient shields protect against injuries by cushioning blows that might otherwise damage teeth or lead to jaw fractures (American Dental Association, 1993). Children should wear a mouth protector when participating in activities that may involve falls, head contact, tooth clenching, or flying equipment. These activities range from skateboarding to basketball, football, or soccer (American Dental Association, 1993). See Chapter 14 for a discussion of dental emergencies. Custom-made mouth protectors constructed by the dentist are more expensive than stock mouth protectors purchased in stores, but their better fit makes them more comfortable and less likely to interfere with speech and breathing.

Dental Health Education. Health education curricula need to be designed to foster attitudes and behaviors among children that promote personal oral hygiene practices and awareness of the risks of dental disease. The school nurse is in an excellent position to educate children about dental health as well as to detect problems such as untreated caries, inflamed gums, or malocclusion. The nurse should look for signs of smokeless tobacco use (irritation of the gums at the tobacco placement site, gum recession, and stained teeth) and should take this opportunity to explain to the child the risks of using tobacco. The use of snuff and chewing tobacco carries multiple dangers, including a greatly increased risk of oral cancer and heart disease. As little as 3 to 4 months of smokeless tobacco use can cause periodontal disease and leukoplakias (precancerous lesions). Abrasives and sugars in smokeless tobaccos also lead to greater tooth abrasion and decay. (American Dental Association, 1993). Children with dental problems should be referred to a dentist for further evaluation and treatment.

Resources. The American Dental Association and the American Society of Dentistry for Children are excellent sources of material about the care of children's teeth (see Dental Care Resources in Appendix H for addresses).

Adjustment to School

Most children are eager to start school, particularly if they have older siblings. They even look forward to bringing home their books and doing "real" homework. This enthusiasm usually fades quickly, however. Most children adjust well to first grade, enjoying the opportunities it provides for peer interaction and stimulating experiences. However, first grade may be the child's first experience being away from home. For these children, starting school may be a frightening experience. Even children who have attended preschool have some anxiety about beginning first grade. Adjustment to school depends on a variety of factors, including the child's physical and emotional maturity, the child's experiences, and the parents' ability to support the child and accept the separation (see Chapter 6).

Influence of Peers. School is often the first experience a child has with a large number of children of the same age. From peers children learn how to cooperate, compete, bargain, and follow rules. Peer approval is of major importance as the child looks to his friends for recognition and support. The influence of peers becomes stronger as the child grows older.

Influence of Teachers. Teachers have a significant influence on the social and intellectual development of children. An effective teacher makes learning fun and capitalizes on the child's interests and talents. Teachers guide the child's learning by rewarding him for success and helping him learn from and deal with failures. The teacher plays an important role in preventing feelings of inferiority in the child. By structuring the learning environment so that the child experiences success, the teacher bolsters feelings of industry.

The student–teacher relationship is a key factor in school success. Effective teachers motivate students by being warm and understanding, showing interest, and communicating on the child's level. Children value the opinion of such teachers and will work to gain their approval. Favorite teachers serve as role models and are often objects of hero worship by their students.

Even excellent teachers cannot do an effective job alone. They need the support of parents and school administration to maximize the learning potentials of children.

The Parents' Role. Parents play a key role in their children's academic success. By taking an active interest in children's progress and encouraging them to do their best, parents can foster learning. Positive reinforcement should be given for honest efforts, not just good grades. Parents should enforce rules that encourage self-discipline and good study habits (e.g., no TV until homework is finished). The child must create and adhere to a schedule for completing large assignments to prevent last-minute panic. If the child does not have a desk or another private place for homework, the kitchen table or another quiet, well-lighted area should be made available during study time. The TV should be turned off during study time, and distractions should be kept to a minimum. Adequate sleep is important for school performance. Parents may need to enforce bedtime rules to meet the child's needs. Rewarding children for meeting deadlines and for being organized encourages them to take responsibility for their learning and fosters skills that are important for success in jobs as adults.

Parents need to communicate with teachers and stay informed about their children's progress. Visiting the classroom and attending parent–teacher conferences and school activities are important. Showing respect for the teacher and supporting his efforts facilitates learning.

School Phobia

School phobia affects 3% to 5% of school-age children. The child with school phobia becomes anxious even at the thought of leaving home for school. Complaints of abdominal pain, nausea, vomiting, anorexia, and headache occur when it is time to go to school and resolve quickly once the child is allowed to remain home (Leung, 1989). Symptoms do not occur on weekends or holidays unless they are related to going other places, such as Sunday school. These children want to go to school and often earn good grades, but fear, depression, and anxiety prevent them from going.

Traditionally, school phobia has been attributed to separation anxiety (the result of an overdependent parent–child relationship). A child with separation anxiety is not afraid to go to school, but is afraid to leave home (Eisenberg, 1958; Leung, 1989; Strawbridge & Gable, 1989). Research suggests that childhood depression is the cause of school phobia (Bernstein et al., 1990). Other factors that encourage the development of school phobia include bullying at school, an overly critical teacher, and rejection by peers. Events such as sudden marital discord, a family move, or arrival of a new sibling can precipitate fear of going to school. School phobia should not be confused with truancy, which is a deliberate, conscious attempt to avoid school to do other, more enjoyable activities.

School phobia affects boys and girls equally. Almost all children with school phobia have average or above average intelligence. School phobia occurs most often at the start of school, between ages 5 and 7, or at puberty and the start of high school, between ages 11 and 14 (Turner-Boutle, 1984).

Helping a Child Overcome School Phobia. Prompt return to school is the key to treatment of school phobia. The child should be treated with sympathy and understanding, but with a firm expectation of school attendance. The longer the child is allowed to avoid school, the more severe the symptoms are likely to become. Physical causes for the symptoms should be ruled out by examination by a physician. Once the child has returned to school, treatment is focused on determining and alleviating the cause of the phobia. The child should be gently questioned about factors at school that cause worry or fear. Specific causes, such as a bully or an overly critical teacher, should be dealt with immediately. Parents must support each other because the child may play one parent against the other to avoid school. Parents should not express anxiety over the child's symptoms, but should merely state, "If children are well enough to be up around the house, they are well enough to be in school." If a child stays home, she should not be allowed to watch TV, play games, or stay in bed. Positive reinforcement for school attendance is essential. Encouraging and maintaining peer contacts and emphasizing the positive aspects of school are helpful. The principal and teacher should be told about the situation so that they can cooperate with the treatment plan. If symptoms are severe, a limited period of part-time or modified school attendance may be necessary. For example, part of the day may be spent in the counselor's or school nurse's office, with assignments obtained from the teacher. Parents should be told that school phobia is considered a family problem, but that neither the child nor the parents are to blame (Leung, 1989).

"Latchkey" Children

As the number of working mothers and single parents increases, so does the number of children who are left at home without adult supervision for all or part of the day. More than 2 million United States children who are 5 to 13 years old return home from school to an empty house **(latchkey children).** An additional half million are alone at home before school in the morning (Berman et al.,

1992). The number of latchkey children may be underestimated because of parents' reluctance to admit that their children have to care for themselves. Parents often feel guilty about leaving children alone and may feel concern for their children's safety. These children are at increased risk for accidents as well as for injuries caused by intruders. Fear, loneliness, lack of homework supervision, and poor nutrition are potential problems for latchkey children. Studies have suggested that these children are more likely to succumb to peer pressure in the use of alcohol, tobacco, and marijuana (Richardson et al., 1989; Steinberg, 1986). On the other hand, these problems do not always occur, and children may even benefit from self-care. Some children thrive on the challenge of being on their own, assuming greater responsibility, and becoming increasingly self-reliant, independent, and resourceful.

Support and Safety. Nurses can help families by offering support and education to parents and children to reduce the risks for self-care children. Parents need to know how to prepare their children for self-care, teaching them specific strategies for staying safe at home alone (see Chapter 13). Nurses can serve as child advocates by working to develop expanded after-school child care programs in the community. A number of communities have established after-school telephone help lines to provide information, support, and assistance to self-care children. Phone Friend and Grandma, Please are two programs that have materials available for those wishing to establish similar programs. A number of books are also available for parents and children (see Latchkey Children: Books and Other Resources in Appendix H).

Discipline

Because school-age children possess a strong sense of justice and believe in the importance of rules, they want and expect limits to be set on their behavior. Firm, consistent limits increase children's sense of security and reinforce the message that an adult cares about them. Realistic expectations, clearly defined rules, and logical consequences help children to develop self-discipline and increased self-esteem. The goal of discipline is to educate children to take responsibility for their actions. If children are to learn to take this responsibility, they must be involved in the process of understanding and even establishing rules, limits, and consequences (Adelman and Taylor, 1990). Examples of effective discipline techniques for school-age children include:

- *At the beginning of the year, the den leader asks the Cub Scouts what rules they think should exist at den meetings and what the consequences should be if someone breaks a rule.* It is not unusual for the children's rules to be more stringent than rules that the adult would have suggested. Involving children in making the rules helps them to understand the importance of limits and increases motivation to follow the rules that they have established.
- *The teacher prevents a discipline problem from emerging by asking a hyperactive student to be a helper in the classroom.* Providing the child with a concrete activity increases the child's self-esteem by letting him know that he is capable and has something to offer. Such "contributory activities" help the child to become more successful at school (Brooks, 1992).
- *The parent uses the technique of "grounding" when the child breaks a rule.* An effective variation of grounding is called job grounding. Rather than grounding the child for a specified period, the parent grounds the child until he has finished a job assigned by the parent. During job grounding, the parent must not nag the child about the job, discuss the reason for the grounding, or interact with the child. The child may not have friends over, talk on the telephone, or watch TV. As soon as the job is completed satisfactorily, the grounding is over (Christopherson, 1992).

Teachers' discipline efforts are often thwarted when parents do not support them or show no concern about their children's misbehavior. Teamwork between parents and teachers is essential for effective discipline. Regular parent-teacher conferences help make discipline effective (see Chapter 16).

Stress

Today's children are subjected to stress as no generation has been before. Alarming increases in drug abuse, childhood suicide, child abduction and murder, and school failure attest to the overwhelming stress that children experience. Rapid, bewildering social change and ever-increasing demands for achievement often pressure children to grow up too quickly.

Research has shown that patterns of reacting to stress established in childhood are often carried over into adulthood (Elkind, 1981; Matthews, 1981). Stressed children may not show serious symptoms during childhood, but may develop patterns of emotional response that can lead to serious illness as adults. Manifestations of stress are listed in the accompanying box.

Sources of Stress for Children

Growing up is stressful, even for well-adjusted children with loving, supportive families. Children experience stress from societal change, school, competitive athletics, rushed schedules, and the media.

Middle-class children, particularly, are pressured to grow up quickly. Achievement-oriented parents, focused on success and financial gain, often view children as extensions of themselves and unwittingly expect too much of their children. Pressure on children to succeed, to win, and to be the best and brightest is great, especially when parents value academic achievement. Children are often pressured into a frenzied schedule of music, dance, sports, and art lessons and may have little time for family meals or playing with friends. Self-esteem and peer relationships often suffer.

Economically deprived children must cope with an even greater burden of stress. Faced with the dangers of violence, drug and alcohol addiction, and gangs, these children must fight daily for survival. Children from lower-income families travel dangerous streets to and from school and suffer from the insecurity and uncertainty of poverty. Families are the fastest growing segment of the homeless population. The National Coalition for the Homeless estimates that 750,000 school-age children are homeless and that as many as 60% of homeless children do not attend school. These children face tremendous chronic stress. Many are developmentally delayed, do not receive immunizations or basic health care, suffer from malnutrition, contract sexually transmitted diseases, are victims of trauma or assault, and many die as a result of their dangerous surroundings (Berne et al., 1990; Raferty, 1989).

School Pressures. School can be a source of stress for children. Some children are unable to cope with the competitive, test-regulated curricula of school. They find it difficult to keep up with the unrelenting academic pressure. A survey of 8000 students showed that fifth and ninth graders ranked school performance as number one in importance in their lives. Further, 16% of the fifth graders and 9% of the ninth graders surveyed thought that someday they might kill themselves because of school concerns (Search Institute of Minneapolis, 1985, as cited in Busen, 1988). Children who are expected to perform beyond their mental abilities may see themselves as failures (Elkind, 1981). School imposes chronic stress on these children, and they tend to dislike school and stay home whenever they can. They are often tardy and may abuse alcohol and drugs. Eventually, they may drop out of school. These children rarely return to complete their education.

Other children, particularly those who are academically gifted, find school stressful because it is tedious. Boredom can be stressful. Meaningless, repetitive schoolwork can cause bright, talented children to become chronically fatigued, inattentive, and careless.

Physical Threats. Children also face other types of stress at school. Violence and theft in schools are national problems. Fears of being beaten up or held up are commonly voiced by school-age children. The child who leaves a bike unlocked or a watch or jacket unattended quickly learns the hazards of such carelessness. Students who abuse drugs or participate in gang activity create a pervasive attitude of wariness and fear and are a real source of stress for children.

Competitive Sports. Participation in competitive sports is stressful for some children. Fear of failure, especially in front of a cheering crowd, can be overwhelming. Some parents contribute to competitive stress by overemphasizing the importance of winning. Because of their own needs or interests, some parents push their children to participate in organized sports at an early age. Many young children are forced into sports that require physical skills beyond their ability (Elkind, 1981). Overscheduling athletic activities can make children more vulnerable to the pressure of competition (Busen, 1988).

Tight Schedules and "Adaptation Overload." As the number of single parents and working mothers increases, so does the stress on children who must adapt to parents' work schedules. Many children are rushed from home to school to carpool to daycare or a babysitter. It is not unusual for children to spend a long day outside of the home, adapting to several environments, all with different expectations (Busen, 1988). Children must draw on their energy reserves to exercise self-control in these varying situations and may not be able to cope. Fatigue and exhaustion from such demands often result in behavioral problems and regression. Chronic hurrying is an

Manifestations of Stress

How children perceive stress influences its effects. It is not just the stress, but how the child perceives and responds to the stress that determines whether the child experiences symptoms of stress.

Intervention is needed when a child shows the following signs of stress:

- Unhappiness, moodiness
- Irritability, increased aggressive behavior
- Fatigue, inability to concentrate
- Hyperactivity
- Changes in eating or sleeping habits
- Physical complaints (nausea, headaches, stomachaches)
- Bedwetting
- Substance abuse
- Diminished school performance
- Suicidal behavior

enormous source of stress for children. Young children (2–8 years) tend to perceive hurrying as a rejection, a sign that their parents do not really care about them. Children find such rejection threatening and often develop stress symptoms as a result (Elkind, 1981). Older children can understand that parents' work schedules necessitate after-school care, but they too are stressed by insufficient time to relax and are susceptible to adaptation overload. When parents routinely place their own needs ahead of the child's, hurrying can produce real damage (Elkind, 1981).

Family Pressures. Fragmentation of the family, mobility of people in our society, and deterioration of social institutions, such as religion, place tremendous stresses on children today (Hluchy, 1981, as cited in Elkind, 1981). David Elkind, noted child psychologist and author of *The Hurried Child,* said:

> *Children are forced to take on the physical, psychological, and social trappings of adulthood before they are prepared to deal with them. We dress our children in miniature adult costumes (often with designer labels), we expose them to gratuitous sex and violence, and expect them to cope with an increasingly bewildering social environment—divorce, single parenthood, and homosexuality. Through all of these pressures the child senses that it is important for him or her to cope without admitting the confusion and pain that accompany such changes. This pressure to cope without cracking is a stress in itself.*

Overhearing parents quarrel produces anxiety and fear in children and erodes a child's sense of security. Some parents, although physically present, may be emotionally unavailable to children because of their own stresses. Divorce and separation are especially painful. Changes frequently caused by divorce, such as moving to a new house, attending a new school and, usually the most stressful of all, separation from one of the parents, can cause great stress for children.

Influence of the Media. The media are a common source of stress for today's children. TV programs and movies often give children information that they are intellectually and emotionally unprepared to handle (Elkind, 1981). Sexual and violent material portraying loss of control may frighten children because it suggests that they may not be able to master their own sexual and aggressive impulses. TV exposes children to vivid portrayals of the problems of today's society for many hours of their day. It also tends to isolate children from their parents and peers. Hours spent watching TV can limit children's participation in more creative play as well as contact and interaction with others.

Interventions and Anticipatory Guidance

The nurse is in an ideal position to help parents and children to identify factors that produce stress and to suggest ways to cope with its effects. Parents may need guidance about realistic expectations of their children. Parents who understand the negative effects of hurrying children are more likely to set healthier, more realistic schedules for the family. Parents should watch for behavior changes in their children that may indicate signs of stress and offer appropriate reassurance. If parents are asking too much of their children, they can either reduce their demands or increase their supports (Elkind, 1981). If there is a significant tension in the home, parents can try to resolve conflicts by negotiating rather than continuing to build an emotionally charged atmosphere. Parents should examine the child's schedule to make sure the child is not overburdened with school and extracurricular activities. Most importantly, parents should be available to listen whenever the child wants to talk (Elkind, 1993).

Close communication with teachers is important to prevent and deal with school-related stress. Becoming interested in and involved with the child's schoolwork conveys support and caring. Parents need to become active in parent–teacher associations and other community organizations to find solutions to the problems of violence and crime in the schools.

Children should be allowed to decide whether to participate in competitive athletics. It is important for parents to talk to coaches to determine what is expected of their children. Corrective instruction rather than punishment should be given for errors. Focusing on having fun and on the excitement of the game rather than on winning decreases competitive stress (Busen, 1988). Parents should serve as role models for good sportsmanship.

Limiting the number of hours that children watch TV and helping them to select appropriate programs can decrease its negative effects. Watching TV with children and discussing the content of programs is also helpful.

Children need to have time just to play. Parents should recognize that play is the child's work. Whether it is shooting baskets in the driveway, working on a collection, or building a model, play reduces stress for children. Toys and games that provide the greatest opportunity to use imagination are the best stress relievers. Most children love animals. Spending time playing with and caring for pets can be relaxing and fun. Children who are given the time and encouragement to play are better able to deal with the stresses of life (see Chapter 9).

One of the most effective antidotes for childhood stress is a loving, attentive parent who takes the time to listen. A sympathetic adult who understands the stresses of childhood can offer valuable support. Discussion and modeling of ways to deal with the inevitable stresses of life can teach the child valuable lessons for living in today's society.

TABLE 7–2 *Health Screening, Health Maintenance, and Anticipatory Guidance for School-Age Children*

6–7 YEARS	8–10 YEARS	10–12 YEARS
Immunization		
DTP #5, OPV #4 to be given between 4–6 years, at or before school entry. DTP is not given to children ≥ 7 years (use Td instead). Review immunization record; administer appropriate immunizations if not up to date. Review previous reactions and contraindications.	Review immunization record; administer appropriate immunizations if not up to date.	MMR #2 at entry to middle school unless second dose was previously given. Td booster between ages 11–16, then every 10 years. HBV given to 11- to 12-year-olds who have not previously received three doses of HBV vaccine.
Safety		
Seat belts, fire and bicycle safety. Does child know how to swim? Is water play supervised at all times? Does child play sports? Is the sports program well supervised and is protective gear mandatory (e.g., helmets for T-ball, shin guards for soccer)? Teach child safety around swings, skateboards, playground equipment. Protect child from sunburn with sunscreen.	Seat belts. Teach child not to ride in back of pickup trucks. Teach child safety around lawn tractors, farm equipment. Does child know how to swim? Does child take risks that concern or frighten parents? Does child know what to do if approached by a stranger? Sex education: Make child aware of "good touching" and "bad touching." Discuss dangers of fireworks, matches, campfires. Wear a helmet when riding a bicycle or horse.	Car safety belts. Has there been any involvement in or discussion of drugs, smoking, alcohol? Does child know how to swim? Teach gun safety.
Nutrition		
Assess usual diet: what do meals and snacks consist of? Discuss importance of breakfast to school performance. Discuss food pyramid and importance of a healthy diet. Any concerns about weight?	Appetite increases. Child needs approximately 2400 calories per day. Nutrition education: nutritious snacks, basic cooking skills, meal planning. Assess regularity of meals and snacks.	Assess adequacy of diet and snacks. Is child too busy to eat properly? Assess amount and frequency of junk food, fast food. Teach child to avoid concentrated sweets.
Vision, Hearing, and Speech		
Assess vision with Snellen and hearing with audiometry every 2 years. If child has been screened elsewhere, what were the results? Assess parents' and teacher's perceptions of child's vision and hearing. Is child's speech clear? Any dysfluency?	Assess vision with Snellen and hearing with audiometry every 2 years. Have corrective lenses been prescribed? Does child wear them? Teach child and parents not to remove earwax with cotton-tipped applicators or hairpins.	Assess vision with Snellen and hearing with audiometry every 2 years. Address parental concerns. Discuss effect on hearing of listening to loud music with headphones.

KEY CONCEPTS

- The school age years, from 6 to 12, are characterized by slow, steady physical growth and rapid social and cognitive development. Average weight gain in the school-age child is 2.5 kg (5.5 lb) per year, and the increase in height is approximately 5.5 cm (2 inches) per year. During the early school-age period, boys are approximately 1 inch taller and 2 lb heavier than girls.
- During the school-age years, children gradually move away from home and parents as a primary source of support, and they enter the wider world of peers and school.
- Physical changes include increased height and weight, increased muscle mass, maturation of body systems, and increased antibody production. During the school-age period, all 20 primary teeth are lost and are replaced by 28 of the 32 permanent teeth.
- Pubertal changes begin at around age 9 for girls and age 11 for boys. The average age of menarche is 12. The average age for puberty in boys is 14.

TABLE 7-2 *Health Screening, Health Maintenance, and Anticipatory Guidance for School-Age Children (continued)*

6–7 YEARS	8–10 YEARS	10–12 YEARS
Dental Care		
Does child brush teeth and have regular dental checkups? Does parent assist child with flossing? Dental visit every 6 months to 1 year.	Does child brush teeth and have regular dental checkups? Many cavities? Malocclusion? Discuss importance of well-balanced diet, limited sweets. Does child brush and floss twice daily? Discuss importance of good oral hygiene with braces.	Does child brush and floss twice daily? Discuss importance of dental visit every 6 months to 1 year.
Screening		
Plot height and weight on growth charts. Screen blood pressure yearly. Bacteriuria screen for girls. Perform annual TB testing for high-risk children (otherwise tested in infancy, preschool, adolescence). Screen blood cholesterol level if family history of hyperlipidemia or early myocardial infarction.	Plot height and weight on growth charts. Assess if weight gain follows the curve (high-risk period for obesity). Screen blood pressure yearly. Bacteriuria screen for girls. Annual TB testing for high-risk children. Hemoglobin or hematocrit and urinalysis once during school-age period and more often if indicated.	Plot height and weight on growth charts. Assess for scoliosis. Screen blood pressure yearly. Bacteriuria screen for girls. Annual TB testing for high-risk children.
Teaching and Counseling		
Discuss TV viewing. Advise parents that child's TV viewing be limited to 2 hours per day. How does child get along with other children? How much time does he spend playing with other children? Does she have a best friend? Is gender identity fixed? If child has not started school, assess parental and child reactions to approaching school entry, parents' perceptions of child's readiness for school.	Assess parents' and child's reactions to school. How is child doing in school? If there are difficulties, have they been addressed by the school and parents? How many days has child been absent from school? Reasons? Child care arrangements for before and after school? Have sexuality and sexual development been discussed with child? Any signs of puberty yet? Does child understand what is happening and what will happen in the future?	Assess child's stress level. Help parents and child identify factors that produce stress and suggest ways to cope with its effects. Discuss dangers of drug and alcohol use and sexual activity.

Abbreviations: DTP, Diphtheria and tetanus toxoids with pertussis vaccine; OPV, oral poliovirus vaccine; OTP, ; Td, tetanus–diphtheria toxoid; MMR, measles, mumps, and rubella; HBV, hepatitis B virus vaccine.

- School-age children enjoy a variety of activities. Cooperative play and team sports are typical of this age group.
- According to Erikson, the developmental task of this period is the development of a sense of industry.
- The child develops a conscience and internalizes cultural and social values. The child is able to understand and obey rules.
- Thinking becomes less egocentric as children learn to consider viewpoints different from their own. School-age children can solve problems, form hypotheses, and make judgments based on reason.
- Sources of stress for school-age children include societal change, school, competitive athletics, rushed schedules, and the media. Teaching children coping strategies can reduce the effects of stress.
- Dental care is increasingly important as the primary teeth are replaced by permanent teeth. Common dental problems of school-age children include caries, periodontal disease, and malocclusion.

REFERENCES

Adelman, H. S., & Taylor, L. (1990). Intrinsic motivation and school misbehavior: Some intervention implications. *Journal of Learning Disabilities, 23*, 541.

Algranati, P. S. (1992). *The pediatric patient: An approach to history and physical examination*. Baltimore: Williams and Wilkins.

American Academy of Pediatrics, Council on Nutrition. (1986). Fluoride supplementation. *Pediatrics, 77*, 758–761.

American Dental Association. (1988, July 4). Research shows caries disappearing in children. *ADA News*, Chicago: Author.

American Dental Association. (1993). *Your child's teeth*. Chicago: Author.

Bailey, D. (1978). The growing child and the need for physical activity. In M. Smart, & R. Smart. *School age children: Development and relationships*. New York: Macmillan.

Berman, B. D., Winkleby, M., Chesterman, E., & Boyce, W. T. (1992). After-school child care and self-esteem in school age children. *Pediatrics, 89*(4), 654–659.

Berne, A. S., Dato, C., Mason, D. I., & Rafferty, M. (1990). A nursing model for addressing the health needs of homeless families. *Image: Journal of Nursing Scholarship, 22*(1), 8–13.

Bernstein, G. A., Peder, H., Svingen, P. H., & Garfinkel, B. D. (1990). School phobia: Patterns of family functioning. *Journal of the American Academy of Child and Adolescent Psychiatry, 29*(1), 24–30.

Brooks, R. B. (1992). Self-esteem during the school years: Its normal development and hazardous decline. *Pediatric Clinics of North America, 39*(3), 537–550.

Burt, B. A. (Ed.). (1989). Cost-effectiveness of caries prevention in dental public health: Results of the workshop. *Journal of Public Health Dentistry, 49*, 331–340.

Busen, N. (1988). Societal values: A cause of stress in children. *Journal of Pediatric Health Care, 2*(6), 300–306.

Carlson, V. B. (1989). *Spiritual dimensions of nursing practice*. Philadelphia: W. B. Saunders.

Christopherson, E. R. (1992). Discipline. *Pediatric Clinics of North America, 39*(3), 395–411.

Coble, P., Kupfer, D., Reynolds, C., & Houck, P. (1987). EEG sleep of healthy children 6 to 12 years of age. In C. Guilleminault (Ed.), *Sleep and its disorders in children*. New York: Raven Press.

Dworkin, P. H. (1989). School failure. *Pediatric Review, 10*, 309.

Eisenberg, L. (1958). School phobia: A study in the communication of anxiety. *American Journal of Psychiatry, 114*(7), 712–718.

Elkind, D. (1981). *The hurried child*. Reading, MA: Addison-Wesley.

Elkind, D. (1993). *Parenting your teenager*. New York: Ballantine Books.

Erikson, E. (1963). *Childhood and society* (2nd ed.). New York: Norton.

Ferber, R. (1987). Circadian and schedule disturbances. In C. Guilleminault (Ed.), *Sleep and its disorders in children*. New York: Raven Press.

Goldman, R. (1965). *Readiness for religion* (p. 8). London: Routledge and Kegan Paul.

Griffin, A. L. & Goepferd, S. J. (1991). Preventive oral health care for the infant, child, and adolescent. *Pediatric Clinics of North America, 38*(5), 1209–1226.

Jarvis, C. (1992). *Physical examination and health assessment*. Philadelphia: W. B. Saunders.

Leung, A. K. (1989). School phobia: Sometimes a child or teenager has good reason. *Postgraduate Medicine, 85*(1), 281–289.

Leverett, D. H., Adair, S., Proskin, H. M. (1988). Dental fluorosis among children in fluoridated and non-fluoridated communities [abstract, special issue]. *Journal of Dental Research, 67*, 230.

Matthews, K. A. (1981). Antecedents of the type A coronary-prone behavior pattern. In S. S. Brehn, S. M. Kassen, & G. X. Gibbons (Eds.), *Developmental Social Psychology* (pp. 235–248). New York: Oxford.

Nelms, B. C. (1990). They need more exercise. *Journal of Pediatric Health Care, 4*(4), 167–168.

Park, B. Z., Kinney, M. B., & Steffensen, J. E. (1992). Putting teeth into your physical exam: Part 1. Children and adolescents. *Journal of Family Practice, 35*(4), 459–462.

Piaget, J. (1962). *Play, dreams, and imitation in childhood*. (C. Gattegno & F. M. Hodgson, Trans.) New York: W. W. Norton.

Raferty, M. (1989). Standing up for America's homeless. *American Journal of Nursing, 12*, 1614–1617.

Richardson, J. L., Dwyer, K., & McGuigan, K. (1989). Substance use among eighth-grade students who take care of themselves after school. *Pediatrics, 84*, 556–566.

Schuster, G. S., & Ashburn, S. S. (1992). *The process of human development* (3rd ed.). Philadelphia: J. B. Lippincott.

Shelley, J. A. (1982). *The spiritual needs of children*. Downers Grove, IL: Intervarsity Press.

Strawbridge, G. W. & Gable, J. F. (1989). *Journal of the American Academy of Physicians Assistants, 2*(5), 368–372.

Steinberg, L. (1986). Latchkey children and susceptibility to peer pressure: An ecological analysis. *Developmental Psychology, 22*, 433–439.

Subcommittee on Fluoride of the Committee to Coordinate Environmental Health and Related Programs. (1991). *Review of fluoride: Benefits and risks*. Washington, DC: U.S. Department of Health and Human Services, Public Health Service.

Turner-Boutle, T. (1984). School phobia. *Nursing Times, 80*(33), 55–58.

BIBLIOGRAPHY

American Dental Association, Council on Dental Therapeutics. (1984). Fluoride compounds. In *Accepted dental therapeutics* (40th ed.). Chicago: Author.

Ames, L. B., & Ilg, F. L. (1979). *Your six year old: Loving and defiant.* New York: Delacorte Press.

Caplan, G. (1974). *Support systems and community mental health.* Englewood Cliffs, NJ: Behavioral Publications.

Castiglia, P. T. (1991). Moral development. *Journal of Pediatric Health Care, 5*(6), 324–326.

Centers for Disease Control. (1988). *Fluoridation census 1985.* Atlanta: Centers for Disease Control.

Corbin, C., & Pangrazi, R. (1992). Are American children and youth fit? *Research Quarterly for Exercise and Sport, 63*(2), 96–106.

Doak, S., & Hobbie, C. (1991). Latchkey children. *Journal of Pediatric Health Care, 5*(2), 110–111.

Dobson, J. (1979). *Hide or seek: How to build self-esteem in your child,* Old Tappan, NJ: Fleming H. Revell.

Duska, R., & Whelan, M. (1975). *Moral development: A guide to Piaget and Kohlberg.* New York: Paulist Press.

Erikson, E. (1968). Identity: *Youth in crisis.* New York: W. W. Norton.

Featherstone, J. D. B. (1987). The mechanisms of dental decay. *Nutrition Today, 22*(3), 10–16.

Fonterix, P., & O'Shea, B. (1990). Latchkey children. *Nursing Times, 86*(42), 55–57.

Furman, W. (1987). Acquaintanceship in middle childhood. *Developmental Psychology, 23*(4), 563–570.

Graham, M. V., & Uphold, C. R. (1992). Health perceptions and behaviors of school-aged boys and girls. *Journal of Community Health Nursing, 9,* 77–86.

Grey, M., & Hayman, L. L. (1987). Assessing stress in children: Research and clinical implications. *Journal of Pediatric Nursing, 2*(31), 316–327.

Gutin, B., Basch, C., & Shea, S. (1990). Blood pressure, fitness, and fatness in 5- and 6-year-old children. *JAMA, 264*(9), 1123–1127.

Hartup, W. (1989). Social relationships and their developmental significance. *American Psychologist, 44,* 120–126.

Healthy people 2000: National health promotion and disease prevention objectives (full report, with commentary) (1991). (DHHS publication no. [PHS] 91-50212). Washington, DC: U.S. Department of Health and Human Services, Public Health Service.

Horowitz, H. S. (1980). Combination of caries preventive agents and procedures. *Journal of Dental Research, 59,* 2183–2189.

Kaufman, A. (1989). School phobia. *The Practitioner, 233,* 1165–1167.

Klein, S. P., Bohannan, H. M., Bell, R. M., Disney, J. A., Fock, C. B., & Graves, R. C. (1985). The cost and effectiveness of school-based preventive dental care. *American Journal of Public Health, 75*(4), 382–391.

Levy, S. M. (1986). Expansion of the proper use of systemic fluoride supplements. *Journal of the American Dental Association, 112,* 30–34.

Levy, S. M., & Muchow, G. (1992). Provider compliance with recommended dietary fluoride supplement protocol. *American Journal of Public Health, 82*(2), 281–283.

Lewis, C. E., Siegal, J. M., & Lewis, M. A. (1984). Feeling bad: Exploring sources of distress among pre-adolescent children. *American Journal of Public Health, 74,* 117–122.

Mayberry, W. (1990). Self-esteem in children: Considerations for measurement and intervention. *American Journal of Occupational Therapy, 44*(8), 729–734.

McAnanly, E. (1986). School phobia: The importance of prompt intervention. *Journal of School Health, 56*(10), 433–436.

National Institute of Dental Research. (1981). *The prevalence of dental caries in United States children: The national dental caries prevalence survey.* (NIH Publication No. 82–2245) Washington, DC: National Institute of Dental Research.

Noller, K., & Ingrisano, D. (1984). Cross sectional study of gross and fine motor development. *Physical Therapy, 64*(3), 308–316.

Padilla, M. L., (1989). Latchkey children: A review of the literature. *Child Welfare, 68,* 445.

Parker, D. F., & Bar-Or, O. (1991). Juvenile obesity: The importance of exercise and getting children to do it. *The Physician and Sportsmedicine, 19*(6), 113–121.

Peterson, F. L. (1987, October–November). Promoting dental health in elementary school children. *Health Education,* 18–22.

Price, A. H. & Parry, J. A. (1982). *101 Ways to build your child's self esteem.* Wauwatosa, WI: American Baby Books.

Rebich, T. R. (1985). School-based preventive dental care: A different view. *American Journal of Public Health, 75*(4), 392–394.

Ryan-Wenger, N. M. (1992). A taxonomy of children's coping strategies: A step toward theory development. *American Journal of Orthopsychiatry, 62,* 256–263.

Seffrin, J., & Seffrin, S. (1979). Dental health education contributing to high level wellness. *Health Values: Achieving High Level Wellness, 3,* 212–216.

Seigler, R. S. (1989). Mechanisms of cognitive development. *Annual Review of Psychology, 40,* 353–379.

Smardo, F. A. (1985). Dental health of young children: How can we help them cope? *Health Values: Achieving High Level Wellness, 9*(3), 15–19.

Steinberg, L. (1986). Latchkey children and susceptibility to peer pressure: An ecological analysis. *Developmental Psychology, 22*(4), 433–439.

Wellman, H. M. & Gelma, S. A. (1992). Cognitive development: Foundational theories of core domains. *Annual Review of Psychology, 43,* 337–375.

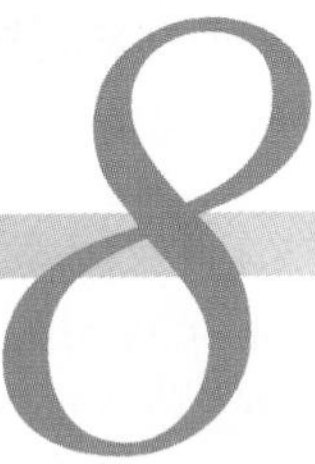

The Adolescent

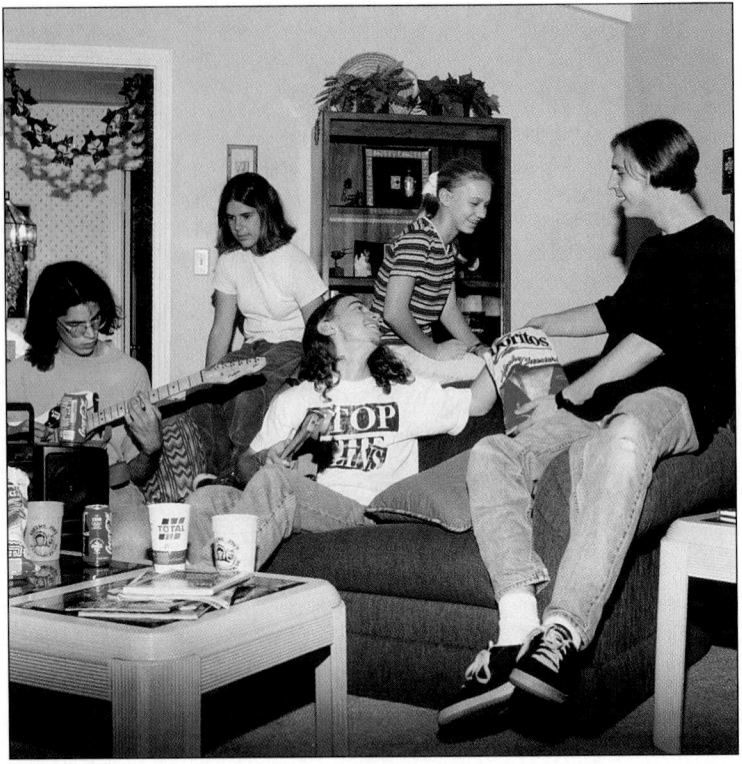

CHAPTER OVERVIEW

LEARNING OBJECTIVES

After studying this chapter, you should be able to:

- Describe the normal growth and development of the adolescent.
- Identify the sexual maturity rating/Tanner stages and recognize deviations from normal.
- Describe the developmental tasks of adolescence.
- Describe the concept of identity formation in relation to adolescent psychosocial development.
- Describe appropriate health-promoting behaviors for adolescents and young adults.
- Provide adolescents and their families anticipatory guidance with respect to risk-taking behaviors.
- Discuss the incidence of adolescent violence and strategies to deal with aggressive behavior.
- Discuss adolescent sexuality and effective contraceptive methods.

KEY TERMS

adolescence: the biological and psychosocial transition from childhood to adulthood

autonomy: independent will and the capacity to be self-governing

egocentrism: concerned with oneself; the lack of differentiation between one's own views and those of others

identity formation: the acquisition of psychosocial, sexual, and vocational identity

primary sexual characteristics: internal and external reproductive organs in males and females (i.e., uterus, fallopian tubes, testes, spermatic cord)

puberty: the period of time during which adolescents experience a growth spurt, develop secondary sex characteristics, and *achieve* reproductive maturity

pubescence: the period of time *prior* to sexual maturity characterized by the development of breast tissue and pubic hair in females and genital growth and pubic hair in males

reproductive maturity: the establishment of menstruation/ovulation in females and the development of spermatogenesis in males

risk-taking behaviors: behaviors that predispose the adolescent to physical or psychosocial harm

secondary sexual characteristics: physical characteristics of males and females influenced by reproductive hormones, but having no direct role in reproduction (i.e., voice, body shape, pubic hair distribution)

sexual maturity rating (SMR): stages of sexual maturation based on pubic hair and breast development in girls and pubic hair and genital development in boys

Adolescence spans ages 11 to 21 years; the developmental tasks of early adolescence, as well as the beginning stages of sexual maturation, may overlap with the school age years. Adolescence is a time of change for teenagers and their families, a transition from childhood to adulthood. Included in this transition are dramatic physical, cognitive, psychosocial, and psychosexual changes that are exciting and at the same time frightening.

The adolescent tries on and tests out many new roles during this time as part of the important developmental task of identity formation. The peer group is of the utmost importance as adolescents experiment with these new roles outside the confines of the family unit. When identity formation is complete, the young adult emancipates from the family and establishes independence.

Parents as well as adolescents need the nurse's support and guidance in understanding and facilitating health-promoting behaviors to make this transition successfully. Nurses can assist adolescents and their families in the areas of health promotion, disease prevention, and management of common problems by making use of effective communication strategies, knowledge of normal growth and development, anticipatory guidance, and early identification of potential problems.

GROWTH AND DEVELOPMENT OF THE ADOLESCENT

The rapid rate of physical growth during adolescence is second only to that of infancy. Adolescents come in many shapes and sizes, and the changes that take place during these years are obvious and dramatic. With physical change comes the development of secondary sexual characteristics and an intense interest in the opposite sex. Adolescents move from the same sex friendships of childhood to the capacity for intimate, long-lasting relationships as young adults. Sexual orientation and gender identity are often recognized during adolescence as the teenager engages in exploration and self-discovery. Growth and development of the adolescent is summarized in Table 8–1.

According to Erikson, the major developmental task of adolescence is the development of one's identity and the establishment of **autonomy** (Erikson, 1968). The adolescent is able to accomplish these tasks by the acquisition of abstract reasoning, which allows for analytical thinking, problem solving, and planning for the future.

Physical Growth and Development

Physical development during the adolescent years is characterized by dramatic changes in size and appearance. The majority of physical growth and development occurs between ages 11 and 15 years with some additional physical maturation between ages 15 and 21 years. Boys increase in muscle mass and girls increase in fat deposits.

TABLE 8–1 *Summary of Growth and Development: The Adolescent*

PHYSICAL	MOTOR	PSYCHOSOCIAL
Early Adolescence (11–14 Years) Girls: Breast tissue develops. Girls generally taller and slightly heavier than boys. Begin to put on fat. PHV: 8.3 cm/year. Menarche, pubic hair, axillary hair. Boys: PHV: 9.4 cm/year. Testes enlarge. Gynecomastia. Spermatogenesis. Boys may appear chunky before PHV. Both: Cardiovascular pump less mature. Appetite increases in response to rapid growth.	Increase in gross muscle mass and fine motor coordination. Prone to ligamental tears. Awkward, gangly during and immediately after PHV. Physical contact sports recommended after PHV. Watch for exercise-induced asthma.	Often shy, awkward. More confident with same sex. Self-conscious. Low self-esteem common. Begin rebellious behavior. Struggle over dependence/independence issues.
Middle Adolescence (15–17 Years) Girls: Increase in percent of total body fat. Average height gain: 6 to 10.4 cm/year. Increase in breast size. Increase in pubic hair. Sexual maturation occurs. Develop "hourglass" body contour. Growth decelerates. Appetite declines. Boys: Genitalia enlarge. Gynecomastia begins to decline. Voice begins to change as larynx enlarges. Muscle mass increases. Facial hair. Rapid growth in height. 2 to 3 years after PHV. Appetite intense. Both: Dentition complete. Incidence of gingivitis. Malocclusions common in 50% of adolescents. Sweat gland function increases. Acne peaks. Sensory and language development complete. Increasing capacity of cardiovascular pump.	Increased coordination in fine and gross muscle. More adept at sports. Greater physical endurance. Greater skill at drawing, sewing, etc.	Impulsive, impatient. Conflict with parents increases. Limit testing. Sexual experimentation begins. Narcissistic, moody. Intensely private. Peer group of utmost importance.

By age 20 years, girls have twice the body fat of boys, and boys have one-third greater muscle mass than girls (American Academy of Pediatrics, Committee on Sports Medicine, 1991). Because of greater muscle mass, fully developed adolescent boys tend to be larger and stronger than adolescent girls.

Psychosexual Development, Hormonal Changes, and Sexual Maturation. Physical development, hormonal changes, and sexual maturation occurring during adolescence correspond with Freud's final stage of psychosexual development: the genital stage (see Chapter 2 for discussion of Freud's stages of psychosexual development). The genital stage

TABLE 8–1 *Summary of Growth and Development: The Adolescent (continued)*

PHYSICAL	MOTOR	PSYCHOSOCIAL
Late Adolescence (18–21 Years) Girls: Physically mature. Sexual maturation complete. Boys: Physically mature, although boys may continue to increase in height and weight. Rapid growth decelerates. Sexual maturation complete. Gynecomastia resolves. Both: Cardiovascular pump mature. Appetite relatively stable. Verbal and written expression becomes more sophisticated with additional education and experience.	Endurance for motor activity increases, especially with fitness training. Boys may continue to increase in muscle bulk for competitive sports.	Less emotionally labile. Idealistic but more realistic with respect to partner selection and goals. May continue sexual experimentation. Independent, yet maintains family ties. Engaged in education/employment.

begins with the production of sex hormones and maturation of the reproductive system. Sexual tension and energy is manifested in the development of sexual relationships with others, and sexual gratification is sought. Freud's theory suggests that personality development is closely related to psychosexual development, with emphasis on aggressive and sexual impulses as determining factors of personality. Freud's belief in male dominance, sexual repression, and the Oedipus/Electra complex make the psychosexual theory of development highly controversial even today.

Girls generally reach physical maturation before boys with the onset and establishment of menstruation (menarche). The average age of menarche in females is between age 9 and 15 years with the approximate average 12.8 years (Hatcher et al., 1994). Most young women achieve **reproductive maturity** 2 to 5 years after the onset of menstruation. During the 2 to 5 years before reproductive maturity, the female sex hormones gradually increase, ovulation occurs more frequently, and menstrual periods become more regular. Girls experience epiphyseal closure of long bones as the result of estrogen secretion with regularly established menstrual cycles (see Chapter 27 for a discussion of problems related to menstruation).

Ultimately, the height, weight, and body build of adolescents is influenced by diet, exercise, and hereditary factors. Over the past three decades, adolescents have reached a greater proportion of height and weight as compared to their ancestors, and the age of puberty has declined.

Physical growth of boys and girls is directly related to sexual maturation and occurs in a relatively predictable sequence. The development of breast tissue, pubic hair, and genitalia is influenced by the secretion of sex hormones: estrogen in girls and testosterone in boys. Hormonal secretion at the time of puberty is the result of a complex regulatory process between the environment, the central nervous system, the hypothalamus, the pituitary gland, the gonads, and the adrenal glands. **Puberty** is a biological process that brings about the period of peak height velocity (PHV) or the "growth spurt," the changes in body composition, and the development of **primary** and **secondary sexual characteristics** in both sexes. Although variable in both sexes, the PHV (rapid period of linear growth) occurs at approximately age 12 years in girls and age 13.5 years in boys. Table 8–2 describes five distinct stages of **sexual maturity rating (SMR)** based on breast and pubic hair development in girls and genital and pubic hair development in boys and includes approximate age ranges for early, middle, and late puberty (Tanner, 1962). The beginning Tanner stages frequently occur in the school age child (see Chapter 7), and Tanner stages 3 to 5 occur in adolescence.

> Knowledge of Tanner staging is essential for nurses to assess normal growth and development and to provide adolescents and their parents with anticipatory guidance regarding sexual development. However, nurses must remember that sexual maturation and physical development are *highly variable* and that Tanner stages may overlap with one another. Description of the adolescent's sexual maturity rating provides greater information about the child's physical development than does chronological age (age in years).

TABLE 8–2 *Sexual Maturity Rating (SMR): Tanner Stages of Adolescent Sexual Development*

BOYS

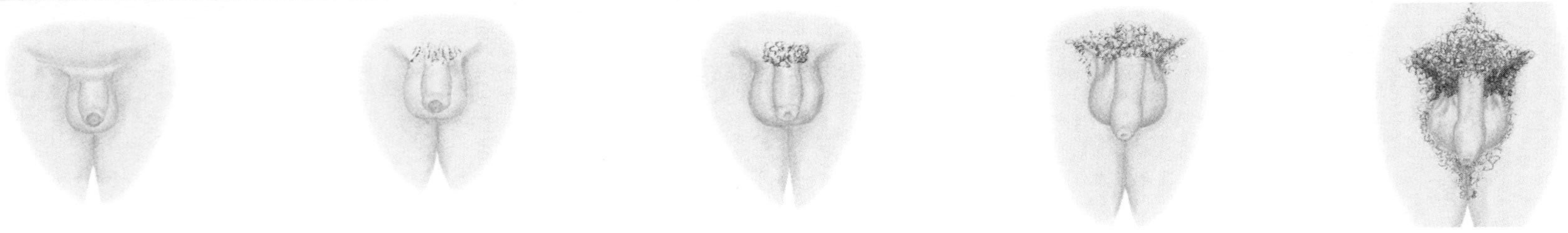

Stage 1	Stage 2	Stage 3	Stage 4	Stage 5
Pubic Hair: None	*Pubic Hair:* Slight, long, straight, slightly pigmented at the base of the penis	*Pubic Hair:* Darker in color, starts to curl, small amount	*Pubic Hair:* Coarse, curly, similar to adult but less quantity	*Pubic Hair:* Adult distribution spread to inner thighs
Penis: Preadolescent	*Penis:* Slight enlargement	*Penis:* Longer	*Penis:* Larger, glans and breadth increase in size	*Penis:* Adult in size and shape
Testes: Preadolescent	*Testes:* Enlarged scrotum, pink, slight alteration in texture	*Testes:* Larger	*Testes:* Larger, scrotum darker	*Testes:* Adult

Early puberty: Testes, 9.5 to 13.5 years; penis, 10.5 to 14.5 years; pubic hair, 12 to 12.5 years

Middle puberty: Testes, 13.5 to 14.5 years; penis, 13.5 to 15 years; pubic hair, 12.5 to 14.5 years

Late puberty: Testes, 13.5 to 17 years; penis, 13.5 to 16 years; pubic hair, 13.5 to 16.5 years

BREAST DEVELOPMENT IN GIRLS*

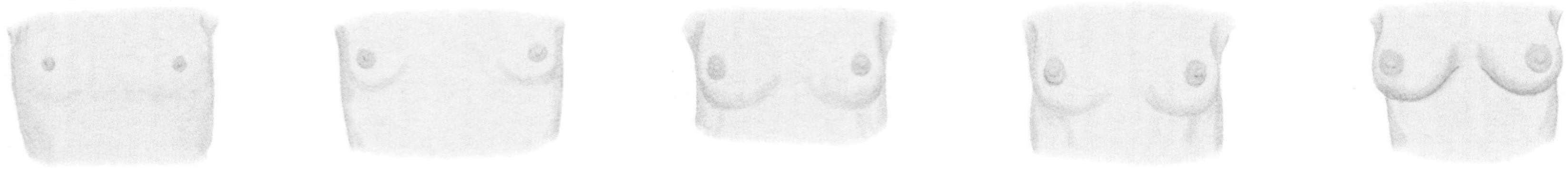

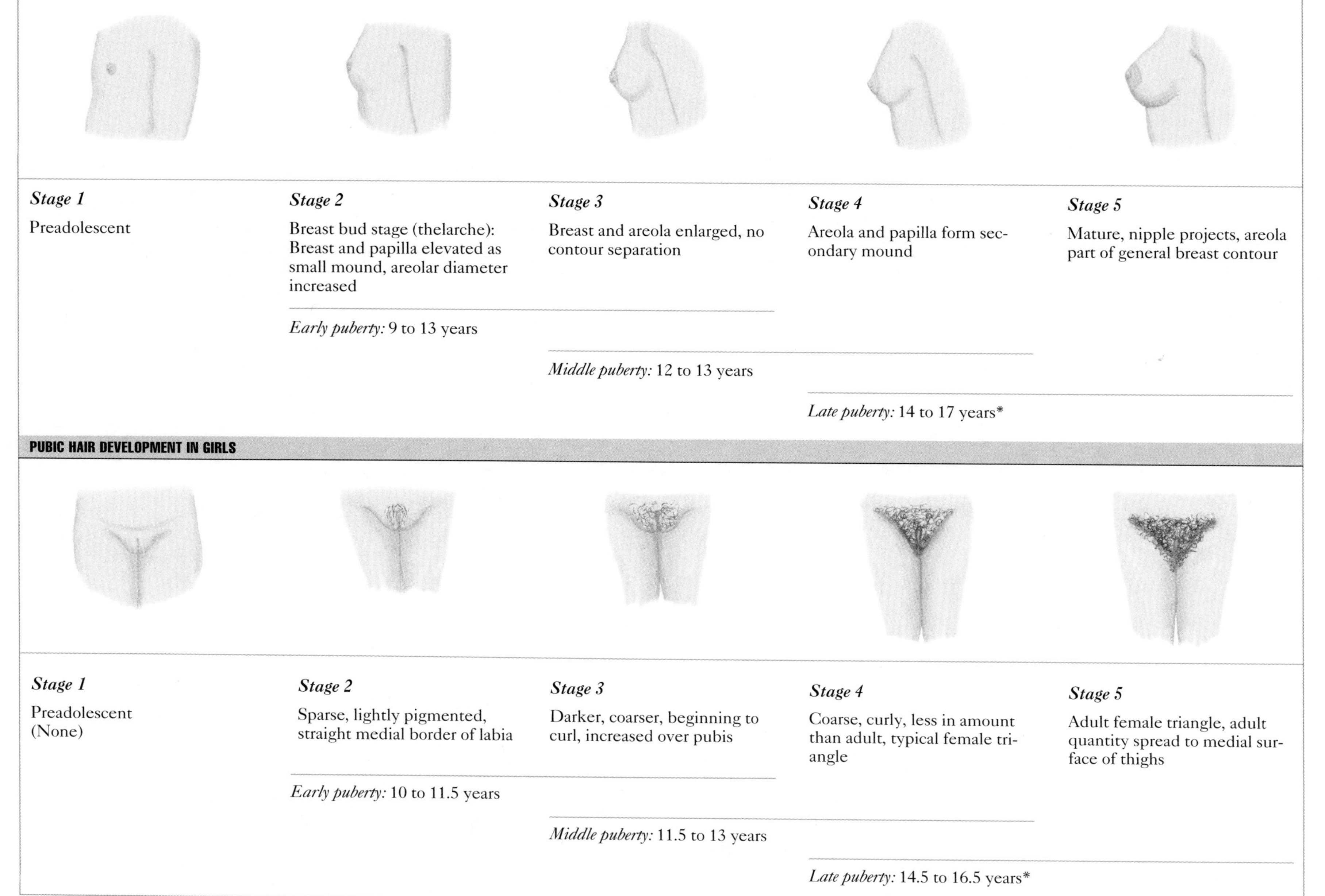

Stage 1
Preadolescent
Stage 2
Breast bud stage (thelarche): Breast and papilla elevated as small mound, areolar diameter increased
Stage 3
Breast and areola enlarged, no contour separation
Stage 4
Areola and papilla form secondary mound
Stage 5
Mature, nipple projects, areola part of general breast contour
Early puberty: 9 to 13 years
Middle puberty: 12 to 13 years
Late puberty: 14 to 17 years*
PUBIC HAIR DEVELOPMENT IN GIRLS
Stage 1
Preadolescent (None)
Stage 2
Sparse, lightly pigmented, straight medial border of labia
Stage 3
Darker, coarser, beginning to curl, increased over pubis
Stage 4
Coarse, curly, less in amount than adult, typical female triangle
Stage 5
Adult female triangle, adult quantity spread to medial surface of thighs
Early puberty: 10 to 11.5 years
Middle puberty: 11.5 to 13 years
Late puberty: 14.5 to 16.5 years*

*Breast and pubic hair development may continue into late adolescence and increase with pregnancy.

Adapted from Tanner, J. M. (1962). *Growth at adolescence* (2nd ed.). Oxford, Blackwell Scientific Publications; and Marshall, W. A., & Tanner, J. (1969). Variations in pattern of pubertal changes in girls. *Archives of Disease in Children. 44*, 291–303. Adapted with permission from Blackwell Scientific Publications and The BMJ Publishing Group.

However, failure to begin breast development by age 13 years in girls and failure to increase testicular size by 2.5 cm at age 14 years in boys indicates delayed puberty; such children should be referred for medical evaluation (Kulin & Reiter, 1992).

Female Sexual Maturation. Sexual maturation in girls begins with the appearance of breast buds (thelarche), which is the first sign of ovarian function. The thelarche occurs at approximately age 9 to 11 years and is followed by the growth of pubic hair. The PHV is reached during the thelarche, usually in Tanner stage 2 or 3. Linear growth slows and menarche begins approximately 1 year after the PHV. As pubic hair increases in amount and becomes dark, coarse, and curly, axillary hair develops and the apocrine sweat glands reach secretory capacity in approximate Tanner stage 3 or 4. Frequent showers and the need for deodorant become important to the adolescent. With increasing hormonal activity, girls develop a more adult body contour by age 14 to 15 years (see Table 8–2). As breasts mature the nipples become projectile and the pubic hair extends to the medial thighs; the young female is estimated at Tanner stage 5. Ovulation may be established and conception can occur.

For sexually active teens oral contraceptives are usually not prescribed until Tanner stage 5 when ovulation and menstruation are more likely to be regular.

Male Sexual Maturation. The first sign of pubertal changes in boys is testicular enlargement in response to testosterone secretion, which usually occurs in Tanner stage 2. There is also some slight pubic hair and some alteration in the smooth skin texture of the scrotum. As testosterone secretion increases, the penis as well as the testes and scrotum, enlarge. The PHV usually occurs during Tanner stages 3 and 4, and the voice deepens and "cracks" as the cartilage in the larynx enlarges. Axillary hair develops, and the eccrine and apocrine sweat glands are stimulated in response to stressful and/or emotional stimulation (Lee, 1980). Secretions from the apocrine glands are metabolized by skin surface bacteria, and body odor develops. Gynecomastia (male breast enlargement) occurs in about 60% of young males around age 13 to 14 years and may be unilateral or bilateral (Kreipe, 1992). This phenomena is often disturbing to boys, and they need considerable reassurance that the breast tissue will decrease. During Tanner stages 4 and 5 increasing levels of testosterone cause sebaceous glands to enlarge and excessive sebum may result in acne. The voice continues to deepen, facial hair appears at the corners of the upper lip and chin, and ejaculation may occur. Nurses need to provide anticipatory guidance to adolescent boys regarding involuntary nocturnal emissions of seminal fluid ("wet dreams") and assure them that this occurrence is normal. By Tanner stage 5 genital maturation is complete, spermatogenesis is well established, facial hair is present on the sides of the face, and the male physique is adult-like in appearance. Gynecomastia significantly decreases or disappears, much to the adolescent male's relief.

Motor Development

Adolescents often engage in various forms of motor activity from aerobic exercise to football. Motor activities such as sports and dancing provide an outlet for the adolescent's energy as well as an opportunity for competition, teamwork, and social relationships. Adolescents increase in large muscle mass and in coordination of gross and fine muscle groups. With practice, adolescents become more adept at athletics and also at art, music, and sewing. Because of the rapid growth during Tanner stages 3 and 4, boys need to be cautioned about playing contact sports; they are more prone to ligamental tears and damage to the growth plates of the long bones (Pendergrast & Strong, 1992). However, bones are not completely calcified until after puberty and are still fairly resistant to breaks in the young adolescent. Participants in sports activities should be grouped according to their size and their SMR rather than their chronological age. A small, thin, late-maturing boy is less capable of competing with an early-maturing, muscular classmate and injuries are more likely to occur. Physical contact sports such as football are not recommended until after the PHV when greater muscle mass has been achieved (Greydanus, 1990).

Nurses (particularly those in schools) may be helpful in assessing the growth and development of adolescents and counseling them into sports activities in which they can succeed, rather than those in which they will meet with physical and psychological failure. See box for nursing goals for the preparticipation athletic physical examination (Russell, 1992).

Nursing Goals for Preparticipation Sports Physical Examination

- Assess the adolescent athlete's general health.
- Detect conditions that limit participation and/or predispose to injury.
- Assess the adolescent athlete's physical and psychosocial maturity.
- Determine fitness related to performance abilities.
- Assess legal insurance requirements for participation.
- Provide wellness counseling and anticipatory guidance.

The development of the cardiovascular pump plays an essential role in the adolescent's participation in gross motor activities. The cardiopulmonary capacity increases during adolescence and is relatively mature in the late adolescent. The cardiovascular pump is not as efficient in young adolescents, and the lungs are smaller. Adolescents generally cannot run as fast or as long as the young adult. The cardiopulmonary capacity increases with fitness training *after* the PHV, but before puberty fitness training is less likely to have a significant effect on the aerobic capacity of the adolescent (Pendergrast & Strong, 1992). Physical fitness is determined by the athlete's aerobic power, body composition, joint flexibility, and strength of skeletal muscles.

All adolescent athletes need adequate equipment, appropriate training schedules, frequent rest periods, and adequate fluids to prevent injury, dehydration, and exhaustion.

Cognitive and Sensory Development

Cognitive development influences every aspect of adolescent psychosocial development. Cognition moves from concrete to abstract thinking during the three phases of adolescent development (see Table 8–3).

According to Piaget, the last stage of cognitive development is characterized by formal operations, or the ability to think abstractly. Early abstract thinking encompasses inductive/deductive reasoning, the ability to connect separate events, and the ability to understand later consequences. Abstract thinking in late adolescence is increasingly logical, and young adults are capable of scientific reasoning, understanding complex concepts, and using analytical methods. Because of logical reasoning, adolescents are able to differentiate between others' perceptions and their own, and to view social situations from a societal perspective.

Nurses and other adults need to consider the adolescent's cognitive capacity when doing any counseling or education.

For example, sex education for ninth graders is very different than for college freshmen. The college freshman should be able to appreciate the later consequences of sexual behavior whereas the young adolescent is focused on the here and now. Ask the ninth grader and the college freshman how an unwanted baby will affect their lives and compare their answers.

For a variety of reasons (including poor comprehension ability, lack of education, and chronic substance abuse), some older adolescents remain concrete thinkers. Nurses and educators must know their audience and address them appropriately. Counseling a group of adolescent substance abusers may be ineffective if the consequence of their behavior is tied to the future when their thinking is in the present.

Sensory Maturation

The eyes and ears of adolescents are fully developed and, with the exception of refractive errors and occasional minor infections of the eyes, ears, and sinuses, the sensory system remains quite healthy. Myopia occurs in early adolescence between ages 11 and 13 years.

Because of increased participation in competitive sports and outdoor activities, eye injuries are common in adolescence. Males are more prone to eye injuries than females. Adolescents should always be required to wear safety or protective equipment when competing in sports or participating in any activity that may compromise eye safety.

Language Development and Communication

With the acquisition of formal operational thought and adequate intellectual capacity, adolescents are able to understand abstract concepts, process complex thoughts, and express themselves verbally. Adolescents who read extensively are generally more articulate and have a greater vocabulary than other adolescents. Social development and self-confidence play a significant role in how well adolescents express themselves verbally to others. Shy, introverted adolescents may have difficulty speaking to a group or to members of the opposite sex, but may be able to demonstrate expressive writing skills. Conversely, extroverted, social adolescents who have no trouble with verbal expression may lack the reading and writing skills for effective written communication.

Computer technology has added to the adolescent's avenues for creative expression. Adolescents are capable of expressing ideas in symbols and abstract concepts, and many enjoy interpreting or even developing complex computer programs. Computers have a symbolic language of their own that some adolescents find fascinating. The teen's mastery of computer technology often exceeds that of the parents. As well as teaching teens basic computer literacy, many high schools have computer clubs where students who excel in computer languages share ideas and knowledge of computer information systems.

Communicating with adolescents sometimes presents a challenge to parents and other adults. Although adolescents are capable of verbal expression, they are also intensely private and may not wish to divulge their thoughts and feelings to others. Developmentally, the verbally expressive 12-year-old may turn into a relatively uncommunicative 14-year-old. Conflict with parents is known to increase tension with regard to communication.

TABLE 8–3 *Adolescent Psychosocial Development*

	EARLY ADOLESCENCE (11 TO 14 YEARS)	MIDDLE ADOLESCENCE (15 TO 17 YEARS)	LATE ADOLESCENCE (18 TO 21 YEARS)
Cognitive Development	**Concrete Thinking, limited abstract thought** Appreciates here and now. Little sense of later consequences.	**Early Abstract Thought** Use of inductive/deductive reasoning. Ability to understand later consequences of actions. Ability to connect separate events and to project into the future. Self-absorbed/introspective; daydreaming, fantasy.	**Abstract Reasoning** Ability to abstract and conceptualize. Idealism about life, love, society. Concern for society, politics, religion.
		Developmental Tasks	
Identity/Self-Perception	Reacts to imaginary audience, personal fable present. Self-conscious about bodily changes. Reacts to peers; conformity. Often experiences low self-esteem.	State of flux over body image. Narcissistic, introspective. Often moody, impulsive, impatient. Values group identity over family. Can be manipulative for self-gain. Begins to think of future.	Realistic body image. Generally positive outlook on future. Able to consider others' needs, less narcissistic. Able to reject group pressure in favor of own interests.
Emancipation from Family/Independence	Transition from obedient to rebellious. Ambivalence about independence. Flux from child to adult. Rejection of parental rules, but has desire to please adults. Self-esteem declines when punished for poor behavior. Hero worship, crushes common with both sexes.	Independent, private. Limit testing maximal. Overt rebellion, withdrawal. Role-playing common, roles easily abandoned (moratorium). Separation from parents. Child-parent conflict often intense.	Emancipation from parents, but maintenance of parental ties. Future directed. Adult-like commitments to relationships/roles. Consideration of family. Educational/vocational goals related to physical and financial emancipation from parent.

Parents need encouragement to maintain open communication with their teenager while not appearing too intrusive. Plying adolescents with questions or going through their belongings causes feelings of invasion and a lack of trust. Adolescents get more out of discussions in which they participate than lectures, and are more likely to respond positively to adults who listen and appear interested in what they have to say.

Nurses who work with adolescents must develop communication skills that include assuring confidentiality, making no assumptions, remaining nonjudgmental, and posing open-ended questions. Questions such as "Tell me about your plans for the future" will glean more information than "Do you plan to go to college?" "Do you live with your parents?" makes an assumption about the living situation that could make the adolescent feel uncomfortable. "Describe where you live and who lives with you" gives the adolescent an opportunity to discuss the living situation in a broader context.

One method of assessing psychosocial development and encouraging adolescent communication is the use of the Home, Education/vocation, Activities, Drugs, Sexuality, Suicide/depression, and Savagery (HEADSSS) approach (Goldenring & Cohen, 1988; J. Goldenring, personal communication, August 17, 1994). Following the HEADSSS approach, the nurse assesses all areas important to adolescent psychosocial development, with special attention to any problem areas that might be indicated.

TABLE 8–3 *Adolescent Psychosocial Development (continued)*

	EARLY ADOLESCENCE (11 TO 14 YEARS)	MIDDLE ADOLESCENCE (15 TO 17 YEARS)	LATE ADOLESCENCE (18 TO 21 YEARS)
Education/Vocation	Goals unrealistic, changing. Structured school setting. Role models important.	Begins to identify skills and interests. Self-esteem often tied to school achievements and popularity. Begins to consider long-term consequences of school performance. Role-play with after school activities and part-time jobs.	Realistic career plans. Less flux about future goals. Commitment to work and school, but may have changing career choices.
Sexuality Social/Peers	Same sex best friend. Group activity same sex. Concern about "normal" body changes. Boy-girl fantasy, often with peers and media stars. Sexual experimentation may occur, but is not as common as middle adolescence.	Peer acceptance at utmost. Intense preoccupation with physical appeal and body image. Intense interest in opposite sex. Sexual experimentation common. Relationships generally short-term. Serial partners. Role of partner often unrealistic. Decision about hetero-sexual/homosexual preference.	More commitment to intimate relationships. Long-term relationships. More realistic concept of partner's role. Peer group less important. Mate selection possible. Some continuation of sexual experimentation. Serial monogamous relationships for those uncommitted.
		Professional Nursing Approach	
• Enjoy teens • Be patient • Be flexible • Know adolescent development • Be open • Listen	Open, direct, supportive. Set limits, give concrete choices. Encourage self-responsibility and measures to enhance self-esteem. Orient to reality.	Open, objective; negotiate choices. Consider how teen will look to peers. Encourage problem solving. Praise good decisions. Keep criticism to a minimum. Be an advocate, but don't take sides against parent. Set firm limits. Maintain confidentiality.	Encourage mutual decision making. Act as a resource and role model. Consider hidden agendas. Explore feelings about health care choices. Allow for questions and analysis of health care options.

See the accompanying box for the HEADSSS format with suggested questions to include when interviewing adolescents. Keep in mind that the HEADSSS format is fairly comprehensive and may take more than one visit to complete.

Psychosocial Development

Identity formation is the major **developmental task** of adolescence; others include the formation of a sexual and vocational identity and the ability to emancipate from the family or to become independent. Energy is focused within the self, and the adolescent is described as egocentric or self-absorbed. Frustrated parents often describe teenagers during this phase as self-centered, lazy, or irresponsible when they just need time to think, concentrate on themselves, and determine who they are going to be. Erikson (1968) describes the conflict of this phase of psychosocial development as identity formation versus role confusion; this phase corresponds with Freud's genital stage of psychosexual development (see Chapter 2 for information on developmental theories).

Being in a transition period from childhood to adulthood, adolescents try on new roles and experiment with the environment until finding a role that fits. The phase of experimentation is termed the "moratorium," meaning a period of delay granted to someone not yet ready to make more than a tentative commitment (Erikson, 1968). The lack of commitment is illustrated by the adolescent's

HEADSSS Interview Technique

HOME

Where do you live? How many people live with you?

Tell me about who lives with you. Who is close to you at home?

Do you consider home to be a safe place? Do you avoid going home? If yes, why?

EDUCATION/VOCATION

Are you currently in school? If so, what is the last grade you completed?

Describe what you like and don't like about school.

What kind of grades do you make in school?

Have you ever been held back in school or skipped any grades?

Have you ever been in any kind of trouble at school? What happened?

Are you working? Tell me about what you do.

Do you make enough money to pay for the things you need or want?

Describe a typical day at work or school.

ACTIVITIES

Describe what you like to do in your spare time.

Who is your best friend? Tell me about what you like to do together.

Are you dating? Anyone special? At what age did you start to date?

How do you get to and from your activities?

DRUGS

Tell me about *any* drugs that you are currently taking. Aspirin, prescription drugs, cigarettes, marijuana, coffee or other caffeine like colas? Beer, wine, wine coolers? What do you usually drink, especially on the weekends?

Street Drugs? Crack, marijuana, cocaine.

Have you ever been arrested for drinking? Tell me about any legal or school problems involving drugs or alcohol. Describe what happened.

Who does drugs and/or alcohol in your home?

SEX

Many young people begin to have sexual experiences; tell me about yours.

At what age did you have your first sexual experience?

Are you sexually active with the same partner? What kind of sex do you have?

Tell me when was the last time you had a sexual relationship. Birth control used?

Have you ever been treated for any sexually transmitted diseases? Describe that treatment if you can.

SUICIDE/DEPRESSION

Do you have someone that you can talk to when you have problems? Tell me a little about that person.

Do you ever feel so sad that you feel like life isn't worth living? Describe your feelings.

What do you do when you feel sad, hopeless, frustrated?

Did you ever form a plan for doing away with yourself? Describe that plan.

Have you ever been hospitalized or take medication for feelings of depression? Has anyone in your family ever had mental problems? If yes, tell me about those family members.

SAVAGERY

Describe how you feel when you are angry. How do you usually handle anger?

How often do you get into physical or verbal fights? When was the last time you hit someone? Do you ever carry a weapon? What kind? Where do you use the weapon?

Have you ever been expelled from school because of violence? Describe what happened.

Are there gangs in your school, neighborhood? Tell me about these gangs. How do you feel about gangs?

Adapted with permission from Goldenring, J., & Cohen, E. (1988). Getting into adolescent heads. *Contemporary Pediatrics*, 7, 76. Also from J. Goldenring, personal communication, August 17, 1994.

changing interests from year to year. Parents may invest in expensive sports equipment or a musical instrument one year only to find it abandoned the next.

The peer group plays an essential role in adolescent identity formation. Teenagers take their cues on appearance, social behavior, and language from the peer group. The peer group serves as a safe haven as adolescents emotionally move away from the family and struggle to determine who they are. The peer group validates acceptable behavior, and teenagers feel secure in trying on new roles with peer group approval. It is not unusual for teens to spend all day with friends in school and all evening rehashing the day's events over the phone. Changes in the adolescent's body image, psychosocial development, and peer group acceptance are closely related. Early and middle adolescents are particularly audience conscious and feel that they are the focus of everyone's attention. A bad hair day or a blemish may throw the adolescent into despair. Clothing, hairstyles, and material possessions that are accepted by the group gain the utmost importance. Nurses should counsel parents to negotiate choices with teens but always consider how the child will be judged by peers.

Early and middle adolescence is the period when teens are prone to gang formation and activities. Peer modeling and peer acceptance, being of the utmost importance, lead some adolescents to form gangs that provide a collective identity. Gang membership confers identity, a sense of power, and most importantly, a sense of belonging that may be lacking in the adolescent's life (Castiglia, 1993). Peer pressure, companionship, and protection are the most frequently reported reasons for joining gangs, particularly those associated with violent or criminal acts. Loyalty is demanded, and behavior is monitored and regulated by gang members. Of great concern is the escalating violence associated with gangs and the decreasing age of the participants. Early adolescents (age 11 to 14 years) are recruited by gangs for drug trafficking and violent acts with the belief that children are invulnerable to legal action because of the judicial system's lack of resources and lack of adjudication of minors (see Chapter 13 for additional information on gangs).

There are marked developmental differences between early and late adolescence. Each age group has unique reactions to the developmental tasks, which are influenced by the adolescent's cognitive thinking as described in Table 8–3. According to Swiss psychologist Jean Piaget (1969), adolescent cognition is characterized by the transition from concrete operational thought to formal operational thought, the ability to think logically and use deductive and abstract reasoning (see Chapters 2 and 7 for further information on Piaget's theory of cognition). Acquisition of formal operational thinking allows the adolescent to draw on past experience and apply knowledge to the future by drawing on logical consequences from a set of observations. Adolescents are capable of using abstract symbols such as those derived from higher order mathematics, making and testing hypotheses, and considering and arguing philosophical issues. Problem solving and decision making skills become more highly developed, although adolescents may still be conflicted about idealism versus reality.

Early Adolescence. The early adolescent (11 to 14 years) has intense feelings about body image and the many physical changes taking place. Less confident with members of the opposite sex, early adolescents tend to group together and have best friends of the same sex. One only has to visit the local mall or movie theater to see groups of young teens of the same sex, observing but rarely speaking to groups of the opposite sex.

The early adolescent is very egocentric and may go from obedience to rebellion with respect to parental authority. Parents are often shocked at the sudden turn of events and are hurt by the teen's rejection. Providing parents with anticipatory guidance regarding age-specific developmental changes is a primary nursing function. For example, the happy-go-lucky 11-year-old may turn into the shy, self-absorbed 12-year-old who only seems comfortable in the presence of friends. Young teens, who are developmentally **egocentric,** fail to differentiate between how others see them and their own mental preoccupations, thinking everyone is as obsessed with them as they are with themselves. Elkind (1967) describes this phenomenon as the reaction to the imaginary audience. The belief in the imaginary audience is probably why young teens are so self-conscious; they believe everyone is critical of them and indeed teens are very critical of each other, especially someone who is different. Self-conscious behavior may also be the result of the physical and emotional transition to middle adolescence. The early adolescent is losing the familiar role of the child but does not yet feel comfortable with the role of the adult. Ambivalence toward independence is common, and the teen who feels too grown up for a good night kiss still falls asleep with a favored teddy bear.

Elkind (1967) believes that because young teens are so audience conscious, they see themselves as unique and tell themselves a "personal fable" that supports feelings of invulnerability. Early to middle adolescence is characterized by behavior that suggests that adolescents believe negative consequences only happen to others. Adolescent suicide attempts serve as a dramatic message to others, but young teens often do not realize the very final consequences of their actions.

> Nurses should counsel parents that *all* adolescent suicidal gestures should be taken very seriously. Many adolescents do not know what type of drug ingestion or action will actually harm them. The suicidal gestures may appear minor to adults, but the actions may have serious intent.

Suicide is the third most common cause of death among American adolescents (CDC, 1995). The death rate for adolescent suicide increased 200% between 1960 and 1987. More than 5,000 teens kill themselves yearly; for every completed suicide, there are an estimated 50 to 220 suicide attempts, many of which are unreported (National Center for Health Statistics [NCHS], 1990). The identification of adolescents at risk for suicide is a problem of growing concern. Depression is a common finding among suicidal youth; other risk factors include declining mental health, poor impulse control, poor school performance, family disorganization, conduct disorders, substance abuse, and recent stress. More obvious markers include prior suicide attempts, previous mental health care, and the lack of a primary health care placement (Slap, Vorters, Chaudhuri, & Centor, 1989). Nurses must be aware that youth identified as at risk for suicide and their families should be targeted for supportive guidance and counseling before a crisis situation. (See Chapter 41 for more in-depth information on suicide and nursing interventions.)

Middle Adolescence. Middle adolescence (15 to 17 years) is often described by parents as the most frustrating period of adolescent development. The imaginary audience is gradually replaced by the real audience, and teens become even more introspective and narcissistic. Conformity to peer group norms becomes even more important, and conflicts between teenagers and parents often escalate. Testing of limits, sulky withdrawal, and overt rebellion may occur over conflicts with regard to curfews, friends, activities, appearance, cars, and money. It is important for nurses to counsel parents to negotiate choices where possible and set limits that are perceived as reasonable by the adolescent. Consistent discipline and structure actually make adolescents feel more secure and assist them with decision making. With parental guidance, adolescents are able to make decisions that will result in desirable outcomes. However, adults must keep in mind that middle adolescents are impulsive and impatient. Parental concern may be seen as interference rather than guidance and be met with resistance and resentment.

Feelings about self-image and social relationships are intense. Middle adolescence is a transition period from same sex friendships to an extreme interest in the opposite sex. Independent dating occurs and sexual experimentation is common. According to Hatcher et al., (1994) the average age of first time intercourse is between 14 and 16 years, but varies widely with respect to gender, culture, and socioeconomic status. Sexual activity is often related to peer pressure and self-esteem issues. Adolescents with the poorest self-esteem are more vulnerable and are apt to engage in negative risk-taking activities associated with sexuality. Decisions about sexual activity are often impulsive and made with little regard to later consequences or prior preparation. Nurses may help by providing accurate information to assist adolescents in making appropriate sexual choices. Parents need encouragement to maintain open communication and guide teenagers in sexual decision making. Parental guidance regarding sexual behavior is not an easy task during middle adolescence, when privacy is of extreme importance and communication with parents tends to decrease. Additionally, some parents may find sexual behavior a difficult topic to discuss and often avoid communication with teens regarding sexual issues.

In the initial stages of establishing a vocational identity, adolescents are more likely to experience role diffusion and have unrealistic expectations of themselves. Some adolescents will identify a role that holds their interest, while others will experiment with many roles, moving quickly from one role to another. Overidentification with glamorous roles takes precedence over reality and is enriched by daydreams and fantasy. It is not unusual for a 15-year-old girl to spend time with her friends describing her future as a favored media star, while failing to fold the laundry or do the dishes.

During middle adolescence, some teens acquire part-time jobs and identify various skills and interests. Part-time jobs are often a source of income for material possessions and activities not provided by parents. Such experiences help adolescents to set realistic expectations about work, increase independence, and develop a positive sense of self-esteem. Those who are successful in the work world demonstrate a sense of responsibility and tend to have more positive social interactions. However, some adolescents may allow work to interfere with educational activity and have difficulty setting priorities. School nurses, in collaboration with parents and teachers, are in an excellent position to identify working students and to assist them in setting realistic guidelines for work and education.

> Nurses working with middle adolescents face a definite challenge. It is important to be approachable, objective, and to encourage confidence, yet maintain parental authority and child advocacy. The nurse does not want to come between adolescents and their parents but wants to encourage them to work as a mutually respected unit.

Late Adolescence (18 to 21 Years). Late adolescence is characterized by the ability to think abstractly, conceptualize verbally, and express one's thoughts and feelings about various aspects of life. Late adolescents tend to be idealistic about love, social issues, ethics, and lifestyles until their experiences modify their beliefs. Conformity becomes less important as teens progress through late adolescence. With the development of one's unique identity, self-esteem increases and adolescents are able to resist group pressure if it's not in their best interest. There is less turbulence with parents unless values clash, and relationships with both friends and family are maintained.

Emancipation (leaving home) is a major issue; late adolescents prepare themselves to meet this task by education and/or vocational training. The identification of realistic career goals is important, but many adolescents are not quite ready to make lifelong commitments. Changing career goals is not uncommon, but the nurse should observe for those adolescents who have set no career goals, demonstrate apathy about the future, and appear only committed to the present. Boredom and apathy are often symptoms of a greater problem with depression. Lack of goal orientation is related to high-risk behaviors and a sense of failure (Prothrow-Stith, 1991).

Social relationships are more mature although partner selection often continues to fluctuate. Friendships developed in late adolescence may last a lifetime, and expectations of friends and lovers become more realistic and less self-serving. The ability to consider others' needs increases, and recognition of societal needs is more apparent as the adolescent moves from adolescence to adulthood.

Failure to achieve identity formation may leave adolescents in role confusion and impede the successful mastery of the tasks of young adulthood. A positive ego identity depends on the adolescent's ability to accept the past, learn from experience, and become engaged in the future. Most adolescents move through the identity versus role confusion stage of development with minimal difficulty. Research has shown that American teenagers are positive in their outlook on life, maintain a strong work ethic, and are goal oriented (Offer, Ostrov, & Howard, 1989).

Moral and Spiritual Development

Children develop moral reasoning in a sequential manner as described by American psychologist Lawrence Kohlberg (1984). As adolescents move from concrete to analytical thinking they advance to Kohlberg's stage 4 conventional level or enter Kohlberg's stage 5 postconventional level of moral development. Adolescents who remain concrete thinkers may never advance beyond Kohlberg's stage 3 of moral reasoning: conformity to please others and avoid punishment. The teenager's sense of justice is developed by interpersonal relationships with peers, family, and other adult role models. Behaviors that are modeled and rewarded, such as helping the less fortunate and showing loyalty to friends, contribute to the development of a conscience, which operates as a moral guide for subsequent behavior. The middle to late teen can appreciate that stealing from others is wrong regardless of whether one is caught and punished.

Adolescents and young adults develop a respect for law and order and a society-maintaining orientation (Kohlberg stage 4). Young adults may even advance to the societal-perspective stage (Kohlberg stage 5), which honors the moral rules of right and wrong, contractual agreements, majority opinion, and overall utility or the greatest good for the greatest number. (See Chapter 2 for all stages of Kohlberg's theory of moral development.)

Older adolescents and young adults question the values of family and society and challenge existing moral codes before integrating their experiences and beliefs into a personal moral framework. Once the moral framework is developed, interpersonal relationships tend to be with those whose values and beliefs are similar.

The development of the adolescent's ability to understand religious concepts parallels cognitive development (Ratcliff, 1985). Young adolescents in the stage of concrete operational thought are able to think logically. Concrete operational children deal well with the observable, but also begin to see other points of view and to examine what they have learned. The young adolescent will accept religious teaching and examine how religious concepts relate to everyday life. Young adolescents are especially inclined to look to God for guidance when troubled.

Middle to late adolescents are capable of analytical thought and may begin to question the religious affiliation of the family, much as they question other family values. Older adolescents may explore different kinds of religion and share religious activities with the peer group.

HEALTH PROMOTION FOR THE ADOLESCENT AND FAMILY

Adolescence is generally a period of wellness. Young people may seek health care for school/sports physicals, skin conditions (acne, contact dermatitis), acute minor illness (colds and flu), conditions related to sexuality (birth control, pregnancy, and sexually transmitted diseases [STDs]), and management of chronic illness (diabetes, epilepsy). Health promotion and disease prevention is achieved through adequate nutrition, rest, balanced exercise, and proper immunization against disease.

Table 8–5 at the end of this chapter presents an overview of health screening, health maintenance, and anticipatory guidance activities for adolescents.

Nutrition

The acceleration of height, weight and muscle mass, and sexual maturation during adolescence requires an increase in nutritional requirements that include protein, calories, zinc, calcium, and iron (see Chapter 12 for more information on RDAs.) Periods of intense growth (PHV) require increased caloric intake, and the adolescent appears constantly hungry. Snacks and regular meals must contain adequate nutrients to meet the body's anabolic needs. Although teens appear to be eating all the time, their selection of food is not always healthy, and "fast" food and "junk" food may be preferred over nutritious food. The social aspect of food consumption gains importance, and adolescents may prefer to eat meals with peers at social gatherings and restaurants of their choice. Parental supervision of meals declines as the adolescent increases time away from home and engages in extracurricular activities with peers. Skipping breakfast, frequent snacking, and eating what the peer group eats are common practices. Parents need to provide nutritional meals and snacks in the home, and nurses can be helpful in assisting adolescents to select foods that are acceptable to peers, yet low in saturated fats and empty calories. Adolescents are generally interested in nutrition and the effects food has on their bodies.

Body image is of particular importance to adolescents. The media reinforces the belief that "thin is in." Adolescents hold themselves to standards set by the entertainment and advertising worlds, which emphasize fitness, glamor, and sexuality. Products that promise a quick weight loss or enhanced muscle mass with a lean physique are appealing to adolescents. A recent study suggests that young, white, adolescent females are particularly concerned about being overweight as opposed to adolescent males; 43% of females reported trying to lose weight as compared to only 15% of their male counterparts (Centers for Disease Control [CDC], 1992). Weight management techniques may include fasting, diet pills and laxatives, self-induced vomiting, and fad diets as opposed to low fat/low calorie nutritionally sound diets and increased aerobic exercise. Adolescents may not realize that unsound nutritional habits often follow for a lifetime, or that growth and development may be delayed or permanently impaired. School nurses are in an excellent position to identify adolescents who suffer from nutritional problems and provide counseling and/or referral for adolescents and their families. (See Chapter 41 for information on eating disorders.)

Sleep and Rest

Along with increasingly independent activities, adolescents show a propensity for staying up late (particularly if working on a school project or attending a weekend party) and having difficulty waking up in the morning. Setting one's own bedtime and sleeping late on weekends are behaviors associated with gaining independence. Hours of sleep may vary from 6 to 8 hours during the week to 12 hours on the weekends, but an overall approximate of 8 hours per night is recommended for adolescents and young adults.

Rapid physical growth and increased activities contribute to the adolescent's fatigue, and frustrated parents may complain that their teenager has energy for everything but household/family chores. Nurses can educate teens and their parents to set realistic schedules that allow for adequate rest and relaxation. Some teens may find themselves so overscheduled that they develop sleep disturbances from excess fatigue and anxiety. Adult sleep cycles are formed during adolescence, and sleep disturbances continue into the adult years. Persistent difficulty in falling asleep, wakefulness during the night, and/or early waking may be signs of emotional problems associated with tension, anxiety, or depression, and warrant referral.

Exercise and Activity

Although adolescents are often involved in many activities, these activities don't always promote physical fitness. A recent study found that over half of the female students in the sample did not enroll in physical education classes, and that by grade 12, only 10.9% of male students reported daily attendance (CDC, 1992). Only one-third of the students who did participate in physical education reported exercising 20 minutes or more in classes three to five times a week. Regular exercise is known to enhance physical and emotional development, and to promote healthy sleep patterns. Healthy diet and exercise habits formed during adolescence can follow into adulthood and significantly reduce the risk of cardiovascular disease.

Adolescence is an ideal time to initiate an exercise program as a team sport or as an individual activity. Exercise need not always involve an athletic activity but should provide for a program that gradually increases exercise over a 1 to 3 week period with a goal of 30 to 60 minute sessions three to four times per week to enhance cardiovascular fitness (Rocchini, 1992). Nurses can assist adolescents in designing an exercise program that allows for gradual fitness and provides for warm-up and cool-down sessions. Exercise programs are highly personal and should be structured for enjoyment with consideration of physical capabilities and limitations.

Safety

Injuries claim more lives during adolescence than all other causes combined. The predominance of injuries during adolescence results from a combination of factors: physical growth, psychomotor function, physical coordination, energy, impulsivity, peer pressure, and inexperience. Impulsivity, inexperience, and peer pressure may place adolescents in unsafe situations. Feelings of invulnerability ("It can't happen to me") persist, and little thought may be given to the negative consequences of certain behaviors. Alcohol and other drugs that impair judgment are known to contribute to fatal accidents among adolescents, especially those involving firearms and motor vehicles. The sad fact is most serious or fatal accidents involving adolescents are preventable. Nurses must educate adolescents and their families about safety issues and accident prevention. Nurses in school and community action programs are becoming

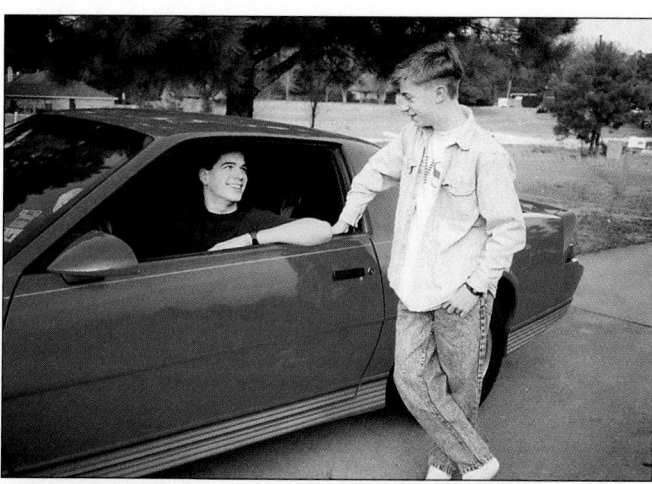

◀ As adolescents struggle toward maturity, their peer group is of utmost importance to them. The group is a haven of acceptance and support while they establish independence from their family. Group norms dictate appropriate appearance, social behaviors, and language that members must follow to remain accepted.

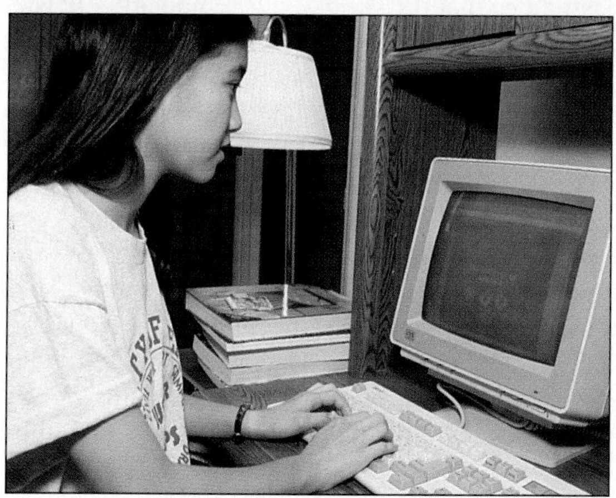

◀ Computers in school and in many homes provide the adolescent with opportunities for learning, creative expression, communication, and entertainment. Adolescents often enjoy "surfing" the Internet, which can provide them with information not readily available locally. Parents must monitor their computer connections, however, for these networks sometimes allow access to people and activities that conflict with family values.

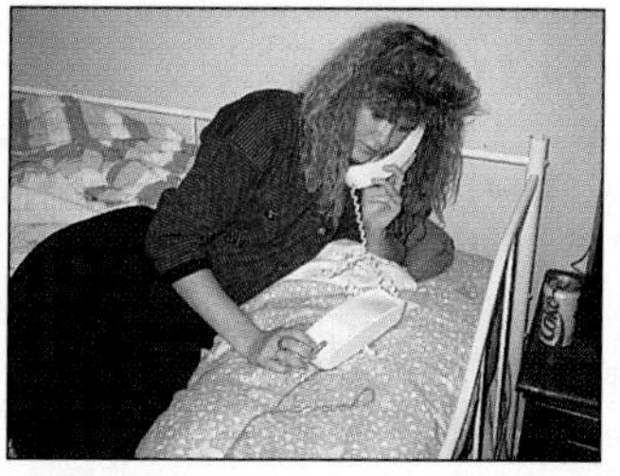

◀ The telephone provides a vital link between adolescents and their peer group. Other family members are often very frustrated because teens are always on the telephone, and virtually all incoming calls are for them.

Relationships with the opposite sex are more mature by late adolescence. Late adolescents have more realistic expectations of both themselves and those who are important to them. They devote many hours and much anxiety toward making events such as prom night memorable for a lifetime. Some adolescents may be left out because they are "unpopular" or shy, or do not have the financial resources to participate in these special events. ▶

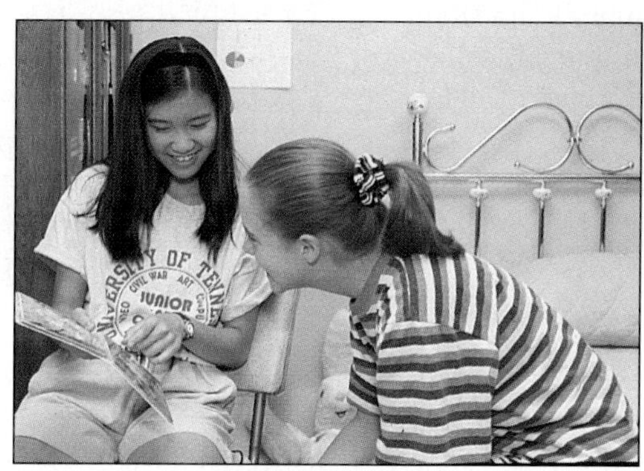

Teens often just "hang out" together rather than participating in planned activities. Although teens often have friends of both sexes, they are more comfortable sharing many hopes, dreams, secrets, and even embarrassing incidents with a friend of the same sex. ▶

Figure 8–1
Growth and development of the adolescent.

more focused in the prevention of firearm and traumatic head injuries.

Firearm education should be included in anticipatory guidance for adolescents and their families. Violence associated with firearms is escalating in our communities and is identified as a major public health concern. For more information on **adolescent violence** and guns, see Chapter 13.

Nurses are taking an important role in the prevention of traumatic head injuries. The National Association of Pediatric Nurses and Practitioners (NAPNAP) has identified head trauma prevention as an area of concentration (Swartz, 1994). Nurses can be effective in providing helmet safety education to children and their families in schools, hospitals, public health clinics, private practices, and community groups. Helmet use has been shown to be significant in preventing head injuries in various sports in which adolescents participate (Rivara, 1994). Although helmet use is mandated in some sports, helmets should be used routinely in any sport that provides a potential source of head trauma.

Helmet safety standards vary, and adolescents and their parents should thoroughly investigate the safety standards set for helmets used in specific sports activities. Helmets recommended for one sport (bicycling) are not necessarily appropriate for another sport (hockey). Sizing and fit should be considerations when using helmets for more than one child. Padding can be added to increase security and removed or adjusted as the adolescent grows. Helmets used in a serious crash or accident should be replaced (Swartz, 1994).

There are no federal laws mandating helmet use. State legislation varies, and helmet use may be mandated by organizations such as schools based on perceived need and economic resources. The key to preventing traumatic head injuries lies with education on the risks of the activity and the benefits of helmet use. Nurses can play a key role in providing the needed education. Many local, state, and national resources, such as the American Automobile Association (AAA), the National Head Injury Foundation, and the National Safety Kids Campaign, provide educational materials for health providers, parents, and children on the prevention of head trauma.

For additional information on safety issues, see Chapter 13.

Dental Care

The incidence of dental caries decreases in adolescence but the need for fluoridated water or fluoride supplements continues until age 16 years. Most permanent teeth are erupted with the possible exception of the third molars (wisdom teeth), which erupt by late adolescence or remain impacted and require surgical removal. Several dental conditions are prevalent during the adolescent years: gingivitis, malocclusion, and dental trauma. Gingivitis is the inflammation and breakdown of the gingival epithelium; gums appear pale and swollen and bleed easily. Increased hormonal activity at the time of puberty, diets high in sugar and simple carbohydrates, and the use of dental braces and appliances that make cleansing less effective are thought to contribute to gingivitis.

Malocclusion (improper contact) occurs in approximately 50% of adolescents due to facial and mandibular bone growth and dental crowding. Treatment varies but generally requires dental devices such as braces to correct tooth position and redirect facial growth. Adolescents may be self-conscious if their peers are no longer in braces and need reassurance that the condition is temporary. For economic reasons, some adolescents are unable to correct malocclusions and suffer the consequences indefinitely. Nurses may be of help in referring adolescents with no dental care to free clinics or agencies providing dental care at low cost. People with uncorrected malocclusions are at greater risk for dental trauma. By middle adolescence, dental injuries approximate 15% to 25%, and boys are most affected, usually secondary to contact sports. Most cases of dental trauma should be referred to a dentist immediately. Dental trauma that involves fractured teeth, fractures of the jaw, or lacerations of the gums or oral mucosa are considered dental emergencies and should be treated as such.

Complete avulsion of a tooth (tooth knocked out of the mouth) may require replantation. The sooner the replantation occurs, the greater the success of the procedure. If the tooth can be recovered, it should be rinsed in lukewarm tap water and placed in the tooth socket. The tooth should not be scrubbed, and cleaning agents and disinfectants should be avoided. If the tooth cannot be repositioned, it should be placed in a container of milk and the child should proceed to the dentist *immediately* (Krasner, 1990). The best prognosis occurs if the injury is treated within 30 minutes. School and clinic nurses may be the first health professionals to see a child with a complete tooth avulsion. Nurses need to be educated in emergency dental care so that proper procedures can be followed for the most successful dental outcome.

Immunization

Adolescents who were never immunized or are lacking in immunization documentation should receive immunizations according to guidelines from the Advisory Committee on Immunization Practices at the CDC (see Chapter 22).

Other Issues

Body Piercing. Ear piercing has been popular with teens for many years, and nose, navel, and nipple piercing are emerging as current fads. Generally, body piercing is harmless but nurses should caution teens about performing these procedures under less than sterile conditions and educate teens about complications such as bleeding, infection, keloid formation, and allergies to metal. Piercing procedures should be performed by qualified personnel *always* using sterile needles.

Tattoos. Tattoos are increasingly popular among mainstream adolescents and are no longer necessarily a mark of gang membership (Armstrong, 1994). Like clothing and hairstyles, tattoos serve to define one's identity. Unfortunately, tattoos are often the result of an impulsive decision and are performed by amateurs who are less than qualified to do the procedure. Because of the invasiveness of the tattoo procedure, it should be considered a health-risk situation. Little regulation exists in the tattoo industry, and nurses should educate adolescents about the risks of blood-borne infections, skin infections, and allergic reactions to dyes used in the tattoo process. Additionally, nurses need to be informed about tattoo removal to provide correct information to adolescents and their families. Impulsive decisions to tattoo are often regretted, and teens and/or their parents may want the tattoo removed. Laser therapy is available for tattoo removal but is costly and not usually covered by insurance. Amateur tattoos are removed quite easily, but studio tattoos using red and green dyes are still quite difficult to remove. Tattoo removal requires several visits, and adolescents need to be tolerant of the tattoo's presence during the removal process.

Suntanning. There is no such thing as a "good" tan. However, it is difficult to convince adolescents that tanning is not only harmful to their skin, but is also a risk factor for developing skin cancer later in life. The media (advertising, movies, and television) promote the image of beach glamour: young, well-built, and tanned. Although most companies that manufacture tanning products promote the sun protection factor (SPF) in their products, the advertised image remains a bronzed, attractive young person.

> Most exposure to ultraviolet radiation occurs during childhood and adolescence, and skin cancers could be prevented with the appropriate and consistent use of sunscreens and sunblocks.

Nurses should educate teens about the benefits and side effects of different sun protection products and encourage use not only for water sports but for all activities that involve sun exposure. Teens involved in athletic activities are often exposed to the sun for long periods of time without protection. Teenagers may be cognizant of body exposure at a beach but may forget about the exposure of body parts during a long tennis match or a baseball game, especially on a cloudy day, when up to 80% of the sun's radiation reaches the ground. Nurses should caution teens receiving any type of medication about the side effects related to sun exposure. Some medications may potentiate the sun's UV rays, resulting in quicker burning. Side effects of sunscreen products include itching, burning, and redness immediately or up to 24 hours after the product is applied. Some people are allergic or sensitive to the sunscreen agent (such as PABA, PABA esters, cinnamates, anthranilates, or benzophenones) and/or other ingredients used, such as fragrances or preservatives. Sunscreen use should be discontinued if an allergic dermatitis is noted and another type of sunscreen may be tried. There are numerous products on the market with various ingredients that have sunscreening capabilities. Sun damage can be prevented and simple measures can minimize the effects of ultraviolet radiation on the skin.

Risk-Taking Behaviors

Adolescent **risk-taking behavior,** with both positive and negative consequences, is considered to be a part of normal growth and development. Opportunities that involve self-challenge are normal transitional risk-taking behaviors and are associated with secondary gains, such as increased self-confidence, stress tolerance, and self-initiative. Normal risk-taking may be illustrated by learning how to snow ski; there is the potential for physical harm, but also for increased self-confidence, skill, and enjoyment. Maladaptive behaviors that have virtually no secondary gains are considered self-destructive. Most adolescents experiment with alcohol and other drugs of abuse: however, chronic substance abuse has no secondary gains and therefore is considered maladaptive (see Chapter 41 for further discussion of substance abuse).

In their efforts to excel in athletics, adolescents may be tempted to use performance-enhancing drugs such as stimulants (amphetamines) or ergogenics (anabolic steroids). The short-term effects of these drugs may enhance athletic performance by making individuals more psychologically energized and aggressive, but the long-term effects may be harmful and even life-threatening. Most anabolic steroids are obtained on the "black market" and are used primarily by male athletes who participate in football or weightlifting. When combined with proper diet and exercise, anabolic steroids may cause an increase in muscle strength and body mass. In addition to the drug-induced physical changes, the mood-enhancing

TABLE 8–4 *Methods of Adolescent Contraception*

METHOD	FAILURE RATE*	ADVANTAGES	DISADVANTAGES
Chance (no protection)	85%	No cost. Requires no preparation.	High failure rate. No disease prevention.
Abstinence (no sex)	0%	No cost. Disease prevention.	Unrealistic for sexually active teens.
Withdrawal (withdrawal of penis from vagina before ejaculation)	19%	No cost. Requires no preparation.	High failure rate. Requires control and motivation by male. No disease prevention.
Periodic Abstinence (rhythm; no sex during fertile/ovulation period)	20%	No cost. Natural family planning.	High failure rate. Requires motivation and predictable menstrual cycle. No disease prevention.
Condom (latex penile sheath to trap sperm)	12%	Inexpensive. Allows for planning. Effective with spermicide. Disease prevention. Readily available. Available over-the-counter.	Moderate failure rate. Requires planning. Best used with spermicide. Requires new condom with each successive intercourse.
Diaphragm (rubber cup covers cervix to prevent sperm from entering; used with spermicide)	18%	Allows for planning. May be inserted before sexual intercourse. Once fitted, relatively inexpensive. Disease prevention.	Requires planning. Messy creams and jelly. Requires motivation and consistency of use. Requires medical intervention and prescription. Requires knowledge for insertion and use. Must be left in for 8 hours after sex; more spermicide must be applied for each successive intercourse.

quality of anabolic steroids is thought to contribute to the athlete's sense of well-being and invulnerability (Goldberg, Bents, & Bosworth, 1991). Among the more serious side effects of anabolic steroids are impaired kidney function and the development of malignant tumors. Nurses are in an excellent position to caution adolescent athletes against the use of performance-enhancing drugs and other products, such as protein powders, vitamins, and energy drinks, without careful supervision by medical personnel.

Because of limited experience, adolescents sometimes engage in risk-taking behaviors with little thought to negative outcomes. Experience modifies behavior, and adolescents learn from their mistakes. It is sometimes difficult for parents and other adults to sit back and watch the results of adolescent decision making. However, in order to grow and move forward, adolescents need to accept responsibility for their actions. Nurses and other adults should recognize the adolescent's natural drive toward risk-taking and educate adolescents to consider outcomes of risk-taking behaviors.

Sexual Activity

Adolescent sexuality is a term used to describe the thoughts, feelings, and behaviors related to the adolescent's sexual identity. Middle adolescence typically marks the initial period of dating and experimentation with heterosexual and homosexual behaviors, although in some cultures sexual experimentation occurs much earlier. Initially, group dating may be popular, but this is quickly replaced by dating in couples, who may be sexual partners. Intimate relationships in middle adolescence are usually short-lived as adolescents experiment with their sexual identity. Although mature, intimate relationships

TABLE 8–4 *Methods of Adolescent Contraception (continued)*

METHOD	FAILURE RATE*	ADVANTAGES	DISADVANTAGES
Spermicides (creams, jelly, foam, suppositories placed in vagina to kill sperm before it enters cervix)	21%	Available over-the-counter. Effective if used with barrier method. Disease prevention. Relatively inexpensive. Allows for planning.	Requires planning. High failure rate if used alone. Messy. Must reapply with each successive intercourse.
Oral Contraceptives (combination products: suppress ovulation, increase thickness of cervical mucus, decrease thickness of uterine lining)	0.1%	Not tied to sexual activity. Highly effective. Allows for planning.	Medical intervention and prescription needed. Requires knowledge for use. Expensive for teens. Side effects of medication: *especially* weight gain, break-through bleeding during cycles (varies with pill and patient). No disease prevention.
Contraceptive Implants (six subdermal implants of progestin [Norplant]: suppresses ovulation, increases thickness of cervical mucus)	.04%	Not tied to sexual activity. Long-term (5-year) contraception. Highly effective. No estrogen; safe for drug addicts, those with selected cardiac disease and lactating females. No planning required once implants are in place.	Expensive (now approved by Medicaid for low-income women) Requires medical intervention for insertion/removal. May be visible under the skin. Side effects of progestin: irregular, heavy, or no bleeding; headaches; acne; depression.
Injectable Contraceptive (Depo-Provera [DMPA], injectable progestin given every 3 months: suppresses ovulation for 14 to 16 weeks)	0.3%	Highly effective. Not tied to sexual activity. No estrogen. No planning once injection has been received for 3 months. Stops menses in 50% of users. Can be used with lactating females, those with selected cardiac disease, and drug addicts.	Requires medical intervention. May have delay in fertility after use. Side effects of progestin: irregular, heavy, or no bleeding; headaches; weight gain; depression. Expensive.

*Failure rates are based on the percentage of women experiencing an accidental pregnancy in the first year of use of reported contraceptive method. Adolescent failure rates are much higher than those rated in this table because adolescents rarely maintain consistent compliance.

Adapted with permission from Hatcher, J., et al. (1994). The essentials of contraception: Effectiveness, safety, and personal considerations. *Contraceptive technology* (p. 113). New York: Irvington Publishers, Inc.

are rare during this stage of development, middle adolescents are generally not promiscuous, but move rapidly from one relationship to another (Stevens-Simon, 1993). Of greatest concern to parents during the adolescent's stage of sexual experimentation are unwanted pregnancy, STDs, and the teen's feelings of despair over failed relationships. Adolescents themselves are often impervious to the possibility of negative consequences of their sexual experimentation and believe that "it can't happen to me."

The Alan Guttmacher Institute (1994) estimates that approximately 1,000,000 pregnancies (1 in 10) occur among American adolescents between ages 15 and 19 years annually. The United States has the highest teen pregnancy rate of any country in the western world. Statistics on adolescent pregnancy have remained relatively stable despite over 30 years of available birth control. Pregnancies are increasing among young teens while decreasing among older teens. The reasons for the shift in the age of teen pregnancy are earlier maturation of adolescent females, earlier age of sexual experimentation, ignorance about contraception, and cultural acceptance of single mothers. Teens from minority backgrounds and those living in poverty are more vulnerable to adolescent pregnancy and are more inclined to keep the baby after delivery. Approximately 40% of teen pregnancies are terminated by elective abortion, the majority of those abortions among teens living *above* the poverty level (Alexander & Guyer, 1993).

According to Hatcher et al. (1994), the average age of first-time sexual experience in females is 16 years; in males, 14 to 15 years. There is a wide variation in the age of first-time sexual intercourse, and the variation is often culturally driven. African American adolescents are known to engage in sexual intercourse earlier than white and Hispanic adolescents, African American

TABLE 8–5 *Health Screening, Health Maintenance, and Anticipatory Guidance for Adolescents*

11–14 YEARS	15–17 YEARS	18–21 YEARS
Immunization		
May need second immunization of MMR #2 before entrance to middle or junior high school. Series according to ACIP guidelines for unimmunized teens or teens with no documentation of immunizations. Td booster between ages 11–16 years, then every 10 years. HBV if not already vaccinated.	HBV if not already vaccinated. Varicella vaccine if adolescent has not had prior infection with chicken pox.	HIB, pneumococci, tetanus, influenza, and hepatitis B to HIV + adolescents. No OPV, IPV, or live measles vaccines to pregnant teens. HBV if not already vaccinated.
Safety		
Counsel about seat belts, emergency numbers, and bicycle safety. Need for proper equipment during exercise and sports activities. Sunscreens, diet, and fluids during exercise. Water/pool safety. Firearm and neighborhood safety. Safety issues with body piercing and tattoos.	Counsel about safety issues associated with sexual activity, drugs, and alcohol. Water safety/diving accidents. Neighborhood safety. Seat belts, driving any motor vehicle. Drugs and alcohol associated with driving. Firearm safety. Proper use of safety equipment with sports. Proper use of 911 emergency number. Safety issues when babysitting. Resisting peer pressure.	Counsel about safety issues associated with travel, school, and work. Child care. Use of 911, CPR, and Heimlich maneuver in emergencies. Sexual activity and safe sex practices. Alcohol and drug use, needle sharing. Firearm/neighborhood safety.
Nutrition		
Appetite increases in response to body's needs for protein, calcium, iron, and zinc. Concerns about weight, body build. Assess usual diet for basic nutrients. Assess height to weight ratio before and after "growth spurt." Counsel to avoid concentrated sweets and high fat foods for snacks. Assess food and fluids in relation to sports.	Assess usual diet, perception of body image in relation to peers. Discuss basics of nutrition relative to dieting. Assess potential for eating disorders: overeating, undereating, binging and purging. Assess eating as a coping mechanism. Assess consumption of fast and junk food. Assess food and fluids in relation to sports.	Need for calories declines. Need for calories and protein increases with sports activities. Need for calories, calcium, iron, and protein increases during pregnancy. Fad diets, junk food, and fast food continue. Assess basic cooking and meal planning skills. Assist in choosing nutritious, low fat foods in restaurants and other facilities.
Screening		
Vision screening yearly, refractive errors common. Counsel regarding proper use and care of glasses and contacts. Blood pressure. Sports physicals. Height and weight, obesity screen. TB testing if high risk.	Vision screening and need for prescriptive lens change as necessary. Blood pressure, height and weight. Sports physicals. Hemoglobin, hematocrit, urinalysis at age 15 years. TB testing if high risk. Pelvic exam and Pap smear for sexually active females. VDRL and STD cultures as appropriate for sexually active males and females. Self-breast exam. Pap smear for adolescent females seeking contraception regardless of sexual activity. Testicular screening for cancer begins at age 15 years in males.	Vision screening every two years or as needed. TB testing if high risk, hemoglobin, hematocrit, and urinalysis at age 19 years. Height, weight, and blood pressure. Cardiac risk appraisal. Pre-employment or school physical. Gonorrhea and chlamydia cultures, VDRL for sexually active females. Pelvic exam and Pap smear. Gonorrhea and chlamydia cultures and VDRL in sexually active males. HIV, hepatitis B, TB screening as appropriate. Self-breast exam, testicular screening.

TABLE 8–5 *Health Screening, Health Maintenance, and Anticipatory Guidance for Adolescents (continued)*

11–14 YEARS	15–17 YEARS	18–21 YEARS
Dental Care		
Brushing, flossing, regular check-ups every 6 months. Need for braces and low cost dental facilities. Oral hygiene. Fluoridated water needed or fluoride supplements. Ask about diet, sweets? Cavities? Use of dental sealants?	Fluoride until age 16 years. Gingivitis common, need for flossing. Correction of malocclusions. Provide emergency care for avulsed or fractured teeth. Ask about diet, cavities. Oral hygiene necessary with braces.	Less prone to dental accidents. Brush and floss twice daily. Braces usually off. Dental visit every 6 months.
Sleep		
Requires 8 hours or more. Growth may be fatiguing. More difficulty waking in morning. May nap after school if tired and no activities planned.	Requires 8 hours often, gets less as activities increase. Difficult to wake up in morning. Likes to stay up late with friends. Up late for TV shows.	Requires 8 hours, some less. Sleep time varies. Up later at night, weekend. Early to bed for work. Up late with studies.
Exercise		
May fatigue quickly with exercise. Assess exercise program for safety, cardiovascular fitness, rest, fluids, and psychological well-being. Counsel adolescent and parents about appropriate sports before, during, and after "growth spurt."	May fatigue quickly without endurance training. Assess diet, exercise, and overall physical fitness. Counsel regarding sports competition and stress. Encourage a balance in sport activities and studies. Consider physical stature and psychosocial readiness when selecting sport activities.	Capacity for endurance increases. Develop an appropriate long-term diet, exercise program. Assess cardiovascular risk factors. Encourage a balance in sport activities with work and studies.

Abbreviations: HBV, Hepatitis B virus vaccine; Td, tetanus toxoid.

males initiating sexual activity at the earliest age (Fisher, 1991).

Research suggests that "abstinence only" programs are ineffective and do not significantly delay the initiation or frequency of premarital intercourse among teens (Christopher & Roosa, 1990). Abstinence focused pregnancy programs given in combination with reproductive information and family planning methods are more effective in reducing early sexual involvement (Howard & Mitchell, 1993). Approximately 80% of all adolescent pregnancies occur within one year of initiating sexual intercourse, and one in five pregnancies occur within the first month (Woods, 1991; Ringdahl, 1992). Young women are sexually active for 6 to 12 months prior to seeking birth control and two-thirds do not use birth control routinely. Contraceptive practices are often influenced by the adolescent's limited cognitive abilities or lack of abstract thinking. Adolescents who feel invulnerable to pregnancy often cannot internalize information on sexual behavior, conception, and birth control. Lack of self-esteem and peer pressure also play a role in determining adolescent sexual behavior. Teens may use sex to feel loved or desired, and fear abandonment by a partner if sex is refused. Some teens lack correct reproductive information and don't plan ahead for sexual encounters. Sexual activity is often impulsive, erratic, and unplanned as the relationships are relatively short-term.

Current research shows that common predictors of adolescent pregnancy include academic failure, low self-esteem, limited parental support, poverty, peer pressure, and a helpless/hopeless outlook (Schwartz, 1992). Economically, teenage pregnancy is devastating to the mother, child, and society at large. In 1992, the General Accounting Office reported that low-income families begun by teenage mothers received $34 billion a year in health and welfare benefits. Approximately two thirds of teenage mothers do not graduate from high school, obtain less work experience, receive lower wages, and earn less per year than women who give birth later in life (Greene & Cromer, 1991). The teen mother's lack of basic academic skills makes job opportunities limited and perpetuates the cycle of poverty that is both the cause and consequence of teen pregnancy. The product of a teen pregnancy is often a premature (less than 37 weeks' gestation) or low-birthweight infant (less than 2500 grams). The lack of prenatal care, STDs, poor nutrition, smoking, and substance abuse are factors that contribute to prematurity, intrauterine growth retardation, and low-birthweight infants. Approximately 25% of low-birthweight infants are born to teen mothers; these infants have a neonatal mortality 50 times greater than normal weight infants (Tsang, 1993). In the postneonatal period, infants of normal birthweight born to teen mothers under age 17 years have twice the mortality rate of children born to older women. Studies suggest that environmental factors such as poverty and the lack of knowledge of child development, child supervision, and primary health care services contribute to the increased incidence of illness, injury, and mortality among infants and young children (Stevens-Simon & McAnarney, 1991).

Nurses are in a position in schools and community clinics to identify teens at risk for pregnancy and to provide guidance with appropriate information and referral in a confidential atmosphere. Nurses should strongly encourage adolescents to discuss sexuality, sexual behavior, and contraception with their parents whenever possible, but must guarantee confidentiality of communication.

The nurse's professional role is to ensure that adolescents have the knowledge, skills, and opportunities that enable them to make responsible decisions regarding sexual behavior. Education regarding sexuality and contraception should be oriented to the developmental level of the individual or group. Additionally, primary prevention must be emphasized by assisting adolescents to develop coping strategies to meet their needs in ways other than through sexual behavior.

Adolescent Contraception. Complete protection from pregnancy and STDs is through sexual abstinence. However, because approximately half of adolescents between ages 15 and 19 years are sexually active, nurses need to feel comfortable with managing health concerns related to sexuality. Comprehensive health care is essential in providing services for sexually active adolescents. Health care providers should include screening and management of STDs, contraceptive services, and psychosocial counseling (see Chapter 22 for more information on STDs). The accompanying box lists factors to be considered in assisting teens to select birth control methods.

Factors to Consider in the Selection of Adolescent Contraception

- Cognitive development (concrete vs abstract thinking)
- Clarification of attitudes and values
- Sexual maturity rating (SMR)
- Communication with partner
- Use of more than one method
- Frequency of intercourse
- Appropriate information (three messages per visit)
- Problem solving abilities (appeal to logic and feelings of power over body)
- Communication with parents or other adults
- Physical/mental health
- Motivation of both partners
- Concrete, graphic instruction on all methods
- Number and gender of partners
- Encouragement that abstinence is OK

Adolescents use withdrawal, condoms, and oral contraceptive pills (OCPs) as the most frequent methods of birth control. **Adolescent contraceptive** methods, typical efficacy, and the advantages and disadvantages of each method used by teens are listed in Table 8–4. Most adolescents rarely maintain consistent compliance, and failure rates are much higher than those described in the table.

Condoms are becoming more popular with adolescents as awareness of human immunodeficiency virus (HIV) transmission has increased. Condoms are relatively inexpensive, readily available, yet only moderately effective (9 to 12% failure rate if used consistently and properly). It is estimated that only 3 out of 10 sexually active teens use condoms regularly (Moscicki & Millstein, 1993).

When educating adolescents about birth control methods, it is ideal to see partners together. Open communication between partners is essential, and decisions about contraception should be mutual. Male as well as female adolescents need to assume responsibility for sexual behavior. Regardless of the selected method of birth control, all adolescents need frequent follow-up to maintain consistent contraception behaviors. Counseling teens about sexuality and contraception requires nurses who are open, forthright, and respectful of the decisions teens make about sexual activity.

KEY CONCEPTS

- Adolescence is a transition period from childhood to adulthood marked by important biological and psychological changes.
- Biological development during adolescence is variable, and primary and secondary sexual characteristics are acquired by the influence of reproductive hormones in males and females.
- Sexual maturity ratings (SMR/Tanner stages) are somewhat variable but predictable stages of sexual maturation based on pubic hair and breast development in females and pubic hair and genital development in males.
- According to Erikson, the major developmental task in adolescence is the development of an identity/self-perception. Other developmental tasks include the development of a sexual identity, a vocational/educational identity, and independence/autonomy.
- Early and middle adolescents are egocentric and concerned with themselves.
- Cognitive thinking during adolescence moves from concrete to abstract reasoning.
- According to Kohlberg, adolescents and young adults develop a respect for law and order and a society-maintaining orientation.
- Adolescents question the values of family and society before integrating their experiences and beliefs into a personal moral framework.
- Adolescents may be emotionally labile, with extreme highs and extreme lows.
- Physical growth during adolescence is second only to infancy.
- Poor eating habits and lack of aerobic exercise contribute to obesity and decreased overall physical fitness.
- Suntanning, body piercing, and tattooing are behaviors associated with identity formation.
- Risk-taking behavior is considered part of normal growth and development.
- Safety issues related to sports activity, sexual activity, firearms, and the use of motor vehicles should be emphasized.
- Sexual maturation precipitates sexual activity; teen pregnancy and sexually transmitted diseases are related issues.

REFERENCES

Alan Guttmacher Institute. (1994). *Sex and America's teenagers.* New York: Author.

Alexander, C., & Guyer, B. (1993). Adolescent pregnancy: Occurrence and consequences. *Pediatric Annals, 22*(2), 85–88.

American Academy of Pediatrics. Committee on Sports Medicine (1991). *Sports medicine: Health care for young athletes.* Elkgrove, IL: American Academy of Pediatrics.

Armstrong, M. (1994). Adolescents and tattoos: Marks of identity or deviancy? *Dermatology Nursing, 6*(2), 119–124.

Castiglia, P. (1993). Gangs. *Journal of Pediatric Health Care, 7*(1), 39–41.

Centers for Disease Control (1992). Body-weight perceptions and selected weight management goals and practices of high school students—United States, 1990. *Morbidity and Mortality Weekly Report, 40,* 741, 747–750.

Centers for Disease Control. (1995). *Morbidity and Mortality Weekly Report, 44*(15), 289–291.

Christopher, F., & Roosa, M. (1990). An evaluation of an adolescent pregnancy prevention program: Is "just say no" enough? *Family Relations, 39,* 68–72.

Elkind, D. (1967). Egocentrism in adolescence. *Child Development, 38,* 1025–1034.

Erikson, E. (1968). *Identity: Youth and crisis.* New York: W. W. Norton.

Fisher, M. (1991). Adolescent sexuality: Overview and implications for the pediatrician. *Pediatric Annals, 20*(6), 285–289.

Goldberg, L., Bents, R., & Bosworth, E. (1991). Anabolic steroid education and athletes: Do scare tactics work? *Pediatrics, 87*(3), 283–286.

Goldenring, J., & Cohen, E. (1988). Getting into adolescent heads. *Contemporary Pediatrics, 7,*75–90.

Greene, E., & Cromer, S. (1991). Adolescent pregnancy. *North Carolina Medical Journal, 52*(10), 494–495.

Greydanus, D. (1990). Pediatrics and the teenage athlete: The sports specific physical examination. *Adolescent Health Update, 2*(3), 2–5.

Hatcher, J., et al. (1994). *Contraceptive technology* (16th ed.). New York: Irvington Publishers.

Howard, M., & Mitchell, M. (1993). Preventing teenage pregnancy: Some questions to be answered and some answers to be questioned. *Pediatric Annals, 22*(2), 109–118.

Kohlberg, L. (1984). *Essays on moral development, 2,* San Francisco: Harper & Row.

Krasner, P. (1990). The treatment of avulsed teeth. *Journal of Pediatric Health Care, 4*(2), 86–90.

Kreipe, R. (1992). Normal somatic adolescent growth and development. In W. McAnarney, R. Kreipe, D. Orr, & G. Comerci (Eds.), *Textbook of adolescent medicine* (pp. 44–67). Philadelphia: W. B. Saunders Co.

Kulin, H., & Reiter, E. (1992). Delayed pubertal development. In W. McAnarney, R. Kreipe, D. Orr, & G. Comerci (Eds.), *Textbook of adolescent medicine* (p. 509). Philadelphia: W. B. Saunders.

Lee, P. A. (1980). Normal ages of pubertal events among American males and females. *Journal of Adolescent Health Care, 1*(1), 26–29.

Marshall, W. A., & Tanner, J. (1969). Variations in pattern of pubertal changes in girls. *Archives of Disease in Children, 44,* 291–303.

Moscicki, A., & Millstein, S. (1993). Risks of human immunodeficiency virus infection among adolescents attending three diverse clinics. *Journal of Pediatrics, 122*(5), (Part 1), 813–820.

National Center for Health Statistics. (1990). *Vital Statistics of the United States, 1987, Vol. II, Mortality, Part A.* (DHHS Publication No. PHS-90-1101). Public Health Service, Washington, DC.

Offer, D., Ostrov, E., & Howard, K. (1989). Adolescence: What is normal? *American Journal of Diseases in Children, 143*(6), 731–736.

Pendergrast, R., & Strong, W. (1992). Sports medicine. In W. McAnarney, R. Kreipe, D. Orr, & G. Comerci (Eds.), *Textbook of adolescent medicine* (pp. 767–772). Philadelphia: W. B. Saunders Co.

Piaget, J. (1969). *The theory of stages in cognitive development.* New York: McGraw-Hill.

Prothrow-Stith, D. (1991). *Deadly consequences.* New York: HarperCollins.

Ratcliff, D. (1985). The development of children's religious concepts: Research review. *Journal of Psychology and Christianity, 4*(1), 35–43.

Ringdahl, E. (1992). The role of the family physician in preventing teenage pregnancy. *American Family Physician, 45*(5), 2215–2220.

Rivara, F. (1994). Epidemiology and prevention of pediatric traumatic brain injury. *Pediatric Annals, 23,* 12–17.

Rocchini, A. (1992). Cardiovascular risk factors and prevention. In W. McAnarney, R. Kreipe, D. Orr, & G. Comerci (Eds.), *Textbook of adolescent medicine* (pp. 365–373). Philadelphia: W. B. Saunders.

Russell, J. A. (1992, October). *Sports medicine: Management of injuries in exercise and athletics.* Paper presented at the Texas Nurse Practitioner Conference, Houston.

Schwartz, P. (1992). Teenage pregnancy: Everyone's responsibility. *Journal of the Medical Association of Georgia, 81*(7), 377–380.

Slap, G., Vorter, D., Chaudhuri, B., & Centor, R. (1989). Risk factors for attempted suicide during adolescence. *Pediatrics, 84*(5), 762–771.

Stevens-Simon, C. (1993). Clinical applications of adolescent female sexual development. *The Nurse Practitioner, 18*(12), 18–27.

Stevens-Simon, C., & McAnarney, E. (1991). Adolescent pregnancy: Continuing challenges. In D. Greydanus & M. Wolraich (Eds.), *Behavioral pediatrics.* New York: Springer-Verlag.

Swartz, M. (1994). Promoting helmet use in recreational sports. *Journal of Pediatric Health Care, 8*(3), 138–139.

Tanner, J. (1962). *Growth at adolescence* (2nd ed.). Oxford: Blackwell Scientific Publications.

Tsang, R. (1993). Teenage pregnancy is preventable—a challenge to our society. *Pediatric Annals, 22*(2), 133–135.

Woods, E. (1991). Contraceptive choices for adolescents. *Pediatric Annals, 20*(6), 313–321.

BIBLIOGRAPHY

American Academy of Pediatrics. Committee on Adolescence (1992). Firearms and adolescents. *Pediatrics, 89*(4), 784–787.

Bidwell, R., & Deisher, R. (1991). Adolescent sexuality: Current issues. *Pediatric Annals, 20*(6), 293–297.

Bolus, J. (1994). Teaching teens about condoms. *RN, 3,* 44–47.

Bullough, B., & Bullough, V. (1991). Contraceptive for teenagers. *Journal of Pediatric Health Care, 5*(5), 237–244.

Busen, N. (1992). Counseling the high-risk adolescent. *Journal of Pediatric Health Care, 6*(4), 194–199.

Cates, W. (1991). Teenagers and sexual risk taking: The best of times and the worst of times. *Journal of Adolescent Health Care, 12*(2), 84.

Clore, E. (1993). A guide for the testicular self-examination. *Journal of Pediatric Health Care, 7*(6), 264–268.

Eastman, M., & Rozen, S. (1994). *Taming the dragon in your child: Solutions for breaking the cycle of family anger.* New York: John Wiley & Sons.

Ebmeier, C., Lough, M. A., Huth, M., & Autio, L. (1991). Hospitalized school-aged children express ideas, feelings, and behaviors toward God. *Journal of Pediatric Nursing, 6*(5), 337–348.

Fay, M. (1992). *Children and religion: Making choices in a secular age.* New York: Simon & Schuster, Fireside Books.

Fenwick, E., & Smith, T. (1994). *Adolescence: The survival guide for parents and teenagers.* New York: Darling Kindersley.

Levine, M., Carey, W., & Cracker, A. (1992). *Developmental-behavioral pediatrics.* Philadelphia: W. B. Saunders.

Lindsay, J. (1988). *Teen parenting.* Buena Park, CA: Morning Glory Press.

Madaras, L., & Madaras, A. (1993). *My body my self.* New York: New Market Press.

Madaras, L., & Madaras, A. (1993). *My feelings my self.* New York: New Market Press.

Muscari, M. (1992). The "acting-out" adolescent: Identification and management. *Pediatric Nursing, 18*(4), 362–366.

Prothrow-Stith, D. (1992). Television violence promotes youth violence. In B. Leone (Ed.), *Youth violence* (pp. 70–78). San Diego: Greenhaven.

Roye, C. (1993). Pap smear screening for adolescents: Rationale, technique, and follow-up. *Journal of Pediatric Health Care, 7*(5), 199–206.

Shafer, M. A. (1990). The pediatrician and teen sports. *Adolescent Health Update, 2*(3), 1–3.

Smith, K., Turner, J., & Jacobsen, R. (1987). Health concerns of adolescents. *Pediatric Nursing, 13*(5), 311–314.

Spivak, H., Prothrow-Stith, D., & Housman, A. (1988). Dying is no accident. *The Pediatric Clinics of North America, 35*(6), 1339–1347.

Stringham, P., & Weitzman, M. (1988). Violence counseling in the routine health care of adolescents. *Journal of Adolescent Medicine, 9*(5), 389–393.

Turecki, S., & Wernick, S. (1994). *The emotional problems of normal children: How parents can understand and help.* New York: Bantam Books.

Wadler, G., & Hainline, B. (1989). *Drugs and the athlete.* Philadelphia: F. A. Davis.

Wall-Hass, C. (1991). Nurses' attitudes toward sexuality in adolescent patients. *Pediatric Nursing, 17*(6), 549–555.

Wheeler, E., & Brown, S. (1994). *Violence in our schools, hospitals and public places: A prevention and management guide.* Ventura, CA: Pathfinder Publishing.

UNIT III

SPECIAL CONSIDERATIONS IN CARING FOR CHILDREN

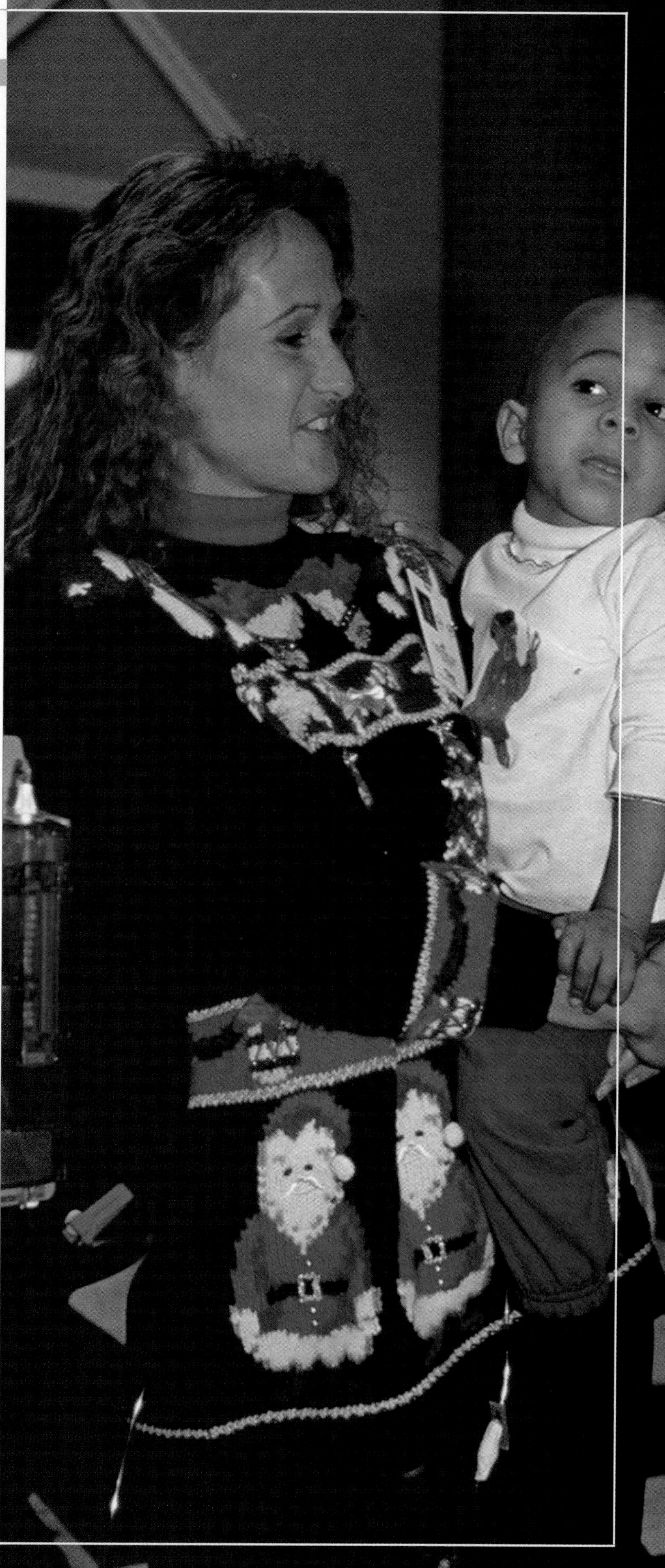

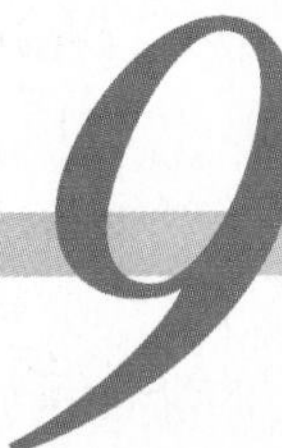

The Child and Play

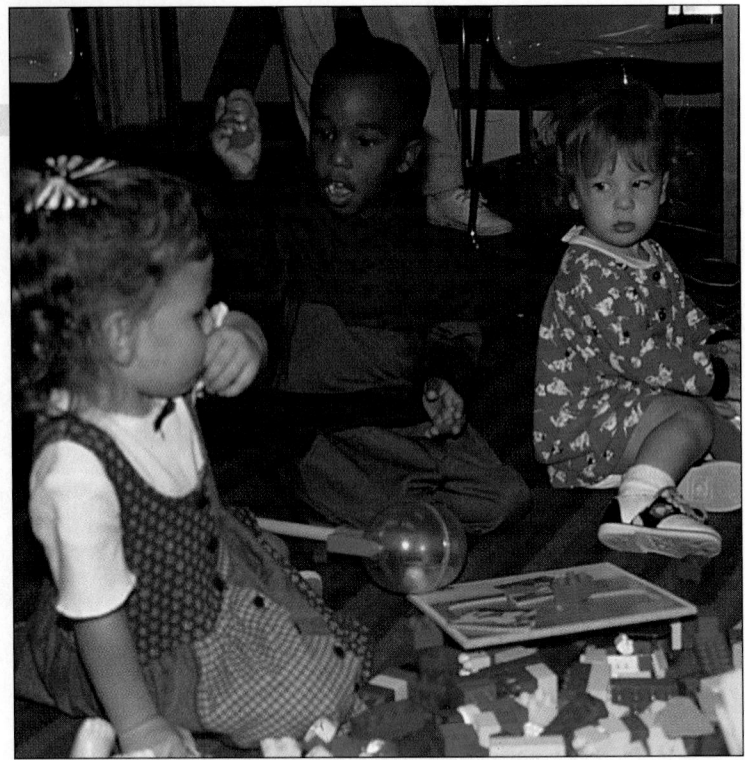

CHAPTER OVERVIEW

LEARNING OBJECTIVES

After studying this chapter, you should be able to:

- Define play.
- Describe the categories of play.
- Explain how play enhances the child's growth and development.
- Describe play according to developmental levels.
- Describe therapeutic play.
- Describe the role of the nurse in therapeutic play.

KEY TERMS

dramatic play: allows children to act out roles and experiences that may have happened to them, that they are fearful will happen to them, or that they observed happening to someone else

expressive play: provides children opportunities to express feelings and energy in appropriate and active ways

familiarization play: the providing of materials that are commonly associated with health care situations and using them in creative and playful activities

surrogate play: offering to play for a child who is too ill or immobilized or who lacks physical stamina to sustain play interactions on his or her own

symbolic play: uses games and interactions that represent an issue or concern to be addressed

therapeutic play: guided play that promotes the psychophysiologic well-being of a child

Play is often called the work of children. However, Webster's unabridged dictionary defines play as an opposition to work. In fact, we know that play is not work in the traditional sense. Rather, it is those tasks, done to amuse oneself, that have behavioral, social, and/or psychomotor rewards. It is inner-directed, and the rewards come from within the individual (Ellis, 1979). It is fun and spontaneous—something we sometimes want to do purely for the joy of it. We all seem to know what play is, although it may mean different things to different people.

Play is also an important part of the developmental process. Play is how children learn about shape, color, cause and effect, and themselves. In addition to cognitive thinking, play helps the child learn social interaction and psychomotor skills. It is a way of communicating joy, fear, sorrow, and anxiety.

The nurse caring for an ill child has numerous opportunities to play with the child. In fact, it is virtually impossible for the nurse to care for a child or infant without engaging in some form of play. Sometimes the nurse will play with a young patient just because being with a child makes us want to play. But play also helps the nurse communicate with the child, develop trust, increase compliance, decrease fear and anxiety, and generally make the office visit or hospital experience a little more pleasant. Play may be structured or unstructured, planned or unplanned, but in all of its varieties it can serve important purposes.

CATEGORIES OF PLAY

It is very difficult to put play into well defined categories. The different forms or categories of play may overlap. A child may be playing with medical equipment to express fear of a procedure and to feel more comfortable with the equipment. While this play is focusing on the above objective, it is also providing diversion and may be increasing the child's psychomotor skills.

An understanding of play in its many forms can assist in understanding the importance of its presence when caring for children of all ages. Chance (1979) classified play as *physical, manipulative, symbolic,* and *games.* Gaynard et al. (1990) also mentions symbolic play and includes *expressive, dramatic, familiarization,* and *surrogate play.*

Physical Play

Physical play involves physical action. Children are demonstrating physical play when they run and jump and play games such as chase, hide and seek, and tag. This particular type of play has a social nature because it can easily involve other children. It is spontaneous and fun. Physical play can also provide distraction and exercise.

In the hospital or clinic setting physical play can provide an opportunity for the child to release aggression, anger, and frustration. Because the hospital is not a playground, it is more difficult to provide safe areas where children can experience the freedom to safely move about. Riding toys, hoops for throwing bean bags through, inflatable punching figures, and Velcro dart boards can all provide safe physical activity and an opportunity for the nurse to interact with the child.

Expressive Play

Expressive play is similar to physical play in some ways. It provides children opportunities to express feelings and energy in appropriate and active ways. Materials frequently used in expressive play include tempera paints, water colors, crayons, colored pencils and markers, drawing paper, finger paints, clay, water, sponges, bean bags, pounding benches, punching bags, rhythm instruments, shaving cream, pudding, and gelatin (Fig. 9–1).

Providing choices is important since an activity that appeals to one child may be of no interest to another. Always be prepared with several options. Nurses can take an active role in expressive play by using paper and paint alongside the child or directly interacting in throwing bean bags at a target with the child's consent.

Expressive play, such as hammering on this toy, allows the child to actively communicate his feelings or dissipate energy in an acceptable and safe way. ▶

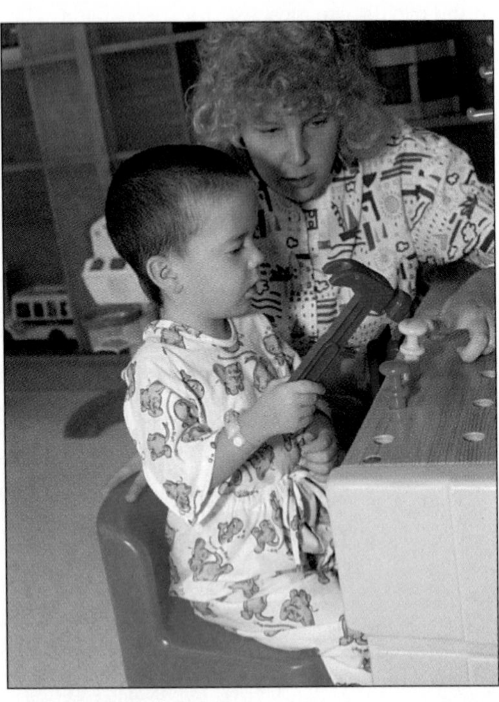

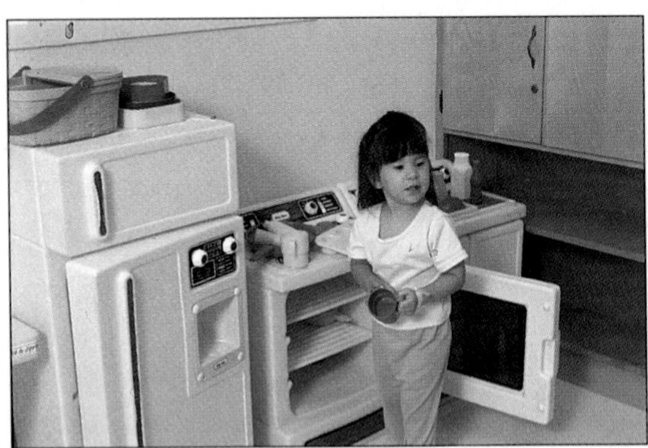

Symbolic play consists of activities that the child uses to express his or her perception of reality. This little girl is acting out a familiar adult scenario as she manipulates child-size toys that represent kitchen equipment.

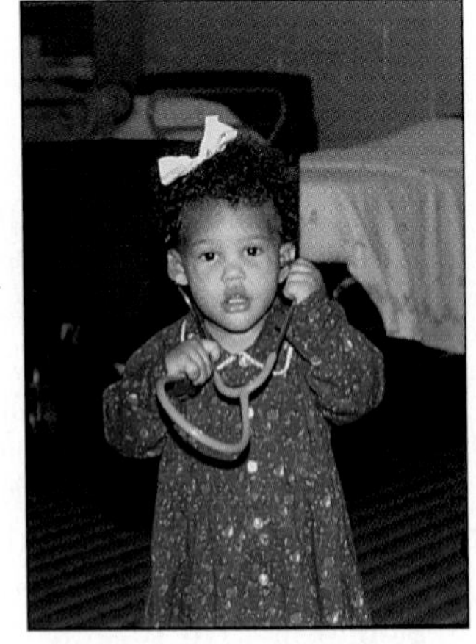

Playing safely with medical equipment (familiarization play) lessens its unfamiliarity to the child and can allay fears. A less fearful child is likely to be more cooperative and less traumatized by necessary care. (Courtesy of University of Texas at Arlington School of Nursing, Arlington, Texas) ▶

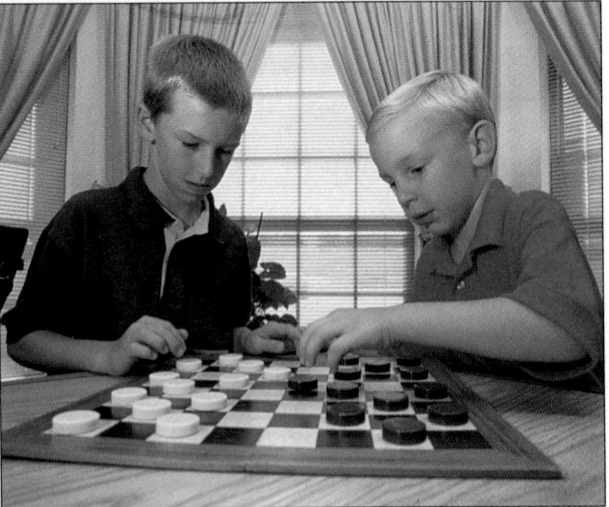

Games with rules, such as board games, help children learn boundaries, teamwork, taking turns, and competition. (Courtesy of Cook Children's Medical Center, Fort Worth, Texas)

Figure 9–1

Manipulative Play

Manipulative play is the child's way of controlling or mastering the environment. Children manipulate the environment and other people. This type of play starts in infancy. Infants "play" with their parents by dropping a rattle, waiting for the parent to pick it up, and dropping it again. This brings enjoyment to both the infant and the parent and brings the infant and parent together in a game of sorts. Children turn and move objects such as puzzles and gadgets in order to better understand how they work.

Many of the activities associated with manipulative play can be easily provided in the hospital or clinic setting. Children will spend hours working on a puzzle or trying to put together a fort or house using interlocking blocks. These activities provide a means of psychomotor stimulation, increase the child's self-esteem, and provide distraction and a means of interacting with peers and the staff.

Symbolic Play

Symbolic play, as its title suggests, uses games and interactions that represent an issue or concern to be addressed. Garvey (1979) identified three elements of symbolic play: one or more objects, a theme or plan, and roles. As the child plays he incorporates some object (a syringe), uses a theme (getting an injection), and then plays the roles each player will have (child, nurse).

Because there are no rules in symbolic play the child can use this play not only to reinforce or learn the good things in life, but also to alter those things which are painful. The child who is in an abusive family may pretend to be a mother who loves and cuddles her child rather than one who verbally or physically abuses the child. Or, in play this same child might act out the abuse she is receiving by hitting or screaming at her pretend child.

Parents are often struck by their children's perception of the reality of the family. Children will mimic their parents as they play games of make believe which are linked to reality (see Fig. 9–1). They will also play games of make believe in which they become the heroes they have read about or seen on television. At certain developmental stages they may come to believe that they actually can fly or disappear.

Symbolic play can be incorporated into the health care setting when coping with fear of separation, a common fear particularly in hospitalized young children. Simple games for infants and young children are peek-a-boo, hiding toys under containers and finding them, rolling cars and balls back and forth using corners and obstacles to obstruct the view at times. These play activities symbolize the action of leaving and returning and demonstrate separation and reunion similar to a parent leaving and returning to a hospitalized child.

Dramatic Play

Dramatic play allows children to act out roles and experiences that may have happened to them, that they are fearful will happen, or that they have observed in others. This type of play can be spontaneous or guided, and it often includes medical or nursing equipment. It is especially valuable for children who have or will experience multiple procedures or hospitalizations.

Hospitals and clinics with child life specialists on staff usually have a medical play area as part of the activity room. Nurses may provide opportunities for spontaneous as well as guided dramatic play. A toy medical bag can be bought or one can be created using real equipment and supplies. Recommended supplies for a general medical kit include stethoscope, blood pressure cuff, syringes without needles, Band-Aids, gauze, tape, tongue depressor, gloves, thermometer, and a cloth doll to function as the patient. Children enjoy exploring and using the contents in spontaneous play, reenacting their experience or making up experiences. The nurse may choose to just observe such spontaneous play or be an active participant with the child. There will be occasions when nurses will want to structure the dramatic play to review a specific treatment or procedure. In guided play situations, the nurse directs the focus of the play. Specialized play kits may be developed for specific procedures, such as central line care, casting, bone marrow aspirations, lumbar punctures, and surgery, using supplies related to the hospital or clinic setting.

Familiarization Play

Familiarization play allows children to handle and explore health care materials in nonthreatening and fun ways (see Fig. 9–1). This type of play is especially helpful, but not limited to, preparing children for procedures and the whole experience of hospitalization.

Examples of familiarization activities include using sponge mouthswabs as painting and gluing tools; making jewelry from Band-Aids, tape, gauze, and lid tops; creating mobiles and collages with health care supplies; making finger puppets using plaster casting material; filling a basin with water and using tubing, syringes, medicine cups, and bulb syringes for water play; decorating beds, wheelchairs, and IV poles with health care supplies; and using syringes for painting activities.

Games

Games include rules and usually are played by more than one person, although some games can be played by oneself. For example the card game solitaire is played by one person, as are many video games. Games with rules rarely occur before age 4 years and are most common with the school age child (Piaget, 1962). Games continue throughout life as adults play board games, cards, and sports.

Through games children learn to play by the rules and to take turns. One common way children accomplish this is through board games. Young children often make up games with unique sets of rules, which may change each time the game is played. Older children have games with specific rules; younger children tend to change the rules.

Surrogate Play

Surrogate play can be used with children who are too ill, are immobilized, or lack the physical stamina to sustain play interactions on their own. In such cases the nurse might offer to play for the child and/or help parents understand how to play for their child. This provides an alternative activity for a bedridden child who needs more stimulation and interaction than that provided by television.

During surrogate play, patient participation can range from passively observing to being moderately active. The patient may offer nonverbal directions with nods of the head or some verbal instructions. Surrogate play activities include entertaining with puppets, dolls, or family and animal figures; reading books; expressive art projects such as decorating the room, window painting, modeling clay, and button making; musical activities, such as singing or playing an instrument; building block creations; and model assembly.

FUNCTIONS OF PLAY

Play enhances the child's growth and development. Some of the more common functions of play are physical development, cognitive development, emotional development, social development, and moral development.

Physical Development

Play aids in the development of both fine and gross motor activity. Children repeat certain body movements purely for pleasure, and these movements in turn aid in the development of body control. For example, an infant will first hit at a rattle, then will attempt to grasp it, and eventually will be able to pick up that same rattle. Next the infant will shake the rattle or perhaps bring it to the mouth.

The parent and child may make a game of repeating sounds such as "ma ma" or "da da," which increases the child's language ability. Repeating rhymes and songs can be a fun way for children to increase their vocabulary. Children love to color on a paper with a crayon and will scribble before being able to draw pictures and to color. This aids the child in eventually learning how to write the alphabet letters and numerals.

> The principle that states that all growth and development is predictable and progressive can be applied to play. Play will also progress from simple to complex.

Cognitive Development

Play is a key element in the cognitive development of children. Once a child has learned a general concept, further experiences with that concept expand from that beginning knowledge. Piaget gives the example of an infant learning to swing an object and then subsequently swinging other objects (Piaget, 1962). This could apply, for example, to things to be eaten, read, or ridden. Progression takes place as the child begins to have certain experiences and to test beliefs and to understand the world around him or her.

Children can increase their problem-solving abilities through games and puzzles. The child involved in pretend play can stimulate several types of learning. Language abilities are strengthened as the child models significant others in role playing. The child must organize thoughts and be able to communicate with others involved in the play scenario that is being set. Children observed playing house will create elaborate details of what the characters do and say.

Children also increase their understanding of size, shape, and texture through play. They begin to understand relationships as they attempt to put a square peg into a round hole, for example. Books and videos increase a child's vocabulary while increasing understanding of the world.

Emotional Development

Children who are experiencing an anxiety-producing situation are often helped through role playing. Play can be a way of coping with emotional conflict. Play can be a way to determine what is real and what is not. Children may escape through play into a world of fantasy and make-believe in order to make sense out of a sometimes senseless world. Play can also increase a child's self-awareness as he explores an event or situation through role playing or symbolic play.

As significant others in a child's life respond to the child's initiation of play, the child begins to learn that he or she is important and cared for. Whether the play is initiated by the child or the adult, when a significant person plays a board game with a child, shares a bike ride, plays baseball, or reads a story, the child gets the message "You are more important than any other thing at this time." The child's self-esteem is increased. The parent sends a message to the infant in the way daily care is given. From these early interactions, the child develops a vision of the world and his control over it.

Social Development

The newborn cannot distinguish self from others and therefore is very narcissistic. As the infant begins to play with others and things, a realization of self and others begins to develop. The infant begins to experience the joy of interaction with others and soon initiates behavior that

TABLE 9–1 *Age-Related Activities and Toys*

GENERAL ACTIVITIES	TOYS AND SPECIFIC TYPES OF PLAY
Infant	
The infant enjoys watching other members of the family, being rocked, being taken for a walk in a stroller, time spent in a swing, supervised time on a blanket on the floor, crawling, walking, and being sung and read to. Play is narcissistic; it is difficult, if not impossible, to direct play. Human interaction is the most important component of play.	Oral movements (playing with the nipple of the bottle, lip movements unrelated to sucking); peek-a-boo; playing with the caretaker's fingers, hair, face, and the infant's own body parts; and playing in water Soft stuffed animals, crib mobiles, squeeze toys, rattles, busy boxes, mirrors, musical toys, water toys during the bath, blocks, safe kitchen utensils, push toys (after they begin to walk) Contrasting colors for young infants (black and white mobiles) Large picture books
Toddler	
The toddler fills and empties containers, begins dramatic play, has increased use of motor skills, enjoys feeling different textures, explores the home environment, imitates others, likes to be read to and to look at books and television that are age appropriate. Toys should meet the child's need for activity and inquisitiveness. This age group also enjoys manipulating small objects such as toy people, cars, and animals.	Continued exploring of the body parts of self and others; mechanical toys; objects of different textures such as clay, sand, finger paints, and bubbles; push-pull toys; large ball; sand and water play; blocks; painting; coloring with large crayons; nesting toys; large puzzles; trucks; dolls Therapeutic play can begin at this age.
Preschooler	
Dramatic play is prominent. This age likes to run, jump, hop, and in general increase motor skills. The child likes to build and create things whether it be sand castles or mud pies. Play is simple and imaginative. Simple collections begin.	Riding toys, building materials such as sand and blocks, dolls, drawing materials, crayons, cars, puzzles, books, appropriate television and videos, nonsense rhymes, singing games, pretending to be something or somebody, dressing up, finger paints, clay, cutting, pasting, simple board and card games
School-Age Child	
Play becomes organized with more direction. The early school age child continues dramatic play with increased creativity but loses some spontaneity. Awareness of rules when playing games. Begins to compete in sports.	Collections, drawing, construction, dolls, pets, guessing games, board games, riddles, physical games, competitive play, reading, bike riding, hobbies, sewing, listening to the radio, television and videos, cooking
Adolescent	
Games and athletics are the most common forms of play. Strict rules are in place. Competition is important.	Sports, videos, movies, reading, parties, hobbies, listening to their favorite music on video or compact disc, experimenting with makeup and hairstyles

involves others. The infant discovers that when she coos, mother coos back. The child will soon expect this response and make a game of playing with mother.

Playing make-believe aids the child in trying on different roles. When the child plays "restaurant" or "hospital," the rules that govern these settings are experimented with. Research has shown that children who played "school" adjusted easier in kindergarten than did other children (Chance, 1979).

Of course most games, from board games to sports, involve interaction with others. The child learns boundaries, taking turns, teamwork, and competition. Children also learn how to negotiate with different personalities and the feelings associated with winning and losing. They learn to share and to take turns.

Moral Development

When children engage in play with their peers and their families, they begin to learn which behaviors are acceptable and which are not. Quickly they learn that taking turns is rewarded and cheating is not. Group play assists the child in recognizing the importance of teamwork, sharing, and being aware of the feelings of others.

TYPES OF PLAY

As the child develops, there is more interaction with people. Certain types of play are associated with, but not limited to, specific age groups. Table 9–1 lists play activities and toys appropriate for various age groups.

Solitary Play. Solitary play is characterized by independent play (Fig. 9–2). The child plays alone with toys very different from those chosen by other children in the area. This type of play begins in infancy and is common in toddlers because of their limited social, cognitive, and physical skills. However, it is important for all age groups to have some time to play by themselves.

Parallel Play. Parallel play is usually associated with the play of toddlers, although it can be found in any age group.

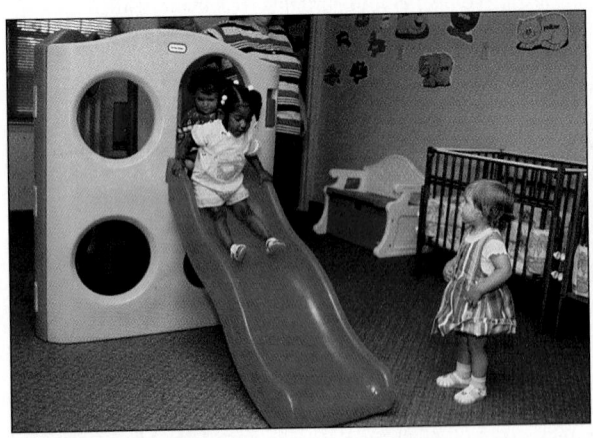

The little girl at right demonstrates onlooker play. She is interested in what is going on and observes another girl playing on the slide. However, she makes no attempt to join the youngster on the slide.

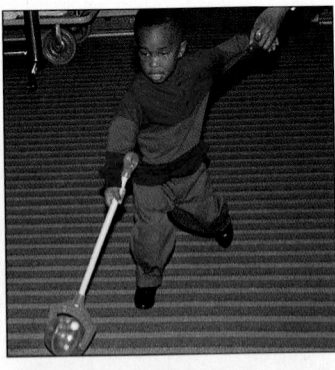

◀ When engaging in solitary play, the child is playing apart from other children and with different types of toys. (Courtesy of University of Texas at Arlington School of Nursing, Arlington, Texas)

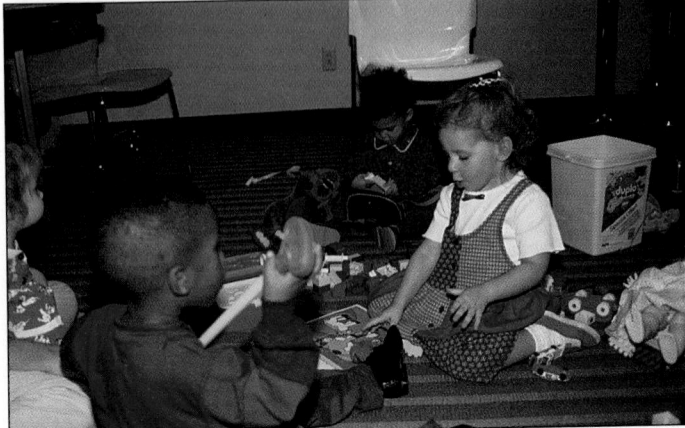

Parallel play occurs when children play side by side with similar toys, but there is no organized group activity. The children play *beside* each other but not *with* each other. (Courtesy of University of Texas at Arlington School of Nursing, Arlington, Texas) ▶

Figure 9–2

Children play side by side with similar toys, but there is a lack of group activity (see Fig. 9–2).

Associative Play. Associative play is characterized by group play without group goals. Children in this type of play do not set group rules, and although they may all be playing with the same types of toys and may even trade toys, there is a lack of formal organization. This type of play can begin during toddlerhood and moves into the preschool age.

Cooperative Play. Cooperative play begins in the late preschool years. This type of play is organized and has group goals. There is usually at least one leader, and children are definitely in or out of the group.

Onlooker Play. Onlooker play is present when the child observes others playing. Although the child may ask questions of the players, there is no attempt to join the play (see Fig. 9–2). This type of play usually starts during the toddler years, but can be observed at any age.

PLAYROOMS IN HEALTH CARE SETTINGS

Hospitals and clinics often provide play rooms where children may go to play with toys, participate in age-appropriate arts and crafts, and socialize with other children. This area should always be seen by children as a safe place where procedures and treatments do not take place. Children, when their condition is stable, may be taken to the play room in their beds and wheelchairs (Fig. 9–3). A separate activity area should be provided, when possible, for adolescents where they may listen to music, play video games, and visit with their peers.

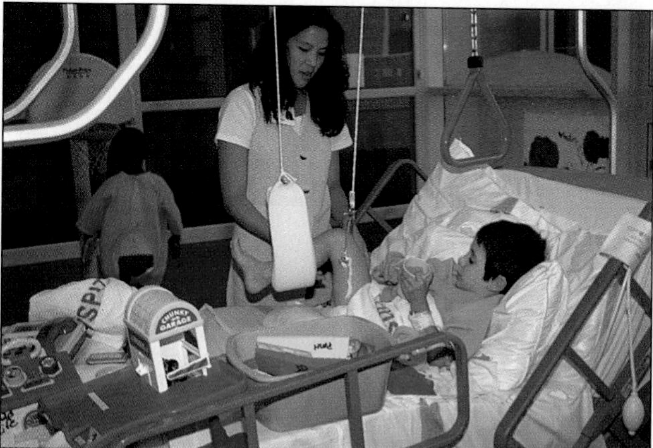

Figure 9–3

Being in traction is no reason not to enjoy the hospital's play facilities. The play therapist wheels this child in his bed to the playroom to give him a change of surroundings and allow him to interact with her and with other children. Because his mobility will be limited for a significant length of time, it is especially important to provide diversion. (Courtesy of Parkland Memorial Hospital, Dallas, Texas)

> The playroom should never be used to give treatments or medication. It should be seen as a "safe place" where the child can go to play.

THERAPEUTIC PLAY

When a child is hospitalized, one component of the child's plan of care is the use of **therapeutic play.** Therapeutic play differs from normative play in its design and intent. It is guided by members of the health team, and activities are planned to meet the physical and psychological needs of the child. Therapeutic play can provide an emotional outlet, instruct, or improve physiologic abilities (Vessey & Mahon, 1990). Supervised play with medical equipment can often decrease fear and separate reality from fantasy.

Child life specialists or play therapists are available in many hospitals and share their expertise in the area of child growth and development and the use of play. Child life programs have as their goal the maintenance of normal living patterns, the minimizing of psychological trauma, and the promotion of optimal development of the child and family. Nurses should also be involved in this type of activity either in conjunction with the child life specialist or individually when a child life specialist is not available. Interpretation of the child's play behavior and some types of play therapy require guidance by a skilled health care worker.

Dramatic Play

Emotional outlet play is often called dramatic play. During this type of play the child acts out or dramatizes real life stressors. This might include emotional stressors such as abuse or neglect or a painful physical stressor such as a bone marrow aspiration. The child who is hospitalized and is separated from family and friends might use a wooden hammer and pegs to express anger over the separation. A child who has been sexually abused might not be able to communicate verbally the experience but may be able to use an anatomically correct doll to show what happened.

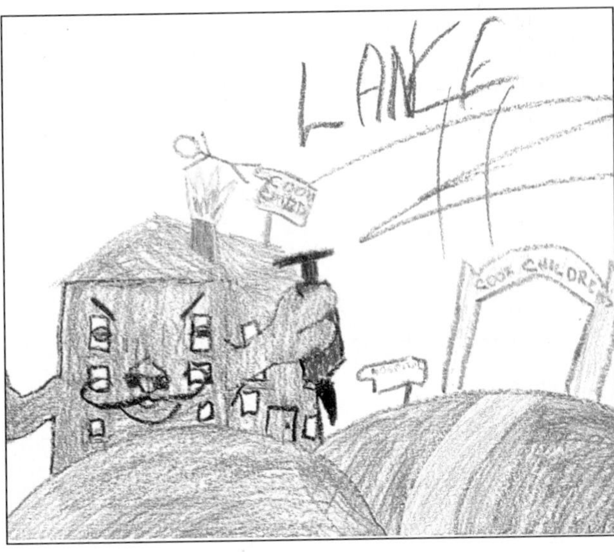

Art materials allow children to express their thoughts and feelings about health care procedures.

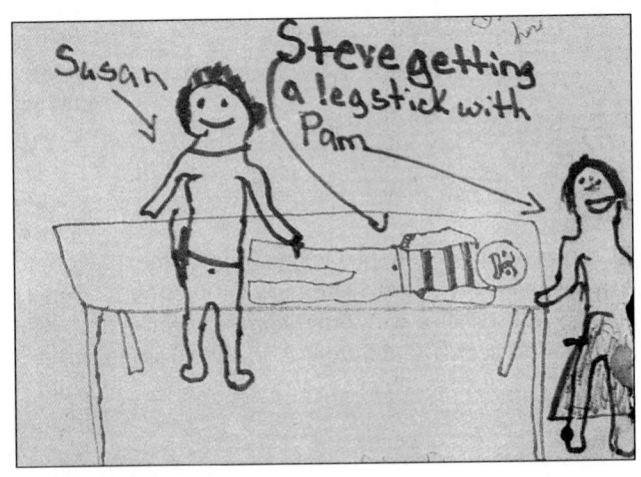

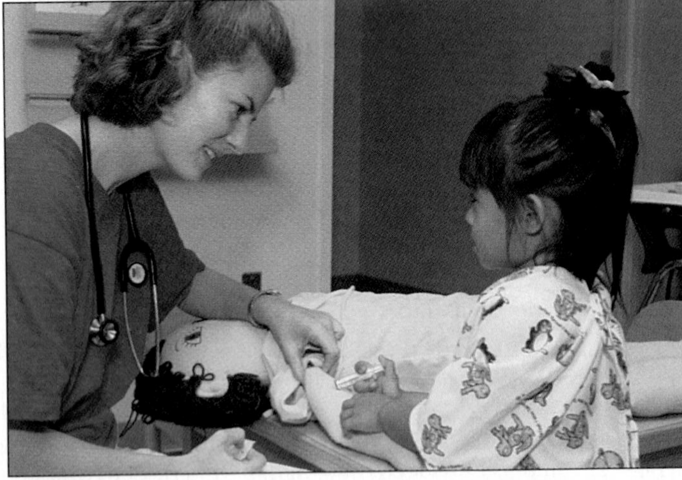

◄ Giving a doll an injection can help a child work through anxiety and anger about injections she may be receiving.

Figure 9–4
Therapeutic play can be used to teach children about medical procedures or help them work through their feelings about what has happened to them in the health care setting. Child life specialists or play therapists are often members of the team in children's hospitals to provide expert guidance for therapeutic play.

There are many commercially crafted toys available for dramatic play. Anatomically correct dolls and puppets are available. Some dolls have removable parts that enable the child to see the various organs of the body.

Children can express their inner beliefs and perceptions through drawing (DiLeo, 1970). It is not unusual to see a child draw a very big bed with a tiny child on it surrounded by large hovering adults or a huge syringe with a long needle. Children often express their thoughts and feelings through the use of paper and crayons or colored markers (Fig. 9–4).

Supervised needle play is an appropriate intervention with the child who has to undergo frequent blood work, injections, intravenous therapy, or any other therapy involving needles. Safety when using needle play is always important, and the child's growth and development level should be evaluated before using this type of directed play. An adult is always present during needle play. The child can give a doll an injection and can thereby work through anger and anxiety. Wooden hammers and pegboards, Nerf balls, and boxing gloves are all avenues for release of stress and/or anger.

Teaching Through Play

Play can also be used to teach the child. It can be used in preoperative teaching and teaching before a new, painful, or extensive procedure (see Fig. 9–4). The child's cognitive level should be assessed before this type of teaching, and the play should be appropriate to the child's level.

Numerous books are available to assist in this area. Hospital equipment is often used in this type of play. The nurse might demonstrate taking a blood pressure on the child's stuffed animal before putting the cuff on the child. A breathing treatment might be "given" to the child's doll before the child is given the treatment. The nurse might use drawings and diagrams to explain procedures or surgery.

Some hospitals have preoperative visits during which children come and meet the people who will be taking care of them and the physical surroundings. They may see the scrubs and masks worn by the surgical staff and a typical room. Children and parents can ask questions and meet other children and parents who are going through the same experience. The visit usually includes a tour of the operating and recovery rooms and is followed by a snack.

Enhancing Compliance Through Play

Children with illnesses that require a therapeutic activity that is unpleasant or painful often are noncompliant. It is a challenge to develop a plan that will stimulate and engage the child in the activity. The nurse should include age-appropriate growth and development activities when planning care. The school age child who loves competition and games is going to be more likely to increase range of motion of an arm if points can be made each time he throws a Nerf ball through a hoop.

Deep breathing exercises can be enhanced by allowing the child to blow bubbles, a whistle, or a pinwheel, or to simulate blowing out the nurse's pen light. Range of motion can be accomplished by throwing Nerf balls, bean bags, and paper balls. The child who needs to increase his intake can sometimes be motivated to drink more fluids if he can graph the amount taken in and receive a reward if he reaches a selected goal. The child is included in planning, and rewards and goals are identified. Colorful stickers, baseball cards, small toys, and special pencils can be used as awards.

Unstructured Play

In addition to therapeutic play, it is also important for the nurse to encourage unstructured play in the hospital setting. Through unstructured play children can control events, ideas, and relationships. Because play is controlled by the individual, the child has a sense of control (Bolig, Fernie, & Klein, 1986).

Hospitals that do not have a special room set aside for play should be encouraged to provide developmentally appropriate toys, games, and books. These items can be kept in a special box that is accessible to the nursing staff.

Evaluation of Play

Therapeutic play should be reflected in the child's nursing care plan in the nursing interventions. During the evaluation step of the nursing process, the nurse looks at the outcome criteria to determine if the goals have been met. The nurse is asking if play enhanced the care of the child. Did the child hold her arm still while the needle for intravenous fluids was inserted? Is the child coughing and deep breathing every 2 hours? Is the child relating feelings of fear over the separation from her parent? Is the child eating or sleeping? If the patient goals have been achieved, then the interventions were appropriate and effective.

KEY CONCEPTS

- Play has many definitions but it is basically done for fun, is inner directed, and has behavioral, social, and psychomotor rewards.
- Some of the categories of play include physical, manipulative, symbolic, games, expressive, dramatic, familiarization, and surrogate.
- Play enhances the child's growth and development through physical, cognitive, emotional, social, and moral development.
- Solitary play begins in infancy and is common in toddlers. Parallel play is usually associated with toddlers, and onlooker play usually starts during the toddler years. Associative play can begin in toddlerhood and moves into the preschool age. Cooperative play begins in the late preschool years.
- Therapeutic play can provide an emotional outlet, instruct, or improve physiologic abilities.
- Play can be incorporated into nursing care when teaching and when providing a therapeutic activity that the child finds unpleasant or painful. Compliance can be increased when the child can make deep breathing and range of motion exercises fun activities.

REFERENCES

Bolig, R., Fernie, D., & Klein, E. (1986). Unstructured play in hospital settings: An internal locus of control rationale. *Children's Health Care: Journal of the Association for the Care of Children's Health, 15*(2), 101–107.

Chance, P. (Ed.). (1979). *Learning through play.* New York: Gardner Press.

DiLeo, J. (1970). *Young children and their drawings.* New York: Brunner/Mazel.

Ellis, M. (1979). What is play? In Paul Chance (Ed.). *Learning through play* (p. 13). New York: Gardner Press.

Garvey, C. (1979). What is play? In Paul Chance (Ed.). *Learning through play,* (p. 5). New York: Gardner Press.

Gaynard, L., et al. (1990). *Psychosocial care of children in hospitals: Clinical practice manual from the ACCH Child Life Research Project.* Bethesda, MD: Association for the Care of Children's Health.

Piaget, J. (1962). *Play, dreams and imitation in childhood.* New York: W. W. Norton.

Vessey, J., & Mahon, M. (1990). Therapeutic play and the hospitalized child. *Journal of Pediatric Nursing, 5*(5), 328–333.

BIBLIOGRAPHY

Barnes, L. (1992). Don't forget to play! *Maternal Child Nursing, 17,* 183.

Bunker, L., Johnson, C., & Parker, J. (1982). *Motivating kids through play.* West Point, NY: Leisure Press.

Casanova, U. (1989). Play is the work of childhood. *Instructor, 3,* 22–23.

Frankiel, R. (1993). Hide-and-seek in the playroom: On object loss and transference in child treatment. *Psychoanalytic Review, 80*(3), 341–359.

Frick-Helms, S. (1993). You make the diagnosis. *Nursing Diagnosis, 4*(4), 166–168.

Hart, R., Mather, P., Slack, J., & Powell, M. (1992). *Therapeutic play activities for hospitalized children.* Bethesda, MD: Association for the Care of Children's Health.

Herron, R., & Sutton-Smith, B. (1971). *Child's play.* New York: John Wiley & Sons.

Hill, E. (1986). *Where's Spot?* New York: G. P. Putnam's Sons.

Hyde, D. (1970). *Piaget and conceptual development.* London: Holt, Rinehart, and Winston.

Kapsch, L. (1991). A culture of one: Case study of play therapy with an abused child. *Journal of Pediatric Nursing, 6*(6), 368–373.

LeVieux-Anglin, L., & Sawyer, E. (1993). Incorporating play interventions into nursing care. *Pediatric Nursing. 19*(5), 459–463.

Lewis, J. (1993). Childhood play in normality, pathology, and therapy. *American Orthopsychiatric Association, 63*(1), 6–15.

Loranger, N. (1992). Play intervention strategies for the Hispanic toddler with separation anxiety. *Pediatric Nursing, 18*(6), 571–575.

McCue, K. (1988). Medical play: An expanded perspective. *Children's Health Care, 16*(3), 157–161.

Piaget, J. (1962). *Dreams and imitation in childhood.* New York: W. W. Norton.

Pulaski, M. (1971). *Understanding Piaget.* New York: Harper & Row.

Sadler, C. (1990). Child's play. *Nursing Times, 86*(11), 16–17.

Schuster, C., & Ashburn, S. (1992). *The process of human development.* Philadelphia: J. B. Lippincott.

Summers, K. (1991). Providing for play in the care of children. *Pediatric Nursing, 17*(3), 266–267.

Tillay Johnson, M. (1994). The doll clinic: A preschooler's guide to less fearful health care. *Journal of Pediatric Health Care, 8,* 291–292.

10

Communicating With Children

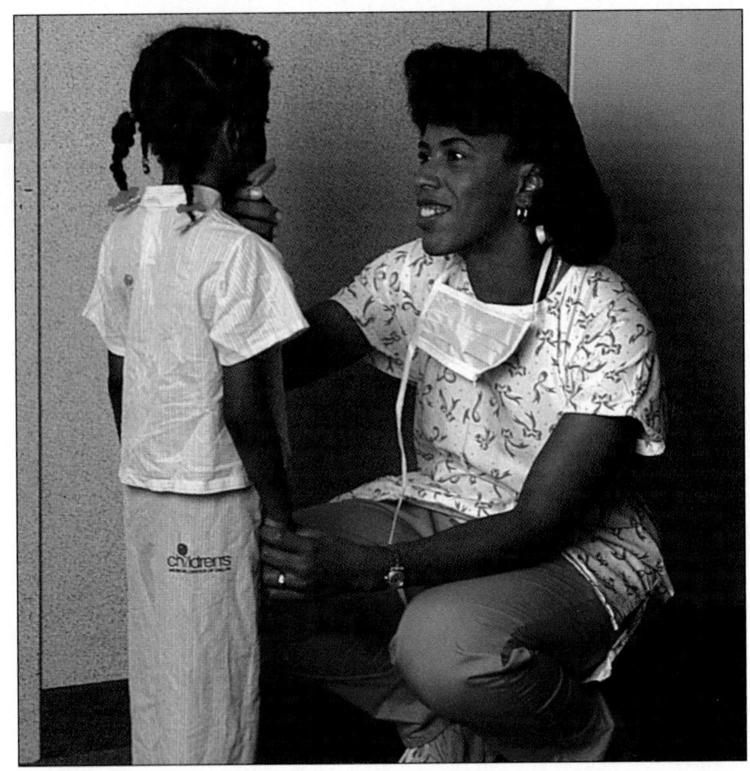

CHAPTER OVERVIEW

LEARNING OBJECTIVES

After studying this chapter, you should be able to:

- Describe six components of effective communication with children.
- Describe communication strategies that assist nurses in working effectively with children.
- Explain the importance of avoiding communication pitfalls in working with children.
- Describe effective family-centered communication strategies.
- Describe effective strategies for communicating with children with special needs.

KEY TERMS

active listening: the ability to empathetically listen in order to gain better understanding of the actual as well as implied message

communication: the act of transmitting and receiving information

empathy: the ability to remain objective while seeing from another's perspective

empowerment: providing the family with the appropriate tools (education, information, support) that enable them to fully participate in decision making and the care of their child

family-centered care: the recognition and incorporation of the family in planning, implementing, and evaluating the plan of care

preparation: providing the child with information in advance of procedures, treatments, and/or events in order to facilitate coping

professional boundaries: self-awareness that allows an individual to recognize the differences between professional and personal relationships and maintain these in work settings

self-esteem: the personal value that an individual places on himself or herself

sensory information: sharing concepts with children using techniques that incorporate sight, taste, touch, smell, and hearing

win/win solution: establishment of a common goal, as resolution to a conflict, that both parties can support

To be effective in working with children and their families, the nurse must develop keen communication skills. Parents and other family members play a crucial role in the lives of pediatric patients; the nurse needs to establish a rapport with the family in order to identify mutual goals and facilitate positive patient outcomes. Good verbal communication skills must be accompanied by an awareness of body language, eye contact, and tone of voice when listening to young patients and their families, as well as when assessing one's own communication style.

This chapter discusses the various components of communication, both verbal and nonverbal. Included are strategies for establishing and maintaining open communication with family members. Communication techniques appropriate to the child's age and developmental abilities are also described, as are techniques for transcultural communication and strategies for children with special needs. All of these techniques will help the nurse establish a therapeutic relationship with the child and family.

COMPONENTS OF EFFECTIVE COMMUNICATION

Communication is much more than words going from one person's mouth to another's ears. In addition to the words themselves, messages are conveyed by the tone and quality of voice, eye contact, physical proximity, visual cues, and overall body language.

Touch

Touch can be a positive, supportive technique effective from birth through adulthood. In infancy messages of love, security, and comfort are conveyed through holding, cuddling, gentle stroking, and patting. Infants cannot comprehend the meaning of words they hear, but they can feel, interpret, and respond to gentle, loving, supportive hands caring for them. Toddlers and preschoolers find being held and rocked as well as gentle stroking of the head, back, arms, and legs very soothing and comforting (Fig. 10–1). School-age children and adolescents appreciate giving and receiving hugs as well as a reassuring pat on the back or a gentle hand resting on their hand. Requesting permission from patients is recommended for any contact beyond a casual touch. Warmth, comfort, reassurance, security, trust, caring, and support may all be conveyed through touch.

Physical Proximity and Environment

Children's familiarity and comfort with their physical surroundings affects communication. As expected, children are most at ease in their home environments. Once they enter the clinic, emergency department, or patient care unit, they are in an unfamiliar environment and anxiety is heightened. Hospital and clinic staff have a tremendous advantage in knowing their clinic or unit as a familiar workplace. Try to imagine a child's first impression of the triage desk, the reception desk, the admitting office, the treatment room, the hospital room. The child's perspective is probably very different from that of an adult. Creat-

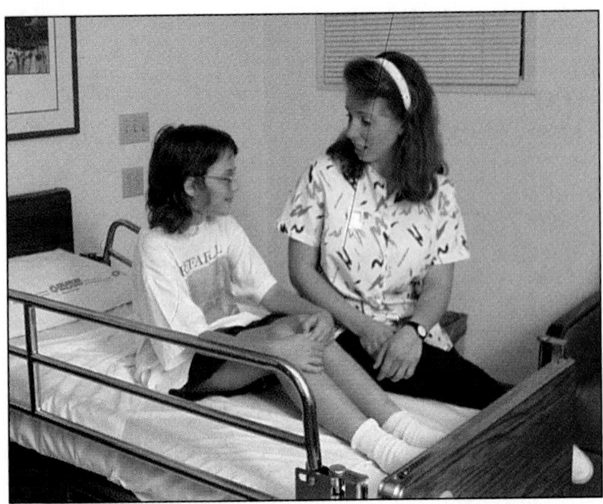

It is easier for a child to communicate with a nurse who is at eye level and at a comfortable conversational distance. The nurse may need to squat or even sit on the floor to talk with very young children.

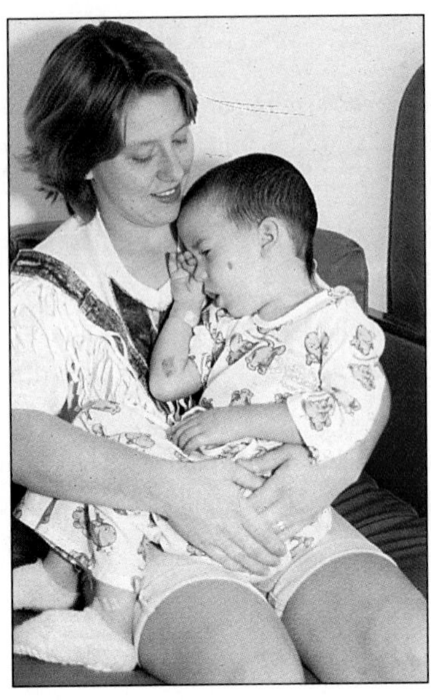

◄ Touch is a powerful means of communicating. Toddlers and preschoolers often find touch in the form of cuddling and stroking to be soothing. Even older children who prize their independence find that a parent's hug or pat on the back helps them feel more secure.

Figure 10–1
Communication with children is enhanced by direct eye contact and by body language that conveys attentiveness and openness.

ing a physical environment that is inviting and child-friendly makes a statement that children are welcome, gives a positive message to everyone entering, and creates a supportive atmosphere (Olds, Daniel, & Hall, 1987). Creating a supportive, inviting environment for children includes the use of child size furniture, colorful banners and posters, developmentally appropriate toys, and art displayed at a child's eye level.

In gauging conversation space, keep vertical and horizontal distances minimal (see Fig. 10–1). (Marion, 1986). Individuals have different comfort zones for physical distance. The nurse should be aware of this and move cautiously when meeting new children and families, respecting each individual's personal space. The nurse should pull over a chair from across the room to sit closer to the child and family. This puts the nurse at eye level. Standing over the child and family could be viewed as intimidating. The nurse may also stoop, squat, or sit on the floor by the child if a chair is not accessible. The important concept is to be at eye level while remaining at a comfortable distance for the child and family.

Privacy should not be overlooked nor its importance underestimated. Make sure a room is available for conducting private conversations away from roommates or family members and visitors. This is particularly critical when working with adolescents. There may be sensitive topics adolescents will not want to discuss with parents present. The nurse's skill and ease with parents of adolescents will increase the trust adolescents have for the nurse. Hallway conversations, particularly outside a patient's room, should be avoided because patients and parents may hear only select words or phrases and misinterpret their meaning. This may lead to unnecessary stress and potentiate the development of mistrust between the health care providers and the patient/family.

Listening

Messages given must be received for communication to be complete. Therefore, listening is an essential component of the communication process.

Stephen Covey suggests we should "first seek to understand, then to be understood" (Covey, 1989). By practicing **active listening** skills, nurses can be effective listeners. Active listening skills include:

1. *Attentiveness.* Be intentional about giving the speaker your undivided attention. Eliminate distractions whenever possible. *Examples: Maintain eye contact. Close the door. Eliminate potential distractions (television, computer, video games) when possible.*
2. *Clarification Through Reflection.* Using similar words, express back to the speaker what was heard and understood about the content of the message. *Example: When the patient/family says "I hate the food that comes on my tray," an appropriate response would be "You are unhappy with the food you've been given?"*
3. *Empathy.* Identify and acknowledge feelings expressed in the message. *Example: Child is crying after a procedure. "I know it is uncomfortable to have this procedure. It is OK to cry. You did a great job holding still."*
4. *Impartiality.* Listen with an open mind in order to understand and avoid prejudicing what is heard with

personal bias. *Example: An adolescent expresses concern to you that she's having difficulty with relationships at school. She feels disconnected socially because she's a lesbian. Be a supportive listener. Help her identify ways to connect with peers and interact with her as you would interact with all your patients, regardless of your personal values and beliefs.*

Children must also learn to be effective listeners. In working with children, it is the nurse's responsibility to ensure that messages are accurately comprehended. Characteristics to be aware of when communicating with children are their level of growth and development, age, sex, health status, personality, communication behavior, and intellectual abilities. These characteristics can provide insights into how a child may respond to various messages. Such insight can be a foundation for selecting the content, structure, and form of the message most likely to achieve the child's comprehension (Haynes & Shulman, 1994).

Children's receptive communication skills are generally more advanced than their verbal communication skills (Garbarino et al., 1990).

> Children are capable of comprehending more than would be expected based on their verbal skills.

Focus on talking with children rather than to them, to enhance effectiveness of communication and maximize normal language patterns that contribute to language development.

> Develop conversations with children. Ask open-ended questions to encourage conversations rather than questions requiring yes/no responses.

The nurse must be prepared to listen with eyes as well as with ears. Communication of information will not always be audible, so be alert to subtle cues of body language and closeness. Only then can one fully understand the messages of children. For example, when you enter the room to complete an initial assessment of a 4-year-old child, you observe her turning away from you and beginning to suck her thumb. The child is giving you information about her basic security and comfort level, and she hasn't said a word.

Visual Communication

Eye contact is a communication connector. Making eye contact helps confirm attention and interest between the individuals communicating.

Clothing, physical appearance, and objects being held are visual communicators. Children may react to an individual's presence based on a white lab coat, a bushy beard, a syringe in hand, or a video game in hand. Think ahead and anticipate visuals a child may find startling, as well as those that may be pleasing, and make appropriate adjustments when possible. For example, it is routine practice for nurses to bring a medication in a syringe for insertion into an intravenous line. Unless the purpose of the syringe is immediately explained, children may immediately assume they are about to receive an injection.

Some children, as well as some adults, are visual learners. They learn best when they can see or read instructions, demonstrations, diagrams, or information.

> Using various methods of presenting and sharing information will increase comprehension.

Photographs, videotapes, dolls, computer programs, charts, and graphs can more vividly represent a concept than written or spoken words alone. Remember to select teaching tools and materials that appropriately match the growth and developmental levels of your patients.

Tone of Voice

The spoken word is what comes to mind most often when considering communication. Actually, it is not only what is said that influences communication, but also how it is said. The tone and quality of voice often communicate more than words themselves.

Because infants' comprehension of verbal language is extremely limited, their impressions are based on tone and quality of voice. Infants are able to discriminate parental voices from those of strangers and are more responsive to familiar voices (Cataldo, 1983). Soft, smooth voice quality is more comforting and soothing to infants than loud, startling, harsh voices. Infants can sense by tone of voice whether their caregiver is angry, frustrated, calm, or happy. Awareness of infants' sensitivities to these messages can be gained by observing their body language. They are relaxed when they hear a calm, happy caregiver and tense and rigid when they hear an angry, frustrated caregiver.

Children can detect anger, frustration, joy, and other feelings voices convey, even when the accompanying words are incongruent. This can be very confusing for children. The nurse should strive to make words and their intended meanings match.

Verbal communication extends beyond actual words. All audible sounds convey meaning. An infant's primary mode of audible communication is crying. Crying is a cue to check basic needs, including hunger, pain, discomfort (e.g., wet diaper), or temperature. Cooing and babbling, also heard during the first year of life, generally convey messages of comfort and contentment. As children develop and mature they will have increasing vocabularies to express their ideas, thoughts, and feelings verbally.

Choice of words is critical in verbal communication. The nurse should avoid talking down to children but should not expect them to understand adult words and phrases. Health care terminology should be used selectively and jargon should be avoided. More specific examples will be shared later in this chapter under strategies for explaining procedures and treatments.

Body Language

From the gentle caress of holding an infant to sitting with an adolescent listening intently to her story, body language is a communication factor. Open body stance and positioning invite communication and interaction, whereas closed body stance and positioning impedes communication and interaction.

Using an open body posture will improve the nurse's understanding of children and the children's understanding of the nurse. It is important for nurses to learn to read the body language of children as well as to increase awareness of their own body language. Table 10–1 offers comparison of open and closed body postures.

TABLE 10–1 *Open and Closed Body Postures*

OPEN	CLOSED
Leaning toward other person(s)	Leaning away from other person(s)
Arms loose at the sides	Arms folded across chest
Frequent eye contact	No eye contact
Hands moving freely	Hands on hips
Soft stance, body swaying slightly	Rigid stance
Head up	Head bowed
Calm, slow movements	Constant motion, squirming
Smiling, friendly facial cues	Frowning, negative facial cues
Conversing at eye level	Conversing at diagonal eye level

Timing

Recognizing the appropriate time to communicate information is a developed skill. A distraught child whose parents have just left for work is not ready for a diabetic teaching session. The session will be much more productive and the information better comprehended if the child has a chance to make the transition. The child's needs must be met first rather than the convenience of a schedule.

FAMILY-CENTERED COMMUNICATIONS

Any discussion about effective ways to communicate with children must also include discussion on how to effectively communicate with families. In health care, the importance of practicing family-centered care is often discussed.

> The ability to establish open lines of communication with the family is one of the first and most essential steps toward achievement of a family-centered care environment.

Family-centered care reflects a belief that the family is intricately involved in the care of the child. Family-centered care is achieved when health care professionals can create partnerships with families, recognizing that the family is essential to the child and that the family has the right to fully participate in planning, implementing, and evaluating the child's plan of care. Commitment to family-centered care means that the nurse respects the family's cultural, educational, and socioeconomic variations and can use the strengths found in these variations. It also means that the nurse truly believes that the child's care and recovery is greatly enhanced when the family fully participates in the child's care (Fig. 10–2).

The following are key components essential to establishing open lines of communication in a family-centered care environment.

Establishment of Rapport. Critical to establishing good rapport with families is the nurse's ability to convey respect and concern in a genuine manner upon the first encounter. The family needs to know the nurse is interested in their well-being, nonjudgmental in approach, and willing to assist them in effectively caring for their child.

Identification of Needs and Establishment of Expectations. The thorough needs assessment of the patient and family should include information about problem solving skills, cultural needs, coping behaviors, and patient routines. A thorough assessment requires the nurse to obtain information from the patient as well as the family. This enables the nurse to gain better insights from all perspectives and facilitates the development of a more comprehensive plan of care. The nurse should also describe routines as well as provide information about what the patient and family can expect during their visit.

> "Mrs. Brown, I value your input as well as that of your child. Hearing Michael explain his understanding of his diabetic dietary restrictions in his own words will help us to gain better insight into how to best manage his care. Let's take a few minutes to hear from Michael and then we can talk about your perspective."

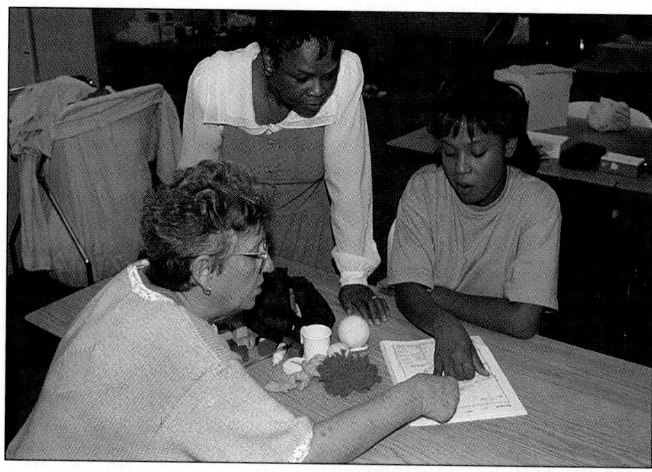

◀ The nurse explains a child's test results to his mother and grandmother. Including all important family members in the child's health care reflects a commitment to family-centered care. (Courtesy of University of Texas at Arlington School of Nursing, Arlington, Texas)

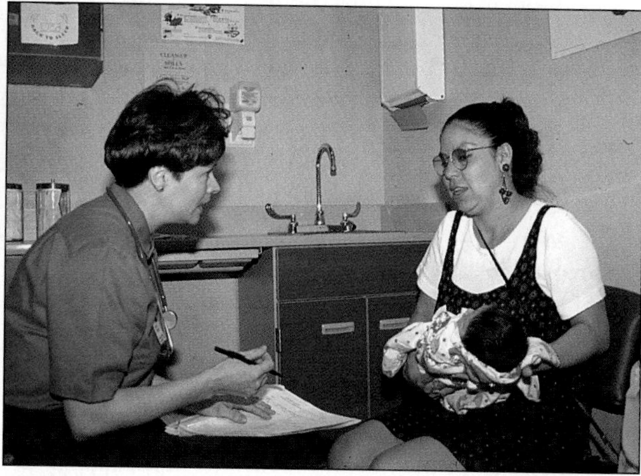

This nurse practitioner has learned Spanish to better communicate with her many Spanish-speaking clients. Speaking with family members in their own language encourages the family to remain in the health care system. The nurse is also using eye contact and has positioned herself at the mother's eye level. (Courtesy of Dallas County Hospital District Community Oriented Primary Care Clinic, Dallas, Texas) ▶

Figure 10–2

The child's ongoing health care, both preventive and during illness, is enhanced by participation of family.

Availability and Openness to Questions. A nurse who does not take time to see how a patient and family is doing, such as by leaving a room immediately after a treatment or administration of a medication, will not encourage or invite families to feel comfortable in asking questions. Families want and need unrushed and uninterrupted time with the nurse. Sometimes this can only be accomplished by purposefully scheduling it into the day.

> Encouraging families to write down their questions will enable them to take full advantage of their time with the nurse: "I know you have a lot of questions and are very anxious to learn more about your son's condition. I have another patient who has an immediate need, but I will be available in 10 minutes to meet with you. In the meantime, here is a parent handbook that gives general information about seizures. Please feel free to review it and write down any questions that we can discuss when I return."

Family Education and Empowerment. Educating families about their child's condition, ensuring their continued involvement in planning and evaluating the plan of care, and teaching them the skills to participate empowers the family. Families need support as they gain confidence in their skills and guidance to assist them as they navigate through the health care experience. Communication is enhanced when families feel competent and confident in their abilities.

Feedback from Patients and Families. The nurse must be alert for verbal as well as nonverbal cues. Routinely checking with the family about their experiences, satisfaction with communications, teaching sessions, and health care goals is an effective way to ensure that appropriate feedback is obtained. It is important that the nurse explain how this feedback will be used to further enhance the delivery of care. Listen and observe carefully to make sure that what the family is saying is truly what they are feeling. For example, while the nurse is teaching the mother of a 2-year-old who was recently diagnosed with diabetes mellitus, the mother reports that although she is the primary caregiver of her child, the child's grandmother frequently cares for the child while she is at work. The nurse therefore notifies the other team members and alters the diabetes care teaching plan to include the child's grandmother.

Effective Management of Conflict. When a situation of conflict occurs, it should be addressed in an expedient manner to prevent further breakdown in communication. The accompanying box offers several strategies to use in managing conflict situations.

Strategies for Managing Conflict

- *Understand the parent's perspective (walk in their shoes).* Think about how it would feel to be a parent of a child in the hospital where your values and beliefs are exposed and scrutinized. Try to gain a better understanding of the other person's perspective through encouraging them to share their perspective.
- *Determine a common goal and stay focused on it.* Determine the end result agreed upon by both and work toward it. By staying focused on the common goal, the parties involved are more likely to find workable strategies to achieve the identified goal.
- *Seek win/win solutions.* Conflict should not be about who is right and who is wrong. Effective management of conflict focuses on finding a solution whereby both "win." Through establishing a *common* goal, both parties win when this goal is achieved.
- *Utilize active listening skills.* Critical to resolving situations of conflict is the ability to listen and understand what the other person is saying *and* feeling. In active listening, the receiver actively and empathetically listens to gain better understanding of the actual as well as implied message.
- *Openly express your feelings.* Talking about feelings is much more constructive than acting them out.

  Example: Nurse: "I am very concerned about Jamie's safety when you leave his side rails down."
- *Avoid blaming.* Each party owns part of the problem. Pointing fingers and blaming others will not solve the problem. Instead, identify the part of the problem that each party owns and work together to resolve it. Seek win/win solutions.
- *Summarize the decision.* At the end of the discussion, summarize what has been decided and identify who is responsible for follow-up. This will ensure that everyone is clear about the decision and facilitates accountability for implementing solutions.

Table 10–2 offers a discussion regarding the importance of choosing words carefully to make families feel welcome and to further facilitate family-centered care.

Transcultural Communication: Bridging the Gap

Situations of conflict can arise when the nurse and patient/family come from differing cultural backgrounds that could influence one's approach to care. As the demographics in the United States continue to change, health care professionals will be challenged to become more cross-cultural in approach if they want to continue to be effective in their relationship with patients and families. It is important for health care professionals to be aware of their own values and beliefs and to recognize how these influence their interactions with others. It is equally important to be aware and respectful of patient's and family's values and beliefs and how this can affect how they behave and respond, especially in a health care environment. In working with patients and families, the initial assessment should include an examination of the patient's and family's values, beliefs, and traditions and how this might affect their communication style, methods of decision making, and other behaviors related to health care practices.

During the initial interview, the nurse should ascertain the following information related to the patient and family:

- Decision making practices: Are decisions made by individuals or collectively as a group?
- Child rearing practices: Who are the primary caregivers? What are their disciplinary practices?
- Family support: What is the family structure? Who does the patient and family turn to for support?
- Communication practices: How is the information communicated to the remainder of the family?
- Health and illness practices: Do they seek out professional help or rely on other resources for treatment and advice?

Once this information is obtained, use this knowledge to individualize your treatment plan and approach to best meet the patient's and family's needs.

- The parents of a child with an Orthodox Jewish religious background request a kosher diet. The nurse facilitates the routine delivery of kosher meals and communicates the family's wishes to the rest of the team members so that they may also respect the family's customs.
- The family of a child who suffered a severe brain injury requests the services of a healer. The nurse enables the family to arrange the visit through coordination of the child's daily schedule to provide an uninterrupted visit with the healer.

To be more effective in working with clients from differing backgrounds, the nurse must be aware of his or her personal values and beliefs as well as the values and beliefs of others. In a cross-cultural environment, it is criti-

TABLE 10–2 *Choosing Words Carefully*

POOR WORDS	RATIONALE	BETTER WORDS	RATIONALE
policies *allowed* *not permitted*	Convey attitude that hospital personnel have authority over parents in matters concerning their children	*guidelines* *working together* *welcome*	Convey openness and appreciation for position and importance of families
noncompliant *uncooperative* *difficult* (referring to parents and other family members)	Imply that health care providers make the decisions and give instructions that families must follow without giving input	*partners* *colleagues* *joint decision-makers* *experts about their child*	Acknowledge that families bring important information and insight, and that families and professionals form a team
dysfunctional *in denial* *overprotective* *uninvolved* *uncaring* (labeling families)	Pronounce a judgment that may not incorporate a full understanding of a family's situation, reactions, or perspective	*coping* (describing family's reactions with care and respect)	Leave room to build a more complete and appreciative understanding of families over time

cal that one is aware of one's biases in order to be sensitive and respectful of another's point of view. Effectiveness will be enhanced when the nurse has knowledge and understanding, as well as sensitivity and respect for the cultural differences of others (Lynch & Hanson, 1992). Gaining an understanding of a patient's and family's perspective can be a strong foundation toward the development of an effective therapeutic relationship. Refer to the section entitled Communicating With Children Who Have Special Needs for further suggestions on how to communicate with a child who speaks another language and how to work with an interpreter.

Therapeutic Relationships: Maintaining Professional Boundaries

The importance of establishing supportive, therapeutic relationships with patients and families, as well as communication strategies that can help foster this family-centered approach to care, has been addressed. It is necessary to also discuss the importance of identifying and maintaining **professional boundaries.** Because nurses are caring, nurturing people and the profession demands that nurses sometimes become intimately involved in the lives of the people for which they care, maintaining the balance between being related in a meaningful way but professionally separate is at times very difficult. However, the key to establishing a supportive therapeutic relationship lies in the ability to successfully maintain this balance. When sight of this boundary is lost and the nurse becomes too emotionally involved, effectiveness as an objective professional resource decreases (Barnsteiner & Gillis-Donovan, 1990). This greatly diminishes the ability to effectively guide families in meeting the health care needs of their children.

> Maintaining professional boundaries requires that the nurse must constantly be aware of the fine line between being empathetic and being overinvolved.

The accompanying box lists some behaviors that could be warning signs of overinvolvement.

An example of nurse overinvolvement may be the exclusion of parents in the care of their child. The possibility for a nurse to assume a "parenting" role is particularly heightened when the parents, for whatever reason, are unable to visit frequently (Barnsteiner & Gillis-Donovan, 1990).

Warning Signs of Overinvolvement

- Buying gifts for individual patients or families
- Sharing home phone number
- Competing with other staff for the patient/family's affection
- Inviting patient/family to social gatherings
- Accepting invitations to family gatherings (e.g., birthday parties, weddings)
- Visiting and/or spending time with patient/family during off-duty time
- Revealing personal information
- Loaning or borrowing money
- Making decisions for the family about their child's care

TABLE 10-3 *Developmental Milestones and Their Relationship to Communication Approaches*

DEVELOPMENT	LANGUAGE DEVELOPMENT	EMOTIONAL DEVELOPMENT	COGNITIVE DEVELOPMENT	SUGGESTED COMMUNICATION APPROACH
Infancy (0–12 Months) The infant experiences the world through senses of hearing, seeing, smelling, tasting, and touching.	Crying. Babbling. Cooing. Single word production. Able to name some simple objects.	Dependent on others. High need for cuddling and security. Responsive to environment (sounds, visual stimuli, etc.). Distinguishes between happy and angry voices as well as familiar and strange voices. Beginning to experience separation anxiety.	Interactions are largely reflexive. Begins to see repetition of activities and movements. Begins to intentionally initiate interactions. Short attention span (1–2 minutes).	Use calm, soft, soothing voice. Be responsive to cries. Engage in turn-taking vocalizations (adult imitates baby sounds). Talk and read regularly to babies. Prepare infant as you are about to perform care. Talk to infant about what you are about to do to him or her. Use a slow approach and allow child time to get to know you.
Toddler (1–2 Years) The toddler experiences the world through senses of hearing, seeing, smelling, tasting, and touching.	Two-word combinations emerge. Participates in turn taking in communication (speaker/listener). "No" becomes a favorite word. Able to use gestures and verbalize simple wants and needs.	Strong need for security objects. Separation/stranger anxiety heightened. Participates in parallel play. Thrives on routines. Beginning development of independence; "Want to do by self." Still very dependent on significant adults.	Experiments with objects. Participates in active exploration. Begins to experiment with variations in activities. Begins to identify cause and effect relationships. Short attention span (3–5 minutes).	Learn the toddler's words for common items and use them in conversations. Describe activities and procedures as they are about to be done. Use picture books. Use play for demonstrations. Be responsive to child's receptivity toward you and approach cautiously. Preparation should occur immediately prior to the event.
Preschool (3–5 Years) Many words used are not fully understood by child.	Further development and expansion of word combination (able to speak in full sentences). Upward growth in correct grammatical usage. Uses pronouns. Clearer articulation of sounds. Vocabulary rapidly expanding.	Likes to imitate activities and make choices. Strives for independence but needs adult support and encouragment. Demonstrates purposeful attention-seeking behaviors. Learns cooperation and turn taking in game playing.	Begins developing the concepts of time, space, and quantity. Magical thinking becomes prominent. World view seen only from child's perspective. Short attention span (5–10 minutes).	Seek opportunities to offer choices. Use play to explain procedures and activities. Speak in simple sentences and explore relative concepts. Use picture and story books, puppets.

	May know words without understanding meaning.	Needs clearly set limits and boundaries.		Describe activities and procedures as they are about to be done. Be concise; limit length of explanations (less than 5 minutes). Engage in preparatory activities 1–3 hours prior to the event.
School Age (6–11 Years) Communicates thoughts and appreciates viewpoints of others; words with multiple meanings and words describing things they have not experienced are not thoroughly understood.	Expanding vocabulary enabling child to describe concepts, thoughts, and feelings. Development of conversational skills.	Interacts well with others. Understands rules to games. Very interested in learning. Builds close friendships. Beginning to accept responsibility for own actions. Competition emerges. Still dependent on adults to meet needs.	Able to grasp concepts of classification, conversation. Concrete thinking emerges. Becomes very oriented to "rules." Able to process information in serial format. Lengthened attention span (10–30 minutes).	Use photographs, books, diagrams, charts, videos to explain. Make explanations sequential. Engage in conversations that encourage critical thinking. Establish limits and set consequences. Use medical play techniques. Introduce preparatory materials 1–5 days in advance of the event.
Adolescent (12 Years and Older) The adolescent is able to create theories and generate many explanations to situations; beginning of communicating like an adult.	Able to verbalize and comprehend most adult concepts.	Beginning to accept responsibility for own actions. Perception of "imaginary audiences." Needs independence. Competitive drive. Strong need for group identification. Frequently has small group of very close friends. Questions authority. Strong need for privacy.	Able to think logically and abstractly. Attention span extends up to 60 minutes.	Engage in conversations about adolescent's interests. Use photographs, books, diagrams, charts, videos to explain. Use collaborative approach and foster/support independence. Introduce preparatory materials up to 1 week in advance of the event. Be respectful of privacy needs.

Feelings of incompetency, fear, and loss of control may be displayed by family members as anger, withdrawal, or dissatisfaction. What is important in working with families is to promote the parent's feelings of competency through education and empowerment. Keep them well informed of the child's care through frequent phone calls and involvement in decision making. The nurse should promote their confidence, enhance their self-esteem, and foster their independence through teaching them the skills necessary to care for their child.

Critical to our effectiveness as caregivers working with families in caring for their child is our ability to recognize and maintain professional boundaries. This is accomplished when the nurse is able to recognize his or her own personal and professional needs. Self-awareness about the motives behind actions will greatly enhance the nurse's ability to understand the needs of patients and families and to give families the tools to effectively manage the care of their child.

COMMUNICATION STRATEGIES FOR NURSES

The communication techniques described earlier in this chapter provide the nurse with a foundation to communicate effectively with children. Practical application of these techniques in conjunction with the following strategies fosters effective, supportive, and caring interactions between nurses and children. These interactions can facilitate a positive health care experience for children and families.

Determining the Best Communication Approach

The most important communication strategy for nurses working with children is to determine the best communication approach based on each child's age and developmental abilities. This is dependent on the nurse's understanding of developmental milestones and the nurse's ability to assess the child's comprehension and communication skills. This assessment needs to include an evaluation of the child's cognitive and emotional development as well as language abilities. Table 10–3 presents an overview of developmental milestones related to child communication skills and some suggested approaches to facilitate successful interactions. For more details about assessment of growth and development in children, refer to the other related chapters in this text. The remainder of this chapter will focus on other strategies that nurses can use to most effectively interact with their pediatric patients.

Play

Communicating with children can be greatly facilitated through the use of play.

> Approaching children at their developmental level with familiar forms of play increases their comfort and allows the nurse to be seen in a more positive, less threatening role.

Because play is an everyday part of children's lives and a method they use to communicate, they are less likely to be inhibited when participating in play interactions. Children may express thoughts and feelings through play that they may be unable to verbalize.

Please refer to Chapter 9 for a more in-depth discussion of play.

Storytelling

Storytelling is an innovative and creative communication strategy. It is a skill acquired and refined through practice. Familiarity with stories and frequency in using storytelling techniques helps increase confidence and competence in the storyteller (see Storytelling Strategies box). Storytelling can be a routine part of a nurse's day, from establishing rapport to approaching challenging or uncomfortable topics such as loss, death, fear, grief, and anger. Two roles are played during storytelling—the teller and the listener. Assessment of individual situations is necessary to determine whether the adult or child will be the teller and the other the listener or, in the case of a shared story, each may have a turn at both roles.

Storytelling Strategies

- Capturing a story on paper or on videotape as told by a child or group of children.
- Telling a yarn story with two or more people; a long piece of yarn with knots tied at varied intervals is slid loosely through the hands of the teller until a knot is felt, at which time the yarn is passed to the next person, who continues the story.
- Sentence completion, either verbal or written, with topics like "If I were in charge of the hospital . . . ," "I wish . . . ," "When I get home I will . . . ," "My family . . ."
- Reading stories with themes related to issues a patient is facing. The children's section of the local public library is an excellent resource.

Explaining Procedures and Treatments

Effective communication with children in a health care setting includes the nurse's ability to prepare children for procedures, treatments, and/or events that may be frightening and/or painful (Petrillo & Sanger, 1980). **Preparation** in advance of a procedure, which includes an explanation of reasons for the procedure, as well as the expected sequence of events and outcomes, can greatly reduce the child's fears and anxieties. Preparation enables the child to experience some mastery over the events in his or her life, gives the child time to develop effective coping behaviors, and fosters a level of trust in those who care for him or her.

> Adequate preparation is the key to helping a child have a successful, positive health care experience.

The Association for the Care of Children's Health (ACCH), in their book entitled *Psychosocial Care of Children in Hospitals* (Gaynard et al., 1990), describes "Key Elements of Communicating Complete and Accurate Information." They are as follows:

1. *Learn the Procedure.* To adequately explain a procedure, the nurse must have an understanding of what is involved. What pieces of equipment will be used? Where will it take place? Essentially learn what the child can expect to happen during the procedure.
2. *Determine What Information to Share With the Child and Family.* The preparation should only include information about what the child will experience or perceive directly. Consultation with the family will allow the nurse to find out words and terminology used by the child. Table 10–4 offers other concrete suggestions in choosing appropriate language for nurses to use in working with children.

   In general, the younger the child, the closer to the event the preparation should occur. For example, a 3-year-old will generally be very anxious and therefore should be prepared immediately before, whereas a teenager would benefit from a longer preparation time so that he or she can develop strategies for dealing with the situation. See Table 10–3 for age-related attention span guidelines.
3. *Provide Sensory Information.* Allowing children to see, hear, feel, taste, smell, and experience similar sensations during their preparation will greatly enhance their preparedness and diminish their anxieties. For example, in preparing a child for an intravenous line insertion, show the child the catheter. Explain the purpose of the tourniquet and allow the child to put it on himself or herself and on the arm of a doll if desired. Let the child smell an alcohol swab and feel its coolness when applied to the skin. Show the child the treatment room and allow him or her to sit on the treatment table where the procedure will be performed.
4. *Explain the Sequence of Events.* Part of preparation should include a description of the sequence in which events will occur. Being able to break the procedure down into sequential steps allows children to appropriately anticipate and gives them a sense of being in control as well as a better understanding of how many more steps there are before the procedure is over.
5. *Explain How Long the Procedure Will Last.* Whenever possible allow the child to have simulated "play" experiences, such as allowing the child to perform the procedure on a doll or stuffed animal. This gives them a real sense of time as well as firsthand experience with the sequence of events. If a concrete demonstration is not possible, explain the timing in terms that the child can understand, e.g., "The procedure will last as long as it takes to sing your favorite song."
6. *Monitor Accuracy of Information—Feedback.* Feedback can be used to modify or reinforce future preparation sessions. This also allows you time to correct any misunderstandings the child may have and offers an opportunity for the child to verbally process and express feelings about the experience.

The goal in explaining procedures and treatments to children is to promote understanding, ensure adequate preparation, and reduce anxieties and fears (Petrillo & Sanger, 1980). Open, honest communication about treatments and procedures and attentiveness to the learning needs of the child will greatly facilitate the achievement of these goals.

Strategies for Enhancing Self-esteem

Stanley Coopersmith (1967) defined **self-esteem** as a "personal judgement of worthiness that is expressed in the attitudes the individual holds toward himself or herself." Development of self-esteem begins early when infants start to realize they are separate beings, realize they affect the world around them, and accept their environment as either responsive or nonresponsive to their needs (Sieving & Zirbel-Donisch, 1990).

> Communication practices play an important role in the development of children's self-esteem.

The words adults choose, the tone of voice, the place, and the timing of message delivery all influence the child's interpretation of the message. The interpretation may be positive, negative, or neutral. To enhance the child's self-esteem, adults should be striving for the positive.

Nurses are in an excellent position to model communication practices that enhance self-esteem. Table 10–5 offers comparisons of helpful and harmful communication practices.

TABLE 10–4 *Considerations in Choosing Language*

POTENTIALLY AMBIGUOUS	CLEARER
The doctor will give you some "dye." To make me die?	The doctor will put some medicine in the tube that will help her be able to see your _________ more clearly.
Dressing; dressing change Why are they going to undress me? Do I have to change my clothes?	Bandages; clean, new bandages
Stool collection Why do they want to collect little chairs?	Use child's familiar term, such as "poop" or "BM" or "doody."
Urine You're in?	Use child's familiar term, such as "pee."
Shot When people get shot, they're really badly hurt.	Medicine through a (small, tiny) needle
CAT scan Will there be cats?	Describe in simple terms, and explain what the letters of the common name stand for.
PICU Pick you?	Explain as above.
I.C.U. I see you?	Explain as above.
I.V. Ivy?	Explain as above.
Stretcher Stretch her? Stretch who?	Bed on wheels
Special; funny (words that are usually positive descriptors) It doesn't look/feel special to me.	Odd; different; unusual; strange
Gas; sleeping gas Is someone going to pour gasoline into the mask?	Medicine, called anesthesia. It is a kind of air you will breathe through a mask like this—to help you sleep during your operation so you won't feel anything. It is a different kind of sleep. (Explain differences.)
Put you to sleep Like my cat was put to sleep? It never came back.	Give you medicine that will help you go into a very deep sleep. You won't feel anything until the operation is over. Then the doctor will stop giving you the medicine, so you can wake up.
Move you to the floor Why are they going to put me on the ground? OR (or treatment room) table People aren't supposed to get up on tables.	Unit; ward. (Explain why the child is being transferred, and where.) A narrow bed
Take a picture (X-rays, CT and MRI machines are far larger than a familiar camera, move differently, and don't yield a familiar end product.)	A picture inside of you. (Describe appearance, sounds, and movement of the equipment.)
Flush your I.V. Flush it down the toilet?	Explain

TABLE 10–4 *Considerations in Choosing Language (continued)*

Words can be experienced as "hard" or "soft" according to how much they increase the perceived threat of a situation. For example, consider the following word choices.	
HARDER	**SOFTER**
This part will hurt.	It (you) may feel (or feel very) sore, achy, scratchy, tight, snug, full, or . . . (other manageable, descriptive term). (Words such as scratch, poke, or sting might be familiar for some children and frightening to others.)
The medicine will burn.	Some children say they feel very warm.
The room will be very cold.	Some children say they feel very cold.
The medicine will taste (or smell bad).	The medicine may taste (or smell) different than anything you have tasted before. After you take it, will you tell me how it was for you?
Cut, open you up, slice, make a hole	The doctor will make an opening. (Use concrete comparisons, such as "your little finger" or "a paper clip" *if* the opening will indeed be small.)
As big as . . . (e.g., size of an incision or of a catheter) As long as . . . (e.g., for duration of a procedure) As much as . . . (These are open-ended and "extending" expressions.)	Smaller than . . . For less time than it takes you to . . . Less than . . . (These expressions help to confine, familiarize, imply the manageability of an event or of equipment.)
The unfamiliar usage or complexity of some common medical words or expressions can be confusing and frightening.	
POTENTIALLY UNFAMILIAR	**CONCRETE EXPLANATION**
Take your vitals (or your vital signs)	Measure your temperature; see how warm your body is; see how fast and strongly your heart is working. (Nothing is "taken" from the child.)
Electrodes, leads	Sticky like a Band-Aid, with a small wet spot in the center, and small strings that attach to the snap (monitor electrodes); paste like wet sand, with strings with tiny metal cups that stick to the paste (EEG electrodes). The paste washes off easily afterwards; the strings go into a box that will make a picture of how your heart (or brain) is working. (Show child electrodes and leads before using. Let child handle them and apply them to a doll or to self.)
Hang your (I.V.) medication	Bring in a new medicine in a bag, and attach it to the little tube already in your arm. The needle goes into the tube, not into your arm, so you won't feel it.
N.P.O.	Nothing to eat. Your stomach needs to be empty. (Explain why.) You can eat and drink again as soon as . . . (Explain with concrete descriptions.)
Anesthesia	The doctor will give you medicine—you may hear it called "anesthesia." It will help you go into a very deep sleep. You will not feel anything at all. The doctors know just the right amount of medicine to give you so you will stay asleep through your operation. When the operation is over the doctor stops giving you that medicine and helps you wake up.

Note: Words or phrases that are helpful to one child may be threatening for another. Health care providers must listen carefully and be sensitive to the child's use of and response to language.

Adapted with permission of the Association for the Care of Children's Health, 7910 Woodmont Ave., Suite 300, Bethesda, MD 20814, from Gaynard, L., Wolfer J., Goldberger, J., Thompson, R., Redburn, L., & Laidley, L. (1990). *Psychosocial care of children in hospitals: A clinical practice manual from ACCH Child Life Research Project.* Bethesda, MD: The Association for the Care of Children's Health.

TABLE 10–5 *Self-Esteem in Children: Communication Practices*

THAT ENHANCE SELF-ESTEEM	THAT HARM SELF-ESTEEM
Praise efforts and accomplishments	Criticize efforts and accomplishments
Use active listening skills	Too busy to listen
Encourage expression of feelings	Tell children how they should feel
Acknowledge feelings	Give no support for dealing with feelings
Use developmentally based discipline	Physical punishment
Use "I" statements	Use "You" statements
Be nonjudgmental	Judging
Set clearly defined limits and reinforce them	No known limits or boundaries
Sharing quality time together	Giving time grudgingly
Honesty	Dishonesty
Describe behaviors observed when praising and disciplining	Use coercion and power as discipline
Complimenting	Belittling, blaming, shaming
Smiling	Using sarcastic, caustic, or cruel "humor"
Touching and hugging	Not coming near child even when the child is open to touching, holding, or hugging. Touches only when performing a task.
Rocking	Touching and holding only when performing a task. No comforting through rocking.

COMMUNICATING WITH CHILDREN WHO HAVE SPECIAL NEEDS

The opportunity to interact with children who have special communication needs presents an exciting challenge for nurses. It requires particular attention in working with patients and families to identify successful alternative methods of communicating. This is critical so that the child can accurately express his or her wants and needs; in addition, the nurse can offer the child comfort and understanding through adequate preparation and reassurance. Successfully meeting this challenge will present a rewarding experience for the nurse and a positive, supportive experience for the patient and family.

> It is vital in working with children with special needs for the nurse to carefully assess each child's physical, mental, and developmental abilities and determine the most effective methods of communication.

The Child With a Visual Impairment

- Obtain a thorough assessment of the child's self-help skills and abilities (include toileting, bathing, dressing, feeding, and mobility).
- Orient the child to his or her surroundings. Walk him or her around the room and unit several times, indicating landmarks (such as doors, closets, bedside tables, windows) as you guide him or her by the hand. Explain sounds that the child may frequently hear (such as monitors, alarms, nurse call bell).
- Encourage parents to stay with the child. They can facilitate communication and greatly enhance comfort in this unfamiliar environment.
- Keep furniture and other items in the same consistent place. This aids in the child's orientation to the room and fosters independence.
- Keep the nurse call bell in the same place and within reach of the patient.
- Identify yourself when entering the room and tell the child when you are departing.
- Carefully and fully explain all procedures.
- Allow the child to handle equipment while explaining the procedure to enhance understanding.

The Child With a Hearing Impairment

- Thoroughly assess the child's self-help skills and abilities.
- Identify family's method of communication and if you can, adopt it.
- Encourage family member to stay with child at all times to decrease stress of hospitalization and facilitate communication.
- If sign language is used, learn most frequently used signs and use them whenever able.
- Develop a communication board. This is a board with pictures of most commonly used items or needs (i.e., television, cup, toothbrush, toilet, shower).
- Determine child's use of a hearing aid. If child uses one, make sure batteries are working and the hearing aid is clean and appropriately intact.
- When entering the room, do so cautiously and gently touch patient before speaking.
- Always face the child when speaking. If child is a lip reader, this will greatly enhance his or her ability to understand you.
- Do not shout or exaggerate speech. This will distort your face and can be very confusing. Rather talk in a normal tone and at a regular pace.
- Remember nonverbals can speak as loud, if not louder, than verbals (a frown or worried face can say more than words).
- When performing a procedure that requires standing behind the child, such as when giving an enema or

assisting with a spinal tap, have another person stand in front of the child and explain the procedure as it is being performed.

- Whenever possible use play strategies to help communicate and demonstrate procedures. See sections on "Play" and "Explaining Procedures and Treatments."

The Child Who Speaks Another Language

- Thoroughly assess the child's abilities in speaking and understanding both languages.
- Ask the family if they would like an interpreter, and involve them in the selection. Whenever possible, avoid using children as interpreters due to the psychological stress this can place on a child (Lynch & Hanson, 1992).
- Determine the availability of an interpreter. This could be another adult family member, friend of the family, or other individual with proficiency in both languages.
- Use an interpreter whenever possible, but especially when explaining procedures, determining understanding, teaching new skills, and assessing needs.
- Use a communication board with the names of items in both languages.
- Learn words and names of commonly used items in the child's language and use them whenever possible. This not only aids in communication, but also demonstrates sincere interest in learning the language and demonstrates respect for the culture.
- Learn as much about the child's culture as possible and develop plans of care that demonstrate respect for the culture. Sincere attempts to learn to communicate with the child and family demonstrate your concern for their well-being.
- Use play strategies whenever possible. Play seems to be a universal language.

The Aphonic Child

- Thoroughly assess the child's self-help skills and abilities.
- Determine the child/family's method of communicating and adopt these as much as possible.
- Encourage parents to stay to decrease anxiety and foster communication.
- Determine use of sign language or other augmented communication devices.
- Use a communication board.
- Be attentive to and maximize the child's nonverbal communication. Facial grimaces, frowns, smiles, and nods are effective means of communicating responses and expressing likes and dislikes.
- If appropriate, encourage the child to use writing boards (dry erase, chalk, or pads of paper) to write needs, wants, questions, and concerns.

The Child With a Profound Neurologic Impairment

- Because hearing, vision, and language abilities are often hard to determine in this population, it is important to assume the child can hear, see, and comprehend something in what is said. Because of this, use a friendly tone of voice that conveys warmth and respect.
- Address the child when entering and exiting the room. Gently touch the patient while saying his or her name.
- Speak softly, calmly, and slowly to allow the child time to process what you are saying.
- While in the room with the child, talk to the child. Do not talk over the child as if he or she were not there.
- Explain all procedures as they are about to be done.

  Example: *"Jenny, I am going to wash your arm now."*

  Example: *"Jenny, now I am going to take your temperature by putting the thermometer under your arm."*

  Example: *"Jenny, Kristi, another nurse, is here to help me lift you into your chair."*

- Talk to the patient about activities and objects in the room, things that the child might see, hear, smell, touch, taste, or sense.

  Example: *"It is a sunny day today, can you feel the warm sunshine shining on you through the window?"*

- When asking questions of a child, make sure to allow the child adequate time to respond. Be careful to only ask questions of children who are capable of responding.
- Ascertain the child's ability to respond to simple questions. Some children can respond to yes/no questions by squeezing a hand and blinking eyes (once for yes and twice for no).
- Be extremely attentive to any signs or gestures (facial grimaces, smiling, eye movements) that may convey responses to likes or dislikes. This may be the child's only means of communicating.
- As with all children with special communication needs, thoroughly document and communicate to others who interact with the child any special techniques that work. This will greatly enhance continuity and more fully facilitate the child's ability to communicate.

KEY CONCEPTS

- Components of effective communication with children involve verbal as well as nonverbal interactions. Essential components include touch, physical proximity and environment, listening, eye contact and visual cues, timing, tone of voice, and overall body language.
- Communication strategies that assist nurses in working effectively with children include determining the best communication approach based on age and developmental abilities, using play and storytelling, explaining procedures and treatments, and modeling communication practices to enhance self-esteem.
- Communication pitfalls, such as using jargon, talking down to individuals or beyond their developmental level, and avoidance or denial of a problem, can lead to a breakdown in the relationship between the nurse and the patient and family.
- Family-centered communication strategies include establishment of rapport, identification of needs and establishment of expectations, availability and openness to questions, family education, and empowerment, feedback from patients and families, effective conflict management, transcultural communication, and maintaining professional boundaries.
- In working with children with special needs, it is important that the nurse carefully assess each child's physical, mental, and developmental abilities and determine the most effective methods of communication.

REFERENCES

Barnsteiner, J. H., & Gillis-Donovan, J. (1990). Being related and separate: A standard for therapeutic relationships. *Maternal-Child Nursing, 15,* 223–228.

Cataldo, C. Z. (1983). *Infant and toddler programs.* Reading, MA: Addison–Wesley.

Coopersmith, S. (1967). *The antecedents of self-esteem.* San Francisco: Wilti Freeman.

Covey, S. R. (1989). *The seven habits of highly effective people.* New York: Simon & Schuster.

Garbarino, J., Stott, F. M., & Faculty of the Erikson Institute. (1990). *What children can tell us: Eliciting, interpreting and evaluating information from children.* San Francisco: Jossey-Bass.

Gaynard L., Wolfer, J., Goldberger, J., Thompson, R., Redburn, L., & Laidley, L. (1990). *Psychosocial care of children in hospitals: A clinical practice manual from ACCH Child Life Research Project.* Bethesda, MD: The Association for the Care of Children's Health.

Haynes, W. O., & Shulman, B. B. (1994). *Communication development: Foundations, processes, and clinical applications.* Englewood Cliffs, NJ: Prentice Hall.

Lynch, E. W., & Hanson, M. J. (1992). *Developing cross-cultural competence: A guide for working with young children and their families.* Baltimore: Paul H. Brookes.

Marion, M. (1986). *Guidance of young children.* Columbus, OH: Charles E. Merrill.

Olds, A. R., Daniel, P. A., & Hall, J. H. (1987). *Child health care facilities.* Bethesda, MD: Association for the Care of Children's Health.

Petrillo, D., & Sanger, S. (1980). *Emotional care of hospitalized children.* Philadelphia: J. B. Lippincott.

Sieving, R. E., & Zirbel-Donisch, S. T. (1990). Development and enhancement of self-esteem in children. *Journal of Pediatric Health Care, 4*(6), 290–296.

BIBLIOGRAPHY

Als, H., et al. (1994). Individualized development care for the very low-weight preterm infant: Medical and neurofunctional effects. *Journal of American Medical Association, 272*(11), 853–858.

Baerz, K. L. (1991). Effective communication with autistic children. *Rehabilitation Nursing, 16*(2), 88–93.

Baretich, D. M., Stephenson, P. A., & Igoe, J. B. (1989). Using art to understand children's perceptions of roles in physician's office visits. *Pediatric Nursing, 15*(4), 355–360.

Brown, J., & Ritchie, J. A. (1989). Nurses' perceptions of their relationships with parents. *Maternal-Child Nursing, 18*(2), 79–95.

Cameron, C. O., Juszczak, L., & Wallace, N. (1984). Using creative arts to help children cope with altered body image. *Children's Health Care, 12*(3), 108–112.

Carson, D. K., Gravley, J. E., & Council, J. R. (1992). Children's prehospitalization conceptions of illness, cognitive development and personal adjustment. *Children's Health Care, 21*(2), 103–110.

Davis, H. (1993). *Counselling parents of children with chronic illness or disability.* Baltimore: Paul H. Brookes.

Douglas, T. (1989). A real case for nonverbal communication in nursing practice. *Washington Nurse, 19*(10), 12–14.

Edelman, L., Greenland, B., & Mills, B. L. (1993). *Family-centered communication skills.* St. Paul, MN: Pathfinder Resources.

Fosson, A., & deQuan, M. M. (1984). Reassuring and talking with hospitalized children. *Children's Health Care, 13*(1), 37–44.

Fosson, A., & Husband, E. (1984). Bibliotherapy for hospitalized children. *Southern Medical Journal, 77*(3), 342–346.

Foster, S. H. (1990). *The communication competence of infants and young children: A modular approach.* New York: Longman.

Free, T. A. (1984). Paternalism in pediatric care. *Maternal-Child Nursing, 9,* 9–14.

Freedman, M. (1991). Therapeutic use of storytelling for older children who are critically ill. *Children's Health Care, 20*(4), 208–215.

Gill, K. M. (1993). Health professionals' attitudes toward parent participation in hospitalized children's care. *Children's Health Care, 22*(4), 257–271.

Hall, S. S., & Weatherly, K. S. (1989). Using sign language with tracheotomized infants and children. *Pediatric Nursing, 15*(4), 362–367.

Hanson, J. L., et al. (1994). *Hospitals moving forward with family-centered care.* Bethesda, MD: Institute for Family-Centered Care.

Heiney, S. P. (1991). Helping children through painful procedures. *American Journal of Nursing, 91*(11), 20–24.

Heinrich, K. T. (1992). What to do when a patient becomes too special. *Nursing92, 22*(11), 63–64.

Hudson, C. J., Leeper, J. D., Strickland, M. P., & Jessee, P. (1987). Storytelling: A measure of anxiety in hospitalized children. *Children's Health Care, 16*(2), 118–122.

Inman, C. E. (1991). Analyzed interaction in a children's oncology clinic: The child's view and parents' opinion of the effect of medical encounters. *Journal of Advanced Nursing, 16,* 782–793.

Jeppson, E. S., & Thomas, J. (1995). *Essential allies: Families as advisors.* Bethesda, MD: Institute for Family-Centered Care.

Jerome, A. M., & Ferraro-McDuffie, A. R. (1992). Nurse self-awareness in therapeutic relationships. *Pediatric Nursing, 18*(2), 153–156.

Johnson, B. H. (1990). The changing role of families in health care. *Children's Health Care, 19*(4), 234–241.

Johnson, B. H., Jeppson, E. S., & Redburn, L. (1992). *Caring for children and families: Guidelines for hospitals.* Bethesda, MD: The Association for the Care of Children's Health.

Kirkman-Liff, B., & Mandragon, D. (1991). Language of interview: Relevance for research of Southwest Hispanics. *American Journal of Public Health, 81*(11), 1399–1404.

LaMontagne, L. L. (1993). Bolstering personal control in child patients through coping interventions. *Pediatric Nursing, 19*(3), 235–237.

Lash, M., & Wertlieb, D. (1993). A model for family-centered service coordination for children who are disabled by traumatic injuries. *The ACCH Advocate, 1*(1), 19–41.

Leff, P. T., Chan, J. M., & Walizer, E. M. (1991). Self-understanding and reaching out to sick children and their families: An ongoing professional challenge. *Children's Health Care, 20*(4), 230–239.

MacDonald, J. D., & Carroll, J. Y. (1992). A partnership model for communicating with infants at risk. *Infants and Young Children, 4*(3), 20–30.

McClowry, S. G. (1993). Pediatric nursing psychosocial care: A vision beyond hospitalization. *Pediatric Nursing, 19*(2), 146–148.

Meadows, J. L. (1991). *Multicultural communication.* Binghamton, NY: The Haworth Press.

Nadel, J., & Camaioni, L. (1993). *New perspectives in early communication development.* New York: Routledge.

Pennington, S., Gafner, G., Schilit, R., & Bechtel, B. (1993). Addressing ethical boundaries among nurses. *Nursing Management, 24*(6), 36–39.

Piaget, J. (1962). *Play, dreams and imitation in childhood.* New York: W. W. Norton.

Pontious, S. L. (1982). Practical Piaget: Helping children understand. *American Journal of Nursing, 82*(1), 114–117.

Revell, G. M., & Liptak, G. S. (1991). Understanding the child with special health care needs: A developmental perspective. *Journal of Pediatric Nursing, 6*(4), 258–268.

Robinson, C. A. (1987). Preschool children's conceptualizations of health and illness. *Children's Health Care, 16*(2), 89–96.

Sabbeth, B. F., & Leventhal, J. M. (1988). Trial balloons: When families of ill children express needs in veiled ways. *Children's Health Care, 17*(2), 87–92.

Slusher, I. L., & McClure, M. J. (1992). Infant stimulation during hospitalization. *Journal of Pediatric Nursing, 7*(4), 276–279.

Smith, J., & Felice, M. (1980). Interviewing adolescent patients: Some guidelines for the clinician. *Pediatric Annals, 9*(6), 38–44.

Striker, S. (1986). *Please touch: How to stimulate your child's creative development.* New York: Simon & Schuster.

Taylor, D. (1990). The little girl who couldn't smile. *Nursing90, 20*(2), 136.

Thornton, S. M., & Frankenburg, W. K., (Eds.). (1983). *Child health care communications: Enhancing interactions among professionals, parents and children.* Skillman, NJ: Johnson & Johnson Baby Products Company.

VIDEO BIBLIOGRAPHY

Communicating with children: Supportive interactions in hospitals. (1991). Bethesda, MD: The Association for the Care of Children's Health. 1 hour, 55 minutes with study guide.

Communication with preverbal infants and young children. Boulder, CO: The University of Colorado Health Science Center School of Nursing. 29 minutes. Distributed by Learner Managed Designs, Inc.

Designing for family-centered care. Hall, J. (Executive Producer) & Atkins, P. (Producer/Director). (1995). Bethesda, MD: Institute for Family-Centered Care.

Mickey's field trips: The hospital. Walt Disney Media Company, Cornet MTI Films Inc. 10 minutes, 32 seconds.

Mr. Rogers: Having an operation. (1976). Family Communications, Inc. 16 minutes, 25 seconds.

Mr. Rogers: Going to the doctor. (1986). Family Communications, Inc. 14 minutes, 54 seconds.

The process of communication: Facilitating interactions with young children with severe disabilities in mainstream early childhood programs. (1993). Boulder, CO: The University of Colorado Health Science Center School of Nursing. 10 minutes. Distributed by Learner Managed Designs, Inc.

11

Physical Assessment

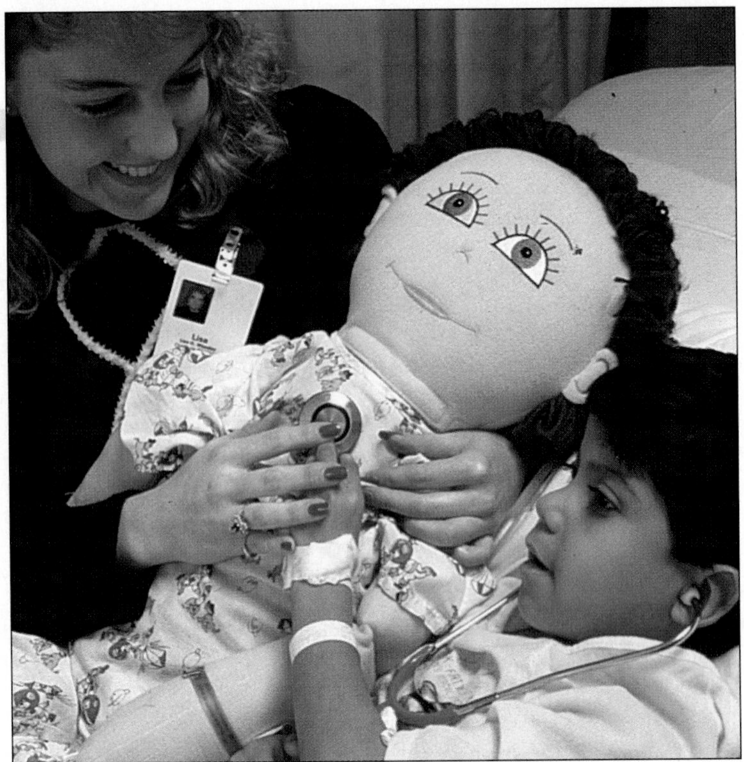

CHAPTER OVERVIEW

LEARNING OBJECTIVES

After studying this chapter, you should be able to:

- Apply principles of anatomy and physiology to the systematic physical assessment of the child.
- Describe the major components of a pediatric history.
- Identify the principal techniques for doing a physical examination.
- Use a systematic and developmentally appropriate approach for examining a child.
- Describe the general sequence of the physical examination of an infant, a young child, the school-age child, and the adolescent.
- Describe normal findings of a physical examination.
- State common terms used in describing findings of a physical examination.
- Record findings in a systematic way.

KEY TERMS

auscultation: the art of listening to sounds produced by the body; frequently using a stethoscope to magnify body sounds

development: changes that occur over time in function, psychosocial, and cognitive behavior

growth: measurable physical and physiologic changes that occur over time

history: the collection of subjective data to describe past and present health status

inspection: the art of careful observations to identify physical findings

palpation: the art of touching to determine such factors as texture, temperature, moisture, and organ location

percussion: the art of tapping the body to determine density, location, and size of organs

systematic assessment: following an organized method to collect data

Nurses perform physical assessments of infants and children in various settings: the clinic, the hospital, the school, and the home. The physical examination may be part of a well-child assessment; it may be the admission examination provided when a child is admitted to the hospital; or it may be part of an initial assessment provided by a nurse working in home health care. The physical examination provides the nurse with objective and subjective information about the child. The child's health status is determined and, based on the information obtained, the nurse is able to make judgments about the child's state of health and the need for nursing care.

As is true when providing any nursing care for infants and children, a growth and development approach is used. Knowledge of growth and development assists the nurse in the preparation of the child and throughout the examination. Parents should be involved as much as possible, and the child should be encouraged to handle and play with those instruments used in the examination that are safe, such as the stethoscope.

GENERAL APPROACHES TO PHYSICAL ASSESSMENT

The physical examination is often the first direct contact between the nurse and the child. It is important to establish a trusting relationship between the child and the examiner. Throughout the examination the nurse should be sensitive to the cultural needs and differences among children. A quiet, private environment should be provided for the history and physical examination. The classic **systematic approach** to the physical examination is to begin at the head and proceed through the entire body to the toes. However, when examining a child, the physical assessment must be tailored to the child's age and developmental level.

The Infant, 1 to 6 Months. Infants from age 1 to 6 months are responsive to human faces, are increasingly interested in their environment, and do not mind being undressed, making their examination relatively easy. If the infant is nursing or asleep in the parent's arms, auscultate the heart, lungs, and abdomen without waking the baby. If the baby is awake, it is possible to lay the baby on the examining table with the parent close to do the examination. Incorporate evaluation of the primitive reflexes—palmar grasp, plantar grasp, placing, stepping, and tonic neck—as body parts are examined. Leave all uncomfortable procedures, such as abduction of the hips, the speculum exam of the tympanic membranes, and eliciting the moro reflex, until last. Undress the infant, leaving the diaper on a male child, before beginning the examination. Calmly talking to the infant using a soft voice, distracting with a rattle, or using a pacifier help refocus an unhappy infant.

The Infant, 6 to 12 Months. Follow the procedures used with the infant from birth to 6 months. Keep in mind that infants 6 months and older are more difficult to examine because of their anxiety toward others they do not recognize. Offering a child of this age a toy or object for distraction may be useful. It is easier to do as much of the exam with the child held on the parent's lap as possible. Leave ear, oral, and other uncomfortable procedures until last.

The Toddler. The toddler is the most challenging age to examine and have "cooperate." To form a supportive relationship with the parent and toddler, begin by sitting or standing by the parent. Provide a few toys and books to encourage the child to explore and to facilitate relaxation of the child. Fears can be decreased by allowing the child to handle objects used during the examination (see photos, pp. 208–210). Communicating with the child using age-appropriate words to describe what is about to be done can help to decrease fear. Portions of the examination can be done before the child is totally undressed. The order of the exam must be flexible, and painful or frightening procedures should be left to last. Resistance is often encountered with a child in this age group. Assure the parent that the child's response to the examination is normal for this age. The parent is the best assistant and can be asked to hold the child's outstretched arms against the child's head or abdomen while the examiner uses her body to immobilize the lower half of the child's body.

The Preschooler. The preschool child is usually more cooperative. However, these children like their parents nearby. The preschool child is happy to show the nurse that he can undress himself and can be expected to cooperate. The nurse may proceed to do the examination beginning at the head and moving to the toes. It is still advisable to save the more invasive procedures, such as the speculum ear exam and the oral exam, until the end of the examination. Reinforce the child's interest in the examination by allowing the child to participate in the exam and by praising him.

The School-Age Child. To establish trust with the school-age child, address questions the child can answer directly to the child. Children in elementary school will talk about school, favorite friends, and activities. Older school-age children may have to be encouraged to talk about their school performance and activities. The parent is encouraged to support and reinforce the child's participation in the examination. The examination proceeds from head to toe. Children of this age prefer a simple drape over their underpants, and the examiner should be sensitive to the modesty needs of this age group. This is a wonderful opportunity to teach the child about the body and personal care. Answer questions openly and in simple terms.

The Adolescent. Adolescents are most comfortable with a straightforward, uncondescending approach. Decisions about who should be present for the examination should be openly discussed with the adolescent. The order of the examination is the same as for the school-age child. It is best to incorporate the genital examination into the middle of the examination. If possible proceed from the abdominal exam to the genital exam, to allow ample time for questions and discussions about this part of the examination. The physical examination is a wonderful opportunity to assure the pubertal child about normal developmental stages and to answer concerns children this age frequently have about what is happening to their bodies. The adolescent is expected to undress and wear a gown during the examination. Draping the adolescent appropriately when different regions are being assessed and explaining procedures promote trust and a sense of dignity in the adolescent patient (Schwartz et al., 1990).

TECHNIQUES OF THE PHYSICAL EXAMINATION

When performing the physical assessment, the nurse uses the four basic techniques of **inspection, palpation, percussion,** and **auscultation** carried out in that order. When examining the abdomen the sequence is altered; auscultation is performed after inspection, then percussion, and lastly palpation. The sequence of the abdominal examination is changed so as not to alter bowel sounds before determining their presence and characteristics and to determine the size of abdominal organs before palpation.

Inspection. The majority of information gathered during the physical examination is determined by the ability to systematically and deliberately make visual observations. The nurse first surveys an entire area of the body and then focuses on specifics, such as color, shape, size, or movement. Inspection can be both direct and indirect. Direct inspection relies on the examiner's senses of sight and hearing, whereas indirect inspection is accomplished with the use of special equipment, such as an otoscope, to examine a specific body area.

Palpation. During palpation the nurse uses the sense of touch to make judgments about pulsations and vibrations and to locate structures and masses. Palpation allows the nurse to determine characteristics such as size, texture, warmth, mobility, and tenderness of various areas of the body.

Different parts of the hands are used to detect different characteristics. The fingertips are used to palpate the breast, lymph nodes, and pulses. The back of the hand is used to assess temperature. The palm of the hand is used to detect vibrations.

The type of palpation used is governed by the structure to be examined and the need to avoid any unnecessary discomfort to the patient. Light palpation is accomplished by gently applying fingertip pressure to depress the skin surface approximately $\frac{1}{2}$ to $\frac{3}{4}$ inches and moving the fingertips in a circular motion.

Deep palpation is used to detect abdominal masses and is performed after light palpation. The surface is depressed approximately $1\frac{1}{2}$ to 2 inches to detect underlying masses. Bimanual palpation uses both hands; the examiner superimposes one hand over the other to increase pressure or places one hand below the other to capture and trap a mass or structure between them, such as the kidneys or spleen.

Percussion. To percuss, the nurse uses quick, sharp tapping of the fingers or hands to produce sounds. Percussion is performed to locate the position, size, and density of underlying structures. There are three basic methods: mediate or indirect, in which the finger of one hand is placed against the body surface and the finger of the other hand acts as the hammer; immediate, which is striking the finger of one hand directly against the body; and fist percussion, in which the ulnar aspect of the fist is used to deliver a firm blow directly to the area. The method used depends on the area to be percussed. The nurse uses quick, light blows to create vibrations that penetrate approximately 2 inches below the surface. Sounds identified by percussion are classified as flat, dull, resonant, and tympanic (see box).

Sounds Identified When Percussing

Flat: High-pitched, soft intensity sound elicited by percussing over solid masses such as bone or muscle

Dull: Medium-pitched, medium intensity sound elicited when percussing over high-density structures such as the liver

Resonance: Low-pitched, loud intensity sound elicited over a hollow organ such as the lungs

Tympany: High-pitched, loud intensity sound heard over air-filled body parts such as the bowel or stomach

Auscultation. Auscultation is the art of listening to body sounds created in the lungs, heart, blood vessels, and abdominal viscera. The most common way to auscultate is to use a stethoscope. Most sounds auscultated result from air or fluid movement within the body. The diaphragm of the stethoscope is most effective in assessing high-pitched sounds such as heart and breath sounds. The bell of the stethoscope is most effective in hearing low-pitched sounds such as blood pressure and vascular sounds. To perform auscultation the environment must be quiet and the stethoscope placed on the skin in the appropriate area. Sounds heard are described in terms of pitch, intensity, duration, and quality.

Smell. The nurse uses the sense of smell to detect body odors while examining the patient. Attention to odors such as body odor and the odor of urine or feces is important. In addition, certain odors are useful in identifying disease states; for example, the odor of acetone may be present in a patient with diabetes (Jarvis, 1992).

GENERAL APPEARANCE

During the first contact with the child and parent the examiner develops an initial impression by making a general survey of the patient. The nurse will determine age, sex, and race, and will identify clues concerning the child's behavior and health status. Clues to distress or abuse in children include dress (appropriate for the weather, ragged and excessively dirty clothing, or the latest "fad"); grooming and personal hygiene (dirty teeth, broken and dirty fingernails, matted and dirty hair); body type, posture, and movements (crouching in a corner, slow concentrated

Health Screening for a 2-Year-Old

INTRODUCTION

Community-based clinics promote optimum health in their clients. Children and their parents can develop an ongoing relationship with a provider, which encourages them to return for needed care in both health and illness. This 2-year-old girl is having a routine checkup at the clinic today.

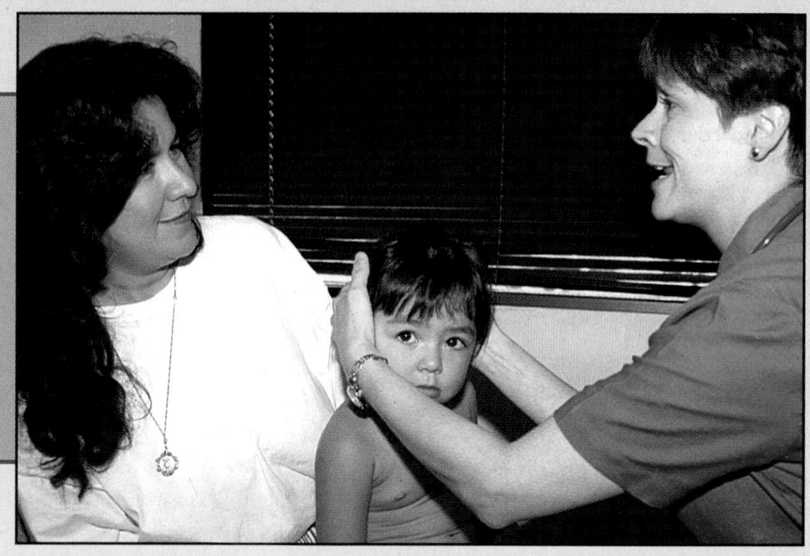

Communication and enlisting the trust of the child are vital elements in a successful physical examination. The girl remains in the security of her mother's arms as the nurse assesses her head. The little girl's anterior fontanelle is not quite fully closed. The nurse reassures her mother that, although the fontanelle is usually closed by 18 months of age, her child's open fontanelle likely represents a normal variation. Note that the nurse is at the mother's eye level and makes eye contact with her, promoting effective communication.

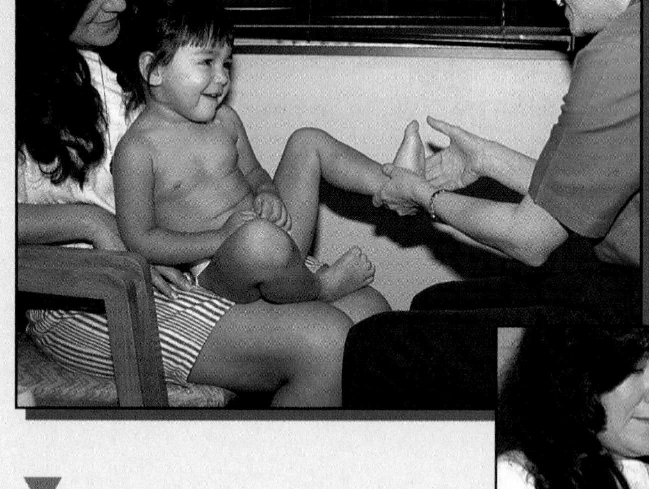

The nurse examines the child's feet for the presence of normal or abnormal reflexes and for straightness.

To limit the child's stress, the nurse creates an "examination table" by placing her knees next to the mother's knees. The child then lies across their laps as the nurse examines her thorax and abdomen.

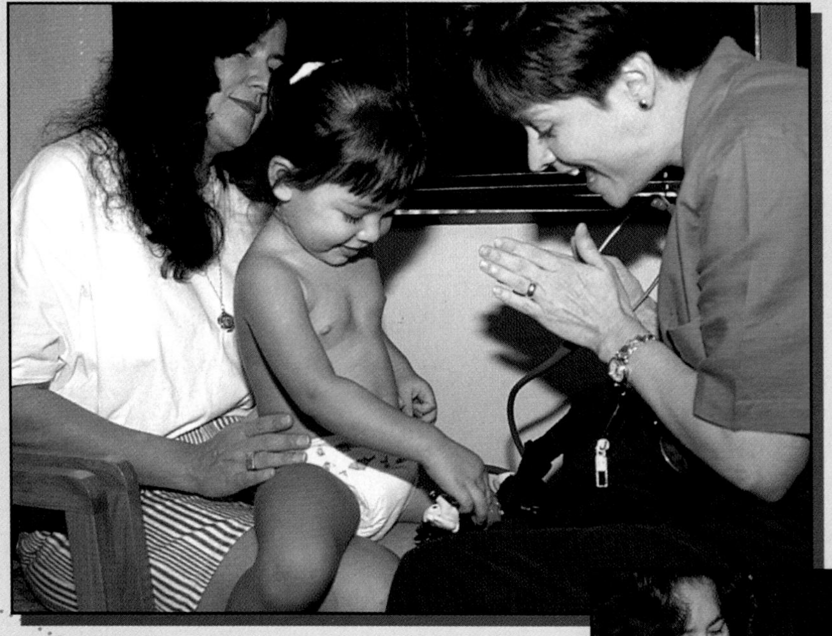

Allowing the child to check Mickey Mouse with a stethoscope before auscultating her chest enlists the child's cooperation and reduces her stress. This is especially important for assessments that are best done when the child is quiet. As the nurse auscultates her chest, the child is distracted by handling Mickey. Toddlers must be prepared for procedures immediately before they occur because their attention span is so short.

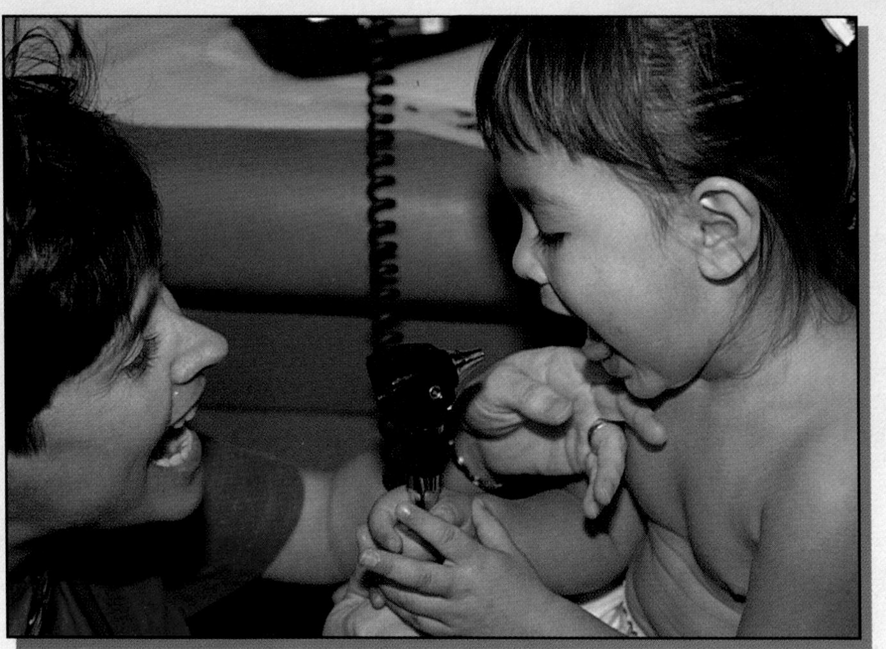

"Pant like a puppy!" the nurse tells the child as she examines her mouth and throat. Incorporating play and fun into exams promotes the child's trust in the nurse as well as enlisting her cooperation.

CONTINUED

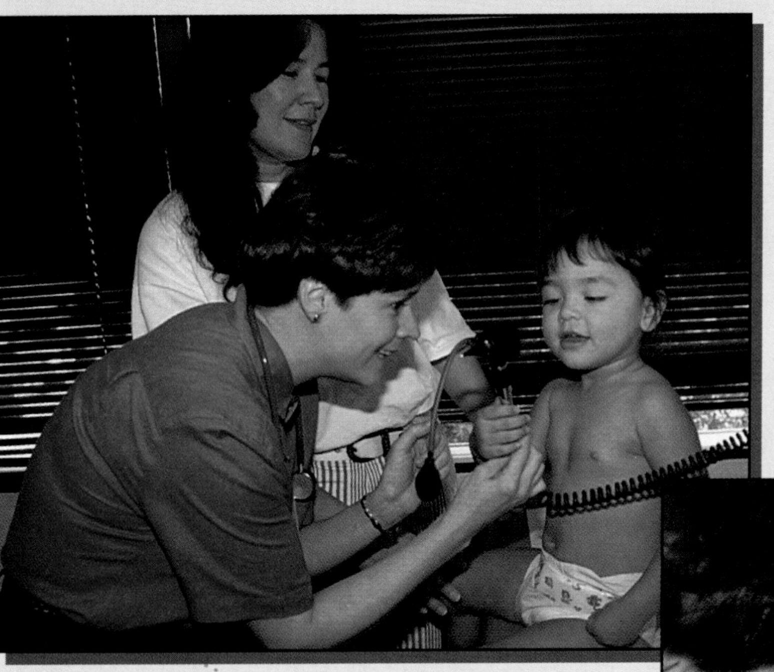

As in other examinations, the nurse helps the child examine the otoscope just before she uses it to examine her ears.

The nurse deftly examines the child's ears, pulling her pinna down and back. Ear examinations are especially important during the toddler years to identify fluid accumulation in the middle ear, which can interfere with hearing and speech development.

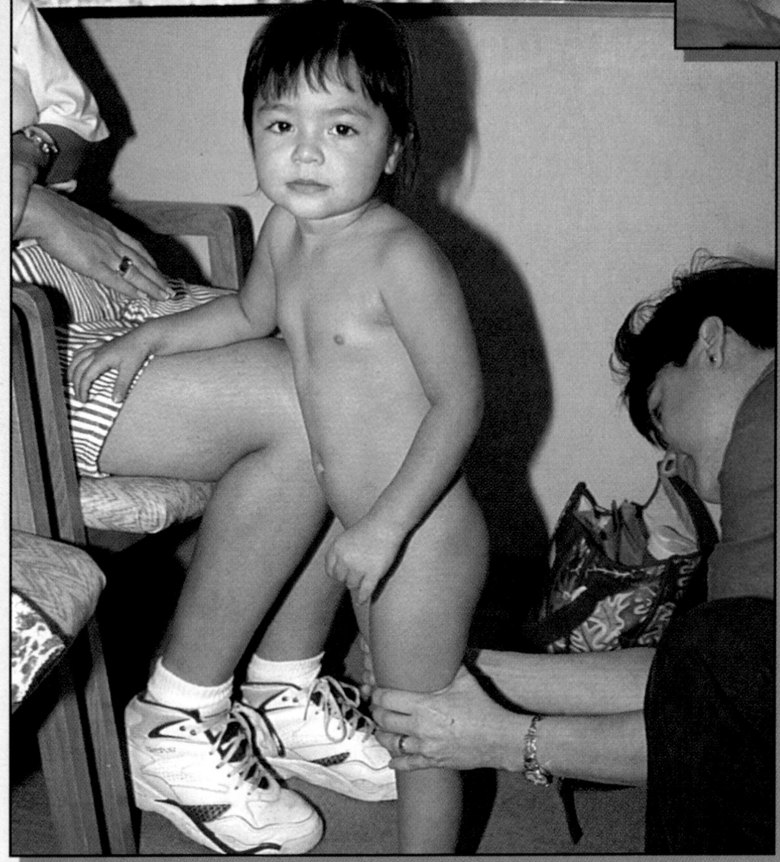

Photos courtesy of Dallas County Hospital District Community Oriented Primary Care Clinic.

The nurse concludes the examination by checking the unclothed child for normal genital development, straightness of her spine and extremities, and evidence of previously undiagnosed hip dysplasia. She observes the child's gait to identify problems in motor development.

CONCLUSION

The nurse determines that this little girl's development is appropriate for her age. She is tall, as is her mother, so the cherubic toddler appearance is less apparent than it might otherwise be at her age. The nurse shares her findings as she does the examination and summarizes them for the mother at the end. Because the child is developing normally, she does not need to return to the clinic for a checkup until she is 3 years old.

movements, image distortion [i.e., being thin and describing self as fat]); speech and communication (answering questions in one syllable only, looking to others to respond first, seeking approval of answers); facial characteristics and expressions (predominance of fearful, anxious, tearful, sad, or angry appearance); and overall psychological state (labile, demanding, bizarre, and overly dramatic or condescending). Because each child is a unique human being, there will be individual differences in behavior and health status related to growth and development. During the general survey the examiner should continually note the parent–child interaction and how the parent responds to the child's needs and behavior.

HISTORY TAKING

> Taking an accurate history of the child is the single most important component of the physical examination.

Practitioners obtain three different types of health histories: the complete or initial history, the well interim history, and the episodic or problem-oriented history.

In the *complete or initial history*, data is gathered about the child from the time of conception to the current status of the child. The content of the complete history is outlined in the accompanying box.

In the *well interim history*, data is gathered about the child from the last well visit to the current visit. When doing a well interim history, the examiner assumes that there is a database in place. In a *problem-oriented or episodic history*, information is gathered about a current problem. Information about the specific problem is then added to an already existing database.

To collect information about a specific problem, the nurse elicits the following information:

PROBLEM-ORIENTED HISTORY

Chief complaint: Use the child's own words.
Bodily location: Place the problem somewhere on the body.
Quality: What the problem is like for the child.
Quantity: The intensity of the problem for the child.
Chronology: When the problem began, periodicity and frequency, course of symptoms.
Setting: Where the problem occurs.
Aggravating and alleviating factors: What makes it better or worse.
Associated manifestations: Other related information.

Recording of Data

The information gathered during the history is documented in a concise fashion that provides all the necessary information from pregnancy to the current status of the child. Milestones in **growth** and **development,** immunizations, and family status are always included in the child's history.

VITAL SIGNS

> Vital signs are taken on every child on every visit in ambulatory settings and are monitored throughout the day in a child who is hospitalized.

Assessment of vital signs (temperature, pulse, respirations, and blood pressure) is an important method for measuring and monitoring vital body functions. Measuring of vital signs provides the basis for decisions concerning the overall health and illness of the child. In children, changes in vital signs are important signs of changes in health status. (See Chapter 18 for vital signs procedures.) Table 11–1 describes normal vital signs by age.

Temperature. The method for measuring children's temperature may vary from one setting to another. Some parents are comfortable taking a rectal or axillary temperature; health care providers may use a mercury, a tympanic membrane sensor, an electronic, or a digital thermometer. Currently parents are encouraged to take an axillary temperature as opposed to a rectal temperature because of the invasive nature of rectal temperatures, the risk of injury, and their questionable accuracy with febrile children since feces retain body heat for hours after fever has diminished. Axillary temperatures, when taken correctly, provide accurate information concerning changes in the child's health status. Tympanic temperature measurements are frequently used in health care agencies because they can be performed quickly and involve less cross-contamination of patients. When recording a tympanic temperature, include the side on which the temperature was elicited; there can be variation from one ear to the other on the same child. An oral thermometer may be used with older children. (See Chapter 18 for a discussion of various methods of assessing temperature.)

Pulse. Arterial pulses are palpated to determine pulse rate and rhythm and to evaluate blood flow, arterial wall elasticity, and vessel patency. Palpate the apical impulse in infants and children under age 6 years to determine the position of the heart in the anterior precordium. In the acute care setting an apical impulse is always palpated on every child. Changes in the location of the apical impulse from the fourth or fifth left intercostal space may indicate dextrocardia or mediastinal shift. Note the location of the apical impulse in all children. Simultaneously palpate and compare femoral, radial, and carotid pulses on children of any age. The nurse may also compare a carotid pulse with a femoral or radial pulse to determine the presence of a

The Complete History

The content of the complete or initial history includes:

1. **Statistical information:** name, age, address, telephone number, Social Security number, names of parents or guardians, and source of support.
2. **Client profile:** When the child eats and sleeps, educational level, developmental level, race and nationality, religion, economic status, and health status perception. If an interpreter was used to gather the health history the person's name is included in the data, usually in this section of the history. Include a statement about the reliability of informant such as an older sibling answering questions concerning a younger sibling, or an aunt or uncle answering questions regarding a child visiting them.
3. **Past health history:** Birth history, growth and development, common childhood illnesses, immunizations, previous hospitalizations, accidents or injuries, allergies or allergic reactions, and the exact symptoms the allergy produced. Ask about medications taken on a daily basis or for an acute episode of an illness. List all medications being taken, including dose and frequency. Name both prescription and over-the-counter medications. Ask if the child has ever had a blood transfusion or has received any blood products. For any hospitalizations, serious illnesses, and injuries, the nurse should obtain the following information:
   a. Reason for admission
   b. Place of admission
   c. Length of stay
   d. Surgical procedures
   e. Outcomes
   f. Other
4. **Family history:** The person taking the history should seek information concerning the health status of the child's mother, father, siblings, and specific blood relatives such as aunts, uncles, and grandparents. If deceased, include the age and cause of death. The purpose is to determine constitutional and hereditary factors that are likely to affect the child's health.
5. **Lifestyle and life patterns:** How the child interacts with the social, psychological, physical, and cultural environment. Growth and development, use of street drugs and smoking, roles and relationships, and family life information is important.
6. **Review of systems:** A systematic review of the major anatomic and physiologic parts. A head to toe review that emphasizes the health function and maintenance of each body part, in this order:
   a. General appearance
   b. Head
   c. Hair
   d. Face
   e. Eyes
   f. Ears
   g. Nose and sinuses
   h. Mouth
   i. Throat
   j. Neck
   k. Lungs
   l. Heart
   m. Breasts
   n. Abdomen
   o. Kidneys and bladder
   p. Bowels, rectum, and anus
   q. Genitalia
   r. Extremities

TABLE 11–1 *Normal Vital Signs by Age*

AGE	TEMPERATURE*		PULSE RATE (bpm)	RESPIRATORY RATE (breaths/min)	BLOOD PRESSURE (mmHg)
	FARENHEIT	CELSIUS			
Newborn	96.8–99 (axillary)	36–37.2 (axillary)	120–160	30–60	Systolic: 46–92 Diastolic: 38–71
3 Years	97.5–98.6 (axillary)	36.4–37 (axillary)	80–125	20–30	Systolic: 72–110 Diastolic: 40–73
10 Years	97.5–98.6 (oral)	36.4–37 (oral)	70–110†	16–22	Systolic: 83–121 Diastolic: 45–79
16 Years	97.5–98.6 (oral)	36.4–37 (oral)	55–90	15–90	Systolic: 93–131‡ Diastolic: 49–85

*The normal range of the child's temperature will depend on the method used. Temperatures are subject to circadian rhythms in all ages.

†After age 12 years, a boy's pulse is 5 bpm slower than a girl's.

‡After age 14 years, blood pressure in boys is higher than in girls.

gap in opposite pulses. In infants the nurse notes the pulsating anterior fontanel. Anxiety, fever, exercise, inflammatory illnesses, shock, and congestive heart failure can increase the pulse significantly in infants and children. The resting heart rate changes with increasing age. (See Table 11–1 for average heart rate, respirations, blood pressure, and temperature for infants, children, and adolescents at rest.)

The rhythm of the heartbeat is assessed for equal spacing between consecutive beats. Irregular cardiac rhythms in children are not uncommon. Irregular rhythms in children are commonly related to changes in rhythm that occur in response to respiratory inspiration and expiration.

Respirations. The rate, depth, and ease of respiration are observed in the child; respirations vary with age. (See Table 11–1 for average respiratory rates for infants, children, and adolescents.) The respiratory rate, like the heart rate, is significantly influenced by emotion and exercise. In infants, the rate may be counted by observing abdominal excursion and in children, thoracic excursion. Since the movements are irregular, the rate should be counted for 1 minute in infants and young children. Respiratory rates are best counted when the child is not paying attention to the examiner. Respirations should be counted while the examiner continues to keep fingers on a pulse or the stethoscope on the chest, as though checking the pulses. This will ensure that the child is unaware that respirations are being counted.

The depth and rhythm of respiration is determined subjectively and compared with norms observed in a particular age group. Ease or difficulty of respiration is in part a subjective determination. Respirations should be quiet and appear effortless. Stridorous respirations—a crowing noise heard on inspiration—in a child are a worrisome sign and may be related to croup or epiglottitis.

Blood Pressure. See Chapter 18 for a description of the procedure to obtain blood pressure in children.

Blood pressures are taken on all children at every ambulatory visit and at least daily and often more frequently, depending on the child's condition, in an acute care setting. The appropriate size cuff must be used to auscultate the blood pressure. Blood pressure measurements in healthy ambulatory children are compared with standard norms. (See Table 11–1 for the effects of age on vital signs.) Blood pressure is monitored more closely on any child you suspect may have a condition that affects blood pressure, such as hypertension, cardiovascular disease, kidney diseases, or liver disease.

The size of the cuff is important; cuffs that are too small will cause falsely elevated values and those that are too large will cause inaccurate low values. The cuff should cover two-thirds of the distance between the antecubital fossa and the shoulder. Several determinations may be required to obtain values unaffected by anxiety. Instructing the child that the balloon will gently squeeze the arm or give the arm a "hug" will usually decrease anxiety. The child can also assist with taking a blood pressure on a doll, a stuffed animal, or on the parent to alleviate anxiety (Jarvis, 1992).

ANTHROPOMETRIC MEASUREMENT

Anthropometrics measure the human body and assess nutritional status as well as growth and development. Weight, height, and head circumference are always measured in children and are compared to average standards for age group and sex. Midarm muscle circumference, skinfold thickness, and weight provide information about three body tissues (subcutaneous tissue, muscle, and fat) altered by nutrition. Anthropometric measurements are of most value when they are evaluated serially so that trends can be monitored.

Taking height and weight measurements is a routine procedure that provides valuable information about the health of a child. Children grow and develop very rapidly, and this growth and development must be constantly evaluated. Physical measurements of a child reflect the rate of growth; a failure in growth, an acceleration in growth, or any change in growth pattern may be the first clue to serious problems. Falling off her own growth curve is the most significant indicator of a problem in a child. Measurements must be taken correctly and accurately and are taken at every visit from birth to adulthood.

Height. The methods of measurement of a child vary with age. Length of infants and toddlers is best measured with the child lying down on a flat measuring board until able to stand independently. The child's head is held secure to the headboard and the movable end stretched to touch the child's heel. If a measuring board is not available for the infant and young child it is possible to position the child's body on a flat surface, mark the point where the heel touches the surface, and then mark the point where the tip of the head is lying on the surface, taking care to assure that the child's legs and body are straight on the surface. Remove the child and measure the distance between the two points with a measuring tape. Measuring the length of the child in this manner is not as accurate as using a measuring board.

When a child is able to cooperate and stand without support, around age 2 years, the examiner should stand the child in stocking feet next to a standard measuring tape that begins at the child's heel and is not displaced by room molding (Fig. 11–1). A flat, hard surface is used to reach from the top of the child's head to the tape so that guessing or adding height because of the hair does not occur.

The standing child's height is measured while in stocking feet. A flat surface is lowered to the top of his head, compressing hair for greatest accuracy. The child's height is then compared to the norms for his age, as seen in the chart attached to the measuring board. (Courtesy of University of Texas at Arlington School of Nursing) ▶

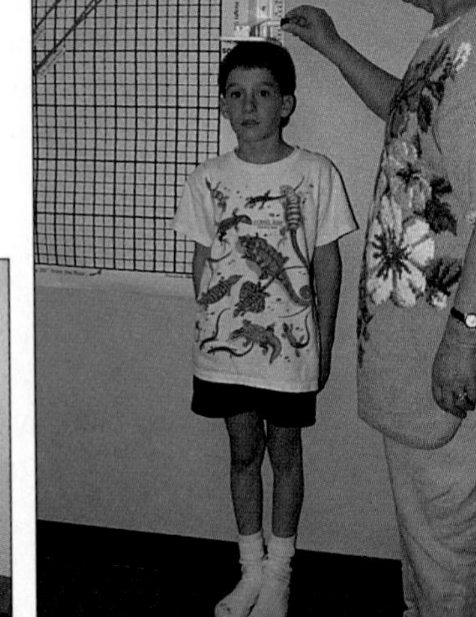

When weighing a child on a balance beam scale, the scale is first balanced with a pad on it, then the child is placed in the tray. The weights are moved until the beam again balances and the weight is noted. Because of the child's movement, there will be slight up-and-down motion of the beam even when it is balanced. (Courtesy of Dallas County Hospital District Community Oriented Primary Care Clinic, Dallas, Texas) ▶

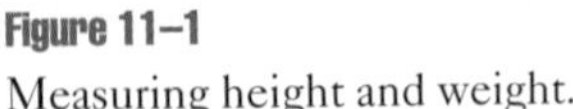

Figure 11–1
Measuring height and weight.

Once the measurement is taken, it must be plotted on a standardized growth chart (see Appendix C at end of book). Height and weight are evaluated by determining whether the child is following a predictable percentile curve on a growth chart. In a child, height and weight are related to hereditary factors and will vary from child to child.

Weight. The method and equipment for weighing varies with age. All scales must be balanced first before weighing. Infants are placed in a lying position on a regular baby scale with all their clothing removed. Older children who are able to stand or walk without support may be weighed on the adult standing scale. Remove all clothing except underwear on the older child.

Weight is plotted on a standardized growth chart (see Appendix) in a similar fashion as height. There are some general rules concerning weight measurements. Infants will gain 1 ounce per day for the first 6 months of life. After that, growth is slower, and from age 2 to 10 years the child gains an average of about 1 pound every 2 months, or 6 pounds a year.

Head Circumference. Head circumference is measured on all children from birth to age 36 months and plotted on a standard growth chart on all visits. Children over age 3 years with any questionable head size, such as hydrocephaly or microcephaly, will have their head circumference measured at every visit. To measure the head circumference, a nonstretching measuring tape is wrapped above the supraorbital ridges and over the most prominent part of the occiput (Fig. 11–2).

The head circumference is plotted on a standardized growth chart. During the first 6 months of life the head circumference normally increases by 1.5 cm each month and by 0.5 cm per month between 6 and 12 months. Head circumference can reflect an abnormal rate of development, give some indication of nutritional status, and possibly indicate an undetected tumor growth.

Chest Circumference. Chest circumference is routinely measured only in the newborn. The head circumference is larger than the chest circumference in the newborn. Chest circumference is almost equal to head circumference after age 1 year. To measure chest circumference the measuring tape is wrapped around the chest at the nipple line. The measurement is taken between inspiration and expiration.

Midarm Circumference. Midarm circumference reflects muscle mass and fat. To measure midarm circumference, the midpoint on the arm between the acrominal process and the olecranon process is determined. Then with the arm hanging loosely at the side, the child's arm is measured at the midpoint with a tape measure (see Figure 11–2). The measurement is recorded in centimeters. With a decrease in fat or muscle atrophy, the midarm circumference decreases. It will increase with weight gain.

Triceps Skinfold. Triceps skinfold indicates total body fat because at least half of body fat is directly below the skin. Metal calipers are used to obtain this measurement. On the nondominant arm the midpoint of the arm is determined using the method described for midarm circumference measurement. With the arm hanging loosely at the

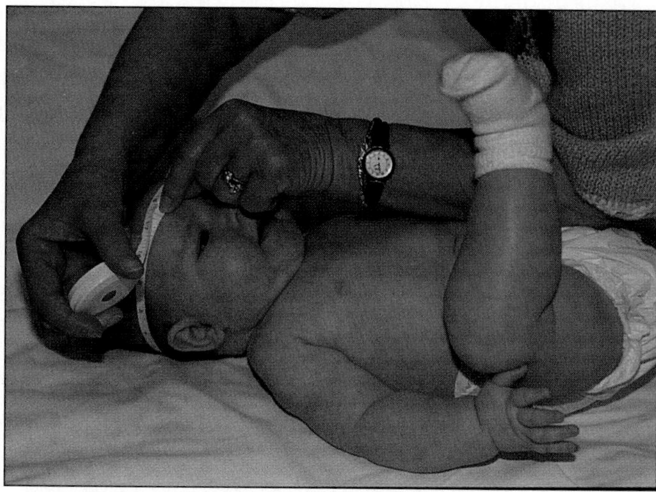

◀ The head circumference is measured from birth through age 36 months. The nurse uses a nonstretching tape and measures in a "hatband" position, just above the eyebrows and around the occipital prominence in the back. Chest circumference is also routinely measured in the newborn, and is usually smaller than the newborn's head circumference. (Courtesy of University of Texas at Arlington School of Nursing)

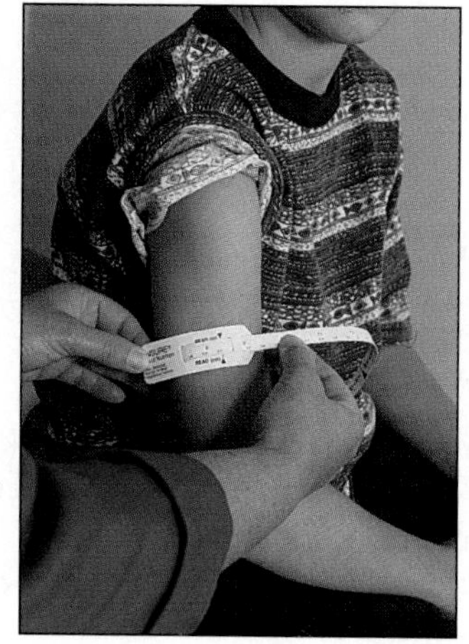

Midarm circumference is measured at a point halfway ▶ between the acromial process of the shoulder and the olecranon process of the elbow. (Courtesy of University of Texas at Arlington School of Nursing)

Figure 11–2
Measuring head, neck, and midarm circumference.

side, a fold of skin at the midpoint on the posterior aspect of the arm is grasped. To avoid error, the child is asked to flex the arm muscle after the examiner grasps the skin. If contraction is felt, then muscle as well as fat has been grasped. Apply the caliper and take a reading after waiting for 3 seconds. With long-term undernutrition and malnutrition fat stores decrease.

Growth Charts

An accurate record of an infant's or child's overall general pattern of growth is best determined by serial measurements over months or years. The National Center for Health Statistics publishes growth charts for length-for-age or stature-for-age, weight-for-age, head circumference-for-age (to 36 months), and weight-for-length or weight-for-stature from birth to puberty.

There are separate charts for girls and boys for two different age groups (see growth charts in Appendix C). To plot height, weight, and head circumference on growth charts, the exact age of the child is determined on the horizontal plane of the chart; on the vertical plane of the chart, the length in inches or centimeters or the weight in pounds or kilograms is determined. The chart is marked where the two lines intersect. The percentile lines on these charts indicate the number of normal North American children expected to fall above and below the index child's measurements (Barkauskas et al., 1994).

SKIN, HAIR, AND NAILS

Skin

Assessment of the skin includes inspection and palpation. The entire skin surface is examined; this examination may be combined with assessment of other areas of the body.

Inspection. Color and pigmentation of the skin is observed. The color of the skin is due to the amount of melanin and can range from pink to black. In dark skinned infants and children it is best to determine the normal skin color and then compare any color change with the normal skin color. The accompanying box defines skin color terminology.

> In dark-skinned infants and children, erythema will appear dusky red or violet, cyanosis will appear black, and jaundice will appear diffusely darker (Hurwitz, 1993).

Palpation. The skin is palpated to determine moisture, temperature, turgor, edema, and lesions.

Skin Color Terminology

Vitiligo: Areas of depigmentation
Nevi: Areas of increased pigmentation
Jaundice: A yellow discoloration of the skin best seen in the sclera of the eyes
Cyanosis: A blue discoloration of the skin, best seen in all races in the mucous membranes of the mouth, particularly under the tongue
Carotenemia: An orange color of the skin, best seen on the soles of the feet and palms of the hands
Pallor: Loss of skin color
Erythema: Diffusely red
Mottling: Discolored areas of the skin

Moisture is determined by lightly stroking the skin surface and body creases. The external skin on exposed areas is normally dryer than unexposed areas of the skin.

Temperature is determined by using the back of the hand, as it is more sensitive to skin changes. Each side of the body is compared with the other.

Normal *texture* of the skin is described as being smooth and soft. Scars or excessive scar tissue should be noted.

Turgor is determined by grasping the skin between the thumb and index finger and quickly releasing (Fig. 11–3). The skin normally returns to place without excessive skin markings. When the skin "tents" when released, this indicates dehydration. The best place to test for tissue turgor on a child is on the abdomen and upper arm.

Edema, the accumulation of excessive salt and water in the interstitial spaces, is identified by pressing the thumb into areas of the body that may appear puffy. The extremities and buttocks are classic areas to palpate for edema in the child. Periorbital edema is observed on the eyelids.

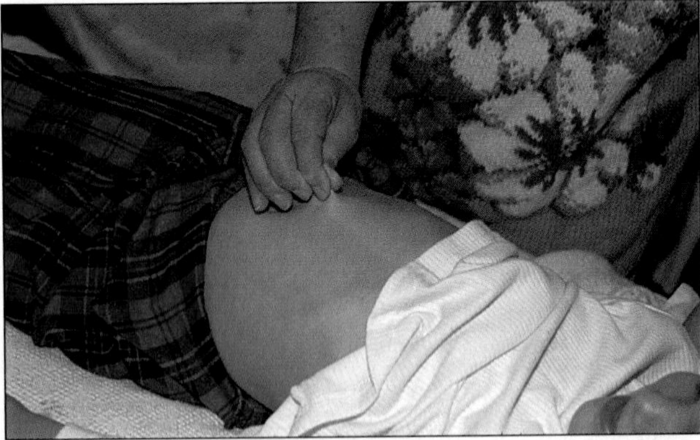

Figure 11–3
Skin turgor is best tested by grasping the abdominal skin between the thumb and forefinger, and quickly releasing it. "Tenting" (persistent elevation of the skin when released) suggests dehydration. (Courtesy of University of Texas at Arlington School of Nursing, Arlington, Texas)

Lesions are identified, noting configuration, distribution, color, and size. Skin lesions are identified as primary skin lesions, arising from normal skin; secondary skin lesions, occurring from modification in a primary skin lesion; and purpuric lesions, those associated with red blood cells (Weston & Lane, 1991).

Configuration of a skin lesion refers to the arrangement or position of several lesions in relation to each other or to the arrangement of a single lesion. Distribution refers to the body location and the symmetry or asymmetry of lesions.

Hair

Hair normally covers the entire body except for the palms, soles, and parts of the genitalia. Hair is examined for texture, changes in color, unusual distribution, and cleanliness.

Scalp hair has a wider range of normal textures, including straight, curly, or kinky. The hair is usually shiny, silky, and strong. The examiner should keep in mind the age and development of the child. Fine downy hair would be normal for a newborn, whereas in an older child it would lead the examiner to consider nutrition and endocrine abnormalities. Brittle hair, identified when the hairs break off easily when bent between the fingers, might indicate endocrine and nutritional abnormalities.

The color of the hair may be anything from pale blond to black. Changes in color may be due to depigmentation or may be a hereditary factor.

Distribution of the hair over the head is identified. In most children the hair begins in a whorl and then is distributed over the head. Some children may have more than one whorl. Scalp hair does not grow beyond the nape of the neck or down to the eyebrows. *Hirsutism* is defined as excessive hair growth, *alopecia* is unusual hair loss.

The hair is separated and examined for cleanliness, signs of trauma, lesions, or scaling. The scalp should be clean and free of any infestations. Head lice (*Pediculosis capitis*) are found most commonly on the scalp, and nits (ova) adhere to the hair shaft (Simon & Janner, 1990).

Nails

Nails are inspected and palpated for shape and contour. The nail surface is normally flat or slightly convex. The edges of the nails should be smooth, rounded, and clean. Clubbing of fingernails can be identified by looking at the index finger; the angle at the nail base and the finger should be less than 160°. On palpation, the base of the fingernail should be firm. On touching the index fingernails

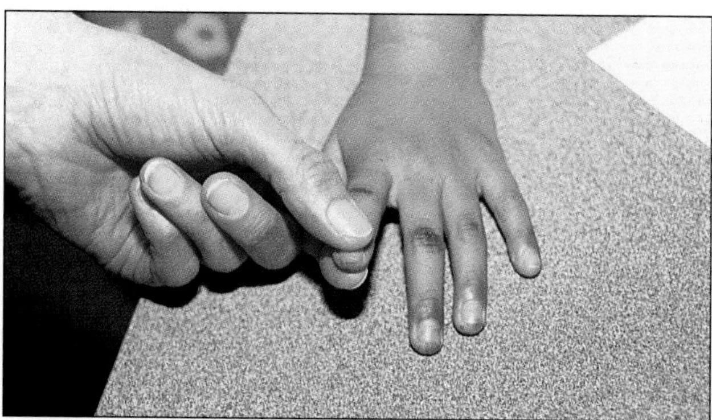

Figure 11–4
To assess capillary refill, press the edge of the nail and release it. The nail should blanch with pressure, and color should return within one or two seconds. Delay of capillary refill longer than 3 seconds suggests impairment of peripheral circulation. Note that this child also has bruises on her knuckles. (Courtesy of Parkland Memorial Hospital, Dallas, Texas)

back to back, a diamond of light below the knuckle and above where the fingernails touch will be present. In early clubbing the diamond shape is decreased or not apparent (see Fig. 29–2).

Capillary refill of the nails is assessed by pressing on the nail edge and releasing (Fig. 11–4); the nail will blanch and color return to the nail within 1 or 2 seconds. Delayed capillary refill, greater than 3 seconds, is a worrisome sign of beginning peripheral arterial or venous shutdown (Zitelli & Davis, 1987).

LYMPH NODES

Lymph nodes are inspected and palpated. Lymph tissue is found all over the body and must be evaluated as the examiner assesses body systems. Always assess for enlarged lymph nodes in the head and neck, the axillary region, the arms, and the inguinal region (see the accompanying box).

> Examination of lymph nodes should be incorporated into the examination when that part of the anatomy is being assessed.

When an enlarged lymph node or a mass is found during examination the characteristics listed in the accompanying box should be used to describe your findings.

To palpate for most lymph nodes the examiner uses the distal portion of the fingers and gently but firmly moves the fingers in a circular motion to determine the characteristics described above.

Characteristics of Enlarged Lymph Nodes and Masses

Location: Identify the anatomic location of the enlarged lymph node or mass. Use imaginary body lines or body axes to assist in locating findings.

Size: Describe using three dimensions: length, width, and thickness. Describe the shape: round or irregular.

Surface characteristics: On palpation describe the surface as smooth, nodular, or irregular.

Consistency: On palpation describe as hard, soft, firm, resilient, spongy, or cystic.

Symmetry: Use paired anatomic structures.

Fixed/mobile: If mass is fixed, identify whether it is fixed to underlying or overlying tissue. If mobile, describe in centimeters and in what direction.

Tenderness/pain: Describe whether the tenderness or pain is present on direct palpation, referred or rebound tenderness, or if the pain is present without stimulation.

Erythema: Describe the extent of any color change.

Heat: Palpate with the back of the hand to determine the extent of any heat.

Pulsative nature: Describe pulsations, if present, particularly when they are in an area where you would not expect to see pulsations. All pulsating masses are auscultated for bruits.

Increased vascularity: Describe prominence of overlying veins or the presence of cyanosis of the area.

Transillumination: If the mass is in an anatomic structure that can be transilluminated, describe the results of the procedure.

Lymph nodes that are enlarged, warm, firm, and fluctuant are a sign of infection.

Two areas of the body where you can find normal enlarged lymph nodes are in the cervical area and inguinal area. These lymph nodes are less than 1 cm in size and are cool, movable, and nontender.

> In young children "shotty" lymph nodes can be found. These are lymph nodes that are less than 3 mm in diameter and are also cool, movable, and nontender. They can be found anywhere on the body and are usually a sign of past infection in the area drained by the "shotty" lymph node (Alexander & Brown, 1974).

Common Skin Lesions

COMMON PRIMARY SKIN LESIONS

Flat circumscribed discolorations of the skin:

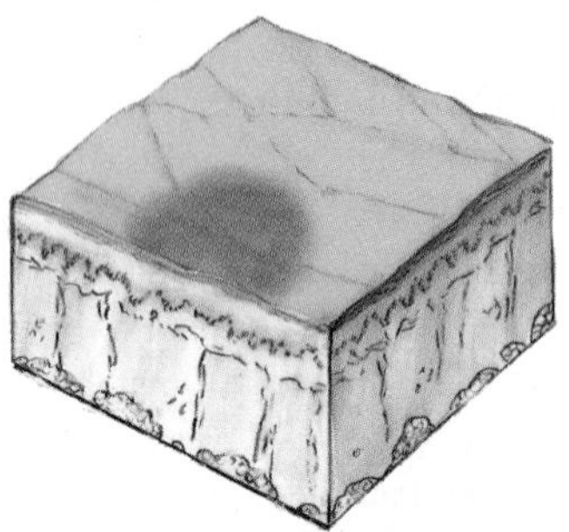

Macule (less than 1 cm)
Patch (greater than 1 cm)

Elevated circumscribed solid lesions:

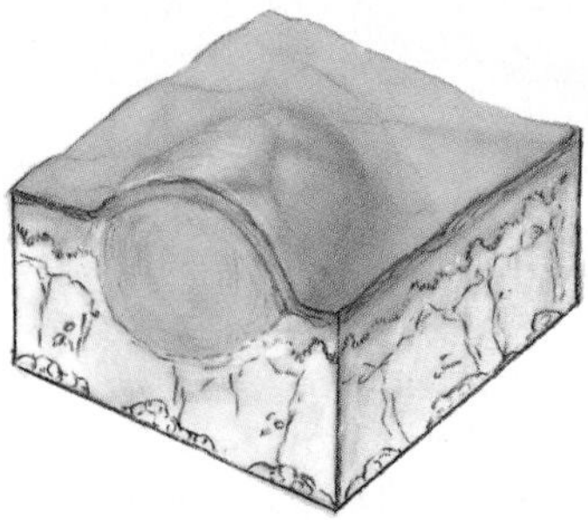

Papule (less than 1 cm)
Plaque (greater than 1 cm)

Solid lesion that can be level with, above, or beneath the skin:

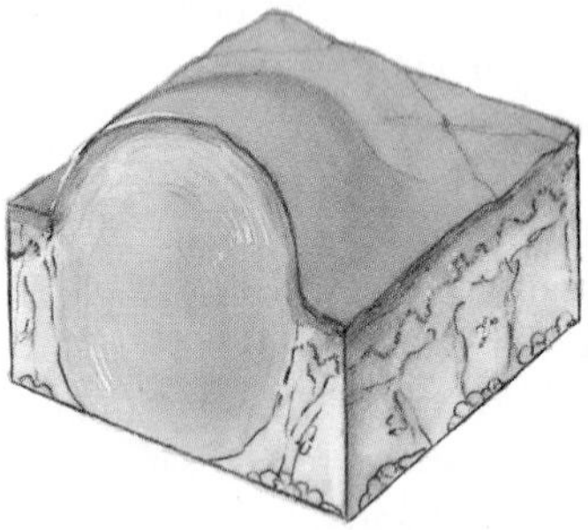

Nodule (less than 1 cm)
Tumor (greater than 1 cm)

Elevated fluid-filled lesions:

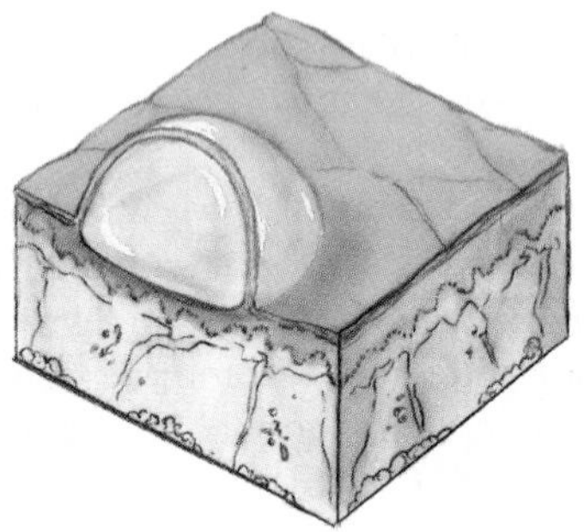

Vesicle (less than 1 cm)
Bulla (greater than 1 cm)

Erythematous, irregular shaped skin edema:

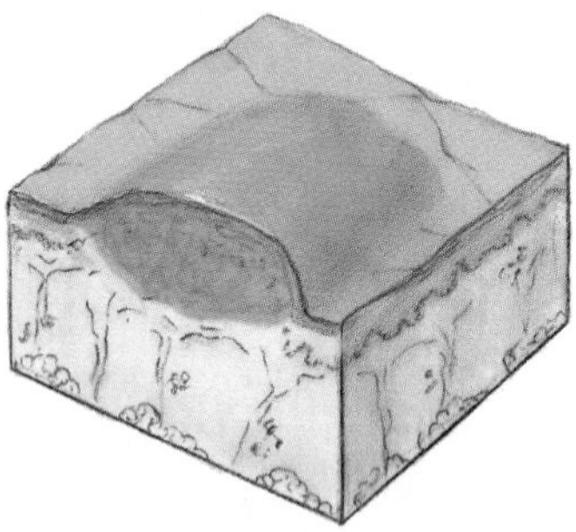

Wheal (variable size)

Vesicle containing purulent exudate:

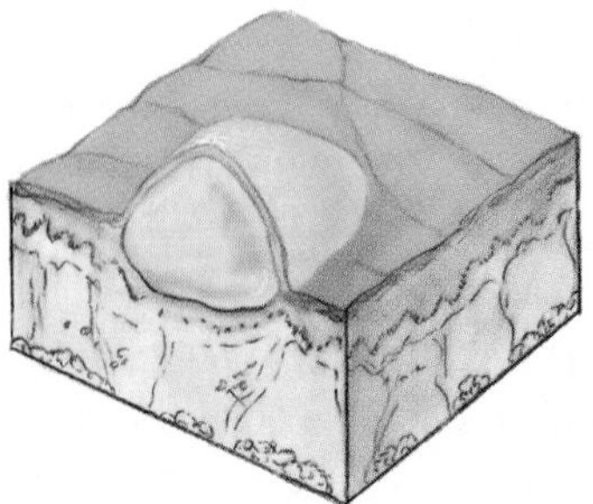

Pustule

Common Skin Lesions (continued)

COMMON SECONDARY LESIONS

All secondary skin lesions will vary in size.

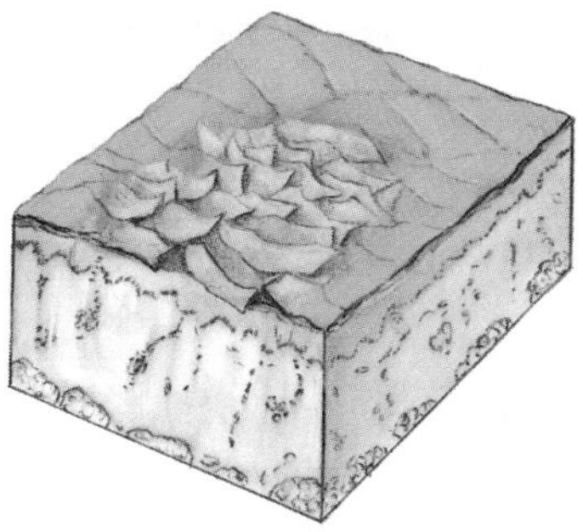

Scale:
Thin flakes of exfoliated epidermis

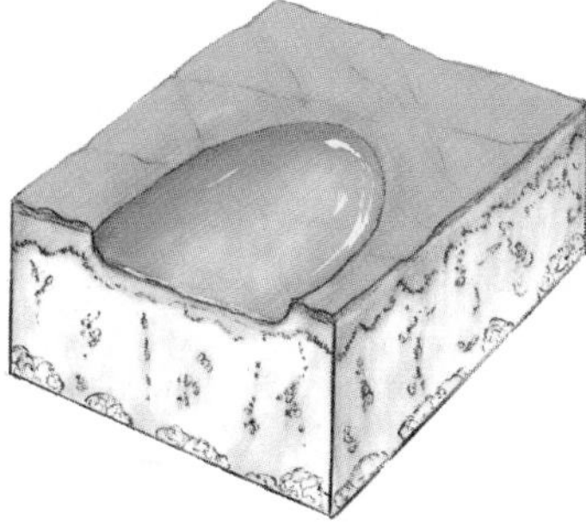

Erosion:
Loss of the superficial epidermis

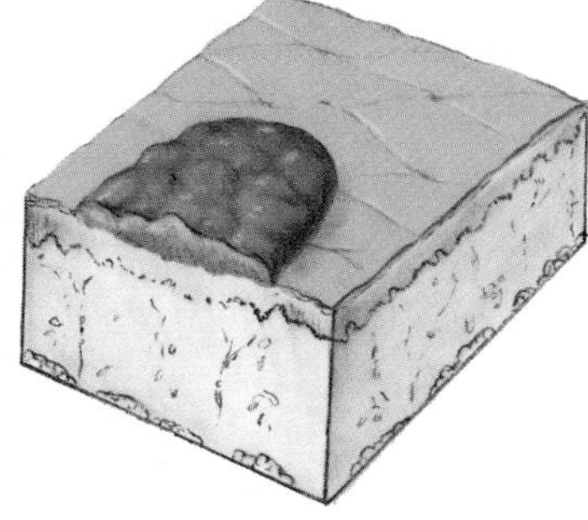

Crust:
Dried serum, purulent exudate, or blood

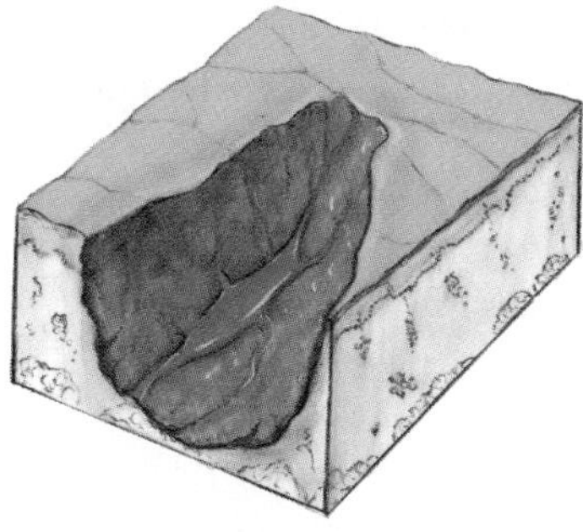

Ulcer:
Loss of the skin surface that may extend to dermis and subcutaneous tissue

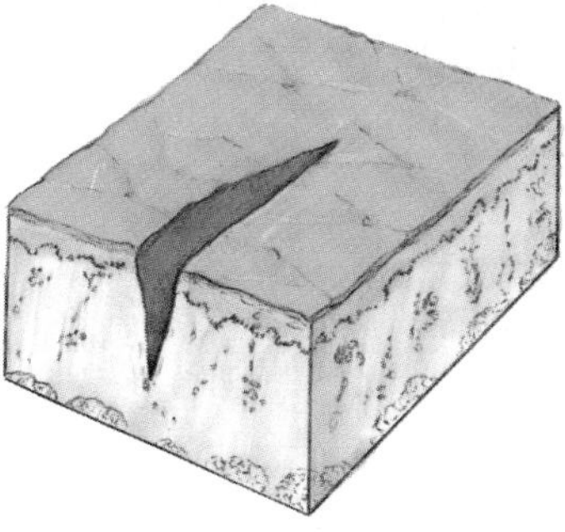

Fissure:
Linear crack in the skin

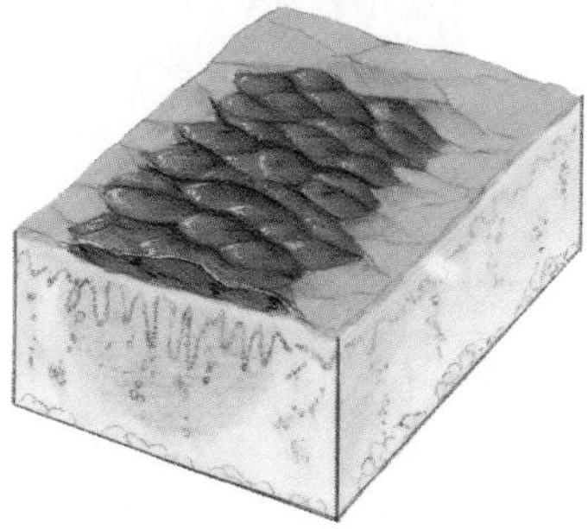

Lichenification:
Thickening of all layers with accentuated skin markings

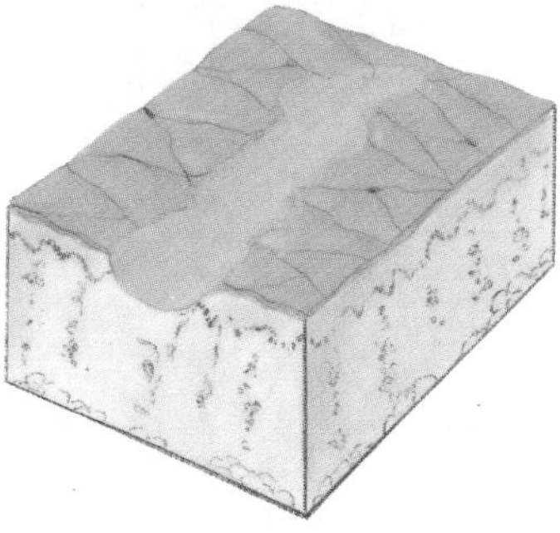

Striae:
Thin white or purple stripes commonly found on the abdomen

Purpuric Lesions

Purpuric lesions occur when red blood cells are outside the vascular channels and located in the adjacent dermis.

Petechia: Flat, round, deep red or purplish mass (less than 3 mm or 0.1 in)
Purpura: Large skin deposit or blood or heme pigment (greater than 1 cm)
Ecchymosis: Mass of variable size and shape, initially purplish, fading to green, yellow, then brown

Illustrations from Jarvis, C. (1996). *Physical examination and health assessment,* 2nd ed. (pp. 249–252). Philadelphia: W. B. Saunders.

Palpating Lymph Nodes

LYMPH NODES OF THE HEAD AND NECK

Flex the head forward or bend toward side being examined.

Submental: Under the chin.
Submandibular: Tuck the head toward the side to be palpated and cup fingertips under the mandible and pull upward and outward over the mandible.
Tonsillar: Behind the temporomandibular joint and under the angle of the jaw.
Superficial cervical: Superficial to the sternomastoid.
Deep cervical: Hook thumb and fingers around either side of the sternomastoid muscle, starting below the chin, and work down to the clavicle.
Posterior cervical: Along the anterior edge of the trapezius.
Preauricle/parotid: Run the side of the finger down the face in front.
Postauricle: Behind the ear.
Occipital: Palpate along the occipital bone.

LYMPH NODES OF THE AXILLARY REGION AND ARM

Roll the tissues against the chest wall and muscles of the axillae.

Epitrochlear: On medial surface of arm about 3 cm above elbow. Reach around behind the arm and feel in the groove between biceps and triceps muscles, about 3 cm above medial epicondyle.
Axillary, pectoral (anterior) group: Along lower border of pectoralis major inside anterior axillary fold.
Axillary, subscapular (posterior) group: Along lateral border of scapula; felt deep in posterior axillary fold.
Axillary, lateral group: Deep along upper humerus and midaxillary line.
Infraclavicular and supraclavicular: Below and behind clavicle. Left supraclavicular lymph node is called "sentinal" node in children because it is sometimes enlarged with Wilms tumors.

LYMPH NODES OF THE INGUINAL AREA

Horizontal: High in the anterior thigh below inguinal ligament.
Vertical: Clustered near upper part of saphenous vein.

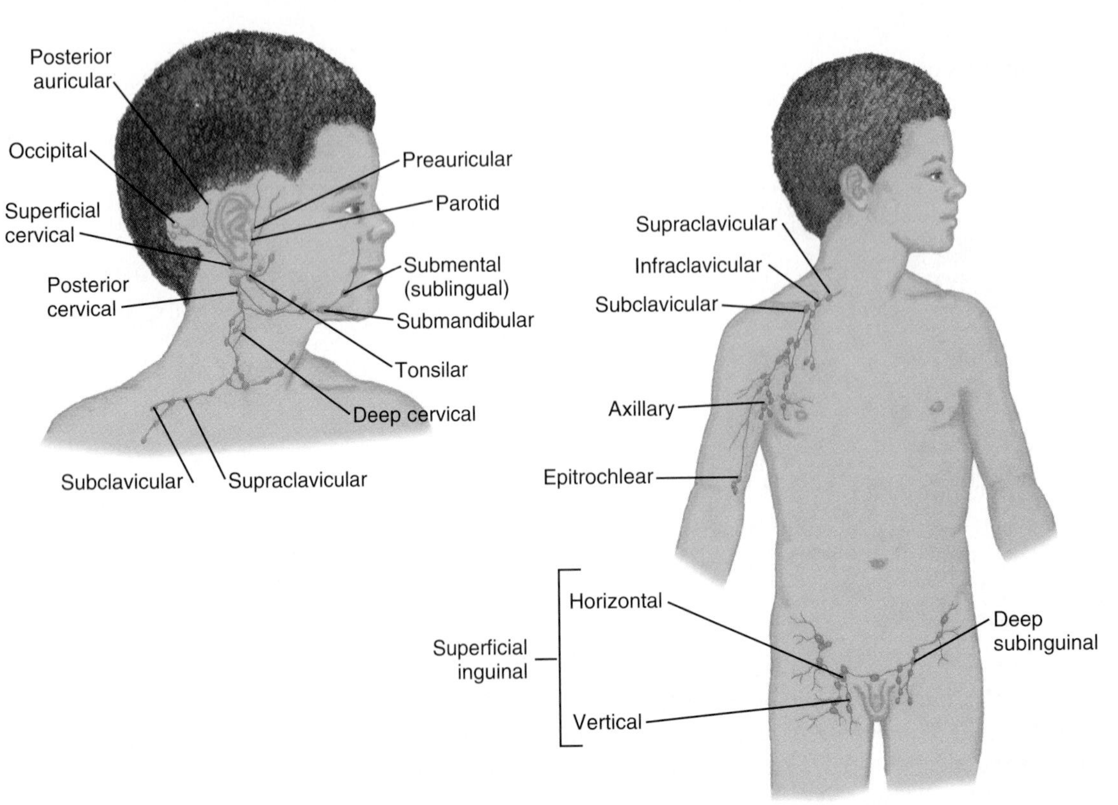

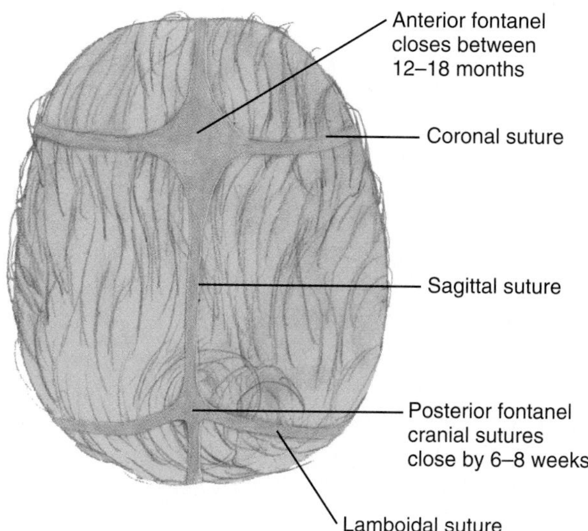

Figure 11–5

Fontanels are inspected and palpated for size, tenseness, and pulsation.

HEAD, FACE, AND NECK

Head

The head is inspected and palpated. In order to examine the head the examiner must see and feel it all. The head is evaluated from the front, from behind the child, and from the sides. The head is examined for symmetry, paralysis, weakness, and movement.

Symmetry is determined by looking at and feeling the entire head. If any lumps or bumps are seen or felt, notation is made of the exact location and size and density. The suture lines in infants should be palpated. Sutures are felt as prominent ridges in the newborn but usually flatten by 6 months.

Paralysis and weakness of the head is directly related to the condition of the neck muscles. That is, paralysis and weakness of the head will occur when there is paralysis or weakness of the neck muscles.

Head movement is determined by observing the child move his or her head. Head control is observed with the child in a lying position and while the examiner grasps the child's hands and pulls the infant into a sitting position. An infant younger than age 4 months may show some head lag; however, when the infant is in a upright position he or she should be able to maintain the head in a upright position for several seconds. Head lag after age 6 months may be an indication of poor muscular development. The head should be put through a full range of motion by asking the older child to look up, down, and sideways. The inability to move the head or hold the head in an upright position after age 4 months may be related to paralysis or weakness of the neck muscles.

HEAD SHAPE TERMINOLOGY

Normocephalic: Normal size head.
Microcephalic: Small size head for body size and age.
Hydrocephalic: Enlarged head; indicates excessive fluid in the cranial cavity.
Bossing: Frontal enlargement.

Fontanels are inspected and palpated for size, tenseness, and pulsation (Fig. 11–5). The posterior fontanel is closed by age 6 to 8 weeks. The anterior fontanel should be soft, flat, and pulsatile with the child in a sitting position. Measure the width and length of an open anterior fontanel. The anterior fontanel should be less than 5 cm in length and width after age 12 months and should be completely closed by age 12 to 18 months. A sunken fontanel is associated with dehydration, and a bulging fontanel can be associated with increasing intracranial pressure in the infant (Greenberger & Hinthorn, 1993).

Neck

In the child the neck is inspected and palpated for symmetry, size, and shape. The neck should be viewed from the front, behind, and both sides. *Symmetry, size, and shape* of the neck is directly related to use or disuse of the neck muscles. Webbing of the neck, the presence of an extra fold of skin posteriorly, is associated with some chromosomal abnormalities such as trisomy 21 and Down syndrome.

While palpating the neck of the child the *thyroid gland* is palpated by identifying the isthmus of the thyroid across the trachea. To identify an enlarged thyroid in a child the examiner gently displaces the thyroid gland in a lateral position and palpates thyroid tissue with the opposite thumb and fingers. The lobe may be more palpable when the child swallows (Fig. 11–6).

Face

The face of the child is inspected and palpated for dysmorphic features. Spacing and symmetry of the eyelids, eyebrows, palpebral fissures, nasolabial folds, mouth, and nose are noted in the child. The face is observed for any changes in color or the presence of edema such as cellulitis. The eyes are examined for size, position, and configuration. Hypertelorism are eyes set unusually wide apart; hypotelorism are eyes set unusually close together. The child's nostrils are oval in shape and equal in size, and there should be no evidence of a hypoplastic philtrum (shallow crease or absence of a crease below the nose). The lips are equal on either side of the midline. The

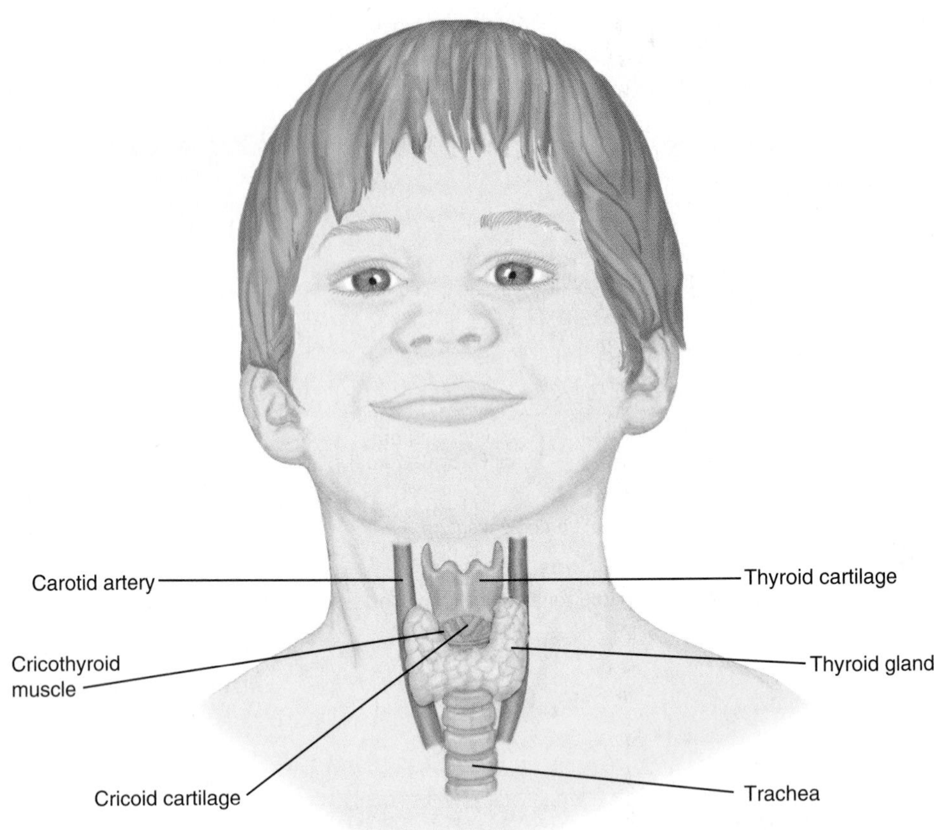

Figure 11–6
The thyroid gland is palpated by identifying the isthmus of the thyroid across the trachea.

child's ears are inspected for alignment. Low set ears are identified when the auricle of the ear does not cross or touch the eye–occiput line. The position of the auricle should be almost vertical, with no more than a 10° lateral posterior angle (Fig. 11–7).

Cranial nerve V (trigeminal) and cranial nerve VII (facial) functions are examined while assessing the face. Cranial nerve V is evaluated by observing chewing or sucking, evaluating strength of the tempomandibular joint, and by touching the child's forehead and cheeks with a piece of cotton. The child should move his head or bat the object away. Cranial nerve VII is evaluated by having the child frown, smile, or make a face while observing for symmetry of movement. Having the child puff out his cheeks or whistle can also be used to evaluate cranial nerve VII (Jarvis, 1992).

NOSE, MOUTH, AND THROAT

Nose

The examiner should wear clean gloves when doing the nasal examination. Note any drainage coming from the nose, describing amount, color, and consistency.

The external nose is inspected and palpated. Patency can be determined by occluding one nostril and having the child sniff. Repeat on the other side. The external nose is observed for symmetry, deformity, inflammation, or skin lesions. The "allergic salute," frequent wiping of the nose because of drainage, produces a transverse crease on the nose of a child and indicates that the child has allergies. Palpate the entire external nose for septal deviation or other deformities. The sense of smell is mediated by cranial nerve I. This can be evaluated by having the patient close her eyes, occlude one nostril, and identify familiar odors such as cinnamon, peppermint, orange, or cherry.

The nasal cavity can be examined by using a short wide-tipped speculum on the otoscope and inserting it into the nasal vestibule, being careful not to put pressure on the nasal septum. The nasal mucosa is inspected for color and moisture. Nasal mucosa is normally smooth, moist, and has a bright pink color. In children with allergies the mucosa is pale and appears boggy. With infectious diseases the mucosa is erythematous and swollen; the nasal drainage may be yellow or green. The nasal septum is examined for intactness and any deviation.

The *frontal and maxillary sinuses* are inspected and palpated (Fig. 11–8). The areas over the sinuses are examined for color and swelling. Puffiness and redness over the

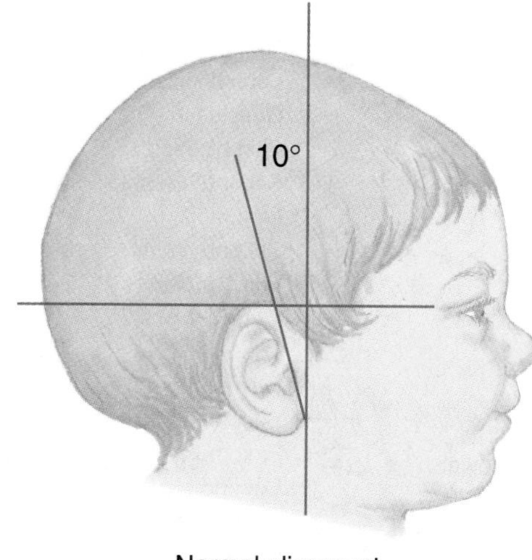

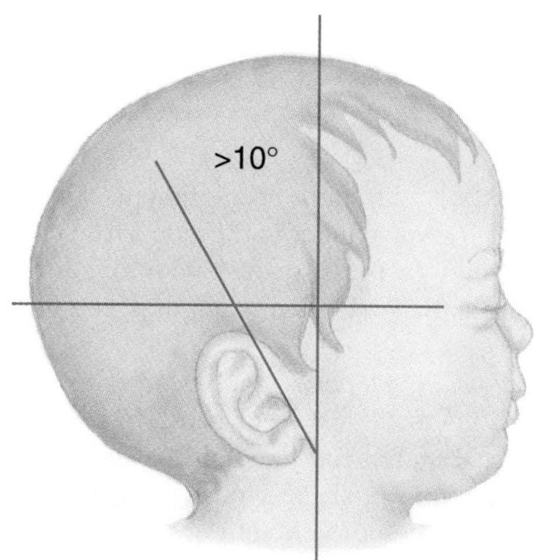

Figure 11–7
The child's ears are inspected for alignment. Low-set ears could indicate mental retardation or renal anomalies.

sinuses and dark circles under the eyes may indicate an inflammatory process in children. The frontal sinuses are palpated by pressing over the sinuses below the eyebrow. The maxillary sinuses are palpated by pressing upward with the thumbs under the maxillary bones.

Mouth and Throat

Assessment of the mouth in a young child should be performed at the end of the physical examination because it may create anxiety in the child. The examination should proceed from the anterior structures to the internal structures of the mouth.

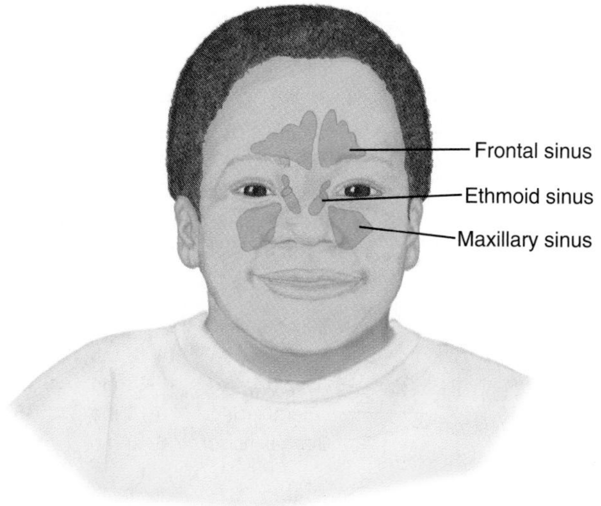

Figure 11–8
The frontal, ethmoid, and maxillary sinuses.

The *philtrum,* the little notch between the nose and upper lip, should be intact. In children with dysmorphic features the philtrum is invisible or incompletely "dug out."

The examiner should wear clean gloves when doing the oral exam. A tongue blade and a good penlight are used to assist with illumination of the oral cavity. The mouth and internal structures are examined using inspection, palpation, and the sense of smell.

Lips are inspected for color, moisture, cracking, or the presence of any lesions. The alveolar frenulum, which attaches the lips to the gums, should be intact. The lips are palpated to determine the presence of any masses.

The *buccal mucosa* is examined by holding the cheeks open with a tongue blade and examining for color, nodules, or lesions. Significant mouth odors should be noted. For many children this part of the exam can be unpleasant. To facilitate the child's cooperation it may be necessary to demonstrate on a doll or on the parent what you are going to do or allow the child to place the tongue blade in the parent's mouth. The buccal mucosa is described as pink, smooth, and moist. Dark skinned children may have patch areas of hyperpigmentation. The opening of the *parotid gland* is found as a small dimple on the buccal mucosa opposite the upper second molar. The entire surface of the buccal mucosa is palpated for changes in consistency or masses.

Teeth are inspected for number, cavities, tooth formation, and occlusion. The number and characteristics of the teeth will change with growth and development (Fig. 11–9). The eruption of deciduous teeth begins around the sixth month of extrauterine life; all 20 deciduous teeth are present by age 28 months. Have the child close the mouth, and note the position of the teeth. The upper teeth will protrude slightly over the lower teeth. The color

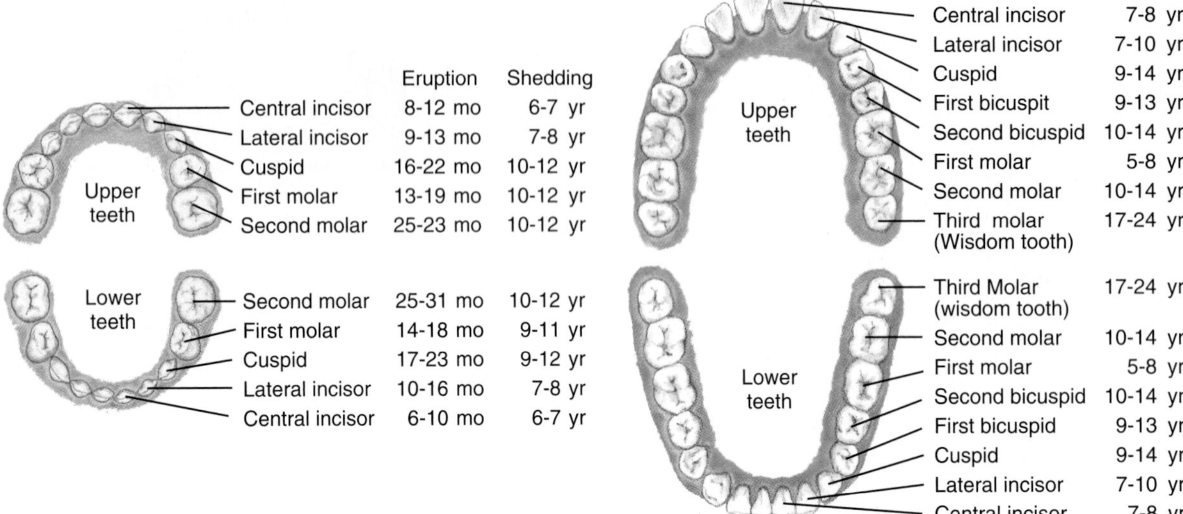

Figure 11–9
Sequence of eruption of primary and secondary teeth.

and shape of each tooth should be noted. The color of the crown is white with some variations from person to person. Permanent teeth are larger and have a darker color than deciduous teeth. Brown and black discoloration of the teeth is usually due to dental caries. Chronic use of certain medications (i.e., tetracycline and iron) may stain teeth. With excessive fluoride ingestion the enamel of the permanent teeth may appear mottled. The shape of the tooth will be determined by age, development, and the amount of wear. The teeth should be palpated for mobility by placing the thumb behind the tooth and the finger in front and gently trying to move the tooth (Barkauskas et al., 1994).

The *gums* (gingiva) are inspected and palpated for color and swelling. The gum surface will have a pink, stippled appearance and will feel firm. Dark skinned children may have a dark pigmented line along the gingival margin.

The floor of the mouth can be inspected by asking the child to lift the tongue to the roof of the mouth. Observe the frenulum, sublingual ridge, and Wharton ducts that lie on either side of the frenulum. The color of the floor of the mouth will be pink.

The *tongue* is inspected and palpated. The dorsum of the tongue should appear dull red, moist, and glistening, with a white coat. The anterior portion of the tongue should have a slightly roughened appearance with papillae and small fissures. The tongue is palpated for indurations or ulcerations. While palpating the mouth of a young child, biting can be prevented by holding the cheeks.

Cranial nerve XII (hypoglossal) is examined by asking the child to stick out the tongue as though he is going to lick a lollipop and observe for any deviation of the tongue to one side. Strength of the tongue can be determined by placing your finger in the side of the cheek and asking the child to press against your finger with his tongue. You should feel equal strength of the tongue on each side.

The *hard palate, soft palate,* and *uvula* are examined by asking the child to tilt his head back. Inspect the hard palate for shape and color. The hard palate is whitish in color and has a convex shape with transverse rugae. Palpate the hard palate for the height of the arch and intactness. Allow the infant to suck on your gloved finger while palpating the hard palate to determine strength of the sucking reflex. The soft palate is continuous with the hard palate and is concave and pinker in color. The uvula varies in length and thickness and is located in midline as a continuation of the soft palate. Cranial nerves IX (glossopharyngeal) and X (vagus) are evaluated at this time. The child is asked to say "ah"; normally, the soft palate rises symmetrically while the uvula remains in midline.

A tongue blade is used to depress the tongue and observe the *oropharynx.* This can be an unpleasant part of the exam for the child. To minimize discomfort, slide the tongue blade along the side of the tongue until you reach the soft palate, then compress the tongue to elicit the gag reflex (cranial nerve X) and observe the back of the throat. The tonsillar pillars are inspected with particular notation of size and color of tonsils. The tonsils are pink in color. Size of tonsils will vary; large tonsils in young children are common. Tonsils may have crypts where food particles collect. With inflammatory processes the crypts may contain exudate. A child whose parents complain of her snoring or a child who wakes herself up by snoring may have grossly enlarged tonsils. The posterior wall of the pharynx should be smooth and glistening pink; the wall may have small irregular spots of lymphatic tissue and small blood vessels (Seidel, 1995).

EYES

The eyes are inspected and palpated as well as evaluated for visual acuity and extraocular muscle function.

Visual Acuity

Visual acuity can be difficult to evaluate in a young child; it develops over a period of time and requires cooperation of the child. Equipment needed for evaluating visual acuity in a child are an eye cover and visual charts such as those described in the accompanying box. The chart chosen will be determined by the age and development of the child. The infant from birth to age 1 or 2 months will gaze at black and white contrasting figures and faces. At age 4 weeks or older an infant will fix on a bright colored object and follow it.

A child age 2 years may be able to identify pictures from a distance of 15 feet using Allen cards, depending on verbal ability. Each eye is tested separately. The child should be able to name three of seven cards in a maximum of five tries.

Preschool children can be tested using the HOTV chart at 10 feet. A card with HOTV is given to the child to hold, one eye is covered, the child is instructed to keep the eye covered and to match the letters on the chart at 10 feet with the letters held in her lap or on a table directly in front of her.

Older children's visual acuity can be tested using the Snellen chart. Place the chart on a wall 20 feet away from the child. There should be no glare on the chart and it should be well illuminated. No other materials should be around or near the chart. Both eyes are tested first, then each eye separately. If the child has corrective lenses the procedure should be repeated with the corrective lenses on. Unless the child is known to have very poor vision, testing is begun at the distance on the chart for 40 feet. A child must miss half plus one of the symbols on a line of the chart in order to determine at what level he cannot see. The visual acuity would then be designated as the smallest line at which the child is able to identify more than half of the symbols on a line. For corrective lenses, note the last date the child was examined for a prescription. Findings are recorded by noting the distance of the line correctly read for both eyes, i.e., right eye 20/20 and left eye 20/20. This means that the child has correctly interpreted the letters on the chart for 20 feet at a distance of 20 feet, which correlates to what the average child can see at that distance. If the child correctly identifies the letters on the line labeled 40 feet, this means that that child can see at 20 feet what the average child can see at 40 feet. Visual acuity changes with age and varies according to the test used:

Birth: Fixates on objects (8 to 12 in), 20/100–20/200
4 months: 20/50–20/80
1 year: 20/40–20/70
4 years: 20/30–20/40
5 years: 20/20 to 20/30

Color Vision

Color vision is evaluated using Ishihara's charts, a series of polychromatic cards. These cards have a pattern of colored pictures imbedded in the charts. Boys between ages 4 and 8 are asked to touch or identify the imbedded pictures.

Peripheral Vision

Visual fields are evaluated in older children to determine peripheral vision. The examiner's face is positioned directly in front and on the level of the child, about 2 feet away. The visual fields should roughly mirror the examiner's. Cover one eye and have the child mimic by covering the opposite eye. Slowly a puppet or some other test object is brought from the periphery into the field of vision. It is best to come from a position slightly behind the head and slowly bring the object from the periphery into the field of vision. The child is asked to say "now" when she sees the object (Fig. 11–10). Testing for visual acuity and visual fields evaluates cranial nerve II, the optic nerve, which mediates vision.

Binocular Vision and Strabismus

Extraocular muscle function is evaluated to test binocular vision and the presence of strabismus. Strabismus, or "crossed eyes," is the abnormal or incomplete development of binocular visual alignment. Three tests are performed: the corneal light reflex (Hirschberg) test, field of vision test, and the cover/uncover (alternate cover) test.

Corneal Light Reflex Test. The corneal light reflex is assessed by shining a light directly into the irises of the eyes from a distance of about 40.5 cm (16 inches). The reflection of the light should appear in exactly the same spot on both eyes. If the light falls off center in one eye, then the eyes are malaligned. Children with epicanthal folds (Fig. 11–11) may give a false impression of malalignment (pseudostrabismus).

Types of Eye Charts

Snellen chart: A standardized chart with graduated letters for testing far vision of children at 20 feet. Used with children over age 6 years.

Tumbling E (Snellen E): A standardized chart using the letter E in various directions, used with preschoolers age 3 to 6 years, for testing far vision at 20 feet. Also available for a distance of 10 feet.

Illiterate chart: A standardized chart with pictures, can be used with children age 3 to 6 years, for testing far vision at a distance of 20 feet.

HOTV chart: A standardized chart with graduated letters using HOTV. Designed for use at 10 feet with children age 3 to 6 years.

Allen cards: Picture cards of familiar objects for testing children $2\frac{1}{2}$ years and older. Vision is tested at a distance of 15 feet. If cooperative, may be used in children as young as 24 months.

Jaeger chart: Standardized chart with graduated letters for testing near vision at 12–14 inches from the eyes. Used with children over age 6 years.

Ishihara chart: A series of polychromatic cards with a pattern of dots printed against a background of many colored dots. Designed to test only boys for color vision between ages 4 and 8 years.

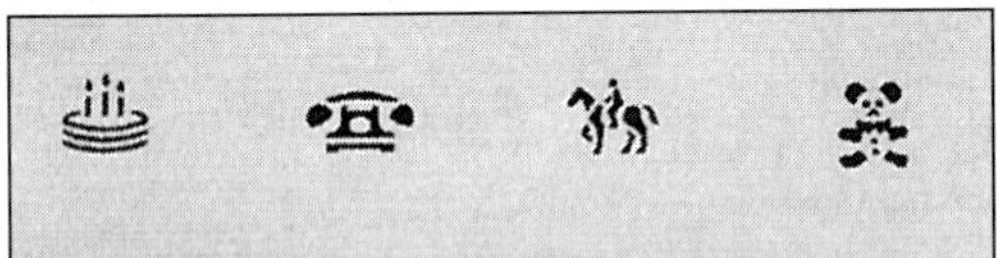

Allen cards, for testing preliterate children. (From Cassin, B. [1995]. *Fundamentals for ophthalmic technical personnel* [p. 160]. Philadelphia: W. B. Saunders.)

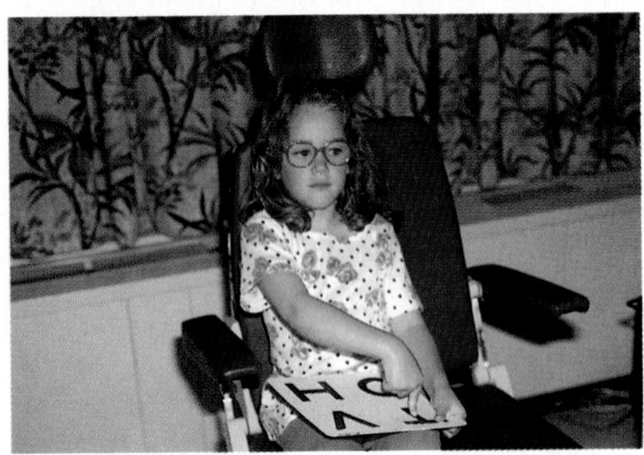

HOTV chart, for children ages 3 to 6 years. The letters H O T V are presented at a distance, and the child points to the corresponding letter on the card resting on her lap. (From Albert & Jakobiec [1994]. *Principles and practice of ophthalmology,* Vol. 4 [p. 2722]. Philadelphia: W. B. Saunders.)

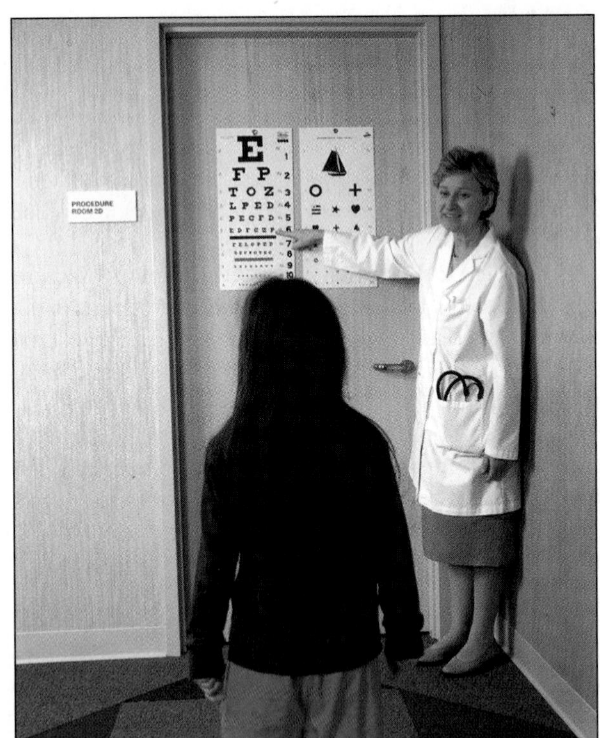

The standard Snellen E chart can be used for an older child who can read letters. The picture chart to the right of the Snellen chart can be used to assess vision in 3- to 6-year-olds. (From Jarvis, C. [1996]. *Physical examination and health assessment* [2nd ed., p. 329]. Philadelphia: W. B. Saunders.)

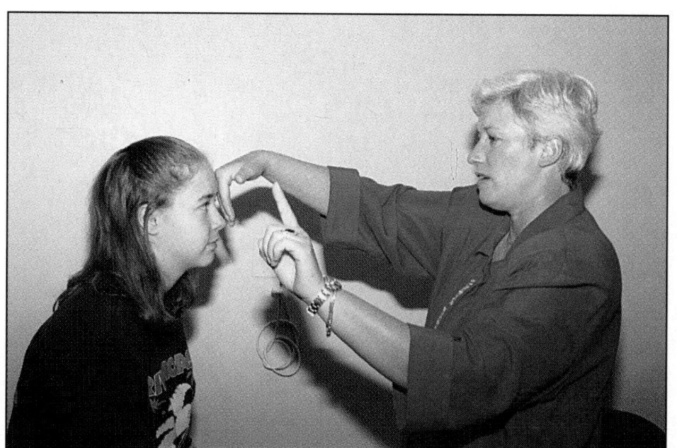

Figure 11–10
Visual fields (cranial nerve II) are tested in each eye separately. One eye is covered as the child stares straight ahead. An object is slowly moved from the side of the head into the field of vision. The child says "now" when the object is first seen.

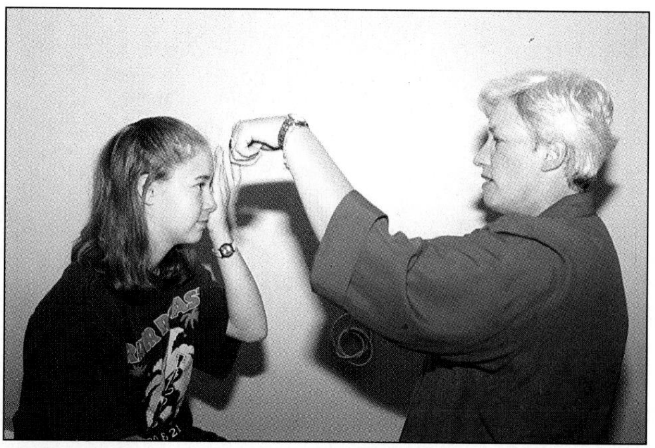

Figure 11–12
The cover/uncover test detects small degrees of deviated eye alignment. With one eye covered, the child gazes straight ahead with the uncovered eye. The cover is then removed and the eye should continue to stare straight ahead. Movement in either eye suggests muscle weakness. Extraocular muscle function is controlled by cranial nerves II, IV, and VI.

Field of Vision Test. The six cardinal fields of vision are tested by holding the child's chin so that the head does not move and asking the child to follow a puppet or a familiar object held approximately 12 inches away from the face with her eyes to each of the six cardinal positions. As the object is moved into the extreme of each cardinal position, it is held momentarily in that position before proceeding back to the center. The eyes will track in a parallel fashion to each position. As the eyes are in the extreme of each position it is possible to note *end-stage nystagmus,* or a gentle oscillation of the eye, which is considered normal.

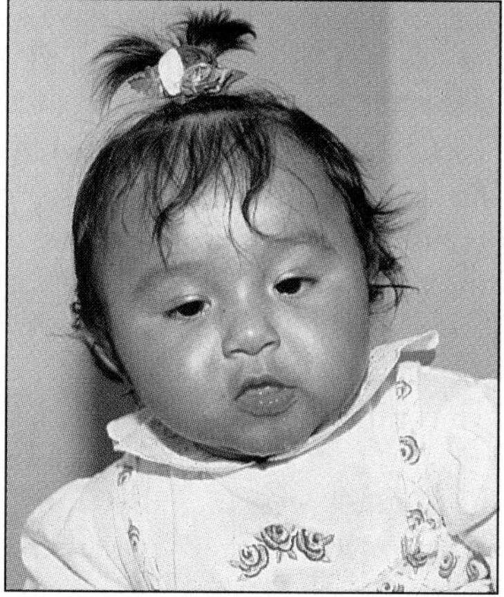

Figure 11–11
The eyes of a child with epicanthal folds may appear to be malaligned when the eyes are actually aligned properly. This characteristic is called *pseudostrabismus,* and is quite common in Asian children. (Courtesy of Dallas County Hospital District Community Oriented Primary Care Clinic, Dallas, Texas)

Young children under age 2 or 3 years may not be able too cooperate with this test.

Cover/Uncover Test. The cover/uncover test is used to detect small degrees of deviated alignment by interrupting fusion of the eyes as they gaze at a fixed object. One eye is covered with an opaque card while the child stares straight ahead, at which time the examiner observes the uncovered eye. A steady fixed gaze is maintained in the uncovered eye. Next the eye is uncovered and observed for any movement; it should continue to stare straight ahead (Fig. 11–12). The procedure is repeated with the opposite eye. Any movement in either eye in the process of covering or uncovering may indicate muscle weakness. Testing for extraocular muscle function in children under age 5 years is critical to determine if any muscle imbalance is present so that it can be corrected at an early age to preserve vision. Extraocular muscle function evaluates three cranial nerves: cranial nerve VI, the abducent, which innervates the lateral rectus muscle (responsible for abducting the eye); cranial nerve IV, the trochlear nerve, which innervates the superior oblique muscle (responsible for down and inward movement of the eye); and cranial nerve III, the oculomotor nerve, which innervates the superior, inferior, and medial rectus and the inferior oblique muscles (Nelson et al., 1991).

External Eye

The external eye (Fig. 11–13) is evaluated for position and placement. It is noted whether the eyes are set wide apart or close together. *Epicanthal folds* are vertical folds that

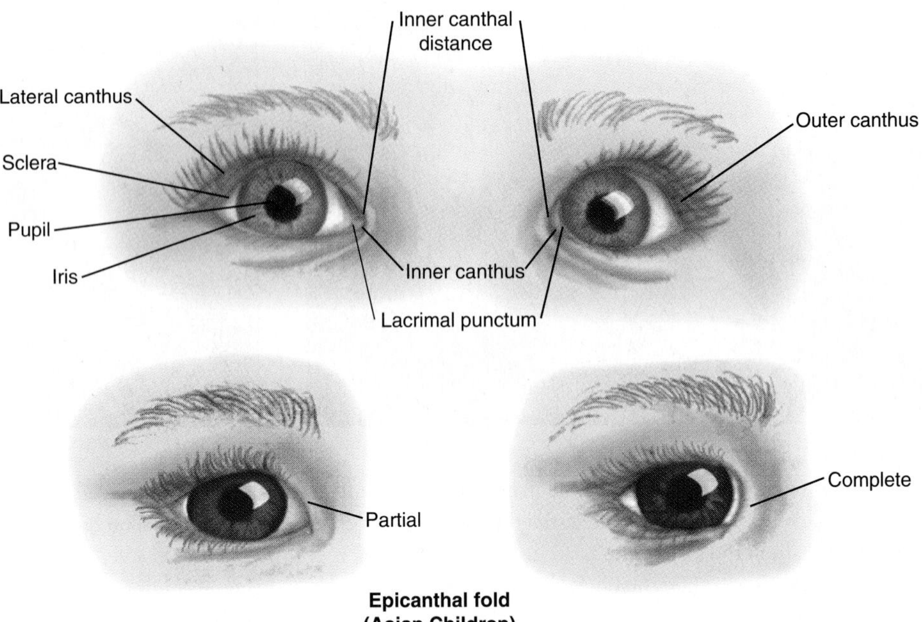

Figure 11–13
External structures of the eye.

partially or completely cover the inner canthi. Epicanthal folds are seen in Asian children and in some non-Asian children (see Fig. 11–11). The slant of the eyes is determined by drawing an imaginary line across the inner canthi.

The *eyebrows* are inspected for symmetry and hair growth. The *eyelashes* are inspected for even distribution.

The *lacrimal apparatus* is assessed by asking the child to look down. The outer part of the upper lid is palpated along the bony orbit for any discomfort, swelling, or the presence of any redness. The puncta (tear duct) on the inner canthus of the eye is palpated for obstruction in the infant.

The eye globe is palpated for firmness and can be gently pushed into the orbit without causing discomfort. Palpation of the eye may cause anxiety in small children and should not be done unless there is a serious concern about the size of the eye.

Eyelids are inspected for color, swelling, discharge, and lesions. The position of the eyelids is noted on the globe. With the eyelids open, the upper lid normally falls below the superior limbus, but does not cover any of the pupil of the eye. The lower lids normally fall just at the inferior limbus. The limbus is where the sclera of the eye meets the color portion of the iris. When closed, the eyelids approximate each other completely and there should be no tremor, fasciculations, or tics.

There are two portions of the *conjunctiva* to evaluate. The palpebral portion of the conjunctiva lines the lids. The palpebral conjunctiva is examined by pulling down as the child looks up. It is normally clear, with a pink color, and may have several small blood vessels visible. The upper lid can be inspected by everting the upper eyelid over a cotton-tipped applicator. Eversion of the upper eyelid is not normally done because eye manipulation may cause apprehension in a child. The bulbar portion of the conjunctivae is transparent and lies over the sclerae, allowing the white of the sclerae to be clearly visible.

The following anterior structures of the eye are inspected: sclerae, cornea and lens, anterior chamber, and irises. The sclerae are white. Dark skinned children may have small brown macules or they may have a gray-blue or "muddy" color, particularly at the limbus of the eye, which is normal. The corneas are clear and transparent. The shining of a light across the cornea obliquely highlights any abnormal irregularities on the corneal surface. Illuminate the anterior chamber by shining a light across the eye from the temporal side to illuminate the entire iris without producing a shadow. The irises are round, regular shaped, and clear. The color of the irises are similar; however, it is not uncommon to have some variation between them.

Pupils appear round, regular, and of equal size in both eyes. *Pupillary light reflex* is tested by darkening the room and asking the child to gaze into the distance. A light is brought from the side (temporally) and the change in the size of the pupil is noted. Shining a light directly into a pupil will cause the pupil to constrict (direct light reflex). The procedure is repeated while the opposite eye is observed. The opposite eye will constrict (consensual light reflex) in response to the light being shone in the other eye. Pupil size should be the same in both eyes (in some children, pupils of unequal size are normal, but in general, unequal pupils call for a consideration of central nervous system injury). The speed by which the pupils constrict should be equal. Accommodation can be tested by asking the child to focus on a distant object. The pupils normally dilate. An object such as a puppet or a finger brought into the line of vision about 7 to 8 cm from the nose should cause pupillar constriction and convergence of the axes of the eyes (Nelson et al., 1991).

A recording of "PERRLA" means that the pupils are equal in size, round in shape, and reactive to light and accommodation.

Ophthalmoscopic Examination

The ophthalmoscopic examination requires a cooperative child, practice, and patience. Lights in the room will need to be dim. Most children will enjoy playing with the light of the "flashlight" and watching the light as you move it around the room and facilitates their cooperation. Minimally all practitioners will view the red reflex. The procedure for examining the red reflex is to darken the room, position the child in front of the examiner, and ask the child to gaze straight ahead. The child is approached from a distance of 30.5 cm (12 inches) on the temporal side of the eye. The ophthalmoscope is gradually moved across the eye until it crosses the pupil. When the light from the ophthalmoscope focuses on the pupil, the pupil will glow back with a bright red color. The child's right eye is examined with the examiner's right hand and right eye, the left eye with the left hand and left eye. The retina, choroid, optic disk, macula, fovea centralis, and retinal vessels are also visualized with the ophthalmoscope.

EARS

Assessment of the ears includes testing for hearing acuity, inspection and palpation of the external ear, and visualization of the internal ear using the otoscope.

Hearing Acuity

Infant Assessment. In an infant, hearing is assessed by asking the mother to speak to the infant from behind and observing the infant's response to the mother's voice. The examiner can stand behind the infant and ring a bell or make a sound the infant is familiar with and observe the infant turning to locate the sound. A very young infant, younger than age 4 months, may demonstrate a startle reflex to loud sounds.

Preschool and School-Age Assessment by Audiometer. In preschool and school-age children the audiometer gives a precise (quantitative) assessment of the child's ability to hear. The child is placed in a soundproof room and is asked to identify tones played at a level the child can hear. Two tests are used to evaluate hearing using the audiometer: the sweep test and the pure tone hearing test. The *sweep test* is used to screen for hearing losses. Headphones are placed on the child's ears and sounds of a different pitch (Hz) are introduced into each ear separately at a specific level of loudness (decibel level). The child is instructed to raise his hand in response to recognizing the sound.

The *pure tone test* is used to determine the exact extent of the hearing loss. A pitch is introduced into each ear and the exact level of loudness (decibel level) is determined at which the child hears each tone by moving the decibel level up by 5 decibels and then down 5 decibels until each tone is correctly identified.

School-Age and Adolescent Assessment: The Whisper Test. The whisper test is performed on school-age children and adolescents. The child is asked to cover one ear or occlude one ear canal and to repeat what is heard as the examiner stands about 0.3 m (1 foot) behind or to the side of the child.

For a preschool child the examiner stands in front of the child approximately 0.6 to 0.9 m (2 to 3 feet) and gives the child a command such as "Please put the toy on the floor."

Conduction Tests (Tuning Fork Hearing Tests). Tuning fork tests are qualitative tests to determine the ability to hear by air conduction and by bone conduction (Fig. 11–14). In the normal child air conduction is greater than bone conduction. The *Rinne* hearing test is used to determine if air conduction is greater than bone conduction (AC > BC). To perform this test, the tuning fork is struck on the back of the hand or on the fatty part of the hand to activate the sound. Bone conduction is tested by placing the tuning fork on the child's mastoid process and the child is asked to tell the examiner when she no longer hears the tone. Air conduction is assessed as the tuning fork is quickly removed from the mastoid process and held in front of the ear canal and the child is asked to tell when she no longer hears the tone. The examiner counts the seconds for each test. Air conduction should be greater than bone conduction by a ratio of two to one.

The *Weber* hearing test determines the child's ability to hear by bone conduction. The tuning fork is activated and placed on the middle of the skull or directly in the midline on the top of the forehead, and the child is asked

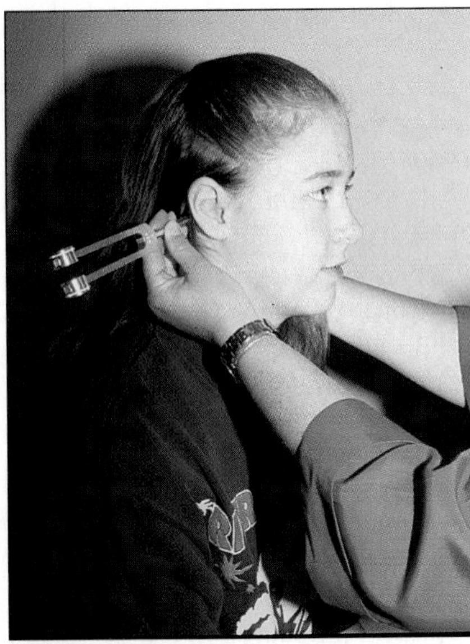

◀ Rinne Test, Step I. The Rinne test uses a tuning fork to compare hearing by bone conduction and air conduction. In the first step, the tuning fork is struck to activate the sound and then placed on the mastoid process. The child is asked to tell you when the sound ceases as you count the seconds (bone conduction).

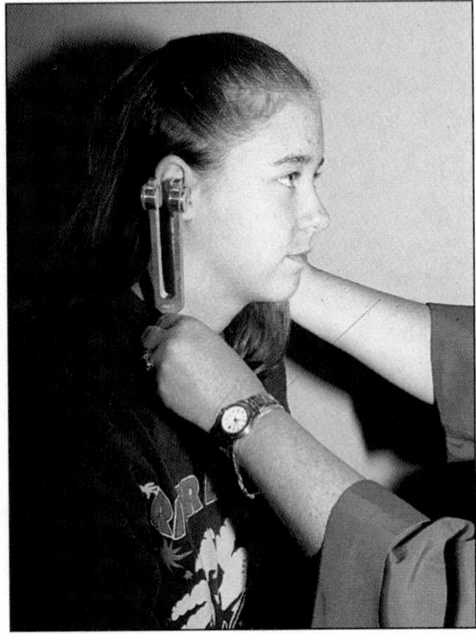

◀ Rinne Test, Step II. The fork is then quickly inverted and placed in front of the ear canal, and the child is again asked to tell you when the sound ceases as you count the seconds (air conduction). The sound is normally heard twice as long by air conduction as by bone conduction.

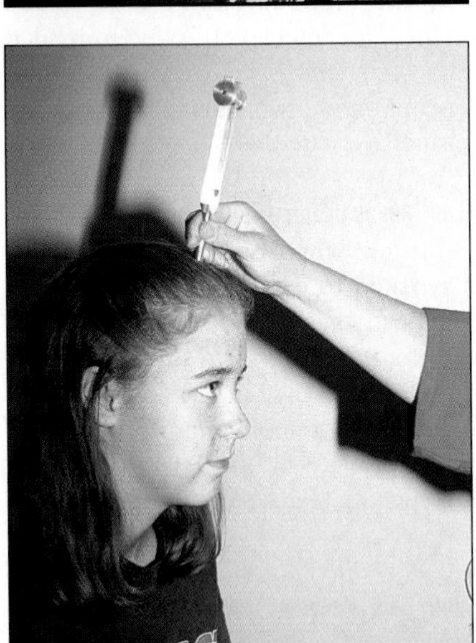

◀ Weber Test. Bone conduction of sound is further assessed by placing a vibrating tuning fork on the head in the midline. The child is asked if the sound is louder in one ear than in the other. Sound should be equal in both ears if bone conduction is equal. Hearing tests evaluate cranial nerve VIII function.

Figure 11–14
Hearing tests using the tuning fork: Rinne and Weber tests.

if the tone sounds louder in one ear than the other. Sound is transmitted by bone conduction equally well to both ears.

Testing the child's hearing evaluates cranial nerve VIII (acoustic) (Fuller & Schalley-Ayers, 1994).

The External Ear

The external ear is inspected and palpated. Ear placement and position were evaluated when assessing the face. (See the section of inspection of the face.) The external ear is examined for any malformations or unusual markings (Fig. 11–15). Any discharge coming from the auditory meatus is noted, and its amount and characteristics are described. Soft yellow-brown cerumen (earwax) is normally seen in the external auditory meatus.

The bony prominence of the mastoid process behind the ear is palpated for tenderness. The auricles are gently pulled to determine if discomfort is created.

Otoscopic Examination

The *tympanic membrane* is examined by using the otoscope (Fig. 11–16). Many children may be apprehensive about this examination. If necessary, a small child is positioned on the parent's lap and the child's arms are

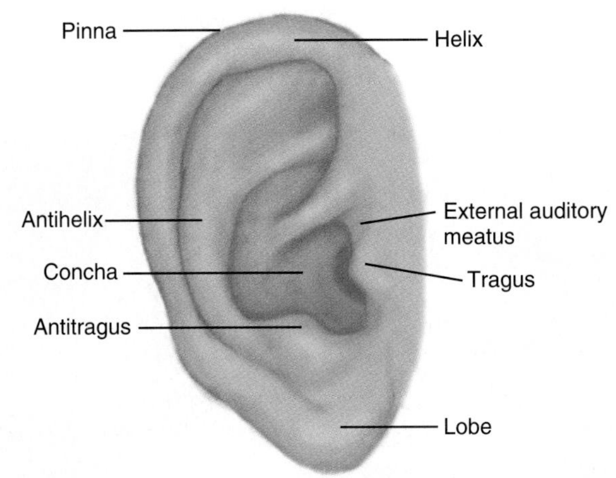

Figure 11–15
Landmarks of the external ear.

secured. The largest speculum that will fit comfortably into the ear canal is used. In a child younger than age 3 years the ear canal is straightened by pulling the pinna of the ear down and back. If a child is age 3 years or older, the pinna is pulled up and back. As much of the canal as possible should be visualized before inserting the speculum into the auditory meatus. The canal is inspected for any lesions and the presence of cerumen. The tympanic membrane is inspected for landmarks, color, and mobility. With an insufflation bulb, a puff of air is injected into the canal and the tympanic membrane is observed for movement. Normally the tympanic membrane moves inward with a slight puff and outward with a slight release.

THORAX AND LUNGS

Assessment of the thorax and lungs consists of inspection, palpation, percussion, and auscultation, in that order. To assist with localizing findings on the thorax, anatomic landmarks such as the ribs and intercostal spaces are determined and imaginary lines are drawn on the surface (Fig. 11–17). Location of lung tissue will depend on the age and development of the child. On the anterior chest lung tissue of an infant can be located from the apex, above the clavicle, to the level of the fifth rib in the midclavicular line. By age 6 years lung tissue is assessed from the apex to the level of the sixth rib in the midclavicular line. Laterally lung tissue is assessed from the axilla to the level of the eighth rib. Posteriorly lungs are assessed from the level of the first thoracic vertebra to the tenth thoracic vertebra.

Inspection

The child's shirt or clothing covering the chest is removed. In adolescent females the breasts should be kept covered, exposing only when necessary. Inspection of the chest includes observing the child for any cough, stridor, grunting, hoarseness, snoring, wheezing, and type and amount of any sputum if present. *Respiratory rate and pattern* are observed. In young children and infants breathing is more diaphragmatic or abdominal. (See Table 11–1 for the effect of age on vital signs.) Expansion of the chest wall should be symmetrical during respiration. Respirations should be easy, regular, and without apparent distress.

Thoracic configuration is evaluated by determining the shape and symmetry of the chest from the front, sides, and back. Two common alterations in structure in the anterior chest are *pectus carinatum* (pigeon breast) and *pectus excavatum* (funnel breast) (Fig. 11–18).

Palpation

Palpation of the chest begins with the posterior chest. To alleviate fear in a young child the examiner stands in a position that allows the child to see her at all times. The posterior chest is palpated for areas of tenderness, tactile fremitus, and chest excursion.

To palpate for tenderness the examiner touches the entire thorax with the palmar aspects of the fingers to elicit any points of discomfort or pain and to note any masses or edema (Fig. 11–19).

To evaluate for *tactile fremitus* the examiner palpates the chest wall while the child speaks the words "ninety-nine." Vibrations felt on the chest wall are the result of vibrations that are produced in the vocal cords and transmitted to the chest wall via the respiratory tract.

Percussion of the chest is performed by advanced practitioners to determine changes in sound produced by the density of the underlying tissues.

Auscultation

Auscultation of the chest is done to determine the characteristics of breath sounds heard with a stethoscope. Breath sounds heard with the stethoscope are made by the flow of air through the respiratory tree and are characterized by intensity, pitch, quality, and duration (Table 11–2).

It is best to listen to breath sounds with the child sitting upright, if possible. Infants and toddlers can be held in the parent's lap; have the parent assist with removal of clothing and positioning of the child (Fig. 11–20). Position yourself to the side, allowing the child to observe your movements.

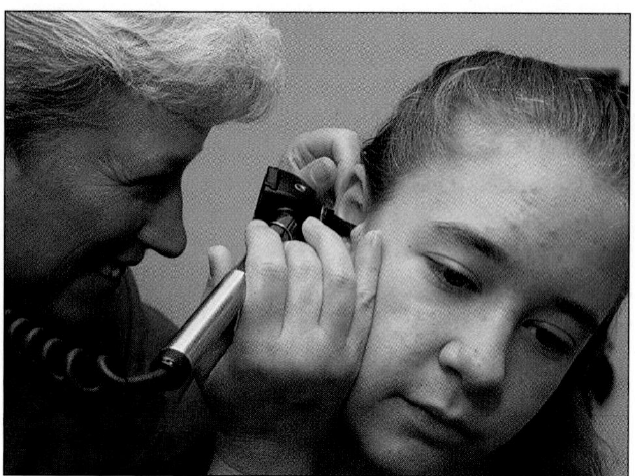

◀ To straighten the ear canal for assessment, the nurse pulls the child's pinna up and back if he or she is over age 3 years.

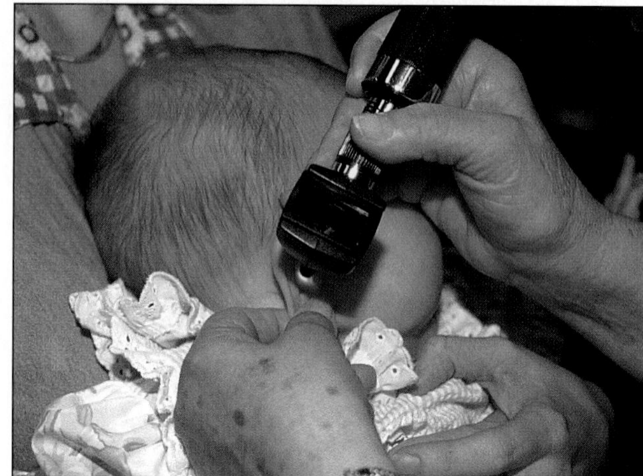

For children under age 3 years, the pinna is pulled down ▶ and back.

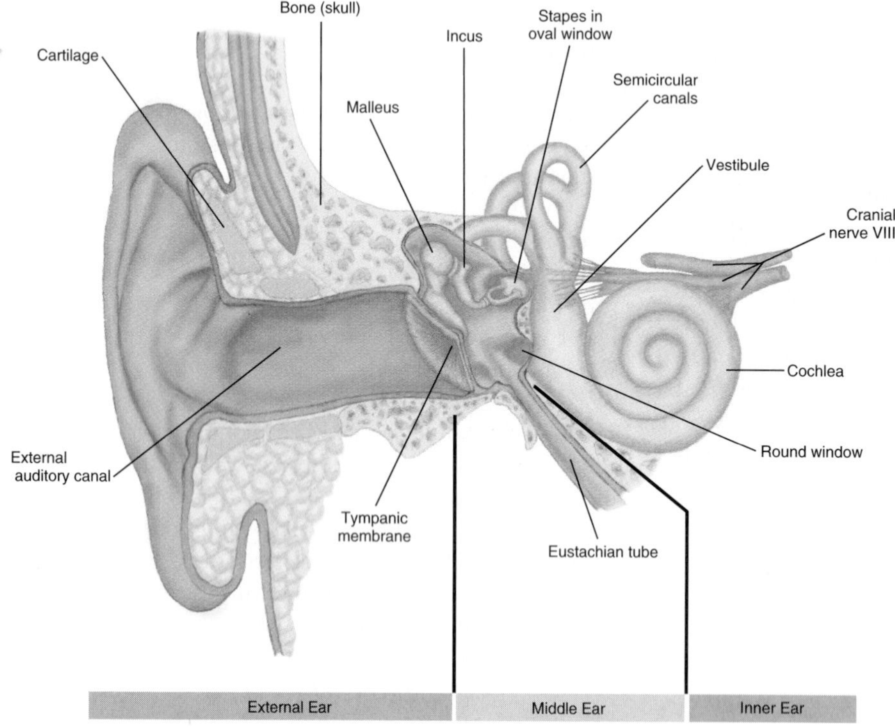

◀ Structures of the ear.

Landmarks of the tympanic membrane. ▶

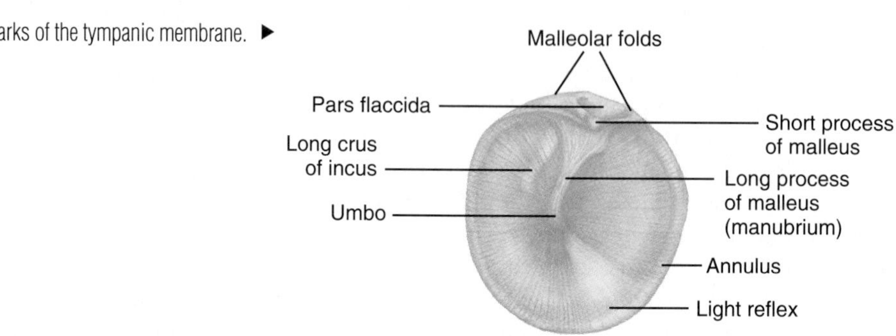

Figure 11–16

Inspection of the tympanic membrane using the otoscope. The auditory canal is inspected before inserting the otoscope to visualize the child's tympanic membrane.

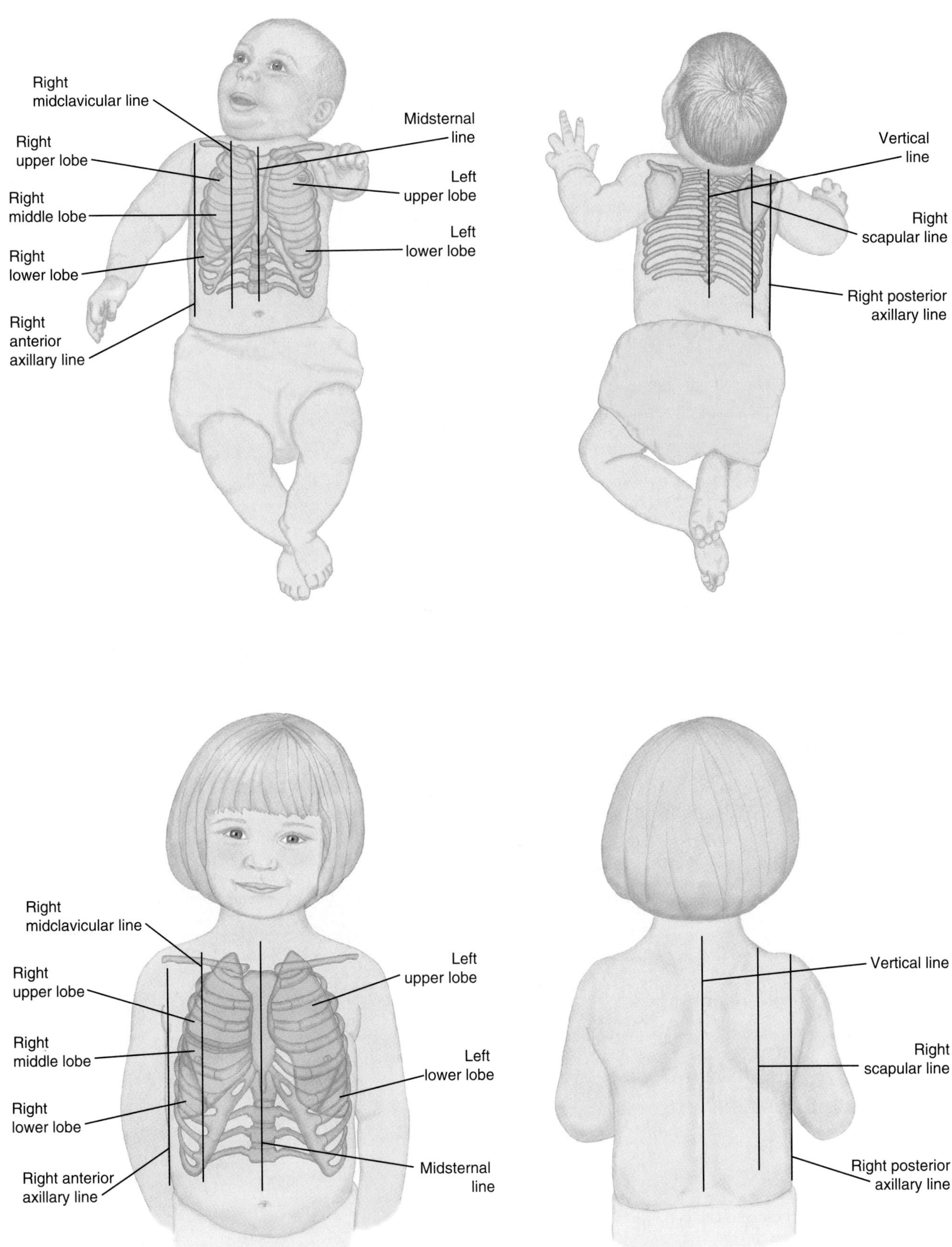

Figure 11–17

Anatomic landmarks of the thorax in infants and children.

Normal Infant

The chest of the normal infant is approximately round or barrel-shaped in cross-section. A barrel chest in a child older than 6 years suggests a chronic pulmonary disease such as asthma or cystic fibrosis.

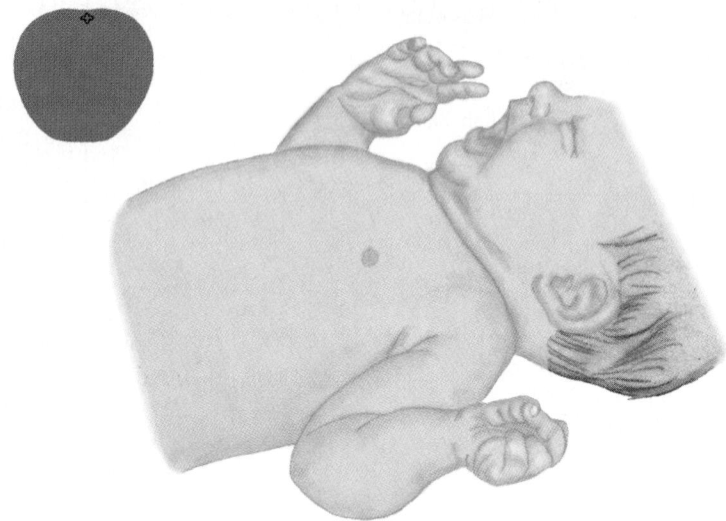

Funnel Chest (Pectus Excavatum)

A funnel chest has a depression in the lower portion of the sternum. Compression of the heart and great vessels may cause murmurs.

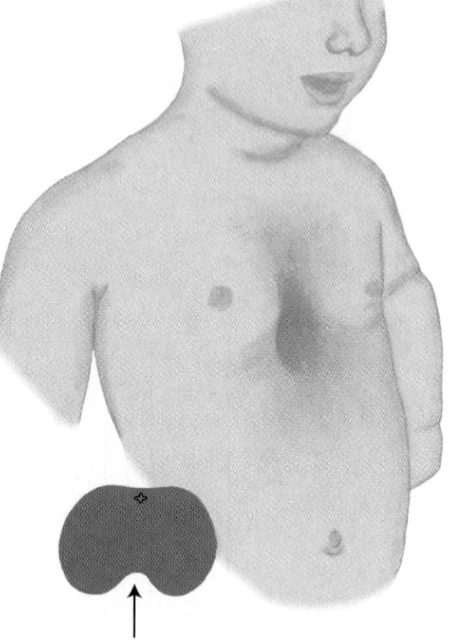

Pigeon Chest (Pectus Carinatum)

In pigeon chest, the sternum is displaced anteriorly, increasing the anteroposterior diameter. Grooves in the chest wall accentuate the deformity.

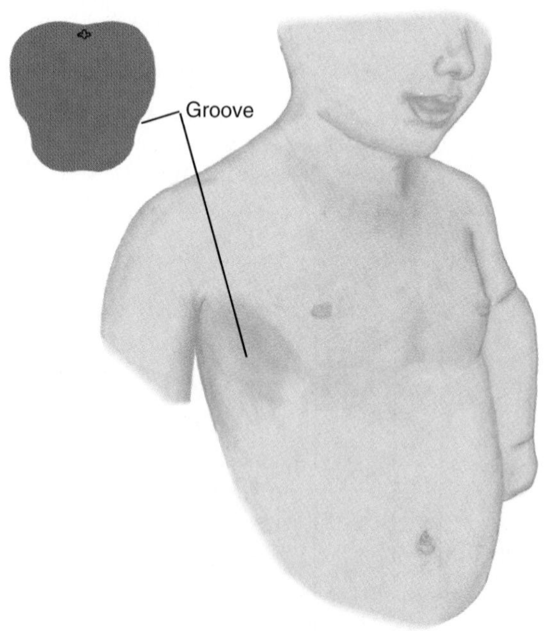

Figure 11–18
Common alterations in chest configuration.

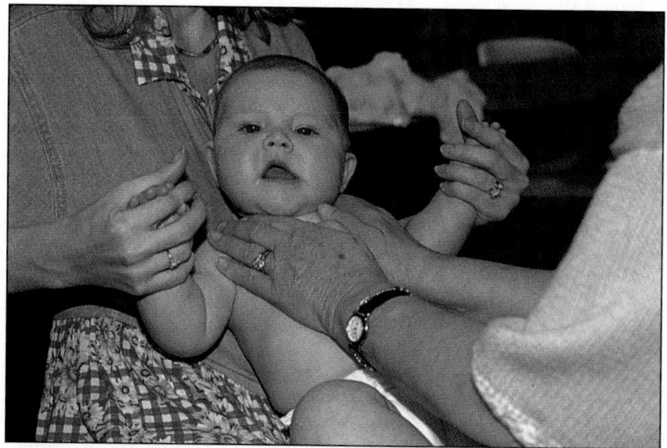

Figure 11–19
The nurse palpates the child's posterior and anterior chest to identify areas of fremitus, tenderness, symmetry, and depth and equality of expansion. When palpating any area, warm hands increase the child's comfort. (Courtesy of University of Texas at Arlington School of Nursing, Arlington, Texas)

Before touching the chest, allow the young child to hold or play with the stethoscope. Warm the stethoscope before placing it on the child's chest. An anxious or frightened child may cry during this part of the examination. Distracting the child or having the young child focus on another activity may facilitate listening. For the inconsolable child, listen to breath sounds between each cry. If the young child is sleeping or comfortable in the parent's arms, listen to the chest first before proceeding to the rest of the exam.

The position of the child for listening to the posterior thorax is with the head bent forward and hands folded in front. To listen laterally, have the child raise the arms overhead while sitting erect. To auscultate the anterior chest, have the child sit erect with the shoulders back.

The examiner begins on the posterior thorax and has the child open the mouth and breathe in and out while he listens with the diaphragm of the stethoscope. Having the young child blow bubbles, pretend to blow out birthday candles, or blow a tissue will increase breath sounds. Compressing the hand holding the stethoscope on the chest wall and placing the other hand on the opposite side of the chest accentuates expiration and makes end-expiratory sounds (e.g., wheezes) easier to hear. The sequence for listening to breath sounds is posterior chest, right and left lateral chest, and anterior chest (Fig. 11–21).

Adventitious Breath Sounds. In addition to hearing normal breath sounds it is possible to hear adventitious sounds with the stethoscope. Adventitious sounds are additional sounds heard when there is an abnormal clinical state. Adventitious sounds are described by their quality, whether they are continuous or discontinuous, where they occur in the respiratory phase, and the effects of coughing. When adventitious sounds are heard, they are described as to their location, timing, and intensity. Table 11–3 describes the origin and characteristics of adventitious sounds (Bates, 1991).

HEART

The techniques used for assessing the heart are inspection, palpation, and auscultation. The sequence of this examination depends on the age, growth, and development of the child being examined. For an infant or young child the examiner may want to listen to the child's heart while the parent is holding the child, before doing other parts of the examination. Infants and children have varying independent and dependent needs on the parent and may be fearful of the examination. Percussion of the heart primarily indicates the size and shape of the heart and is not routinely done. The heart is assessed with the child in a supine position, left lateral recumbent, and sitting up and leaning forward slightly.

TABLE 11–2 *Characteristics of Breath Sounds*

CHARACTERISTICS	TRACHEAL	BRONCHIAL	BRONCHOVESICULAR	VESICULAR
Intensity	Very loud	Loud	Moderate	Soft
Pitch	Very high	High	Moderate	Low
I:E Ratio	1:1	1:3	1:1	3:1
Description	Harsh	Tubular	Rustling, but tubular	Gentle rustling
Normal locations	Extrathoracic trachea	Manubrium	Over mainstem bronchi	Most of peripheral lung
Diagram Inspiration Expiration	/\	/\	/\	/\

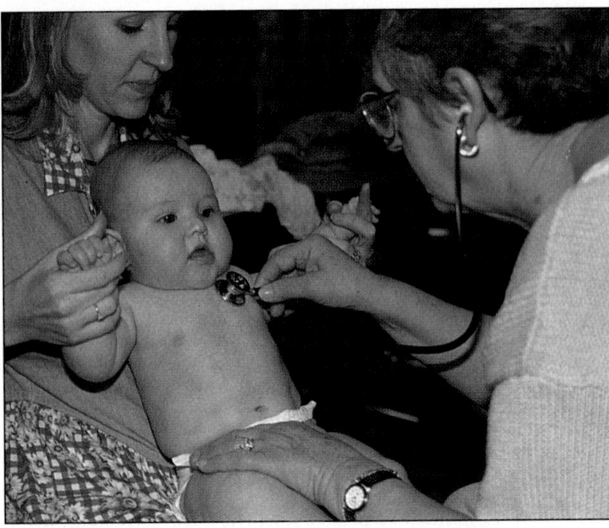

◀ Infants and toddlers can be held sitting upright in the parent's lap while the nurse listens to breath sounds.

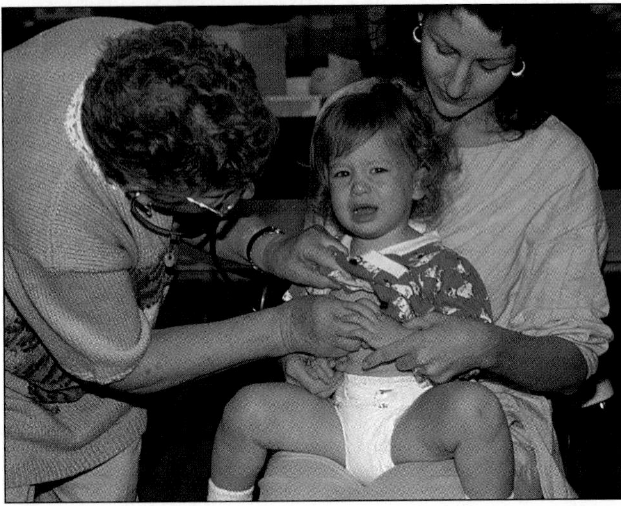

If the child is upset, you may have to listen to breath ▶ sounds between cries. Keeping her in the comfort of her mother's arms lessens her distress.

Figure 11–20
The nurse auscultates the child's chest with a stethoscope in an orderly way to hear heart and breath sounds. Auscultation is best performed when the child is quiet, so do this part of the examination first if the child is quiet or asleep. To allay the child's fears and make the examination more comfortable, allow the child to play with the stethoscope first and warm the instrument. The child also can be distracted with a toy while listening. (Photos courtesy of University of Texas at Arlington School of Nursing, Arlington, Texas)

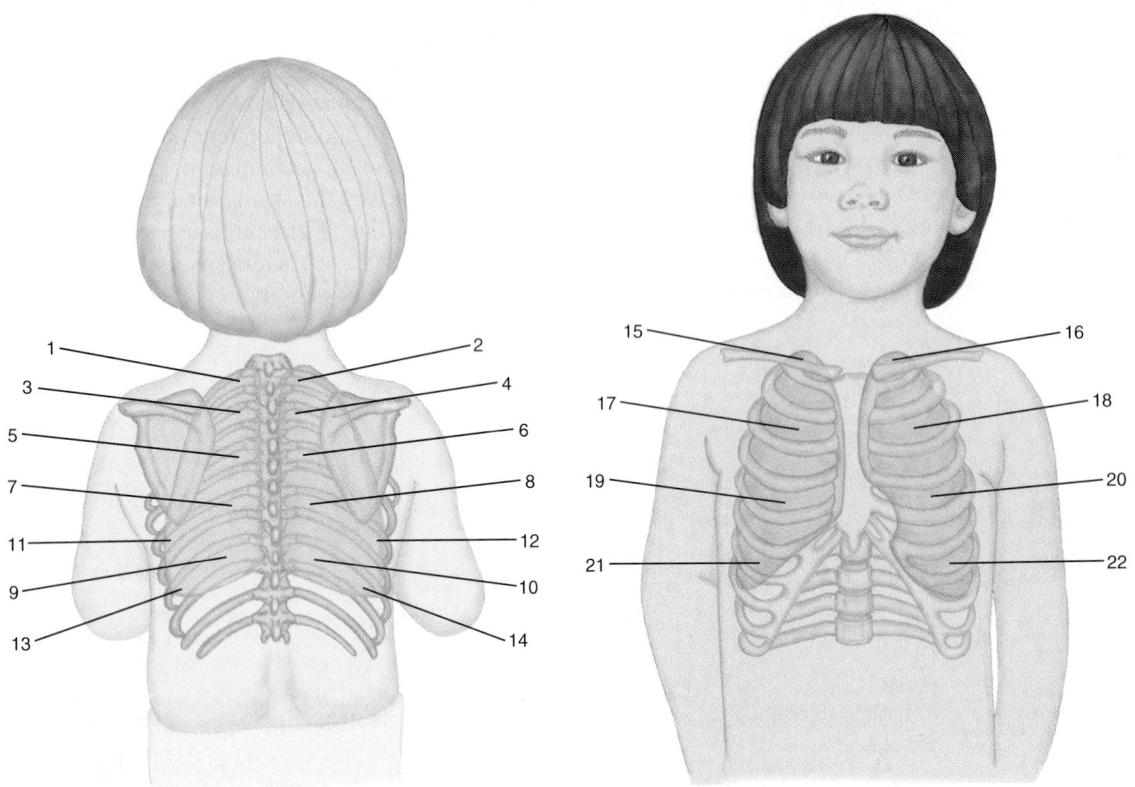

Figure 11–21
Sequence for listening to breath sounds.

TABLE 11–3 *Origin and Characteristics of Adventitious Breath Sounds**

SOUND	DESCRIPTION	MECHANISM	CLINICAL EXAMPLE
Discontinuous Sounds			
Crackles—fine (rales, crepitations); heard when fluid is in airways.	Discontinuous, high-pitched, short crackling, popping sounds heard during inspiration that are not cleared by coughing. You can simulate this sound by rolling a strand of hair between your fingers near your ear, or by moistening your thumb and index finger and separating them near your ear. Described as discrete (short), discontinuous.	Inhaled air collides with previously deflated airways; airways suddenly pop open, creating crackling sound as gas pressures between the two compartments equalize.	*Late inspiratory crackles* occur with restrictive disease: pneumonia, congestive heart failure, and interstitial fibrosis. *Early inspiratory crackles* occur with obstructive disease: chronic bronchitis and asthma.
Pleural friction rub.	A very superficial sound that is coarse and low-pitched; it has a grating quality as if two pieces of leather are being rubbed together. Sounds just like crackles, but close to the ear. Sounds louder if you push the stethoscope harder onto the chest wall.	Caused when pleurae become inflamed and lose their normal lubricating fluid. Their opposing roughened pleural surfaces rub together during respiration. Heard best in anterolateral wall where there is greatest lung mobility.	Pleuritis, accompanied by pain with breathing. (Rub disappears after a few days if pleural fluid accumulates and separates pleurae.)
Continuous Sounds			
Wheeze—high-pitched; heard when there is a narrowing of the air passages due to fluid, swelling, spasm, and tumors.	High-pitched, musical squeaking sounds that predominate in expiration but may occur in both expiration and inspiration. Coughing frequently will change the character of the sound.	Air squeezed or compressed through passageways narrowed almost to closure by collapsing, swelling, secretions, or tumors. The passageway walls oscillate in apposition between the closed and barely open positions. The resulting sound is similar to a vibrating reed.	Obstructive lung disease such as asthma.
Wheeze—low-pitched (sonorous rhonchi)	Low-pitched, musical snoring, moaning sounds. They are heard throughout the cycle, although they are more prominent on expiration. May clear somewhat by coughing.	Airflow obstruction as described by the vibrating reed mechanism above. The pitch of the wheeze cannot be correlated to the size of the passageway that generates it.	Bronchitis.

*Although nothing in clinical practice seems to differ more than the nomenclature of adventitious sounds, most authorities concur on two categories: (1) discontinuous, discrete crackling sounds; and (2) continuous, coarse, or wheezing sounds.

Inspection

The anterior chest is systematically inspected, paying special attention to the following five areas: second right intercostal space (aortic area), second left intercostal space (pulmonic area), left sternal border (right ventricular area), fifth left intercostal space in the midclavicular line (apex), and just below the xiphoid process (epigastric area). The areas will differ at different ages (Fig. 11–22).

During infancy the heart is more horizontal in the thorax and the apex is one or two intercostal spaces above the fifth intercostal space and lateral to the midclavicular line. The second intercostal space is located by identifying the sternal angle. The second rib is attached to the sternum just below or at the sternal angle. The second intercostal space is below the second rib. Other ribs and intercostal spaces are identified by their relationship to the second rib.

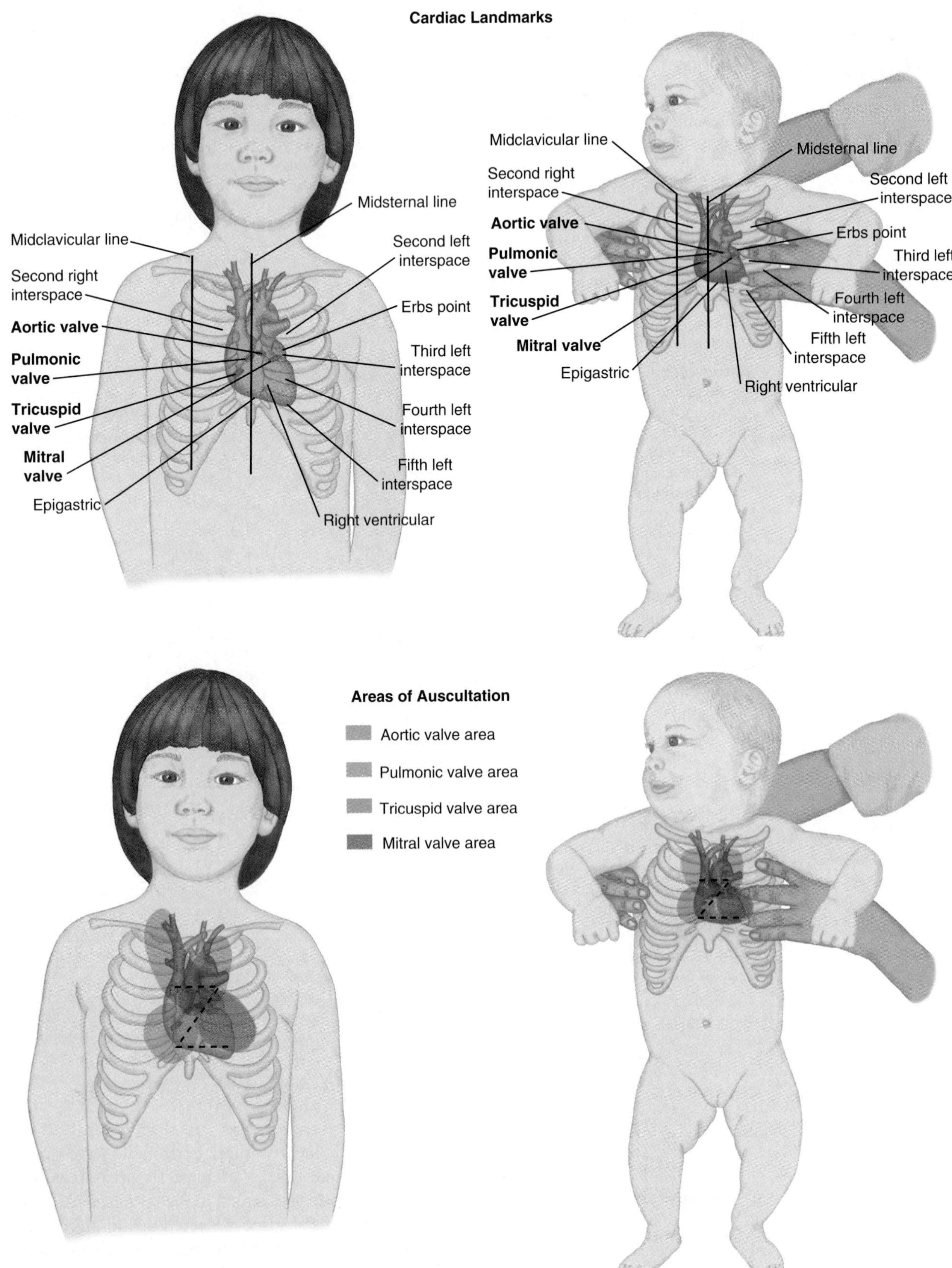

Figure 11–22

Location of the heart within the thorax in the infant and the older child, showing landmarks and areas of auscultation.

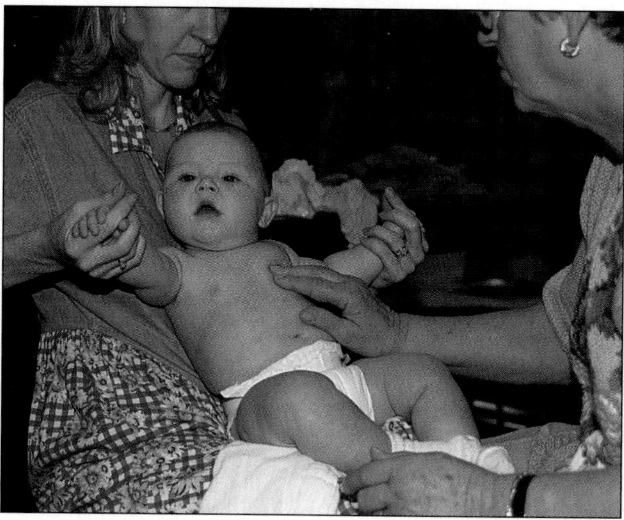

◀ The nurse uses her fingertips to identify areas of tenderness, masses, or edema on the chest. The fingertips are also used to palpate pulsations and to identify the point of maximal impulse (PMI) where light tapping of the heart is best felt.

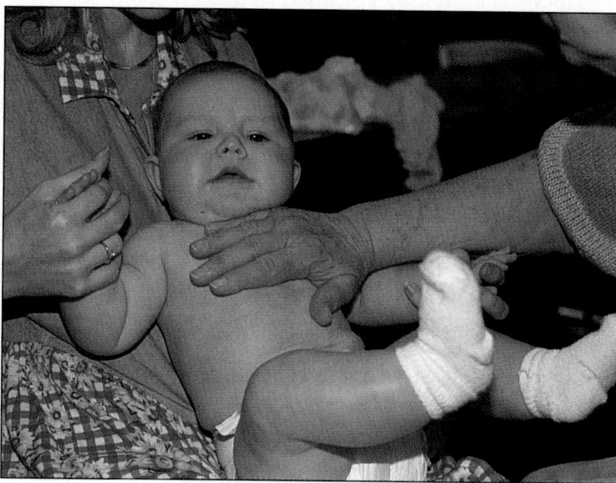

The palmar surface of the hand is used to palpate each area of the precordium to identify thrills, which are palpable vibrations of the heart. ▶

Figure 11–23

Palpation of the chest. (Photos courtesy of University of Texas at Arlington School of Nursing.)

The precordium (anterior chest overlying the heart and great vessels) is inspected for *bulges, lifts, heaves,* and *apical impulse.* The apical impulse is the light tapping of the anterior chest wall every time the heart beats. The location of the apical impulse will change gradually as the child matures and by age 7 years can be seen at the fifth intercostal space in the midclavicular line.

Palpation

The precordium is then palpated at each individual area with the fingertips for the presence of any pulsations (Fig. 11–23). The examiner will identify the exact location of the apical pulse. The apical impulse is sometimes identified as the point of maximal impulse (PMI), or the point where the light tapping of the heart is felt the best. The examiner will then palpate each individual area of the precordium using the palmar aspect of the hand to feel for *thrills.* Thrills are palpable vibrations of the heart (see Fig. 11–23).

Auscultation

Auscultation of the heart is done by listening both with the bell and the diaphragm of the stethoscope with the child lying down, in a left lateral recumbent position, and sitting up. To auscultate heart sounds the examiner uses a systematic approach. Sounds heard with the stethoscope are predominantly the sounds produced with the closing of the heart valves. The four traditional areas for listening to the heart sounds are aortic valve area, second right intercostal space; pulmonic valve area, second left intercostal space; tricuspid valve area, left lower sternal border; and mitral valve area, fifth intercostal space at the left midclavicular line (see Fig. 11–22). The position for listening to these areas will be slightly different depending on the age of the child. It is best to listen to the heart sounds by inching the stethoscope across the precordium in a "Z" pattern, from the base of the heart across and down, or from the apex upward. All areas are listened to with both the bell and the diaphragm of the stethoscope.

Sounds produced by the closing of the valves can be heard all over the precordium, so it will be necessary to concentrate on one heart sound at a time.

The heart sounds are divided into two components: the first heart sound (S_1) and the second heart sound (S_2). S_1 is heard best at the apex of the heart and S_2 is heard best at the base. S_1, phonetically described as *Lub,* is produced by the closing of the mitral and tricuspid valves. S_2, phonetically described as *Dub,* is produced by the closing of the aortic and pulmonic valves and is heard best at the base of the heart.

The routine for assessing heart sounds is as follows:

ROUTINE FOR ASSESSING HEART SOUNDS

1. Identify the rate and rhythm.
2. Identify S_1 and S_2.
3. Assess S_1 and S_2 separately to determine where they are heard best.
4. Listen for extra heart sounds.
5. Identify murmurs.

Normal Rate and Rhythm. The normal rate of a child's heart will be different for different ages (see Table 11–1). Children's heart rates will often increase with inspiration and slow down during expiration. Having the child hold his breath as you continue to listen will decrease the irregular rhythm associated with respirations.

S_1 and S_2. S_1 is best heard at the apex and is usually heard as one sound. It is lower in pitch and longer than S_2 and signals the beginning of diastole. S_2 is heard best at the base of the heart and is louder than S_1 at the base of the heart. S_2 signals the beginning of diastole.

The physiologic splitting of S_2, an audible pause between the closing of the aortic and pulmonic valves, is frequently heard in children of all ages and is considered a normal event. Splitting of S_2 can be heard best at the pulmonic area because ejection times on the right side of the heart are slightly longer than on the left side. Splitting of S_2 is greatest at the peak of inspiration and decreases or goes away during expiration.

Extra Heart Sounds, Including Murmurs. Extra sounds, heard over and above the normal heart sounds, may be described as opening snaps, ejection clicks, mid-to-late systolic clicks, and murmurs. Snaps and clicks are short, high-pitched sounds heard with valve disorders and do not vary with respirations. *Murmurs* are blowing, swooshing sounds that occur because of some disruption in the blood flow into, through, or out of the heart. Heart murmurs that are innocent or functional are frequently heard in children.

Most innocent murmurs in children are soft, systolic, medium pitch, heard best at the left sternal border, and do not radiate (Swartz, 1989).

PERIPHERAL VASCULAR SYSTEM

Arterial pulses are examined for decreased or absent pulses. Pulses are palpated, noting rate, rhythm, elasticity of vessel wall, and equal force. Pulse force should be symmetric and should be the same for upper and lower extremities (Fig. 11–24).

In children it is necessary to compare opposite pulses. Compare one femoral pulse with the opposite carotid pulse for equality, and compare one lower extremity pulse with an upper extremity pulse for equality.

BREAST

Breast tissue will be inspected and palpated. Developmental differences occur in response to circulating hormones and affect the appearance of breast tissue. In infants of both sexes the breasts may appear engorged due to maternal estrogen crossing the placenta. *Thelarche,* breast development, marks the beginning of puberty in preadolescent girls and can occur as early as age 8 years.

Nipples are inspected for position and appearance. In infants the nipple is flat and symmetrical with darker areola pigmentation. In the preadolescent and adolescent female Tanner's sexual maturity rating is used to evaluate developmental levels (see Table 8–2). Position of the nipples should be symmetrical, and they should be pointed in the same direction. Nipples may appear to be inverted or everted. An inverted nipple is significant if the inversion is of recent origin. The skin of the breast should be smooth and free of any dimpling. It is common to see some asymmetry during growth.

All adolescent females should be taught how to do a self-examination of the breast once they have reached *menarche.* Teaching the adolescent how to do this self-examination and reinforcing its importance at every visit is an important role for the nurse. Many adolescents do not do breast self-exams because of lack of knowledge or fear of finding something wrong. Once the adolescent is familiar with how her breasts look and feel, the natural and normal changes that occur in the breast as a result of hormones can be easily identified. The examination of the tissue that supports and constructs the breast is divided into three parts: the visual examination, the shower examination, and the examination done while lying down.

The visual examination is done while looking in the mirror with arms at the side, arms over the head, and flexing the chest muscles by rolling the shoulders forward. Tell her to look for unusual lowering of one breast, unusual increase in the size of one breast, puckering of the skin of the breast, swelling of the upper arm, lump in the breast, discharge or bleeding from the nipple, new dimpling of nipple or breast, enlarged lymph nodes at the neck or under the arm, and change in skin of the nipple.

The shower examination is done by soaping the breasts and pressing the pads of the middle fingers in a firm and smooth circular motion against the chest wall. Palpate no more than 1 inch at a time and begin at the outer aspects of the breast and move in smaller concentric

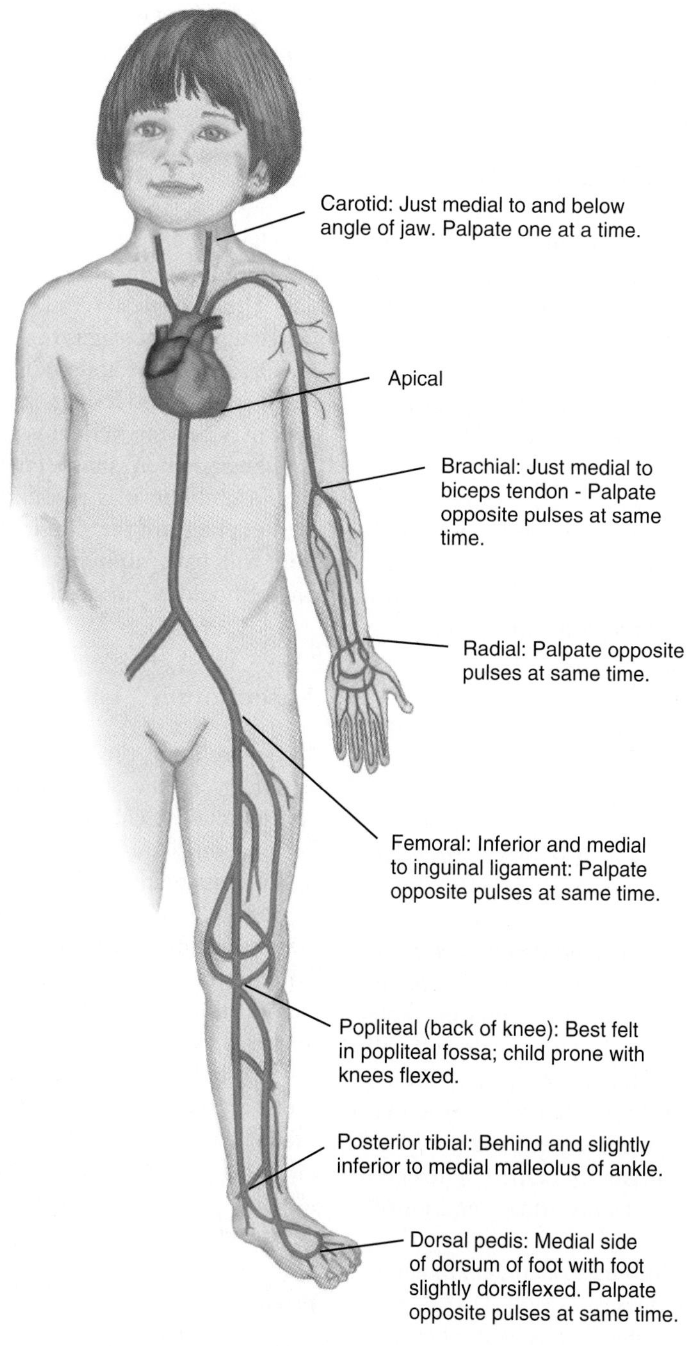
Carotid: Just medial to and below angle of jaw. Palpate one at a time.
Apical
Brachial: Just medial to biceps tendon - Palpate opposite pulses at same time.
Radial: Palpate opposite pulses at same time.
Femoral: Inferior and medial to inguinal ligament: Palpate opposite pulses at same time.
Popliteal (back of knee): Best felt in popliteal fossa; child prone with knees flexed.
Posterior tibial: Behind and slightly inferior to medial malleolus of ankle.
Dorsal pedis: Medial side of dorsum of foot with foot slightly dorsiflexed. Palpate opposite pulses at same time.

Grading Arterial Pulses

Examine the child for decreased or absent arterial pulses. Note rate, rhythm, and elasticity of vessel wall. The force of each pulse is graded on a 4-point scale:

- 4 + bouncing
- 3 + increased
- 2 + expected
- 1 + weak or diminished
- 0 + absent

Figure 11–24

Location of arterial pulses.

circles until all the breast tissue is felt. Palpate the axillary region, under the breast, and the tissue above and under the collarbone (clavicle). The nipple is gently squeezed between the fingers for any discharge.

The adolescent is asked to lie down with the arm on the side to be examined extended above the head, and a small folded towel is placed under the shoulder of the breast to be examined. The fingertip exam is done in a circular pattern, beginning at the center of the nipple and moving counterclockwise in a circular motion over the breast and the area around the breast. The procedure is repeated on the opposite breast.

The adolescent female is taught to do the self-examination of her breasts 3 to 4 days after menses in the menstrual cycle, as the breasts are least tender and sensitive at that time.

The breast tissue and the axillas of the adolescent male are palpated by the examiner using the same technique. In the male the examiner expects to feel a thin layer of fatty tissue overlying the muscle. During puberty some males will experience *gynecomastia*, an enlargement of breast tissue, felt as a smooth, firm, movable disc. It frequently affects only one breast and is temporary (Fuller, 1994).

ABDOMEN

The comfort of the child should be considered during the abdominal examination. An empty bladder, a warm room, and positioning of the child supine on the examining table with a pillow under the head and knees flexed will enhance abdominal relaxation. For an infant and young child it is possible to do most of the abdominal examination while the child is lying in the parent's lap. For an older child the genitalia and breasts are draped. The child or parent should be questioned about urinary and bowel patterns.

The abdomen is divided into four quadrants to correlate with underlying anatomic structures (Fig. 11–25). The sequence of assessment techniques is changed when the abdomen is assessed because bowel sounds are disturbed by percussion and palpation. The abdomen is first inspected, then auscultated, then percussed, and lastly palpated.

Inspection

Inspection of the abdomen is done to determine contour, symmetry, characteristics of the umbilicus and skin, pulsations or movement, and hair distribution. *Contour* is the profile of the abdomen from the rib margin to the pubic bone and is best determined by looking tangentially across the abdomen. The contour is described as flat, scaphoid, rounded, or protuberant (Fig. 11–26). The contour of the abdomen gives an overall description of the nutritional state.

The abdomen should be *symmetrical* bilaterally. The examiner looks for distentions, bulging, visible mass, or asymmetric shape.

The *umbilicus* is normally midline and inverted. There should be no signs of discoloration, inflammation, or hernia. The umbilical cord is inspected throughout the neonatal period for signs of infection or bleeding.

The *skin* of the abdomen is inspected for color and the presence of scars, lesions, and striae. A fine venous network may be seen in infants and small children.

The abdomen is inspected for *pulsations and movement.* In thin children it is possible to see the pulsations from the aorta beneath the skin in the epigastric area. Most children will have abdominal movement with respirations. There should be no visible peristalsis of the abdomen.

Auscultation

Auscultation of the abdomen follows inspection. The diaphragm of the stethoscope is held lightly against the skin to note the character and frequency of bowel sounds. Bowel sounds are high-pitched, gurgling sounds heard in all four quadrants. They are heard irregularly and can occur from 5 to 34 times a minute. The examiner begins in the lower right quadrant and listens in all four quadrants. To determine that there are no bowel sounds, the examiner must listen up to 5 minutes in an area where no bowel sounds are heard.

The bell of the stethoscope is used to listen for bruits over the aortic, renal, iliac, and femoral arteries. The examiner also listens in the epigastric region and around the umbilicus for a venous hum, which is described as a soft, low-pitched, continuous sound.

Percussion

Percussion of the abdomen by advanced practitioners is done to determine tympany, liver span, and splenic dullness.

Palpation

Palpation of the abdomen is done to determine the presence of any mass or tenderness and to judge the size, consistency, and location of certain organs.

The examiner should warm her hands before palpating the abdomen. Palpation of the infant and young child's abdomen can be done in the parent's lap by laying

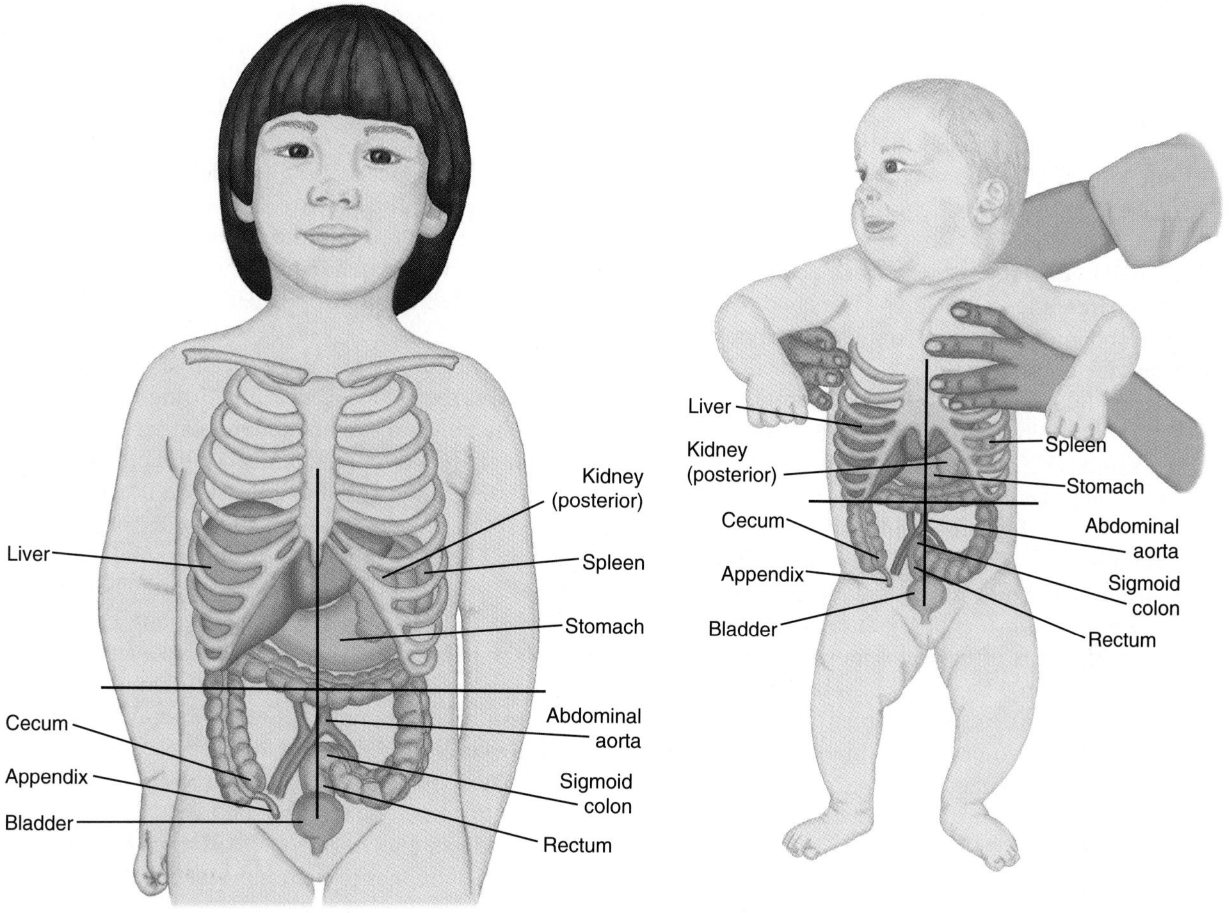

Liver
Kidney (posterior)
Spleen
Stomach
Cecum
Abdominal aorta
Appendix
Sigmoid colon
Bladder
Rectum
Liver
Kidney (posterior)
Spleen
Stomach
Cecum
Abdominal aorta
Appendix
Sigmoid colon
Bladder
Rectum

Figure 11–25
Abdominal quadrants and structures.

Flat: Thin child
Scaphoid: Emaciated or malnourished child
Rounded: Normal appearance of abdomen in a young child
Protuberant: Recent distention with flatus; or extremely obese child (If adolescent female, may indicate pregnancy.)

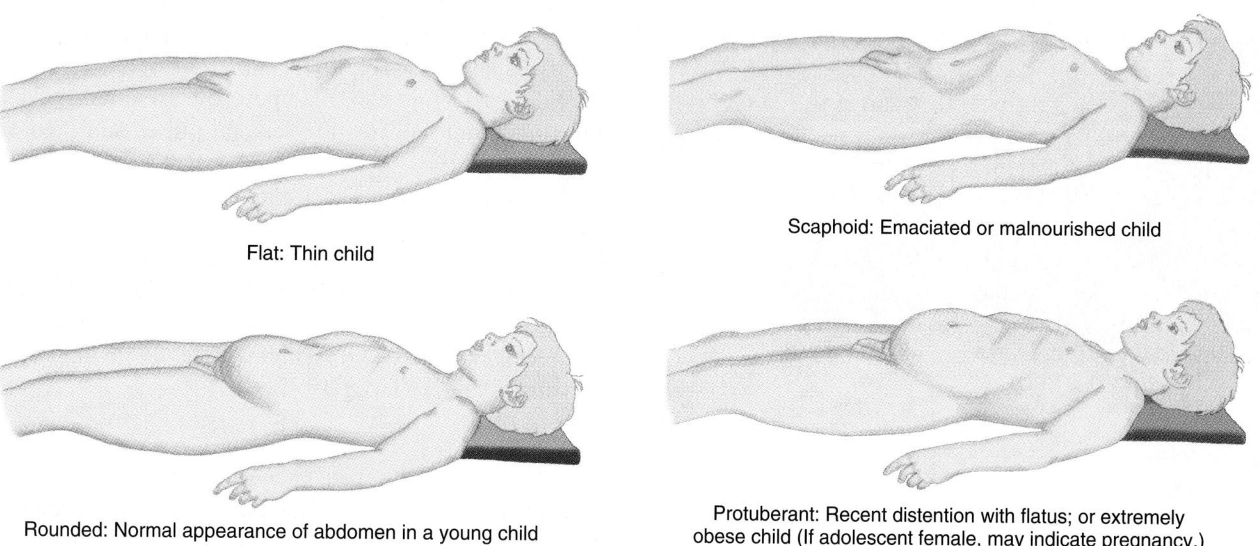

Figure 11–26
Abdominal contours. The contour of the abdomen provides an indication of the overall nutritional state.

the child's head and thorax across the parent's legs and extending the abdomen and legs across the examiner's legs. The child should be prepared for palpation of the abdomen by flexing the knees.

Fear and anxiety may cause the child to resist when the examiner touches the abdomen. Distracting the young child with a toy or talking is helpful. By beginning with light palpation you establish that this will not "hurt."

Ask an older child who is anxious or ticklish to assist you with this part of the examination. The child places her hand on the abdomen and the examiner places her hand, with fingers touching the abdomen, on top of the child's hand and asks the child to push as the examiner pushes (Fig. 11–27). This allows the child some control as you begin the examination and reduces the sensation of tickling. Ask the child to take deep breaths while palpating to assist with relaxation of the abdominal muscles.

The examiner begins with light palpation of all four quadrants using light and even pressure and pressing the palmar surface of the fingers no more than 1 cm into the abdomen. The hand is lifted while moving from area to area. Sudden jabs should be avoided. As the examiner circles around the abdomen, the abdomen should feel soft and smooth. Light palpation is useful in identifying areas of tenderness and muscular resistance. Guarding, resistance, or tenderness should alert the examiner to move cautiously with deeper palpation.

Tenseness can be either voluntary or involuntary. In a child tenseness and rigidity may be due to fear and anxiety. Distracting the child or waiting for the child to breathe will assist with determining whether the tenseness is voluntary or involuntary. The examiner gently indents the fingers into the abdominal wall during inspiration. The abdomen should feel soft with even pressure. Rigidity, a constant boardlike hardness of the abdomen, is usually associated with an acute inflammation of the peritoneum.

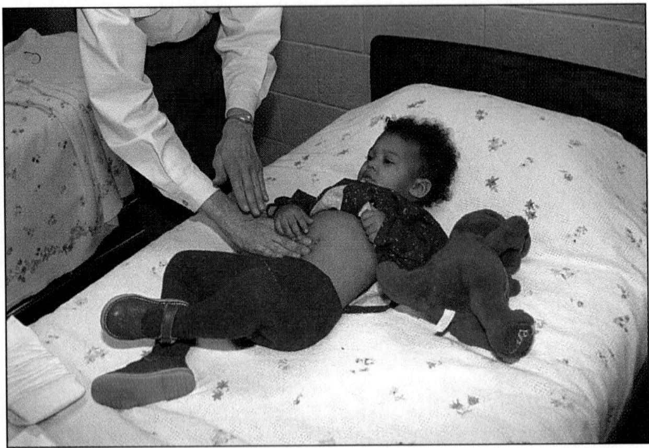

Figure 11–27
Palpating the abdomen often causes the sensation of tickling in both children and adults. Have the child push downward with you as you palpate to reduce this sensation. Also, the child's knees should be flexed to reduce tension of the abdominal muscles, making the examination easier. (Courtesy of University of Texas at Arlington School of Nursing, Arlington, Texas)

Using the same techniques described above, the abdomen is deeply palpated. The examiner pushes down about 5 to 8 cm into the abdominal wall beginning in the right lower quadrant. The entire abdomen is deeply palpated to identify palpable organs and identify masses.

To palpate the liver's edge, begin at the level of the umbilicus in the midclavicular line, using the side of the hand to indent into the abdomen about 5 to 8 cm. With deep penetration of the abdominal wall the hand is gently inverted toward the costal margin. Then progress upward with the same maneuver until the border of the liver is palpated. The edge of the liver is felt as soft, smooth, and with a sharp border that moves downward when the child takes a deep breath. In infants and young children it is possible to begin at the costal margin and using the palmar aspects of the fingers indent into the abdominal wall about 5 to 8 cm. The examiner should move down from the costal margin until the hand falls off the edge of the liver border. The liver edge may be palpated at 1 to 3 cm below the costal margin in infants and toddlers.

Palpation of the spleen and kidneys is done by the advanced practitioner to determine size and the presence of masses or enlargement.

When areas of tenderness are elicited during palpation, a special procedure for identifying rebound tenderness is used. A site away from the identified tenderness is chosen. The examiner places a hand perpendicular to the abdomen and pushes down slowly and deeply into the abdomen and then lifts the hand up quickly. The sudden release of the pressure will cause severe pain and muscle rigidity when there is peritoneal inflammation.

While palpating the abdomen, the examiner checks skin turgor and palpates the femoral pulses and inguinal lymph nodes.

The child is turned over and the buttocks inspected. The buttocks in children are full with symmetric folds. There should be no evidence of scars or ecchymosis on the buttocks. The sacrococcygeal area is examined for the presence of any dimples or tufts of hair. If it is necessary to do a rectal examination on a child, it should be done with the patient supine (Jarvis, 1992).

MALE GENITALIA

The approach to the examination of the male genitals will depend on the growth and development of the child being examined. In an infant, toddler, and young child it is important to tell the child what the nurse is going to do and concur with the parent or guardian that it is appropriate for the nurse to examine the genitalia of the child.

It is normal for the adolescent boy to be apprehensive about the genital examination. Concerns arise from modesty, fear of pain, negative judgment, or a previous uncomfortable experience. A matter-of-fact approach and direct communication will facilitate this part of the physical examination. The genital examination is performed during or immediately after the abdominal examination. In the adolescent the physical examination should not conclude with the genital examination so as to allow further opportunity for communication. A good practice is to conclude the physical examination with the musculoskeletal and neurologic examination after the genital examination has been completed.

Gloves should be worn during every genital examination. The examiner begins by inspecting the *penis.* The size of the penis is directly related to age and growth and development. In infants and young boys the penis is approximately 2 to 3 cm. Genital hair distribution is noted. The adolescent shows a wide variation in normal development of the genitals. Tanner's stages are used for determining the level of development in the adolescent (see Table 8–2).

The skin on the penis normally appears wrinkled, hairless, and without lesions. In the adolescent a prominent dorsal vein may be apparent. Any indurations on the penile shaft should be noted. In the circumcised male the glans looks smooth and without lesions. In an uncircumcised infant the glans may not be visible. By the time the male is age 5 or 6 years the foreskin should be easily retracted behind the corona of the glans. The adolescent is asked to retract the foreskin behind the corona of the glans.

The *meatus* is evaluated by compressing the glans between the thumb and forefinger anteroposteriorly. The adolescent may be requested to compress the glans to visualize the meatus. The meatus in the male has a slit-like or tear-shaped configuration and is located on the ventral surface just millimeters from the tip of the glans. The meatus opening is pink, smooth, and without discharge.

The *scrotum* is inspected for size and configuration, which will change with growth and development. In the infant and young male the proximal portion of the scrotum is wider and the distal portion narrower. In the adolescent male the proximal portion is narrower and the distal portion is wider. Asymmetry of the scrotum is normal with the left half slightly lower than the right. The scrotum is movable and will move closer to or away from the body in response to environmental temperature to maintain optimal temperature of the testes.

The contents of the scrotum are palpated. The cremasteric reflex in young males may cause the testes to withdraw into the inguinal canal, making palpating them more difficult. If the boy is old enough, have him sit in a cross-legged or "tailor" position, which will help prevent the cremasteric reflex by stretching the muscle, thereby preventing its contraction. Before beginning the abdominal examination, warm your hands, block the inguinal canal with one hand, and palpate for the scrotal contents (Fig. 11–28). Using the thumb and first two fingers, each *testis* and *epididymis* are palpated. The testes are smooth, rubbery, and free of nodules on palpation. The size of the testes will change with growth and development. Tanner's growth and development stages are used for appropriate interpretation. Because of the high incidence of testicular tumors in young men, adolescents should be taught to do testicular self-examinations.

FEMALE GENITALIA

In general the anogenital examination in prepubescent girls is limited to visual inspection and gentle palpation of the external area. Internal specula examinations are not routine in prepubescent children. Appearance of the external genitalia in females varies from child to child and with growth and development. A relaxed, caring attitude will reassure both child and parent. To assure privacy, the child is draped appropriately to reinforce modesty and decrease anxiety. The examiner should communicate with the child what will be done and concur with the parent or guardian that it is appropriate to examine the genitalia. There will be difference in tone, relaxation, and appearance of the genitalia with the child in different positions. Generally the young female genital examination is performed with the child supine, gently drawing the legs up onto the abdomen to expose the genitalia.

The examiner gloves and begins by inspecting the mons pubis and labia majora. The skin should be smooth and clean; pubic hair distribution is noted. Tanner's stages are used to determine appropriate growth and development (see Table 8–2).

In the newborn the labia majora and minora may be edematous, with the labia minora often more prominent. In the infant the hymen may protrude and may appear thick and vascular and the clitoris may appear relatively large. The presence of an opening of the hymen is determined. The hymen is centrally located and about 0.5 cm in diameter.

In the young girl and adolescent, the labia majora may be gaping or closed, shriveled or full, and appear dry or moist depending on the age and development of the child. The labia majora are usually symmetrical (Fig. 11–29).

The labia major are spread gently with the fingers and the labia minora, the clitoris, the urethral orifice, and the vaginal introitus are inspected and palpated. The *labia*

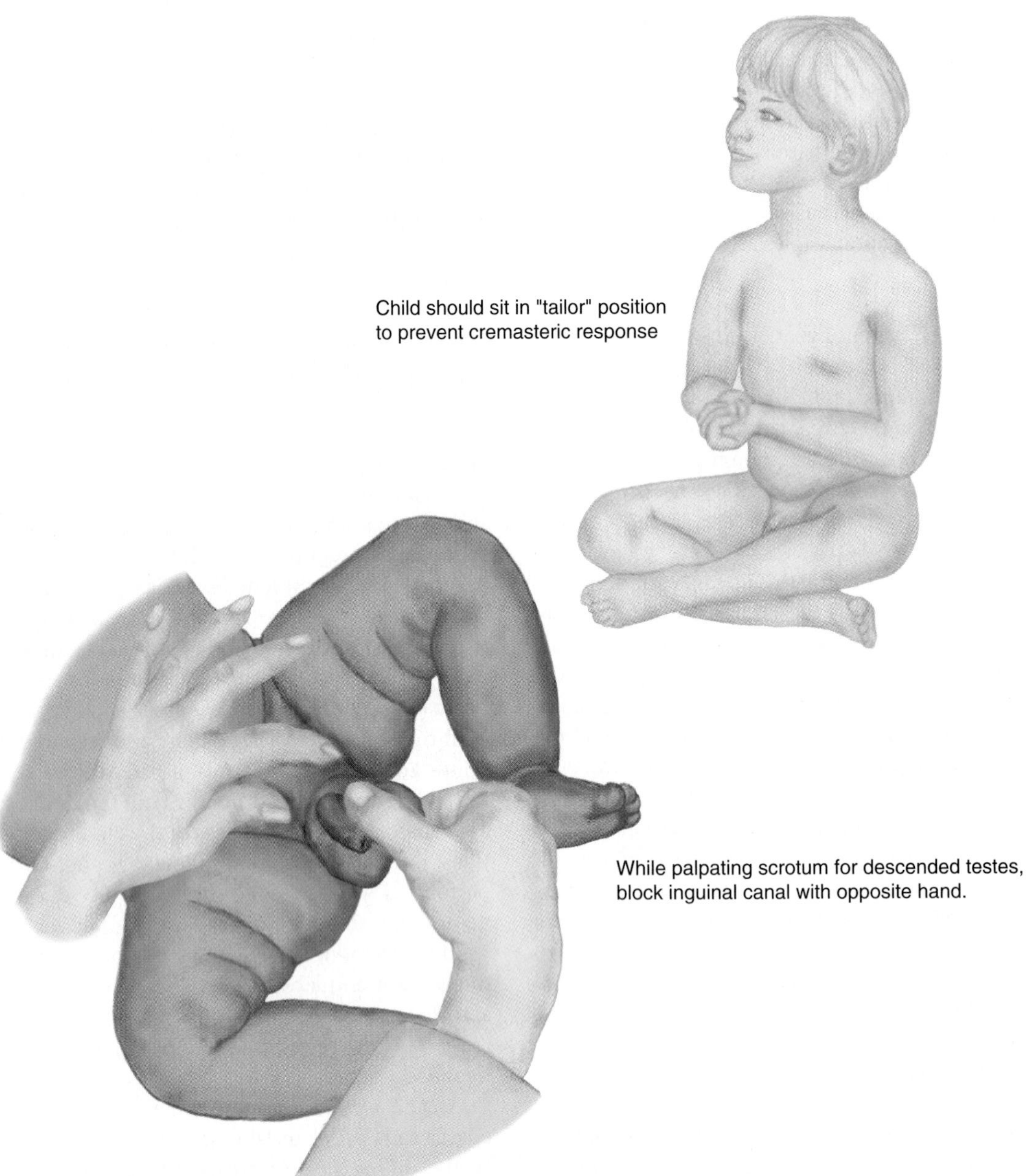

Child should sit in "tailor" position
to prevent cremasteric response
While palpating scrotum for descended testes,
block inguinal canal with opposite hand.

Figure 11–28

When you are examining a boy's scrotum, the cremasteric reflex may cause the testes to withdraw into the inguinal canals. To prevent this reflex, have the boy sit in a tailor position if possible. Use one hand to block the inguinal canals and the other to palpate.

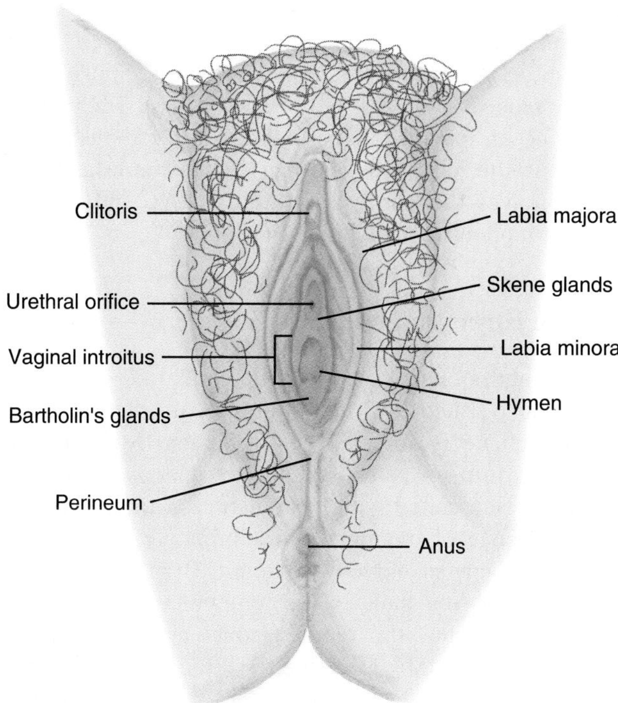

Figure 11–29
Postpubertal female genitalia.

minora should appear symmetric, dark pink, and moist. On palpation the tissue should be soft and homogeneous with no tenderness.

With the labia majora spread, by looking superiorly the *clitoris* can be inspected for size and length, which will vary with growth and development.

Progressing inferiorly, the *urethral meatus* is located. The urethral meatus may be close to or inside the vaginal introitus. It is usually in the midline. The opening may appear as an irregular opening or slit, depending on the characteristics of the hymen. This tissue is usually moist.

The *vaginal introitus* may be a thin vertical slit or a large orifice with irregular edges, depending on the characteristics of the hymen. The hymen may or may not be stretched across the vaginal opening. By menarche the opening should be at least 1 cm wide. The tissue is usually moist. The amount and characteristics of any discharge from the vagina will depend on the circulating hormones in the female. A normal vaginal discharge is odorless and may be cloudy or clear, or thick or thin.

Normally *Skene's glands,* located just inferior to the urethral meatus, are not seen or felt and have no discharge. Any discharge from Skene's glands is an indication of an infection. *Bartholin's glands,* located in the posterolateral portion of the labia majora, are inspected and palpated. There should be no swelling or tenderness of Bartholin's glands.

A speculum examination of the internal reproductive organs is not indicated for young girls. The adolescent girl has special needs during the genital examination, which is performed by advanced practitioners.

MUSCULOSKELETAL SYSTEM

The musculoskeletal system is comprised of the bones, joints, cartilage, ligaments, and muscles. Joint motions are defined as flexion, extension, abduction, adduction, internal rotation, external rotation, and circumduction. The major focus of the musculoskeletal examination will be on the upper and lower extremities and the spinal column. The evaluation of the musculoskeletal system begins with observation of the child during play or while the history is being taken. Observation of the child climbing, jumping, hopping, rising from a sitting position, and manipulating toys and other objects provides evidence of the function of joints, range of motion, bone stability, and muscle strength. Assessment of fine motor and gross motor ability is accomplished during the Denver Developmental Screening Test for the child under age 5 years. (See Chapter 2 and Appendix D.)

General inspection begins with a visual scanning of the body using a cephalocaudal (head to toe) organization. The child can be examined in shorts or underwear. The two sides of the body are compared for symmetry, contour, size, and involuntary movement. The two sides are inspected for areas of swelling or edema and ecchymoses or other discolorations. The structural relationship of the feet to the legs, the hips to the pelvis, the upper extremities, shoulder girdle, and upper trunk are evaluated.

Common deformities of the extremities are *varus* and *valgus* deformities. With the reference point of the midline of the body, a varus deformity of the leg is a lateral deviation of the leg from the midline. A valgus deformity of the leg is a deviation of the leg toward the midline (see Chapter 37).

Deformities of the spine are *scoliosis, kyphosis,* and *lordosis,* which are discussed in Chapter 37.

Infants. During infancy symmetric flexion of the arms and legs is noted. Limbs should be freely movable and there should be symmetry of the axillary, gluteal, femoral, and popliteal creases. The hands are inspected, noting shape, number, and position of fingers and palmar creases. The clavicle should feel smooth, regular, and without crepitus. By age 2 months the infant can lift the head while prone. Range of motion is observed through spontaneous movement of the extremities. When the infant is lifted with the hands of the nurse under the axillae, the infant with normal muscle strength wedges securely between the hands. The hips are checked for congenital dislocation. The *Ortolani and Barlow maneuvers* are performed by a trained examiner on every visit until the infant is 1 year old (see Chapter 37).

Toddlers, Preschool-, and School-Age Children. The examiner may want to start with the hands and arms by checking for range of motion and presence of pain while the child is sitting. Children are willing to show their hands and it is an excellent way to make contact with the child.

The child should stand in order for the examiner to observe the posture from behind. The shoulders should be level and the scapulae symmetric. In young children it is common to observe lordosis. Anteriorly the examiner begins with the feet and observes for adduction and pronation of the foot. Pronation (pes planus) is common between ages 12 and 30 months because of the broad-based stance of the young child. Adduction, toeing in, is demonstrated when the child walks on the lateral side of the foot. Adduction tends to correct itself by age 3 years, as long as the foot is flexible. *Genu varum* (bowleg) is present when a space of more than 2.5 cm is measured between the knees when the medial malleoli are held together. Genu varum is normal for 1 year after the child has begun to walk. *Genu valgum* are present when there is more than 2.5 cm between the medial malleoli when the knees are held together. Genu valgum is present between age 2 and 3½ years. The child is instructed to stand on one leg and then the other while the examiner watches from behind. The iliac crest should stay level when the weight is shifted. (See Fig. 37–6.)

Adolescents. The sequence described above is followed with special attention to the spine. Adolescents frequently have kyphosis (Fig. 37–2) because of poor posture. Routine screening for scoliosis is begun at age 12 years. The child is clothed only in underpants and if an older girl, a bra is also worn. The examiner stands behind the child and observes alignment of the spine. A line drawn from the spinous process of the first thoracic vertebrae straight down the vertebra should fall through the gluteal cleft (see Chapter 37, p. xxx). The spinal processes should be palpated for alignment. The examiner places the hands under each scapulae and notes alignment. The scapulae should be symmetric. The hands are placed on each iliac crest and alignment is noted. They should also be symmetric. With the arms at the side, the position of the hands should be equal on both sides of the body. The child should be instructed to slowly bend forward and touch the toes. The concave curve of the lumbar spine becomes convex with forward flexion. The examiner should observe the presence of a rib or lumbar hump. The child should be observed from the front, behind, and side to detect the presence of a hump.

Range of Motion

The child's ability to perform active range of motion should be noted. The equality of movement for each joint and contralateral joints should be noted. There should be no pain, limitation of movement, spastic movement, joint instability, deformity, or crepitation during movement. Passive range of motion is performed on joints where limitations occur. Passive range of motion is accomplished by anchoring the joint with one hand while the other hand slowly moves the joint to its limit. Active and passive range of motion should be the same.

Muscle Strength and Mass

The strength of each muscle group should be evaluated. The child is asked to flex the muscle and then resist as opposing force is applied against flexion. Muscle tone should be firm on palpation. The evaluation of muscle strength is integrated with examination of the associated joint for range of motion when appropriate. The motor segment of cranial nerve V (trigeminal) is evaluated by applying opposing force to the temporalis muscle while the child clenches the teeth. Cranial nerve XI (spinal accessory) is tested by assessing the strength of the sternocleidomastoid and trapezius muscles with rotation of the head side to side and chin to shoulder. Table 11–4 describes the grading of muscle strength.

Measurement of muscle mass is done when atrophy or hypertrophy is suspected. Muscles are best measured at their greatest circumference. Using the joint as a landmark, measurement is taken from the joint to a point on the extremity. A comparison with the opposite muscle is made. One measurement is not as significant as a series of measurements to determine changes in size of muscles.

Joints

Each joint is palpated for temperature, tenderness, swelling, crepitation, or masses. In children fatigue, stiffness, or weakness along with heat and redness are frequently associated with disorders of the joints. Children will usually not move a joint if they are experiencing pain.

TABLE 11–4 *Grading Muscle Strength*

	SCALE	
	GRADE	**% NORMAL**
No evidence of contractility	0	0
Slight contractility, no movement	1	10
Full range of motion with passive range of motion	2	25
Full range of motion with gravity	3	50
Full range of motion against gravity, some resistance	4	75
Full range of motion against gravity, full resistance	5	100

TABLE 11–5 *Gross Motor Development in the Infant: Progression to Walking*

ACTIVITY	AGE
Raises head and holds position.	2 weeks to 2 months
Prone infant moves all extremities, kicking arms and legs.	2 months
Draws up knees and raises abdomen off table. Rocks back and forth while up on hands and knees. Rolls over.	3 to 6 months
Sits alone, using hands for support (tripod fashion).	By 7 months
Lurches forward and pulls legs to chest in "inch worm" fashion. Some infants move backward in same fashion. Creeping and rolling.	By 9th month
Crawls in one-sided manner (moves arm and leg on same side of body, then other side).	6 to 9 months
Crawls in regular fashion alternating arm and opposite leg.	6 to 9 months
Begins to pull up.	By 11 months
Attempts to walk with support or holding on to something stable.	By 12 months
Momentarily lets go and maintains balance for a few seconds.	Once comfortable standing and holding on
Takes first steps (a broad stance with arms flexed for balance).	Once standing balance accomplished
Sits from a standing posture.	By 12 months
Walks alone.	By 15 months

Gait

Assessment of gait and the ability to ambulate is an essential part of both the musculoskeletal and neurologic assessments. The developmental acquisition of the ability to walk follows a prescribed sequence in infants and toddlers (Table 11–5). (See also the photo story in Chapter 4, pp. 80–81.)

Gait is assessed in two phases: stance and swing. The stance phase begins when the heel strikes the floor; then the weight is transferred to the ball of the foot, and the toes push off the floor. The swing phase consists of acceleration, swing through, and deceleration. One foot is in stance while the other is in swing. The gait of the walking child should be assessed for the following characteristics (Hoekelman, 1992):

- Phase (conformity)
- Cadence (symmetry, regular rhythm; strike length symmetry, length of swing)
- Pelvic posture (related to phases)
- Arm swing (symmetry, length of swing)

NEUROLOGIC SYSTEM

The purpose of the neurologic examination in the child and adolescent is to determine if there is any nervous system malfunction and to ascertain the extent of nervous system development and functioning. If neurologic deficits exist it is important to determine the degree, type, and location of nervous system lesions. In the child, it is significant to determine the degree to which the nervous system is functioning so that the healthy portion of the nervous system can be used for habilitation or rehabilitation. For the child under age 5 years, the best evaluation of neurologic functioning can be determined by using the Denver Developmental Screening Test II (see Chapter 2 and Appendix xx). For the child over age 5 years, the sequence of the neurologic examination should be adapted according to the child's understanding and cooperation.

Testing cerebral function, cranial nerves, and cerebellar function gives a picture of the nervous system functioning at the horizontal levels above the spinal cord. The age and development of the child will determine the sequence of the neurologic examination. The infant and younger child will not be able to cooperate with neurologic testing. A review of attainment of developmental milestones will help to establish the rate and consistency of development of the infant and younger child. The 3 or 4-year-old will cooperate with testing when it is approached as a game.

Cerebral Function

Evaluation of cognitive function focuses on appearance, behavior, orientation, speech patterns, memory, logic, and affect. It is essential to obtain information from the primary caregiver about changes in the child's behavior, personality, and appearance and age-appropriate school performance. Evaluation of cognitive function of the older child and adolescent is based on observation of level of consciousness, awareness, thought processes, and communication.

The level of consciousness of the older child and adolescent is determined by the degree of response to sensory stimuli. The child is described as being alert, lethargic, obtunded, stuporous, or comatose.

The older child and adolescent has the ability to understand, think, feel emotions, and appreciate sensory information about self and surroundings. Awareness is evaluated by observing the older child's or adolescent's level of orientation in relation to person, place, and time. The child is described as being oriented to person, place, and time.

Evaluation of thought processes include evaluation of abstract thinking, problem solving (simple calculations and concentration), insight, memory (recent and remote), and judgment. The child's school performance may or may not be an accurate indicator of thought processes. Factors that may influence thought processes are attention span, communication, perceptual problems, and emotional withdrawal and depression.

Language ability is evaluated through speech patterns and the ability to comprehend language. The child is questioned about reading and writing ability. Is his speech intelligible? Does the child answer questions appropriately for his age and development? The child is described as being able to speak fluently, name objects correctly, and write his name and address.

Some specific tests to evaluate cerebral function are described in the accompanying box.

Cranial Nerves

Assessment of the cranial nerves (Table 11–6) should be done during that part of the examination when the system each nerve affects is assessed. The use of games, such as making faces or performing tests on a parent or the examiner, will enhance cooperation.

Cerebellar Function

The cerebellum controls balance and coordination; proprioception evaluates laterality and orientation in space. The techniques used will vary with age and development. The child should attempt the technique and show continued improvement with maturation.

Proprioception, balance, and coordination are tested by having the child perform the movements described and illustrated in the accompanying box.

Motor System

Muscle size, muscle tone, involuntary movements, and muscle strength are assessed during the musculoskeletal examination.

Muscles are inspected and palpated while at rest for size, consistency, and possible atrophy. The examiner notes symmetry of posture, and of muscle contours and outlines. The fine muscles of each hand are evaluated for wasting, fasciculations, and fine tremors of individual muscle fibers.

Muscle tone is evaluated by palpating the muscles at rest and resistance to passive movement.

The muscles are inspected for involuntary movements such as slow dystonic twistings, irregular and jerky choreiform movements, quick myoclonic contractions, tics, and tremors.

Muscle strength is tested first without resistance and then against resistance. Corresponding muscles are compared on each side. The major joints are tested for flexion, extension, and other movements.

Specific Cerebral Function Tests

Sound recognition: With eyes closed, ask the child to identify familiar sounds.

Auditory/verbal comprehension: Does child answer questions and carry out instructions appropriate for age?

Recognition of body parts and sidedness: Does the child recognize the parts of the body? Does the child know right from left?

Performance of skilled motor acts: Can the child drink from a cup, button clothes, use a common tool?

Visual object recognition: Ask the child to identify a familiar toy or object (wrist watch).

Visual/verbal comprehension: Can the child read appropriately and explain the meaning?

Motor speech: Does the child imitate different sounds and phrases?

Automatic speech: Ask the child to repeat series learned, i.e., nursery rhyme or days of the week.

Volition speech: Does the child answer questions relevantly?

Writing: Have the child write his name, or the name of an object.

TABLE 11–6 *Assessing Cranial Nerves*

CRANIAL NERVE	PROCEDURE
Cranial nerves are tested during that part of the exam when the system in which it is found is assessed.	
I (Olfactory nerve)	Can the child identify familiar odors with the eyes closed? Each side of the nose is tested separately.
II (Optic nerve)	Visual acuity is tested using the Snellen chart, HOTV chart for young children, or the tumbling E for very young children. Each eye is tested separately, and then both eyes together. If corrective lenses are worn, the eyes are tested both with and without correction.
III, IV, and VI (Oculomotor, trochlear, abducens nerves)	The child is asked to follow a toy or examiner's finger as they move in all directions of gaze (six cardinal fields of gaze).
V (Trigeminal nerve)	Is the child able to identify a wisp of cotton on the face? Corneal reflex is tested by observing for blinking when you approach the face closely. The masseter and temporal muscles strength can be evaluated by having the child bite down on a tongue blade as you try to remove it.
VII (Facial Nerve)	Have the child imitate you as you frown, wrinkle your forehead, smile, and raise your eyebrow. Ask the child to try to keep the eyes closed while you attempt to open them to test the strength of the eyelid muscles. The sensory portion of the facial nerve can be evaluated by having the child identify the taste of sugar and salt placed on the anterior part of the tongue on each side.
VIII (Acoustic nerve)	Cochlear nerve tests are tests for hearing. Audiometric testing is a quantitative evaluation of hearing. The Weber (lateralization) and Rinne (air and bone conduction) tests are qualitative evaluations of hearing.
IX (Glossopharyngeal nerve) X (Vagus nerve)	The glossopharyngeal and vagus nerves are tested together. With a tongue depressor, the gag reflex is tested by touching the posterior pharyngeal wall. The palatal reflex is tested by stroking each side of the mucous membrane of the uvula. The side touched should rise. Normal function of the vagus nerve is revealed by the child's ability to swallow and to speak clearly.
XI (Accessory nerve)	Palpate and note the strength of the trapezius and sternomastoid muscles against resistance or have the child shrug the shoulders against resistance.
XII (Hypoglossal nerve)	Have the child stick out the tongue and note any lateral deviation when it is protruded. The strength of the tongue is assessed by having the child push against your finger pressed against the cheek with their tongue.

Sensory System

Sensory testing depends on the child's perception and interpretation of the stimuli and on the age and development of the child. Tests to be performed should first be done with a child in an educational practice session before being done in a testing situation. Sensory testing compares both sides of the body, corresponding extremities, and the sensitivity of the distal and proximal parts of each extremity for each form of sensation. Sensory testing is performed to determine if sensory changes involve one entire side of the body, are dermatomal in distribution, or are confined to the peripheral nerves.

Cortical and discriminatory forms of sensation are complex somatic sensory impressions that require interpretation by the cerebral cortex. The sensations tested in a child will depend on the age and development of the child being tested.

Tests for sensory function are described on page 252 in the box entitled Cerebellar Function: Tests of Balance and Coordination.

Reflex Status

The major portion of brain growth occurs in the first year of life. Primitive reflexes in the newborn are inhibited when more advanced cortical functions and voluntary control take over as the child matures and grows. Motor maturation proceeds in a cephalocaudal direction. The ability to elicit a reflex requires an intact afferent nerve fiber, functional synapses in the spinal cord, intact motor nerve fibers, functional neuromuscular junctions, and competent muscle fibers. The right and left side responses are compared; responses should be equal.

Cerebellar Function: Tests of Balance and Coordination

Balance and coordination are tested by having the child perform the following movements:

- **Finger-to-nose test.** Child performs first with one hand, then with the other; first with eyes open, then with eyes closed. Ask child to first touch her finger to her nose and then to your finger as you change the position of your finger. Repeat this action with increasing rapidity. The tests are performed with each hand.

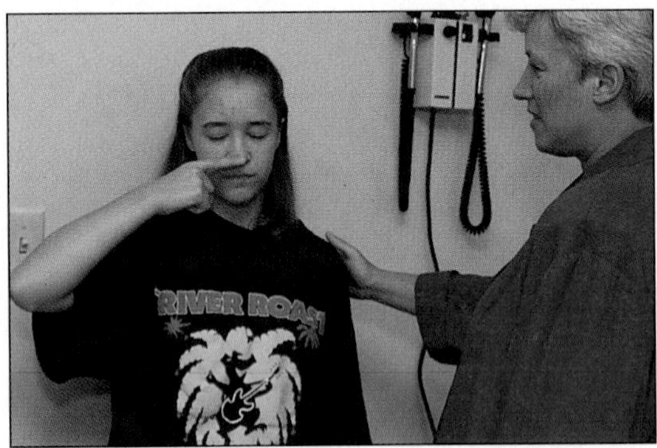

- **Rapid alternating movements.** Ask the child to rapidly pat his knee with the palms and backs of his hands, by pronating and supinating his hands (demonstrate first). Then, ask the child to touch his thumb to each of his fingers in rapid succession (demonstrate first).

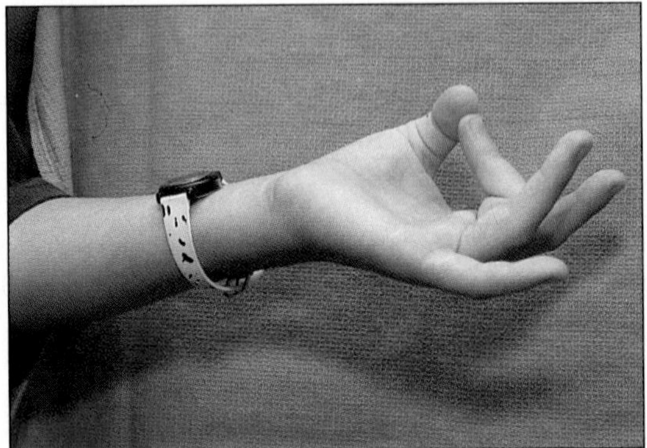

- Ask the child to stand erect first with the eyes open and then with the eyes closed. Stand near the child to prevent injury in case she should begin to fall.

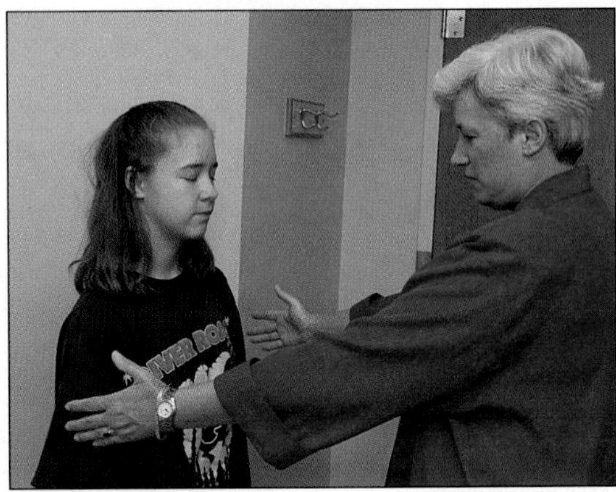

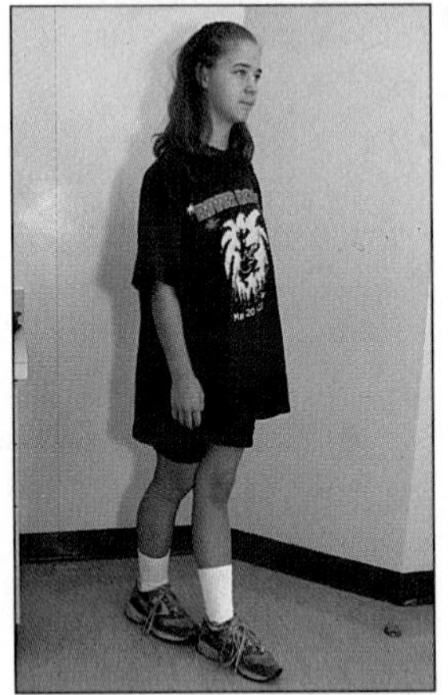

- Ask the child to walk in tandem fashion, placing her heel immediately in front of her opposite foot's toe and alternating while walking a straight line.

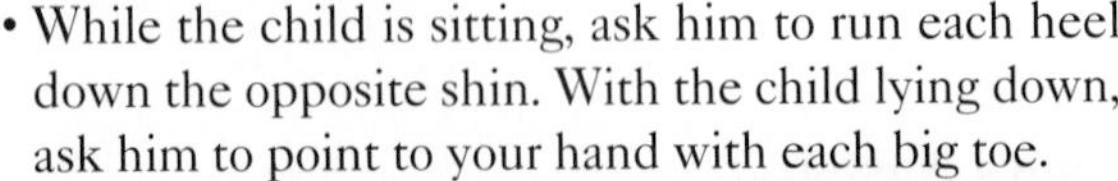

- While the child is sitting, ask him to run each heel down the opposite shin. With the child lying down, ask him to point to your hand with each big toe.

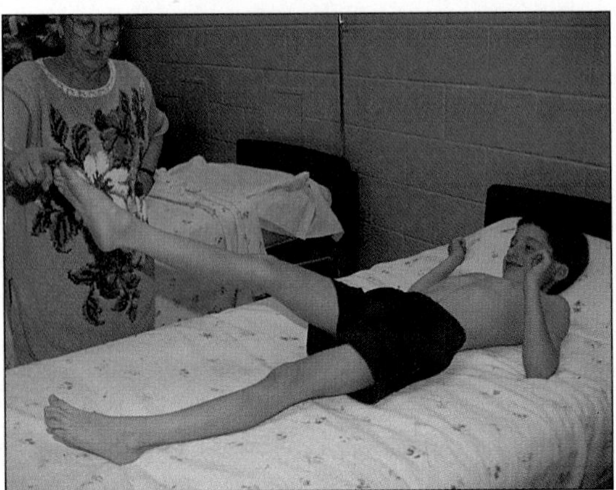

Tests for Evaluating Sensory Function

PRIMARY FORMS OF SENSATION

Sequence: Check the hands, forearms, upper arms, trunk, thighs, lower legs, and feet for the following:

Superficial tactile sensation: Touch the child with a wisp of cotton.

Superficial pain: Touch the child with a pin or other sharp object. Be careful not to injure or frighten the child.

Sensitivity to temperature: Touch the various parts of the body with test tubes containing warm and cold water. This test is not frequently done with children because of the difficulty of keeping water warm or cold enough for the child to distinguish the difference.

Sensitivity to vibration: Hold a vibrating tuning fork to the bony prominences, noting the child's ability to perceive the vibration and tell you when the vibration stops.

Deep pressure pain: Press the tip of your fingernail against the fingernail of the child. The child will feel discomfort. You may also squeeze the Achilles tendons, calf, and forearm muscles, noting sensitivity.

Motion and position: Hold the sides of the toes, thumbs, and fingers by grasping them between your index finger and thumb. Move the fingers and toes passively and ask the child to tell the final position of the digit.

CORTICAL AND DISCRIMINATORY FORMS OF SENSATION

These forms of sensation are complex somatic sensory impressions that require interpretation by the cerebral cortex. The following sensations can be evaluated depending on the age and development of the child being tested.

Two-point discrimination: With the child's eyes closed, various parts of the body are touched simultaneously with two sharp objects. The examiner may alter touching the child with one point or two points. Different areas of the body differ in the distance by which the child can differentiate one from two points. This is more appropriate for older children.

Point localization: With the eyes closed, can the child locate the spot where they were touched?

Texture discrimination: Can the child recognize the difference in the feel of materials such as cotton, wool, and silk with her hands?

Stereognostic function: Can the child identify familiar objects placed in each hand? Place several objects in a paper bag and have the child identify them with each hand and show you the object.

Graphesthesia: Write letters or numbers on the palms or the back with a blunt point and ask the child to identify what was written. Numbers are easier for a young child to recognize than letters.

Extinction phenomenon: Touch opposite sides of the body in identical areas simultaneously. With the eyes closed, can the child tell you that she has been touched on both sides? Older children only.

Commonly elicited reflexes are described and illustrated in Table 11–7.

A stick figure is used to record findings of reflexes.

Neurologic "Soft" Signs

Neurologic "soft" signs are findings that indicate the child's inability to perform certain activities related to the child's age. They may provide subtle clues to an underlying central nervous system deficit or neurologic maturation delay. Examples of "soft" signs include short attention span; minimal lack of coordination; clumsiness; frequent falling; hyperkinesis, both voluntary and involuntary; uneven perceptual development; incomplete laterality, no side clearly dominant; language disturbances; articulation disorders; dyslexia; motor outflow (motor movements involving more muscles than intended); and mirroring movements of the extremities, for example, when one-hand performs a function, the other is also in motion. Although these findings may fall in a gray area, they should be documented when observed. Children with multiple soft signs are often found to have learning problems (Seidel, 1995).

TABLE 11–7 *Evaluating Common Reflexes*

Deep Tendon Reflexes	*Deep tendon reflexes* are elicited by tapping briskly on a tendon or a bony prominence, evoking a sudden stretching of certain muscles and their resulting contraction. For an adequate response, the limb should be relaxed and the muscle partially stretched. The reflex is stimulated by directing a sharp blow of the reflex hammer onto the muscle's insertion tendon.
Biceps Reflex 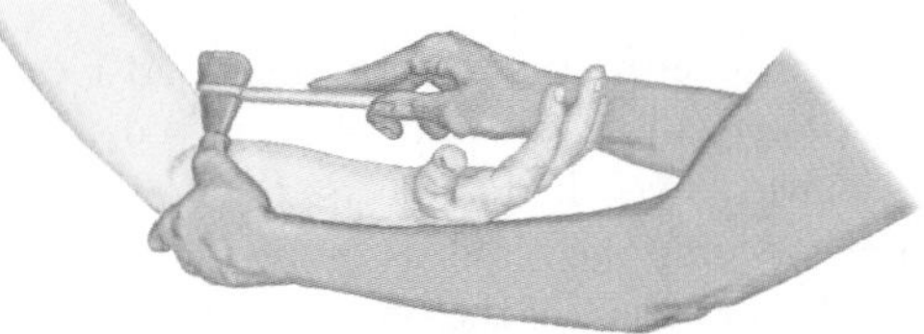	The child's arm should be flexed up to 45° at the elbow. The biceps tendon in the antecubital fossa is palpated. The thumb is then placed on the biceps tendon and a blow is struck on the thumb. The response will be a visible or palpable flexion of the forearm.
Triceps Reflex 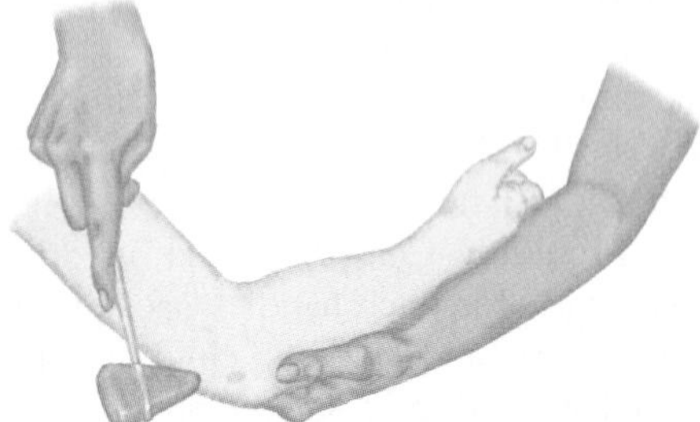	The arm is suspended by holding the upper arm and instructing the child to just let the arm "go limp." Alternatively, the forearm can be supported on the examiner's arm. The triceps tendon is struck directly just above the elbow. The response will be extension of the forearm.
Brachioradialis Reflex 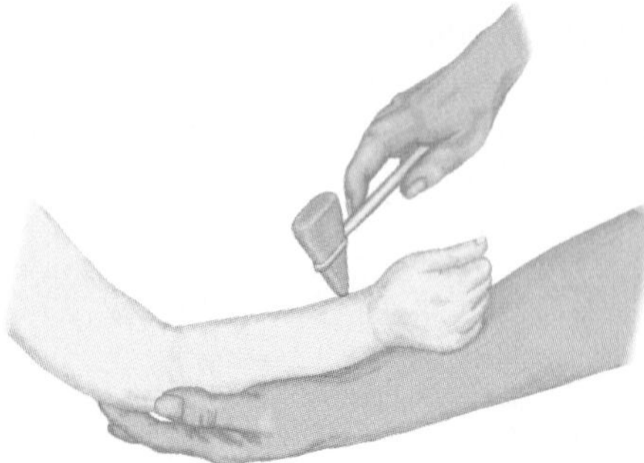	The child's arm is supported on the examiner's arm and the elbow flexed up to 45°. The brachoradial tendon is struck 1–2 inches above the radial styloid process with the reflex hammer. The response will be pronation and flexion of the elbow.
Patellar Reflex 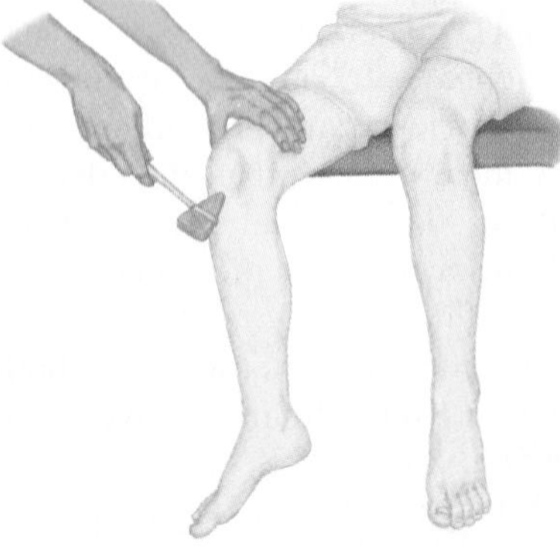	The lower leg is allowed to dangle free by flexing the child's knee up to 90°. Support the upper leg with the hand, and strike the patellar tendon just below the patella. The response will be extension of the lower leg.

TABLE 11–7 *Evaluating Common Reflexes (continued)*

Achilles Reflex 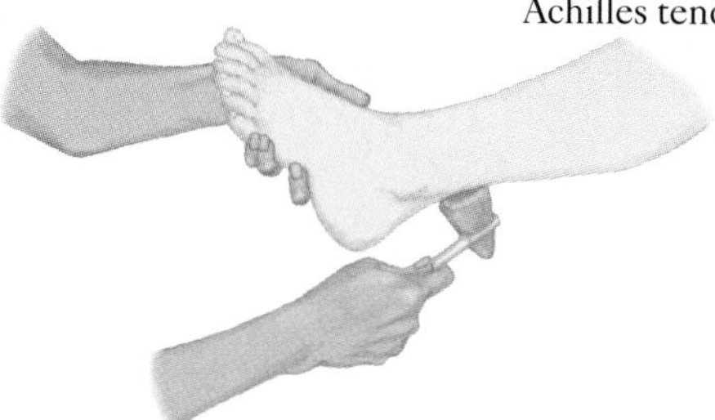	The hip is externally rotated and the foot is held in dorsiflexion. The Achilles tendon is struck directly. The response will be plantar flexion of the foot. An alternative method to elicit this reflex is to have the child kneel on a chair with the toes pointing toward the floor and strike the Achilles tendon directly.
Clonus Reflex	Eliciting a *clonus*, a continued, rapid flexion and extension of the foot and hand, is attempted in children. Clonus is elicited by suddenly and briskly dorsiflexing the foot or hand and applying sustained and moderate pressure. No rhythmic oscillating movements should be palpated.
Superficial Reflexes	*Superficial reflexes* are tested by stroking the skin with an object that is moderately sharp, but not sharp enough to break the skin. The receptors are in the skin rather than the muscles.
Upper and Lower Abdominal Reflexes and Cremasteric Reflex 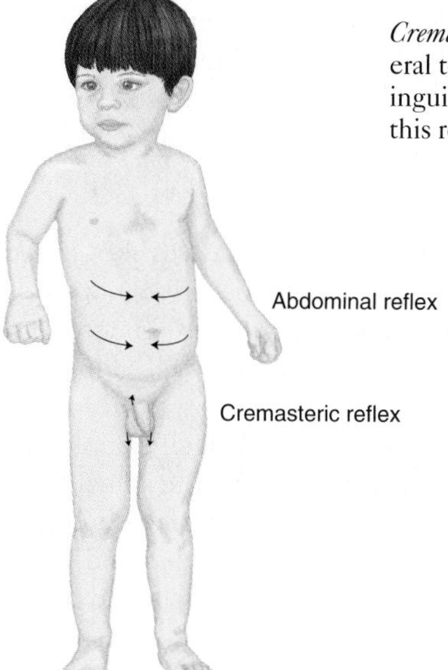	*Upper and Lower Abdominal Reflexes.* While the child is in a supine position and with the abdomen exposed and knees slightly bent, the skin of the abdomen is stroked. Movement of stroking is from the side of the abdomen toward the midline at both the upper and lower abdominal level. The response will be ipsilateral contraction of the abdominal muscle with an observable movement of the umbilicus toward the side being stroked. 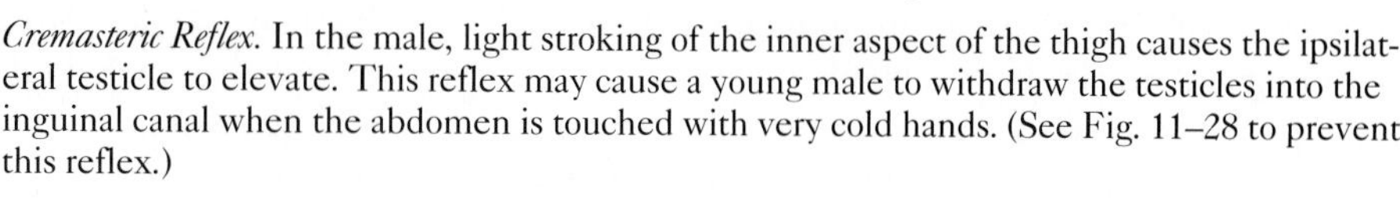 *Cremasteric Reflex.* In the male, light stroking of the inner aspect of the thigh causes the ipsilateral testicle to elevate. This reflex may cause a young male to withdraw the testicles into the inguinal canal when the abdomen is touched with very cold hands. (See Fig. 11–28 to prevent this reflex.)
Plantar Reflex (Babinski Reflex) 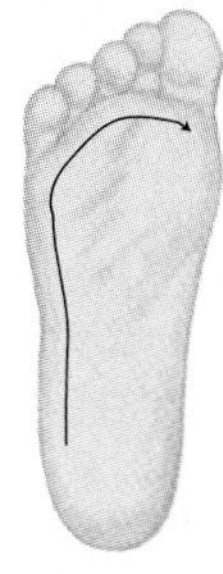	The lateral aspect of the sole of the foot, from the heel to the ball of the foot, is stroked in a movement curving medially across the ball. A fingernail or the wooden end of an applicator stick may be used. The response in an infant will be dorsiflexion, fanning of the toes, and hyperextension of the great toe. Once a child is walking the response will be plantar flexion of the toes. Some children will withdraw from this stimulus by flexing the hip and the knee.
Gluteal Reflex	When the buttocks are separated the skin tenses at the gluteal area.

SUMMARY

The examiner should develop creative approaches to complete the physical examination of different aged children. When the physical examination has been completed the examiner should ask the parents if they have any questions concerning the examination. Examination findings are documented in a complete and concise manner. Deviations from normal and risk factors should be identified and documented. The history and physical examination provides both the subjective and objective data for identifying health and illness states of the child.

KEY CONCEPTS

- A systemic approach to the physical examination is to begin at the head and proceed through the entire body to the toes. In children the physical examination must be tailored to the child's age and developmental level.
- The order of the examination should be flexible, and intrusive and frightening procedures should be done at the end of the examination.
- An accurate history is the single most important component of the physical examination.
- Vital signs should be taken on every visit in ambulatory settings and monitored on a routine basis in the hospitalized child.
- Assessment of vital signs is an important method for measuring and monitoring vital body functions.
- Anthropometrics measure the human body and assess nutritional status as well as growth and development; they are of most value when they are evaluated serially so that trends can be evaluated.
- The skin is observed for color and palpated to determine moisture, temperature, turgor, edema, and lesions.
- The general appearance of the child is observed for signs of abuse, both physical and psychologic.
- Examination of the lymph nodes is incorporated into the examination when that part of the anatomy is being assessed.
- The head is inspected for symmetry, movement, control, and shape.
- The fontanels are inspected and palpated for size, tenseness, and pulsation.
- Spacing and symmetry of the eyelids, eyebrows, palpebral fissures, nasolabial folds, mouth, and nose are inspected.
- The nasal mucosa is inspected for color and moisture.
- Assessment of the mouth in a young child should be performed at the end of the examination because it may cause anxiety.
- The chart chosen to evaluate visual acuity is determined by the age and development of the child.
- Assessment of the thorax and lungs consists of inspection, palpation, percussion, and auscultation.
- Auscultation of the heart is done by listening with both the bell and the diaphragm of the stethoscope with the child lying down, in the left lateral recumbent position, and sitting up.
- An empty bladder, a warm room, and the child supine with a pillow under the head and with the knees flexed will enhance abdominal relaxation.
- Examination of the genitalia may evoke concerns regarding modesty, fear of pain, negative judgment, or a previous uncomfortable experience. A matter-of-fact approach and direct communication will help create a positive experience.
- The major focus of the musculoskeletal examination is the upper and lower extremities and the spinal column.
- The neurologic examination is done to determine if there is any nervous system malfunction and to ascertain current nervous system development and functioning.

REFERENCES

Alexander, M. M., & Brown, M. S. (1974). *Pediatric history taking and physical diagnosis for nurses.* New York: McGraw-Hill.

Barkauskas, V. H., et al. (1994). *Health and physical assessment.* St. Louis: Mosby–Year Book.

Bates, B. (1991). *A guide to physical examination* (5th ed.). Philadelphia: J. B. Lippincott.

Chadwick, D. L., et al. (1989). *Color atlas of child sexual abuse.* Chicago: Year Book Medical.

Fuller, J., & Schaller-Ayers, J. (1994). *Health assessment: A nursing approach* (2nd ed.). Philadelphia: J. B. Lippincott.

Greenberger, N. J., & Hinthorn, D. R. (1993). *History taking and physical examination.* St. Louis: Mosby–Year Book.

Hoekelman, R. A. (Ed.). (1992). *Primary pediatric care* (2nd ed.). St. Louis: Mosby–Year Book.

Hurwitz, S. (1993). *Clinical pediatric dermatology* (2nd ed.). Philadelphia: W. B. Saunders.

Jarvis, C. (1992). *Physical examination and health assessment.* Philadelphia: W. B. Saunders.

Nelson, L. B., et al. (1991). *Pediatric ophthalmology* (3rd ed.). Philadelphia: W. B. Saunders.

Seidel, H. B. (1995). *Mosby's guide to physical examination* (2nd ed.). St. Louis: Mosby–Year Book.

Simon, C., & Janner, M. (1990). *Color atlas of pediatric diseases* (2nd ed.). Philadelphia: B. C. Decker.

Swartz, M. H., William, E., Charney, E., Curry, T. A., & Ludwig, S. (1990). *Pediatric primary care* (2nd ed.). Chicago: Year Book Medical Publishers.

Weston, W. L., & Lane, A. T. (1991). *Color textbook of pediatric dermatology*. St. Louis: Mosby–Year Book.

Zitelli, B. J., & Davis, H. W. (1987). *Atlas of pediatric physical diagnosis*. St. Louis: C. V. Mosby.

BIBLIOGRAPHY

Boisvert, J. T., Reidy, S. J., & Lulu, J. (1995). Overview of pediatric arrhythmias. *Nursing Clinics of North America, 30*(2), 365–379.

Burns, C. (1992). A new assessment model and tool for pediatric nurse practitioners. *Journal of Pediatric Health Care, 6*(2), 73–81.

Catterall, A. (1991). A method of assessment of the clubfoot deformity. *Clinical Orthopedics, 264*, 48–53.

Clore, E. R., & Corey, A. (1991). Hair loss in children and adolescents. *Journal of Pediatric Health Care, 5*(5), 245–250.

Cusick, B. D., & Stuberg, W. A. (1992). Assessment of lower-extremity alignment in the transverse plane: Implications for management of children with neuromotor dysfunction. *Physical Therapy, 72*(1), 3–15.

Gladstein, J., Holden, E. W., Peralta, L., & Raven, M. (1993). Diagnoses and symptom patterns in children presenting to a pediatric headache clinic. *Headache, 33*(9), 497–500.

Graham, M. V., & Uphold, C. (1994). *Clinical guidelines in child health*. Gainesville, FL: Barmarrae Books.

Hayman, L. L., & Ryan, E. A. (1994). The cardiovascular health profile: Implications for health promotion and disease prevention. *Pediatric Nursing, 20*(5), 509–515.

Kaleida, P. H., & Stool, S. E. (1992). Assessment of otoscopists' accuracy regarding middle-ear effusion. Otoscopic validation. *American Journal of Diseases of Children, 146*(4), 433–435.

Malasanos, L., Barkauskas, V., Moss, M., & Stoltenberg-Allen, K. (1986). *Health assessment* (3rd ed.). St. Louis: Mosby.

Miola, E. S. (1994). The otoscope: An update on assessment skills. *Journal of Pediatric Nursing 9*(4), 283–286.

Morton, P. F. (1993). *Health assessment in nursing* (2nd ed.). Springhouse, PA: Springhouse.

Newberger, E. H. (1990). Pediatric interview assessment of child abuse. Challenges and opportunities. *Pediatric Clinics of North America, 37*(4), 943–954.

Pollack, M. M. (1993). Outcome assessment. *Critical Care Medicine, 21*(9 Suppl), S395–S396.

Schreiner, B., & Brondum, L. A. (1994). Nutrition in pediatric primary care: Assessment and common problems. *Nursing Practice Forum, 5*(1), 13–23.

Smythe, J. F., Teixeira, O. H., Vlad, P., Demers, P. P., & Feldman, W. (1990). Initial evaluation of heart murmurs: Are laboratory tests necessary? *Pediatrics, 86*(4), 497–500.

Tan, T. Q., Seilheimer, D. K., & Kaplan, S. L. (1995). Pediatric lung abscess: Clinical management and outcome. *Pediatric Infectious Disease Journal 14*(1), 51–55.

Teo, S., Hanson R, Van Asperen, P., Giles, H., Fasher, B., Davis A. M., Kristidis, P. (1995). Improving asthma documentation in a pediatric emergency department. *Journal of Paediatric and Child Health, 31*(2), 130–133.

van der Net, J., van der Hoeven, H., Esseveld, F., de Wilde, E. J., Kuis, W., Helders, P. J. (1995). Musculoskeletal disorders in juvenile onset mixed connective tissue disease. *Journal of Rheumatology, 22*(4), 751–757.

12

Nutrition

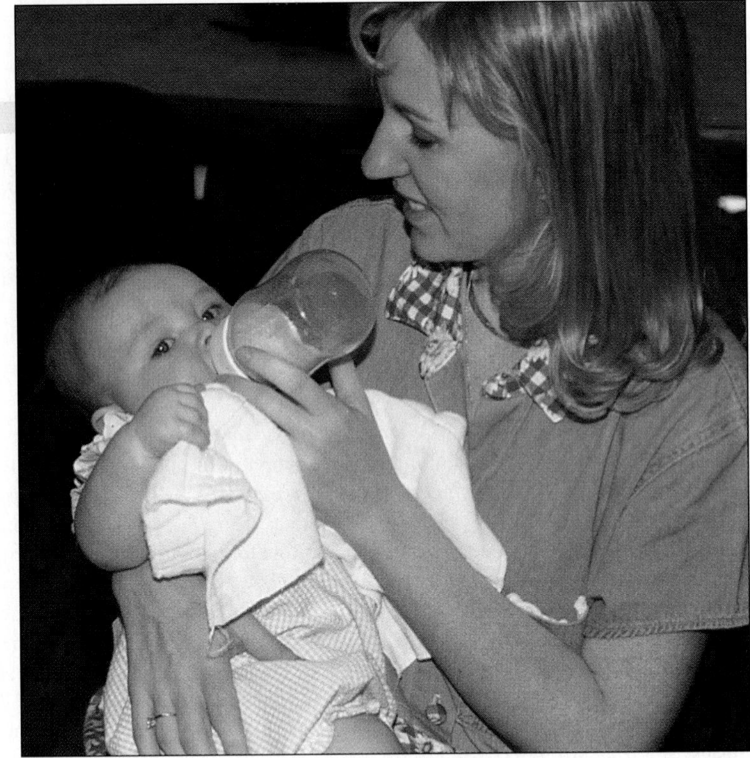

CHAPTER OVERVIEW

LEARNING OBJECTIVES

After studying this chapter, you should be able to:

- Explain the Food Guide Pyramid.
- Discuss the six basic nutrients.
- Describe the roles of protein and carbohydrates.
- Discuss breast-feeding, bottle feeding, and weaning.
- Describe vitamin and mineral supplementation for the infant.
- Explain the introduction of solids into the infant's diet.
- Describe the special nutritional needs of low–birth-weight infants.
- Discuss the components of nutritional assessment.
- Describe an increased nutritional requirement of the adolescent.
- Describe the components of assessment for an obese child.
- List the most common foods causing allergies.

KEY TERMS

anthropometric measurements: measurement of height, weight, head circumference, skinfold thickness, and arm circumference

body mass index (BMI): body weight (kg) divided by height squared used as an index of relative weight and obesity

complex carbohydrates: classed as complex because they are large molecules with many bonds that must be broken so that monosaccharides can be released and absorbed; include starch, glycogen, and cellulose

food jags: the refusal of previously liked foods or the requesting of a particular food at every meal

nutrients: foods that supply the body with elements necessary for metabolism

physiologic anorexia: normal loss of appetite

recommended dietary allowance (RDA): recommendations for the average amounts of nutrients that should be consumed daily by healthy people in the United States

WIC: Special Supplemental Food Program for Women, Infants, and Children with the purpose of improving the nutritional status of pregnant and breast-feeding women and children up to age 5 years from low-income families

Social and economic changes have increased the risk of nutritional deficits in children. Increased fragmentation of the family, unemployment, homelessness, and inadequate access to information and aid are all factors underlying the need for greater emphasis on the nutritional needs of infants and children.

Nurses must have an understanding of the nutritional requirements of infants and children in order to assess the needs of their clients and to plan care, including teaching and referral. Children themselves have become more aware of their nutritional needs as schools and the food industry have provided educational programs for this age-group. Still, overnutrition and undernutrition remain problems in the United States.

NUTRIENTS

To provide care for infants and children, the nurse must have an understanding of the nutritional needs of the body. The body is nourished by food. Foods are comprised of six basic **nutrients:** carbohydrates, protein, fat, vitamins, minerals, and water. Carbohydrates, fat, and protein provide energy, which is required by the cells of the body to transport all substances across the cell membrane, to synthesize substances within the cell, and to dispose of waste products. Common sources of carbohydrates, fats, and protein are listed in the accompanying box.

Carbohydrates

Carbohydrates should be the major dietary source of energy. Foods that are good sources of carbohydrates are relatively inexpensive and easily obtained. During digestion, carbohydrates are broken down to glucose and other sugars, which are absorbed into the bloodstream and used by the cells for energy. Glucose is an essential energy source for the brain and red blood cells. In the body, small amounts of carbohydrates are stored as glycogen in the liver, and in cardiac, skeletal, and smooth muscles, and larger amounts are stored as fat in adipose tissue. Insufficient calorie intake causes the body to break down protein and fat for energy and glucose production. There is no recommended dietary allowance for carbohydrates. The National Research Council recommends that after infancy at least 50% to 60% of the energy requirement should be provided by carbohydrates, especially complex carbohydrates (Food and Nutrition Board, 1989). Common sources of carbohydrates are listed in the box.

The *simplest carbohydrates* are monosaccharides, which are absorbed without further digestion. Included in this group are glucose, fructose, galactose, and mannose. Mannose is a 6-carbon sugar derived from some legumes. Glucose is abundant in many fruits, such as grapes, oranges, and dates, and in some vegetables, including fresh corn and carrots. Fructose is found naturally in honey and fruits. Galactose is found primarily in milk, although legumes also contain some galactose.

Most **complex carbohydrates** are found in starch from cereal grains, roots, vegetables, and legumes. The more mature the vegetable, the higher the starch content.

Common Sources of Nutrients

CARBOHYDRATES	FATS	PROTEINS
Breads	Butter	Meat
Cereals	Margarine	Poultry
Pasta	Shortening	Fish
Dried peas and legumes	Oils	Milk
Vegetables	Cream	Cheese
Rice	Cheeses	Eggs
Fruits	Nuts	Legumes
	Meats	

Fats

Fats should serve as the secondary source of energy by providing 30% or less of daily calorie intake. Of this amount 10% should be saturated, 10% polyunsaturated, and 10% monounsaturated fatty acids. Dietary fat allows the absorption of the fat-soluble vitamins (A, D, E, and K) and adds flavor to foods. The layer of fat beneath the skin plays a part in the regulation of body temperature. Fat is a component of cell membranes and acts as a protective padding of the internal organs. When excess calories are consumed, dietary fats are stored as excess body fat. Common sources of fat are listed in the box.

Cholesterol is not a fat but a fat-like substance classified as a lipid. Cholesterol is essential in the structure of all cells and is a major component of brain and nerve cells. It is found only in animal foods.

Proteins

Dietary *protein* is necessary for building and maintaining body tissues. Proteins are involved in homeostasis by working with other elements in the blood to maintain fluid balance. Many vitamins and minerals are bound to protein carriers for transport. Proteins, as antibodies, aid in the regulation of the body's immune system. Common sources of protein are listed in the box.

Water

Water is essential for life. It transports nutrients to cells and waste products away from the cells. It assists in the regulation of body temperature and in chemical reactions. Water lubricates joints and provides form and structure to the cells and the medium for body fluids. Water is found in most foods, including solids.

The percentage of body weight provided by water is 75% at birth. In the adult, water is 60% to 65% of the total body weight. There is an excess of extracellular fluid at birth. This high percentage of extracellular fluid (blood plasma, interstitial fluid, and lymph) predisposes the infant to a more rapid loss of total body fluid than the older child or adult and places the infant at increased risk to become dehydrated. See Chapter 24 for a further discussion of dehydration and fluid and electrolyte requirements.

Water requirements can be estimated by a variety of methods. The child's activity level and ambient temperature influence the amount of water needed.

Vitamins and Minerals

Vitamins and *minerals* are necessary in the regulation of metabolic processes. They are present in a wide variety of foods. Vitamins and minerals are added to processed formulas and to other foods such as cereals. It is generally not necessary for children to receive supplementation after infancy unless they are at nutritional risk (anorexia, chronic diseases).

Iron is the only mineral supplement recommended for healthy infants. *Vitamin K* is given at birth to prevent hemorrhagic disease. The *vitamin D* content of human milk is low and rickets can occur in breast-fed infants who are deeply pigmented or do not have adequate exposure to sunlight. These infants should receive vitamin D supplementation. *Fluoride* supplementation in the breast-fed infant shortly after birth is recommended by the American Academy of Pediatrics (AAP). This recommendation is controversial and the AAP acknowledges that fluoride supplementation could be initiated at 6 months (American Academy of Pediatrics, 1993). If powdered or concentrated formula is used, fluoride supplements should be given only if the community water contains less than 0.3 ppm of fluoride. Ready-to-feed formulas are prepared with water low in fluoride, and infants using these formulas should receive fluoride supplements. This supplementation should continue into childhood if there is insufficient fluoride in the drinking water.

Healthy infants and children consuming adequate amounts of fruits, vegetables, animal protein sources, cereals or bread, and dairy products fortified with vitamin D do not need vitamin and mineral supplementation. Children eating only vegetables and no dairy products or eggs require a supplemental source of vitamin B_{12} (American Academy of Pediatrics, 1993).

A preterm infant should receive a multivitamin supplement until he is consuming 300 kcal per day or weighs 2.5 kg. Iron supplementation is usually delayed until after the first few weeks of life. These recommendations may vary depending on the protocol of the institution and neonatologist.

DIGESTION

The role of the digestive system is to break down foods into smaller molecules so that cells can utilize them. Digestion begins in the mouth with mechanical and enzyme breakdown of food. Active chemical digestion begins in the stomach. The stomach normally empties in 1 to 4 hours depending on the kind and amount of food eaten. If carbohydrates are eaten alone, they leave the stomach most rapidly, followed by protein and fat. Within the intestinal lumen enzymes break down proteins into amino acids, carbohydrates into simple sugars, and fats into fatty acids and glycerol. Products of digestion (amino acids, sugars, fatty acids), vitamins, minerals, and fluids are absorbed through the intestinal mucosa and then enter the bloodstream for transport to body cells.

DIETARY GUIDELINES

Food Guide Pyramid. The guidelines for a healthful diet for Americans age 2 years or older were published by the United States Department of Agriculture (USDA) in 1992. The guidelines recommend that a variety of foods be eaten to get the energy, protein, vitamins, minerals, and fiber needed for good health. The diet should be low in fat, saturated fat, and cholesterol. There should be ample vegetables, fruits, and grain products to provide needed vitamins, minerals, fiber, and complex carbohydrates. Sugars, salt, and sodium should be used in moderation (see box).

The Food Guide Pyramid was developed by the USDA to show what should be eaten each day (Fig. 12–1). The pyramid focuses on eating a variety of foods to get the required nutrients and adequate energy. The importance of grains, fruits, and vegetables is evident in the pyramid. Five food groups are shown in the lower section of the pyramid. Foods in each group provide some, but not all, of the nutrients needed. No one food group is more important than another. All are needed in different proportions.

At the top of the pyramid fats, oils, and sweets are shown. These foods supply calories but little or no vitamins and minerals. These foods should be eaten sparingly. The fat and sugar symbols, throughout the pyramid, indicate fats and sugars naturally found in the various food groups. These fats and sugars are not "bad," or necessary to avoid, if one consumes the servings of each food group recommended within the pyramid.

*Dietary Guidelines for Americans**

- Eat a variety of foods.
- Maintain desirable weight.
- Avoid too much fat, saturated fat, and cholesterol.
- Eat foods with adequate starch and fiber.
- Avoid too much sugar.
- Avoid too much sodium.

*These guidelines apply to children age 2 years and older.

Adapted from guidelines issued by the United States Department of Agriculture and the Department of Health and Human Services.

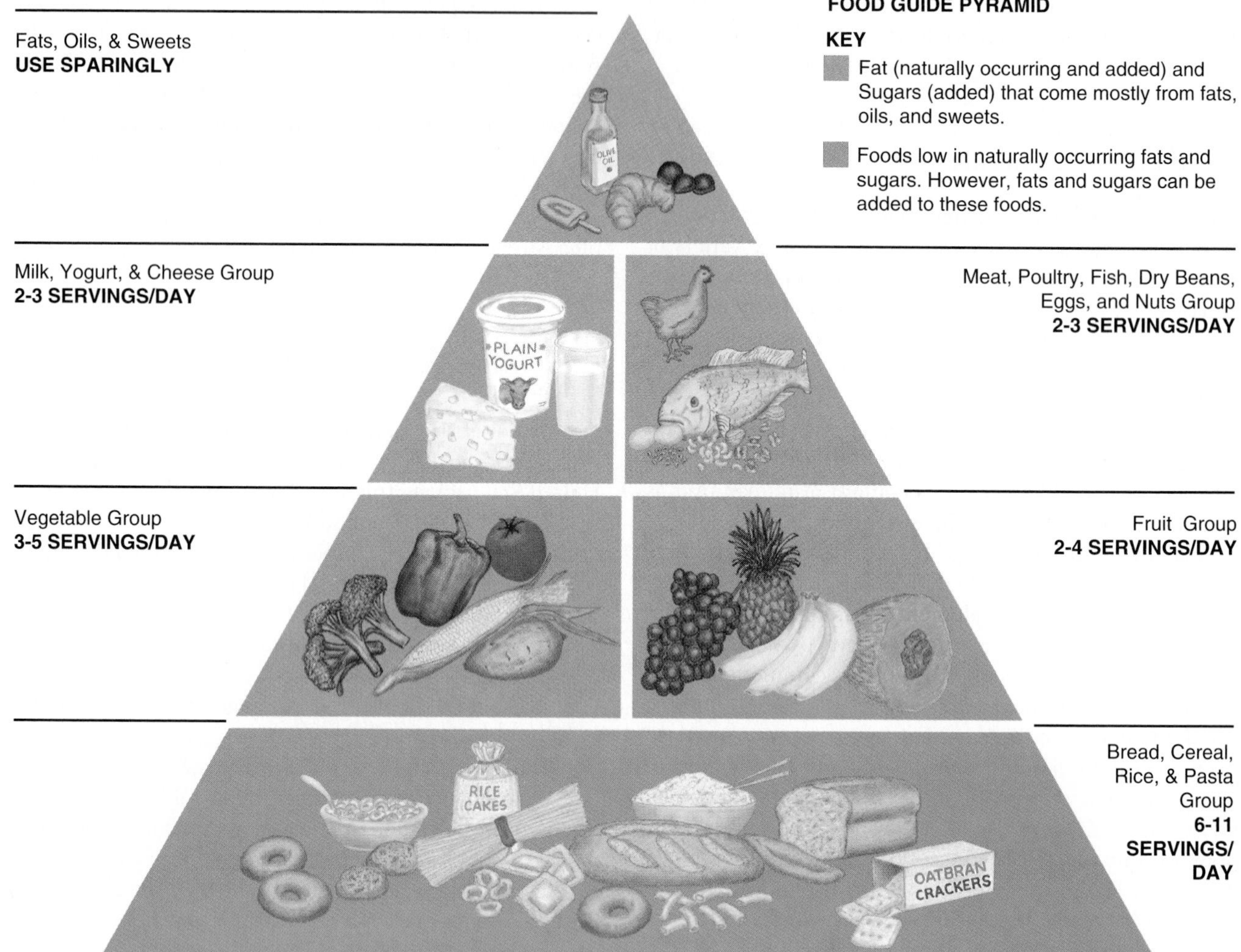

Figure 12–1

The Food Guide Pyramid shows the variety of foods needed for a healthy diet. Serving sizes are tailored to the age and energy needs of the individual child. For toddlers and preschoolers, serving size can be based on 1 tablespoon of solid food per year of age. Very active children and those going through a rapid growth spurt will have higher energy needs. (U.S. Department of Agriculture, U.S. Department of Health and Human Services)

Energy. *Energy* is measured in calories. Energy or calorie needs depend on the person's age, sex, height, weight, and level of physical activity. Food energy is measured in kilocalories (kcal), the amount of heat necessary to raise 1 kilogram of water 1° Centigrade. Carbohydrates and proteins each render 4 kcal/g of energy, and fats render 9 kcal/g. Table 12–1 shows the **Recommended Dietary Allowances (RDA)** for energy and protein for children.

Calories and Servings. The RDAs for energy and protein vary according to age. (See Table 12–1). They are determined by basal metabolism, rate of growth, and activity. Other recommended nutrient intakes are shown in Table

TABLE 12–1 *Recommended Dietary Allowances for Energy and Protein*

	CALORIES		PROTEIN	
AGE	DAILY	PER kg	DAILY	PER kg
1–3 years	1,300	102	16 g	1.2
4–6 years	1,800	90	24 g	1.1
7–10 years	2,000	70	28 g	1.0
11–14 years (female)	2,200	47	46 g	
11–14 years (male)	2,500	55	45 g	

Reprinted with permission from *Recommended Dietary Allowances: 10th Edition.* Copyright 1989 by the National Academy of Sciences. Courtesy of the National Academy Press, Washington, D.C.

TABLE 12–2 *Summary of the Recommended Daily Nutrient Intakes*

	INFANTS UNDER 13 MONTHS	CHILDREN 13 MONTHS TO 10 YEARS	CHILDREN 11–18 YEARS	PREGNANT OR LACTATING FEMALES
Protein (g)	13–14	16–28	44–59	60–65
Vitamin A (μg RE)	375	400–700	800–1000	800–1300
Vitamin D (μg)	7.5–10	10	10	10
Vitamin E (μg α-TE)	3–4	6–7	8–10	10–12
Vitamin K (μg)	5–10	15–30	45–65	65
Vitamin C (mg)	30–35	40–45	50–60	70–95
Thiamin (mg)	0.3–0.4	0.7–1.0	1.1–1.5	1.5–1.6
Riboflavin (mg)	0.4–0.5	0.8–1.2	1.3–1.8	1.6–1.8
Niacin (mg)	5–6	9–13	15–20	17–20
Vitamin B6 (mg)	0.3–0.6	1–1.4	1.4–2.0	2.1–2.2
Folate (μg)	25–35	50–100	150–200	260–400
Vitamin B12 (μg)	0.3–0.5	0.7–1.4	2.0	2.2–2.6
Calcium (mg)	400–600	800	1,200	1,200
Phosphorus (mg)	300–500	800	1,200	1,200
Magnesium (mg)	40–60	80–170	270–400	320–355
Iron (mg)	6–10	10	12–15	15–30
Zinc (mg)	5	10	12–15	15–19
Iodine (μg)	40–50	70–120	150	175–200
Selenium (μg)	10–15	20–30	40–50	65–75

See Appendix L for the complete Recommended Dietary Allowances of the National Research Council. (From "Designed for the Maintenance of Good Nutrition of Practically All Healthy People in the United States," "Estimated Safe and Adequate Daily Dietary Intakes of Selected Vitamins and Minerals," "Estimated Sodium, Chloride, and Potassium Minimum Requirements of Healthy Persons," Food and Nutrition Board, National Academy of Sciences, in Williams, S. R. [1994]. *Essentials of Nutrition and Diet Therapy* [6th ed.]. St. Louis: Mosby-Year Book, Inc.)

12–2 and Appendix L. Recommended Dietary Allowances are used as an assessment guide, and their use should be limited to healthy infants and children. Very active children and those going through rapid growth spurts have higher energy needs than more sedate children and/or those who are at periods when growth is slower.

CULTURAL AND RELIGIOUS INFLUENCES ON DIET

Dietary intake is profoundly affected by both cultural and religious beliefs. An understanding of these patterns will assist the nurse in both the assessment and implementation of nutrition-related behaviors. Hospitalized children who become stressed by being in a new and strange environment do not need the added stress of unfamiliar foods. Information regarding a child's food preferences can be obtained during a dietary history. Table 12–3 indicates common food practices of selected ethnic groups.

A child's religious beliefs may also have an impact on the types of foods eaten and the way in which they are served. Within religious groups there may be a variety of dietary observances. Table 12–4 can be used as a guide to some of the more common dietary restrictions related to religious beliefs, but the nurse should assist and encourage the child and/or family in communicating specific dietary needs.

THE NURSING PROCESS IN RELATION TO CHILDHOOD NUTRITION

Assessment

A nutritional assessment is an essential component of the health examination of infants and children. This assessment should include anthropometric data, biochemical data, clinical examination, and dietary history. From these data a plan of care can be developed. In addition, children at risk can be identified and areas of prevention pursued through teaching and further evaluation and follow-up.

Anthropometric Data. *Height* and *head circumference* reflect past nutrition or chronic nutritional problems. Present nutritional status is better reflected by *weight, skinfold thickness*, and *midarm circumference*. The nurse should always be aware of the role that birth weight, ethnic, familial, and

Text continued on page 268

TABLE 12-3 *Cultural Food Practices*

FOODS	PREPARATION
Spanish-American/Mexican Dietary Habits*	
Meats: Chicken, pork chops, wieners, cold cuts, and hamburger.	Used only once or twice a week.
Other Proteins: Eggs, beans.	Eggs used frequently and usually fried. In rural areas, chickens are kept for their eggs. Beans usually eaten mashed and refried with lard.
Vegetables: Potatoes, red and green chilies, fresh and canned tomatoes, pumpkin, corn, field greens, onions, carrots.	Potatoes are a basic item, usually fried; may be used three times a day. Chilies are popular at each meal. Fresh tomatoes are very popular. Other vegetables used frequently.
Fruits: Bananas, melons, peaches, canned fruit cocktail, oranges, apples.	Oranges, apples used occasionally as snacks. Others are the more popular fruits.
Cereals and breads: Oatmeal, enriched white flour, packaged breakfast cereals, macaroni, white bread, tortillas, sweet rolls.	Sugar-coated packaged cereals are popular; oatmeal used occasionally. Macaroni is fried and served with beans and potatoes. Tortillas are homemade daily. Both purchased and homemade breads are used frequently. Purchased sandwich bread is a status symbol.
Milk: Limited availability, expensive.	
Cheese: Limited amounts used.	
Fats: Lard, salt pork, bacon fat.	Used liberally. Most foods are fried.
Beverages: Soft drinks; other sweets very popular.	
Cuban Dietary Habits	
Meats: Beef, pork, lamb, veal, poultry, sausages.	Pork is either roasted or fried. Beef and chicken are used in soups, stewed, roasted, broiled, or barbecued. The sausages are used with beans.
Fish: All varieties of fish (fresh, salted, smoked, and canned).	Fried, boiled, marinated, roasted, or grilled.
Other proteins: Beans (black, red, kidney, navy, yellow, lima, green); split peas; eggs.	Black beans with rice and roast pork is a favorite dish and is eaten on Christmas day. Eggs are eaten daily; fried, scrambled, or in dessert.
Vegetables: Native tubers such as *yuca, ñame, malanga* (white and yellow), *boniato* (white yams), *chayote, berenjena,* plantain, potatoes, lettuce, tomatoes, carrots.	The tubers are boiled and served with *mojo* (made with sour orange, crushed garlic, sliced onions, and hot oil), or mashed with butter and milk. Fried ripe or green plantains are a favorite side dish.
Fruits: Anona, *mamey, guanábana, chirimoya,* papaya, banana, *zapote, marañón,* mangoes, grapefruit, oranges (sweet and sour), coconuts, *caimito.*	Eaten fresh, in juice, or in desserts such as pastes, jellies, puddings.
Cereals: Rice, cornmeal, cornstarch; imported breakfast cereals, such as oatmeal, corn flakes.	The favorite is white (long grain) steamed rice; sometimes *bijol* is added to make it yellow as in *arroz con pollo* (yellow rice with chicken). White rice is eaten daily for dinner and supper.
Milk: Fresh cow's milk (whole, skimmed), condensed, evaporated, dry; sour cream; goat's milk for the sick, usually.	Adults use it in coffee; children use as beverage. Also used in cream sauces, gravies, desserts, etc.
Cheese: Gouda, cream, *queso de mano.*	The native cheese is *queso de mano* (hard cheese) made from milk, lactate of calcium, and salt, which looks like compressed cottage cheese; usually eaten with guava paste.
Fats: Pork lard, olive oil, peanut oil, soy oil, butter, margarine, and shortening.	Pork lard is most popular. Oil is used in salads and beans.
Desserts: Fruits, ice cream, cakes, pies, custards, puddings; guava, prune and mango pastes; *morón* cookies, *terrejas, boniatillo, buñuelos, cafiroleta.*	Eaten after each meal and also as snacks. *Raspadura* is very sweet and the most typical native dessert.
Seasonings: Oil, vinegar, cumin, oregano, *bijol,* salt, pepper, garlic, onion, green peppers.	
Beverages: Coffee, beer, wines, tea, carbonated beverages.	Dark strong coffee served demitasse, with or without sugar.
Greek Dietary Habits	
Meats: Lamb is main meat. Some beef, goat, mutton, pork products; poultry is popular.	Meat is either cut into small pieces or ground. Poultry is cooked into broth. Lamb is cooked on skewers or cut up and browned in oil or fat with rice or flour and vegetables.
Fish: Salt-water fish (fresh, smoked or salted), shellfish, smoked roe, squid, and octopus.	Fish is fried or steamed with vegetables. Used frequently.
Other proteins: Eggs, white beans, and legumes.	Legumes are boiled, mashed, or stewed and eaten either hot or cold. Soup made of dried beans, onions, celery, and carrots is a national dish. Eggs are popular.

TABLE 12–3 *Cultural Food Practices (continued)*

FOODS	PREPARATION
Vegetables: Cabbage, cauliflower, cucumbers, eggplant, greens, okra, onions, peppers, some potatoes, vine leaves, zucchini, tomatoes, salad greens.	Vegetables are boiled or fried in a small amount of olive oil and served hot or cold. Many vegetables are stuffed. Potatoes or vegetables are cooked with meat or fish. Lemon juice is used to dress salads and cold foods.
Fruits: Apricots, cherries, dates, oranges, lemons, figs, grapes, melons, nuts, plums, peaches, pears, quinces, and raisins.	Fruits in season are eaten raw, grapes are pressed into wine or dried as raisins. Fruit for dessert.
Cereals and breads: Maize, rice, and wheat.	Maize is used in polenta; rice is an ingredient for *pilawi* and stuffing for vegetables; wheat is made into bread. Bread used abundantly, and white is preferred.
Milk: Cow's, goat's, and sheep's milk.	Milk is boiled for children. Fermented milk or *yaourti* is eaten as dessert or with pastry.
Cheese: Soft and mild, hard and dry cheeses.	Cheese is popular.
Fats: Olive oil, seed oils, salted black olives, and little butter.	Olive oil is used to dress salads and hot or cold vegetables and in cooking.
Seasonings: Caraway and pumpkin seeds, herbs, honey, nuts (hazel, pignolia, and pistachio), and sesame.	Seeds are eaten between meals, and nuts are served as dessert.
Beverages: Coffee and wine.	Coffee (American) is the beverage served in the mornings. At other meals it is made and served Turkish style. Wine is served at meals.
Japanese Dietary Habits	
Meats: The Buddhist tradition of not eating meat conforms with the physical necessities of agriculture. The Japanese consume very little meat, except beef. Since World War II, however, protein intake has steadily increased.	Quantity is small. Usually cut into small pieces and served mixed with vegetables and cereal products.
Fish: Liked and one of the staple foods.	Prefer fish, shellfish, and other marine life to meats of all types. Certain kinds of raw fish are considered great delicacies. Others cooked or dried.
Other proteins: Soybean preparations used freely. Eggs used when available.	Variety of soybean preparations.
Vegetables: Prefer plants such as seaweed, bamboo shoots, onions, large radishes, dried mushrooms (*shiitake*), and beans. Potatoes and others when available.	Pickled is the favorite form. Others cooked with meat or fish.
Fruits: Principal fruit is *nasi* (tastes somewhat like pear, shaped like an apple; yellow, rough skin). Some persimmons and mulberries. Tangerines in mountain regions. Postwar increase in variety.	Dessert.
Cereals and breads: Rice is main food. Some barley, oats, and rye.	Rice is mixed with barley by farmers and the poorer classes. Wheat bread, especially in urban communities.
Milk: Enjoy when available; mainly import evaporated or dry milk powder.	Mostly for children.
Cheese: Very little.	
Fats: Soy oil. Rice oil. Suet when available. Practically no butter or cream.	Used in cooking.
Seasonings: Salt, *sake* (liquor distilled from rice).	
Beverages: Tea, *sake.*	Tea freely used when affordable.
Chinese Dietary Habits	
Meats: Pork (favorite), lamb, goat, and poultry. Entire animal is eaten, including organs, brain, spinal cord, skin, and coagulated blood.	Quantity is small and is usually cut into small thin slices about 2 inches long and cooked in sesame or peanut oil with soy sauce, spices, and a little water and served mixed with vegetables. Many methods for preserving and drying. Sweet and pungent pork or duck is a favorite (meat cubes rolled in batter and fried in oil, then simmered in sauce made of pineapple, green peppers, molasses, brown sugar, vinegar, and seasonings).
Fish: Fish and shellfish liked.	Fish is frequently baked with native spices or prepared in sweet-and-sour dishes. Many dried.

(continued)

TABLE 12–3 *Cultural Food Practices (continued)*

FOODS	PREPARATION
Other proteins: Hen, duck, and pigeon eggs in abundance when affordable; soybean products; legumes.	Eggs are preserved and dried; also combined with chicken, mushrooms, and bean sprouts and served with soy sauce (looks like vegetable omelet), termed *egg foo yong.* Egg roll served at beginning of meal is made of shrimp or meat and chopped vegetables rolled in thin dough and fried in deep fat. Soybeans used as sauce, as milk for infants in China, and in many products. Legumes as substitute for meat.
Vegetables: Many plants such as carrots, onions, leeks, peas, cabbage, white turnips, corn, cucumbers, green and yellow beans, squash, shepherd's purse, radish leaves, sprouts (bean, bamboo, etc.), some white but more sweet potatoes.	Cut into uniform pieces and simmered or steamed with eggs or meat or added to meat and widely used in soups.
Fruits: Kumquat is favorite.	Preserved dessert.
Cereals and breads: Rice used freely. Some wheat, barley, corn, and millet seed. Noodles are popular. Rice is main dish; others are side dishes.	Rice is used as main dish, plain or fried. Millet seed is made into cakes or used in a gruel. Noodles are small and fried. Steamed bread is eaten at breakfast.
Milk: Very little and generally not used. Given to children and invalids.	
Cheese: Little used.	
Fats: Chief oil is peanut oil. Some soy oil, rice oil, sesame oil, or lard. Practically no butter or cream.	Used in cooking.
Seasonings: Sesame seed, salt, ginger, garlic, fresh herbs, red pepper.	
Beverage: Tea is the national beverage.	Beverage at all meals, when affordable.
Laotian Dietary Habits [†]	
Meats: Pork, beef, chicken, rabbit, wild pig, buffalo, deer, snake, and elephant.	Eaten fresh, dried, or salted. Prepared by frying, boiling, baking, or broiling, mixed with vegetables and spices. Hmong and Mien might also eat monkey and bear.
Fish: Numerous varieties of freshwater fish and shellfish. Saltwater fish available in cities.	Eaten fresh, fermented, dried, or salted. *Padek,* a fermented fish paste made from small whole fish, salt, and rice bran, is frequently eaten by lowland Lao but not by the Hmong and the Mien.
Other proteins: Eggs, peanuts, black-eyed peas, kidney beans.	Soybean products not eaten by the Lao. Soybean curd (tofu) sometimes eaten by Hmong. Legumes often used in desserts.
Vegetables: Wide variety of vegetables, including pumpkin, squash, squash blossoms and young shoots, tomato, cabbage, spinach, green papaya, bamboo shoots, mushrooms, watercress, cucumber, and corn. See also Vietnamese vegetables.	Eaten raw, as juice, or cooked with meat or fish. Preserved by drying or pickling.
Fruits: See Vietnamese fruits. Wide variety consumed.	Usually eaten fresh or as juice. Tamarinds sometimes salted and eaten as a snack.
Cereals and breads: Glutinous (sticky) rice, wheat, rice or bean thread noodles, French bread.	Sticky rice is rinsed several times and then soaked overnight. The soaking water is discarded, and the rice is steamed. It is eaten with the fingers at meals or as a snack. The Hmong eat regular rice. Bread is eaten plain, with paté or coconut milk.
Milk: Sweetened condensed milk.	Sometimes diluted and used as infant formula. Also as a beverage for adults.
Fats: Lard.	
Seasonings: Padek, chili, lemon grass, coconut milk, coriander, tamarind, curry, monosodium glutamate, red and black pepper, salt, fish sauce, browned ground rice, mint.	*Padek* and chilies are characteristic seasonings of the lowland Lao.
Beverages: Soybean drink, sugar cane drink, tea, coconut juice, fruit or vegetable juice, beer, wine.	

TABLE 12-3 *Cultural Food Practices (continued)*

FOODS	PREPARATION
Vietnamese Dietary Habits[†]	
Meats: Pork, beef, chicken, sausage, chicken feet, ox tails, liver, stomach.	Pork is most common. Chicken is consumed only on special occasions. Meats are usually cut into small pieces and fried, boiled, or steamed. (See also Chinese Dietary Habits.)
Fish: Numerous types of freshwater and saltwater fish and shellfish.	Eaten fresh, dried, salted, or fermented. Chinese like to steam fish, while Vietnamese like it fried and dipped in fish sauce.
Other proteins: Eggs, soybeans, peanuts, other legumes.	Soybeans eaten in processed forms such as soy sauce, soybean milk, and soybean curd (tofu). Peanuts eaten in soups or as a snack. Legumes eaten in desserts (Chinese influence) or in soups.
Vegetables: Wide variety of vegetables, including bamboo shoots, bok choy, broccoli, carrots, cauliflower, napa cabbage, mustard greens, bittermelon, wintermelon, green beans, eggplant, corn, water chestnuts, (see also Laotian vegetables).	Eaten fresh, dried, or pickled. Usually eaten with meat or fish. Vietnamese eat raw vegetables more often than Chinese-Vietnamese.
Fruits: Wide variety of fruits, including bananas, mangoes, papayas, pineapples, melons, oranges, pears, grapefruit, longans, and tamarinds.	Usually eaten fresh. Sometimes cook pear or papaya to make a sweet soup for dessert.
Cereals and breads: Short-grain, long-grain, and glutinous rice (See Laotian Dietary Habits), bean thread, wheat and rice noodles, French bread.	Rice is often eaten with every meal. It is rinsed several times before steaming. Bread eaten plain or with pork, paté, or sweetened condensed milk.
Milk: Sweetened condensed milk.	Served in coffee, with hot water, or on bread. Also sometimes used as infant formula.
Fats: Lard, peanut oil.	
Seasonings: Oyster sauce, soy sauce, monosodium glutamate, black pepper, ginger, garlic, green onion, coriander, sesame oil (Chinese influence), curry (Indian influence), mint, dill, red pepper, lemon grass, vinegar, lemon, *nuoc mam* sauce.	Vietnamese food tends to be hotter than Chinese food. *Nuoc mam* sauce is a fish sauce, a thin extract made from fermented fish and salt.
Beverages: Tea, coffee, soft drinks, soybean milk, sugar-cane drink, beer, and wine.	Tea is the most common beverage. Beer and wine are only for the men.
Cambodian Dietary Habits[†]	
Meats: Pork, beef, chicken, deer, wild pig, buffalo, rabbit.	Eaten fresh, dried, or salted. Prepared by frying, boiling, baking, with spices. Not eaten as frequently as fish. Pork and chicken are expensive.
Fish: Numerous types of freshwater and saltwater fish and shellfish.	Very common food. *Prahoc,* a salted fermented fish paste, is a characteristic Cambodian food eaten with rice and raw vegetables. Fish also eaten fresh, smoked, or dried.
Other proteins: Eggs, peanuts, soybeans, other legumes.	Eggs are expensive and thus are not eaten often. Soybeans eaten only by Chinese Cambodians. Legumes eaten in desserts.
Vegetables: See Laotian and Vietnamese vegetables.	Eaten raw with *prahoc* or cut up small and cooked with other protein foods.
Fruits: See Vietnamese fruits.	Eaten raw as dessert or snack.
Cereals and breads: Long-grain, short-grain, glutinous (see Laotian Dietary Habits), and black, sweet rice; rice and egg noodles, French bread.	Glutinous and black, sweet rice used in desserts. French bread found mostly in cities.
Milk: Sweetened condensed milk.	Sometimes eaten on bread or used as infant formula.
Fats: Lard.	
Seasonings: Prahoc, red pepper, vinegar, garlic, ginger, curry salt, monosodium glutamate, lemon, coconut milk, and coriander.	*Prahoc* is a characteristic seasoning. Food is generally not as hot as Laotian food.
Beverages: Tea, coffee, soft drink, beer, soybean drinks, sugar-cane drink.	

*Adapted from *Cultural Food Patterns in the U.S.A.* Chicago, American Dietetic Association, 1976.

[†]Developed by Andrea Carlson, M.S., R.D.

From Mahan, L., & Arlin, M. (1992). *Krause's food, nutrition and diet therapy* (8th ed). Philadelphia: W.B. Saunders.

TABLE 12–4 *Religious Beliefs Affecting Diet*

Baptist, Church of Christ, Church of God, Pentecostal	Most groups discourage alcohol and some coffee and tea.
Buddhism	Some groups are strict vegetarian. Discourage use of alcohol, coffee, and tea.
Eastern Orthodox (Greek Orthodox, Russian Orthodox, Armenian)	May fast Wednesdays, Fridays during Lent, before Christmas, or for 6 hours before Communion (seriously ill are exempted). May avoid meat, dairy products, and olive oil during fast (seriously ill are exempted).
Episcopal	May abstain from meat on Fridays. May fast during Lent or before Communion.
Friends (Quaker)	Most avoid alcohol and practice moderation.
Hinduism	Many vegetarian. Mandatory abstinence from alcohol for some groups. No beef or pork. Prefer fresh, cooked foods.
Jehovah's Witness	No foods to which blood has been added. May eat meats that have been drained.
Judaism	Strict Kosher dietary laws are not followed by all of the Jewish faith. Strict Kosher prohibits pork, shellfish, and the eating of meat and dairy products at same meal or with same dishes. Milk products served first can be followed by meat in a few minutes; however, the reverse is not true. Fast for 24 hours on holy day of Yom Kippur (seriously ill are exempted). Matzo replaces leavened bread during Passover.
Mormon	No alcohol, tobacco, and hot drinks (tea and coffee). Sparing use of meats.
Muslim (Islamic, Moslem) and Black Muslim	Pork prohibited. May oppose alcohol and traditional black American foods (corn bread, collard greens).
Roman Catholic	Fast and abstain from meat on Ash Wednesday and Good Friday. (Abstaining from meat on all Fridays during Lent is highly recommended; seriously ill are exempted.) Children are not expected to fast.
Seventh-Day Adventist	No alcohol, coffee, tea, narcotics, or stimulants. Some abstain from pork, other meat, and shellfish.

Adapted from Carpenito, L. (1995). *Nursing diagnosis: Application to clinical practice.* Philadelphia: J.B. Lippincott.

environmental factors play when evaluating **anthropometric measurements.** Infants and children should be measured during each preventive health care visit. (Reference to the AAPs Recommendations For Preventive Health Care.)

Weight and *height* can be plotted on grids to determine if the child is within the normal parameters for age. The nurse should also look at trends and be alerted to sudden loss or gain that does not coincide with normal growth and development trends. Children who are above the 95th percentile or below the fifth percentile need further evaluation.

Differences in skeletal size and the proportion of lean body mass can explain variations in body weight among children the same height. The *skinfold thickness measurement* is a means of measuring this difference. Skinfolds over the triceps and below the scapula are the most accurate sites for measurement because the most complete standards and methods of evaluation are available for these sites.

Midarm circumference measurements are usually used when actual body composition is needed. The upper arm circumference is measured halfway between the acromion process of the scapula and the tip of the elbow. The midarm muscle area gives an indication of the lean body mass and indicates the skeletal protein reserves, which are important in growing children.

Biochemical Data. Biochemical data measurements can be obtained from the examination of plasma, blood cells, urine, or tissues such as liver, bone, and hair. Although biochemical tests are the most objective measurement of nutritional status, their accuracy is affected by many factors, making them complicated to perform. In addition,

TABLE 12–5 *Physical Signs Indicative or Suggestive of Malnutrition*

NORMAL APPEARANCE	SIGNS ASSOCIATED WITH MALNUTRITION	POSSIBLE DISORDER OR NUTRIENT DEFICIENCY	POSSIBLE NON-NUTRITIONAL PROBLEM
Hair Shiny; firm; not easily plucked.	Lack of natural shine; dull and dry. Thin and sparse. Dyspigmented. Flag sign. Easily plucked (no pain).	Kwashiorkor and, less commonly, marasmus.	Excessive bleaching of hair. Alopecia.
Face Skin color uniform; smooth, healthy appearance; not swollen.	Nasolabial seborrhea (scaling of skin around nostrils). Swollen face (moon face). Paleness.	Riboflavin. Kwashiorkor	Acne vulgaris.
Eyes Bright, clear, shiny; no sores at corners of eyelids; membranes a healthy pink and moist; no prominent blood vessels or mound of tissue or sclera.	Pale conjunctiva.	Anemia (e.g., iron)	Bloodshot eyes from exposure to weather, lack of sleep, smoke, or alcohol.
	Bitot's spots. Conjunctival xerosis (dryness). Corneal xerosis (dullness). Keratomalacia (softening of cornea).	Vitamin A.	
	Redness and fissuring of eyelid corners.	Riboflavin, pyridoxine.	
	Corneal arcus (white ring around eye). Xanthelasma (small yellowish lumps around eyes).	Hyperlipidemia.	
Lips Smooth, not chapped or swollen.	Angular cheilosis (white or pink lesions at corners of mouth).	Riboflavin.	Excessive salivation.
Tongue Deep red in appearance; not swollen or smooth.	Magenta tongue (purplish). Filiform papillae atrophy or hypertrophy—red tongue.	Riboflavin. Folic acid. Niacin.	Leucoplakia.
Teeth No cavities; no pain; bright.	Mottled enamel. Caries (cavities). Missing teeth.	Fluorosis. Excessive sugar.	Malocclusion. Periodontal disease. Health habits.
Gums Healthy; red; do not bleed; not swollen.	Spongy, bleeding. Receding gums.	Vitamin C.	Periodontal disease.
Glands Face not swollen.	Thyroid enlargement (front of neck swollen).	Iodine.	Allergic or inflammatory enlargement of thyroid.
	Parotid enlargement (cheeks become swollen).	Starvation. Bulimia.	
Nervous System Psychological stability; normal reflexes.	Psychomotor changes. Mental confusion.	Kwashiorkor. Thiamine.	
	Sensory loss. Motor weakness. Loss of position sense. Loss of vibration. Loss of ankle and knee jerks. Burning and tingling of hands and feet (paresthesia).	Thiamine.	

From Mahan, L., & Arlin, M. (1992). *Krause's food, nutrition and diet therapy* (8th ed). Philadelphia: W.B. Saunders.

TABLE 12–6 *24-Hour Recall Form and Food Group Evaluation*

FOOD AND FLUID INTAKE FROM TIME OF AWAKENING UNTIL THE NEXT MORNING							
	FOOD AND DRINK CONSUMED		NUMBER OF SERVINGS IN THE FOOD GROUPS				
TIME	NAME AND TYPE	AMOUNT	MILK GROUP	MEAT GROUP	FRUITS AND VEGETABLES	BREADS AND CEREALS	FATS, SWEETS, AND ALCOHOLIC BEVERAGES
	Totals						
RECOMMENDED NUMBER OF SERVINGS DAILY							
		AMOUNT	MILK GROUP	MEAT GROUP	FRUITS AND VEGETABLES	BREADS AND CEREALS	FATS, SWEETS, AND ALCOHOLIC BEVERAGES*
Children age 6 or under			2–3	2	3	4	Avoid too many
Adolescent			3–4	2–3	3–5	6–11	Avoid too many
Adult			2–3	2–3	3–5	6–11	Avoid too many
Pregnant or Lactating			3–4	2–3	3–5	6–11	Avoid too many
			MILK GROUP	MEAT GROUP	FRUITS AND VEGETABLES	BREADS AND CEREALS	FATS, SWEETS, AND ALCOHOLIC BEVERAGES
Evaluation L = low A = adequate E = excessive							

*Servings of high calorie, low-nutrient items, such as sugar, candy, and soda pop. Excessive amounts in this group usually mean excessive fat, sugar, and energy intake.

From Mahan, L., & Arlin, M. (1992). *Krause's food, nutrition and diet therapy* (8th ed). Philadelphia: W. B. Saunders.

biochemical measurements to evaluate all nutrients are not available. Blood urea nitrogen, protein, albumin, prealbumin, glucose, triglycerides, and cholesterol are a few of the biochemical measurements available.

Clinical Evaluation. The clinical evaluation includes a physical examination and complete history. Special attention is paid to the areas where signs of nutritional deficiencies appear: skin, hair, teeth, gums, lips, tongue, and eyes. Table 12–5 lists some of the physical signs suggestive of malnutrition. Clinical symptoms usually are not within themselves diagnostic but are confirmed by biochemical tests and diet histories. There may be more than one deficiency. (See also the section on Failure to Thrive in Chapter 41.)

Dietary History. Obtaining an accurate history of dietary intake is a difficult task. The knowledge that what the child is eating is being recorded can influence what the parent feeds the child and/or what the child eats. Children often cannot remember what they have eaten. If the child or parent is not committed to the process, incomplete information may be obtained. However, it is still a useful assessment process and should be used. Patient teaching should include an understanding of the importance of recording the child's dietary intake and the need for accuracy. Common methods of assessing dietary intake include the following:

- 24-hour recall
- food frequency questionnaire
- food diary

TABLE 12–7 *A General Food Frequency Questionnaire*

For the frequency of food use, the following pattern of questions may be useful. However, you may have to modify questions after learning some information from the 24-hour recall. For instance, if the patient has said he or she had a glass of milk yesterday, you wouldn't ask "Do you drink milk?" but rather "How much milk do you drink?" Record answers as 1/day, 1/wk, 3/mo, for example, or as accurately as possible. It may just have to be noted as "occasionally" or "rarely."

1. Do you drink milk? If so, how much? ________ What kind? Whole ________ Skim ________ Low-fat ________
2. Do you use fat? If so, what kind? ________ How much? ________
3. How many times do you eat meat? ________ eggs ________ cheese ________ beans ________
4. Do you eat snack foods? If so, which ones? ________ How often? ________ How much? ________
5. What vegetables do you eat? (in each group) How often?
   a. Broccoli ________ green peppers ________ cooked greens ________ carrots ________ sweet potato ________
   b. Tomatoes ________ raw cabbage ________
   c. Asparagus ________ beets ________ cauliflower ________ corn ________ cooked cabbage ________ celery ________ peas ________ lettuce ________
6. What fruits and how often?
   a. Apples or applesauce ________ apricots ________ banana ________ berries ________ cherries ________ grapes or grape juice ________ peaches ________ pears ________ pineapple ________ plums ________ prunes ________
   b. Oranges ________ orange juice ________ grapefruit ________ grapefruit juice ________
7. Bread and cereal products
   a. How much bread do you usually eat with each meal? ________ between meals ________
   b. Do you eat cereal (daily, weekly) cooked ________ dry ________
   c. How often do you eat foods such as macaroni, spaghetti, noodles, etc. ________
   d. Do you eat whole grain breads and cereals? ________ how often? ________
8. Do you use salt? ________ Do you salt your food before tasting it? ________ Do you cook with salt? ________ Do you "crave" salt or salty foods? ________
9. How many tsp of sugar do you use/day (1 packet = 1 tsp)? ________ (Be sure to ask patient about sugar on cereal, fruit, toast and in coffee, tea, etc.)
10. Do you eat desserts? ________ If so, how often? ________
11. Do you drink sugar-containing beverages such as soda pop? ________ How often? ________
12. How often do you eat candy or cookies? ________
13. Do you drink water? ________ How often during the day? ________ How much each time? ________ How much would you say you drink each day? ________
14. Do you use sugar substitutes in packet form or in drinks? ________ What is your use? ________ How often? ________
15. Do you drink alcohol? ________ How often? ________ How much? ________ Beer, wine, liquor? ________

From Mahan, L., & Arlin, M. (1992). *Krause's food, nutrition and diet therapy* (8th ed). Philadelphia: W. B. Saunders.

Twenty-Four-Hour Recall. The most frequently used intake assessment method is the *24-hour recall method.* The child or parent is asked to recall everything eaten during the past 24 hours. A questionnaire may be used or the nurse may conduct an interview asking the pertinent questions (Table 12–6).

The child or parent may have difficulty remembering the kinds and amounts of food eaten. Or, they may have had an atypical day on the previous day and/or they may not feel comfortable relating what was eaten the day being evaluated. How the child or parent sees the nurse may influence the response; they may say what they think the interviewer wants to hear. Asking for information in relation to meals eaten as opposed to food groups may increase the accuracy of the assessment.

Food Frequency Questionnaire. The *food frequency questionnaire* gathers information on intake of particular foods or food groups on a daily, weekly, or monthly basis. This tool can be used to validate the 24-hour recall data (Table 12–7). Like all methods of assessment, this requires the interviewer to be nonjudgmental and objective. Putting the information into a questionnaire may be less threatening to a child and/or family and will save time.

Food Diary. When keeping a *food diary,* the child or parent records everything consumed during a specified time period. Various sources recommend different lengths of time for keeping the diary; 3-day to 7-day records may be used. As in all nursing care, the nurse must evaluate what is a reasonable time to expect the family and/or child to keep the records. The time, place, and people present when the food was eaten may also be recorded. This provides the nurse with additional information, which may identify trends and other information related to the child's eating behaviors.

Nursing Diagnosis and Planning

The following nursing diagnoses and expected outcomes are examples that may be appropriate following nutritional assessment.

Nursing Diagnoses

- Altered Nutrition: Less Than Body Requirements related to inability to absorb nutrients
- Altered Nutrition: Less Than Body Requirements related to insufficient intake

Expected Outcomes: The infant/child will:

- experience no further weight loss
- have an age-appropriate caloric intake
- retain foods without emesis

Nursing Diagnosis

Altered Nutrition: More Than Body Requirements related to imbalance of intake and activity

Expected Outcome: The infant/child will lose an age-appropriate amount of weight per week until desired weight is attained.

Implementation

The following sections (The Infant through The Adolescent) discuss nursing measures to encourage proper nutrition in children.

THE INFANT

The infant has high nutritional needs related to rapid growth. Energy (calorie) intake requirements are high. During the first year of life body weight triples, brain weight doubles, and length increases 50%. This is the first of two "growth spurts" that occur during childhood. The other is during adolescence, which will be discussed later in this chapter. See Chapter 4 for further discussion of the infant.

Breast-Feeding

The Committees on Nutrition of both the AAP and the Canadian Paediatric Society strongly recommend breast-feeding for full-term infants (AAP, 1993). In spite of this recommendation, there has been a decline in breast-feeding. The decline seems to be greatest in young primiparas with less than a college education (Ryan et al., 1991). It has been noted that 50% of newborns are breast-fed in the hospital, by age 5 to 6 months only 18% are breast-fed (AAP, 1993). Much of this decline is attributed to shorter hospital stays and lack of adequate support for the breast-feeding mother. This need has been met in some areas of the country by follow-up calls and visits (Moore et al., 1991). Some mothers also choose to stop breast-feeding when they return to the workplace.

Human milk has several advantages over cow's milk, which forms the base for most infant formulas. Human milk changes to meet the changing nutrient and energy needs of the infant. Human milk and colostrum contain immunologic and antibacterial components not present in cow's milk. There is less risk of allergies because cow's milk has certain proteins that human milk lacks. This may cause allergies in allergy-prone infants. Human milk is more easily digested, convenient, and economical.

Nutrients in Breast Milk versus Cow's Milk

Protein. Whey proteins constitute 60% of the protein in human milk and are easily digested by the infant. Casein, the main protein in cow's milk, is a tough, hard-to-digest curd. Some commercial formulas increase the percentage of whey to make the curd more easily digested.

Carbohydrate. The lactose count is higher in human milk than cow's milk. Lactose promotes the growth of normal bacterial flora in the intestines.

Fat. Fat provides approximately 50% of the energy from human milk and 40% to 50% from formulas. Whereas human milk contains cholesterol, some formulas are made with vegetable oils and contain little or no cholesterol.

The fat content of breast milk varies during the feeding and the time of day. The milk produced at the end of a feeding (hindmilk) and in the middle of the day has a higher fat content.

Vitamins. Vitamin C must be added to commercial formulas to meet the levels found in human milk. Vitamin D content is low in breast milk, and breast-fed infants may need supplementation, especially if they have limited exposure to sunlight.

Minerals. Full-term infants who are exclusively breast-fed generally have adequate iron stores until they are age 5 to 6 months. Iron stores in premature and multiple birth infants are depleted at a younger age—2 to 3 months. Solid foods in combination with breast milk or iron-fortified formula provide sufficient iron for normal infants.

There is not agreement on whether breast-fed infants need a fluoride supplement if the drinking water supply is inadequate (AAP, 1993). Parents should follow the recommendation of their health care provider.

Assisting the Breast-Feeding Mother

Mothers who breast-feed need instruction and support as they begin. They are more likely to succeed if they are given practical information (Hill, 1991). The infant should receive at least six feedings per 24 hours and should sleep between feedings.

> An infant who is receiving adequate intake should have at least six wet diapers over a 24-hour period.

The infant should gain an average of $\frac{1}{2}$ ounce per day. An infant who does not regain birth weight by age 3 weeks

Tips for Storing Breast Milk

- Milk may be stored 3–5 days in refrigerator or as long as 3 months in a separate freezer compartment.
- Bottles used to store breast milk should be sterilized (Sterilization can be done in the dishwasher) until the infant is about 4 months old.
- Breast milk should be thawed either in the refrigerator or by holding it under warm running water.
- Breast milk should not be boiled or thawed in the microwave oven. These methods destroy the infection-fighting properties of the milk (Winthrop, 1995).

or has continuous weight loss after 10 days should be evaluated.

Collecting and Storing Breast Milk. Mothers who must return to work need added information to make this transition. Areas of instruction should include milk expression and storage. Expressed breast milk is relatively free from bacterial contamination, but it can become contaminated when artificially collected and stored. Hands and collection equipment should be clean and the milk stored in a refrigerator. Milk not used within 48 hours should be frozen. Thawed milk should not be refrozen. (See box, Tips for Storing Breast Milk.)

Breast-Feeding Techniques. The breast-feeding mother often needs assistance with the technique for successful breast-feeding. There are several positions that both the mother and infant may assume. Several techniques to help the infant latch on to the breast may be taught. Most maternity textbooks provide ready references with detailed information about this subject. The pediatric nurse may encounter mothers of newborns on the pediatric unit and therefore should have current knowledge of proper breast-feeding techniques (see the accompanying box).

The mother should be aware that the first milk ingested, called foremilk, quenches the infant's thirst and later milk, called hindmilk, is higher in fat and leads to weight gain and greater satisfaction between feedings. Infants who nurse for short periods and then fall asleep may not be nursing long enough to receive the hindmilk. This may cause the infant to want to feed too frequently, resulting in frustration for both the infant and the mother.

Discharge Teaching for Breast-Feeding Mothers

Successful breast-feeding often depends on the support shown the mother. Some facilities provide home visits and/or may call to assess the mother's needs. The nurse should inquire how often the infant is nursing and the time spent on each breast. The mother should be asked if her milk has come in and if she is engorged and/or her nipples are sore.

Mothers may also be referred to a lactation consultant or support groups such as the La Leche League. It is becoming increasingly more common for hospitals to have nurses on staff who have become certified as lactation consultants. La Leche Leagues are available in most communities and are listed in the telephone directory. Lactation specialists are prepared to deal with more difficult problems. Significant others are included in teaching to provide a support system for the mother.

Bottle Feeding

Formula

Infant formula does not have the immunologic properties and digestibility of human milk, but it does meet the energy and nutrient requirements of infants. The Infant Formula Act of 1980, which was revised in 1986, establishes the standards for infant formulas. It also requires that the label show the quantity of each nutrient.

There are many reasons why some mothers choose to use formula. Some mothers simply do not want to breastfeed. Others may use formula to supplement an omitted breast-feeding. Formula may be used if the mother's milk is inadequate or there are medical reasons why the mother cannot breast-feed. Maternal infectious disease, inborn errors, or other conditions causing intolerance to components of milk, and maternal disorders requiring medications that might harm the infant are all contraindications to breast-feeding (AAP, 1993). Mothers who choose not to breast-feed should never be forced to breast-feed or made to feel guilty because of their choice. Rather, support should be given for whatever feeding choice is selected.

Formulas are available as three types:

- concentrated liquid, which is diluted with water according to instructions
- powder, which is mixed with water according to instructions
- ready-to-use, which can be poured directly into a bottle

It is very important that the mother understand preparation instructions and care of any leftover formula. Many manufacturers print instructions in several languages. Some health care providers discourage the use of powdered formula until the infant is past age 6 weeks.

Ready-to-use formula should be refrigerated once it is opened and discarded after 24 hours. It is helpful to write the date and time opened on formula bottles.

Although the commercially prepared formulas have many similarities, there are also differences. Some more

TEACHING GUIDELINES *for Breast Feeding*

1. Wash hands. Wash nipples with warm water, no soap.
2. There are three basic positions:
   a. The *cradle position* is achieved by cradling the infant in one arm, head resting in the bend of the elbows. The infant's lower arm is tucked out of the way and the infant's mouth is close to the breast. The mother can be sitting up in bed with pillows supporting the back or sitting in a chair.
   b. The *lying down position* is attained by having the mother lie on her side in bed with the infant lying on his side also.
   c. A pillow is needed to be successful with the *football hold.* The mother is seated in a chair and a pillow placed next to her on the nursing side. The pillow supports the elbow and the infant's buttocks, and should bring the infant's head up to the level of the breast.

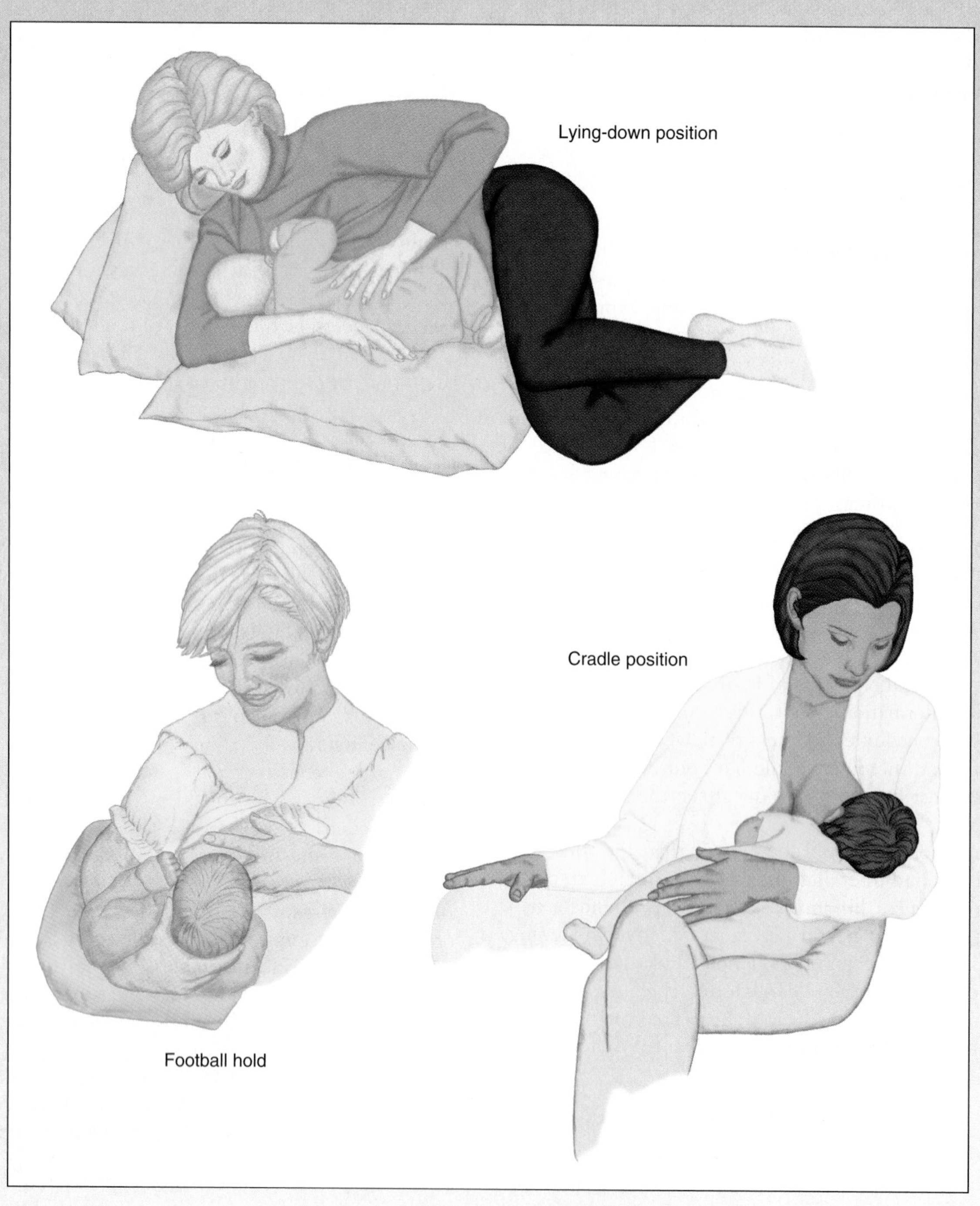

Teaching Guidelines for Breast-Feeding (continued)

3. Stroke the infant's cheek with the nipple.
4. The infant's mouth should be opened wide, as with a yawn, and should cover the entire areola, or a large amount of the areola. If necessary, apply pressure to the infant's chin with your index finger to open the infant's mouth more widely. The breast needs to be placed far back into the infant's mouth to drain the breast adequately. Your hand position is important: hold your hand in a "C" position around your breast with the thumb on top behind the areola and the fingers against the chest wall, and supporting the underside of the breast.
5. Both breasts are used: the first breast for about 10 minutes, the other breast for about 6 minutes. At the next feeding the infant starts to feed on the breast used to finish the preceding feeding.
6. Retract breast tissue from the infant's nose during sucking. Break suction by placing finger in corner of infant's mouth.
7. The neonate is nursed shortly after birth and approximately every 2 to 3 hours thereafter.
8. Infants should be burped after each breast and at the end of the feeding.
9. Nipples often become tender during the first week of nursing, but should not become sore. Soreness and prolonged feedings are most often the result of a baby who is not latched onto the breast properly.

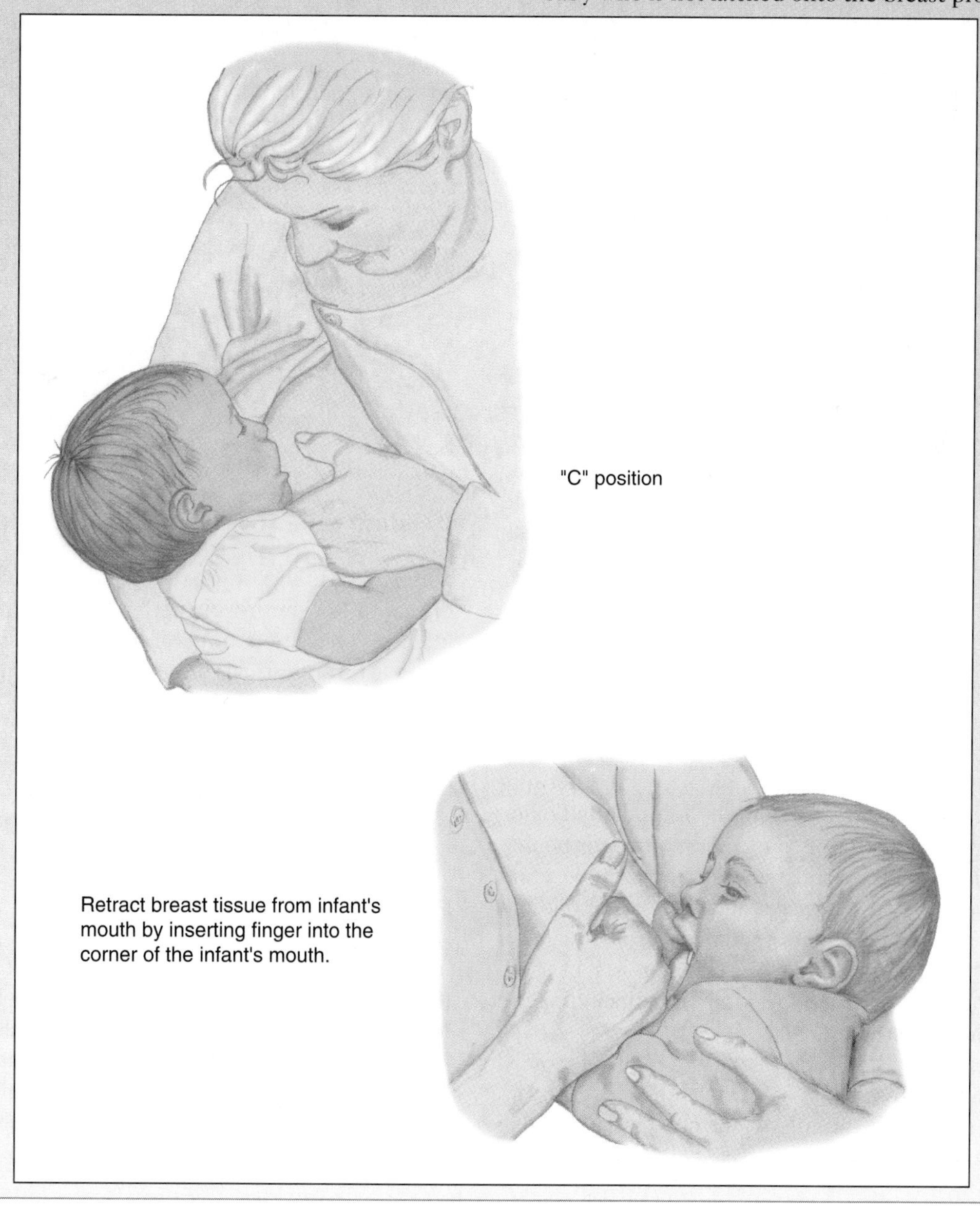
"C" position
Retract breast tissue from infant's mouth by inserting finger into the corner of the infant's mouth.

commonly used brands are Enfamil, SMA, Similac, Gerber, and Good Start. Advance and Follow-Up formulas are for older infants. Advance has fewer calories per ounce but is still fortified with vitamins and minerals. Although these formulas are suitable for the infant after age 6 months, it is not necessary to change to a different formula when the child reaches that age. Most clinicians recommend that the infant continue on the same formula until age 12 months. The AAP Committee on Nutrition recommends that all formulas be fortified with iron (AAP, 1989). Formulas come with low iron (1.5 mg/L) and regular iron (12 mg/L). There is currently controversy surrounding the use of low iron formulas (AAP News, 1995).

Soy Formulas. Infants who cannot tolerate milk protein or lactose may be given soy formulas (ProSobee, Isomil, Nursoy, Soyalac). These formulas may also be used by vegetarians and infants with IgE-mediated reaction to cow's milk proteins. However, soy milks may be allergenic in infants allergic to cow's milk protein (Miskelly et al., 1988). These formulas are generally preferred over the protein hydrolysate formulas because they are better tasting and less expensive, and there has been more experience with these formulas.

Protein Hydrolysate Formulas. Protein hydrolysate formulas were developed for infants who cannot digest intact protein or are severely allergic to intact protein. These formulas, which include Nutramigen and Progestimil, are more expensive than other formulas. Parents should be encouraged to buy small amounts until it is certain that their infant can tolerate the formula. They are mainly used for infants who cannot tolerate milk and soy-based formulas.

Protein hydrolysate formulas may also contain varying amounts of medium-chain triglycerides (MCT) to facilitate absorption of fat. Infants with cystic fibrosis, fat malabsorption, short gut syndrome, and severe chronic diarrhea benefit from this addition.

Preparation of Formula

The two most common methods of sterilization of infant's formula are aseptic sterilization and terminal sterilization. In the aseptic method, the bottles, nipples, and other supplies are sterilized separately from the formula by boiling for 20 minutes. In the terminal method, formula is poured into unsterilized bottles and they are sterilized together for 25 minutes. However, bottles and formula are not routinely sterilized where sanitary conditions are adequate. In this case the clean technique, which consists of good handwashing and washing of all equipment, including the cans of formula, is used.

Instructions on the labels should be followed closely. Some products are packaged with directions in several languages. Warming the formula is not necessary, although many parents prefer to do so. Nursing babies who get only an occasional bottle of formula may prefer it warm. The bottle may be warmed by letting it stand in a container of hot water for several minutes or by holding it under warm tap water. See the Teaching Guidelines for Bottle Feeding box as well as Chapter 3.

> Bottles should not be warmed in the microwave to prevent accidental burning either through a bottle exploding or the development of "hot spots," which cannot be felt by touching the outside of the bottle.

> Leftover formula should not be rewarmed for future feedings because of the risk of bacterial growth.

Cow's Milk

Cow's milk (whole, skim, 1%, and 2%) is not recommended in the first 12 months. Cow's milk contains too little iron, and its high renal solute load and unmodified derivatives can put small infants at risk for dehydration. The tough, hard curd is difficult for infants to digest. In addition, skim milk and reduced fat milk deprive the infant of needed calories and essential fatty acids. The incidences of allergy and iron deficiency anemia are higher with cow's milk.

> Cow's milk, skim milk, 1% to 2% fat milk, and evaporated milk formulas are not recommended in the first 12 months of life (AAP, 1992).

Feeding the Low-Birth-Weight Infant

The ability to ingest, digest, absorb, and utilize nutrients differs in low-birth-weight (LBW) infants from full-term infants. The immaturity of the gastrointestinal system alters gastrointestinal motility and enzyme availability. Gastric emptying is delayed due to the small stomach capacity and impaired gut motility of the LBW infant. The LBW infant is easily fatigued and has difficulty sucking because of the inability to coordinate sucking, swallowing, and respirations. This also increases the risk of aspiration.

Human Milk. The requirements for energy, protein, minerals, and selected vitamins are usually higher in these infants than in term infants. However, the growth demands of the LBW infant may exceed the contents of human milk for protein and some minerals and vitamins. Mixtures of whey-predominant protein, carbohydrate, calcium, phosphate, trace minerals, and vitamins have been commercially developed to add to milk from mothers to fill these deficiencies.

TEACHING GUIDELINES *for Bottle Feeding*

SUPPLIES

- Six bottles and 12 nipples. The type does not matter, but all should be the same to avoid frustrating the infant.
- Bottle brush (used to reach all crevices).
- Dishwasher basket (for securing the pieces in the dishwasher).

PREPARATION

- Use commercial formula rather than cow's, goat's, or soy milk. These types of milk lack the nutrients necessary for growth.
- Do not use "raw" or unpasteurized milk. This type of milk contains bacteria that can make the infant ill.
- Tap water does not need to be boiled before it is mixed with formula. Boiling can concentrate the minerals that are found in the water supply.
- If well water is used to mix formula, it should be checked for safety before use.
- Formula does not need to be sterilized. It is sterilized during the manufacturing process. It needs to be refrigerated.
- It is not necessary to heat bottles before feeding them to the infant.
- Bottles should never be heated in a microwave oven. Hot spots can occur in the formula and cause burns. Heating also changes the nutritional composition of the formula.

FEEDING

- Hold the infant close with the head elevated.
- A quivering motion during sucking indicates that the nipple has collapsed. Remove the bottle from the infant's mouth to break the vacuum.
- Low flow despite vigorous sucking indicates that the nipple opening is clogged or the screw cap is too tight. Loosen the cap and see if the flow improves. If not, inspect the nipple opening.
- Do not "prop" the bottle or put the infant to bed with a bottle in his mouth. Bottle propping prevents close contact and increases chances of aspiration and middle ear infections. These practices also allow sugar to accumulate around the teeth and may lead to milk bottle caries.

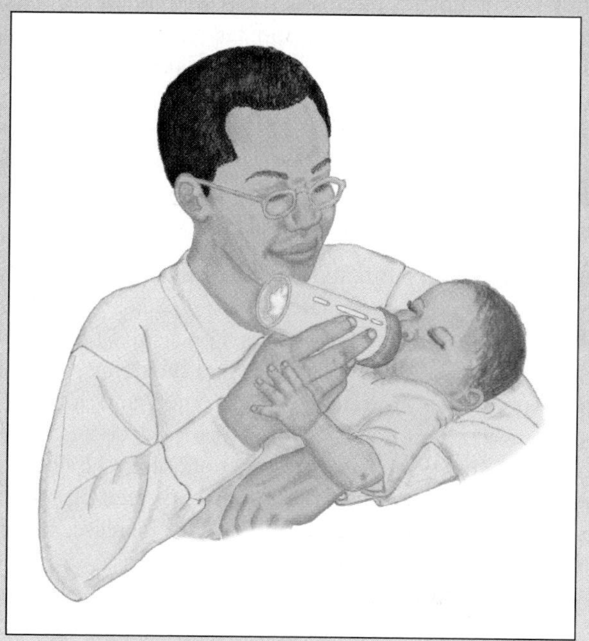

STORING INFANT FORMULA

- Unopened formula should be stored in a cool, dry place and used before the expiration date printed on the can.
- Refrigerate opened cans of formula. If unrefrigerated formula is not used within 2 hours, discard it.
- Opened cans of formula (ready-to-feed or concentrate) should be used within 24 hours.
- Do not save the remainder of a bottle for later. Formula becomes contaminated with bacteria from the infant's mouth, and using it later could lead to illness.
- Formula should not be frozen.

Adapted from Heslin, J. A. (1988). *No-nonsense nutrition for your baby's first year.* Englewood Cliffs, NJ: Prentice-Hall; and Heslin, J. (1992). If you bottlefeed . . . *American Baby, 54*(5), B10–B14.

Formula. Special formulas have been developed to meet the needs of the LBW infant. These formulas provide whey-predominant proteins, carbohydrate mixtures of lactose and glucose polymers, and fat mixtures containing combinations of MCT and relatively unsaturated long-chain triglycerides. Some of the formulas are "Preemie" SMA 24, Similac Special Care 24, and Enfamil Premature 24. The content of these formulas varies, and they should be selected according to the needs of the infant under the direction of a pediatrician or dietitian.

Methods of Feeding. Infants weighing less than 1500 grams are typically fed glucose, fat, and amino acids *parenterally* (IV). *Enteral* (e.g., oral, gastric, or nasogastric) *feedings* are introduced slowly because of the high incidence of respiratory problems, limited gastric capacity, and intestinal hypomotility. Parenteral feedings can be decreased as enteral feedings increase, thus maintaining the infant's nutritional needs through the use of both feeding routes. As the infant's coordination and energy increase, nipple feedings may be slowly added.

The use of *enteral feeding* is based on gestational age, weight, and clinical state. The infant who is at least 32 to 34 weeks gestational age (coordination of sucking, swallowing, and respirations) may be fed through a nipple. Before the infant develops suck/swallow coordination and/or if the infant has respiratory problems, intragastric or jejunal continuous drip feedings may be used. The infant is typically fed every 2 to 3 hours.

If he can tolerate being held, the infant receiving enteral or parenteral feedings should be held and offered a pacifier. This will assist in meeting the infant's needs for touch and sucking.

Introduction of Solid Foods

Human milk or commercial formula meets the nutritional requirements for the first 6 months of life. The infant goes through a so-called transitional period during which prepared foods are introduced and given together with human milk or formula. This usually occurs between ages 4 and 6 months. The growth and development of each infant varies, and there are milestones that indicate the infant's readiness for solid foods (see box). The early introduction of solid food is associated with a higher incidence of food allergy. In addition, the solids the infant eats cannot be adequately digested and the nutrients in breast or formula milk will not be taken in because the infant's appetite has been satisfied. In contrast, failure to offer solids by age 6 months may result in difficulty accepting solid feedings at a later time (AAP, 1993).

Solids should be introduced one at a time in small amounts (1 teaspoon to 2 tablespoons) for several days before introducing a new food. This is done to avoid confusion should a food intolerance be present. The order of introduction is not critical, but rice cereal is most often recommended as a first food because it is high in iron, is easily digested, and has a low allergenic probability. Other commercially available cereals include oatmeal, barley, mixed grain, and cereals with added fruit. When foods are first being introduced, mixed grain and cereals with added fruit should be avoided. Foods should never be mixed with formula and fed through a nipple with a large hole. This deprives the child of the chewing experience as well as changing the texture and taste of the food. There may be medical conditions in which an exception to this rule is made (gastroesophageal reflux).

Readiness for Introduction of Solids

- Infant can sit.
- Birth weight has doubled and infant weighs at least 13 pounds.
- Can reach for an object and maintain balance.
- Reaches for objects and brings to mouth.
- Indicates a desire for food by opening mouth and leaning forward.
- Extrusion reflex has disappeared (4–5 months).
- Moves food to back of mouth and swallows during spoon feedings.

Solids should be introduced one at a time over a week. The infant should be given 1 teaspoon to 2 tablespoons during this period. The amount is gradually increased. As solids increase, the intake of milk decreases. By 12 months the infant should be taking 24 ounces of milk per 24 hours.

There are several commercially prepared fruits and vegetables. In addition, fruits and vegetables can easily be steamed or boiled and then pureed in a blender or food processor at home. It is usually necessary to add a small amount of water during the blending process. As with cereals, mixed fruits should be avoided until the infant is older and has tolerated individual foods.

Although most sources indicate that the order of introduction of foods is arbitrary, the introduction of meat usually follows cereal, fruit, and vegetables after age 6 months. The infant may be given ground liver, lean beef, or a variety of commercially prepared meats.

Salt and sugar should not be added to commercially or home-prepared foods. Parents should avoid using canned foods or home-prepared foods that contain large amounts of sugar and salt. Feeding honey to infants under age 12 months has been associated with botulism and should therefore be avoided.

> Foods such as hot dogs, nuts, grapes, carrots, popcorn, peanuts, and hard, round candies should be avoided because of the risk of choking.

Juices

Citrus fruits and juices are introduced after age 6 months. This later introduction reduces the chance of allergies. In infants with a history of allergies, orange and tomato juice should be delayed until age 1 year. Some prepared foods and dinners contain orange juice and tomato juice. Parents should be taught to read labels. Juice is not warmed because vitamin C is destroyed by heating. Juices should be kept in a covered container in the refrigerator to prevent the loss of the vitamin. Juices should not be given in the bottle to avoid the development of nursing-bottle caries.

Water

Sufficient water is provided in breast milk and in prepared formula during the nursing period. When solid foods are introduced, it may be necessary to add water because some foods have a high renal solute load (strained meats, high meat dinners). Infants should be offered water as part of a feeding or during the day. Additional water is necessary when intake is low or the infant is experiencing fluid loss because of illness (fever, respiratory disease).

Finger Foods

Between age 8 and 10 months the infant can be introduced to finger foods. At this time the pincer grasp is developing and the infant can pick up foods. The infant will have a palmar grasp before this time and soft foods can be given, but the infant will mainly "play" with the food. This can be a positive experience that enables the infant to feel different textures and increase fine motor skills.

Finger foods should be bite-sized pieces of soft food. Arrowroot biscuits, cheese sticks, slices of canned peaches or pears, slices of bananas, and breads can be offered. As the child's fine motor skills increase, he may enjoy eating some of the dry cereals, such as Cheerios.

Snacks

When the infant is on a three meals a day schedule, small snacks are an appropriate addition to the nutritional intake. Because infants have small stomachs, they may not be content to wait until the next meal before eating. This usually occurs between ages 6 and 9 months. Snacks should be nutritious, and parents should resist the urge to give the infant a bottle to satisfy her hunger. Some of the finger foods listed above are good nutritious snacks. If the infant is not hungry at mealtime, the snack should be given in a smaller portion or eliminated.

Weaning

Weaning is the replacement of breast or bottle feedings with drinking from a cup. Infants usually have a decreasing interest in the breast or bottle starting between ages 6 and 12 months. This varies from infant to infant but, if solids and a cup have been introduced, the infant will probably begin to indicate a readiness for the cup. When weaning is begun after age 18 months, the infant may resist because of increased attachment to the breast or bottle.

Behaviors that might indicate a readiness to begin weaning include:

- throwing the bottle down
- chewing on the nipple
- taking only a few ounces of formula
- refusing the breast or dawdling

Weaning should not take place during times of change or stress (e.g., illness, starting child care, new baby). It is a gradual process and should start with the replacement of one bottle or breast-feeding at a time. If breast-feeding must be terminated before age 6 months, it should be replaced with bottle feedings to meet the infant's sucking needs. The older infant who has learned to use a cup may not need to use a bottle.

The first bottle or breast-feeding eliminated should be the one the infant is least interested in. Initially the infant may only accept the cup after drinking some formula from the bottle or milk from the breast. The infant is next offered the cup before the feeding. In approximately 1 week another feeding can be eliminated if the infant is not resisting the change. The bedtime feeding is usually the last feeding to be eliminated.

> Infants who are being weaned should receive formula in the cup. Whole milk should not be given before age 12 months.

The child is giving up time that had been spent being held in his parent's arms. The parent needs to respond to the infant's continued need to be held and cuddled. Infants should not be allowed to carry bottles around as toys, to take them to bed, or to use them as pacifiers. Infants who indicate sucking needs should be given pacifiers.

Food Assistance Programs

The Special Supplemental Food Program for Women, Infants, and Children (WIC) was established to improve the nutritional state of low-income, pregnant and breastfeeding women and their children up to age 5 years. The WIC program provides supplemental cereal, eggs, juice, cheese, milk, and iron-fortified infant formula and cereal each month. In addition to the food, families are provided with nutritional education and regular health examinations of the mother and children.

Food Allergies

Food allergies can occur at any age, but the incidence for development of certain food allergies is increased before age 1 year. Some of the more common foods allergies are milk, egg, soy products, peanut, chocolate, corn, and wheat. Cow's milk protein intolerance is the most common food allergy during infancy but usually does not last past age 3 years.

Some of the common clinical manifestations of food allergies are abdominal pain, diarrhea, nasal congestion, cough, wheezing, vomiting, and rashes. Many children will "outgrow" their allergic response to certain foods; for example, 70% to 80% of infants with a milk allergy will tolerate milk by age 4 years. Children who develop food allergies after age 3 years tend not to outgrow them.

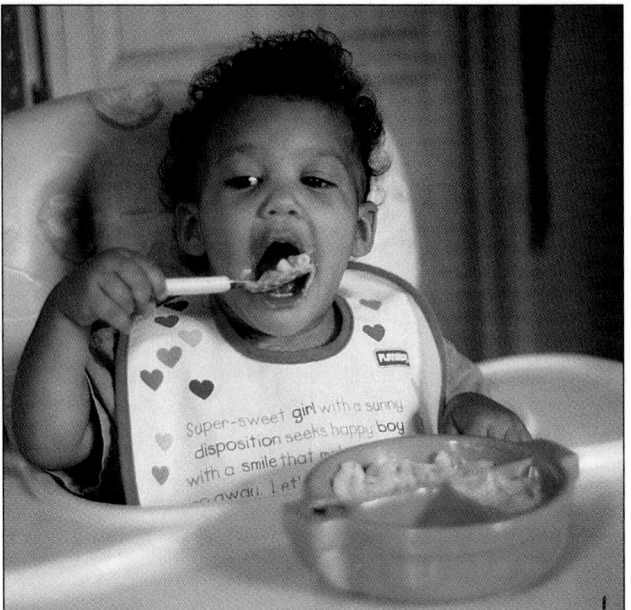

Figure 12–2
By age 1 year most children are eating the same foods as the rest of the family. Toddlers should be offered three meals and two healthy snacks a day. Most 2-year-olds can drink from a cup and use a spoon well if given the opportunity to practice.

THE TODDLER AND PRESCHOOLER

The rate of growth slows during the toddler and preschool period and so does the child's appetite. This is sometimes referred to as "physiologic anorexia." Protein and calorie needs per kilogram of body weight are decreased. The food experiences the child has during this period can have a lasting effect on how food and meals are viewed. The family is the primary influence at this time, although the media plays an important role through television. Children should be discouraged from eating while watching television, and family mealtimes should be encouraged.

Nutritional Requirements

Recommended dietary allowances per day for *energy* and *protein* vary according to the child's age (see Table 12–1). Fat and cholesterol intake should not be restricted in children under age 2 years (AAP, 1986). There are many nutritional similarities between the toddler and the preschooler. The caloric and protein requirements drop slightly during the preschool period. Children this age who eat well-balanced diets should not suffer from iron deficiency. However, if milk remains the primary food, it will replace foods rich in iron, vitamins, and minerals such as dark green leafy vegetables, meats, and legumes. Three servings from the milk group each day are more than adequate for this age child. Refer to Chapter 32 for further discussion of iron deficiency anemia. The child who is healthy does not need vitamin supplementation. However, giving a daily children's multivitamin containing 100% of the RDA is not harmful.

After 2 years of age, low-fat (2%) milk may be given. Milk intake should be limited to 2 to 3 cups per day. Yogurt and cheese are other milk-group sources. Poultry, fish, and lean meat are good sources of iron. Low-sugar breakfast cereals are sources of iron and vitamins. Snacks of fruits and vegetables assist in meeting the child's nutritional requirements.

Solid Foods

Children at this age are increasing their proficiency in using a spoon and cup. By age 2 years children can hold a cup in one hand and use a spoon well (Fig. 12–2). By age 12 months most children are eating the same foods prepared for the rest of the family. The child should be offered three meals and two snacks each day.

By age 3 to 4 years the child begins to use the fork. The child continues to develop fine motor skills and by the end of the preschool period should be beginning to use a knife for cutting.

One method to determine serving size for children is 1 tablespoon of solid food per year of age. Children may be more likely to try new foods and to eat nutritious meals if smaller portions are served. Foods with different textures, colors, consistencies, tastes, and temperatures should be encouraged. The child should sit in a chair that allows easy access to the food; the dishes should be small, nonbreakable, and, when possible, steady enough to prevent spilling. Thick, short handled spoons and forks and shallow bowls increase the toddler's ability to be successful when eating.

Foods that could be aspirated should continue to be avoided during the toddler period. Soft drinks and candy should be discouraged. Sugar is a source of calories and is naturally present in breast milk as lactose, as fructose in fruits, and as maltose in grain products. However, a diet with too much sugar can replace other more nutritious foods and increase tooth decay. Artificial sweeteners and foods that contain artificial sweeteners are not recommended for children under age 2 years.

Age-Related Nutritional Challenges

Food Jags. The volume of food the child eats may vary from day to day. The child may want the same food at every meal for several days and then suddenly reject the food completely. Children this age may refuse foods because of odor and temperature. They may not like mixing foods and therefore may not eat casseroles. This rationale does not seem to apply to foods like pizza, spaghetti, and macaroni and cheese. Many children prefer juices over milk and water. Just as too much milk is not good, neither is too much juice, because it can replace other foods and their nutrients. Parents and older siblings can affect how a child sees a food and should be careful about making negative comments about a certain food. Children should be assisted in developing tastes for new foods through role modeling and making the foods available.

Physiologic Anorexia. Parents should be taught appropriate ways to approach the child who is experiencing physiologic anorexia (see box). Children should not be allowed to "fill up" with snacks, milk, and juices. Small portions should be offered so the child does not feel overwhelmed by the amount of food. Mealtimes should be pleasant and not a time to discuss discipline problems or even the child's poor appetite. Children should never be made to sit at the table after the rest of the family has departed. This will only create a negative association with mealtime. Parents need to maintain a balance between ignoring their child's nutritional intake and making it the focus of their parenting.

The nurse can encourage parents to focus more on the weekly nutritional intake of their child, rather than looking at one day. Frequently children are the best judge of what they need and they may eat primarily fruit one day and peanut butter the next. It does tend to balance out over a week.

Increasing Nutritious Intake

- Limit to two nutritious snacks per day and give only at toddler's request.
- Limit to 6 ounces of juice per day.
- Introduce to finger foods at age 8–10 months and continue to make these types of food available.
- Limit to 16–24 ounces of milk per day.
- Keep mealtimes pleasant.
- Do not force feed.
- Do not feed children who can feed themselves.

THE SCHOOL-AGE CHILD

Growth continues at a slow but regular pace, but the school-age child begins to have an increase in appetite. During the later school-age years energy needs increase. This age-group tends to have few eating idiosyncrasies and generally enjoys eating to satisfy appetite and as a social function. Children who developed dislikes for certain foods during earlier periods may continue to refuse those foods. This age child is influenced by family patterns and the limitations their activities put on them. They may rush through a meal in order to go out to play or watch a favorite program on television.

Nutritional Requirements

The caloric and protein requirements begin to increase at age 11 years because of the preadolescence growth spurt. The requirements for males and females also begin to vary at this age. A gradual increase of food intake will also take place.

Age-Related Nutritional Challenges

At this age the child's schedule changes and more time is spent away from home. Most children eat lunch at school, and they usually have a choice of foods. Even if the parent packs a lunch for the child to take to school, there are no guarantees that the child will eat the lunch. Children sometimes trade foods with other children or may not eat a particular item. It is also during this period that the child becomes more active in clubs, sports, and other activities that interrupt the normal meal schedule.

The federal government funds The School Lunch Program, which provides approximately one-third of the RDAs for a child. This program provides lunches for low-income children at either free or reduced rates. Some schools also offer breakfast and milk programs.

School-age children usually request a snack after school and in the evening. Parents should be encouraged

Nutritious Snacks

Fresh fruit
Celery sticks with peanut butter or cheese spread
Yogurt
Bagels
Carrot sticks
Graham crackers
Pretzels
Puddings

to provide their child with healthy choices for snacks (see box). By not buying foods high in calories and low in nutrients the parent can remove the temptation for the child to choose the less healthy foods.

Unpredictable schedules, advertising, easy access to fast food, and peer pressure can all have an effect on the foods a child chooses. The child can begin to prefer "junk foods," which do not contain nutritional value. Most of these foods are high in fat and sugar. The family plays an important role in modeling good eating habits for the child. Schools also have a responsibility to provide nutritious meals for children.

THE ADOLESCENT

Adolescence is a period of rapid growth. There is an increase in height, weight, and muscle mass. Children this age tend to be concerned about their weight, complexion, sexual development, and acceptance by their peers. These issues together with the adolescent's increasing independence can have nutritional implications.

Nutritional Requirements

The RDAs for adolescents are based on extrapolations from recommendations for children and adults. Because not only age but also physical maturity must be considered, it is difficult to do studies. For this reason, the recommendations for energy and protein are stated during three different ages (Table 12–8).

Iron requirements increase during adolescence. This increase is related to the rapid growth. Iron deficiency anemia in adolescence is usually related to the depletion of marginal stores by increased demand and the adolescent's nutritional habits. In girls there is an increased need for iron related to menstrual losses as well as growth.

Age-Related Nutritional Challenges

The adolescent's food habits are influenced by many factors (see box). Unfortunately this happens at a time when the body has increased nutritional needs. Adolescents are at risk to not meet the RDAs for vitamin A, vitamin B_6, riboflavin, iron, calcium, and zinc (Mahan & Arlin, 1992). Boys tend to have fewer deficiencies than girls because they take in more food and are less likely to be dieting. Milk is frequently replaced by soft drinks. Fast foods and "junk foods" sometimes become the mainstay of the adolescent's diet. Some sources indicate that up to 50% of the adolescent's intake is through snacks.

TABLE 12–8 *Recommended Energy and Protein Allowance for Adolescents*

AGE	CALORIES		PROTEIN	
(years)	DAILY	PER kg	DAILY	PER kg
Females				
11–14	2,200	47	46	0.29
15–18	2,200	40	44	0.26
19–24	2,200	38	46	0.28
Males				
11–14	2,500	55	45	0.28
15–18	3,000	45	59	0.33
19–24	2,900	40	58	0.33

Reprinted with permission from *Recommended Dietary Allowances: 10th Edition.* Copyright 1989 by the National Academy of Sciences. Courtesy of the National Academy Press, Washington, D.C.

Nutritional Guidance for the Adolescent

The nurse must have an understanding of growth and development to be successful in counseling adolescents and their parents in the area of nutrition. The adolescent's increasing need for independence and for freedom to make choices should guide the nurse in planning for teaching in this area. The adolescent should always be involved in the planning.

The nurse should assess the adolescent's present diet and determine habits and eating patterns. Included in this

Influences on the Adolescent's Diet

- Busy schedule (sports, activities, jobs)
- Body image concerns, which can lead to undereating
- Often skip breakfast
- Often eat away from home
- Frequently eat fast food
- Beginning to buy and prepare own food
- Peer pressure
- Psychologic and emotional problems

assessment should be identification of the frequency of intake of the food groups and those foods the adolescent does not eat. Based on this information, nutritious foods for meals can be identified and a plan developed.

The nurse can also assist the adolescent by identifying nutritious fast foods and snacks. An awareness of nutritious fast foods can also aid the adolescent in meal selection. Many fast food chains now have salads with nonfat or low fat dressings, grilled chicken sandwiches, pasta, and nonfat yogurt. Fat and salt content has been reduced and vegetable fats have replaced animal fats at some restaurants. Adolescents should be guided in mixing an occasional hamburger and fries with a regular selection of more nutritious foods. Permission should be given to eat foods that may be somewhat untraditional at a particular meal (i.e., pizza for breakfast).

Evaluation

Through use of assessment methods and tools the status of the child is evaluated. As outcomes are evaluated, the plan of care must be carefully viewed. Does the child and/or family have an understanding of the nutritional goals? Are the nutritional requirements being provided for the child? If not, is the problem one of education, finances, or culture? Was the child's cultural background a factor when the diet was recommended? Are there psychosocial and psychologic problems affecting the child and/or family? If so, what effect does this have on the child's intake? Based on the evaluation, the plan of care is adjusted.

OBESITY

When intake of food exceeds expenditure, the excess is stored as fat. Obesity is an excessive accumulation of fat in the body. There is an increase of weight beyond that considered desirable with regard to age, height, and bone structure.

Obesity can be a precursor of cardiovascular disease, hypertension, and diabetes. Because the obese child develops increased numbers of fat cells, which are carried into adulthood, the prevention of obesity in childhood can reduce the risk of obesity in adulthood and play a role in the prevention of hypertension and cardiovascular disease.

Etiology and Prognosis

Both genetic and environmental factors have been linked to childhood obesity. It is very difficult to separate these two factors in a family in which the parents are obese. When a parent lacks nutritional knowledge, it is reflected in the meals and snacks provided in the home. The child is at risk to develop the same habits. As the child's independence increases, this becomes more evident. Unstructured meals and "meals on the run" and at fast food restaurants can also lack the proper nutrition and be high in calories. Lack of exercise also contributes to obesity.

Genetic obesity does occur in some animals and may be true in humans. More research is needed in this area. The child who is given food for reward or punishment attaches more to eating than gaining nutrition. Some people still have the belief that a fat baby is a healthy baby. This type of thinking leads to overfeeding.

Although the child may experience an initial weight loss, the long-term success rate for the elimination of obesity is poor. Positive outcomes are increased when the child has a support system and understands the importance of diet and exercise.

Prevention

The American Academy of Pediatrics (1993) suggests that the following measures are reasonable ways to prevent obesity:

- breast-feeding
- delay in the introduction of solids
- feeding as a response to hunger, not as a pacifier
- eating when hungry and not basing food consumption on the clock
- promotion of physical exercise.

NURSING CARE OF THE CHILD WITH OBESITY

Assessment

The child who is obese looks overweight. In addition, the child's weight and height should be graphed to determine at which percentile he falls. Children who fall above the 20th percentile for ideal body height and weight should be evaluated. A caliper measurement of skinfold thickness should be taken and compared to the established guidelines. The best site for measurement is the triceps. The **body mass index (BMI)** provides another measurement of body fat that takes into account the child who is highly muscled.

A dietary history should be taken. The child's eating habits and patterns should be evaluated. The child and/or parent should keep a food diary for 1 week. The diary should include the (1) time; (2) place; (3) type and amount of food; and (4) reason for eating. The general dietary habits of the family should also be assessed.

A psychosocial history of the child and family should be taken. The possibility of disease as a contributing factor must be evaluated. Increased weight gain has been associated with central nervous system tumors, hypothyroidism, Cushing syndrome, and Turner syndrome.

The child's exercise or lack of it is also assessed. The amount of time spent watching television and playing video games is pertinent. It should be determined if the child is participating in any regularly scheduled exercise.

Nursing Diagnosis and Planning

The following nursing diagnosis and expected outcomes offer an example that may be appropriate in the treatment of obesity in the child or adolescent.

Nursing Diagnosis

- Altered Nutrition: More Than Body Requirements related to excessive intake

Expected Outcomes: The child/adolescent will

- develop and implement an exercise plan
- alter diet to allow for weight loss while maintaining normal growth patterns

Implementation

One of the key elements of successful weight reduction in the child or adolescent is ownership by the child of whatever plan is proposed. Care should be taken to avoid a power struggle between the parent and child. Obviously the young child will need more parental involvement than the older child or adolescent. The family should be willing to support the child but should not take on the role of watchdog.

Diet and Exercise. The caloric requirements will vary depending on the age and sex of the child. By changing the child's lifestyle to include exercise and nutritional foods in smaller servings, the possibility of success is increased. The family and child are taught how to select and prepare foods that are tasteful and how to restrict serving size. The child's favorite foods should be identified and incorporated whenever possible. Since snacks are an important aspect in childhood nutrition, nutritious snacks should be identified.

Television time should be limited. Children should be involved in regular physical exercise at school and at home. Children can be encouraged to ride their bicycles or to walk rather than ride to a friend's house to play. Planned physical activities should be part of the child's after-school routine and on weekends.

Some older children and adolescents may find success in a support group such as Weight Watchers and Overeaters Anonymous. Some centers have a special group for children. There may be other support groups associated with schools, summer camps, and children's hospitals in the community.

For a discussion of other eating alterations such as anorexia nervosa and bulimia nervosa, refer to Chapter 41.

Evaluation

The child's weight loss is assessed at regular predetermined intervals. The log or diary is reviewed and areas of concern discussed. This is also an excellent time for positive feedback related to changes in eating behaviors and adherence to an exercise program. Feelings and goals should also be discussed. If the child is having difficulty losing weight, the plan should be assessed to determine if it is appropriate for the needs of that child.

KEY CONCEPTS

- The six basic nutrients are carbohydrates, protein, fat, vitamins, minerals, and water.
- Carbohydrates should be the major source of energy.
- Protein is necessary for building and maintaining body tissue.
- Infants receiving commercial iron-containing formulas do not need vitamin and mineral supplementation in the first 6 months of life, or in the second 6 months if appropriate solids are added to the diet.
- The Food Guide Pyramid guidelines recommend that a low fat, low saturated fat, and low cholesterol diet be eaten together with ample vegetables, fruits, and grains.
- Components of a nutritional assessment are anthropometric data, biochemical data, clinical examination, and dietary history.
- Human milk meets the nutrient and energy needs of the infant and contains immunologic and antibacterial components not found in cow's milk.
- Solid foods are usually introduced between ages 4 and 6 months in small amounts, one at a time, based on the infant's growth and development.
- The low–birth-weight infant has difficulty digesting, absorbing, and utilizing nutrients. The infant may need to receive parenteral or enteral feedings.
- Weaning usually begins between ages 6 and 12 months. It should never take place during stress and the infant should receive formula in the cup until age 12 months.
- Food jags and physiologic anorexia are common occurrences in the young child.
- The most common food allergies include milk, eggs, soy products, peanuts, chocolate, corn, and wheat.
- Adolescents have increased iron requirements.
- Assessment of the child who is obese should include a dietary history, a psychosocial history, a physical examination, and assessment of the child's exercise habits.

REFERENCES

American Academy of Pediatrics Committee on Nutrition. (1986). Prudent life-style for children: Dietary fat and cholesterol. *Pediatrics, 78,* 521–525.

American Academy of Pediatrics Committee on Nutrition. (1989). Iron-fortified infant formulas. *Pediatrics, 84,* 1114–1115.

American Academy of Pediatrics Committee on Nutrition. (1992). The use of whole cow's milk in infancy. *Pediatrics, 89,* 1105–1109.

American Academy of Pediatrics Committee on Nutrition. (1993). *Pediatric nutrition handbook.* Elk Grove Village, IL: American Academy of Pediatrics.

Hill, P. (1991). The enigma of insufficient milk supply. *Maternal-Child Nursing, 16,* 312–316.

Institute of Medicine. National Academy of Sciences. Food and Nutrition Board. (1989). *National Research Council, NAS: Recommended Dietary Allowances.* Washington, DC: National Academy Press.

Institute of Medicine. National Academy of Sciences. Food and Nutrition Board. (1991). *Nutrition during lactation.* Washington, DC: National Academy Press.

Mahan, L., & Arlin, M. (1992). *Krause's food, nutrition and diet therapy* (8th ed.). Philadelphia: W. B. Saunders.

Miskelly, F., Burr, M., Vaughan-Williams, E., Fehily, A., Butland, B., & Merrett, T. (1988). Infant feeding and allergy. *Archives of Disease in Childhood, 63,* 388–393.

Moore, E., Bianchi-Gray, M., & Stephens, L. (1991). A community hospital-based breast-feeding counseling service. *Pediatric Nursing, 17*(4), 383–389.

Ryan, A., Rush, D., Krieger, F., & Lewandoski, G. (1991). Recent declines in breast feeding in the United States, 1984 through 1989. *Pediatrics, 88,* 719–727.

United States Department of Agriculture & United States Department of Health and Human Services. (1992). *Dietary guidelines for Americans.* Hyattsville, MD: U.S. Government Printing Office.

BIBLIOGRAPHY

Basch, C., Shea, S., Arliss, R., Contento, L., Rips, J., Gutin, P., Irigoyen, M., & Zybert, P. (1990). Validation of mothers' reports of dietary intake by four- to seven-year-old children. *American Journal of Public Health, 81*(11), 1314–1317.

Bidlack, W., & Taylor, S. (1992). The fear of healthy eating: Understanding the paranoia. *Journal of Pediatric Health Care, 6*(6), 355–360.

Davis, J., & Sherer, K. (1994). *Applied nutrition and diet therapy for nurses.* Philadelphia: W. B. Saunders.

Hardy, S., & Kleinman, R. (1994). Fat and cholesterol in the diet of infants and young children: Implications for growth, development, and long-term health. *Journal of Pediatrics, 125*(5 Pt 2), 923–927.

Jonides, L. (1990). Childhood obesity: An update. *Journal of Pediatric Health Care, 4*(5), 244–251.

Jopling, J. (1992). Getting families to "eat right." *Contemporary Pediatrics, 5,* 97–118.

Nemethy, M., & Clore, R. (1990). Microwave heating of infant formula and breast milk. *Journal of Pediatric Health Care, 4,* 131–135.

Oski, F. (1993). Infant nutrition, physical growth, breastfeeding, and general nutrition. *Current Opinion in Pediatrics, 5,* 385–388.

Schreiner, B., & Brondum, L. (1994). Nutrition in pediatric primary care: Assessment and common problems. *Nurse Practitioner Forum, 5*(1), 13–23.

Thompson, F., & Dennison, B. (1994). Dietary sources of fats and cholesterol in US children aged 2 through 5. *American Journal of Public Health, 84*(5), 799–806.

United States Department of Health and Human Services. (1990). *Healthy people 2000.* Washington, DC: US Government Printing Office.

United States Department of Health and Human Services. (1988). *The Surgeon General's report on nutrition and health.* Washington, DC: US Government Printing Office.

Ziegler, E., Fomon, S. (1989). Potential renal solute load of infant formulas. *Journal of Nutrition, 119,* 1785–1788.

Ziegler, L. (1990). Milks and formulas for older infants. *Journal of Pediatrics, 117*(suppl), S76–S79.

13

Safety

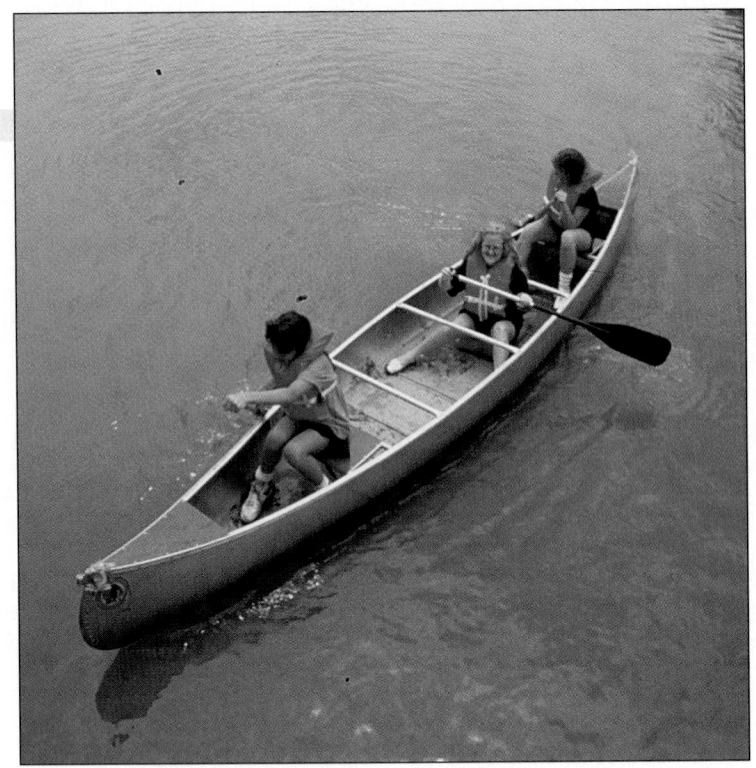

CHAPTER OVERVIEW

LEARNING OBJECTIVES

After studying this chapter, you should be able to:

- Describe the magnitude of childhood injuries in the United States.
- Describe the normal developmental characteristics of children that make them vulnerable to injury.
- List specific injury risks for each developmental level and discuss appropriate anticipatory safety principles to address each risk identified.
- Describe effective safety educational approaches for each stage of childhood development.
- Describe the various ways that nurses can help to prevent childhood injuries.
- Describe appropriate methods to restrain children in motor vehicles.

KEY TERMS

asphyxiation: a state of suffocation that severely compromises oxygen delivery to the body.

aspiration: accidentally drawing foreign objects into the nose, throat, or lungs on inspiration.

inertial forces: the external forces of motion that are exerted on the body during impact with blunt energies.

injury control: interventions that reduce the incidence or severity of injury events.

injury prevention: activities or educational efforts to promote or increase an individual's awareness of safety issues.

Injury is the most significant, yet underrecognized public health threat facing children today. Unintentional injury results in more deaths of children 1 to 14 years of age than all childhood diseases combined. Each year, an estimated 8000 children die as the result of preventable injury (National SafeKids Campaign, 1993). This trend continues into adulthood. Injury remains the leading cause of death and disability of Americans until the age of 44 years (American College of Surgeons Committee on Trauma, 1993).

The number of childhood deaths is staggering, but it is only a fraction of the number of children who suffer permanent disability as a result of injury (Fig. 13–1). For each injury-related death, 45 children are hospitalized and 1300 children require emergency treatment. Thousands more children are treated at home.

The economic burden to society is equally staggering, reaching billions of dollars yearly. What cannot be quantified is the emotional loss, suffering, and pain a child or family must endure once an injury has occurred.

Until a few years ago, injuries were commonly referred to as accidents or random acts of fate. Today, the public attitude is changing. It is now known that most childhood injuries are preventable and predictable. Increased awareness and basic safety interventions can and have saved children from needless death and thousands more from permanent disability. Nurses and other health care professionals are in a key position to reduce the number of childhood injuries. Safety education and awareness may not prevent every bump, bruise, or cut, but simple safety guidance can help to lower the risk of serious injury in children.

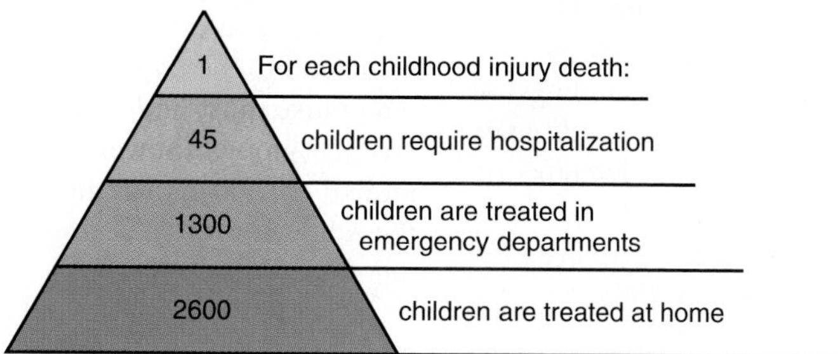

Figure 13–1
Childhood injury pyramid. (Data from Guyer, B., & Gallagher, S. [1985]. Approach to the epidemiology of childhood injuries. *Pediatric Clinics of North America, 32*[1], 5–15.)

CHILDHOOD INJURIES: ETIOLOGY AND PREVENTION

All children are at risk for injury because of their normal curiosity, impulsiveness, and impatience. Everywhere they venture, they are exposed to potentially hazardous situations. Developmentally, children are vulnerable to injury for the following reasons:

- Children are naturally curious and enjoy exploring their surroundings.
- Children are driven to test and master new skills.
- Children frequently attempt activities before they have developed the cognitive and physical skills required to safely accomplish the task.
- Children often assert themselves and challenge rules.
- Children develop a strong desire for peer approval as they grow older.

All children are at risk for injury because of their normal curiosity, impulsiveness, and desire to master new skills.

From the moment infants enter the world, they interact with the environment with increasing frequency, exposing themselves to more and more potentially dangerous situations. Children often experience these situations without a clear understanding of causal relationships or a reasonable fear of the possible danger. Normal growth and development predispose all children to some degree of injury risk, but select populations of children are at increased risk for injury.

Boys, minorities, and children from low-income families are at increased risk for injury.

Boys are more likely to suffer injuries than girls. There are many factors contributing to this trend, ranging from inborn differences of behavior, to early cultural assignment of traditional sex roles, to subtle differences in socialization for risk-taking behaviors (Wilson et al., 1991).

Low-income and minority children are much more likely to die as a result of injury than children with more economic resources. Injury death rates for African American children are almost double those for white children. Some minority children and those living in low-income areas tend to live in crowded and unsafe surroundings. A low-income family struggling to meet basic needs may lack access to safety devices such as smoke detectors or child car safety seats. Regardless of sex, race, or socioeconomic class, all children have the right to grow up in a safe environment (National SafeKids Campaign, 1993).

Injury Prevention. **Injury prevention** is a relatively new focus of health promotion. The term accident, with its implied meaning of random chance or lack of responsibility, is being replaced with the idea that injuries have causes that can be modified to prevent or lessen their frequency and severity. Safety education is a critical component of injury prevention. It increases awareness, attempts to modify human behavior, and reinforces changes implemented through legal mandates (i.e., seat belt laws) or product modification (i.e., crib design, air bags.).

Nurses need to become proactive in childhood injury prevention (increasing awareness of safety issues). Nurses who care for children are acutely aware of the devastating effects and complex problems injuries cause. From their experiences, they become well-informed advocates for childhood safety. Nurses can participate in the prevention activities outlined in the accompanying box.

COMMUNITY HEALTH ***What Nurses Can Do to Prevent Childhood Injuries***

- Model safety practices in the home, work, and community.
- Educate parents and children through anticipatory safety guidance to help reduce needless injuries.
- Support legislative efforts that advocate prevention measures.
- Collaborate with other health care providers to promote safety and injury prevention.
- Participate in school and community safety programs.

A DEVELOPMENTAL APPROACH TO SAFETY PROMOTION

Children are constantly changing as they develop. Their abilities to react and respond to others, coordinate their movements, plan ahead, and judge the consequences of their actions change as their physical, psychosocial, and cognitive skills develop.

Anticipatory Guidance. To be most effective in providing anticipatory safety guidance, educational strategies must be geared to the child's level of growth and development. The nurse must understand the risks associated with various age groups (Sewell & Gaines, 1993). Knowledge of growth and development also helps the nurse to choose the educational strategy appropriate to a child's developmental level.

Early in the parenting role, parents need to know how to provide a safe environment for their children as well as what behaviors they can expect at various developmental levels. Anticipatory guidance builds on the safety principles of the previous stage. Awareness of a child's changing capabilities allows the parent to be more alert and reactive to safety hazards that the child is likely to encounter. This awareness is especially important for first-time parents.

Some parents, when learning of the potential hazards surrounding their children, have a natural inclination to overprotect them. However, children learn from their mistakes as part of the developmental process. The role of parents is to promote their child's autonomy with a healthy respect for safety risks so that dangers can be eliminated or minimized. Additionally, parents must teach their children safety-conscious behaviors.

Children imitate adult behavior from an early age, so parents should be encouraged to model safe behaviors and habits.

Simply telling parents to "watch your children" or to "childproof" the home, or telling a child to "be careful," has little educational impact. Educational efforts are much more likely to be effective if they are focused on specific problems with specific solutions, rather than broad or vague advice.

Assessment of Safety Knowledge. Once developmental injury risks for the child's age have been identified, the child's or parent's current level of safety knowledge should be assessed. This assessment can be accomplished by direct questioning or general observation of behaviors exhibited by the child or parent. Assessment serves a dual purpose: it allows the nurse to identify specific educational needs and to reinforce positive safety behaviors.

Teaching Strategies. Teaching can be formal or informal, simple or elaborate, as long as it provides relevant safety information and coincides with the child's or parent's cognitive abilities. For children younger than 5 or 6 years, it is advisable to incorporate the parent into the teaching process so that the parents can assist with reinforcement or questions the child later has about the safety issue. With younger children, who are easily distracted, the information should be presented in short sessions.

GIVING POSITIVE INSTRUCTIONS Instruct children about what they should do, not what they should not do, to educate from a positive perspective.

Parents are often the primary target for safety education. They want to protect their children from harm, but simply lack all or part of the information to do so.

Many local and national organizations have safety information available for distribution. This information can be used to supplement the teaching process. Prepared materials range from pamphlets, booklets, posters, and audiovisuals to entire teaching programs that can assist in providing injury prevention education to all age groups. Some programs offer the materials free of cost. See Appendix H for a partial listing of organizations that provide safety information.

INFANT SAFETY

Infants are totally dependent on others for safety and protection. They are especially vulnerable to serious injury because of their relatively large head size. Motor development progresses to the point where they quickly master new skills to learn more about their environment. They begin to impulsively reach out and move toward interesting objects around them.

Because of an infant's dependence, parents and caregivers are the primary recipients of anticipatory safety guidance. Beginning the first day of life, safety must be considered and incorporated into the infant's world. The task of providing a safe environment for a rapidly growing infant is challenging. Potential safety hazards multiply as the baby learns to creep, crawl, climb, and explore. For this reason, parental responsibility is great. Some parents may not have a complete awareness of the safety issues that must be addressed to protect the infant from injury.

Car Safety

Injuries associated with automobile accidents constitute the single greatest threat to an infant's life and health. Restraining seats are the only practical means of reducing this risk. The crushing forces of a crash or sudden stop, even at low speed, can cause serious injury to the infant. Without a car safety seat, an infant involved in a collision or sudden stop becomes an unguided missile, colliding with the interior of the car or, worse, ejected from the vehicle. In a collision, infants are usually thrust headfirst, placing them at greater risk for head, facial, or spinal injuries because of the weight of the head, high center of gravity, and open fontanel (Halpern, 1987).

Proper use of car restraints or safety seats is the single most important protective measure that parents can use to prevent motor vehicle injuries.

When correctly installed and secured, child safety seats are effective in reducing the risk of death by 71% and the risk of hospitalization by 67% (Kahane, 1989). As of 1985, the use of child safety restraints for children under the age of 4 years was mandated in all 50 states.

Infant safety in motor vehicles depends entirely on adults. Parents must be informed that they cannot protect their child from injury in a crash by cradling or holding the infant in their laps. Adults are neither strong nor quick enough to prevent the sudden forward motions or overcome the **inertial forces** (external forces of motion caused by impact) exerted in a crash. An unrestrained adult is propelled forward, trapping and crushing the infant between the adult's body and the hard surfaces inside the car on impact. The only way to prevent injuries and death to an infant in a car is to use a car safety seat for each trip, no matter how short.

A lifelong practice begins with the newborn's first ride home. Getting a child accustomed to using a safety seat at a young age establishes a safety habit and may reduce resistance later (see Fig. 13–2).

> Infants who weigh up to 20 pounds should be restrained in a car seat in a semireclined, rear-facing position to allow the seat and infant's spine to bear the forces of impact should a collision occur.

Harness straps should be snugly adjusted to prevent movement of the infant, decreasing the risk of slipping out of the seat or strangulation by loose straps. Infants should not be wrapped in blankets or dressed in bulky clothing because the extra cushioning prevents a snug fit of the crotch strap in the safety seat. A loose strap could allow the infant's body to move downward, increasing the risk of strangulation.

Infants and children should not be restrained in the front-seat of cars equipped with passenger-side air bags. When deployed, the air bag can severely jolt the car safety seat and harm the infant. Optimally, infants and small children should be restrained in the middle back-seat, the most protected location in the vehicle during a collision. All car safety seats should be secured to the framework of the vehicle according to the manufacturer's directions. Failure to adequately secure the car safety seat increases the possibility of serious injury to the infant in the event of a collision.

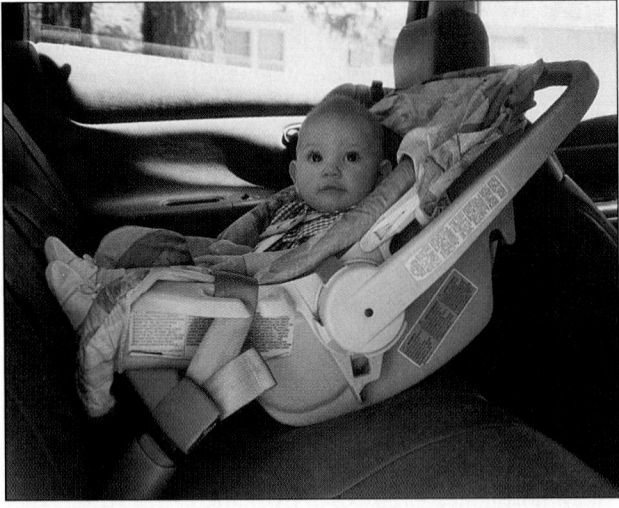

Figure 13–2
The infant rides facing the rear of the vehicle, ideally in the middle of the back seat. The infant seat is secured to the vehicle with the seat belts; straps on the car seat adjust to accommodate the growing baby. The smaller infant will need a rolled blanket to prevent excess head movement.

Providing a Safe Environment

During infancy and early childhood, when children are typically limited to the home environment, safety in and around the home is a top priority. With the exception of injuries and deaths related to motor vehicle crashes, the majority of childhood injuries occur in the home.

Parents or caregivers with preschool or younger children need to make the home environment safe for a growing, inquisitive child. Parents must assume responsibility for preventing falls, burns, suffocation, firearm injuries, drownings, and poisonings.

Parents who entrust the care of their children to others, such as daycare centers, should be conscious of the same injury risks. Parents must consider safety as a factor when selecting appropriate daycare for their child.

With children who are hospitalized, parents entrust the care of their children to health care providers. Health care providers must be equally aware of injury risks in the hospital environment. The accompanying box highlights safety measures for hospitalized children.

Fire Safety

House fires kill approximately 1200 children from birth to 14 years each year and account for 90% of all childhood burn deaths. House fire death rates are especially high in low-income areas and in the southern United States (Wilson et al., 1991). This finding is disturbing because most of these deaths can be prevented. According to the United States Fire Administration, the majority of child fire deaths occur in homes without working smoke detectors.

Infants lack independent mobility and cannot escape from smoke and flames on their own. Parents must assume a greater responsibility in preventive measures to avoid house fires and related burn injuries. Anticipatory guidance should emphasize the preventive measures summarized in the accompanying box.

Burn Safety

Infants are especially vulnerable to inflicted burns, particularly scald burns. Their limited mobility makes it impossible for them to escape from immersion in hot water. Parents should be instructed to decrease the setting on hot water heaters to 120°F. Infant skin is thin, causing burns

Safety Measures for Hospitalized Children

- To prevent falls, siderails on cribs and beds should be kept raised and locked in position unless an adult is next to the bed.
- Fire doors and doors that lead to stairways should be equipped with a door alarm to prevent children from wandering into an area from which they could fall.
- Electric sockets in patient care areas and hallways should be covered with appropriate protectors or guards.
- Housekeeping closets and supplies in patient care areas should be locked or attended. Buckets of water or cleaning solutions should never be left unattended.
- Needle boxes should be mounted in locations that are inaccessible to children.
- Cribs must be positioned away from curtain or blind cords. Wires and tubing attached to a child (i.e., intravenous tubing, oxygen tubing) should be secured so that entanglement and strangulation do not occur. Children with this type of equipment need frequent monitoring.
- Medicines and many toxic chemicals are readily accessible in a hospital setting. Health care providers must ensure that these items are inaccessible to children.

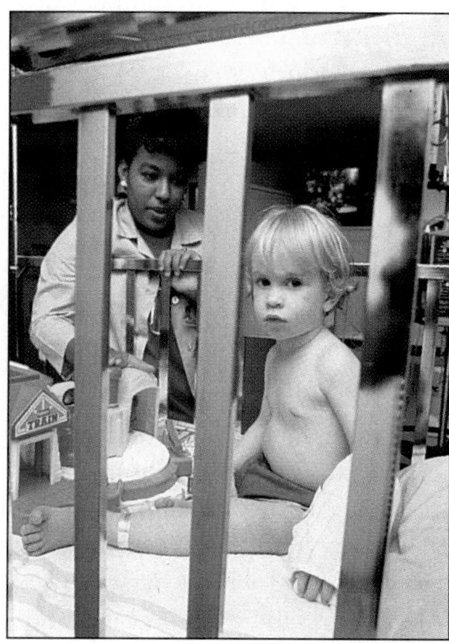

- Small (mouth size) pieces of equipment (e.g., syringe caps, needles, caps from ends of IV tubing, rubber tips from syringes, bandaids left on fingers, etc.) need to be kept away from young children and their immediate area (beds, bedside tables, sink counters, etc.) to prevent possible choking.

TEACHING GUIDELINES *for Residential Fire Prevention and Safety*

- Smoke detectors should be installed on all levels of the home, outside the kitchen, and outside each bedroom. Batteries should be routinely changed and tested for proper functioning.
- Parents should be encouraged to plot several escape routes from each area of the home and to designate a place where all family members should meet immediately after leaving the home. Parents should develop specific escape routes for each small child in the home. Chain or rope ladders should be kept in each bedroom on upper floors to permit rapid escape. Overnight guests should be informed of the family's fire plan.
- Many fire departments offer special window decals to assist with early identification of a child's room in the event of a fire.
- Auxiliary heaters should be placed on noncombustible pads and positioned away from walls or furniture. They should not be used while the family is sleeping.
- Infants' night clothing should be made of flame-resistant material.
- Infants or small children should never be left alone in the home without adult supervision.
- Fire extinguishers should be installed in the home, particularly in the kitchen, bedroom, and garage, where fires are likely to occur. Fire extinguishers should *not* be put above the stove; if a fire occurred on a burner, the extinguisher couldn't be reached.
- Home heating systems should be inspected and cleaned annually to reduce fire risks.
- Electric appliances and cords should be checked regularly for wear, loose connections, and frayed wires.

to occur faster at lower temperatures. With water temperature settings of 140°F, it only takes 3 seconds for the child to suffer serious burns. When the temperature is lowered 20°, it takes 8 to 10 minutes of submersion to cause the same degree of burn injury. Water should be tested by an adult before the infant is submerged to decrease the risk of accidental scald injuries. Older siblings who assist with the bathing of an infant should always be supervised by an adult to prevent accidental burn injuries.

Reducing water heater temperatures to 120°F helps to prevent severe scald injuries in children.

Burn injuries in infants can also be caused by a variety of other sources. Exposure to sunlight can result in serious sunburn to their delicate skin. Parents should be encouraged to liberally apply sunblock and sunscreens and to protect the face and head with a hat when exposing the infant or toddler to sunlight, even for brief periods.

Parents should be advised to avoid smoking, drinking hot liquids, or cooking while holding an infant. As infants begin to crawl around on the floor, open electric sockets should be covered with appropriate socket protectors. Open stoves or fireplaces are especially intriguing to an exploring infant and should be outfitted with a guard or grid. Cool mist vaporizers should be used rather than steam vaporizers to prevent scald injuries to a curious infant.

TEACHING GUIDELINES *for Crib Safety*

- The distance between slats must be no more than $2\frac{3}{8}$ inches wide to prevent entrapment of the infant's head or body.
- The interior of the crib must snugly accommodate a standard size mattress so that the gap is minimal, less than the width of two adult fingers. Excessive space could allow the infant to become wedged, potentially suffocating.
- Decorative enhancements on the crib are not recommended because they can break apart and become aspirated by the infant. Design cutouts can trap an infant's arm or neck, causing death or serious injury.
- Corner post or finials that rise above the end panels can snag garments and inadvertently strangle infants.
- The drop side must be impossible for an infant to release. Activating the drop side must take either a strong force (at least 10 lb) or a distinct action at each locking device.
- Wood surfaces should be free of splinters, cracks, and lead-based paint.

Safe Baby Furnishings

Baby furniture, although seemingly benign, can present lethal hazards to a growing infant. Parents should be aware of safety considerations when planning or decorating the infant's room. Governmental regulations were implemented in 1973, based on the recommendations of the United States Consumer Product Safety Commission, regulating crib design and production to prevent needless injury. Crib safety considerations are outlined in the accompanying box. These regulations also apply to the use of cribs in the hospital. Parents need to be aware that older furniture that has been handed down may not meet current safety regulations. Older cribs can have slats that are distanced so that an infant could entrap his head, or the paint may contain lead.

Hanging toys or mobiles placed over the crib should be positioned well out of the infant's reach to prevent entanglement and strangulation. Large toys in the crib should be avoided because an older infant may use them as steps to climb over the side, resulting in a serious fall injury. Cribs should be positioned away from curtains or blinds to prevent accidental entanglement in dangling cords.

Preventing Falls

Infants are often placed on surfaces at heights that are convenient for the adult, such as on changing tables, counters, or furniture. These surfaces often have no restraining barriers. Infants begin to roll over as early as 2 months, and as they begin to scoot or crawl, fall injuries from these elevations are common. There must be constant adult supervision when infants are placed at such heights (Fig. 13–3). If the parent or nurse must move away from the infant, he should either take the infant with him or, if supplies are close, place his hand on the infant while reaching. At home, parents may choose to place their child on the floor for changing diapers, etc.

Falls from infant seats or out of high chairs are common and can be prevented with supervision and the use of safety restraining straps to limit the mobility of the infant (Fig. 13-3). The distance of the fall is not as great, but the same principle applies when the infant is in a stroller. If unrestrained, an infant can pull herself up and fall from the stroller onto the underlying surface, resulting in a potentially serious head injury.

As infants begin to crawl, falls can be prevented by using gates at the top and bottom of stairs. Infant walkers are dangerous, and their use should be discouraged. They allow infants mobility and the freedom to explore sur-

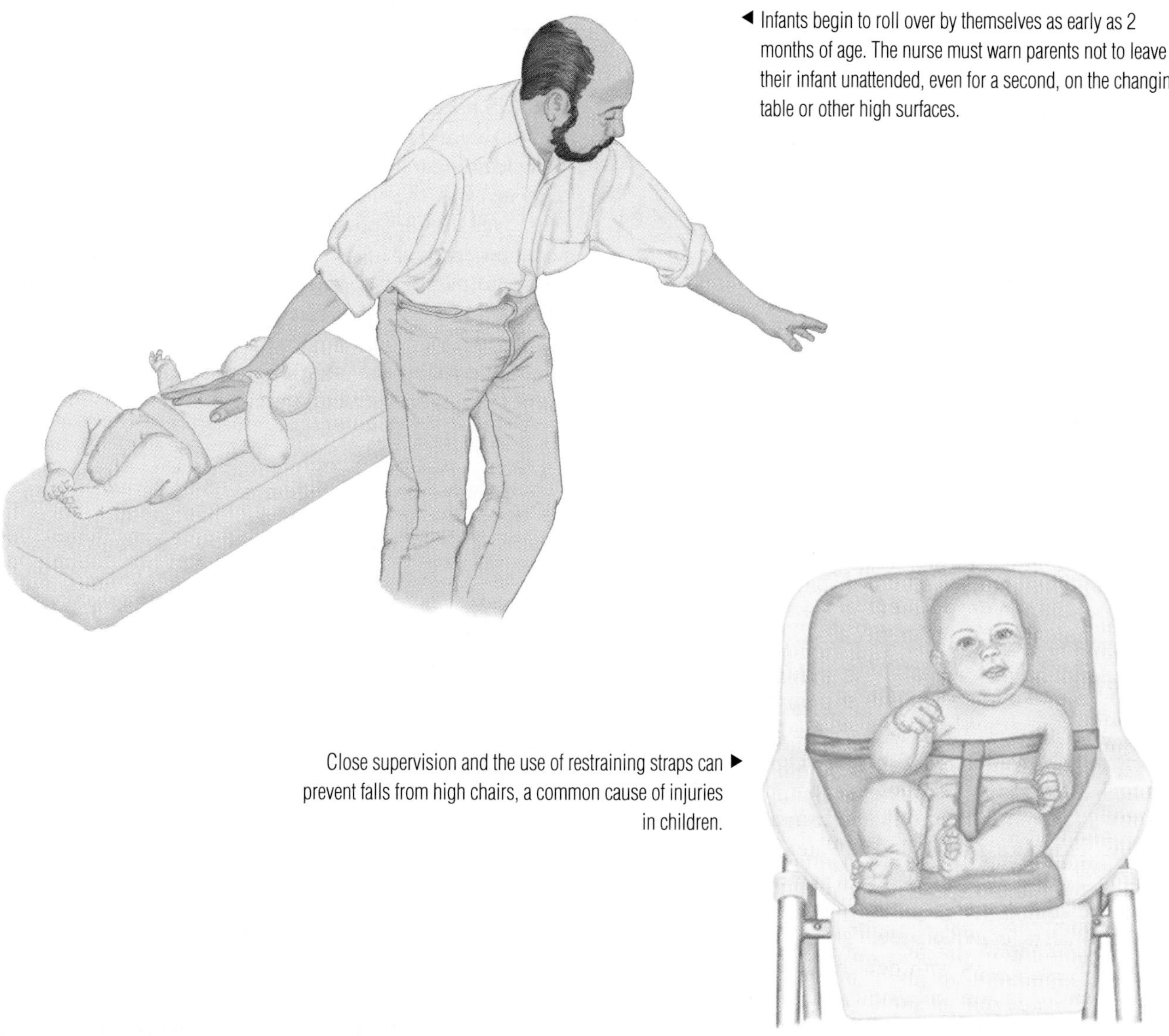

◀ Infants begin to roll over by themselves as early as 2 months of age. The nurse must warn parents not to leave their infant unattended, even for a second, on the changing table or other high surfaces.

Close supervision and the use of restraining straps can ▶ prevent falls from high chairs, a common cause of injuries in children.

Figure 13–3
Safety education for parents of infants should emphasize the need for constant supervision and the use of restraining devices to prevent falls.

roundings before they have developed the ability to interpret heights or protect themselves from falls.

Educating parents about an infant's risk of falls helps them to recognize and take simple steps to prevent fall injuries.

Preventing Suffocation and Choking

Asphyxiation (suffocation) occurs when air cannot get into or out of the lungs and oxygen supplies are consequently depleted. Carbon dioxide levels then increase, causing life-threatening disruption of cardiac and cerebral functioning. Choking occurs when substances or objects are **aspirated** into the airway or into the branches of the lower airways, causing partial or complete obstruction of the lungs. Strangulation is typically thought of as a constriction of the neck, but also includes blockage of the nose and mouth by airtight materials, such as plastic. This blockage prevents air exchange. All plastic bags or covers should be stored out of the infant's reach.

Choking is a major concern in the first few months of an infant's life, when aspiration of feedings or vomit can occur easily because of the immature swallowing mechanism. Parents should be taught to position the infant on his side after feedings and to avoid placing a small infant in bed with a bottle propped in his mouth.

As infants grow, they begin to explore the world around them by placing anything and everything in their mouths. Size, shape, and consistency are major determinants of whether a food or object is likely to be aspirated by an infant.

Small children put anything and everything in their mouths. Choking hazards for infants and small children include food, small household items, and detachable parts of toys.

Food that is round or similar to the size of the airway is especially dangerous. Dangerous foods include sliced hot dogs, hard candy, peanuts, grapes, and chewing gum. These foods should be avoided until the child is able to chew thoroughly before swallowing. Food should be cut into small pieces and the child should be supervised. Playing, singing, or other activities should be strongly discouraged while eating to avoid choking. Infants are equally endangered by rattles, pieces of toys, ribbons from stuffed animals and common household objects, such as coins, buttons, pins, or beads, found on the floor or within their reach.

Latex balloons are choking hazards that should never be given to infants or small children.

Anticipatory guidance for parents includes performing a thorough inspection of the infant's surroundings to remove all potential items that the infant could grasp, place in her mouth, and choke on. Parents can be encouraged to crawl through the home to gain a better perspective of the infant's environment. Parents can then substitute safe objects for exploration.

Ornaments or toys with detachable parts are not recommended for infants because of the aspiration risk. In 1979, the Consumer Product Safety Commission established a toy standard to prevent choking hazards in nonfood products targeted for children younger than 3 years of age. Parents should take extra care to note the presence of small detachable parts on toys before allowing the infant to play with the item. Although the government regulates the size of parts on infant's toys, older children's toys are not regulated by the same standard. As the infant explores an older sibling's or a playmate's territory, adult supervision is important.

To prevent strangulation injuries, parents should be cautioned against placing a pacifier on a string or cord around the infant's neck, putting an infant to sleep with a bib in place, or positioning a crib near blinds or curtain cords. Crib slats should comply with the $2\frac{3}{8}$-inch width requirement to prevent head entrapment.

In addition to inspecting and providing a safe environment for the infant, parents should be encouraged to complete a course on cardiopulmonary resuscitation (CPR) so that if an incident occurs, they will be able to immediately administer lifesaving interventions competently.

TODDLER SAFETY

Toddlers are adventurous and eager to explore the world around them. They are constantly on the move, progressively learning to run, jump, and climb. It is challenging to keep up with the unlimited energy of the toddler or to foresee all of the possible dangers. Understanding the developmental changes a toddler undergoes helps the nurse and parent to appreciate why this stage of development is the most injury-prone stage of a child's life (see Chapter 5). Constant supervision is challenging for parents, but remains the most important step in preventing injuries in this energetic age group.

Car Safety

Motor vehicle injuries continue to be a significant threat to the toddler. Although toddlers begin to develop more independent behaviors, they are still solely reliant on an adult for protection while traveling in a car. Once a toddler is able to sit up alone, car safety seats can be adjusted to face forward in an upright position (Fig. 13–4). Safety straps should continue to be adjusted to provide a snug fit. The car safety seat is suitable for the growing toddler until she reaches a weight of 40 lb. Car doors should be locked while the car is in motion to prevent a curious toddler from opening the door.

Toddlers should be restrained in an upright, forward-facing position in a car safety seat until they weigh 40 lb (usually 3–5 years of age).

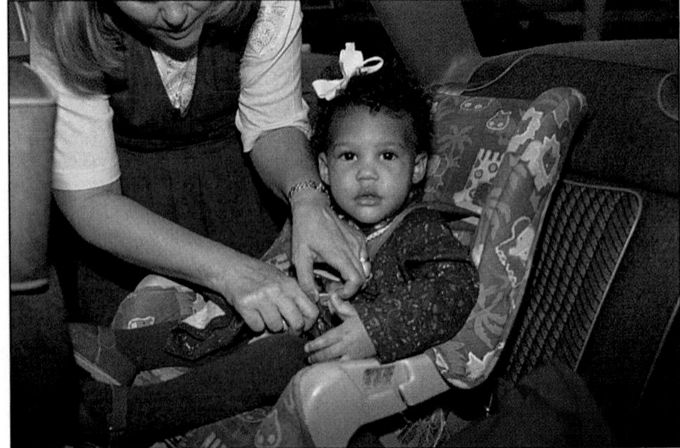

Figure 13–4
When an older infant easily sits alone, the car safety seat can be adjusted to a forward-facing, upright position. This seat is appropriate for the toddler until she reaches about 40 pounds. The safety straps should be adjusted to provide a snug fit, and the seat should be placed in the back seat of the car, ideally in the middle rear seat.

Key educational points for parental teaching include emphasizing the importance of properly restraining the toddler each time he rides in the car. Parents should be encouraged to model safe behavior by consistently wearing their seat belts because children begin to imitate their parents at an early age. Studies have demonstrated a secondary benefit of child car safety seats: a restrained child exhibits better behavior than an unrestrained child. A restrained child is less likely to fight or cause other distracting behaviors (Christophersen, 1977).

As the toddler's cognitive and fine motor skills develop, her curiosity will enable her to learn how to wiggle free of the restraining system, despite releases that are designed to be difficult for a child to operate. Parents must insist on compliance in spite of temper tantrums, which are characteristic of this developmental stage.

Because of the short physical stature of the toddler, adults should visually inspect the area surrounding the automobile before placing it in gear. A toddler near the car may not be visible and can sustain serious crushing injuries if run over by the car or trapped between the car and a stationary object. There is always the potential for a toddler to dart out on foot or on a tricycle into oncoming traffic. Parents should closely supervise play activities and remain in close proximity to the toddler to prevent these types of injuries. Automatic garage doors should have safety settings that are adjusted to raise if a toddler becomes entrapped between the closing door and the floor.

Toddlers or infants should never be left unattended, even for a moment, in a car. Exposure to extreme heat or cold temperatures is dangerous in this age group. An anticipated brief moment unattended could become a prolonged interval during which the child is exposed to temperature extremes, with serious consequences. Injuries have occurred when parents have left cars running for various reasons and curious toddlers have disengaged the gears, causing the car to roll and collide with other objects. Parents must be made aware of the dangers of leaving children unattended in a car.

Fire and Burn Safety

Toddlers, with their increased mobility and developing fine motor skills, can reach hot water, open fires, or hot objects placed on counters, and stoves above their eye level. They may pull objects off of stoves, pull down cords attached to small appliances, open oven doors, and place electric cords or frayed wires into their mouths. They may drink liquids that are dangerously hot. Parents should be encouraged to remain in the kitchen when preparing a meal and reminded to use the back burners on the stove and to turn pot handles inward and toward the middle of the stove to reduce the toddler's risk of burn injuries. Dangling cords from irons or other small appliances should not be accessible to toddlers. Open fires and heaters are also inviting. Sturdy guards fixed to the wall prevent young children from getting too close to these burn hazards.

Toddlers depend on adults for their protection in the event of a house fire. Anticipatory guidance should stress the importance of smoke detectors and escape plans. Additionally, the curious toddler is fascinated with matches and lighters; therefore, they must be kept out of reach. Parents should not use them to distract or amuse the toddler.

Preventing Falls

Toddlers move quickly and climb everywhere. Vulnerability to fall injuries is increased because they are able to get themselves into a variety of dangerous and compromising situations in and out of the home. Toddlers can fall from playground equipment, off of tricycles, and out of windows. Falls from above the first floor of a building can result in serious injuries to the child. A chair next to a kitchen counter or table allows the toddler easy access to dangerously high places. With climbing and exploration a normal aspect of the developmental process, safety education for the parent emphasizes constant supervision and some anticipatory planning, such as moving furniture, installing screen guards, or restricting access to potential climbing hazards. Additionally, parents should consider other interventions to prevent fall injuries in toddlers (see accompanying box).

Water Safety

Children younger than 4 years of age are at especially high risk for water-related injuries.

> Drowning is the third leading cause of death for children younger than 4 years (Wilson et al., 1991). Close, constant supervision is the most essential aspect of safety promotion to prevent childhood drowning.

Toddlers love to play in water. Most drownings occur when a child is left alone in a bathtub or falls into a residential pool. Even for a child who survives a submersion injury, the risk of permanent brain and lung damage is great. Parents should be educated never to leave a child alone in or near a bathtub, pail of water, wading or swimming pool, or any other body of water even for a moment. A toddler can drown in as little as 1 inch of water. Toilet lids should remain closed. The young toddler may inadvertently fall headfirst into a toilet or bucket, but lack the upper-body strength and coordination to remove himself from submersion. Prevention of drowning requires constant parental supervision of the toddler and his activities.

TEACHING GUIDELINES *for Prevention of Injuries from Falls*

- Install window locks on all windows. Never allow a young child to sit on a window sill.
- Avoid placing furniture directly under windows to discourage young climbers.
- Lock doors to any dangerous areas, such as cellars, basements, or garages. Inexpensive door alarms can be purchased and installed to alert parents that a child has opened a restricted door.
- Place gates at both the top and the bottom of stairways. Slide gates are preferable to folding or collapsible gates. Folding gates have the potential to strangle or entrap a child.
- Install window guards and stops on all windows above the first floor.
- Secure safety straps in strollers, high chairs, and shopping carts. Never allow a child to stand while in any of these.
- Inspect balconies and high porches to ensure that railings are strong and in good condition. Rails should be spaced so that a child's head or body cannot become entrapped.
- Install rubber, skidproof mats in the bath and shower to prevent falls.
- Do not permit young children to play or sleep on the upper bunk of a bunk bed.

Parents should carefully assess their immediate neighborhood for residential pools or other bodies of water, all of which create a potential hazard to a wandering toddler. Pool submersion happens quickly, often without splashing to alert anyone that a child is in trouble. Many communities have enacted regulations governing residential pools, both in-ground and aboveground. Adults must comply with these regulations. Parents who own pools must take precautions to reduce the likelihood that their child will enter the family pool or spa without adult supervision. Barriers are not childproof, but they provide layers of protection for the child who strays from supervision. Barriers also provide extra seconds to locate a child before an injury occurs. Most submersion incidents happen less than 5 minutes after the child is seen by an adult.

Parents with pools or spas or who reside near residential or apartment pools or other bodies of water should be encouraged to complete a course on CPR. Immediate resuscitation is critical to decrease the possibility of a devastating neurologic injury.

Recommendations by the United States Consumer Product Safety Commission to promote water safety and reduce fatal or devastating submersion incidents in young children are shown in the accompanying box (U.S. Consumer Product Safety Commission, 1993a, 1993b).

Preventing Poisoning

Each year, more than 2 million children are poisoned. National averages show that by the time a child reaches 5 years of age, the chance that he has ingested a potentially toxic substance is greater than 40%. Most poisonings occur in the child's home (Centers for Disease Control, 1990). Children younger than 5 years are the most common victims, and children 1 to 3 years old are at the highest risk. Small children open drawers or cabinets and climb everywhere. With exploration, everything eventually finds its way to the child's mouth, even if it does not smell or taste good. Small children who are thirsty or hungry will ingest poisons that look or smell inviting. Some containers that hold toxic substances held a common food or drink at one time. Parents need to be educated on how to poison-proof the home. Potential toxic products need to be stored safely for the child's benefit rather than the convenience of the adult. Any nonfood item is a potential poison: prescription and over-the-counter medication, alcohol, polishes, insecticides, antifreeze, drain cleaners, plants, bleaches, and cosmetics.

All medicines, poisons, and household products must be stored out of the reach of small children.

Parents and caregivers have the responsibility to prevent a child's access to poisons. Child-resistant locks or catches should be placed on all cupboards that contain poisons. Parents should be taught the appropriate actions to take if an ingestion occurs: immediately contacting a Poison Control Center or a physician. Parents should keep syrup of ipecac in the home and be familiar with its administration. However, they should not give syrup of ipecac to a child unless instructed to do so by the Poison Control Center or a physician. See the accompanying box.

Common household products and cleaners can be toxic if ingested, and they should be used only in the presence of an adult. If the parent needs to leave the area where cleaning supplies are being used, she should take the toddler with her or remove the substance from the area. The accompanying box shows considerations for poison-proofing a child's surroundings.

Medications often come in interesting shapes and colors that are appealing to children. Parents and caregivers should not refer to medicine as candy. Because young children often mimic their parents, adults should be discouraged from taking medicine in the child's presence.

TEACHING GUIDELINES *for Pools and Children: Drowning Prevention*

DESIGN AND ACCESS

Fencing

- A fence or barrier should be at least 4 feet high and must completely surround the pool. A wall of a house may serve as part of the barrier.
- If the house is part of the barrier, the doors leading to the pool area should be protected with an alarm. Some pools may even be covered with a power safety cover.
- The fence or barrier should be free of footholds or handholds that can assist the young child in climbing it. With chain-link fences, the diamond-shaped openings should not be larger than $1\frac{3}{4}$ inches in diameter.
- Vertical slats of fences should be less than 4 inches apart to prevent a child from squeezing through.

Gates

- Gates should be self-closing, with self-latching mechanisms in proper working order.
- The latching mechanisms to the gates should be out of reach of young children.

Doors

- All exit doors from the house to the pool should be protected by an audible alarm. Adults can disarm the alarm temporarily for a single opening of the door by the use of a keypad or switch that is located out of the reach of children.

Steps and Ladders

- Steps and ladders leading to aboveground pools must be secured, locked, or removed when the pool is not in use.

Pool Covers

- Pool covers should be completely removed when the pool is being used.
- Standing water must be removed from pool covers to prevent drownings.
- A power cover should be closed when the pool is not in use, even for only short periods.

SUPERVISION

- Young children must never be left alone in or around pools, even for a moment. An adult should always be available to monitor pool activity.
- Caregivers must be instructed about potential hazards to young children in and around the pool.
- Caregivers should never rely on flotation devices or swimming lessons to protect a child.

EMERGENCY PROCEDURES

- Parents and caregivers need to have cardiopulmonary resuscitation training.
- Parents or caregivers should initiate cardiopulmonary resuscitation immediately and not wait for emergency rescue personnel to arrive.
- A telephone should be available at poolside at all times.
- Emergency numbers should be posted on or near the pool telephone.
- Rescue equipment should be available poolside.

POOL RULES

- Parents should instruct caregivers about pool hazards and the use of protective devices such as door alarms and latches. The need for constant adult supervision must be emphasized.
- An unsupervised child should never be left near a pool. During social gatherings at or near a pool, a designated watcher should be appointed to protect young children. When adults become preoccupied, children are at risk.
- If a child is missing, the pool area should be checked first. Seconds count in preventing deaths. It is important to go to the ledge and scan the entire pool, bottom, and surface and also to move objects or floats in the water that may obscure the view.
- Young children should not be allowed in a pool without an adult.
- Children should not be considered "drown-proof" because they have had swimming lessons. Children must always be watched closely while in and around water.
- Flotation devices are not a substitute for supervision.
- Toys should be removed from the pool area when not in use. Toys attract young children to the pool area.
- Gates leading to pool areas should never be propped open.
- Older children should be taught to swim with a buddy, never alone.
- Children should be taught not to run or push when in the pool area.

Data from U.S. Consumer Product Safety Commission. (1993a). *Children and pools: A safety checklist* (Publication No. 357). Washington, DC: Author.

Guidelines for the Administration of Syrup of Ipecac

Indications:

Ingestion of potentially toxic substance in the awake, alert child. Most effective in the first hour after the ingestion of the toxic substance. Administration should be followed by 10 to 20 ml/kg of clear fluids.

Dosages by Age:

younger than 6 months: none
6 to 12 months: 10 ml; do not repeat
1 to 12 years: 15 ml; may repeat once if vomiting has not occurred in 20 minutes
older than 12 years: 30 ml; may repeat once if vomiting has not occurred in 20 minutes

Contraindications:

Nontoxic substances, acids, alkalis, petroleum distillates, hydrocarbons, loss of gag reflexes, coma, or seizures. (See Chapter 14, p. 314.)

The same precautions should be taken when small children go to a grandparent's home to visit. Ingestions sometimes occur when a guest visits and the curious toddler finds medications in a purse or overnight bag. Childproof caps slow the toddler, but are not an absolute barrier. Labeling poisons with characteristic symbols, such as the skull and crossbones or "Mr. Yuk," helps to provide visual cues to young children; however, labels are not absolute deterrents for a determined child. The best way to prevent toxic ingestions is with careful storage of all potential poisons in a place that is inaccessible to children.

PRESCHOOLER SAFETY

Preschoolers are active and inquisitive. They have increased self-control, but still have an immature understanding of danger. Safety becomes even more challenging for the parent because the preschooler is no longer content with his own backyard. The preschooler is mesmerized by cartoons depicting make-believe situations. They see cartoon characters engaged in daring endeavors and walking away unharmed. Because of their magical thinking, preschoolers may believe that these feats are possible and may attempt them (see Chapter 6).

Safety education can now be directed toward the child as well as the parent. Preschoolers are at an ideal age to learn simple safety practices because they can follow verbal directions and their attention span is lengthening (Zuckerman & Duby, 1985). They have a strong rhythmic

TEACHING GUIDELINES *for Childhood Poison Prevention*

- Keep all poisons, medicines, cleaners, and toxic substances out of the reach of children. Cabinets or storage areas should be routinely cleaned out, with old or unused products discarded by flushing them down the toilet or drain. Never discard poisons in a wastebasket.
- Parents should be familiar with poisons commonly found in or near the home, including detergents, drain cleaner, dishwashing soap, furniture polish, cleaning agents, window cleaners, all medicines, vitamins, children's medications, sprays, powders, cosmetics, fingernail preparations, hair care products, sachets, mothballs, rodent poisons, fertilizers, gasoline, paints, glues, insecticides, cigarette butts, plants, and shrubs.
- Poisons should be stored in areas that are secured with locks or protected by child-resistant safety latches.
- Medicines and all harmful substances should be purchased in child-resistant packages.
- Alcoholic beverages should be kept out of the reach of children or locked in a separate cabinet. Parents should be discouraged from giving sips of alcohol to children because small amounts can be toxic to young children.
- Children should not be allowed to chew on plants or shrubs.
- Ashtrays should be kept empty and out of the reach of small children.
- Handbags and overnight luggage of guests in the home often contain medicines or other toxic substances and should be kept out of a child's reach.
- Poisons or harmful substances should always be stored in the original container. Parents should be discouraged from placing toxic substances in food or beverage containers for storage.
- Children should be taught to ask an adult before they touch a nonfood substance.
- Parents should poison-proof all areas of the home, especially the following areas: kitchen, bathroom, pantry, bedroom, garage, basement, and work areas. Grandparents and other caregivers should be encouraged to do the same.
- The telephone number of the local Poison Control Center should be posted for immediate access in the event of a poisoning. Parents should be instructed, when contacting the Poison Control Center, to have on hand the substance with the label for prompt identification of toxic ingredients.

sense, and songs and rhymes about safety can enhance the learning process. Instruction should be simple, with one concept introduced at a time. Short stories, puppet shows, songs, coloring activities, and role-playing games are all suitable learning activities that help preschoolers to learn safety-conscious behaviors.

Even though a preschooler begins to assert his independence, he is not able to solve problems with adult reasoning. Anticipatory guidance for parents addresses the conflict between the preschooler's growing autonomy and the restrictions that must be enforced. Parents must remain firm and consistent in applying the rules for safety. Parents should begin to discuss why the restrictions are necessary to help the child to anticipate the consequences of dangerous actions.

Car Safety

Child car safety seats are suitable for children until they weigh 40 lb. Typically, the average girl reaches this weight at about 5 years and the average boy at about $4\frac{1}{2}$ years. However, the preschooler may outgrow the seat before he reaches the weight limit because the harness system becomes too tight (Wilson et al., 1991). As they outgrow the car seat, preschoolers often develop a burning desire to see or reach out of the car window. Children should not sit in the front seat of a car equipped with air bags.

Once a child has outgrown her child car safety seat, a booster seat is strongly recommended (Fig. 13–5). Although they are preferable to no restraints at all, standard seat belts alone can contribute to injury because they fit poorly over the small frame of the preschooler. The standard shoulder harness often crosses the child's face or neck, and the lap belt is positioned across the midabdomen rather than across the bony structure of the pelvis. Booster seats are designed to raise the child high enough so that the restraining straps are correctly positioned over the child's smaller body frame.

A booster seat is recommended for a preschooler who weighs more than 40 pounds. It raises the child to properly accommodate the seat belt system of the car.

Parents continue to have the primary responsibility for ensuring that a child is safely restrained before the vehicle is started and in motion. Parents must insist that children remain restrained at all times and that seat belts are used correctly. Although it may seem fun and relatively harmless, riding in the open bed of a pickup truck or in the cargo area of a van or station wagon is a potentially deadly situation in the event of a crash. It is outlawed in some states. Nurses should investigate local laws to provide accurate information to families who may be faced with this dilemma or are unaware of the associated dangers.

Children should never be allowed to ride in the bed of a pickup truck or unrestrained in the cargo area of a van or station wagon.

Fire and Burn Safety

Preschoolers imitate adults in all types of daily routines and activities. They may attempt these activities before they are able to safely manage the appliance (e.g., stove, iron, oven), increasing the risk of burn injuries. Matches and lighters continue to fascinate preschoolers. With their increased fine motor skills, preschoolers may be able to ignite a flame. Teaching a preschooler that lighters and matches are adult tools and instructing them to tell an adult immediately if they find these items can prevent burn injuries.

Children should never be allowed to play with matches or lighters.

Children younger than 5 years are at the greatest risk for burn deaths in a house fire. They often panic and hide in closets or under beds rather than escaping safely. Parents should practice with their children to teach them what to do in the event of a house fire. Preschoolers should become familiar with the sounds emitted by the smoke alarms and taught to crawl under smoke and to check doors for heat. In addition, parents should be encouraged to practice family fire drills on a routine basis so that the child learns to escape rapidly.

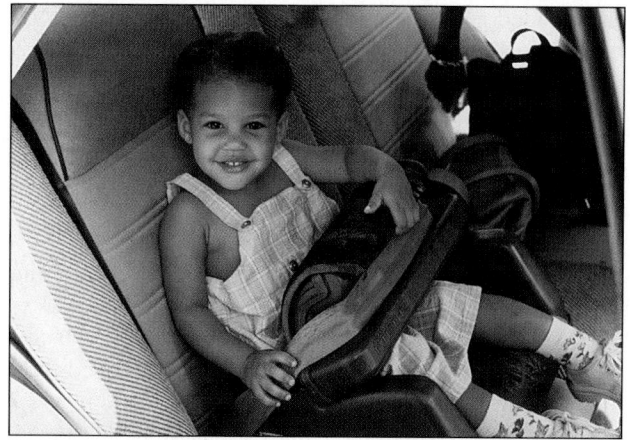

Figure 13–5
A booster seat with an abdominal shield is strongly recommended for children who have outgrown a child safety seat. Booster seats raise the young child high enough to allow the car seat belts to be correctly positioned over the child's chest and pelvis.

Preschoolers are at an ideal age to learn what to do if their clothing ignites in flames. Preschoolers should be instructed to stop immediately if their clothes catch on fire and to cover their face and mouth with their hands. They should then drop to the ground and roll to smother the flames. This simple command (stop, drop, and roll) can help prevent severe burn injuries. Teaching specific behaviors educates children to remain calm and not panic.

Firearm Safety

Many guns are kept in the home loaded and readily accessible to young children. Parents should be encouraged to critically evaluate their need for a firearm in the home. Do the potential devastating risks outweigh any benefits of keeping a weapon in the home? Parents who choose to keep a gun in the home should receive anticipatory guidance about injury prevention. Guns kept in the home should always be unloaded, stored with trigger guards in place, securely locked in metal vaults, and inaccessible to all children (Brady, 1994). Gun owners should also complete an extensive training course on the safe handling and proper operation of a firearm. Total responsibility for preventing firearm injuries to children falls on adults who choose to own a gun (Patterson & Smith, 1987).

Guns must be stored unloaded, with trigger guards engaged, secured under lock and key, and absolutely INACCESSIBLE to ALL children. If a child finds a gun, he should be taught to leave the area immediately and tell an adult.

Too often, tragic incidents occur when a child finds and plays with a loaded gun, thinking it is a toy, or discovers a loaded gun in a relative's or playmate's home. Children must be taught what to do if they find a gun. This teaching should begin at a young age and must be reinforced throughout the growing years. Three key safety points should be emphasized:

- If a child finds a gun, he should stop and must not touch the gun.
- The child should immediately leave the area.
- The child should find an adult right away and tell the adult.

The child should also be taught never to attempt to take a gun away from someone, but leave the area immediately (National Rifle Association, 1992).

Children are exposed to guns with alarming frequency through television and movies and in their play activities. Toy guns are often designed to resemble real guns. Play involving guns is popular and often accepted, especially in male-dominated activities. Parents are instrumental in helping their children to distinguish between the make-believe world and real-life situations, in which the consequences of firearms can be devastating. At the very least, parents need to teach children never to point a toy gun at another person.

Equally important for safety consideration are non-powder rifles (e.g., BB guns, air rifles). They are not toys and are capable of causing serious injury, and should be used only with adult supervision. Because of the deadly consequences to children, the American Academy of Pediatrics supports the removal of guns from a child's environment.

Older children and adolescents may use guns for recreational hunting. It is the responsibility of parents to ensure that gun safety is taught. Lack of knowledge regarding the responsible and safe use of firearms places the individual at increased risk of injury and death.

Personal Safety

Preschoolers have an interest in establishing relationships with others as they expand the boundaries of their world. With the child's increasing assertion of independence, parents are less able to provide the constant protection they once did.

Teaching children about personal safety encourages them to develop skills to detect danger and teaches appropriate ways to handle threatening situations. Strangers are often portrayed as evil characters, when in reality their appearance and approach may be nonthreatening and friendly. Distinguishing a stranger from a well-intentioned person is challenging and often difficult for the preschooler. Basic guidelines that a child needs to know about personal safety include saying no, getting away, and telling an adult. Guidelines to help children define what types of situations to avoid are described in the accompanying box.

Children need to know how to access emergency help if they need it. Parents should help their children to learn to identify safety officials and how to dial 911 or other locally appropriate emergency numbers. Children need to respond to emergency operators with their full name, address, parent's name, and other appropriate information, and should remain on the phone until help arrives. Parents can practice this safety skill with their children to ensure proper reactions in an emergency and to help the child to understand what constitutes an emergency situation.

Sexual Abuse. Sexual abuse is another threat to personal safety. Preventing sexual abuse begins with teaching children the normal, healthy boundaries of their bodies and what constitutes inappropriate behavior. Often the victimizers are known and trusted by the child. Abusers frequently intimidate the child into silence with threats of personal harm or suggestions that the child initiated the behavior. Children need to know that no matter how great the threat, if someone is touching their body in an inap-

TEACHING GUIDELINES *for Childhood Personal Safety*

- Children should be taught who a stranger is. A stranger is someone the child does not know. The child may recognize the person, but he is considered a stranger unless the parents know him by name (e.g., mail carrier, garbage collector). A stranger can be a man or woman and young or old. A stranger can wear jeans or dress up in a suit and tie. Children should be taught that adults do not usually ask children for help, such as directions or help in locating a pet.
- Children should be taught to refuse offers of toys, treats, or special activities from anyone without their parents' permission.
- Children should be taught that if they are grabbed or harassed, they should make as much noise as possible, yelling loudly to draw attention.
- Children should be taught not to accept rides with anyone if not approved by the parent. Even if the person says that there is an emergency situation or parental consent, the child must refuse. Teach children that if someone is hurt or there is an emergency, someone they know will come to get them, not a stranger. The parents and child may develop a secret code to help identify someone who has legitimately been sent to pick up the child.
- Children should be discouraged from speaking to strangers.
- Parents need to remain with their children in public places (e.g., stores) and keep the child in constant view. Small children should not be allowed to use public restrooms alone.
- Parents need to be familiar with their child's friends and the general neighborhood. Children need to remain on well-traveled sidewalks, avoiding shortcuts, deserted streets, alleys, or fields.
- Parents should encourage their children to walk and play with friends instead of alone. They should play in open areas.
- Older children should be taught how to write down the license plate number of anyone that offers them rides, follows them, or hangs around playgrounds.
- Parents need to have frank discussions with their preschoolers at an early age concerning sexual abuse or inappropriate behavior so that a child will be comfortable confiding in the parent. Children should be taught that any area normally covered by a swimsuit is off-limits for touching. If touching does occur, they should tell a parent as soon as possible.
- Children should be taught to tell an adult immediately if inappropriate behavior does occur. They should know that they need to tell as many adults as it takes until someone listens and stops the inappropriate behavior.
- Parents need to teach their children that no one has the right to take their picture without the parents' approval or permission.
- Parents should be encouraged to teach their children how to be assertive and say "no" when someone does something that frightens them or is inappropriate.
- Children need to know their full name, address, and parents' names as early as possible. Knowing the telephone number, including the area code, is also helpful.

propriate way, they should always tell an adult. If that adult cannot help them, they should tell as many adults as necessary until the inappropriate behavior is stopped.

Children should be taught the personal boundaries of their bodies and to tell an adult if the boundaries are violated in any way.

Playground Safety

Playgrounds are a natural environment for children to run, jump, climb, and test their physical limits in a secure setting. However, some play areas contain significant injury risks for children. Nearly 200,000 children are injured on playgrounds every year. Seventy percent of these injuries occur in public parks and schoolyards. Falls from equipment are the major cause of serious playground injuries (Tinsworth & Kramer, 1990).

PLAYGROUND SAFETY RULES FOR CHILDREN

- Never walk or run near a moving swing.
- Always sit, and never stand, while swinging.
- Always swing alone, never double or triple.
- Climb up ladders of the slide, never up the slide itself.
- Do not push anyone while on play equipment.
- Do not stand on or suddenly jump off a seesaw.

Children are inventive and can be expected to use playground equipment in many unintended ways. Adult supervision helps to curb the more daring maneuvers and reduce injuries. Along with supervision, equipment design, layout, and maintenance are equally important for the promotion of overall playground safety.

Children should be taught to observe basic safety rules to ensure injury-free play on the playground.

SCHOOL-AGE SAFETY

School-age children can be divided into early school age (5–9 years) and middle school age (10–12 years). The approaches to safety education vary as the child grows older. Physically, this age is a period of great activity, with the child moving from the home environment and into the community. The school-age child experiences less fear in her play activities and frequently imitates real life by using tools and household items. This age group enjoys helping with adult routines and chores around the home.

Safety education is best accomplished by simply stating safety rules and providing reinforcement through short projects and immediate rewards. Role-playing activities and error-detection picture games are excellent ways to reinforce safety lessons. This age group is inquisitive and will frequently ask questions. Responses to their questions should contain concrete rationales. The school-age child can begin to think about safety rules and behaviors with respect to her experiences and can apply the rules in future situations (Sewell & Gaines, 1993).

Children in the middle school-age years enjoy reading and begin to develop abstract thinking. They strive to gain peer acceptance, and peer relationships become increasingly important. In this developmental stage, the child begins to take off on his own, attempting more and more daring actions. There is a tendency to disobey rules simply because they exist. Educational approaches to safety include those applied in the early school-age period, in addition to reading activities, crossword puzzles, and find-a-word games (Sewell & Gaines, 1993). Group projects with safety topics help to foster independent thinking while providing interactions with the child's peer group.

Car Safety

The school-age child is large enough to use the vehicle's three-point restraining system. Compliance often is determined by family values, with use or nonuse reflecting parental practices. For the younger, smaller child, correct positioning of the seat belt is important. Parents should help with adjustment of the belts so that the lap belt fits snugly over the bony pelvis and the shoulder harness is positioned across the chest. Although this placement is not optimal, the shoulder harness can be placed behind the shoulder if it crosses the face or soft tissue of the neck. Once the child is big enough, the seat belts should be positioned correctly.

Fire and Burn Safety

Parents should continue to reinforce safety procedures associated with fire safety. Routine fire drills should be practiced in the home. Repetition of family drills helps to ensure that the child will respond correctly and automatically to smoke alarms. Children of this age can better comprehend cause and effect relationships, so they can understand why they should not play with potentially flammable substances.

> Fire safety includes knowing two specific escape routes from each area in the home, how to access 911, and how to safely leave a burning house by crawling under the smoke. A meeting area outside the home should be designated. All family members should be instructed never to return inside a burning building. Fire drills should be practiced to establish automatic responses in a crisis situation.

School-age children are eager to help parents with daily chores such as cooking or ironing. Parents need to invest the time to teach their children how to properly use tools and appliances and must establish guidelines to avoid burn injuries as a result of the inexperience of the child. The older child with younger siblings may create potentially dangerous situations while helping with daily chores or tasks because he lacks the insight to fully anticipate the actions of the younger children. Parents should set guidelines and supervise activities that could result in burn injuries.

Fireworks create another burn hazard for children. Each summer, many children are seriously burned or permanently scarred by fireworks. Despite their patriotic association, fireworks are a safety hazard. To prevent serious burn injuries, the federal government, under the Federal Hazardous Substance Act, prohibits the sale of the more dangerous fireworks to the general public. However, there is always a degree of risk associated with any fireworks. There are no absolutely safe fireworks for children or adults. Fireworks are best left to the experts and viewed from a safe distance. Encourage families to enjoy the many community-sponsored fireworks displays.

Bicycle, Rollerblade, and Skateboard Safety

Mastering the ability to ride a bicycle is a milestone in a child's life, leading to independence. The bicycle is typically considered a toy, but is actually a vehicle that is capable of speedy transportation. It is also a major cause of death and serious head trauma in children. Bicycles are associated with more childhood injuries than any other consumer product except the automobile. Each year, about 400 children younger than 15 are killed, with another 400,000 requiring hospitalization or emergency department treatment. Of the children who are treated in the emergency department, more than one-third sustain head injuries, many permanently disabling (Wilson et al., 1991). For this reason, the public health community supports the mandatory use of bicycle helmets. Research has demonstrated that the use of a helmet can reduce the incidence of head injury by as much as 85% by absorbing the shock of the crash and cushioning the child's head (Thompson et al., 1989).

Bicycle safety practices actually begin when the child learns to ride a tricycle and progressively build as the child becomes more skilled and begins to ride a bicycle. A helmet and other safety accessories are essential for protection, but they are only an adjunct to the child's skill level and knowledge of the rules of the road. The challenge of balancing a bicycle, combined with the capability of starting and stopping without falling, is a learned skill, requiring sophisticated motor skills (Wilson, et al., 1991). A young cyclist is unpredictable and may be preoccupied with managing the bicycle itself. For this reason, parents should set limits on where, when, and how far the child may ride, until the child can competently maneuver the bicycle.

Rollerblades and skateboards are recreational activities that are popular with school-age children. Balancing, stopping, and turning are challenging and require similar motor skills to bicycling. As the child begins to learn these skills, falls are frequent and protective gear is essential. Helmets and protective pads covering the knees and elbows help to protect the most vulnerable areas of the child's body from serious injury. Key educational points and an overview of safety principles are described in the accompanying box.

Pedestrian Safety

Children between the ages of 5 and 9 years are at the greatest risk for auto–pedestrian injuries. The tremendous forces of impact and the lack of protection for the pedestrian can lead to severe injury. Children are commonly struck when they dart into traffic, especially where parked cars obscure the driver's view of the child (e.g., crossing the street in front of a school bus, playing near cars in driveways or yards). Several factors predispose this age group to such injuries. Their smaller physical stature limits their visibility to drivers until too late. Additionally, this age group has the misconception that if they can see the car, the driver must be able to see them and will be able to stop instantly. Focused on play activities, they often impulsively dart into the street, oblivious to boundaries and potential traffic dangers. Even if a car sounds its horn, this age group cannot accurately determine the source of the sound (Guyer et al., 1985).

Children learn traffic safety by watching and doing. Exposure to traffic increases as the child begins to walk to and from school and friends' houses. Parents have the responsibility to practice pedestrian safety hundreds of times before the child is allowed to venture across streets alone.

PEDESTRIAN SAFETY GUIDELINES

- Children should not be allowed to run into the street without looking first. They should learn to stop at the curb or edge of the road to check for traffic before crossing the street.
- Children should check for traffic by listening and looking, first to the left, then to the right, and finally to the left again.
- Children need to learn how to read traffic lights and crosswalk signs, and should be familiar with the right turn on red rule. They should understand the importance of waiting until all traffic is clear before crossing the street.
- Children should walk on sidewalks whenever possible. If there are no sidewalks, they should walk facing traffic on the left side of the street.
- Children should not walk at night, but if they must do so, they should wear bright, reflective clothing.

Water Safety

The school-age child learns to swim well enough to keep his head above water for a short time at about the age of 8. The length of time he can keep his head above water and swimming ability increase with age and experience. The incidence of drowning decreases in this age group; however, adult supervision is still needed to prevent a water-related injury. Children in this age group often overestimate their swimming capabilities and endurance. As their swimming abilities improve, anticipatory guidance can be directed toward general swimming safety. Children should be taught to stay away from canals and the fast-moving waters of creeks or rivers. Children need to be taught to wade into shallow water or to jump feetfirst into water of unknown depth to prevent neck injuries. Safety near the water includes never running, pushing, or jumping on others who are in the water.

When boating with children, an adult must make sure that they are wearing correctly sized floatation devices

TEACHING GUIDELINES *for Bicycle, Rollerblade, and Skateboard Safety*

- Children should always wear a helmet when riding a bike, on rollerblades, or on a skateboard. This safety practice should begin when the child begins to learn these activities.
- Helmets should fit properly and snugly on the head. Helmets need to be lightweight, ventilated, and decorated with reflective trim.
- Children should be taught not to ride at dusk or in the dark. They should always call home for a ride if it is after dark.
- Children should never ride two on a bicycle.
- Children should not ride barefoot, in thongs, or in slippers. Stereo headsets should be avoided while riding a bicycle because they can diminish hearing capabilities.
- Children should be encouraged to stay on sidewalks, paths, or driveways until they have mastered advanced biking skills and know the rules of the road.
- While riding or rollerblading, children should avoid uneven road surfaces, gravel, potholes, or bumps.

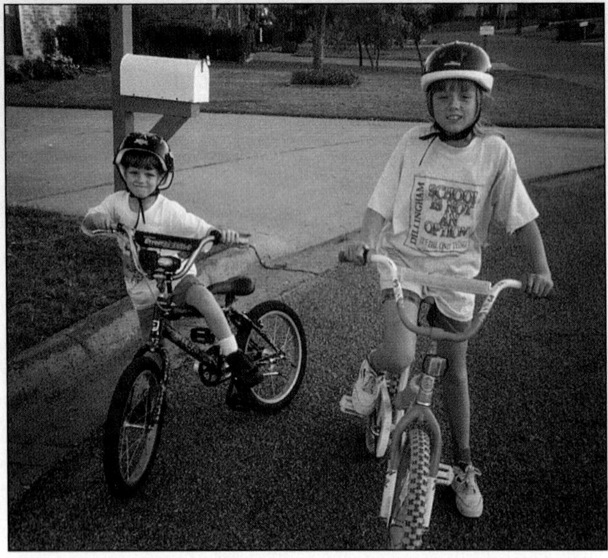

- Bicycles should be equipped with reflectors and lights. Children should routinely inspect their own bicycles with their parents' help to ensure that they are functioning properly (brakes, tires, lights, etc.).
- Parents should be taught the importance of proper sizing when purchasing a bicycle for their child. Oversized bicycles are responsible for many injuries.

  The child should be able to place the balls of both feet on the ground when sitting on the seat with the hands on the handlebars.

  The child should be able to straddle the center bar with both feet flat on the ground. There should be about 1 inch of clearance between the crotch and the bar.

  The handlebars should be within easy reach for the child.

Rules of the Road

- Children younger than 8 years should ride only with adult supervision, and never in the street. Rollerblading or skateboarding should be limited to areas where there is no car traffic.
- Children should not ride bicycles on roads with heavy traffic.
- A bicycle should be ridden on the right side of the road, with the traffic. Bike riders must obey all traffic laws, traffic signs, and lights.
- Children should learn the appropriate hand signals and use them every time before turning.
- Bicycles should be walked across busy intersections, not ridden.
- Children need to learn to stop, look left, look right, and look left again before entering a street or leaving a driveway, alley, or parking lot.
- Children should stop at all intersections, marked and unmarked.
- Children riding bicycles should obey all stop signs and red lights.
- Children should look back and yield to traffic coming from behind before turning left at intersections.
- Basic bicycle safety rules apply to rollerblading and skateboarding.

(Fig. 13–6). Older children should be taught what to do in the event of a water emergency, even how to perform CPR. However, swimming lessons and emergency training never replace the need for close adult supervision for this age group.

Animal Safety

Each year, thousands of children require first aid or emergency department treatment because of an animal bite. Children between the ages of 7 and 12 years are at the greatest risk, with dog bites being the most common source of these injuries (Beck & Jones, 1985). However, children of all ages and all types of animals, domestic and wild, should be considered when providing anticipatory guidance to children or families about animal safety. Animals are just as curious about children as children are about them. Children often become excited and approach and play with animals too aggressively. In the event of an attack, children are frequently unable to protect themselves. Because of their short stature, children often sus-

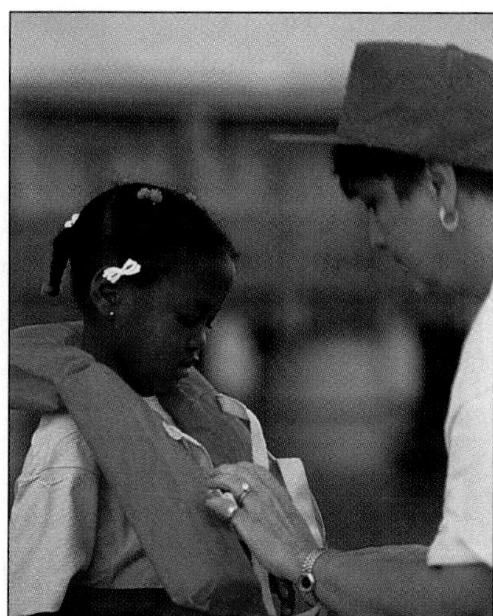

Figure 13–6
Proper size and application of a flotation vest ensures that it will support an unconscious child's head above the water level. When boating, adults should make sure that any children on board are wearing flotation devices. Adults should wear flotation vests themselves, both to ensure their own safety and to model safety conscious behavior for children. (Courtesy of Children's Medical Center, Dallas, Texas)

tain bite injuries to the head, neck, and face, especially the upper lip. Because of their anatomic locations, these injuries can be potentially serious or permanently disfiguring.

Parents whose children will be in contact with animals need to invest the time to teach and reinforce appropriate behaviors. They also must establish limitations of child–animal interactions to promote safety. Young children require supervision around all animals and must be taught to approach unfamiliar animals only when an adult is present. Depending on the potential for exposure to various types of animals (i.e., wild, farm, domestic, rabid, marine), anticipatory safety education should be geared to the geographic risks. The accompanying box highlights considerations for providing anticipatory guidance about animal safety.

ADOLESCENT SAFETY

Adolescence is a period of transition marked by rapid changes in physical, social, and cognitive abilities. Surges of energy and confidence often lead to impulsive actions and behaviors that contribute to the adolescent's vulnerability to injury. The natural urge of adolescents to experiment and be independent, a perception of immortality, and the influence of peers, all contribute to their predisposition to injury (see Chapter 8).

Effective safety promotion among the adolescent population begins with an understanding of their vulnerabilities. Injuries continue to be the leading cause of death for adolescents, with the most vulnerable period between the ages of 15 and 24 years. With such a threat to the health of adolescents, safety promotion is urgent for this age group.

Safety education should be approached by providing factual information with supportive explanations. Allowing adolescents to discuss and debate the facts is the most effective means to reach this age group (Sewell & Gaines, 1993). Nurses can be instrumental in helping to promote safe behaviors in the adolescent. Expressing a genuine interest in them as individuals and listening in a nonjudgmental way are important steps to gain their confidence and trust.

Helping the adolescent to recognize that he has choices when faced with difficult or potentially dangerous situations is an important component of safety promotion with this age group. Drugs and alcohol are well documented as contributing factors in most adolescent injuries. These substances are available to younger teenagers than ever before. Evaluation for abuse should be considered when injuries occur.

The adolescent period is also a frightening time for parents because they are aware of the risks predisposing the adolescent to injury or death. Parents may request guidance from health care professionals in setting appropriate limits and establishing methods of effective enforcement. Parents should be encouraged to model the safe behaviors that they expect from the adolescent.

TEACHING GUIDELINES *for Animal Safety*

- Adults should avoid adopting aggressive breeds of domestic pets when young children are likely to come in contact with them.
- All domesticated animals should be vaccinated against rabies.
- Children should be taught to avoid teasing or playing roughly with animals, even family pets. Parents should teach and demonstrate appropriate ways to interact with animals, emphasizing gentle play or petting.
- Children should be cautioned to avoid approaching fenced or chained animals.
- Children should be cautioned to avoid playing with or attempting to take food away from any animal while it is eating.
- Ferrets are particularly aggressive and should be avoided as pets in homes with small children.
- Large animals, such as farm animals, should be approached from the front to avoid the powerful hind legs, which can kick the child.
- If attacked by a large animal, children should drop to the ground and crawl rapidly toward safety.

Car Safety

The privilege of driving a car signifies a passage into adulthood and provides a means of greater freedom to explore and experience the world. Driving is a complex activity, and proficiency requires skill, judgment, and experience. The adolescent's lack of judgment, opposition to authority, and need to express her independence often result in a disregard for sound defensive driving practices. Risk-taking behaviors appear to play a major role in the high incidence of car-related injuries and deaths among teenagers. The young, inexperienced driver tends to drive faster and take greater chances while operating a car. Teenagers may refuse to wear seat belts, often viewing this behavior as childish (Grossman & Rivera, 1992).

There is an alarming association between the use of alcohol and motor vehicle crashes in adolescents. Despite legal drinking age laws, alcohol is easily accessible to adolescents. The greater social activity of the teenager, combined with the availability of alcohol, increases the occurrence of impaired driving. The adolescent's inexperience with both alcohol and driving is a potentially lethal combination.

Nurses can promote car safety by supporting driver education programs for teenagers. Additionally, many schools and community organizations have developed drinking and driving prevention programs that are helpful in presenting the facts to adolescents. Nurses should support these programs and continue to advocate the use of seat belts in adolescents, explaining their protective capabilities in the event of a crash. Nurses should encourage teens and their parents to set up a ride home agreement to discourage any driving after drinking alcohol. Adolescents need to know that they have an option available to them if they find themselves in this situation. Dealing with the consequences of drinking is much better than facing the consequences of injuries and damage that motor vehicle crashes cause.

Water Safety

Drowning is a needless cause of death in the adolescent population. The majority of these drowning deaths occur in lakes, rivers, and ponds, with the rest occurring in public or private swimming pools. Diving injuries resulting in spinal cord trauma are also a concern for this age group (Spyker, 1985).

Risk-taking behaviors contribute greatly to the incidence of drowning and spinal cord injuries. Adolescents have the ability to travel to areas that are free of adult supervision. Frequently, alcohol and drugs are contributing factors. Given the combination of freedom and alcohol, adolescents may inadvertently place themselves at risk for these types of injuries by exceeding the limits for safe swimming and diving.

Safety promotion includes the encouragement of swimming lessons, water safety classes, and the completion of a CPR course. An important safety lesson is the feetfirst principle. Adolescents need to know how alcohol and drugs impair their ability to perform activities in which they are usually competent.

> To prevent devastating spinal cord injuries, adolescents should be taught to enter water feetfirst as opposed to headfirst when jumping into water of unknown depths.

Violence

Violence is a growing threat to the health and well-being of youth and society as a whole. Violence has rapidly become a major cause of death and injury among adolescents and young adults (see Chapter 1). Violent crimes have increased among adolescents and young adults from ages 10 through 25 years, regardless of gender or race. Absolute rates were highest among males and African Americans (Rachuba, Stanton, & Howard, 1995). Faced with this escalating epidemic of violence, society is urgently seeking an understanding of contributing factors, with appropriate interventions directed at decreasing these alarming statistics.

Factors contributing to the trend of violence are multiple and complex. Interventions to prevent violence will require the collaboration of many professional and community organizations. Limited economic resources, low self-esteem, and racism can create deep-seated anger that may reduce an individual's threshold for violence (Prothrow-Stith & Spivak, 1992). However, there are major societal issues that are far beyond the capabilities of health care alone, other than to help establish and identify populations who are at risk. Contributing factors related to behavior provide the greatest opportunity for interventions initiated by health care professionals. The accompanying box highlights factors that are believed to contribute to violence in the adolescent.

Nurses working with children, adolescents, and their families have the opportunity to include violence prevention as a component of anticipatory guidance. Ideally, this prevention should begin when the child is young. Violence is a learned behavior. It is often reinforced by the actions of those closest to the child and the ever-increasing exposure to violence on TV. Assessing how a family deals with anger and resolves conflict provides insight into the way the child will likely react to similar situations. A family with violent tendencies should be referred to a counselor. Learning to react to anger or stress with nonviolent actions through conflict resolution is the goal for the youth. Unfortunately, intervention cannot be a one-time educational session. Efforts must be reinforced in multiple facets of the adolescent's life, such as in school, youth organizations, church, and home.

Parents need to be aware of the amount and type of violence that their children are exposed to on TV. There

Factors Contributing to Adolescent Violence

- Low socioeconomic status.
- Crowded, urban housing.
- Single-parent family or limited parental supervision.
- History of family violence or child abuse.
- Accessibility to guns.
- Peer pressure or gang involvement.
- Limited education.
- Racism.
- Drug or alcohol use or abuse.
- Low self-esteem and hopelessness about the future.
- Aggression.

is growing evidence suggesting that exposure to media violence and its portrayal as an acceptable and successful means to solve problems may influence real-life behavior (AAP News, 1995). It is unrealistic to expect parents to isolate their children from all media violence, but they can be encouraged to limit their children's TV viewing and discuss the implications of violence with their children.

The availability of firearms is related to the increase of violent acts. In a survey of students in grades 9 through 12 conducted by the U.S. Centers for Disease Control and Prevention, it was found that 22.1% had carried a weapon within the 30 days preceding the survey (Centers for Disease Control and Prevention, 1995). Guns are found in one out of every two American homes. Children of all ages are involved in firearm incidents. For this reason, guns in the home are a serious health hazard to children. Guns and knives are becoming part of teenage culture, especially in the urban setting. Carrying a weapon establishes a feeling of control or power or may be a response to fear of those with power. Regardless of the reasons, firearms in the hands of youth are impulsively used, before the ramifications of such actions can be logically considered.

As society urgently seeks a solution to the growing problem of violence, health care professionals must become advocates of violence prevention. Opportunities for youth to discover and use less violent means to express themselves or resolve day-to-day issues should be taught and promoted. Given the tragic effects of violence on the safety and health of American children, nurses should participate in efforts to resolve the complex issues of violence in our society.

Gangs

American cities have been plagued by youth gangs since the late 1700s. Until recently, gangs were typically found in large cities. Unfortunately, the number of gangs has grown to epidemic proportions, and gangs have become entrenched in communities throughout the United States. Members of established gangs are estimated to number between 125,000 and 250,000, with another 750,000 youths aspiring to become gang members (Hay, 1992).

Not all groups of youths are gangs. Adolescents associate with peers to gain a sense of identity and belonging, fulfilling normal developmental needs. A gang is defined as a number of individuals who band together to form a highly developed subculture. As a result of this affiliation and peer influence, they engage in unacceptable, violent, illegal, or antisocial activities (Rollins, 1993). Youth gangs and their negative behaviors have become more apparent in recent years, attracting more and more young people who are seeking to make sense out of their perceived chaotic situation. Associating with a gang, even if it is involved in criminal activity, gives them a sense of acceptance and understanding. Gangs offer excitement, structure, and protection, or serve as a source of income for

Signs of Gang Involvement

- Association with new friends while ignoring old friends. The child usually will not talk about new friends or what they do together.
- Change in hairstyle or clothing. Association with other youths with the same styles. Usually some of the clothing, such as a hat or jacket, has the gang's initials or "street" name on it. Parents may note tatoos on the body.
- Unexplained source of money or possessions (e.g., stereos, jewelry, cars).
- Indications of drug, alcohol, or inhalant abuse (e.g., paint or correction fluid on the clothes, the smell of chemicals on the breath or clothes).
- Change in attitude about activities such as sports, Scouts, or church. Discipline problems at school, in public, or at home. Youth no longer accepts parents' authority and challenges it frequently.
- Problems at school, such as failing classes, skipping school, or causing problems in class.
- Fear of the police.
- Unexplained signs of fighting, such as bruises, cuts, or complaints of pain.
- Graffiti on or around residence or possessions.
- Threats by rival gang members. Sometimes a family member is a victim of a drive-by shooting before the family realizes the youth is involved in a gang.

their members. Some youths simply join out of fear or intimidation of the established gang (Rollins, 1993).

Gangs establish their identities through graffiti, clothing styles or colors, hand signals, permanent markings such as tattoos, and defined territories. Gangs typically participate in illegal or aggressive acts to establish themselves as the dominant group.

In analyzing the growing gang phenomenon, it is evident that there are no simple solutions to counteract the complex problem of youth gangs. Addressing the problem will take a committed community-wide effort to curb the number of gangs and their activities. Preventing young people from joining gangs is a top priority. Once an adolescent becomes a member, it is difficult to sever the bonds of the gang (Rollins, 1993). The challenge facing communities is the development and promotion of other options that are less destructive to youths and will meet their developmental needs.

Nurses working with adolescents can participate in gang prevention efforts by early identification of gang participation, alternate options, and referrals to other agencies or resources in the community. Interventions with gang members will require the collaboration of many professional groups in the community (Rollins, 1993).

Often parents turn to nurses for support and guidance when their child is involved with a gang. Helping parents to recognize and understand the reasons why youths turn to gangs enables parents to counter those influences. If warning signs are identified early, the adolescent can be directed away from gang activity. Parents who have reason to believe that their child is involved with a gang should be encouraged to act quickly to prevent further involvement. Nurses can provide guidance to the concerned parents, referring them to appropriate agencies or groups within the community. Indicators of potential gang involvement are outlined in the box on page 307.

KEY CONCEPTS

- Injuries are the leading cause of death and disability in children. No child is immune to childhood injuries and related deaths.
- As children grow, their physical and cognitive skills develop, enabling them to aggressively explore the world around them. Children are curious, creative, and bound to come across dangerous situations.
- Childhood injuries and deaths are predictable and preventable. Understanding the developmental milestones of each age group is important for promoting safety awareness for parents, caregivers, and children.
- The key to preventing injuries is improved safety awareness and adult supervision. Promoting safety in children of all ages provides a valuable foundation for a safe, healthy lifestyle.
- Nurses can speak out supporting legislative issues related to childhood safety and contribute to the design or development of products that promote childhood safety.

REFERENCES

American College of Surgeons. Committee on Trauma. (1993). *Resources for optimal care of the injured patient: 1993* (pp. 13–15). Chicago: Author.

Beck, A. M., and Jones, B. A. (1985). Unreported dog bites in children. *Public Health Reports, 100*(3), 315–321.

Brady, M. (1994). Educating youths and their parents about the prevention of firearm injury. *Journal of Pediatric Health Care, 8*(3), 120–129.

Centers for Disease Control. (1990). Childhood injuries in the United States. *American Journal of Diseases of Children,* 144, 627–646.

Centers for Disease Control. (1995). Youth risk behavior surveillance—United States, 1993. *MMWR, 44*(55–7), 1–16.

Christophersen, E. R. (1977). Children's behavior during automobile rides: Do car seats make a difference? *Pediatrics, 60,* 69–72.

Grossman, D. C., and Rivera, F. P. (1992). Injury control in childhood. *Pediatric Clinics of North America, 39*(3), 471–485.

Guyer, B., Talbot, A. M., Pless, I. B. (1985). Pedestrian injuries to children and youth. *Pediatric Clinics of North America, 32*(1), 163–174.

Halpern, J. S. (1987). The misuse of child safety restraints. *Journal of Emergency Nursing, 13*(6), 365–368.

Hay, S. (1992). Building gang prevention bridges to parents and families. In *Tools to involve parents in gang prevention.* Washington, DC: National Crime Prevention Council.

Kahane, C. J. (1989). An evaluation of child passenger safety: The effectiveness and benefits of safety seats (summary), DOT-HS 806-899). Washington, DC: U.S. Department of Transportation.

Morbidity and Mortality Weekly Report. (1995). 44(551), U. S. Department of Health and Human Services, Public Health Service, Centers for Disease Control and Prevention.

National Rifle Association. (1992). *The Eddie Eagle Gun Safety Program.* Washington, DC: Author.

National SafeKids Campaign. (1993). *Investing in children's safety: A national agenda for childhood injury prevention.* Washington, DC: Author.

Patterson, P., and Smith, L. (1987). Firearms in the home and child safety. *American Journal of Diseases of Children, 141,* 221–223.

Prothrow-Stith, D., and Spivak, H. R. (1992). Violence. In McAnarney, E. R., Kreipe, R. E., Orr, D. P., Comerci, G. D. (Eds.), *Textbook of adolescent medicine* (pp. 1113–1118). Philadelphia: W. B. Saunders.

Rachula, L., Stanton, B., and Howard D. (1995). Violent crime in the United States. *Archives of Pediatric Adolescent Medicine, 149,* 953–960.

Rollins, J. A. (1993). Nurses as gangbusters: A response to gang violence in America. *Pediatric Nursing, 19*(6), 559–567.

Sewell, K. H., and Gaines, S. K. (1993). A developmental approach to childhood safety education. *Pediatric Nursing, 19*(5), 464–466.

Spence, A. (1995). Family instability leaves children vulnerable. *AAP News 11*(8), 10–12.

Spyker, D. A. (1985). Submersion injury epidemiology, prevention and management. *Pediatric Clinics of North America, 32*(1), 113–125.

Thompson, R. S., et al. (1989). A case-control study of the effectiveness of bicycle safety helmets. *New England Journal of Medicine, 320*(21), 1361–1367.

Tinsworth, D. K., and Kramer, J. T. (1990). Playground equipment-related injuries and deaths. Washington, DC: U.S. Consumer Product Safety Administration.

U.S. Consumer Product Safety Commission. (1993a). *Children and pools: A safety checklist* (Publication No. 357). Washington, DC: Author.

U.S. Consumer Product Safety Commission. (1993b). *New splash! for safety: Drowning prevention for parents with pools.* Washington, DC: Author.

Wilson, M. H., Baker, S. P., Tevet, S. P., Shock, S., and Garbarino, J. (1991). *Saving children: A guide to injury prevention.* New York: Oxford University Press.

Zuckerman, B. S., and Duby, J. C. (1985). Developmental approach to injury prevention. *Pediatric Clinics of North America, 32*(1), 17–29.

BIBLIOGRAPHY

American Academy of Pediatrics, Committee on Injury and Poison Prevention. (1991a). Children and fireworks. *Pediatrics, 88*(3), 154–155.

American Academy of Pediatrics, Committee on Injury and Poison Prevention. (1991b). Children in pickup trucks. *Pediatrics, 88*(2), 393.

American Medical Association, Council on Scientific Affairs. (1989). Firearm injuries and deaths: A critical public health issue. *Public Health Reports,* 104, 111–120.

Arneson, S. W., and Triplett, J. L. (1990). Riding with bucklebear: An automobile safety program for preschoolers. *Journal of Pediatric Nursing, 5*(2), 115–122.

Brent, D. A., Perper, J. A., Allman, C. J., Moritz, G. M., Wartella, M. E., and Zelenak, P. (1991). The presence and accessibility of firearms in the homes of adolescent suicides: A case study. *Journal of American Medical Association, 266,* 2989–2995.

Castiglia, P. T. (1993). Gangs. *Journal of Pediatric Health Care,* 7(1), 39–41.

Crawley, T., and Velsor-Fredrick, B. (1991). The cost to our children: The issue of gun control. *Journal of Pediatric Nursing, 6*(5), 350–351.

Dowd, M. D., Knapp, J. F., and Fitzmaurice, H. S. (1992). Pediatric firearm injuries, Kansas City, 1992: A population based study. *Pediatrics, 94*(6), 867–873.

Eichelberger, M. R. (1993). *Pediatric trauma prevention, acute care, rehabilitation.* St. Louis: Mosby–Year Book.

Ellerby, P., and Ward, P. M. (1989). Development of a pediatric injury prevention program for the emergency department. *Journal of Emergency Nursing, 15*(3), 224–228.

Fulginiti, V. A. (1992). Violence and children in the United States. *American Journal of Diseases of Children, 146,* 671–672.

Fresby, M. L., and Hill, J. H. (1991). A community response to childhood drownings: A model for accident prevention. *Critical Care Nursing Clinics of North America 3*(2), 373–379.

Gratz, R. R. (1992). School injuries: What we know, what we need. *Journal of Pediatric Health Care, 6*(5), 256–262.

Israeloff, R. (1994). How to teach street smarts. *Parents 69*(9), 84–86.

Jones, N. E. (1992). Prevention of childhood injuries: Part II. Recreational injuries. *Pediatric Nursing, 18*(6), 619–621.

Kitchen, L., Lynch, F. P., and Murphy, P. A. (1990). Pediatric risks for injury. *Emergency Care Quarterly, 5*(4), 82–87.

Leven, N. (1993). How to protect your family from fire. *Geico Direct,* 15–17.

National Fire Protection Association. (1993). *Community awareness kit: Get out, stay out. Your fire safe response.* Quincy, MA: Author.

National SafeKids Campaign. (1991). *Safe kids are no accident: How to protect your child from injury.* Washington, DC: Author.

Price, S. C. (1993). Warning labels: Do they really work? *Childhood Injury Prevention Quarterly, 4*(3), 2–6.

Price, S. C. (1992). Child pedestrian injuries: A complex problem with no easy solution. *Childhood Injury Prevention Quarterly, 3*(4), 2–7.

Swartz, M. (1992). Playground safety. *Journal of Pediatric Health Care, 6*(3), 161–162.

Swartz, M. K. (1994). Promoting helmet use in recreational sports. *Journal of Pediatric Health Care, 8*(3), 138–139.

Takata, S., and Zevitz, R. (1990). Divergent perceptions of group delinquency in a midwestern community: Racine's gang problem. *Youth and Society, 21*(3), 282–305.

Turner, E. S. (1992). How safe are our playgrounds? CPSC issues new guidelines but critics find them lacking. *Childhood Injury Prevention Quarterly, 3*(2), 11–15.

Webster, D. W., Wilson, M. E., Duggan, A. K., and Pakula, L. C. (1992). Parents' beliefs about preventing gun injuries to children. *Pediatrics, 89,* 908–914.

Westerverlt, V. D., and McDonald, J. A. (1994). Counseling parents about guns in the home. *Archives of Pediatric and Adolescent Medicine, 148,* 109–110.

Wilson, P. D., and Testani-Delfour, L. (1993). Bicycle safety program: Targeting injury prevention through education. *Pediatric Nursing, 19*(4), 343–346.

14

Emergency Care of the Child and Family

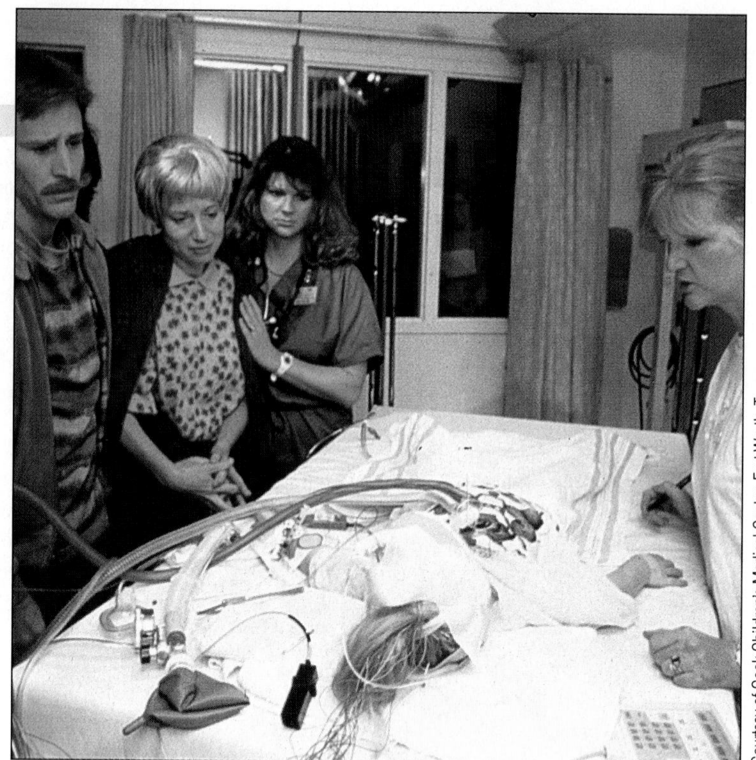

Courtesy of Cook Children's Medical Center, Fort Worth, Texas

CHAPTER OVERVIEW

LEARNING OBJECTIVES

After studying this chapter, you should be able to:

- Name four general principles that encourage cooperation and help to make examination and treatment of children in emergency settings more comfortable for the child and the family.
- List the developmental issues that are significant in caring for infants, toddlers, school-age children, and adolescents.

- Compare the airway anatomy of a child with that of an adult, and explain the significance of the differences in managing the pediatric airway.
- Assess the early signs of shock in infants and children, recognizing that heart rate and skin signs are more critical in early recognition of shock than blood pressure.
- Define triage and list the three most important factors to assess in obtaining an overall impression of an infant's or child's general condition during triage.
- Describe the general guidelines for cardiopulmonary resuscitation in infants and children, and discuss what additional precautions and procedures are required for infants and children with traumatic injuries.
- List three possible indications that a child brought into the emergency care setting has been neglected or abused, and discuss the nurse's responsibility in reporting possible neglect or abuse.
- Identify several possible roles for nurses in prevention of submersion injuries, traumatic injuries, and ingestions of poisons.

KEY TERMS

ABCDEs: Airway, Breathing, Circulation, Disability, and Exposure. When assessing children, it is important to remember to assess each one of these areas.

airway management: correct positioning of airway, and appropriate interventions used to assure patency of the airway, and adequate oxygenation and ventilation.

cardiopulmonary resuscitation (CPR): performed when a patient's respiratory and cardiovascular systems require support, as in the pulseless, nonbreathing patient. Airway management, ventilation, and chest compressions are provided to improve tissue perfusion until the patient can receive definitive care.

dental emergency: injury or infection of a tooth or teeth, when the length of time to definitive care is critical for the care of the tooth or to alleviate pain.

emergency: a psychological, medical, or traumatic condition that requires immediate care or care within an hour to prevent further deterioration.

envenomation: injection of venom by an animal (usually snakes, lizards, spiders, scorpions, etc.) into a human body.

hypothermia: cooling of body temperature to subnormal levels. Temperature levels considered to be dangerous to infants and children are core body temperatures below 96° F.

ingestion: swallowing of a potentially toxic substance, such as a large amount of medication, petroleum products, or toxic plants.

shock: inadequate tissue perfusion, usually caused by illness or injury, that causes respiratory or cardiovascular compromise.

submersion injury: injury resulting from a near-drowning incident. Such an injury may be immediately apparent or may appear up to 48 hours after the submersion incident.

trauma: injury from an external cause, such as a motor vehicle accident, gunshot wound, or stabbing. Trauma may be self-inflicted, may be deliberately inflicted or accidental, and may be physical or psychological.

trauma score: a numeric score assessed by health care providers to determine the condition of patients. The score usually results from adding, subtracting, dividing, or multiplying numbers representing physiologic parameters or specific types of injuries. These scores are used for field triage and are assessed serially to determine whether a patient's condition is improving or deteriorating.

triage: a sorting process used to decide the urgency of a patient's illness or injury and allocate appropriate resources effectively. The purpose of triage is to assure that the most seriously ill or injured patients receive the highest level of care possible.

There are very few experiences as frightening to a family as a child's sudden illness or injury. Caring for children and families in the emergency setting therefore provides special challenges for the health care team. Nurses play an important role in emergency settings because they are most often responsible for the initial contact, triage, and continuing care throughout an emergency visit. The goal of emergency nursing care is not only to address the physical problems of the patient, but also to support the coping mechanisms of the child and family and to create an atmosphere where the family unit is valued and kept intact as much as possible.

CLINICAL REFERENCE PAGES

GENERAL GUIDELINES FOR EMERGENCY NURSING CARE

Many factors play a role in the psychological effects of an emergency on both the child and family: fears of separation, pain, and alteration in body image. In addition, there is a lack of familiarity with the setting, the staff of the health care facility, the equipment, and the procedures being performed. Some general attitudes and simple interventions can help to make examination and treatment of children in the emergency setting more comfortable for the child and for the family (Seidel & Henderson, 1992).

1. **Communicate an attitude of calm confidence.** This may be difficult when the situation is critical, but families in crisis look to nurses for reassurance and expect to see competent, professional behavior. Speak quietly and calmly to the child and to the parents, and remain firmly in charge. Remember to talk to the family often throughout the visit—silence is a form of communication that is easily misinterpreted. The parents must be kept informed of any untoward delays.
2. **Establish a trusting relationship with the child and family.** Make eye contact with the child and family when you speak to them. To establish a trusting relationship, check back with the family and provide periodic updates if the child and family are separated. When parents are confident that they are being kept informed, they are less likely to make demands for additional attention and information. When you speak to the child and family use simple, nonmedical terms and remember that children (and sometimes adults) may have inaccurate ideas of how their bodies function and the location of body parts (Gellert, 1978).
3. **Try to avoid separating the child and parents.** Include the parents as partners in their child's treatment as much as possible. Unless the child does not want a parent in the room (as in the case of some adolescents), a parent can help to calm the child, and many examinations and procedures can be performed with the child on a parent's lap (Ross & SA, 1988). Sometimes parents may not know exactly how to be of assistance in these situations. It may be helpful to explain how a parent might help, such as "I think he might stay calmer if you hold his hand and tell him a story while I clean this burn" or "Try counting to ten with her while I start this intravenous line."
4. **Designate one staff member as caretaker of the child and liaison to the parents whenever possible.** In the unfamiliar emergency setting, it is less confusing for the child and family to have one contact person. Consistency is helpful in a crisis situation, as the child and family may feel overwhelmed in the busy and sometimes confusing emergency department environment.
5. **Tell the truth.** To establish a trusting relationship, it is important to be as honest as possible. If a procedure will be painful, tell the child (usually briefly beforehand)—only then can the child believe you if you assure them that a procedure will *not* be painful. Keeping a child informed of what will occur by describing sensations ("This will feel cold and wet as I clean your arm") has been shown to be more helpful than describing the actual procedure (Johnson, Kirchhoff, & Endress, 1976).
6. **Provide incentives and rewards.** Provide positive feedback when either the child or the parents are being helpful. Children from ages 3 to 12 years especially appreciate concrete rewards for good behavior, such as stickers, fancy bandages, or inexpensive toys (Henderson & Brownstein, 1994). Adults also appreciate being thanked for their patience and for their assistance in the care of their child. All of these techniques will help to create as positive an experience as possible.

There will be instances, however, when the child's and family's coping mechanisms break down, resulting in inappropriate behavior. If violence or abusive behavior are an issue, assistance from law enforcement or hospital security officers should be obtained. For an emotional crisis that does not involve abusive or aggressive behavior, however, some simple rules apply:

- Encourage the person in crisis to move to a quiet place. Observers and stimuli from other sources tend to aggravate a crisis.
- Encourage the patient or parent to talk about feelings rather than the "facts" of the situation. Use reflective statements.
- Avoid defensiveness, explanation, or justification of your own or others' behavior.
- Speak in simple sentences. Use sentences of no more than five words, with words no longer than five letters (e.g., "Let's sit down over here," "Let me help," "Please let go of that.").

When coping with families in distress, a good general rule is to try to listen rather than talk. Resist the tendency to give advice until a specific problem has been identified by the patient or family, and even then give advice only when solutions are solicited (Aguilera, 1990). Simply being present for patients and families, and empathizing with them, is a useful intervention. When coping mechanisms break down entirely, however, some direction will be necessary. Consulting social services, spiritual counselors (i.e., chaplain), or crisis intervention professionals may be helpful.

COMMON PEDIATRIC EMERGENCY MEDICATIONS

DRUGS AND INDICATIONS	DOSE	COMMON SIDE EFFECTS	NURSING IMPLICATIONS
Adenosine Treatment of supraventricular tachycardia.	0.1–0.2 mg/kg. Maximum single dose: 12 mg.	Extremely short half-life (10 seconds) minimizes duration of side effects and makes it relatively safe.	Give by rapid IV bolus. Monitor heart rate and electrocardiogram (ECG) continuously throughout therapy.
Atropine Sulfate Treatment of symptomatic bradycardia.	0.02 mg/kg. Minimum dose: 0.1 mg. Maximum single dose: 0.5 mg in child, 1.0 mg in adolescent.	Tachycardia. Low doses may cause paradoxical bradycardia in infants, so minimum dose (0.1 mg/kg) must be administered.	Will produce pupil dilation, but will not affect the pupil constrictive response to light, so pupils should constrict briskly even after atropine administration.
Bretylium Treatment of ventricular tachycardia and prophylaxis against ventricular fibrillation. May be administered if defibrillation and lidocaine are ineffective in correcting ventricular fibrillation.	5 mg/kg; may be increased to 10 mg/kg if fibrillation persists after an additional defibrillation attempt.	Postural hypotension; nausea and vomiting (rapid IV infusion to conscious patients). Transient increase in arrhythmias and hypertension may occur 1 hour after initial administration.	Administer undiluted by rapid IV infusion. Do not dilute bretylium for IM injection. ECG and blood pressure should be monitored continuously during administration. There are no data on the usefulness of bretylium in the pediatric age-group.
Calcium Chloride 10% Treatment of hypocalcemia, hypomagnesemia, hyperkalemia, and calcium channel blocker overdose.	20 mg/kg.	May cause bradycardia and even cardiac asystole, especially if patient is receiving digoxin. Can sclerose peripheral veins and produce severe chemical burn if medication infiltrates into tissues.	Give slowly through a small-bore needle in a large vein. Do not administer through a scalp vein. Do not give IM or SC. Calcium forms in insoluble precipitate in the presence of sodium bicarbonate.
Dopamine Hydrochloride Treatment of hypotension or poor peripheral perfusion in the pediatric patient with adequate intravascular volume and a stable cardiac rhythm.	2–20 mcg/kg/min.	Tachycardia, arrhythmias, and hypertension. High infusion rates (>20 mcg/kg/min) may produce severe peripheral vasoconstriction and ischemia.	Should be delivered through a large-bore catheter or central venous catheter. Extravasation can cause local ischemia and tissue necrosis. Do not mix with sodium bicarbonate—inactivated by alkaline pH.
Dobutamine Hydrochloride Treatment of hypoperfusion, severe congestive heart failure, or cardiogenic shock.	2–20 mcg/kg/min. Has a short plasma half-life and must be delivered by a constant infusion controlled by an infusion pump. (6 mg dopamine times the child's body weight in kg to sufficient diluent to create a solution totaling 100 ml; infusions of 1 ml/hr of this mixture deliver 1.0 mcg/kg/min).	Tachycardia, tachyarrhythmias, or ectopic beats. Nausea, vomiting, hypertension, and hypotension are less frequent side effects. Extravasation may cause tissue necrosis.	Titrate to desired effect. Monitor blood pressure, pulse, respirations, and hemodynamic status every 5–15 minutes during and after administration. Must be administered by a constant infusion via large-bore venous catheter regulated by an infusion pump. High doses should be administered via central venous catheter.
Epinephrine for Bradycardia	IV/Intraosseous (IO): 0.01 mg/kg (1:10,000, 0.1 ml/kg). Endotracheal (ET): 0.1 mg/kg (1:1,000, 0.1 ml/kg).	Tachycardia, arrhythmias.	Monitor blood pressure, respirations, and pulse every 5 minutes during and after administration. Be aware of total dose of preservative administered (if preservatives are present in epinephrine preparation) when high doses are administered.

Table continued on following page

COMMON PEDIATRIC EMERGENCY MEDICATIONS *(continued)*

DRUGS AND INDICATIONS	DOSE	COMMON SIDE EFFECTS	NURSING IMPLICATIONS
Epinephrine for Asystolic or Pulseless Arrest	*First dose:* IV/IO: 0.01 mg/kg (1:10,000, 0.1 ml/kg) ET: 0.1 mg/kg (1:1,000, 0.1 ml/kg) IV/IO: doses as high as 0.2 mg/kg of 1:1000 may be effective. *Subsequent doses:* IV/IO/ET: 0.1 mg/kg (1:1000, 0.1 ml/kg). Repeat every 3–5 min. IV/IO doses as high as 0.2 mg/kg of 1:1000 may be effective.	Tachycardia, arrhythmias. High dose infusions may cause profound vasoconstriction that compromises extremity and skin perfusion.	Be aware of total dose of preservative administered (if preservatives are present in epinephrine preparation) when high doses are used.
Lidocaine Treatment of recurrent ventricular tachycardia, ventricular fibrillation, or ventricular ectopy.	1 mg/kg. *Lidocaine infusion:* 20–50 μg/kg/min.	Excessive plasma concentrations may cause myocardial and circulatory depression and possible CNS symptoms (drowsiness, disorientation, seizures).	Monitor ECG continuously and pulse and blood pressure frequently during administration. Risk of toxicity is increased in children with low cardiac output or severe congestive heart failure.
Naloxone Used to reverse the effects of narcotics.	If ≤ 5 years or < 20 kg: 0.1 mg/kg. If > age 5 years or > 20 kg: 2.0 mg/kg.	Even at high doses, naloxone is safe. Use with caution immediately after birth to infants of addicted mothers, because it may precipitate abrupt narcotic withdrawal and seizures in these infants.	Titrate to desired effect. Monitor respiratory rate and depth, pulse, ECG, blood pressure, and level of consciousness frequently until effects of narcotic wear off. Short duration of action may result in recurrence of symptoms of intoxication.
Sodium Bicarbonate For treatment of severe acidosis associated with cardiac arrest, unstable hemodynamic state, or hyperkalemia.	1 mEq/kg per dose or 0.3 × kg × base deficit.	Excessive administration may result in metabolic alkalosis.	Acidosis during resuscitation should be corrected through restoration of effective ventilation and systemic perfusion. Infuse slowly and only if ventilation is adequate. Should not be administered into the tracheobronchial tree. IV tubing must be irrigated with normal saline before and after infusions of sodium bicarbonate.
Syrup of Ipecac To induce vomiting in early management of overdose or poisoning of noncaustic substances in conscious patients.	Age 6–12 months: 10 ml. Do not repeat. Age 1–12 years: 15 ml; may repeat one time if vomiting does not occur. Over age 12 years: 30 ml; may repeat one time if vomiting does not occur.	Sedation, diarrhea. Arrhythmias, myocarditis (if drug is absorbed or overdosage ingested).	Assess level of consciousness before giving ipecac. Contraindicated in semiconscious, unconscious, or seizing patients or after ingestion of caustic substances. Safety not established in infants < age 6 months. Administer clear fluids, 10–20 ml/kg, after giving ipecac. Do not give with activated charcoal (will reduce emetic effect). Do not confuse syrup with fluid extract, which is 14 times more concentrated.

GROWTH AND DEVELOPMENT ISSUES IN EMERGENCY CARE

Emergency nursing care of children must address both the physiologic and psychologic differences in children by age. Paying close attention to developmental issues will assist in obtaining a more accurate assessment and can affect the course of care. See Unit I and Chapters 15 and 18 for detailed information on approaches to use with children of difference ages. A few simple age-related guidelines for children in emergency care follow.

The Infant

An infant experiences the world through the senses; hunger, satiation, cold, warmth, quiet, and noise have the greatest effect on the child's comfort or discomfort. An infant has not learned patience and has little tolerance for discomfort. In particular, an older infant (ages 9 to 18 months) may experience both separation and stranger anxiety. Keep the infant in the parent's lap or arms as much as possible for examination and treatment. This may not be possible in a critical situation, but nurses should always keep in mind that the separation of parent and child is very painful for both and should reunite them when feasible. Some helpful interventions to comfort infants during painful procedures are:

- Allow the use of a pacifier.
- Use a quiet, soothing voice.
- Touch, rock, or cuddle the infant. Holding the infant securely may also be comforting.
- Keep the infant warm; if he must be left undressed, use warming lights to assure a comfortable temperature.
- Around age 6 months, infants may become afraid of strangers. Do not take an infant's apparent distrust personally—it is just a healthy stage in ego development.

Remember that infants do feel pain and should be provided with as much comfort and consideration as a full-grown child or an adult (McGrath & Craig, 1989). (See Chapter 20 for additional information on pain.)

The Toddler

Toddlers are just beginning to explore the world, and seem to have limitless energy and curiosity. They are also beginning to have a clearer image of themselves as autonomous and distinct human beings. For this reason, they do not respond well to restrictions and will tend to push any limits imposed. This can be a problem in the emergency setting because some nursing care will involve securing and restraining the toddler. The toddler may feel less afraid and may resist less during procedures if you do the following:

- Give treatments and perform procedures with the toddler sitting up on the stretcher or examining table or on the parent's lap whenever possible to decrease the sense of vulnerability.
- Perform the most distressing/intrusive parts of the examination last.
- Reassure the family as much as possible—the child will benefit from their confidence.
- Allow the child to have familiar objects ("transitional objects") such as a blanket, doll, or toy to help him feel safe (Henderson & Brownstein, 1994).
- Keep frightening objects out of the child's line of vision.

The Preschool Child

The preschool child is talking and beginning to be more independent. This outward appearance of organization is somewhat misleading, however—this is also the age of fear and fantasy. Preschool children have nightmares, and may have exaggerated ideas and impressions. They are also confused about the concept of responsibility and tend to blame themselves for illnesses and injuries. In the emergency setting, it is important to remember the following:

- Encourage the preschool child to talk about how she became ill or injured. If she is inappropriately taking responsibility for the illness or injury, try to provide reassurance that she is not to blame for the situation.
- Remember that preschool children may seem to understand more than they actually do. Health care providers often overestimate understanding in a child of this age.
- Explain a procedure or treatment a few seconds rather than minutes beforehand—allowing the child time to think about it may result in frightening fantasies or exaggerations.
- Talk to preschool children throughout procedures, describing the sensations they are feeling or will feel.
- Distract the child with noises or bright objects. Counting with some preschool children may help to calm them during procedures.
- Avoid shaming the preschool child for crying, struggling, or fighting during a procedure. Reassurance that he tried his best will help to build a positive self-image.
- Use less frightening and more positive terms such as "make better" and "help," and avoid terms such as "shot" and "cut."
- Use adhesive bandages over small wounds and injection sites. Preschool children may imagine their blood leaking out through puncture wounds.

The preschool child may be more willing than the toddler to be separated from parents; keep this separation as brief as possible, however. Include the parents in treatments, and provide instruction on how to calm the child if they seem unsure. Do not ask them to restrain the child, as this may be confusing to the child and difficult for the parents.

The School-Age Child

Once children begin to go to school, they become interested in learning and gradually develop reasoning skills, including some abstract thinking. They are able to understand the cause of illness and injury, and are much less apt to fantasize and exaggerate. The vocabulary of school-age children can be quite extensive, and they can understand simple explanations of procedures. They are also able to make decisions about their own care. By this time, they have also developed techniques of their own to help them through painful times. Some helpful nursing interventions for the school-age child include:

- Offer simple choices whenever possible to help the child feel more in control. The school-age child is capable of deciding in which arm to have an injection or in which hand to hold a nebulizer.
- Talk directly to the child, explaining procedures in simple terms. When explaining treatments or care options to the parent, include the child.
- Ask the child about her understanding of your explanations, and allow time for questions.
- Give rewards such as a sticker, or inexpensive toy after a procedure, regardless of the child's behavior. Think of this as a reward for undergoing the procedure, not as a judgment of "good" or "bad" behavior.
- Address the child's fears or concerns directly, rather than treating them as foolish or inconsequential.

The Adolescent

Adolescence is the period in which a child goes through puberty and begins to take on an adult appearance. Children this age are also beginning to explore the adult world and develop their own unique identities. Coping with extraordinary changes in their physical appearance, they are often concerned with whether they are "normal" and whether others have similar thoughts and feelings. Although this is an age of risk-taking, they may be quite fearful of death. Adolescents are prone to very serious injury due to risk-taking. Although they are aware of the possibility of their own death, they avoid thinking about the reality of death. This is an age of extremes: teenagers may either exaggerate or underplay the seriousness of their illness or injury. In caring for the adolescent, the following guidelines apply:

- Preserve the patient's modesty; this includes offering adolescents a choice as to whether they want their parents present or not.
- Consider the legal issues of the right to privacy for pregnant adolescents and adolescents with sexually transmitted diseases.
- Provide an opportunity for questions.
- Listen to the adolescent's concerns nonjudgmentally, and without belittling her. It is often a temptation to develop a teasing relationship with an adolescent, but this has potential for harm—the adolescent is easily embarrassed.
- Explain procedures or treatments carefully, and allow choices. Adolescents are capable of complex abstract thinking, and can make intelligent and reasoned decisions about their own care.

Each child must be treated as an individual; although there are similarities in children by age-groups, one toddler may be much more mature than another, and one adolescent may lean more toward school-age behaviors while another may be very adultlike in her behavior.

THE FAMILY OF A CHILD IN EMERGENCY CARE

For the family, there are added stressors resulting directly and indirectly from the child's illness. How a child perceives an illness or injury is often related to the parents' attitude, so caring for the child requires assessment and intervention with the family.

The most common emotions experienced by parents of children cared for in emergencies are fear and anxiety. Parents are afraid that:

- Their child may die. This is the greatest source of anxiety and may be present even when this is highly unlikely, as in the case of minor illnesses or injuries. This anxiety is often the underlying cause of parents' anger toward health care providers.
- Their child may experience pain. As a rule, parents try very hard to protect children from pain. Even when pain may be necessary, it is difficult for parents to understand and to accept.
- The child's body may be permanently altered. Parents often fear that their children will have permanent scars or bodily changes.

Another common emotion of parents is guilt. Parents may feel guilty because:

- They feel responsible for their child's illness or injury.
- They are submitting their child to a painful experience.
- They do not have enough knowledge to make educated decisions about their child's care.

In addition, parents may have had negative experiences with health care providers in the past and may have other concerns about siblings, financial arrangements, and work schedules.

The particular causes of stress for a family in an emergency situation are unique to the circumstances and to the family involved. All of the stressors combined may stretch parents' coping mechanisms to the limit, and may result in anger, withdrawal, or tearfulness. Another manifestation of stress may be hyperactivity—making numerous phone calls, repeating questions, and involving a large number of people in decision-making processes.

Nursing care of the family should include interventions designed to promote their coping mechanisms.

It is far easier and less time consuming to intervene early and provide support for appropriate coping mechanisms than it is to intervene after a patient's or parent's emotional decompensation.

EMERGENCY ASSESSMENT OF INFANTS AND CHILDREN

In the emergency setting, assessment of the ill or injured child must be rapid and accurate. Early identification of abnormal findings is essential. Initial evidence of life-threatening conditions may be very subtle, with few signs of impending respiratory or cardiopulmonary arrest. It is particularly important to make as many initial observations as possible without touching the patient, so that assessments can reflect the baseline, resting condition of the child. Remember also to observe the relationship between the parent(s) and child during the examination process.

Initial observation in the emergency setting is usually performed by the *triage* nurse, who makes the decision of the level of care needed for the pediatric patient. This is an important skill that improves with experience. Much of this "initial" assessment is based on an overall sense of how the child looks—sick or well. Because children do not try to cover up either how they feel or how they look, you receive a fairly accurate impression of illness or wellness immediately. Emergency assessment of the pediatric patient is summarized in Table 14–1. Three essential factors combine to form this first impression: skin color, respiratory rate and effort, and response to the environment (Henderson & Brownstein, 1994).

If results of all three of these assessments appear to be normal, a more thorough and in-depth evaluation can follow. If your general impression is that the child is seriously ill, however, you must intervene immediately, and any further evaluation must be combined with intervention. Because the two most common pathways to mortality in children are respiratory failure and shock, interventions would include providing respiratory and circulatory support (see the section Cardiopulmonary Resuscitation of the Pediatric Patient).

INITIAL OBSERVATION FOR TRIAGE

- Is the child's breathing rapid or shallow, or is he using accessory muscles? When a child is having difficulty breathing, accessory muscles will be used to aid in breathing. Substernal, intercostal, or subclavicular retractions are all signs of serious breathing difficulties. Nasal flaring, head bobbing, grunting, stridor, and prolonged expirations signal increased work of breathing. Are abnormal breath sounds present? What is the child's position of comfort?
- Skin color: Is the child's skin pale, mottled, or cyanotic? Abnormal skin color could result from the two greatest threats to a child's life: respiratory distress or failure, or inadequate tissue perfusion (shock).
- Response to the environment: Although response to the environment is more difficult to evaluate in the preverbal child, this is an important component of the assessment. A well child should look around, fixate on objects, and appear to recognize caretakers. An anxious-appearing child may be in respiratory distress; a flaccid, disinterested child may be in respiratory failure or frank shock. Is the child alert, interactive, crying, sleepy, or limp?

For an infant or young child, most of the examination required for general *triage* can be performed with the child on his parent's lap (Seidel & Henderson, 1992). For the initial rapid assessment, it is not necessary to touch the child at all. Once you have decided that immediate intervention is not needed, proceed with further assessment. Both medical and trauma assessments include assessment of **airway, breathing,** and **circulation.**

The ABCs: Assessment of Airway, Breathing, and Circulation

Airway Assessment. Although it will ultimately be important to determine the etiology of respiratory distress or failure in an ill child, it is more important to recognize symptoms and signs of respiratory distress; in the emergency setting, initial treatment will be the same regardless of the cause.

Children are at greater risk of airway problems than adults because of some differences in airway anatomy:

- The child's airway is narrower than an adult's, and is therefore more easily obstructed by small foreign bodies, small amounts of mucus, or edema. Infants are preferential nasal breathers for the first several months of life; therefore, nasal secretions can cause respiratory compromise.

TABLE 14-1 *Approach to Pediatric Assessment*

ASSESSMENT	INTERVENTION
A—Airway: patency, positioning for air entry, audible sounds, airway obstruction (blood, mucus, edema).	A—Allow the child to maintain a position of comfort or position the airway (jaw thrust or head tilt–chin lift); use airway adjuncts, as required.
B—Breathing: increased or decreased work of breathing; nasal flaring; use of accessory muscles of respiration; pattern; quality.	B—Provide supplemental oxygen; initiate assisted ventilation with bag-valve-mask and intubate as indicated; provide gastric decompression by use of an oro or nasogastric tube.
C—Circulation: color of skin and capillary refill; strength of peripheral and central pulses; skin temperature.	C—Obtain vascular access; initiate volume replacement; perform chest compressions; defibrillate or provide synchronized cardioversion; initiate drug therapy.
D—Disability: activity level or level of consciousness; response to the environment; pupillary response.	D—Treat the underlying cause (e.g., signs of increased intracranial pressure; fluid or blood volume deficit, hypoxia).
E—Expose: to identify underlying injuries or additional signs of illness.	E—Remove all clothing, including diapers.
F—Fahrenheit: initiate measures to keep the child warm.	F—Maintain normothermic environment; initiate supplemental warming measures.
G—Get vital signs: evaluate the child's vital signs, including temperature, for abnormal findings; obtain weight in kgs.	G—Continuously monitor the child's vital signs, including temperature; weigh child, obtain estimated weight if child's condition prohibits measured weight.
H—Head-to-toe assessment: perform a complete head-to-toe assessment and obtain a history; during triage assessment the head-to-toe (secondary assessment) may need to relate to the chief complaint.	H—Continuously monitor the child for changes in condition; assess for any unusual odors.
I—Inspect the back and isolate: observe the back for obvious or hidden injuries; assess for communicable illness or susceptibility to illness (immunocompromised patients).	I—Reassess the back as indicated; provide isolation as indicated.

Reprinted with permission from Emergency Nurses Association. In: *Emergency Nursing Pediatric Course,* Park Ridge, IL: Author; 1993.

- Cartilage of the larynx is relatively soft and the trachea is thinner and more flexible than an adult's. The airway is more easily obstructed by flexion or hyperextension of the neck.
- The submandibular area is softer and can be more easily compressed to occlude the airway.
- The tongue is relatively large in relation to the oral cavity, and can more easily fall into the airway in the unconscious pediatric patient.
- The larynx is higher and more anterior, increasing the risk of obstruction and aspiration.
- Deciduous teeth are poorly anchored and easily dislodged.
- The chest wall is thin, softer, and more compliant. Rib alignment is more horizontal. The younger child is more susceptible to respiratory distress and failure. Retractions commonly occur with respiratory distress and can compromise the ability to increase tidal volume.
- The diaphragm is the predominant muscle of respiration. Pressure above or below the diaphragm can impede respiratory effort.
- Infants and children have a higher metabolic rate and increased oxygen demand. Hypoxia occurs more rapidly.
- Children are more susceptible to infectious diseases, which also contribute to the increased risk of airway obstruction in pediatric patients. Edema and mucus in a narrow airway cause incrementally more obstruction than in a wider one (Chameides, 1994).

Airway assessment in pediatric patients should include special attention to breath sounds (often audible to the naked ear) as well as snoring, stridor, wheezing, and grunting. Snoring is caused by obstruction in the upper airway (often the tongue relaxing against the posterior pharynx) and may be heard in a child with decreased mental status. Stridor is a high-pitched sound, which may be heard on inspiration (laryngeal obstruction) or on both inspiration and expiration (midtracheal obstruction). Wheezing, a high-pitched musical sound heard primarily on expiration, is a sign of obstruction of the *lower* airway. Crackles or rales are fine popping noises heard on inspiration; they usually indicate that there is fluid in the lungs, as in pneumonia (Henderson & Brownstein, 1994).

Breathing Assessment. The rate and depth of breathing, as well as the respiratory effort made by the child, indicate the work of breathing. Abdominal breathing is normal in the infant or young child, so you should observe the rise and fall of the abdomen. A rapid respiratory rate with shallow breathing indicates respiratory distress. Very slow breathing in an ill child is an ominous sign, indicating respiratory failure—the child may no longer have the energy for adequate ventilation.

The use of accessory muscles for breathing invariably indicates respiratory distress. The chest wall of a child is relatively weak and unstable, so retractions occur with increased work of breathing. Assessment of breathing should include observing the child for intercostal, substernal, suprasternal, supraclavicular, and infraclavicular retractions. As a child becomes exhausted, retractions may diminish; this usually indicates respiratory failure.

Nasal flaring with inspiration is another form of accessory muscle use. Grunting, a sound made by expiration against partially closed vocal cords, may also be present with respiratory distress. This is the body's effort to improve oxygenation by generating positive end-expiratory pressure and is a sign of hypoxemia.

Observe the child's preferred body posture. A child in respiratory distress will be upright with the jaw thrust forward, leaning forward on outstretched arms—the "tripod" position. This position helps to maximize airway opening and the use of accessory muscles of respiration.

Once the work of breathing has been carefully observed, listening to the chest may provide some useful information. Children have small chests, and breath sounds may be transmitted throughout the chest, so the child's chest should be auscultated at both sides of the body at the midaxillary line and over the trachea to confirm equality of breath sounds and to distinguish upper from lower airway noises.

Normal respiratory rates for children vary by age, and are faster than for adults. A respiratory rate over 60 breaths per minute, however, is abnormal for any age. Another important adjunct for respiratory assessment is the pulse oximetry reading (see Chapter 18).

> A slow respiratory rate is of great concern; a child who seems to be breathing at a rate normal for an adult is almost certainly hypoventilating. This may signal imminent respiratory arrest.

Circulation: Assessment of the Cardiovascular System. Cardiovascular assessment of the pediatric patient includes observing the child's skin color and temperature, checking capillary refill, determining heart rate, and measuring blood pressure. A child can compensate more effectively for fluid loss than an adult through increased heart rate and peripheral vasoconstriction. These are early signs of cardiovascular compromise in a pediatric patient that suggest the need for immediate intervention to prevent decompensation. A systolic blood pressure below 70 mmHg in a child is an indication of uncompensated *shock*, which may require immediate and aggressive intervention (Chameides, 1994). Children can maintain a normal blood pressure until up to 25% of their circulating blood volume is lost.

Neurologic Assessment: Level of Consciousness

The infant or child's level of consciousness is an essential component of the initial assessment. This assessment can only be made when the child is awake; if the child is sleeping, ask the parent to awaken the child gently to establish arousability.

Most methods of assessing level of consciousness in adults include some form of verbal feedback on the part of the patient, which of course is not possible in a preverbal child. There are other ways to assess the neurologic status, however. One method for children is AVPU (Chameides, 1994). This is a means of documenting the response of the child:

> **NEUROLOGIC ASSESSMENT BY A.V.P.U.**
>
> **A**lert
> **V**erbal (responds to verbal stimuli)
> **P**ainful stimuli (responds to painful stimuli)
> **U**nresponsive

This method gives a global assessment and includes documentation of the type of stimuli used to evoke responses or lack of response. More thorough and sophisticated means of assessment are used at a later point, but this method is usually adequate in the emergency setting. The Glasgow Coma Scale, commonly used in neurologic assessment of the adult patient, may also be used, but this is only useful in the revised version adapted for children; however, this scale has not been tested for validity in children (Table 14–2).

Additional Assessments

Vital Signs. Vital signs are useful in the triage assessment of the pediatric patient, but do not serve as reliable an indicator as in adult assessment, because their significance is more difficult to interpret due to age variations.

When taking the vital signs of children, observe the respiratory rate first, then assess the pulse; obtain the

TABLE 14–2 *Glasgow Coma Scale Modified for Children*

CHILD	INFANT
Eyes	
4 Opens eyes spontaneously	Opens eyes spontaneously
3 Opens eyes to speech	Opens eyes to speech
2 Opens eyes to pain	Opens eyes to pain
1 **No response**	**No response**
_____ = Score (Eyes)	
Motor	
6 Obeys commands	Spontaneous movements
5 Localizes	Withdraws to touch
4 Withdraws	Withdraws to pain
3 Flexion	Flexion (decorticate)
2 Extension	Extension (decerebrate)
1 **No response**	**No response**
_____ = Score (Motor)	
Verbal	
5 Oriented	Coos and babbles
4 Confused	Irritable cry
3 Inappropriate words	Cries to pain
2 Incomprehensible words	Moans to pain
1 **No response**	**No response**
_____ = Score (Verbal)	
_____ = Total Score (Eyes, Motor, Verbal) Scores will range from 3–15	

Reprinted from James, H. E., Anas, N. G., Perkin, R. M. (1985). *Brain Insults in Infants and Children*. Orlando, FL: Grune & Stratton.

blood pressure last, since it is the most upsetting for children. Both the respiratory and heart rates should be taken for one full minute, because subtle differences are important in the child. Note that normal respiratory and heart rates are faster than an adult's, while the blood pressure is lower on average. See Table 11–1 in Chapter 11 for normal vital signs by age.

History. A brief history should be taken, as some knowledge of prior illness and/or injury may affect the emergency care of the child. A format often used for pediatric patients is AMPLE:

A	Allergies
M	Medications taken, immunization history
P	Prior illness and/or injury
L	Last meal, eating habits
E	Events leading up to this illness—exposure to other children, mechanism of injury, etc.

This mnemonic gives sufficient information to determine whether the child's medical history will play an important role in assessment and treatment of the current illness or injury. In emergency departments where children are cared for, a list of immunizations and the appropriate ages should be posted in a convenient location for easy reference (see Appendix A).

Weight. Determining the weight of the child is absolutely essential in emergency care because all medication dosages and fluid amounts are calculated according to the child's weight in kilograms. A child should be weighed, but a chart with ages and weights of children may be used if it is not possible to use a scale. Another way to determine the child's weight and medication dosages is through the use of a length-based tape, such as the Broselow tape. A length-based tape is placed on a gurney or stretcher next to the child, and the child's length is measured. The length is keyed to emergency medication dosages, usually listed on the tape. Fluid bolus volumes and defibrillation dosages are also indicated. Pediatric airway, bag-valve-mask, laryngoscope, endotracheal tube, nasogastric tube, urinary catheter, chest tube, and intravenous catheter sizes may also be printed on the tape.

When all else fails, it is sometimes easiest to remember three estimated average weights for children under age 6 years, and estimate the child's weight from there:

2 Years:	10 kg
4 Years:	20 kg
6 Years:	30 kg

Parent–Child Relationship. Rapid triage assessment of the pediatric patient should also include observation of the child in relation to his parents. If the relationship does not appear to be close, comfortable, and trusting, the nurse may want to explore further. Especially when there is trauma, the nurse may want to consider possible causes and manifestations of dysfunctional parent–child relationships, such as **child abuse** or neglect (Henderson & Brownstein, 1994).

CARDIOPULMONARY RESUSCITATION OF THE PEDIATRIC PATIENT

Early recognition of and intervention for respiratory distress and compensated shock can be lifesaving for the pediatric patient. Assistance with ventilation and administration of fluids may prevent further deterioration in the child's condition. Once the child progresses to respiratory failure and shock, **cardiopulmonary resuscitation (CPR)** is an absolute necessity (Fig. 14–1). Resuscitation of pediatric patients requires attention to the differences between adults and children. General guidelines for CPR begin with the ABCs.

Airway and Breathing

Once it has been determined that an infant or child is in respiratory distress or failure, or is unresponsive, the

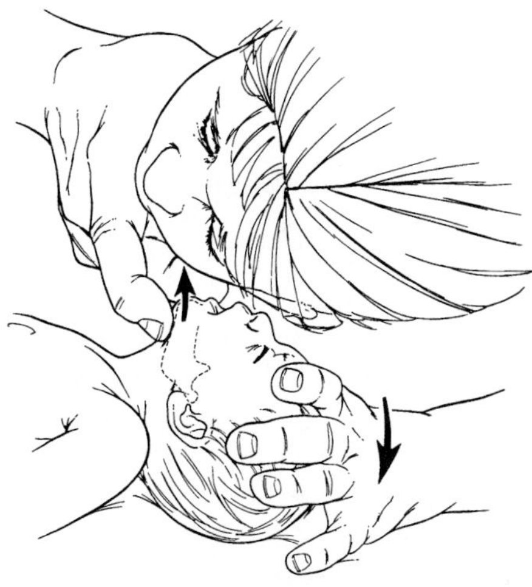

A. Opening the airway with the head tilt-chin lift maneuver. One hand is used to tilt the head, extending the neck. The index finger of the rescuer's other hand lifts the mandible outward by lifting on the chin. Head tilt should not be performed if cervical spine injury is suspected.

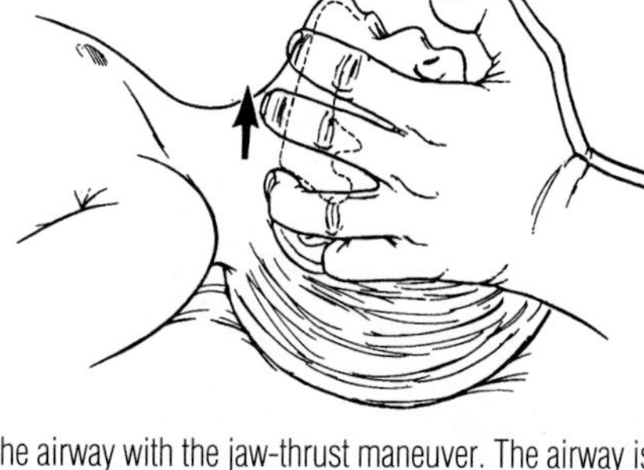

B. Opening the airway with the jaw-thrust maneuver. The airway is opened by lifting the angle of the mandible. The rescuer uses two or three fingers of each hand to lift the jaw while the remaining fingers guide the jaw upward and outward.

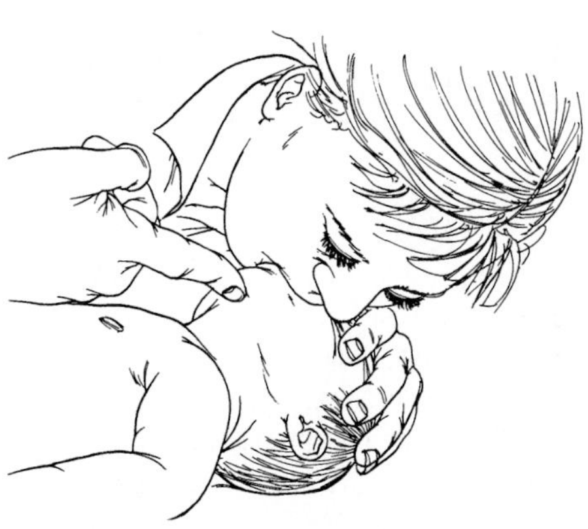

C. Rescue breathing in an infant. The rescuer's mouth covers the infant's nose and mouth, creating a seal. One hand performs head tilt while the other hand lifts the infant's jaw. Avoid head tilt if the infant has sustained head or neck trauma.

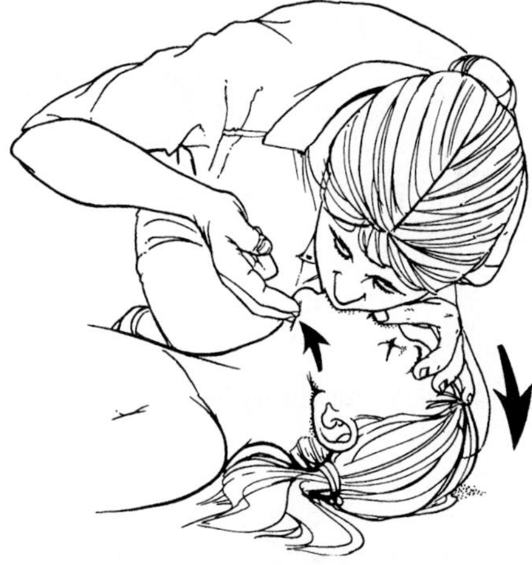

D. Rescue breathing in a child. The rescuer's mouth covers the mouth of the child, creating a mouth-to-mouth seal. One hand maintains head tilt; the thumb and forefinger of the same hand are used to pinch the child's nose. If head or neck trauma is suspected, immobilize the head in neutral position and *do not* perform head tilt.

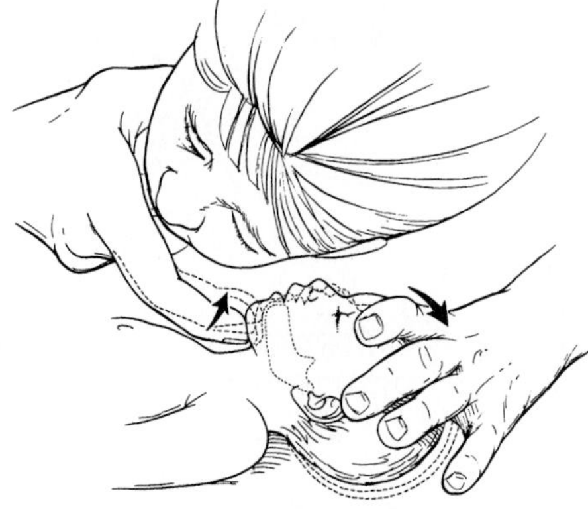

E. Movement of victim's head into positions of progressive neck extension until position of optimum airway patency (and effective ventilation) is achieved. Such manipulation of the head should *not* be performed if head, neck, or cervical spine injury is suspected.

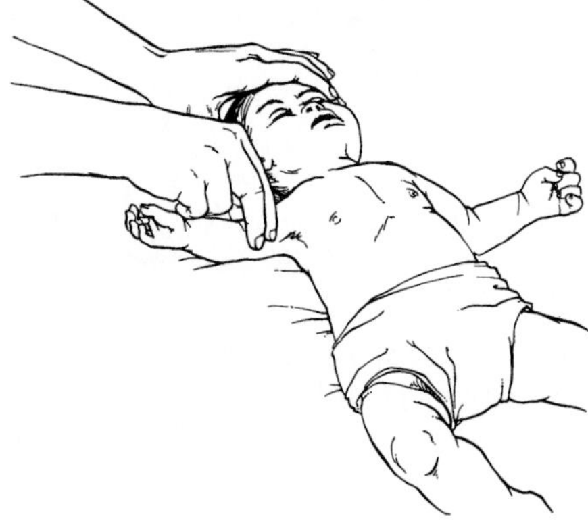

F. Palpating the brachial artery pulse in an infant.

Figure 14–1

Cardiopulmonary resuscitation for infants and children. (Reproduced with permission. *Textbook of Basic Life Support for Healthcare Providers*, 1994. Copyright American Heart Association.)

Illustration continued on following page

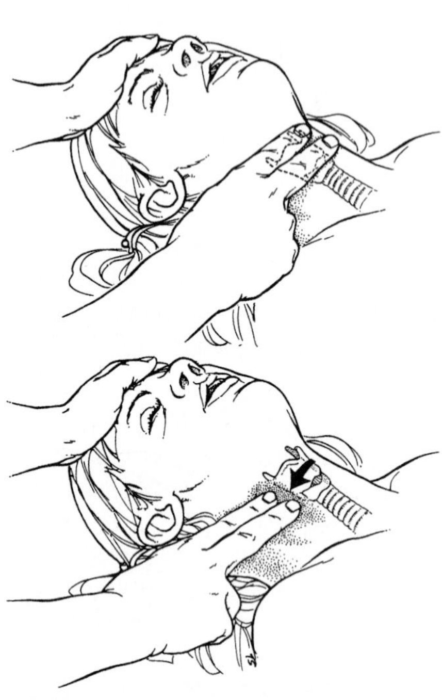

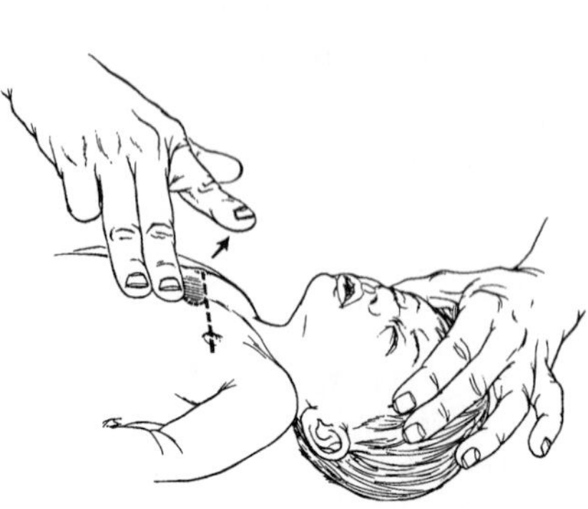

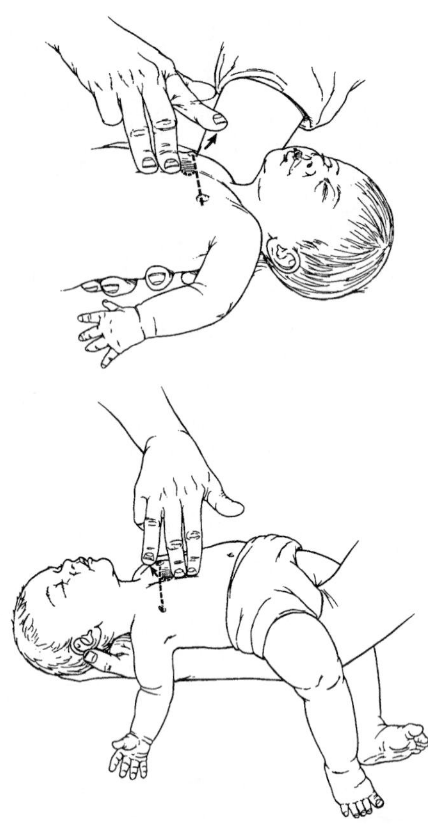

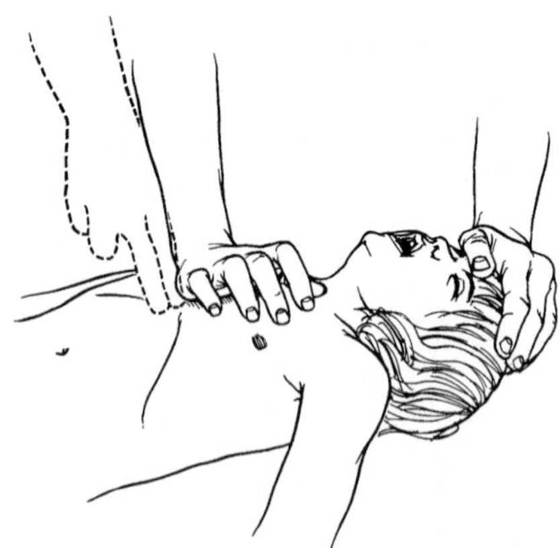

G. Locating and palpating the carotid artery pulse in the child.

H. Cardiac compressions. Top, Infant supine on palm of the rescuer's hand. Bottom, Performing CPR while carrying the infant or small child. Note that the head is kept level with the torso. (Compare Fig. I)

I. Locating proper finger position for chest compression in infant. Note that the rescuer's other hand is used to maintain head position to facilitate ventilation.

J. Locating hand position for chest compression in child. Note that the rescuer's other hand is used to maintain head position to facilitate ventilation.

Figure 14–1
Continued

patient's airway should be carefully positioned. The airway is opened with the head-tilt/chin-lift maneuver. If neck injury is suspected, head tilt should be avoided and the airway should be opened with a jaw-thrust maneuver. Because of the flexibility of the trachea of infants, and the relatively larger size of the head, the neutral, or "sniffing," position is maintained to assure maximal airway opening. In older children, look for chest rise, listen, and feel for exhaled breath against your cheek; when the patient is not breathing or ventilation is not adequate after the airway is positioned correctly, give two slow breaths by means of a bag-valve-mask device, watching for the rise and fall of the chest. Endotracheal intubation is necessary if the patient cannot be ventilated adequately with these measures.

Remember to stop inflation of the lungs when the chest just begins to rise, and to allow enough time for exhalation (longer than inhalation).

A pressure gauge should be attached to the bag and mask device in order to deliver the breaths at the correct pressure, especially for infants and young children. Gastric decompression by use of an oro or nasogastric tube is indicated during assisted ventilation.

If you are unable to inflate the lungs, the airway may be blocked, and obstructed airway maneuvers or medication to open the lower airways will be necessary. It is important to choose the appropriate size mask and the correct volume bag. The mask should cover the child's mouth and nose but not place pressure on the eyes. A good fit is needed to ensure a seal around the face and under the chin.

Obstructed Airway Management. Airway obstruction is a life-threatening emergency; when ventilation is not possible, the infant or child will die in a very short time. *Management of airway obstruction* depends on the cause and on the age of the patient. Definitive treatment will depend on diagnosis.

Aspiration is common among children, with more than 90% of deaths from foreign body aspirations in the pediatric age-group occurring in children under age 5 years (Chameides, 1994).

When a pediatric patient's airway is obstructed, and the child is coughing or is able to breathe adequately despite partial obstruction, he should be allowed to maintain whatever position is comfortable until specialized care is available and definitive care can be provided.

When a child is unable to ventilate adequately and aspiration of a foreign body is suspected as the cause, initiate maneuvers to remove the obstruction. Although there is still controversy about how to clear the airway of a foreign body, the American Heart Association recommends the use of the Heimlich maneuver in a conscious child older than age 1 year, and five abdominal thrusts for the unconscious child older than age 1 year (Fig. 14–2).

Infants are small and portable, and gravity may be of assistance in expelling a foreign body. Hold the infant in a downward slanting position and give five back blows to attempt removal of the foreign body. Back blows are followed by five chest thrusts, using two fingers on the lower third of the sternum. The oropharynx should be inspected for the foreign body. Note that in infants chest thrusts are recommended in preference to abdominal thrusts because of the potential for injury to the abdomen in infants (see Fig. 14–1).

If no foreign body is observed, rescue breathing should be attempted once again. The cycle then continues until the foreign body is expelled or until more advanced techniques are available. Blind finger sweeps are not recommended for infants and children due to the risk of forcing the object further down into the airway. If obstruction continues after these maneuvers, direct laryngoscopy and the use of a Magill forceps to remove the foreign body would be the next step; as a last resort, a tracheostomy is established. When the lower airway is obstructed due to a disease process such as asthma, medication to open the airway may be necessary.

Circulation

Feel for the pulse—in the child over age 1 year, palpate the carotid artery. For a child under age 1 year, use the brachial artery because the infant's relatively short, fat neck makes palpation of the carotid artery difficult. If no pulse is palpated or if the infant's heart rate is less than 60 beats/min, begin chest compressions.

Table 14–3 summarizes basic life support (BLS) maneuvers for infants and children.

Obtain venous access for fluid resuscitation and administration of medications. Usually a peripheral vein can be cannulated. If venous access cannot be obtained within 90 seconds, an intraosseous line should be considered—the medial tibia, a fingerbreadth below the tibial tuberosity, is the site of choice for insertion. Epinephrine is the drug of choice for management of cardiac arrest and can be given via the endotracheal tube when necessary. Atropine is used to diminish vagally mediated bradycardia. Naloxone is given if there is suspicion of narcotic ingestion. Sodium bicarbonate is given on the basis of arterial blood gas results, and dextrose may be used on the basis of blood glucose results or for patients unresponsive to resuscitative efforts. Pediatric patients should be given 20 mL/kg IV fluid, usually normal saline or lactated Ringer's solution, as an initial bolus for shock; the patient should be reassessed and additional boluses given as needed.

Although cardiac rhythm disturbances in children are rare, rapid heart rates can occur, including sinus tachycardia, supraventricular tachycardia (SVT), and ventricular tachycardia. Cardiac output is a function of stroke volume

THE INFANT: BACK BLOWS AND CHEST THRUSTS

The following sequence is used to clear a foreign-body obstruction from the airway of an infant. Back blows are delivered while the infant is supported in the prone position (face down) straddling the rescuer's forearm, with the head lower than the trunk. Chest thrusts are delivered while the infant is supine, held on the rescuer's forearm, with the infant's head lower than the body. The rescuer should perform the following steps to relieve airway obstruction in the *conscious* infant:

1. Hold the infant face down, resting on the forearm. Support the infant's head by firmly holding the jaw. Rest your forearm on your thigh to support the infant. The infant's head should be lower than the trunk.
2. Deliver up to five back blows forcefully between the infant's shoulder blades, using the heel of the hand (Fig. A).

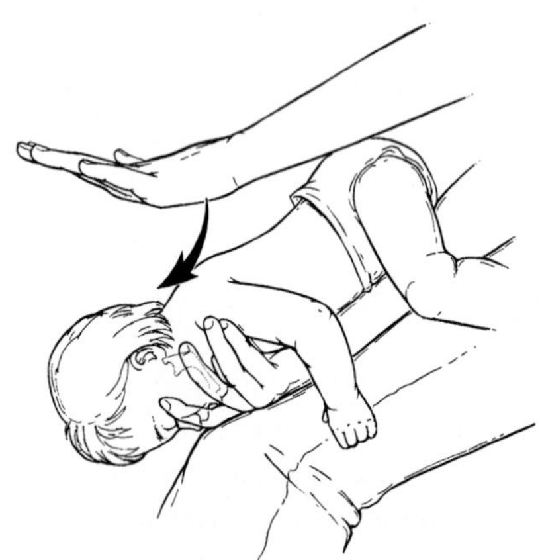

A. Back blows to relieve foreign-body airway obstruction in the infant.

3. After delivering the back blows, place your free hand on the infant's back, holding the infant's head. The infant is effectively sandwiched between your two hands and arms. One hand supports the head and neck, jaw, and chest while the other supports the back.
4. Turn the infant while the head and neck are carefully supported, and hold the infant in the supine position, draped on the thigh. The infant's head should remain lower than the trunk.
5. Give up to five quick downward chest thrusts in the same location and manner as chest compressions—two fingers placed on the lower half of the sternum, approximately one finger's breadth below the nipples (Fig. B). If the rescuer's hands are small or the infant is large, these maneuvers may be hard to perform. If so, place the infant supine on the lap, with the head lower than the trunk and the head firmly supported. After you have given up to five back blows, turn the infant as a unit to the supine position and give up to five chest thrusts.

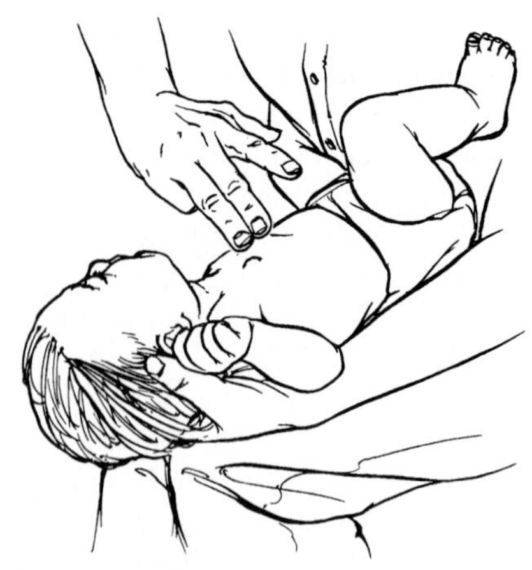

B. Chest thrusts to relieve foreign-body airway obstruction in the infant.

6. Open the airway by grasping both the tongue and lower jaw and lifting the mandible (tongue-jaw lift). Remove the foreign body if you see it (see below).

Steps 1 through 6 should be repeated until the object is expelled or the infant loses consciousness. If the infant loses consciousness, open the airway using a tongue-jaw lift and remove the foreign object if you see it and attempt rescue breathing and relief of airway obstruction.

If the victim is or becomes unconscious:

1. Open the infant's airway. If the loss of consciousness is witnessed, and foreign-body obstruction is suspected, lift the chin using a tongue-jaw lift and remove the object with a finger sweep if you see it.
2. Attempt rescue breathing.
3. If the first attempt is unsuccessful, reposition the head and reattempt ventilation.
4. If ventilation is unsuccessful, give five back blows and five chest thrusts.
5. Open the mouth using a tongue-jaw lift and remove the foreign object if you see it.
6. Repeat steps 2 through 4 until ventilation is successful (chest rises).
7. Activate the EMS system after approximately 1 minute, then resume efforts.
8. If the victim resumes effective breathing, place in the recovery position and monitor closely until rescue personnel arrive.

Figure 14–2

Procedures for clearing airway obstruction in infants and children. (Reproduced with permission. *Textbook of Basic Life Support for Healthcare Providers*, 1994. Copyright American Heart Association.)

Illustration continued on following page

THE CHILD: THE HEIMLICH MANEUVER

Abdominal Thrusts With Victim Conscious (Standing or Sitting)

Perform the following steps to relieve complete airway obstruction in the *conscious* victim:

1. Stand behind the victim, arms directly under the victim's axillae encircling the victim's torso.
2. Place the thumb side of one fist against the victim's abdomen in the midline slightly above the navel and well below the tip of the xiphoid process.
3. Grasp the fist with the other hand and exert a series of quick upward thrusts (Fig. C). Do not touch the xiphoid process or the lower margins of the rib cage because force applied to these structures may damage internal organs.

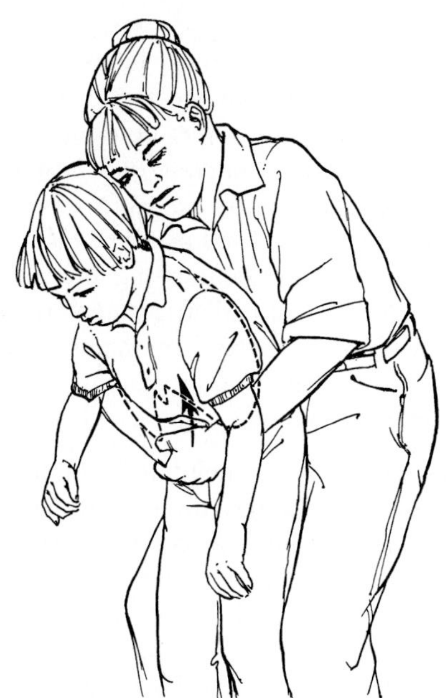

C. Abdominal thrusts with victim standing or sitting (conscious).

4. Each thrust should be a separate, distinct movement, intended to relieve the obstruction. Continue abdominal thrusts until the foreign body is expelled or the patient loses consciousness.
5. If the victim loses consciousness, open the airway using a tongue-jaw lift and remove the obstructing object with a finger sweep if you see it.
6. Attempt rescue breathing. If the chest fails to rise, reposition the head and reattempt rescue breathing again. If the airway remains obstructed in the unconscious victim, repeat the Heimlich maneuver (see below).

Abdominal Thrusts for the Victim Who Is Unconscious or Who Becomes Unconscious

The rescuer should perform the following steps:

1. Place the victim supine.
2. If the loss of consciousness is witnessed and foreign-body airway obstruction is suspected, open the airway using a tongue-jaw lift and remove the object with a finger sweep if you see it.
3. Attempt rescue breathing. If ventilation is unsuccessful, reposition the head and reattempt ventilation. If ventilation is still unsuccessful, continue with steps 4 through 8 below.
4. Kneel beside the victim or straddle the victim's hips.
5. Place the heel of one hand on the child's abdomen in the midline slightly above the navel and well below the rib cage and xiphoid process. Place the other hand on the top of the first.
6. Press both hands into the abdomen with a quick upward thrust (Fig. D). Each thrust is directed upward in the midline and should not be directed to either side of the abdomen. Perform a series of five thrusts. Each thrust should be a separate and distinct movement.

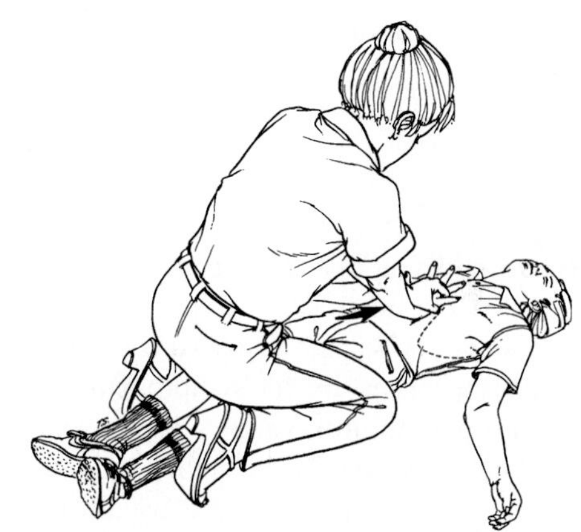

D. Abdominal thrusts with victim lying (conscious or unconscious).

7. Open the airway by grasping both the tongue and lower jaw and lifting the mandible (tongue-jaw lift). If you see the foreign body, remove it using a finger sweep.
8. Repeat steps 3 through 7 until ventilation is successful.

Figure 14–2
Continued

TABLE 14–3 *Summary of Basic Life Support Maneuvers in Infants and Children*

MANEUVER	INFANT (<1 YEAR)	CHILD (1 TO 8 YEARS)
Airway	Head tilt–chin lift (if trauma is present, use jaw-thrust)	Head tilt–chin tilt (if trauma is present, use jaw-thrust)
Breathing		
Initial	Two breaths at 1 to 1½ s/breath	Two breaths at 1 to 1½ s/breath
Subsequent	20 breaths/min (approximate)	20 breaths/min (approximate)
Circulation		
Pulse check	Brachial/femoral	Carotid
Compression area	Lower half of sternum	Lower half of sternum
Compressed width	2 or 3 fingers	Heel of 1 hand
Depth	Approximately one-third to one-half the depth of the chest	Approximately one-third to one-half the depth of the chest
Rate	At least 100/min	100/min
Compression-ventilation ratio	5:1 (pause for ventilation)	5:1 (pause for ventilation)
Foreign Body Airway Obstruction	Back blows/chest thrusts	Heimlich maneuver

Reproduced with permission. *Textbook of Pediatric Advanced Life Support,* 1994. Copyright American Heart Association.

and heart rate, and a rapid rate can cause decreased cardiac output. Sinus tachycardia usually requires observation and determination of the cause. Cardioversion at 0.5 to 1.0 joules/kg may be necessary for symptomatic SVT (heart rate >200 beats per minute); Valsalva maneuvers or adenosine would be considered for the stable patient. Ventricular tachycardia in a pediatric patient is usually the result of congenital abnormalities or chronic cardiac disease, and requires complex interventions.

Resuscitation of the pediatric patient requires a team effort; training and rehearsal, such as mock codes, are very helpful, as are national courses now available such as the Pediatric Advanced Life Support (PALS) provided by the American Heart Association.

PEDIATRIC TRAUMA

Injury is the number one cause of death of children between ages 1 and 19 years in the United States. Motor vehicle injuries are the leading cause of death, followed by homicide and suicide (Guyer & Ellers, 1990; Ray & Yuwiler, 1991). Annually, 16 million children are treated in emergency departments; an estimated 600,000 children are hospitalized, 22,000 die of their injuries, and 50,000 survive but have permanent disabilities (Gausche, 1995; Ray & Yuwiler, 1991). Of the 600,000 hospital admissions, 23% are caused by respiratory illness, followed by injury with 20% of the admissions (Bernardo & Kelley, 1994). Note that the term “injury” is used in preference to “accident” when describing *trauma,* since some trauma is not accidental, and much of it is preventable.

Injury prevention and education is essential to lower the incidence of trauma in the pediatric population. Successful prevention and education steps include bicycle helmet programs, safety caps and locking up of medications, and eliminating potential hazards such as old refrigerators. Information about injury prevention should be provided to all minor trauma patients on discharge from the emergency department (see Chapter 13).

Mechanism of Injury

Knowing the mechanism of injury helps to identify common injury patterns and predict patient needs and outcomes. The mechanism of injury determines the type of injuring force—kinetic energy—which results in tissue response. As the kinetic energy is displaced into the body, it causes traumatic injury (Cardona, 1988). The trauma can result from either blunt or penetrating force. Blunt trauma is responsible for 87% of pediatric trauma (motor vehicle accidents and falls), whereas penetrating trauma constitutes only 10% of injury. The remaining 3% are categorized as submersion and other injuries (Gausche, 1995).

Blunt Trauma. Injuries sustained from blunt trauma are often less apparent and may be more serious than those from penetrating trauma. A common cause of blunt trauma is acceleration-deceleration force, often from motor vehicle accidents or falls (Bernardo & Waggoner, 1992). Just before a motor vehicle collision, both the occupant and the vehicle are traveling at the same speed. When the vehicle meets an opposing force, the speed of both the occupant and the vehicle rapidly decelerate. When this occurs, three collisions take place: the moving auto collides with the opposing object, the occupant's body collides with the interior portion of the auto, and the occupant's internal organs and tissues collide with rigid internal structures (Cardona, 1988).

Unrestrained occupants in a motor vehicle accident suffer a higher incidence of injury than restrained occupants (Cardona, 1988). Children who are unrestrained in a vehicle can become missiles, thrown around the vehicle, pinned under the dashboard, or ejected from the vehicle. This principle is the same for children riding unrestrained in the back of open pick-up trucks; they become missiles ejected out of the vehicle into oncoming traffic or onto the road. Children who are held on an adult's lap during a motor vehicle accident can be instantly crushed between the rigid part of the auto and the moving adult.

Restraining devices in vehicles offer some protection, but also have some consequences for the pediatric patient.

Because of differences in developmental anatomy, children can suffer injuries when placed in adult restraining mechanisms. Children ages 4 to 9 years are of shorter sitting height when compared to adults, and a larger proportion of their bodies is located above the safety belt. This may cause more forward motion during impact and increase the potential for head injury from striking the dashboard. The child may also jackknife over a lap belt during impact, causing abdominal injuries (Agran, Winn, & Dunkle, 1989). The adult shoulder restraint may cross the child's face or neck, leading to potential airway injury (Agran, Castillo, & Winn, 1992). Infants and children in car seats are susceptible to high cervical injuries during sudden deceleration because:

- The combination of the child's small body and relatively heavy head result in flexion-extension injuries.
- The child's spinal mobility is greater because of looser spinal ligaments.
- Infants have underdeveloped cervical musculature.
- The child's cervical spine has a higher fulcrum of movement at C2–3, and the child is therefore more susceptible to high cervical spine injuries (Fuchs et al., 1989).

Fifty thousand children are also injured as pedestrians each year—the largest number are between ages 4 and 9. Eighty percent of these injuries occur during the daylight hours as the child darts out into the middle of the street between parked cars (Cardona, 1988). When a child is hit by an auto, a triad of injuries, referred to as Waddell's triad, occurs (Fig. 14–3). This one traumatic event results in three different injuries:

1. The child is initially struck by the bumper and hood of the car.
2. The child is then propelled into the air, landing on the ground (Halpern, 1989).
3. As the child is propelled like a missile to the ground, the large size and weight of the child's head results in injury to the contralateral side of the head (Cardona, 1988).

The first two impacts result in potential chest, abdomen, or femur injuries; the third injury is a skull fracture or other head injury.

Penetrating Trauma. Penetrating injury is produced when energy from a foreign object (such as a knife or bullet) is dissipated into the surrounding tissue (Cardona, 1988). Damage to the body tissue is a direct result of the penetrating object and, in the case of a bullet, there may be damage resulting from shock waves, cavitation, and pulsation of the cavity and surrounding tissue as a result of the bullet's passage (Bernardo & Kelley, 1994). The severity of an injury depends on the anatomic area penetrated, the length of the penetrating object, the type of gun and bullet, the distance from bullet to impact, and the angle of penetration (Bernardo & Kelley, 1994). With gunshot wounds, what may seem like a fairly innocuous wound may actually be very severe, depending on the amount of damage occurring after initial penetration.

Multiple Trauma. A multiple trauma patient has injuries to more than one body system. Initial assessment of and quick intervention for the multiple trauma patient is a collaborative effort from the prehospital setting to the trauma center emergency department, to the critical care units, through the rehabilitation phase. This continuous line of care begins with contact between the health care providers at the scene of the accident with medical direction. Ideally, a critically injured pediatric patient should be rapidly transported to a facility with the personnel, equipment, and the commitment to provide care to children; any delay could have a negative impact on patient outcome.

Obtaining a History of the Injury. Determination of the degree and severity of injuries is truly both an art and a science. Diagnosis depends on the mechanism of injury as well as the presenting signs and symptoms. Because assessment proceeds simultaneously with intervention, the discussion here will be limited to consideration of the mechanism of injury, which is explored briefly dur-

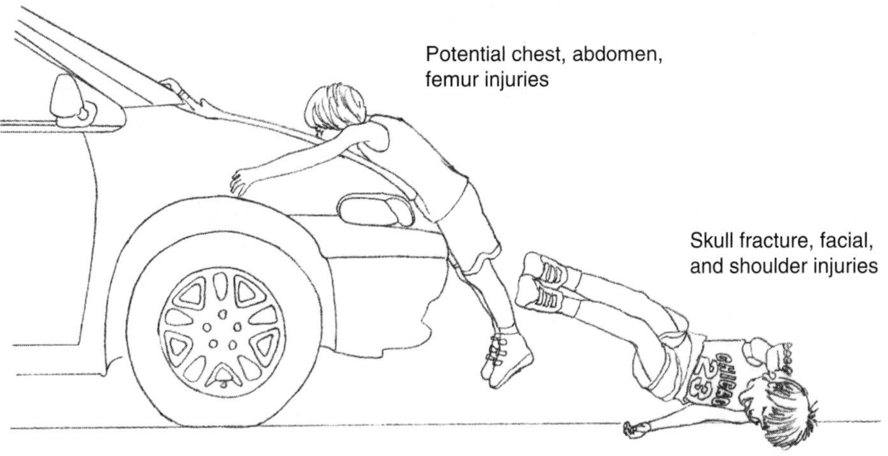

Figure 14–3
Waddell's triad of injuries.

HISTORY OF INJURY QUESTIONS

For a victim of a motor vehicle accident:

Was the child wearing a seat belt or in a child's car seat?
What was the speed of the motor vehicle?
With what did the motor vehicle collide?
At what point on the motor vehicle was the location of impact?
Where was the victim seated in the motor vehicle?
How much damage was done to the motor vehicle?

For a victim of a fall:

How far did the child fall?
How did the child land (on what part of the body)?
On what type of ground did the child land?
Was the child's fall broken by any objects?

For a victim of a penetrating injury:

How long and how wide was the blade of the knife?
How far away was the gun when it was fired?
What type of gun was used and what was the caliber of the gun?

ing the primary survey and explored in greater depth during the secondary survey. Obtaining a good history of the event will help to determine the precise mechanism of injury and potential injuries. Nurses can obtain a good history by asking specific questions.

Obtaining information about the mechanism of injury gives some information as to what types of injuries can be expected and the potential severity of those injuries. Thorough evaluation depends on a systematic trauma evaluation, which takes place along with lifesaving intervention.

Trauma Scoring

Various kinds of scoring are performed and documented by nursing staff; these are used as an objective measure of the severity of the injury caused by a traumatic event. Tools have been developed for field triage, quality assurance, and epidemiologic surveillance (Cardona, 1988). Most of the scoring systems that have been developed are for the assessment of injury to adults, and do not take the anatomic differences of children into account. The accompanying box presents a sample of **trauma scoring** systems.

Patient Assessment and Management

Preparation

At the trauma center, and even in the emergency department of the community hospital, the presence of qualified trauma team members to assess and treat the trauma patient is crucial. A trauma team generally consists of skilled surgeons, physicians, nurses, social workers, and other health professionals, each with a specific role and duties during trauma resuscitation. The team is usually assembled after notification of pending arrival by prehospital personnel, and the trauma room is readied with personnel and equipment (i.e., emergency medications, endotracheal tubes, catheters, fluid warmer, and O negative blood in the blood bank). Trauma units often have carefully orchestrated protocols. For instance, the recording nurse and circulating nurse may be stationed at the right and left of the patient, respectively.

All multiple trauma patients require a rapid, complete, and thorough assessment to determine injuries sustained. Assessment and intervention must proceed at the same time in the trauma patient—the two cannot be separated. The assessment is composed of two parts. The primary assessment, or survey, includes identification of any life-threatening injuries and rapid intervention. The secondary survey involves a more detailed head-to-toe evaluation of the trauma patient and initiation of needed diagnostic and therapeutic interventions.

Primary Survey

The goal of the primary survey is to assess and to intervene in life-threatening injuries. First, the ABCDs (airway, breathing, circulation, and disability) are evaluated.

Trauma Scoring Systems

TRAUMA SCORE (TS)

Adult scoring tool sometimes used with children.
Assesses respiratory rate and effort, blood pressure, and capillary refill.
Includes the Glasgow Coma Scale (GCS).

REVISED TRAUMA SCORE (RTS)

Comprises the GCS, blood pressure, and respiratory rate.

PEDIATRIC TRAUMA SCORE (PTS)

Adapted for the pediatric patient.
Assesses weight, airway control, central nervous system response, systolic blood pressure, open wounds, and skeletal deformities, which help predict the outcomes for death or survival (Cooper et al., 1992).

MODIFIED GLASGOW COMA SCALE (SEE TABLE 14–2)

Developed for neurologic assessment of pediatric patients.
Based on adult GCS but takes into account a child's preverbal communication.
Objective tool for monitoring child's neurologic function through the continuum of care (Fitzmaurice, 1992).

A—Airway. The pediatric multiple trauma patient should be brought in on a pediatric immobilization board and remain on it when there is concern that there may be injury to the spinal cord (Fig. 14–4). The first priority is to open and maintain the airway, using the chin life-jaw thrust maneuver to prevent movement of the cervical spine. Because the child's lower airway is narrow and easily obstructed by edema and mucus, frequent observation is necessary; oral suctioning may be required to keep the airway clear (Gausche, 1995). If a cervical collar is used, correct sizing is essential to maintain stabilization: the chin must rest securely in the chin holder, the collar must be below the ears, and the lower end should not extend below the upper part of the sternum (Bernardo & Waggoner, 1992). The cervical immobilization device and spinal immobilization device (long backboard) must remain in place until spinal injury has been ruled out.

In some cases, a child is brought to the emergency setting in the car seat; cervical immobilization can be maintained without removing the child from the seat. Rolled towels should be used on either side of the child's head and secured with tape. If otherwise stable, the child may remain in the car seat until x-rays have shown there is no injury to the cervical spine.

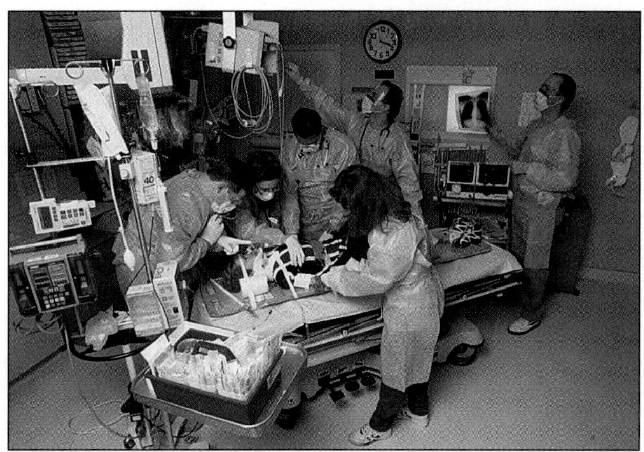

Figure 14–4
The child with multiple trauma injuries must remain on an immobilization board (long backboard) with a cervical immobilization device in place until being evaluated for spinal injuries. (Courtesy of Children's Medical Center, Dallas, Texas)

B—Breathing. Ventilation and oxygenation of the patient should be evaluated; check the rate, rhythm, and depth of respirations, auscultating breath sounds in the midaxillary line. Pulse oximetry readings provide helpful information, but should be used with close observation of the patient's general condition, including color and work of breathing (Bernardo & Kelley, 1994).

> Use supplemental oxygen for any child with multiple trauma—there is no contraindication for this. A rate of 4 to 6 liters of oxygen via nasal cannula or 10 to 12 liters by mask is the usual dosage.

Start the flow of oxygen after placing the cannula or mask on the child's face, as the flow of air may bother children initially (Bernardo & Waggoner, 1992). If the child is alert and does not tolerate the mask, blow-by oxygen using only the tubing, or using a plastic cup with the end of the tubing inserted, may be less threatening to a child.

If ventilation is inadequate or absent, ventilation using a bag-valve-mask with a reservoir with high flow oxygen should be instituted. If there is altered level of consciousness, an oropharyngeal or a nasopharyngeal airway can be used to maintain airway patency, although these should only be used for a child over age 1 year and without signs of facial trauma (Gausche, 1995). The length of the oropharyngeal airway should be equal to the distance from the corner of the child's mouth to the angle of the mandible. An incorrect size may obstruct the child's airway. The nasopharyngeal airway should be equal in size to the distance from the nares to the tragus of the ear. When there is severe head injury, such as basilar or cribriform plate fracture, a nasopharyngeal airway should not be used, as it may cause further injury by entering the cranial vault during insertion. When a bag-valve-mask device is used, sufficient gastric distension may occur in the pediatric patient to interfere with respiratory excursion. If this occurs, a nasal-oral gastric tube may be placed for gastric decompression (Semonin-Holleran & Rouse, 1991).

When there is altered level of consciousness, lack of spontaneous respirations, or severe head injury, endotracheal intubation may be necessary to provide airway control, oxygenation, and hyperventilation. Spinal immobilization must be maintained throughout this procedure as long as there is uncertainty about the presence of spinal cord injury. Hyperventilate the patient before this procedure. Medication is often used to prevent movement, counteract the slowing of the heart rate caused by vagal stimulation, and provide amnesia for the patient. While observing the child for respiratory difficulty, check the neck for jugular vein distension or tracheal deviation (the cervical collar may be opened for this assessment and then closed, keeping the neck in alignment). Respiratory difficulty may also be caused by injury to the chest. Observe the chest for contusions, penetrations, abrasions, and paradoxical movement. With penetrating injury, insertion of a chest tube or intervention for cardiac tamponade may be necessary.

Although facial trauma is rare in children under age 5 years because the face is relatively small in relation to the head, nasal and mandibular fractures are seen occasionally (Barkin, 1992). As the child grows, the increasing prominence of the face also causes increases in the incidence of facial trauma. Other factors resulting in the lower incidence of facial trauma in small children include the following:

- The facial bones of children are less brittle and more elastic than those of adults.
- Children have smaller sinus cavities, so facial bones have better support than adults'.
- Fat pads over the upper and lower jaws create a cushioning effect.

Severe facial trauma may be life-threatening mainly because of the potential to obstruct ventilation—both fractures and soft tissue injury may cause narrowing of the airway. Facial trauma in children is treated as in adults. Nursing intervention mainly includes assuring an adequate airway and breathing, observing for possible progressive obstruction, and keeping the injured areas clean to prevent infection. Insertion of tubes (such as nasogastric and nasotracheal) through the nares should be avoided when facial fractures are suspected, because of possible faulty insertion into the cranial vault through fractured facial bones.

Specialists should be available for initial diagnosis and treatment of suspected facial fractures in children, and for follow-up. Close follow-up in the initial stages and over several years is usually required because facial fractures in the younger age-group may become progressively more disfiguring as the child grows (Barkin, 1992).

C—Circulation. Cardiovascular assessment of the pediatric patient focuses on early recognition and treatment of hypovolemia (Gausche, 1995). Blood loss in pediatric patients is usually caused by abdominal or chest injury or severe injuries to extremities; head trauma alone is almost never the root cause of shock unless there is substantial bleeding from lacerations (Bernardo & Waggoner, 1992). Because of the smaller amount of fluid volume in the pediatric patient, however, even a small amount of blood loss may be significant. Children can maintain blood pressure, even with a 25% to 30% blood loss, by increased heart rate and vasoconstriction. The early indicators of shock in children are tachycardia, decreased capillary refill (greater than 2 seconds), mottled skin, apprehension, pallor, and cool extremities. A decrease in blood pressure is a very late and ominous sign, indicating that the child is unable to compensate for the fluid loss. Decreased level of consciousness, dusky skin color, cool clammy extremities, weak and thready pulses, poor capillary filling, tachycardia, tachypnea, and hypotension are late signs, indicating that cardiac arrest is imminent. Cardiac monitoring and frequent cardiovascular assessments are necessary during the acute stage. During this stage, any external hemorrhage is noted and controlled, and intravenous or other access to the circulatory system is obtained. Two large-bore IV lines should be initiated, if possible. An intraosseous line should be initiated if three attempts at IV access are unsuccessful.

Extremities are also rapidly evaluated as a part of the primary survey, and fractures should be splinted. Pulses in the affected extremity should be evaluated on initial presentation, and before and after it is splinted. Evaluation should include assessment of motor (Can the child move the extremity? Is there pain?), circulatory (Is there a pulse and good capillary refill?), and neural function (Is sensation to the area intact?). If neurovascular or circulatory compromise are present, immediate intervention is necessary.

D—Disability. During the primary survey phase a brief neurologic examination is performed, establishing level of consciousness along with pupillary size and reactivity and muscle movement. AVPU may be used to assess mental status. Sudden changes such as agitation or somnolence may indicate hypoxia or decreased cerebral perfusion. The primary survey is conducted simultaneously with resuscitation; continual reassessment is necessary.

Secondary Survey

The secondary survey includes head-to-toe assessment evaluating all body systems along with continued attention to the ABCs and mental status and frequent re-evaluation of cardiovascular status and fluid intervention.

Neurologic System. Pediatric head injury is common due to the size of the child's head and relative malleability of the skull. The physical examination should include palpation of the child's scalp for lacerations and/or impaled objects. The presence of otorrhea and rhinorrhea that test positive for glucose are indicative of cerebrospinal fluid leakage. Because the anterior fontanelle does not close until 12–18 months, infants are able to compensate for intracranial swelling for several hours. Observe closely and continuously for changes in level of consciousness (Soud, 1992). When head injury is present, mild hyperventilation is recommended to counteract increased intracranial pressure. If the patient is in shock, the amount of fluid infused must be carefully monitored; there is a risk of increased intracranial pressure from fluid overload. (See Chapter 40 for additional coverage of head injury.)

Chest. In children under age 14 years, blunt chest trauma is more frequent than penetrating chest trauma, although violent injuries such as gunshot wounds and stabbings increase the number of penetrating injuries in adolescence. The most serious thoracic injuries include hemothorax and/or pneumothorax, tension pneumothorax, flail chest, and cardiac tamponade.

Observe the chest carefully for areas of discoloration and penetrating injuries, and note any abnormalities for further observation and intervention. With any penetrating injury, pneumothorax, hemothorax, or cardiac tamponade should be suspected. Although rib fractures from blunt trauma are rare in children due to the flexibility of the chest wall, lung contusion may cause respiratory difficulty during hospitalization.

Total or partial collapse of the lung may occur when blood or air leaks into the pleural space from a tear or puncture in the lung tissue (pneumothorax or hemothorax) (Jutzi-Kosmos, 1990). Pneumothorax may occur after blunt chest trauma with or without rib fractures or from penetrating trauma. Collapse of the lung can be seen on x-ray, and there will be decreased breath sounds on the affected side. If the pneumothorax is small, the child may be asymptomatic. If the pneumothorax is clinically significant, the child will have signs of hypoxemia, such as tachycardia, increased respiratory rate, and decreased oxygen saturation on the pulse oximeter. If this condition is not corrected by rapid decompression with a chest tube, it may lead to a tension pneumothorax.

Tension pneumothorax occurs when air enters the pleural cavity and cannot escape, leading to increased intrathoracic pressure. This, in turn, causes collapse of the affected lung, shift of the mediastinum, and tracheal deviation to the opposite side. Because this cascade affects ventilation, oxygenation, and cardiac output, the patient may have a cardiac arrest if there is not rapid intervention. Hemothorax is the accumulation of blood in the pleural space. With a mechanism similar to the tension pneumothorax, the patient will have compromised ventilation and shock without rapid insertion of a chest tube and decompression of the hemothorax.

Flail chest occurs when fractures of the chest wall free a segment to move independently, compromising ventilation. This occurs when three or more ribs are fractured, often from blunt trauma. Treatment includes stabilization of the chest wall and the use of a ventilator; the patient should be observed for underlying chest injuries such as pneumothorax, hemothorax, and lung contusion.

Cardiac tamponade can occur from blunt or penetrating injuries. Injury to the heart or great vessels causes leakage of blood into the pericardial sac. As the pericardial sac fills with blood, the heart muscle cannot pump effectively. Ventricular filling is decreased so cardiac output also decreases. Assessment for cardiac tamponade includes measurement of blood pressure, pulse pressure, and auscultation of heart sounds, which will be muffled.

Pulmonary contusion results from blunt trauma to the chest wall. The energy is transferred from the chest wall to the lung tissue, causing injury and resulting edema. Hours or days after the injury, the patient will experience difficulty breathing, hypoxemia, and clouding of the lung tissue on x-ray. Oxygen by mask or cannula is always necessary; more aggressive interventions such as breathing treatments or use of a ventilator may also be required.

Cardiac contusion is caused by blunt trauma to the chest. Damage to cardiac tissue may alter electrical conduction and mechanical contractility. Patients should be placed on a cardiac monitor and observed for tachycardia, rhythm disturbances, chest pain, murmurs, rales, hypotension, and tenderness over the precordium.

Abdomen and Genitourinary Tract. Palpate the child's abdomen and flanks, and observe for bruising, abrasions, contusions, masses, or presence of pain. Auscultate the abdomen for the presence of bowel sounds. Younger children have protruding abdomens due to underdeveloped abdominal musculature, less fat surrounding and protecting the kidneys, and relatively larger, anteriorly positioned kidneys (Bernardo & Kelley, 1994). The flexible lower rib cage also adds to the child's vulnerability to blunt trauma (Fitzmaurice, 1992).

Careful assessment of the abdomen involves inspection and palpation, looking for abrasions and ecchymoses, distension, and tenderness (Gausche, 1995). Gastric dilation may occur due to crying, air swallowing, or prolonged bag-valve-mask ventilation, complicating the evaluation of the abdomen. A nasogastric tube may be placed to decompress the stomach if there is no head trauma; otherwise, an oral gastric tube can be inserted. If there are symptoms of abdominal pain and/or signs of lower abdominal mass, a urinary catheter may be placed to decompress the bladder and obtain a urine sample (Foltin, 1992). Diagnostic peritoneal lavage is rarely used in the pediatric patient. An abdominal computed tomography scan is the diagnostic tool generally used (Donnellan, 1990). A very small number (8%) of hospital admissions are for children with abdominal injuries, and fewer than 15% of these require operative intervention (Cooper, Barlow, & DiScala, 1992).

Renal injury is suspected if there is evidence of trauma to the flank, back, lower chest, or abdomen and the presence of a pelvic fracture. Hematuria is the hallmark of a renal injury, so the urine of all trauma patients should be tested as soon as possible (Donnellan, 1990).

Musculoskeletal System. Obvious fractures are assessed for in the secondary survey, along with the circulation to all extremities. In the secondary survey, assess the symmetry of extremities and motor function. The ligaments, muscles, and tendons of children are relatively strong and able to withstand injury, so children may be more prone to fractures than to sprains or tears in ligaments (Bernardo & Waggoner, 1992). If the child is awake and alert, the motor function of upper extremities may be evaluated by holding a brightly colored object above the child, encouraging her to reach for it. To evaluate the motor function of the lower extremities, rub the bottom of her foot to elicit a response. Children under age 18 months will still have a Babinski reflex present (Cardona, 1988).

Orthopedic injuries are rarely life-threatening, but improper interventions can jeopardize the viability of an extremity. Certain orthopedic injuries are unique to the pediatric population (see Chapter 36):

- Growth plate injuries from compression, torsion, or other mechanisms can result in growth arrest or growth disruption.
- A greenstick fracture is an incomplete fracture often seen in young children because of their soft bones.
- Radial head subluxation or nursemaid's elbow is also seen in young children. It is caused by the sudden pulling on a pronated arm, as when a mother pulls her child away from danger or lifts the child by one arm.

Children with this injury will generally present to the emergency department with a nonfunctional pronated arm.

Integumentary System. Observation for multiple trauma includes undressing the child entirely to expose all potential injuries. Infants younger than age 6 months have less subcutaneous fat to insulate themselves and are not able to regulate temperature effectively, so a radiant warmer should be used to assist in maintaining body temperature, especially when exposing the child. Warm blankets, warm IV fluids, and warm blood products are also helpful.

Interventions

Intervention for the seriously injured trauma patient proceeds simultaneously with assessment. Oxygen is always administered, at 4 liters via nasal cannula or 6 to 10 liters by mask.

> Any seriously injured child with a rapid heart rate and abnormal skin signs should be considered to be in compensated shock—even when the blood pressure is normal—and the nurse should prepare for fluid resuscitation.

With most trauma patients, two large-bore IV lines are started for administration of fluids; blood is drawn for laboratory analysis at the time these lines are started, if possible. In young children, subclavian lines are rarely used because of the small size of the chest and the increased risk of lung perforation. Many hospitals have specific protocols directing the type of lines and length of time allowed before cutdowns, arterial lines, and/or intraosseous lines are attempted. Intraosseous access is rapid and effective, and is recommended for children under age 6 years when intravenous access is not rapidly obtainable. A strong needle such as a bone marrow aspiration needle, spinal needle, or intraosseous needle is inserted into the proximal tibia, the distal femur, or the distal tibia, and fluid is directly administered into the bone marrow. Fluids and medications are absorbed rapidly via this route. An initial fluid bolus for a child is 20 mg/kg of lactated Ringer's solution, followed by assessment; if the child's condition does not improve, this is repeated, followed by colloids or blood according to the trauma protocols of the hospital. Dextrose 5% is not given to children because it is a hypertonic solution and may cause damage to blood cells if given in quantity.

A nasogastric tube is usually inserted unless there is facial trauma; the tube is connected to low suction to assure gastric decompression and decrease the risk of vomiting and aspiration. A urinary catheter is also inserted in most seriously injured patients to determine urine output. A suprapubic tap may be performed in certain cases, but externally applied urine bags or condom catheters are rarely used.

> If blood is found at the meatus, a urinary catheter should not be inserted, as there may be disruption in the urinary tract. A urologist should be consulted immediately.

Other interventions for trauma patients will depend on the type and severity of injuries, and may include insertion of chest tubes and a variety of surgical procedures and diagnostic tests.

Diagnostic Tests for the Multiple Trauma Patient

Once the patient has arrived in the emergency setting and has undergone an initial evaluation and interventions, many diagnostic tests are performed to assist in the evaluation process.

Standard trauma protocols for laboratory tests usually include a complete blood count (CBC) with differential, coagulation profiles, serum electrolytes, blood urea nitrogen (BUN), creatinine, glucose, amylase, lipase, serum glutamic-oxaloacetic transaminase (SGOT),* serum glutamic-pyruvate transaminase (SGPT),* blood type and crossmatch, and urinalysis. Arterial blood gases are obtained if there are signs of shock or respiratory distress.

Radiologic films are also obtained. The cross-table lateral cervical spine x-ray is the first x-ray obtained. Anteroposterior and open mouth views may also be obtained. The purpose is to check the alignment and intactness of all seven cervical vertebra. Other x-rays will be ordered on the basis of physical assessment. A chest x-ray may be ordered to check endotracheal tube placement, presence of pneumothorax, rib fracture, clavicle fractures, and the intactness of the diaphragm. Other x-rays are ordered based on the child's condition.

Nursing Care of the Child and Family

The most critical aspect of nursing care of the pediatric trauma patient is continuous assessment of respiratory and circulatory status. These patients must be observed for the early signs of shock, and intervention must proceed immediately to prevent rapid and irreversible deterioration. Preparing for the many procedures and examinations required and observing the equipment used for monitoring should not interfere with close and continuous observation of the patient's signs and symptoms.

Nursing care of the child also requires care of the family. When the family arrives at the hospital, one staff member should be identified as their contact person and should provide regular updates. The family should be allowed to

*SGOT is also known as AST (aspartate aminotransferase). SGPT is also known as ALT (alanine aminotransferase).

be with the patient as soon as possible, if they so desire. Even when the child is in critical condition, parents should be allowed in, however briefly, attended by a staff member who will be responsible for them. Hospital staff are often uncomfortable about parental presence in a critical situation, but all agree that they would want to be there if it were their child. Remember that consent must be obtained from the families of patients for all procedures, unless the intervention is required to save the life of the child.

Assessing for Child Abuse. No discussion of pediatric trauma is complete without mentioning the possibility of child maltreatment as a cause of the injury. Nurses working in emergency settings play an important role in both the assessment and reporting of child maltreatment. In acute care settings, there is rarely time to assess parent–child interactions or to observe at length the behavioral indicators of the child, although these may provide important information (see Chapter 41). Some of the most important indicators that raise the suspicion of child maltreatment in the emergency setting include:

- a history inconsistent with physical findings
- activity reportedly leading to the trauma that seems inconsistent with the age of the child
- delay in seeking treatment for the trauma
- a history of other emergency visits.

There may also be physical findings that should raise the level of suspicion:

- bruises or fractures in various stages of healing noted on x-ray
- injuries rarely found in children (such as long bone or rib fractures) when the history is not appropriate for the injury
- patterns of injury indicating that a specific object caused injury (i.e., belt marks, cigarette burns).

These indicators should be carefully assessed in the context of the injury and in relation to the affect of the child and family. Observe the family's reaction to the child and staff, keeping in mind that people may behave very differently depending on culture, ethnicity, experience, and psychological makeup. Above all, do not assume an investigative role—that is law enforcement's responsibility. Nurses are required to report suspicion of child maltreatment, however, so be careful to document any observations in detail. It may help to remember that over 90% of parents who have abused their children feel ashamed of doing so, but are unable to control the impulse. When child maltreatment is suspected, the intervention of child protective services is essential to assure the safety of the child to prevent further injury.

Nursing Care During Recovery. Regardless of the cause of the injury, the majority of pediatric trauma patients do well, unless the injuries are extremely severe; their cardiovascular systems are strong, and their bodies are growing, allowing them to compensate for even the most serious injuries. Even children with severe head injuries have far more favorable chances of recovery than do adults. These patients and their families have a great need for nursing support to recover from both the physical and psychological effects of trauma; the need for rehabilitation must be considered from the moment the patient arrives in the emergency setting.

SUBMERSION INJURIES (NEAR DROWNING)

Drowning is the second leading cause of accidental death in children. "Drowning" is defined as submersion that results in asphyxia and death within 24 hours. If the child survives longer than 24 hours after submersion, the event is referred to as "near drowning."

PATHOPHYSIOLOGY *of Submersion Injury*

Hypoxia is responsible for the injury to organ systems when drowning occurs. The extent of damage depends on length of submersion, extent of hypothermia, and the physiologic response of the victim.

Drowning progresses in a predictable sequence of events. The drowning child panics and struggles in the water and attempts to hold his breath. Then the child usually swallows a small amount of water, vomits, and aspirates the vomitus. This either causes laryngospasm, leading to hypoxia, seizures, and death (dry drowning), or the child becomes unconscious from hypoxia, loses airway reflexes, and aspirates large amounts of water into the lungs and stomach (wet drowning). As hypoxia and acidosis progress, cardiopulmonary arrest occurs. The majority of submerged children aspirate water.

Submersion also results in hypothermia. Children lose body heat quickly in cold water because of their relatively large surface area. Severe hypothermia offers some protection to the brain. The diving reflex is stimulated when the face is submerged in cold water. This neurologic reflex shunts blood away from the periphery, increasing blood flow to the brain and heart. The diving reflex may be stronger in young children than in adults. Irreversible brain damage usually occurs after 4 to 6 minutes of submersion, but some children have had a complete recovery after lengthy submersion (10 to 40 minutes) in very cold water.

One of the most important nursing responsibilities related to drowning is prevention of injury, including water safety education and training, support of legislative efforts to pass drowning prevention measures, and teaching of CPR. Nurses must emphasize the importance of adequate adult supervision when children are in or around water. (See Chapter 13 for further discussion of drowning prevention.)

Etiology. Most drownings occur in residential swimming pools. Children can become submerged in any body of water, including hot tubs, spas, bathtubs, toilets, and even buckets. Open water sites, such as lakes, rivers, and oceans, are more likely to be the site of accidents among teenagers. Alcohol is often a factor in teenage drownings.

Incidence. Each year approximately 4,000 children die from drowning. Near drowning accounts for three to four times as many injuries as drowning. Forty percent of drowning victims are under age 4 years. Boys are five times more likely than girls to die from drowning. Drowning is more likely to occur in the summertime, on weekends, and between 4 and 6 p.m.

Clinical Manifestations. The child's condition after near drowning varies with the extent of injury:

Conscious with Adequate Respirations

- May have mild hypothermia
- Slight changes on chest x-ray
- Slight arterial blood gas changes

Unconscious with Adequate Respirations

- May be obtunded or stuporous; purposeful response to painful stimuli
- May have mild to moderate hypothermia
- Abnormal chest x-ray, mild to moderate respiratory distress
- Arterial blood gas abnormalities

Unconscious with Absent or Inadequate Respirations

- Comatose, abnormal response to pain
- Seizures, shock
- Marked arterial blood gas abnormalities, metabolic acidosis
- Hyperkalemia, hyperglycemia
- May develop disseminated intravascular coagulation

Complete Cardiopulmonary Arrest

Therapeutic Management. Treatment begins at the scene of the accident with rescue and removal from the water. The prehospital care the child receives may significantly affect the chances for a normal recovery. Prompt initiation of CPR and activation of the emergency medical system is imperative.

As with other types of trauma, management begins with the ABCs (airway, breathing, circulation), including spinal immobilization when spinal injury is a possibility. When the child is in both cardiac and respiratory arrest, CPR must be initiated using BLS procedures (see pp. 321–322). Often the victim of submersion injury has a heartbeat but is not breathing. In such a case the goal of resuscitation is resumption of respiration. Every child with submersion injury is considered hypoxic—the major task is to assure adequate ventilation and oxygenation. When the brain is deprived of oxygen for even a short period of time, irreversible brain damage may occur. The child's airway is opened, with care being taken to protect the neck from movement if cervical injury is suspected. The oropharynx should be suctioned to remove mucus and fluid. Oxygen is given by mask at 10 L/minute. If the respiratory rate is inadequate and/or breathing is shallow, ventilation is assisted with a bag-valve-mask device using 100% oxygen. Overinflation of the lungs should be carefully avoided to prevent causing a pneumothorax—the lungs should be inflated until the chest just begins to rise. Elevating the head of the bed to 30° may help to lower intracranial pressure; this should be done only if there is no spinal injury or shock. Intubation may be necessary for unconscious and nonbreathing children.

A cardiac monitor is used for ongoing assessment of heart rate and rhythm. The child's cardiovascular status must be assessed at regular intervals in addition to observing the rhythm on the cardiac monitor because presence of a cardiac rhythm does not ensure perfusion of the tissues.

Hypothermia. For mild *hypothermia* (33° to 35° C), the child should be kept covered with warm blankets, and warming lights should be used if available. More severe hypothermia may require aggressive measures such as warming of resuscitation fluids, warm baths, and lavage with warm fluids. Warming measures may lead to decreased blood pressure due to vasodilation. Blood pressure must be monitored closely.

Pulse oximetry should be used to determine oxygenation, and arterial blood gases should be measured on all patients with significant injury. Sodium bicarbonate to correct acidosis should be used only on the basis of blood gas analysis. A baseline chest x-ray should be obtained when the patient is relatively stable. Pulmonary edema is usually diagnosed after a few hours; it is not usually present in the first hour after a submersion incident.

Shock. Two intravenous lines should be started immediately in critically ill submersion injury patients. Lactated Ringer's or normal saline solution should be given on the basis of clinical assessment: rapid heart rate, altered level of consciousness, and abnormal skin signs may signal impending shock. A fluid bolus of 20 ml/kg should be given rapidly when shock is suspected. Assessment should follow the fluid bolus, and the same amount may be given again immediately if perfusion has not improved. All fluids given should be closely monitored to prevent fluid overload. Urine output should be checked hourly. If a urinary catheter is not inserted, a urine bag can be placed on the child, or diapers can be weighed.

Gastric Distension. Both air and water may be swallowed during a submersion incident. Air may also be forced into the stomach with resuscitative efforts. Because gastric distension resulting from air and water in the stomach may prevent full expansion of the lungs, a nasogastric tube should be inserted to ensure full respiratory excursion and prevent aspiration of stomach contents from vomiting. A toxicology screen should be ordered for suctioned stomach contents when substance abuse is suspected.

Diagnostic Tests and Laboratory Procedures

Measurement of Urine Output. The kidneys may be damaged by hypoxia during the submersion incident. Urine output is measured to determine adequacy of renal function—normal urine output is 1 to 2 ml/kg/hr. A urinary catheter may be inserted and the urine output measured every 15 to 20 minutes during the first few hours.

Blood Tests. Standard blood analyses for submersion injuries include: hemoglobin and hematocrit, CBC, serum electrolytes, BUN, creatinine level, and serum amylase. An arterial blood gas sample may be obtained. If the patient is in shock or has experienced significant trauma, typing and crossmatching of two to four units of blood should be included. When substance abuse is a possibility, a toxicology screen may be ordered on blood, urine, and stomach contents. Unless there has been a lengthy hypoxic period, laboratory findings may be close to normal during resuscitation.

Blood should be obtained for laboratory analysis while the intravenous line is being inserted, when possible. Even when the history indicates a short submersion period, the patient should be observed for at least 6 hours or be admitted to the hospital for further observation.

NURSING CARE OF THE CHILD WITH SUBMERSION INJURIES

Nursing care of the child with submersion injury requires obtaining an accurate history, assuring adequacy of the airway and tissue perfusion, and maintaining body temperature.

Assessment

Assessment of the child with a submersion injury focuses on the respiratory system. Airway and breathing are the first priorities. Observe the child for rate and depth of respiration and work of breathing. Cardiovascular assessment should include assessment of capillary refill and heart rate. The child's temperature should be taken as soon as possible, as hypothermia is common in cold water submersion. Assess the child's mental and neurologic status. (See Chapter 40 for discussion of neurologic assessment.)

An accurate history of the injury is important, although often difficult to obtain. Whether the submersion incident occurred in salt or fresh water is irrelevant in terms of early treatment, but subsequent intensive care may vary somewhat depending on the immersion fluid.

Nursing Diagnosis and Planning

Nursing Diagnosis

- Impaired Gas Exchange (Actual or Potential) related to bronchospasm, aspiration of fluid, surfactant elimination, or pulmonary edema.

Expected Outcome: The child will maintain a Pco_2 lower than 50 mmHg and a Po_2 higher than 90 mmHg.

Nursing Diagnosis

- Altered Cerebral Tissue Perfusion related to severe anoxia and increased intrancranial pressure caused by fluid shifts with freshwater aspiration.

Expected Outcome: The child will maintain a systolic blood pressure greater than 70 mmHg.

Nursing Diagnosis

- Fluid Volume Excess or Deficit related to volume shifts from interstitial to intravascular space.

Expected Outcome: The child will maintain urine output greater than 1 to 2 ml/kg/hr.

Nursing Diagnosis

- Hypothermia related to prolonged exposure.

Expected Outcome: The child will maintain body temperature within normal limits.

Nursing Diagnosis

- Ineffective Family Coping related to child's critical status.

Expected Outcomes: The family will:

- verbalize feelings and concerns appropriately.
- exhibit an attitude of confidence in care.
- demonstrate an understanding of the child's condition and therapeutic interventions.

Implementation

After the initial assessment has been completed, the nurse will monitor for changes from the baseline, anticipate the development of complications, and implement appropriate medical and nursing interventions.

Respiratory System. Because hypoxia is the main problem, with potential for damage to all major organ systems, attention to the pulmonary system is a priority. The nurse listens for adventitious breath sounds, which may signal the development of complications such as pulmonary edema, atelectasis, or pneumonia. Persistent hypoxemia, dyspnea, tachycardia, and respiratory alkalosis may also signal these pulmonary complications. If the child is intubated, the nurse maintains the airway and observes for signs of tube displacement or pneumothorax. A nasogastric tube is inserted after the airway is protected to decompress the stomach. This will allow for easier ventilation and reduce the risk of aspiration.

Cardiovascular System. Cardiovascular assessment includes vital sign measurement, assessment of perfusion, level of consciousness, skin temperature, color, and urine output. Although peripheral perfusion can be assessed by pulses and blood pressure, particular attention is given to end organ perfusion (kidneys and brain). The well perfused child will be alert with age-appropriate behavior, have a capillary refill time of less than 2 seconds, and urine output of 1 ml/kg/hr. The nurse prepares for and/or inserts intravenous/intraosseous lines and administers fluid volume replacement.

Neurologic System. The neurologic system is assessed and monitored frequently. Common parameters include level of consciousness, pupillary response, movement of extremities, reflexes, and vital signs. The nurse should anticipate signs and symptoms of increased intracranial pressure 48 to 72 hours after the submersion event. Conventional measures to prevent increased intracranial pressure such as positioning the head in the midline, elevating the head of the bed 30°, and preventing or managing elevated body temperature are instituted as ordered and as needed.

Genitourinary System. The nurse will also assess the child's renal status. Renal insufficiency should be anticipated as a result of hypoxia. Urine output, specific gravity, pH, glucose, protein, ketones, BUN, and serum creatinine are major indicators of renal function.

Fluids and Electrolytes. As a result of ingestion of large amounts of water during the near drowning event, the child is at risk for developing alterations in fluid and electrolyte balance. The nurse will carefully monitor urine output, laboratory data, and physical signs and symptoms. Hyponatremia and water intoxication should be anticipated. The nurse should observe for changes in central nervous system functioning, especially seizures, as the serum sodium level drops.

Infection Control. The acutely ill child is at risk for local and/or systemic infection. Intubation and ventilation tubes, invasive monitoring lines, and urinary catheters are possible sources for infection. If infection is present, antibiotic therapy will be started. The child's response to the therapy will be monitored.

Gastrointestinal System. The gastrointestinal system may suffer the effects of hypoxia as well. Blood supply to the bowel may be decreased. Stress ulcers and gastrointestinal bleeding are not uncommon. The nurse is responsible for monitoring gastrointestinal function in terms of what goes in (NPO, oral or enteral feedings), what goes on inside (bowel sounds and residual feedings), and what comes out (presence or absence of blood; amount, color, and consistency of stool).

Nutritional Status. The increased metabolic demands of the child, along with disruption of gastrointestinal functioning, may result in a nutritional deficit. The nurse is responsible for ongoing assessment of nutritional status and implementation of nutritional therapy in the form of enteral feedings or total parenteral nutrition. If enteral feedings are ordered, the nurse will monitor weight gain, residuals, amount and consistency of stools, and vomiting to ascertain tolerance of the feedings. If total parenteral nutrition is ordered, the nurse will check the label with the order, administer the fluid as ordered, and monitor for any side effects. Blood chemistries will be followed as well.

Emotional Care of the Family

Because children brought in to the emergency department with CPR in progress rarely have a good outcome, an important element of nursing care is also psychological intervention and support for the child's family.

The most important nursing interventions with the family of any critically ill or injured child initially include attention to the physical needs of the family and provision of information and hope. The family should have privacy, access to a bathroom and a telephone, and an identified staff member to contact when they have questions (Lenaghan, 1988).

> The highest ranked need of families in most research studies is the need for hope. The need for privacy and comfort are also consistently identified as extremely important by the families of critically ill and injured children; these needs are usually ranked higher than the need for psychological support from nursing staff.

In most cases, families should be allowed to see their child in the treatment area, especially if the child is likely to die and the family may not have an opportunity to see him alive again (Henderson & Brownstein, 1994). It is very important to be honest with the family. If the child is in full arrest, a simple statement such as, "Your child (use the child's name if possible) is not breathing, and has no heartbeat. We are supporting his breathing and helping his heart to beat right now." This statement is far better than "We're doing everything we can," which leaves much more room for doubt. If the parents are to be brought into the resuscitation room, one person should be in charge of them, bringing them in and escorting them out at appropriate times.

Parents may react in many different ways, according to their cultures, religious beliefs, and individual personalities. Remember that denial can be protective initially, and allow the family to accept information gradually. Ask the family if they want other family members or clergy contacted. Religious rites, including baptism, may be very important to the families. A list of clergy from a variety of religions should be readily available for use by the nursing staff.

It is always important to provide hope for the family. At times the only hope may be that the child is not suffering or did not suffer. If the child survives the incident, the parents will have ample time to adjust to the worst news, so it is not necessary to insist on their acceptance at this point. There have been many miraculous recoveries of lengthy submersions, although these are usually in very cold water. In the emergency setting, however, it is impossible to predict the ultimate outcome for a child; a realistically positive attitude, with acknowledgment of the strong possibility of long-term effects for the child, is the most reasonable approach.

Evaluation

Has the child's neurologic status returned to its predrowning state? Is the child's urine output greater than 1 to 2 ml/kg/hr? Do the parents verbalize their feelings and concerns appropriately?

INGESTIONS AND POISONINGS

The combination of curiosity, lack of fear, and evolving motor ability place all children at risk for toxic exposure and **ingestion.** There are differences, however, in types of incident by age-group. Younger children (age 1 through 5 years) are indiscriminately curious, and can innocently ingest a toxic substance in a matter of seconds, although the amount of substance ingested tends to be small (Tennenbein, 1992). As children grow, they gradually learn from parents to avoid dangerous substances, but accidental ingestions and exposures may still occur, and often in larger amounts. In adolescence, the risk is higher for deliberate ingestion; according to the American Association of Poison Control Centers, children between ages 13 and 19 years have three times as many reported fatalities from poisonings as children under age 6 years. Twenty-five percent of pediatric poisonings require emergency intervention; while 75% can be managed at home with advice from a poison control center and/or primary care provider (Dean, 1992).

Incidence. The most common age of poisoning in young children is age 2 years and under, with the greatest incidence occurring at age 1 year. Seventy-six percent of poisonings occur as a result of oral ingestion. Ocular or topical exposure, inhalation, or envenomation account for the remainder of poisoning incidents. Young children are most often poisoned by ingestion of household products, plants, or medications such as acetaminophen (Tylenol), aspirin, vitamins, or minerals. Adolescents have a much higher incidence of ingestion of psychopharmacologic drugs (tranquilizers, sedatives, antidepressants).

Diagnostic Evaluation. Assessment and treatment of toxic exposure and ingestion go hand in hand. Although identification of the type and amount of the exposure is important, the patient must initially be treated on the basis of physical signs and symptoms.

An accurate history of the ingestion is useful in planning care for the patient. History given by the patient, parent, friend, or caretaker may not always be accurate or complete—there are often areas of confusion as well as a reluctance to provide information that may be damaging to themselves or others. It may be helpful to interview all those involved individually if they are available. The most useful questions are listed below.

TOXIC INGESTION QUESTIONS

What substance did the patient ingest?
How much of the substance did the patient ingest?
What time did the ingestion occur?
How has the patient's condition changed from the time of ingestion?
Was any intervention done after the ingestion?
Is it possible the ingestion was intentional? (For adolescents)

(Dean, 1992)

Most ingestions seen in emergency settings occur acutely, and the child is brought in immediately, or when parents realize this event has occurred. An exception to this is lead poisoning. Although lead poisoning is relatively common, it is rarely identified in the emergency setting. A child who has unusual neurologic signs or symptoms, neuropathy, footdrop, or anemia that cannot be attributed to other causes may be suffering from lead poisoning. This most often occurs when a child ingests or inhales paint chips or powder of lead-based paint. Other common sources of lead include dust or soil contaminated by emissions from lead smelters, some vinyl mini blinds, improperly glazed pottery, and paint from peeling walls or dust from remodeling in older buildings. A careful history may assist in the diagnosis of lead poisoning, but accurate diagnosis is made by testing blood lead levels. The child is generally admitted to the hospital; chelation therapy is administered on an inpatient basis to remove lead from the blood and tissue.

The information obtained in the history of the ingestion will be combined with the patient's presenting physical assessment to provide a complete picture of the event and to plan treatment. Laboratory analysis provides definitive diagnosis.

Therapeutic Management. The first step in treatment of a toxic exposure or ingestion is to assess the ABCs and to stabilize the patient. Oxygen may be given and breathing supported with a bag-valve-mask device if necessary. If there is altered level of consciousness, endotracheal intubation may be necessary to protect the airway. When the child has ingested a sufficient amount of a substance to cause rapid deterioration in mental status, an intubation tray should be at the bedside even when he is awake and

TABLE 14–4 *Commonly Ingested Poisonous Substances*

SUBSTANCE	PATHOPHYSIOLOGY	CLINICAL MANIFESTATIONS	TREATMENT
Acetaminophen (Tylenol, many over-the-counter products) Toxic dose: uncertain, do not exceed recommended levels. Seriousness of the ingestion is determined by the amount ingested and the length of time before intervention.	Cellular necrosis of the liver resulting in liver dysfunction and, in some cases, liver failure. Children < age 6 years seem to be more resistant to development of hepatotoxicity than older children and adults.	*First stage* (first 24 hours): malaise, nausea, vomiting, sweating, pallor, weakness. *Second stage* (1 to 3 days): latent period with a rise in liver enzymes (AST, ALT) and bilirubin, right upper quadrant pain, prolonged prothrombin time. *Third stage* (1 week): jaundice, liver necrosis, possible death from hepatic failure.	Induce vomiting or gastric lavage, depending on amount ingested. Administer activated charcoal or antidote: acetylcysteine (Mucomyst). Give po with juice or cola or via NG tube (offensive odor). Do not give charcoal if antidote is anticipated, as charcoal will make antidote ineffective. IV fluids. Sodium-restricted, high-calorie, high-protein diet.
Salicylates (aspirin, many over-the-counter products, oil of wintergreen) Most common cause of drug poisoning in children. Toxic dose: Single dose exceeding 200–280 mg/kg. Peak gastric absorption occurs within 2 hours of ingestion.	*First stage:* Stimulation of respiratory center, leading to respiratory alkalosis, hyperglycemia. *Second stage:* Loss of potassium, increase in metabolic rate and accumulation of ketones leading to metabolic acidosis, hypokalemia, and dehydration. Inhibition of prothrombin formation, decreased platelet levels and adhesiveness, and capillary fragility.	Gastrointestinal (GI) effects: nausea, vomiting, thirst. Central nervous system (CNS) effects: hyperventilation, confusion, seizures, coma, respiratory failure, circulatory collapse. Renal effects: oliguria. Hematopoietic effects: bleeding tendencies. Metabolic effects: sweating, dehydration, fever, hyponatremia, hypokalemia, dehydration, hypoglycemia.	Induce vomiting with syrup of ipecac or perform gastric lavage; administer activated charcoal to decrease absorption. IV fluids, sodium bicarbonate (enhances excretion), electrolytes; volume expanders as needed to support circulation. Vitamin K for bleeding tendencies. Glucose for hypoglycemia. Dialysis in severe cases if child unresponsive to therapy.
Corrosives (toilet and drain cleaners, bleach, ammonia) Extent of damage depends on the causticity of the substance and the amount ingested.	Severe chemical burns of mouth, throat, esophagus. Alkali substances can continue to cause damage after initial contact. If damage is severe, long-term care is needed, including repeated esophageal dilatations and surgical repair of esophagus, sometimes with colon tissue transplant (done when child is older).	Whitish burns of mouth and pharynx, color darkens (red, swollen, and oozing as ulcerations form and tissue erodes). Edema, difficulty swallowing, drooling. Respiratory distress, pain. Difficulty swallowing; subsequent healing of burns can produce esophageal strictures. Severe burns causing perforation can lead to vascular collapse and shock.	Do not induce vomiting: do not lavage. Activated charcoal may be given. Dilute with small amounts of water orally (take care not to stimulate vomiting). Flood external areas with large amounts of water. Endoscopy to diagnose esophageal burns. Tracheostomy if severe respiratory distress; possible gastrostomy, possible esophageal dilatations to prevent strictures and to maintain patency of esophagus. IV fluids while NPO. Analgesics, steroids, antibiotics, NG tube feedings.
Hydrocarbons (gasoline, kerosene, paint thinner, lighter fluid, turpentine, furniture polish)	Chemical pneumonitis from aspiration of hydrocarbon. Pneumonia and acute hemorrhagic necrotizing disease, usually in 24 hours.	Burning sensation in mouth and pharynx. Characteristic petroleum breath odor. Nausea, vomiting, anorexia, CNS depression, fever.	Do not induce vomiting. Support ventilation; administer oxygen, antibiotics, IV fluids.

TABLE 14–4 *Commonly Ingested Poisonous Substances (continued)*

SUBSTANCE	PATHOPHYSIOLOGY	CLINICAL MANIFESTATIONS	TREATMENT
Lead (paint chips, soil contaminated with lead, lead solder used in plumbing, vinyl mini blinds, improperly glazed pottery) Diet high in fat and low in iron and calcium increases lead absorption. Erythrocyte protoporphyrin (EP) levels are used to screen children for lead levels and anemia: EP ≤ 9 µg/dl are considered normal. > 9 µg/dl: more frequent screening indicated; > 15 µg/dl: nutritional and educational interventions and environmental investigation; > 20 µg/dl: pharmacologic treatment.	GI tract is the major route of absorption. Lead is deposited in the blood, bone, and soft tissue. Major toxic effects occur in the bone marrow, nervous system, and kidney. Amount of lead ingested, size of the particle, and repeated ingestion over time contribute to severity of lead poisoning.	Symptoms may be vague with insidious onset. CNS effects: irritability, lethargy, hyperactivity, cognitive and perceptual-motor difficulties, clumsiness, seizures, coma, and death (associated with blood level of >100 µg/dl). Hematopoietic effects: anemia. GI effects: anorexia, nausea, vomiting, constipation, lead line along gums. Skeletal effects: increased density of long bones, lead line in long bones. Renal effects: glycosuria, proteinuria, possible acute or chronic renal failure. Kidney damage is reversible early in the disease, but with continued lead exposure, permanent kidney damage may occur.	Remove child from lead source, hospitalize. Administer chelating agents: EDTA (usually in combination with BAL; given IM for 5 days (causes lead to be deposited in bone and excreted via kidneys); monitor kidney function because EDTA is nephrotoxic; monitor calcium levels because EDTA enhances excretion of calcium. Calcium, phosphorus, and vitamin D aid lead excretion. Anticonvulsants, oral or IM iron. Follow-up lead levels to monitor progress (lead is excreted more slowly than it accumulates in the body).
Iron (vitamin supplements with iron) Second most commonly ingested poisonous substance in children.	Corrosive effect on the GI mucosa; may leave deposits in the liver.	*First stage:* (1–4 hours): bloody stools, vomiting (hematemesis), abdominal pain. *Second stage* (8–12 hours): symptoms subside, child remains asymptomatic for 12 to 36 hours. *Third stage:* fever, metabolic acidosis, shock, seizures, coma.	Induce vomiting. Administer IV fluids and sodium bicarbonate. Deferoxamine chelation therapy for severe intoxication (with severe overdose, the urine will be pink or red after deferoxamine administration).
Carbon Monoxide Most often from improperly ventilated heaters; also from poorly ventilated vehicles. The cause of the exposure should be determined and eliminated.	An odorless, colorless gas that binds to receptors on hemoglobin more effectively than does oxygen, thereby causing hypoxia.	Headache, visual disturbances. Altered level of consciousness, cherry red lips and cheeks, nausea, and vomiting.	100% oxygen by rebreathing mask. Serum carboxyhemoglobin levels, hyperbaric chamber treatment may be necessary for patients with high carboxyhemoglobin levels. Other interventions are based on signs and symptoms.
Narcotics and Sedative-Hypnotics Occurs most often in adolescence, but may also occur at any age when a family member is a substance abuser.	Respiratory and CNS depression.	CNS and respiratory depression, hypotension.	Respiratory support, gastric emptying, and activated charcoal. Blood gas analysis may be ordered if patient is hypoventilating. Naloxone is given for narcotic overdose in all age-groups.

alert (Dean, 1992). If the patient is in shock, or shows signs of compensated shock, fluid resuscitation should be initiated. Cardiac rhythm disturbances can result from many ingested substances, so placement of a cardiac monitor and pulse oximeter are also indicated. An intravenous line should be established for any patient with a significant ingestion because medications or fluid resuscitation may be necessary.

Care of the patient who has been exposed to or ingested a toxic substance depends on the amount ingested and the toxicity of the ingested substance (Table 14–4). After initial stabilization of the patient, absorption of the ingested poison should be decreased (Tennenbein, 1992). Several methods are commonly used for removal of toxic substances: dilution of the toxin, administration of syrup of ipecac, gastric lavage, and administration of activated charcoal (AC).

Dilution of the Toxin. Dilution is used for acid or alkali ingestions; milk or water is usually recommended. Since these caustic substances will continue to cause damage until neutralized, **emesis should not be induced.**

Syrup of Ipecac. There is an ongoing controversy as to whether the value of syrup of ipecac and gastric lavage outweighs the risk (Tennenbein, 1992). Ipecac produces vomiting and rapid stomach emptying, primarily through gastric irritation and secondarily through central stimulation of the medullary chemoreceptor trigger zone (Dean, 1992). Ipecac should be followed with 6 to 12 ounces of clear fluid. Emesis generally occurs within 20 minutes and may last for several hours. Ipecac is available without prescription, and should be cautiously administered to any child under age 1 year; between age 6 months and 1 year, ipecac may be recommended in certain cases (Dean, 1992). Absolute contraindications for ipecac are:

- decreased level of consciousness (due to risk of aspiration)
- ingestion of a corrosive or petroleum-based substance
- ingestion of drugs that result in rapid deterioration of the mental status.

Gastric Lavage. Gastric lavage is used for gastric emptying in the first 1 to 2 hours after the ingestion. This method is selected when the toxic ingestion has potentially serious complications such as seizures, decreased level of consciousness, respiratory depression, and cardiac effects. Lavage should not be used following ingestion of corrosives, because of the danger of esophageal perforation. The child is placed on his left side, with the head lowered about 10° in the Trendelenburg position. Depending on the size of the child, a 16 to 32 French nasal or orogastric tube is inserted, small amounts of normal saline are given through the tube, and are removed along with the substance. This process is repeated until the fluid return is clear (Barkin, 1992). The returned fluid should be observed for any type of pill fragments or toxic substance. Activated charcoal is given after the completion of the lavage process.

Activated Charcoal. Activated charcoal is a charcoal substance with a porous surface that binds to the toxin and passes through the gastrointestinal system. It is generally administered after the use of ipecac and/or gastric lavage. It is also used when the ingestion has occurred longer than 2 hours prior to presentation to the emergency setting (Dean, 1992). Activated charcoal can bind to the toxin at any point along the gastrointestinal tract. The longer the time between activated charcoal administration and the time the toxin was ingested, however, the less effective it will be. If the patient has received ipecac, ongoing vomiting may delay administration and retention of activated charcoal. Activated charcoal is prepared with or without sorbitol, which is added to act as a cathartic, facilitating transport of the toxin through the gastrointestinal tract; it also makes the charcoal more palatable. Mixing the activated charcoal with chocolate milk also sometimes makes it easier to drink. Often, children refuse to drink the activated charcoal, and it must be administered via a nasogastric tube. Activated charcoal administration may be repeated to prevent reabsorption of the toxin from fluid secreted in the biliary tract. Caution must be taken when administering activated charcoal with sorbitol, especially with multiple doses, because this may lead to severe diarrhea and potential fluid and electrolyte problems in children. The dose is generally 1 g/kg in children (Barkin, 1992).

Antidotes. Specific antidotes may be used to inhibit the absorption of the toxin at the receptor site or reduce the concentration. Examples of commonly used antidotes are acetylcysteine (Mucomyst) for acetaminophen ingestion and naloxone for narcotics. (See also Table 14–4.)

Laboratory and Diagnostic Tests. Laboratory tests are performed to assess serum levels of the substance and the effect of the toxin on body systems. Regional poison control centers and clinical pharmacists should be included as members of the treatment team. Blood glucose level may be tested initially by means of a reagent strip. Measurement of serum glucose level and toxicologic analysis of urine, serum, and stomach contents are the most common laboratory tests ordered for toxic exposure or ingestion. Blood gases may be required if the patient is hypoventilating.

NURSING CARE OF THE CHILD WHO HAS INGESTED A TOXIC SUBSTANCE

Assessment

Accurate and rapid assessment of the poisoned child may mean the difference between life and death. The child's condition, beginning with respiratory function, should be assessed. Rate, depth, and effort of breathing are noted. Vital signs are taken and re-evaluated frequently. Respiratory and/or circulatory support are initiated as needed. Because shock is a result of ingestion of many toxic substances, blood pressure, tissue perfusion, and urine output are carefully monitored. The nurse should observe and document the child's mental status frequently to determine any changes in level of consciousness. Changes in pupil size or reactivity as well as occurrence of seizures are assessed.

The nurse should take the responsibility for assessing the cause of poisoning. A poisoning incident is extremely distressing to parents, and detailed questioning should be deferred until the child's condition is stabilized. If the ingestion was purposeful, psychological consultation and referral should be provided.

Nursing Diagnosis and Planning

Nursing Diagnosis

- Risk for Injury related to insufficient parental knowledge about first aid for toxic ingestion and accidental poisonings

Expected Outcome: The child will receive appropriate treatment by parents if accidental poisoning occurs.

Nursing Diagnosis

- Ineffective Breathing Pattern related to effects of toxic substances

Expected Outcome: The child will maintain adequate oxygenation and ventilation as evidenced by normal arterial blood gases and serum pH or pulse oximetry.

Nursing Diagnosis

- Risk for Fluid Volume Deficit related to effects of ingested substances, treatment modalities, or decreased fluid intake

Expected Outcome: The child will maintain a urine output of 1 to 2 ml/kg/hr, with age-appropriate specific gravity.

Nursing Diagnosis

- Ineffective Family Coping related to sudden hospitalization and emergency aspects of illness

Expected Outcomes: The family will:

- demonstrate an understanding of the child's condition and treatment.
- verbalize feelings and concerns appropriately.
- remain with the child as much as possible.

Nursing Diagnosis

- Risk for Poisoning related to insufficient parental knowledge about poisoning prevention

Expected Outcomes:

- The child will not ingest potentially toxic substances.
- The parents make the necessary changes in the home environment to prevent poisoning.

Implementation

Stabilization of the patient, as described above, is the nurse's first priority in caring for the child who has ingested a poisonous substance. Nursing care also includes reducing the child's and the family's fear and anxiety, providing preventive teaching concerning the storage of poisons and supervision of children, and removal of the poison from the child's skin and mucous membranes to reduce further injury.

Parents are usually overwhelmed by feelings of self-blame, fear, and anger when their child has ingested a poisonous substance. Providing an opportunity for them to express their feelings in a nonjudgmental atmosphere helps parents cope with this experience. Aspects of treatment such as induction of vomiting, placement of a nasogastric tube, or support of ventilation are disturbing and frightening to parents. The nurse offers support by explaining treatment and keeping the parents informed about the status of their child.

Ideally, nurses intervene with parents before a poisoning incident occurs. Discussion of safe storage of medications and other potentially toxic substances as well as age-appropriate supervision of children are essential aspects of poison prevention. (See Chapter 13 for discussion of poison prevention.) Parents should be instructed to keep two bottles of syrup of ipecac available in the home and to be familiar with its use and proper dosage. This and other injury prevention information should be readily available in emergency care settings and should be given to families when a child is discharged. Education through community programs to prevent poisoning and reduce drug abuse should be directed to young children as well as to adolescents, parents, and caretakers.

Evaluation

Do parents verbalize common household hazards that can result in child poisoning?

Are preventive measures in place in the home? Is ipecac available in the home?

Do parents verbalize the appropriate actions to take when a child has been poisoned?

ANIMAL, HUMAN, AND SNAKE BITES

Incidence. Animal bites in the pediatric age-group are most often from domestic animals and have the highest incidence in school-age male children (Barkin, 1992; Gershman, Sacks, & Wright, 1994; Sinclair & Zhou, 1995). Most bites are from dogs, usually a dog familiar to the victim (Wiggins, Akelman, & Weiss, 1994). Larger dogs can cause serious damage—their teeth can exert up to 450 pounds of pressure per square inch (Barkin, 1992). Chows, Dobermans, German shepherds, pit bulls, and Rottweilers have all caused serious bite injuries to children (Avner & Baker, 1991; Clark et al., 1991; Gershman, Sacks, & Wright, 1994).

Cats are the most common family pets, and although a cat bite is less likely to cause serious injury initially, it is more likely to become infected than a dog bite. Bites from pet birds, rats, ferrets, pigs, hamsters, turtles, fish, alligators, snakes, horses, and many other animals have been seen in emergency settings, as well as all varieties of wild animals such as raccoons, skunks, coyotes, and others.

In the United States, there are two groups of poisonous snakes: pit vipers (Crotalidae), such as rattlesnakes, water moccasins, and copperheads, and coral snakes (Elapidae). Each year there are 45,000 reported snakebites—less than 20% of these are from venomous snakes (Gold & Wingert, 1994). Almost half (45%) of the bites from venomous snakes are dry bites, delivering no venom (Gold & Wingert, 1994; Semonin-Holleran, 1993). Annually, there are 9 to 15 fatalities from snakebites, mostly children and the elderly (Gold & Wingert, 1994).

Etiology

Animal and Human Bites. Both animal and human bites involve soft tissue damage from crushing, lacerations, and puncture wounds (Tuggle, Taylor, & Stevens, 1993). All animal bites have potential for infection. Although human bites are relatively rare, they carry the greatest risk of infection (Barkin, 1992).

> There is increased risk for serious infection from animal bites found in the following locations:
> - Scalp and face of infants
> - Hands, wrists, feet
> - Tendons and joints

Snake Bites. Envenomations of children on land are usually from snakes, scorpions, and spiders (see Chapter 34 for a discussion of scorpions, spiders, and hymenoptera). Envenomation may also result from marine animals such as jellyfish, sea urchins, and stingrays, although these will not be included in this discussion. Fatalities from **envenomation** are rare; most occur from snakebites.

Clinical Manifestations. Treatment depends on the seriousness and cause of the bite. Serious injury may result from any type of bite, but most dog bites are not life-threatening. Human bites are more serious because of the risk of infection and may be differentiated from dog bites by the distance between the canines; in human bites the distance is generally greater than 3 cm. A human bite is horseshoe-shaped, and rarely breaks the skin (Kelley, 1994).

Snake Bites. To determine the cause of envenomation, medical staff in emergency settings should have some knowledge of the venomous snakes likely to be encountered in the surrounding geographic area, although envenomation may also occur from exotic pets. In general,

- Venomous snakes have vertically elliptic pupils; facial pit between their eyes and nostril; rattle and fangs.
- Nonvenomous snakes have round pupils; no pit, rattle, or fangs (Barkin, 1992).

Whether or not the snake can be positively identified, treatment of the patient should be on the basis of physical assessment and symptoms. The following are the most common signs and symptoms suggesting envenomation:

Local Signs and Symptoms

- Bite marks that look like fang marks
- Burning at the site
- Ecchymosis
- Pain or numbness
- Swelling and erythema

Systemic Signs and Symptoms of Severe Envenomation

- Nausea and vomiting
- Sweating, chills
- Numbness, paresthesia of the tongue and perioral region
- Hypotension
- Epistaxis

> Systemic signs and symptoms may develop within 15 minutes of severe envenomation. When a substantial amount of venom has been injected, and when treatment is delayed, envenomation can progress to disseminated intravascular coagulation, respiratory failure, renal failure, seizures, shock, and death.

Therapeutic Management

Animal Bites. Emergency care for animal bites depends on the type of bite, but usually includes thorough irrigation and debridement. Tetanus prophylaxis may be given if the child's immunization is not up to date, or if documentation is unavailable. Antibiotics may be ordered if there is a high probability of infection. Smaller bite wounds are often left open, rather than being sutured, as puncture wounds and wounds closed with sutures have more potential for infection. Treatment of the child for rabies may be necessary, depending on the specifics of the situation.

Snake Bites. Three factors influence the severity of bite from a venomous snake:

1. Age, size and general health of the victim
2. Size of the snake (larger snakes produce more venom)
3. Location of the injury (peripheral injuries account for 90% of the bites and are less severe)

When assessing the patient with a snakebite, identification of the type of snake is helpful, but this is not always possible. In most cases, an expert in the treatment of snake bites should be consulted. Although traditional emergency treatment of envenomation once included use of a tourniquet, incision, and extraction of the venom, this is no longer recommended (Gold & Wingert, 1994). First aid now includes immobilization of the extremity and prompt administration of sufficient quantities of antivenin. Snake venom is absorbed through the lymph system; thus, decreasing the child's activity may aid in decreasing the systemic spread of the venom (Semonin-Holleran, 1993). An intravenous line should be established if envenomation is suspected, for administration of antivenin and possible fluid resuscitation.

When there are no signs or symptoms of envenomation within 4 hours of the bite, it can be considered a dry bite. For mild envenomation (fang marks and local swelling), the patient is observed and may or may not be given antivenin. Moderate to severe envenomations will require antivenin. A small test dose of antivenin is given subcutaneously prior to the full dose to assess hypersensitivity. All patients with venomous bites are admitted to the hospital. Laboratory studies include CBC, platelet count, coagulation studies, electrolytes, and renal function.

NURSING CARE OF THE CHILD WITH AN ANIMAL, HUMAN, OR SNAKE BITE

When there are severe bites, significant envenomation, or anaphylaxis, nursing interventions for bites and envenomations begin with attention to the ABCs and support of vital functions. When there is envenomation, nursing care includes keeping the patient as calm as possible to help prevent spread of the toxin or venom. Few hospitals have sufficient antivenin for severe envenomation, so nurses should make sure of the availability of protocols that include the location of centers to contact for additional antivenim.

The injury site of all bites should be carefully cleaned, and the child should be given tetanus prophylaxis if immunizations are not up to date. When the bite or envenomation is located on an extremity, the extremity should be immobilized. Any jewelry on the affected digit or extremity should be removed immediately—as swelling occurs, the jewelry may be constricting and have to be cut off or bent during removal.

If antivenin is to be administered, obtain a careful history of allergies, as some antivenins are made from horse serum. Document the type and location of the injury, the length of time since the injury, and the signs and symptoms resulting from the injury. The cause of any bite should be carefully explored. There may be a question of inadequate supervision or inadequate containment of potentially dangerous animals. When the injury appears to be a human bite, child abuse or neglect should be considered a possibility and reported when necessary. Notification of the local animal control agency is required for animal bites in most states, and documentation of rabies immunization status of the animal, if available, should be indicated in nursing notes. Quarantine of the animal responsible for the attack may be necessary if the animal can be found.

Discharge instructions should include observation for signs and symptoms of infection and wound care; injury prevention education should be provided for all patients. Parents should be given information about how to teach their children to avoid dog bites.

DENTAL EMERGENCIES

Incidence and Etiology. Injury to the teeth, particularly the anterior teeth, is common in children. Toddlers, because of their lack of coordination, receive dental injuries from falling from or onto furniture. School-age children are more likely to have their teeth injured on playgrounds and in the course of sports activities.

The first teeth begin to erupt at about age 6 months. By about age 2 years, a child has all 20 primary teeth. Permanent teeth come in at about age 5 or 6 years; by adolescence, a child usually has the full complement of 32 permanent teeth, although the eruption of wisdom teeth may be somewhat delayed. Injury to primary and permanent teeth is considered equally serious. Teeth are imbedded in the bones of the maxilla and mandible. Injuries to teeth are generally divided into the following categories:

Concussion	Tooth is not displaced, but pressure may cause pain.
Subluxation	The tooth is moveable within the socket, but is displaced less than 2 mm. There is no damage to the socket.
Intrusion	The tooth is pushed into its socket with injury to the underlying structures.
Extrusion	An upper tooth is dislodged downward from the socket, or a lower tooth is dislodged upward.
Luxation	Lateral movement of the tooth with tearing of the periodontal ligament.
Avulsion	The tooth is no longer in the socket, and the socket itself may be damaged.

Therapeutic Management. Dental emergencies require specialized care, which is often difficult to obtain immediately. Survival of the tooth depends on the periodontal ligament attachment, so concussion, subluxation, lateral luxation, and extrusion, in which the periodontal ligament is still attached, have a better prognosis than complete avulsion of a tooth. Intrusion of a tooth may damage underlying structures to a greater extent and diminish chances for tooth survival.

Time is of the essence in caring for dental injuries. When there is injury to a child's mouth, observe for missing teeth. If a missing tooth cannot be found in the oral cavity, consider possible aspiration (especially when there is difficulty breathing); x-rays may be needed to determine the location of the tooth. To determine whether other teeth are loose or malpositioned, gently palpate (using standard infection precautions) the teeth for movement. If a tooth is loose in the socket, do not remove it. If the position is not correct, repositioning may be necessary when a specialist is available. Many loosened teeth return to normal position if left alone (Sheehy, 1992).

In general, primary teeth are not replanted, as damage to the developing tooth bud may occur. Complete avulsion of a permanent tooth requires care of the socket and of the tooth itself. Survival of an avulsed tooth is dependent to a large extent on the length of time it is out of the mouth. Irreversible damage to the periodontal ligament due to dehydration of the open socket may occur after 60 minutes.

Emergency care by the dentist will include cleaning of the tooth and socket, placement of the tooth in the socket, and splinting of the tooth. Tetanus immunization may be given if needed, and an antibiotic may be prescribed.

NURSING CARE OF THE CHILD WITH A DENTAL INJURY

Parents calling for emergency advice should be instructed to keep the tooth moist in the child's mouth if possible (in front of the lower incisors or under the tongue, for instance). Alternatively, the tooth can be kept in the parent's mouth. If this is not possible, the tooth may be immersed in saline, water, or milk. The teeth should not be cleaned or scrubbed. Although some recommend replacing the tooth in the socket immediately, a parent may replace the tooth backwards, or the tooth or socket may not be clean or free of debris or clots; these problems would decrease the chances of tooth survival. The child should see a dentist if possible or go to an emergency facility for care without delay.

Parents should be given careful discharge instructions and appropriate referrals for continuing care. When appropriate, reassure the family that first teeth are replaced by the second set of teeth, and that there are many ways to assure a good cosmetic outcome even when there is loss of a permanent tooth.

SUMMARY

Nursing care of ill and injured children may seem more complicated than care of adults because of the smaller sizes of children, the different equipment and dosages needed for their care, and age-related psychological differences. Familiarity with the issues related to growth and development of the child, continuing education in pediatric emergency care, and careful organization of pediatric equipment, supplies, referrals, and reference lists can help to decrease anxiety in health care providers and improve the care of children in emergency settings.

KEY CONCEPTS

- Airway management is the most critical element in pediatric emergency care. Emergency assessment and triage should include airway assessment and intervention. Without adequate oxygenation and ventilation, there is little hope of a patient's survival.
- Shock must be recognized early in the pediatric patient, and should always be considered a possibility when there is an increase in heart rate, breathing, or changes in color, temperature, or moisture of the infant's or child's skin.
- Care of the family and developmental stage of the child should always be considered when providing nursing interventions in the emergency setting. The parents' reactions and developmental factors of the child affect compliance, cooperation, and anxiety levels.
- Trauma assessment of the pediatric patient includes the standard primary and secondary survey and intervention, but must also include assessment of skin signs, use of appropriate age-related tools for determining the level of consciousness, and prevention of or intervention for hypothermia.
- Injury prevention plays an important role in the nursing care of pediatric patients. Motor vehicle injuries, submersion injuries, ingestions, and poisonings are largely preventable. Nurses can play an important role in offering anticipatory guidance and in providing injury prevention materials and instruction to pediatric patients and their families.

REFERENCES

Agran, P., Castillo, D., & Winn, D. (1992). Comparison of motor vehicle occupant injuries in restrained and unrestrained 4-to 14-year-olds. *Accident Analysis and Prevention, 24*(4), 349–355.

Agran, P., Winn, D., & Dunkle, D. (1989). Injuries among 4- to 9-year-old restrained motor vehicle occupants by seat location and crash impact site. *American Journal of Diseases of Children, 143*(11), 1317–1321.

Aguilera, D. (1990). *Crisis intervention: Theory and methodology.* St. Louis: C. V. Mosby.

American Academy of Pediatrics. (1992). Access to emergency medical care. *Pediatrics. 90*(4), 67–68.

Avner, J. R., & Baker, M. D. (1991). Dog bites in urban children [see comments]. *Pediatrics, 88*(1), 55–57.

Barkin, R. (1992). *Pediatric emergency medicine: Concepts and clinical practice.* St. Louis: Mosby–Year Book.

Bernardo, L., & Kelley, S. (1994). Care of the multiply injured child. In S. Kelley (Ed.). *Pediatric emergency nursing.* Norwalk, CT: Appleton & Lange.

Bernardo, L., & Waggoner, T. (1992). Pediatric trauma. In S. Sheehy (Ed.). *Emergency nursing: principles and practice.* St. Louis: C. V. Mosby.

Cardona, V. D. (1988). *Trauma nursing.* Philadelphia: W. B. Saunders.

Chameides, L. (Ed.). (1994). *Textbook of pediatric advanced life support.* Dallas: American Heart Association.

Clark, M. A., Sandusky, G. E., Hawley, D. A., Pless, J. E., Fardal, P. M., & Tate, L. R. (1991). Fatal and near-fatal animal bite injuries. *Journal of Forensic Science, 36*(4), 1256–1261.

Coburn, M., & Pfeifer, J. (1995). Non-operative management of splenic and hepatic trauma in the multiply injured pediatric and adolescent patient. *Archives of Surgery, 130*(3), 328–338.

Cooper, A., Barlow, B., Davidson, L., Relethford, J., O'Meara, J., & Mottley, L. (1992). Epidemiology of pediatric trauma: Importance of population-based statistics. *Journal of Pediatric Surgery, 27*(2), 149–153; discussion 153–154.

Cooper, A., Barlow, B., & DiScala, C. (1992). Morality and thoracoabdominal injury: The pediatric perspective. *Journal of Pediatric Surgery, 27.*

Dean, B. (1992). Ingestions and poisoning. In *Pediatric Nursing.*

Donnellan, W. (1990). Pediatric trauma. In S. Kitt & J. Kaiser (Eds.). *Emergency nursing: A physiologic and clinical perspective* (pp. 545–574). Philadelphia: W. B. Saunders.

Emergency Nurses Association. (1995). Emergency Nurses Association Policy Statement. Park Ridge, IL.

Fitzmaurice, L. (1992). Approach to multiple trauma. In R. Barkin, et al. (Eds.). *Pediatric emergency medicine, concepts and clinical practice.* St. Louis: C. V. Mosby.

Foltin, G. (1992). Abdominal trauma. In R. Barkin, S. McClellan, J. Knapp et al. (Eds.). *Pediatric emergency medicine, concepts and clinical practice.* St. Louis: C. V. Mosby.

Fuchs, S., et al. (1989). Cervical spine fractures sustained by young children in forward-facing car seats. *Pediatrics, 84,* 352.

Gausche, M. (1995). Pediatric trauma. In J. Siedel & D. Henderson (Eds.). *Pre-hospital care of pediatric patients.* Boston: Jones and Bartlett.

Gellert E. (1978). What do I have inside me? How children view their bodies. In E. Gellert (Ed.). *Psychosocial aspects of pediatric care.* New York: Grune & Stratton.

Gershman, K. A., Sacks, J. J., & Wright, J. C. (1994). Which dogs bite? A case-control study of risk factors. *Pediatrics, 93*(6 Pt 1), 913–917.

Gold, B. S., & Wingert, W. A. (1994). Snake venom poisoning in the United States: A review of therapeutic practice [see comments]. *Southern Medical Journal, 87*(6), 579–589.

Guyer, B., & Ellers, B. (1990). Childhood injuries in the United States. Mortality, morbidity, and cost. *American Journal of Diseases in Children, 144*(6), 649–652.

Haller, J., Papa, P., Drugas G., & Colombani, P. (1994). Nonoperative management of solid organ injuries in children. Is it safe? *Annals of Surgery, 219*(6), 625–631.

Halpern, J. (1989). Mechanisms and patterns of trauma. *Journal of Trauma, 15,* 380.

Henderson, D., & Brownstein, D. (1994). *Pediatric emergency nursing manual.* New York: Springer.

Hoff, B. (1979). Multisystem failure: A review with special reference to drowning. *Critical Care Medicine, 7*(7), 308–320.

Johnson, J., Kirchhoff, K., & Endress, M. (1976). Easing children's fright during health care procedures. *American Journal of Maternal Child Nursing* (7), 206–210.

Jutzi-Kosmos, C. (1990). Assessment of multiple trauma and thoracic trauma. In S. Kitt & J. Kaiser (Eds.). *Emergency nursing, a physiologic and clinical perspective.* Philadelphia: W. B. Saunders.

Kelley, S. (1994). *Pediatric emergency nursing* (2nd ed.). Norwalk, CT: Appleton & Lange.

Lenaghan, P. (1988). Nursing interventions after sudden death in the emergency department. In *Emergency Nurses Association Scientific Assembly.* Boston: Emergency Nurses Association.

McGrath, N. (1996). Head injury. In J. Seidel & D. Henderson (Eds.). *Pre-hospital care of the pediatric emergencies.* Boston: Jones & Bartlett.

McGrath, P., & Craig, K. (1989). Developmental and psychological factors in children's pain. *Pediatric Clinics of North America, 36*(4), 823–836.

Ray, L., & Yuwiler, J. (1991). *Child and adolescent fatal injury data book.* San Diego: Children's Safety Network.

Ross, D., & Ross, S. A. (1988). *Childhood pain: Current issues, research, and management.* Baltimore: Urban & Schwarzenberg.

Seidel, J., & Henderson, D. (1992). Approach to the pediatric patient in the emergency department. In R. Barkin (Ed.). *Pediatric emergency medicine: Concepts and clinical practice.* St. Louis: Mosby–Year Book.

Semonin-Holleran, R. (1993). Taking the sting out of summer. *RN, 56*(7), 40–46.

Semonin-Holleran, R., & Rouse, M. (1991). Biomedical technology: Using it during patient transport. *J Air Med Transp, 10*(5), 7–12.

Sheehy, S. (Ed.). (1992). *Emergency nursing.* St. Louis: C. V. Mosby.

Sinclair, C. L., & Zhou, C. (1995). Descriptive epidemiology of animal bites in Indiana, 1990–92—a rationale for intervention. *Public Health Reports, 110*(1), 64–67.

Soud, T. (1992). Airway, breathing, circulation, and disability: What is different about kids? *Journal of Emergency Nursing, 18*(2), 107–116.

Tennenbein, M. (1992). General management principles of poisoning. In R. Barkin et al. (Eds.). *Pediatric emergency medicine, concepts and clinical practice.* St. Louis: C. V. Mosby.

Tuggle, D. W., Taylor, D. V., & Stevens, R. J. (1993). Dog bites in children. *Journal of Pediatric Surgery, 28*(7), 912–914.

Wiggins, M. E., Akelman, E., & Weiss, A. P. (1994). The management of dog bites and dog bite infections to the hand. *Orthopedics, 17*(7), 617–623.

15

The Ill Child in the Hospital and Other Care Settings

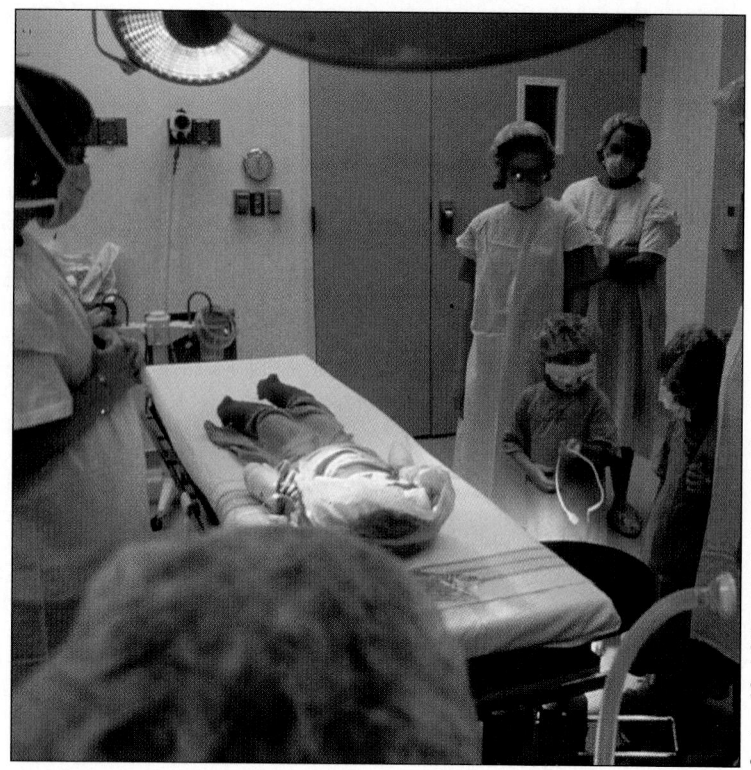

Courtesy of Cook Children's Medical Center, Fort Worth, Texas

CHAPTER OVERVIEW

LEARNING OBJECTIVES

After studying this chapter, you should be able to:

- Discuss the nurse's role in various settings where care is given to ill children.
- List common stressors affecting hospitalized children.
- Describe the child's response to illness.
- Discuss the stages of separation anxiety.
- Describe the factors that affect the child's response to hospitalization and treatment.
- Discuss the psychologic responses of families to the illness of a child in the family.

KEY TERMS

denial: a defense mechanism in which unpleasant realities are denied and kept out of conscious awareness.

egocentric: preoccupied with one's own interests and needs.

regression: defense mechanism in which conflict or frustration is resolved by returning to a behavior that was successful in an earlier stage of development.

separation anxiety: distress and apprehension caused by being removed from parents, home, or familiar surroundings.

situational crisis: unanticipated event that poses a threat to an individual's psychosocial or psychologic well-being.

Because of current trends within health care, the care of ill children is moving from the traditional acute hospital setting to community-based settings and to the home. Children who are hospitalized are more acutely ill than in the past, and their stay is shorter. In addition, the child who is hospitalized is more likely to have a chronic or terminal disease. These changes do not mean that the need for pediatric nurses has diminished; their role is changing and expanding. Pediatric nurses will continue to care for children in hospitals, but also in schools, clinics, and the home.

Prevention will continue to be a key component of pediatric nursing care and will increase in importance. In all areas of practice, pediatric nurses will need to add a teaching and prevention component to their nursing interventions to provide holistic care.

All children experience some form of illness. The ways in which stressors and developmental needs are addressed are important factors in how the immediate crisis is resolved and how future illnesses will be viewed. The nurse spends more time with an ill child than any other health care worker. For this reason, the nurse has a unique opportunity to influence that child's physical and emotional health.

The nurse is often the first person a child sees when he enters the health care system. The nurse plays a major role in assessing the child's individual needs and in planning and implementing his care.

How a child reacts to illness is influenced by his age, cognitive development, preparation, coping skills, and culture. Previous experience with the health care system and the parent's reaction to the illness also affect the child.

Each child is unique, and it is often difficult to predict how a child will react to an illness. However, certain responses seem to occur in varying degrees in all children. Fear of the unknown, separation anxiety, fear of pain or mutilation, loss of control, anger, guilt, and regression are all commonly observed responses to illness or hospitalization. Adults often experience some of the same responses, although to a lesser degree.

Care of the ill child is complex, and the needs of the child and family are many.

SETTINGS OF CARE

The Hospital

Entering the hospital is somewhat like visiting a foreign country. The language, culture, activities, and expectations may be unfamiliar to the child and the family. The nurse acts as a "tour guide" and provides a safe environment, both physically and emotionally. Being the guide includes activities as diverse as explaining the jargon (NPO, IV, vitals), explaining procedures that are often painful, and facilitating the parent's access to the ethics committee. Above all, the nurse must educate the child and family about the disease process, management of the disease, hospital procedures, and discharge issues.

Hospitalizations can be categorized according to length of stay, planned versus unplanned, surgical versus medical, and outpatient (day) versus inpatient. Although there is some overlap, these categories provide a method of examining the child's experience.

Another variable is the type of facility. Children may be hospitalized in a pediatric hospital, a pediatric unit within a general hospital, or a general hospital that occasionally admits children. Pediatric units within a general hospital or hospitals that do not have a specific pediatric unit may not have as many child-oriented services as a pediatric hospital. Special play areas and child-size equipment and fixtures often are not available in general hospitals. Some of the staff who do not routinely care for children may not be comfortable in that role.

The nurse is aware of these challenges and can provide support for the child and the family, for example, by taking extra time when the child is admitted to explain routines and procedures or by placing the child close to the nurse's station. This support might include moving a cot into the room for the parent and ordering special foods for the child. Sometimes it means removing food from a tray that is about to be served so that the child is not overwhelmed by the large servings intended for an adult. Ultimately, it means being sensitive to the needs of the child and the family.

24-Hour Observation

Children can become ill quickly and can recover quickly. For this reason, they may need acute care for a short time (e.g., children who are dehydrated or are having an episode of acute asthma). At the end of 24 hours, the child is evaluated to determine if she needs further hospitalization or if she can be discharged with instructions.

The Nurse's Role. The nurse must prepare the child and family for discharge and assess the parents' capacity to care for the child at home. Instructions should be written, and the parent should be encouraged to ask questions. The parent should be told when to notify the primary health care provider in the event the child's condition changes. An awareness of cultural differences enhances the nurse's assessment ability. For example, is the parent smiling because he feels content, or is he embarrassed to ask a question? Is she nodding because she understands, or is she embarrassed to say that she cannot read?

Emergency Hospitalization

An emergency admission can be traumatic because there is limited time for preparation. The admission can be the result of trauma or acute sudden illness. The family may arrive at the hospital with little money, clothing, or other resources. The siblings may also be present, competing with the sick child for the parent's attention. In addition to caring for the sick child, the staff may be called on to help meet the family's basic need for food, clothing, and a place to stay. A social service referral is appropriate in such situations.

The Nurse's Role. Because of the intense level of activity in emergency departments, care of the family is often overlooked. The family may fear that their child will die or be permanently disabled. Although nurses may see many similar situations each day in which the children do well, they must be sensitive to the family's fears and keep them informed of the child's condition and care.

Having parents present can affect the way a child reacts to a stressful situation. In most cases, the child is more secure and relaxed if at least one parent remains with her. In the past, it was the practice to keep parents out of the room until the child's condition was stabilized. The staff believed that they were protecting the parent, but the parent was wondering if he would ever see his child again. In most situations, the parents can decide whether they want to be with the child. If the parent's behavior impairs the ability of the staff to care for the child, he is asked to wait outside the room and is kept informed.

Time for preparation of the child is usually limited in an emergency situation. Nurses must seize every opportunity to prepare the child for the care she is receiving. Holding the child, touching her, talking softly, distracting her, and involving her in the procedure are methods of support used in emergency situations. After the child is stable, the nurse returns to her and uses therapeutic communication appropriate for her developmental age to help her to talk about the event. A child life specialist may also help the child to express her feelings. The use of dolls, puppets, and hospital equipment can aid the child in communicating her feelings.

Chapter 14 provides more detailed information about caring for children and their families in an emergency setting.

CLARIFYING FEELINGS ***Scenario:*** A 7-year-old boy is admitted to the medical-surgical unit after spending several hours in the emergency department because of acute asthma. Although his mother brought him to the hospital, she had his younger brother and sister with her and could not remain with him in the room. He is quiet, and you notice that he watches every move you make.

You might say: "Some kids say it's scary to come to the hospital and especially to be in the emergency room, with the bright lights and everyone rushing around. If you'd like, I can spend a little time with you, and we can talk about being in the hospital."

Outpatient and Day Facilities

Outpatient facilities have evolved in an effort to keep children out of the hospital unless absolutely necessary. The outpatient facility may be part of a hospital or freestanding. The child arrives in the morning; undergoes a procedure, test, or surgery; and goes home by that evening. Common procedures performed during such admissions include tympanostomy tubes, hernia repair, tonsillectomy, cystoscopy and bronchoscopy.

This mode of care has three main advantages: (1) it minimizes separation of the child from the family; (2) it decreases the risk of infection; and (3) it decreases cost. One disadvantage is that outpatient facilities that are not connected to a hospital may not be equipped for overnight stays. If the child experiences complications that require continued observation and treatment, she may need to be transferred to a hospital. This situation can be upsetting to the child and the family.

The Nurse's Role. Although the procedure may be short, teaching the child and the parent is as important as in the acute care setting. When possible, a tour of the facility before the procedure can decrease fear of the unknown. Parents have indicated that although they like the idea of outpatient care, it is frightening to take their child home. Assessment of the parent can assist the nurse in deciding whether the parent is capable of handling the home care of the child or if home health care is needed. At the very least, a follow-up phone call to the home should be required. Parents should also be encouraged to call the facility if they have any concerns, and they should be given other resources to contact after the facility closes. Families who live far from the health care facility may want to spend the night at a nearby hotel or consider an overnight admission.

Rehabilitative Care

After a serious illness or trauma, changes may occur in the child's ability to function. After the acute situation has resolved, the child may be admitted to a rehabilitation hospital. Through the collaborative efforts of nursing, medicine, physical therapy, occupational therapy, and other staff, a treatment plan is developed in which the child, family, and health professionals work to help the child regain her previous abilities. Children with neurologic injuries, such as head injuries, or children with serious burns may thrive in this environment, which usually resembles a home environment with the facilities available for the child to relearn the activities of daily living.

The Nurse's Role. Nurses in this setting must balance nurturing and firm discipline as they help the child to reclaim his independence. Parents often need encouragement and support because they are torn between doing for their child and watching the child struggle to do things independently. Overprotection is a common reaction of parents, and they can be assisted in identifying the child's developmental need to master the environment. The focus should be on what the child can do rather than on his limitations.

The Medical-Surgical Unit

Children admitted to the hospital unit are usually acutely ill or have a chronic disease or disability that requires frequent, often long-term, hospitalizations. The care of the child with a chronic disease is discussed in Chapter 17. The average length of hospital stay of the acutely ill child has been shortened significantly, and the need for teaching has increased in proportion to the shortened length of hospitalization.

The Nurse's Role. Preparation for a planned hospitalization is essential. Some hospitals provide the opportunity for the child to visit the hospital before admission, and many pediatric hospitals host preoperative parties to introduce children to the strange sights and sounds experienced during a surgical experience. Many children's books about the experience of illness and hospitalization are available through public libraries. In addition, some children's hospitals have libraries. Parents should answer questions honestly and encourage the child to talk about the hospitalization. Videos are also available for the family to view together and then discuss.

The Intensive Care Unit

When a child is admitted to the intensive care unit (ICU), both he and his parents experience increased stress because of the seriousness of the admitting diagnosis and the highly technical, unfamiliar environment. In addition, the child often is experiencing pain, uncomfortable procedures, noise, and constant lighting. In many instances, he cannot eat or talk. Meanwhile, the child's parents are experiencing a parent's worst fear, the possible loss of a child.

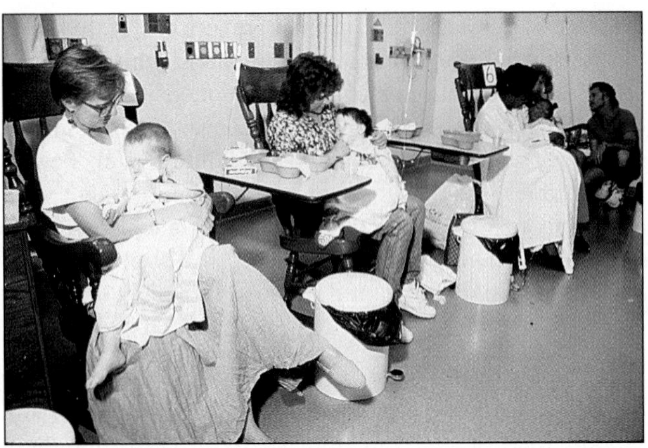

Figure 15–1
When nursing care centers on the family, hospital rules must be altered. These parents are holding their children and rocking them in a postanesthesia care unit, normally a place that is off-limits to those not on the staff. (Courtesy of Cook Children's Medical Center, Fort Worth, Texas)

The Nurse's Role. The child and family require intense emotional support. All of the normal responses to hospitalization are magnified and need to be assessed. When possible, planned admissions to the ICU (e.g., for cardiac surgery) should be preceded by visits to the unit.

The parent should be encouraged to remain with the child and should be kept informed of the child's condition (Fig. 15–1). Procedures, equipment, and treatments should be explained to both the child and the parent. If the parent leaves and the child's condition changes or a new tube or piece of equipment has been added, the parent should be prepared for the change before seeing the child. Parents should be encouraged to provide care for the child and to touch him as much as possible. Active listening by the nurse is essential.

Siblings of the seriously ill hospitalized child can easily be overlooked. Siblings may need to talk, to be comforted, or to have the hospital experience explained. Often family members want to help, but do not know what to do. Suggesting that a grandparent or other relative relieve a parent so that she has time with the sibling of the ill child can help both the parent and the child. Parents may feel pulled between the ill child and the rest of the family. Helping the parent by discussing their options can relieve stress and may lead to a solution.

School-Based Clinics

There have been school-based clinics for more than 25 years, but with the recent changes in health care delivery, this setting is being viewed as a site for expanding primary care. These clinics play an important role in providing care for children in remote rural communities and in underserved inner-city areas. The current clinics are typically staffed by school nurses, nurse practitioners, physicians, social workers, and other health care providers. It is expected that this area of practice will continue to grow, and many believe that a school-based clinic is the perfect setting to provide primary care for selected groups of children and adolescents.

Prevention remains the focus as children are taught health habits that may prevent the need for them to enter the acute care setting. The need for immunizations is identified, and immunizations can be given. Screening results that in the past needed referral can be handled on-site in many cases. Through the use of such clinics, medical services can be obtained in a timely manner and expensive emergency department visits can be avoided. It makes sense for a child who is experiencing an earache at school to be seen on-site, treated, and sent home if his condition warrants. The child's compliance with treatment can be monitored, and a follow-up visit can be scheduled to determine whether treatment has been effective. One clinic documented that school absences decreased significantly when a school-based clinic was started (Pietrobono, 1994). Funding for school-based clinics is increasing, and these clinics will continue to be a focus as the delivery of health care moves out of the acute care setting and into the community.

The Nurse's Role. Nurses in this setting must be sensitive to parental concerns about certain topics in health care, especially areas related to sexuality (e.g., birth control, sexually transmitted diseases, abortion). Community involvement and support can dispel concerns and assist in setting guidelines for such clinics. School-based nurses must also be team members who act in collaboration with other health care workers and have a strong preventive health background as well as the ability to think critically.

The school-based clinic provides a setting for parental education in the areas of preventive health, growth and development, anticipatory guidance, and care of acutely ill children. The rights and wishes of the parents are respected. Respecting the parent's wishes can be a challenge when the value systems of the health care provider and the parent are different. Although the pediatric nurse is a patient advocate, caution must be exercised unless the child is being harmed.

Community Clinics

Community health clinics provide primary care for children and their families. In these settings, nurses, nurse practitioners, and physicians provide case management of illness and health promotion. Because most children enter this setting when they are experiencing an illness, preventive care is integrated into the care of the child. Support services and groups (e.g., social services, dental clinic, daycare) may meet or may be located in the same center.

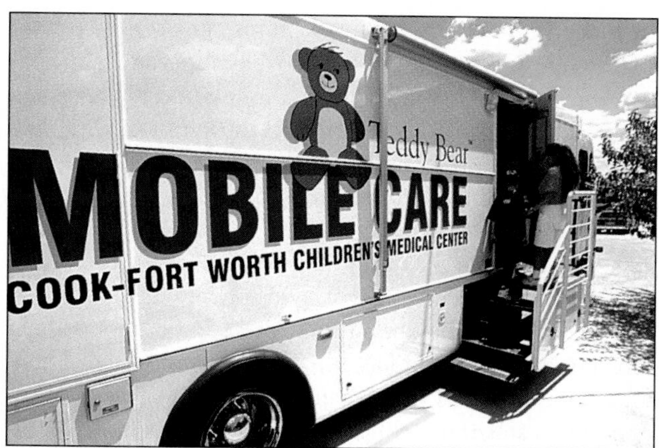

Figure 15–2
Nurses today help take health care on the road to provide services to those who otherwise might not obtain them. This mobile van is stationed at a public school, where it offers health screenings and prevention services to children. (Courtesy of Cook Children's Medical Center, Fort Worth, Texas)

Referrals are also made to medical specialists and other health care providers.

The Nurse's Role. Although many of the children at community health clinics are ill, nurses must use the opportunity to take a health history to assess such areas as immunization, nutrition, anticipatory guidance, and growth and development. If the child is ill at the time of the visit, the nurse can set an appointment for the child to return for immunizations or other care that cannot be given when the child is ill.

In some urban areas, nurses are involved in primary prevention (Fig. 15–2). Information and education are offered on childhood immunization, the signs and symptoms of childhood illnesses, injury prevention, and parenting skills. Demonstration projects have proved that support and education have reduced hospitalization and emergency department visits, increased compliance with prescribed medical care, and improved health outcomes for the entire family (Struk, 1994).

Home Care

Pediatric home care is the provision of skilled care within the child's home. Nurses in this setting are part of a multidisciplinary team that usually includes physical therapists, speech therapists, occupational therapists, and social workers. The care is directed by a physician. Children receiving respiratory therapy, having dressing changes, receiving total parenteral nutrition, or requiring skilled care because of a chronic illness or an injury may be cared for in the home.

The Nurse's Role. Nurses who work in home care should have previous hospital experience in their practice area. The nurse must be able to make independent decisions and think critically, and should have good clinical, documentation, communication, and teaching skills. The nurse must have an understanding of various cultures and socioeconomic backgrounds to meet the needs of each child and family.

Although the separation of the child from the family is not a problem in home health care, the child may experience many of the other effects of illness, such as fear of the unknown, loss of control, anger, guilt, and regression. In addition, care is taking place in the family's domain, and the nurse is a guest in the home. The family may have to adjust to unfamiliar noises and equipment, such as special beds, ventilators, or intravenous pumps, in the living room. They may feel that they have lost all of their privacy and that they cannot "be themselves" because someone outside of the family is frequently there. Awareness of the needs of the siblings is also a nursing goal in this setting.

The nurse's role as teacher is especially important in this setting because many of the tasks that the nurse might perform in the hospital are delegated to the family, with the nurse monitoring the care. The nurse acts as a case manager and coordinator of care.

STRESSORS ASSOCIATED WITH ILLNESS AND HOSPITALIZATION

Much of the research on the effects of hospitalization on children has been based on adult assumptions of what the child is experiencing and on children's self-reports. Several categories have been identified: separation, physical harm or bodily injury, fear of the unknown, uncertainty about limits, and loss of control (Visintainer & Wolfer, 1975). It has been suggested that previous experience may not reduce fear, but rather replace fear of the unknown with fear of the known (Hart & Bossert, 1994).

Although preschoolers and young school-age children experience separation anxiety, it is most significant in infants and toddlers, especially from the ages of 6 to 30 months. In times of stress, anxiety related to separation increases.

Each age group has its own fears related to pain and injury. During the last decade, there has been an expansion of knowledge about pain and its treatment. Previously, many practitioners had erroneous beliefs about children and pain. Children learn quickly to associate health care activities and professionals with pain and injury. The fear is usually focused on "shots." Chapter 20 discusses issues related to pain.

A child's feeling of having control over a situation has been shown to affect his distress reactions to medical events (LaMontagne, 1993). In other words, if children believe that they have personal control over a situation, they are more likely to feel confident and master the task, whether it is holding still while a needle is inserted or lying still while tomography is performed.

Hospitalization puts all children at high risk for fears related to their unfamiliarity with the people, surroundings, and events. The child has not developed a trust of the health care provider and therefore does not know what to expect. Dependent on his age, the child may have real or imagined fears: Will the nurse know when I am hungry or hurting? Will the nurse hurt me?

The Infant and Toddler

Separation Anxiety. Infants and toddlers, especially between the ages of 6 and 30 months, experience **separation anxiety.** Separation is this age group's major stressor, and it is traumatic to both the child and the parent.

The child experiences several stages as she reacts to the separation.

STAGES OF SEPARATION

Protest: Child is agitated, resists caregivers, cries, and is inconsolable.

Despair: Child experiences hopelessness and becomes quiet, withdrawn, and apathetic.

Detachment: Child becomes interested in the environment, plays, and seems to form relationships with caregivers and other children. If parents reappear, the child may ignore them.

In the initial phase, known as protest, the child demonstrates her distress by crying and rejecting anyone other than her parent (Fig. 15–3). The child appears angry and upset. During the despair phase, the child experiences hopelessness and becomes quiet and withdrawn. Crying decreases, and the child becomes apathetic. If the separation from the parent continues, the child enters the detachment phase. During this phase, the child again becomes interested in the environment and begins to play. This phase may be misinterpreted as a positive sign showing that the child has adjusted to the hospitalization. In reality, the child has "given up." If the parents return during this stage, the child may ignore them, and the parents may think that the child does not want to see them. This reaction by the child is a coping mechanism to protect her from further emotional pain related to the separation.

Nurses in the acute care setting see the first two stages of separation—protest and despair—much more frequently than the final stage—detachment—which is more common in long-term separations. Parents may misunderstand their child's behavior and wonder why she is acting so differently. They may even perceive the child's reaction as a behavior problem. Parents need to be reassured that this reaction is a normal response to separation and that most children will not suffer any permanent effects from the event. As an understanding of separation anxiety has evolved, changes in visiting times have changed from being structured to permitting "rooming-in" (Fig. 15–3).

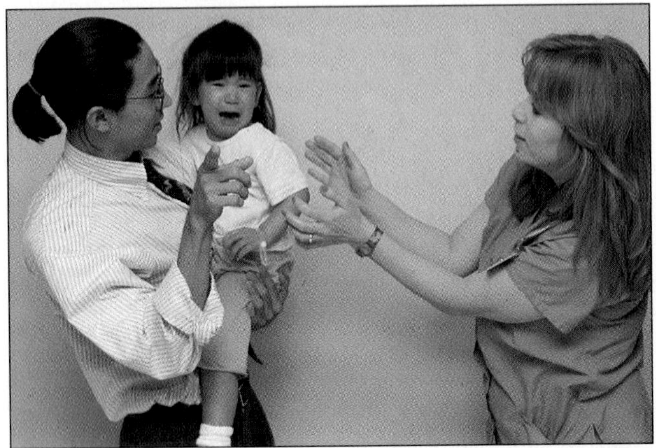

◀ Between the ages of 6 and 30 months, a child is expected to have separation anxiety. The child initially reacts with protest, as this girl is doing. If separation continues, the child becomes quiet and withdrawn (despair phase). In the final phase, detachment, the child may ignore the parents.

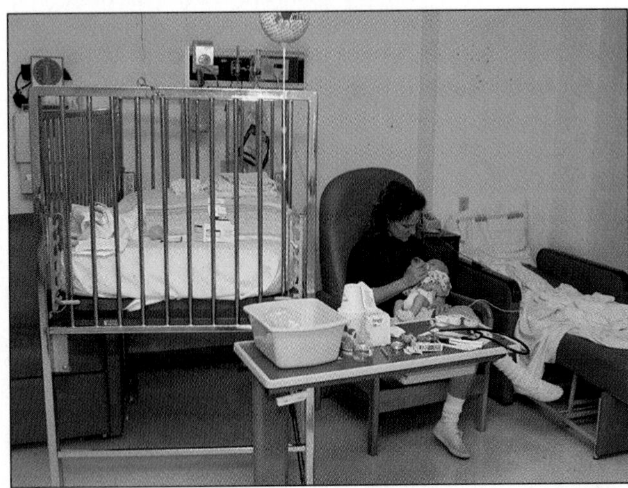

Hospitals try to reduce the stress of hospitalization for both parents and the child by having rooming-in arrangements. Rooming-in promotes parental attachment and provides many opportunities to teach parents how to care for their child's needs. ▶

Figure 15–3

Separation is one of the stressors of hospitalization that affects both child and parent. (Courtesy of T. C. Thompson, Children's Hospital of Chattanooga, Tennessee)

It is generally believed that if separation can be avoided, the child will be much more resilient during a hospitalization. Infants and toddlers go through the stages of separation. The older the child in this age group, the more elaborate the protest. The child not only cries, but also may cling to the parent, kick, and generally create a scene. Parents need to understand that this behavior is a sign of healthy parent–child attachment. The toddler may resist bedtime and eating and may have temper tantrums more frequently than normal for this age. There may also be signs of regression in toileting and eating. Parents should be told that regression is normal and encouraged to reinforce appropriate behavior and allow the regression.

RESPONDING TO PARENTAL CONCERN *Scenario:* A parent asks whether someone needs to be with their toddler all of the time while he is in the hospital because both parents work and they have other children.

You might say: "We encourage parents to stay with their children when they are in the hospital. However, if you have to leave, we will spend time with Tommy and check on him frequently. You may call us at any time, day or night. When you return, perhaps you could bring a favorite toy or stuffed animal and something that reminds him of you, such as a picture or a piece of clothing. He will feel more secure if he has something familiar to keep with him."

Fear of Injury and Pain. The reaction of infants and toddlers to pain and bodily injury is affected by previous experiences, separation from parents, restraint, and preparation. The young child views injury and pain in a concrete manner. Nurses who have worked with toddlers know that most children of this age react to any intrusive procedure, whether it is painful or not. A more extensive discussion of pain in infants and toddlers is given in Chapter 20.

Loss of Control. According to Erikson, the major task of the toddler period is autonomy. Control is a major issue with this age group. The toddler experiences the environment through all of his senses, and loves to explore the environment. At the same time, he needs sameness (rituals and routines). The toddler must know that his routines and rituals will be there when he needs to be replenished. Because of the growth and development changes taking place in the toddler, familiar rituals and routines (e.g., eating, sleeping, playing) provide reassurance and stability.

Hospitalization, with its own set of rituals and routines, can severely disrupt the life of a toddler. The child may be confined to a crib, and the crib may have a cover over it. Because of safety issues, the child is not allowed to run in the halls. If the parents are unable to be with the child, the way he is put to bed or bathed may be unfamiliar. When children are not given the time to do things themselves, their sense of control and autonomy is weakened. They are frustrated and may have temper tantrums. Choices, even simple ones, can return some control to the child.

This lack of control is often exhibited in behaviors related to feeding, toileting, playing, and bedtime. It is important to remember that each of these activities may have associated rituals and routines. The child may also show some regression in these areas.

The Preschooler

Separation Anxiety. Separation anxiety occurs in this age group, but it is generally less obvious and less serious than in the toddler. Although the preschooler may already be spending some time away from her parents at a daycare center or preschool, illness adds a stressor that makes separation more difficult.

As stress increases, the preschooler's ability to separate from her parent decreases.

The preschooler experiences the same protest response as the toddler, but tends to be less direct. The nurse may find a preschooler quietly crying with his back to the door because he has been told to "act like a big boy." He may refuse to eat or take his medication, and may be generally uncooperative. He may repeatedly ask when his parents will be coming for a visit, or if he has a phone, he may constantly call his parents. All of these behaviors are signs that the child is having difficulty coping with the situation.

Fear of Injury and Pain. The preschooler fears mutilation. If he must have surgery affecting a limb or other body part, there will be increased fear. The preschooler has a general lack of understanding of body integrity. Children of this age are also afraid of intrusive procedures and because of their literal interpretation of words, they often imagine things to be much worse than they are (see Chapter 10). Finally, the child's active imagination can go wild when he is ill. The preschooler may believe that he is ill because of something he did or thought, or perhaps just because he touched something or someone. Specific reactions of the preschooler to pain are further discussed in Chapter 20.

GIVING CHOICES *Scenario:* A 5-year-old boy refused to have his dressing changed by the nurse who cared for him during the previous shift. She said that he cried, pulled up the covers, and said that she was "mean." This behavior is unusual for him, and you suspect that he is being told to do too many things and has not been given choices.

You might say: "Vin, I know there have been many changes for you since you came to the hospital. Today, we are going to decide together what is going to happen. I see you have selected a video to watch. Would you like me to change your dressing before you watch the video, or after?"

This approach gives the preschooler a choice and some control while maintaining boundaries.

Loss of Control. The preschooler has attained a good deal of independence in self-care. He has been given more independence at home, preschool, or day care, and may expect that to continue in the hospital. He likes to wander about the unit and may not be happy when restricted to his bed or room. Like the toddler, a preschooler likes familiar routines and rituals and may show some regression if he is not allowed to maintain some areas of control.

The School-Age Child

Separation. The school-age child is accustomed to periods of separation from her parents, but just as in the preschooler, as stressors are added, the separation becomes more difficult. The younger school-age child already may have been experiencing separation anxiety related to starting school.

Older children may be more concerned with missing school and the fear that their friends will forget them. However, the adjustment to an unfamiliar environment and the regression seen in ill children increases the likelihood that some separation anxiety will take place.

Fear of Injury and Pain. The school-age child is concerned with body disability and death. He is more relaxed about having a physical examination or having his eyes or ears examined, but is uncomfortable with any type of sexual examination. These children want to know the reasons for procedures and tests, and ask relevant questions about their illness. Because at this age a child can understand cause and effect, he can relate his actions to becoming ill. Their parents may tell them that if they do not get enough rest, wear warm clothes, or eat nutritious meals, they will get a cold. If they become ill, they associate their actions with the disease. For further discussion of pain in the school-age child, see Chapter 20.

Loss of Control. School-age children are movers and shakers. They control their self-care and are typically highly social. They like being involved, and most children fill their days with many activities. Illness can change all of these things. If the child has physical limitations, he can feel helpless and dependent (Fig. 15–4).

Friends are important to this age group, and school-age children may think that their friends will forget them while they are ill. They are also accustomed to making choices about meals and activities. By capitalizing on the child's abilities and needs, the nurse can encourage the child to become involved in his own care. School-age children can select their menus, assist with some treatments, keep their rooms neat, and visit with younger children when it is appropriate for both children. With these opportunities for independence, children retain a sense of control, enhance their self-esteem, and continue to work toward achieving a sense of industry.

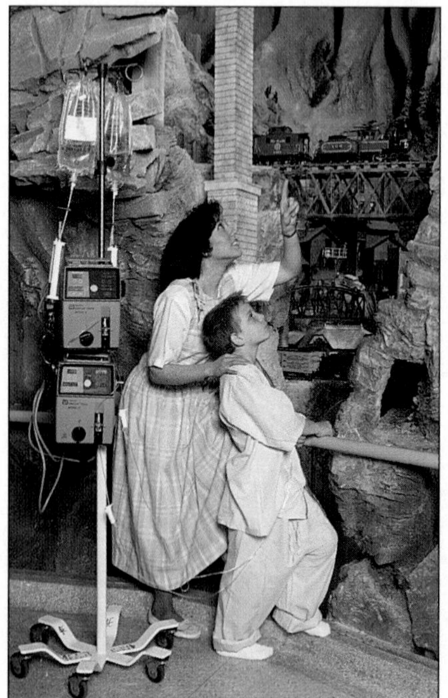

◀ This multilevel trainscape in a children's hospital provides children and adults alike with a welcome respite from real-life stresses. (Courtesy of Children's Medical Center, Dallas, Texas)

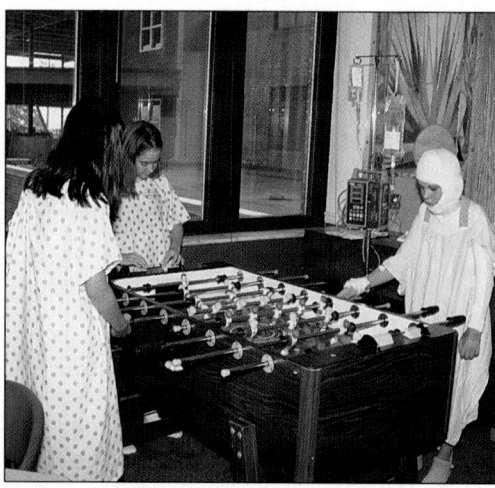

◀ Hospitalized teens need to interact with their peers, as they do when they are well. A lounge area that is separate from the playroom used by younger children fulfills this need.

Figure 15–4
Activities for the hospitalized child are important for growth and development, stress relief, socialization, and a sense of control.

The Adolescent

Separation. Adolescents often are not sure whether they want their parents with them when they are hospitalized. Some enjoy the freedom and the period of independence. Others, in response to the stress of illness, become more dependent and want their parents near them. A third group cannot decide what they want, and this situation can be frustrating to the parents. All of these responses are consistent with the normal growth and development of an adolescent.

Because of the importance of the peer group, separation from friends is a source of anxiety to the adolescent. Ideally, the peer group will support their ill friend (Fig. 15–4). Some adolescents are reluctant to visit friends in the hospital either because of their own health fears or because the reality of illness in someone their age is difficult for them to handle. The hospitalized adolescent may be upset if his friends simply go on with their lives, excluding him. Special activity areas and other opportunities for the adolescent to meet and interact with other hospitalized adolescents are important.

Fear of Injury and Pain. To the adolescent, appearance is crucial. Therefore, if illness or injury changes how the adolescent perceives himself, it can have a major impact on him. Even children who have seemingly adjusted to a chronic disease during their earlier years may have difficulty during adolescence simply because they do not want to be different. The diabetic adolescent may not want to eat different foods or take time out from an activity to give himself an injection. Adolescents do not want attention drawn to them, so they may eat the wrong foods and skip their medication.

The adolescent may also give the impression that she is not afraid, even though she is terrified. Adolescents may think that it is not "cool" if they are not in control. They may question everything, or they may appear overly confident. Because of their concern with their bodies, they are guarded when any areas connected with sexual development are examined. Nurses need to be sensitive to the adolescent's concerns and reassure them that they are normal if in fact they are. Some adolescents also believe that they are invincible and that nothing can hurt them or cause death. This belief can cause them to take risks and to be noncompliant because they may not see the consequences of their behavior.

Because of the importance of this topic, Chapter 20 is devoted to a discussion of pain in children. See Chapter 8 for growth and development implications related to the adolescent.

Loss of Control. Control is important to the adolescent. Some of the challenges in caring for an ill adolescent stem from control issues. An understanding of this issue is key when caring for this age group. If the adolescent is given some control, endless power struggles can be avoided. Behaviors exhibited by the adolescent in response to this loss of control may include anger, withdrawal, and general uncooperativeness.

This issue can cause a major conflict between the adolescent and her parents. Parents often feel like Ping-Pong balls as they are bounced back and forth by their child who wants their help one minute and rejects it the next. Parents who do not understand the growth and development implications of this behavior can become frustrated and angry. Education of parents increases understanding and facilitates communication between parents and their child.

Adolescents may also feel that they are losing control of their social lives as they sit on the perimeter of activities. Time to plan for the separation (e.g., scheduled surgery) allows a greater sense of control than an unplanned hospitalization (e.g., trauma).

Fear of the Unknown

The sights and sounds of the hospital unit can be frightening and confusing to the child. The child may have many questions: Why are the nurses wearing masks? Why does that alarm keep ringing? Am I dying? Why are they putting tubes in me? Why am I under a plastic tent?

The child's routines and rituals may have been disrupted, and the child may wonder what will happen next. An understanding of these fears can assist the nurse in structuring care and teaching in a way that avoids unnecessary anxiety.

A designated safe area can enhance the security of the child. For example, procedures that are intrusive or may cause discomfort or anxiety are not performed in the child's room, but in the treatment room.

Regression

The child may **regress** regarding toileting or may cry for a bottle even though he has been weaned for several months. He may require increased attention at bedtime or have temper tantrums. The older child may react even to short periods of separation by clinging or crying, or may have fears about shadows on the walls or noises in the halls.

Parents may be overly concerned about regression. They should be told that the child may continue the behavior at home. The child may need increased emotional support while the parent slowly returns the child to her normal routine. If the child has regressed in the area of toileting, the parent should wait until the child has returned to a daily routine and then begin the toilet training again. Behavior that is appropriate for the child's age should be reinforced.

CLARIFICATION OF BEHAVIOR "I know that you are concerned because David has been soiling his pants since he has been in the hospital. This soiling is a normal reaction to the stress of being ill and in the hospital. When he returns home and things return to normal for him, he will resume his previous schedule."

Guilt and Shame

Because their thinking is **egocentric** and magical, preschoolers may believe that their illness is somehow related to a thought or deed. This belief can lead to feelings of guilt and shame and increased stress at a time when the child is already attempting to cope with several other stressors. Because the child typically does not share these feelings with adults, parents and caregivers must be aware of the possibility of this type of thinking in this age group. The nurse's role is to assess the child for this type of thinking and, through therapeutic communication, assist the child in identifying his unfounded fears and beliefs. The child may be able to relate what he perceives to be happening to him. The use of puppets can help children to deal with their feelings. Helping the child to identify a perceived punishment issue and then reassuring him that he did nothing to cause the illness can result in a tremendous decrease in anxiety.

FACTORS AFFECTING A CHILD'S RESPONSE TO ILLNESS AND HOSPITALIZATION

Each child responds to illness or hospitalization differently. The phrase "perception is everything" certainly

Developmental Approaches to the Hospitalized Child

NEONATE

Anticipate needs and fulfill them in a timely manner.
Provide opportunities for sucking and oral stimulation, using a pacifier if NPO.
Provide swaddling and soft talking to soothe.
If very ill, provide a quiet, soothing environment.
When stimulation is appropriate, provide stimulation for each sense (e.g., mobiles, music, smell, soft stuffed animals). Use contrasting colors and textures.
Follow painful procedures with holding and cuddling.
Model appropriate behaviors to family members regarding stimulation, touch, verbalization, and feeding.
Provide consistency in caregivers when parents are not available.
Collaborate with parents on ways to provide home care.
Involve the parents in the care of their infant as much as possible.
Encourage parents to room-in if possible.

INFANT

The same as neonate for the younger infant.
The older infant will begin to anticipate painful procedures and fight.
Expect and inform parents about regression.
Limit the number of caregivers to whom the infant must adjust.
Request that parents bring the infant's security object (e.g., blanket, stuffed animal).
Encourage parents to be present during procedures.

TODDLER

Expect regression, and inform parents about behaviors.
Follow home routines and rituals.
Involve parents in the care of the toddler.
Provide for rooming-in if possible.
Allow opportunities for mobility when it can be done safely.
Employ all possible methods of pain control when the child must have a painful procedure.
Anticipate temper tantrums when the child's frustration level is high.
Maintain a safe environment for physical acting out and temper tantrums.
Encourage the child to be independent (e.g., feed self, use potty chair, put on socks).
Provide support when the toddler needs to be dependent (e.g., hold after a procedure, comfort if parents leave).
Approach with a positive attitude ("I am going to give you your medicine").

PRESCHOOLER

Provide safe ways to act out aggression (e.g., punching bags, painting, clay).
Take time for communication. Answer questions with simple, concrete explanations. Explain all procedures honestly.
Expect egocentric behavior.
Provide for a safe and secure environment (e.g., nightlight, view of others, objects from home).
Be consistent.

applies to the ill child. How a child perceives the incident will affect his response before, during, and after the illness or hospitalization. How a child reacts is often related to the parents' response to the illness and the child's age, level of cognitive development, preparation, previous experiences, and coping skills.

If the child has had a previous illness or hospitalization, how that event unfolded and the child's response to it affect how the child views future occurrences. Children with chronic diseases who experience multiple hospitalizations have a different perception of illness than the child who has an occasional cold (see Chapter 17). A visit to a pediatrician's office may show the different reactions children have in response to their experiences. Some older children have more negative responses as they begin to associate certain people, colors, and surroundings with what they perceive as an unpleasant experience.

Age and Cognitive Development

The child's developmental age affects how she reacts to illness, and it needs to be taken into consideration when planning nursing care. Preparing a toddler for hospitalization or a procedure differs from preparing a school-age child. The content, the time frame, the setting, and the method of preparation are all based on the child's growth and development. It is imperative that pediatric nurses have a clear understanding of the cognitive abilities of each age group (see the accompanying box).

Parental Response to Illness or Hospitalization

Children have sharp observation skills and know when their parents are anxious and upset. This anxiety is trans-

Ask the parents how the child usually copes in new situations.
Tell the child that he did not cause the illness.
Involve parents in care, and follow home routines.
Place the child with other children of the same age if possible.
Provide for play activities in the playroom and in the room.
Accept regression if it occurs, and explain it to parents.
Encourage the child to be independent (e.g., feeding, dressing, toileting).

SCHOOL-AGE CHILD

Inform the child of limits (no water fights, wheelchair races, leaving the unit, etc.).
Involve the child in planning and implementing care (e.g., choose from menu, assist with some procedures).
Explain all procedures, and allow the child time for questions and answers. Use medical and scientific terminology and diagrams or body outlines to explain the procedure.
Accept regression, but encourage independence.
Provide privacy.
Encourage the child to assist in keeping room and belongings in order.
Assist the child in contacting friends. Encourage parents to contact the teacher and have school friends send cards and letters.
If the child's condition supports visits and calls from friends, encourage this contact.
Provide for the educational needs of the child by encouraging parents to bring in work and scheduling study times. If the child will have a prolonged period of hospital or home care, provide for a teacher to work with the child. Some hospitals have a hospital-based teacher.

ADOLESCENT

Provide privacy for care and visiting.
Encourage the adolescent to wear street clothes and perform normal grooming.
Encourage questions about appearance and the effects of illness on the adolescent's future.
Use scientific and medical terminology to prepare the adolescent for procedures.
Use body outlines and diagrams, and give the rationale for the procedure.
When possible, provide for a special activity area that is limited to adolescent use. Introduce the child to other adolescents on unit.
Encourage peers to call and visit if the adolescent's condition can tolerate this action.
Assist parents in communicating, supporting, and guiding their adolescent children by providing them with growth and development information.
Allow favorite foods to be brought in if the adolescent does not require a special diet.
Approach the adolescent with caring, understanding, and acceptance.
Provide for educational needs (see school age).

ferred to the child, and the child's anxiety then increases. If the parents talk outside the child's room or within hearing range, but in whispers, the child begins to imagine what her parents are saying. All children, but especially the preschooler, who has such an active imagination, can invent elaborate stories to explain what is happening.

The parent who does not answer the child's questions or who does not tell her the truth for fear it will frighten her only confuses the child and weakens the trust the child has in the parent. The child wants to believe that someone is in control and that she can trust that person. Some parents cannot be honest with their children because of their own fears and insecurities. All of these issues must be assessed by the nurse.

Preparation of the Child and Family. Stress has been defined as a nonspecific response of the body to any demand made on it. Perceived stressors, the conditioning factors brought to the situation, and the coping mechanisms used to adapt all affect how each person adapts to a stress-producing situation (Selye, 1974). Preparing for an event, in this case hospitalization, can decrease stress in several ways. During preparation, the child's and the parent's perceptions of the event can be explored. In addition, previous experiences that might affect the impending hospitalization and the use of previous coping strategies can be identified and discussed.

The depth and method of preparation vary among children and are based on an understanding of the child's individual needs. Variables that should be considered include the child's age and developmental level, involvement of the family, timing, the child's physiologic status and psychological status, setting, sociocultural factors, and the child's experiences with illness and hospitalization (Manion, 1990).

The preparation sessions should be planned. Teaching is more effective if trust is developed between the nurse and the child and parent. Honesty and age-appropriate language for the child are imperative. When possible, all of the senses should be involved. The child should be allowed to see the intensive care area before being admitted, to take the blood pressure of a stuffed animal, or to handle the mask that will be used in surgery. The nurse should avoid using medical terminology that children and their parents may not understand. Literal interpretation of some words may be confusing and scary to some children, especially the preschooler (see Chapter 10). Some children assume that certain procedures include pain. Explanation and the opportunity to handle equipment, when possible, can help a child to master the fear of hospitalization and treatment.

Coping Skills of the Child and Family. Coping is the process of contending with difficulties in an effort to overcome or work through them. How the child copes with illness or hospitalization is related to her age, her perception of the event, previous hospitalizations and encounters with the health care profession, support from significant others, and the child's and parent's coping skills.

The child's coping behaviors include words, descriptions, phrases, and actions that children use to help them through stressful situations (Corbo-Richert et al., 1993). The child may also cope by ignoring or negating the event. The younger child is more likely to use emotional expression, whereas the older child and adolescent are more likely to withdraw or practice more self-control behaviors. For example, whereas the younger child might scream and kick during a procedure, the older child might remain stoic and say that it did not hurt, even though it did, to appear brave and meet either self-imposed or parental expectations.

Breathing (e.g., blowing bubbles, pinwheels, party blowers) helps with relaxation and offers a focus for the child. Teaching coping mechanisms and practicing them before a procedure can help a child to feel more in control as well as successful. Distraction (e.g., waterwheels, games, books) and imagery (e.g., tapes, scenarios) for older children are effective tools for coping. Parents, nurses, and child life therapists may all serve as facilitators for these techniques.

Psychological Benefits of Hospitalization

Some think that hospitalization causes only negative psychological effects. The stress of illness and hospitalization can actually be growth enhancing by promoting a child's coping skills and bolstering his self-esteem. Children can increase their self-confidence as a result of overcoming the anxiety related to hospitalization and perhaps by mastering some self-care skills. They feel good about their recovery or increased ability to cope with any disability they have. In addition, hospitalization offers an opportunity for children to ask questions and obtain new information. Some even become interested in a career in health care while observing professionals caring for them. Hospitalization can also be an opportunity to teach parents about children's growth and development, improve parenting skills, and assess the child's immunization record.

NURSING CARE OF THE HOSPITALIZED CHILD

Assessment

Admission. The admission procedure sets the tone for the hospitalization. It should not be a series of questions, but rather a time of collaboration between the nurse and the family. The time the family has spent in the emergency department, the seriousness of the illness, other family needs (e.g., other children with parents or left with neighbors), and many other factors may affect the interview process.

T. C. THOMPSON CHILDREN'S HOSPITAL
ADMISSION SHEET

Dear Parent,
Welcome to Children's Hospital. We want to work with you to plan the care that your child will receive. You can help us by completing pages 1 and 2 of this form. The information will help us learn about your child's illness or condition and about his/her general health. Your nurse will review your answers and together we will develop a plan for your child's care.

Person completing form ______________ Relationship to patient ____________ Legal guardian: ☐ Yes ☐ No

I brought my child to the hospital because ______________________________

My doctor told me this about my child's illness ______________________________

My child was in Children's or ______________ Hospital before because of ____________ Date ____________

My usual doctor is ______________ My language: ☐ English ☐ other ____________

While my child is in the hospital, I can be reached at: (____) ____________ I will be staying with my child in the hospital. ☐ Yes ☐ No

DISCHARGE PLANNING INFORMATION

I live in ______________ (city) ☐ house ☐ apartment ☐ other ____________

Please circle: electric / gas / wood / kerosene / other well water / city water

I have been receiving help from: ☐ Home health ______________ (name) ☐ Visiting nurse ☐ Birth defects center ☐ CSS ☐ other ______________

I may need help with my child at home, after discharge. ☐ Yes ☐ No

My child has been exposed to these illnesses in the past 3 weeks:

☐ measles ☐ chickenpox ☐ mumps ☐ rubella ☐ none

My child's immunizations are: ☐ up to date ☐ not up to date ☐ unknown

My child is in school/daycare at ______________ School ______________ Grade ________

Does he/she enjoy going to school? ☐ Yes ☐ No

Please list each medication your child takes. If there are problems taking the drug, please describe those also. While your child is in the hospital, ALL medications will be provided unless your doctor tells us differently. If you brought medications with you, please show them to your nurse.

Name	Amount	Schedule	Last taken	Reason for taking

Allergies/adverse reactions to medications: ☐ None

Medicine: ____________ Reaction: ____________

Medicine: ____________ Reaction: ____________

Medicine: ____________ Reaction: ____________

Medicine: ____________ Reaction: ____________

Other allergies: (i.e., food, environmental)

____________ Reaction: ____________

____________ Reaction: ____________

____________ Reaction: ____________

____________ Reaction: ____________

Previous blood transfusion: ☐ No ☐ Yes Date: ____________

Reactions: ______________________________

____

ADDRESSOGRAPH

Figure 15–5

Sample hospital admission interview form. (Courtesy of T. C. Thompson Children's Hospital of Chattanooga, Tennessee)

Illustration continued on following page

Please circle your answer and use the space provided to describe or provide more information.

My child uses a: ☐ pacifier ☐ bottle ☐ cup ☐ special nipple-feeding tube Type ______

My child ate/drank ______ at ______ (time)

My child's diet formula: breast formula baby food table (regular) vegetarian kosher other ______

Yes	No	
____	____	Recent weight loss? Gain? Amount ______
____	____	Changes in appetite or thirst? How? ______
____	____	Difficulty with eating or swallowing? ______
____	____	Special likes/dislikes ______ Wets bed? ______
____	____	My child is potty trained. Word for bowel movement? ______ Word for urine? ______
____	____	Diarrhea or constipation? Laxatives/other aids ______

Special needs ______

Find your child's age group and check what your child can do.

0-10 Months	10 Months - 2.5 Years	2.5-5 Years	5 -11 Years	11 Years and Older
☐ Smiles spontaneously	☐ Use words "Dada", "Mama"	☐ States own name	☐ Writes own name	☐ States how he/she became sick and in hospital
☐ Vocalizes laughs	☐ Drinks from a cup	☐ Dresses self with supervision	☐ Adds 4 + 3 =	☐ States special interests/hobbies
☐ Holds head steady	☐ Indicates wants without crying	☐ Correctly identifies two colors	☐ States name of one friend	☐ Multiplies 9 × 7 =
☐ Turns head toward voice	☐ Stands alone well	☐ Follows two-step command: "Pick up the toy and put it away"	☐ States why he/she is in hospital	☐ States duties at home/work
☐ Resists toy pull	☐ Walks alone well		☐ States one positive thing about self	☐ States one positive thing about self
☐ Sits without support	☐ Uses two-word phrases	☐ Balances on one foot for 5 seconds	☐ Maintains eye contact	☐ Reads this sentence: I am a patient at Children's Hospital.
☐ Works for toy out of reach	☐ Follows one-step command: "Give me the toy"	☐ Copies: 0+	☐ Reads this sentence: The flower is red.	
☐ Stands holding on	☐ Uses spoon, spilling little	☐ Makes eye contact		☐ Able to state name of two friends
☐ Plays pat-a-cake	☐ Points to one named body part	☐ Defines: "house, book, car"	Comments: ______	
☐ Walks holding on	☐ Scribbles			

Any difficulty with hearing? ☐ Yes ☐ No

Difficulty seeing? ☐ Yes ☐ No Wears glasses/contacts? ______ Type ______ Do you have them with you? ______

Difficulty learning new things? ☐ Yes ☐ No

The easiest way for my child to learn new things ______

My child responds to pain or discomfort by ______

My child has chronic pain ☐ Yes ☐ No How often? ______ How severe? ☐ Mild ☐ Moderate ☐ Severe

Do you do anything special that helps? ______ Usual medication for pain ______

What changes has this illness/condition caused in your child's life? ______

What has your child/you and your family done to respond to these changes? ______

How does your child react to new experiences in general? ______

Are there any recent changes in family life that may affect this hospitalization? ______

Are there other children in the family? ______

Who else lives in your household? ______

Do you have family or friends in the area? ______

Whom do you define as your family or support team? ______

Security item? ______ Night light? ______

Being in the hospital is stressful for many people. These are things you can do to make it easier for me or for my child ______

______

I want you to be aware of these cultural or spiritual needs ______

______

How would you like to participate in your child's care? ☐ bath ☐ bedmaking ☐ feeding ☐ giving oral medications ☐ other ______

Signature ______

Reviewed and discussed with parents ______ , RN

Figure 15–5

Continued

ACKNOWLEDGING PARENTAL STRESS "Mrs. Smith, I know you're concerned about your other children. Would you like to call your neighbor before I ask you some questions about Heidi and her illness?"

Most hospitals provide an admission interview form (Fig. 15–5). Some of the information is essential for providing immediate care, and some can be collected later. By recognizing the needs of the family, the nurse can structure each admission to fit that particular child and family. If the parent has entered the system through the emergency department, he may have answered some of the questions previously. By looking at the forms from other departments, repetition can be avoided. However, data about allergies, medications taken at home, the history of the illness, and other relevant details must be repeated.

Information should be collected only if there is intent to use it. It is important to determine the best time to interview the parent, based on the condition of the child and family. Setting priorities is a critical component of the admission process.

Although hospitals have policies and procedures for admission, the routine may need to be altered based on the child's condition. For example, a severely dehydrated child should have an intravenous infusion started, and a child in pain should be medicated before any other interventions are performed. On the other hand, the primary needs of the child and family may be emotional. A parent who has just been told that her child may have a terminal disease may have difficulty remembering the dates of the child's immunizations. In this situation, the nurse should provide the parent with support and assistance in mobilizing coping mechanisms and support systems rather than focusing on data gathering.

Initial Assessment. The initial assessment determines the need for any immediate or emergency care that must be provided before other information can be obtained. After the child is made comfortable (Fig. 15–6), a more thorough assessment of the body systems and a health and psychosocial history can be obtained.

Baseline Data. For all types of admissions, a complete physical assessment is performed by the nurse and an admission data sheet is completed. The format of the admission data sheet varies from hospital to hospital, but most contain much of the same information: history; allergies; nutritional, sleep, elimination, and psychosocial information; and the initial physical assessment.

The physical assessment should be thorough, and special attention should be given to the body system involved in the child's admission. Many admission forms have an outline of the child's body to indicate any bruises, scratches, or other markings on the skin to provide specific objective data. The process of interviewing, taking a history, and physical assessment is explained in Chapter 11.

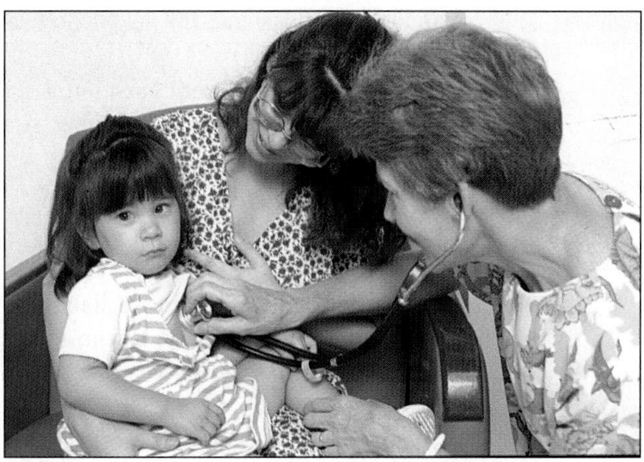

Figure 15–6
To reduce the stress of unfamiliar surroundings and people, the nurse assesses this child while she remains in the security of her mother's arms. (Courtesy of T. C. Thompson, Children's Hospital, Chattanooga, Tennessee)

Information about assessment of communication, nutrition, and pain is provided in Chapters 10, 12, and 20, respectively.

Ask the parents whether there is anyone they need to notify of the child's hospitalization. This question helps to mobilize the support system for the family.

Data collected at admission are used to formulate nursing diagnoses and the child's plan of care, and should be placed in the body of the child's chart. The information should not merely be placed at the back of the chart and forgotten.

Nursing Diagnoses

The following nursing diagnoses are examples that may be appropriate following assessment of a child who is hospitalized.

- Altered Nutrition: Less Than Body Requirements related to unfamiliar foods, separation from caregiver, strange environment, or disease process.
- Ineffective Individual Coping related to anxiety of hospitalization.
- Anxiety related to fear of the unknown and separation from significant others and familiar surroundings.
- Anxiety related to procedures and treatment.
- Diversional Activity Deficit related to separation from normal activities and peers.
- Altered Family Processes related to hospitalization of a child.
- Self Care Deficit related to physical disability, change in environment, and regression.
- Sleep Pattern Disturbance related to unfamiliar environment, separation from caregiver, or discomfort.

Planning, Implementation, and Evaluation: The Hospitalized Child

NURSING DIAGNOSIS • Altered Nutrition: Less Than Body Requirements related to unfamiliar foods, separation from caregiver, strange environment, or disease process.

Expected Outcome: • The child's nutritional intake will meet the metabolic needs for the age group.

Intervention	Rationale
1. Assess the child's current nutritional intake, and identify the normal nutritional requirements for the child's age. Obtain height and weight and plot on growth chart.	Assessment data form a baseline, and normal nutritional requirements are the foundation for formulating a plan of care.
2. Identify the cause of the child's anorexia.	Identification of the cause of anorexia can assist in the elimination of the problem.
3. Obtain a nutrition history of the child, including favorite foods and eating rituals.	Identification of normal nutrition habits will aid in providing the child with familiar foods and eating routines that will reduce anxiety associated with unfamiliar surroundings.
4. Encourage parents to bring foods from home and to be with the child during meals.	Simulates the home environment and increases the likelihood that the child will eat.
5. Allow the child to select food from the menu.	Gives the child control and provides an opportunity to select foods that the child likes and will eat.
6. Offer frequent, nutritious snacks, and encourage parents to do the same.	Children may eat junk food and then refuse nutritious foods offered at mealtimes.
7. Offer small portions. Use small dishes, cups, and glasses.	Children may be overwhelmed by large portions and refuse to eat any of the food (see Chapter 12 and also Chapters 4, 5, 6, 7, 8 for further discussion of portions).
8. If parents cannot be available during meals, allow the child to eat with other children.	Other children may distract the child and decrease separation anxiety.
9. Request a nutritional consultation.	Dietitians can assist in planning age-appropriate nutritious meals.
10. Respect the child's cultural and religious dietary requests.	Religious and cultural preferences may restrict a child's food choices. Efforts should be made to meet the individual needs of each child.

See Chapter 12 for further discussion of the nutritional needs of children.

Evaluation: The child maintains baseline body weight during hospitalization, and nutritional intake is appropriate for the child's age and body weight. Goals should be realistic based on the child's health status.

NURSING DIAGNOSIS • Ineffective Individual Coping related to anxiety associated with hospitalization.

Expected Outcome: • The child will maintain the current level of toilet training.

Intervention	Rationale
1. Follow home routines of elimination.	Compliance will increase and anxiety will be decreased if the child is able to maintain normal routines and rituals.
2. Inquire about the child's terms for elimination.	Communication will be enhanced if both parties have an understanding of what they are asking.
3. Do not scold the child if she is incontinent.	If the incontinence is caused by anxiety, scolding will only increase the anxiety.
4. Explain to parents that some regression is normal in hospitalized children and that most children resume their normal routines soon after discharge.	Parents may be concerned by the child's regression and may increase the child's anxiety by focusing on the child's incontinence.
5. Discourage parents from beginning toilet training during hospitalization.	Toilet training can add another stressor at a difficult time.

Expected Outcome: • The child experiences no incontinence or urine or stool while hospitalized.

NURSING DIAGNOSIS • Anxiety related to fear of the unknown and separation from significant others and familiar surroundings.

Expected Outcome: • The child will display decreased indicators of distress (e.g., crying, withdrawal).

Intervention	Rationale
1. Orient the child and parent to the hospital and the routines of the unit.	A familiarity with the environment and its expectations will decrease anxiety related to fear of the unknown.
2. Prepare the child and parent for all procedures.	Preparation for an event decreases anxiety and fear.
3. Encourage parents to stay with the child when possible and to be involved in the care of the child.	Supports the parental role and decreases the anxiety of the child related to separation.
4. Hold, rock, and cuddle the infant or young child.	Increases feelings of security and trust.
5. If the parents cannot stay with the child, provide for a consistent caregiver.	Continuity of care provides the child with a consistent person with whom he can develop a trusting relationship.
6. Follow home routines and rituals when possible.	Familiar routines help the child to predict events and reduce anxiety caused by the unfamiliar setting.
7. Encourage the parents to be honest with the child when they leave and to inform the nurse where they can be reached and when they will return. Encourage the parents to call while they are gone. The older child can talk on the phone with his parents.	Trust is increased when parents and caregivers are honest with the child. If parents just disappear, the child will feel anger, abandonment, and acute anxiety. By keeping open the lines of communication, the parent's anxiety is decreased.
8. Encourage parents to bring a transitional object (e.g., blanket, teddy bear) and to provide reminders of parents if they cannot be with the child (e.g., pictures, scarf, handkerchief).	Transition objects give the child a feeling of security. Both transition objects and reminders of the parents comfort the child and help decrease the anxiety related to separation.

Intervention	Rationale
9. Take the child to the playroom and introduce him to other children when appropriate.	Provides a form of distraction and assists the child in adapting to the environment.
10. For the older child, arrange for peer contact through visits, phone calls, and letters.	The older child may fear that his peers may replace him. By maintaining contact and sharing information with peers, the child maintains his sense of importance and security.
11. Offer choices and allow the child to make decisions when appropriate.	Increases the child's sense of control.
12. Involve the child in his care when appropriate.	Increases the child's self-esteem.
13. Encourage the child to wear his own clothes and decorate his room.	Gives the child an opportunity to express himself and feel more comfortable in the environment.
14. Provide opportunities for the older child to express his feelings about his illness and hospitalization.	Fear and anxiety can be decreased if the child has an opportunity to communicate his feelings, have them validated, and participate in problem-solving techniques.

Evaluation: The child plays and communicates with other children and staff, performs self-care when appropriate, and separates from parents with increased ease.

NURSING DIAGNOSIS • Diversional Activity Deficit related to separation from normal activities and peers.

Expected Outcome: • The child becomes involved in play activities.

Intervention	Rationale
1. Plan for play activities. Spend time with the child reading, playing board games, drawing, or working on a journal.	Play is a normal part of a child's life. Play is a means of communication. It can decrease stress and boredom and act as a means of releasing anger associated with the illness.
2. Plan diversional activities based on the child's age, developmental level, interests, limitations, and safety.	Play is a part of a child's development. The needs of each age group are different (see Chapter 9).
3. Have parents bring the child's favorite toys from home.	Familiar toys can act as transition objects for the child and decrease anxiety by giving the child a sense of security.
4. Communicate with a child life specialist about the identified needs of the child (e.g., fear, anxiety, anger, boredom, lack of information).	Child life specialists can work with the child to identify her fears and concerns, provide an avenue for release of feelings, and teach her about procedures or surgery.
5. Provide opportunities for the child to meet other children. Assign the child a roommate of the same age, sex, and physical capabilities when possible.	Peer activities are especially important to the older child and the adolescent. Children who have more in common are more likely to interact.
6. Encourage peers to visit, call, and send cards and letters.	Spending time with friends and reading cards and letters can provide distraction for the hospitalized child.

Intervention	Rationale
7. Document the child's response to play.	Observation of play can provide information about the child's developmental level, psychosocial skills, level of anxiety, and adjustment to hospitalization.
8. If the child is too ill, play for the child.	Children who are too ill to play often benefit from watching someone else play (e.g., parents, siblings, nurse).

Evaluation: The child engages in play with other children in the playroom or in his room.

NURSING DIAGNOSIS • Altered Family Processes related to hospitalization of a child.

Expected Outcome: • The parents will participate in the care of the child and maintain mutual support of each member of the family.

Intervention	Rationale
1. Assess the physical and emotional needs of the family.	Assists in identifying factors that might interfere with an appropriate adjustment to the child's illness.
2. Orient the parents to the hospital and provide information related to their physical needs (e.g., food, sleep, bathing).	The physical needs of the parents must be met for them to meet the child's and their own emotional needs. Meeting these needs indicates support for the parents from the health care giver.
3. Encourage the family to express their feelings and to ask questions about the child's illness.	Decreases anxiety and clarifies misconceptions.
4. Provide the family with information about the child's condition, treatment, and support systems.	Gives the parents a sense of control and decreases their anxiety.
5. Identify with the family the ways in which they are coping.	Individuals are not always aware of their coping mechanisms, and the nurse should evaluate the effectiveness of the family's coping mechanisms.
6. Refer the family to other professionals (e.g., social worker, clinical psychologist, clinical specialist, psychiatrist, clergy) when their problems are not within the scope of nursing.	Early identification of family problems can decrease the possibility of escalation of the problems. Collaboration with other professionals can bring a holistic approach to the care of the child and family.
Home Care Teaching 1. Assess the family's knowledge. 2. Provide information about the illness or trauma and expected outcomes. Tell the parents when they should consult the primary care physician or nurse. 3. Explain medications to be given at home, and provide written information about times, route, side effects, and any special care to be taken when giving the medication.	A systematic approach should be used to assist the family in their readjustment to the home environment.

Intervention	Rationale
4. Explain any special nutritional needs.	A systematic approach should be used to assist the family in their readjustment to the home environment.
5. Identify specific activities in which the child may and sometimes should participate.	
6. Provide a date when the child may return to school.	
7. Explain, demonstrate, and request a return demonstration of any treatments or procedures that will be done at home. This teaching should be an ongoing process and not left until the time of discharge because learning takes place at different rates.	
8. Provide the parents with a date to bring the child back to the hospital, clinic, or office for follow-up care.	
9. Provide the parents with information about any referral agency needed for the child or family.	

Evaluation:
- The family members support each other and seek other resources when necessary.
- The child is cared for by the family, who assists the child in moving from a sick role to a well role.

NURSING DIAGNOSIS
- Self Care Deficit related to physical disability, change in environment, and regression.

Expected Outcome:
- The child will participate physically in age-appropriate feeding, dressing, toileting, and bathing activities.

Intervention	Rationale
1. Assess the child's usual self-care activities.	Provides a baseline of the child's actual abilities rather than age-expected criteria, which may be inaccurate if the child has a chronic illness or other factors that have caused delays.
2. Encourage the child to participate in self-care according to his developmental abilities.	Increases the child's self-esteem and feeling of control.
3. Teach the child self-care behaviors and provide opportunities to relearn or adapt to an activity.	Limitations may be placed on the child because of immobility, sensory alterations, or cognitive deficits. The child's sense of self-worth increases when his abilities are used to their maximum.
4. Assist the child when his ability to perform self-care is limited because of fatigue, discomfort, or other factors related to the disease process.	The disease process may limit the child's ability to physically or mentally perform self-care.
5. Explain to the parents that regression is a response to illness and may affect the child's ability to perform self-care.	Regression may be a defense mechanism to a threatening situation (i.e., illness and hospitalization).

Intervention	Rationale
6. Provide the necessary equipment for self-care, and place it within easy reach.	Decreases the complexity of providing self-care by making the environment easier to manipulate.
7. Offer choices, and include them in the plan of care.	Reduces the child's feelings of powerlessness and promotes self-worth and a feeling of control.

Evaluation: The child feeds, toilets, and bathes herself at the same level as before illness when appropriate for the child's condition.

NURSING DIAGNOSIS • Sleep Pattern Disturbance related to unfamiliar environment, separation from caregiver, or discomfort.

Expected Outcome: • The child will maintain a balance of sleep and activity.

Intervention	Rationale
1. Determine the child's usual sleep routine, including time, hygiene practices, and rituals, such as rocking, stories, or snacks.	An understanding of the child's normal sleep patterns will assist in planning care. Maintaining a routine decreases anxiety and increases the child's ability to sleep.
2. Decrease the child's level of anxiety or discomfort (see the diagnosis related to anxiety in this care plan and see Chapter 20 for information on relief of pain).	Inability to sleep can be caused by anxiety or discomfort.
3. Plan care to allow time for periods of sleep. Care can be organized so that vital signs can be taken and other procedures performed when medication is given.	Allows for uninterrupted sleep. Children who are awakened a short time after they have fallen asleep often have difficulty going back to sleep.
4. Post a sign on the door when the child is asleep to prevent other staff and visitors from waking the child. Unplug the phone, turn off the TV, close the door unless the child must be observed, and pull the blinds.	Environmental distractions can be major sleep interruptions.
5. If the parents are not with the child, explain to the child that you will be nearby and will check on her during the night. Provide a nightlight.	Feelings of security are increased if the child understands that someone is watching out for her.

Evaluation: The child takes naps and sleeps an appropriate amount of time based on her age requirements. See Chapters 4, 5, 6, 7, and 8 for further discussion of age-related sleep requirements.

THE FAMILY OF AN ILL CHILD

Parents

When a child becomes ill, it may cause a **situational crisis** for the family. If the illness leads to hospitalization, either planned or unplanned, the anxiety in the family increases. Ill children become the central focus of the parents. The parents' need for information and knowledge and their desire to be with the child are important to them (Fisher, 1994; Fig. 15–7).

Parents may wonder why their family is facing the crisis of a childhood illness or may believe that if they had sought treatment earlier, the child would not be so ill. A parent may delay taking a child who has had a low-grade fever and vague symptoms to a physician. If the symptoms are a sign of a serious illness, the parent may feel guilty for

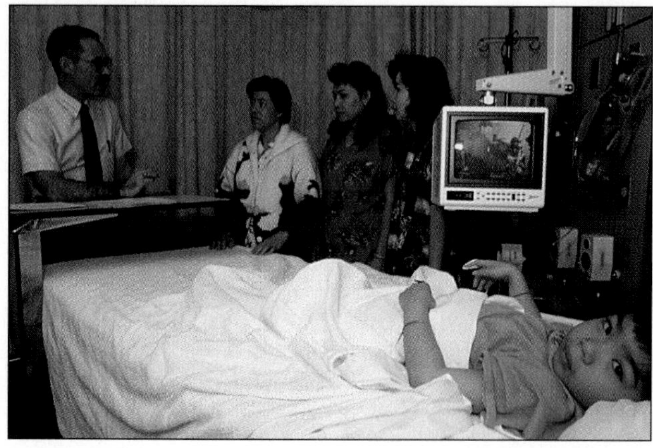

Figure 15–7
Sometimes the family of a hospitalized child may not speak the prevailing language. Translators on call at many hospitals help such parents communicate with hospital personnel and provide a familiar link to the parents' and child's culture and language. (Courtesy of Cook Children's Medical Center, Fort Worth, Texas)

not seeking care earlier. It is important to be aware of parents' feelings and to listen closely to what is being said. The nurse can then assist the parent in working through their feelings of guilt.

Parents have varied responses to a child's illness. They may initially deny that their child is ill, especially if the illness is serious. The period of **denial** may be followed by anger. The anger may be directed at the nurse, another family member, or sometimes at God. When the immediate crisis is over, a period of depression may occur. At this point, the parents are usually both physically and psychologically exhausted. Often, they have been spending long hours at the hospital while working and trying to care for the other children in the family.

The parental role often changes when the child is admitted to the hospital. The parent who had been in control before the admission is now in an unfamiliar environment. Parents may be confused as to what they can and cannot do. Can they bathe their child? Can they even hold their child, or will they disturb the tubes? When the parent is not given permission to perform some of the care, both the child and the parent suffer.

> The parents are the experts about their child. They need to participate in the planning and care of their child.

The needs of fathers are sometimes forgotten because they may not be as visible as those of mothers. The father may come to the hospital only after he has worked and then, after a short visit, may need to go home to be with other children. He may not be there when the primary care physician makes rounds, and therefore receives most of his medical information from someone else. The father may think that he needs to be the strong one in the family and not show his fear and anxiety. In some families, the mother works outside the home while the father stays with the child. In either case, an awareness of each parent's role will assist the nurse in identifying the individual needs of the parents.

Because of dual roles, long separations, increased stress, and numerous other factors, the parents' marriage may be strained. This situation is especially likely in marriages that are already at risk. Even when both partners are at the hospital, they may not have any time alone.

Many children have stepmothers and stepfathers. In such cases both sets of parents need recognition, support, and education. How the family copes with the illness of a child depends on its coping strategies. A family that is already in crisis or one without support systems (e.g., family, friends, church) will have more difficulty adjusting to the change than a family that is organized and adjusted. A family that deals successfully with the crisis is strengthened by the experience.

For further discussion of the effects of illness on the family, see Chapter 16 and the care plan for nursing diagnoses (pp. 388–391). For a discussion of the family with a child with a chronic illness, see Chapter 17.

Siblings

The illness or hospitalization of a brother or sister can be difficult for children. The siblings of the ill child may experience jealousy, insecurity, resentment, confusion, and anxiety. It is often difficult for children to understand why their ill sibling is getting all of the attention and why their parents seem so preoccupied and have so little time for them. They may worry that if their sibling could get sick, so could they. The preschool child who is engaged in magical thinking may worry that he somehow caused his sister's illness. All of these thoughts and feelings are compounded by the fact that children have difficulty expressing their feelings and may hold everything within themselves. Some children are at greater risk than others. The amount of stress the sibling experiences varies according to the type of sibling relationship, the residence of the well sibling during the hospitalization, the frequency of sibling visitation, and the amount of parental behavior change as perceived by the ill child's sibling (Simon, 1993).

The accompanying box lists factors that may affect siblings of a hospitalized or ill child, and provides guidelines for meeting the needs of the siblings. A detailed discussion of siblings can be found in Chapters 16 and 17.

Caring for the Siblings of an Ill or Hospitalized Child

FACTORS THAT ADD TO THE STRESS OF SIBLINGS

- Age younger than 10 years.
- Emotionally close to the hospitalized child.
- Receiving only a limited explanation of the experience.
- Afraid of getting the illness themselves.
- Cared for outside their own home.
- Perceive their parents as acting differently toward them.
- Sibling of progressively ill child.

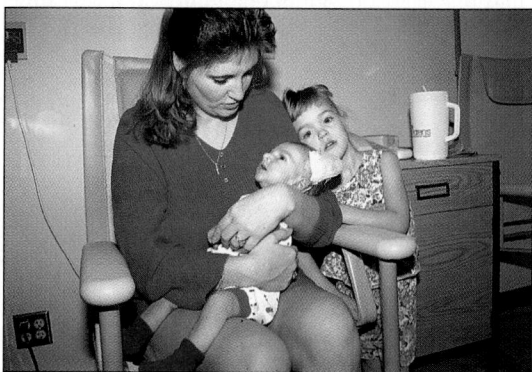

Her brother's repeated hospitalizations for problems associated with a diaphragmatic hernia have been difficult for this girl. Siblings of ill children may experience jealousy, insecurity, resentment, confusion, and anxiety. The nurse can help this child to cope by paying attention to her when she is providing care to the infant. (Courtesy of Children's Medical Center, Dallas, Texas)

NURSING CARE GUIDELINES FOR MEETING THE NEEDS OF SIBLINGS

- Encourage caregivers to have the ill child retell what happened. This experience may be uncomfortable for the adult, but it helps the sibling to put the illness or accident in perspective.
- If the sibling suggests that he feels guilty, address the child's concerns directly. If the feelings of guilt continue, suggest a consultation with a counselor.
- Give parents educational materials, and show them how to use them with the sibling.
- Schedule a time for the sibling to visit. Prepare the sibling for the medical equipment and any changes in the ill child's appearance that may cause concern.
- If the sibling cannot visit, send photographs.
- Encourage the sibling to talk with the patient on the telephone.

Adapted from Craft, M., Wyatt, N., & Sandell, B. (1985). Behavior and feeling changes in siblings of hospitalized children. *Clinical Pediatrics, 24*(7), 374–378.

NURSING CARE OF THE FAMILY

Through the use of family-centered care, the child is considered and treated in the context of the family and the family is recognized as the primary and continuing provider of care for the child. Although it is sometimes necessary to plan care without involving the family, it is difficult to do so.

Assessment

Several factors are identified in Chapter 16 that affect a family's adjustment to illness and hospitalization (see p. 387). Each of these factors should be assessed as well as the history of the child's admission. Was the admission an emergency? Have there been previous admissions, and how did the parents perceive those hospitalizations? How serious is the illness or trauma? Are there unknown factors such as the cause of the disease or the prognosis of the child? Special attention should also be given to any information obtained in the admission interview.

Nursing Diagnoses

- Parental role conflict related to lack of knowledge of expected role, change in environment and culture, and separation from other family members.
- Anxiety and fear related to the crisis of illness and hospitalization.
- Family health maintenance, altered, related to situational crisis.
- Home maintenance management, impaired, after discharge related to knowledge deficit and lack of support.

See Chapter 16 for a care plan outlining nursing care for the family of an ill child and information about nursing care of the siblings.

KEY CONCEPTS

- Pediatric nurses may care for children in the hospital, community, or home. Each setting requires special interventions.
- Common stressors affecting hospitalized children include fear of the unknown, separation anxiety, fear of pain or mutilation, and loss of control.
- Children may experience anger, guilt, and regression in response to illness.
- The stages of separation anxiety are protest, despair, and detachment.
- The more stressed a child becomes, the more difficult it is for him to separate from his parent.
- A child's reaction to pain and fear of injury is related to the child's previous experiences, separation from parents, restraint, and amount of preparation.
- Children who feel that they have control over their illness and hospitalization are more likely to feel confident and to be cooperative.
- Regression is a common response to illness and hospitalization. The child returns to an earlier form of behavior.
- How a child reacts to illness and hospitalization is affected by her perception of the event, age, cognitive ability, preparation, previous experiences, coping skills, and the parent's response.
- Nursing care of the ill child is directed toward meeting the child's needs related to self-care, separation anxiety, growth and development, diversion, family, control, and pain.
- Parents may experience guilt, denial, anger, and depression when their child is hospitalized.

REFERENCES

Corbo-Richert, B., Caty, S., & Barnes, C. (1993). Coping behaviors of children hospitalized for cardiac surgery: A secondary analysis. *American Journal of Maternal-Child Nursing, 21,* 27–36.

Craft, M., Wyatt, N., & Sandell, B. (1985). Behavior and feeling changes in siblings of hospitalized children. *Clinical Pediatrics, 24*(7), 374–378.

Fisher, M. (1994). Identified needs of parents in a pediatric intensive care unit. *Critical Care Nurse, 14*(3), 82–90.

Hart, D., & Bossert, E. (1994). Self-reported fears of hospitalized school-age children. *Journal of Pediatric Nursing, 9*(2), 83–89.

LaMontagne, L. (1993). Bolstering personal control in child patients through coping interventions. *Pediatric Nursing, 19*(3), 235–237.

Manion, J. (1990). Preparing children for hospitalization, procedures, or surgery. In M. Craft & J. Denehy (Eds.), *Nursing Interventions for Infants and Children.* Philadelphia: W. B. Saunders.

Pietrobono, J. (1994). Taking health care where the kids are. *Texas Medicine,* 14–23.

Selye, H. (1974). *Stress Without Distress.* New York: J. B. Lippincott.

Simon, K. (1993). Perceived stress of nonhospitalized children during the hospitalization of a sibling. *Journal of Pediatric Nursing: Nursing Care of Children and Families, 8*(5), 298–304.

Struk, C. (1994). Women and children: Infant mortality, urban programs, and home care. *Nursing Clinics of North America, 29*(3), 395–408.

Visintainer, M., & Wolfer, J. (1975). Psychological preparation for surgical pediatric patient: The effect on children's and parents' stress response and adjustment. *Pediatrics, 56*(2), 187–202.

BIBLIOGRAPHY

Baker, N. (1994). Avoiding collisions with challenging families. *American Journal of Maternal-Child Nursing, 19*(2), 97–101.

Biddinger, L. (1993). Bruner's theory of instruction and preprocedural anxiety in the pediatric population. *Issues in Comprehensive Pediatric Nursing, 16*(3), 147–154.

Biester, D. (1994). Schools and health: A partnership for a healthier future. *Journal of Pediatric Nursing, 9*(6), 414–416.

Bossert, E. (1994). Factors influencing the coping of hospitalized school-age children. *Journal of Pediatric Nursing: Nursing Care of Children and Families, 9*(5), 299–306.

Brennon, A. (1994). Caring for children during procedures: A review of the literature. *Pediatric Nursing, 20*(5), 451–461.

Brewster, A. (1982). Chronically ill hospitalized children's concepts of their illness. *Pediatrics, 69*(3), 355–362.

Coffman, S., Levitt, M., & Guacci-Franco, N. (1993). Mothers' stress and close relationships: Correlates with infant health status. *Pediatric Nursing, 19*(2), 135–140.

Craft, M. (1993). Siblings of hospitalized children: Assessment and intervention. *Journal of Pediatric Nursing: Nursing Care of Children and Families, 8*(5), 289–297.

Durham, E., & Frost-Hartzer, P. (1994). Relaxation therapy for children and families. *Journal of Maternal Child Nursing, 19*(4), 222–225.

Ellerton, M., Ritchie, J., & Caty, S. (1994). Factors influencing young children's coping behaviors during stressful healthcare encounters. *Maternal Child Nursing Journal, 22*(3), 74–82.

Fisher, M. (1994). Identified needs of parents in a pediatric intensive care unit. *Critical Care Nurse, 14*(3), 82–90.

Grey, M. (1993). Stressors and children's health. *Journal of Pediatric Nursing, 8*(2), 85–99.

Heuer, L. (1993). Parental stressors in a pediatric intensive care unit. *Pediatric Nursing, 19*(2), 128–133.

Jones, D., (1994). Effect of parental participation on hospitalized child behavior. *Issues in Comprehensive Pediatric Nursing, 17*(2), 81–92.

Kashani, J., Canfield, L., Borduin, C., Soltys, S., & Reid, J. (1994). Perceived family and social support: Impact on children. *Journal of the American Academy of Child and Adolescent Psychiatry, 33*(6), 819–823.

McGraw, T. (1994). Preparing children for the operating room: Psychological issues. *Canadian Journal of Anaesthesia, 41*(11), 1094–1103.

Melnyk, B. (1994). Coping with unplanned childhood hospitalization: Effects of informational interventions on mothers and children. *Nursing Research, 43*(1), 50–55.

Nugent, K. (1989). Routine care: Promoting development in hospitalized infants. *Journal of Maternal Child Nursing, 14*(5), 318–321.

Page, N. (1994). Visitation in the pediatric intensive care unit: Controversy and compromise. *AACN Clinical Issues in Critical Care Nursing, 5*(3), 289–295.

Schepp, K. (1991). Factors influencing the coping effort of mothers of hospitalized children. *Nursing Research, 40*(1), 42–46.

Youngblut, J., & Shiao, S. (1993). Child and family reactions during and after pediatric ICU hospitalization: A pilot study. *Heart and Lung: Journal of Critical Care, 22*(1), 46–54.

Ziegler, D., & Prior, M. (1994). Preparation for surgery and adjustment to hospitalization. *Nursing Clinics of North America, 29*(4), 655–669.

16

Family-Centered Nursing Care

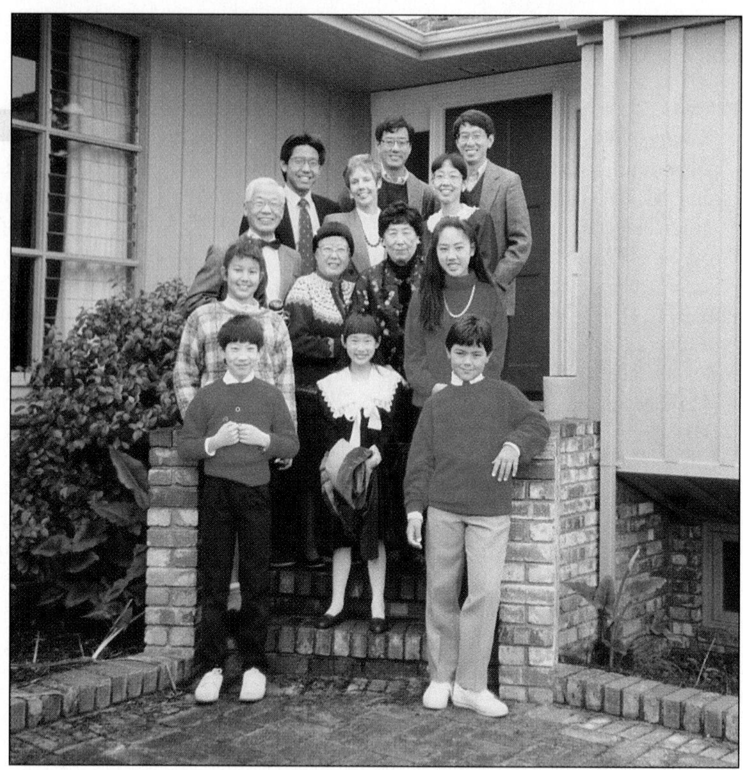

CHAPTER OVERVIEW

LEARNING OBJECTIVES

After studying this chapter, you should be able to:

- Identify the importance of family in the care of ill children.
- Assess the structure and function of a family.
- Discuss how family systems theory provides a framework for organizing nursing care.
- List important factors in parenting.
- Identify the family characteristics and health beliefs and practices of six different cultures.
- Differentiate between functional and dysfunctional families.
- Evaluate the effects of an ill child on the family.
- List internal and external coping behaviors used by families.

KEY TERMS

coping: efforts directed toward managing and solving various problems, events, and stressors.

culture: sum of the customs, habits, and traditions of a particular ethnic or social group.

discipline: the structure an adult sets for a child's life designed to allow him to happily and effectively fit into the real world.

family: two or more emotionally involved people living in close proximity and having reciprocal obligations with a sense of commonness, caring, and commitment (Friedman, 1986).

situational crisis: a period of vulnerability or disorganization after a specific event.

stress: any situation or condition, positive or negative, requiring adjustment on the part of the individual, family, or group.

No other factor influences the child as profoundly as the family. The family protects and promotes the child's growth, development, health, and well-being. The family provides the child with love, affection, and a sense of belonging, and nurtures feelings of self-esteem and self-worth. Every area of a child's life is affected by the family.

Nurses caring for children must consider the whole family the client rather than just the child. The child's needs cannot be adequately met in isolation from the family. This chapter emphasizes the importance of empowering the family in the role of care provider of an ill child. The child's recovery depends on the parents and other family members—their level of stress, effectiveness in coping, and degree of hope, and the amount of physical and emotional support they give to the child. The nurse cares for the child in the context of a dynamic family system, assessing and responding to needs of the family as a unit.

Today, the family is under greater stress than ever before. Although dramatic changes in family structure, roles, and tasks have occurred in recent years, the basic functions of the family remain the same. Children need stable families to grow into happy, functioning adults. It is the responsibility of the nurse to support families and to encourage healthy coping patterns as families experience the crisis of illness.

DEFINITION OF FAMILY

Family structures in the United States have changed considerably in the last 30 years. In 1970, traditional nuclear families made up 40% of all households, but only 26% of all households in 1991 (Saluter, 1992). In addition, roles have changed within the nuclear family. The role of provider, once almost exclusively assigned to the father, is now often shared by both parents, and many fathers are more active in nurturing and disciplining their children.

The growing number of nontraditional families includes single-parent families, blended families, adoptive families, unmarried couples with children, and multigenerational families. Different family structures can produce varying stressors. For example, the single-parent family has as many demands for resources such as time and money as the two-parent family. However, there is only one parent to meet these demands. The number of single-parent families increased from 12.9% of all families in 1970 to 29% in 1991, mostly as a result of the increase in the divorce rate and the increase in births to single mothers (Saluter, 1992). Single-parent households also result from the death of one parent and from separation without divorce. Mothers head nearly 90% of single-parent households. In 1970, 12% of all children under 18 years of age in the United States lived in single-parent households. By 1993 this figure had risen to 27% (U.S. Bureau of the Census, 1996).

Divorce and remarriage have increased the number of blended families, those with stepparents and stepchildren. These families may have some role conflict as the children of one parent seek to adapt to the new parent and vice versa. The number of unmarried couples has also increased, and 40% of these households include children (Saluter, 1992). The multigenerational family, with at least three generations in the same household, is another variation of the family. A growing number of households are being headed by grandparents because of the inability of the parents to care for the children. The mother or father may be present physically, but absent emotionally, or the parent may be absent physically for short or extended periods. If the grandparents are elderly, and sometimes even if they are not, the strain of raising children a second time may cause tremendous physical, financial, and emotional stress.

Nurses should be aware of these variations in family structure to avoid assuming that a family has a traditional structure. Making such an assumption can place a value judgment on the family and close off communication.

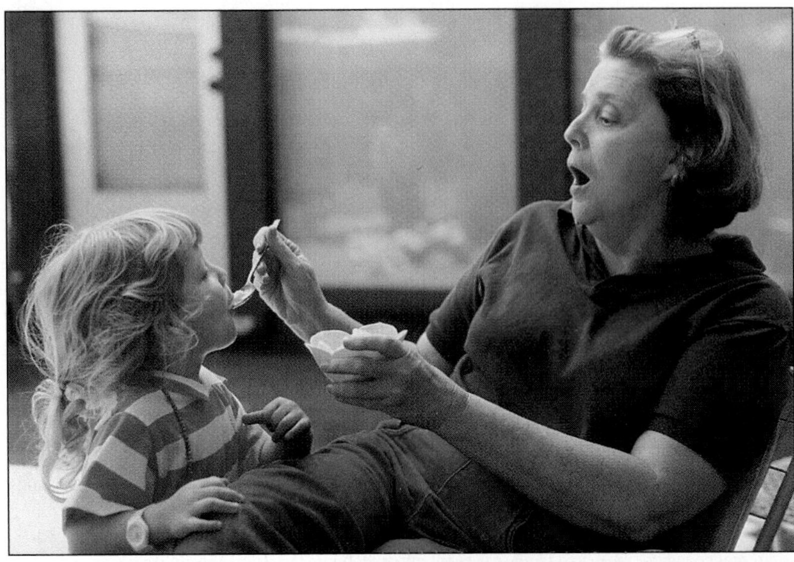

◀ Busy parents may rely on grandparents for child care or for an additional measure of love and attention for their children. Some grandparents raise grandchildren because of their own children's inability to do so.

Fathers are the primary child care providers in a growing number of families. Fathers who are not the primary caregivers often participate more actively in caring for their children than the fathers of previous generations.

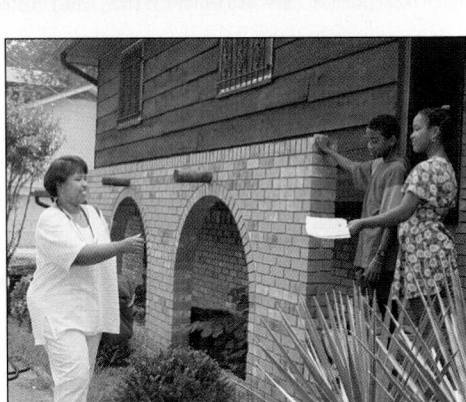

A single parent often experiences ▶ financial and time constraints. Children in single-parent families are often given more responsibility to care for themselves and younger siblings.

Figure 16–1

The nurse caring for a child needs to know the child's family structure and the identity of the child's primary caregiver. This background is the context in which the nurse provides care. The nurse who is concerned with family support will be able to provide the family with information about local community resources. For example, in some communities, after-school programs and "warm lines" are available to help latchkey children with schoolwork and alleviate some of the loneliness or fear these children have.

Considering these changes, the broad definition of **family** used in this chapter is as follows:

> A family is composed of two or more people emotionally involved, living in close proximity, and having reciprocal obligations with a sense of commonness, caring, and commitment (Friedman, 1986).

Five Major Functions of the Family. Marilyn Friedman, professor of family nursing and author of *Family Nursing: Theory and Assessment* (1986), defined five major functions of families:

1. *Affective Function (Personality Maintenance):* To meet the psychological needs of family members: trust and nurturance, intimacy, belonging and bonding, identity, and mutual respect.
2. *Socialization (Social Placement) Function:* To guide children to be productive members of society, and to transmit cultural beliefs to the next generation.
3. *Reproductive Function:* To ensure family continuity and societal survival.
4. *Economic Function:* To provide and effectively allocate economic resources.
5. *Health Care Function:* To provide the physical necessities of life (e.g., food, clothing, shelter, health care); to recognize illness in family members and provide care; and to foster a healthy lifestyle or environment based on preventive medical and dental health practices.

Many people believe that any one or a combination of these five functions cannot be fulfilled by families outside the traditional structure. Many believe that the traditional family structure and traditional family values are in danger of becoming extinct. Because families are the foundation of any society, some are concerned that disintegration of families will lead to the downfall of American society. Poverty, ignorance, and social problems, such as domestic violence, drug or alcohol use, and premature sexual activity, can affect family function. It is important for the nurse to recognize when a child's family is not fulfilling one or more of the five major functions of families.

FAMILY THEORIES AND MODELS

Scholars use different theories or models to explain the dynamics of family relations. For the last 20 years, the most commonly discussed theory in family literature has been von Bertalanffy's systems theory. According to von Bertalanffy (1968), any system is characterized by wholeness, feedback, equifinality, and boundaries (see accompanying box). A family can be viewed as a system.

A direct offshoot of von Bertalanffy's general systems theory is family systems theory. The family systems theory developed by Bowen (1976) is widely accepted today. Bowen described four processes that occur within families: differentiation of self, multigeneration transmission process, triangulation, and family projection process (see box, Systems Theories: An Overview).

PARENTING AND DISCIPLINE

Parenting Styles

There are three major styles of parenting: authoritarian (dictatorial), authoritative (democratic), and permissive (laissez-faire). These three styles represent a continuum of control exerted by the parents over the child, with the authoritarian parent exerting the most control and the permissive parent exerting the least (Fig. 16–2).

Authoritarian parents are rigid in their rules. They expect absolute obedience from the child without any questioning about the reasons behind the rule. They also expect the child to accept the family beliefs and principles without question. Any sign of questioning or disobedience is dealt with by severe punishment, often physical. Withdrawal of love and approval is also a common punishment.

Children raised with this style of parenting are typically shy and withdrawn because of a lack of self-confidence. If the parents are somewhat affectionate, the child may be sensitive, submissive, honest, and dependable. However, if affection has been withheld, the child commonly exhibits rebellious, antisocial behavior.

Authoritative parents tend to show respect for the opinions of each of their children by allowing them to be different. Although there are rules in the household, the parents permit discussion if the children do not understand or agree with the rules. The parents make it clear to the children that although they (the parents) are the ultimate authority, some negotiation and compromise may take place.

This style of parenting tends to result in children who have high self-esteem and are independent, inquisitive, happy, assertive, and highly interactive.

Permissive parents have little or no control over the behavior of their children. If any rules exist in the home, they are inconsistent and unclear. Underlying reasons for rules may be given, but children are generally allowed to decide whether they will follow the rule, and to what extent. Limits are not set, and **discipline** is inconsistent. Parents may make empty threats of punishment. The children learn that they can get away with any behavior. Role reversal occurs: the children are more like the parents, and the parents are like the children.

Children who come from this type of home are typically disrespectful, disobedient, aggressive, irresponsible, and defiant. They are insecure because of a lack of guidelines to direct their behavior. However, these children tend to be creative and spontaneous.

Parent–Child Relationship Factors

As indicated in the discussion of family theories, no family member lives in isolation. The quality of the parent–child relationship is affected by the parents' age, experience, and self-confidence; the stability of the marital relationship; and the unique characteristics of the child compared with the parents' expectations of the child.

Parental Characteristics. Parental self-confidence appears to be an important predictor of parental competence. A study of 48 clinically depressed and 38 nondepressed mothers of 3- to 13-month old infants showed that mothers who believe that they are effective parents are more competent, regardless of whether they are depressed. Mothers who perceived themselves as effective also perceived their infants as less difficult in temperament (Teti & Gelfand, 1991). Parental age and previous experience also appear to be important factors. Research has shown that older mothers are more responsive to their infants than younger mothers (Ragozin et al., 1991). In addition, parents who have had previous experience with children, whether through younger siblings, a career, or previous children, are better able to cope with parenthood.

Parenting is the single greatest commitment in adult life and is a difficult job. Nurses have many opportunities to provide support for parents. The nurse should find at least one area in which to compliment the parents and build their confidence.

Characteristics of the Child. Characteristics that may affect the parent–child relationship include the child's physical appearance, sex, and temperament. At birth, the infant's

Systems Theories: An Overview

VON BERTALANFFY'S SYSTEMS THEORY: AN OVERVIEW

Systems theory gives nurses a way to organize their thinking about families. It helps nurses understand how families function and what happens when something goes wrong. Theories help to organize facts in some sort of pattern. One analogy is a coat rack. A pile of clothes on the floor has no organization. However, if they are hung on a coat rack, they can be organized. For instance, the shirts can be placed on one hook, the sweaters on another, the scarves on another, and the jackets on another. The theory is like a coat rack; it provides one way to organize facts.

The following terms and definitions help to organize facts and ideas about families:

Wholeness

A change in one family member will affect every other member of the family as well as the family structure itself.

Example: The father loses his job and becomes depressed. His mood makes everyone in the family nervous. The mother has to get a job to support the family. She becomes tired and irritable. The children act out by misbehaving in school.

Feedback

The process by which family members relate to each other and their community while maintaining the family's function (self-regulation).

Example: A child misbehaves in school. The principal telephones the parents to arrange a conference (feedback to the parents). The parents talk to the principal and then discipline the child (feedback to the child).

Equifinality

The process by which a family goal can be achieved from several starting points.

Example: Cohesiveness (a family goal) can be achieved if the family members contribute to a fund for a trip that they decide to take together. They talk about the trip, gather brochures, and plan their itinerary.

Boundaries

The invisible lines of demarcation separating the external and internal environments of individual family members, subsets of the family (e.g., parents), and family units. The boundaries vary in permeability and flexibility, and control the amount of energy and information exchanged (Scott, 1993).

Example: A family that never socializes with other families and has family secrets has rigid closed family boundaries. A family that never refuses visitors when they desire privacy has rigid open boundaries.

BOWEN'S FAMILY SYSTEMS THEORY

Differentiation of Self

The degree to which a person can distinguish between the feeling process (emotional system) and the thought process (intellectual system). People with low differentiation are controlled by emotions that direct their decisions and behavior. They are less adaptable than highly differentiated people, are more prone to physical or emotional illness, have weak self-identity, and tend to form highly dependent and emotional relationships. People who are highly differentiated tend to be guided by reason and rational decision making and are less impulsive in their behavior.

Multigeneration Transmission Process

The level of self-differentiation is determined by how the family members socialize the child as he is growing up. When the child becomes an adult, he tends to socialize his children in the same way—one possible explanation for why child abuse and criminal behavior tend to recur in subsequent generations.

Triangulation

The process by which two family members who are experiencing anxiety coerce a third member into joining their struggle or problem to decrease their level of anxiety. In families with lower levels of differentiation, there is more anxiety, and triangles are more commonly formed. This pattern is commonly seen by nurses dealing with families in highly anxious situations. If there are two parents, they may disagree about some treatment choice. One or both parents may attempt to subtly coerce the child into taking "their side" against the other parent. This process is called "triangulating in" the child. The nurse has to be aware of this subconscious strategy and refuse to be drawn into the disagreement or to take sides.

Family Projection Process

A process whereby the anxiety of one of the parents is decreased by becoming overly involved with one of the children. The parent defines what the child is like by projecting attributes onto the child that may have little to do with the child's real character. Eventually, the child becomes what the parent has projected (e.g., rebellious, a loner, an overachiever). Adolescence can be traumatic for these children because it is the time when they search for their identity. A child who has not had an opportunity to explore her unique talents and personality in early childhood will be more confused in adolescence.

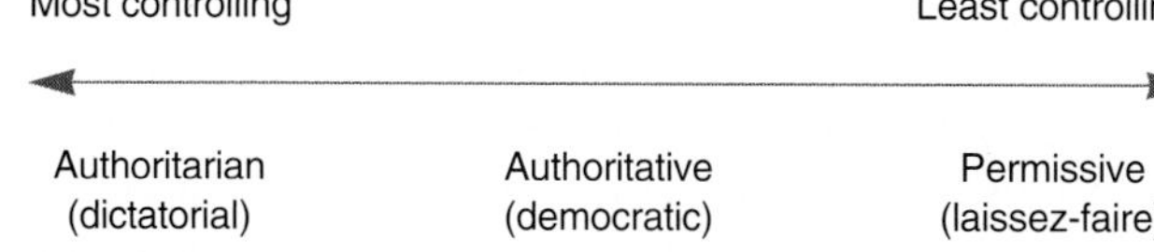

Figure 16–2
Continuum of control in parenting styles.

physical appearance may not meet the parents' expectations, or the infant may resemble a disliked relative. As a result, the parent may subconsciously reject the child. If the parents desired a baby of a particular sex, they may be disappointed. If parents are not given the opportunity to talk about this disappointment, they may reject the infant.

Temperament and Parental Expectations. Thomas and Chess (1977) discovered that most infants (about 70%) exhibit clear temperaments even at birth. These temperaments are classified as follows:

Easy: These children are even-tempered, predictable, and regular in their habits. They react positively to new stimuli. About 40% of children fall into this group.

Difficult: These children are highly active, irritable, moody, and irregular in their habits. They adapt slowly to new stimuli and often express intense negative emotions.

Slow-to-warm-up: These children are inactive, moody, and moderately irregular in their habits. They adapt slowly to new stimuli and express mildly intense negative emotions.

Thomas and Chess derived these three classifications from the nine characteristics of temperament they identified in children (see accompanying box). Some studies have shown that it is not the actual temperament of the child, but rather the fit between the child's temperament and the parents' expectations that determines the parent–child relationship. If the child is different from what the parent expected, there will be conflict. However, in a recent study of 77 mothers of 3- and 4-year-olds, the difficult temperament caused distress in mothers. The mothers' relationships with their children negatively affected their day-to-day lives, including their marital relationships (Sheeber & Johnson, 1992).

Nine Characteristics of Temperament in Children

1. **Level of Activity:** The intensity and frequency of motion during play, eating, bathing, dressing, or sleeping.
2. **Rhythmicity:** Regularity of biologic functions (i.e., sleep patterns, eating patterns, elimination patterns).
3. **Approach/Withdrawal:** The initial response of a child to a new stimulus, such as an unfamiliar person, unfamiliar food, or new toys.
4. **Adaptability:** Ease or difficulty in adjustment to a new stimulus.
5. **Intensity of Response:** The amount of energy with which the child responds to a new stimulus.
6. **Threshold of Responsiveness:** The amount or intensity of stimulation necessary to evoke a response in the child.
7. **Mood:** Frequency of cheerfulness, pleasantness, and friendly behavior versus unhappiness, unpleasantness, and unfriendly behavior.
8. **Distractibility:** How easily the child's attention can be diverted from an activity by external stimuli.
9. **Attention Span/Persistence:** How long the child pursues an activity and continues despite frustration and obstacles.

Data from Thomas, A., & Chess, S. (1977). *Temperament and development.* New York: Brunner-Mazel.

Discipline

Children's behavior offers challenges to even the most educated and experienced parents. The manner in which parents respond to a child's behavior has a profound effect on the child's self-esteem and future interactions with others. Children learn to view themselves in the same way that the parent views them. Thus, if the parent views the child as wild, the child begins to view himself as wild, and soon his actions consistently reinforce his self-image. In this way, the child will not disappoint the parent. This pattern is called a self-fulfilling prophecy and is a cyclic process.

Discipline is often confused with punishment. The word discipline is derived from the word disciple, which means "to learn." Howard (1991) defined **discipline** as:

> *the structure that the adult sets up for a child's life that is designed to allow him or her to fit into the real world happily and effectively. The discipline set up by the parents is the foundation for the development of the child's own self-discipline later. It is within this structure that the child has real choices for behavior that take into account other people and are within the child's control* (Howard, 1991, p. 1352).

Discipline is designed to teach a child how to function effectively within society. It is the foundation for self-discipline. The primary goal of a parent should be to help the child to feel lovable and capable. This goal is best accomplished by the parent setting limits to enhance a sense of security in the child until he can incorporate the family's values and is capable of self-discipline.

Ways to Promote a Child's Socialization and Self-Esteem

PROMOTING A CHILD'S SENSE OF BEING LOVABLE

- Spend guaranteed time with the child.
- Be nonjudgmental and nondirective.
- Play with the child.
- Attend to the child through eye contact, touch, and active listening.
- Ignore minor transgressions.
- Convey positive regard; label the act, not the child.
- Offer positive feedback for positive behavior.
- Demonstrate emotional congruence between verbal and nonverbal messages.
- Warn the child 5 minutes before changing the activity.
- Offer thank you messages.
- Give apologies, but not for punishment.

PROMOTING A CHILD'S SENSE OF BEING CAPABLE

- Establish and maintain routines.
- Role model for the child.
- Make instructions short, simple, and clear.
- Progressively increase expectations as the child ages.
- Allow role-taking opportunities.
- Offer praise and reward.
- Ensure appropriate consequences that are natural and logical.
- Promise, but do not threaten.
- Carry out consequences immediately.
- Allow the child to make choices.

Adapted from Howard, B. (1991). Discipline in early childhood. *Pediatric Clinics of North America, 38*(6), 1351–1369.

When a child is hospitalized, the nurse has the opportunity to aid in the socialization of the child to some degree. The nurse can help the parent to learn how to effectively discipline a child through both formal instruction and informal role modeling. The accompanying box lists ways in which a parent or nurse can facilitate a child's socialization and increase his self-esteem.

Dealing With Misbehavior

A child's misbehavior may be defined as behavior outside the norms of acceptance within the family. Misbehavior presents one of the greatest challenges of parenting. It stretches the limits of tolerance in all parents, even the most patient. It can have minor consequences, such as short-term frustration, or major consequences, such as child abuse. To prevent these negative consequences, the nurse can help to teach parents various strategies to deal with misbehavior.

Time-Out. Time-out is a method of removing the attention given to a child who is misbehaving. The child is placed in a nonstimulating environment where the parent can unobtrusively see her. For example, a chair could be placed facing a wall in a hall or bathroom. The child is told to sit on the chair for a predetermined time, usually 1 minute per year of age. If the child cries or fights, the timing is not begun until the child is quiet. The use of a kitchen timer with a bell is effective because the child knows when the time begins and when it has elapsed. At that time, the child is permitted to get up. After the child has calmed and the time is completed, it may be appropriate to discuss the behavior that prompted the time-out at a level appropriate to the child's age.

Corporal Punishment. Corporal punishment usually takes the form of spanking. It is highly controversial. The problems cited include the following:

- The decrease in misbehavior is short term.
- Children learn that violence is acceptable.
- Children become accustomed to the pain, so some parents may feel that more severe pain is needed.
- Parents may experience rage and lose control, causing harm to the child.

Corporal punishment can lead to child abuse if the disciplinarian loses control. It can also lead to false accusations of child abuse by either the child or other adults. Because of the high cost and low benefit of this form of punishment, parents should think seriously before using it.

Behavior Modification. The behavior modification technique of discipline rewards positive behavior and ignores negative behavior. This technique requires parents to choose selected behaviors, preferably only one at a time, that they desire to extinguish. They choose others that they want to encourage. The basic technique is useful for any age from toddlerhood through adolescence. For a young child, the selected positive behaviors are marked on a chart and explained to the child. For an older child, a contract can be written. The negative behaviors are kept in mind by the parents, but are not recorded where the child can see them. A system of rewards is established. Stickers or stars on a chart for young children and tokens for older children are effective ways to record the behaviors. Children should receive a predetermined reward, for example, a movie, book, or outing, after he successfully performs the behavior a set number of times. This system should continue for several months until the behavior becomes a habit for the child. Then a new behavior can be substituted for the unwanted behavior. Children gain a sense of mastery and actually enjoy the process, often viewing it as a game. Negative behaviors are simply ignored. Consistency is the key to success for this technique, and many parents find this method difficult. Behavior modification theory states that certain negative behaviors are performed solely for gaining attention. Therefore, if the parent refuses to give the child attention for the behavior, the child soon gives up that strategy. Parents need to be warned that children frequently test the seriousness of this attempt by increasing their negative behavior soon after the parents begin ignoring it. This behavior is called a response burst. If this technique is to be successful, the parents need to ignore the negative behavior every time.

Reasoning. Reasoning is a technique that involves explaining why a behavior is not permitted. Because toddlers and preschoolers are egocentric, this technique is not effective for them. They are incapable of "putting themselves in someone else's shoes." When this technique is used with older children, it is important to focus on the behavior and not the child. The child should not be made to feel guilt and shame because these feelings are counterproductive and can damage the child's self-esteem. The parent can focus on the behavior most effectively by using "I" rather than "you" messages.

Eight-year-old Scott takes a toy from his younger brother.

Effective "I" message aimed at the behavior: "I feel angry when I see you take that toy from your brother. He was playing with it first."

Ineffective "you" message aimed at the child: "You are a very bad boy for taking that toy away from your brother."

Consequences. This technique helps children to learn the direct result of their misbehavior and can be used for toddlers through adolescents. If children are required to suffer the consequences of their behavior and the consequences are meaningful to them, then they will not repeat the behavior. There are three categories of consequences:

- *Natural:* Consequences that occur spontaneously. For example, a child loses a favorite toy after leaving it outside. The parent reminds the child that if he had brought the toy inside and put it away, he would not have lost it. Now the toy is gone. The parent does not replace it.
- *Logical:* Consequences that are directly related to the misbehavior. For example, when two children are fighting over a toy, the parent removes the toy from both of them for a day.
- *Unrelated:* Consequences that are imposed purposely. For example, a child comes in late for dinner and, as a consequence, is not allowed to watch TV that evening.

Marital Conflict and Divorce

Although divorce is traumatic to children, research has shown that children are even more traumatized by a home filled with ongoing conflict. In the majority of cases, divorce is highly disruptive to all members of the family. Divorce can be the outcome of many years of unresolved family conflict. It can result in disputes over child custody, visitation, and child support; changes in housing, lifestyle, cultural expectations, friends, and extended family relationships; diminished self-esteem; and changes in the physical, emotional, or spiritual health of the child and other family members.

For children, divorce is loss and needs to be grieved. Parents can have a successful divorce after a failed marriage. Nurses can help children through the grieving process through therapeutic play, such as drawing, puppet play, and sand play. Principles of active listening are valuable. Nurses can also help newly divorced or separated parents through listening, encouragement, and referrals to support groups or counselors.

CULTURAL CHARACTERISTICS OF FAMILIES

Culture—the deposit of knowledge, beliefs, values, and possessions of a group—influences family roles, communication patterns, decision-making patterns, child-rearing practices, rites, and rituals. The meanings and practices attached to health and illness are defined by cultural values. For this reason, nurses need to know how to assess the effect of the family's culture on their health practices to provide optimal nursing care. Stereotypes do not apply to everyone from a particular culture. Each family is unique and needs to be assessed individually. When assessing the child's family from a cultural perspective, the nurse should consider:

- Ethnic affiliation.
- Family and child-rearing patterns.
- Religious and spiritual beliefs.
- Nutrition and food patterns.
- Ethnic health care practices.
- Health-promoting practices.

Table 16–1 summarizes the characteristics of family relationships and the health beliefs and practices of some cultural groups. These descriptions are generalizations, and every family is unique.

Religious beliefs often have a strong influence on families as they face the crisis of illness. A family's belief in infant baptism affects the decision of the nurse to call in a member of the clergy when an infant is critically ill. Specific beliefs about the causes, treatment, and cure of illness are important for the nurse to know to empower the

TABLE 16–1 *Cultural Differences in Families*

	FAMILY RELATIONSHIPS	HEALTH BELIEFS/PRACTICES
American	Mothers perceive the baby as a separate being. Baby has the ability to "tell" the mother its needs. Parents stimulate activity in the infant. Wide variety of parenting styles. Increasing acceptance of nontraditional family structures.	Believe in germ and stress theories. Value modesty and privacy. Health is a state of physical and emotional well-being, the ability to think and act the way one desires. Increasing interest in health-promoting lifestyles and alternative health care.
Japanese	Mother perceives a baby as extension of herself. Suppress emotions. Respect elders. Close extended family. Value self-control and self-sufficiency.	Stoicism: do not show pain. Use of Eastern medicine techniques (e.g., acupuncture, acupressure, massage).
Native American	Obstinate children are respected; docile children are considered weak. Close extended family relationships. Elders are respected. Nonverbal communication used. Most keep native language.	Eye contact is avoided because eyes are the "windows to one's spirit." Health is a state of harmony with nature and the universe. Strong belief in supernatural influence on health. May carry objects to protect against witchcraft. Illness is a price that is paid for a past or future deed. Medicine man is highly respected, altruistic, and empowered by supernatural; he uses herbs and rituals.
Asian-American	Family is highly valued. Close extended family. Elders respected. Place high value on honor (face). Self-control and self-sufficiency are valued. Emotions suppressed.	Health is a balance between energy forces of yin (cold) and yang (hot). Eastern medicine used. Belief in reincarnation. Stoicism may make pain assessment difficult.
African-American	Close extended family. Many single mothers as heads of family. Strong sense of community. Loyalty to race valued. Distrust of majority group.	Self-care and folk medicine prevalent. May "test" health care workers before actively seeking care. Religious rituals, such as prayer, used. Black minister is highly influential. Illness may be seen as "will of God." Health is viewed as harmony with nature.
Hispanic American, Mexican-American	Men considered breadwinners, women homemakers. Men are seen as strong (macho). Close extended family (includes godparents). Children highly valued. Catholicism is predominant religion. Most keep native language.	Strong association between religion and health. Good health is seen as reward, and poor health is seen as punishment. Illness is imbalance between hot and cold. "Hot" diseases are treated with "cold" foods (does not refer to temperature). Curandero, a folk healer, is usually consulted for health care before an American health care worker. Belief that the patient is the passive recipient of disease, which is caused by an external force.

Data in part from Spector, R. (1991). *Cultural diversity in health and illness* (3rd ed.). Norwalk, CT: Appleton & Lange.

family to deal with the immediate crisis. Table 16–2 describes how some religious beliefs affect health care.

Poverty. People who live below the poverty level represent an entire subculture. Inadequate financial resources have obvious effects on the health care function of families (Friedman, 1986). Factors include the ability to provide food, clothing, shelter, and health care; the ability to recognize illness in family members and provide care; and the ability to foster a healthy lifestyle or environment based on preventive medical and dental health practices. Studies indicate that blacks are about three times and Hispanics more than two times as likely as whites to live below the poverty level (U.S. Department of Health and Human Services, 1990). Regardless of race or ethnic group, people in female-headed households with no husband are twice as likely as people in male-headed households with no wife to be poor. The lower the family income, the less frequent are dental visits. Both blacks and the economically disadvantaged are more likely than others to perceive their health as "fair" or "poor" and to lose days from work. Children from low-income families miss more school days than do children from middle- and upper-income families (U.S. Department of Health and Human Services, 1990).

Maternal and infant mortality rates have decreased during the last 40 years, but the infant mortality rate during the first year of life is still high. The rate of death for infants under 1 year of age has decreased by an average of more than 3% per year from 1950 to 1991. The provisional infant mortality rate for the United States in 1994 hit a record low of 7.9 infant deaths per 1000 live births (National Center for Health Statistics, 1995b). For minority children younger than 1 year, the death rate is 2.4 times that of whites (National Center for Health Statistics, 1995a).

Poverty is blamed for many problems, including malnutrition, crime, high stress, and domestic violence (Kantor & Straus, 1990; Straus & Smith, 1990). Some of these correlations may be valid; however, some have been too readily adapted as simple explanations for complex problems. For many years, it was believed that child abuse was more prominent among poverty-stricken populations. Research later found this belief to be false. Child abuse knows no socioeconomic boundaries.

FAMILY STRUCTURE AND FUNCTION

Family health is concerned with the physical, mental, and spiritual well-being of the family as a unit, not only with the well-being of the individuals within the family. Nurses caring for children need to look at the whole family as the client rather than the child alone. Children are profoundly affected in every area of life by the way they are treated within their families.

In assessing family health, the nurse first must determine the structure of the family. The structure is the actual physical composition of the family, the family's environment, and the occupations and education of its members. Next, the nurse needs to determine how well the family is fulfilling its five major functions as described by Friedman (1986). See the accompanying checklist of structural and functional components that the nurse can use in assessing the strengths and weaknesses of the family.

Health problems can arise from structural problems, such as too few or too many people sharing the same living quarters. If too few people are present, children may be left unattended, whereas too many people can lead to overcrowding, stress, and the spread of communicable diseases. Environmental problems include impure drinking water, inadequate sewage facilities, damaged electric wiring and outlets, and inadequate sleeping conditions. Other environmental factors, such as rodents, crime, and noise, can affect health. Occupation and education can affect health through lack of adequate supervision of children; inability to purchase physical necessities, such as food; exposure to hazards, such as lead or toxic substances, which are carried home on the skin and clothes; and stress from employment dissatisfaction.

Healthy vs. Dysfunctional Families

Although a lack of health can be found in any combination of the five functions, the problems that are most devastating and difficult to treat arise from deficits in the affective and socialization functions. Typically, these are the functions referred to when the popular term "dysfunctional family" is used. To the degree that the family is not meeting the five functions, the family is dysfunctional.

One relatively quick and easy way to assess the family's functioning is to give each parent (separately) the Family APGAR questionnaire (Smilkstein, 1978). The questionnaire contains five items with three responses for each item (Table 16–3). A score of 7 to 10 suggests a highly functional family, and a score of 4 to 6 suggests a moderately functional family. A score of 0 to 3 suggests a severely dysfunctional family. The test has been used since 1978 and takes only a few minutes to complete.

Although traits of healthy families vary, some traits are fairly consistent. Curran (1985) surveyed 551 professionals who work with families. The 15 most frequently identified traits of a healthy family are listed in the accompanying box.

Some of the results of family dysfunction are abuse, neglect, codependency, mental health problems, family conflict and stress, and divorce (see Chapter 41).

Family Conflict. Family conflict is unavoidable because it is a natural result of perceived unequal exchange or imbalance of resources by individual members. Conflict should not be viewed as bad or disruptive because it is the management of the conflict, not the conflict itself, that may be problematic. Conflict can produce growth and improved family functioning if the outcome is resolution as opposed to dissolution or continued conflict. The goal is effective management and resolution of the conflict.

Three ingredients are required to resolve conflict:

1. Open communication.
2. Accurate perceptions about the nature and degree of conflict.
3. Constructive efforts to resolve the conflict, such as willingness to consider the view of the other, consider alternate solutions, and compromise.

Dysfunctional families have problems in any one or a combination of these areas. They tend to become trapped

TABLE 16–2 *Religious Beliefs Affecting Health Care*

RELIGION AND BASIC BELIEFS	PRACTICES
Christian Science Based on scientific system of healing. Beliefs based on Bible, science, and health with key to scriptures. Seek to overcome evil through prayer, belief, and Christian acts. Healing is divinely natural, not miraculous.	*Birth:* Use physician or midwife during childbirth. No baptism ceremony. *Dietary habits:* Alcohol and tobacco are considered drugs and are not used. Coffee and tea may also be declined. *Death:* Autopsy and donation of organs are usually declined. *Health care:* May refuse medical treatment. View health in a spiritual framework. Seek exemption from immunizations, but obey legal requirements. When Christian Science believer is hospitalized, parent or client may request that a Christian Science practitioner be notified to come.
Jehovah's Witness Believe in God and Son Jesus Christ. Expected to follow the example of Jesus Christ in daily living. Expected to preach house to house about the good news of God. Bible is doctrinal authority. No distinction made between clergy and laity.	*Baptism:* No infant baptism. Baptism by immersion of adults. *Dietary habits:* Use of tobacco and alcohol discouraged. *Death:* Autopsy decided by persons involved. Burial and cremation acceptable. *Birth control and abortion:* Use of birth control is a personal decision. Abortion opposed based on Exodus 21:22-23. *Health care:* Blood transfusions not allowed. May accept alternatives to transfusions, such as use of nonblood plasma expanders, careful surgical technique to minimize blood loss, and use of autologous transfusions. Nurses should check unconscious clients for identification that state that the person does not want a transfusion. Jehovah's Witnesses are prepared to die rather than break God's law. Respect the health care given by physicians, but look to God and His laws as the final authority for their decisions.
The Church of Jesus Christ of Latter-Day Saints (Mormon) Restorationism: True church of Christ ended with the first generation of apostles, but was restored with the founding of Mormon Church. Articles of faith: Mormon doctrine states that individuals are saved if they are obedient to God's divine ordinances (faith, repentance, baptism by immersion and laying on of hands, observance of Lord's Supper on Sunday). Word of God can be found in the Bible, Book of Mormon, Doctrine, and Covenants, Pearl of Great Price, and current revelations. Christ will return to rule in Zion, located in America.	*Baptism:* By immersion. Considered essential for the living and the dead. If a child older than 8 is very ill, whether baptized or unbaptized, a member of the church's priesthood should be called. *Holy Communion:* Hospitalized client may desire to have a member of the church's priesthood administer the sacrament. *Anointing of the sick:* Mormons frequently are anointed and given a blessing before going to the hospital and after admission by laying on of hands. *Dietary habits:* Tobacco and caffeine are not used. Mormons eat meat (limited), but encourage the intake of fruits, grains, and herbs. *Death:* Prefer burial of the body. A church elder should be notified to assist the family. *Birth control and abortion:* Abortion is opposed unless the life of the mother is in danger. Only natural methods of birth control are recom-

TABLE 16–2 *Religious Beliefs Affecting Health Care (continued)*

RELIGION AND BASIC BELIEFS	PRACTICES
The Church of Jesus Christ of Latter-Day Saints (Mormon) (continued)	mended. Other means are used only when the physical or emotional health of the mother is at stake. *Other practices:* Believe in the healing power of "laying on of hands." Cleanliness is very important. Believe in healthy living and adhere to health care requirements. Families are of great importance, so visiting should be encouraged. The church maintains a welfare system to assist those in need.
Roman Catholic Beliefs based on Bible, Apostolic tradition, and contemporary revelation. Faith and good works are necessary for salvation.	*Baptism:* Infant baptism by affusion (sprinkling of water on head). Original sin is believed to be "washed away." If death is imminent or a fetus is aborted, anyone can perform the baptism by sprinkling water on the forehead, saying "I baptize thee in the name of the Father, Son, and Holy Spirit." Anointing of the sick encouraged for anyone who is ill or injured. Always done if prognosis is poor. *Dietary practices:* Fasting and abstinence from meat optional during Lent. No meat on Fridays and during Lent strongly encouraged. Children and ill adults exempt from all fasting. *Death:* Organ donation permitted.
Hinduism Belief in reincarnation and Karma, Yoga. Nonviolent approach to living. Various deities worshiped: Vishnu, Shiva, Ganesh, Surya, Durgam Shati. Congregation worship is not customary.	*Diet:* Dietary restrictions vary according to sect. *Death:* Death rituals specify practices and who can touch corpse. *Other practices:* Oppose artificial insemination. Circumcision is observed by ritual.
Islam Sunni (90%), Shiite (10%). Belief in one God. Based on the teaching of Muhammad. Five Pillars of Islam. Compulsory prayers are said at dawn, noon, afternoon, after sunset, and after nightfall.	*Diet:* Prohibit eating pork and the use of alcohol. Fast during Ramadan (ninth month of Muslim year). *Death:* Oppose autopsy and organ donation. Death ritual prescribes the handling of corpse by only family and friends.
Judaism Beliefs are based on the Old Testament, the Torah, and the Talmud, the oral and written laws of faith. Belief in one God who is approached directly. Believe Messiah is still to come. Believe Jews are God's chosen people.	*Circumcision:* A symbol of God's covenant with Israel. Done on eighth day after birth. *Bar Mitzvah:* Ceremonial rite of passage for boys (approximately 13 years of age) into manhood. *Death:* Remains are washed according to rite by members of the Ritual Burial Society. Burial occurs as soon as possible.

Data from Carson, V. B. (1989). *Spiritual dimensions of nursing practice* (pp. 100–102). Philadelphia: W. B. Saunders. Betz, C. L., Hunsberger, M., & Wright, S. (1994). *Family centered nursing care of children* (2nd ed., pp. 2230–2236). Philadelphia: W. B. Saunders.

Checklist for Assessing Family Strengths and Weaknesses

STRUCTURE

Family Composition

______ Family members living in the home
______ Family members living outside the home but who have significant influence

Home and Community Environment

______ Physical features
______ Sleeping arrangements
______ Utilities
______ Safety features
______ Type of neighborhood
______ Proximity of the home to needed facilities

Occupation and Education

______ Type of activity
______ Hours away from home
______ Exposure to hazards
______ Employment satisfaction
______ Economic security

FUNCTION

Affective

Nurturance
______ Given and received by both parents and children
______ Outcomes are trust and intimacy
______ Clear communication patterns; congruent verbal and nonverbal messages

Mutual respect
______ Rights of each member respected
______ Conflict management

Bonding and identification
______ Sharing of joys and sorrows
______ Sensitivity and responsiveness to needs

Separateness and connectedness
______ Each member has sense of belonging and identity

Socialization

______ Parenting style
______ Discipline strategies
______ Cultural beliefs and practices

Reproductive

______ Family planning strategies, including current method of birth control

Economic

______ Adequacy of resources to meet basic needs

Health Care

______ Lifestyle practices (e.g., nutrition, sleep, exercise, recreation, drug habits)
______ Environmental practices (cleanliness and safety)
______ Medically based practices (physical examinations, immunizations)
______ Dental health practices

in patterns in which they maintain conflicts rather than resolving them. The conflicts create stress, and the family must cope with the resultant stress.

Coping With Stress. Curran (1985) views the family as a delicately balanced system. Stressors are forces, either inside or outside the family, that contribute to fluctuations in the balance of the family system. The top 10 stressors in families identified by Curran are listed in the accompanying box. Families respond in some manner to these stressors. Some families are able to mobilize their strengths and resources, thus effectively adapting to the stressors. Other families fall apart. Nurses should be able to recognize exactly how a specific family responds to stress. Curran identified patterns of families who were coping effectively:

- Recognizing that stress is temporary and may be positive.
- Working together to find solutions.
- Developing new rules, including prioritizing time and sharing responsibility.
- Expecting that some stress is normal.
- Feeling accomplishment in dealing with stress.

Families who dealt ineffectively with stress exhibited the following patterns:

- Feeling guilt for permitting stress to exist.
- Looking for a place to lay blame rather than a solution to the problem.
- Giving in to stress and giving up trying to master it.
- Focusing on family problems rather than on strengths.
- Feeling weaker rather than stronger after a normal stress experience.
- Growing to dislike family life as a result of the accumulation of stress.

TABLE 16–3 *The Family APGAR (Adaptation, Partnership, Growth, Affection, Resolve) Questionnaire*

	ALMOST ALWAYS	SOME OF THE TIME	HARDLY EVER
I am satisfied with the help that I receive from my family when something is troubling me.	______	______	______
I am satisfied with the way my family discusses items of common interest and shares problem solving with me.	______	______	______
I find that my family accepts my wishes to take on new activities or make changes in my lifestyle.	______	______	______
I am satisfied with the way my family expresses affection and responds to my feelings, such as anger, sorrow, and love.	______	______	______
I am satisfied with the way my family and I spend time together.	______	______	______

Scoring

The patient checks one of three choices, which are scored as follows: 2 points for almost always, 1 point for some of the time, and 0 for hardly ever. The scores for the five questions are then totaled. A score of 7 to 10 suggests a highly functional family. A score of 4 to 6 suggests a moderately dysfunctional family. A score of 0 to 3 suggests a severely dysfunctional family.

What the Questionnaire Measures

Adaptation: How resources are shared, or the member's satisfaction with the assistance received when family resources are needed.

Partnership: How decisions are shared, or the member's satisfaction with mutuality in family communication and problem solving.

Growth: How nurturing is shared, or the member's satisfaction with the freedom available within the family to change roles and attain physical and emotional growth or maturation.

Affection: How emotional experiences are shared, or the member's satisfaction with the intimacy and emotional interaction within the family.

Resolve: How time is shared, or the member's satisfaction with the time commitment that has been made to the family by its members.

From Smilkstein, G. (1978). The family apgar: A proposal for a family function test and its use by physicians. *Journal of Family Practice, 6*(6), 1231–1239. Reprinted by permission of Appleton & Lange, Inc.

Traits of a Healthy Family

- Communicates and listens
- Affirms and supports one another
- Teaches respect for others
- Develops a sense of trust
- Has a sense of play and humor
- Exhibits a sense of shared responsibility
- Teaches a sense of right and wrong
- Has a strong sense of family in which rituals and traditions abound
- Has a balance of interaction among members
- Has a shared religious core
- Respects the privacy of members
- Values service to others
- Fosters family meal time and conversation
- Shares leisure time
- Admits to and seeks help with problems

Adapted from Curran, D. (1985). *Stress and the healthy family*. Minneapolis, MN: Winston.

Top Ten Stressors in Families

1. Economics/finances/budgets
2. Children's behavior/discipline/sibling fighting
3. Insufficient couple time
4. Lack of shared responsibility in the family
5. Communicating with children
6. Insufficient "me" time
7. Guilt for not accomplishing more
8. Spousal relationship (e.g., communication, friendship, sex)
9. Insufficient family play time
10. Overscheduled family calendar

Adapted from Curran, D. (1985). *Stress and the healthy family*. Minneapolis, MN: Winston.

SITUATIONAL CRISIS: THE ILL CHILD

When a child becomes ill, the event is a crisis known as a **situational crisis** for the entire family: the ill child, the parents, the siblings, and the extended family. There is a threat to the integrity of the family because the child may die. There may be a fear of death or permanent disability. The fear of the unknown is often overwhelming. The parents may feel helpless because the child may be experiencing physical pain or discomfort. In addition, because of health care costs, the family may have anxiety about finances.

A family's reaction to a child's illness is influenced by the family's history, culture, environment, and beliefs. The severity of the illness, its chronicity, the suddenness of onset, and the prognosis also affect family reactions. If the child requires hospitalization, the stress is magnified, particularly if the family has never experienced the illness of a child. Parents often have role confusion because they no longer feel in control of what happens to their child. Often one parent, frequently the mother, takes on added decision-making responsibilities if the other parent cannot stay at the hospital. If there are other children at home, the parents must arrange for child care and transportation for them. One or both parents may have depression secondary to exhaustion, fear, guilt, grief, or loss of control.

The hospital environment offers many stressors as well. Simply not knowing the location of the restrooms and cafeteria can add stress. Many parents are unfamiliar with hospital culture. They must learn the various roles of the staff, what is expected of whom, and what role they are to play in the hospital. The hospital even has its own language. Nurses become so accustomed to terms such as IV, Foley, cath, PRN, and NPO that they forget that parents may not know what they are talking about. All of these factors add to parental stress.

Also, because the nurses have so much power over the child and parents by virtue of their knowledge and authority, parents often feel vulnerable. They want to please and not anger the nurses because they fear possible recrimination should they "make waves." Although this fear may make life more pleasant for the nurses, it is not therapeutic for the parents. They should be given permission to get angry, ask questions, and express doubts.

Some parents react in the opposite way. Rather than being quiet and pleasant, they question everything. The nurse may become irritated and feel threatened by this behavior, especially if she feels insecure. However, the nurse should understand that the underlying reason for the parental questioning is an attempt to maintain some control over the situation. The nurse should make every attempt to answer all questions in a pleasant, sincere manner.

EFFECTIVE COMMUNICATION WITH PARENTS Parents are often overwhelmed with everything that is happening to them and their child in the hospital. They might ask a question about the IV that seems obvious to the nurse such as, "How is that fluid getting into my child?"

Ineffective response: "There is a plastic catheter threaded into the vein leading to the heart. The D5 and a quarter normal saline is infusing into his bloodstream to hydrate him and provide a mechanism for IV meds."

Effective response: "The fluid in this bag runs through this tube and enters Johnny's bloodstream right here (pointing to each part of equipment as it is mentioned). Let me draw you a picture. IV stands for intravenous. Intra means inside, and venous means vein. There is a small needle at the end of this tube that we used to insert the tube into his vein. (Draw a picture.) The needle will stay in his vein until he no longer needs the fluid. We are giving him this fluid because he can't drink anything right now. This fluid will keep him from getting dehydrated. Does that make sense? If you have any more questions, I'd be happy to try to answer them for you." It is important never to make the parent feel foolish for asking a question.

Effects of Illness on Siblings. Siblings of the ill child are often at risk for being neglected. The focus of attention for parents and nurses is the ill child. Siblings feel this neglect and may feel anger, resentment, or possibly guilt that they did something to cause their sibling's illness. They may respond to these feelings by acting out, becoming quiet and withdrawn, developing physical symptoms, or having social problems at school.

If given the opportunity, nurses can assist siblings directly by giving the child permission to talk about and express his feelings about the sick child. For example, the hospital nurse could take the sibling to the playroom and sit down and color or play dolls with the child. While playing, the nurse can explain how brothers or sisters of sick children often feel like their mommy and daddy are paying more attention to the sick child than to them. If the child responds positively, then the nurse can ask the child to draw a picture about how he feels. Through active listening, the nurse can then help the child explore these feelings and provide strategies to deal with the situation. Providing reassurance that the child's parents still care for him often comforts the child.

Because parents are overwhelmed by the stress of the child's illness, they may have difficulty recognizing the effect of the illness on the siblings. Nurses can explain that the response of the siblings is normal and suggest that the parents seek support from extended family members or friends. Lightening the burden of some ordinary household chores can allow the parent to spend more time with the sibling.

Coping Strategies. Some families adjust quickly to extreme crises, whereas other families become chaotic with relatively

Factors Affecting Adjustment to Situational Crises

- Previous functional patterns
- Perceived meaning of the crisis event
- Available support systems
- Reactions to the child
- Available resources
- Concurrent stresses in the family
- Coping mechanisms

Data from Cohen, F. (1984). Coping. In J. D. Matarazzo, S. Weiss, J. Herd, & S. Weiss (Eds.), *Behavioral health: A handbook of health enhancement and disease prevention* (pp. 261–274). New York: Wiley.

minor crises. Family functional patterns that existed before the crisis are probably the best indicators of how the family will respond to a crisis. Other factors that affect the family's adjustment to a crisis are listed in the accompanying box.

Cohen (1984) stated that "the key question may not be which coping strategies an individual uses but rather how many are in his or her repertoire or how flexible the person is in employing different strategies." The same principle applies to families.

Family coping strategies can be divided into internal (intrafamilial) and external (extrafamilial), as listed in the accompanying box.

NURSING CARE OF THE FAMILY

Nurses often come in contact with families when they are experiencing a health crisis and are in need of health restoration. The following sample care plan illustrates this type of care. The setting is a pediatric unit, and the child has been on the unit for 4 hours. She has an IV and is in isolation.

Assessment

A 2-year-old girl is admitted for possible bacterial meningitis. The family is Mexican-American and speaks both Spanish and English. Both the mother and father are in the room, sitting beside the crib. The mother is holding the child's hand, and the father is watching TV. He is sitting beside the mother, but not touching either the mother or the child. The mother is wearing a necklace bearing a cross. The chart states the religion as Catholic, and they have a 6-month-old son at home staying with a grandmother. During the initial interview, the parents give brief responses and avoid eye contact. They share little information. The mother's eyes are puffy and red, and she gently rubs the child's arm. As you begin to assess the child, you notice that both parents and the child are watching you closely.

Nursing Diagnoses

- Parental role conflict related to lack of knowledge of expected role, change in environment and culture, and separation from other family members.
- Anxiety and fear related to the crisis of illness and hospitalization of a 2-year-old.
- Risk for alteration in family health maintenance related to a situational crisis.
- Risk for impaired home maintenance management after discharge related to knowledge deficit and lack of support.

Coping Strategies of Families

INTERNAL COPING STRATEGIES

- Reliance on the family group
- Use of humor
- Greater sharing of feelings, thoughts, time, and activities
- Controlling the meaning of the problem (reframing)
- Attributing a spiritual purpose to the event
- Optimism
- Selective ignoring of negatives
- Making the event less important
- Joint problem solving
- Role flexibility

EXTERNAL COPING STRATEGIES

- Seeking information
- Increasing links to the community
- Using social support systems (e.g., family, friends, experts, co-workers, professional services)
- Joining self-help groups
- Seeking spiritual support

Data from Cohen, F. (1984). Coping. In J. D. Matarazzo, S. Weiss, J. Herd, & S. Weiss (Eds.), *Behavioral health: A handbook of health enhancement and disease prevention* (pp. 261–274). New York: Wiley.

Planning, Implementation, and Evaluation: Nursing Care of the Family

NURSING DIAGNOSIS

- Parental role conflict related to lack of knowledge of expected role, change in environment and culture, and separation from other family members.

Expected Outcome:

- Parents will maintain their parental role function as evidenced by being the primary decision makers and providing care for their child in partnership with the nurse.

Intervention	Rationale
1. Offer information about rooming-in options to parents during orientation to the unit.	The parents will feel more comfortable in resuming their parental role if they are made to feel welcome and given permission to parent their child.
2. Encourage parental care of the child. Include the parents in setting goals.	
3. Ask the parents advice about caring for their child, such as the child's normal routines and rituals and parental disciplinary methods.	
4. Ask what foods the child would prefer.	Remember the cultural importance of hot–cold, wet–dry balance in some cultures, and place high priority on the parents' suggestions.
5. Make the environment comfortable for the parents. Offer them coffee, pillows, and blankets, and give them a tour of the unit.	
6. If there are Spanish-speaking nurses available, they should be assigned to this family.	Sensitivity to cultural differences helps families to feel more comfortable in an unfamiliar environment. They may feel free to express their beliefs and practices if you have invited them to do so in a nonjudgmental manner.
7. Ask the parents if they would like to invite their curandero (a person whose healing powers are believed to be a gift from God) to the hospital. Be open to their beliefs, which may be different from yours.	
8. After the 24- to 48-hour isolation period, encourage the family to bring objects from home that will make them and the child feel more comfortable.	
9. Ask whether there is anything you or the hospital staff can do to make the parents more comfortable.	Making them feel comfortable communicates that you care.
10. Offer to show parents where the hospital chapel is located, and offer to take them there.	
11. Offer to call the hospital priest if they would like to see him.	
12. After the isolation period, tell the family that other family members may visit the child.	Family is important in the Mexican-American culture. Inviting them to include the family shows sensitivity and concern for their needs.
13. Provide parents with a phone.	
14. Ask open-ended questions about the family.	
15. Show an interest in the family (e.g., ask to see pictures).	Allowing the parents to talk gives them an opportunity to express their anxiety.

Evaluation:
- Parents act as primary decision makers in consultation with the health care team.
- Parents actively participate in the care of their ill child.

NURSING DIAGNOSIS
- Anxiety and fear related to the crisis of illness and hospitalization of a 2-year-old.

Expected Outcome:
- All members of the family, including the 2-year-old, will show a reduction in anxiety and fear as evidenced by a calm affect, eye contact with the nurse during conversations, participation in the care of the child rather than vigilant observation, and spontaneous discussions with the nurse.

Intervention	Rationale
1. After assessing the parents' knowledge, educate the parents about the cause of illness, signs and symptoms, treatment, and prognosis. Use terms that the parents can understand. Evaluate their knowledge by gently asking questions without "quizzing" them.	Knowledge helps to decrease anxiety. Quizzing would be intimidating.
2. Provide a little information at a time to prevent overload.	Remember that people can only retain a small amount of new information when in a crisis.
3. Tell parents what you are going to do before you do it, and then again while you do it.	Decreasing uncertainty decreases anxiety.
4. Instruct the parents about all medications, and explain how they will help their child.	
5. Explain the purpose for all procedures (e.g., x-rays) and equipment (e.g., monitors).	
6. Do not appear rushed. Spend time with the family and child.	
7. Interpret medical terms used by the staff.	
8. Interpret the child's behavior (e.g., possible regression, protest, negativism), and offer strategies to deal with the behavior.	Hospitalization is an ideal time to instruct parents about parenting and growth and development.
9. Respect the family's need for privacy and space.	
10. Be alert to nonverbal signs of anxiety, fear, sadness, anger, a need for privacy, or a need to talk.	
11. Help parents to express their fears and concerns by asking open-ended questions, clarifying, reflecting, validating, and avoiding blocking statements. Do not make judgments or offer quick fixes.	The use of therapeutic communication helps people to identify and clarify their concerns and decreases anxiety.
12. Introduce parents to the staff.	
13. Ask parents if they have the finances to eat meals in the cafeteria. If not, arrange for a social service consult.	Knowing that someone cares decreases fear. Adequate nutrition enhances coping ability.

Intervention	Rationale
14. Ask parents if they have transportation to and from the hospital. If not, help them to make arrangements.	Even simple problems can seem enormous during a crisis.
15. Support the family's use of effective coping strategies.	Signs of ineffective coping can indicate the need for a referral.
16. Be alert to signs of ineffective coping. Avoid projecting your methods of coping onto the parents.	
17. Be optimistic, and help the family to see that this stress is temporary.	

Evaluation: • All members of the family, including the 2-year-old, demonstrate nonverbal behaviors indicating minimal anxiety and fear. Examples of such behavior include calm affect, smiling, laughing, appropriate use of humor, eye contact with the nurse and physician while conversing, nonfurrowed eyebrows, spontaneous discussions with the nurse, relaxed body posture, and participation rather than vigilant observation of the nurse while he cares for the child.

NURSING DIAGNOSIS • Risk for alteration in family health maintenance related to a situational crisis.

Expected Outcome: • All family members will maintain their health as evidenced by the appearance of being well rested, absence of illness, and adequate energy to perform daily activities.

Intervention	Rationale
1. Explain to the parents that if they do not take care of themselves, they may become ill.	Parents cannot help the child if they are ill.
2. Suggest that the parents get adequate rest, fresh air, exercise, and nutrition. Offer to check on the child at regular intervals (e.g., every 15 minutes) when the parent leaves or takes a nap.	Parents often forget about their needs when a child is ill. They may even feel guilty for thinking about themselves.
3. Provide sleeping facilities at the hospital if possible, and make the parents as comfortable as possible.	
4. Suggest that other family members visit to allow some time at home for each parent. Help the family to set up a schedule based on their needs and the needs of the 6-month-old.	
5. Assure parents that the child will receive good care in their absence.	
6. Provide parents with the hospital phone number, and tell them that they can call at any time to check on their child's condition.	
7. Provide parents with a list of nearby restaurants, and encourage them to eat regular, nutritious meals away from the hospital if possible.	

Evaluation:
- Family members have adequate energy to perform daily activities; absence of illness; and appearance of being well rested.

NURSING DIAGNOSIS
- Risk for impaired home maintenance management after discharge related to knowledge deficit and lack of support.

Expected Outcome:
- The family will effectively manage the care of the 2-year-old child after discharge as evidenced by verbalization of home care needs, potential strategies to meet the stated needs, demonstration of any skills that may be needed at home, keeping follow-up appointments, and seeking appropriate help.

Intervention	Rationale
1. Assess the family's knowledge.	Home care can be frightening to parents because they no longer have nurses available to help them.
2. Teach the family any skills that may be needed after discharge (i.e., seizure care, cardiopulmonary resuscitation [CPR]).	
3. Teach the family about discharge medications: action, side effects, dosage, and schedule.	
4. After assessing the family's reading ability, provide written materials in their primary language so the family can refer to the written information later.	A great deal of instruction at once is overwhelming and may not be retained. This situation can be avoided by beginning discharge teaching during early hospitalization, by providing written material, and by making referrals.
5. Take time to sit down with the parents and explain home care. Ask them whether they have any questions or concerns.	
6. Educate parents about the expected progress of the disease (i.e., signs to look for to detect problems, course of action).	
7. Provide the phone numbers of the physician and any agency that the family may need.	
8. Prepare parents for the child's post-hospital behavior, such as possible regression.	
9. Include parents in decisions about referrals, and contact the needed agencies (e.g., community health nurse, home health care).	
10. Allow parents to schedule a follow-up appointment with the physician.	
11. Inform parents of community agencies that may be of service to them.	

Evaluation:
- The family discusses with the nurse their home care needs and potential strategies to meet the stated needs.
- Family members demonstrate any skills that may be needed at home.
- The family seeks help when appropriate and keeps follow-up appointments.

KEY CONCEPTS

- Empowering the family in the role of care provider is important to the child's recovery.
- Assessing the structure and function of the family is a basic part of caring for an ill child.
- Family systems theory provides one framework in which the nurse can organize care.
- Important factors in parenting include the style of parenting, the parent–child relationship, marital conflict, and the method of handling misbehavior.
- Understanding the family's cultural health beliefs and practices is essential in providing effective nursing care.
- Identifying functional versus dysfunctional family patterns can help the nurse to avoid conflict and confusion in implementing effective strategies in the care of the child.
- The effects of an ill child on a family may include fear, helplessness, anxiety, role confusion, and general stress in the parents. The siblings of the ill child may experience confusion, anger, resentment, and guilt.
- Coping strategies can be either effective or ineffective, healthy or unhealthy. A knowledge of generally effective, healthy internal and external coping strategies can help the nurse to offer the family specific suggestions for coping.

REFERENCES

Betz, C. L., Hunsberger, M., & Wright, S. (1994). *Family centered nursing care of children* (2nd ed.). Philadelphia: W. B. Saunders.

Bowen, M. (1976). Theory in the practice of psychotherapy. In P. J. Guerin (Ed.), *Family therapy theory and practice* (pp. 42–89). New York: Gardner Press.

Chess, S., & Thomas, A. (1983). Individuality: Dynamics of individual behavioral development. In M. Levine (Ed.), *Developmental-behavioral Pediatrics*. Philadelphia: W. B. Saunders.

Chess, S., & Thomas, A. (1985). Temperamental differences: A critical concept in child health care. *Pediatric Nursing, 11*(3), 167–171.

Cohen, F. (1984). Coping. In J. D. Matarazzo, S. Weiss, J. Herd, & S. Weiss (Eds.), *Behavioral health: A handbook of health enhancement and disease prevention* (pp. 261–274). New York: Wiley.

Curran, D. (1983). *Traits of a healthy family*. Minneapolis: Winston.

Curran, D. (1985). *Stress and the healthy family*. Minneapolis: Winston.

Friedman, M. (1986). *Family Nursing: Theory and assessment*. Norwalk, CT: Appleton-Century-Crofts.

Howard, B. (1991). Discipline in early childhood. *Pediatric Clinics of North America, 38*(6), 1351–1369.

Kantor, G. K., & Straus, M. A. (1990). The drunken bum theory of wife beating. In M. A. Straus & R. J. Gelles (Eds.), *Physical violence in American families*. New Brunswick, NJ: Transaction.

National Center for Health Statistics. (1995a). Advance report of final mortality statistics, 1992. *Monthly Vital Statistics, 43*(6), suppl.

National Center for Health Statistics. (1995b). Births, marriages, divorces, and deaths for 1994. *Monthly Vital Statistics Report, 43*(12).

Ragozin, A., Basham, R. B., Crnic, K. A., Greenberg, M. T., & Robinson, N. M. (1982). Effects of maternal age on parenting role. *Developmental Psychology, 18*, 627–634.

Saluter, S. (1992, December). Marital status and living arrangements: March 1992. In *Current population reports, population characteristics*. (Series P-20, No. 468). Washington, DC: U.S. Department of Commerce Administrative Bureau of the Census.

Scott, A. (1993). A beginning theory of personal space boundaries. *Perspectives in Psychiatric Care, 29*(2), 12–21.

Sheeber, L., & Johnson, J. (1992). Child temperament, maternal adjustment, and changes in family life style. *American Journal of Orthopsychiatry, 62*(2), 178–185.

Smikstein, G. (1978). The family apgar: A proposal for a family function test and its use by physicians. *Journal of Family Practice, 6*(6), 1231–1239.

Spector, R. (1991). *Cultural diversity in health and illness* (3rd ed.). Norwalk, CT: Appleton & Lange.

Straus, M. A., & Smith, C. (1990). Family patterns and child abuse. In M. A. Straus & R. J. Gelles (Eds.), *Physical violence in American families*. New Brunswick, NJ: Transaction.

Teti, D., & Gelfand, F. (1991). Behavioral competence among mothers of infants in the first year: The mediational role of maternal self-efficacy. *Child Development, 62*(5), 918–929.

Thomas, A., & Chess, S. (1977). *Temperament and development*. New York: Brunner-Mazel.

U.S. Bureau of the Census. (1996). Living arrangements of children under 18 years old: 1960–present [on-line]. Available: http://www.census.gov/population/socdeme/ms1a/history1.prno.

U.S. Department of Health and Human Services, Public Health Service, Health Resources Administration. (1990). *Health status of the disadvantaged chartbook 1990* (DHHS Publication No. [HRSA] HRS-P-DV90-1). Washington, DC: Author.

von Bertalanffy, L. (1968). *General systems theory*. New York: Braziller.

BIBLIOGRAPHY

Beckman, J. (1978). Couples' decision-making processes regarding fertility. In K. Tauber, L. Burgess, & J. Sweet (Eds.), *Social Demography*. New York: Academy Press.

Berkey, K., & Hanson, S. (1991). *Pocket guide: Family assessment and intervention*. St. Louis: Mosby–Year Book.

Borrine, M., Handal, P., Brown, N., & Searight, H. (1991). Family conflict and adolescent adjustment in intact, divorced, and blended families. *Journal of Consulting and Clinical Psychology, 59*(5), 753–755.

Carson, V. B. (1989). *Spiritual dimensions of nursing practice*. Philadelphia: W. B. Saunders.

Gillis, C., Highley, B., Roberts, B., Martinson, I. (1989). *Toward a science of family nursing*. Menlo Park, CA: Addison-Wesley.

Janosik, E., & Green, E. (1992). *Family life: Process and practice*. Boston: Jones & Bartlett.

Johnson, S. (1986). *Nursing assessment and strategies for the family at risk: High-risk parenting* (2nd ed.). Philadelphia: J. B. Lippincott.

Ross, B., & Cobb, K. (1990). *Family nursing: A nursing process approach*. Redwood City, CA: Addison-Wesley.

Saluter, S. (1992, December). Marital status and living arrangements: March 1992. In *Current population reports, population characteristics* (Series P-20, No. 468). Washington, DC: U.S. Department of Commerce Administrative Bureau of the Census.

Sprenkle, D., & Cyrus, C. (1983). Abandonment: The stress of divorce. In C. R. Figley & H. K. McCubbin (Eds.), *Stress and the family: Vol. II. Coping with Catastrophe* (pp. 53–75). New York: Brunner-Mazel.

Wallerstein, J. (1991). The long-term effects of divorce on children: A review. *Journal of the American Academy of Child and Adolescent Psychiatry, 30*(31), 349–360.

Wallerstein, J., & Kelly, J. (1980). *Surviving the breakup: How children and parents cope with divorce*. New York: Basic Books.

17

The Child With a Chronic or Terminal Illness

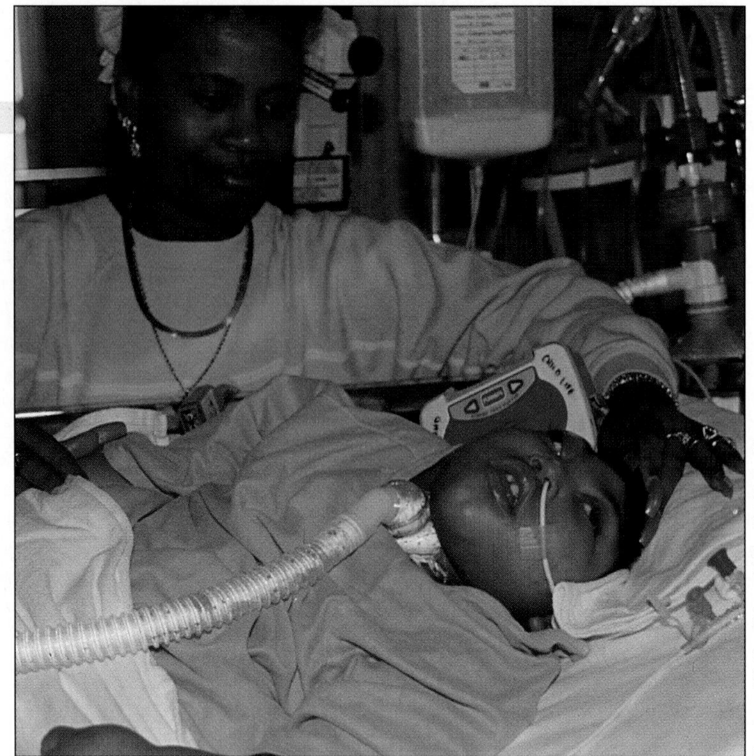

Courtesy of Parkland Memorial Hospital, Dallas, Texas

CHAPTER OVERVIEW

LEARNING OBJECTIVES

After reading this chapter, you should be able to:

- Define chronic illness.
- Discuss the effects of a chronic illness on the child and family.
- Discuss concerns and needs of the child and family dealing with a chronic illness.
- Discuss the concepts of death and dying as they relate to the pediatric patient.
- Define the stages of death and dying.
- Explain concerns and needs of the child and family facing an impending death.
- Discuss the patient's and family's responses to death and dying.
- Describe the nurse's response to death and dying in the pediatric population.
- Use the nursing process to describe nursing care of the chronically ill and dying child.

KEY TERMS

anticipatory grief: the processes of mourning, coping, interacting, planning, and psychosocial reorganizing that are begun in part as a response to the impending loss of a loved one (Rando, 1986)

bereavement: the objective condition or state of loss (Rando, 1986)

chronic illness/condition: a condition or illness that is long-term and either without cure or with residual characteristics that result in limitations upon activities of daily living (Jessop & Stein, 1988)

chronic sorrow: recurrent feelings of grief, loss, and fear related to the child's condition and the loss of the ideal, healthy child (Fraley, 1990)

family-centered nursing care: a philosophy of care that recognizes the family as the constant in a child's life, as well as the need for personnel and service systems to encourage, respect, and support family competencies (Johnson et al., 1989)

grief: a psychophysiologic process that occurs in response to a specific loss (Rando, 1986)

hospice care: a system of specialized and comprehensive care that provides support and assistance to patients (and their families) affected by terminal illness. The purpose of the care is to rehumanize the dying experience while providing the means for the patient and family to live as comfortably and as fully as possible. This is accomplished through the provision of respectful, noninvasive care, pain and symptom control, and emotional, physical, psychological, and spiritual support services.

illness trajectory: the impact of a disease or condition upon all family members, the physiologic progression of the disease, and the work organization done by the family as part of the coping process (Strauss et al., 1985).

normalization: responses of the family of a child with a chronic illness that are used to negate the illness and/or abnormal behaviors in order to maintain valued social roles (Hymovich & Hagopian, 1992)

palliative treatment: medical treatments or procedures that aim to promote patient comfort and quality of life, not to cure the underlying disease (Clark & McGee, 1992)

terminal care: a philosophy of care for the dying child in a hospital setting that is based on the tenet that the remaining time is precious for both the patient and the family. During terminal care, procedures and treatments deemed necessary for comfort and pain relief are arranged so as not to disrupt the family. Such care is provided on a 24-hour basis and reflects the needs and desires of the family (Gibbons, 1986)

Rapid advances in medicine have changed the face of chronic illness in childhood. Children with chronic illnesses are living longer, and increasing numbers of children are living with illnesses previously considered to be fatal. Both quality of life and longevity have been enhanced owing to earlier, improved diagnostic testing, as well as improved treatment modalities.

Family involvement in the care of children with chronic illnesses has also changed over the past 10 to 20 years. These changes are reflected in policies concerning sibling visitation and overnight privileges for parents, the family's provision of physical care previously handled only by those with medical training, the provision of terminal care in the hospital setting, the availability of free-standing in-patient hospice units for children, and the delivery of hospice care in the home. Currently, the emphasis in pediatric care is to provide and maintain the most normal, nonstressful, and supportive environment possible for the child undergoing any medical procedure or experiencing even a brief hospitalization. (Chapter 15 provides a more detailed look at the effects of hospitalization on the child.)

The realm of home care is expanding at a dramatic rate. Procedures once considered too risky or difficult to perform outside of the hospital are now being routinely provided in the home setting. Antibiotics, antifungals, gamma globulin, and narcotic drips are administered at home, as is parenteral nutrition. Ventilator-dependent children are also being cared for at home.

The public schools have also been affected by the changing face of chronic illness in the pediatric population. Federal laws dictate an array of services that must be provided to children with special health care needs, including children as young as 3 years of age. The hospital-based nurse must assist in educating the school nurse regarding the illness, expected progression, treatment, and any physical changes or disabilities that may result from either the illness or treatment.

CHRONIC ILLNESS DEFINED

A **chronic illness** or condition is one that is long-term and either without cure or with residual characteristics that result in limitations upon activities of daily living (ADLs) and the need for either adaptation in function or special assistance. Severity among these conditions varies. Many chronic conditions, such as bleeding disorders, diabetes, or sickle cell disease, although not physically apparent, have a tremendous impact on the patient and family. Likewise, a condition that exists only for a short time, yet results in death, may have serious, long-term effects upon the family. It is estimated that 10% to 15% of the pediatric population lives with a chronic illness; 10% of this group (or 1% to 2% of the general population) have conditions severe enough to interfere with normal life activities (Hobbs et al., 1985). The accompanying box lists some common chronic illnesses of childhood.

Common Chronic Conditions of Childhood

Asthma (reactive airway disease)
Bleeding disorders (i.e., hemophilia)
Bronchopulmonary dysplasia
Cancer
Cerebral palsy
Congenital heart disease
Chronic renal failure
Cystic fibrosis
Diabetes mellitus
Down syndrome
Epilepsy
Human immunodeficiency virus (HIV) and acquired immunodeficiency syndrome (AIDS)
Hydrocephalus
Juvenile rheumatoid arthritis
Lupus erythematosus
Muscular dystrophy
Neural tube defects
Phenylketonuria
Sickle cell disease

THE FAMILY OF THE CHILD WITH SPECIAL HEALTH CARE NEEDS

Impact on the Family

Increased technology, insurance provisions, and allocation of health care have all had an impact on the role of the family in caring for the child with a chronic illness. It has been confirmed that pediatric patients can be safely cared for (including provision of psychosocial support) in the home setting. This type of care is the most cost-effective and most desirable for both child and family.

Although improved quality of life, longevity, and an increased involvement in the provision of actual physical care are positive developments, they are accompanied by certain difficulties. Despite recent medical advances, the child and family must live with an ongoing physical problem that requires continued attention and adaptation. Strauss et al. (1985) refer to this as the **illness trajectory:** the impact of the disease upon all family members, the physiologic unfolding of the disease, and the work organization done by the patient and family in order to cope with the disease.

Chronic illness is a stressful and situational crisis for families. A situational crisis is an unexpected crisis in the family's developmental process. Like a developmental crisis, it disrupts the family's equilibrium, and the usual problem solving mechanisms are found not to be adequate to handle the crisis (Aguilera & Messick, 1990). Coping and adaptive abilities are challenged as the family attempts to regain equilibrium. However, various studies show that, in response to such a crisis, some families reorganize and actually become stronger. These families are considered to be resilient; that is, they exhibit specific traits and the ability to recover from adversity (see box).

Resilient families exhibit many important traits; however, the predominant trait is family cohesiveness (Patterson, 1991). This cohesion is achieved by active efforts to remain intact, not only through sharing the new responsibilities related to the chronic condition, but also through sharing the enjoyable activities of family life. Social integration and support are important factors in these activities.

Traits of the Resilient Family System

- Balancing the illness with other family needs
- Maintaining clear family boundaries
- Developing communication competence
- Attributing positive meaning to the experience
- Maintaining family flexibility
- Maintaining a commitment to the family as a unit
- Engaging in active coping efforts
- Maintaining social integration
- Developing collaborative relationships with professionals

From Patterson, J. M. (1991). Family resilience to the challenge of a child's disability. *Pediatric Annals, 20*(9), 491–499.

Maintaining social integration involves balancing the needs of the family with the needs imposed by the child's condition. Resilient families are careful in allocating resources, including money, time, and energy, as they balance various needs. This ensures that the other children in the family are not neglected or overindulged, and that the condition-related needs of the ill child are balanced with normal growth and development needs, without overprotection. In resilient families, the child's condition-related needs are incorporated into the family's daily life rather than becoming the focus around which the activities of the entire family revolve. This helps to achieve and maintain the new normalcy imposed by the illness. In such a family setting, baseball practices, school activities, ballet recitals, and other activities do not stop for either the ill child or the well sibling. Rather, medical appointments and treatments are arranged around these activities insofar as it is possible. When conflicts do arise, parents (or other family members or friends) alternate responsibility for maintaining the activities of the patient and siblings.

Sharing caregiving and encouraging parental involvement with well siblings helps maintain appropriate family boundaries. When one parent becomes primarily involved with meeting the needs of the ill child, both parental and marital relationships suffer. To keep these boundaries intact, resilient families pay specific attention to the marital relationship. They also work to avoid showing favoritism toward the ill child. Boundary problems of a different sort can arise when the need for outside provision of care and assistance increases. External family boundaries can be negatively affected in these instances. Such difficulties can be minimized by adopting an assertive role in managing the child's care and by maintaining professional relationships with caregivers.

Resilient families work consistently to ensure appropriate communication patterns. Communication may be more difficult owing to the addition of new, disorder-related language (medical or otherwise), an increased need for problem solving communication, and, most importantly, the need to express emotions. The task of accepting the validity of all emotions and learning suitable means of expressing those emotions may be most difficult. However, many families report that the experience of living with a chronic illness brings about positive life changes, such as increased empathy, increased family unity, and new meanings of life.

Even when positive meaning is attached to a child's chronic illness, a high level of flexibility is required of family members with regard to roles, family rules, and expectations of each other. This flexibility is also required of the health care team, both for the benefit of the family and as a means of achieving a positive, collaborative relationship between the team and the family. The team of health care professionals becomes an integral part of the family's life, and the quality of their relationship can affect how the entire family adapts to and copes with the child's condition.

For resilient families, coping is an active process that entails learning about their child's illness and the resources available to them. These families do not sit idly by, letting others meet their child's needs. The nurse and other members of the health care team have an important role in helping families learn how to meet their child's special health care needs.

At times of extreme stress, such as during periods of relapse, unexpected physical setbacks, worsening of the condition, and/or death, families may slip into less effective patterns. Gentle reminders and encouragement may be all that a family needs to help them resume the behaviors that foster resiliency, despite the many stressors and uncertainties of a chronic illness. Concerns and needs listed as greatest among parents of a child with a chronic illness include the following (Phillips, 1990):

- understanding how the illness affects their child physically and emotionally
- finding ways to provide for their child's emotional, social, and intellectual needs
- identifying and utilizing appropriate resources for assistance and health care planning for their child
- improving communication among the child's health-care providers

The Grief Process

Although much of the research concerning chronic disorders has focused on individual disorders, the effects of chronic illness can be generalized, and a variety of common responses have been recognized (Mahon, 1992). The most important aspect of a chronic illness is that it affects not only the patient but the entire family as well. This necessitates consistent utilization of **family-centered nursing care**—care that recognizes the family as the constant in a child's life, as well as encouraging, respecting, and supporting the family competencies (Johnson et al., 1989). Responses will be seen among all family members, and will vary according to the family member's relationship and involvement with the patient, age, developmental level, and previous experience with a medical problem. Chronic disorders involve the loss of health and result in **grief.** Common responses to a chronic disorder include the five stages of the grieving process delineated by Kubler-Ross (1969) (see box). These include denial and shock, anger and resentment, bargaining, sadness or depression, and acceptance. Individuals require varying periods of time to work through and resolve feelings before proceeding to the next stage. There may be some fluctuation between these five stages before the stage of acceptance is reached.

Kubler-Ross's Five Stages of Dying

First stage: Denial and Isolation
Second Stage: Anger
Third Stage: Bargaining
Fourth Stage: Depression
Fifth Stage: Acceptance

Acceptance of a chronic illness can occur even in the face of apparent denial, denial that might appear to be sustained throughout the course of the disease. As a coping or protective mechanism, denial may be adaptive for one person, but maladaptive for another (Lazarus, 1981). Because children have less variable protective mechanisms, denial may be utilized frequently. An individual who has a positive, optimistic outlook and who focuses on concerns and tasks of the day, rather than on fears about the illness, is utilizing adaptive denial as a protective mechanism. The time frame for denial is important. In the short term, true denial, although often considered to be maladaptive, can actually be adaptive, as it is universally experienced at the onset of a chronic illness as a normal stage of grieving. Persistence of such denial over the course of the illness, however, is maladaptive (Walker et al., 1993).

As adjustment to the disorder progresses, many parents experience **chronic sorrow,** defined as the recurrent feelings of grief, loss, and fear related to the child's disorder and the loss of the ideal, healthy child. As identified and defined by Fraley (1990), chronic sorrow is considered to be a normal process and involves grief that may never resolve. It is important to recognize grief as a normal, healthy mechanism and chronic grief as a normal process, both for the child with a chronic illness and for the family. The first step in supporting families and helping them deal with chronic sorrow is to listen to and recognize the pain of their chronic sorrow. They can then be assisted in recognizing and acknowledging the normalcy of such pain. Although families should be encouraged to acknowledge and express their feelings of chronic sorrow, they should also be encouraged to verbalize and demonstrate realistic hopes and dreams. One parent's reflections on the challenge of raising a child with a disability are presented in the piece "Welcome to Holland" (see box).

Many organizations, both general in nature and disease-specific, offer family support and assistance, and the nurse should help the family to utilize these services fully. This is particularly important when observation and

Welcome to Holland

by Emily Perl Kingsley

I am often asked to describe the experience of raising a child with a disability—to try to help people who have not shared that unique experience to understand it, to imagine how it would feel. It's like this. . . .

When you're going to have a baby, it's like planning a fabulous vacation trip—to Italy. You buy a bunch of guidebooks and make your wonderful plans. The Coliseum. Michelangelo's David. The gondolas in Venice. You may learn some handy phrases in Italian. It's all very exciting.

After months of eager anticipation, the day finally arrives. You pack your bags and off you go. Several hours later, the plane lands. The stewardess comes in and says, "Welcome to Holland." "HOLLAND?!?" you say. What do you mean Holland? I signed up for Italy! I'm supposed to be in Italy. All my life I've dreamed of going to Italy.

But there's been a change in the flight plan. They've landed in Holland, and there you must stay.

The important thing is that they haven't taken you to a horrible, disgusting, filthy place, full of pestilence, famine, and disease. It's just a different place.

So you must go out and buy new guidebooks. And you must learn a whole new language. And you will meet a whole new group of people you never would have met.

It's just a *different* place. It's slower paced than Italy, less flashy than Italy. But after you've been there for a while and you catch your breath, you look around . . . and you begin to notice that Holland has windmills . . . and Holland has tulips. Holland even has Rembrandts.

But everyone you know is busy coming and going from Italy . . . and they're all bragging about what a wonderful time they had there. And for the rest of your life you will say, "Yes, that's where I was supposed to go. That's what I had planned."

And the pain of that will never, ever, ever, ever go away because the loss of that dream is a very very significant loss.

But . . . if you spend your life mourning the fact that you didn't get to Italy, you may never be free to enjoy the very special, the very lovely things . . . about Holland.

assessment of family behaviors indicate problems that may require professional support or care. In caring for children with special health care needs and their families, one factor that is often overlooked and that is difficult to acknowledge is that death can occur unexpectedly, or sooner than planned. It is important to consider this even when the child's condition is viewed as chronic but not terminal. Grief support includes helping the family deal with chronic grief and the **anticipatory grief** of a terminal situation, as well as offering **bereavement** support once the child has died. Anticipatory grief is the process of mourning, coping, interacting, planning, and psychosocial reorganization that is begun as a response to impending loss of a loved one (Rando, 1986). This type of support requires an understanding of the family's knowledge base, coping skills, and personal beliefs, as well as recognition of and attention to actual grief-related problems. Grief support is thoroughly covered in the section of this chapter devoted to care of the child with a terminal condition.

THE CHILD WITH SPECIAL HEALTH CARE NEEDS

Growth and Development Concerns

Children with chronic disorders have many different concerns and needs related to their conditions, not the least of which is successful navigation of the stages of growth and development. The response of these children is influenced by their age at onset of the disorder, as well as by distinct growth and development considerations (see box). Nursing care must be planned accordingly. (See Chapter 2 for a more complete discussion of the normal stages of growth and development.) Eleven areas of concern have been identified for children with an illness or condition that requires hospitalization (Petrillo & Sanger, 1980), including:

- an imperfect body
- the degree of the condition requiring hospitalization
- threatened or real hospitalization
- spending time with unfamiliar people
- difficulty maintaining contact with siblings and peers
- the possibility of painful procedures
- guilt toward self or parents for hospitalization
- unfamiliar routines and environment
- the forced helplessness of parents
- the forced dependency of the child
- the need for the child to relate to the health care team, who may appear frightening

Often, chronic conditions span several years and developmental stages. Regardless of the growth and development stage, concerns related to self-esteem, self-reliance, and autonomy are often prevalent among children with chronic conditions. Many such children experience altered body awareness and image as a result of physical changes related to the illness or treatment, and this frequently has a negative impact on their self-esteem. Control and autonomy may be decreased owing to hospitalizations and treatment regimens that offer few, if any, decision-making opportunities for the patient. Social activities and adjustment may be limited as a result of hospitalization or the effects of the illness or treatment, or both. Such effects may include altered appearance, decreased physical ability, or increased susceptibility to infection. These factors may profoundly affect a child's acquisition of age-appropriate growth and development skills, especially when the patient is an adolescent. Issues concerning self-esteem and autonomy must be understood and dealt with as they relate to each stage of growth and development. This is necessary in order to minimize the effects of illness and hospitalization and to maximize the patient's potential at any given age.

Despite the best efforts and interventions of family and staff, a variety of changes and effects are frequently seen among children with a chronic illness. Most are minimal, last only briefly, and are actually expected as a part of the "normal" course of a chronic condition. For example, among older infants and toddlers, stranger anxiety may be heightened or may reappear months after previous resolution. Temporary regressive behavior is common from older infancy through the young school-age years. Regression is utilized very frequently and effectively by toddlers as they attempt to cope with the stress of a serious illness. Despite its frequent occurrence, regression may be extremely unsettling, as it entails the loss of recently acquired skills. Common regressive behaviors include reverting back to the baby bottle and/or thumb sucking, a decline in toileting skills or an increase in incidences of bed-wetting, and an increased use of "baby talk" or communication techniques more appropriate for younger ages.

Another possible difficulty is almost total lack of communication on the part of a child whose communication skills were previously age-appropriate or beyond. This often occurs exclusively in the clinic or hospital setting, with regular patterns of communication being utilized at home. Among older preschoolers, a lack of communication may be a form of withdrawal or an expression of stubbornness and a refusal to cooperate. This particular problem may also be seen in school-age children and adolescents and is related to issues involving independence and self-esteem.

The Infant

From infancy to 1 year of age, a child strives to develop a sense of trust, faith, and optimism in those around him. Initially, infants depend on their parents to meet their basic and social needs, subsequently developing their sense of attachment and trust as their needs are consis-

The Illness Experience: The Child and Adolescent

INFANT

Developmental Task: Achievement of awareness of being separate from significant other

Impact of Illness: Potential distortion of differentiation of self from parent/significant others

Cognitive Age/Stage: Sensorimotor (birth–2 yr)

Major Fears: Separation, strangers

Interventions: Provide consistent caretakers. Minimize separation from parents/significant others. Decrease parental anxiety, which is projected to infant. Maintain crib/nursery as "safe place" where no invasive procedures are performed.

TODDLER

Developmental Task: Initiation of autonomy

Impact of Illness: Interference with/loss of developing sense of control, independence

Cognitive Age/Stage: Preoperational (2–7 yr): egocentric, magical, little concept of body integrity

Major Fears: Separation, loss of control

Concept of Illness: Phenomenism (2–7 years): Perceives external, unrelated, concrete phenomena as cause of illness, e.g., "being sick because you don't feel well." Contagion: Perceives cause of illness as proximity between two events that occurs by "magic," e.g., "getting a cold because you are near someone who has a cold."

Interventions: Minimize separation from parents/significant others. Keep security objects at hand. Provide simple, brief explanations. Explain and maintain consistent limits. Encourage participation in daily care. Provide opportunities for play.

PRESCHOOLER

Developmental Task: Creation of a sense of initiative

Impact of Illness: Interference/loss of accomplishments such as walking, talking, controlling basic bodily functions

Cognitive Age/Stage: Preoperational thought: egocentric, magical, tendency to use and repeat words they don't understand, providing own explanations and definitions. Literal translation of words. Inability to abstract.

Major Fears: Bodily injury and mutilation; loss of control; the unknown; the dark; being left alone.

Concept of Illness: Phenomenism; contagion.

Interventions: Provide simple, concrete explanations. Advance preparation is important: days for major events, hours for minor events. Verbal explanations are usually insufficient, so use pictures, models, actual equipment, medical play.

SCHOOL-AGE CHILD

Developmental Task: Sense of industry

Impact of Illness: Potential feelings of inadequacy/inferiority if autonomy and independence are compromised.

Cognitive Age/Stage: Concrete operational thought (7–10+ years): beginning of logical thought but tendency to be literal.

Major Fears: Loss of control; bodily injury and mutilation; failure to live up to expectations of important others; death.

Concept of Illness: Contamination: Perceives cause as a person, object, or action external to the child that is "bad" or "harmful" to the body, e.g., "getting a cold because you didn't wear a hat." Internalization: Perceives illness as having an external cause but being located inside the body, e.g., "getting a cold by breathing in air and bacteria."

Interventions: Provide choices whenever possible to increase the child's sense of control. Stress contact with peer group. Use diagrams, pictures, and models for explanations because thinking is concrete. Emphasize the "normal" things the child can do, since the child does not want to be seen as different. Reassure child he/she has done nothing wrong; hospitalization, etc. is not "punishment."

ADOLESCENT

Developmental Task: Achieving of a sense of identity

Impact of Illness: Potential alteration/relinquishment of newly acquired roles and responsibilities.

Cognitive Age/Stage: Formal operational thought (11+ years): beginning of ability to think abstractly. Existence of some magical thinking (e.g., feeling guilty for illness) and egocentrism

Major Fears: Loss of control; altered body image; separation from peer group

Concept of Illness: Physiologic: Perceives cause as malfunctioning or nonfunctioning organ or process; can explain illness in sequence of events. Psychophysiologic: Realizes that psychologic actions and attitudes affect health and illness.

Interventions: Allow adolescent to be an integral part of decision making regarding care. Give information sensitively, since this age group reacts to content of information as well as the manner in which it is delivered. Allow as many choices and as much control as possible. Be honest about treatment and consequences. Stress what the adolescent can do for him or herself and the importance of cooperation and compliance. Assist in maintaining contact with peer group.

Developed by Martha Blechar Gibbons in Chapter 3: Psychosocial Aspects of Serious Illness in Childhood and Adolescence of *Hospice Care for Children* by Ann Armstrong-Dailey and Sarah Zarbock Goltzer. New York: Oxford University Press, 1993. Data on concept of illness for table obtained from Bibace, R., & Walsh, ME: Development of children's concepts of illness. *Pediatrics, 66*:912–918, 1980.

tently met. Accomplishing this developmental task may be extremely difficult for the infant being cared for in a medical setting filled with large numbers of strangers who represent only inconsistency, fear, and pain. The infant's illness and treatment may lead to disruption of eating and sleeping patterns, frequent exposure to painful or noxious stimuli, and weakening of the parent-infant bond as a result of separation. Under these conditions, the provision of comfort and security at the time of need is of paramount importance to the infant, especially in the absence of the parents. The health care team must be prepared to meet the infant's needs. In doing so, the caregivers provide a sense of safety and comfort for both the child and parents, and the trust in the health care team that the family develops will also help to ensure compliance with the prescribed treatment regimen. The infant's sense of security may be further enhanced by providing something familiar in the environment, whether it be a blanket, pacifier, stuffed animal, background music, or other item.

Issues of self-esteem and autonomy are important at this age even though the child's level of cognitive development may not allow full understanding or verbalization of such needs. Development of trust and a positive relationship with a caregiver enables the child to feel comfortable enough to attend physically to the external sensory stimuli and experiences required to complete other tasks of growth and development. This also provides necessary autonomy for the child. Growth includes not only physical growth, but also mastery of physical skills, such as hand coordination (grasping, clapping), rolling over, sitting up, and the like. The positive reinforcement supplied by others in response to such skill mastery promotes self-esteem in the child.

The Toddler

A primary developmental task of the child age 1 to 3 years is development of a sense of autonomy. Illness and hospitalization may lead to feelings of loss of control for patients of any age. For toddlers, such loss of control may also be accompanied by feelings of shame, doubt, and helplessness. Moreover, the regressive activities often seen in ill children this age can involve the loss of recently acquired achievements and skills and may be alarming to the child. With short-term illnesses or hospitalizations, these feelings generally resolve quickly, without lingering negative implications for normal growth and development. Chronic illnesses and repeated or long-term hospitalizations, however, may perpetuate such feelings and interfere with the child's development of a sense of autonomy in relation to self and environment. This, in turn, can have a negative impact on the child's self-esteem.

A sense of security and control in such situations can be facilitated by maintaining home routines, such as family rituals (eating at a certain time, prayer before meals, etc.), patterns of activity (play and nap times), and bedtime routines (including provision of a favorite comfort item and nightlight). Such an approach, which promotes a sense of security, may enable the child to cope more effectively with the stresses associated with the chronic condition. Frequently, such interventions provide sufficient emotional support to allow the toddler to continue her expected developmental progression.

The Preschooler

During ages 3 to 6 years, the child develops a sense of initiative. Tasks are undertaken and the world is explored very enthusiastically. Illness and hospitalization can interfere, both physically and emotionally, with the child's ability to start a task and work through to completion. Physical changes or disabilities, as well as common regression patterns, may not only hamper a child physically, but may also affect self-esteem, causing self-doubt and concern about abilities, even when the physical capacity for performing a certain activity has not been affected by the illness or condition. Self-esteem may be easily disturbed in the child at this age due to an increasing awareness of body image and integrity. Increased concerns relating to injuries and wholeness of the body are common. Minor injuries, such as scratches or bruises, may be very alarming at this time, and fears of mutilation may exist, particularly when the child misunderstands the purpose or nature of medical procedures and equipment. This response on the part of the child calls for simple yet realistic explanations of procedures, the manner in which they will be accomplished, the level of discomfort to be expected, and any resulting physical damage.

In explaining procedures to preschoolers, the caregiver must be mindful of how literal children this age are in their interpretations. One preschool child who underwent frequent blood draws expressed her initial fears of the procedure in an explicit drawing in which her arm was pictured with a twig-like structure protruding from it. This picture was drawn in response to being told "O.K., now, you will feel a little stick in your arm." No doubt the fear that resulted from her interpretation of the information provided about the procedure persisted far longer than the actual discomfort of the phlebotomy! No matter how minor the intervention or injury, caregivers must consistently assess and validate the magnitude assigned to it by the child, adjusting their approach to care accordingly.

At this age, children also develop a sense of conscience, often experiencing guilt with regard to their activities or imaginings. This guilt may surface in relation to illness, as children this age may fear that their illness was caused by something they said or did. Frequent reassurance must be offered so that the child understands that the illness did not occur because of anything said or done by him or any other person. Such a conversation may best be initiated by staff, as the child may be so frightened by the thought of more pain, injury, or discomfort that they might not verbalize their fears.

The School-Age Child

A sense of industry normally develops during the ages of 6 to 12 years. With the sense of autonomy and initiative in place, the child is ready to engage in tasks that can and will be followed through to completion. Illness, hospitalization, and physical disabilities may interfere with a child's ability to engage in task completion. This can lead to feelings of inferiority and diminished self-esteem as a result of the child's belief that she does not and cannot meet expected standards. The tasks that children of this age are attempting to learn are all fundamental to successful adulthood. Modifications may be necessary as a result of illness or disability, but it is essential that these tasks be attempted and completed. School-age children may require frequent encouragement to continue their efforts to complete a selected task. It may also be necessary to offer continual reassurance as to the validity of their efforts (even when modifications are necessary) and the quality or value of the outcome.

One task of children this age that is often underestimated or overlooked is the acquisition of basic social skills, including cooperation, competition, accommodation, and compromise. Because many of these skills are learned through the social interaction that naturally occurs during play or school activities, frequent hospitalizations may interfere with this socialization process. The benefits of social interaction for the school-age child, particularly one who is ill, are numerous. Not only is play valuable because of the social skills learned, but it is also fun, it offers relief from stress, and it can even heighten a child's sense of control and preparedness. Moreover, positive social interactions allow the school-age child to recognize peers as individuals and to accept others despite differences in appearance, values, characteristics, and behaviors. These social skills are particularly helpful in enabling children with a chronic illness or disorder to accept physical differences in themselves and in others they encounter in the health care environment.

The Adolescent

The primary developmental task for adolescents is the development of a sense of identity and of independence from their parents. A rapidly changing and growing body causes adolescents to question all that they have known and trusted about themselves. Most children this age are preoccupied with how they appear and what they appear to be in the eyes and opinions of others. This may be true even when the opinions of others may be in opposition to the young person's own beliefs and self-concepts. Anything that sets adolescents apart from their peers, especially something as obvious and invasive as illness or physical differences, is likely to be considered a massive barrier to successful achievement of their desired role identity. Negative patterns, beliefs, and roles already in place, or those assumed at this time in reaction to the illness and special needs, may be difficult to change. Nevertheless, it is important for caregivers to help the adolescent choose healthy, appropriate beliefs and behaviors regarding their life with a chronic condition and any resulting disabilities.

In establishing independence, adolescents often turn away from their parents a great deal of the time, even in situations in which they need and actually desire their parents' help and support. It is especially important, then, for the adolescent with a chronic illness to establish a meaningful relationship with an adult caregiver who may assume the role of a substitute peer in communication and companionship, yet also provide mature, appropriate guidance.

Parental Responses to Developmental Issues

Regardless of the developmental stage or the number of years that a chronic illness has existed, the basic tenets of child rearing and development still apply. As with the well child, discipline and consistency are very important. (One mother of a 3-year-old with neuroblastoma who was seen at our health care facility would frequently remind both the ill child and her sibling that cancer is no excuse for bad manners!) Experiencing a chronic illness is confusing, especially for children whose cognitive ability is not sufficiently developed to allow the comprehension that could ease stress somewhat. When the changes in their world begin to affect the only virtual constant they know—their family unit—patients often reflect this in their behavior. Negative behavior may result from the stress of the illness or the changes in their family and environment, or both. Previously existing negative behaviors may worsen. This can all make treatment, including a positive relationship and compliance with the medical team, difficult. Future behavior and long-term development may be affected as well. At the time their child is diagnosed, parents should be instructed about the need to maintain any previous rules and expectations for their child. They may also need to be reminded that all children, both well and ill, need to grow up in an environment conducive to the development of self-esteem, self-reliance, and autonomy (Sinnema, 1990).

NURSING CARE OF THE CHILD WITH A CHRONIC ILLNESS

The goal for any child with a chronic illness is to achieve and maintain **normalization:** responses that are used to negate the illness and/or abnormal behaviors in order to maintain valued social roles and to obtain the highest level of health and function possible, physically, emotionally, and psychosocially (Hymovich & Hagopian, 1992). The aim is similar for the family system, including parents, siblings, and extended family members. The objective for the family is to remain intact, achieve and maintain normalization, and to maximize function throughout the course of the illness. In order to assist the patient and family to reach these goals, all care provided by members of the health care team must be implemented utilizing a family-centered approach.

Goals for the Child:

- To achieve and maintain normalization
- To obtain the highest level of health and function possible physically, emotionally, psychosocially.

Goals for the Family:

- To remain intact
- To achieve and maintain normalization
- To maximize function throughout the course of the illness

Nursing diagnosis and care of the child with a chronic illness may be very complex because of goals that are both physical and psychosocial in nature. Care takes place in a psychosocial environment complicated by a span of years and a rapidly changing picture of growth and development. This span of years and developmental stages means the nurse must be prepared for a changing assessment regardless of whether problems are physical or psychosocial. Nursing care should include assisting the child and family to accept, understand, and incorporate the illness appropriately into each stage of growth and development, regardless of the child's age and development at diagnosis.

Planning and implementation of nursing care is based on several factors. The child's actual condition is, of course, the first consideration. The nurse should not generalize across broad illness categories, such as cancer, respiratory conditions, cardiac problems, etc. Each specific illness within a broad category will include specific implications, including subsequent disabilities. Patient and family needs, coping mechanisms, and available resources are the other influencing factors.

As with assessment and diagnosis, effective implementation involves the entire family. Evaluation will be an ongoing process, often done on a daily basis owing to the nature of a chronic condition. Unexpected setbacks, such as a relapse, critical infection, undesirable response to medication, lack of physical progression, or the need to undergo a medical or surgical procedure unexpectedly or sooner than anticipated, may be a part of the standard progression of a chronic illness. Goals may need to be revised frequently. These facts may be stressful and difficult, even for the most "seasoned" patient and family. Continuous support and reassurance of the patient and family are necessary throughout the course of a chronic illness.

Education

In discussing nursing care of the child with special health care needs, it should be recognized that the education component can take on a critical level of importance. Education is directed toward the child and the family and addresses both psychosocial issues and clinical issues, such as physical care of the child. With an illness that spans a number of years, the education process will be ongoing and may change frequently with the child's advancing age and/or altered physical condition.

A special consideration with respect to the education process involves the use of a child life specialist (Fig. 17–1). Educational methods that can be utilized by either nursing or childlife specialists include medical play, medical art, therapeutic play, and therapeutic art (see Chapter 9). All are similar in that they present the child with an opportunity for increased self-expression of ideas or situa-

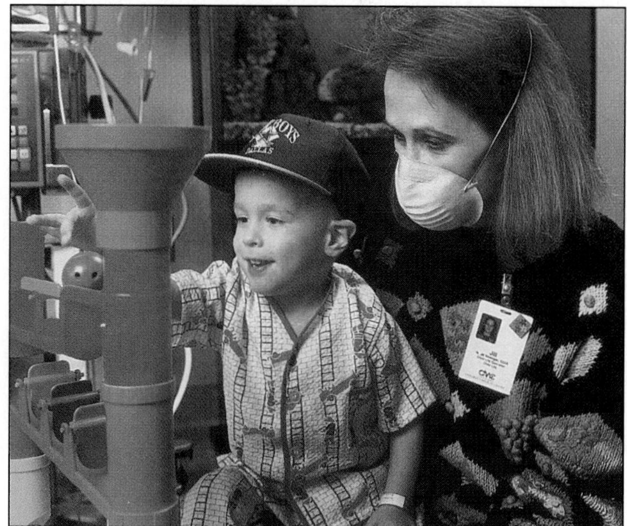

Figure 17–1

The nurse or a child life specialist can use therapeutic play, medical play, and therapeutic art to enhance self-expression and education, as well as growth and development, in the child with a chronic illness. (Courtesy of Norm Tindell for Cook Children's Medical Center, Fort Worth, Texas)

tions that may present difficulties for the child. This leads to externalization of previously hidden feelings and mastery of difficult and troublesome situations (Thompson & Standford, 1981). The most important aspect of each of these activities is that, although they may be offered or initiated by an adult, they are voluntarily maintained by the child (McCue, 1988). A detailed discussion of medical and therapeutic play can be found in Chapter 9.

Communication

Communication with the pediatric patient is frequently more difficult than the actual physical care of the child. Often, it is also the most important factor in determining the success of teaching efforts and in establishing a good relationship with the patient. This holds true for either a chronic or terminal illness. Appropriate communication is based on the child's age and development and always involves honesty, as well as compassion. Following these principles helps to decrease the child's fears and misunderstandings and to increase confidence in the nurses and other members of the health care team. Increased compliance and cooperation is an additional benefit. If fears and misunderstanding are not decreased initially, and the child's trust is not gained by the caregivers, it can be very difficult to establish them at a later date. This may be especially true when the nursing care involves unpleasant or painful medications and treatments.

Communication that utilizes honesty, compassion, and age-appropriate patterns is important in educating the child about clinical and psychosocial issues. In order to prevent misinterpretations and misunderstandings, it is helpful to ask the child to explain what they know and understand. The nurse or caregiver should also strive to understand what the child is really asking. The classic example of miscommunication can be found in the child who asks where he comes from, only to have the entire reproduction story explained, when all he really wanted to know was whether his family is from Texas or Oklahoma! Clarification of the question can help to avoid overinforming a child, or possibly frightening them unnecessarily or hindering them from asking future questions.

Honesty and trust must be maintained at all times in the care of the child, and these elements should likewise be encouraged among the family and other members of the health care team. This may cause problems for some individuals, family, or staff, especially when faced with the difficult questions that often arise when caring for a chronically or terminally ill child. The most difficult and feared questions, are of course, "Am I going to die?" and "Why did I get sick?" or "Why do I have to die?" These are followed closely by questions concerning the death of other patients whom the child knows and with whom they have developed a close relationship. Children are often reluctant to even ask questions of adults at all, much less questions whose answers they fear. Many times the answer is actually already known by the child. The question becomes a test and a benchmark in the child's relationship with the adult involved, whether it be a parent or staff. In the case of a chronic or terminal condition, honesty may engender an increased level of emotional pain, something not always handled well. As with adults, children require honesty in order to establish trust. However, children may not be able to comprehend the use of dishonesty as a means of protecting them against discomfort or unpleasantness. Once aware of dishonesty, children may feel that they cannot and will not trust those who have been deceitful. This may have disastrous effects, particularly when one is trying to reassure and gain cooperation from the child. Many times, a chronic condition may progress to the point of impending death, at which point the child's trust can be paramount to achieving comfort and peace. These issues are discussed in greater detail in later sections of this chapter devoted to care of the child facing impending death. For further discussion of communication, refer to Chapter 10.

THE NURSING PROCESS

Assessment

Family-centered care mandates assessment of the entire family system, which may be an overwhelming task given the variety of factors involved. All family members have unique qualities, each of which has a bearing on the way they function and interact with others. This applies whether the member is functioning as an individual or as a member of a group. Existing coping mechanisms must be assessed. If they are inappropriate, suggestions and support for changing to healthy, beneficial mechanisms should be offered. Additionally, the family's response to the child's illness and their level of recognition of the impact the illness has upon the entire family system should be explored. Evaluating perceptions of the illness will include discovering what each individual actually understands about the disease process and the treatment regimen and determining whether any altered processes are the result of misinformation or misinterpretation. Learning about existing support systems is also necessary. Such support not only assists the family to cope, but may also shape the family's method of coping, responses, and beliefs. Given the ongoing challenges of a chronic condition and the often frequent changes in the patient's physical status, education should be viewed as a continual process. This ensures that the family shares an accurate knowledge base if and when they assume physical care for the patient.

The child's level of development and abilities (physical and cognitive) must be assessed jointly by the patient, family, and interdisciplinary team. This baseline assessment of skills and abilities helps to ensure consistency of expectations and to gauge the level of assistance that will be required. Psychosocial abilities should also be assessed, including family patterns of communication and behavior, as well as emotional concerns. As previously mentioned, issues of self-esteem, self-reliance, and autonomy are primary concerns for the child with a chronic illness.

The child with a chronic illness is considered to be at risk for self-esteem problems related to physical changes which are frequently the result of either the condition or the treatment, or both. Even in the case of apparently minor changes, there can be altered body awareness and body image, with a resultant negative impact on self-esteem. The nurse must carefully assess the child's perception of the physical change, as well as the child's evaluation of how that change has or will affect her life. This assessment must take into consideration the special concerns prevalent at each different stage of growth and development. It must also be remembered that this assessment, perhaps more than any other, may change with the passing years. A child of 8 years of age may be very comfortable with and well adjusted to a physical change or disability, yet may experience difficulties with the same circumstances upon becoming a young adolescent.

Coping and adaptive abilities must be assessed, along with the family's progress in the process of normalization. This information will guide the health care team to explore any possible sources of difficulties in the family process. As these areas are examined over the course of a chronic condition, it is also important to keep in mind the illness trajectory. As the condition unfolds and the patient's condition changes, so will the impact upon the family and the work that will be necessary to complete in order to cope. In turn, this means that the family process will likely fluctuate in its normalcy and appropriateness.

Nursing Diagnoses

- Altered Growth and Development related to chronic illness or disability
- Body Image Disturbance related to actual or perceived physical differences or disabilities caused by an illness
- Altered Family Processes related to care of the child with a chronic illness

Planning, Implementation, and Evaluation: The Child With a Chronic Illness

NURSING DIAGNOSIS • Altered Growth and Development related to chronic illness or disability

Expected Outcome: The child will experience minimal disturbance of normal growth and development (physical, cognitive, and psychosocial) as evidenced by:

- Minimal delays documented by an appropriate developmental screening tool
- Ability to interact in an age-appropriate manner—socially, physically, and cognitively—to the degree allowed by any existing disability
- Ability to perform the usual age-appropriate ADLs as allowed by any existing disability

Intervention	Rationale
1. Educate patient and family about the physical condition, expected physical changes and/or disabilities, and prescribed treatment. Education should be offered in a manner appropriate for the child's cognitive abilities rather than her chronological age.	This encourages a sense of control, and acceptance, of physical changes related to the condition, as well as increased compliance with the prescribed treatment regimen. Many children with a chronic condition are wise beyond their years with a cognitive ability that does not necessarily correspond with their chronological age. Among such children, even those as young as 6 years of age may be able to discuss medical matters, such as lab values or the results of a diagnostic procedure, knowledgeably.
2. Set reasonable goals for improving and maximizing abilities in relation to any existing disability. This should be a group effort involving the patient, family, and interdisciplinary team.	Goal setting assists patients to increase their abilities and self-esteem through opportunities for successful task accomplishment. This may also increase a sense of situational control.

Intervention	Rationale
3. Assist child to develop a sense of pride in existing abilities and to gain the desire to achieve physical abilities.	Focus upon activities or skills once enjoyed. There can also be the setting of achievable, once considered goals. The patient with a prosthesis can strive toward once more becoming an accomplished skier . . . on one leg! Or, the patient can establish a goal of learning to drive an automatic instead of a standard-shift automobile, receiving a driver's license along with his peers.
4. Encourage and provide opportunities for autonomy and situational control by offering as many choices as possible. Include the child in age-appropriate decisions regarding treatment. Control can be offered in the form of choices, such as whether to be admitted to the hospital before or after lunch, or whether to reserve the time after a treatment for a family celebration or a special time of sharing between patient and parent. Older patients may be given the option of driving themselves to the clinic provided this is physically possible in terms of the treatment planned that day.	Autonomy and situational control are often lost as a result of limitations imposed by the condition and/or treatment. The child often cannot have a say in accepting a treatment or determining the type of treatment received, but she can be made to feel a part of the decision making process. Situational control and autonomy are positively connected to self-esteem. Choices are not always possible, but when they are, no matter how small, they should be offered.
	The setting of a goal and the reasons for achieving it will be facilitated if the goal has meaning for the patient, not just for the family or staff. A chronically or terminally ill child's goals may not always be what the healthy child would choose at that age, but if such goals are safe, reasonable and attainable, they may be very appropriate for that child's situation.
5. Encourage and provide opportunities for normal, age-appropriate ADLs/self-care. Provide assistive devices and education in their proper use.	This serves to encourage independence and provides an opportunity for practice and improvement of abilities.
6. During hospital stays, provide regular street clothes (when possible) and items from home for grooming, eating, recreation, etc.	This promotes normalization despite an illness or disability and helps to minimize disturbance of the patient's usual routines. It also serves to maintain and maximize the child's sense of control.
7. Provide age-appropriate activities and encourage the child to continue regular peer interaction (sports, school clubs/activities, church, social groups, etc.). This should be done both in and out of the hospital to the degree allowed by the child's physical condition/treatment. When possible, clinic visits, treatments, and hospitalizations should be arranged so as not to interfere with social, school, or church events. During hospitalizations, support and encourage the completion of school work, as well as peer visits/activities (Fig. 17–2).	This encourages development and maintenance of age-appropriate activities and developmental skills and contributes positively to the child's self-esteem and autonomy.
Misunderstandings and fear regarding the child's condition and/or medical setting may decrease involvement of the patient's well peers. Education can be offered through school visits by a nurse and child life therapist. Involvement can also be encouraged by including well peers in special events that occur during hospitalizations.	

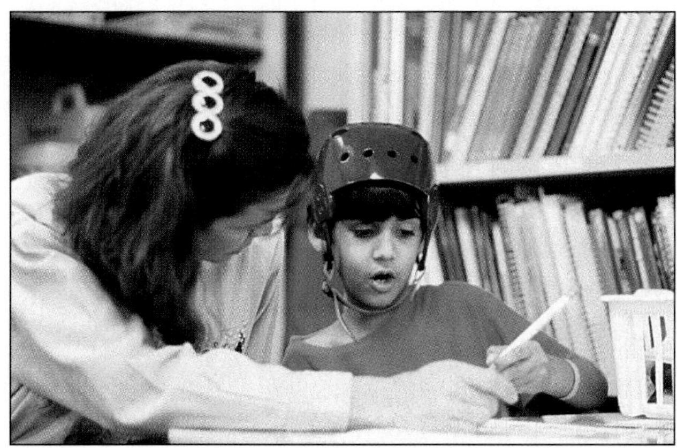

Figure 17–2
As more children with chronic conditions are living longer, it is common for them to attend public school. However, because these children are likely to be hospitalized frequently, hospitals often provide an area where teachers can help them keep up with their studies. (Courtesy of Cook Children's Medical Center, Fort Worth, Texas)

Intervention	Rationale
8. Encourage the patient to participate in the general or disease-specific support groups found at most pediatric hospitals. It may be appropriate to offer the strongest encouragement when the child is initially diagnosed (i.e., when she is likely to have increased fears and concerns). Participation in support groups should be encouraged; however, the decision not to join must be accepted if that is the patient's choice. Disease-specific camps, where all campers share the same problem, are also available; examples include camps for children with renal, endocrine, neurologic, pulmonary, hematologic, or oncologic conditions.	Tremendous and valuable support can be derived from peers who are experiencing a similar medical situation. In such a setting, there is acceptance and understanding not frequently found among those who are well. However, because comfort levels and the type of support needed vary, such support groups may not be the best or only answer for every child.

Evaluation:

- The child exhibits minimal developmental delays.
- The child exhibits age-appropriate social, physical and cognitive interaction.
- The child performs age-appropriate ADLs, as allowed by existing disability.

NURSING DIAGNOSIS

- Body image disturbance: related to actual or perceived physical differences or disabilities caused by an illness

Expected Outcome: The child will exhibit minimal disturbance of body image and adaptation to the illness and related physical changes or disabilities, as evidenced by:

- Expression of all attitudes and feelings (positive and negative) concerning the condition, physical change, or disability
- Expression of acceptance regarding the condition, physical changes, and/or disability
- Maintenance of as much independence as possible and as allowed by physical changes and/or disability
- Maintenance of a well-groomed physical appearance

Intervention	Rationale
1. Encourage and provide opportunities for child to verbalize all feelings, positive and negative, regarding the illness, physical change, or disability. Emphasize the normalcy of negative emotions.	Negative emotions will occur. These should be expressed and dealt with by the health care team and family in an accepting, nonjudgmental fashion in order to assist the child to progress to a positive accepting attitude.
2. Educate child regarding physical changes or disability, expected limitations or progression of disease, duration, required assistive devices and newly required self-care skills.	Misperceptions concerning physical changes or disability may hamper acquisition of a positive, accepting attitude, compliance with the prescribed treatment, and acquisition of newly required skills.
3. Encourage and assist patient to achieve as much independence as allowed by the physical change or disability.	Independence in self-care promotes a positive self-esteem and sense of control.
4. Provide constant reassurance as to the child's self-worth and ability to be autonomous, despite a physical change or disability. Teach child and family the actual self-care skills necessitated by the physical change or disability.	The presence of an ongoing physical difference/disability can cause poor self-esteem. It may also cause many doubts regarding the child's ability to become and remain self-reliant and autonomous. These skills must be taught, encouraged, and supported.
5. Focus positively upon the unchanged physical attributes of the child and the intact physical abilities. Teach and encourage the child and family to do likewise.	Achieving and maintaining a positive body image (with resulting positive self-esteem) is often difficult when physical changes have resulted from a condition, treatment, or assistive device.
6. Assist child to utilize aesthetic devices, such as wigs, special clothing, and make-up. Educate child and family about more extensive measures, such as prosthetics, and reconstructive surgery. Support any decision made with regard to use of such measures.	Physical changes, such as hair loss or scarring, may be considered by adults to be minor when compared to changes, such as limb loss or salvage, that result in disability. But they are often considered by the child to be severe, resulting in negative emotions and poor self-esteem.
7. Teach and encourage positive, accepting attitudes about physical differences. Foster new ideas regarding what constitutes physical attractiveness.	Minimizing or disguising physical changes is often necessary to foster a positive self-image. These adaptations may also be necessary to assist others to accept one's physical differences more easily. However, it is important for children and adults to learn to accept physical differences and to consider different standards of physical attractiveness.
There are many programs available that are designed to help patients adapt to physical changes, for instance, by offering advice about headcoverings and makeup for the cancer patient ("Look Good, Feel Better," the American Cancer Society) or fashion alternatives for those with braces or prosthetics. Disease-specific support groups provide information concerning available programs.	
8. Encourage and assist patient to utilize special support groups and special camps for children with similar health problems or disabilities. Accept and respect the decision of patients who choose not to participate in such support groups.	This helps provide peer interaction, possibly on a more comfortable, familiar level. Such programs may also provide activities that foster positive self-esteem. Realize that individual comfort levels will vary, as will the type and amount of support required by each child. Support groups may not be the best or only answer for every patient.

Intervention	Rationale
9. Refer the patient or family to appropriate personnel to manage coping or adjustment difficulties requiring therapeutic or nonprofessional intervention.	Some children experience serious problems, such as depression. Early intervention may lead to acceptance, adjustment, and resolution of such problems.

Evaluation:
- The child openly expresses feelings, both negative and positive, regarding the condition, physical changes, and/or disability.
- The child expresses an attitude of acceptance regarding the condition, physical changes, and/or disability.
- The child maintains independence as allowed by the physical change and/or disability.
- The child maintains a well-groomed appearance.

NURSING DIAGNOSIS
- Altered Family Process related to care of the child with a chronic illness

Expected Outcome: The child and family will experience minimal disturbance of appropriate family process, as evidenced by:
- Positive adjustment to and acceptance of the illness
- Appropriate parenting and parent/child interaction
- Effective family coping

Intervention	Rationale
1. Educate family about the patient's condition, including expected disease progression, physical changes or disabilities, and treatment options. Assist family to achieve a positive, realistic view of patient in relation to the condition.	This enables and encourages appropriate interaction with the health care team and compliance with the treatment plan, in addition to decreasing fears and misconceptions.
2. Assist family to identify fears and emotions pertaining to patient's illness. Emphasize that all feelings are normal and that appropriate verbalization is a positive and healthy part of coping.	Verbalization of feelings, with positive feedback, can help to decrease stress and facilitate resolution of negative emotions.
3. Act as a role model for appropriate, accepting, positive attitudes and behaviors concerning the patient.	Grief over the loss of a healthy child, discomfort with providing medical care, or a physical disability may hamper positive adjustment and acceptance. A positive role model may facilitate adjustment.
4. Refer the family and/or patient to additional resources (social worker, clergy, professional counselor) when necessary (i.e., if problems are beyond the nurse's scope or upon the family's request).	Situations requiring psychosocial assistance that is beyond the scope of nursing practice are not always indicators of family dysfunction requiring mental health intervention. However, when such intervention is indicated, early referral leads to a greater opportunity for positive outcomes.

Evaluation:
- The child and family exhibit a positive adjustment to the illness.
- The child and/or family exhibit appropriate parenting and parent/child interaction.
- The child and family exhibit effective family coping.

Care of the Parents

The concerns and needs listed as greatest among parents of a child with a chronic illness include (Phillips, 1990):

- understanding how the illness affects their child physically and emotionally
- finding ways to provide for their child's emotional, social, and intellectual needs
- identifying and utilizing appropriate resources for assistance
- health care planning for their child
- improving communication among the child's health care providers

Grief Education and Support. Nursing care should include education about the child's condition and treatment as well as education concerning the grief process resulting from a chronic condition. The nurse must assist all family members, including the patient, to understand and express the emotional responses of the grief process. Taking time to provide care and support in this area is as important as physical care of the patient. Many adults have not experienced illness and/or death prior to their child's diagnosis and are not accustomed to the idea of grief, much less grief as a normal, healthy process. The nurse must educate the family about the importance of this process and provide opportunities for grieving. This is done through conversation and listening and by being present for all family members as the need arises.

Cultural and Religious Beliefs. In order to provide caring and comprehensive grief support, the nurse must be aware of the impact of culture and religion upon the grief process in both illness and death. Culture and religion influence a number of variables, including the meaning of death and illness, as well as customs observed by the family at such times. Family life patterns (as they relate to authority, family roles, and available assistance) and the family's expectations of the health care team are also affected (Lawson, 1990). When faced with an unfamiliar culture or religion, nurses must acquaint themselves with standard beliefs and practices. The health care team's acceptance of these beliefs and practices should be communicated. The importance of such beliefs and practices to the family must also be validated by the health care team. It must not be assumed that an individual or family belongs to a particular religion solely on the basis of their cultural background. If in doubt, question the family, stressing that this is merely to provide the most comprehensive, appropriate care possible. The family services department or the education department should be able to provide extensive information concerning culture and religion in the health care setting. Table 17–1 presents a synopsis of beliefs among the major cultures and religions.

Referrals. To the degree possible, it is the job of the nurse not only to meet the physical, emotional, psychosocial, and intellectual needs and concerns of the patient, but also to meet those of the family as well. In addition, this means assisting the family to provide for the patient's needs themselves. Regardless of culture or religion, in some cases, the nurse may not be able to provide the necessary support owing to lack of time or expertise. At such times, the family should be referred to other personnel, such as a chaplain or social worker. If they cannot provide assistance, these personnel are generally in a better position to make a referral to outside professionals or services. The social service department will also be able to provide information concerning other resources needed by the family. These may include financial information, such as insurance and public assistance, housing and transportation assistance, as well as assistance with medical care and supplies. (See Appendix H for a list of general and disease-specific support organizations.)

> The health care team must not be the only providers of support. Nurses can assist families to find other sources of support, such as other parents, parent support groups, clergy, extended family, friends, and helping professionals (Fraley, 1990).

The Nurse as Liaison. The nurse acts as a liaison for the family in many different situations. However, the most important liaison work is that which links the family with other members of the health care team, particularly the physician. Acting in this capacity, the nurse can ensure that the family receives correct information and has a solid understanding of their child's condition and resulting needs. This facilitates health care planning by the family, helps to ensure a good relationship and appropriate communication with the health care team, and increases compliance with the prescribed treatment plan.

Care of the Siblings

For the sibling, as with the patient, concerns and needs in relation to the chronic illness will vary according to age and development. Fluctuations are common when the condition spans a number of years. Research has shown that siblings' areas of concern reflect those of the patient and parents. These include family communication, behavior management, and protection of the patient in public (Gallo et al., 1991). Other concerns include anxiety about the patient's condition and current health status. Regardless of whether the child is past the age of magical thinking, siblings frequently have feelings of guilt regarding their role in the patient's illness. What child with a sibling has not had thoughts as to what life would be like if only they did not have to share their material possessions and their parent's love with another child? The sibling should be reassured about the normalcy of such feelings, as well

TABLE 17–1 *Cultural and Religious Variations in Grief and Death*

RELIGIOUS ATTITUDES	GRIEF EXPRESSION	DEATH RITUALS	RESOURCES FOR SUPPORT
Japanese/Chinese			
Very protective of people's feelings. Believe in afterlife. Decedents return to "Nirvana." Deceased infants become little "Buddhas."	Not publicly expressive.	Chanting ceremony at bedside after death. Accepting clothes of deceased may not be appropriate. Japanese prepare gift food packs for mourners.	Families.
Indochinese			
After death soul lives in land of "tian." Deceased baby returns in body of another child. Stillborns are "marked" on soles of the feet. Assign number to baby instead of name for first few days of life.	May weep/wail aloud.	May cover baby's head after death as a sign of respect for soul believed to be housed in the head. Mourning attire consists of a white outfit worn by women mourners. Black armband worn by men.	Families.
African Americans			
Commonly recognized western concept of heaven/hell. Deceased do not watch over earthlings.	Very expressive.	Funeral rite is an informal gathering including prayers, scripture reading, songs, crying/screaming.	Minister, family, friends, church. Strong family kinship.
Mexican Americans			
Illness/death are God's will.	Very expressive.	Dependent on religious beliefs.	Families.
Native Americans			
No life after death—return to ancestors. Navajos are fearful of death; will burn decedent's possessions. Beliefs in spirits and need to be in harmony with nature.	May/may not be publicly expressive.	May take form of beasts chanting, monotonous singing over the dead to frighten away evil spirits.	Families, Shaman, tribal group.
Arabs			
Anticipatory grief work not acceptable. Children are integral part of family activities.	Express grief openly. Much touching of decedent's body.	Remain with body till transported. Do life review at decedent's bedside.	Family.

Developed and used with permission of Dr. Roy Martin, D.Min., Chaplain, Director of Family Services, Cook Children's Medical Center, Fort Worth, Texas.

as the fact that the illness is definitely not the result of anything said or done by the well sibling.

Nursing care of the sibling involves education about the patient's condition, treatment, physical changes and/or disabilities, and expected disease progression. The hospital setting—rules, equipment, and personnel—must also be explained.

Siblings may also be anxious about family relations owing to emotional stressors (with the resulting changes in behavior) and physical separation (Mahon, 1992). As with the patient, it should be expected that siblings may also experience regression in their developmental stage and activities. Parents frequently do not expect such behavioral changes from the sibling and may need to be reminded that this is a normal coping mechanism for all children, both ill and well, in the face of a stressful event. With these types of anxieties and resulting behavioral changes, special emphasis should also be placed on educa-

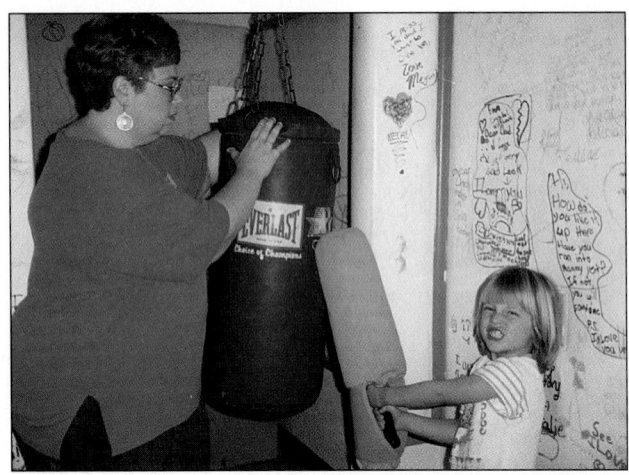

Figure 17–3
Chronic illness is stressful for the siblings of an ill child, whose emotional needs may be overlooked. Siblings should be given the opportunity to express negative feelings, such as anger and jealousy. This can be accomplished through art and play therapy, and through physical outlets, such as striking a punching bag, as this little girl is doing.

tion in the area of psychosocial and emotional concerns as well as appropriate behaviors. Even preschoolers can be assisted to learn appropriate communication techniques and behaviors. Such communication and behavior help well siblings to deal with their problems and anxieties effectively.

It is important to help the sibling understand that illness creates stress that often results in difficult emotions, such as anger and jealousy. These emotions are a normal part of life in general, although they are often perceived as being negative, harmful emotions. Children must be allowed to experience and express each of these feelings (Fig. 17–3). This significant and difficult task becomes all the more important in the case of chronic illness. The physical and emotional needs of the patient are generally well tended to, as are the emotional needs of the parent. However, it may be all too easy to exclude the sibling and neglect their emotional needs, leading to an additional set of stress-producing problems to be dealt with by the entire family.

Siblings often experience a significant change in their relationship with the patient as a result of the condition (Rollins, 1990). It is often helpful for the nurse and family to include the sibling as much as possible in the life and activities of the patient, whether hospitalized or receiving outpatient care. The family should be educated regarding the pros and cons of sibling involvement. The level of sibling involvement, however, is always determined by the family. Many families choose to minimize siblings' time and involvement in the medical setting as a means of keeping their lives as normal and uninterrupted as possible. Spiritual or cultural beliefs may affect this decision. Other families attempt to maintain the existing level of closeness and may choose complete involvement, including the presence of the sibling during the day and for overnight visits if allowed by the institution. Regardless of their choice or the reasons behind it, the family's decision must always be supported.

When extensive involvement is chosen, it is important for the nurse to ensure that the sibling is appropriately educated in order to decrease misunderstanding and fear. As with the patient, medical play, therapeutic play, and therapeutic art are excellent means of educating the sibling. These techniques can be used by the nurse and/or child life specialist to allay fears and misunderstandings about the patient's condition and medical treatment. They are also an excellent mechanism for support, allowing the child to acquire an understanding of their often intense, confusing, and varied emotional responses while venting them in a healthy, appropriate manner. Involvement with the health care team and a sense of connection with the patient are also provided.

It should also be recognized that this type of extensive involvement brings with it additional risks. The sibling will frequently be exposed to the intense physical and emotional experiences of the patient, which can certainly have emotional consequences for the sibling. There must be close attention from staff and family in order to detect problems of this type. If problems do arise, the necessary support and intervention should be provided by appropriate team members (medical, nursing, child life, and family services personnel).

> Nurses striving to teach and include siblings in the hospital life of the patient should collaborate with the child life specialist. This interaction can help the entire family discover, explore, and resolve feelings that might otherwise be problematic for both patient and sibling(s).

The relationship between patient and sibling may be altered due to normal but unintentional feelings of resentment, jealousy, and competition as the ill child receives increased amounts of attention. This may be accentuated if the sibling spends extended time at the hospital, thus witnessing the extra attention given to the patient. Siblings may experience guilt and shame about such feelings. The nursing staff and/or child life specialist can devote individual attention to the sibling, apart from the patient, as a means of providing sibling support. The opportunity to verbalize emotions and interact with a caring, nonjudgmental individual may help siblings to understand and accept the normalcy of their feelings. Additionally, a sibling support group is a resource available at many hospitals.

Nurses can provide immeasurable sibling support by focusing just a few minutes of time on simple items, such as the sibling's day at school or a recent achievement or, most importantly, how the sibling is feeling, both physically and emotionally.

An important aspect of sibling support is to remember them at special times when the patient is recognized, such as birthdays or graduations. The ill child often receives extra attention, including gifts, from family and friends during the course of the illness, and special events may be recognized by a large number of staff. Often, siblings associate illness with this extra attention and gifts, subsequently experiencing real or imagined illness themselves as a bid for similar attention. Remembering the sibling with a small gift on special occasions or when the patient is receiving a gift can be a helpful and supportive gesture. This, along with individual attention from staff, may subsequently help to decrease feelings of guilt and resentment, as well as to affirm the sibling's importance. It is helpful for nurses to remind parents and other family members of such interventions throughout the course of the illness. In most circumstances, a good rule of thumb is to have family and friends bring a gift to siblings whenever the patient is to receive a gift. This can be particularly important at diagnosis, during a relapse, or in terminal illness situations.

Despite all of the difficulties and concerns mentioned, research indicates that well siblings of children with a chronic illness are not uniformly at risk for maladjustment and do not experience significant behavioral or social competence problems (Gallo et al., 1992). However, with the significant stress that accompanies a chronic illness, the potential for problems certainly exists. Support of the well sibling then, is as integral a part of nursing care as is care of the actual patient.

THE TERMINALLY ILL OR DYING CHILD

The Child's Concept of Death

An understanding of death and dying in relation to childhood is necessary when caring for the child approaching death. The established and accepted guidelines concerning children's concepts of death are based upon the stages of growth and development. As discussed by Waechter (1984) and Wass (1985), these concepts correlate with age and cognition (Table 17–2). It is also recognized that a child's concept of death is affected by intellectual, social, and psychological life experiences (Bowden, 1993).

TABLE 17–2 *The Child's Concept of Death*

AGE	COGNITIVE STAGE	CONCEPT
Infant/toddler (0–2 yrs)	Sensorimotor	Death as the loss of caretaker
Early childhood (2–7 yrs)	Preoperational	Death as a reversible and temporary separation
Middle childhood/ school-age (7–11/12 yrs)	Concrete operational	Death as sad and irreversible, but not necessarily inevitable
Adolescence (12+ yrs)	Formal operations	Death as inevitable and irreversible, but often a distant event

Infants and Toddlers. Infants and toddlers view death in relation to the loss of a caretaker and the subsequent emptiness in their lives. They are also affected by the loss of comforting measures, as when they experience pain, cold, etc. Consequently, time with primary caregivers is quite important. As they approach death, they often sense the severity of their condition through their parents' nonverbal communication. Children of this age may react to the dying process based upon the feelings of sadness, anger, and anxiety conveyed in the responses and behaviors of their parents. Reactions will be expressed through crying, attachment to their primary caregiver, and separation anxiety.

Preschoolers. Preschoolers view death as a separation or departure and believe it to be only temporary. Death is also seen as reversible. Magical thinking and egocentricity at this age often lead to guilt and shame as children may believe that their thoughts or actions caused the death. The child's first exposure to death is frequently a dead animal, such as an insect, bird, or pet. Preschoolers facing an impending death frequently view their condition as punishment for behaviors or thoughts. They respond with guilt, anger, sadness, and fear. Their self-imposed guilt may cause them to believe that others, including parents, see them as "bad" and are angry with them. Feelings are kept inside and the children may withdraw from everyone, including those whom they love and on whom they depend. Children may direct their anger at those they care about, and the intensity of their anger frightens them. Great patience and understanding are required of their parents and nurses, particularly when emotions are labile and subject to frequent, acute changes. Indeed, all children feel greater security when adults maintain discipline and suitable, customary limits. This is especially true for the dying child of preschool age who is experiencing multiple changes and discrepancies in his daily life.

School-Age. By the school-age years, death begins to be understood as a sad and irreversible event, yet still may be considered inevitable only for adults. By the age of 10 years or so, children begin to understand that they, too, can die. Some associated feelings of guilt often persist for children this age. They may continue to believe that thoughts or actions can cause death, or that death serves as a punishment for wrong-doing. The school-age child has increased cognition and other resources necessary to cope with the dying process, but these same abilities may lead to additional questions and fears. The child may wonder why he has the illness and must die so young. Fear about the process of dying and what follows also may arise. Even in children who have a foundation of faith and spiritual beliefs, this fear may persist because they do not have a concrete knowledge of what heaven or the hereafter is like. They may also fear being without the love and support of the parents they have always known. Moreover, school-age children may feel vulnerable and doubt their ability to cope with the knowledge of their impending death, as well as the experience itself.

Adolescent. Most adolescents have a fully developed understanding of death as inevitable and irreversible. However, owing to an increasingly independent frame of reference, many adolescents view death as a distant event and may consider themselves resistant to death. Although adolescents may have a cognitive understanding of death and dying, they do not necessarily have an emotional acceptance. Adolescents who are attempting to separate from their parents often test and break rules as they stride toward independence. This may cause guilt for the dying child, especially when contemplating the spiritual aspects of life and death.

Adolescents may become isolated from their peers as a result of an illness. The terminal illness or disability of a peer forces adolescents to abruptly and unwillingly face and question their own mortality and wholeness. Discomfort with this is very often the cause of infrequent visitation or no visits at all on the part of even close friends. Adolescents may also become isolated from caring adults, family, and staff owing to the feeling that adults do not understand them. Consequently, many feel lonesome and become afraid that they will die without the love and support that they need and desire. Realizing that they face death at an age when their lives are just beginning, many adolescents respond with bitterness and sadness. This may be particularly true when they consider the adult experiences that will be denied them. Such bitterness and sadness may lead to depression.

The Response to Death and Dying

The process of dying, as well as the actual death of a child, is widely acknowledged as being a unique and complex situation. The responses of all involved—patient, family, and staff—will be affected by various factors, such as personal and spiritual beliefs, previous experiences with illness and death, as well as experiences during the current situation. An individual's progression through the stages of grief and death are also important, as is the relationship with the dying child. The stages of grief and dying, as delineated by Kubler-Ross (1969) are recapped in the box on p. 398. At any given time, the patient, parents, and siblings may all be experiencing a different stage of grief and expressing that grief in very different ways.

The Child's Response

The responses of dying children at every age indicate that, like the adult, their primary concerns relate to comfort, safety, and not being alone (Foley & Whittam, 1990). These concerns are frequently more intense and problematic with school-age children and adolescents. The child's responses to death and dying will be multiple and varied, not always fully correlating with their chronological cognition and development. The often traumatizing experiences of a chronic condition and its treatment tend to make children more mature and wise beyond their years. Additionally, children with a terminal illness may reach a point where they consider their illness and treatment worse than death. Relief is frequently evident as the dying child works through the five stages of grief and dying. Responses and actions of the dying child may also be affected by the behaviors and feelings of those around them, particularly family and staff. Progression through the five stages is often accomplished rapidly in order to achieve the necessary acceptance and closure.

The child's response to dying and her resulting actions are often more precocious than would be expected, particularly among those of preschool age. Precocious actions and those of a spiritual nature are often considered by family or staff to be inappropriate or unbelievable, and may be attributed to physical alterations, such as a low hemoglobin level, altered neurologic status, or medications, such as analgesics or sedatives.

Spiritual beliefs may influence the child and be reflected in their conversation and actions. Children may speak of seeing or even interacting with angels or the higher being recognized by their particular faith. They may also speak of going to heaven to be with the angels or other spiritual beings. Moreover, it is not uncommon for children to speak of going to play or be with a child or relative who has already died. This type of conversation may take place only days or hours before death, with the child giving specifics as to when they will see or be with the deceased individual. One such conversation was initiated by a 4-year-old with cancer only 2 days before his death. In response to the boy's insistence that he would soon play with his former playmate (an oncology patient who had died previously), the hospital staff and parents attempted to remind him of the other child's death, thinking he was in denial or had forgotten. The boy could not be dissuaded, however, and did indeed die on the day he said he would once again be able to play with his friend. Another preschool child was very determined to play in the playroom for a longer time than usual late one night. When staff and parents attempted to convince him to go back to his room, noting that he could play again in the morning, the boy insisted that no, he would not be able to go to the playroom the next day. The child died during the night.

Precocious actions also tend to be observed with regard to closure, including the recognition of psychosocial issues that must be resolved before death and a corresponding emphasis upon these issues. Dying children often experience a heightened sense of understanding and awareness, particularly as death nears. Many know when they will die, and death often occurs after they are successful in achieving closure of some type. Closure may be a special event in their life or that of a loved one, such as a graduation, holiday, or birthday. Frequently, closure also entails resolution of unfinished business, such as interacting with a loved one who has been absent or correcting a wrong. Increased awareness and/or the need for closure are often communicated in a manner difficult to understand.

Correspondingly difficult to understand is the concept of "allowing" the child to die. For most children, this means giving them permission to die. A predominant issue of childhood is that, as a child, one should obey the directives given by parents. This is based on the knowledge that parents know best and provide guidance so that their children will do that which is safe and correct. Additionally, as noted by Kubler-Ross (1983), children are not afraid of death, but rather of abandonment. Children who are enveloped with hope, joy, and love will maintain their grasp upon their precious and fragile lives. Accordingly, most children, particularly those who are younger, need verbal permission to die, as well as reassurance that it is safe to do so. Such reassurance should include a description of what and who to expect as they die and in the time afterward. Children may also need reassurance that the family, friends, and loved ones who are left behind will be all right and that they will take care of each other. Equally important to children of all ages is the need to be remembered. They should have the knowledge and reassurance that, regardless of how brief their life, they will never be forgotten by those loved ones with whom they have shared their life (Gibbons, 1993).

The Parents' Response

When a child is initially diagnosed with any condition that is potentially fatal, every parent faces and begins to cope with the *possibility* of their child's death. When they are informed that nothing more can be done medically, parents face the *reality* of their child's death. The stages of grief worked through in relation to the illness must now be experienced in relation to the death of their child. Resolution into acceptance does not always occur. Some parents may find it difficult or unacceptable to discontinue treatment. They may choose to continue treatment of a curative rather than a palliative nature. However, such a choice does not always indicate denial. It may simply represent a particular belief system based on spiritual or personal convictions. From a legal, emotional, and psychosocial standpoint, the family's decision must be upheld and supported. Regardless of treatment choices, the paramount concern of all parents is the possibility of their child experiencing pain (Foley & Whittam, 1990).

Parents will exhibit the need to talk about their child and the experience of their child's illness and death. They talk in order to assimilate the experience, but more importantly, they talk to remember their child.

When a chronic condition has existed for an extended period of time, the parents' initial reaction to their child's death is often relief that the child is no longer suffering and that the uncertainty of their situation has ended. Many times, this relief and feeling of peace may begin before death, when a definite resolution is known to be imminent. This relief may correlate with numbness, followed by intense sadness and a sense of profound loss and emptiness. The grief of a child's grandparent is similar to that of her parents, yet three-fold. The grandparent must grieve for their grandchild, for themselves, and for their own child, the parent (Ponzetti, 1992).

The Siblings' Response

As with their response to the illness itself, siblings' responses to death and dying, as well as their progression through the stages of grief, will vary according to age and development. Although children usually experience all five stages of grief/dying, this may not necessarily occur in the given sequence. Frequently, children move between the stages in a seemingly random fashion, often experiencing a stage several times. This process is an appropriate coping mechanism for the child based upon their cognitive and developmental needs and abilities. Issues and worries over having caused the illness and/or death may resurface, even if they were dealt with successfully earlier in the illness. Without appropriate guidance and assistance, these issues may persist. Siblings may experience many other emotions, many of which are the same as those of their parents. However, owing to their level of cognition and development, they may not be as well equipped to understand, to cope, and to work their way through the grief process successfully.

Smith (1991) believes that grief is similar among people of all ages. There are three important tasks necessary to process the grief itself and to integrate the loss: (1) to understand that the person is no longer there (and will not return), (2) to feel the emotions, and (3) to reinvest in life. Successful completion of these tasks will become a part of the surviving child's normal growth and development. This will require continued support and assistance as the child advances in age.

Unresolved grief is recognized as a contributing factor in many problems of adulthood. It is now acknowledged that children work through the grief process differently than adults, and that they often require special assistance to complete the process. There are now many centers across the country available specifically to provide grief support for the child who has experienced the death of a significant loved one.

The most important aspect of providing support for the grieving child is to acknowledge that the loss of his sibling is just as significant as the parents' loss of their child. It is common practice for the health care team to send sympathy cards and other correspondence to parents after their child's death. This can be taken an important step further by also addressing cards, phone calls, and other gestures of sympathy to siblings individually. Such validation of their grief can be a first and important step in their successful navigation of the grief process.

NURSING CARE OF THE TERMINALLY ILL OR DYING CHILD

Despite medical advances and current technology, many chronic disorders ultimately lead to death. Providing nursing care to the child with a fatal illness who is nearing death and to family members requires a heightened level of understanding, compassion, and support. A family's coping abilities are often tested beyond measure. Nursing care includes assisting the family to withstand the tremendous pressures and to meet the emotional demands of the situation (Fig. 17–4). Preparedness for the impending death of a child cannot be accomplished without essential nursing support and education, which is directed not only toward the dying process, but toward the lifetime of grief, healing, and recovery faced by the surviving family (Gyulay, 1989).

A common reproach of children and families is that the expansive education and emotional support that they received during the course of a terminal illness declines substantially as death becomes more imminent (Gibbons, 1993).

Professional Boundaries. Nurses must be cognizant of potential stresses, not only for the child and family, but also for themselves. Caring for the child who is approaching death can be very rewarding, but it may also be a severe test of the nurse's personal and professional coping skills. Compassion is a must, but there must also be an awareness and maintenance of professional boundaries. This is necessary in order for the nurse to provide clinically sound, compassionate care while also maintaining sound emotional, physical, and spiritual health.

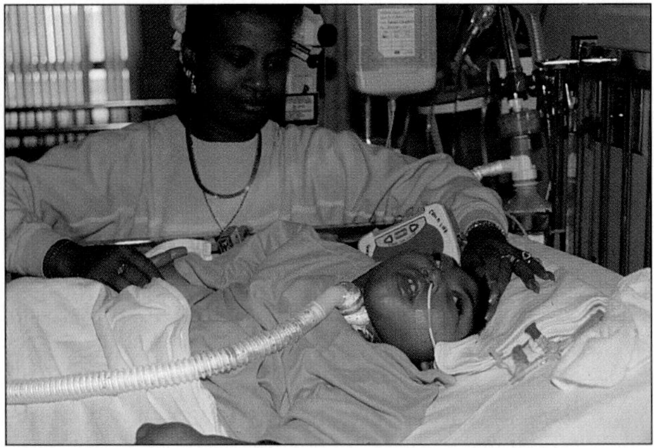

Figure 17–4
The family of the child with a terminal condition requires a high level of compassion and support from the nurse. This child has anencephaly (absence of most of the brain), a birth defect that is usually fatal before birth or in the first few days after birth. His grandmother is his primary caregiver. His nursing care includes not only physical care, but also support of the grandmother's caregiving and assistance with the grieving process. (Courtesy of Parkland Memorial Hospital, Dallas, Texas)

Nurses must understand and accept their personal feelings and beliefs concerning death in order to provide professional care and support. Unresolved difficulties may interfere with nursing care.

Communication

Staff and family must be aware of the communication needs and patterns of the dying child. This requires openness and acceptance on the part of all involved. Nurses and parents should assure the child that they will not be abandoned or alone, and that they will always have the presence of their loved ones. Children should emphatically be assured that the illness and approaching death are not the result of anything they have or have not done or said. Children must also be assured that their emotions and actions are not wrong and that they are loved and accepted, no matter what. Children, parents, and siblings need assistance to understand their often varied, intense emotions, especially such emotions as anger and guilt, which are often perceived negatively. Parents, in particular, need opportunities away from the patient to express their grief and anger. This helps to minimize or prevent the child from feeling responsible for the parents' difficult emotions. It also contributes to an environment that is as soothing, comfortable, and stress-free as possible where parents can have uninterrupted time with their child and the opportunity to provide whatever level of physical care they wish to handle.

Regardless of age, most dying children will follow the rules and patterns of communication set by those closest to them. As death approaches, the essential element of communication between child and family can decline in both extent and effectiveness. Therefore, one of the most important responsibilities of nursing care is to facilitate dynamic, purposeful communication (Bluebond-Langner, 1978). The nurse should take into account how communication was handled at particularly stressful times, such as the time of diagnosis, relapse, or periods of disease exacerbation. Generally, what has been effective in the past will continue to be effective. However, blanket assumptions should be avoided, and each circumstance should be evaluated carefully to ensure the best communication possible for the child and family.

The most common issue that arises in relation to a child's impending death is whether or not to *inform* the child of the prognosis. Bluebond-Langner (1978) asserts that children either instinctively know or will discover the prognosis, whether or not it is revealed by an adult. She proposes that the question should be whether to *acknowledge* the prognosis to the child. Needs of the patient, parents, and staff frequently conflict, but the needs of all must be considered. The suggested approach is to adopt a policy that allows the patient to maintain open awareness and communication with those who choose to do so. This makes it possible to meet the child's need for someone to know and to acknowledge that she is dying while simultaneously allowing mutual pretense and decreased communication to be maintained by those who prefer that approach. This flexible system has been found to be effective, and is prevalent among dying children and those who care for them.

Despite the use of this system, nurses may be caught between children who wish to talk about their death and parents who would forbid any such conversation. When faced with this type of situation, the nurse should remember that dying children of every age must attend to unfinished business. Failure to communicate with them openly and honestly can hinder their efforts toward task completion (Gibbons, 1993). As the caregiver and primary patient advocate, the nurse should first meet the needs of the patient. Any skirting of the issues or dishonesty with the patient may destroy the nurse-patient relationship, possibly denying the patient a much-needed source of comfort and support. Nurses can inform the parents that they will not initiate any discussion with the patient but that they need and intend to respond openly and honestly when such a discussion is initiated by the child. This allows nurses to respect the wishes of the parents and to provide assistance or support when needed by the child.

Honesty and simplicity are the keys to communicating with dying children. The nurse should tell them what they are asking about and what they want to know, on their own terms (Bluebond-Langner, 1978).

In terms of nurse-patient communication, it is important never to underestimate the power and necessity of providing communication and support in the manner and at the level desired by the dying child. Words are not always necessary. Presence, simply sitting with the child, and/or light touch, such as holding a hand, may be all the child requires. The silence itself may be a therapeutic intervention, or it may help to open the door for desired verbal communication.

The Family's Beliefs and Practices

Nursing care must impart consistent respect and acceptance in order to support parents appropriately during their most difficult time, the death of their child. This must occur regardless of any differences between the beliefs and practices of the family and the nurse; personal, spiritual, and cultural.

Personal, spiritual, and ethical beliefs must often be put aside by the nurse in order to provide care and support in an accepting and nonjudgmental fashion.

The nurse will encounter different beliefs and practices surrounding death and the grief process. These may include prayer cloths, holy water or oil, religious pictures, icons or other objects, extemporaneous prayer gatherings, preparation and serving of certain foods, and the like. Some may be troublesome to deal with because of concerns as to whether the practice is in the best interest of the child, or even safe at all. Parents' last-ditch attempts may include the use of unproven medications or treatments, such as those being utilized in other countries. Although difficult to justify in our world of the Federal Drug Administration–approved medical care, many of these attempts are not physically harmful to the child. Indeed, they may actually be emotionally beneficial to both parent and child, for such efforts affirm the fact that everything possible was tried, a notion that may be very important to patients and families. These efforts may also instill hope, which under no circumstances should be taken from the child or parents. At times, however, such medication or treatment may be harmful to the child, as with intramuscular injections that are painful or treatments that may cause bleeding in a child with a low platelet count. In such instances, the staff may decide not to administer the treatment. Their decision and the rationale for it must be explained compassionately, yet firmly, always noting that this is done in the best interest of the child.

Cultural and spiritual beliefs about death may influence patterns of grief and behavior both before and after death. Nurses should familiarize themselves with beliefs of the child and family in order to provide sensitive and appropriate care and support.

Often, treatment decisions that do not offer any hope of increased comfort and quality of life and that are not based on cultural or spiritual beliefs are made by parents. These often do not seem to be in the best interest of the child. For instance, parents may refuse pain medication for their child because they want him to be alert, at any cost. Likewise, a parent may rescind a "do not resuscitate" (DNR) order in the case of cardiac arrest, mandating a full code situation even when there is clearly no hope of long-term survival for the child. Some settings are using the words "comfort and care only" rather than "do not resuscitate." Situations of this type must be dealt with individually, based upon existing facts and opinions. The withholding of pain medication may be more easily resolved than the question as to whether a child should be resuscitated, and there are laws that address some of these situations. Either of these circumstances may be the cause of emotional, spiritual, and professional distress for the nurse. This may be particularly true if the action is in conflict with the nurse's beliefs and perceived as being useless for the child. The nurse must cope with and resolve these types of situations in order to provide the necessary, appropriate care. If unable to do so, the nurse should always be given the option of not participating in the care of the patient. These types of circumstances generally do not go unnoticed by the child, and may contribute to a care environment that is stressful. Nurses cannot always prevent these situations or resolve them to the satisfaction of everyone involved. They can, however, provide care, communication, and a level of support that will minimize stress and involvement of the patient.

Pain Control

For all involved—patient, family, and staff—the most pressing and emotional issue relating to the dying child is usually pain control. The nurse should educate the child and family regarding pain control and then provide constant, consistent reassurance that everything will be done to guarantee the continued comfort of the child. Families and older children may express concerns about addiction in the same breath as concerns that pain relief will not be adequate. Without belittling the feelings of those involved, the nurse should remind the family of the terminal nature of the situation, reassuring them that their concerns regarding addiction are unnecessary and inappropriate under the circumstances. When there is a physical reason for pain medication, such as with a terminal condition, addiction does not and will not occur. Questions regarding increasing doses of narcotics and addiction may arise just as frequently in the care of a pediatric patient as they do in the care of an adult patient. The child and family should be informed that the pain associated with terminal conditions may escalate acutely and frequently, with a corresponding decrease in the child's response to narcotics. It should also be emphasized that any necessary increase in medication dosage or change in regimen will always occur in response to escalating pain. The child and family must always know and believe that pain will be handled in a manner that provides comfort as well as the optimal environment for meeting their psychosocial and spiritual needs. (For further information and discussion, refer to Chapter 20.)

Pain control can be achieved either enterally or parenterally. Although more children than adults tend to have central intravenous lines, such access is not exclusively utilized or necessary for pain or other symptom control. Oral morphine is usually the first medication of choice for the management of severe cancer pain. The development of oral, controlled-release morphine preparations, along with a highly concentrated immediate-release liquid preparation, has made possible improved pain control for children without the use of parenteral medications. Babul and Darke (1993) have noted that, although the effective use of controlled-release morphine is well documented in adults, its use in the pediatric population has been limited to open-label studies in patients with various types of pain, including that caused by cancer (Atchison et al., 1991; Brookoff et al., 1989; Goldman & Bowman, 1990; Poulain, 1989; Richter, et al., 1989; Rogers, 1990; and Teresi et al., 1990). Although clinical trials are needed to fully evaluate the use of these morphine preparations in children, anecdotal reports as well as the results of these various studies, indicate that such preparations can be used successfully in the management of severe pain associated with cancer and other terminal diseases.

Parents must be instructed that the time-release form of morphine must be swallowed whole and cannot be crushed.

Frequently, the use of oral pain medications is not possible because of the patient's inability to swallow (related to age and/or the loss of swallow function) or the presence of recurrent vomiting. Under these circumstances, rectal administration of oral medication is an option. Research on this mode of administration in the pediatric population has focused largely on seizure medications (Anonymous, 1990 and 1992; Cox, 1993). Anecdotal use and research indicate that, for certain oral seizure medications, rectal administration is both appropriate and efficacious (Keane, 1993). More research has been conducted on adults regarding the rectal administration of many oral medications, including timed-release morphine (McCaffery et al., 1992; Rigamonti & Bruera, 1991; van Hoogdalem et al., 1991 [Parts I and II]; Wilkinson et al., 1992). Such research, as well as anecdotal use, supports rectal administration when it is no longer feasible to utilize the oral route of administration and when parental administration is not feasible or desirable. Despite the lack of similar research in the pediatric population, anecdotal experience with children (primarily in a hospice care setting) has indicated similar results.

Although there is a similar lack of information and research, the same is also true regarding the use of adjuvant medications for pain control in the dying child (Geller et al., 1987; Heilgenstein & Steif, 1989; Yee & Berde, 1994). Additional approaches to pain control include analgesic nerve blocks, noninvasive techniques (imagery, hypnosis), and neurosurgical procedures (Miser & Miser, 1993).

Careful record keeping of all pain medications given, especially the use of immediate-release liquid morphine for breakthrough pain, should be a collaborative effort between family and staff, with the result being the best pain management possible for the child. Personalized medication sheets (similar to those used in the hospital) with room for recording new medications and/or dose changes can make the task of medication administration easier and less daunting for families. Others may prefer to use a notebook to keep a narrative record.

When parenteral medications are required, administration is generally simple owing to the availability of central IV access devices and IV pumps that are "user friendly" for both families and staff. In children without venous access, subcutaneous morphine or Dilaudid has been used in some settings with good results. Some narcotics are beginning to be used intranasally, and epidural medications can be used for severe pain.

When central access is utilized, it is not unusual for those overseeing the patient's care to adopt a very flexible attitude regarding the changing of dressings and implanted port needles. This approach differs greatly from the rigorous standards imposed when the child is participating in aggressive curative treatment. Many families are grateful for the more relaxed approach, which generally means one less worrisome or painful experience for their child. However, some families and children prefer to maintain the established dressing change routine, possibly because of concerns about infection or the appearance of "giving up." The option of a flexible attitude regarding this matter should always be offered, along with reassurance that the chosen option will in no way be harmful to the child. The child and family should be permitted to make the decision that best suits their needs; the health care staff then can provide any physical or emotional care required to support their decision.

Hospice Care

For many terminally ill children and their families, a nonhospital environment, involving either an inpatient or a home hospice program, may be the preferred choice for meeting their various needs during the dying process. **Hospice care** is a specialized and comprehensive system of care that provides support and assistance to patients (and their families) who are in the last phase of a terminal illness. This phase is generally considered to be the last 6 months of a patient's life. Children's Hospice International (CHI) is an organization devoted solely to the needs of pediatric hospice patients and their families. Founded in 1983, this nonprofit organization provides support and resources to children with life-threatening conditions and their families. They also provide education, training, and technical assistance to health care professionals (Armstrong-Dailey & Goltzer, 1993).

The use of hospice care for pediatric patients, either in a home setting or an inpatient setting, is increasing. In part, this is due to the wide range of support services offered by hospice programs. Although nursing support is perhaps the primary reason hospice care is feasible, it is only a small component of the array of services available through a comprehensive hospice program. For instance, social workers provide a number of social services that assist families with a wide range of difficulties. These include, but are not limited to, identifying sources of financial assistance, locating and bringing home family members who are in the armed services or living at a distance, planning a funeral, and facilitating legal affairs. The accessibility of equipment that can easily be managed by the layperson has also contributed to the increased use in hospice care. Such equipment includes hospital beds; bedside commodes; assistive devices, such as walkers and bath chairs; oxygen administration set-ups; and other respiratory equipment.

In general, death usually occurs peacefully for children, but hospice care and death in the home setting affords a more natural, relaxed backdrop than the traditional hospital setting. This is because the child is able to have close at hand family, pets, friends, and the comfort of their own room. Although children dying at home do not usually experience any final outburst of pain or long periods of intense suffering, any necessary pain control may be achieved more easily in the home because the child is more relaxed in familiar surroundings and may have more activities available to help keep her mind off the illness (Tartler, 1993).

Just as home hospice care has been increasingly utilized for the pediatric population, so, too, has inpatient hospice care. Inpatient hospice care may be provided in a free-standing setting or as a separate unit within an acute care setting. Families may choose inpatient hospice for a variety of reasons:

- physical care requirements and emotional burdens that are too great for family caregivers to manage
- the presence of physical symptoms requiring aggressive management, or of extensive pain requiring intensive and complex medication control (Lombardi, 1993)

Brief periods of inpatient hospice care may also be used to meet a family's respite care needs, providing an environment that is less threatening and more home-like than that available in a regular hospital or medical center.

Hospice should always be an alternative offered to families, along with the information necessary for making an educated choice. In some cases, a family will choose home-based hospice care, only to admit the child to a hospital during the final hours or days of life. This choice, which always remains available to families, may be based on fears about pain control, adequate physical care of the child, or concerns over handling the emotional aspect of a death at home. Parents may be particularly anxious as to how successfully siblings will cope with living in their home once a death has occurred there. These types of fears should be discussed by the health care team and family early in the hospice experience and then dealt with appropriately. However, regardless of such discussions, families may still opt for hospitalization when death nears. As previously mentioned, the family's choices must be accepted and supported, regardless of the type or frequency of changes in decision making.

THE NURSING PROCESS

Assessment

Nursing care of the dying child and family is based upon a complex set of issues. Circumstances affecting the child, parents, and siblings must be assessed and taken into consideration. These include the family's relationship and involvement with the child, cognition, developmental stage, and previous experiences with illness and death, as well as experiences during the current condition. The individual's progression through the stages of grief and dying must also be explored. These stages were experienced in relation to the grief caused by the chronic illness; and they must now be experienced in relation to the impending death.

Anxiety can negatively affect the child physically, resulting in heightened pain and/or other physical symptoms, such as dyspnea. Negative affects can also be seen psychosocially, for both child and family. Anxiety and concerns exhibited during the current condition should be assessed, particularly at times of increased stress, such as at diagnosis, or during disease exacerbations or relapses. Coping and adaptive mechanisms of the child and family should also be assessed.

Nursing Diagnoses

- Anticipatory Grieving: related to the impending death of a child
- Anxiety related to diagnosis and/or impending death

Planning, Implementation, and Evaluation: The Terminally Ill or Dying Child

NURSING DIAGNOSIS • Anticipatory Grieving related to the impending death of a child

Expected Outcome: The child and family will experience appropriate progression through the five stages of grief as evidenced by:

- Verbalization of an understanding of the five stages of grief
- Verbalization of all emotions in an appropriate manner
- Verbalization of feelings by each family member in a communication style most comfortable for each individual
- Behaviors indicating acceptance of the child's impending death
- Provision of care and support by the family in the manner desired by the child: emotional, physical and psychosocial

Intervention	Rationale
1. Explain the five stages of grief and their necessity for healthy grieving, including resolution to acceptance.	An understanding of the normal grief process may be lacking. An explanation should facilitate grief progression and guide behaviors in each stage.

Intervention	Rationale
2. Identify the stage of grief being experienced and provide each family member with the opportunity to verbalize feelings corresponding to that stage. Provide positive feedback for appropriate progression.	Verbalization of feelings and positive feedback will guide behaviors and facilitate continuing progression.
3. Educate family as to grief stage progression characteristic of children (patient and any siblings). Encourage patience with the extended time frame of grief for the child.	Understanding the ways in which children's coping mechanisms differ from those of adults will facilitate acceptance and understanding by parents.
4. Offer all family members the opportunity to verbalize and act out, as necessary, all emotions in an appropriate manner.	Venting of emotions helps to decrease stress and to facilitate resolution of anger.
5. Exhibit a nonjudgmental attitude toward and acceptance of verbalization and behaviors.	An attitude of acceptance will convey care and support. It will also encourage appropriate, needed expression of all emotions, both negative and positive.
6. Encourage open, honest communication with the patient to the degree requested by the child. Demonstrate appropriate communication techniques.	Appropriate communication with the patient will provide comfort and support. It will also ease closure and resolution of problems for the patient.
7. Offer family members the opportunity to participate in the patient's physical care, as desired by both parties. Demonstrate care in a gentle, supportive fashion.	Many individuals fear the atmosphere of dying and the provision of physical care. Learning by example will lessen fears and enhance provision of care.

Evaluation:
- The child (when cognitively appropriate) and family will verbalize an understanding of the five stages of grief.
- The child and family will verbalize all emotions in an appropriate manner and in a communication style most comfortable for each individual.
- The child and family will exhibit behaviors indicative of acceptance regarding the impending death.
- The family will provide physical, emotional, and psychosocial care and support in the manner and environment desired by the child.

NURSING DIAGNOSIS
- Anxiety related to diagnosis and/or impending death

Expected Outcome: The child and family will experience minimal fear as evidenced by:
- Open verbalization of all feelings and emotions
- Open verbalization of questions concerning diagnosis and prognosis
- Expression of physical, emotional, and spiritual comfort by the child
- Expression of emotional and spiritual comfort by the family

Intervention	Rationale
1. Educate patient and family about the terminal phase of illness, including what to expect physically, emotionally, spiritually, and how such needs will be met. Offer alternatives, such as hospice care.	Misconceptions may lead to increased fear and anxiety. Expression of such feelings by family members may distress an otherwise comfortable child.
2. Assure patient and family that the patient will be safe and comfortable, and that she will not be alone. Provide frequent reassurance as needed.	Fears about the child's comfort and security are the most common; frequent reassurances are often necessary as the disease and/or symptoms worsen.

Intervention	Rationale
3. Provide as much privacy as possible for the child dying in the hospital setting. Allow and encourage parents and siblings to stay with the patient as desired by the family unit. Regulate visitation by those outside the immediate family and friends as necessary.	Families may require extended time for closure. Although well-meaning, the number of visitors, which often increases as death nears, may interfere with needed family time. It may be difficult for the family to regulate visitors due to concerns over hurt feelings, etc. If so, the staff must help by regulating visitors as a means of ensuring the family's privacy.
4. Provide extensive opportunities for the family to care for the child. Teach them the necessary physical skills. Allow the family to decline provision of care when it is physically distressing or painful.	Children are usually most comfortable when cared for by family members. However, in some instances, the child and family may be more comfortable and less anxious if certain care is provided by the staff.

Evaluation:
- The child and family will openly and appropriately verbalize all feelings and emotions.
- The child and family will openly verbalize questions concerning diagnosis and prognosis.
- The child will exhibit physical, emotional, and spiritual comfort.

Nursing Care During the Process of Dying and at the Time of Death

Care needs of the actively dying child are not unlike the needs of the chronically or seriously ill child. Much of the care is directed by the physical, emotional, and spiritual needs of the child and family. The goal of nursing care in this situation is to provide time for the child and family during which there are minimal disruptions. Whether the death is occurring at home, in the hospital, or at an inpatient hospice unit, the child's room should be secluded, comfortable, and quiet. Appropriate surroundings contribute significantly toward creating a meaningful time for the child and family.

Privacy for the Child and Family. Disruptions by staff and even by friends or extended family should be discouraged and minimized to the degree possible. Often, the request will come for private time between the dying child, parents, and siblings. Occasionally, this may cause others, such as grandparents, to become distraught and/or insistent upon their presence with the child. In a hospital or inpatient hospice setting, this can be less difficult to handle. In such an environment, the nurse can more easily treat the matter as a request he or she is appropriately responsible for enforcing. In the home environment, the nurse has no such authority, yet there is still responsibility to the patient and family. Here, the nurse must attempt to communicate the desires of the family to others. There must also be education as to the importance of meeting such desires and needs for privacy.

Regardless of whether privacy requirements are expressed in relation to emotional or spiritual needs, they will exist for physical reasons. The dying child's endurance will be greatly diminished with increased needs for daytime napping and extended nighttime sleep. The child may also experience difficulties with sleep, such as sleep deprivation, frequent wakefulness, or nightmares. Privacy and careful control of visitors (amount and frequency) will help to ensure as much normalcy and quality in sleep as possible. Also helpful is the knowledge that loved ones are present or close by. In the home or inpatient hospice setting, where privacy may not be as great a problem, open doors and/or an intercom system (such as a baby monitor) can help to reassure the child that loved ones are close by and always available.

Changes in Family Routines. Because the periods of sleep required by the child will become increasingly frequent and prolonged, the availability of loved ones becomes much more important. Minimal wakefulness and alertness mean that family time and activities need to be geared around such times (Gyulay, 1989). Regardless of the duration—moments, minutes, or hours—these intervals spent with the child can become treasured memories and should be facilitated as much as possible by the nurse. Special care must be taken to explain to siblings the reasons for rearranging life around the patient's wakeful times. They must also be allowed to have their time with the patient. Most importantly, their feelings should be explored and emotional support provided.

Family Concerns About Oral Intake. Heightened emotional support is often necessary for the entire family with regard to nutrition and oral intake for the dying child. The child's lack of desire for and actual lack of oral intake are a normal part of the dying process. Yet this can be one of the most difficult aspects of dying with which families must cope. Parents, as well as siblings, may worry that the patient will starve to death and that this will add to any other physical discomfort. The available literature, however, contradicts this notion that the absence of oral intake contributes to discomfort in the dying process (Rousseau, 1992). The nurse should educate each family member about this finding, reminding them that there will be a point before death—often days before, or (rarely) weeks before—when intake will cease as a result of loss of the swallow function. There will be a need for enhanced emotional support for all concerned when the lack of oral intake continues for an extended time.

Fluids and Oral Care. A lack of oral intake has some implications for the nurse in the physical care of the child. Any feelings of dry mouth and thirst (usually minimal) resulting from the reduced intake can be eased with small amounts of ice chips or fluids, given when desired and requested by the child. In light of decreased swallow function and the possibility of aspiration, water would appear to be the best choice. However, given the terminal situation, physical and emotional comfort can be enhanced by meeting the requests of the child. Many children continue to drink their favorite fluid, such as milk or root beer, up until the time of death. A lack of strength or coordination may make drinking from a glass or straw difficult. In such cases, fluids can be squirted into the child's mouth easily and tidily with a medicine dropper or syringe. A catheter-tip syringe may be an even better choice, as the child may find it easier to close his mouth around the syringe's wide opening and long tip. However, care must be taken with such a wide opening not to deliver too much fluid and cause choking. Many children also find it easy to drink from the cups used to assist toddlers as they first learn to drink. These usually have easy-to-grip handles, a secure lid, and a small spout that requires little strength for sucking out fluids. Use of such cups may also give the child a small sense of independence and control, which are often lost in the process of dying.

If oral discomfort occurs as a result of the lack of fluids, several interventions may prove useful and appropriate. Provision of good oral care will help to minimize discomfort, swelling, and infection. Sponge swabs can be used to clean the lips and mouth, but lemon and glycerin swabs should be avoided as they are too drying. Dryness can be further minimized through the use of artificial saliva preparations, which can be swished if the child is able and then swallowed or spit out. These preparations may also be applied with the sponge swabs, along with agents to reduce inflammation or pain. Lip balm or petroleum jelly products can be applied for dry, chapped lips. Good oral care will help to minimize odor and unsightliness, which may be distressing to the child and family. Providing such care may also give the family an opportunity for much needed physical contact with the child and a feeling of usefulness. For these reasons, provision of this and other physical care should be encouraged until the time of death, regardless of whether the child is alert enough to notice or to experience a physical benefit.

Responsiveness of the Child and Communication. The state of a child's awareness or wakefulness until the time of death is frequently an overwhelming concern for family members. This aspect of dying will always vary from person to person, in both children and adults. The child may become unresponsive in the days or hours before death, or there may be intermittent responsiveness until the actual moment of death. The nurse should explain this to the family and should remind them that hearing is the last sense to cease before death. For this reason, verbal communication and physical touch should be encouraged until death occurs, and even after, as desired by the family. Occasionally, such actions are difficult owing to personal fears or beliefs. The absence of either verbal communication or physical touch may not necessarily be emotionally harmful to either child or family. There may simply be a different comfort level in relation to the dying process, or a different degree of personal space or expression of emotions, either verbal or physical. The nurse should investigate the cause and offer assistance only when it is indicated that the lack of such interaction is having a negative effect. No matter what the type or level of touch and communication, family members should be reassured that a heightened sense of awareness as to the presence of loved ones exists among those who are dying, regardless of how young they are. This information may impart an added sense of comfort and security.

Physical Indicators of Imminent Death. Security and comfort may also come from knowing that there are usually reliable physical indicators when death is imminent. This phase may last a few hours or a few days. Heart rate increases, with a concomitant decrease in the strength and quality of peripheral pulses. There is also a decrease in blood pressure. Pulses and blood pressure may become nonpalpable, a state that can exist for numerous hours. Cardiac changes generally occur before respiratory changes, but this is not always true. Even if mild respiratory changes occur without significant cardiac changes, it is important to remember how quickly and acutely a cardiac transition can occur. There have been cases in which apparently innocuous respiratory variations were present, with normal heart rate and blood pressure, and death ensued within less than 30 minutes.

Respiratory changes, which usually follow a typical pattern and are both visible and audible, are more readily assessed by family members. There is a decline in the effectiveness of the respiratory effort, which may be evidenced by rapid, shallow respirations. Increased work of breathing, along with apnea, may also be manifested. The respiratory picture may fluctuate between the two states. Respirations may cease after rapid, increasingly shallow breaths. Cessation may occur after a continuing increase in the amount and length of apneic episodes, coupled with a tremendous increase in the work of breathing (referred to as Cheyne-Stokes or agonal respirations). Respirations may become more audible, and may be accompanied by an expiratory sigh. This often resembles moaning and may cause alarm as to the presence of pain. If the child is otherwise without verbal or physical indications of pain, parents and family members should be reassured that the child's pain level is well controlled. The nurse can reinforce this information by educating the family as to the cause of the sounds and noting their correlation with each breath.

All of these variations in the respiratory patterns will result in either hypoxia or hypercapnia. The agitation of hypoxia should be treated with oxygen in order to provide physical comfort for the child and emotional comfort for the family. If the nurse is uncertain as to whether the agitation results from hypoxia or pain, the patient should be treated for pain as well as given oxygen. A rising carbon dioxide level may actually contribute to a peaceful and comfortable death through its sedative and analgesic qualities.

Continuing respiratory and cardiac changes may lead to cool extremities and cyanosis. These most often begin with the lower extremities and progress upward to the face. All of these changes, although potentially distressing, are usually well handled with adequate preparation and education.

Perhaps most distressing is the noisy breathing caused by the rattling of secretions in the upper airway. This occurs when the child has lost the strength and ability to clear airway secretions. It is often referred to as the "death rattle." Even with preparation, this can be extremely difficult for family. Scopolamine is very effective in not only drying the secretions, but also in relaxing the smooth muscles of the tracheobronchial tree. Scopolamine can be given intramuscularly. However, recently, anecdotal success has been achieved with the use of transdermal and sublingual scopolamine. Oral or rectal medications, such as diphenhydramine and glycopyrrolate, have also been shown to be effective. Pharyngeal suctioning can be helpful, but may need to be done frequently and can be a source of discomfort for the child. Until a prescribed medication takes effect, it may be helpful to position the child on her side to facilitate drainage of the secretions. A cloth should be placed appropriately and the family prepared in the event that secretions drain from the mouth. The child is very rarely aware of this respiratory occurrence, so the focus of care should be symptom management to ensure the emotional comfort of the family.

When respirations have ceased, there may be a short delay before the heart stops beating. There may also be a final gasping noise after the respirations and heartbeat have stopped. Reassure the family that this is a normal event, and not painful.

Care of the Family After Death. After death has occurred, the family should have the opportunity to spend as much time with the child as is desired. This can be done before cleaning of the body if the family desires, although cleaning is preferably done first because of the drainage, bleeding, and/or spontaneous elimination of body wastes that often occur at the time of death. Before the body is bathed, the family often appreciates the opportunity to make hand and foot prints and/or cut a lock of hair as a remembrance of the child. The family should be invited to assist in the bathing if they so desire, as provision of this final act of physical care may be a special means of closure.

Frequently, siblings or other children are interested in this procedure. Adults may find this to be distressing, whether or not they wish to assist in the procedure. Encourage the family to allow the child's participation, noting that this may facilitate closure, as well as correct or prevent fears and misconceptions about death or the deceased child. Remember, what children imagine is very often more frightening than reality! Educating the child's siblings and answering their questions should always be a part of postmortem care. Frequently, the emotions and questions a child expresses mirror those of the adults but are not expressed by the adults because of their own fears. When possible, the question of participation in postmortem care, both for the adults and children, should be resolved before the patient's death. This may help to prevent an unexpected and additional stress at the time of death. The nurse should respect whatever decisions are made and offer an explanation as to what the care will involve even if the family chooses not to participate.

Inform the family that the child can go to the funeral home either in a hospital gown or their own clothes, reassuring them that the clothes will be returned after the child is dressed for burial. If the family will not be participating in postmortem care, this is a good time to choose clothing and a personal item, such as a blanket or toy. These will also be returned. Sibling participation in this process is another good closure mechanism. As the family prepares to hold the deceased child, remember to inform the family that physical changes after death may occur very quickly, including cooling of the body temperature, cyanosis or paleness, and stiffening of the body. Attempt to prevent further drainage of any body fluids, particularly if the child will be held by family. Prepare them emotionally and provide towels if preventive measures are not possible or are ineffective.

The nurse should allow privacy for the family, reminding them that she will be close by and will return as needed or desired. Always offer clergy support even if there has been no such involvement previously. If no personal clergy has been identified or one is not available, remind the family of the availability of hospital or hospice personnel. If a funeral home has not been chosen, clergy or social services personnel are usually good sources for assistance.

The Nurse's Response to the Dying Child

Individuals, including health care providers, who have little experience in dealing with the reality and crisis of death may not be equipped to sustain friends, family, or themselves in grief (Gibbons, 1986). This may hold serious implications for the nurse who works in an area where death is frequently seen. Caring for dying children and their families can be stressful and emotionally demanding, regardless of one's previous experience with death or one's ethical, professional, and spiritual belief systems. Even the nurse who works closely and frequently with dying children is not immune to the pressures and responses experienced in such an environment. The demands of chronic and/or terminal illness may require increased emotional and psychosocial strength, as well as clinical expertise. The nurse must pay strict attention to personal emotional health and well-being.

The nurse's response to the dying process and death of a child will correlate to a certain degree with the stages of grief/dying. As the nurse becomes more accustomed to the reality and frequency of death, each stage may not be experienced. Length of treatment and personal factors often cause the nurse to become more involved and/or closer to one child or another, possibly resulting in a more intense response or a delay in appropriate resolution of the grief stages. In providing competent and caring nursing care, it may be difficult to maintain the appropriate boundaries between personal involvement and professional care. A nurse who is more detached and professional may be able to more easily provide care on a continuing basis. However, sincere, consistent, personal involvement and availability is necessary in providing care to the dying child (Gibbons, 1993). Regardless of the depth of involvement, level of professionalism, or the number of deaths encountered, every nurse who cares for the dying child will experience loss and grief. Consequently, he or she will need support through the difficult times. It is important that both staff nurses and management recognize and acknowledge this fact. All must work together to provide mutual support. This can be done through active, organized support programs, along with simple acts of respect, concern, and care among nursing colleagues. Care of the caregiver is also an integral part of caring for the child with a chronic or terminal illness.

KEY CONCEPTS

- Children with chronic conditions are living longer, and there are more children living with conditions that were once considered fatal. Despite improvement in quality of life and longevity, chronic illness is a stressful and situational crisis for families, one that requires ongoing attention and adaptation.
- The most important aspect of a chronic illness is that it affects not only the patient, but also the entire family.
- Families dealing with a chronic illness have many varied concerns and needs, including meeting the physical and emotional needs of the patient, providing care for the rest of the family, and meeting financial burdens. The family must strive to meet the physical, emotional, psychosocial, and spiritual needs of each of its members.
- Some families normalize, reorganize, and become stronger in the face of chronic illness. These families are considered to be resilient.
- The stages of grief, as well as of death and dying, are applicable to pediatric patients, but there are special considerations for both patient and family. The child's concepts of death and dying are based upon his stage of growth and development. They are further affected by age, cognition, and experiences of life—intellectual, social, and psychosocial. This is true for both the patient and the well sibling. Thus, there will be fluctuations when the illness persists for a number of years.
- The dying child, like the dying adult, desires the comfort, safety, and presence of loved ones.
- Parents must move from the reality of *fearing* the death of a child to *acknowledging* the impending death of a child. Pain is the greatest concern of parents caring for a dying child.
- Although the grief of parents is often more intense, the grief of siblings can be more difficult to deal with for both the child and family. This is because of the sibling's lesser cognitive abilities and changing developmental needs and capabilities.
- Grief is similar for all families (adults and children); the grief must be processed and the loss integrated. It must be understood that the person who has died is gone, and the resulting emotions must be experienced. The family must reinvest in life and go forward with their lives.
- Nursing care of the terminally ill or dying child can be extremely stressful and demanding. It requires strict attention to one's own physical, emotional, and spiritual health. Care of the caregiver is imperative if the nurse is to provide physical and psychosocial care for families at such a difficult time.

REFERENCES

Aguilera, D. C., & Messick, J. M. (1990). *Crisis intervention: Theory and methodology*, (6th ed.). St. Louis: Mosby–Year Book.

Anonymous. (1990). Rectal diazepam for acute seizures. *Emergency Medicine, 22*(15), 35.

Anonymous. (1992). Rectal doxepin and carbamazepine. *Nurses Drug Alert, 16*(12), 92.

Armstrong-Dailey, A., & Goltzer, S. (1993). *Hospice care for children.* New York: Oxford University Press.

Atchison, N. E., Szyfelbein, S. K., Osgood, P. F., et al. (1991). MS Contin: Time-released pain relief for burn patients. *Journal of Pain and Symptom Management, 3,* 156.

Babul, N., & Darke, A. (1993). Evaluation and use of opioid analgesics in pediatric cancer pain. *Journal of Palliative Care, 9*(4), 19–25.

Bluebond-Langner, M. (1978). *The private worlds of dying children.* Princeton: Princeton University Press.

Bowden, V. R. (1993). Children's literature: The death experience. *Pediatric Nursing, 19*(1), 17–21.

Brookoff, D., Polomano, R., & Callans, D. (1989). Management of sickle cell pain with controlled-release morphine. *Proceedings of the Eighth Annual Scientific Meeting, American Pain Society,* p. 54.

Clark, J. C., & McGee, R. F. (1992). *Core Curriculum for Oncology Nursing* (2nd ed.). Philadelphia: W. B. Saunders.

Cox, D. (1993). Diazepam use for seizures. *Emergency, 25*(9), 22–27.

Foley, G. V., & Whittam, E. H. (1990). Care of the child dying with cancer: (Part I). *CA, 48*(6), 327–354.

Fraley, A. M. (1990). Chronic sorrow: A parental response. *Journal of Pediatric Nursing, 5*(4), 268–273.

Gallo, A. M., Breitmayer, B. J., Knafl, K. A., & Zoeller, L. H. (1991). Stigma in childhood chronic illness: A well sibling perspective. *Pediatric Nursing, 17*(1), 21–25.

Gallo, A. M., Breitmayer, B. J., Knafl, K. A., & Zoeller, L. H. (1992). Well siblings of children with chronic illness: Parents' reports of their psychological adjustment. *Pediatric Nursing, 18*(1), 23–27.

Geller, B., Cooper, T. B., & Schluchter, M. D. (1987). Child and adolescent nortriptyline single dose pharmacokinetic parameters: Final report. *Journal of Clinical Psychopharmacology,* 7(6), 321–324.

Gibbons, M. B. (1993). Psychosocial aspects of serious illness in childhood and adolescence. In A. Armstrong-Dailey & S. Goltzer (Eds.). *Hospice care for children.* New York: Oxford University Press.

Gibbons, M. B. (1986). When the dying patient is a child: A challenge for the living. In M. J. Hockenberry & D. K. Coody, (Eds.), *Pediatric oncology and hematology: Perspectives on care* (pp. 493–508). St. Louis: Mosby–Year Book.

Goldman, A., & Bowman, A. (1990). The role of oral controlled-release morphine for pain relief in children with cancer. *Palliative Medicine, 4,* 279–285.

Gyulay, J. (1989). Home care for the dying child. *Issues in Comprehensive Nursing, 12,* 33–69.

Heilgenstein, E., & Steif, B. L. (1989). Tricyclics for pain. *Journal of the American Academy of Child and Adolescent Psychiatry, 28*(5), 804–805.

Hobbs, N., Perrin, J. M., & Ireys, H. T. (1985). *Chronically ill children and their families.* San Francisco: Jossey-Bass.

Hymovich, D. P., & Hagopian, G. A. (1992). *Chronic illness in children and adults: A psychosocial approach.* Philadelphia: W. B. Saunders.

Jessop, D. J., & Stein, R. K. (1988). Essential concepts in the care of children with chronic illness. *Pediatrician, 15,* 5–12.

Johnson, B., McGonigel, M., & Kaufmann, R. (1989). *Guidelines and recommended practice for the individualized family service plan.* Washington, DC: Association for the Care of Children's Health.

Keane, E. F. (1993). Another way to administer antiepileptic medications in infants and children. *American Journal of Maternal Child Nursing, 18*(5), 270–274.

Kubler-Ross, E. (1983). *On children and death.* New York: Macmillan.

Kubler-Ross, E. (1969). *On death and dying.* New York: Macmillan.

Lawson, L. V. (1990). Culturally sensitive support for the grieving parents. *Maternal-Child Nursing, 15,* 76–80.

Lazarus, R. (1981). The costs and benefits of denial. In J. J. Spinetta, & P. Deasy-Spinetta, (Eds.), *Living with childhood cancer.* St. Louis: C. V. Mosby.

Lombardi, N. (1993). Palliative care in an inpatient hospital setting. In A. Armstrong-Dailey & S. Goltzer (Eds.), *Hospice care for children.* New York: Oxford University Press.

Mahon, M. M. (1992). Chronic conditions and the family. In P. L. Jackson & J. A. Vessey, (Eds.), *Primary care of the child with a chronic condition* (pp. 12–25). St. Louis: Mosby–Year Book.

McCaffery, M., Martin, L., & Ferrell, B. R. (1992). Analgesic administration via rectum or stoma. *The Journal of Enterostomal Nursing, 19*(4), 114–121.

McCue, K. (1988). Medical play: An expanded perspective. *Children's Health Care, 16*(3), 157–161.

Miser, J. S., & Miser, A. W. (1993). Pain and symptom control. In A. Armstrong-Dailey & S. Goltzer (Eds.), *Hospice care for children.* New York: Oxford University Press.

Patterson, J. M. (1991). Family resilience to the challenge of a child's disability. *Pediatric Annals, 20*(9), 491–499.

Petrillo, M., & Sanger, S. (1980). *Emotional care of hospitalized children.* Philadelphia: J. B. Lippincott.

Phillips, M. (1990). Support groups for parents of chronically ill children. *Pediatric Nursing, 16*(4), 404–406.

Ponzetti, J. J. (1992). Bereaved families: A comparison of parents' and grandparents' reactions to the death of a child. *Omega, 25*(1), 63–71.

Poulain, P. (1989). Slow release morphine tablets for children with cancer pain. In: *Pain in children. Minisymposium: Caring for children with pain.* Maastricht, The Netherlands, June 2, p. 21.

Rando, T. A. (1986). *Loss and anticipatory grief.* Lexington, MA: D. C. Heath and Company.

Richter, R., Sittl, R., Fengler, R., Beck, J., & Sorge, J. (1989). First results of a German multicenter study concerning pain therapy in incurable pediatric patients (Abstr. 13). *Journal of Pain and Symptom Management, 4*(4), S5.

Rigamonti, C., Bruera, E. (1991). Rectal, buccal, and sublingual narcotics for the management of cancer pain. *Journal of Palliative Care, 7*(1), 30–35.

Rogers, A. G. (1990). The successful use of controlled-release morphine. *Journal of Pain and Symptom Management, 5*(5), 331–332.

Rollins, J. A. (1990). Childhood cancer: Siblings draw and tell. *Pediatric Nursing, 16*(1), 21–23.

Rousseau, P. C. (1992). Why give IV fluids to the dying? *Patient Care*, July 15, pp. 71–74.

Sinnema, G. (1990). Resilience among children with special health-care needs and their families. *Pediatric Annals, 20*(9), 483–486.

Smith, I. (1991). Preschool children play out their grief. *Death Studies, 15,* 169–176.

Strauss, A., Fagerhaugh, S., Suczek, B., & Weiner, C. (1985). *Social organization of medical work.* Chicago: University of Chicago Press.

Tartler, A. R. (1993). Family dynamics. In A. Armstrong-Dailey & S. Goltzer (Eds.), *Hospice care for children.* New York: Oxford University Press.

Teresi, M., Wickland, B. M., McMillan, S., Rucknagel, D. L., Kalinyak, K. A., Payne, R., & deAlacron, P. A. (1990). Comparison of controlled-release oral morphine to continuous IV morphine in the control of pain in sickle cell crisis (Abstr. 15). *American Journal of Pediatric Hematology Oncology, 12*(1), 109.

Thompson, R. H., & Standford, G. (1981). *Child life in hospitals: theory and practice.* Springfield: Charles C Thomas.

van Hoogdalem, E. J., de Boer, A. G., & Breimer, D. D. (1991). Pharmacokinetics of rectal drug administration (Part I). *Clinical Pharmacokinetics 21*(1), 11–26.

van Hoogdalem, E. J., de Boer, A. G., and Breimer, D. D. (1991). Pharmacokinetics of rectal drug administration (Part II). *Clinical Pharmacokinetics, 21*(2), 110–128.

Waechter, E. H. (1984). Dying children: Patterns of coping. In H. Wass, & C. A. Corr (Eds.), *Childhood and death* (pp. 51–68). New York: Hemisphere Publishing.

Walker, C. L., Wells, L., Heiney, S., Hymovich, D. P., & Weekes, D. P. (1993). Nursing management of psychosocial care needs. In G. V. Foley, D. Fochtman, & K. H. Mooney (Eds.), *Nursing care of the child with cancer.* Philadelphia: W. B. Saunders.

Wass, H. (1985). Concepts of death: A developmental perspective. *Issues in Comprehensive Pediatric Nursing, 8*(1–6), 3–25.

Wilkinson, T. J., Robinson, B. A., & Begg, E. J. (1992). Pharmacokinetics and efficacy of rectal versus oral sustained-release morphine in cancer patients. *Cancer, Chemotherapy and Pharmacology, 31,* 251–254.

Yee, J. D., & Berde, C. B. (1994). Dextroamphetamine or methylphenidate as adjuvants to opioid analgesia for adolescents with cancer. *Journal of Pain and Symptom Management, 9*(2), 122–125.

BIBLIOGRAPHY

Adams, D. W., & Deveau, E. J. (1984). *Coping with childhood cancer: Where do we go from here?* Virginia: Reston Publishing.

Altshuler, A., & Seidl, A. (1977). Teen meetings: A way to help adolescents cope with hospitalizations. *MCN: The American Journal of Maternal Child Nursing.* November/December, 348–353.

American Academy of Pediatrics Committee on Bioethics. (1994). Guidelines on foregoing life-sustaining medical treatment. *Pediatric Nursing, 20*(5), 517–521.

Austin, J. K. (1990). Assessment of coping mechanisms used by parents and children with chronic illness. *MCN: The American Journal of Maternal Child Nursing, 15,* 98–102.

Bakewell-Sachs, S., & Porth, S. (1995). Discharge planning and home care of the technology-dependent infant, *JOGNN, 24*(1), 77–83.

Birenbaum, L. K. (1989). The relationship between parent-sibling communication and coping of siblings with the death experience. *Journal of Pediatric Oncology Nursing, 6*(3), 86–91.

Bombeck, E. (1989). *I want to grow hair, I want to grow up, I want to go to Boise: Children surviving cancer.* New York: Harper and Row.

Breirmayer, B. J., Gallo, A. M., Knafl, K. A., & Zoeller, L. H. (1992). Social competence of school-aged children with chronic illness. *Journal of Pediatric Nursing,* 7(3), 181–197.

Brown, P. G. (1989). Families who have a child diagnosed with cancer: What the medical caregivers can do to help them and themselves. *Issues in Comprehensive Nursing 12,* 247–260.

Buckingham, R. W. (1989). *Care of the dying child: A practical guide for those who help others.* New York: Continuum Publishing.

Callahan, M., & Kelley, P. (1992). *Final gifts.* New York: Poseidon Press.

Chesler, M. A., & Babarin, O. A. (1987). *Childhood cancer and the family: Meeting the challenge of stress and support.* New York: Brunner/Mazel.

Clubb, R. L. (1991). Chronic sorrow: Adaptation patterns of parent with chronically ill children. *Pediatric Nursing, 17*(5), 461–465.

Craft, M. J. (1989). Siblings of hospitalized children. Assessment and intervention. *Journal of Pediatric Nursing, 8*(5), 289–297.

Deford, F. (1983). *Alex: The life of a child.* New York: Viking Press.

Diamond, J. (1996). Family centered care for children with chronic illness. *Journal of Pediatric Health Care, 8,* 196–198.

Doka, K. J. (1995). *Children mourning: Mourning children.* Washington, DC: Hospice Foundation of America.

Faux, S. A. (1989). Siblings of children with chronic physical and cognitive disabilities. *Journal of Pediatric Nursing, 8*(5), 305–317.

Fleming, J., Challella, M., Eland, J., Hornick, R., Johnson, P., Martinson, I., Nativio, D., Nokes, K., Riddle, I., Steele, N., Sudela, K., Thomas, R., Turner, Q., Wheeler, B., & Young, A. (1994). Impact on the family of children who are technology dependent and cared for in the home. *Pediatric Nursing, 20*(4), 379–388.

Gallo, A. M., Breitmayer, B. J., Knafle, K. A., & Zoeller, L. H. (1989). Mothers' perceptions of sibling adjustment and family life in childhood chronic illness. *Journal of Pediatric Nursing, 8*(5), 318–324.

Hammer, M., Nichols, D. J., & Armstrong, L. (1992). A ritual of remembrance. *MCN: The American Journal of Maternal Child Nursing, 17,* 310–313.

Heiney, S. P., Hasan, L., & Price, K. (1993). Developing and implementing a bereavement program for a children's hospital. *Journal of Pediatric Nursing, 8*(6), 385–391.

Heiney, S. P., Wells, L. M., Ettiinger, R. S., Ettiginger, S., & Cannon, B. (1989). Effects of group therapy on parents of children with cancer. *Journal of Pediatric Oncology Nursing, 6*(3), 63–69.

Hockenberry-Eaton, M. J., & Cotanch, P. H. (1989). Evaluation of a child's perceived self-competence during treatment for cancer. *Journal of Pediatric Oncology Nursing, 6*(3), 55–62.

Johnson, L. C., Rincon, B., Gober, C., & Rexin, D. (1993). The development of a comprehensive bereavement program to assist families experiencing pediatric loss. *Journal of Pediatrics, 8*(3), 142–146.

Johnston, C. E., & Marder, L. R., (1994). Parenting the child with a chronic condition: An emotional experience. *Pediatric Nursing, 20*(6), 611–614.

Komp, D. M. (1992). *A window to heaven: When children see life in death.* Grand Rapids: Zondervan Publishing.

Komp, D. M. (1993). *A child shall lead them: Lessons of hope from children with cancer.* Grand Rapids: Zondervan Publishing.

Komp, D. M. (1994). *Hope springs from mended places: Images of grace in the shadows of life.* Grand Rapids: Zondervan Publishing.

Kovar, S. J. (1993a). *My wonderful journey to heaven.* Grand Rapids: Zondervan Publishing.

Kovar, S. J. (1993b). *My journey of hope.* Grand Rapids: Zondervan Publishing.

Kruger, S. (1992). Parents in crisis: Helping them cope with a seriously ill child. *Journal of Pediatric Nursing,* 7(2), 133–140.

Kubler-Ross, E. (1983). *Children and death.* New York: Macmillan.

Kushner, H. S. (1981). *When bad things happen to good people.* New York: Avon Books.

Kruckenberg, C. (1989). *What was good about today?* New York: Madron Press.

Leder, S. N. (1992). Life events, social support, and children's coping after the death of a parent and sibling death. *Journal of Pediatric Nursing,* 7(2), 110–119.

Linn, E. (1990). *150 facts about grieving children.* Nevada: The Publisher's Mark.

Mahon, M. M. (1994). Death of a sibling: Primary care interventions. *Pediatric Nursing, 20*(3), 293–295, 328.

Menten, T. (1991). *Gentle closings: How to say good-bye to someone you love.* Philadelphia: Running Press.

Menten, T. (1994). *After good-bye: How to begin again after the death of someone you love.* Philadelphia: Running Press.

Menten, T. (1995). *Where is heaven? Children's wisdom on facing death.* Philadelphia: Running Press.

Miles, A. (1990). Caring for a family when a child dies. *Pediatric Nursing, 16*(4), 346–347.

Morse, M., & Perry, P. (1990). *Closer to the light.* New York: Ivy Books.

Newacheck, P. W., & Stoddard, J. J., (1994). Prevalence and impact of multiple childhood chronic illnesses. *Journal of Pediatrics, 124,* 40–48.

Papadatou, D., & Papadatou, C. (1991). *Children and death.* New York: Hemisphere Publishing.

Patterson, J. M., Jernell, J., Leonard, B. J., & Titus, J. C., (1994). Caring for medically fragile children at home: The parent-professional relationship. *Journal of Pediatric Nursing, 9*(2), 98–106.

Phillips, M., & Brostoff, M. (1989). Working collaboratively with parents of disabled children. *Pediatric Nursing, 15*(2), 180–185.

Rabin, N. B. (1994). School reentry and the child with a chronic illness: The role of the pediatric nurse practitioner. *Journal of Pediatric Health Care, 8,* 227–232.

Rawlins, P. S., & Horner, M. M. (1988). Does membership in a support group alter needs of chronically ill children? *Pediatric Nursing, 14*(1), 70–72.

Ray, L. D., & Ritchie, J. (1993). Caring for chronically ill children at home: Factors that influence parent's coping. *Journal of Pediatric Nursing, 8*(4), 217–225.

Schepp, K. S. (1992). Correlates of mothers who prefer control over their hospitalized children's care. *Journal of Pediatric Nursing, 7*(2), 83–89.

Simon, K. (1989). Perceived stress of non-hospitalized children during the hospitalization of a sibling. *Journal of Pediatric Nursing, 8*(5), 298–304.

Smigielski, P. A., & Parton, E. (1992). A home health record for children with chronic health conditions. *Journal of Pediatric Health Care, 6,* 121–126.

Sokol, M. (1995). Creating a community of caring for families with special needs. *JOGN, 24*(1), 64–69.

Teague, B. R., Felming, J. W., Castle, A., Kiernan, B. S., Lobo, M. L., Riggs, S., & Wolfe, J. G. (1993). "High tech" home care for children with chronic health conditions: A pilot study. *Journal of Pediatric Nursing, 8*(4), 226–232.

Turner-Henson, A., Holaday, B., Corser, N., Ogletree, G., & Swan, J. H., (1994). The experiences of discrimination: Challenges for chronically ill children. *Pediatric Nursing, 20*(6), 271–577.

Walker, C. L. (1989). Sibling bereavement and grief responses. *Journal of Pediatric Nursing, 8*(5), 325–334.

Ward, M. (1992). The family and chronic sorrow. Role theory approach. *Journal of Pediatric Nursing, 17*(3), 205–210.

Wells, P., DeBoard-Burns, M. B., Cook, R. C., & Mitchell, J. (1994). Growing up in the hospital: Part I, let's focus on the child. *Journal of Pediatric Nursing, 9*(2), 66–72.

Woods, N. F., Yates, B. C., & Primomo, J. (1989). Supporting families during chronic illness. *Image: Journal of Nursing Scholarship, 21*(1), 46–50.

Yoder, L. (1994). Comfort and consolation: A nursing perspective on parental bereavement. *Pediatric Nursing, 20*(5), 473–477.

Yoos, L. (1987). Chronic childhood illnesses: Developmental issues. *Pediatric Nursing, 13*(1), 25–28.

18

Application of Nursing Principles to Pediatrics

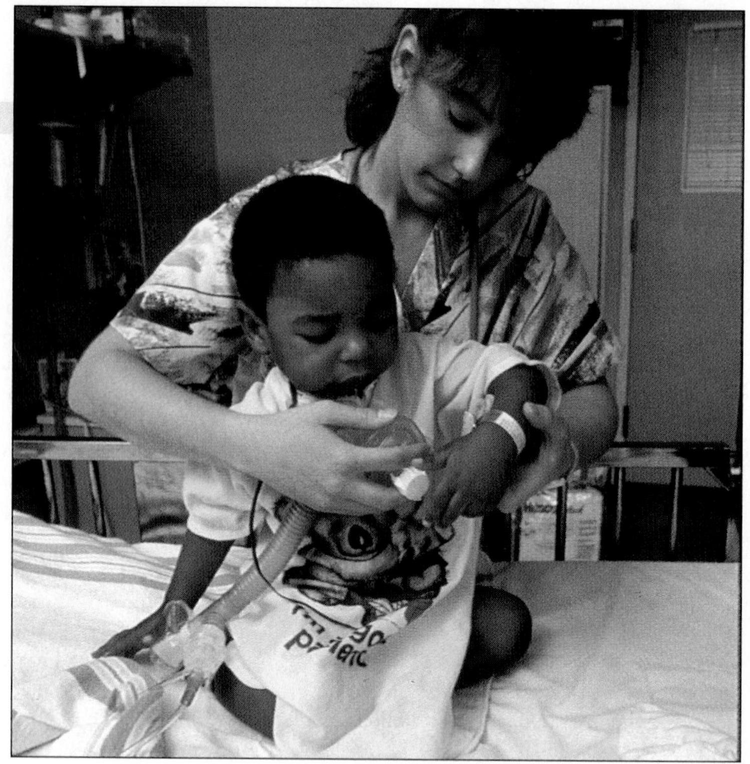

Courtesy of Cook Children's Medical Center, Fort Worth, Texas

CHAPTER OVERVIEW

LEARNING OBJECTIVES

After studying this chapter, you should be able to:

- Describe preparation of children and families for selected procedures.
- Describe anatomic and physiologic differences in children and adults for selected procedures.
- Describe unique psychosocial considerations for children undergoing selected procedures.
- Describe techniques useful in eliciting cooperation from the child undergoing selected procedures.
- Describe nursing actions and rationales for performing selected procedures.
- Explain selected procedures step-by-step.

KEY TERMS

antipyretic: an agent that reduces or relieves fever

apical pulse rate: heart rate determined by placing the stethoscope over the point of maximum intensity (PMI) and counting for 1 minute

auscultate: to listen to body sounds (e.g., heart sounds, breath sounds)

diarrhea: an increase in the volume of stool output and/or a change in the consistency of stool compared to the individual's normal stool pattern

enteral: by way of the alimentary canal (e.g., enteral feeding)

epiglottitis: inflammation of the epiglottis

hypoxia: reduced or inadequate cellular oxygenation

informed consent: a requirement, both legal and ethical, that the patient and the parent/guardian completely understand proposed procedures and/or treatments, including their benefits and risks

Standard Precautions: infection control guidelines developed by the National Center for Infectious Disease (NCID) and the Hospital Control Practices Advisory Committee (HICPAC) to prevent the spread of infectious organisms from blood, body fluids, secretions and excretions, mucous membranes, and nonintact skin (see Appendix G)

Children require preparation before and accurate information about *any* procedure that is performed. This is essential to promote a sense of security, decrease fear, promote cooperation, and improve coping skills. Parents also need preparation, as their anxiety may be transferred to the child (Thompson, 1994).

The responsibility of the nurse caring for a child undergoing a procedure is twofold: to help the child and parents through the procedure effectively and to ensure that the procedure is done as efficiently as possible (Brennan, 1994). The nurse may implement strategies to help the child and parents through all phases of a procedure, including the anticipation and preparation for the procedure, the actual procedure, and the period following the procedure. Teaching prior to performing procedures also helps to increase the knowledge base of the child and family.

GENERAL GUIDELINES FOR PREPARING CHILDREN FOR PROCEDURES

A thorough individualized assessment is essential when preparing children and families for procedures, especially those that are painful, threatening, and/or invasive. This process should include an assessment of the age and developmental level of the child, personality, existing level of knowledge, present level of understanding, past experience, coping skills, and family situation (Brennan, 1994). The nurse can then match explanations and teaching to the specific needs of that child and family.

Ideally, the nurse should review the procedure prior to giving explanations and performing the procedure. This is especially important if the procedure is one that is seldom performed, new, or unfamiliar. Equipment should be gathered and checked prior to attempting any procedure. This also provides an opportunity for the nurse to request sedation, gather extra supplies, and obtain assistance, as necessary.

Explanations of procedures should be simple and concise. They may include a demonstration of equipment, as well as a description of anything the child will feel, hear, see, and smell (Broome, 1990). Time should be allowed for questions and for the child to become familiar with the equipment, if possible. Role playing may be used to allow the child to examine and handle equipment that will be a part of the procedure. A developmentally appropriate approach must always be used.

The child's privacy should be assured before beginning any procedure. This may be done by closing the door to the room and drawing a curtain around the bed or, optimally, taking the child to a treatment room. Visitors should be asked to leave and parents may also opt to leave at this point, although parental participation is always supported and encouraged.

> If available, a treatment room is preferred for procedures. This is a private area away from the "safe haven" of a child's hospital room where invasive procedures may be performed with the appropriate equipment readily accessible (Fig. 18–1).

Tell the child what is expected of him. For example, if he must hold an extremity still for the placement of an IV catheter, he must know that *before* the procedure is begun. He should be asked if he will be able to do this, if not, assistance can be obtained to help him remember to do so. *Never* threaten a child or tell him you will "hold him down" if he does not cooperate. The nurse must have realistic expectations, based on the child's developmental level and past experience, of the child's capacity for cooperation.

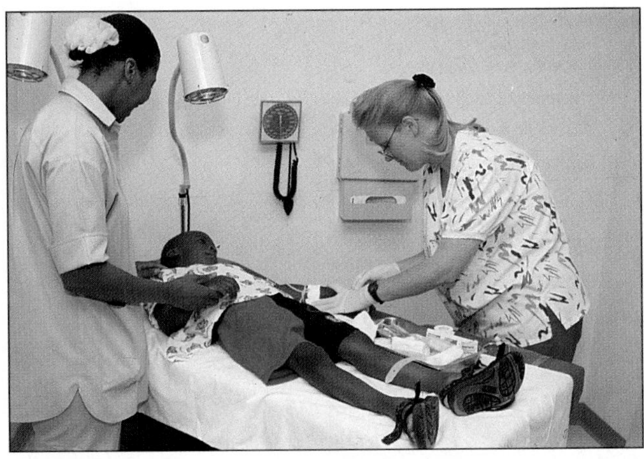

Figure 18–1
A child should feel that his or her hospital room is a safe haven, so a treatment room is used for invasive or painful procedures. The parent is present, not to restrain the child, but to provide emotional support.

Parents should be involved as much as they desire and is possible during procedures. In some cases, for example, a child may be much more cooperative in taking medications if her mother administers them. Often, by explaining what the parents will be seeing and what they can be doing, the nurse helps them feel comfortable in staying with and supporting their child. The nurse should recognize, however, that parents may be very uncomfortable in remaining with their child during a painful or invasive procedure. They should be "given permission" to step out of the room, if they so desire, and should be assured that they will be called if they are needed or as soon as the procedure is completed.

The accompanying box lists tips for interacting with a child before, during, and after a procedure.

Consent for Procedures. Some procedures require **informed consent.** This consent meets both the legal and ethical requirement to inform the child, if appropriate, and the parents of the benefits and risks of the proposed procedure or treatment and must be obtained from the parent or legal guardian *prior* to performing the procedure. Informed consent must be obtained for any surgical or diagnostic invasive procedures, particularly those that involve risk to the child. Examples are lumbar punctures, chest tube insertion, and bone marrow aspirations. Other procedures, such as IV insertions, specimen collection, and medication and oxygen administration, are covered under the general consent to treat that is signed upon admission. It is now also customary to obtain *assent* from children 7 years of age and older. This means that the child has been fully informed about the procedure and concurs with those individuals giving the informed consent. Laws on informed consent vary from state to state, so nurses should become familiar with the laws and policies of their institution. (See Chapter 1 for specific information related to legal issues.)

Tips for Preparing and Supporting Children Undergoing Procedures

BEFORE THE PROCEDURE

1. Offer the child ways of coping with pain or discomfort. For example, some children can use coping strategies, such as guided imagery. Others might try using a radio, increasing the volume as the discomfort level increases. Give the child permission to cry or yell if he needs to.
2. Use developmentally appropriate words when discussing the procedure and expectations.
3. Give the child as much choice over what will happen as is possible. For example, when possible, the child might be allowed to choose an injection site or a site for IV catheter placement.

DURING THE PROCEDURE

1. Talk to the child during the procedure, if she desires. If the child is using a coping strategy, such as guided imagery, however, talking will be a distraction and will decrease the child's ability to cope with what is happening to her.
2. Keep the child informed of the procedure's progress.
3. Tell the child when the procedure is nearly completed and the "worst is over."

AFTER THE PROCEDURE

1. *Praise* the child for *attempts* at cooperation, even if the child did not do anything you asked. Trying counts! Specifically, praise the child for accomplishing an expected task.
2. Provide an opportunity for the child to vent his feelings about the procedure. Remember, it's OK for feelings of anger to be expressed when appropriate. Tell the child that you understand that he does not want to talk with you right now and that you will return later.
3. If parents were not present during the procedure, reunite the child with the parents and allow them to provide comfort and support.
4. Reward the child using age-appropriate methods, such as stickers.
5. Document the preparation process and procedure performance, who performed the procedure, the child's tolerance of the procedure, and outcomes.

Consents should be obtained by the person performing the procedure. It is the nurse's responsibility to check that the consent is signed and witnessed and to respond to questions relating to the procedure.

Occasionally, an emergency or life-threatening situation arises during which the parent or legal guardian may not be able to be contacted for consent. In this case, administrative consent may be obtained to allow physicians to perform the indicated procedures. (Refer to Chapter 1 for legal issues related to informed and emergency consent.)

TRANSPORTING INFANTS AND CHILDREN

At times, it may be necessary for a child or infant to be transported to other areas within the hospital unit, or even outside the unit. This may be done in response to worsening of or improvement in the child's condition, to allow increased parental involvement in the child's care (e.g., rooming-in privileges), for specialized care (e.g., rehabilitation), or for diagnostic testing. An infant or child may also be transported to different areas on the same unit (treatment room, playroom).

The method of transportation should take into consideration the age and development of the child, the physical condition, the destination, and safety factors. Specialized equipment may need to accompany the child. Any special accommodations need to be arranged prior to the planned transfer.

Infants who are being transported within the unit can be held in several positions (Fig. 18–2). Infants may be cradled in the arms by holding them in a horizontal position, supporting the back and grasping the thigh. When using the football hold, the head of the infant is carried on the nurse's arm with the nurse's hand supporting the head and the body of the infant held between the nurse's body and elbow. In a third position, the infant is held upright against the chest of the nurse. The buttocks of the infant rest on the nurse's forearm and the infant's head and shoulders are supported by the nurse's other arm to prevent the infant from falling backward. Even in infants with well-developed head control, this extra support is necessary to prevent falling in the event the infant makes a sudden move.

Infants and toddlers can also be transported to other areas while in their bassinet or crib. The rails should always be up, and with older infants and toddlers, the protective top should be in place. Strollers and wagons may also be used for transfer of older infants and toddlers to other areas on the unit (Fig. 18–2). Safety belts should be utilized, the

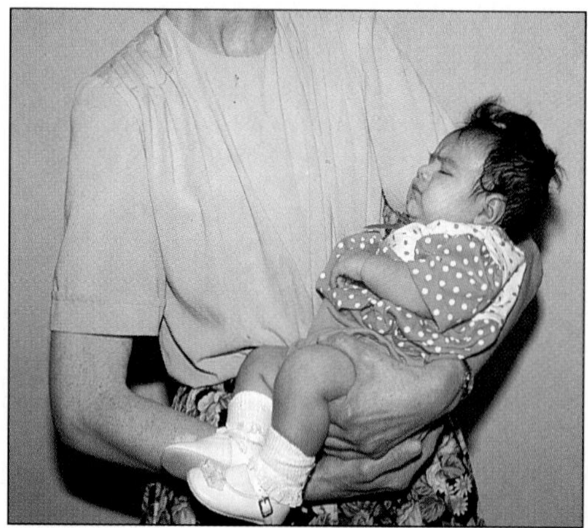

◀ The cradle carry is useful for infants up to about 2 to 3 months of age. The nurse's left hand firmly grasps the infant's thigh in case she suddenly moves.

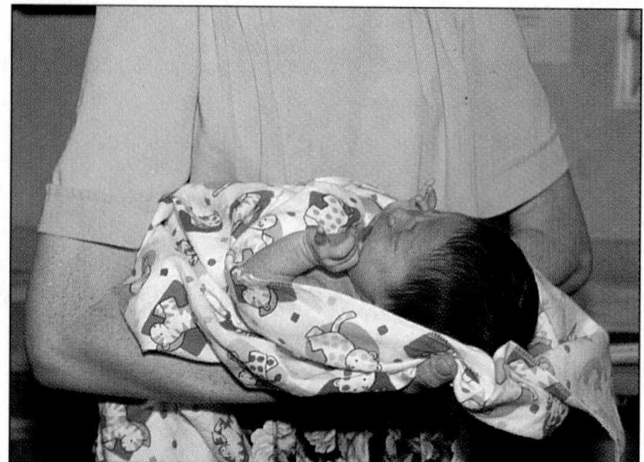

The football hold is appropriate for infants 2 months of age or younger because the method provides head support and protection, yet leaves the opposite arm free.

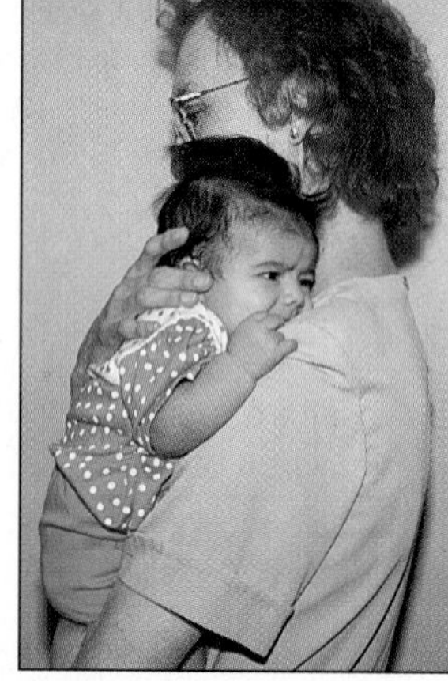

The over-the-shoulder carry can be used until the infant is 6 to 7 months old. The nurse supports the head of this 2-month-old infant because the child does not have reliable head and neck control yet. ▶

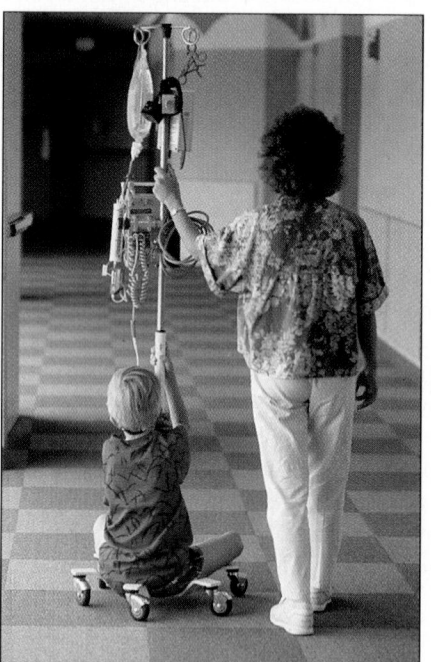

This older child enjoys riding his IV pole.

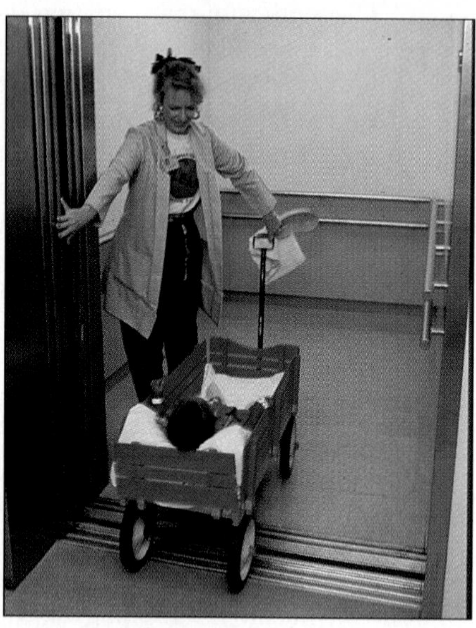

◀ Small children often enjoy being transported in a wagon.

Figure 18–2

Methods of transporting infants and children. The infant should be carried securely, planning for any sudden movement. Transport can be fun for young children, especially when it is on wheels. The child's safety must be a primary consideration, of course. (Infant transport photos courtesy of Dallas County Hospital District Community-Oriented Primary Care Clinic, Dallas, Texas. Wagon photo courtesy of Cook Children's Medical Center, Fort Worth, Texas. IV transport photo courtesy of Children's Medical Center, Dallas, Texas)

sides of the wagon should be raised, and the infant or toddler should never be left unattended. In all methods of transfer, equipment can be pushed along with the transporting vehicle, or, in some cases, stored beneath the transport vehicle (e.g., bassinets with shelves). Equipment should not be placed in the transporting unit with infants.

Older children can be transported in the same manner as adults (i.e., in wheelchairs or on stretchers). Alternatively, preschoolers may enjoy a ride in a wagon or other, less conventional means of transport (Fig. 18–2). As with younger children, safety belts should be in place, the sides of the transport unit should be up, and the child should not be left unattended. Any necessary equipment should accompany the child.

BATHING INFANTS AND CHILDREN

Safety principles must be strictly observed when assisting in or bathing any child. This is necessary to prevent falls, burns, or aspiration of water. The nurse must always take care to note any other conditions, such as paralysis, surgical incisions, loss of sensation, or alterations in skin integrity, that may require special consideration. Newborn infants may be immersed in water after the umbilical stump has healed (see Chapter 3). Water should be warm, but not hot. A bath thermometer may be used to check the temperature of the water, which should not exceed 100°F. If a thermometer is not available, a temperature that is comfortable when tested on the inside of the wrist or elbow is appropriate.

Prior to bathing any child, the nurse should assess the family's preferences and home practices. These include the time of day usually set aside for the bath, bathing rituals, special equipment, any product allergies, and the type of bath preferred. The nurse can also use this time to assess the amount of assistance needed and to address any learning needs related to hygiene. Because this is one of the few areas over which parents may be allowed to retain control, it is important to allow them to make as many decisions as possible. This also allows parents to maintain a part of their home routine with their child.

A young infant who cannot sit unaided may be bathed either by sponge bath or in a tub. It is important that the infant's body be supported by the nurse at all times during the bath (Fig. 18–3). Older infants and toddlers may be bathed in either a bedside tub or regular bathtub.

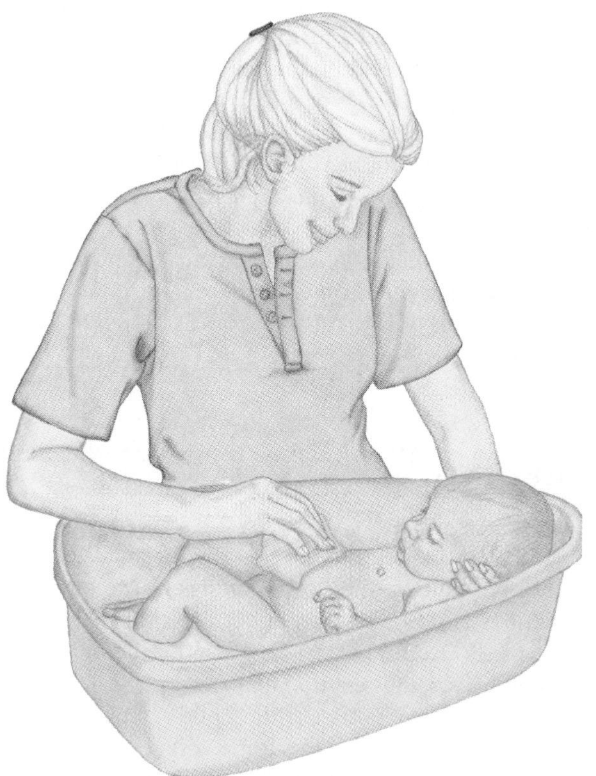

Using hand to support infant's neck and head

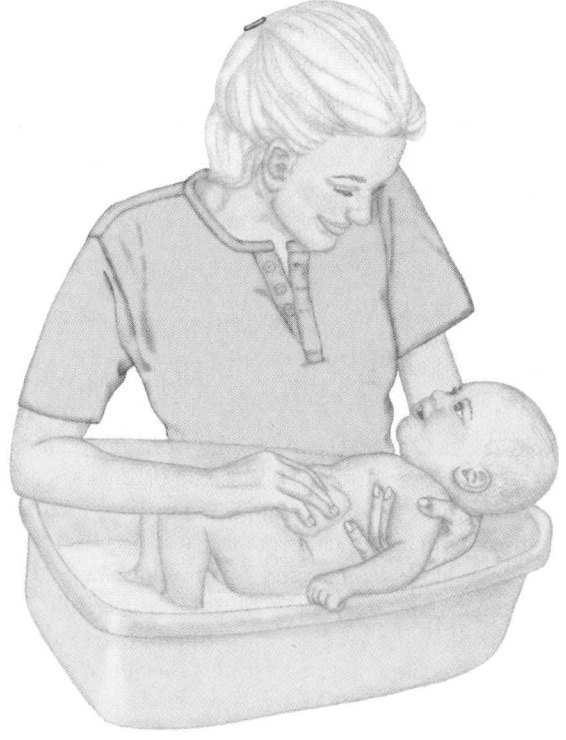

Using arm to support infant's neck and head

Figure 18–3

When giving an infant a tub bath, the nurse supports the infant's body at all times.

Never leave an infant or small child unattended in the bath. Older children may choose a shower, if facilities are available. The nurse should use judgment in deciding how much supervision an older child requires in bathing. It is important to provide for privacy for any child who has reached school age.

Special Considerations. Bed baths are frequently used for hospitalized children. The technique for bathing a child differs little from that used in bathing an adult. The nurse should perform the same assessment as with any patient and should provide assistance, as necessary. The room temperature should be adjusted to a comfortable setting and the curtain should be drawn around the bed. As with any bed bath, the nurse should begin with the face and proceed in a head-to-toe progression. Fresh water should be obtained when it is time to rinse the child. Care needs to be taken to dry each body section as it is rinsed in order to prevent chilling. The child should also be draped adequately for privacy and warmth. The bath may be followed with application of lotion or deodorant, etc., if desired. Avoid the use of talcum powder because of the risk of chemical pneumonia if it is inhaled into the lungs (Schmitt, 1992).

Some bathing restrictions may apply to patients with surgical incisions, skin traction, IV catheters, casts, urinary catheters, artificial airways, and feeding tubes. Some children are also restricted in position and mobility. For example, children who have undergone orthopedic or neurosurgical procedures must frequently remain in a supine position. Other children may be intolerant to position changes because of underlying physiological conditions or injury. It is imperative to assess for these special needs prior to beginning the bath.

Documentation. Documentation includes the type of bath, child/family participation, procedure tolerance, and any abnormal findings noted, such as bruising, rashes, or excoriation. Any lotions or other skin preparations used should also be documented.

Parent Teaching. General principles of hygiene and safety may need to be reinforced with some parents. (See Chapter 3 for instructions for care of the newborn infant.) Special bathing needs, such as infant bathtubs, safety bars, or tub grips, should be included as part of discharge teaching and preparation. After about 1 year of age, a child may be safely bathed in a regular tub. Appropriate supervision should be maintained at all times, however, to prevent injury or accidental drowning.

ORAL HYGIENE

Babies' gums need to be wiped with a wet cloth after each feeding to remove excess food and bacteria. After teeth erupt, a soft, damp cloth or piece of gauze, or a soft child's toothbrush, may be used. This should be done following each feeding and before bed. Young children need supervision when performing oral care at least until they are 6 years of age or older (Schmitt, 1992). Teeth should be brushed at least twice a day with a soft child's toothbrush and a *small* (pea-sized) amount of toothpaste. Older children may not need direct supervision, but may require reinforcement in order to perform oral care correctly. Children may ingest excessive amounts of fluoride if they are allowed to use large amounts of toothpaste or if they eat the toothpaste. Using the recommended amount of toothpaste and encouraging the child not to swallow the toothpaste will prevent fluorosis (Schmitt, 1992).

Immunosuppressed children, in particular, require excellent oral hygiene. Soft toothbrushes, sponge-covered toothettes, or moistened gauze sponges may be used for dental care in the child who is at risk for gingival bleeding.

Flossing the teeth is a useful mechanism for cleaning teeth. This should begin when all the child's primary teeth are in or when the child's molars begin to touch (Schmitt, 1992).

Parent Teaching. Discharge teaching in the area of oral hygiene is very important but is often forgotten. Many parents do not realize that infants' gums and teeth can and should be cleaned. Children should have their first visit to a dentist by the time the first teeth erupt and no later than $2\frac{1}{2}$ years of age. Thereafter, they should be seen on a regular basis for checkups.

Frequent bottle feeding increases the risk of dental caries. Parents should be discouraged from putting a child to bed with a bottle of formula, juice, or sweetened drinks (Schmitt, 1992).

Good nutrition influences dental health and vice versa. Dental teaching often provides means for educating the child and family more about proper nutrition and health maintenance.

FEEDING

Mealtimes may be difficult for the hospitalized child. Changes in routine, diet, surroundings, as well as dietary restrictions and illness, may affect the child's ability and desire to eat. Refusal to eat may also be the only control the child has over his environment.

It is important to assess the child's preferences and dislikes on admission. Mealtime rituals and routines should also be noted. Serving favorite and preferred foods can increase consumption. Nutritious snacks should also be offered as a way to ensure appropriate caloric intake.

The type and form of food chosen should be appropriate to the child's age and developmental status. (Refer to Chapter 12 for a discussion of food types appropriate for each age group.) The nurse must also consider any special needs of the child when choosing food types and forms. For example, the child with an impaired gag reflex cannot tolerate the same foods as other children. Likewise, the child with nausea should not be offered favorite foods, as these may then be associated with the nausea when she is feeling better.

Feeding a hospitalized infant seldom differs from feeding an infant at home. As long as the infant is healthy and growing, formula and any solids that have been introduced usually remain the same. Feeding schedules and routines should mimic home schedules and routines when possible. The choice of bottle or nipple should also remain the same, when possible. Parents should be encouraged to participate as fully as possible in this aspect of care. This reinforces the special bond that develops between the child and his parents. Infants should be held during feedings unless contraindicated by their medical condition. Bottles *should never be propped up* because of the risk of aspiration. Frequent burping during and after feedings may reduce the incidence of spitting up. Following the feeding, the infant can be positioned on the right side to facilitate the flow of the feeding toward the lower end of the stomach and to allow any swallowed air to rise to the esophagus.

Toddlers and preschoolers often use food as a source of control. They often exhibit "food jags," during which they will only eat one or two items for a period of several days. Finger foods are usually most appropriate for this age group, but pieces should be small and appropriate in size and texture so as to decrease the risk of aspiration. Certain foods, such as hot dogs, popcorn, peanuts, grapes, and the like, should be avoided. Seasoning should be mild, and food preferences should always be assessed prior to ordering a meal in order to ensure adequate intake. Young children should never be allowed to eat unsupervised. They should be secured at a table, in a high chair, or in bed using a bedside table during meals (see Chapter 13, Fig. 13–3). "Roaming" should be discouraged. Allow the child to feed herself, if possible, and restrict the feeding time to 15 to 20 minutes. Discontinue the meal if the child begins to play with the food. Parents may be encouraged to bring the child's own utensils, bottles, or cups to the hospital to simulate the usual mealtime routines as closely as possible.

Older children and adolescents seldom have difficulty expressing their dietary preferences. Difficulty may arise, however, when children this age are placed on a restricted or special diet. For example, the diabetic child often has difficulty maintaining dietary restrictions in the face of peer pressure. Support and clear limit setting are often needed to ensure compliance.

Intake and Output. For some children, it may be necessary to keep accurate intake and output (I & O) measurements. All intake, both oral and parenteral, should be measured and recorded. All output, including that from urine; stool; drainage from tubes, stomas, or fistulas; and emesis, should be measured and recorded.

Parental education is very important, particularly if the hospital admission is related to eating disorders or accidents, such as food aspiration. Parents should receive careful instruction on any food restrictions or special diets. For example, a child with phenylketonuria (PKU) or diabetes is at high risk for injury if the diet is not followed closely.

VITAL SIGNS

The procedure for taking vital signs in an infant or child is essentially the same as that in adults. Vital signs should be assessed when the infant or child is quiet. If this is not possible, specific activity, such as crying, should be documented.

Measuring Temperature

Temperature measurement is a simple, objective, and reliable indicator of illness and is an integral part of pediatric assessment. There are a variety of methods by which a child's temperature may be obtained. These include oral, rectal, axillary, and tympanic temperatures using glass, electronic, digital, and tympanic membrane thermometers. Whatever method is chosen, the child's temperature should be measured at the same site and with the same temperature-measuring device in order to maintain consistency and to allow for reliable comparison and tracking of temperatures over time (Davis, 1993).

Axillary temperature measurements should be taken in infants and in children younger than 4 to 6 years of age, as well as in any child who is uncooperative, immunosuppressed, or neurologically impaired, or who has had oral surgery. The thermometer should be placed in the axilla and the child's arm pressed close to his body for a minimum of 5 minutes (Fig. 18–4). Axillary temperatures are approximately 1° lower than the body's core temperature.

Oral temperatures may be taken in most children 6 years of age or older, including adolescents. The thermometer should be placed under the tongue in the right or left sublingual space. The mouth should remain closed during the time the thermometer is in place, usually a minimum of 3 minutes. If a glass thermometer is used, the patient must be instructed not to bite on the thermometer. Liquids should be avoided for 30 minutes prior to oral temperature assessment. Oral temperatures may be inaccurate because of oral intake, oxygen administration, nebulized treatments, and other activities, such as crying (Pontious et al., 1994).

Because of the risk of rectal perforation, particularly in young infants, and the intrusive and upsetting nature of the procedure, *rectal temperatures* are taken only when there is no other feasible route. The child is positioned

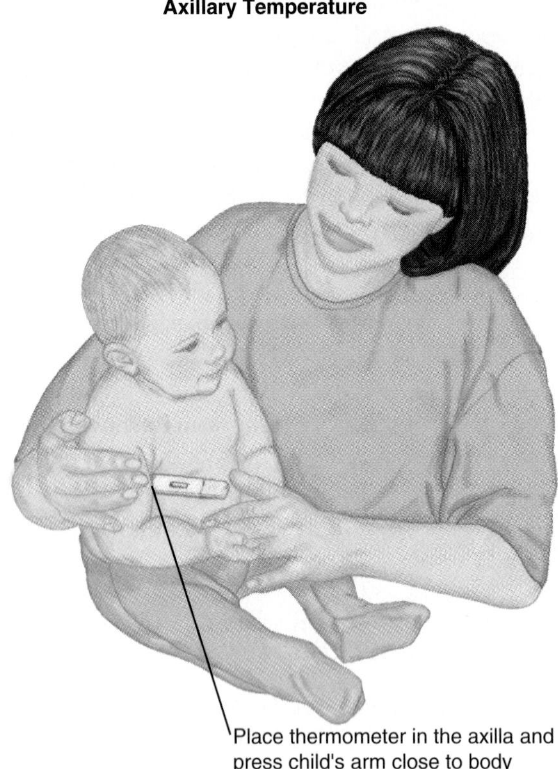
Axillary Temperature
Place thermometer in the axilla and press child's arm close to body

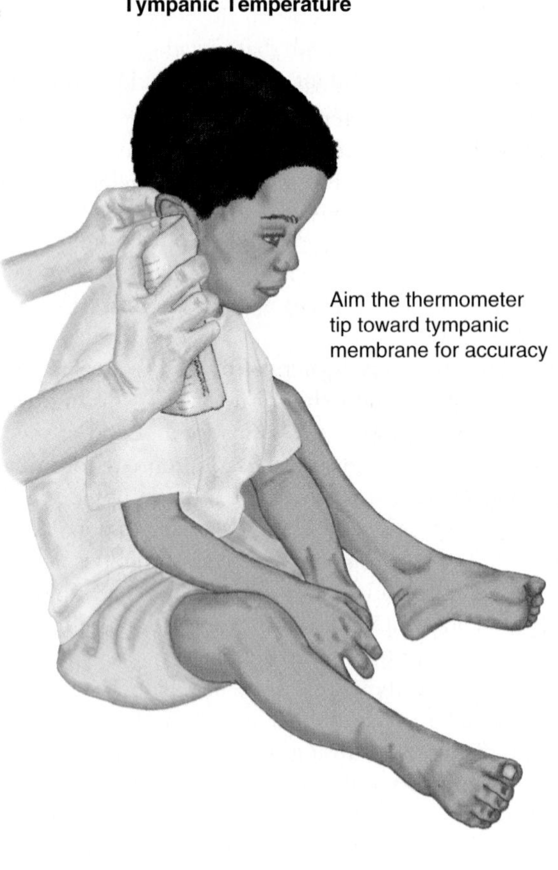
Tympanic Temperature
Aim the thermometer tip toward tympanic membrane for accuracy

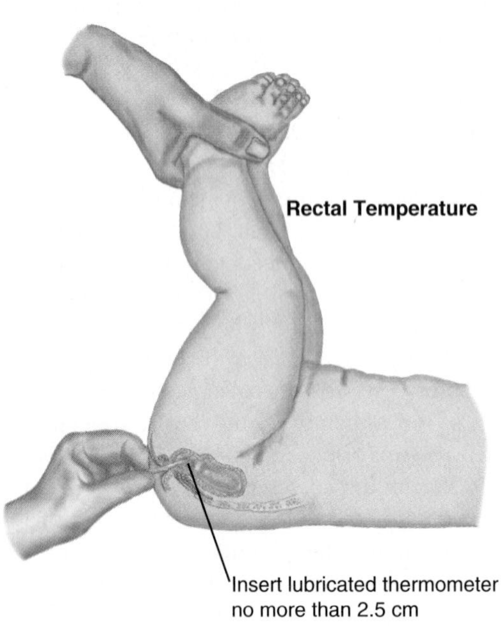
Rectal Temperature
Insert lubricated thermometer no more than 2.5 cm

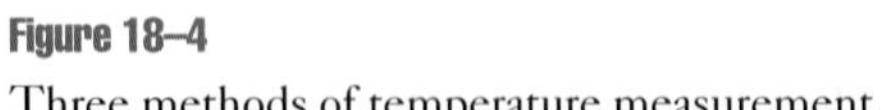

Figure 18–4

Three methods of temperature measurement.

supine, prone, or side-lying, the lubricated thermometer is inserted *no more than a maximum of 1.0 to 2.5 cm, depending on the size and age of the child* (Fig. 18–4), for 3 to 5 minutes. Glass thermometers are never recommended for rectal temperatures.

CONTRAINDICATIONS

Rectal temperatures are always contraindicated in the neonate, immunosuppressed child, or any child who has had rectal surgery, diarrhea, or a bleeding disorder.

Although there is no universal agreement on the length of time thermometers should be left in place, 5 minutes is usually recommended for the axillary method, 3 minutes for oral temperatures, and 3 to 5 minutes for rectal temperatures. These times may vary according to the type of thermometer used. In addition, the instrument type and site of measurement influence the accuracy and reliability of temperature readings (Pontious et al., 1994).

Digital thermometers are commercially available which run on a button battery and measure the temperature quickly, usually in less than 30 seconds. These may be used for oral, axillary, or rectal temperatures. Disposable covers should be used for obtaining temperatures to prevent cross-contamination.

Tympanic temperature measurement is now frequently used in pediatric practice (Fig. 18–4) and is also available for home use. These measurements are more quickly obtained, usually within a few seconds. Tympanic temperatures strongly correlate with oral and rectal temperatures. The use of the "ear tug," putting posterior traction on the pinna to completely expose the tympanic membrane, has been shown to enhance the accuracy of tympanic temperature measurements (Wells et al., 1995).

Normal temperatures by age are shown inside the front cover of the book.

PROCEDURE: *Measuring Temperature*

Determine the most appropriate temperature measuring technique for the child's age and condition and perform the procedure.

Preparing the Child and Family. Inform the child and family of the purpose of the procedure and assure them that minimal (if any) discomfort is involved.

Equipment

- Thermometer: mercury, electronic, or tympanic
- Nonsterile gloves
- Water-soluble lubricant
- Hospital-approved or manufacturer-approved cleaning solution for equipment

STEP-BY-STEP PROCEDURE

1. Select the appropriate method for obtaining the temperature measurement based on the child's age and condition.
2. Provide an explanation of the procedure to the child and family.
3. Assist the child into a position of comfort. The child may remain on the parent's lap if preferred.
4. Wash hands.
5. Don gloves. Maintain **Standard Precautions.**
6. Obtain the child's temperature using method chosen.
7. Offer praise to the child for cooperating.
8. Document and report core temperatures of less than 36°C (96.8°F) or greater than 38.5°C (101.4°F).
9. Reassess the child's temperature every ½ to 1 hour, or as directed.

DOCUMENTATION

Document the method chosen for temperature measurement in the patient's medical record. Include the measurement obtained and any action taken.

Parent Teaching

Some parents may need to learn how to take the child's temperature at home. The nurse may demonstrate how it is done and then observe the parent in performing the procedure. Make sure the parent is comfortable with the procedure and is able to read the thermometer accurately. There are a variety of thermometer types available. Digital thermometers are relatively inexpensive and may be used to take oral, rectal, and axillary temperatures. The numbers are displayed on a small screen and are much easier to read accurately than glass thermometers.

The average body temperature, when measured orally, is 98.6°F (37°C). Mild elevations may occur as the result of exercise, excessive clothing, hot baths, hot weather, warm food, or warm drinks. If one of those conditions may have had an effect on the child's temperature, it should be measured in ½ hour. The child has a fever if the temperature is greater than 100.4°F (38.0°C) when measured rectally, greater than 99.5°F (37.5°C) when measured orally, or greater than 98.6°F (37°C) when measured by the axillary method. In general, the height of the fever is not an indication of the seriousness of the illness. What is important is how the child is acting. If the child has a fever and is acting sick, notify the health caretaker (Schmitt, 1992).

Measuring Pulse

Apical pulse rate measurements are recommended for infants and children younger than 2 years of age and any child who has an irregular heart rate or known congenital heart disease (Fig. 18–5). Apical heart rates must be determined prior to administration of certain medications, such as digoxin. Radial pulse measurements are appropriate for children older than 2 years of age. (See the inside front cover for normal pulse measurements.)

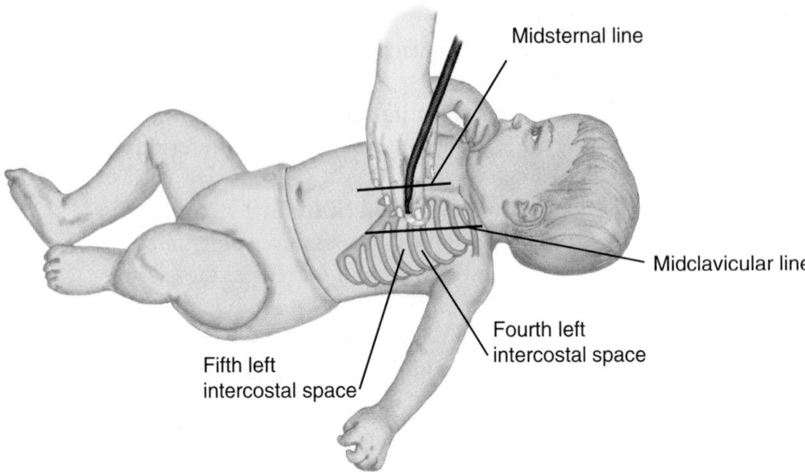
Apical pulse is lateral to the left MCL and fourth ICS
in children <7 years of age and to the left MCL and fifth ICS
in children >7 years of age.
Midsternal line
Midclavicular line
Fourth left
intercostal space
Fifth left
intercostal space

Figure 18–5
Apical pulse measurement is the preferred method for infants and children younger than 2 years of age, as well as for any child with an irregular heart rate or congenital heart disease. *MCL*, midclavicular line; *ICS*, intercostal space.

PROCEDURE: *Measuring Pulse*

Preparing the Child and Family. Inform the child and family of the purpose of the procedure. Children who are fearful should be allowed to examine or handle the stethoscope.

Equipment
- Stethoscope

STEP-BY-STEP PROCEDURE

For measuring apical pulse in infants and children younger than 2 years of age, or any child with an irregular heart rate or known congenital heart disease:

1. Place the stethoscope at the point of maximum intensity (PMI), which is usually located at the fourth to fifth intercostal space at the midclavicular line.
2. Count the pulse for a full minute for any child with an irregular heart rate. Rates greater than 90 beats per minute tend to be undercounted, whether the rhythm is regular or irregular (Margolius et al., 1991).

Counting the apical heart rate for a full minute is the most accurate measurement of the true heart rate and should be used when (1) assessing the patient for the first time, (2) when the patient is unstable or has an irregular rhythm, or (3) when treatment decisions need to be made which are based on the heart rate. A shorter counting interval may be accurate for stable patients who have normal rates and rhythms or for whom a baseline has already been established (Sneed & Hollerbach, 1995).

For measuring radial pulses in children older than 2 years of age:

1. Place the index and middle fingers on the radial pulse (thumb side).
2. Press gently to avoid occlusion of the pulse. If the radial pulse is irregular, thready, or difficult to locate, an apical pulse should be taken.

Parent Teaching

Some parents may need to be taught how to determine their child's heart rate accurately, as well as the acceptable range for their child. Special considerations relating to notification of the physician by parents may need to be made for children who are taking certain medications, such as digoxin.

DOCUMENTATION

Document the method chosen for pulse measurement in the patient's medical record. Include in the documentation the measurement obtained and any action taken.

Evaluating Respirations

Infants often have irregular respiratory rates that change with stimulation, crying, and feeding. Some infants will initially exhibit a Cheyne-Stokes type of respiratory pattern, but this should disappear by 4 weeks of age. Table 11–1 shows normal rates.

PROCEDURE: *Evaluating Respirations*

Preparing the Child and Family. Inform the child and family of the purpose of the procedure. It is best to do this in a low-key manner to avoid exciting the child.

Equipment

None necessary

STEP-BY-STEP PROCEDURE

1. Observe the child's respiratory rate and effort for 1 full minute while the child is quiet. Abdominal movement is normally observed in infants and young children, whereas thoracic movement can be noted in older children and adolescents.
2. Evaluate the quality of respirations, symmetry of chest movement with each breath, and any noisy respirations (crackles, wheezes, friction rubs, etc.).
3. Observe the child for any signs of respiratory distress, such as nasal flaring, grunting, stridor, retractions, increased work of breathing, cyanosis, or apneic periods.

DOCUMENTATION

Document and report any deviations from the expected norm.

Parent Teaching

Parents may not be aware that younger children are primarily diaphragmatic breathers, necessitating observation of the rise and fall of the abdomen, rather than the chest. The importance of diversional activities during the counting should be stressed, as should the importance of counting respirations for 1 full minute.

Measuring Blood Pressure

Blood pressure is usually assessed at least once per shift in the hospitalized child. Unless a problem is suspected, however, blood pressure may not be assessed more than once per year during routine physical examinations.

Cuff size should be based on a midpoint limb circumference. Blood pressure measurement will differ according to the type of measurement technique and the site selected. (See inside front cover for normal rates.)

- Choosing the appropriate cuff size is extremely important (see Table 18.1 for recommendations). An inappropriate cuff size will yield a blood pressure that is either too high or too low.
- Electronic measurements are frequently obtained, but hypertension or hypotension that has been assessed electronically *should always be verified* with a manual cuff.

TABLE 18–1 *Recommended Blood Pressure Cuff Sizes*

ARM CIRCUMFERENCE (cm)	CUFF NAME	BLADDER WIDTH (cm)	BLADDER LENGTH (cm)
5–7.5	Newborn	3	5
7.5–13	Infant	5	8
13–20	Child	8	13
24–32	Adult	13	24
32–42	Wide Adult	17	32
42–50	Thigh	20	42

PROCEDURE: *Measuring Blood Pressure*

Blood pressures may be measured in the upper arm, lower arm, thigh, calf, or ankle (Fig. 18–6). Be sure to select an appropriate-size cuff for the extremity chosen. Measurements should be taken in the same limb, in the same place, and with the patient in the same position to ensure consistency. When using electronic devices to measure blood pressure, the manufacturer's guidelines should be followed closely to ensure accuracy. For most devices, the first reading is considered to be a "priming" reading, whereas the second reading is considered to be the true blood pressure.

Preparing the Child and Family. Inform the child and family of the purpose of the procedure. Allow the child to handle the equipment while offering an explanation as to how it is used.

Equipment

- Measuring cuff
- Stethoscope

STEP-BY-STEP PROCEDURE

1. Position the limb or body part at the level of the heart.
2. Inflate the cuff to about 20 mm Hg past the point where the distal pulse disappears.
3. Place the diaphragm of the stethoscope over the pulse.
4. Slowly deflate the cuff, noting when the pulse is first heard (systolic pressure) and when the sound becomes muffled or disappears (diastolic pressure).

In young children, it may not be possible to **auscultate** the diastolic pressure. The systolic blood pressure may be heard down to a measurement of zero. If this is the case, the blood pressure should be documented as the systolic number over pulse (e.g., 90/P).

When it is impossible to auscultate a blood pressure in infants and toddlers: In this instance, the pulse may be palpated. The cuff is inflated as with an auscultated pressure, but the nurse palpates where the pulse should be

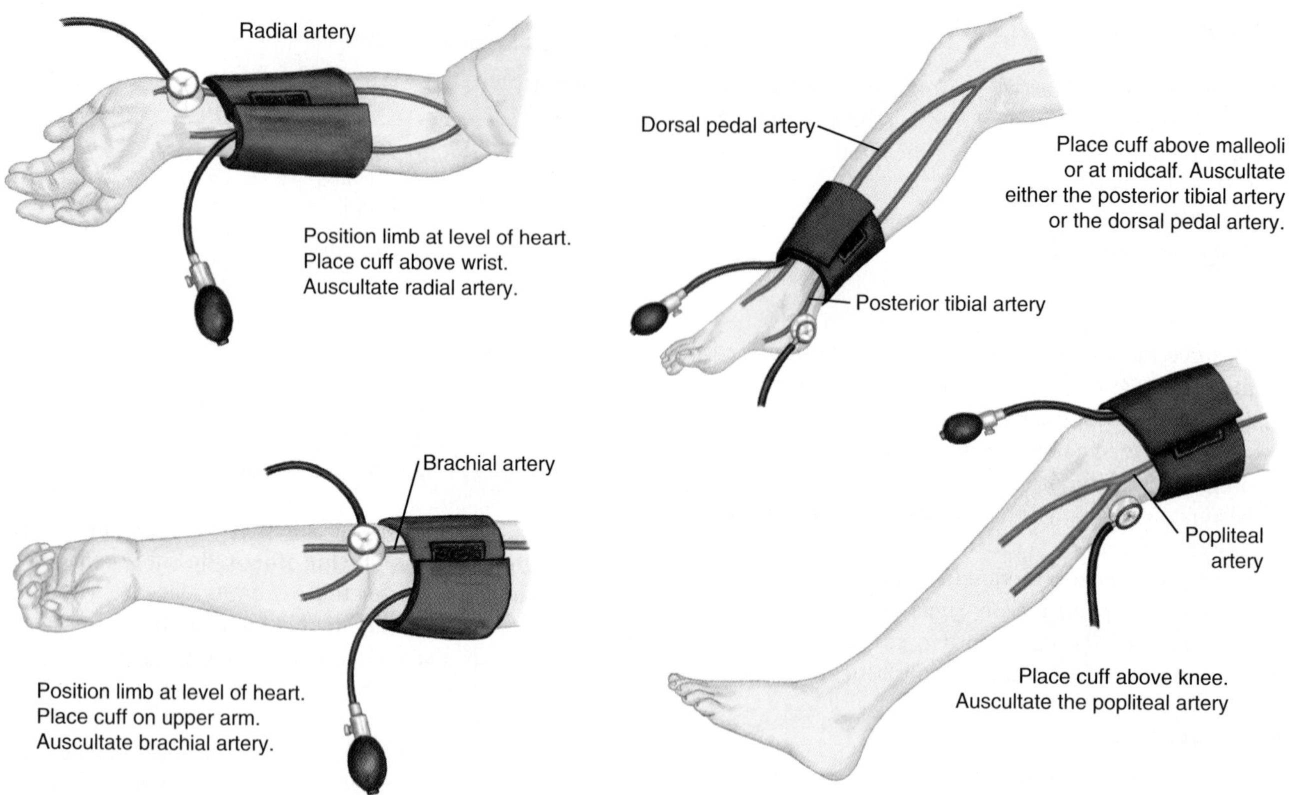

Figure 18–6

Blood pressures may be measured in the upper arm, lower arm, thigh, calf, or ankle. It is important that an appropriate-size cuff be used to obtain accurate results (see Table 18–1).

using the index and middle fingers. Note when the pulse is first felt. This is the systolic measurement. This form of measurement is always documented as systolic pressure over pulse (e.g., 90/P).

DOCUMENTATION

Document blood pressure measurements and note any changes from previous readings. *For young children in whom the lower (diastolic) pressure cannot be auscultated,* blood pressure is documented as the systolic number over pulse (e.g., 90/P). *When the pulse is palpated in infants and toddlers,* blood pressure is always documented as systolic pressure over pulse (e.g., 90/P).

Parent Teaching

If the child's condition requires home monitoring of the blood pressure, the parent may be taught this procedure. Guidelines regarding size of the cuff and methods that may be used to involve the child who might resist this procedure should be provided. For instance, parents might make a smaller cuff for the child's favorite doll or stuffed animal in order to involve the child.

Special Considerations. Some children may require continuous cardiorespiratory monitoring. Many types of monitors are available commercially that can provide a continuous measurement of heart rate, respiratory rate, blood pressure, and temperature. It is not uncommon for children who are acutely ill or who are undergoing procedures to be placed on a monitor to assist the health care providers in detecting subtle changes in the child's condition. The procedure and indications for attaching a child to a cardiorespiratory monitor are no different from those appropriate for an adult. Monitors will sound an alarm to warn of changes in the child's cardiorespiratory status. Remember that "false" alarms can occur. Always look at the patient and perform an assessment prior to intervening. A flat line on the electrocardiogram (ECG) does not always signal a cardiac arrest. It can be just a loose monitor lead. Check the manufacturer's recommendations for attaching leads and monitoring selected vital signs.

SPECIMEN COLLECTION

Specimens are collected from children for the same reasons they are collected from adults, but children often require more of an explanation of the reasons and procedure for specimen collection. The explanations should be given in age-appropriate language, and the child should be prepared for any sensations that may be experienced.

Regardless of the type of specimen to be obtained, Standard Precautions must be maintained (see Appendix G). The use of gloves, gowns, masks, eye protection, and handwashing provides a means of protection for individuals coming in contact with potentially infectious materials. Use of equipment for Standard Precautions will vary according to the degree of "potential splash." Any time there is a chance for contamination, *use Standard Precautions*. Follow procedures for handling biologic hazards as directed by individual facilities, based on Standard Precautions.

Urine Specimens

Older children and adolescents are often cooperative in the collection of urine specimens. Most can use a bedpan, urinal, or specimen cup with little difficulty.

Younger children and preschoolers often have difficulty voiding upon request. The nurse should take care to use familiar terms, such as "pee-pee," "tinkle," or "potty" when telling the child what is needed. Parents are often very helpful in obtaining a specimen from children this age. Parents may also be successful in obtaining specimens from older toddlers who are in the process of being toilet-trained. However, infants and young toddlers are unable to void on request. Because they are not toilet-trained, specimen collection devices are needed.

If the specimen must be collected under special conditions (as in the case of a midstream urine sample), the nurse should carefully explain to the child what preparation is needed and ensure that he understands all directions. An adult may need to accompany the child during the collection. A young child may be able to sit on the toilet but may be unable to manipulate a specimen cup. The parent or nurse can hold the cup while the child voids. For a boy who wishes to stand while voiding, the cup can be held in the stream as he voids. If the specimen is to be carried to another room or down a hallway, a paper bag or other container should be provided for transport.

See the accompanying box for tips on urine specimen collection.

Tips for Obtaining Urine Specimens

- If blood and urine specimens need to be obtained from an incontinent child, place a collection bag ("wee bag") *prior* to drawing the blood. Infants and toddlers will often void during a painful procedure.
- Wiping an infant's abdomen with an alcohol pad and fanning it dry may facilitate voiding (Ellis, 1989).
- Applying pressure over the suprapubic area or stroking along the spine of older infants will often induce voiding.
- Urine for certain tests, such as specific gravity, may be obtained from a diaper. Tear the inner lining of the diaper after the infant has voided and place the diaper's absorbent material inside a syringe from which the plunger has been removed. Replace the plunger and use it to compress the material, thus squeezing the urine out the end of the syringe.
- After placing a collection bag on an incontinent child, place a small slit in the diaper and gently pull the bag through it. This facilitates visualization of urine and also avoids unnecessary "pull" on the specimen bag.

PROCEDURE: *Urine Specimen Collection from the Incontinent Child*

Although many methods have been used to collect urine from incontinent children (such as placing plastic wrap in a diaper to catch urine), the most reliable is the urine "wee" bag. This collection device is a plastic bag that has an opening that is lined with adhesive so that it may be attached to the perineum (Fig. 18–7). It is available in two sizes (infant and pediatric) to accommodate almost any child. Twenty-four hour collection bags are also available. These bags have a tube that extends from the end of the bag that allows for each void to be removed from the bag.

In some situations, absorbent material from the disposable diaper saturated with urine may be placed in a 10-ml syringe from which the plunger has been removed. The plunger is then reinserted into the barrel of the syringe and the urine is expressed from the syringe for the specimen.

Preparing the Child and Family. Care should be taken to provide the child with privacy. The child may be more relaxed if a parent is present during the procedure.

Equipment

- Nonsterile gloves
- Urine collection bag
- Sterile specimen cup
- Mild soap, warm water, and a washcloth
- Diaper, towel
- Label
- Requisition form

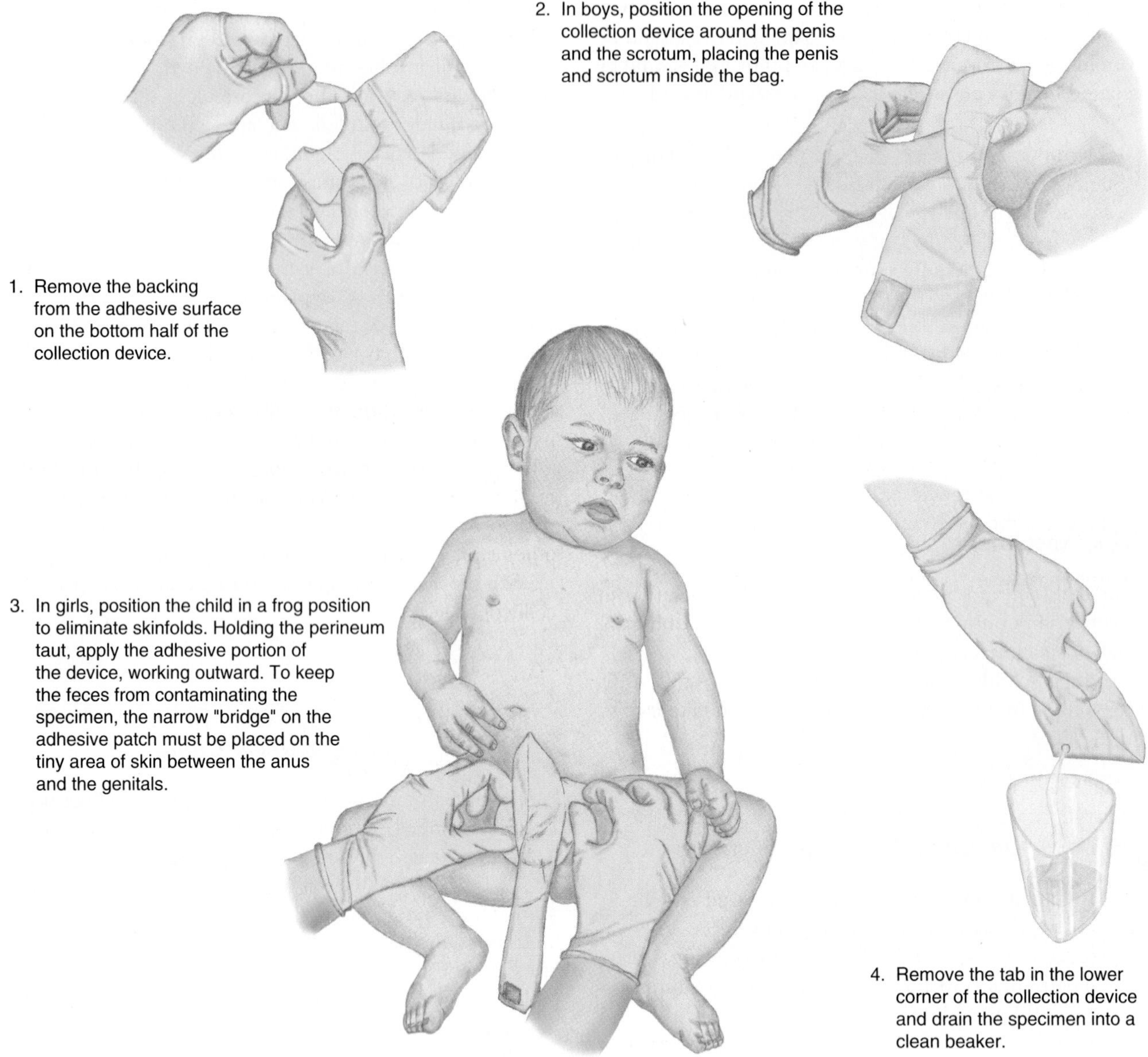

2. In boys, position the opening of the collection device around the penis and the scrotum, placing the penis and scrotum inside the bag.
1. Remove the backing from the adhesive surface on the bottom half of the collection device.
3. In girls, position the child in a frog position to eliminate skinfolds. Holding the perineum taut, apply the adhesive portion of the device, working outward. To keep the feces from contaminating the specimen, the narrow "bridge" on the adhesive patch must be placed on the tiny area of skin between the anus and the genitals.
4. Remove the tab in the lower corner of the collection device and drain the specimen into a clean beaker.

Figure 18–7

Guidelines for using a urine collection device, or "wee bag," to collect urine from an incontinent child.

STEP-BY-STEP PROCEDURE

1. The perineum should always be cleansed (by the same method used for urinary catheterization) prior to placing the bag on the child. Cleaning the perineum will remove any lotions, or ointments and will help the bag to adhere. Studies have shown, however, that cleaning the perineum does not necessarily decrease contamination of the urine specimen (McDonald et al., 1985; Lohr et al., 1989).

   For girls: The perineum should be cleaned front-to-back and from the urinary meatus to the labia majora (in-to-out).

   For boys: The penis should be cleansed from the tip of the penis in a circular motion.
2. After the perineum has been cleansed, it should be dried thoroughly. This will also help the bag to adhere.
3. Place the child in a frog-like position in order to eliminate skin folds that may interfere with bag adherence.

4. *With girls:* Hold the perineum taut and apply the adhesive portion of the bag, working outward. Cut a slit in the disposable diaper and pull the end of the empty bag through the slit so that the bag protrudes from the diaper. Pressure from the diaper is prevented and the bag is less likely to loosen and leak.
   With boys: Place the penis and scrotum inside the bag.
5. After attaching the bag, a diaper may be reapplied.
6. Check the bag every 30 minutes. As soon as urine is noticed in the bag, it should be removed gently from the perineum.
7. Transfer the urine into a sterile specimen cup. Most bags have a small tab that can be removed to allow the urine to be poured. If the bag does not have a tab, the outside of the bag may be cleansed with an alcohol pad and the urine withdrawn with a needle and syringe for placement in the appropriate container.
8. Label the urine specimen with the patient's name and date and time of collection and deliver it promptly, together with a requisition form, to the laboratory. Urine for culture that cannot be tested within 30 minutes should be refrigerated or placed in a sterile container with a preservative.

DOCUMENTATION

Record the collection of the specimen in the child's chart. Include the date and time of collection and the amount, color, and appearance of the urine.

Parent Teaching

Instruct the parents how to collect a specimen. Parents may keep the urine that is collected at home in the refrigerator until they are asked to bring it to the laboratory. Care should be taken to keep the specimen chilled during transport (i.e., placed in a cooler or plastic bag packed with ice).

Urinary Catheterization

The basic procedure for urinary catheterization is much the same in children as in adults.

PROCEDURE: *Urinary Catheterization*

Catheterization kits often contain all the necessary equipment. They may or may not, however, include an appropriate-size catheter or a closed drainage bag. The catheter should be small enough to allow it to be inserted easily into the urinary meatus, but large enough to prevent leakage of urine. Although feeding tubes are frequently used as catheters for infants, urinary catheters are available in sizes as small as no. 6 French. See the accompanying box for appropriate catheter sizes.

Urinary Catheter Sizes According to Age

Infants 1 year of age or younger: No. 5 French feeding tube or No. 6 French Foley
Children 1 to 2 years of age: No. 8 French Foley
Children 10 years of age or younger: No. 8–10 French (Brown and Ioli, 1993)
Older children: No. 12 to 14 French

Some children, particularly those who undergo multiple urinary catheterizations (e.g., children with spina bifida), are at high risk for developing latex sensitivity. Patients with documented or suspected latex allergies should be identified as early as possible and should be provided with a latex-free environment.

Preparing the Child and Family. Preparation for the procedure should be done using age-appropriate methods, and the child should be prepared for what she will feel and what must be done to "help." It may be helpful to demonstrate the procedure on a teaching doll. Teach the child to take slow deep breaths during the procedure and have her practice this prior to the procedure. The assistance of another adult is often necessary with younger children.

Equipment

- Catheterization kit
- Appropriate-size catheter
- Closed drainage bag
- Requisition form
- Label
- Sterile gloves
- Sterile specimen cap

STEP-BY-STEP PROCEDURE

The procedure is the same as for an adult. However, special care should be taken in the following areas:

1. Recruit an assistant to help restrain the child and provide emotional support.
2. Make sure the area is well lighted and all necessary equipment is gathered before beginning the procedure. Obtain extra sterile gloves in case of contamination.
3. Take extra care to be gentle when cleansing the meatus or glans penis.
4. See box above to determine the size of catheter needed. See the earlier section, "Preparing the Child and Family," for suggested preparation hints.
5. In female patients, direct the catheter slightly upward, insert gently through the meatus 1 to 2 inches, or until urine appears. In males, hold penis at 90° angle from

body and gently insert catheter 2 to 3 inches, or until urine appears.
6. Never force the catheter. The older child can assist in relaxing the external sphincter by bearing down.

DOCUMENTATION

Record the date and time the procedure was done, as well as the size of catheter used and the amount, color, and appearance of the urine. Note how the infant or child tolerated the procedure. Deliver labeled specimen promptly, together with requisition form, to the laboratory.

Stool Specimens

Stool may be obtained for testing for the presence of such things as fat, blood, bacteria, parasites, or reducing substances. If a stool specimen from an incontinent child is needed, it may often be scraped from a diaper and placed in an appropriate container. If the stool is watery, a piece of gauze may be placed in the diaper to absorb some of the stool, or a "wee" bag may be placed over the anus in an attempt to collect a specimen.

In the continent child, a bedpan or a specimen collector designed to be placed in the toilet can be used. Because older children may be embarrassed about providing such a sample, the nurse should use a calm, matter-of-fact manner when explaining the reason the specimen is needed, as well as the procedure for handling the specimen.

Blood Specimens

Blood collected for testing can be obtained from children in a variety of ways. Because blood collection is an invasive procedure, it should be performed in a treatment room, if one is available.

The collection of blood is very distressing to a child. The use of EMLA, a topical anesthetic cream, can reduce the discomfort felt by the child. (See Chapter 20 for a discussion of EMLA.) Some children who require long-term venous access for nutrition or medications may have a central intravenous catheter or port in place. These may also be utilized to obtain blood for laboratory studies. However, this procedure may be performed *only* by specially trained, licensed personnel.

PROCEDURE: *Venipuncture*

Venipuncture in children is often performed using a butterfly catheter. The most commonly used sites are the veins of the hand and antecubital area. Standard Precautions are always maintained when collecting blood specimens.

Preparing the Child and Family. The child should be prepared for the procedure using explanations presented in age-appropriate language. She should know what she will hear and feel. It is often necessary to obtain help to restrain the child during the procedure. Parents may or may not wish to remain in the room.

Equipment

- 23- or 25-gauge butterfly catheter
- Gloves
- Alcohol and/or povidone-iodine (Betadine) swabs or pads
- Tourniquet (*Note:* Most tourniquets are composed of rubber tubing that is $\frac{1}{2}$ to 1 inch in length. Although rubber bands have been used as tourniquets in infants, these are not preferred, as they may abrade the skin.)
- Syringe(s)
- Labels
- Appropriate collection containers
- Requisition form

STEP-BY-STEP PROCEDURE

Conventional Method

1. Restrain the child's arm by having one nurse place one hand under the arm of the child (usually at the shoulder) and the other hand on the child's hand (Fig. 18–8). The sampling nurse is then able to draw the blood with less likelihood of missing the vein.
2. Apply a tourniquet tight enough to restrict blood flow toward the heart, but not so tight as to cause pain or to restrict arterial blood flow. Tourniquets are used to slow venous blood return to the heart and cause dis-

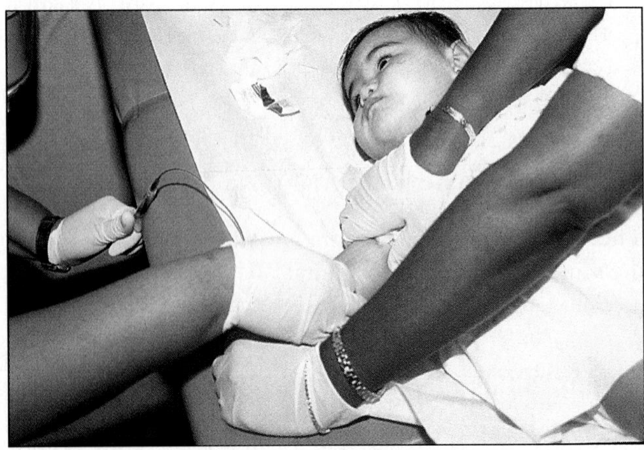

Figure 18–8
The vein of the antecubital area is a site commonly used for venipuncture in children. One nurse restrains the child's arm while another nurse draws the blood sample. A butterfly needle is often used; the needle is inserted into the vein with the bevel up. When blood flows and reaches the end of the catheter, the syringe is attached and the sample is gently drawn into the syringe. (Courtesy of Dallas County Hospital District Community-Oriented Primary Care Clinic, Dallas, Texas)

tension of the veins, thus making them more visible. The tourniquet should be looped when applied to facilitate easy removal. A tourniquet should be left in place no longer than 2 minutes to prevent hemoconcentration.
3. Lightly pat or rub the sample site to help the veins become more visible.
4. Using a circular motion, cleanse the puncture site with alcohol and allow to dry. If the child is immunocompromised, Betadine should be used to cleanse the skin.
5. Insert the needle of the butterfly catheter into the vein, bevel side up.
6. When blood begins to flow into the catheter, avoid the temptation of placing the syringe on the end of the catheter and attempting to speed up the blood flow by pulling back the plunger.
7. When blood reaches the end of the catheter, attach the syringe and slowly draw the appropriate amount of blood into the syringe.
8. After obtaining the required amount of blood, withdraw the needle and apply pressure to the puncture site until bleeding has stopped (Garza & Becan-McBride, 1993).

Alternate "Drip" Method

Another method of obtaining venous blood is the dorsal hand vein procedure or "drip" method (Clagg, 1989).

1. Hold the child's wrist between the index and middle fingers and stabilize the child's fingers with the thumb. The index and middle finger act as a tourniquet.
2. Insert a 21- or 23-gauge needle, bevel up, into the vein.
3. As blood flows through the hub of the needle, allow it to drip into the specimen containers.
4. If blood flow slows, the pressure of the finger "tourniquet" may be released slightly and then reapplied. The needle may also be rotated slightly, but it should never be moved in and out to increase blood flow (Garza & Becan-McBride, 1993).
5. After the specimen is collected, the child should be comforted and praised for his cooperation. Parents are often the best people to provide comfort.
6. Band-Aids are important, as they help to prevent bleeding from the puncture site. Specially colored or cartoon-character Band-Aids are available commercially and are appropriate for children's "boo-boos." The nurse may also give the child a reward, such as a sticker.

DOCUMENTATION

Label the specimen with the child's name and record the date and time of collection, the amount of blood collected, the site used for puncture, and the reason blood was drawn (diagnostic test). Note the child's reaction to the procedure and the number of attempts made before a specimen was obtained.

Parent Teaching

Encourage and assist parents to comfort and hold the child. Praise the child for her help.

Jugular Venipuncture

Jugular and femoral venipuncture are performed by a physician, with the nurse assisting and monitoring the child.

Blood specimens from infants and young children may be obtained from the large superficial external jugular vein. Place the child in a mummy restraint (see Fig. 18–11), allowing enough area at the top edge of the restraint to permit access to the jugular vein. If a restraint is not used, the arms and legs can be held by a second nurse. The child's head is hyperextended to the side opposite the site, over the edge of a table or a small pillow (Fig. 18–9). Pressure should be applied to the side for 3 to 5 minutes or until bleeding stops. Care should be taken not to overextend the head to the point of causing airway problems.

Femoral Venipuncture

Another site to obtain blood is the femoral veins. The child is supine in the frog position to expose the groin area (see Fig.18–9). One nurse stands above the child's head, holding the child's arms with the elbows and the legs with the hands. A cloth diaper should be placed over the infant's perineal area and tucked under the buttocks with the site exposed. This is to protect the area in case the child urinates. Apply pressure to the site with a dry, sterile gauze square after specimen is obtained.

Heelsticks and Fingersticks

When a small blood sample is needed, a disposable pediatric lancet (inserted ≤ 2.4 mm deep) can be used for a fingerstick or heelstick. For fingersticks, the third or ring finger of the nondominant hand should be used. The puncture should be made just to the side of the fingerpad rather than the tip. There are few nerve endings, and the areas are highly vascular. The heel is used in infants; it is warmed first to increase blood flow. Care must be taken to avoid hitting bones in the foot, which could lead to infection and possible osteomyelitis. The heel is not used once the infant is walking because it is more difficult to puncture due to calluses.

PROCEDURE: *Heelsticks*

The heels of infants under 12 months of age and those not yet walking are good sites for obtaining blood (Fig. 18–10). When using this area, only the outer aspects of the heel should be used. These areas may be identified by drawing imaginary lines from the middle of the great toe and from a

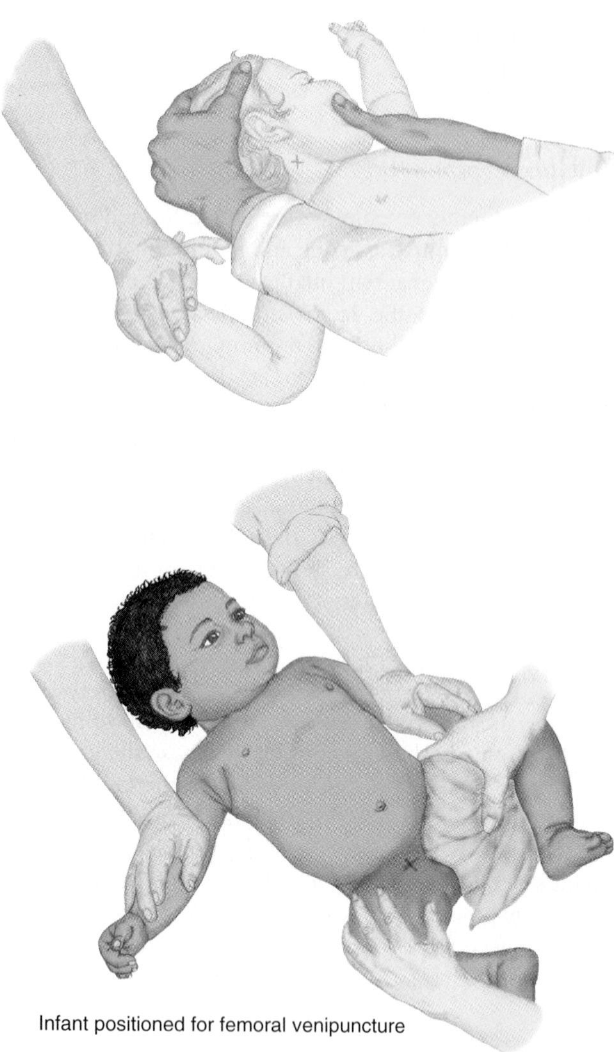

Infant positioned for jugular venipuncture
Infant positioned for femoral venipuncture

Figure 18–9
Two additional sites for obtaining blood specimens from infants and young children are the large superficial external jugular vein and one of the femoral veins.

point between the fourth and fifth toes to the heel, running parallel to the lateral aspect of the heel. It is important to stay within these areas to avoid hitting bone. If bone is hit, it may lead to infection and, possibly, osteomyelitis.

Preparing the Child and Family. The child should be prepared for the procedure using explanations presented in age-appropriate language. He should know what he will hear and feel. It is often necessary to obtain help to restrain the child during the procedure. Parents may wish to leave the room to avoid being associated with a painful procedure.

Equipment

- Disposable lancets or microlancets
- Alcohol or povidone-iodine (Betadine) swabs
- Specimen containers/labels
- Requisition forms
- Sterile 2 × 2 gauze pads
- Gloves
- Warmer (or a warm washcloth)

STEP-BY-STEP PROCEDURE

1. The heel should be warmed to increase blood flow. This may be done with commercially available warmers or with a warmed washcloth. The item used to warm the heel should not exceed 42°C (107.6°F) to avoid burns. The warmer should be left in place 3–10 minutes.
2. After the heel has been warmed, select a site within the "safe" area. Previously used sites should not be repunctured. Areas that are bruised or abraded should also be avoided.
3. Clean the skin with alcohol. The alcohol should be allowed to dry or should be wiped with a sterile gauze to avoid contamination of the specimen.
4. Using a pediatric lancet, puncture the skin to a depth of 2.4 mm or less (Garza & Becan-McBride, 1993). A pediatric lancet has a set depth for puncture. Metal lancets or needles should never be used for skin punctures.
5. The heel may be lightly massaged during specimen collection.

Excessive massage or "milking" should be avoided so as to prevent hemolysis.

6. After the necessary amount of blood is collected, apply pressure with a sterile gauze or cotton ball. Band-Aids should never be applied to the heels of an infant.

DOCUMENTATION

Label the specimen with the patient's name and record the date, time, amount of blood collected, site used for puncture, and reason the blood was drawn (diagnostic test). Note the child's reaction to the procedure and whether more than one stick was necessary.

PROCEDURE: *Fingersticks*

Preparing the Child and Family. The child should be prepared for the procedure using explanations presented with age-appropriate language. He should know what he will hear and feel. It is often necessary to get help to restrain the child during the procedure. Parents may or may not wish to remain in the room.

Equipment

Same as for heelsticks.

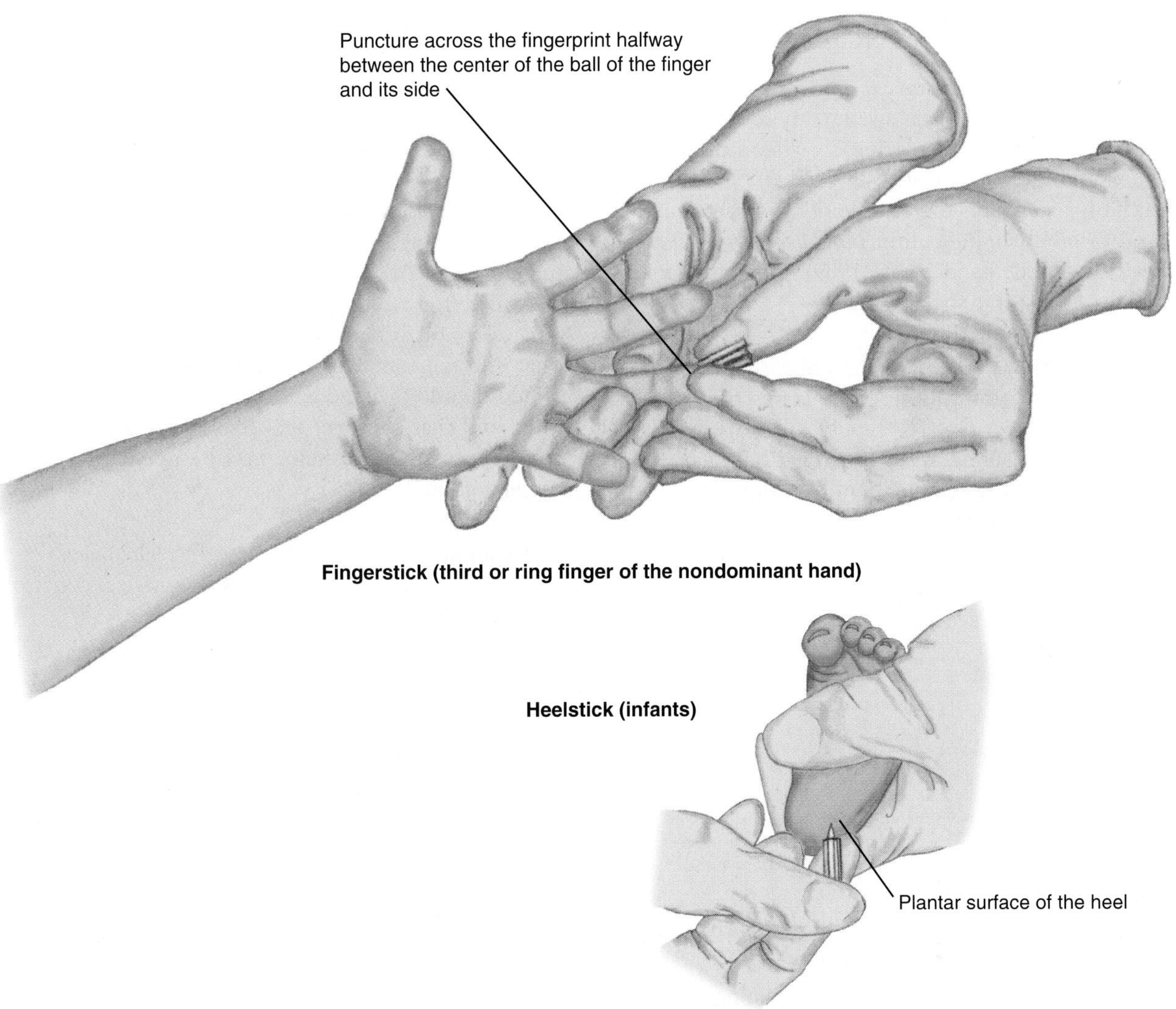

Figure 18–10
Fingerstick and heelstick methods for obtaining blood samples.

STEP-BY-STEP PROCEDURE

1. If possible, the third or ring finger of the nondominant hand should be used to obtain the specimen (see Fig. 18–10). A bruised, edematous, or abraded finger should never be used. Old puncture sites should be avoided.
2. As with heelsticks, fingers may be warmed prior to obtaining a blood specimen.
3. Using the lancet, make a puncture across the fingerprint halfway between the center of the ball of the finger and its side (Garza & Becan-McBride, 1993).
4. The first drop of blood should be wiped away with a sterile gauze.
5. The finger may be gently massaged from its base to the tip to ensure good blood flow.
6. Collect the blood in the appropriate container(s).
7. Apply pressure with sterile gauze until bleeding stops.

Sputum Specimens

Sputum specimens are most commonly obtained to identify or rule out a respiratory infection. When obtaining any specimen, maintain standard precautions. If splashing is anticipated, masks and goggles or protective eyewear should be worn in addition to gloves.

Sputum in the older child is usually easy to obtain. Most older children and adolescents can cough deeply and produce a sputum sample, which can then be placed in the appropriate container. Specimens are easily obtained from children with artificial airways by attaching a mucous or suction trap to a suction catheter and suctioning the airway in order to obtain the specimen.

PROCEDURE: *Nasal Washing*

Younger children and infants can seldom produce a deep cough on demand and often swallow those secretions. A cough may be elicited by placing a suction catheter into the back of the throat. It is usually necessary, however, to utilize lavage to obtain the sample. This method should be used when obtaining cultures for respiratory syncytial virus (RSV) (Nederhand et al., 1989). Other specimens may be obtained using special swabs.

Preparing the Child and Family. The child should be prepared for the procedure using explanations presented in age-appropriate language. He should know what he will hear and feel. It may be necessary to get help to restrain the child during the procedure. Parents can help by holding or restraining the child.

Equipment

- Butterfly catheter
- Syringe
- Sterile saline
- Gloves
- Sterile specimen container
- Labels
- Requisition forms

STEP-BY-STEP PROCEDURE

1. Cut the "butterfly" (needle and wings) off the butterfly catheter and discard.
2. Attach a syringe (without needle) containing 1 to 3 ml of sterile saline to the catheter.
3. Place the child in a supine position and place the catheter into one nostril.
4. Instill the saline into the nostril and immediately withdraw into the syringe.
5. Place the saline into a sterile, labeled container.
6. A small, sterile bulb syringe may also be used to aspirate secretions.

DOCUMENTATION

Document the amount of saline instilled and the method of collection used. Note the date, time, amount, color, and consistency of secretions.

Throat Culture

Throat cultures are frequently used to identify the causative agent of "sore throats" or tonsillitis in children.

A throat culture should never be attempted in a child in whom the diagnosis of **epiglottitis** *is suspected.* Prior to obtaining the specimen, the throat should be assessed visually for the presence of erythema or exudate.

Preparing the Child and Family. The procedure should be explained using explanations presented in age-appropriate language. The procedure should not be done immediatley after the child has taken medication, eaten, or had something to drink. The child should be prepared for what she will need to do and what she will feel. She should be told that she will need to open her mouth very wide, and that she may feel like she needs to cough or gag. If necessary, assistance may be needed to restrain a younger child.

Equipment

- Tongue depressor
- Swabs
- Collection containers
- Gloves

STEP-BY-STEP PROCEDURE

1. An older child can sit in a chair or sit upright in bed for the throat culture. A younger child should be placed in a supine position on a bed or examining table.
2. Have the child open her mouth and say "Ahhh." Eliciting a cry from an infant will give optimal access to the pharyngeal area.
3. Insert a tongue depressor into the mouth with the nondominant hand so that it covers the anterior half of the tongue.
4. Depress the tongue to allow visualization of the pharyngeal area.
5. Swab the area quickly, avoiding the tongue, buccal mucosa, and palate. Only one swab should be used for each culture.
6. Place the swabs in the appropriate culture media and transport them to the laboratory.
7. If possible, offer the child cool fluids to drink following the procedure.

DOCUMENTATION

Record the date, time, and appearance of specimen. Note the child's response to the procedure.

Parent Teaching

Assist parents to support and comfort the child during and after the procedure.

Lumbar Puncture

Lumbar punctures are performed in order to examine the cerebrospinal fluid (CSF) for bacteria or abnormal cells, to measure pressure within the cerebrospinal cavities, or to inject certain medications (i.e., for pain control, to prevent or eradicate specific diseases, or as a contrast for scans).

PROCEDURE: *Lumbar Puncture*

Because a lumbar puncture is frequently performed when a child is acutely ill (as with meningitis, leukemia), this stressful procedure becomes even more stressful for the child and family. The nurse must provide a great deal of support and education for the child and his family. The physician will explain what is planned and will obtain an informed consent from the parents or guardians. This procedure is performed by a physician or qualified nurse practitioner. A nurse assists by positioning, restraining, and monitoring the patient.

Preparing the Child and Family. The child should be prepared for what he will need to do and what he will hear and feel. He should be told that he will need to stay very still until the physician is finished and that the nurse will be there to help him remember to hold the position. If time permits, the child should be allowed to practice the position.

Equipment

- Lumbar puncture tray
- Antiseptic cleansing solution (povidone-iodine)
- Sterile gloves
- Additional light source if needed
- Laboratory requisition forms

STEP-BY-STEP PROCEDURE

1. Place the child in the appropriate position. The two positions used for lumbar puncture are the lateral or side-lying position and the sitting position (see box with photos on the following pages). The intraspinal fluid pressure can only be measured if the child is in the lateral position. Both positions can be used in collecting CSF or injecting medications.

   Infants younger than 3 months are placed in the lateral position. Older infants and children can be positioned either in the lateral or sitting position. Restraint is sometimes better obtained in the side-lying position. The positions are sometimes modified, based on experience.
2. If the child is in a side-lying position, secure the child by holding him under his thighs and behind his neck. Extreme care should be taken to avoid airway obstruction. The infant placed in a sitting position can be secured by holding him along his sides with the nurse's thumbs across his shoulder blades. The older child leans over a pillow and the nurse places her arm across his back.
3. Explain to the child that he will feel something cold as his back is washed and may feel a "stick and sting" when the physician injects local anesthetic. EMLA (Chapter 20) may be used for the elimination of pain.
4. Explain to the child that he may feel pressure when the spinal needle is inserted and, possibly, some pain in his leg if medication is injected.
5. During the procedure, provide constant verbal reassurance *unless* the child is utilizing guided imagery. (If he is using guided imagery, being spoken to will ruin his ability to concentrate.)

> The child's respiratory status should be monitored carefully because of the risk of airway obstruction related to neck flexion. A pulse oximeter may be used to monitor oxygen saturation.

6. After the needle is inserted into the vertebral space, flexion may be relaxed. If appropriate, the child should be encouraged to relax and take slow breaths. The nurse should maintain restraint, however, to prevent the child from moving.
7. The physician will obtain CSF samples and may measure CSF pressure.
8. After completing the sampling and measurement, the needle is removed. Explain that the child will feel light pressure and a Band-Aid being applied.
9. The child may need to remain in bed with the head of the bed flat or elevated no more than 15° for 4 to 6 hours.
10. Monitor the child for complaints of headache, fever, or CSF leakage at the puncture site.

DOCUMENTATION

Record the date, time, and name of the physician performing the procedure. Monitor the patient's vital signs as ordered and observe for changes in responsiveness or motor activity, headache, bradycardia, and condition of the puncture site. Note the color, clarity, and pressure of CSF.

Parent Teaching

Assist parents in comforting the child during and after the procedure. Inform parents of the child's need for quiet and fluid intake.

Bone Marrow Aspiration

Bone marrow aspiration is performed in order to obtain specimens of marrow for diagnostic testing, for evaluation of response to treatment modalities, or for transplantation.

Restraining a Child for a Lumbar Puncture

Lumbar punctures (also called L.P.s or spinal taps) are performed for many different reasons to a variety of age groups. A lumbar puncture may be performed in order to examine cerebrospinal fluid, and measure pressure within the cerebrospinal cavities, or inject certain medicines (for the control of pain, for specific diseases, or to introduce contrast for scans). Patients suspected of having meningitis, leukemia, or central nervous system tumors are candidates for the L.P. procedure. The procedure is performed by a physician or qualified nurse practitioner in a standard treatment or exam room. A nurse assists by positioning, restraining, and monitoring the patient.

There are two common positions for L.P.s. The first is lateral—the patient lies sideways, as in photos A through D. The second is sitting up, as in photos E through H. In either position, proper curvature of the spine allows for a hollow spinal needle to be inserted between the 3rd and 4th lumbar vertebrae into the subarachnoid space. The intraspinal pressure can be measured only if the patient is in the lateral position. Spinal fluid can be collected or medicines can be injected in either position.

Correct positioning and good restraint of the child will reduce the trauma during the procedure. It will also allow easier access for the person performing the L.P. Because of the sharp flexion of the neck in these positions, children need to be carefully observed for respiratory depression or bradycardia throughout the procedure. Placing the child on a cardio-respiratory monitor enables close monitoring of the patient's status. If a cardio-respiratory monitor is not available, the child's status should be directly observed by a second nurse. This is especially important for the child held in the lateral position.

INFANT (3 MONTHS AND YOUNGER): LATERAL POSITION

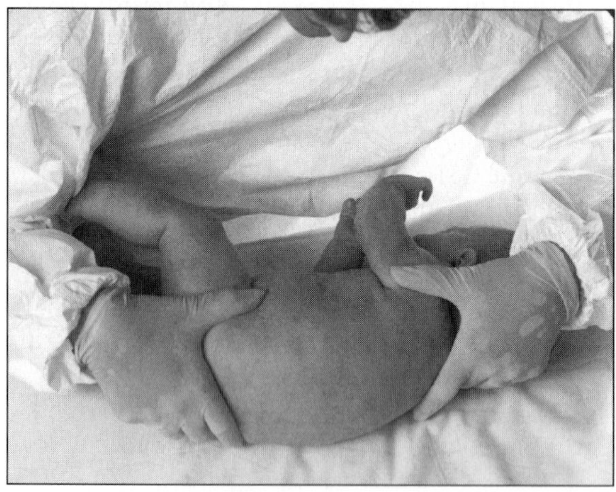

A: The nurse places the infant on his side, placing one hand across the hips, the other hand on the baby's shoulders and back of head.

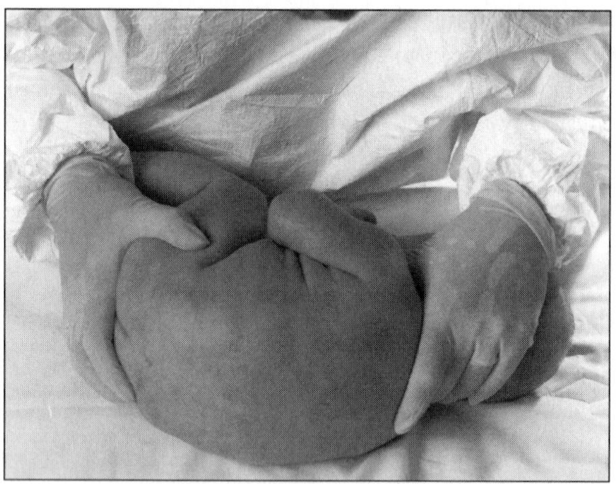

B: For the lumbar puncture: Curl the infant into a tight ball by curving the spinal vertebrae and bringing the baby's knees up to the head. (Note the close proximity of the patient's knees to the elbows.) Meanwhile support the head and neck with the other hand.

Text adapted from Zappa, S. C. (1994). Pediatric practice review: Lumbar punctures: restraining the pediatric patient. In *Nursing in Pediatrics*, (Fall), a publication of Cook Children's Medical Center, Forth Worth, Texas, pp. 22–23. Photographs A–D and G, H © Bob Lukeman. Photographs E and F courtesy of Parkland Memorial Hospital, Dallas, Texas.

CHILD (4 MONTHS AND OLDER): LATERAL POSITION

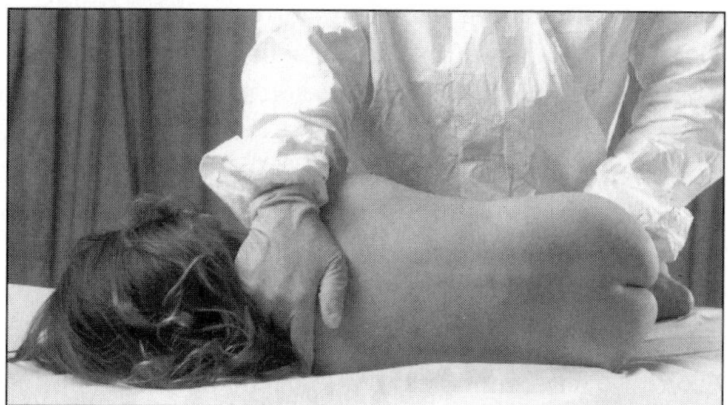

C: The nurse places the child in a side-lying position with one hand behind the child's neck and shoulders, the other hand under the child's bent upper thighs.

D: For the lumbar puncture: Place hand further down under child's neck. The nurse's forearm moves behind the child's head to support the neck. Place other arm further under the child's upper thighs, and curl the body by bringing the knees up to the head. The nurse should support her weight on the edge of the gurney and lightly lean over the child, controlling the arms and legs. Because direct visualization of the patient's respiratory status is limited in this position, a cardio-respiratory monitor must be on the patient or another nurse should be at the bedside.

INFANT (3 MONTHS AND YOUNGER): SITTING POSITION

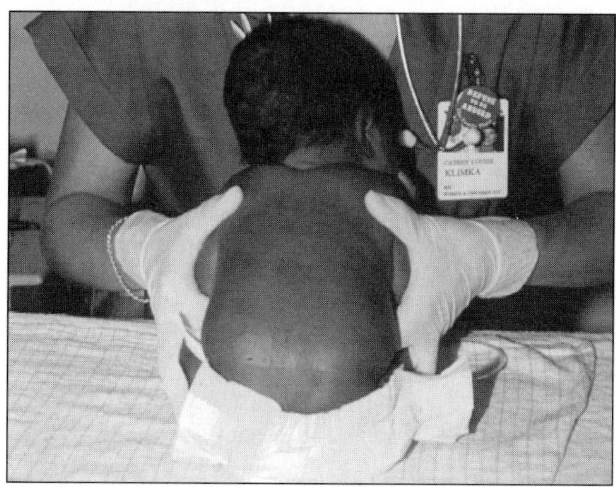

E: The nurse secures the infant in a sitting position with her thumbs across the baby's scapulae.

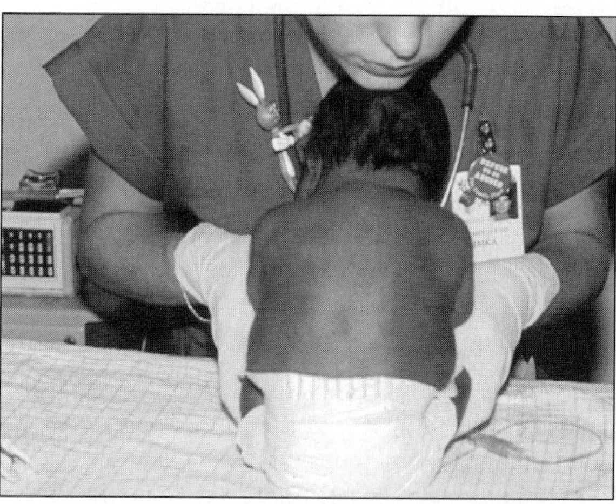

F: The nurse demonstrates an alternative method useful in small infants: She holds the infant in a sitting position with his arms between her thumbs and index fingers, and his legs between her index and middle fingers. She maintains his head in alignment with his spine by steadying it with her chin.

CHILD (4 MONTHS AND OLDER): SITTING POSITION

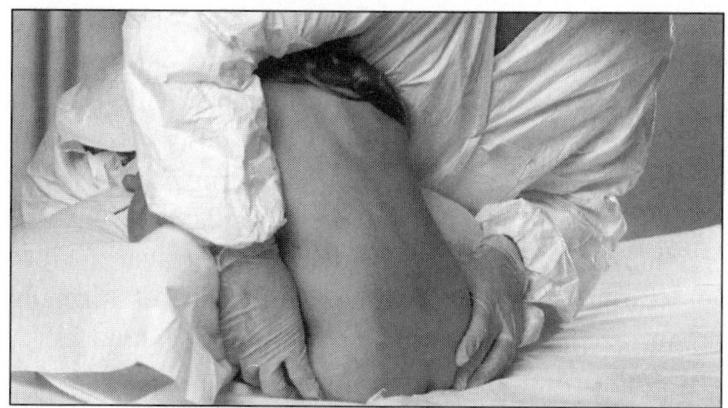

G: Seat the child upright on the stretcher and place a pillow in her lap. Allow the child to lean over a pillow while turning her head to the side. The child can sit cross-legged or can have her legs dangling down straight. The nurse then places one arm behind the head and around the child's upper shoulders and places a hand on each upper thigh.

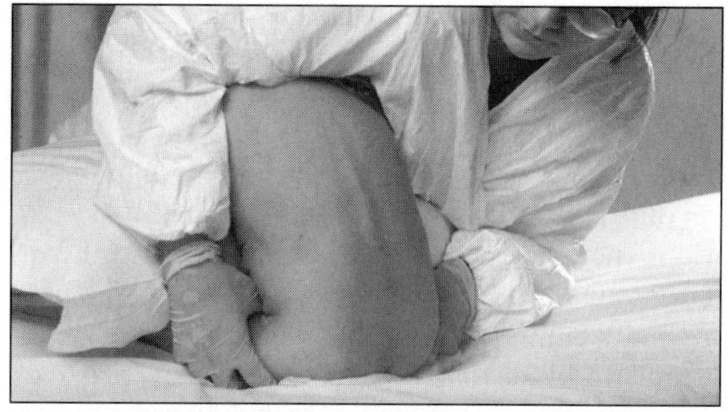

H: For the lumbar puncture: The nurse leans further down over the child using her upper body to hold the child still while bending the child's back into a convex curve. Both hands are used to hold the hips still.

The most common site of bone marrow aspiration is the posterior iliac crest. Other sites include the anterior iliac crest and the tibia.

PROCEDURE: *Bone Marrow Aspiration*

Because the reasons for a bone marrow aspiration are usually to rule out serious disease (such as leukemia) or to assess the progress of cancer treatment, the child and family need a tremendous amount of support and preparation prior to the procedure.

Preparing the Child and Family. The child should be told what she will feel and hear during the procedure. The physician performing the procedure should obtain consent. The child and family should be given the opportunity to ask questions about the procedure. This procedure is usually performed in a treatment room. The child will usually be given pre-procedural sedation.

Equipment

- Bone marrow aspiration tray
- Sterile gloves
- Sterile 2 × 2 gauze
- Tape
- Antiseptic ointment (povidone-iodine)
- Laboratory requisitions/labels

STEP-BY-STEP PROCEDURE

1. Position the child prone with a small pillow under the hips to facilitate access to the posterior iliac crest. If other sites are to be used, alter the position accordingly. The child may also be positioned sitting up the same as for lumbar punctures.
2. A nurse or parent should be positioned at the child's head. Although having parents present during painful procedures is controversial, studies have shown that most children prefer to have a parent present (Hamner & Miles, 1988).
3. Restrain the child adequately to prevent movement during the procedure. If adequate sedation has not been given, a second nurse may be needed to help restrain the child.
4. Explain to the child that she will feel something cold as her hip is washed and may feel a "stick and sting" when the physician injects local anesthetic. EMLA (Chapter 20) may be used for local anesthesia.
5. A needle is inserted into the bone and the marrow is withdrawn by suction. Explain that the child may feel a sharp pain as suction is applied to withdraw the marrow.
6. The marrow is examined for the presence of white marrow spicules. If they are not present, the syringe is reattached to the needle and aspiration is attempted again.
7. After the procedure is complete, the needle is withdrawn and pressure is applied to the site.
8. Cover the site with a pressure bandage or Band-Aid.
9. Return the child to her room and assess the child's vital signs until stable (this is particularly important if she has received pre-procedural sedation). The puncture site should be assessed for signs of bleeding or infection. After the child is fully recovered from sedation and the site shows no signs of complications, she may resume normal activities.

DOCUMENTATION

Record the date, time, and name of the physician performing the procedure. Note the patient's vital signs and the appearance of the specimen and the sampling site. Document the child's response to the procedure.

RESTRAINTS

Restraints are used for a variety of reasons in pediatric practice. Most often, they are used to prevent injury to the child or others, or to temporarily suspend movement during certain procedures to prevent trauma. All possible alternatives to restraint should be considered prior to applying the restraint. These may include utilizing a sitter; behavior modification techniques, such as time-out; or diversional activities, such as reading.

> If restraint is considered for unruly or dangerous behavior, the cause of the behavior should also be examined. Causes may include **hypoxia,** sedation, adverse drug reactions, and mental illness.

The Omnibus Budget Reconciliation Act (OBRA) of 1987 states that restraints should only be utilized as a last resort for the protection of the patient and others. The legislation further specifies that restraints should not be applied merely for the staff's convenience.

Physical restraints include such items as safety vests, mitts, and ankle and wrist restraints. They may require a physician's order stating why the restraint is needed and how long it will be in place. The restraint chosen should be the least restrictive device that will prevent injury (Tammelleo, 1992). The Food and Drug Administration (FDA, 1991), has also made recommendations for the use of restraints (see the accompanying box, Nursing Tips for the Restrained Child). Other methods of protective restraint, such as bubbles placed over a crib, should also be considered. See Figure 18–11 for examples of pediatric restraints.

Prior to placing the restraint, the area to be restrained should be checked for any sign of compromise of the circulatory, integumentary, and neurologic systems. Any orthopedic compromise should also be noted. If these conditions exist, extra monitoring of the restrained extremity will be needed.

Clove hitch restraint

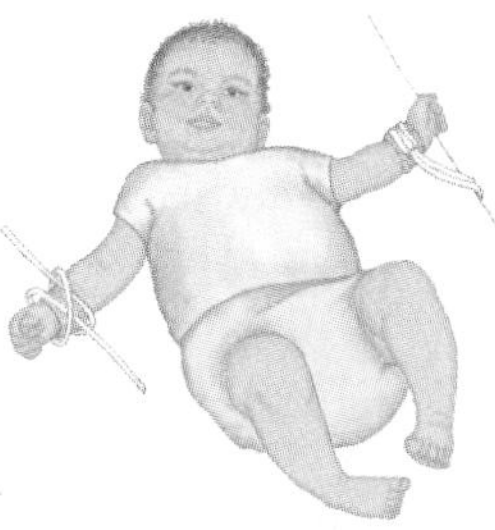

Prevents range of motion of extremities. Use on wrists or ankles.

Elbow restraint

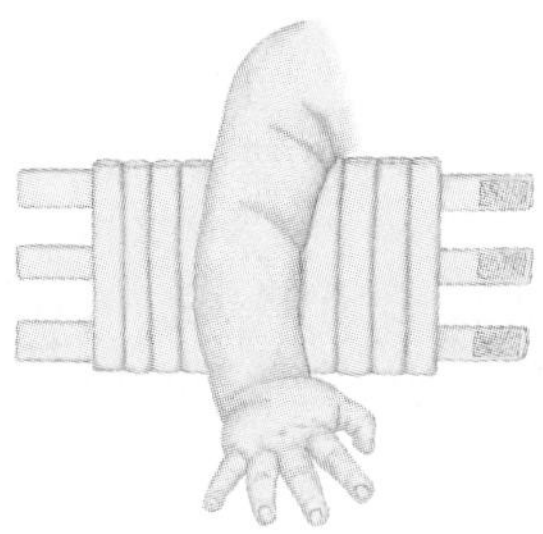

Prevents child from flexing and reaching face, head, IV and other tubes. Position so that it does not rub against the axilla.

Mummy restraint (body restraint)

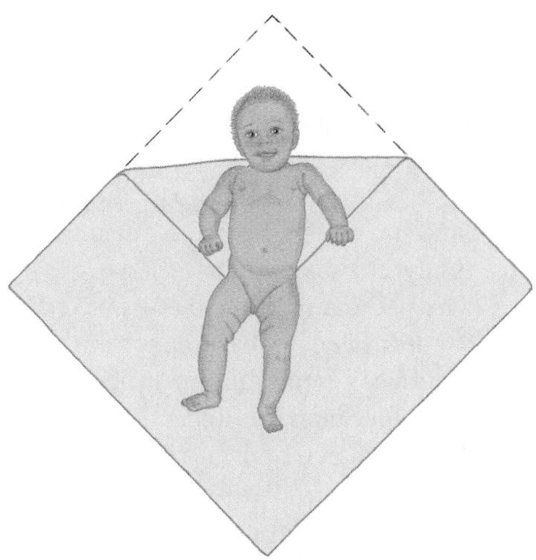

A restraint can be made from a sheet folded into a square of the appropriate size for the infant. Start by folding the top corner under the infant's shoulders and aligning his head with the folded edge.

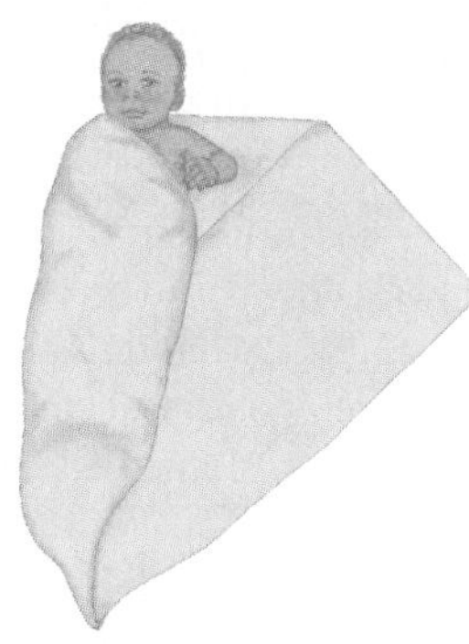

Fold one point of the sheet across the child and tuck it firmly behind his back.

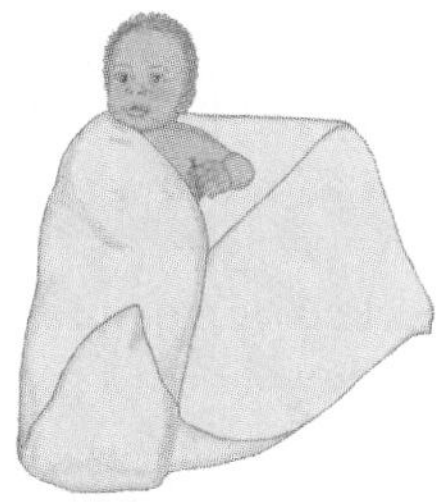

Fold the bottom corner of the sheet up to cover and restrain the infant's feet.

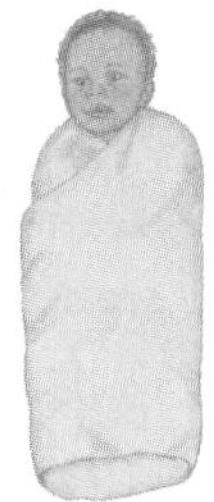

Fold the remaining corner over the child and tuck firmly behind his back.

Jacket restraint

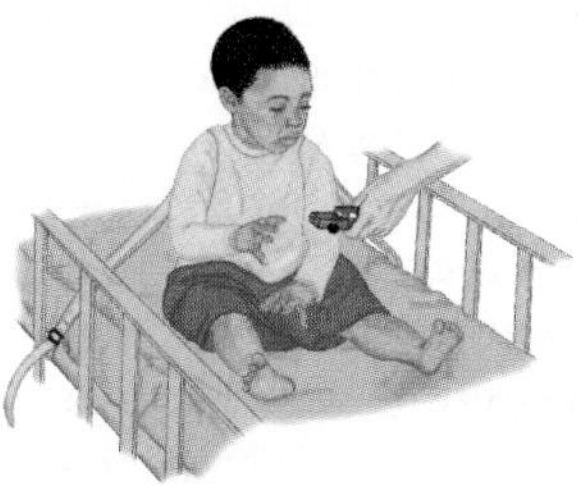

Tied to the back of the child and to the frame of the bed. Used primarily to keep children flat in bed after surgery.

Crib top bubble restraint

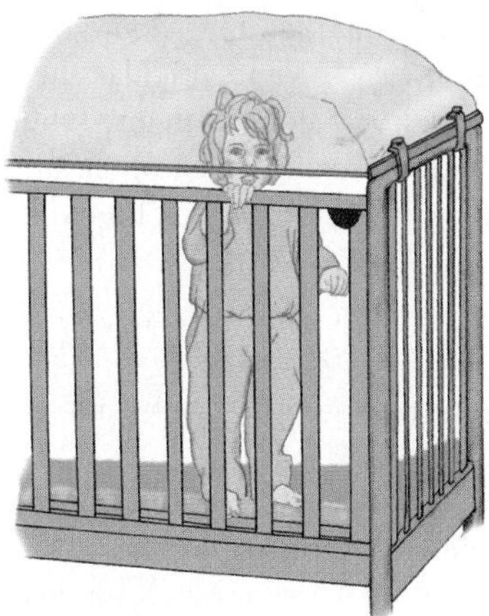

Prevents older infant and younger child from falling and climbing out of bed.

Figure 18–11
Examples of pediatric restraints.

NURSING TIPS FOR THE RESTRAINED CHILD

- Choose the proper device for the child's condition.
- Ensure proper fit of the device.
- Tie knots that can be easily untied for quick access.
- Secure ties to bed frames (not mattresses or side rails) or to the frames of wheelchairs, etc.

When restraints are applied, the child and family should be informed as to why the restraint will be used, where it will be applied, what movement it will prevent, and how long it will be in place. The nurse should tell the child and family how often he or she will be coming in to check on the child. The call button should be readily available to older children so the nurse may be summoned as needed. Developmental needs, such as thumb sucking, should also be considered and met, if possible. (For example, an infant's or toddler's arm can be restrained so that the thumb can still be placed in the mouth.)

Restraints should be checked 15 minutes following initial placement. After that, they should be checked at least every hour, and more often if a child is aggressive or extremely active. The restrained extremity should be checked for temperature, pulses, and capillary refill. Restraints should be removed every 2 hours to allow for range of motion and repositioning. The child should be offered food and bathroom breaks at least every 2 hours.

Documentation. Documentation must include what behavior was noted that led to the restraint and all attempts to calm the patient prior to the restraint application and his response (Tammelleo, 1992). If a decline in condition has led to the need for restraint, that, too, should be well documented (Tammelleo, 1992). Neurovascular checks should be documented every hour, along with any other changes. The removal of restraints, range of motion, and position changes should be documented every 2 hours.

ISOLATION

In 1985 *Universal Precautions* were introduced, which applied blood and body fluid precautions universally to all patients regardless of their diagnosis. This included the use of masks and eye coverings to protect against mucous membrane exposures and the use of individual ventilation devices. In 1987 *Body Substance Isolation* was implemented as an alternative to diagnosis-driven isolation. All moist and potentially infectious body substances (blood, feces, urine, sputum, saliva, wound drainage, and other body fluids) from all patients, regardless of their presumed infection status, were considered infectious and handled with gloves. Unfortunately, this system did not adequately address droplet transmission, transmission of microorganisms from dry skin or environmental sources, or airborne transmission. There are both similarities and differences in the characteristics of Universal Precautions and Body Substance Isolation. One difference is the individual recommendations for glove use and hand washing. The two systems caused confusion and were subject to individual interpretation.

A need for a new system was identified, and the major features of both systems were combined to create *Standard Precautions* (see Appendix G). Standard Precautions apply to:

- Blood
- All body fluids, secretions, and excretions, except sweat, regardless of whether they contain visible blood
- Nonintact skin
- Mucous membranes (Garner, 1996)

Under the new system there are two tiers of precautions. The first precautions (Standard Precautions) are for all hospitalized patients and are not based on diagnosis or presumed infection state. The second-tier precautions are for specific patients and are referred to as Transmission-Based Precautions. They are for patients known or suspected to be infected by pathogens that are transmitted by airborne or droplet transmission or by contact with dry skin or contaminated surfaces (see table in Appendix G). The complete guidelines for Standard Precautions, as well as airborne, droplet, and contact transmission, are quite detailed and extensive. Each facility is responsible for having these guidelines available and implemented.

It is important to remember that when Transmission-Based Precautions are being carried out, the items with which the child comes in contact are also contaminated. These include the bed, linens, IV pump, sink, toys, etc. Therefore, if the nurse is going into the room to reset an IV pump, pick up soiled linens, etc., she must utilize whatever protective equipment is mandated by the type of isolation.

These children often need extra attention to avert boredom. They need additional care paid to diversional activities, such as games, movies, etc. They also need added psychosocial support. Young children, for example, may feel that they are being punished. Finally, visitors may also be hesitant to come into the room and may need additional support.

Family Teaching. Family education is crucial, and it is important to emphasize to parents, other visitors, and other health care providers that these precautions are important and must be followed closely. Commonly, parents state that they are there to visit only that child and do not understand the need to wear special gear. The nurse must take care to acknowledge this, but to also remind the family that some diseases, such as respiratory syncytial virus, may live on inanimate objects, such as clothing, for up to 48 hours and can be spread throughout the hospital or to the home if the precautions are not followed.

FEVER-REDUCING MEASURES

The body's internal thermostat, the hypothalamus, attempts to keep the body's temperature between 96.8° and 100.4°F (36° to 38°C). This is done through a complex series of interactions which gain and lose heat. The body's mechanisms for conserving or producing heat are vasoconstriction and shivering. Heat is lost through radiation, conduction, convection, and evaporation (Enright & Hill, 1989).

Fever is defined as a body temperature greater than 38.0°C (100.4°F) rectally, or greater than 37.8°C (100°F) orally, that results from an insult or a disease during which the body's set-point temperature rises to a higher-than-normal level. After the cause of the fever is removed, the body resets its set-point at the normal level. Mild degrees of fever may or may not require intervention, depending on the underlying cause (Murphy, 1992; Soud, 1993).

There is no sure answer for the best approach to managing fevers secondary to infections. The body's attempt to defend itself against illness is manifested by fever. Therefore, it would be logical to assume that the body's natural defense mechanism would be thwarted if a fever were treated. Some reasons for not choosing to intervene include the following: (1) research studies have not yet clearly categorized fever as friend or foe; (2) most fevers are benign and self-limiting; (3) no data exist to support the theory that permanent damage is caused by a fever of a few degrees' elevation; (4) too rapid cooling can be dangerous and cause permanent damage; (5) fevers with serious etiologies can be masked by treatment; and (6) evidence exists to support the notion that the immune system is boosted by slight temperature elevation (Enright & Hill, 1989).

Fever is uncomfortable and children may become irritable. For every 1°C of temperature elevation, the body's metabolic rate will increase 10% (Bruce & Grove, 1992). Infants and children who have underlying cardiac, respiratory, or neurologic problems, or who are very ill may suffer serious consequences if their fevers are not treated aggressively (Enright & Hill, 1989). Regardless of the cause, the comfort of the child is the primary reason for treating a fever in a normally healthy child. Some children will have seizures associated with fever. These most commonly do not recur after the initial occurrence.

Nursing Interventions. The treatment of fever is dependent on the underlying cause and the degree of risk to the child. Treatment may consist of environmental measures, **antipyretics**, or a combination of interventions. Regardless of the methods used, it is important to explain to the

TABLE 18–2 *Dosage Chart for Children's and Junior Strength Tylenol (Acetaminophen)*

WEIGHT AND AGE	GRAPE SUSPENSION DROPS AND ORIGINAL FRUIT DROPS 80 MG/0.8 ML‡	BUBBLE GUM AND CHERRY SUSPENSION LIQUID AND ORIGINAL GRAPE AND CHERRY ELIXIR 160 MG/5 ML‡	BUBBLE GUM, GRAPE AND FRUIT CHEWABLES 80 MG TABS‡	JUNIOR STRENGTH CAPLETS AND GRAPE AND FRUIT CHEWABLES 160 MG‡
6–11 lb/0–3 months	½ dppr†	***	***	***
12–17 lb/4–11 months	1 dppr†	½ tsp	***	***
18–23 lb/12–23 months	1½ dppr†	¾ tsp	***	***
24–35 lb/2–3 years	2 dppr†	1 tsp	2 tab	***
36–47 lb/4–5 years		1½ tsp	3 tab	***
48–59 lb/6–8 years		2 tsp	4 tab	2 cap/tab
60–71 lb/9–10 years		2½ tsp	5 tab	2½ cap/tab
72–95 lb/11 years		3 tsp	6 tab	3 cap/tab
96 lb and over/12–14 years				4 cap/tab

Note to Parents: Consult a physician if your child's age or weight range is within the orange shaded area. Use only under physician's direction. Consult your physician as your child grows to be sure you are giving the most accurate dose based on your child's weight and age.

†0.8 ml dropperful (dropper enclosed in package)

‡Doses should be administered 4 or 5 times daily or as directed by your doctor. Do not exceed 5 doses in 24 hours.

***Do not use this form in this weight/age unless directed by a physician.

Consult your physician if fever persists for more than 3 days or if pain continues for more than 5 days. In case of accidental overdosage, contact a physician or poison control center immediately.

A calibrated dropper or dosage cup is included in each liquid pacakge.

Note: Do not use with other products containing acetaminophen.

Courtesy of McNeil Consumer Products Company, Division of McNeil-PPC, Inc., Fort Washington, PA 19034.

child and the family the reason for intervention and the method of intervention chosen to reduce the child's temperature (Gildea, 1992).

External cooling is one of the oldest and most common forms of fever management, particularly when the elevated temperature is caused by hyperthermia. External cooling can be accomplished by tepid sponge baths, mechanical cooling blankets, reduction of the environmental temperature, and removal of clothing and blankets.

In febrile illnesses, the body attempts to resist external cooling, resulting in the need for administration of antipyretics in addition to external cooling interventions. Fevers may be treated with antipyretics, such as acetaminophen, aspirin, and NSAIDs. Acetaminophen (Table 18–2) is usually the drug of choice owing to the association between Reye's syndrome and aspirin use in children with viral illnesses, such as influenza and varicella, as well as the limitations of NSAID use in children younger than 12 years of age.

Children with elevated temperatures often experience a loss of appetite. Dehydration can occur owing to decreased oral intake and increased insensible water loss through the lungs and the skin. The need for adequate hydration can be met by offering the child additional oral fluids. For those who refuse oral hydration or who are unable to take in adequate volume, fluids may be given intravenously.

It is important to remember that infants who are being cared for in servocontrolled heating environments must be carefully monitored owing to the potential for accidental dislodgment of the skin temperature probe. This can cause an increase in the heat production of the unit and a resulting increase in the infant's temperature. In addition, the insensible water loss for infants in these controlled units is greatly increased. These additional fluid losses must be considered when calculating fluid replacement.

PROCEDURE: *Sponge Bath*

Infants and children who are hyperthermic respond well to the use of cooling measures, such as sponging and tepid baths. If a cool bath is the intervention chosen, the water temperature should be between 85° and 90°F (29° and 32°C).

> The use of rubbing alcohol is contraindicated because of skin irritation, the risk of neurologic depression from the fumes or absorption through the skin, and too rapid cooling, which can result in shivering.

Preparing the Child and Family. Explain the purpose and the reason for selecting the intervention using developmentally appropriate language. If possible, provide toys or some other distraction for the child. The parent may be present to help comfort or play with the child.

Equipment

- Tepid water
- Washcloths
- Toys

STEP-BY-STEP PROCEDURE

1. Assist the infant or child to sit or lie in a position of comfort in the bed.
2. Using tepid water, wet the washcloths or towels and place them on the child, exposing one area at a time. Tepid water is used because it allows the body temperature to drop gradually, thus avoiding heat-producing responses, such as shivering, which are caused by too rapid cooling.
3. Dry the child, dress her in lightweight clothing or pajamas, and place in a dry bed.
4. Recheck the child's temperature approximately 30 minutes later to assess the effectiveness of the intervention. If shivering occurs, the procedure should be terminated immediately.

When the child is placed in a tub:

5. The child can also be placed in a tub of warm water, with cool water being added until the desired temperature is reached.
6. Gently pour or spray water over the child's back and chest. Continue this for 20 to 30 minutes. Water toys can be used to provide distraction during this nursing intervention.

> An infant or young child should never be left unattended in the tub!

7. Dry the child, dress him in lightweight clothing or pajamas, and place in a dry bed.
8. Recheck the child's temperature approximately 30 minutes later to assess the effectiveness of the intervention. If shivering occurs, the procedure should be terminated immediately.

DOCUMENTATION

Document in the nurses' notes the child's baseline vital signs, hydration status, general appearance, interventions used for fever reduction, the indications for the interventions, the duration, the patient's response, and any problems identified. Any teaching done with the family, as well as their degree of understanding of the information given, should also be documented.

Parent Teaching

Parents often need education about caring for the child with an elevated temperature. Information may include: how to take a temperature, how to read a thermometer, normal temperature parameters, administration of antipyretics, administration of tepid baths, and when to seek professional help. It is important to emphasize in your teaching that ice water and isopropyl alcohol should never be used for sponging or bathing the child with a fever. Ice water and alcohol can cause rapid cooling, peripheral vasoconstriction, and chilling, thus elevating the temperature even further due to shivering (Soud, 1993). Also, the nurse should emphasize the importance of accuracy in dosing, the timing of doses, methods of administration, and appropriate medication choices when giving antipyretics.

Parents need reassurance that fever is a common symptom of illness. A fever rarely poses a threat to the well-being of a child. The way a child looks and acts is more important in evaluating the severity of an illness than is the degree of fever (Soud, 1993).

PROCEDURE: *Using Commercial Cooling Blankets*

Commercial cooling blankets may also be used to control hyperthermia. These units, which can be controlled manually or automatically, lower the body temperature through cold transfer between the blanket and the child. Cooling unit operation varies among manufacturers. Therefore, it is important to read the operation manual prior to using this equipment. Some cooling blankets may be reusable; however, blankets designed for single-patient use are preferred.

Some concerns to be aware of when using a cooling blanket include shivering, frostbite, and skin breakdown.

Preparing the Child and Family. Explain the purpose and the reason for selection of the cooling blanket using developmentally appropriate language. If possible, a parent may be present to help comfort or distract the child.

Equipment

- Cooling blanket
- Sheets or small blankets as needed
- Temperature probe

STEP-BY-STEP PROCEDURE

1. Place the cooling blanket on the bed and cover it with a sheet or thin blanket.
2. Connect the blanket to the cooling unit and set the control mode (manual or automatic) and the desired blanket or body temperature. Temperature parameters should be set according to manufacturer's recommendations and physician's orders.
3. Check the skin condition of the child before, during, and after use of the blanket and document the findings.
4. Cover the child lightly to maintain privacy and reduce shivering.
5. Monitor the child's vital signs frequently to prevent too rapid cooling or overcooling. A temperature probe can be used to monitor the patient's temperature continually during this cooling method.
6. Extremities can be wrapped with towels or baby blankets to reduce shivering.
7. Keep the child completely dry to reduce the risk of frostbite from dampness.
8. Reposition the child on a cooling unit frequently and gently to reduce the risk of skin breakdown.

DOCUMENTATION

Document the type of unit used, control mode and temperature settings selected as well as the condition of the child's skin before, during, and after use.

GAVAGE AND GASTROSTOMY FEEDINGS

Some infants and children are unable to tolerate adequate nutrition orally owing to prematurity, illness, injury, congenital anomalies, previous surgeries, respiratory distress, swallowing disorders, or neurologic impairment. For these children, an alternative method of feeding must be selected. The physician may order **enteral** feedings via an orogastric, nasogastric, or transpyloric route or a gastrostomy tube or gastrostomy button.

Tube Route and Placement. Placement of a gastrostomy tube or gastrostomy button is a surgical procedure performed by the surgeon. Placement of an orogastric, nasogastric, or transpyloric tube is usually done by a nurse. Nasogastric tubes are used most commonly, but patients with head or nasal anomalies or injuries, or infants who are still preferential nose breathers (usually those 4 months of age or younger), will require orogastric tube placement.

A disadvantage of nasal placement of feeding tubes is the potential for interference with respiratory function owing to increased mucus production caused by irritation by the tube. However, nasal placement does make the tube easier to stabilize than oral tube placement (Hill & Rath, 1993).

A transpyloric tube is more difficult to insert than an orogastric or nasogastric tube. It also requires radiographic confirmation of correct placement. Although various methods may be used to secure the tube, the desired position of the tube is often difficult to maintain (Hill & Rath, 1993).

There is controversy regarding measurement of the length of the tube to be inserted. The two most common methods of measurement are: (1) from the nose to the ear and to the end of the xiphoid process; and (2) from the nose to the ear and to a point midway between the xiphoid process and umbilicus. Studies have looked at the role height places in gastric insertion distance and, in low-birth-weight infants, weight. Additional research is needed in this area.

Tube Selection. There are many types and sizes of tubes commercially available. Feeding tubes should be selected according to the child's age, size, the viscosity of the formula, the reason for enteral feeding, and whether an infusion device will be used. By selecting the smallest-bore tube for the infusion, preferably of soft material, the child's discomfort will be decreased. The age, weight, and size of the infant or child determine the size of the tube to be used. Infants require a No. 5–10 French tube, and the size increases proportionately.

Safety Issues. Tube placement must be verified at the time the tube is inserted, any time feeding is interrupted, prior to each bolus feeding, and every 4 to 8 hours during continuous feeding (Metheny, 1993).

The most reliable methods for checking tube placement are auscultation, aspiration of enteral fluid, and pH measurement of the aspirate. Insufflation of air (1–5 ml in infants and small children; 5–20 ml in adolescents) through the tube while auscultating over the epigastrium, stomach, or left upper quadrant for a distinctive "whooshing" or "gurgling" sound will indicate whether the tube is in the stomach. Aspiration of enteral fluid also will indicate whether the tube is in the stomach (pH of 1–4) or in the duodenum (pH of 6–7) (Strong, Gribbon, Durling, & Condon, 1988).

> Do not assume that a feeding tube has remained in its proper position just because the external position has not changed.

Tubes can become dislodged with suctioning, retching, or vomiting (Metheny, 1993). Transpyloric tube placement should be confirmed radiographically prior to initiating feedings and any time the tube position is questioned.

> **CONTRAINDICATIONS** Determine any pre-existing contraindications for the procedure, such as prior surgeries or trauma or congenital anomalies (e.g., choanal atresia, tracheoesophageal fistula, esophageal strictures) which could interfere with passage of the tube. If any of these findings are present, the physician may want to use fluoroscopy to guide tube insertion. DO NOT reinsert a dislodged tube that was placed during or through a surgical repair. Notify the surgeon if this occurs.

PROCEDURE: *Feeding Tube Insertion*

Preparing the Child and Family. Explain the procedure to the patient and family using developmentally appropriate language. Assess their needs and concerns related to the procedure, such as previous experience with tube insertion, ability to assist with the procedure, and need for restraint. Play therapy can be utilized to allay the child's and parents' fears related to the procedure.

Equipment

- Feeding tube of appropriate size and type
- $\frac{1}{4}$- or $\frac{1}{2}$-inch hypoallergenic tape
- Syringe
- Sterile water for oral use
- Stethoscope
- Feeding pump and setup (enteral feeding bag or burette)
- Lubricating jelly (for nasal insertion only)
- pH reagent strips
- Gloves

STEP-BY-STEP PROCEDURE

1. Position the child so that she is on her back or right side with the head of the bed elevated. A small child can also be held in a parent's arms, with the child's head on the parent's shoulder. An older child may sit up in the bed. Restrain if necessary.
2. Wash your hands and don gloves.
3. Measure the length of the catheter to be inserted and mark with waterproof marker or with tape. To determine the appropriate length, see the accompanying box.
4. Lubricate the tube with water or water-soluble lubricant to facilitate passage through the nasopharynx. Follow the manufacturer's recommendations regarding injection of water through the tube and lubricant.

> In neonates and for orogastric placement, use water only.

5. Insert the tube gently but firmly through the mouth or nose and down the throat.

> If obstruction is met or if the tube curls in the mouth, remove the tube and repeat this step. If gasping, coughing, or gagging occur, withdraw the tube and wait for these to subside before proceeding.

6. Continue to advance the tube gently to the predetermined mark.

   For infants: Encourage an infant's swallowing by using a pacifier.

   For cooperative children: Ask the child to swallow repeatedly when the tube reaches the pharynx, or give small sips of water through a straw if not contraindicated.

7. Temporarily secure the tube with tape to check tube position.

Measuring and Inserting Feeding Tubes

CHILD, NASOGASTRIC TUBE

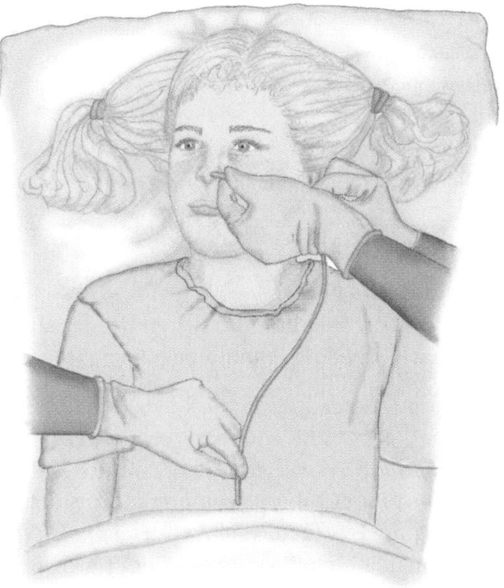

Measuring tube
Measure the distance from the tip of the nose to the earlobe and then down to the xiphoid process. Mark the total measurement with tape or indelible marker.

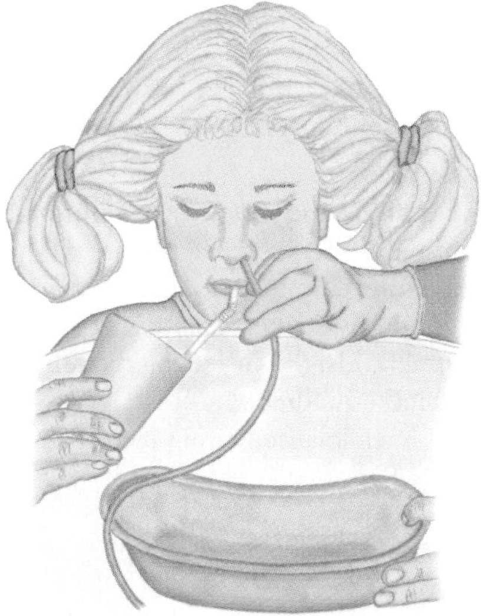

Inserting tube through nose
Insert the tube into the nose and gently advance it along the floor of the naris to the occiput. Pause when the tube enters the oropharynx and ask the child to flex her head forward and sip water. This will ease insertion into the esophagus. Advance the tube 5-10 cm with each swallow. Remove the tube immediately if she gasps for air, as this indicates possible insertion into the airway.

NEONATE, OROGASTRIC TUBE

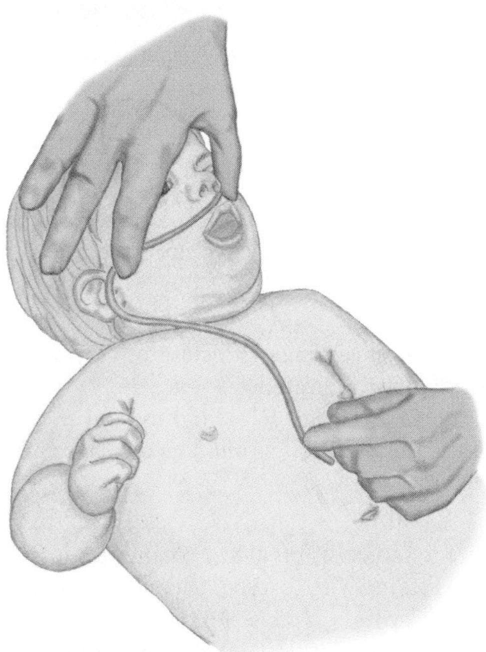

Measuring tube for gavage feeding
Measure the tube from tip of nose to earlobe and to midpoint between end of xiphoid process and umbilicus. The total measurement, NEX (Nose–ear–xiphoid) should be marked on tube with tape or indelible marker.

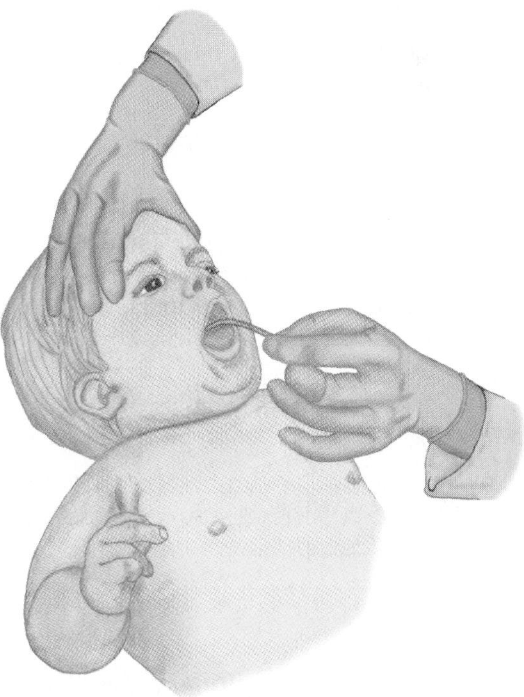

Inserting tube
Insert the lubricated tube to the predetermined mark. Direct the tube toward the back of the throat. Insertion through the mouth helps to stimulate sucking. If possible, encourage swallowing.

8. Attach a syringe to the end of the tube and attempt to aspirate gastric contents. Insufflate 1 to 5 ml of air while auscultating over the stomach area.

> Choking or soundless coughing may indicate placement in the trachea. Accidental placement of a small-diameter tube into the lungs may not be as apparent as with larger tubes, particularly if the child's cough or gag reflex is absent or suppressed (Wilson, 1986).

9. Check the pH of the aspirate to confirm gastric (pH of 1–4 usually) or intestinal placement (pH of 6–7 usually). [**Note:** Administration of antacid and gastric acid inhibitors will alter the pH of the aspirate to near-neutral levels, thus affecting the reliability of the pH test (Metheny, 1988).]

> If a transpyloric tube (TPT) with a guidewire has been used:
>
> - Remove the guidewire by holding the tube at the patient's nostril or corner of mouth and slowly removing it. Keep the patient on the right side to allow gravity to assist in the advancement of the tube into the duodenum.
>
> A plain abdominal film will be ordered by the physician to confirm tube placement in the duodenum.

10. Once tube placement is confirmed, tape the tube securely in place.
11. Label the tube with the date and time of insertion.
12. Refer to your facility's policy/procedure manual for recommended frequency of tube change.

DOCUMENTATION

Document in the nurses' notes the size and type of tube used, route, placement, pH testing results, results of auscultation, date and time of insertion, patient/family teaching, procedure tolerance, and any problems encountered.

Parent Teaching

Parental instruction as to how to insert and check placement of the tube as well as comfort measures that may be helpful, may need to be given by the nurse if the child will be receiving enteral nutrition at home.

PROCEDURE: *Administering Enteral Feedings (via the Orogastric, Nasogastric, or Transpyloric Route)*

Preparing the Child and Family. Explain the procedure to the patient and family using developmentally appropriate language. Assess their needs and concerns related to the procedure, such as previous experience with enteral feedings, ability to assist with the procedure, and need for restraint. Play therapy can be utilized to allay the child's and parents fears related to the procedure.

Equipment

- Stethoscope
- Catheter-tip syringe
- Formula and water at room temperature
- Pacifier (neonates and infants)

STEP-BY-STEP PROCEDURE

Intermittent Feedings (Bolus)

Bolus feedings are used ONLY when the feeding tube is in the stomach. Feedings should be given at room temperature to avoid abdominal discomfort (McGee, 1987).

1. Position the patient and remove the syringe or cap from the tube.
2. Check for proper tube placement and residual volume from the previous feed. Follow the facility's policy/procedure manual or physician's orders for disposition of residual volume.
3. Remove the plunger from the syringe and attach the syringe to the tube.
4. Pour room-temperature formula into the syringe and allow the feeding to flow slowly into the tube (usually over a period of 20–25 minutes).

> Discontinue the feeding if signs of respiratory distress, cyanosis, abdominal distension, or vomiting occur. Notify the physician.

5. After the prescribed volume has been infused, rinse the tube with sterile water and clear the tube by injecting 1–5 ml of air.

> In neonates, the tube may be cleared only with air (1 ml).

6. Discard the used syringe and close or clamp the tube unless otherwise indicated.
7. Leave the patient lying on the right side with the head of the bed elevated for 30 minutes to 1 hour after the feeding.

> During enteral feeds, provide a pacifier for infants to associate sucking with feeding. Older children may be encouraged to sit at a table during meals to promote the normal socialization associated with eating.

Continuous Feedings

1. Position the patient and check tube placement.
2. Fill the feeding bag, volume control set, or syringe and tubing with the prescribed formula.

Provide feeding over a period of 4 hours to avoid accidental overfeeding should the infusion pump malfunction.

3. Attach infusion tubing to the feeding tube and begin the infusion at the prescribed rate.
4. Check tube placement and residual volumes every 4 hours.

Follow the facility's policy/procedure manual or physician's orders regarding disposition of residual volumes.

5. Keep the child positioned on his abdomen or right side to reduce the incidence of reflux and aspiration.

Feeding solutions should not hang for longer than 6–8 hours (McGee, 1987). Check the facility's policy/procedure manual for the prescribed frequency for changing feeding equipment.

DOCUMENTATION

If aspirate was present, record the amount, color, and consistency. Note whether it was re-fed or discarded. Note the type and amount of formula and the child's tolerance of the procedure. Note the position of the child after feeding and whether the tube is clamped or open, which allows venting.

Parent Teaching

Assess the parents' ability to perform enteral feedings. Parents should be encouraged to make this as normal a procedure as possible (e.g., by holding the infant during feedings). Parents should be asked to demonstrate the procedure to the nurse. Assistance at home may be provided by a home health agency.

PROCEDURE: *Administering Gastrostomy Feedings*

The procedure for gastrostomy feedings is much the same as that for orogastric, nasogastric, or transpyloric feedings. The feeding formula should be at room temperature before feeding. The child should be properly positioned during the feeding and maintained in that position for at least 1 hour after the feeding to promote gastric emptying and to reduce the incidence of reflux and aspiration (Huddleston & Ferraro, 1991).

As with any tube feeding, the infant or young child should be held during the feeding, when possible, to associate the feeding with pleasant sensations and socialization, and to promote normal development and bonding. *A pacifier should be offered to infants to stimulate non-nutritive sucking* (McGee, 1987).

Special considerations for patients with gastrostomy tubes or buttons include skin and stoma site care. Assess the site for abnormal findings, such as leakage, redness around the site, drainage, bleeding, and skin breakdown. The skin should be cleaned with soap and water once or twice daily, depending on the condition, and with each spillage (Steele, 1991).

Gastrostomy buttons should be rotated in a full circle during cleaning to facilitate complete cleansing. Buttons offer the added advantage of allowing children to participate in regular childhood activities, such as swimming. Parents also report fewer problems with clothing (Steele, 1991).

Preparing the Child and Family. Explain the procedure to the patient and family using developmentally appropriate language. Assess their needs and concerns related to the procedure, such as previous experience with tube insertion, ability to assist with the procedure, and need for restraint. Play therapy can be utilized to allay the child's and parents' fears related to the procedure.

Equipment

Same as for administering orogastric, nasogastric, and transpyloric feedings

STEP-BY-STEP PROCEDURE

1. The procedure for positioning and feeding is the same as in orogastric, nasogastric, and transpyloric feedings except for the following:
   a. Do not aspirate residual formula.
   b. Note any resistance and follow facility policy.
   c. If the abdomen is distended prior to a feeding, check for residual by suspending an empty syringe attached to the tube and observing backflow of stomach contents.
   d. The tube may be clamped or left open.
   e. Some button gastrostomy tubes have a special tube for decompression. The one-way valve of the button prevents aspiration of gastric contents.
   f. The child with a button requires frequent burping.

Parent Teaching

Parents should be encouraged to make this as normal a procedure as possible (e.g., by holding the infant during feedings). Parents should demonstrate the procedure to the nurse. Assistance at home may be provided by a home health agency.

DOCUMENTATION

Record in the nurses' notes the date and time of the feeding; confirmation of tube placement; the color, consistency, residual volume and disposition of aspirate (refed/discarded); type and volume of feeding and irrigant; child's tolerance of feeding; and any patient/family teaching and their understanding of information given. Watch for signs that the tube or button may need to be replaced, such as leaking, tube occlusion, antireflux valve malfunction, or abnormal tube position. Report these findings to the physician.

Parent Teaching

Many children are discharged home with gastrostomy tubes. Parents must be able to provide all required care. Parent teaching is a major part of the nursing care of a child with a feeding tube. Parents must know how to check tube position, how to administer feedings, how to care for the tube, what symptoms should be reported, and what to do if the tube becomes dislodged. Booklets are available that can assist the family in the care of the child with a gastrostomy tube or button.

Mealtime is considered to be a social time. When possible, parents should feed the child at the same time that others are being fed in order to maintain and nurture normal family relationships (McGee, 1987).

ENEMAS

Enemas may be given when stool needs to be removed from the bowel because of severe constipation or in preparation for a diagnostic procedure or surgery. Giving an enema to an infant or child differs very little from the procedure for an adult. The exceptions are the type and amount of fluid administered and the distance that the enema tip is inserted into the rectum.

Rectal damage and perforation can occur with improper insertion of the enema tip.

Solutions and Volumes. The amount of the enema solution will vary with the age and size of the child. Unless the physician's orders specify a different amount, the values listed in Table 18–3 for volume and depth of enema insertion into the rectum are recommended.

Only isotonic solutions should be used with children. Plain tap water should never be used because it is hypotonic and can cause a rapid fluid shift and fluid overload.

TABLE 18–3 *Recommended Volume and Depth for Enema Insertion, by Age*

	VOLUME	DEPTH OF INSERTION
Infants	120–240	1 inch (2.5 cm)
2–4 years	240–360	2 inches (5.0 cm)
4–10 years	360–480	3 inches (7.5 cm)
11 years and older	480–720	4 inches (10.0 cm)

PROCEDURE: *Administering an Enema*

Preparing the Child and Family. Explain the procedure and its purpose to the child and family in developmentally appropriate language. Determine their previous experience with the procedure and allow the child and family to voice questions and concerns.

Equipment

- Lukewarm enema solution
- Diaper, bedpan, potty chair, or toilet
- Enema bag and tubing
- Lubricant
- Rectal tube of appropriate size
- Gloves
- Towels and washcloths

STEP-BY-STEP PROCEDURE

1. Close the door or the curtain to provide privacy for the child during the procedure.
2. Wash hands and don gloves.
3. Position the child in one of the following positions: (1) prone with knees and hips bent toward the chest, (2) on left side with right leg flexed (Sims position), or (3) sitting on the bedside commode or toilet.
4. Pad the bed with towels. The bedpan may be placed under the buttocks.
5. Remove the plastic tip from the enema bottle/tubing.
6. Prime the tubing and lubricate the tip well.
7. Separate the buttocks and gently insert the catheter tip into the rectum.
8. Slowly administer the solution, allowing it to flow by gravity into the rectum.

If the child shows any signs of distress, stop the flow of the solution immediately.

9. Remove the enema tip and hold the buttocks together for a few minutes (if the child is unable to do so) to assist in retention of the solution.
10. Diaper infants. Toddlers may use the bedpan or "potty" if possible. Older children and adolescents may use the bedpan or bedside commode or be assisted to the bathroom.
11. After evacuation, wash or assist in washing the soiled area.
12. Discard used equipment in the proper receptacle; remove gloves and wash hands.

DOCUMENTATION

Document in the nurses' notes/I & O sheet the following: date and time the enema was given, the type and amount of solution, the amount and characteristics of stool, any unusual findings (blood, mucus, foreign bodies, worms, etc.), and the patient's tolerance of the procedure.

Parent Teaching

Explain the procedure and its purpose to the child and family in developmentally appropriate language. Determine the family's previous experience with the procedure and allow the child and family to voice questions and concerns.

CARE OF OSTOMIES

Urinary and fecal diversion is required when normal methods of elimination are temporarily or permanently halted. Some conditions requiring the creation of a stoma include imperforate anus, Hirschsprung's disease, necrotizing enterocolitis, some cases of intestinal atresia, intussusception, Crohn's disease, and ulcerative colitis. The anatomic location of the stoma will dictate the consistency of the stool. The higher the stoma, the more liquid the stool. Urinary diversion is usually the result of obstructive uropathy, congenital anomalies, or (occasionally) neurogenic bladder. The ureters may be brought out through the abdominal wall (ureterostomy) or connected to a segment of small bowel (ileal conduit).

Nursing Care. Nursing care of the child with an ostomy focuses on (1) minimizing the obstacles the child/family faces in learning to care for the ostomy, (2) encouraging the child and family to be actively involved in the treatment regimen, (3) providing support and guidance, and (4) making appropriate referrals to an enterostomal therapist or other support system.

The actual management and care of pediatric ostomies differs little from that in adults with ostomies. The major difference is the need to use developmentally appropriate terminology to explain the procedure and care of the ostomy to the child and family. A "teaching model," such as a doll with a stoma, may facilitate patient/family education.

In many cases, a pediatric ostomy appliance is fitted soon after surgery. This allows for accurate measurement of stoma output from the pouch. If an appliance has not been applied, a piece of Vaseline gauze and dry dressing can be placed over the stoma and the output measured by weighing the wet dressing and comparing it to the dry weight (1 ml = 1 g). Early application of an ostomy appliance also helps prevent excoriation of surrounding skin.

Young children may pull at the stoma pouch in an attempt to remove it. If this occurs, a cloth diaper or dressing may be used to cover the area. Older children can participate in the care of the stoma, including skin care, application of the appliance, and identification of potential problems. Each child should be evaluated on an individual basis to determine his or her developmental level and desire to assume partial responsibility for the care of his or her stoma.

PROCEDURE: *Care of an Ostomy Without an Appliance*

Preparing the Child and Family. Explain the procedure and its purpose to the child and family in developmentally appropriate language. Determine their previous experience with the procedure and allow the child and family to voice questions and concerns.

Equipment

- Basin of warm water
- A product that aids in removal of adhesive material
- Mild soap
- Skin barrier
- Towels and washcloths
- Skin sealant
- Scissors
- Petroleum gauze
- Diaper
- Gauze
- Gloves

STEP-BY-STEP PROCEDURE

1. Assist the child into a position of comfort.
2. Don gloves (and gown, if indicated) to maintain Standard Precautions.
3. Remove diaper(s) and place in an appropriate receptacle.
4. Remove peristomal skin barrier by gently removing wafer or paste.
5. Gently and thoroughly wash the skin using warm water and a mild soap. Carefully assess the stoma and surrounding skin. Report any abnormal findings, such as discoloration of the stoma (which should be deep pink to cherry red), excessive bleeding, skin rash, or signs of skin breakdown.
6. Assess the stoma output for volume, consistency, and odor in relation to the type and location of the stoma.

Urinary stomas should begin draining immediately after surgery (Petillo, 1987). Output from ileostomies and colostomies will be minimal during the first 48 to 96 hours after surgery.

7. Wipe the peristomal skin with skin sealant.

Use a tightly rolled piece of gauze placed over the stoma to act as a wick during cleaning. The skin must be completely dry before applying the skin barrier to ensure adherence to the skin and to prevent leaks.

8. Apply a protective barrier (wafer or paste/powder). If using a wafer, use the template provided to cut a hole that is slightly larger than the stoma. Paste/powder should be applied in a thick, even coat over the peris-

tomal skin and should extend from the stoma's edge outward in a 3-inch radius.

9. Apply a folded cloth diaper over the stoma and secure it with a regular diaper, tape, or pins.
10. Discard disposable items, soiled linens, and gloves in appropriate receptacles and wash hands.

DOCUMENTATION

Note the condition of the stoma and peristomal skin. The amount and characteristics of the ostomy drainage and the type of dressing applied should also be documented. Note any child/parent teaching and/or psychosocial problems or body image disturbance related to the surgery.

Parent Teaching

Encourage patient/family participation in stoma care as early as possible to ease the transition of the patient into the home setting.

PROCEDURE: *Care of an Ostomy With an Appliance*

Preparing the Child and Family. Explain the procedure and its purpose to the child and family using developmentally appropriate language. Determine their previous experience with the procedure and allow the child and family to voice questions and concerns.

Equipment

- Gloves
- Washcloth, towel, warm water, mild soap.
- Skin barrier (wafer or paste/powder)
- Ostomy pouch with clamp
- Gauze squares (to be held against stoma to absorb fluids/drainage during barrier application)

STEP-BY-STEP PROCEDURE

1. Assist the child into a position of comfort.
2. Don gloves (and gown if indicated) to maintain Standard Precautions.
3. Remove diaper(s) and place in an appropriate receptacle.
4. Remove the pouch and barrier as a single unit and discard in an appropriate receptacle.
5. Gently and thoroughly wash the skin using warm water and a mild soap. Carefully assess the stoma and surrounding skin. Report any abnormal findings, such as discoloration of the stoma (which should be deep pink to cherry red), excessive bleeding, skin rash, or signs of skin breakdown.
6. Assess the stoma output for volume, consistency, and odor in relation to the type and location of the stoma.

> Output from ileostomies and colostomies will be minimal during the first 48 to 96 hours after surgery.

> Urinary stomas should begin draining immediately after surgery (Petillo, 1987).

7. Wipe peristomal skin with skin sealant.

> Use a tightly rolled piece of gauze placed over the stoma to act as a wick during cleaning. The skin must be completely dry before applying the skin barrier to ensure adherence to the skin and to prevent leaks.

8. Apply a protective barrier (wafer or paste/powder). If using a wafer, use the template provided to cut a hole that is slightly larger than the stoma. Paste/powder should be applied in a thick, even coat over the peristomal skin and should extend from the stoma's edge outward in a 3-inch radius (Erickson, 1987).
9. If using a two-piece unit, attach the pouch to the barrier with the center hole over the stoma. Press the entire unit carefully, progressing from the stoma base outward, maintaining smooth, wrinkle-free skin contact.
10. Apply the clamp to the end of the bag. Hold hand over pouch for a minute to secure to skin. Warmth helps pouch to stretch. Apply date and time of change.
11. Discard disposable items, soiled linens, and gloves in appropriate receptacles and wash hands.

> If paste is difficult to remove, dry well, dust with powder, and then remove.

Between Appliance Changes

The pouch may require emptying between appliance changes, usually when it is half full.

13. Open the clamp on the bag and empty the contents into a collection container.
14. Rinse the inside of the pouch with water injected with a 60-ml syringe and allow the fluid to drain into the collection container.
15. Assess the integrity of the skin barrier and observe for any leaks or tears.
16. Dry the outside of the bag with a tissue and reapply the clamp.

DOCUMENTATION

Record in the nurses' notes the date and time of the procedure, the condition of the stoma and peristomal skin, the amount and characteristics of the drainage, the procedure performed, the type of skin preparation used, and any abnormal findings. Note any child/parent teaching that takes place and their level of involvement in the care. Note any psychosocial problems related to body image disturbance.

Parent Teaching

Child/parent teaching should include the reason for the ostomy surgery, the expected stooling pattern and consistency of the stoma output, special nutritional needs and dietary modifications, any medications needed and their effects on the ostomy, signs and symptoms of potential problems, when to notify the physician or enterostomal therapist, supplies needed for care, where to obtain the supplies, support groups, and potential financial aid resources for supplies. The physician or stomal therapist should be notified if the child experiences excessive **diarrhea,** bleeding, absence of stomal output or flatus, prolapse, or skin breakdown.

OXYGEN THERAPY

Hypoxemia, resulting from apnea or inadequate ventilation, occurs more rapidly in children than in adults because of the former's higher metabolic rate and increased oxygen consumption. Early recognition of subtle signs and symptoms of respiratory distress are necessary skills for every nurse.

Cardiopulmonary arrest in children is usually the end result of progressive respiratory distress.

Oxygen is an essential body requirement for any energy-consuming activity or function. For infants and children who are unable to maintain a normal PaO_2, supplemental oxygen may be required. Because oxygen is a drug, it requires a physician's order prior to administration, except in an emergency situation.

Follow your facility's policy for oxygen administration in emergency situations.

Oxygen may be administered by many methods, including a nasal cannula, face mask (simple, non-rebreather, partial rebreather, Venturi, or aerosol), oxygen-hood, or tent (Fig. 18–12). The method of delivery depends on the concentration needed and the ability of the child to cooperate with the chosen method.

In most facilities, a respiratory therapist is responsible for the setup, maintenance, and management of oxygen equipment. However, it is important for the nurse to have a working knowledge of the oxygen delivery system being used.

Oxygen administration systems for pediatric patients differ very little from those used in the adult population. The primary differences are the size of the equipment and the teaching and emotional support required for children/families receiving oxygen. Usually, an oxygen hood is used to provide maximum oxygenation for neonates and infants. Older infants and young toddlers may better tolerate a nasal cannula, blow-by oxygen, or face mask. Nasal cannula, blow-by, and face mask oxygen delivery works well for toddlers and preschoolers. School-age children and adolescents prefer non-rebreather masks in achieving maximum oxygenation.

Children who are already experiencing difficulty breathing may be less than cooperative when an attempt is made to place a mask or cannula on their face. Explain to the child/family in developmentally appropriate language what will happen, why the mask is needed, and how it will feel. Provide assistance, if needed, to keep the oxygen delivery system in place. Check the physician's orders for the percentage of oxygen to be delivered and the method of delivery.

A nasal cannula is a low-flow delivery system that is indicated for infants and children who require modest amounts of supplemental oxygen (up to 40%). Flow rates should not exceed 6 L/min. The loop of the cannula can be enlarged to slip easily over the child's ears. The prongs are placed in the nares and the loop is tightened. If the child is active, the cannula can be taped to the sides of the child's face to maintain proper position. Be aware, however, that a flow rate exceeding 6 L/min may irritate the nasopharynx, cause gastric distention and regurgitation, and may not appreciably improve the child's oxygenation.

The simple face mask and the Venturi mask are indicated for infants and children who require modest amounts of supplemental oxygen (35% to 60%, or a flow rate of 6 to 10 L/min). The Venturi mask can be adjusted to deliver specific concentrations of oxygen (i.e., 24%, 28%, 35%, 40%, or 50%). A minimum flow rate of 6 L/min must be maintained to prevent rebreathing of exhaled carbon dioxide.

Partial and full non-rebreathing masks are simple face masks with an attached reservoir that allows a portion of exhaled gas to remain in the bag and mix with oxygen. These masks are useful for supplying oxygen concentrations of 50% to 60% at a rate of 10 to 12 L/min. A non-rebreather system can deliver almost 100% oxygen at a flow rate of 10 to 15 L/min.

In delivering oxygen by mask, it is important that the correct size of mask be selected to ensure a tight fit. Masks are available in preemie, newborn, infant, child, small adult, and adult sizes. The mask should extend from the bridge of the nose to the cleft of the chin. The mask is then attached to the humidified oxygen source and the flow rate is adjusted to the prescribed level. The mask is placed over the child's face and the nose clip and head strap are adjusted.

Proper fit of an oxygen mask will ensure adequate oxygen delivery.

An oxygen hood or mist tent may be utilized to deliver humidified oxygen to assist in the mobilization of secretions. These apparatuses are particularly useful in the treatment of children with croup, laryngotracheobronchitis, epiglottitis, pneumonia, and bronchiolitis. The mist

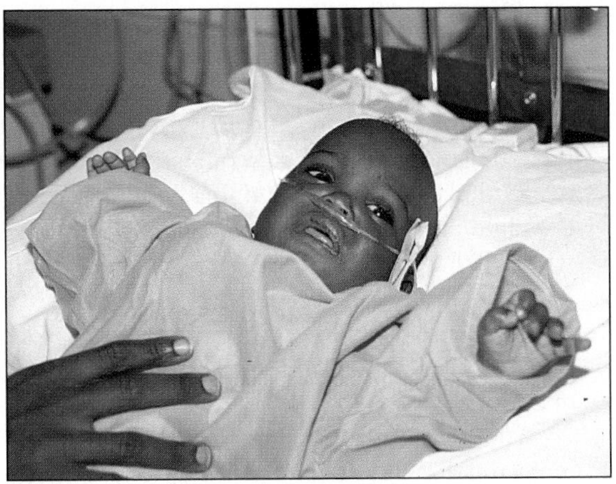

◀ The nasal cannula is useful for administering modest amounts of supplemental oxygen. The prongs are placed in the nares and the loop is slipped over the ears and made snug. The cannula can be taped to the side of the child's face, if needed, to maintain position.

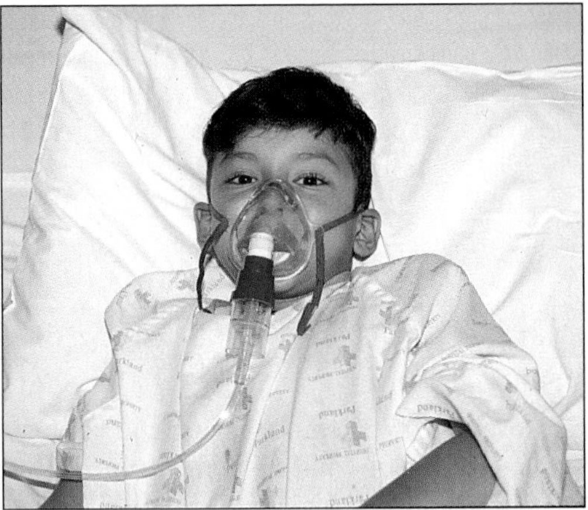

A simple face mask provides oxygen concentrations of 35% to 60% at a flow rate of 6 to 10 L/min. The mask should be long enough to cover the child's nose and mouth, and the elastic band should be adjusted for a snug fit. ▶

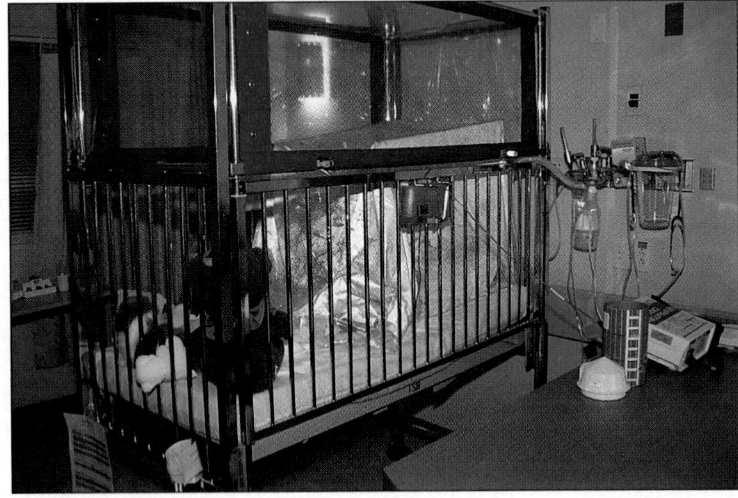

◀ The oxygen mist tent is useful in mobilizing secretions while administering oxygen. The child must be monitored frequently when using this method because hypothermia is possible and the mist obscures the nurse's view of the child. However, it is important not to open the tent unnecessarily because oxygen will escape. Because the child in this crib is an older infant, the bubble top is in place to prevent him from climbing over the crib rail.

Figure 18–12
Administering oxygen to children differs from the procedure in adults in two respects: the choice and size of equipment, and the need to educate and support the child and family. Several methods for administering oxygen to children are shown in these photographs. The choice of methods is based on the concentration of oxygen needed by the child and the child's ability to cooperate with the chosen method. (Courtesy of Parkland Memorial Hospital, Dallas, Texas)

moistens the airways, minimizes fluid loss from the lungs, and provides a cool environment, which aids in temperature reduction. The child's temperature should be monitored frequently to prevent hypothermia.

Oxygen concentrations greater than 40% may be difficult to achieve because oxygen is heavier than air and will escape readily. A canopy can be used to assist in maintaining the desired oxygen concentration (Clarke & Deeds, 1988). Remember that room air will be drawn into the tent any time it is entered, reducing the child's inspired oxygen concentration. Because of this, the tent limits access to the patient. In addition, if humidified oxygen is used, the resulting mist may limit visual observation of the patient, and the child's clothing and linen must be changed frequently. If a concentration of inspired oxygen greater than 30% is required, another method of oxygen delivery will be more effective.

With the use of any oxygen administration system, safety is of great concern. "OXYGEN IN USE/NO SMOKING" signs should be posted outside the patient's door and over the patient's bed. Although most health care facilities are "smoke-free," parents and visitors should be reminded that smoking is not allowed in the room. Toys that have the potential for producing a spark, including those that are battery-powered, should not be allowed.

Documentation. Record in the nurse's notes the date and time; the type of oxygen administration system used; the percentage of oxygen delivered and the flow rate; the patient's vital signs, skin color, respiratory effort, and lung sounds; the patient's response to the procedure, and any teaching done with the child/family.

Parent Teaching. Infants and children often receive home oxygen therapy. Parents or caregivers should be educated regarding the operation of equipment to be used at home, safety factors, cardiopulmonary resuscitation, and support services available.

PULSE OXIMETRY

Pulse oximetry is a sensitive, reliable, noninvasive means of measuring oxygen saturation in the blood. It measures the absorption of light waves as they pass through highly perfused areas of the body, providing the nurse with valuable information and acting as an early warning of hypoxemia (Cote et al., 1988; Carroll, 1993)). Pulse oximetry is a valuable method of assessing oxygenation status in acutely ill infants and children.

There are several advantages to pulse oximetry. It is noninvasive, requires no special site preparation, and, in most cases, provides an accurate measurement in the neonate, infant, child, and adult (Uhing & Dziedzic, 1990). Additionally, the results are immediately available. Despite some limitations, it has significant benefit in the care of the ill child. The immediate feedback provided by pulse oximetry can alert the nurse to changes in oxygenation so that interventions can be instituted rapidly to prevent further problems (Carroll, 1993).

Pulse oximetry is often useful in the care of acutely ill patients. However, monitoring should not be done based on its technical capability. Rather, its use must be balanced against clinical usefulness and cost-effectiveness (Hess & Kacmarek, 1993). Capillary or arterial blood gases may need to be done to document correlation of oxygenation to pulse oximetry readings.

PROCEDURE: *Pulse Oximetry*

Pulse oximeter measurements reflect the oxygen saturation and the perfusion status of the patient. Potential sources for error in measurements include abnormal hemoglobin (e.g., hyperbilirubinemia or carbon dioxide poisoning), peripheral perfusion (e.g., hypotension or hypothermia), ambient light interference, motion artifact, and skin breakdown from the adhesive used to secure the sensor. An opaque shield can be placed over the sensor site to eliminate the effects of ambient light. Skin breakdown can be avoided by using a reusable sensor secured with Coband (Carroll, 1993).

Preparing the Child and Family. Explain to the child/family, using developmentally appropriate language, the indications for the procedure, and what it looks like (e.g., "E.T.-the Extraterrestrial"), in order to enhance understanding and cooperation.

Equipment

- Oximeter
- Sensor (ear clip, finger probe, or adhesive probe)

STEP-BY-STEP PROCEDURE

1. Place the sensor on the index finger (or palm, toe, foot, or ear), as instructed by the manufacturer, and turn on the machine (Fig. 18–13).
2. Set parameters for alarms according to physician's orders.

> Avoid placing the probe on an extremity with an arterial line, blood pressure cuff, or IV line in place. Avoid wrapping the sensor so tightly as to prevent venous flow and cause inaccurate readings.

3. Restrain the extremity, if necessary, to avoid motion artifact.
4. Observe and record the pulse rate and oxygen saturation. The pulse rate on the oximeter should coincide with that of the heart monitor. If the pulse rate is not being detected, reposition the sensor.
5. Remove the sensor from the site at least every 2 hours to check skin condition.

DOCUMENTATION

Note the child's response to the procedure and the pulse oximetry reading obtained, the percentage of oxygen (if in use), and the activity level of the child. Report any abnormal findings to the physician.

> In *most* cases, a pulse oximeter reading of less than 90% should be reported to the physician. However, some children, particularly those with cardiac defects or certain respiratory diseases, such as asthma or cystic fibrosis, may have a lower "normal" pulse oximeter value.

Parent Teaching

Parents should be made aware that an alarm will sound if the child's oxygen saturation falls below the set parameters.

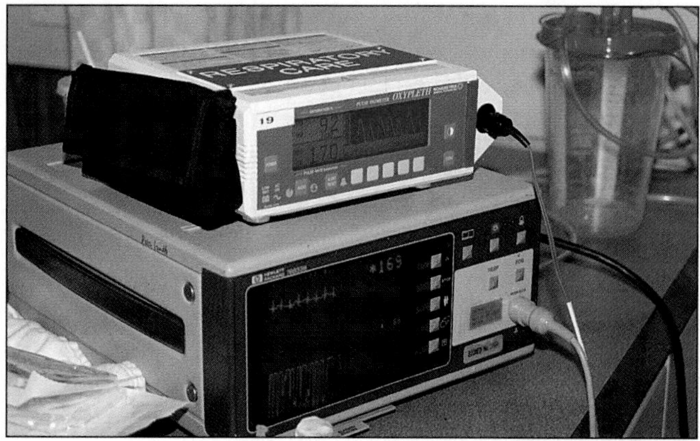

Pulse oximeter. (Courtesy of Parkland Memorial Hospital, Dallas, Texas)

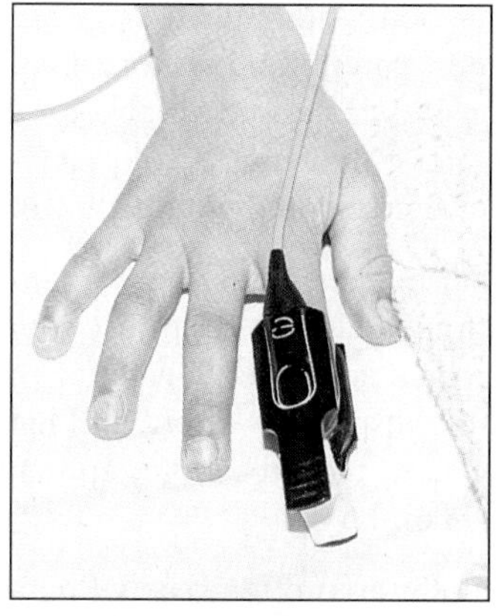

◄ Sensor applied to child's finger.

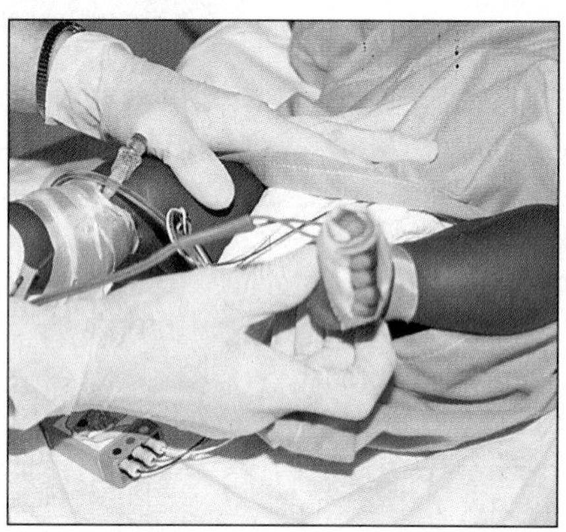

◄ Sensor applied to infant's toe.

Figure 18–13

The pulse oximeter is a reliable, noninvasive way to measure blood oxygen saturation, allowing rapid adjustments in oxygen delivery to meet the child's needs. The sensor is applied to a child's finger or an infant's toe to permit information to be sent to the pulse oximeter.

ARTERIAL BLOOD GASES

Arterial blood gases are used to measure the blood's oxygen content and the body's acid–base balance. Sampling may be done from indwelling arterial catheters or by arterial puncture. The procedure for arterial blood sampling varies between the adult and pediatric population. The differences include the sites used, the size of the equipment, the angle of entry, and the psychosocial interactions with the patient/family. The preferred site in the pediatric population is the radial artery, although alternatives include the brachial, dorsalis pedis, posterior tibial, and temporal arteries (French, 1995). A capillary blood gas measurement can provide similar information, yet is a less painful and invasive procedure.

PROCEDURE: *Sampling Arterial Blood Gases*

Arterial blood gases are drawn by the respiratory therapist, RN, or other personnel trained in performing this procedure. Arterial puncture is painful and often elicits breath-holding, hyperventilation, or crying in the infant and child. Breath-holding, even for short intervals, may produce falsely low pH and PaO_2 levels and falsely high $PaCO_2$ values. Conversely, hyperventilation and crying may produce falsely high pH and PaO_2 levels and falsely low $PaCO_2$ values. Document and report these reactions if they occur during sampling procedures to aid in accurate arterial blood gas interpretation (Suddaby & Sourbeer, 1990).

Preparing the Child and Family. Explain the procedure, its necessity, and its purpose to the child and family using developmentally appropriate language. Allow the parent(s) to remain with the child, if possible, to provide comfort and support. Because arterial sampling is not within the scope of practice for the student or novice nurse, the following procedure is limited to assisting with and restraining for arterial blood gas sampling.

Equipment

- Alcohol prep pads
- 23-gauge butterfly
- 1 cc syringe
- 1:1000 heparin
- 2 × 2 or cotton balls
- Band-Aid

STEP-BY-STEP PROCEDURE

1. The person restraining the child must maintain stability of the extremity, neither allowing twisting of the wrist nor jerking of the shoulder. Care must also be taken not to occlude arterial blood flow by holding the child's arm too tightly.

   For the older child: For the older child who can cooperate to some extent, the restrainer may stand on the sampling side and firmly grip the underside of the lower arm, using the ulna and radius to hold the extremity firmly.

   For the infant or young child: For the infant and young child, the restrainer should stand on the side opposite the sampling site. The restrainer can then reach across the chest of the patient to restrain the extremity and, at the same time, provide verbal comfort and distraction to the child. Increased restraint can be gained by gently lying across the child's chest, if needed. Alternatively, the infant or young child may also be "mummied" in a blanket, sheet, or on a papoose board. Regardless of the technique used, minimizing the child's movement is a crucial aspect of the sampling procedure.
2. The sample is collected using a heparinized tuberculin syringe and butterfly tubing (0.1–0.2 ml of heparin). The excess heparin and air are expelled to avoid alterations in the pH and pCO_2 readings.

> Standard precautions are always used when obtaining blood samples (see Appendix G).

3. The wrist of the patient is positioned with the palm up, but not hyperextended, in order to prevent obliteration of the pulse.
4. The artery is located and the area is prepped with alcohol and/or povidone-iodine solution.
5. The skin is punctured at a 15–45° angle and the needle is advanced until blood appears in the hub or tubing. A sample of blood (0.3–0.5 ml) is withdrawn for blood gas analysis. If other laboratory studies are needed in addition to the arterial blood gas determination, these may be drawn simultaneously to avoid any unnecessary additional sticks.
6. After the sample is obtained, the needle is withdrawn slowly and steadily to decrease incidence of arterial spasm. Standard Precautions should be maintained to ensure the safety of the sampler and the restrainer.
7. Apply direct pressure to the site using a sterile 2 × 2 gauze pad, for at least 5 minutes after the needle is removed to stop the bleeding and reduce hematoma formation.
8. The specimen should be labeled and, unless the analysis is done immediately, the sample should be placed on ice. Failure to do so can result in falsely low pH and falsely high $PaCO_2$ readings owing to continued red blood cell metabolism in the sample.
9. Follow agency policy for transporting biologic hazards.

DOCUMENTATION

On the requisition form and the nurses' notes, record the date and time of the analysis, the patient's temperature, and the percentage of oxygen in use. Include information about the patient's activity level at the time of the sampling (e.g., crying, sleeping) and indicate the sample site. Report test results to the physician.

Parent Teaching

Assist the parents in comforting the child during and after the procedure.

CHEST PHYSIOTHERAPY

Chest physiotherapy (CPT) includes postural drainage, chest percussion and vibration, and coughing and deep breathing exercises. These techniques are utilized to mobilize and eliminate secretions, re-expand the lungs, and promote efficient use of the respiratory muscles. These procedures are used most commonly with patients who have cystic fibrosis, pneumonia, asthma, bronchitis, and obstructive pulmonary disease. CPT is also often used prophylactically in postoperative patients. Contraindications for this treatment include head injury, acute asthma, chest trauma with an unstable chest wall, osteogenesis imperfecta, and lung tumor. The efficacy of CPT has been questioned in recent years (Thornlow, 1995; Andersen, 1991).

In most health care facilities, CPT is the responsibility of the respiratory therapist. However, if respiratory therapy coverage is not available, then the nurse is responsible for this procedure. Many children with chronic pulmonary disease require this treatment at home, so the family must be educated about how to perform this aspect of the child's care. The goal of CPT is to prevent atelectasis and pneumonia.

PROCEDURE: *Chest Physiotherapy and Postural Drainage*

Initiation of CPT requires a physician's order. The order should include the number of treatments per day, and it may specify the areas of the lungs to be treated.

Percussion is rhythmic clapping with cupped hand over the affected portion of the lung or the simulation of this movement using a percussion cup or mechanical percussor or vibrator. *Postural drainage* is positioning of the patient to promote gravity-assisted drainage of the lungs. These two treatments are usually used in conjunction with each other and are carried out three to four times a day, or more often if indicated. Treatments are performed before meals or $1\frac{1}{2}$ hours after meals to decrease the risk of aspiration.

> Children who are receiving continuous feedings should have their feeding interrupted 1 hour prior to the treatment. The "lost volume" can then be replaced in the interim before the next treatment.

The length of the treatment depends on the child's ability to tolerate the procedure, but is usually 20 to 30 minutes. Although there are several positions for postural drainage, it may not be necessary to use all at each session.

Preparing the Child and Family. If the child and family are not familiar with CPT explain the procedure to them using developmentally appropriate language. Show them the equipment and allow time for questions.

Equipment

- Mechanical percussor, vibrator, or rubber cups (if being used instead of hands)
- Gloves
- Stethoscope
- Towel or baby blanket
- Tissues for sputum

STEP-BY-STEP PROCEDURE

1. Assess the child's baseline respiratory status prior to beginning the procedure in order to provide a basis for determining response to the treatment. Prior to treatment, ask the child to cough, or suction the trachea, to remove secretions that may have accumulated in the trachea.
2. Place the child in a postural drainage position (Figs. 18–14 and 18–15).
3. Gently but firmly clap the chest wall with cupped hands (see Figs. 18–14 and 18–15). The sound should be hollow. Percussion cups and mechanical vibrators may be used instead of the hand (see Fig. 18–14). A towel or baby blanket may be used to cover the chest during the treatment.
4. Reposition the child as needed to complete the procedure, maintaining each position for approximately 5 to 10 minutes.
5. Encourage the child to take deep breaths during the treatment. Expiration after these deep breaths will often stimulate coughing.

> Utilize toys, such as pinwheel toys and balloons (with close supervision), or engage the child in blowing soap bubbles to optimize deep breathing and stimulate coughing. Assist with removal of secretions if needed.

6. Assess the child's vital signs and breath sounds after therapy is completed.

DOCUMENTATION

Record the following in the nurses' notes: the date and time of CPT; positions for drainage and length of time each is maintained; chest segments percussed or vibrated; color, amount, and tenacity of any secretions produced; any complications and nursing actions taken; the patient's response to and tolerance of the procedure; and any teaching done with the patient/family and their degree of understanding of the teaching.

Parent Teaching

The parents' ability to perform CPT at home should be assessed. Older children may perform some CPT techniques on themselves. Parents and older children may be taught positions for postural drainage, percussion, and vibration. Observe the parent(s)/child as they demonstrate the procedure. Provide written instructions for parents regarding the child's CPT needs.

Teaching materials are available for families of children requiring CPT at home. Assist the family in obtaining this literature and refer them to appropriate financial resources if needed.

TRACHEOSTOMY CARE

A *tracheostomy* is a surgically created opening (stoma) in the trachea. It is performed in children to bypass an upper airway obstruction, to facilitate pulmonary toilet, or to optimize mechanical ventilation. Tracheostomies may be either temporary or permanent.

Pediatric tracheostomy tubes vary in size and type. The tube most commonly used is made of silastic, which is soft and flexible. It consists of two pieces: the outer cannula, which stays in the trachea to keep the stoma open; and an obturator, which guides the tube into place during tube changes. Some tubes have an inner cannula that can be removed for cleaning (Warnock & Porpora, 1994). Tracheostomy tubes with inner cannulas are often used in children who have increased mucous production and in older children.

Shiley single-lumen tracheostomy tubes are available in a variety of sizes (up to a No. 8 for an adult-sized patient). Tracheostomy tubes with inner cannulas are available in sizes No. 4 and larger.

Tracheostomy care for the infant or child rarely differs from that appropriate for adult patients. The primary differences include the types and sizes of tubes, the ability of the patient to cooperate with procedures, and the parental support and teaching needed to prepare for home care (if indicated).

Because of the risk of aspiration and possible occlusion of the trachea, small toys, toys with small parts, plastic bibs, and plastic bedding should be avoided. In addition, talcum powders and aerosol products should not be used near children with tracheostomies because of the risk of inhalation injury secondary to breathing the particles.

Routine tracheostomy care includes assessing the stoma area for signs of infection and skin breakdown, changing tracheostomy ties, cleaning the tracheostomy site and inner cannula, changing the tracheostomy tube, and suctioning. Tracheostomy care may be given at various intervals, but should be done at least every 8 hours. The tracheostomy tube is usually changed weekly. The tracheostomy is held in place with ties that are made of a durable, nonfraying material. These are changed daily, or more frequently if they become soiled. An assistant should always be present when tracheostomy care is performed.

Keep an extra tracheostomy tube of appropriate size at the bedside (or taped to the head of the bed) for easy access in an emergency.

PROCEDURE: *Cleaning and Care of the Tracheostomy Site and Inner Cannula*

The peristomal area should be assessed for redness, drainage/discharge, and skin breakdown. The site should be kept clean and dry. The area around the tube should be cleaned at the time the tracheostomy ties are changed, or more frequently if needed. Use half-strength hydrogen peroxide and cotton-tipped applicators to gently clean secretions from around the stoma. Some facilities stock commercially packaged tracheostomy care trays, which contain small trays that hold cleaning solution; cotton-tipped applicators; pipe cleaners or a brush for cleaning the inner cannula; forceps; tracheostomy ties; and a sterile dressing. After cleaning the area, pat dry with gauze.

Preparing the Child and Family. Explain the procedure, its purpose, and other pertinent information to the child/parent using developmentally appropriate language.

Obtain assistance when performing tracheostomy care to prevent the tube from being accidentally dislodged.

Equipment

- Small tray to hold cleaning solution
- Cotton-tipped applicators
- Pipe cleaners or brush for cleaning the inner cannula
- Forceps
- Tracheostomy ties
- Sterile dressing (optional)
- Gauze pad
- Gloves (sterile or nonsterile)
- Towel or blanket roll
- Hydrogen peroxide
- Sterile normal saline

STEP-BY-STEP PROCEDURE

1. Position child with a towel or blanket under the shoulders to hyperextend the head and neck in order to expose the site.
2. Wash hands and open the tray, creating a sterile field.
3. Pour equal parts of normal saline and hydrogen peroxide in one small tray and normal saline in the other small tray. Use the large tray for holding cotton-tipped applicators, clean tracheostomy ties, and gauze pad.
4. Don nonsterile gloves and remove the dressing around the tracheostomy, if present. Discard the dressing and gloves according to agency policy. A dressing placed between the skin and the tube can increase the risk for skin breakdown, since it will absorb any secretions. For this reason, it may not be used in some facilities.
5. Don sterile gloves and, using cotton-tipped applicators moistened in half-strength solution, clean the patient's neck under the tracheostomy tube flanges and tracheostomy tape and allow to dry.

If the patient has a tracheostomy without an inner cannula, skip to Step 8.

6. Unlock the inner cannula (if using a 3-piece tracheostomy system) by rotating it counterclockwise. Quickly clean it in half-strength hydrogen peroxide solution using pipe cleaners or brush. (Alternatively, it may be replaced with a new or extra inner cannula, if available.) Rinse the cannula thoroughly in normal saline and inspect it for cleanliness. Repeat the cleaning procedure if necessary.
7. Tap the cleaned inner cannula on the edge of the sterile container to remove excess moisture. Do not dry the outside of the inner cannula because moisture will act as a lubricant during reinsertion.
8. Reinsert the inner cannula into the tracheostomy tube and lock it in place by rotating it clockwise.

   Note: Some facilities require the use of two people to change ties, in which case the following procedure is used. While the assistant wearing sterile gloves gently holds the tube in place, remove the existing tape from the flanges. Clean the skin under the ties and inspect the skin for pressure sores from the ties.

9. Loop the new tracheostomy ties through the flange on one side of the tracheostomy (see Photo Story, p. 478). Bring the ties around the back of the patient's neck and tie them securely to the opposite flange.

Text continued on page 479

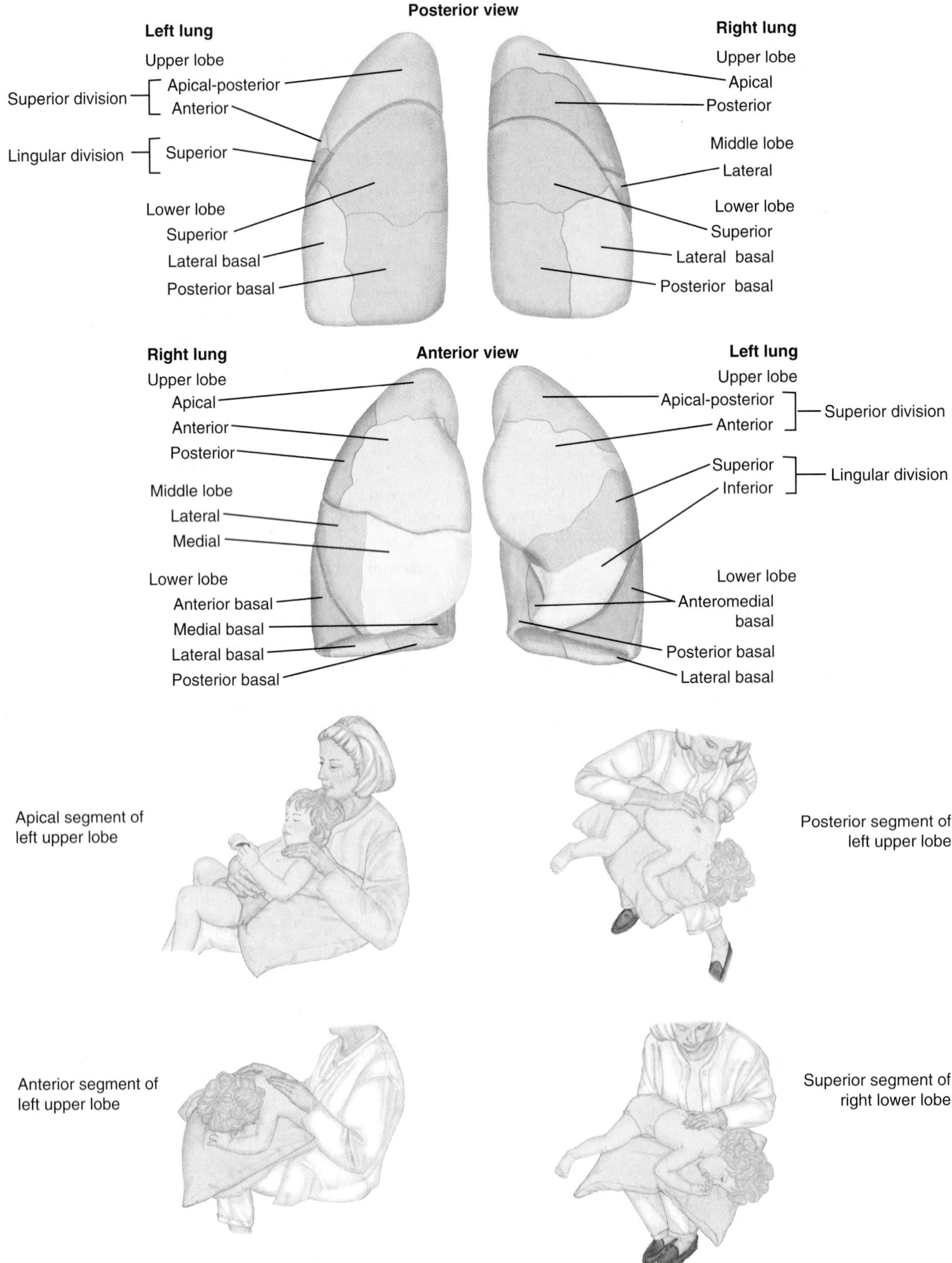

Figure 18–14

An infant or small child can be placed on the nurse's or therapist's lap for chest physiotherapy. Bronchial drainage positions and percussion points for major lung segments are shown. Figure 18–15 shows positions and percussion points for older children.

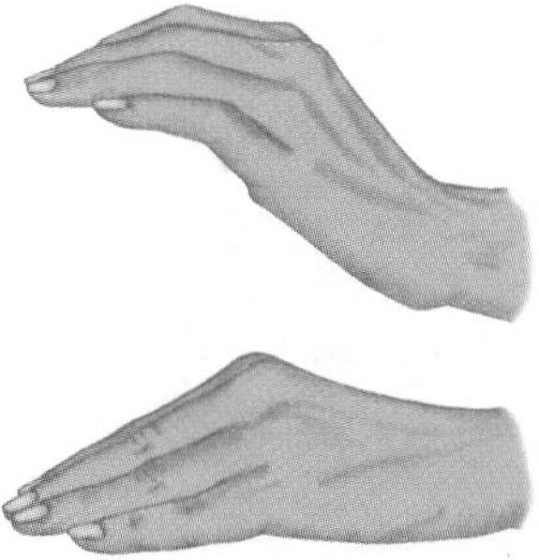
Correct hand position for percussion
Cup the hand to trap a pocket of air that will transmit vibrations through the chest wall to the secretions that need to be dislodged.
Clap the cupped hand in rapid sequence over a lung segment. Elbow should be flexed and the wrist relaxed, while creating a rapid, popping action.

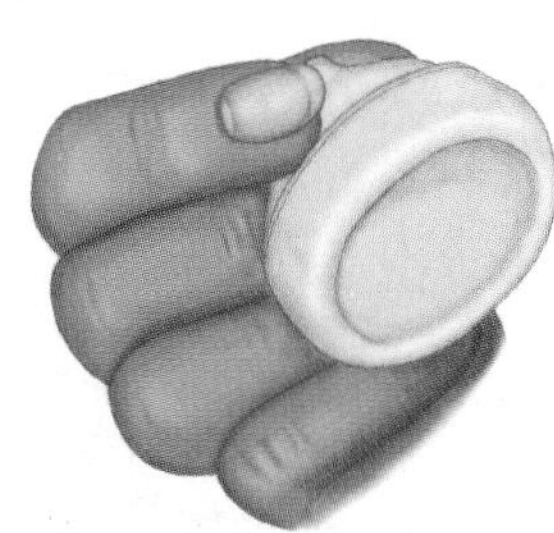
Infant percussion device

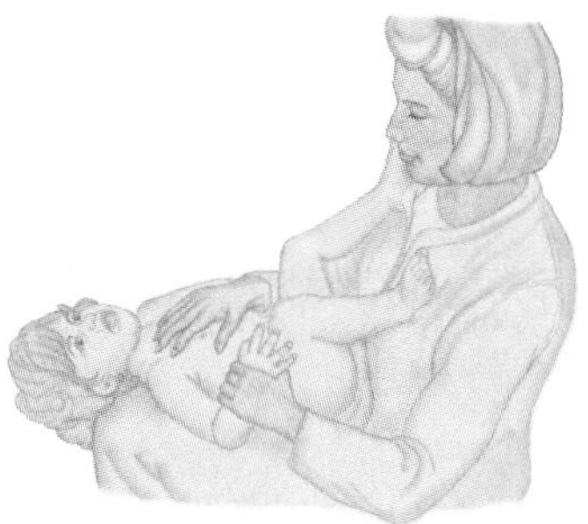
Posterior basal segment of right lower lobe

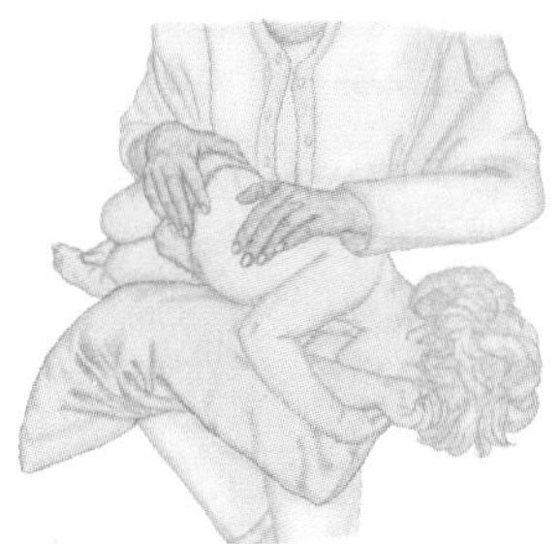
Lateral basal segment of right lower lobe

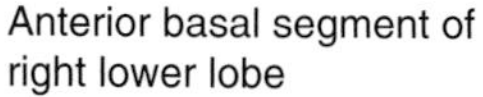

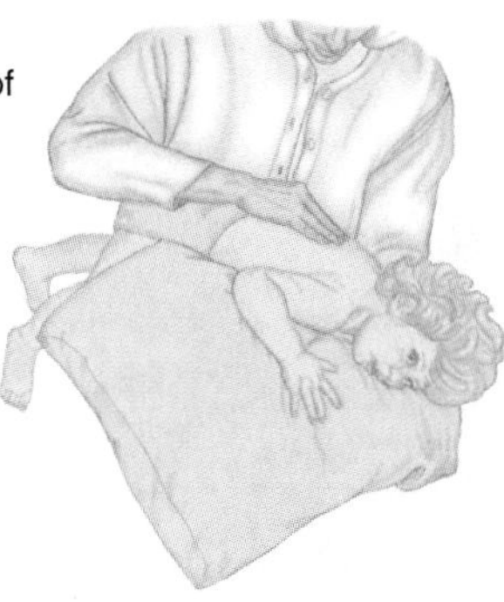
Anterior basal segment of right lower lobe

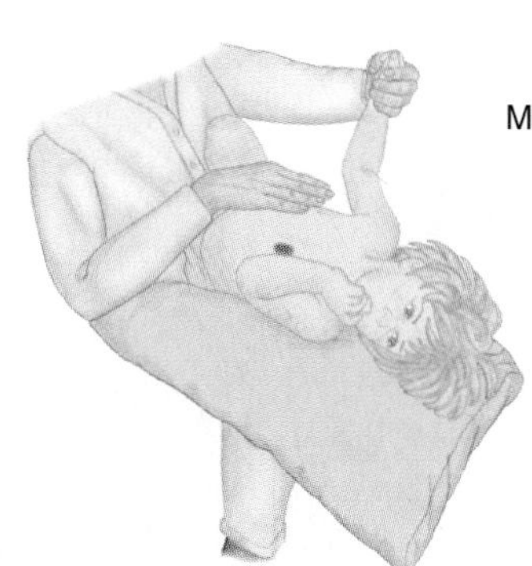
Medial and lateral segments of left middle lobe

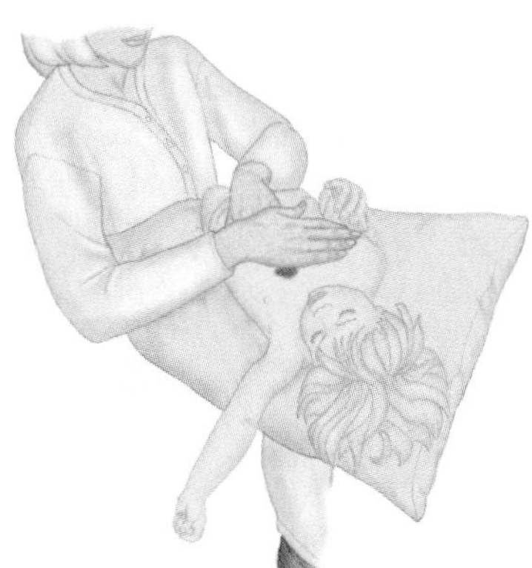
Lingular segments (superior and inferior) of left upper lobe

Figure 18–14
Continued

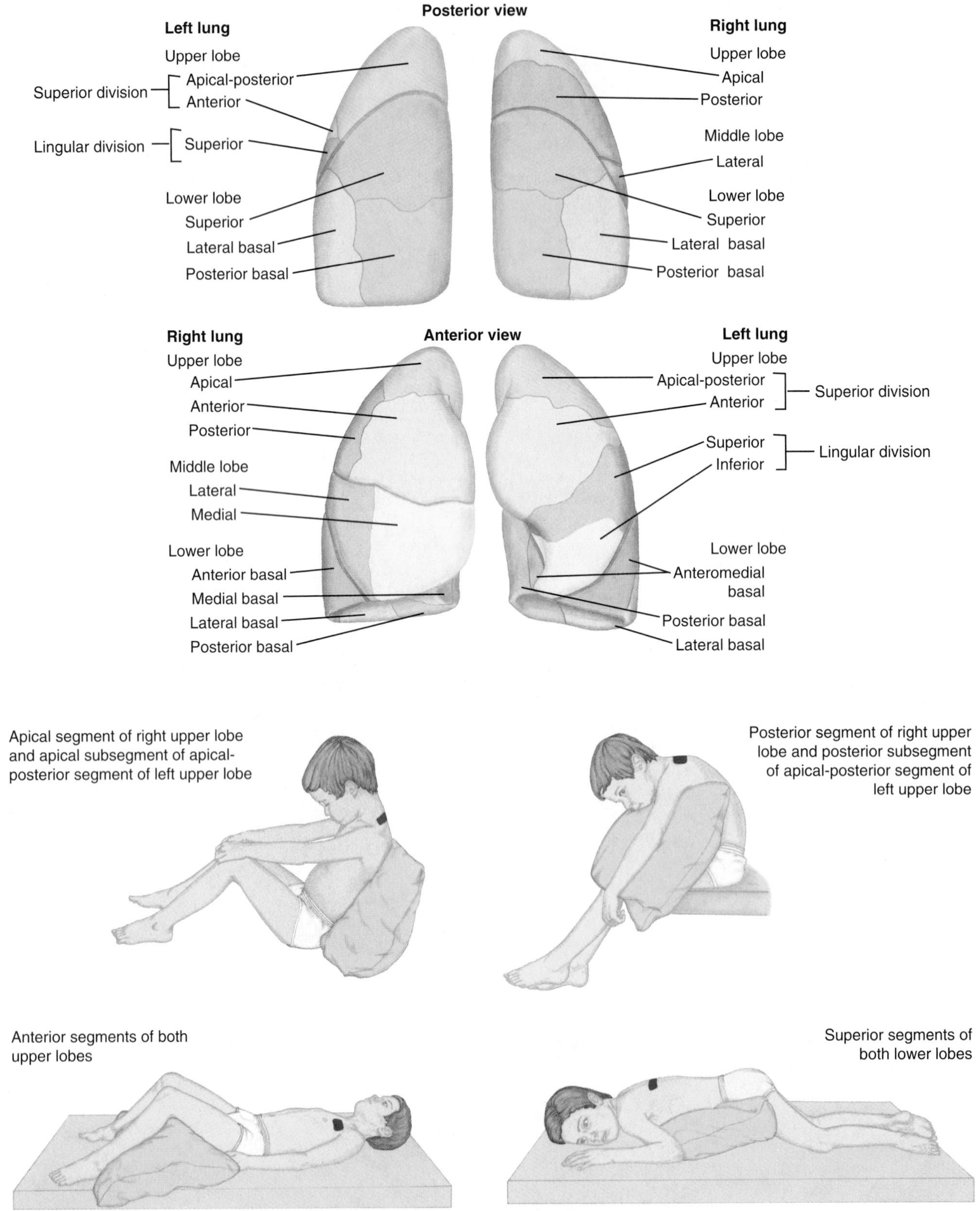

Figure 18–15

Chest physiotherapy for older children. Bronchial drainage positions and percussion points for major lung segments are shown. Figure 18–14 shows positions and percussion points for the infant and small child.

Correct hand position for percussion

Cup the hand to trap a pocket of air that will transmit vibrations through the chest wall to the secretions that need to be dislodged.

Clap the cupped hand in rapid sequence over a lung segment. Elbow should be flexed and the wrist relaxed, while creating a rapid, popping action.

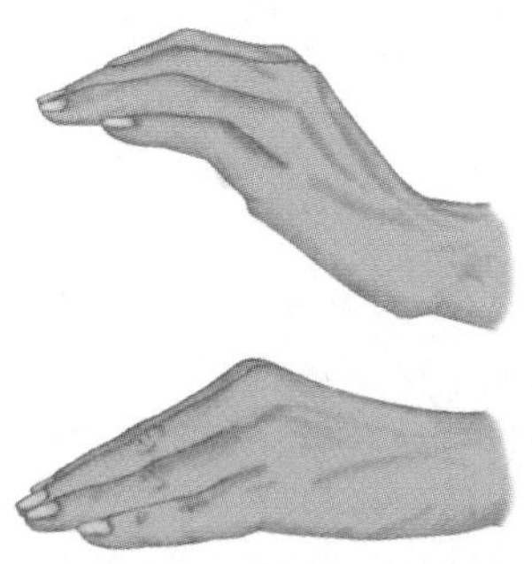

Posterior basal segments of both lower lobes.

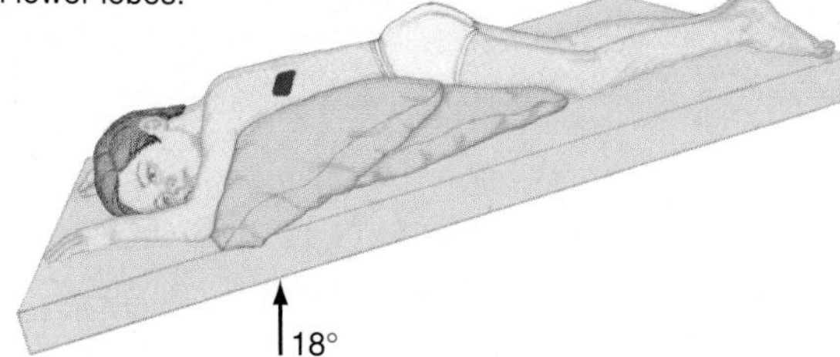

Lateral basal segments of right lower lobe. Left lateral segment would be drained by mirror image of this position (right side down).

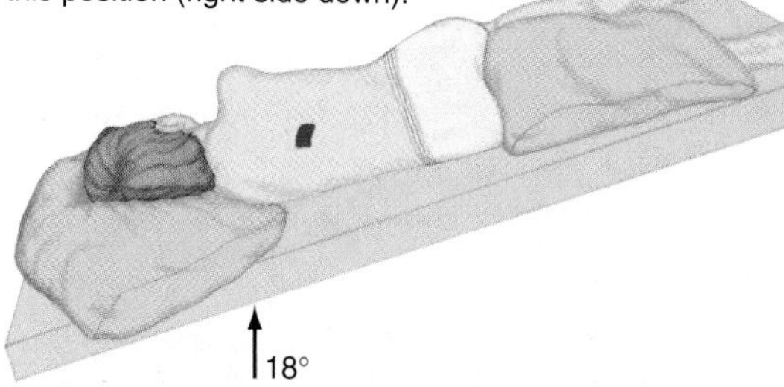

Anterior basal segment of left lower lobe; right anterior basal segment would be drained by mirror image of this position (left side down).

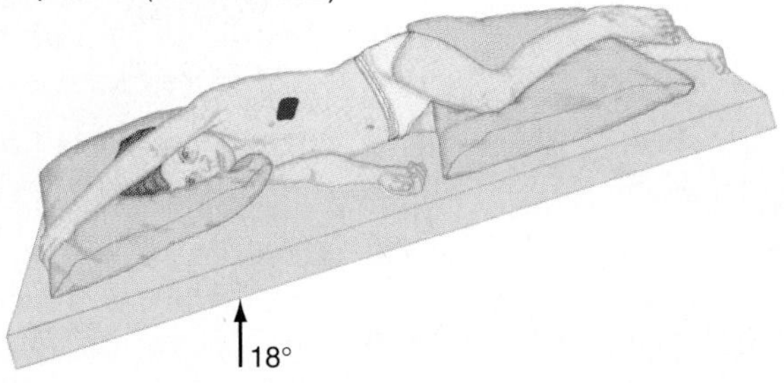

Medial and lateral segments of right middle lobe.

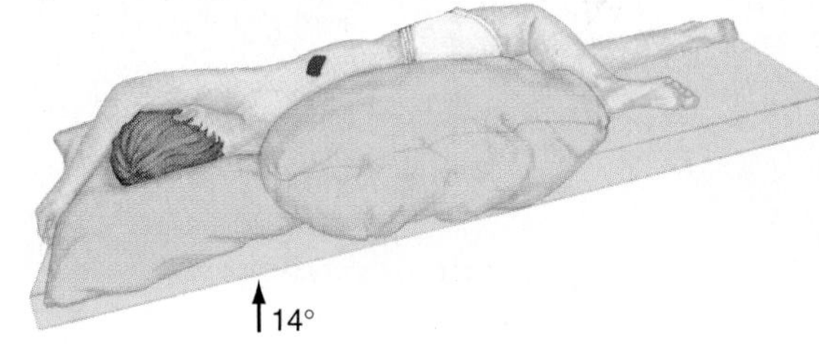

Lingular segments (superior and inferior) of the left upper lobe (homologue of right middle lobe).

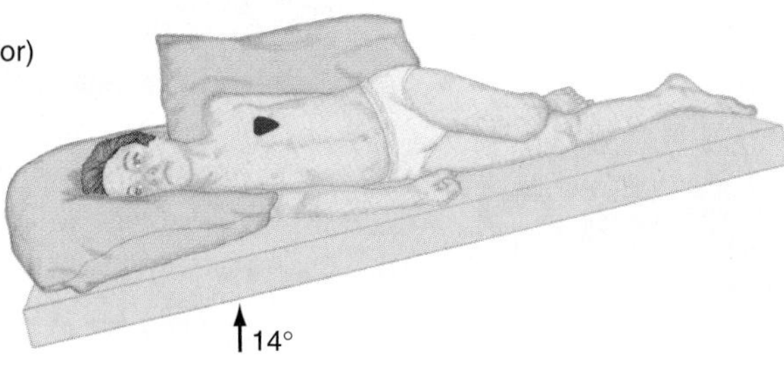

Figure 18–15
Continued

Caring for an Infant With a Tracheostomy

INTRODUCTION

Caring for the child with a tracheostomy can involve several steps, including respiratory therapy treatments, suctioning, and changing the ties that secure the tube. Because many children are discharged from the hospital with tracheostomies, their parents and other home caregivers must be taught these procedures.

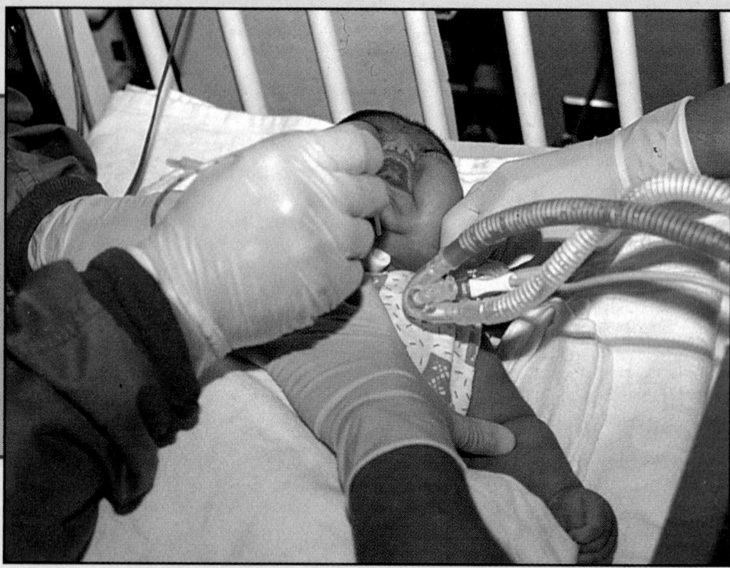

Secretions are removed from this infant's airway with a suction catheter. Appropriate techniques minimize problems with suctioning, such as hypoxia, tissue damage, or infection. The suction catheter is inserted into the tube with the suction turned off. After the appropriate length of tubing is inserted, suction is applied, and the catheter is withdrawn using a twisting motion. Do not suction longer than 5 seconds at a time.

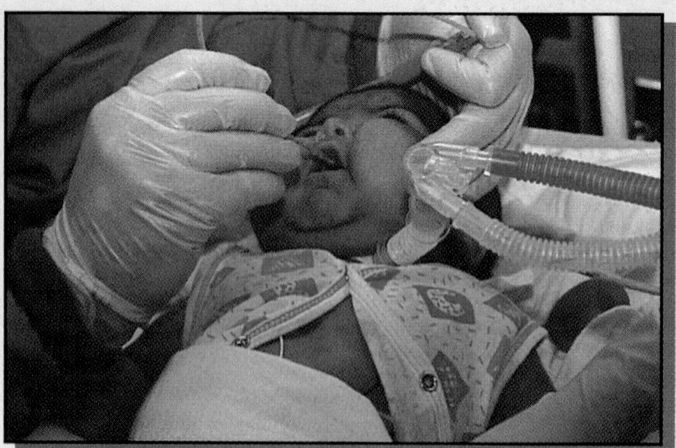

Often the oral cavity requires suctioning as well. The technique is similar to that for suctioning the tracheostomy: the catheter is inserted, then suction is applied while the catheter is withdrawn.

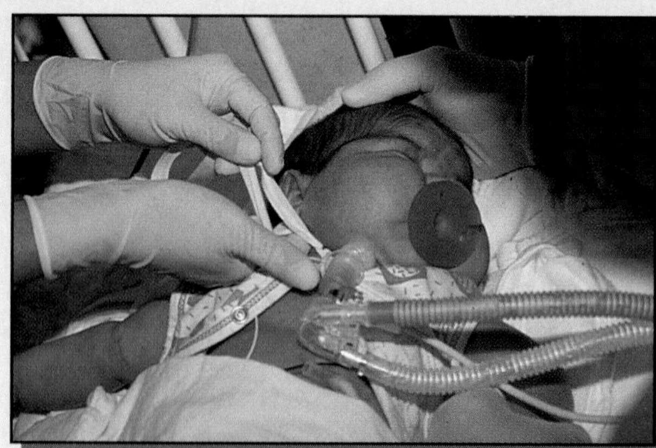

When changing the infant's tracheostomy ties, the nurse has an assistant hold the tube in place to reduce the chance that it will be displaced. The nurse makes sure the ties are snug, but not too tight. When the new ties are in place, the nurse checks their snugness by inserting a finger beneath them.

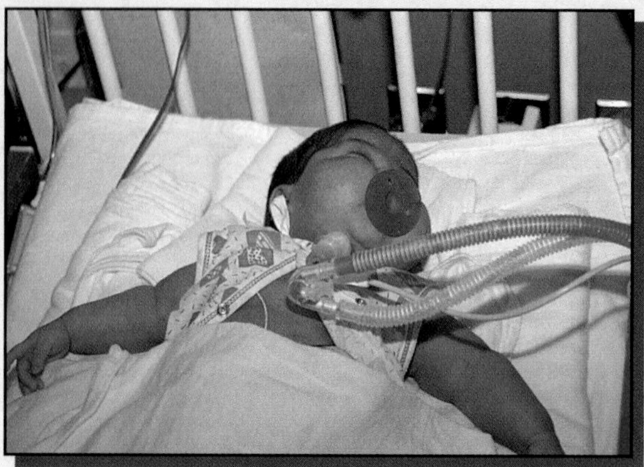

The infant who has a device such as a tracheostomy tube or a gastrostomy feeding tube still needs to suck. A pacifier fulfills this need. Since tracheostomy care often tires the child, she should be allowed to rest afterwards.

Photos courtesy of Parkland Memorial Hospital, Dallas, Texas.

Ties are tight enough if only one finger can be inserted between the ties and neck. Ties should be tied on the side. The back area should be avoided to prevent confusing the tracheostomy ties with bib ties and to avoid putting pressure on the back of the neck. Triple knots are recommended to prevent accidental untying and dislodging of the tracheostomy. Clean and assess the skin under the ties.

10. Carefully cut and remove the soiled tracheostomy ties and any excess clean tracheostomy tape.

> Make sure the tracheostomy tube is secure before leaving the bedside.

11. Discard used supplies in appropriate receptacles.

DOCUMENTATION

Record in the nurses' notes the date, time and type of procedure, condition of the stoma and skin, any abnormal findings or complications and the nursing action taken, the child's tolerance of the procedure, and any patient/family teaching done, as well as their understanding of and involvement in the care.

Parent Teaching

The family's ability to perform the procedure should be assessed. It may be necessary to engage the assistance of a home health agency if the family needs at least temporary assistance and support. More than one family member should be taught tracheostomy care, and the education should begin early in the child's hospitalization. All those caring for the child must also know cardiopulmonary resuscitation (CPR). Instructions should be written, and return demonstration of the technique is imperative. Hemming tape or seambinding which can easily be found in fabric stores, ($\frac{1}{2}$-inch width), can be used for tracheostomy ties (Smith et al. 1991).

PROCEDURE: *Suctioning Tracheostomies*

Patients with tracheostomies require the removal of secretions from the airway by means of a catheter inserted into the airway (see photos, p. 478). Many problems may be encountered during suctioning, such as hypoxia, tissue damage, and infection. These can be minimized by using appropriate techniques and equipment for suctioning.

The suctioning procedure for pediatric patients varies little from that which is used in adults. Suctioning in infants and children requires the use of a smaller suction catheter and lower suction settings than in the adult. Catheter sizes range from No. 5 French to No. 14 French, with smaller sizes being used for smaller tubes. Catheter size should be approximately half the inner diameter of the tracheostomy tube to avoid total airway occlusion. (For suction settings, see the accompanying box.)

Suction Settings for Tracheostomy Care, by Age

Neonates: 60–80 mm/Hg
Infants: 80–100 mm/Hg
Larger children: 100–120 mm/Hg

Assess and document the patient's breath sounds, respiratory rate, and character of respirations every 4 hours. Suction the tracheostomy every 2 to 4 hours or as needed. Always use Standard Precautions.

Preparing the Child and Family. Explain the procedure, its purpose, and other pertinent information to the child/parent using developmentally appropriate language.

Equipment

- Sterile suction catheter
- Sterile gloves
- Normal saline solution

STEP-BY-STEP PROCEDURE

1. Choose a suction catheter of appropriate size and adjust the suction vacuum pressure to the prescribed level.
2. Sterile gloves are put on after equipment is assembled and suction is turned on.
3. Instill normal saline, 0.5 to 2 ml (if being used), to loosen secretions into the trachea. Sterile technique is used.
4. Insert the catheter the length of the tracheostomy tube (measure another tracheotomy tube the same size) *with suction off.* Do not apply suction as the catheter is being inserted.
5. Suctioning deeper than 0.5 to 1 cm beyond the end of the tracheostomy tube is not necessary unless the child is unable to clear secretions because of their thickness or quantity, or is unable to cough them up to the tracheostomy tube (Roemer, 1991).
6. Apply intermittent suction and withdraw the catheter using a twisting motion (Fig. 18–16).

> Limit insertion and suctioning time to 5 seconds to prevent hypoxia (Runton, 1992; Hazinski, 1986). Holding your own breath during suctioning is a good reminder. If you need a breath, then the patient probably does, too.

7. Reoxygenate between suction catheter passes and allow a sufficient recovery time after each pass. This may include allowing the child to rest and take a few breaths, or it may involve bagging.

Bagging of children on ventilatory support (giving oxygen by bag and mask) is imperative (Roemer, 1991).

8. Assess the patient to determine whether secretions are still present. Auscultate to listen for air exchange. Repeat the procedure until the airway sounds clear, rinsing the suction catheter with normal saline between each insertion.

Normal saline lavage may be used if thick secretions are encountered. Refer to your facility's procedure or policy manual regarding this controversial issue.

9. Assess the patient's breath sounds and respiratory rate after suctioning to evaluate the effectiveness of suctioning.
10. Discard the suction tube and gloves in an appropriate container.

DOCUMENTATION

Record in the nurses' notes the date and time the procedure was performed, the amount and characteristics of the secretions obtained, the character of the breath sounds before and after suctioning, the patient's response to the procedure, and any teaching done with the patient/family, as well as their level of understanding/response to the teaching.

Parent Teaching

Early preparation and education is essential for the child and family who will be discharged with a tracheostomy. Families should be included in the teaching plan for tracheostomy care and for CPR, and should be given adequate time to practice and achieve mastery of selected skills prior to discharge.

Parents may be taught to suction, use a humidity collar, and change tracheostomy ties and tubes. The family will need much support and encouragement in order to feel comfortable with these procedures.

The child may take baths, but care should be taken to prevent water from entering the trachea. Showers are not recommended. The tracheostomy can be covered loosely during cold or windy days in order to avoid tracheal spasm.

SURGICAL PROCEDURES

The child undergoing surgery has increased physical and psychological needs. Although each surgical procedure is unique, there is a general body of knowledge that relates to all children experiencing surgery. Surgery can be a very traumatic event for a child.

With the rising cost of health care, managed care contracts, and the need for cost containment in health care, many operative procedures are now being done on an outpatient basis. Ambulatory or same-day surgery utilizes the same standards of care that apply to all routine hospital admissions, but with the added benefit of lower cost.

Preparation for Surgery

A multidisciplinary approach should be used when preparing a child for surgery. The following should be included: parents, nursing staff, child life specialist, the physician, and any other specialty area involved in the individual child's care. Preparation for outpatient procedures is dependent on the type of procedure being done, as well as the age and developmental level of the child. Psychological preparation for an outpatient experience is just as important as it is for an inpatient hospital experience. Indeed, much of the preparation is the same, regardless of whether the surgery will be done as an outpatient or an inpatient, and a multidisciplinary approach to teaching is appropriate for both settings.

The physical and the psychosocial needs of the child and the family should be assessed. Both the child and the family will be anxious, so the nurse needs to be a calming force. An awareness of the stressors of surgery will guide the nurse in providing family-centered care. These stressors include the following (Holden, 1995; Squires, 1995):

- separation from significant others
- pain
- fear of mutilation
- the presence of strangers
- disruptions of routine
- lack of privacy
- disability
- disfigurement

Fear of the unknown is another common fear of children. By assessing the presence of these and other stressors, the nurse can then develop a plan of care.

Preparation for surgery is the foundation for developing the trust of both the child and the family. Formal sessions should be scheduled no more than 1 week before admission. Children younger than 4 years of age seem to do best when information is received no more than 3 days before admission (Squires, 1995). Waiting too long to initiate surgical preparation may give rise to fantasies and increase the child's fear. A short preparation may not provide enough time to answer questions posed by the child or family so that they feel adequately prepared for the surgery.

Although preparation may vary from setting to setting, all teaching should be planned, should use a developmental approach, and should provide information that is simple and truthful. Many hospitals include a tour of the perioperative area. A review of the teaching should be conducted on the day of the surgery. If a child life specialist participates in the preparation, he or she should be present on the day of surgery.

The use of therapeutic play is an essential tool, both in preparation and during the perioperative experience. A discussion of therapeutic play can be found in Chapter 9. Keeping the child busy is especially important if they have a waiting period. Age-appropriate toys should be provided in holding areas or in the child's room if that is the area in which they are waiting.

Parents should explain to the child as clearly as possible why he or she is going to the hospital or surgery center and what will happen during the stay. Nurses can assist the parents in preparing their child. Books on hospitalization or surgery that are geared for children may be obtained from the public library and read to the child in order to better prepare them for the experience. Videotapes are also available.

Children should be reassured that they will not be left alone and that they will not feel the procedure being done.

Regardless of the procedure planned, some preoperative activities are routine. These include:

- no food or drink after a specified time
- a consent for the procedure signed by the parent or guardian
- preoperative medications
- postanesthetic care

Because pediatric patients are at greater risk for dehydration than adult patients, the period during which they can have nothing by mouth (NPO) may be shorter than that imposed on adults. This may vary according to the protocol of the facility. (See the accompanying box for an example of preoperative feeding instructions.) For some procedures, preoperative laboratory tests, such as a complete blood count (CBC) or urinalysis, and a chest x-ray study may be ordered. Additional tests may be ordered as needed.

Most hospitals and surgical centers have preoperative checklists (similar to the ones used in adult care) that assist the nurse in documenting the child's preparation for the procedure. These lists usually include checking the patient's identification, obtaining a signed consent form, laboratory results, administering preanesthetic medication, and other documentation. After the preanesthetic medication has been administered, the parent may hold the child or place him/her on a stretcher with the siderails raised.

Parents should be informed of the anticipated length of the surgery and kept informed of their child's status throughout the surgery.

Sample Preoperative Feeding Instructions

For your child's safety, it is very important that you follow these instructions carefully. If these instructions are not followed, your child's operation or procedure may be canceled or delayed.

1. At 8 p.m.* the evening before surgery, stop all food, including:
   Solid food, candy,† and chewing gum
   Milk, milk products, and formulas‡
   Orange juice and juice containing pulp
2. Breast feeding may continue until 3 hours§ before the time you are to arrive at the hospital.
3. Clear fluids may be continued until 2 hours§ before the time you are to arrive at the hospital.
4. Clear fluids include:

Water	Clear broth
Apple juice	Pedialyte
Clear juice drinks	Ice popsicles
Plain Jell-O	

*Many hospitals use midnight rather than 8 p.m. for the beginning of the NPO period.

†Hard sucking candy is probably of little concern, and the significance of gum chewing remains controversial.

‡The duration for fasting after formulas is uncertain at present, and shorter intervals may be appropriate.

§It usually takes a minimum of 30 minutes to process a day surgery patient, but parents occasionally make subtraction errors when the instructions are not stated using integers.

From Schreiner, M. S. [1994]. Preoperative and postoperative fasting in children. *Pediatric Clinics of North America 41*(1), 118.

Preoperative Anesthesia

Preoperative medication is used primarily to decrease anxiety in the child. In some settings, premedication is not used if the parents are present. It is becoming increasingly common for parents to be present during the anesthetic induction period. When premedication is used, there are many safe and painless methods now available. Some of the common pediatric induction techniques are listed in the accompanying box.

Postanesthesia Care

After the surgery, the child is taken to the postanesthesia care unit (PACU) or recovery room. There, frequent assessments of the child's cardiorespiratory and circulatory systems are performed until the child is fully awake. When the child awakens from surgery, it is important for the parent(s) to be present to comfort and calm their child.

Pediatric Anesthetic Induction Techniques

PREMEDICATIONS—SEDATIVES

Rectal midazolam
Oral benzodiazepine or barbiturate or narcotic
Intranasal benzodiazepine or ketamine
Transmucosal (lollipop) fentanyl

Induction agents—sleep-inducing
Barbiturates: rectal or intravenous
Ketamine: intramuscular or intravenous
Etomidate: intravenous
Propofol: intravenous
Potent inhalational agents

MODIFICATIONS OF MASK INDUCTION

Give the child the option of sitting up, either in a chair or on a lap.
Let the child hold the mask.
Provide a choice of flavored gases.
Conceal the breathing circuit—"Trojan horse"
Halothan Phone—concealed in play phone
Pungent Pacifier—concealed behind a pacifier
Sleepy Bear—concealed with a stuffed animal

MODIFICATIONS OF INTRAVENOUS INDUCTION

Use EMLA cream to place an intravenous cannula.
Use a 25- or 27-gauge "butterfly" needle.
Allow the patient to push a syringe containing the appropriate dose of drug through a preexisting IV access line.
Create diversions (i.e., have the patient count backward from 100, or tell jokes or stories).

From Zuckerberg, A. L. (1994). Perioperative approach to children. *Pediatric Clinics of North America 41*(1) 25.

The child may also want a favorite toy or object. Providing warm blankets and a rocking chair as a comfort measure may assist both the child and the parent. Pain medication should be provided as needed (see Chapter 20). Depending on the procedure performed, the child may be discharged from the hospital or admitted to an inpatient unit for the remainder of the hospital stay.

Postoperative Care

Most facilities have a specific protocol that is followed for postoperative care. After a surgical procedure the child's vital signs are monitored frequently until they are stable. The surgical site is checked for drainage and the child is assessed for pain. The use of patient-controlled analgesia (PCA) and the routine administration of analgesia provide effective pain control. Refer to Chapter 20 for a more detailed discussion of pain management in children.

Atelectasis is a common complication of surgery related to the effects of anesthesia in combination with small tidal volume breathing, somnolence, splinting secondary to pain, and cough suppression caused by pain or opioid analgesics (Yaster et al., 1994). The lungs should be auscultated to determine any abnormal breath sounds or areas of diminished or absent sounds. In addition, early ambulation, deep breathing, and coughing are encouraged. The use of incentive spirometers can increase respiratory movement. The use of games, such as blowing cotton, a windmill, or bubbles, can also facilitate air exchange.

Children generally recuperate more quickly in a familiar environment; as a result, they are discharged as soon as is safely possible following surgery. Because of decreased lengths of stay, discharge planning should begin at the time of admission. Utilizing an organized plan of care, the discharge planner works closely with the child and family to identify needs and resources and then develops an efficient, cost-effective plan for meeting those needs.

Some children will need specialized care in the home following discharge from the hospital. The ability of the family to provide some or all of the care will determine the extent of education provided prior to discharge and the need for involvement of a home health agency after discharge. The family and the nurse must identify the level of knowledge needed and any specific equipment and/or home modifications required to adequately care for the child at home. It is usually the responsibility of the home health agency to make the necessary arrangements for durable or disposable equipment. It is helpful, when possible, for equipment and supplies to be provided by the same agency that provides assistance with home nursing care. Some agencies also will provide education for the family prior to the child's discharge. These issues and delegation of responsibilities need to be addressed as soon as they are identified in order to ensure the child and family the smoothest transition possible from hospital to home.

Common nursing diagnoses associated with the child undergoing surgery include the following:

- Anxiety and fear related to separation from significant other(s), surgery, unfamiliar environment, and personnel
- Pain related to the surgical incision
- Knowledge deficit related to the procedure and expected outcomes
- Altered family processes related to the surgical procedure
- Risk for fluid volume deficit related to NPO status before and after surgery, as well as to nausea and vomiting

Additional Information

The student is referred to Chapter 9 for a discussion of care associated with play, and to Chapter 10 for assistance with communication challenges. Chapter 15 provides information on care related to hospitalization and separation; Chapter 17 describes nursing care as it pertains to certain conditions; Chapter 20 discusses pain-related issues; and Chapter 24 presents nursing care as it relates to fluid volume deficits. To deliver quality care, the child's growth and development needs must be identified by the nurse, along with the care needs associated with the disorder for which surgery is required.

KEY CONCEPTS

- Whenever possible, procedures should be performed in the treatment room, away from the child's room.
- Some procedures require informed consent. Children 7 years of age and older must give assent to some procedures. Because laws on informed consent vary from state to state, nurses must be familiar with the laws and policies of their institution.
- Developmentally appropriate words should be used when preparing children for procedures.
- Children should be praised for attempts at cooperation during a procedure even if they did not follow instructions. Praise them for accomplishing an expected task.
- Documentation of a procedure should include the following: preparation, who performed the procedure, the child's tolerance, the actual procedure, and outcomes.
- Standard Precautions must be maintained in the collection of all specimens.
- Restraints should be used only as a last resort for the protection of the child and others.
- Standard Precautions are used for all hospitalized patients and are not based on diagnosis or presumed infectious state. Transmission-Based Precautions are for patients known or suspected to be infected by pathogens that are transmitted by airborne or droplet transmission or by contact with dry skin or contaminated surfaces.

REFERENCES

Andersen, J. B., & Falk, M. (1991). Chest physiotherapy in the pediatric age group. *Respiratory Care, 36*(6), 546–552.

Brennan, A. (1994). Caring for children during procedures: A review of the literature. *Pediatric Nursing, 20*(5), 451–458.

Broome, M. (1990). Preparation of children for painful procedures. *American Journal of Nursing, 91*(11), 20–24.

Brown, R., & Ioli, J. G. (1993). A pediatric resuscitation poster: Development and multiple uses. *Pediatric Nursing, 19*(1), 56–58.

Bruce, J. L., & Grove, S. K. (1992). Fever: Pathology and treatment. *Critical Care Nurse, 12*(1), 40–49.

Carroll, C. (1993). Clinical applications of pulse oximetry. *Pediatric Nursing, 19*(2), 150–151.

Clagg, M. E. (1989). Venous sample collection from neonates using dorsal hand veins. *Laboratory Medicine*, April 1989.

Clarke, P. C., & Deeds, N. C. (1988). The child in a mist tent. *Pediatric Nursing, 14*(6), 446–450.

Cote, C. J., Goldstein, M. D., Andree, E., et al. (1988). A single-blind study of pulse oximetry in children. *Anesthesiology, 68*, 184–188.

Davis, A. (1993). The accuracy of tympanic measurement in children. *Pediatric Nursing, 19*(3), 267–272.

Ellis, R. (1989). Once more into the void. *Contemporary Pediatrics, 6*(8), 164.

Enright, T., & Hill, M. G. (1989). Treatment of fever. *Focus on Critical Care, 16*(2), 96–102.

Erickson, P. J. (1987). Ostomies: The art of pouching. *Nursing Clinics of North America, 22*(2), 311–320.

Food and Drug Administration. (1991). *Potential hazards with protective restraint devices.* (MDA91–3). Rockville, MD: FDA Medical Alert.

French, J. P. (1995). *Pediatric emergency skills.* St. Louis, MO: C. V. Mosby.

Garner, J. (1966). Guidelines for isolation precautions in hospitals. *American Journal of Infection Control, 24*, 24–52.

Garza, D., & Becan-McBride, K. (1993). *Phlebotomy handbook* (3rd ed.). Norwalk, CT: Appleton & Lange.

Gildea, J. H. (1992). When fever becomes an enemy. *Pediatric Nursing, 18*(2), 165–168.

Hamner, S., & Miles, M. (1988). Coping strategies of children with cancer undergoing bone marrow aspirations. *Journal of the Association of Pediatric Oncology Nursing, 5*(3), 11–15.

Hazinski, M. F. (1986). Pediatric home tracheostomy care: A parent's guide. *Pediatric Nursing, 12*(1), 41–48.

Hess, D., & Kacmarek, R. M. (1993). Techniques and devices for monitoring oxygenation. *Respiratory Care, 38*(6), 646–669.

Hill, A. S., & Rath, L. (1993). The care and feeding of the low-birth-weight infant. *The Journal of Perinatal and Neonatal Nursing, 6*(4), 56–68.

Holden, P. (1995). Psychosocial factors affecting a child's capacity to cope with surgery and recovery. *Seminars in Perioperative Nursing, 4*(2), 75–79.

Huddleston, K. C., & Ferraro, A. R. (1991). Preparing families of children with gastrostomies. *Pediatric Nursing, 17*(2), 153–158.

Lohr, J., Donowitz, L., and Dudley, S. (1989). Bacterial contamination rates in voided urine collections in girls. *Journal of Pediatrics, 114*(1), 91–93.

Margolius, F. R., Sneed, N. V., & Hollerbach, A. D. (1991). Accuracy of apical pulse rate measurement in children. *Nursing Research, 40*, 378–380.

McDonald, N., et al. (1985). Efficacy of chlorhexidine cleansing in reducing contamination of bagged urine specimens. *Canadian Medical Association Journal, 135*, 1211–1213.

McGee, L. (1987). Feeding gastrostomy. *Journal of Enterostomal Therapy, 14*(5), 201–211.

Metheny, N. (1988). Measures to test placement of nasogastric and naso-intestinal feeding tubes: A review. *Nursing Research, 37*(6), 324–329.

Metheny, N. (1993). Minimizing respiratory complications of nasoenteric tube feedings: State of the science. *Heart & Lung, 22*(33), 213–223.

Murphy, K. (1992). Acetaminophen and ibuprofen: Fever control and overdose. *Pediatric Nursing, 18*(4), 428–431, 433.

Nederhand, K., Solon, J., Sweet, J. I., & Conner, S. C. (1989). Respiratory syncytial virus: A nursing perspective. *Pediatric Nursing, 15*(4), 342–345.

Petillo, M. (1987). The patient with a urinary stoma: Nursing management and education. *Nursing Clinics of North America, 22*(2), 263–279.

Pontious, S., Kennedy, A. H., Shelley, S., and Mittrucker, D. (1994). Accuracy and reliability of temperature measurement by instrument and site. *Journal of Pediatric Nursing, 9*(2), 114–123.

Roemer, N. R. (1991). The tracheotomized child: Private duty nursing at home. *Home Healthcare Nurse, 10*(4), 28–32.

Runton, N. (1992). Suctioning artificial airways in children: Appropriate techniques. *Pediatric Nursing, 18*(2), 115–118.

Schmitt, B. (1992). *Instructions for Pediatric Patients.* Philadelphia: W. B. Saunders.

Smith, D., Nix, K., Kemper, J., Liguoni, R., Brantly, D., Rollins, J., Stevens, N., & Clutter, L. (1991). *Comprehensive child and family nursing skills.* St. Louis, MO: Mosby–Year Book.

Sneed, N. V., & Hollerbach, A. D. (1991). Accuracy of apical pulse rate measurement in children. *Nursing Research, 40*, 378–380.

Sneed, N. V., and Hollerbach, A. D. (1995). Measurement error in counting heart rate: Potential sources and solutions. *Critical Care Nurse, 15*(1), 36–40.

Soud, T. (1993). Pediatric update: The febrile child in the emergency department. *Journal of Emergency Nursing, 19*(4), 355–358.

Squires, V. L. (1995). Child-focused perioperative education: Helping children understand and cope with surgery. *Seminars in Perioperative Nursing, 4*(2), 80–87.

Steele, N. F. (1991). The button: Replacement gastrostromy device. *Journal of Pediatric Nursing, 13*(4), 421–424.

Strong, R. M., Gribbon, R., Durling, S., & Condon, S. (1988). Enteral tube feedings utilizing a pH sensor feeding tube. *Nutritional Support Services, 8*(8), 11, 25.

Suddaby, E. C., & Sourbeer, M. O. (1990). Drawing pediatric arterial blood gases. *Critical Care Nurse, 10*(7), 28–31.

Tammelleo, A. D. (1992). Restraints: A legal Catch 22? *RN, 55*(4), 71–72, 75–76.

Thompson, V. (1994). An IV therapy teaching tool for children. *Pediatric Nursing, 20*(4), 351–355.

Thornlow, D. K. (1995). Is chest physiotherapy necessary after cardiac surgery? *Critical Care Nurse, 15*(3), 39–46.

Uhing, M., & Dziedzic, K. (1990). Pulse oximetry in neonatal management. *Respiratory Management, 20(5), 116–120.*

Warnock, C., & Porpora, K. (1994). A pediatric trach card: Transforming research into practice. *Pediatric Nursing 20*(2), 186–188.

Wells, N., King, J., Hedstron, C., & Youngkins, J. (1995). Does tympanic temperature measure up? *Maternal Child Nursing, 20*, 95–100.

Wilson, V. (1986). How to make a feeding tube go down easily. *RN, 49*(11), 40–43.

Yaster, M., Sola, J. E., Pegoli, W., & Paidas, C. N. (1994). The night after surgery: Postoperative management of the pediatric outpatient—Surgical and anesthetic aspects. *Pediatric Clinics of North America 41*(1), 199–219.

19

Medicating Infants and Children

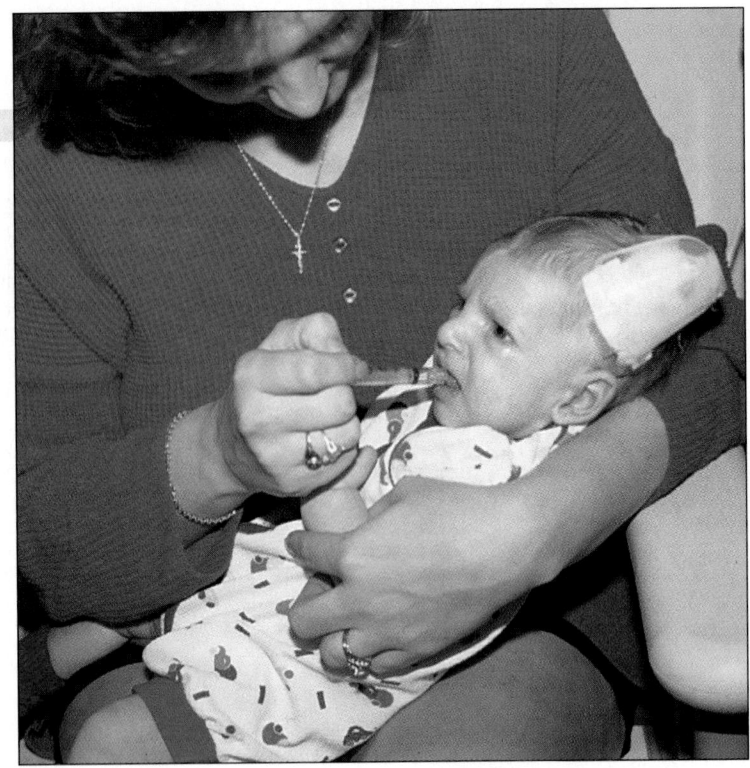

Courtesy of Children's Medical Center, Dallas, Texas

CHAPTER OVERVIEW

LEARNING OBJECTIVES

After studying this chapter, you should be able to:

- Describe different methods of administering medications to children.
- List advantages and disadvantages of each route of pediatric medication administration.
- Describe the physiological differences that must be accounted for when medicating a pediatric patient.
- Describe psychosocial interventions for teaching and successful medication administration for each age group.

KEY TERMS

blood–brain barrier: selective anatomic or physiologic capillary obstruction that prevents potentially harmful substances, such as certain medications, radioactive ions, and viruses, from entering the parenchyma of the brain.

central venous access device: venous access device in which the catheter is centrally placed, usually in the superior vena cava or jugular vein; used for long-term intravenous therapy.

dead space: space in the hub of the syringe and needle; medication remains in the dead space after a medication has been injected (usually 0.2 ml).

epidural medication: medication administered directly into the epidural space in the spine; administered either as a bolus injection or on a continuous basis through an infusion pump.

eutectic mixture of local anesthetics (EMLA): cream used to numb the skin at a depth of 0.5 mm; used before needlesticks.

heparin lock (intermittent infusion port): IV catheter placed and used to administer intravenous medications intermittently.

implanted venous access device (IVAD, infusaport): implanted port or reservoir that is surgically implanted with the catheter tip placed in the superior vena cava; used for long-term intravenous therapy.

metered dose inhaler: handheld device that delivers "puffs" of medication for inhalation.

patient-controlled analgesia: pain medication administered through an infusion pump, either as a continuous (background) infusion, with or without bolus doses, or as a bolus only; allows the patient to retain some control over how often and how much pain medication is administered.

peripherally inserted central line: central line that is inserted peripherally (usually through an antecubital vein) into the superior vena cava.

pharmacokinetics: study of the properties of medications.

sustained-release medication: medication designed to be taken in its complete form; it slowly dissolves and releases medication into the bloodstream over a specified length of time (usually 12–24 hours).

tunneled central line: surgically placed central line held in place by a Dacron cuff located in a subcutaneous tunnel; most commonly placed in the external jugular vein.

Medicating infants and children is one of the nurse's most important responsibilities. The nurse plays a key role in administering medications, supporting the child and family during the experience, and teaching the child and parents about pharmacologic aspects of their care.

Although physicians prescribe medications, it is the nurse who is responsible for their administration. The nurse has a legal responsibility to administer medications safely and accurately. Giving medications to children requires special skill. The nurse must understand the physical characteristics and psychological needs of children in each developmental stage in order to gain the cooperation of the child and to administer the medication in the least traumatic manner. The nurse must use developmentally appropriate strategies to handle children's fears, prevent injury, and enhance coping. Safe administration of medications to children requires an understanding of the dosages of the medications used in pediatrics, as well as the expected actions, possible side effects, and signs of adverse reactions or toxicity. Nurses should utilize reliable sources of information (pharmacists, *Physician's Desk Reference,* drug handbooks) when administering drugs that are unfamiliar or used infrequently and should question orders they do not understand before administering the medication.

Parents must be given information about medications used in their child's treatment and should be encouraged to support their child during the experience. Involving parents in the task of getting children to take medications not only makes the job easier, but also gives the family a sense of self-management and control. If the parents will be asked to administer medications to their child at home, the nurse is responsible for seeing that they are properly instructed before the child is sent home.

This chapter describes the unique physiology of the child (which can influence drug action), methods of approaching the child at different developmental stages, the calculation of pediatric medication doses, techniques for safe medication administration to children, and the teaching and learning needs of children and families.

PHYSIOLOGIC DIFFERENCES

Body Proportions. The child's body proportions are different from those of an adult. The child's height usually increases by about 3.5 times between birth and adulthood. Weight increases by about 20 times, and body surface area (BSA; relationship between height and weight, or the body area exposed to the environment) increases about 7 times. Because the ratio of BSA to weight varies inversely to length, the infant has relatively more surface area than would be expected from weight compared with the adult. Because dosages are often calculated with BSA, this difference is important.

Body Composition. The body water content in children ranges from 85% (premature newborn) to 60% (2 years and older). Most adults have a total body water content of about 50%. Percentages of extracellular (circulating) water are higher in the child (45% compared with 15% in adults). For this reason, children require a higher dose per kilogram of a water-soluble medication to achieve the desired effects (see Chapter 24).

Percentages of fat also change as the child grows. Fat makes up about 16% of an infant's weight. This percentage increases to 23% in a 1-year-old. About 8% to 12% of a preschooler's body weight is composed of fat. Fat makes up about 15% of an adult's body weight. These percentages are estimates, and total body fat varies from child to child. The percentage of body fat is an important consideration when administering fat-soluble medications to children. Because the body fat must be saturated with a fat-soluble medication before blood levels are detectable, doses often must be varied to achieve the desired effects.

Finally, muscle mass is approximately 38% less than in the adult. The infant's body weight is about 25% muscle, whereas the adult's is about 40%. Because of this smaller muscle mass, fewer sites are available for intramuscular (IM) injections. Blood flow to muscles in the young child is erratic and also may affect absorption of injected medications.

Body Systems. Most medications are metabolized in the liver. Because the enzyme systems are less mature in newborn and premature infants, fewer enzymes exist for binding. Maternal hormones also may compete for protein-binding sites in the newborn and interfere with medication binding, allowing more free drug to remain in the bloodstream. For this reason, smaller doses of these medications are needed to achieve the desired effects in newborns. Because fewer binding sites exist, biotransformation may be slower, and toxicity may occur rapidly in newborns and premature infants. Children aged 2 to 6 years have a much greater metabolizing capacity for certain drugs than adults. After age 6 this increased capacity gradually declines to adult values by about puberty (Gladke, 1979). For this reason, larger doses or more frequent administration of certain drugs (such as pain medications) may be needed for young children in order to achieve therapeutic results.

Excretion of most medications occurs through the renal system. The renal system is also immature at birth. The glomerular filtration rate of the newborn is about 30% to 50% of that of an adult. The renal tubules also function less efficiently. Adult rates are reached after the first 6 months of life. Urine pH is lower, and the ability to concentrate urine is less. Because of this renal immaturity, medications may not be filtered out of the circulating blood volume and excreted in the urine (the primary method of medication excretion). As a result, medications may circulate longer and reach toxic blood levels. Likewise, loss of fluid would decrease the child's ability to excrete medications. Therefore, dehydration has a serious effect on drug serum levels.

The **blood–brain barrier** (a selective anatomic or physiologic capillary obstruction that prevents potentially harmful substances from reaching the parenchyma of the brain) is not fully mature until the child is about 2 years of age. This immaturity causes the barrier to be less selective. As a result, encephalopathy may occur with many medications. The relative immaturity of the neurologic system may also lead to paradoxic effects from certain medications (i.e., medications that normally cause sedation in adults have the opposite effect in many children, and cause hyperactivity).

The cardiovascular system is also less developed in the child. The peripheral circulation is less reliable and more responsive to environmental changes. As a result, vasoconstriction or dilation may occur and alter the absorption of an injected medication. The cardiovascular system is also less able to accommodate large or rapid changes in volume, and the child may become fluid overloaded if volumes of intravenous (IV) infusions are not carefully monitored. Finally, the increased amount of circulating volume (extracellular fluid) leads to the need for higher doses of water-soluble medications.

Gastric emptying is slower in infants compared with older children. Peristalsis is often irregular in infants, and the gastrointestinal (GI) tract is longer compared with total body size. Gastric secretions are more alkaline (pH 1–3 compared with 0.9–1.5 in adults). Children, particularly infants, eat more frequently than adults and are more likely to have food and digestive enzymes present in their stomachs. These factors all lead to reduced absorption of oral medications. Some medications, such as enterically coated tablets, which depend on a low pH to break down the outer coating or for activation, may pass through the child's digestive tract unchanged. Acidic medications are more readily absorbed, and basic medications are less readily absorbed. Both of these factors can greatly affect serum drug levels.

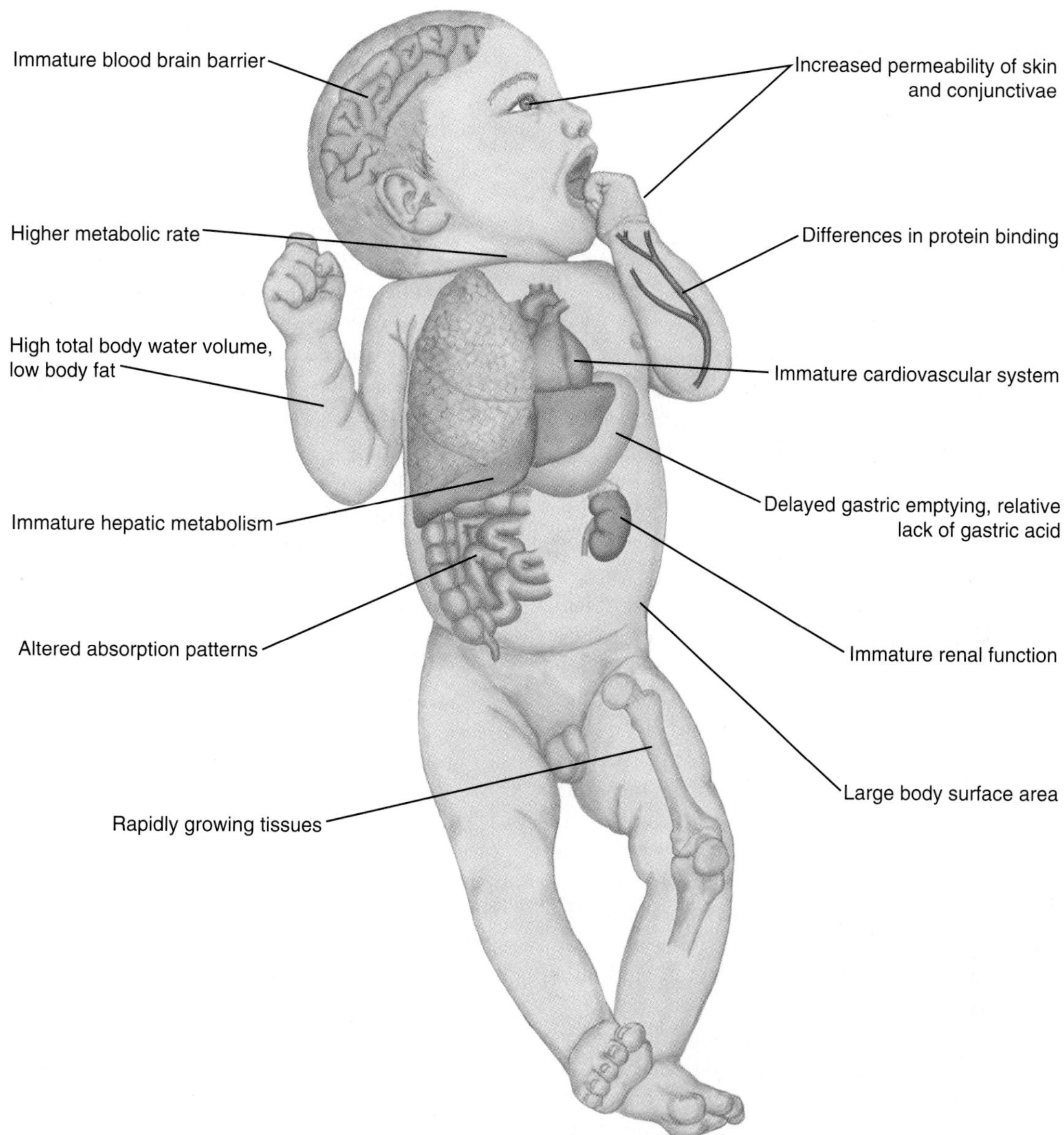

Figure 19–1
Physiologic differences between children and adults affect drug metabolism and distribution. These differences are most extreme in the neonate.

Children have a large BSA (large amount of skin surface). The epidermis is thinner, which allows for more water loss and faster absorption of topical medications and a greater potential for overdose. Skin pH varies with age and may also affect the absorption of topical medications. Finally, a child's skin is more prone to irritation, making contact dermatitis and other allergic reactions more common.

Figure 19–1 reviews some of the physiologic differences in body systems between children and adults. These differences are most dramatic in the neonate.

PSYCHOLOGICAL DIFFERENCES

Growth and developmental principles and differences among age groups must always be taken into consideration when medicating a child.

> The child should always be approached at her developmental level and given age-appropriate explanations and as much choice as possible in the procedure.

Honesty, reward, and praise are important to gain trust and cooperation. Explanations should be honest. The child should be told if a procedure will be painful or uncomfortable. The explanation should be given in terms familiar to the child, such as pinching or bee sting.

Praising the child after the procedure for his attempts at cooperation is important and helps to gain his trust and cooperation for future procedures. Never scold a child for his failure at cooperation.

Restraints may be necessary for safe administration of certain medications, such as injections. Approaches include using a procedure room where another staff member assists in helping the child to remember to hold still; physical restraint devices, such as arm boards; and mummy restraint with a blanket. It is important to explain to the child that the staff person is helping him to remember to hold still. Never tell a child that he will be held down.

Rewards for good behavior often help the child to feel better about the procedure. Rewards should always be safe and appropriate for the child's age. Stickers are often a good choice for younger children. Older children may want a sticker or may choose a small toy or a privilege (e.g., watching a favorite video).

Infants are easier to medicate than toddlers, but more difficult than children who can follow directions. It is important for parents to know why the infant is receiving the medication. It is also important to get help to administer the medication, if necessary, because it may be difficult to restrain a squirming infant. Maintaining a routine and cuddling and comforting the infant before and after the procedure are important.

Toddlers (1–3 years) are prone to magical thinking and may view the administration of medication (especially if painful or intrusive) as a punishment for wrongdoing. They should be given age-appropriate explanations using play, if possible. Cooperation is often gained if the child is allowed to see and handle the instruments before the procedure. Because the toddler may react negatively to restraint, as little restraint as possible should be used. However, assistance from another health care professional may be necessary. Praise and cuddling after the procedure are important. The toddler often needs the cuddling from her mother or other caregiver. Rewards, such as stickers, are also useful for this age group.

Preschoolers (3–5 years) continue to use magical thinking. They fear the unknown and painful procedures. This age group benefits greatly from therapeutic play and participation. They should be given as much control over the procedure and offered as much choice as possible (e.g., "Do you want your medication with juice or milk?"). The preschooler can be asked if she can hold still for a painful procedure. If she cannot, she will tell you. Adhesive bandages are important to children in this age group after an invasive procedure, such as an injection. Preschoolers believe that these bandages "make it better"—an example of magical thinking.

School-age children (6–12 years) fear loss of control, pain, and injury. At this age, a child can understand more complex explanations. He should be given as much choice as possible. He can often cooperate fully, even with painful procedures, but may need a source of distraction (e.g., a radio he can turn up as pain increases) and support (see Chapter 20). He still needs praise, and rewards (e.g., stickers) are still appreciated.

Adolescent patients (13–18 years) fear separation from peers and loss of control. This age group can understand adult explanations and can assist in making decisions about their care. However, adolescents often exhibit a hyperresponse to procedures that may seem inconsistent with their age. It is important to praise their cooperation and find outlets for their frustration (e.g., drawing or writing).

The role of parents in pediatric medication administration is discussed in the accompanying box.

Role of Parents in the Administration of Medication

Often, parents can be helpful in the administration of medication to a pediatric patient. Before the child is medicated, the following information should be obtained from the parent or caregiver:

- Any medication allergies or sensitivities.
- The child's ability to take medications (i.e., he can't swallow pills).
- Any methods the parent uses to administer medication (e.g., mixing it with certain foods).

Parents should receive explanations before any medication administration.

Allow the parents to administer certain medications (oral, otic, ophthalmic) if doing so will ensure successful administration. The nurse is responsible for ensuring that the "five rights" are followed before the administration, but may allow the parent to give the child an oral medication or administer ear drops.

Listen to parents when they express concern that a medication is not effective or is making the child ill. Parents know their children and often can assess subtle changes long before staff notice them.

CALCULATING DOSAGES

Standard doses do not exist for pediatric medications. Instead, doses are calculated based on the child's weight (mg/kg). This practice is the most reliable method of

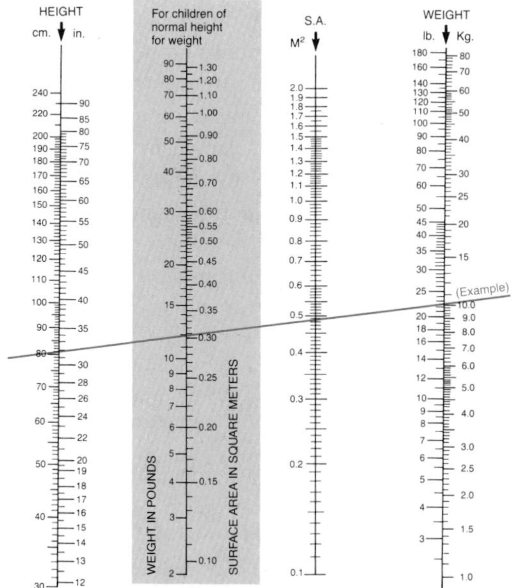

Figure 19–2

Nomogram for calculating body surface area to determine medication dosages for infants and children. (From Behrman, R. E., Kliegman, R. M., & Arvin, A. M. [1996]. *Nelson textbook of pediatrics* [15th ed., p. 2079]. Philadelphia: W. B. Saunders.)

determining doses because it allows for a more precise dose based on weight.

An example of a calculation based on weight follows: For a child weighing less than 20 kg, the dose of amoxicillin should be 20 to 40 mg/kg/day divided every 8 hours. Therefore, a 10-kg child would receive between 200 and 400 mg/day, or 66.67 to 133.33 mg every 8 hours.

Doses may also be calculated based on BSA (mg/m^2) or according to other standardized methods.

To calculate medications based on surface area, the following formula is used:

$$\text{Approximate dose} = \frac{\text{BSA of child (m}^2\text{)}}{1.7} \times \text{adult dose}$$

See also Figure 19–2.

ADMINISTRATION PROCEDURES

Because the margin of safety is minimal in pediatric patients, accuracy is a prime consideration when administering medications (see Checking Prescribed Doses box). Inaccurate dosage calculations may cause errors in decimal point placement. These errors could result in a tenfold or more dosage error. To avoid errors, several procedures should be followed when giving medications to children. These include:

- Use of the "6 rights" of medication administration: right patient, right drug, right dose, right time, right route, and right documentation.
- Always double checking medication calculations before administration.
- Double checking calculations of medications provided by the pharmacy in a unit dose form.
- Having two nurses check the following medications:
  - Insulin
  - Narcotics
  - Chemotherapy
  - Digoxin
  - Anticoagulants
  - K^+ and Ca^{++} salts

Many institutions also require two nurses to check any medication given by continuous infusion and medication syringe pump settings for electrolytes, heparin, and inotropic or vasoactive medications.

Checking Prescribed Doses

Medication doses should always be checked for accuracy before administration:

- Recommended dose in mg/kg/day.
- Number of divided doses recommended (e.g., every 12 hours, every 4 hours).
- Recommended route(s) of administration.

For example, a 20-kg child is to receive an antibiotic that is recommended to be dosed at 100 mg/kg/day divided every 6 hours. Therefore, he would be receiving 2000 mg/day divided into four doses or 500 mg/dose.

If a dose is not within the prescribed limits, the physician should be consulted and the problem reconciled.

Oral Administration

The oral route is the most widespread and economical method of administering medications. It is one of the least reliable methods of administration. This method is affected greatly by the presence or absence of food in the stomach, gastric emptying time, GI motility, and acidity of the stomach. The oral route may also be less predictable because of medication loss to spillage, leaking, or spitting out.

Oral medications are available in liquid (elixir or suspension), tablet or capsule, chewable tablet, or sprinkle (powder) forms. If the child cannot swallow tablets or capsules, the nurse should determine whether the medication is available in a liquid form and if it is not, determine whether it can be crushed.

Before administering oral medications, the nurse should assess the child's gag reflex and ability to swallow. The oral form used should be tailored to the child based on his developmental level and ability to successfully take the form prescribed. An assessment of how the child takes medications at home also helps to determine the proper form. Some older infants and toddlers can successfully take crushed tablets, but refuse liquid forms.

Medication Preparation. When preparing to administer an elixir or suspension, the nurse should ensure that the correct dose is drawn up for administration. Because spoons vary in volume, a calibrated spoon designed for medication administration should be used. Calibrated syringes should be used for doses less than 5 ml or doses that are not in 5-ml increments. Larger volumes may be poured into calibrated plastic medicine cups. Care should be taken to avoid paper measuring cups because volumes tend to vary.

If the medication is to be crushed and mixed with food or is available as a sprinkle or powder, it should be offered with a nonessential food, such as applesauce or pudding, not orange juice or formula, and not with a favorite food, especially if it will alter the flavor of the food. Syrup should be avoided because of the high sugar content (Bindler & Howry, 1991). The medication should be mixed with a small amount (5–10 ml) of food and given to the infant before a feeding. The compatibility of the medication with a food should be determined before a mixture is created. Infants should never receive medications mixed with honey because of the risk of infantile botulism (Bindler & Howry, 1991).

Sustained-release tablets or capsules (designed to be taken whole and to dissolve slowly, releasing medication into the bloodstream over a specified period) should never be crushed. Crushing may cause the dose to be dumped rather than slowly released (Nurses' Drug Alert, 1988). In addition, crushed medication may have an unpleasant taste or odor. The enteric coating prevents the medication from dissolving before passing into the intestinal tract, and crushing may cause mixing of ingredients that should remain separated before administration, or deterioration on exposure to air (Nurses' Drug Alert, 1988).

Medication Administration. The method of administering oral medications should be tailored to the child's age and developmental level. Infants usually receive elixir or suspension forms of oral medications. These may be administered with an empty nipple or oral syringe. The infant's mouth may be opened by applying gentle pressure to his chin. If the nurse is using a nipple, it should be placed in the infant's mouth and the medication added to the empty nipple when the baby begins to suck. An oral syringe should be placed in the infant's mouth along the side of the cheek, and the medication squirted in slowly along the cheek as the infant sucks on the syringe. Aiming the medication toward the back of the throat is dangerous because it may cause choking and aspiration (Fig. 19–3).

Toddlers and preschoolers can easily take liquid medications from an oral syringe or medicine cup. Preschoolers can usually manage chewable tablets without difficulty. Most older children can swallow tablets or capsules. However, it is important to determine whether the child can swallow pills. If she cannot, the nurse should determine whether the medication can be crushed and mixed with food or a small amount of water. If the child cannot swallow tablets or capsules and they cannot be crushed, the nurse should contact the pharmacy to identify another form for administration(elixir or suspension). If the child can swallow tablets and capsules, allow her to choose which tablet to take first and the food it will be mixed with, or the "chaser" (usually water or juice). If the medication is in liquid form, a medicine cup or oral syringe

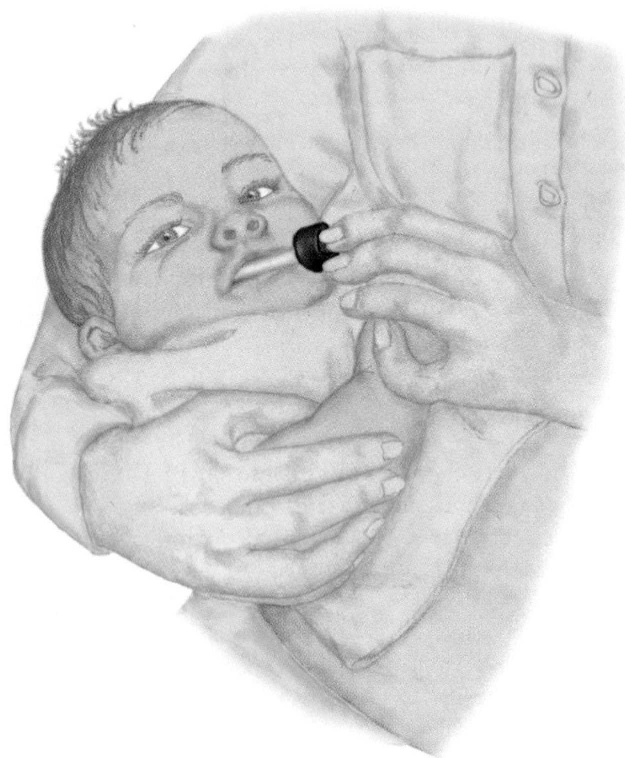

Figure 19–3
A syringe is often used to give liquid oral medication to infants and young children. The adult positions the child on his lap so that the child's back is supported by the adult's nondominant arm. The child's arm that is nearest the adult's body is placed toward the adult's back and waist area. The other arm is restrained with the adult's nondominant hand. The adult's dominant hand is used to administer the medication, injecting it toward the back and side of the mouth to reduce gagging.

may be used to administer the medication. If the child is drinking the medication through a straw, the straw should be cut in half to avoid a loss of medication.

Oral medications should be administered with the child in an upright or slightly recumbent position. It is important for the nurse to use the least amount of force or restraint possible to safely administer the medication to avoid choking and aspiration. If necessary, the child may be restrained by placing him in the nurse's lap with the child's right arm behind the nurse's back, the child's left hand held by the nurse's left hand, and the child's head supported by the nurse's left arm and secured between the nurse's arm and body. The child's legs may also be secured between the nurse's legs, if necessary. If the child objects to the form of the medication, the nurse should try another form. Finally, if the child vomits or spits up after the administration of medication, the physician should be notified. Another dose may need to be reordered depending on how long it has been since administration, the type of medication, and the amount vomited.

Alternate Oral Routes. Oral medications may be administered directly into the GI tract through a feeding tube. If the medication is to be administered through a feeding tube, tube placement should be verified before administration and, depending on the type of tube (i.e., transpyloric), the nurse must determine whether the tube is the proper route for the medication. Placement should be verified by **both** aspirating for stomach contents and auscultating injected air. After the medication is administered, the tube should be flushed with water to ensure that the full length of the tube has been rinsed and will not be clogged by medication and that the medication has reached the GI tract.

Injections

Injected medications have a rapid rate of absorption by diffusion into either plasma or the lymphatic system. Although the rate of absorption is faster and more reliable than the oral route, injections are stressful and threatening to children and are not the first choice of route. Injections are used most often for one-time doses of antibiotics (i.e., penicillin G prophylaxis for rheumatic fever), immunizations, iron, and purified protein derivative (PPD) or allergy skin testing. Injections are potentially more dangerous in infants than in older children because of the decreased muscle mass and variable blood flow to muscles.

Care must be taken to prepare the child for the injection. The reason for the injection and any sensations the child will experience should be described and discussed with the child based on her developmental level. Care should be taken to explain to the child that the injection is not punishment for any wrongdoing. Parents should be offered the option to leave if they feel unable to cope with the procedure. Although most parents prefer to remain with their child during invasive procedures (Baucher et al., 1989), some studies have indicated that toddlers may be less stressed if their caregiver is not present (Broome & Endsley, 1989). If the nurse senses that the parent is uncomfortable, the nurse may need to offer the parent permission to leave by asking if he needs to take a break. It is important to tell the parent how long the procedure is expected to take and that he will be notified if his assistance is needed and when the procedure is completed.

It is usually necessary to restrain the child before administering an injected medication. Restraint helps to avoid administering the injection in the wrong site or breaking or dislodging the needle (Bindler & Howry, 1991). Restraint may be accomplished by swaddling the child or obtaining the assistance of another health care professional. Studies have shown, however, that toddlers are more stressed when restrained in a supine position by an examiner or if other painful procedures are administered before the injection (Broome & Endsley, 1989).

Eland and Anderson (1977) reported that children state that injections are one of their most stressful and painful experiences. Although the child may have experienced more painful procedures, he often perceives a shot as more painful (Gedaly-Duff & Burns, 1992). Several methods are available to help children deal with the pain of an injection. Ice may be applied to the site for 30 seconds to 2 minutes to help numb the area (Gedaly-Duff & Burns, 1992). Topical anesthetic agents such as EMLA have been shown to be effective in reducing injection pain. (See discussion later in this chapter and in Chapter 20.) Children can be taught to deal with the pain of an injection with guided imagery, distraction, or other methods, such as taking a deep breath and blowing out the pain (see Chapter 20). Parents may wish to offer support and comfort to the child, but should not be expected to restrain the child.

Careful documentation of the injection is also important. Documentation should include the amount of medication injected and the site used. If the child will receive several injections, it is important to rotate sites to prevent tissue irritation and possible muscle atrophy and wasting.

Intramuscular Injections. **Dead space** in a syringe (space in the hub of the syringe and needle) must be considered. Most syringes and needle hubs contain approximately 0.2 ml dead space. Therefore, the needle and hub should never be flushed after injection. The air bubble technique for administration is rarely used in pediatric patients, especially when small amounts of medication are given. This technique flushes the hub of the needle with air and administers the medication contained in the hub. This practice adds an additional amount of medication to the prescribed dose and may lead to an overdose of medication. The Z-track method is also seldom used in pediatric patients because it usually involves the administration of

TABLE 19–1 *Preferred Intramuscular Injection Sites in Children*

SITE	KEY POINTS
Vastus lateralis	Located on the anterior lateral thigh. Well developed at birth. Best choice for all age groups, but should always be used in children younger than 3 years. Able to tolerate larger volumes, and not located near vital structures, such as nerves and blood vessels. 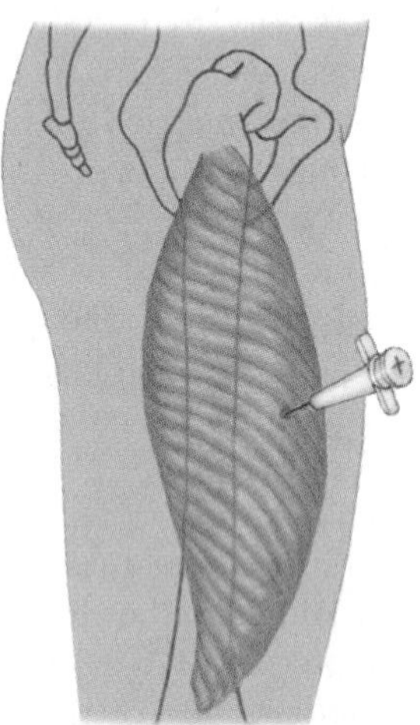 Vastus lateralis
Ventrogluteal	Located by placing the heel of the hand on the greater trochanter with fingers pointed toward the child's head. Place the index finger over the anterior superior iliac spine and the middle finger along the iliac crest posterior as far as possible to form a V. The injection is given in the center of the V. Safe for children older than 18 months because it is free of major blood vessels and nerves. Can generally hold large volumes (up to 2.5 ml in adolescents). Care should be taken to avoid bone and joint. 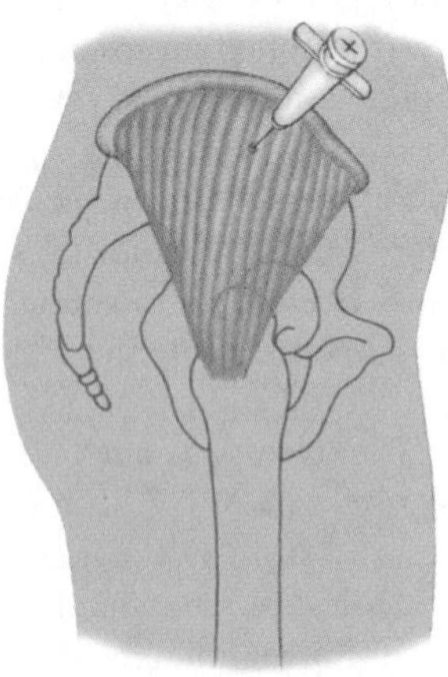 Ventrogluteal
Dorsogluteal	Located by drawing a diagonal line between the posterior superior iliac spine and the greater trochanter of femur. Muscle is found above and lateral to this line. Develops with walking, so should not be used until child has been walking for at least 1 year. The child should be asked to "toe in" to avoid tensing the muscle. Can hold 1 to 2.5 ml but has the slowest and poorest absorption of all sites. 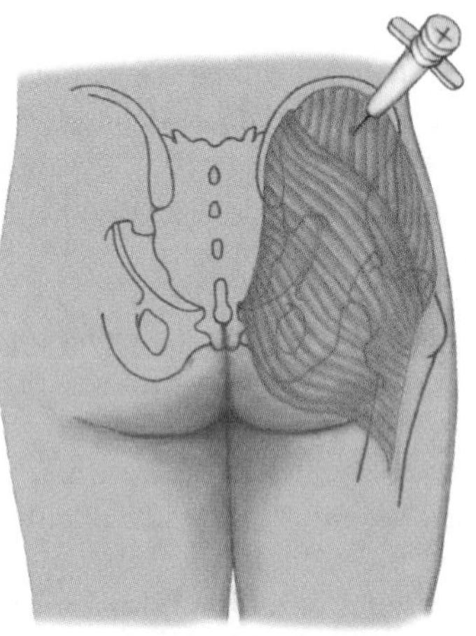 Dorsogluteal
Deltoid	Use part of the muscle located about two fingerwidths below the acromion process. Not used for young children because the small muscle mass cannot hold large volumes of medication or medications that must be injected deep into muscle mass. 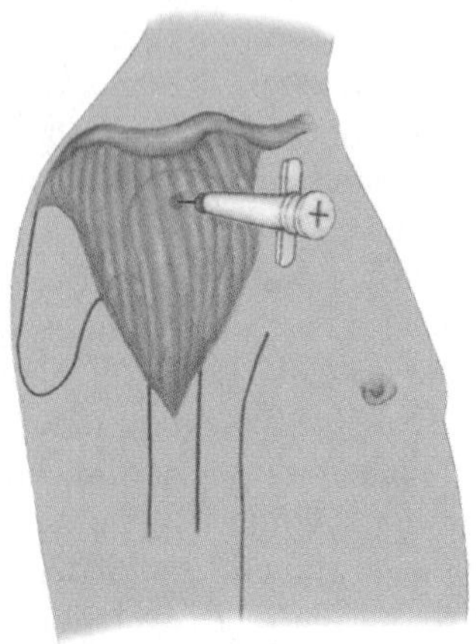 Deltoid

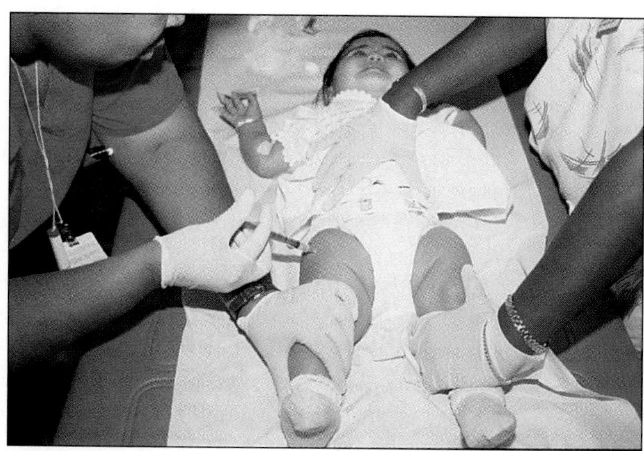

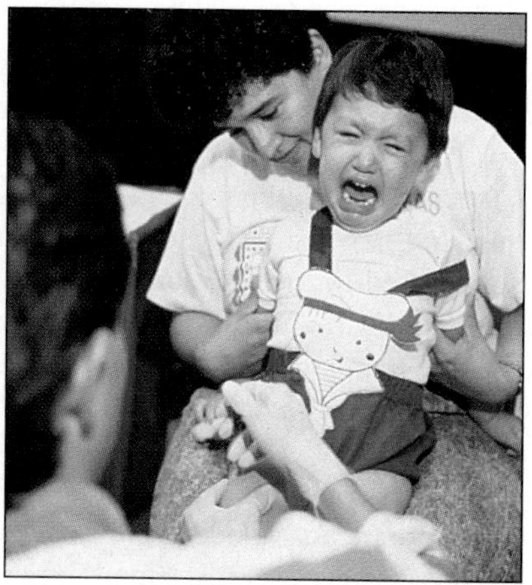

Figure 19–4

The vastus lateralis site for intramuscular injection is located on the anterior thigh, just to the outside of midline, and about halfway between the child's hip and knee. The muscle in this area is well developed and appropriate for intramuscular injections in any age group. The anterior lateral thigh is the only site that should be used for intramuscular injections in children younger than 3 years. Two methods of restraint are shown for IM injection at this site. (Left: Courtesy of Dallas County Hospital District Community Oriented Primary Care Clinic, Dallas, Texas. Right: Courtesy of Cook Children's Medical Center, Fort Worth, Texas.)

an air bubble to lock the medication in. If the Z-track method is used, the dead space in the hub of the needle must be taken into account.

The site must be selected before the child is given an injection. The site should be soft, well vascularized, and healthy. Care must be taken to avoid blood vessels, nerves, or bones, and also to avoid injecting medications intended for IM administration into subcutaneous tissue. Inadvertent injection into any of these areas may result in pain, tissue sloughing, nerve damage, or gangrene (Pagliaro & Pagliaro, 1987). The preferred IM injection sites in children are shown in Table 19–1, and methods of restraint are shown in Figure 19–4.

Needle size and length must be determined before medication is given. The smallest size that will **safely and comfortably** administer the medication should be used. For example, a viscous medication is less painful when injected through a larger-gauge needle. The nurse must also consider the amount of body fat, the distance to the muscle, the size of the muscle, the volume of medication, and the properties of the medication.

Safe volumes for IM injection range from 0.5 ml to 2.5 ml (Bindler & Howry, 1991). The injection is given at a 90° angle with a quick darting motion. The plunger should be aspirated to check for the presence of blood. If blood is noted, the needle should be withdrawn to avoid

GUIDELINES FOR MAXIMUM VOLUMES OF IM MEDICATIONS THAT CAN BE SAFELY INJECTED

	SITE			
AGE	DELTOID	VENTRO-GLUTEAL	DORSO-GLUTEAL	VASTUS LATERALIS
Premature infant	—	—	—	0.5 ml
Neonate	—	—	—	0.5 ml
Infant	—	—	—	1 ml
Young child (3–6 years)	—	1.5 ml	1 ml	1.5 ml
Older child (6–14 years)	0.5 ml	1.5–2.0 ml	1.5–2.0 ml	1.5 ml
Adolescent (age 15–adult)	1 ml	2.0–2.5 ml	2.0–2.5 ml	1.5–2.0 ml

giving the medication IV. If no blood is noted, the injection should be given slowly. Unless contraindicated, the injection site should be massaged after the injection.

Subcutaneous Injections. A subcutaneous injection is given into the tissue that lies just below the skin. This type of administration is used for medications that provide a sustained effect (e.g., heparin, insulin). A subcutaneous injection should be given only into healthy tissue. If circulation is impaired, for example, because of edema, decreased temperature, or shock, a subcutaneous injection should not be used because absorption will be impaired.

Preferred subcutaneous injection sites are the fat pads located above the iliac crests, hips, lateral upper arms, and anterior thighs (Fig. 19–5). Sites should be rotated to avoid the development of abscesses and to facilitate drug absorption. Care should always be taken to document the site of the subcutaneous injection to avoid using the same site and causing tissue irritation.

Subcutaneous injections are usually given with a small (25–27-gauge), short (no more than ½″ in length) needle to ensure that the medication is not inadvertently given IM. Volumes range from 0.5 to 1.5 ml (Pagliaro & Pagliaro, 1987).

The site should be cleansed with alcohol and allowed to dry. The tissue should be pinched up to raise the fatty tissue from the muscle. The angle of needle insertion is usually 45°. The insertion site may be massaged after administration unless contradicted by the injected medication, such as heparin.

If the subcutaneous injections are to be an ongoing procedure (e.g., insulin administration), special attention

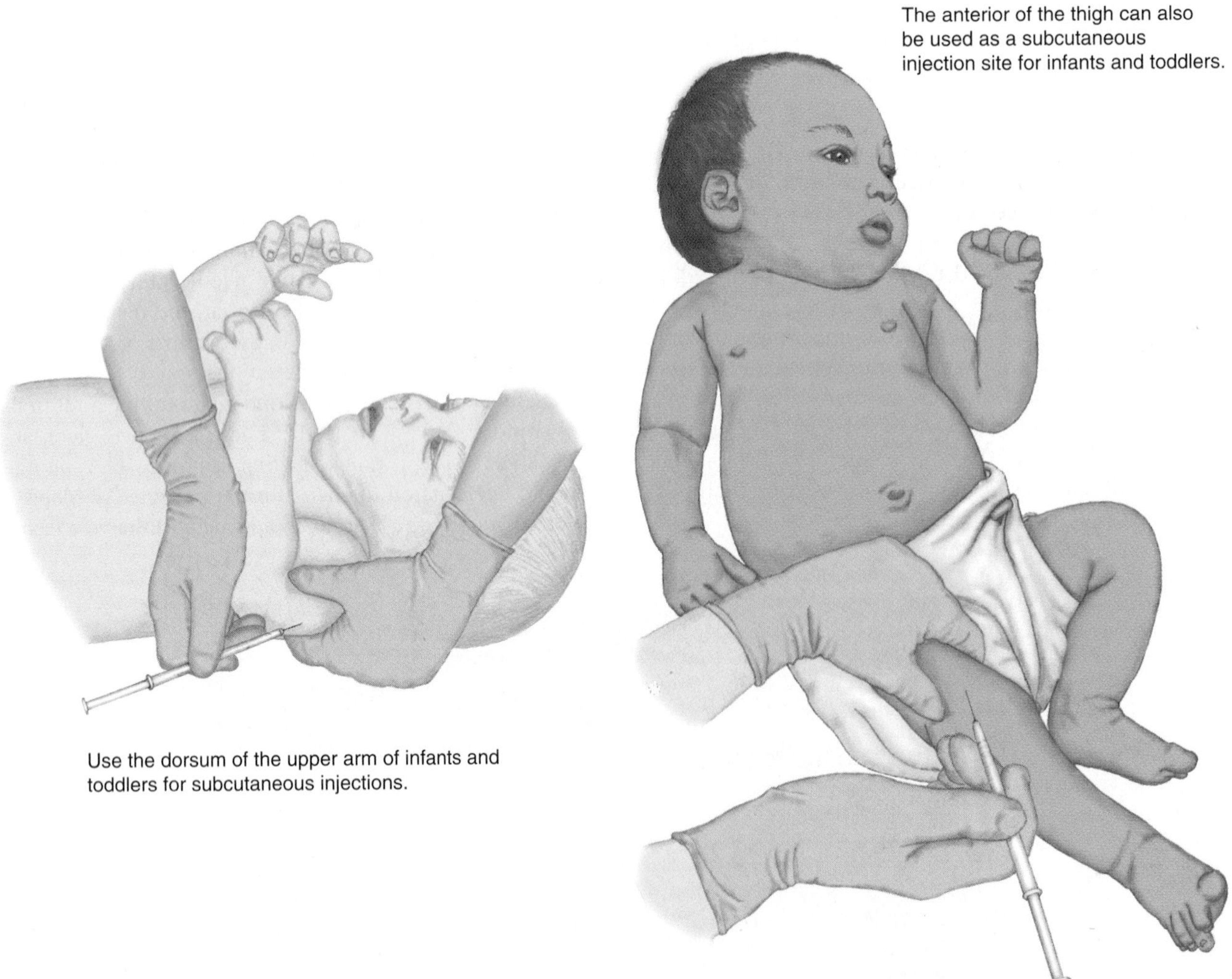

The anterior of the thigh can also be used as a subcutaneous injection site for infants and toddlers.
Use the dorsum of the upper arm of infants and toddlers for subcutaneous injections.

Figure 19–5
Two of the preferred subcutaneous injection sites in children. The fat pads above the iliac crests and hips also may be used.

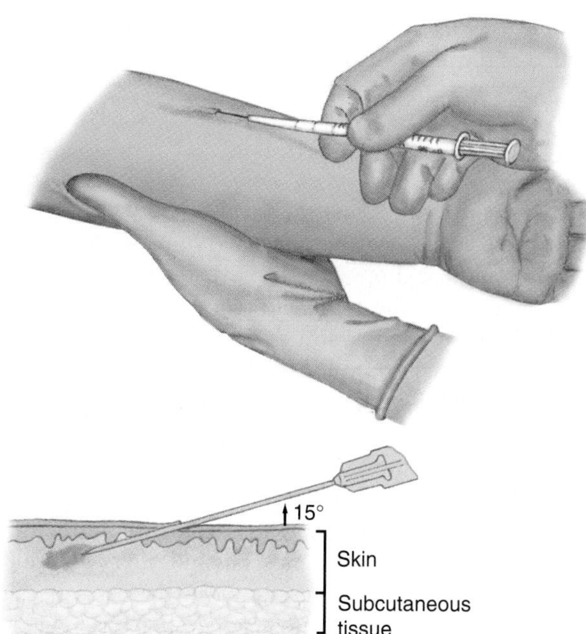

Figure 19–6
Intradermal injection site and technique.

should be paid to patient education. Older children and adolescent patients can usually learn to perform this procedure without difficulty.

Intradermal Injections. Intradermal injections are made just below the outer layer of skin, the epidermis. They are most often used for testing (e.g., allergy, PPD). The sites most often used are the inner aspect of the forearm and the upper back. The needle is small (25–27-gauge) and short ($\frac{1}{2}$–$\frac{5}{8}$inch). The volume is also small (usually 0.1 ml). The needle is inserted at a 15° angle and the medication injected to form a wheal (similar to an insect bite Fig. 19–6). If the injection does not form a wheal, or if bleeding is noted after the injection, administration was probably too deep and should be repeated. If several intradermal injections are made in the same area, each site should be marked with permanent ink for later identification. The child who is to receive multiple injections may benefit significantly from supervised needle play (see Chapter 9). In needle play the child uses a syringe and needle to give shots to a doll. The nurse uses this play to prepare the child for injections and to help him gain a sense of mastery over the experience of receiving an injection. The nurse offers a brief explanation of what will occur and why the child must receive an injection. Through therapeutic play activity the child's anxiety is decreased.

Rectal Administration

The rectal route of administration is unreliable and is not used as often as other routes. It is most often reserved for times when a child cannot tolerate the oral route (e.g., because of nausea and vomiting). It has many possible complications, including the Valsalva response, rectal perforation, and other damage to the rectum or anus.

This route should not be used if the rectum is full of stool. Rectal administration is stressful for children because they fear intrusive procedures. Careful preparation and explanation are essential. The child should know why he is receiving the medication in this form and what he must do to help the nurse. He must also be informed if he must retain the suppository or if it will be expelled.

The child should be positioned on the left side with the right leg flexed. Adequate draping is essential for preschool and older children. The rectal area should be well exposed to prevent injury during administration. Often the child needs help to relax. Distraction and deep breathing exercises may assist the child to relax the external sphincter. The suppository should be well lubricated with a water-soluble lubricant.

The child should be told to take a deep breath or bear down if possible to further relax the sphincter. Then, the suppository is gently inserted past the internal sphincter. The child's rectal vault is not as long as that of an adult, and the distance required to place medication is approximately 1 to 2 cm. After insertion, the buttocks should be held together until the urge to expel the suppository has passed.

Vaginal Administration

Although the vaginal route is not often used in infant, toddler, or preschool girls, it may be required for school-age or adolescent girls. It is most often used to treat candidal infections or possibly for birth control for adolescents. It is essential that an explanation of the procedure, why it is indicated, and what the child needs to do to help is given.

The child should be asked to void and then assisted to a supine position with her knees flexed and hips externally rotated. This position may be achieved easily by having the child place the soles of her feet together and drop her knees laterally until they are lying on the bed. Remember to drape the child and provide for privacy. Using a gloved hand, gently spread the labia so that the vaginal orifice is visualized. If necessary, lubricate the tablet, suppository, or applicator with warm water or water-soluble lubricant. Have the child take a deep breath and gently insert the vaginal tablet, suppository, or applicator approximately 3.5 to 4 inches along the posterior wall of the vagina. To reduce discomfort, the nurse should follow the natural angle of the vagina by pointing the finger or applicator toward the sacrum.

After the procedure is completed, the child may need to remain in a supine position for a period of time. Older school-age children and adolescents can be taught to instill their own vaginal medications. It is important that these children receive good patient education with a return demonstration of the procedure, especially if the instillations are contraceptives.

Ophthalmic Administration

Instillation of ophthalmic preparations is a clean, rather than sterile, procedure. Most pediatric ophthalmic solutions are available as either drops or ophthalmic ointment. If these preparations are refrigerated, they should be allowed to warm to room temperature before instillation.

Before administration, the expiration date should be noted, and drops should be inspected for color changes or cloudiness. Suspensions should always be well shaken before instillation.

The child should receive an explanation of why the medication is ordered, what he will feel, what he must do to help, and what he will experience after the instillation (i.e., blurred vision). Any exudate should be gently removed by wiping the eye with a sterile gauze pad from the inner to outer canthus. A wet compress can help to loosen dried exudate.

The procedure for ophthalmic administration is described in the accompanying box.

Otic Administration

Otic procedures are clean, rather than sterile, procedures except in the case of a ruptured tympanic membrane. Because cold ear drops may cause pain when they come into contact with the tympanic membrane, otic solutions should be allowed to warm to room temperature before administration. The child should have age-appropriate explanations about what she will feel and hear (e.g., "It may sound like there is a butterfly flying inside your ear") and what she must do to help. Assistance in restraining a young child may be necessary.

Any exudate should be gently cleaned from the outer ear with sterile gauze. The nurse should **never** attempt to place anything inside the ear to clean the canal because the risk of rupturing the tympanic membrane is high. The child should be positioned on her side with the affected ear up. The **administering** hand is braced against the child's head above the ear.

Procedure for Administering Ophthalmic Drops and Ointments

1. Assist the child into a supine position with the neck slightly hyperextended (e.g., by placing a rolled towel or small blanket under the shoulder blades).
2. If the drops are to be instilled into the eyes of an infant, obtain assistance in restraining the child's arms and head, as necessary.
3. Instruct an older child to look up toward the top of his head.
4. Gently pull the lower lid down and away from the eye.
5. Place the drops or a ribbon of ointment into the space between the eye and lower lid, taking care not to contaminate the end of the dropper or tube.
6. If both drops and ointment are ordered, the drops should be administered first. If they are placed after the ointment, they will not be absorbed.
7. Have the child look toward his chin as the lower lid is released. Allow him to close his eye, and instruct him to blink as little as possible because much of the instillation may be lost to blinking, thus decreasing the therapeutic effects (Bindler & Howry, 1991).
8. As with any procedure, praise the child for his cooperation and assistance.

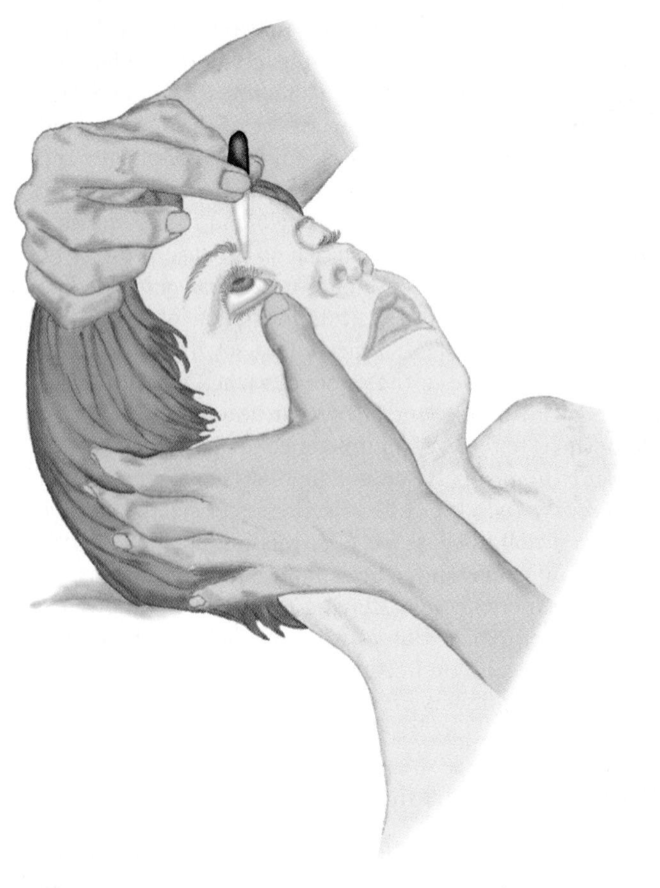

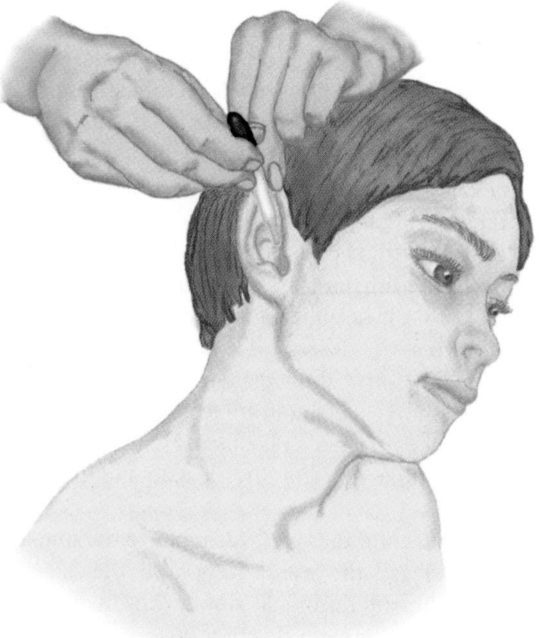

For a child older than 3 years:
pull pinna up and back.

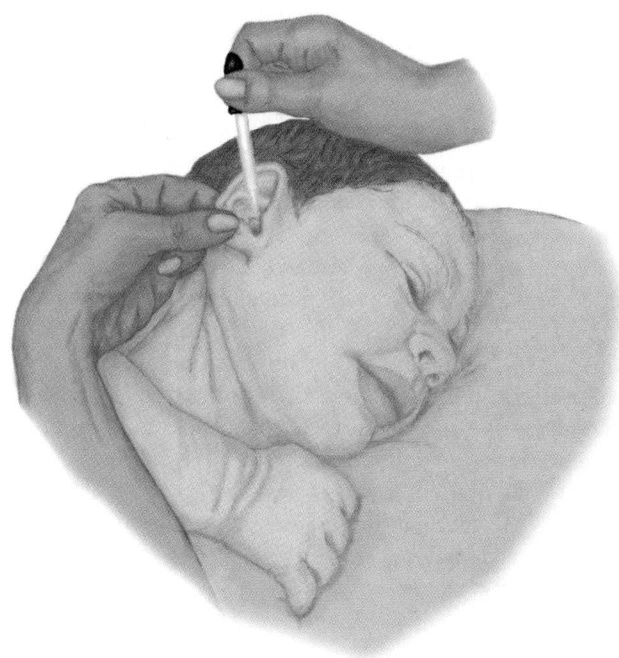

For an infant or a child younger than 3 years:
pull lobe down and back.

Figure 19–7
Administration of ear drops.

ADMINISTRATION OF OTIC DROPS Because of the internal anatomy of the ear, the nurse should remember:

- if the child is 3 years or younger, pull the pinna of the ear back and down.
- if the child is older than 3 years, pull the pinna of the ear back and up.

See Figure 19–7.

After the drops are administered, the tragus (anterior portion) of the ear should be gently massaged to ensure that the drops reach the tympanic membrane. Cotton may be loosely packed into the canal, if ordered. Instruct the child not to remove the cotton or place anything inside the ear. She should also lie on her unaffected side for several minutes after the administration. If medication is to be administered in both ears, the procedure should be repeated in the other ear after a wait of at least one minute.

Nasal Administration

Although the mucous membrane route is generally used only for localized treatment, it has fairly rapid systemic absorption and may be used for the administration of certain systemic medications (i.e., antidiuretic hormone).

When administering nose drops to an infant, the nurse should remove any excess mucous by gently suctioning before administration. Decongestant or saline nose drops should be given 20 to 30 minutes before feedings to make eating easier. Receiving nose drops is stressful for young children, who may feel that they are drowning during the instillation. A thorough explanation of what the child will feel, why the medication has been ordered ("to help unstop your nose"), and what the child needs to do to help is necessary. Assistance with restraint is also necessary with the young child, or mummy restraint or swaddling may be used.

The child is assisted into a supine position with the neck slightly hyperextended by placing a rolled towel or small blanket under the shoulder blades. The head is kept in the midline. The nurse instills the number of drops ordered. The midline positioning allows the drops to reach the ethmoid and sphenoid sinuses. If the child turns his head slightly to the side, the drops will reach the maxillary and frontal sinuses.

After the drops have been instilled, the child remains in a supine position for several minutes to allow the medication to be distributed to the sinuses. The child is instructed not to blow his nose so that the medication can remain. His efforts at cooperation should be praised.

Topical Administration

Because skin is relatively impermeable when intact and has a large surface area, topical administration is generally limited to localized treatment. However, if the medication is applied to abraded skin, over a large area, or over a long period, systemic effects may be noted. Solvents added to the medication to break down skin oils and occlusive dressings also increase absorption. If systemic effects are not desired or if they may be dangerous, the patient should be monitored carefully for signs and symptoms of systemic absorption.

As with all other procedures, the child should have an explanation of what will be done, why it will be done, and what sensations he will experience. The skin should be gently cleaned to remove any exudate, scales, or other residue, and allowed to dry. The amount of medication to be applied should be placed on a sterile pad to avoid contamination of the container. The nurse should wear gloves and apply the ointment or cream as ordered or as recommended by the manufacturer. The site may be covered with a sterile pad, if ordered.

The child should be instructed to avoid touching or scratching the area, and she should be praised for her attempts to cooperate.

Inhalation Therapy

Respiratory medications are used frequently in pediatric patients. They are delivered either as a nebulizer treatment or with a **metered dose inhaler** (MDI; a handheld device that delivers "puffs" of medication for inhalation). Although many inhaled medications have an unpleasant taste or smell, this route is a relatively nonthreatening form of medication delivery (Clark & Pringle, 1990). Monitoring for desired therapeutic effects and systemic effects is essential because most medications used for inhalation have systemic side effects.

Nebulized medications are diluted in normal saline and administered with a handheld small-volume nebulizer (SVN). The SVN device aerosolizes the medication for the child to inhale. Medication may be delivered through mask or through a plastic mouthpiece held between the lips. A mask is preferred for young children because they are seldom able to successfully hold a mouthpiece in place for the required length of time. The child should be encouraged to breathe deeply and slowly during the treatment. The procedure for inhalation therapy is described in the accompanying box.

MDIs offer an inexpensive, portable means of delivering inhaled medications. Many people, particularly children, have difficulty using an MDI correctly. The effectiveness of these medications is increased with the use of an inhalation aid such as a spacer device. These aids may be equipped with a mouthpiece or a mask for young children or those who have difficulty using a mouthpiece.

Although both forms of delivering inhaled medications are effective, the nebulized medication may have greater effectiveness during an acute episode of respiratory distress. It also offers the advantage of being able to be delivered with supplemental oxygen. Nebulized medications may also be delivered to an unconscious or intubated child by inserting the aerosol administration device in-line between the patient and a bag-valve-mask.

Patient education is important to ensure the effectiveness of this form of medication delivery. The technique must be demonstrated and a return demonstration given. The use of the MDI should be reviewed at each return visit.

Procedure for Using an MDI

1. Verify the physician's order for medications(s) to be administered and number of puffs.
2. If one of the medications is an inhaled steroid, it should be administered last.
3. Explain the procedure to the child and parent or caregiver. It is often helpful to demonstrate the use of the inhaler and to explain specifically what the child is expected to do.
4. Place the inhaler in the spacer. Explain to the child that if he inhales too quickly, the spacer will whistle.
5. Explain to the child that he must exhale and place the spacer mouthpiece in his mouth or the spacer mask over his face. He may be more comfortable holding the spacer and helping you.
6. Tell the child that you will squeeze the inhaler and release the medication into the spacer. Then he should inhale slowly. You may need to talk him through this process.
7. Have the child hold his breath for about 10 seconds or until you count slowly to 5.
8. Ask him to exhale and then take another breath from the spacer and hold it for 10 seconds.
9. Repeat with another puff, if ordered.
10. Praise the child for his cooperation.
11. Rinse the inhaler adapter and spacer with cool water. Return the equipment to the medication room or designated area.

INTRAVENOUS THERAPY

Intravenous therapy in children is widely used. The IV route is used to administer fluids and electrolytes, nutrition, blood products, and medications. When used to administer medications, it produces a steadier and more therapeutic blood level and is the only acceptable route for some medications that may be irritating. However, IV therapy poses greater risk because of the danger of fluid overload and possible complications with administration errors.

Intravenous Catheter Insertion

Typically, IV infusions are given through an over-the-needle catheter or a butterfly catheter. The type of catheter chosen often depends on hospital policy. Over-the-needle catheters are generally preferred because of the decreased risk of vein damage and infiltration (Campbell & Jackson, 1991). Over-the-needle catheters are available in even sizes (i.e., 24 and 22 gauge), and butterfly catheters are available in odd sizes (i.e., 23 and 25 gauge).

Venous access sites in children are shown in Figure 19–8. Site selection in the pediatric patient is often determined by the rate and type of fluid to be infused and the availability of veins. The developmental level of the child should also be taken into account. For example, placement of an IV line into the foot of a toddler is often a poor choice. The dominant hand should be avoided if possible (O'Brien, 1991). Scalp veins are often the most accessible in infants. Scalp veins have no valves and may be infused in either direction. IV catheters placed in this area may be secured to allow the infant to move his head without dislodging the IV (Scipien et al., 1990).

Catheter size is also determined by vein size and the type and nature of fluid to be infused. Generally, the smallest catheter that will infuse fluids and medications safely should be used (often a 22- or 24-gauge catheter). For most children, a 20- to 24-gauge catheter provides adequate access (O'Brien, 1991; Campbell & Jackson, 1991).

Before an IV line is started, the child must have an explanation of what will happen (what he will see and feel) and what is needed from him. The child must know what will happen during each step of the procedure. The nurse should assess the child's ability to hold the affected extremity still during the procedure. Parents should receive an explanation of why the catheter will be placed, where it will be placed (if possible), how long it will be in place, and what function it will perform. Parents should also receive an explanation of the purpose of the IV therapy and of any additional equipment (e.g., an infusion pump) used.

Children should be given suggestions for coping with the discomfort. Nonpharmacologic interventions include guided imagery (e.g., putting on an imaginary magic glove that keeps the hand from hurting) and distraction (e.g., music, novelty toys, seek and find books, etc.). Distraction is effective for most children and is easily taught to nurses or parents. Pharmacologic interventions include buffered lidocaine injections (often not used in infants because of the risk of overdose), ice, and topical numbing gels or pastes, such as **EMLA** (eutectic mixture of local anesthetics, a cream used to numb the skin at a depth of 0.5 mm; see the accompanying box). See Chapter 20 for further discussion of pain management techniques.

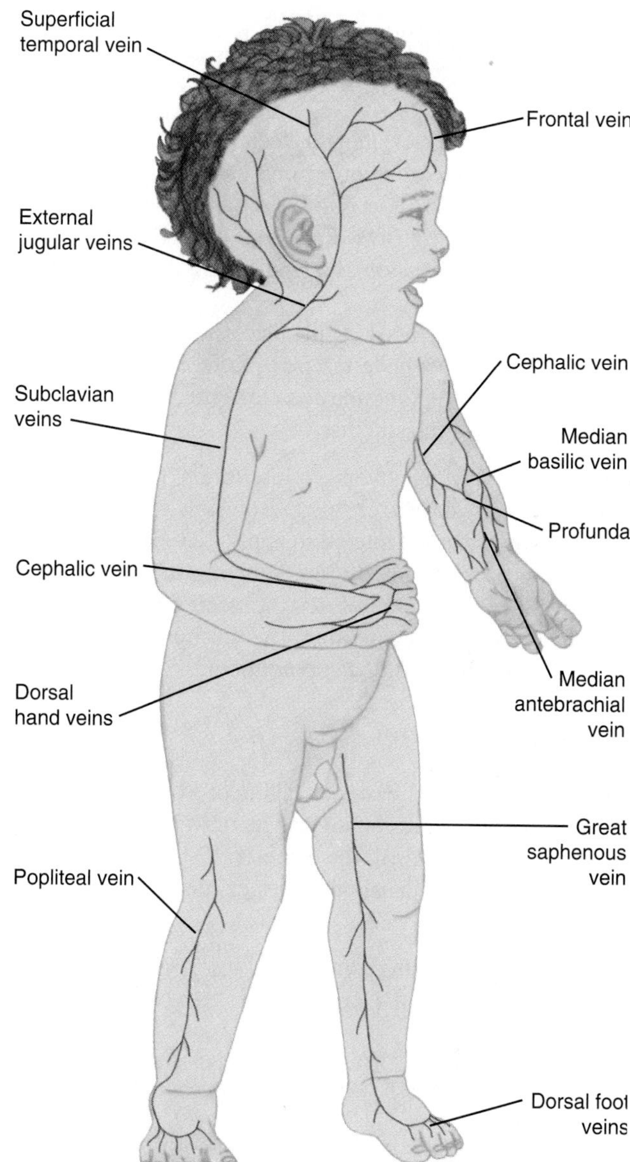

Figure 19–8
Venous access sites in children.

> EMLA should be applied only to intact skin. It should not be used in children with a history of methemoglobinemia (Astra USA, 1993).

Equipment needed includes an IV catheter, tape, occlusive dressing or other sterile dressing, a padded arm board, a tourniquet, and alcohol pads. Povidone-iodine preparations may be used for immunosuppressed patients. The use of an extension set with a T-connector is also recommended. This equipment allows for easier flushing of

Using EMLA Cream Before Performing a Venipuncture

1. Select an intact site and clean it well.
2. Place a liberal amount (one half of 5-g tube or $2\frac{1}{2}$ g) of EMLA cream on the site and cover it with an occlusive dressing (e.g., transparent occlusive dressing). Mound cream; do not rub it in.
3. Leave the EMLA in place for 1–2 hours. EMLA must be left in place at least 60 minutes.
4. Remove the dressing and clean the site.
5. Perform venipuncture.

Parents may be given a prescription for EMLA cream and may be instructed on how to apply it. They must be instructed to apply it at least 1 hour before the scheduled visit. Applying the cream in advance at home alleviates the need for the child and parent to come into the hospital or clinic before their scheduled appointment.

the IV line as well as easier changing of IV tubing. Bacteriostatic normal saline should also be drawn up into a 3-ml syringe and used to flush the catheter. If the venipuncture is also to be used for laboratory specimens, the catheter and T-connector should not be flushed with normal saline before insertion (Bernardo & Bove, 1993). If no blood is to be drawn, flushing the catheter and T-connector with saline may assist in visualizing a blood return (O'Brien, 1991; Bernardo & Bove, 1993). All equipment should be gathered before the nurse enters the room.

Parents should be allowed to remain with the child if they desire. However, they should not be expected to restrain the child during the procedure. The child's ability to hold still during the procedure should be assessed. If he does not feel that he can remain still, the nurse should obtain assistance before attempting to start the IV. Although a variety of restraint devices are available, they do not provide the emotional support of an assistive person. Not only can this person hold the child, but he can also provide emotional support for the child during the procedure (O'Brien, 1991).

The procedure should be explained at each step. The catheter should be placed in the direction of blood flow. The selected site should be assessed for a pulse (to ensure that the vessel is not an artery). When selecting an IV site, the nurse should start with veins of the hand or forearm and work from distal to proximal. If the IV infiltrates, vessels proximal to the IV site can then be used. As the catheter is inserted, it may be helpful to tell the child that he will experience a "big stick" or a pinch, and to take a deep breath and blow out the pain. Catheter placement is confirmed by a blood return and a normal saline flush. If

This boy's IV is secured well enough so he can pretend that he is Magic Johnson as he shoots baskets in the playroom. ▶

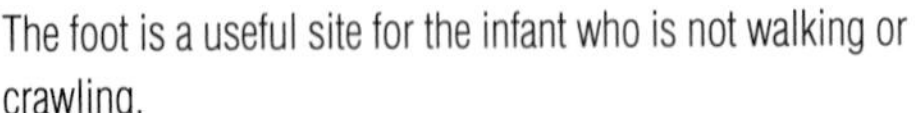
The foot is a useful site for the infant who is not walking or crawling.

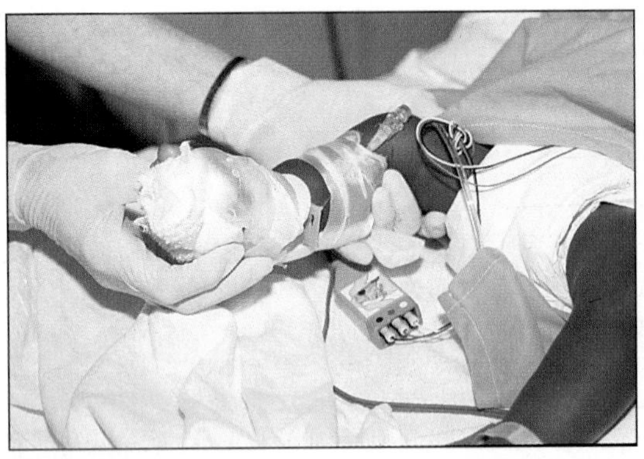

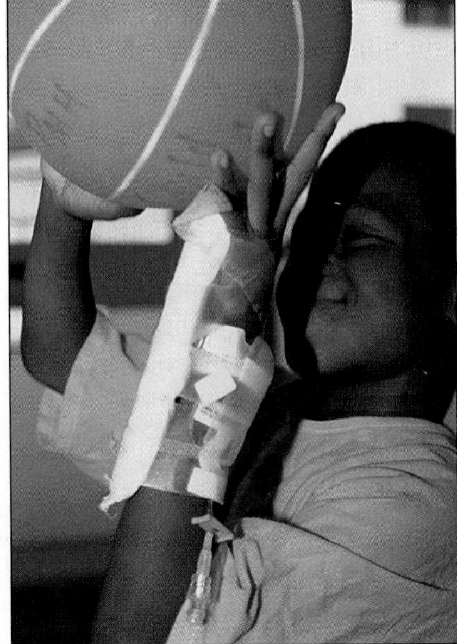

Figure 19–9
Because children's veins are fragile and IV lines may be difficult to place, the site must be well protected to prevent the child from removing the catheter and to tolerate the child's activity. Hand veins may be good for preschoolers and older children because these do not limit walking. A padded arm board gently limits movement of the foot or hand, reducing the risk for infiltration of the IV. A plastic shield allows visualization of the site while protecting it. Saline locks preserve the IV line for administration of medication without the need for constant fluid infusion. (Courtesy of Parkland Memorial Hospital, Dallas, Texas.)

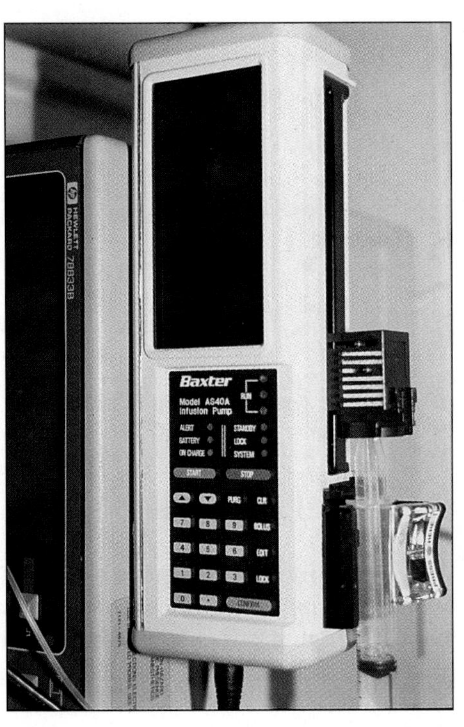

◄ Volumetric infusion pump.

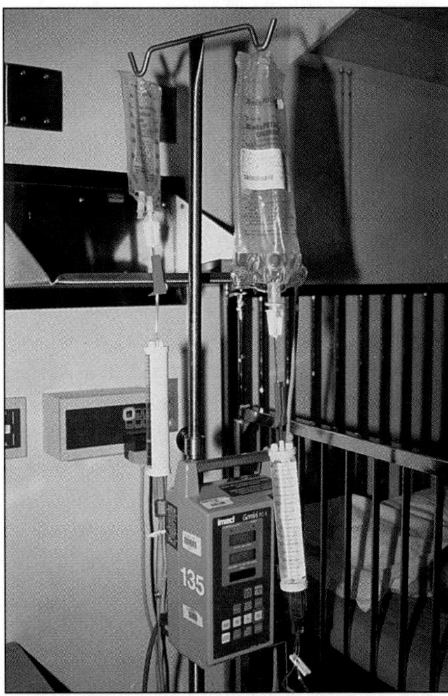

In-line volume control set. ►

Figure 19–10

A syringe infusion pump allows small quantities of solutions to be injected precisely. In this "mode," the syringe filled with IV solution or medication is placed in the pump and the pump is programmed to deliver the appropriate quantity of solution within the correct time. Tubing runs from the tip of the syringe to the child.

The in-line volume control set has two major uses in pediatrics: (1) It provides an additional measure of safety when placed between the large bag of infusion solution and the volumetric pump. The nurse can place a specific volume of fluid in the buretrol chamber (e.g., enough for 2 hours) and clamp the tubing above the volume control set. If the pump malfunctions, the child can receive no more fluid than the amount that was in the volume control set. (2) It is used to administer medication. The medication is diluted appropriately and injected into the volume control set chamber. The volumetric pump is set to infuse the medication from the chamber within the appropriate period. (Courtesy of Parkland Memorial Hospital, Dallas, Texas.)

lab specimens are to be drawn from the catheter, the normal saline flush should not be performed until after the specimens are drawn (Bernardo & Bove, 1993). After the catheter is placed, it should be secured with occlusive dressing or tape with a sterile dressing (Band-Aid) covering the insertion site (Fig. 19–9). Visualization of the site should not be occluded by tape or gauze dressings.

After placement, the IV catheter should be further secured with an arm board. If a bony prominence, such as an elbow or ankle, is to be placed on the arm board, the board should be well padded to avoid interrupting blood flow to the area and causing skin breakdown. The extremity should be secured in an anatomic position to prevent nerve damage. Catheters may be further protected by a plastic shield. This can be a medicine cup that is cut in half and taped on the edges or a commercially available device.

Intravenous Monitoring and Maintenance

Because of the risk of fluid overload, children receiving IV therapy should receive IV fluids through a volumetric infusion pump (Fig. 19–10). An IV counter or controller pump is not appropriate because this device simply counts the number of drops or milliliters that have passed rather than infusing a specific volume over the designated time frame. If available, a pump with a tamperproof design should be used. Another safety feature is the in-line volume control set (Buretrol, Metriset) that is placed between the IV fluid and tubing. This device allows the nurse to place a specific volume of fluid into the volume control set (i.e., enough volume for 1 hour) for infusion and decreases the risk that a large volume of fluid will be inadvertently administered too rapidly.

Sites should be assessed at least every hour or according to hospital policy for signs and symptoms of infiltration. A transparent dressing over the IV site makes assessment easier. The temperature of the site should be assessed as well as the symmetry of the limbs or scalp. The site should be gently touched to determine whether it is soft or taut, or whether the scalp site is boggy. The child may be asked if the site hurts, and nonverbal signs of pain should be noted. If signs of infiltration (e.g., edema, erythema, pain, blanching, coolness, streaking of the skin above the vein) are noted, the infusion should be discontinued immediately and the physician notified. Elevating the extremity may decrease edema. Dry heat may be applied if the infused solution or medication is not a vessicant nor a sclerosing agent. Pediatric IV lines are seldom resited every 72 hours because of the fragility of children's veins. IV fluid bags should be changed every 24 hours. Although Widmer (1993) recommends that IV tubing sets be changed every 48 hours, recent studies have shown that extending this time frame to 72 hours has not significantly increased blood-borne infection rates (Wenzel, 1993). Centers for Disease Control guidelines (1993) recommend that tubing sets used for total parenteral nutrition be changed every 48 hours. Many institutions, however, change TPN tubings every 24 hours in an attempt to further decrease infection rates.

Infusion Rates and Methods

IV medications may be administered as a continuous infusion (e.g., aminophylline, ranitidine) or intermittently (e.g., antibiotics). They may be given in a variety of methods that include IV piggyback, IV retrograde, and IV push. It is imperative that the appropriate method be chosen to meet the needs of the child and fit the restrictions posed by the medication and fluid volume.

At times, the child's IV rate must be adjusted to infuse the medication in the required time frame. In some areas, a physician's order is needed to adjust the IV infusion rate. Before adjusting the rate, the nurse must know the maintenance rates that are appropriate for the child's weight to avoid increasing the rate too much and causing fluid overload. Maintenance rates may be determined according to the following formula for daily fluid requirements:

0–10 kg:	100 ml/kg/day
>10 kg–20 kg:	1000 ml for the first 10 kg of body weight + 50 ml/kg/day for each kg between 10 and 20
>20 kg:	1500 ml for the first 20 kg of body weight + 20 ml/kg/day for each kg > 20

The above formulas give the daily fluid requirements. To determine an hourly rate, take the milliliters per day and divide by 24. Examples are provided in the accompanying box.

Determining an IV Maintenance Rate

Example 1. An 8-kg child:
8 × 100 ml = 800 ml/day
800 ml ÷ 24 hr = 33 ml/hr

Example 2. A 13-kg child:
1000 ml + (3 × 50) = 1150 ml/day
1150 ml ÷ 24 hr = 47.9 or 48 ml/hr

Example 3. A 25-kg child:
1500 ml + (5 × 20) = 1600 ml/day
1600 ml ÷ 24 hr = 66.67 or 67 ml/day

Before increasing the IV rate for medication administration, the nurse must calculate the maintenance rate and adjust the infusion rate accordingly. Likewise, this adjustment should be performed before **decreasing** an IV rate to avoid problems not only with fluid requirements, but also with serum glucose levels. After the IV medication dose has been completed, the nurse must readjust the IV rate to the rate originally ordered.

When administering IV solutions and medications to pediatric patients, the nurse must consider the following:

- Type of IV solution
- Compatibility of the medication and IV solution
- Dilution volume of the medication
- Amount of flush needed
- Administration rate

Some factors, such as the amount of flush needed, are determined by the administration method, type of IV tubing used, and hospital policies and procedures. Specific medication information may be obtained from drug inserts or texts such as the *Guidelines for Administration of Intravenous Medications to Pediatric Patients* (Ford, Leist, & Phelps, 1993).

Intravenous Push Administration

IV push medications are not diluted and are pushed directly into the IV catheter using the port closest to the patient. The volume of medication infused is small (usually < 5 ml), and the effects (both desired and adverse) are immediate.

IV push is most frequently used in emergency situations, when the immediate effects of the medication are desired. An example is the child experiencing a seizure who receives IV lorazepam (Ativan). This method is also used to give pain medications in the immediate postoperative period, to administer sedation and paralytic agents to ventilated patients, and to administer other medications. To administer an IV push medication, the nurse must first ensure that the medication may safely be administered in this way. Compatibility with the infusing solution should be verified, and the administration time should be determined (usually mg/min). Most institutions require two nurses to double check medications ordered to be given by IV push, and many require a physician to be present before certain medications are given by IV push.

The child should be prepared for the procedure by explaining what will be done and what he may feel during the procedure. He should also be reassured that he will not be "stuck" with the needle.

The IV line should be assessed for patency. The IV tubing should be clamped above the injection port closest to the child, and the port should be cleansed with alcohol, or betadine if the line is a central access catheter or the patient is immunosuppressed. If the medication is not compatible with the infusing IV fluid, the tubing should be flushed with approximately 2 ml normal saline flush before and after the administration of the medication. The medication syringe should then be attached to the port and the medication administered at the prescribed rate. IV push medications should never be administered faster than the manufacturer's recommended maximal rate (Bindler & Howry, 1991).

The child must be monitored carefully for the effects of the medication, including undesired side effects. This evaluation may be done by monitoring the child's vital signs (including blood pressure) and reassessing how he feels frequently.

Intravenous Piggyback Administration

IV piggyback medications are more dilute than IV push medications and have a slower administration rate. They frequently are diluted in at least 20 ml IV solution and administered over at least 15 minutes. These medications may be diluted by the pharmacy and sent to the nursing unit in a separate IV bag, or they may be diluted in a volume control set (Buretrol, Volutrol, Soluset) that is in-line in the child's IV tubing. This volume should always be administered through an infusion pump in the pediatric patient to avoid infusing the medication too rapidly or too slowly.

If the medications are to be diluted in the volume control set, the nurse should note the amount of fluid needed for safe dilution of the medication (often stated as the concentration for administration). This amount is the total volume of medication to be administered. Therefore, the volume of the concentrated medication should be subtracted from the total fluid volume required. For example, if the total diluted volume should be 20 ml and the medication was received in a concentrated volume of 2 ml, 18 ml should be placed in the volume control set (Buretrol, Volutrol, Soluset) and 2 ml of medication added to equal 20 ml. When using this method, the nurse must also flush the IV tubing with fluid to complete the delivery of the medication out of the IV tubing and into the patient. The volume needed for the flush varies and must be added when accounting for the total volume infused into the patient for the shift or for 24 hours. Generally, 16 to 20 ml is required to adequately flush the IV tubing.

All flush and medication volumes must be added to recorded intake and calculated into the total volume parameters to avoid fluid overload.

The injection port of the volume control set is cleansed with alcohol, and the medication is added to the required amount of diluent. The volume control set is gently agitated to mix the medication and diluent. The administration time is determined and, if necessary, the flow rate adjusted to infuse the medication (see accompanying box). The volume set to be infused should be the volume **actually** in the volume control set. It is important to set the pump to alarm when the volume is infused so that the nurse may return and add the volume needed to complete the flush. The volume control set should be labeled with the medication added.

Intravenous Retrograde Administration

The IV retrograde method uses smaller volumes of both medication and flush, and generally has a slightly shorter administration time than the piggyback method. The nurse clamps the IV tubing **below the injection port nearest the child.** The medication is then injected into the injection port nearest the child, away from the child (retrograde) and into the tubing above the injection port. The IV pump is then set to deliver the medication volume plus the amount of flush needed to flush the IV tubing from the injection port to the patient.

Some infusion pumps do not allow the pressure created by retrograde infusion. To prevent a problem with back-pressure, low-volume extension tubing, two stopcocks, and two syringes are used for administration of the medication (Fig. 19–11). The syringe containing the medication is attached to the distal stopcock (the stopcock nearest the patient), and an empty syringe is attached to the proximal stopcock. The distal stopcock is turned off to the patient and on to the extension tubing. The IV medication is injected through the distal stopcock into the extension tubing (away from the patient). The empty syringe fills with the displaced fluid from the extension tubing as the medication is injected. The displaced fluid is discarded. The syringes are removed, and sterile injection caps are placed into each stopcock side port. The stopcocks are turned to resume the flow of IV fluid. Extra care must be taken, however, when using the stopcock method to administer retrograde medications. Because the closed system is opened each time a medication is to be administered, special attention must be paid to aseptic technique.

Administering an IV Medication with a Volume Control Set (Buretrol, Soluset, Metriset)

Example 1

Ordered: 150 mg vancomycin
Concentration for administration: 5 mg/ml
Diluted volume required: 30 ml
Amount of flush required: 20 ml
Total volume to be administered: 50 ml
Recommended administration time: 30–60 minutes
Child's IV rate: 52 ml/hr
Child's weight: 15 kg

In this case, the total volume will be administered in slightly less than 1 hour. The IV rate therefore does not need to be altered.

Example 2

Ordered: 450 mg cefazolin sodium
Concentration for administration: 20 mg/ml
Diluted volume required: 22.5 or 23 ml
Amount of flush required: 20 ml
Total volume to be administered: 43 ml
Recommended administration time: 10–60 minutes
Child's IV rate: 20 ml/hr
Child's weight: 15 kg

In this case, the total volume cannot be administered at the current rate and meet the time requirements. Therefore, the IV rate must be increased. To meet the time requirements, the IV rate must be at least 43 ml/hr. This rate is safe for most 15-kg children who have a maintenance rate of 52 ml/hr. **Increase IV rates with caution in the fluid-restricted child.**

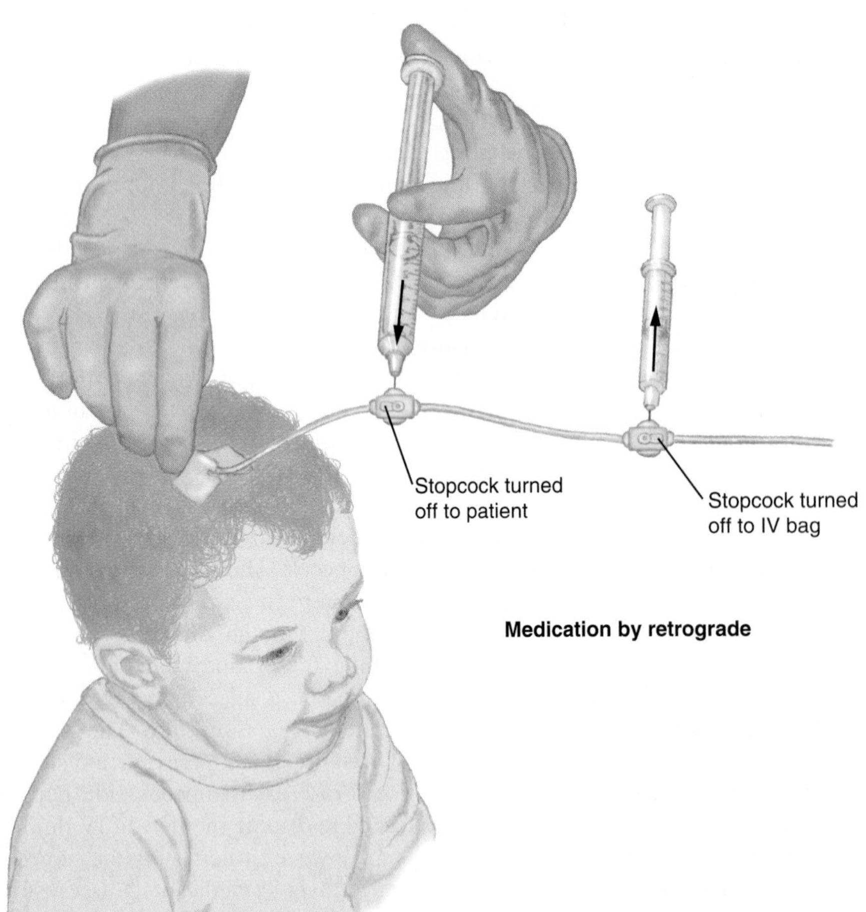

Figure 19–11
Retrograde infusion method used with an infusion pump that cannot accommodate the pressure created by the retrograde infusion.

The nurse must also ensure that stopcocks are secured and kept away from children, who have a tendency to explore and may open the system.

Finally, other systems of retrograde administration involve the placement of a retrograde coil or other special extension tubings.

Intermittent Infusion Ports

Intermittent infusion ports (saline or **heparin locks**) are a form of IV therapy used for intermittent infusions. This device is an IV catheter that is placed, flushed with heparin or normal saline to maintain patency, and then locked with a male adaptor. The port is accessed when needed for fluid or medication infusion. Site care of the device is the same as that for any IV catheter. Frequency of flushing is controversial and determined by personal preference and hospital policy. Routine flushing to maintain patency is performed every 6 hours to every 12 hours. The device may be flushed with saline after medication administration and with heparinized saline solution after blood draws or blood infusions. The use of heparinized saline solution to maintain patency has also become controversial. Research has indicated that saline is as effective as heparin in maintaining patency in 22-gauge catheters, but further studies on 24-gauge catheters are needed (McMullen et al., 1993; Hanrahan et al., 1994; Kleiber et al., 1993).

Central Venous Access Devices

Central venous access devices are venous access devices in which the catheter is centrally placed. These devices are most often used to administer medications, blood products, IV fluids, and parenteral nutrition over the long term to chronically ill children. These devices may be tunneled or nontunneled central catheters and implanted infusion ports. Peripherally inserted central catheters are also being used for children who need IV access for a period longer than peripheral IV catheters can be adequately maintained.

Tunneled central lines are surgically placed lines that are held in place by a Dacron cuff located in a subcutaneous tunnel. They are most commonly placed in the external jugular vein, but also may be placed in the cephalic, axillary-subclavian, femoral, saphenous, or internal jugular veins. The tip of the tunneled catheter is threaded until it rests at the junction of the superior vena cava and right atrium. They are usually flushed with heparin at least every 24 hours and after blood infusions and draws. Short-term or nontunneled central catheters are most frequently placed in the subclavian or femoral veins. These lines involve the placement of a large-gauge catheter that is then sutured into place.

Implanted devices (**infusaports**) consist of a catheter that is connected to a port or reservoir. Like the tunneled catheter, the catheter tip rests at the junction of the superior vena cava and right atrium. The port is under the skin and is accessed with a noncoring needle placed through the skin into the port. The needle is then covered with a bioclusive dressing, and an extension set is attached to the end. When the port is no longer needed for infusions or obtaining blood specimens, the port is flushed with heparin and the needle withdrawn. The child with an implanted port can participate in all typical childhood activities, except those in which there is a potential for high-impact contact with the chest (e.g., competitive football).

Peripherally inserted central catheters (PICC lines) are long catheters made of polyurethane, silicone elastomer, and elastomeric hydrogel and threaded through an introducer placed in the antecubital vein. They are usually placed by specially trained nurses and are used frequently for home antibiotic therapy. After the catheter is threaded so that the tip is located in the superior vena cava, the introducer is removed. The catheter is then covered with a bioclusive dressing, and placement is verified by x-ray. These catheters are usually left in place for several weeks. The major complication of this type of line is phlebitis (Weeks-Lozano, 1991).

SPECIAL METHODS OF ADMINISTRATION OF MEDICATION

Chemotherapy

Chemotherapy is the administration of antineoplastic agents used to treat malignancies. It may be the primary treatment, or it may be used in conjunction with radiation or surgery. The child may receive only one agent or a combination of drugs designed to provide optimal cell cycle destruction.

Chemotherapeutic agents should be administered only by a nurse specially trained in their administration and handling. The child can experience severe cellular damage if the chemotherapeutic agents infiltrate into the tissues (extravasation). Procedure waste products, such as used IV tubing, bags, and other administration devices, should be disposed of in leakproof, puncture-resistant containers. Patient waste products, such as emesis, urine, and stool, must also be disposed of according to hospital guidelines (e.g., double flushing toilets, red-bagging wastes for incineration).

Ribavirin Therapy

Ribavirin (Virazole)™ is a broad-spectrum antiviral agent used for positively identified cases of severe respiratory syncytial virus. It is viral static (prevents the virus from making its end cap) and is administered through a hood or an endotracheal tube through a small-particle-aerosol-generator unit. This unit allows the aerosolized medication to be transformed into an ultrafine mist that is administered 12 to 18 hours per day for 3 to 7 days (average, 5 days).

If the child is intubated, the Food and Drug Administration (FDA) requires informed consent, because the medication may potentially clog ventilator tubing. Ribavirin administration should not be used as a preventive measure and is currently available in the United States for respiratory syncytial virus infection, but is given worldwide for a variety of viral infections (ICN Pharmaceuticals, 1986, 1989).

Currently, there is controversy regarding the administration of ribavirin. The makers of ribavirin offer safety recommendations, and others are available from the National Institute of Occupational Safety and Health (NIOSH). The medication causes conjunctival and upper-airway irritation in caregivers who are exposed to the aerosolized particles. Some hospitals use a double evacuation hood (scavenger device) to decrease the number of particles that escape into the room. When the device is turned off, the tubing is covered with an ultrafilter to prevent particle escape. Because the medication is potentially teratogenic, pregnant or breastfeeding women should not prepare or administer ribavirin or provide direct care of children who are receiving it. Visitors should be notified of the use of ribavirin before they enter the room.

Patient-Controlled Analgesia

Patient-controlled analgesia is a form of medication administration in which the patient retains a certain amount of control over how much pain medication is administered, and when. It is delivered through an IV line connected by a Y port into the main IV line. A medication-filled cassette is placed inside a lockable delivery pump. The medication most often used is morphine; however, fentanyl citrate or hydromorphone hydrochloride (Dilaudid) is sometimes used. The pump may be programmed to deliver a low-dose continuous infusion, a background infusion with rescue boluses, or boluses only. The frequency of boluses is also programmed.

Patient-controlled analgesia should be used only with patients who have the cognitive ability to understand the concept of cause and effect and the purpose of the therapy. The child must have the physical ability to push the button. **Because each child reacts differently to medication and even the correctly prescribed dose may lead to overdose, some practitioners believe that parents should not be allowed to push the button.** If parents are permitted to push the dose button, the nurse must provide thorough education about pain assessment (Gureno & Resinger, 1991).

The child should be monitored carefully for signs of overmedication, especially a depressed respiratory rate or the inability to rouse, and side effects that may accompany narcotic administration (see Chapter 20).

Epidural Administration of Medication

Pain medications may also be administered through an epidural catheter. This form of administration is most useful for patients undergoing abdominal, thoracic, and major orthopedic surgeries. In **epidural medication** administration a catheter is inserted into the epidural space at the lumbar level. This method allows for control of pain without the side effects normally associated with narcotic administration because the medication does not cross the blood–brain barrier.

The patient is placed in a position similar to that used for a lumbar puncture. The insertion site is prepared, and the skin is injected with a local anesthetic. A needle is inserted into the epidural space, and a catheter is threaded into the space for approximately 4 cm. The needle is then removed, and the catheter is secured with occlusive dressing. Although the catheter is usually threaded downward, it may be turned up toward the thoracic area to infiltrate the higher thoracic areas with pain medication. The catheter is then injected with pain medication, usually fentanyl or morphine approved for epidural use.

Nursing care of the patient with an epidural catheter is similar to that of a patient receiving patient-controlled analgesia therapy. The nurse must monitor the patient for adequate pain relief and the presence of undesired side effects as well as for the complications that may accompany the catheter. The patient must always be log-rolled when movement in bed is necessary. He should never be pulled, because it may dislodge the catheter. The catheter site should be monitored for slippage, bleeding, loss of cerebrospinal fluid, or the development of a hematoma at the insertion site. A hematoma is a rare, but serious complication that should be reported immediately. Other side effects include itching, nausea, and vomiting. Itching is treated with naloxone because it is not related to the histamine.

Immunizations

Immunizations have decreased the incidence of many serious infectious childhood diseases. Information about immunizations should be included as part of the routine health promotion teaching for all children. Underimmunization is a problem in the United States. Fear of side effects has led many parents to neglect or refuse immunizations. These fears, however, are unsubstantiated (Cherry, 1990; Hoffman et al., 1987; Ipp et al., 1989).

Although several immunization schedules are available, the most commonly used are those recommended by the American Academy of Pediatrics and by the Immunization Practices Advisory Committee (see Appendix A).

Other schedules are also available for children who were not immunized in infancy (see Chapter 22).

ADMINISTRATION OF BLOOD AND BLOOD PRODUCTS

Patient and parent education is essential whenever a transfusion is administered. Patients and parents must receive all necessary information honestly, consistently, and at a developmentally appropriate level. Information should include why the transfusion is necessary, how long it will take, what the child will feel and hear, and the types of donations. The parent or caregiver should also be asked about the child's transfusion history. The nurse should discuss the risks of receiving versus not receiving the blood product, and should explain each step as it is to be performed. It is important to use clear, concise, age-appropriate terminology.

Information about the types of blood products, the indications and procedures for their administration, and the identification and treatment of transfusion reactions is found in standard medical-surgical nursing texts. The key features of administration of blood products to children are as follows:

- To prevent circulatory hypervolemia, packed red blood cells, rather than whole blood, are usually administered to infants and children.
- Identify child and verify blood (type, Rh factor, donor number, expiration date) with another nurse or physician.
- Take vital signs, including blood pressure, before administering blood and every 15 minutes for the first 2 hours, and then every 30 minutes until the infusion is complete.
- Administer blood with normal saline (dextrose solutions cause hemolysis) on a piggyback setup, through an appropriate filter.
- Use blood within 30 minutes of its arrival from the blood bank. Do not store blood in regular unit refrigeration. Return unused blood to blood bank. Order only as much blood as can be used in 4 hours.
- Infuse blood slowly for the first 15 minutes. The rate should be set to infuse no more than 50 ml or one fifth of the total volume (whichever is smaller) in the first 15 minutes (Smith et al., 1991) because many transfusion reactions are seen during this brief period. If the child has not displayed any signs of a reaction during this time, the rate may be increased to infuse the remainder of the volume within a 4-hour period.
- Cytomegalovirus-negative blood, blood that has tested negative for cytomegalovirus, is used for cytomegalovirus-negative, immunocompromised patients, low–birth-weight neonates, bone marrow transplant recipients, and patients younger than 2 years of age who are receiving chemotherapy.
- Blood that has been irradiated to prevent lymphocyte replication helps to prevent graft-versus-host disease in immunocompromised patients, such as bone marrow transplant recipients; it also is used in neonates.
- Although the FDA requires that the type and crossmatch be less than 48 hours old (National Blood Resource Education Program, 1990), infants younger than 4 months old rarely form red cell antibodies and therefore usually undergo a type and crossmatch only once, the results of which may be used until the infant reaches 4 months of age or is discharged from the hospital (Anderson & Ness, 1994).
- During the administration of blood or blood products, the child and parents should notify the nurse immediately if the child feels "bad" or has fever or chills, headache, nausea, pain at the needle site, or difficulty breathing. Patients often may not know how they are supposed to feel and will not notify the nurse of the signs and symptoms of a transfusion reaction. The child should not be left alone while receiving blood products.
- If a reaction is suspected, stop transfusion immediately and infuse normal saline through new tubing. Notify physician. Continue to monitor vital signs. Monitor urine outputs hourly, send sample of child's blood and urine to laboratory.
- If the child's maintenance IV rate was decreased to avoid fluid overload, the blood sugar level must be monitored with reagent strips (Dextrostix) or another form of measurement because reducing the maintenance IV rate decreases the amount of IV glucose received by the child and may lead to hypoglycemia.
- After the transfusion, the child and family should be praised for their cooperation and help during the procedure.

PATIENT AND FAMILY EDUCATION

Teaching children and their caregivers about medications is an essential part of therapy. In 1990, the U.S. Department of Health and Human Services (U.S. DHHS) reported that one third to one half of Americans do not follow prescribed medication routines properly (U.S. DHHS, 1990). Although a variety of factors appear to be responsible for noncompliance, failure to properly counsel patients about medications is an important reason (U.S. DHHS, 1990).

Teaching the family about medications begins with a thorough assessment that includes a list of all medications the child is currently taking, including over-the-counter medications. Any history of allergies to medications should be noted to prevent potential drug interactions.

Any special learning needs, such as a hearing or speech disability, language barrier, or illiteracy should be noted as well. The nurse must make provisions to accommodate

TEACHING GUIDELINES *for Parents About Home Medications*

Assess the parent's ability and readiness to learn the required content.

Teach the parent or caregiver and the patient (if she is old enough):

- the name of the medication (trade and generic).
- why it was prescribed.
- what it is supposed to do.
- how to take the medication (how much, how often, how long to take it, and techniques for administering the medication).
- determine an acceptable measuring device for home administration of medications.
- demonstrate the use of calibrated droppers or syringes.
- expected or potential side effects and what to do if they occur.
- when the nurse or physician should be notified of side effects.
- any dietary restrictions.
- any activity restrictions.

Problem solve with the family before discharge. This process includes devising acceptable schedules for medication administration, suggesting alternate methods of administering oral medications (e.g., crushing and mixing with food), and identifying foods that may be mixed with the medications.

Emphasis should be placed on taking the medication as ordered. Steps include finishing the full prescribed antibiotic course, not changing dosages without consulting the physician, and returning for follow-up appointments.

Reinforce general safety information, such as keeping medications out of the reach of children and keeping all medications in their original containers.

Validate that learning took place by:

- asking questions (scenarios work well).
- providing a demonstration and asking for a return demonstration.

Document all teaching and the validation of learning.

the child's special needs. For example, teaching information should be presented in a variety of ways (e.g., spoken, written, and illustrated). Written instructions should accompany any verbal instruction.

The accompanying box offers suggestions for teaching parents about home medications.

Special problems should be addressed before the child leaves the hospital or ambulatory setting. This attention before discharge may help prevent medication errors or the failure of the child and family to follow the physician's orders for home treatment.

KEY CONCEPTS

- Standardized dose ranges for many medications have not been established for children.
- A child's body proportions and composition are different from those of adults, and a child's response to medications differs accordingly.
- The nurse must incorporate principles of growth and development into medication administration.
- The margin of safety for medication administration is narrow for pediatric patients.
- Oral medications should be administered according to developmentally appropriate routes.
- Injections are stressful to children and are not usually the first choice of administration route. Care should be taken to choose the appropriate site for the child's size and age and to use the shortest and smallest-gauge needle possible to ensure safe administration of the medication.
- Site selection for venipuncture is often determined by the rate and type of fluid to be infused and the availability and accessibility of veins.
- Children receiving IV infusions should always receive their fluids through a volumetric pump that can be set to deliver a predetermined amount of fluid safely. A volume control set may be used to decrease the chance of fluid overload.
- A baseline assessment must be performed before a blood product is administered to a pediatric patient.
- Informed consent and a written physician's order are required before any blood transfusion, except in cases of life-threatening emergency.
- All blood must be filtered.
- Blood products must be checked before administration to avoid potentially fatal errors.

- Patients must be monitored carefully for any changes in vital signs or physical status that may indicate a transfusion reaction.
- If a transfusion reaction is suspected, the transfusion should be discontinued immediately, the vein kept open with normal saline, and the physician notified.
- Patient and parent education is important to ensure that medications are administered to achieve therapeutic effects and avoid dangerous side effects.

REFERENCES

Anderson, K. C., & Ness, P. M. (1994). *Scientific basis of transfusion medicine.* Philadelphia: W. B. Saunders.

Anonymous. (1989). Measles prevention: Recommendations of the immunization practices advisory committee (ACIP) *MMWR, 38*(S-9), 1–17.

Anonymous. (1988). Medication crushing. *Nurses' Drug Alert, 12*(9), 67.

Astra USA (1993). EMLA cream: Product monograph. Westborough, MA: Author.

Baucher, H., Vinci, R., & Waring, C. (1989). Pediatric procedures: Do parents want to watch? *Pediatrics, 85*(5), 907–909.

Bernardo, L. M., & Bove, M. (1993). *Pediatric emergency nursing procedures.* Boston: Jones and Bartlett.

Betz, C. L., et al. (1994). *Family-centered nursing care of children* (2nd ed., p. 864). Philadelphia: W. B. Saunders.

Bindler, R. M., & Howry, L. B. (1991). *Pediatric drugs and nursing implications.* Norwalk: Appleton and Lange.

Broome, M., & Endsley, R. (1989). Maternal presence, childbearing practices, and children's response to an injection. *Research, Nursing and Health, 12,* 229–235.

Campbell, L. S., & Jackson, K. (1991). Starting intravenous lines in children: Tips for success. *Journal of Emergency Nursing, 17*(3), 177–178.

Centers for Disease Control. (1981). *Guidelines for prevention of intramuscular infections.* Atlanta, GA: Author.

Clark, J. R., & Pringle, R. P. (1990). Pediatric respiratory drugs. *Emergency, 22*(12), 18, 20–23.

Cherry, J. (1990). Pertussis vaccine encephalopathy: It is time to recognize it as the myth that it is. *JAMA, 263*(12), 1679–1690.

Committee on Drugs. (1992). Guidelines for monitoring and management of pediatric patients during and after sedation for diagnostic and therapeutic procedures. *Pediatrics, 89*(6), 1110–1114.

Eland, J. M., & Anderson, J. E. (1977). The experience of pain in children. In Jacox, A. (Ed.), *Pain: A sourcebook for nurses and other health professionals.* Boston: Little, Brown.

Ford, D., Leist, E. R., & Phelps, S. J. (1993). *Guidelines for administration of intravenous medication to pediatric patients* (4th ed.). Bethesda, MD: American Society of Hospital Pharmacists.

Gedaly-Duff, V., & Burns, C. (1992). Reducing children's pain-distress associated with injections using cold: A pilot study. *Journal of the American Academy of Nurse Practitioners, 4*(3), 95–99.

Gladke, E. (1979). The importance of pharmacokinetics for pediatrics. *European Journal of Pediatrics, 13*(85).

Gureno, M. A., & Resinger, C. L. (1991). Patient controlled analgesia for young pediatric patients. *Pediatric Nursing, 17*(3), 251–254.

Hanrahan, K., Kleiber, C., & Fagan, C. A. (1994). Evaluation of saline for IV locks in children. *Pediatric Nursing, 20*(6), 549–552.

Hoffman, H. I., Hunter, J. C., Damus, K., Pakter, J., Peterson, D. R., van Belle, G., & Hasselmeyer, E. G. (1987). Diphtheria-tetanus-pertussis immunization and sudden infant death: Results of the National Institute of Child Health and Human Development Cooperative Epidemiological Study on sudden infant death syndrome. *Pediatrics, 79*(4), 598–611.

ICN Pharmaceuticals. (1986). Virazole (ribavirin) lyophilized for aerosol administration: Product monograph. Costa Mesa, CA: Author.

ICN Pharmaceuticals. (1989). Approved indications for Virazole: Product monograph. Costa Mesa, CA: Author.

Ipp, M. M., Gold, R., Goldbach, M., Maresky, D. C., Saunders, N., Greenberg, S., & Davy, T. (1989). Adverse reactions to diphtheria, tetanus, pertussis-polio vaccination at 18 months of age: Effect of injection site and needle length. *Pediatrics, 83*(5), 679–682.

Kleiber, C., Hanrahan, K., Fagan, C. A., & Zittergruen, M. (1993). Heparin vs. normal saline for peripheral IV's in children. *Pediatric Nursing, 19*(4), 405–409.

McMullen, A., Fioravanti, I. D., Pollack, V., Rideout, K., & Sciera, M. (1993). Heparinized saline or normal saline as flush solution in intermittent intravenous lines in infants and children. *American Journal of Maternal Child Nursing, 18*(2), 78–85.

Pagliaro, L. A., & Pagliaro, A. M. (Eds.). (1987). *Problems in pediatric drug therapy* (2nd ed.). Hamilton, IL: Drug Intelligence Publications.

Scipien, G. M., Chard, M. A., Howe, J., & Barnard, M. U. (1990). *Pediatric nursing care.* St. Louis: C. V. Mosby.

Sievers, T., Yee, J., Foley, M., Blanding, P., & Bude, C. (1991). Midazolam for conscious sedation during pediatric oncology procedures: Safety and recovery parameters. *Pediatrics, 88,* 1172–1179.

Smith, Nix, Kemper, Ligouri, Brantly, Rollins, Stevens, & Clutter. (1991). *Comprehensive child and family nursing skills.* St. Louis: Mosby–Year Book.

Theroux, M. C., West, D. W., Corddry, D. H., Hyde, P. M., Bachrach, S. J., Cronan, K. M., & Kettrick, R. G. (1993). Efficacy of internasal midazolam in facilitating suturing lacerations in preschool children in the emergency department. *Pediatrics, 91*(3), 624–627.

U.S. Department of Health and Human Services. (1990). *Transfusion therapy guidelines for nurses.* (NIH Publication No. 90-2668). Bethesda, MD: National Heart, Lung, and Blood Institute/National Institutes of Health.

Weeks-Lozano, H. (1991). Clinical evaluation of Per Q Cath for both pediatric and adult home infusion therapy. *Journal of Intravenous Nursing, 14*(4), 249–256.

Widmer, A. F. (1993). IV related infections. In R. P. Wenzel (Ed.). *Prevention and control of nosocomial infections* (2nd ed., pp. 556–579). Baltimore, MD: Williams and Wilkins.

BIBLIOGRAPHY

Agency for Health Care Policy and Research (1992). Acute pain management: Operative or medical procedures and trauma. Rockville, MD: U.S. Department of Health and Human Services.

Akcasu, N., & Oswald, D. (1991). A systematic approach to preparing for chemotherapy administration. *Journal of Pediatric Oncology Nursing, 8*(3), 136–138.

Anderson, K. M., & Holland, J. S. (1992). Maintaining the patency of peripherally inserted central catheters with 10 units/cc heparin. *Journal of Intravenous Nursing, 15*(2), 84–88.

Anonymous. (1987). Needle changing with DTP vaccine. *Nurses' Drug Alert, 11*(11), 81.

Anonymous. (1992). *Central venous catheter complications: A nursing perspective.* Bethesda: National Institutes of Health.

Arts, S. E., Abu-Saad, H. H., Champion, G. D., Crawford, M. R., Fisher, R. J., Juniper, K. H., & Ziegler, J. B. (1994). Age related response to lidocaine-prilocaine (EMLA) emulsion and effect of music distraction on the pain of intravenous cannulation. *Pediatrics,* 93(5), 797–801.

Axton, S. E. (1987). A protocol for pediatric IV meds. *AJN, 87*(7), 943A–944B, 946D.

Behrman, R. E., Kliegman, P. M., Nelson, W. E., & Vaughn, V. C. (1992). *Nelson textbook of pediatrics.* Philadelphia: W. B. Saunders.

Brown, J. M. (1989). Peripherally inserted central catheters: Use in home care. *Journal of Intravenous Nursing, 12*(3), 144–150.

Byington, K. C. (1991). Your guide to pediatric drug administration. *Nursing 1991, 21*(8), 82, 84, 86.

Camp-Sorrell, D. (1990). Advanced central venous access. *Journal of Intravenous Nursing, 13*(6), 361–370.

Carey, B. E. (1989). Major complications of central lines in neonates. *Neonatal Network,* 7(6), 17–28.

Centers for Disease Control. (1995). *Epidemiology and prevention of vaccine preventable diseases.* Atlanta: Author.

Clark, J. B., Queener, S. F., & Karb, V. B. (1993). *Pharmacologic basis of nursing practice* (4th ed.). St. Louis: C. V. Mosby.

Chalupka, S., & Gillon-Allard, B. (1989, December). When your patient has an epidural catheter. *RN, 52*(12), 70–77.

Ellerton, M. L., Caty, S., & Ritchie, J. A. (1985). Helping young children master intrusive procedures through play. *Child Health Care, 13*(4), 167–173.

Erlen, J. A. (1987). The child's choice: An essential component in treatment decisions. *Child Health Care, 15*(3), 156–160.

Eskola, J. (1980). Recent advances in the development and use of childhood vaccines. *Current Opinions in Pediatrics, 2*(1), 73–80.

Freiberger, D., Bryant, J., & Marino, B. (1992). The effects of different central venous line dressing changes on bacterial growth in a pediatric oncology population. *Journal of Pediatric Oncology Nursing, 9*(1), 3–7.

Frederick, V. (1991, December). Pediatric IV therapy: Starting therapy. Soothing the patient. *RN, 54*(12), 40–44.

Frey, A. M. (1985). Pediatric dosage calculations. *Nita, 8*(5), 373–379.

Fricks, S. B. (1987). Integrating growth and development content into practice: A nursing process framework. *Nurse Educator, 12*(1), 30–33.

Gillis, A. J. (1990). Nurses' knowledge of growth and developmental principles in meeting psychosocial needs of hospitalized children. *Journal of Pediatric Nursing, 5*(2), 78–87.

Goode, C. J., Titler, M., Rakel, B., Ones, D. S., Kleiber, C., Small, S., & Triola, P. (1991). A metaanalysis of effects of heparin flush and saline flush: Quality and cost implications. *Nursing Research, 40*(6), 324–330.

Gould, T., & Roberts, R. (1979). Therapeutic problems arising from the use of the intravenous route for drug administration. *The Journal of Pediatrics, 95*(3), 465–471.

Griffith, M. R., Taylor, J. A., Daugherty, J. R., & Ray, W. A. (1992). No increased risk for invasive bacterial infection found following diphtheria-tetanus-pertussis immunization. *Pediatrics,* (4, Pt. 1), 640–642.

Griffith, M. R., Ray, W. A., Mortimer, E. A., Fenichel, G. M., & Schaffner, W. (1990). Risk of seizures and encephalopathy after immunization with the diphtheria-tetanus-pertussis vaccine. *JAMA, 263*(12), 1641–1645.

Griffith, M. R., Ray, W. A., Mortimer, E. A., Fenichel, G. M., & Schaffner, W. (1991). Risk of seizures after measles-mumps-rubella immunization. *Pediatrics, 88*(5), 881–885.

Gulanick, M., Gradishar, D., Puzas, M. K., & Gettrust, K. V. (1994). *Ambulatory pediatric nursing.* Albany, NY: Delmar.

Hadaway, L. C. (1990). An overview of vascular access devices inserted via the antecubital area. *Journal of Intravenous Nursing, 13*(5), 197–306.

Haesoon, L., & Evans, H. E. (1987). Evaluation of inhalation aids of metered dose inhalers in asthmatic children. *Chest, 91*(3), 366–369.

Harovas, J., & Anthony, H. (1993). Your guide to trouble-free transfusions. *RN, 56*(11), 26–34.

Hollingsworth, S. (1987). Getting on line. *Nursing Times, 83*(29), 61–62.

Ipp, M., Goldbach, M., Greenberg, S., & Gold, R. (1990). Effect of needle change and air bubble in syringe on minor adverse reactions associated with diphtheria-tetanus toxoids-pertussis-polio vaccination in infants. *Pediatric Infectious Disease Journal, 9*(4), 291–293.

Kelley, S. J. (1994). *Pediatric emergency nursing* (2nd ed.). Norwalk, CT: Appleton and Lange.

Koren, G., Rajchgot, P., Tesoro, A. M., Harding E., Good, F., & MacLeod, S. M. (1983). Improved technique for intravenous drug delivery in children. *American Journal of Intravenous Therapy and Clinical Nutrition, 10*(9), 33–34, 36–38.

Leff, R. (1983). Intravenous administration of medications to the pediatric patient. *National Intravenous Therapy Association, 6*(4), 255–258.

Leff, R. D., & Roberts, R. J. (1984). *Practical aspects of intravenous drug therapy techniques for the practicing nurse, pharmacist, physician*, Iowa City, IA: Author.

Leick-Rude, M. K. (1990). Use of percutaneous Silastic intravenous catheters in high-risk neonates. *Neonatal Network, 9*(1), 17–25.

Loebl, S. A., Spratto, G. R., Matejski, M. P., & Woods, A. L. (1991). *The nurse's drug handbook* (6th ed.). Albany, NY: Delmar.

Lonsway, R. A. (1988). Care of the patient with an epidural catheter. *Journal of Intravenous Nursing, 11*(1), 52–55.

Lunn, J. K., & Wilson, A. (1986). Retrograde medication administration: A predictable and simple system for pediatric drug delivery. *Focus on Critical care, 13*(6), 59–63.

Marcous, C., Fisher, S., & Wong, D. (1990). Central venous access devices in children. *Pediatric Nursing, 16*(2), 123–133.

McCoy, P. A., & Votroubek, W. L. (1990). *Pediatric home care: A comprehensive approach.* Rockville, MD: Aspen.

Merkatz, R., & Couig, M. P. (1992). Helping America take its medicine. *American Journal of Nursing, 92*(6), 59–60, 62.

Metheney, N., Sweeney, M., & Wehrte, A. (1990). Effectiveness of the auscultory method in predicting feeding tube location. *Nursing Research, 42,* 324–331.

Oellrich, R. G., Murphy, M. R., Goldberg, L. A., & Aggarwal, R. (1991). The percutaneous central venous catheter for small or ill infants. *American Journal of Maternal Child Nursing, 16*(2), 92–96.

Rakel, B., Titler, M., Goode, C., Barry-Walker, J., Budreau, G., & Buckwalter, K. (1994). Nasogastric and nasointestinal feeding tube placement: An integrative review of research. *AACN Clinical Issues, 5*(2), 194–206.

Rudy, C. (1992). A drop or a dropper: The risk of overdose. *Journal of Pediatric Nursing, 6*(1), 40, 50–51.

Shim, C. (1987). Inhalation aids of metered dose inhalers. *Chest, 91*(3), 315–316.

Skale, N. (1992). *Manual of pediatric nursing procedures.* Philadelphia: J. B. Lippincott.

Treas, L. S., & Latinis-Bridges, B. (1992). Efficacy of heparin in peripheral venous infusion in neonates. *Journal of Obstetric, Gynecologic, and Neonatal Nursing, 21*(3), 214–219.

Tuten, S. H., & Gueldner, S. H. (1991). Efficacy of sodium chloride versus dilute heparin for maintenance of peripheral intermittent intravenous devices. *Applied Nursing Research, 4*(2), 63–71.

U.S. Department of Health and Human Services (DHHS), Office of the Inspector General. (1990). *Medication regimens: Causes of noncompliance.* Washington, DC: Author.

U.S. Department of Health and Human Services. (1993). *Transfusion alert.* (NIH Publication No. 90-2668). Bethesda, MD: National Heart, Lung, and Blood Institute/National Institutes of Health.

Wachs, T., Watkins, S., & Hickman, R. O. (1987). No more pokes. *Nutritional Support Services, 7*(6), 12–13, 18.

Wink, D. M. (1991). Giving infants and children drugs: Precision + caution = safety. *American Journal of Maternal Child Nursing, 16*(6), 317–321.

20

The Child in Pain

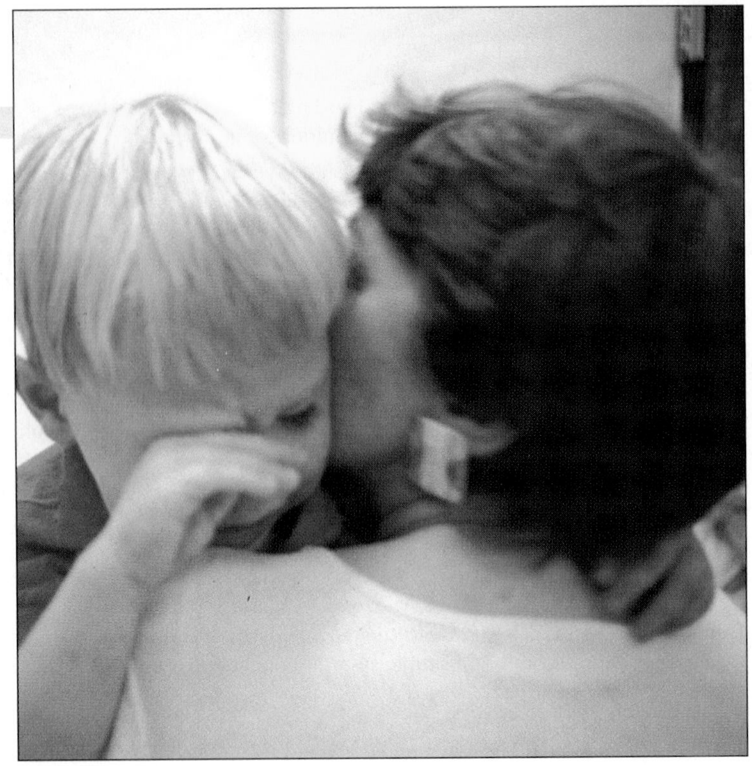

CHAPTER OVERVIEW

LEARNING OBJECTIVES

After studying this chapter, you should be able to:

- Define pain.
- Discuss the gate control theory of pain.
- Discuss the myths and realities of pain.
- Differentiate between acute and chronic pain.
- Explain assessment of pain in children according to developmental levels.
- Describe common pain assessment tools.
- Discuss nonpharmacologic and pharmacologic interventions that may be used to relieve pain in children.
- Use the nursing process to describe nursing care of the child in pain.

KEY TERMS

AHCPR: Agency for Health Care Policy and Research; a federal agency established in 1989

conscious sedation: "light sedation" during which the patient retains airway reflexes and responds to verbal stimuli

epidural: situated within the spinal canal, on or outside the dura mater; synonyms are extradural and peridural

NSAID: nonsteroidal anti-inflammatory drug; an aspirin-like drug that reduces pain and inflammation arising from injured tissue

pain: an unpleasant sensory and emotional experience associated with actual or potential tissue damage or described in terms of such damage

pain threshold level: the level of intensity at which pain becomes appreciable or perceptible

PCA: patient-controlled analgesia; self-administration of an analgesic by a patient instructed in doing so; usually refers to self-dosing with intravenous opioid

TENS: transcutaneous electrical nerve stimulation; a method of producing electroanalgesia through electrodes applied to the skin

There is widespread difficulty defining, identifying, and treating pain in children. Infants and children in pain are often unable to communicate its presence or intensity. In addition, some physicians and nurses have outdated beliefs about pain and pain control in infants and children (see Table 20–1).

As a result of increased research on pain in children, prescription and administration of analgesics in the pediatric population is improving. However, newer resources and strategies for pain management in children are not always implemented, reflecting the need for education. Nurses, who have frequent opportunities to interact with physicians and other health care workers, can make a significant difference in how pain is managed in infants and children.

This chapter provides information on assessing pain in children of different ages, including assessment tools appropriate for various age-groups and cultures. Nonpharmacologic and pharmacologic methods of pain control are presented. Step-by-step nursing care of the child in pain is outlined at the end of the chapter.

DEFINITIONS AND THEORIES OF PAIN

There are many definitions of pain. McCaffrey (1972) defined *pain* as whatever the experiencing person says it is, existing whenever the person says it does. Pain was further defined by the International Association for the Study of Pain (1979) as "an unpleasant sensory and emotional experience associated with actual or potential tissue damage, or described in terms of such damage." Whatever the definition of pain, the fact remains that it is subjective and personal. The problem often encountered in pediatrics is the infant's or child's inability to communicate the presence and/or intensity of his pain.

Gate-Control Theory. The gate-control theory of pain explains how pain impulses travel between the initial site of injury and the brain and the mechanisms that effect pain relief (Melzack & Wall, 1965). The theory states that a gating mechanism at the level of the dorsal horn can facilitate or dampen pain transmission and that stimulation of the larger afferent nerves, which carry benign sensations, can blunt pain. The gating mechanisms are influenced by the relative activity in the sensory fibers. Input from the large fibers closes the gate and input from the small fibers opens the gate. For instance, rubbing an injured part activates large-fiber activity, which decreases the ability of small-fiber activity to open the gate. It is further postulated that cognitive processes such as attention, emotion, and memory influence the gating mechanism and have an impact on the transmission of pain. The gate-control theory provides scientific support for the use of both physiologic and psychological factors when assessing and intervening in pain management.

Acute and Chronic Pain. Children may experience acute as well as chronic pain. Acute pain usually has a sudden onset and continues for a limited time. Acute pain is experienced during and after procedures, postoperatively, from fractures, and from other insults to the body. Chronic pain has an unpredictable time limit while affecting the child's ability to live a normal life. Children with chronic conditions such as juvenile rheumatoid arthritis, sickle cell disease, and cancer experience chronic pain.

RESEARCH ON PAIN IN CHILDREN

Research related to pain in children has been limited in the past. In the late 1980s research in this area began to increase, and the literature reflects this trend. Although there is still much more awareness needed, the prescription and administration of analgesics in the pediatric population is improving (Asprey, 1994).

In 1989, the Agency for Health Care Policy and Research (*AHCPR*) was created to focus on the development of scientifically based practice guidelines for selected problems. One of the targeted areas was pain. The development of the guidelines for caring for children in pain were based on a retrieval and review of articles related to postoperative, procedural, and trauma pain. The research studies were related to the testing of pain assessment tools and pharmacologic and nonpharmacologic pain relief behaviors. Other studies included the description of pain in children, the development of pain assessment tools, and other issues related to pain in children. From this work a document entitled *Clinical Practice Guidelines for Acute Pain Management: Operative or Medical Procedures and Trauma* was published (Agency for Health Care Policy and Research, 1992). This work can serve as a guideline for nurses working with children who are experiencing pain.

There is an identified need for education of physicians about effective pain management, more information about pain management in the neonatal and infant population, more collaboration between nurses and physicians when managing pain in children, and more support for nurses to influence pain management (Margolius et al., 1995).

TABLE 20–1 *Pain and Pain Management in Children: Myths and Realities*

MYTH	REALITY
Neonates do not experience pain due to incomplete myelinization in the peripheral nerves and CNS.	Myelinization is not necessary for pain perception. Pain impulses are carried more slowly in the neonate, but there is a shorter distance for the impulse to travel.
Children have no memory of pain.	Feeding and sleeping differences have been reported in studies of infants who experienced pain, which suggests that the procedure had consequences extending beyond the event (Schechter, 1989).
There is a correct amount of pain for a given injury.	The amount of pain a child experiences cannot be predicted due to cognitive and emotional factors impacting the child (Schechter, 1989).
Children can easily become addicted to narcotic analgesics.	Health care workers often confuse physical dependence with addiction. The actual risk of addiction is very low (Porter & Jick, 1980; Agency for Health Care Policy and Research, Acute Pain Management Guideline Panel, 1992).
Narcotic administration can easily cause respiratory depression.	No data is available to support the belief that children are at higher risk for respiratory depression than adults (Eland, 1990).

MYTHS ABOUT PAIN AND PAIN MANAGEMENT IN CHILDREN

Probably the two beliefs that interfere most with infants and children receiving adequate pain relief are fear of addiction and fear of respiratory distress. Table 20–1 lists and refutes five prevalent myths about pain and pain management in children.

ASSESSMENT OF PAIN IN CHILDREN

Pain in children is multidimensional (Schechter, 1988; Wallace, 1989) and is affected by the following:

- Developmental age (see box)
- Culture and ethnicity
- Previous experience associated with pain
- Type of pain
- Temperament
- Parental response to child's pain
- Sex

When assessing pain in a child, all of the above factors should be considered. Assessment of pain in children is generally more difficult than in adults. Infants and young children cannot verbalize that they are experiencing pain. Although older children may have the ability to verbalize their discomfort, they are often afraid of the cure (injections) or they may have been told to "be brave." Children lack the cognitive ability or the experience to know when and how to verbalize that they are experiencing discomfort. Studies have supported the fact that children are undermedicated for pain (Beyer et al., 1983; Eland & Anderson, 1977; Schechter et al., 1986, Kachoyeanos & Zollo, 1995).

Assessment According to Developmental Levels

NEONATE AND INFANT

- Changes in facial expression, including frowns, grimaces, expressions of surprise, and facial flinching
- Increases in blood pressure and heart rate and decrease in arterial saturation
- High-pitched, tense, harsh crying
- General or total body response in neonate and young infant that becomes more purposeful as infant matures
- Extremities may thrash about; some infants exhibit tremors
- Older infants rub painful area, pull away, or guard the involved part

TODDLER

- Loud crying
- Verbalizes words that indicate discomfort (ouch, hurt, boo-boo)
- Attempts to delay procedures perceived as painful
- Generalized restlessness
- Guards the site
- Touches painful areas
- May run from nurse

PRESCHOOLER

- May think he is being punished for some deed or thought
- Cry, kick
- Describe location and intensity of pain: "ear hurts bad"
- Regression to earlier behaviors (loss of bladder and bowel control)
- Withdrawal
- Deny pain to avoid a possible injection
- May have been told to be "brave" and deny pain even though it is present

SCHOOL-AGE

- Able to describe pain
- Fears bodily harm
- Has an awareness of death
- Stiff body posture
- Withdrawal
- Procrastinates or bargains in order to delay procedure

ADOLESCENT

- Perceives pain at a physical, emotional, and mental level
- Understands cause and effect
- Describes pain
- Increased muscle tension
- Withdrawal and decreased motor activity
- Uses words like sore, ache, pounding to describe pain

Assessment According to Developmental Levels

Neonates and Infants

Because neonates and young infants have immature central nervous systems, with the absence of myelination of pain fibers, many have believed them incapable of perceiving pain. An increasing amount of research has shown evidence to change this way of thinking (Dalla Barba et al., 1991; Gardner, 1994; Phillips, 1995). Because infants are preverbal, pain assessment should be based on physiologic, biochemical, and behavioral responses.

Although biochemical measures indicate hormonal and metabolic changes in infants who are experiencing pain, they are difficult to obtain in the acute care setting. Changes in facial expressions associated with pain include frowns, grimaces, expressions of surprise, and flinching (Mills, 1989). Facial expression is thought by some to be the best indicator of pain in infants. A study by Johnston and Strada (1986) supports this belief. In another study facial expression in combination with short latency to onset of cry and long duration of first cry cycle typified reaction to acute invasive procedures (Grunau et al., 1990).

Physiologic changes are more easily assessed. Increases in blood pressure and heart rate and decreases in arterial oxygen saturation have been associated with pain in neonates. However, the changes can also be linked to other alterations within the infant's body. Sometimes it is difficult to distinguish between pain and agitation. If the child is treated for pain and she is agitated, the intervention will be inappropriate and her agitation may increase (Gardner, 1994). Crying may affect the infant's physiologic response. Rawlings and colleagues (1980) reported that oxygenation will decrease in response to pain, but may increase after vigorous crying. However, during crying, oxygen delivery to cerebral tissues may be compromised even though the oxygen content of the blood remains stable (Brazy, 1988). This can be confusing when evaluating data. The nurse should be aware of these findings and realize that the physiologic changes are just one part of the assessment of pain in the neonate and infant. The nurse should not wait for physiologic changes to occur before intervening when pain is suspected.

Physiologic changes are only one source of information when assessing pain in the infant and neonate and should not be relied on before intervening. Behavioral changes must also be assessed.

Behavioral changes associated with infant pain include crying, facial expression, and motor responses. The length of time an infant cries in response to pain seems to increase as the age of the infant increases. In one study crying lasted 15 to 60 seconds in neonates, 3 minutes in 2-month-olds, and as long as 9 minutes by age 9 months (Mills, 1989). In this same study, 9-month-old infants cried out for mommy and another infant shook his head "no, no." Cries associated with pain are thought to have a sound different from those associated with hunger, discomfort, and stress (Anand & Hickey, 1987). The cry has been described as higher-pitched, tense, and harsh. This assists parents and nurses to differentiate between the cries of infants.

Motor movements associated with pain in the neonate and infant progress from a general body response to more purposeful movements. Infants ages 9 to 12 months can use their hands to push the nurse away if they perceive a painful action about to begin (Mills, 1989). The response of the neonate to painful stimuli (Fig. 20–1) is sometimes described as a total body response. The infant's extremities may thrash about, and some infants exhibit tremors. Older infants may rub the painful area, pull away, or guard the involved body part.

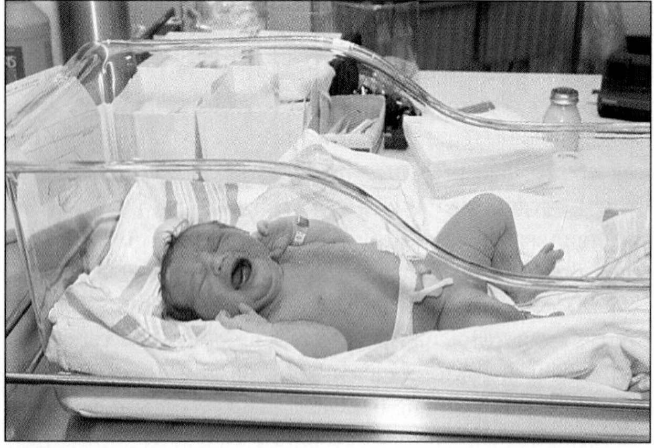

Figure 20–1
Neonates and infants respond to pain with a total body response. Parents can usually distinguish the infant's cry of pain from other cries because it is tense, high-pitched, and harsh-sounding.

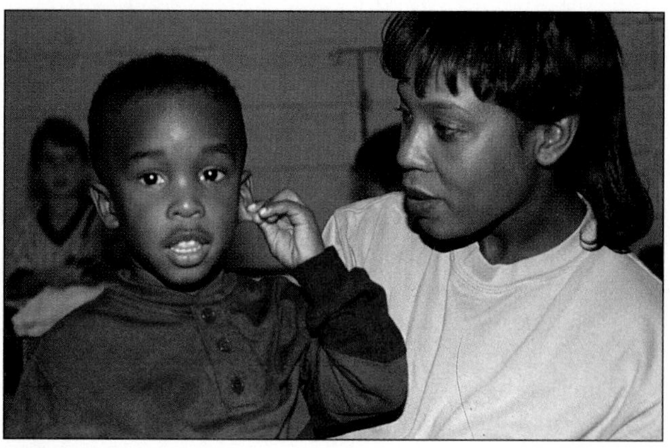

Figure 20–2
Toddlers and preschoolers may express pain by guarding or touching the painful area. Pulling on the ear is a characteristic expression of ear pain that accompanies otitis media. (Courtesy of the University of Texas at Arlington School of Nursing, Arlington, Texas.)

Toddlers

The toddler experiencing pain tends to cry longer than the infant. As verbal abilities become more advanced, the toddler can verbally express displeasure when a painful experience occurs. The toddler asks for parents, verbalizes words that indicate discomfort (ouch, hurt), and may attempt to delay the nurse's attempts to do a procedure that is perceived as painful. The older toddler can often verbalize which part of the body hurts.

Generalized restlessness, guarding the site, and touching the painful area are signs of pain in the toddler (Fig. 20–2). The toddler may associate discomfort with a particular procedure (dressing change) and may run from the nurse when approached. The toddler's face may show anger and fear. He may avoid eye contact and have a look of sadness.

Preschoolers

Preschoolers are egocentric and tend to relate to the here and now. They are unable to relate discomfort to any positive outcome. The preschooler will not understand how debriding a painful burn will ultimately have a positive outcome. The child who is unable to understand why an uncomfortable procedure might be a positive force may find pain disorienting and be affected more profoundly than older children (Schechter, 1988).

The preschooler tends to also think pain will magically go away and that perhaps she is being punished for some previous thought or deed. They also fear body mutilation; males in this age-group have a fear of castration. They may deny pain in order to avoid an injection.

The preschooler may cry and kick to avoid a procedure that she perceives as painful. She may regress to earlier, more comfortable behaviors as a response to discomfort, or may withdraw and not participate in activities on the unit. This age child can describe the location and intensity of the pain.

School-Age Children

School-age children are able to describe pain as it relates to a body part. They have a fear of bodily harm and an awareness of death. Therefore, their reaction to an illness or injury may appear to be an overreaction to the observer who does not understand the developmental level of the child.

As in all age-groups, the school-age child will bring memories of previous pain experiences to the setting, which will affect his response to the present situation. The child's culture, sex, and cognitive abilities will also affect the pain experience.

Nonverbal cues are very important in this age-group. The child may exhibit a stiff body posture, may withdraw, or may be found quietly sobbing in his bed (Fig. 20–3). If the school-age child resists a treatment, cries loudly, or otherwise acts in an aggressive manner, the child may later deny the behavior. He may also make attempts to procrastinate or bargain to delay a procedure that is painful.

Adolescents

Adolescents can perceive pain at a physical, emotional, and mental level. They can think abstractly and understand cause and effect. They have the ability to clearly describe pain, their feelings about pain, and the strategies that help when they experience pain (Savedra et al., 1988).

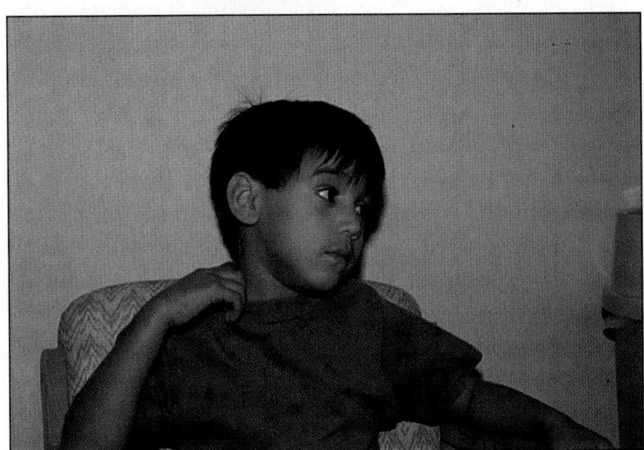

Figure 20–3
School-age children may withdraw and become very quiet when they are ill or in pain. Notice how dull this boy appears. Although he has asthma, his mother knew something else was wrong because he was unusually quiet and withdrawn. (Courtesy of Dallas County Hospital District Community Oriented Primary Care Clinic, Dallas, Texas.)

Having this ability does not mean the adolescent will exercise it. They are often confused by control issues and are uncertain of their role as they move from childhood to adulthood. It is not unusual for some form of regression to also occur.

Because the adolescent is very egocentric, she tends to think that others are also focused on her behavior. This may lead the adolescent to suppress manifestations of pain and to expect the nurse to somehow be aware of the pain she is experiencing. If the nursing staff is unaware of the pain, the adolescent may interpret this as an indication that the pain she is experiencing is indeed minimal and that she should be able to tolerate it (Favaloro & Touzel, 1990).

Adolescents tend to exhibit fewer outward signs of pain than young children. Signs that may be observed in the adolescent include increased muscle tension, withdrawal, and decreased motor activity. Hospitalized adolescents use words such as "sore," "like an ache," "pounding," and "miserable" to describe pain. They complete the statement, "When I have pain, I most often feel . . ." with the following: "sick to my stomach," "scared," "angry," "like crying, but I don't," "like hitting someone," and "like screaming" (Savedra et al., 1988).

Assessment Tools

In order to collect more objective data related to pain assessment, several pain assessment tools have been developed. Self-report and behavioral instruments are available. Validity and reliability has been established on some of these tools. The child benefits when a pain assessment tool is used because the child is given a simple and effective way to communicate the pain he is experiencing. Assessment tools provide more objective data, and there is less chance that the more discrete signs of pain will be overlooked. Unfortunately, they are not always used in the clinical setting.

> The use of a pain assessment tool is imperative in the assessment of pain in children. The tool is part of the child's chart.

Selection of an assessment tool should be based on the child's age and developmental abilities. Self-report tools are effective in children over age 4 years. The Oucher, the Poker Chip Tool, and a faces scale are examples of tools for preschool through school age (Table 20–2). African-American and Hispanic versions of the Oucher have recently been developed. School-age children who have the cognitive ability to understand the concept of order and number can use numerical rating scales, horizontal word-graphic rating scales, or a visual analog scale. In a study of five horizontal pain rating scales, the visual analog scale was the least preferred (Tesler et al., 1991).

TABLE 20–2 *Pain Assessment Tools*

TOOL	DESCRIPTION	AGE
The Oucher (Beyer, 1984, 1986, 1989, 1992)	A poster with two scales: one is numerical for use by children who can count to 100; the other is a photographic scale to be used by children who cannot count to 100. The bottom picture (or 0) is no pain; the top picture (or 100) is the greatest pain (see Fig. 20–4).	3 to 12 years
Poker Chip Tool (Hester, 1979)	Four poker chips are used; each chip represents a piece of hurt. One poker chip represents a little hurt and four chips represent the most hurt the child could have. (See box: Poker Chip Tool Instructions.)	4 to 12 years
The Adolescent and Pediatric Pain Tool: APPT (Savedra et al., 1989; Savedra et al., 1992)	Three-part tool composed of a body outline, an intensity scale, and a pain descriptor word list (see Fig. 20–5).	8 to 17 years
Visual Analog Scale (VAS)	Usually a 10-cm line with one end representing "no pain" and the opposite end "the worst pain."	Older school-age children and adolescents. May be used by younger school-age children but less abstract tools are more appropriate.
Numerical Rating Scale (NRS)	Uses numbers (e.g., 0 to 10 or 0 to 100) to indicate increasing pain.	Child must know numbers.

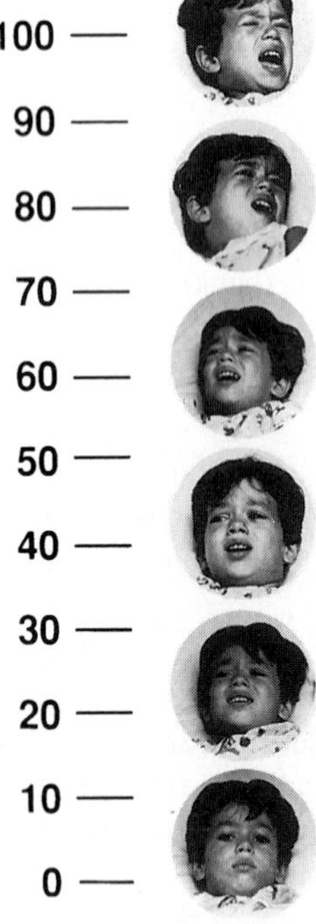

Figure 20–4
The Hispanic version of the Oucher pain scale. (Developed and copyrighted by Antonia M. Villarruel, RN, MS, and Mary J. Denyes, RN, PhD, 1991.)

EXPLAINING THE TOOL Each pain assessment tool will have unique instructions, but the nurse can use communication skills to teach the child the use of the tool. To explain the use of the Word-Graphic Rating Scale, the instructions would be:

"This is a line with words to describe how much pain you may have. This side of the line means no pain and over here the line means the worst possible pain." (Point your finger where "no pain" is, and run your finger along the line to "worst possible pain," as you say it.) "If you have no pain, you would mark this." (Show example.) "If you have some pain, you would mark somewhere along the line, depending on how much pain you have." (Show example.) "The more pain you have, the closer to worst pain you would mark. The worst pain possible is marked like this." (Show example.)

"Show me how much pain you have right now by marking with a straight up-and-down line anywhere along the line."

No pain	Little pain	Medium pain	Large pain	Worst possible pain

Used with permission from the Adolescent and Pediatric Pain Tool in: Savedra, M. C., Tesler, M. D., Holzemer, W. L., & Ward, J. A. (1989). *Adolescent and pediatric pain tool (APPT) preliminary user's manual.* San Francisco: University of California.

CODE ______________

DATE ______________

Adolescent and Pediatric Pain Tool (APPT)

INSTRUCTIONS:

1. Color in the areas on these drawings to show where you have pain. Make the marks as big or small as the place where the pain is.

Right Left Left Right

2. Place a straight, up and down mark on this line to show how much pain you have.

No pain — Little pain — Medium pain — Large pain — Worst possible pain

3. Point to or circle as many of these words that describe your pain.

1	5	10	15
annoying	blistering	awful	off and on
bad	burning	deadly	once in a while
horrible	hot	dying	sneaks up
miserable	6	killing	sometimes
terrible	cramping	11	steady
uncomfortable	crushing	crying	
2	like a pinch	frightening	If you like,
aching	pinching	screaming	you may add
hurting	pressure	terrifying	other words:
like an ache	7	12	
like a hurt	itching	dizzy	___________
sore	like a scratch	sickening	___________
3	like a sting	suffocating	___________
beating	scratching	13	
hitting	stinging	never goes away	
pounding	8	uncontrollable	
punching	shocking	14	
throbbing	shooting	always	
4	splitting	comes and goes	
biting	9	comes on all of a sudden	
cutting	numb	constant	
like a pin	stiff	continuous	
like a sharp knife	swollen	forever	
pin like	tight		
sharp			
stabbing			

For office use only.

BSA: ______

IS: ______

#S (2-9) ____ /37= ____ %

#A (10-12) ____ /11= ____ %

#E (1,13) ____ /8= ____ %

#T (14,15) ____ /11= ____ %

Total ____ /67= ____ %

Figure 20–5

Adolescent and Pediatric Pain Tool, appropriate for use with 8-to 17-year-olds. (From Savedra, M. C., Tesler, M. D., Holzemer, W. L., & Ward, J. A. [1992]. University of California, San Francisco, School of Nursing, San Francisco, CA 94143–0606. Copyright © 1989, 1992. For original tools, write or call 415-476-4040.)

Pain assessment tools are described in Table 20–2; the appropriate age or developmental level of the child is indicated for each tool. Examples of pain assessment tools are provided in Figs. 20–4 and 20–5 and in the box on page 520.

The same scale should be used each time the child is assessed to avoid confusing the child and to provide consistent data. Ideally, the child should be taught how to use the tool before pain is experienced (preoperatively). Obviously, there will be times, such as an emergency admission, when this will not be possible.

The importance of understanding how to appropriately use an assessment tool and then to actually implement its use cannot be overemphasized:

"When using pain assessment tools with children, the tools need to be used in the way that the researchers who developed them intended them to be used. Clinical research was conducted to determine the best ways to introduce them and use them so that the data obtained from the tools were valid. Validity of a tool means that the tool actually measures what it was designed to measure. Measuring any phenomenon in young children is difficult and needs to be done carefully. If instructions are not followed, the information obtained from the child may be meaningless.

The particular tool chosen for each child should be individualized for that child. The nurse should take children's individual needs and preferences into consideration, as well as their cognitive abilities, when choosing a pain assessment tool." (Judith E. Beyer, RN, PhD, Associate Professor, University of Missouri School of Nursing. Beyer developed the Oucher, one of the first instruments designed to measure children's self-reports of pain

Poker Chip Tool Instructions

ENGLISH INSTRUCTIONS

1. Align the chips horizontally in front of the child on the bedside table, a clipboard, or other firm surface.
2. Tell the child, "These are pieces of hurt." Beginning at the chip nearest the child's left side and ending at the one nearest the right side, point to the chips and say, "This (first chip) is a little bit of hurt and this (fourth chip) is the most hurt you could ever have."

   For a young child or for any child who may not fully comprehend the instructions, clarify by saying, "That means this (one) is just a little hurt, this (two) is a little more hurt, this (three) is more yet, and this (four) is the most hurt you could ever have."

   Do not give children an option for zero hurt. Research with the Poker Chip Tool has verified that children without pain will so indicate by responses such as, "I don't have any."
3. Ask the child, "How many pieces of hurt do you have right now?"
4. Clarify the child's answer by words such as, "Oh, you have a little hurt? Tell me about the hurt."
5. Record the number of chips on the Pain Flow Sheet.

SPANISH INSTRUCTIONS

Tell the parent:

"Estas fichas son una manera de medir dolor. Usamos cuatro fichas."

Say to the child:

"Estas son pedazos de dolor: una es un poquito de dolor y cuatro son el dolor maximo que tu puedes sentir. Cuantos pedazos de dolor tienes?"

Used with permission from Nancy O. Hester, University of Colorado Health Sciences Center, School of Nursing, Denver, CO.

Spanish instructions for the Poker Chip Tool initially developed by Jordan-Marsh, M., Hall, D., Yoder, L., Watson, R., McFarlane-Sos, G., & Garcia, M. (1990). *The Harbor-UCLA Medical Center Humor Project for Children.* Los Angeles: Harbor–UCLA Medical Center.

intensity. Dr. Beyer is an author and researcher in the area of Pain Management in Children.)

In addition to the use of a pain assessment tool, the nurse should also:

- Question the child (pain history, word used for pain "owie," "hurt," etc.) (Table 20–3)

TABLE 20–3 *Pain Experience History*

CHILD FORM	PARENT FORM
Tell me what pain is.	What word(s) does your child use in regard to pain?
Tell me about the hurt you've had before.	Describe the pain experiences your child has had before.
Do you tell others when you hurt? If yes, who?	Does your child tell you or others when he is hurting?
What do you do for yourself when you are hurting?	How do you know when your child is in pain?
What do you want others to do for you when you hurt?	How does your child usually react to pain?
What don't you want others to do for you when you hurt?	What do you do for your child when he is hurting?
What helps the most to take your hurt away?	What does your child do for himself when he is hurting?
Is there anything special that you want me to know about you when you hurt? (If yes, have child describe.)	What works best to decrease or take away your child's pain?
	Is there anything special that you would like me to know about your child and pain? (If yes, describe.)

Adapted with permission from Hester, N. O., and Barcus, C. S. (1986). Assessment and management of pain in children. *Pediatrics: Nursing Update, 1,* 2–8.

- Question the parent (pain history, cultural beliefs, other factors affecting child) (Table 20–3)
- Observe behavioral changes (see developmental characteristics)
- Note physiologic changes (pulse, blood pressure, and respirations usually increase and then return to normal).

Physiologic changes may also be caused by fear and anxiety. Because physiologic changes tend to occur during the acute period and then return to normal, they are not valid indicators of chronic pain.

NONPHARMACOLOGIC AND PHARMACOLOGIC PAIN INTERVENTIONS

There are times when nonpharmacologic interventions are the only action needed to relieve discomfort. Some nurses prefer to use medication as the first line of action and thus subject the child to medication that is not needed. At the same time, there are also times when the only way to break the cycle of pain is to give a pharmacologic agent. It is the responsibility of the nurse to determine through the use of assessment which intervention is appropriate.

Nonpharmacologic Interventions

Parents play a very important role in the control of pain in children. They are a resource for determining past effective methods of pain relief with their child. They also aid the nurse in assessing their child's need for intervention. Holding, touching, massage, distraction, and relaxation techniques are all techniques that can be done by the person the child trusts the most, his parent.

The nurse caring for a child in pain can sometimes relieve pain by reducing anxiety and fear of the unknown by preparing the child for all procedures and treatments (see Chapter 15). The use of therapeutic touch can also soothe the child and reduce anxiety and pain.

Distraction

Distraction is one of the most effective ways to relieve pain (Vessey et al., 1994) (Fig. 20–6). Distraction works by refocusing the child from the discomfort to something else. It does not imply total pain relief. The form of distraction chosen should be appropriate for the child's developmental level. Children experiencing severe pain cannot be distracted. In addition, the child who was distracted in the past but for whom distraction is no longer effective should be assessed to determine what has changed about the pain (Eland, 1990). The child's ability to use distraction should not be misinterpreted to mean that the child is not experiencing pain. A child may distract himself to "forget" his pain. Just because a child is watching TV does not mean he is not having pain.

Distraction may be accomplished by music, stories, number games, video games, board games, or even, perhaps, doing multiplication tables or spelling words. If a child has a favorite doll or stuffed animal, it may be used to create a story or a game. Children love to talk about their pets, and the nurse can ask the child to tell his favorite story about the pet. Another distraction technique is to allow the child to help by handing, opening, or holding objects. This technique should only be used when it is safe and there is not a danger of contamination of materials or of a site.

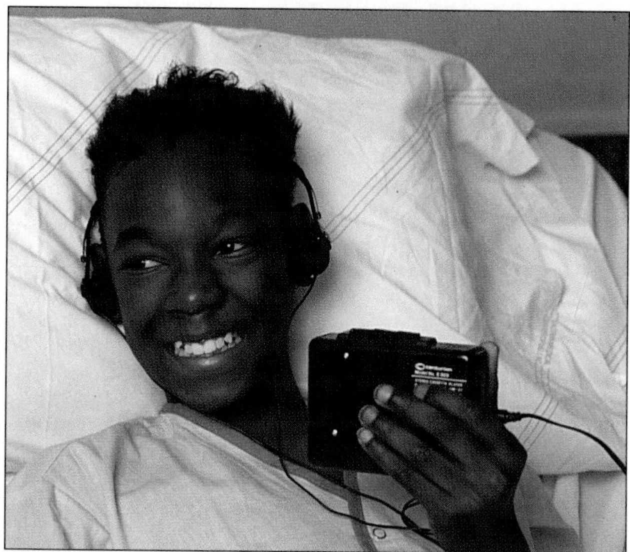

Figure 20–6
Distraction effectively reduces pain by helping the child refocus his attention. This boy listens to the radio through earphones, allowing him to be distracted without annoying others. (Courtesy of Children's Medical Center, Dallas, Texas.)

USING DISTRACTION Imagine how frightening it is for a child to be brought to the emergency department after he has been involved in an accident. Even if the injury is minor by emergency department standards, the fear and pain are going to be very real to the child. Through the use of distraction the nurse can decrease both anxiety and pain. Each child is different and cues can be taken from him as to whether you might hold his hand, touch his head, and so on. Once both the child and nurse are at a point where conversation can become more personal, the nurse can say, "I see you have a baseball shirt on. Do you play baseball?" Assuming the child expresses an interest in the game, you can continue, "Which team is your favorite? What was the most exciting play you saw this year? Have you been to a game?" Be sure that you are comfortable in the topic you are discussing with the child because he will sense if you do not have a genuine interest in the topic. You might interject a personal note: "I love baseball also. When I was a child, it was my biggest treat to go with my father to see the St. Louis Cardinals play." This conversation could go on for 10 to 15 minutes, certainly long enough for sutures to be put in or other minor procedures completed. The child will not be focusing on the procedure, but rather on baseball. The topic is not important; the important thing is focusing the child on something other than the injury.

Relaxation Imagery

Relaxation imagery is a process involving relaxation and a focus on mental images. The child can be encouraged to think of a favorite place and then given permission to go to that place. The nurse, in a quiet, soothing voice, can guide the child on a "make-believe" trip. Breathing techniques can also relax the child. The child is instructed to take several slow, deep breaths while thinking pleasant thoughts. Children often need guidance, and the nurse may suggest remembering a birthday or a special time with family, friends, or a pet.

Biofeedback

Biofeedback is the provision of visual or auditory evidence to the individual that physiologic changes are taking place. Visual feedback in which colors or numbers change or the involvement of computer games are effective ways to use this technique. Biofeedback gives the child a response that she can instantly see and tends to keep the child interested.

Hypnosis

Hypnosis can be defined as focused attention, an altered state of consciousness, or a trance, often accompanied by relaxation (Valente, 1991). Research has shown hypnosis to be effective in the relief of pain and symptoms in children undergoing painful procedures and in those with cancer, burns, sickle cell disease, and nausea and vomiting associated with chemotherapy (Valente, 1991). Nurses need special training to learn this technique. In settings where this is not possible, the child who would benefit from this therapy should be referred to a qualified professional who can provide the service. Children can be taught self-hypnosis.

Transcutaneous Electrical Nerve Stimulator

The transcutaneous electrical nerve stimulator (*TENS*) is a unit that has electrodes that deliver small amounts of electrical energy to the skin. TENS works either by modulating painful input into the spinal cord or by causing endorphin release (Mannheimer & Lampe, 1984). TENS has been used successfully to manage acute and chronic pain.

Pharmacologic Interventions

Many nurses are reluctant to administer analgesics. Some nurses and physicians have the mistaken belief that children will easily become addicted to the analgesic given. Others fear respiratory distress or really do not believe the child is experiencing enough pain to warrant the administration of an analgesic. If a procedure, surgery, trauma, etc., would cause pain in an adult, then it will cause pain in a child. The analgesia ordered may not be the appropriate dosage for that child. Consequently, many children suffer needless pain due to lack of adequate analgesia.

Administration of Analgesics

Analgesics can be administered by various routes: oral, rectal, intravenous, intramuscular, epidural, and intranasal. (See Chapter 19 for discussion of the common routes.) The accompanying box discusses the disadvantages of intramuscular analgesics in children.

The preferred routes of administration of analgesics to children are intravenous or oral.

Disadvantages of Intramuscular Analgesics

Altered tissue absorption leads to peaks and troughs in analgesia.
Children run out of sites quickly.
Intramuscular analgesics have a shorter duration of action than orally administered analgesics.
Contraindicated in children with low platelets.
Children hate them.
Nurses dislike administering them.

Adapted from Eland, J. (1990). Pain in children. *Nursing Clinics of North America, 25*(4), 871–884.

Patient-Controlled Analgesia

One of the most effective ways of administering analgesia is through the use of the patient-controlled analgesia (PCA) pump. It is generally thought that children as young as age 6 years can effectively and safely use a *PCA*. It is thought that children even this young understand the use of the PCA (Gureno & Reisinger, 1991). In some institutions parents or nurses activate the PCA for children under that age. Further research is needed in the use of PCA in the younger child.

The child receives small intravenous doses of the medication when she pushes a button connected to the pump (Fig. 20–7). After each dose there is a period when

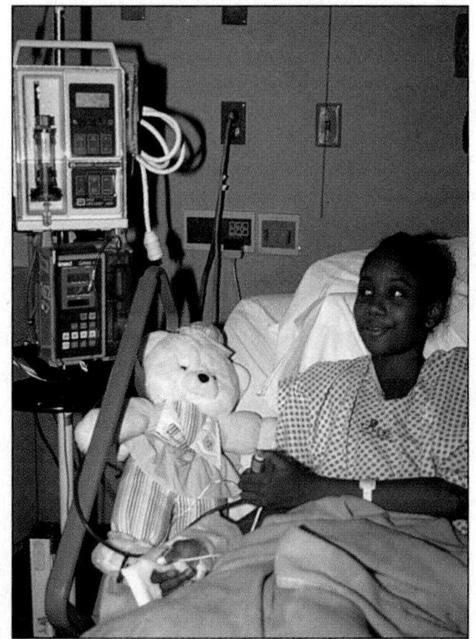

Figure 20–7
Patient-controlled analgesia gives the older child greater control over pain management. The child presses the button when pain medication is needed and the machine delivers a preprogrammed bolus through the IV. The child cannot overdose because the controller has a lock-out feature to prevent excess analgesia. (Courtesy of Children's Medical Center, Dallas, Texas.)

the pump will not release the medication even if the button is pushed. There is also a maximum amount of medication that may be given over a given period of time, usually a 1-hour period. The child is checked frequently to ensure that pain control is effective and that the equipment is functioning correctly.

The child should be monitored carefully for signs of overmedication (especially depressed respiratory rate and/or inability to rouse) and side effects that may accompany narcotic administration. Other side effects of opiates include itching, nausea, and vomiting. Treatment of overdose is naloxone (Narcan). Vital signs should be taken every 15 to 30 minutes when PCA therapy is first initiated and then every 2 to 4 hours thereafter. Policies of many institutions also require that children receiving PCA therapy be placed on continuous pulse oximetry and/or cardiorespiratory monitoring. Oxygen, a bag and mask, and naloxone should be readily available.

Topical Anesthetic Cream

A topical anesthetic cream, lidocaine-prilocaine 5% cream (EMLA), can be used to reduce pain associated with selected procedures: venipuncture, lumbar puncture, suture removal, immunizations, bone marrow aspiration, and removal of foreign bodies from the skin (see also Chapter 19). The use in neonates has not been approved in the United States because of lack of data to support use in this group. The main side effect is skin blanching or redness, which lasts a few hours and actually helps "guide" to the anesthetized area (Zappa, 1994–95).

EMLA cream is applied liberally to intact skin under an occlusive dressing 60 minutes before anesthesia is needed. Mound the cream, do not rub in. The duration of anesthesia is at least 2 hours and not more than 5 hours.

Success in managing pain has been achieved when parents apply the cream at home before scheduled immunizations (Taddio, et al., 1994). EMLA comes with directions in Spanish and English for use by parents. Care should be taken with small children to avoid their removing the dressing and rubbing the cream in their eyes or eating the cream, which looks like cake frosting. Children may still have needle fear, and distraction should be used until they realize the "stick" will not hurt.

Nonsteroidal Anti-inflammatory Drugs

The nonsteroidal anti-inflammatory drugs *(NSAIDs)* are used primarily for pain associated with inflammation, bone pain, and rheumatic conditions because of their ability to inhibit prostaglandin. Aspirin, ibuprofen, and naproxen (Naprosyn) are three of the most common drugs in this category (Table 20–4). Because aspirin has been associated with Reye's syndrome, it is used cautiously in children. Research is needed in the long-term use of ibuprofen and naproxen (Lesko & Mitchell, 1995).

Acetaminophen. Acetaminophen lacks the anti-inflammatory effects of the other NSAIDs and does not inhibit prostaglandin. It is the most commonly used analgesic and is the drug of choice for treatment of fever in children in the United States. It is used in mild to moderate pain management. Short-term use of this drug is safe even in neonates. It does not have the gastric side effects of aspirin, and although it can cause hepatic damage, this is usually related to overdosage (see Table 20–4).

Opioids

Opioids are the preferred drugs in the management of most forms of acute severe pain, including postoperative

TABLE 20–4 *Dosing Data for NSAIDs*

DRUG	USUAL PEDIATRIC DOSE[1]	COMMENTS
Acetaminophen	10–15 mg/kg q 4 hr (see Table 18–2)	Lacks the peripheral anti-inflammatory activity of other NSAIDs.
Aspirin	10–15 mg/kg q 4 hr[2]	The standard against which other NSAIDs are compared. Inhibits platelet aggregation; may cause postoperative bleeding.
Choline magnesium trisalicylate (Trilisate)	25 mg/kg bid	May have minimal antiplatelet activity; also available as oral liquid.
Ibuprofen (Motrin, others)	10 mg/kg q 6–8 hr	Available as several brand names and as generic; also available as oral suspension.
Naproxen (Naprosyn)	5 mg/kg q 12 hr	Also available as oral liquid.

Note: Only the above NSAIDs have FDA approval for use as simple analgesics, but clinical experience has been gained with other drugs as well.

[1]Drug recommendations are limited to NSAIDs where pediatric dosing experience is available.

[2]Contraindicated in presence of fever or other evidence of viral illness.

Adapted from U.S. Department of Health and Human Services. (1992). *Acute pain management in infants, children and adolescents: Operative and medical procedures. Quick Reference Guide for Clinicians* (Publication No. 92-0020). Rockville, MD: Agency for Health Care Policy and Research, Public Health Service.

pain, post-traumatic pain, and sickle cell vaso-occlusive crisis pain, and chronic cancer pain. Opioids are less effective for certain forms of neuropathic pain, such as causalgia and diabetic neuropathy (Shannon & Berde, 1989). Some of the more commonly used opioids are morphine, codeine, meperidine, methadone, and fentanyl (Table 20–5).

Although opioids may be given by most routes, the oral route should be used when it is effective and appropriate for the child. Elixirs are available for children who cannot effectively swallow tablets. The IV route can be used when the oral route is contraindicated. Intravenous opioids may be given by bolus or continuous infusion.

It is important to remember that opioids produce sedation and respiratory depression in addition to analgesia. Other effects include nausea, vasodilation, cough suppression, urine retention, and constipation. Although these effects must be closely monitored, most children can tolerate these drugs if their dosages are monitored. Nausea can usually be controlled through the administration of antiemetics.

Infants and children receiving intravenous and epidural opioids should be placed on a pulse oximeter.

Morphine is the preferred opioid in children. It reaches its peak effect 20 minutes after IV administration. It produces both sedation and analgesia. Maximum respiratory depression occurs 7 minutes after IV administration. Naloxone (Narcan) should be available to reverse the analgesia, sedation, and/or respiratory depression if necessary.

Naloxone HC1 should be used to reverse the effects of morphine when oxygen and stimulation of the child is ineffective.

Meperidine (Demerol) should only be used for short-term pain control in patients who have shown a bold allergy or intolerance to other opioids. The duration of analgesia is shorter than morphine. Some experts believe that meperidine should only be given intravenously in children (Zajac, 1992). Normeperidine, a metabolite of meperidine, has been associated with convulsions and dysphoria, especially with long-term administration of meperidine. Meperidine is most often used postoperatively and in combination with other medications for procedural pain.

TABLE 20–4 *Dosing Data for Opioid Analgesics*

	RECOMMENDED STARTING DOSE (CHILDREN AND ADULTS LESS THAN 50 kg BODY WEIGHT)[1]	
DRUG	**ORAL**	**PARENTERAL**
Morphine[2]	0.3 mg/kg q 3–4 hr	0.1 mg/kg q 3–4 hr
Codeine[3]	1 mg/kg q 3–4 hr[4]	Not recommended
Hydromophone[2] (Dilaudid)	0.06 mg/kg q 3–4 hr	0.015 mg/kg q 3–4 hr
Hydrocodone (in Lorcet, Lortab, Vicodin, others)	0.2 mg/kg q 3–4 hr[4]	Not available
Levorphanol (Levo-Dromoran)	0.04 mg/kg q 6–8 hr	0.02 mg/kg q 6–8 hr
Meperidine (Demerol)	Not recommended	0.75 mg/kg q 2–3 hr
Methadone (Dolophine, others)	0.2 mg/kg q 6–8 hr	0.1 mg/kg q 6–8 hr
Oxycodone (Roxicodone; also in Percocet, Percodan, Tylox, others)	0.2 mg/kg q 3–4 hr[4]	Not available
Opioid Agonist–Antagonist and Partial Agonist		
Buprenorphine (Buprenex)	Not available	0.004 mg/kg q 6–8 hr
Nalbuphine (Nubain)	Not available	0.1 mg/kg q 3–4 hr

Note: Published tables vary in the suggested doses that are equianalgesic to morphine. Clinical response is the criterion that must be applied for each patient; titration to clinical response is necessary. Because there is not complete cross-tolerance among these drugs, it is usually necessary to use a lower than equianalgesic dose when changing drugs and to retitrate a response.

Caution: Recommended doses do not apply to patients with renal or hepatic insufficiency or other conditions affecting drug metabolism and kinetics.

[1]Caution: Doses listed for patients with body weight less than 50 kg cannot be used as initial starting doses in babies less than age 6 months. Consult the *Clinical Practice Guideline for Acute Pain Management: Operative or Medical Procedures and Trauma* (Publication No. 92-0032) section on management of pain in neonates for recommendations.

[2]For morphine, hydromorphone, and oxymorphone, rectal administration is an alternate route for patients unable to take oral medications, but equianalgesic doses may differ from oral and parenteral doses because of pharmacokinetic differences.

[3]Caution: Codeine doses above 65 mg often are not appropriate due to diminishing incremental analgesia with increasing doses but continually increasing constipation and other side effects.

[4]Caution: Doses of aspirin and acetaminophen in combination opioid–NSAID preparations must also be adjusted to the patient's body weight.

Adapted from U.S. Department of Health and Human Services. (1992). *Acute pain management in infants, children and adolescents: Operative and medical procedures. Quick Reference Guide for Clinicians* (Publication No. 92-0020). Rockville, MD: Agency for Health Care Policy and Research, Public Health Service.

The use of meperidine (Demerol), promethazine (Phenergan), and chlorpromazine (Thorazine), known as DPT and/or pediatric cocktail, is discouraged. This combination is thought to be outdated; and can cause significant adverse effects, including respiratory arrest, prolonged sedation, and decreased oxygen saturation (Nahata et al., 1985; Zeltzer et al., 1989; Coté, 1994). It is much safer to use a combination of opioids and benzodiazepines.

Fentanyl and its analogues (sufentanil, alfentanil) have a shorter duration of action than morphine. Because there also is much less histamine released, there is less vasodilation and pruritus. The short duration of effect makes these drugs appropriate for use when a short painful procedure (inserting a chest tube or changing a burn dressing) is to be performed and in patients who are critically ill. Critically ill infants who receive continuous infusion of fentanyl are at high risk for narcotic withdrawal (French & Nocera, 1994).

Methadone is metabolized very slowly and therefore has a prolonged duration of action. It is absorbed well both orally and intravenously. It must be carefully titrated because of its long duration. A constant clinical effect can usually be attained orally by giving the medication every 6 to 8 hours and intravenously in small increments every 4 to 6 hours (Shannon & Berde, 1989).

Codeine is the most commonly given oral opioid for moderate pain. It is usually given in combination with acetaminophen or aspirin. It can cause constipation and gastrointestinal upset.

Hydromorphone (Dilaudid) is very similar to morphine. It is approximately eight times more potent than morphine. It may be used to control chronic pain in cancer patients.

Conscious Sedation

Conscious sedation is a medically controlled state of depressed consciousness that allows protective reflexes to be maintained, retains an independent airway, and permits appropriate response by the patient to physical stimulation or verbal command (American Academy of Pediatrics, Committee on Drugs, 1992). Chloral hydrate, DPT (Demerol, Phenergan, Thorazine), and pentobarbital sodium (Nembutal) have been the drugs used most commonly to achieve this sedation in the past. However, chloral hydrate may cause addictive central nervous system (CNS) depression when given with other CNS depressants (Bindler & Howry, 1991). DPT as mentioned under "Opioids" has several adverse effects and should not be used.

Midazolam (Versed) is a short-acting drug that can be given by multiple routes: parenteral, intranasal, rectal, intramuscular, oral, and sublingual. It can be used for conscious sedation, preoperative sedation, and as an induction agent for general anesthesia. The intranasal route of administration is used in pediatrics for procedures and as an induction to anesthesia (see Chapter 19). Intranasal Versed appears to be safe, with minimal respiratory depression and no effect on blood pressure (Adrian, 1994). Advantages to using Versed include minimal side effects, short duration of sedation, and ability to administer without an IV access.

Nursing Care Plan for the Child in Pain

NURSING DIAGNOSIS

- Pain related to physical, biological, or chemical agents (edema, disease process, surgery, infection, trauma)

Expected Outcome: The child will experience a decrease in pain as evidenced by:

- verbalization of less discomfort through use of assessment tool
- relaxed body posture
- reduced facial grimacing
- decreased crying and behavioral change
- return to activity level experienced prior to discomfort

Intervention	Rationale
1. Observe and document signs of pain in the child (behavioral and physiologic). Note both verbal and nonverbal responses. Assess vital signs.	Assessment of pain in children is based on behavioral and sometimes physiologic changes. Infants and children have difficulty verbalizing pain. Physiologic changes vary in response to pain and should be evaluated together with other data.
2. Assess for factors that might be affecting the child (separation, fear, anxiety, loss of control).	The child's perception of pain and ultimate reaction to pain may be influenced by other factors.

Intervention	Rationale
3. Assessment of pain should be based on the child's developmental stage.	Infants and children at each developmental level have their own way of reacting to and coping with pain.
4. Utilize a developmentally appropriate pain assessment tool (see Table 20–2).	Infants and children have difficulty communicating about their pain and assessment tools provide more objective quantitative information.
5. Note if the child's pain level is different when at rest, ambulating, playing, during procedures, and before and after receiving analgesics.	Pain relief measures can be enhanced by an understanding of cause and effect.
6. Administer the appropriate analgesic (see Tables 20–4 and 20–5). Give by oral or IV route. Avoid injections.	Nonnarcotic analgesics are appropriate for mild to moderate pain. Narcotic analgesics should be given for moderate to severe pain. Children may deny pain in order to avoid an injection.
7. Implement nonpharmacologic pain reduction strategies:	
a. Distraction	a. Distraction interrupts the transmission of pain.
b. Relaxation techniques	b. Also thought to interrupt pain.
c. Cutaneous stimulation	c. Blocks pain transmission.
d. Quiet, calm environment	d. A quiet, calm environment is more conducive to rest, which enhances the effects of analgesia.
e. Reposition	e. A change in position may relieve pressure and/or provide for a more relaxed, comfortable body.
f. Decrease environmental noise/light	f. A quiet, comfortable environment can have a soothing, relaxing effect on the body.
g. Comfort measures (hold, rock, music, books, touch, massage)	g. Decreases anxiety and the skeletal muscle tension that often accompanies pain.
8. Involve parents in care.	The presence of parents may reduce fear and anxiety and thus reduce the amount of pain experienced. Parents also know their child best and can assist in the assessment of pain and its relief.
9. Evaluate and document response to both pharmacologic and nonpharmacologic pain reduction measures. Use a pain management sheet (Stevens, 1990).	Aids in determining the effectiveness of pain relief measures.
10. Observe for side effects of medication.	Respiratory depression is the most serious side effect of opioids. However, it is rare. Other side effects include nausea and vomiting, constipation, sedation, and personality changes.
11. Document the child's response to both pharmacologic and nonpharmacologic interventions. A copy of the pain assessment tool is part of the child's chart for easy reference.	Without documentation the effectiveness of pain reduction measures cannot be evaluated.

Evaluation: The child has a decrease in pain as shown by a relaxed body position, verbalization of the absence of pain, absence of crying, and a return to normal activities.

Home Teaching: When a child is discharged from the hospital or is seen in an outpatient setting, it is imperative that the parents and the child, if appropriate, receive information regarding pain management at home, as outlined below:

- Pain assessment tool together with instructions on use, including a return demonstration
- Pain medication to be given, including dose, route, and schedule, explained and given to parents in writing
- Nonpharmacologic interventions that are appropriate for the child's particular source of discomfort (massage, warm/cold compresses, reposition)
- Instructions to notify primary care physician if pain relief interventions are ineffective or if child shows behavior or physiologic changes not consistent with the expected outcomes for the child
- A phone number where parents can contact a nurse if they have any questions about their child's condition

KEY CONCEPTS

- Pain is an unpleasant sensory and emotional experience associated with actual or potential tissue damage, or described in terms of such damage.
- The gate-control theory of pain postulates that a gating mechanism at the level of the dorsal horn can facilitate or inhibit pain transmission. It further states that stimulation of the larger afferent nerves, which carry benign sensations, can dull pain. The gate-control theory also suggests that a descending control system may enhance or inhibit pain sensations. This theory may explain the effectiveness of the TENS and why anxiety and previous pain experience can affect pain perception.
- Two of the myths that interfere the most with infants and children receiving adequate pain medication are the fear of addiction and the fear of respiratory depression. Neither belief is supported by research.
- Pain assessment in infants and children takes a multidimensional approach. The child and parent should be questioned and behavioral and physiologic changes noted.
- Both pharmacologic and nonpharmacologic measures should be utilized in the treatment of pain in children. Morphine is the opioid of choice for severe pain and acetaminophen for less severe pain. Nonpharmacologic interventions include distraction, relaxation and imagery techniques, hypnosis, TENS, and the use of biofeedback.
- A pain assessment tool should be used for each child to effectively document pain management. The tool should be developmentally correct and must be administered according to instructions for the results to be valid.

REFERENCES

Adrian, E. (1994). Intranasal Versed: The future of pediatric conscious sedation. *Pediatric Nursing, 20*(3), 287–292.

Agency for Health Care Policy and Research. Acute Pain Management Guideline Panel. (1992). *Acute pain management: Operative or medical procedures and trauma. Clinical practice guideline* (AHCPR Pub. No. 92–0032). Rockville, MD: Public Health Service, U.S. Department of Health and Human Services.

Agency for Health Care Policy and Research. (1992). *Acute pain management in infants, children, and adolescents: Operative and medical procedures. Quick reference guide for clinicians* (AHCPR Pub. No. 92–0020). Rockville, MD: Public Health Service, U.S. Department of Health and Human Services.

American Academy of Pediatrics, Committee on Drugs. (1992). Guidelines for monitoring and management of pediatric patients during and after sedation for diagnostic therapeutic procedures. *Pediatrics, 89*(6), 1110–1115.

Anand, K., & Hickey, P. (1987). Pain and its effects in the human neonate and fetus. *New England Journal of Medicine, 317*(21), 1321–1347.

Asprey, J. (1994). Postoperative analgesic prescription and administration in a pediatric population. *Journal of Pediatric Nursing, 9*(3), 150–156.

Beyer, J. (1984). *The Oucher: A user's manual and technical report.* Evanston, IL: Judson Press.

Beyer, J. (1986). Content validity of an instrument to measure young children's perceptions of the intensity of their pain. *Journal of Pediatric Nursing, 1,* 386–395.

Beyer, J. (1989). *The Oucher: A user's manual and technical report.* Denver: University of Colorado Health Sciences Center.

Beyer, J., Ashley, L., Russell, G., & DeGood, D. (1983). Patterns of postoperative analgesic use with adults and children following cardiac surgery. *Pain, 17*, 71–80.

Beyer, J., Denyes, M., & Villarruel, A. (1992). The creation, validation, and continuing development of the Oucher: A measure of pain intensity in children. *Journal of Pediatric Nursing, 7*(5), 335–346.

Bindler, R., & Howry, L. (1991). *Pediatric Drugs and Nursing Implications.* (pp. 130–132). Norwalk, CT: Appleton and Lange.

Brazy, J. (1988). Effects of crying on cerebral blood flow and cytochrome aa3. *Journal of Pediatrics, 112*(3), 457–461.

Coté, C. (1994). Sedation for the pediatric patient. *Pediatric Clinics of North America, 41*(1), 31–51.

Dalla Barba, B., Gatto, C., Valenza, E., Calabro, L., Cavedagni, M., Prandoni, S., & Benini, F. (1991). Pain memory in full-term newborns. *Journal of Pain and Symptom Management.* Second International Symposium on Pediatric Pain. Abstract No. 194.

Eland, J. (1990). Pain in children. *Nursing Clinics of North America, 25*(4), 871–882.

Eland, J. (1991). The use of TENS with children who have cancer pain. *Journal of Pain and Symptom Management, 6*(3), 137–

Eland, J., & Anderson, J. (1977). The experience of pain in children. In A. K. Jacox (Ed.), *Pain: A source book for nurses and other health professionals* (pp. 453–473). Boston: Little, Brown.

Favaloro, R., & Touzel, B. (1990). A comparison of adolescents' and nurses' postoperative pain ratings and perceptions. *Pediatric Nursing, 16*(4), 414–416.

French, J., & Nocera, M. (1994). Drug withdrawal symptoms in children after continuous infusions of fentanyl. *Journal of Pediatric Nursing, 9*(2), 107–112.

Gardner, S. (1994). Pain and pain relief in the neonate. *Maternal-Child Nursing, 19*, 85–90.

Grunau, R., Johnston, C., & Craig, K. (1990). Neonatal facial and cry responses to invasive and non-invasive procedures. *Pain, 42*, 295–305.

Gureno, M., & Reisinger, C. (1991). Patient-controlled analgesia for the young pediatric patient. *Pediatric Nursing, 17*(3), 251–254.

Hester, Nancy. (1979). The preoperational child's reaction to immunization. *Nursing Research, 4*(28):250–254.

Hester, N. O., & Barcus, C. S. (1986). Assessment and management of pain in children. *Pediatrics: Nursing Update, 1*, 2–8.

International Association for the Study of Pain. (1979). Pain terms: A list with definitions and notes on usage. *Pain, 6*, 249.

Johnston, C., & Strada, M. (1986). Acute pain response in infants: A multidimensional description. *Pain, 24*, 373–382.

Kachoyeanos, M., & Zollo, M. B. (1995). Ethics in pain management of infants and children. *Maternal-Child Nursing 20*, 142–147.

Lesko, S., & Mitchell, A. (1995). An assessment of the safety of pediatric ibuprofen. *Journal of the American Medical Association, 273*(12), 929–933.

Mannheimer, J., & Lampe, G. (1984). *Clinical transcutaneous electrical nerve stimulation.* Philadelphia: F. A. Davis.

Margolius, F., Hudson, K., & Michel, Y. (1995). Beliefs and perceptions about children in pain: A survey. *Pediatric Nursing, 21*(2), 111–115.

McCaffrey, M. (1972). *Nursing management of the patient in pain.* Philadelphia: J. B. Lippincott.

Melzack, R., & Wall, P. (1965). Pain mechanisms: A new theory. *Science, 150*, 971–979.

Mills, N. (1989). Pain behaviors in infants and toddlers. *Journal of Pain and Symptom Management, 4*, 184–190.

Nahata, M., Clotz, M., & Krogg, E. (1985). Adverse effects of meperidine, promethazine and chlorpromazine for sedation in pediatric patients. *Clinical Pediatrics, 24*(10), 558–560.

Phillips, P. (1995). Neonatal pain management: A call to action. *Pediatric Nursing, 21*(2), 195–199.

Porter, J., & Jick, H. (1980). Addiction rare in patients treated with narcotics (letter). *New England Journal of Medicine, 302*, 123.

Rawlings, D., Milles, P., & Engel, R. (1980). The effect of transcutaneous PO_2 in term infants. *American Journal of Diseases of Children, 134*, 676–678.

Savedra, M. C., Tesler, M. D., Holzemer, W. L., & Ward, J. (1992). *Adolescent Pediatric Pain Tool: User's manual.* San Francisco: University of California.

Savedra, M., Tesler, M., Holzemer, W., Wilkie, D., & Ward, J. (1989). Pain location: Validity and reliability of body outline markings by hospitalized children and adolescents. *Research in Nursing and Health, 12*, 307–314.

Savedra, M., Tesler, M., & Wegner, C. (1988). How do adolescents describe pain? *Journal of Adolescent Health Care, 9*(4), 315–320.

Schechter, N. (1988). An approach to the child with pain. *Patient Care, 3*, 116–131.

Schechter, N. (1989). The undertreatment of pain in children: An overview. *Pediatric Clinics of North America, 36*, 781–794.

Schechter, N., Allen, D., & Hanson, K. (1986). Status of pediatric pain control: A comparison of hospital analgesic usage in children and adults. *Pediatrics, 77*, 11–15.

Stevens, B. (1990). Development and testing of a pediatric pain management sheet. *Pediatric Nursing, 16*(6), 543–548.

Shannon, M., & Berde, C. (1989). Pharmacologic management of pain in children and adolescents. *Pediatric Clinics of North America, 36*(4), 855–871.

Taddio, A., Nulman, I., Goldbach, M., Ipp, M., & Koren, G. (1994). Use of lidocaine-prilocaine cream for vaccination pain in infants. *Journal of Pediatrics, 124*, 643–648.

Tesler, M., Savedra, M., Holzemer, W., Wilkie, D., Ward, J., & Paul, S. (1991). The word-graphic rating scale as a measure of children's and adolescents' pain intensity. *Research in Nursing and Health, 14*, 361–371.

Valente, S. (1991). Using hypnosis with children for pain management. *Oncology Nursing Forum, 18*(4), 699–704.

Wallace, M. (1989). Temperament: A variable in children's pain management. *Pediatric Nursing, 15*(2), 118–121.

Vessey, J., Carlson, K., & McGill, J. (1994). Use of distraction with children during an acute pain experience. *Nursing Research, 43*(6), 369–372.

Zajac, J. (1992). Pediatric pain management. *Critical Care Nursing Quarterly, 15*(2), 35–51.

Zappa, S. (1994–95). A topical anesthetic and hemophilia care. *Nursing Network/Psychosocial News, Winter*, 6.

Zeltzer, L., Jay, S., & Fisher, D. (1989). The management of pain associated with pediatric procedures. *Pediatric Clinics of North America, 36*(4), 941–964.

BIBLIOGRAPHY

Alfieri, D., & Cagen, D. (1995). Transdermal fentanyl. *Pediatric Nursing, 21*(1), 72–74.

Altimier, L., Norwood, S., Dick, M., Holditch-Davis, D., & Lawless, S. (1994). Postoperative pain management in preverbal children: The prescription and administration of analgesics with and without caudal analgesia. *Journal of Pediatric Nursing, 9*(4), 226–232.

Aradine, C., Beyer, J., & Tompkins, J. (1988). Children's pain perception before and after analgesia: A study of instrument construct validity. *Journal of Pediatric Nursing, 3*(1), 11–23.

Beyer, J., & Aradine, C. (1986). Content validity of an instrument to measure young children's perceptions of the intensity of their pain. *Journal of Pediatric Nursing. 1*(6), 386–395.

Broome, M. (1991). Measurement of pain: Self-report strategies. *Journal of Pediatric Oncology Nursing, 8*(3), 131–133.

Broome, M., & Slack, J. (1990). Influences on nurses' management of pain in children. *Maternal-Child Nursing, 15,* 158–162.

Brown, L. (1987). Physiologic responses to cutaneous pain in neonates. *Neonatal Network. 12,* 18–22.

Cunningham, N. (1990).Ethical perspectives on the perception and treatment of neonatal pain. *The Journal of Perinatal and Neonatal Nursing, 4*(1), 75–83.

Dothit, J. (1990). Psychosocial assessment and management of pediatric pain. *Journal of Emergency Nursing, 16*(3), 168–170.

Elander, G., Hellstrom, G., & Qvarnstromm, B. (1993). Care of infants after major surgery: Observation of behavior and analgesic administration. *Pediatric Nursing, 19*(3), 221–226.

Foster, R., & Hester, N. (1990). The relationship between pain ratings and pharmacologic interventions for children in pain. *Advances in Pain Research Therapy, 15,* 31–36.

French, G., Painter, E., & Coury, D. (1994). Blowing away shot pain: A technique for pain management during immunization. *Pediatrics, 93*(3), 384–388.

Gadish, H., Gonzalez, J., & Hayes, J. (1988). Factors affecting nurses' decisions to administer pediatric pain medication postoperatively. *Journal of Pediatric Nursing, 3*(6), 383–390.

Gedaly-Duff, V., & Ziebarth, D. (1994). Mothers' management of adenoid-tonsillectomy pain in 4- to 8-year olds: A preliminary study. *Pain, 57,* 293–299.

Heiney, S. (1991). Helping children through painful procedures. *American Journal of Nursing, 11,* 20–24.

Howe, C. (1993). A new standard of care for pediatric pain management. *Maternal-Child Nursing, 18,* 325–329.

Hultgren, M. (1990). Assessment of postoperative pain in critically ill infants. *Progress in Cardiovascular Nursing, 5*(3), 104–112.

Johnston, C., & Stevens, B. (1990). Pain assessment in newborns. *The Journal of Perinatal and Neonatal Nursing, 4*(1), 41–52.

Kachoyeanos, M., & Zollo, M. (1995). Ethics in pain management of infants and children. *Maternal-Child Nursing, 20,* 142–147.

Lau, N. (1992a). Pediatric pain management (Part I). *Journal of Pediatric Health Care, 6*(2), 87–92.

Lau, N. (1992b). Pediatric pain management (Part II). *Journal of Pediatric Health Care, 6*(4), 214–219.

Lesko, S., & Mitchell, A. (1995). An assessment of the safety of pediatric ibuprofen: A practitioner-based randomized clinical trial. *The Journal of the American Medical Association, 273,* 929–933.

Mackey, D., & Jordan-Marsh, M. (1991). Innovative assessment of children's pain. *Emergency Nursing, 17*(4), 250–251.

Mahon, S. (1994). Concept analysis of pain: Implications related to nursing diagnosis. *Nursing Diagnosis, 5*(1), 14–25.

Marchette, L., Main, R., Redick, E., Bagg, A., & Leatherland, J. (1991). Pain reduction interventions during neonatal circumcision. *Nursing Research, 40*(4), 241–244.

McCrory, L. (1991). A review of the Second International Symposium on Pediatric Pain. *Pediatric Nursing, 17*(4), 366–370.

Nardone, P., & Schuchard, B. (1991). Parental pain perception of the same-day surgery pediatric patient. *Journal of Nursing Quality Assurance, 5*(3), 59–64.

Robertson, J. (1993). Pediatric pain assessment: Validation of a multidimensional tool. *Pediatric Nursing, 19*(3), 209–213.

Schmidt, K., Eland, J., & Weiler, K. (1994). Pediatric cancer pain management: A survey of nurses' knowledge. *Journal of Pediatric Oncology Nursing, 11*(1), 4–12.

Stein, P. (1995). Indices of pain intensity: Construct validity among preschoolers. *Pediatric Nursing, 21*(2), 119–123.

Taddio, A., Nulman, I., Goldbach, M., Ipp, M., & Koren, G. (1994). Use of lidocaine–prilocaine cream for vaccination pain in infants. *Journal of Pediatrics, 124,* 643–648.

Tyler, D. (1990). Patient-controlled analgesia in adolescents. *Journal of Adolescent Health Care, 11,* 154–158.

Van Cleve, L., & Andrews, S. (1995). Pain responses of hospitalized neonates to venipuncture activities. *Maternal-Child Nursing, 20,* 148–152.

Van Cleve, L., & Savedra, M. (1993). Pain location: Validity and reliability of body outline markings by 4- to 7-year-old children who are hospitalized. *Pediatric Nursing, 19*(3), 217–220.

Vesely, C. (1995). Pediatric patient-controlled analgesia: Enhancing the self-care construct. *Pediatric Nursing, 21*(2), 124–128.

Villarruel, A., & Denyes, M. (1991). Pain assessment in children: Theoretical and empirical validity. *Advances in Nursing Science, 14*(2), 32–41.

Watt-Watson, J., Evernden, C., & Lawson, C. (1990). Parents' perception of their child's acute pain experience. *Journal of Pediatric Nursing, 5*(5), 344–349.

West, N., Oakes, L., Hinds, P., Sanders, L., Holden, R., Williams, S., Fairclough, D., & Bozeman, P. (1994). Measuring pain in pediatric oncology ICU patients. *Journal of Pediatric Oncology Nursing, 11*(2), 64–68.

Zappa, S. (1994). EMLA Cream: A topical anesthetic. *Nursing in Pediatrics, Spring:* 28–31.

Zuckerberg, A. (1994). Reducing perioperative pain and anxiety. *Contemporary Pediatrics, 11,* 40–53.

UNIT IV

CARING FOR CHILDREN WITH HEALTH PROBLEMS

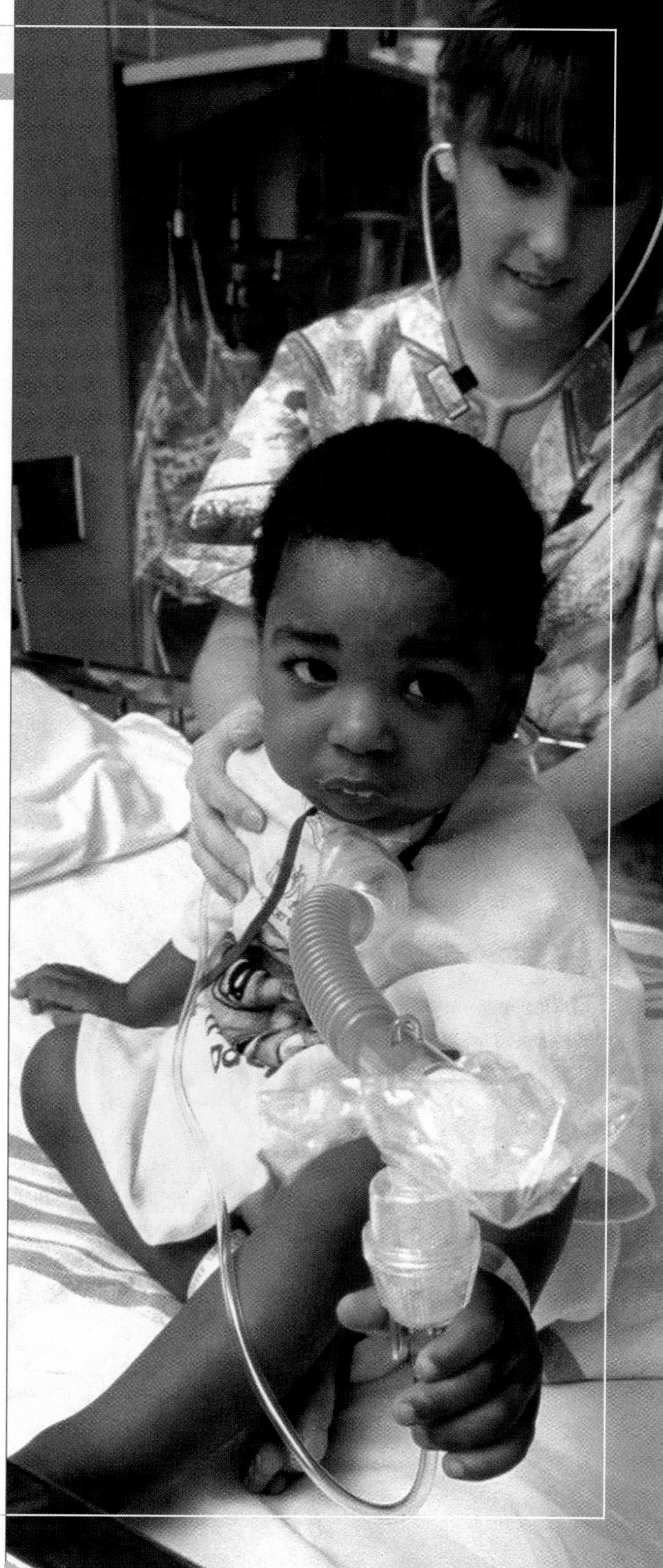

21

The High-Risk Neonate

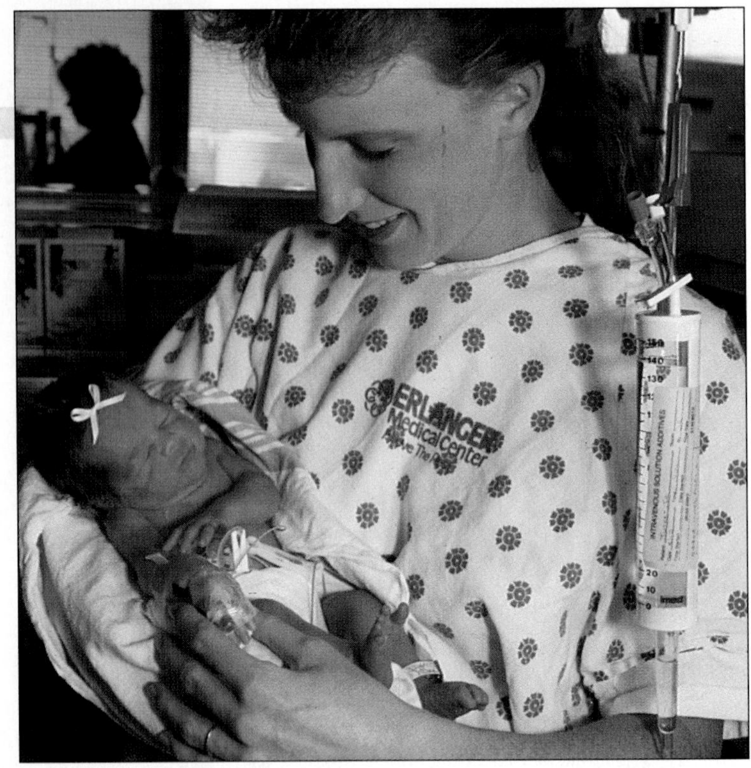

CHAPTER OVERVIEW

LEARNING OBJECTIVES

After studying this chapter, you should be able to:

- Differentiate between normal and abnormal findings on the physical assessment of the neonate.
- List complications associated with prematurity.
- List complications associated with postmaturity.
- Formulate a plan of care for a high-risk infant.
- Identify nursing interventions to support family members who are dealing with the needs of a high-risk infant.
- Identify the components of successful discharge teaching.

KEY TERMS

autosomal recessive: a genetic trait carried on 1 of the 22 pairs of chromosomes not concerned with determination of sex; an autosomal recessive trait is evident in the infant only when it is transmitted by both parents

calcitonin: a hormone, secreted by cells within the thyroid gland, that inhibits bone resorption or breakdown; under normal circumstances, its production is increased when serum calcium concentrations are elevated

cytotoxicity: the degree to which an agent possesses a specific destructive action on certain cells, or the possession of such action

homozygote: an individual who inherited two identical genes for a certain trait

inborn error of metabolism: a genetically determined biochemical disorder in which specific congenital defects in the structure or function of a protein molecule produce a metabolic block that may result in pathologic consequences at birth or later

infarction: the formation of an infarct, which is a localized area of ischemic necrosis produced by occlusion of the arterial supply or the venous drainage of the part

maceration of skin: degenerative changes resulting in discoloration and softening of the skin

microphthalmia: a developmental defect causing moderate or severe reduction in the size of the eye

myelinization: the process by which myelin, a fatty, insulating covering, is formed around the axons of nerve fibers; this process begins during the latter part of fetal life and continues during the first postnatal year

neutral thermal environment: an environmental temperature range within which the infant can maintain normal body temperature with the least amount of metabolic expenditure and oxygen consumption

parathyroid hormone: a hormone produced by the parathyroid glands in response to low serum calcium levels; it increases the breakdown of bone, releasing calcium and phosphorous; increases absorption of calcium from the gastrointestinal tract; and increases reabsorption of calcium in the kidneys

At birth, the neonate begins the first of many physical adaptations to the extrauterine environment. If the infant cannot make this transition completely, the caregiver must intervene quickly if the infant is to survive. Respiratory, cardiac, neurologic, and infectious problems may occur in the first few minutes of life. Problems seen this early are usually life threatening and must be corrected or supported quickly. For other infants, the initial transition is made successfully, but problems occur in the first several days of life.

Because the infant cannot tell the nurse when something is wrong, early, often subtle cues must be read, documented, and reported to the medical team. Cues such as hypotonia, lethargy, irritability, or poor feeding can be early symptoms of serious problems such as sepsis, necrotizing enterocolitis, intracranial hemorrhage, congestive heart failure, or respiratory failure.

Nurses must keep a constant vigil on the infant's status and also care for the parents. Parents, expecting a perfect child, may be met with an infant who does not meet their expectations or who may have a life-threatening illness. Parents may also be faced with physical separation from their child. Often, the child is transferred to another hospital, many miles from the parents' home. When parents visit their infant, they may be intimidated by the caretakers who can perform the physical care needed by their infant. An integral part of the nurse's role is to keep the parents informed of their child's status and encourage their participation in their child's care whenever possible.

This chapter discusses some common problems seen in the newborn nursery or the neonatal intensive care unit (NICU). Much of the discussion centers around preterm infants because they make up the majority of patients in the NICU.

SETTINGS OF CARE

Nurses care for infants in many settings. Labor and delivery nurses care for infants in the delivery room and newborn nursery and often are the first to recognize an infant in distress. Postpartum nurses caring for the mother often come into contact with infants who are rooming-in or visiting with the mother. If they are not vigilant in their assessment, the infant may be discharged with an undiagnosed illness. Because of early discharge of mothers and their newborns, nurses in home health care and community clinics are increasingly coming in contact with infants with special needs.

Not all hospitals are equipped to care for the critically ill neonate. Newborn nurseries are categorized as level 1, level 2, and level 3. Level 1 nurseries provide basic newborn care. Level 2 nurseries provide care for infants with moderate to high-risk problems, such as mild respiratory distress or suspected sepsis. Level 3 nurseries care for extremely high-risk infants. The NICU is equipped with highly technical equipment and requires the expertise of specialized clinicians. Figure 21–1 and the box below list problems experienced by the newborn that may necessitate care in the NICU.

Transport. Not all areas of the country have the specialized care needed by the high-risk neonate available. For this reason, it may be necessary to transfer the pregnant mother or the infant after delivery. It is preferable to make the transfer before birth, but not all infants with problems are identified during the prenatal period.

A special team of nurses, physicians, and respiratory therapists care for the infant during transfer. The infant is transferred in an incubator or radiant warmer in a special ambulance, helicopter, or airplane.

The infant's condition is stabilized before transportation, and the nurse at the birth facility provides the transporting nurse with the information necessary to make a safe trip. The assessment skills of both nurses must be highly developed.

PHYSICAL EXAMINATION OF THE NEWBORN

Assessment

The assessment of the newborn begins with a review of the prenatal and intrapartum history. The infant's history can provide many clues about actual or potential problems. Additional data are obtained through physical examination. The examination of the newborn can be organized by a systems review (Table 21–1). Special emphasis is placed on the neurologic, respiratory, and cardiovascular systems.

Nursing Diagnosis and Planning

Examples of nursing diagnoses and related expected outcomes that might be developed after assessment of the infant are:

- Ineffective Thermoregulation related to prematurity. ***Expected Outcome:*** *A neutral thermal environment (environmental temperature within which an infant can maintain normal body temperature with minimal effort) will be maintained.*

Neonatal Problems that May Necessitate Care in the NICU

Perinatal asphyxia
Birth injuries
Prematurity
Postmaturity
Sepsis
Necrotizing entercolitis
Congenital heart disease
Congenital birth defects

- Abdominal wall defects
- Tracheoesophageal fistula
- Choanal atresia
- Diaphragmatic hernia
- Myelomeningocele
- Exstrophy of the bladder

Intestinal obstruction
Congenital infection
Meconium aspiration syndrome
Persistent pulmonary hypertension
Respiratory distress syndrome
Transient tachypnea of the newborn
Hydrocephalus
Seizure activity
Meningitis
Intracranial hemorrhages
Substance abuse withdrawal
Hyperbilirubinemia
Hydrops fetalis
Osteogenesis imperfecta
Renal failure
Polycythemia
Anemia
Endocrine disorders
Inborn errors of metabolism

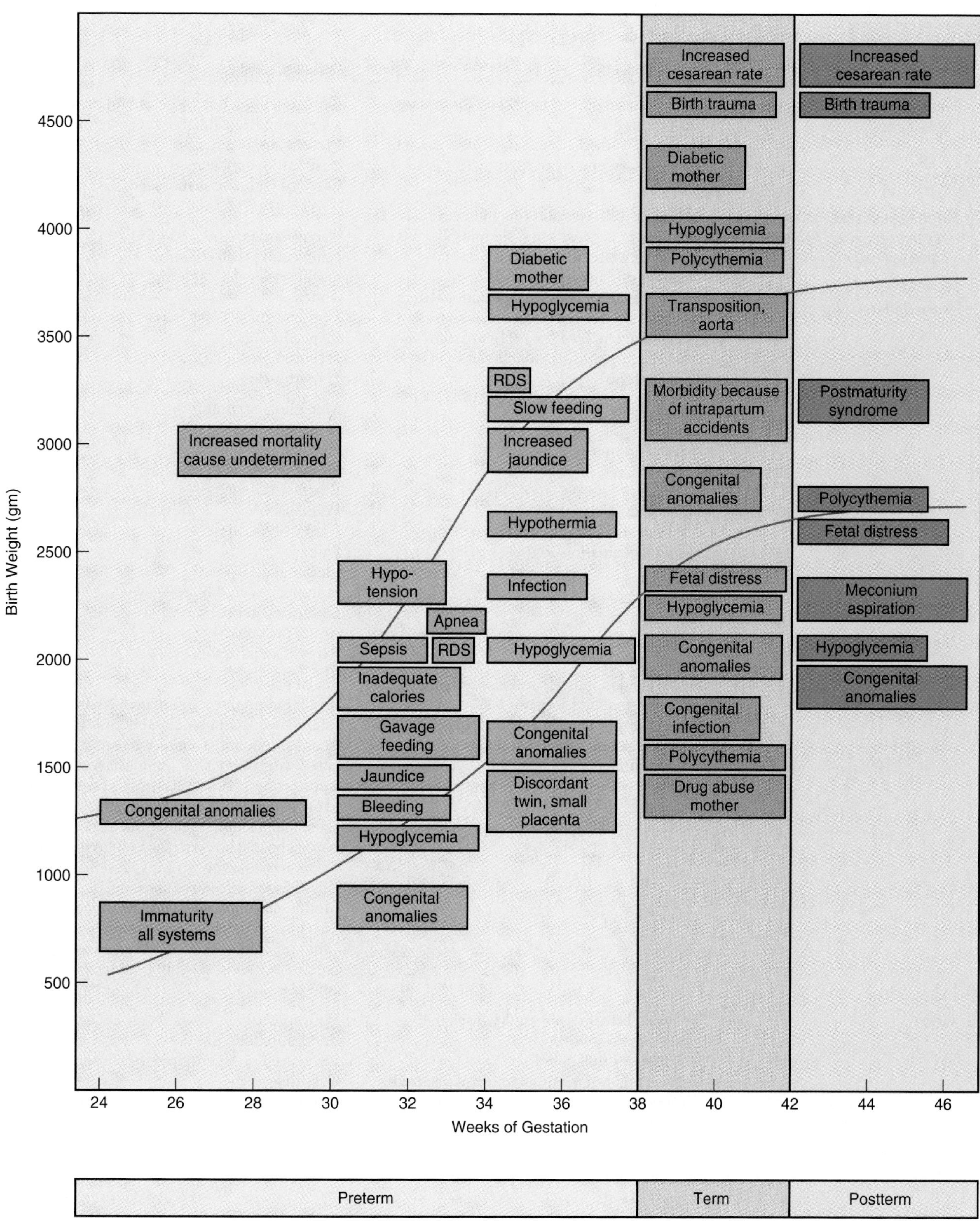

Figure 21–1

Neonatal morbidity by birth weight and gestational age. (From Lubchenco, L. O. [1976]. *The high risk infant* (p. 6). Philadelphia: W. B. Saunders. Modified from Lubchenco, L. O., Hansman, C., & Backstrom, L. [1968]. In J. H. D. Jonxis, H. K. A. Visser, & J.A. Troelstra, [Eds.], *Aspects of prematurity and dysmaturity*. Springfield, IL: Charles C Thomas.)

TABLE 21–1 *Examination of the Newborn by Body System*

	NORMAL FINDINGS	ABNORMAL FINDINGS
Weight, Head Circumference, and Length	Growth parameters appropriate for gestational age Generally normal appearance (placement of features, symmetry of body size)	Growth parameters place the infant small for gestational age or large for gestational age Preterm appearance Postmature appearance Obvious congenital anomalies
Vital Signs (temperature, respiratory rate, pulse, blood pressure) ***Note: Observed resting posture and activity***	Heart rate 120–160/min (may increase with crying or decrease when sleeping) Respiratory rate 30 to 60/min Temperature (axillary) 36°–37.7°C Blood pressure varies with gestational age; systolic: 50–52 mmHg, increasing by 4 days of age to 60–90 mmHg; diastolic: 25–30 mmHg, with a slight rise by 4 days of age (term)	Asymmetry Tachycardia (>160–180/min) Bradycardia (<80–100/min) Tachypnea (>60–80/min) Apnea Hypothermia Hyperthermia Hypotension Hypertension
Skin	Acrocyanosis Milia Nevus flammeus Vernix Lanugo Mongolian spots Erythema toxicum (newborn rash) Mild desquamation	Meconium straining Bruising Excoriation Hemangiomas Blisters Petechiae Central cyanosis Pallor Plethora Jaundice (first 24 hours) Decreased subcutaneous tissue Amniotic bands > 6 café au lait spots
Head and Neck	Head: head molding, caput succedaneum, anterior fontanel soft and flat Eyes: clear corneas, free of discharge Mouth: Epstein's pearls, mucous membranes pink Nose: patent nares, thin white mucus and sneezing Neck: short, 90° rotation	Facial palsy Head: bulging, tense fontanel (hydrocephalus); craniotabes; sunken fontanel; cephalhematoma; craniosynostosis Eyes: subconjunctival hemorrhages, conjunctivitis, clouded cornea, cataracts, narrow palpebral fissures, sunsetting eyes Ears: malposition, preauricular tags, sinuses Nose: choanal atresia, nasal septal dislocation, nasal flaring with inspiration, bloody discharges, excessive sneezing Mouth: cleft lip and palate, natal teeth, asymmetry with crying, macroglossia, micrognathia Neck: skin folds, webbing, torticollis, mass, fistulas
Chest	Enlarged breast tissue, milky discharge Equal breath sounds Respirations unlabored Cardiac point of maximal impulse just to the left of sternum Equal peripheral pulses	Widespread nipples Supernumerary nipples Decreased or asymmetric breath sounds Grunting Retractions Stridor Apnea

TABLE 21–1 *Examination of the Newborn by Body System (continued)*

	NORMAL FINDINGS	ABNORMAL FINDINGS
Chest (continued)		Tachypnea Murmur Hyperactive precordium Tachycardia Bradycardia Bounding femoral pulses Weak or absent femoral pulses
Abdomen	Abdomen flat or slightly rounded Three-vessel umbilical cord Void within 24 hours of birth Stool within 48 hours of birth Normal femoral pulse Liver edge smooth Nonpalpable spleen	Omphalitis, leakage Abdominal distension Abdomen firm or tender to touch Absent bowel sounds Omphalocele Gastroschisis Absent musculature Masses Enlarged liver Enlarged spleen Scaphoid abdomen Bilious vomiting Hematuria Bloody stools Diarrhea Visible bowel loops
Perineum	Female: blood-tinged vaginal discharge, hymenal tag Male: inability to retract foreskin	Hypospadias, epispadias Chordee Hernia Hydrocele Ambiguous genitalia Imperforate anus Extropy of the bladder
Musculoskeletal system	Bowing of legs, return to midline with passive motion	Scoliosis Spina bifida Sacral dimple Polydactyly Syndactyly Clubbed feet Dislocated hips Deformities of the extremities or joints
Nervous System and Behavior	Slightly flexed posture at rest Good arm and leg recoil Drowsy or alert with stimulation Fussy infant quiets with swaddling, holding, or pacifier Normal reflexes: Moro, gag, grasp, suck and swallow Spontaneous movement of all extremities.	Asymmetric, absent, or exaggerated reflexes Hypotonia Hypertonia Stupor Hyperalertness Seizures Staring Jitters Tremors Lethargy Inconsolability, hyperexcitability

- Risk for Infection related to decreased immune function. ***Expected Outcome:*** *The infant will be free of any signs of infection as evidenced by complete blood count (CBC) parameters within normal limits and negative blood culture findings.*
- Anticipatory Grieving by the family related to perceived potential loss of a significant other. ***Expected Outcome:*** *Opportunities for anticipatory grieving are provided.*

Implementation and Evaluation

Implementation and evaluation would follow, depending on the initial assessment and plan. This chapter discusses some of the specific problems experienced by the high-risk neonate.

PREMATURITY

Infants are classified as preterm if birth occurs before the end of the last day of the 37th week of gestation (259th day) as calculated from the onset of the last menstrual period. Any neonate whose birth occurs from the beginning of the first day (260th day) of the 38th week through the end of the last day of the 42nd week (294th day) is considered a term infant. The preterm infant, with its immature organ systems, is at risk for many health care problems.

Etiology. The etiology of preterm labor is not fully understood, but the association between preterm labor and certain risk factors has been identified (see accompanying box).

Risk Factors for Preterm Labor and Birth

History of preterm birth or midtrimester spontaneous abortion
Multiple gestation
Uterine anomaly, incompetent cervix
Urinary tract infection
Hydramnios
Second- or third-trimester bleeding
Diagnosed preterm labor in current pregnancy
Cervical dilation of greater than 2 cm in a parous patient and greater than 1 cm in a nullipara
Low prepregnancy weight (less than 115 lb)

From American Academy of Pediatrics and American College of Obstetricians and Gynecologists. (1992). *Guidelines for perinatal care* (3rd ed., pp. 66–67). Elk Grove Village, IL: Author.

Incidence. In the United States, approximately 8% to 10% of all live births are preterm deliveries. Those preterm births account for 75% of the perinatal morbidity and mortality in the United States.

Clinical Manifestations. The following are potential complications seen in the premature infant:

- Respiratory distress syndrome
- Hypothermia
- Hyperbilirubinemia
- Patent ductus arteriosus
- Apnea
- Sepsis
- Periventricular-intraventricular hemorrhage
- Necrotizing enterocolitis
- Hypocalcemia
- Hypoglycemia
- Anemia of prematurity
- Retinopathy of prematurity

To discuss prematurity, the nurse must understand the initial assessment of the newborn. All newborn infants are classified by birth weight, duration of gestation, and a standard of intrauterine growth. Gestational age provides an estimate of the maturity and development of the neonate's physical systems and thus suggests potential health problems that the neonate may experience. Infants are classified as preterm, term or postterm.

Birth weight and gestational age are used to categorize the neonate by intrauterine growth. This practice increases the sophistication of neonatal assessment by correlating birth weight with gestational age in an attempt to determine the pattern of growth that the fetus experienced in utero. This factor was standardized by determining the average weight of infants born at different gestational ages. A variety of intrauterine growth charts, based on various population groups, have been designed. Most nurseries use the Colorado Intrauterine Growth Chart. The neonate, when compared with this standard, can be categorized as small for gestational age (SGA), appropriate for gestational age (AGA), or large for gestational age (LGA) (Battaglia & Lubchenco, 1967).

Battaglia and Lubchenco developed a graph to display the statistically calculated risk to the infant based on birth weight and gestational age (Fig. 21–1). The gestational age is calculated by the obstetrician through maternal history (menstrual dates) or by an estimate from a fetal ultrasound. This information is not always available or may be incorrect, and the gestational age of the infant, once delivered, must be assessed by other clinical tools. The assessment tool used frequently in nurseries incorporates both neuromuscular and physical criteria to estimate the gestational age of the newborn. The tool was originally developed by Dubowitz and later modified by Ballard, and is often referred to by the primary researcher's name (Ballard et al., 1991; see Chapter 3, Fig. 3–3).

PATHOPHYSIOLOGY *of Prematurity*

Preterm delivery can be the result of an obstetric complication that necessitates delivery, or it can be the result of preterm labor. Preterm premature rupture of the membranes initiates 25% to 30% of preterm deliveries, whereas specific maternal obstetric, medical, or surgical complications result in 20% to 25%. Examples of these complications include maternal diabetes mellitus, hypertension, preeclampsia, placenta previa or abruptio placentae, chorioamnionitis, and intrauterine growth retardation. The remaining 50% of preterm deliveries occur as the result of spontaneous preterm labor with no known etiology (American Academy of Pediatrics and American College of Obstetricians and Gynecologists, 1992).

Preterm delivery results in the birth of an infant whose body systems are still maturing. Even with aggressive intervention by the health care team, the infant may be unable to achieve homeostasis. The premature infant's respiratory system may lack the surfactant necessary to prevent the lungs from collapsing. Small muscle mass and an immature nervous system may also compromise respiratory effort. Other immature organ systems produce other complications. The developing vascular system in the brain is susceptible to significant hemorrhage and anoxic injury. The premature infant may have difficulty maintaining blood pressure, renal perfusion, and oxygenation. The gastrointestinal system may lack the necessary enzymes for protein metabolism, placing the infant at risk for feeding problems. The immune system is deficient, increasing the susceptibility of the preterm infant to infection.

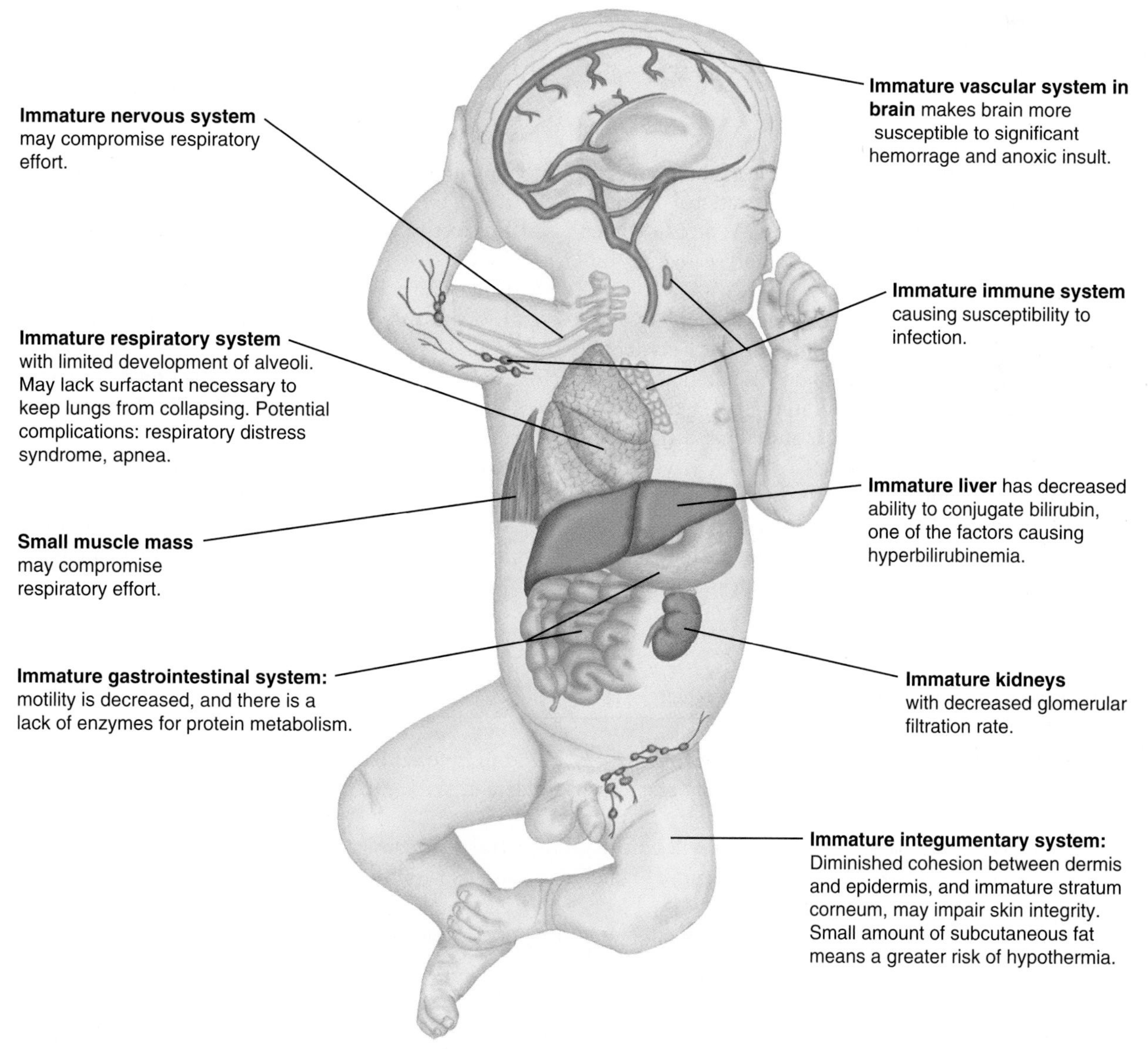

Immature nervous system may compromise respiratory effort.
Immature vascular system in brain makes brain more susceptible to significant hemorrage and anoxic insult.
Immature immune system causing susceptibility to infection.
Immature respiratory system with limited development of alveoli. May lack surfactant necessary to keep lungs from collapsing. Potential complications: respiratory distress syndrome, apnea.
Immature liver has decreased ability to conjugate bilirubin, one of the factors causing hyperbilirubinemia.
Small muscle mass may compromise respiratory effort.
Immature gastrointestinal system: motility is decreased, and there is a lack of enzymes for protein metabolism.
Immature kidneys with decreased glomerular filtration rate.
Immature integumentary system: Diminished cohesion between dermis and epidermis, and immature stratum corneum, may impair skin integrity. Small amount of subcutaneous fat means a greater risk of hypothermia.

This assessment of gestational age and appropriateness of growth alerts the caretaker to the status of the infant and the potential for problems.

Therapeutic Management. Therapeutic management helps the infant to maintain homeostasis. Warmth, through an incubator or radiant warmer, may be required. Enteral nutrition is given to the infant based on his ability to handle the digestive process. If unable to use a nipple, the neonate should be fed with a gastric tube. If he is unable to tolerate any enteral feedings, intravenous (IV) fluids and hyperalimentation are necessary. When required, respiratory support includes oxygen delivery or the use of positive pressure ventilation. Much of the care focuses on the prevention of infection throughout the hospital course. Growth and development should be supported, including involvement of family members to promote parent–infant attachment.

NURSING CARE OF THE PREMATURE INFANT

Assessment

Nursing assessment begins with a review of the perinatal history to identify potential problems. Gestational age and the appropriateness of growth (SGA, AGA, or LGA) are determined. Risk factors for each category can then be reviewed (see Fig. 21–1).

Physical examination should include a complete systems review, including observation for birth defects. Immediate assessment should include auscultation of cardiac and breath sounds and monitoring of vital signs, including temperature. Blood sugar and hematocrit levels should be measured by 1 hour of age.

The preterm infant is at risk for intracranial hemorrhage and infection. Neurologic status is assessed by checking reflexes and evaluating muscle tone. The fontanels are assessed for patency and fullness. Changes in muscle tone and activity can be early indicators of sepsis in the premature infant.

Patent ductus arteriosus is a frequent finding, and cardiac assessment should focus on pulses, blood pressure, and the presence of a murmur.

Respiratory distress, from multiple etiologies, is assessed by checking breath sounds, observing color, evaluating the work of breathing, and reviewing blood gases and oxygen saturations by pulse oximetry.

Skin is assessed for maturity and integrity. Birth injuries are evidenced by skin trauma and limited function of the affected extremity or tissue.

Renal function is assessed by accurate measurement of urine output and careful recording of intake.

The preterm infant is at high risk for hypoglycemia because of inadequate glycogen stores, and metabolic status is assessed by measuring blood glucose levels. Metabolic status can be further compromised by temperature instability, which leads to the depletion of glycogen stores.

Nursing Diagnoses

- Impaired Gas Exchange related to immature development of the lung and chest wall or insufficient amounts of surfactant.
- Impaired Skin Integrity related to immature epidermis.
- Ineffective Thermoregulation related to prematurity.
- Ineffective Infant Feeding Pattern related to immature reflexes.
- Risk for Infection related to decreased immune function.
- Altered Growth and Development related to prematurity and prolonged exposure to the hospital environment.
- Knowledge Deficit (care of the preterm infant) related to lack of exposure to accurate information.
- Risk for Altered Parenting related to situational crisis (preterm birth) or separation from the infant associated with long-term care in the hospital.

Planning, Implementation, and Evaluation: The Premature Newborn

NURSING DIAGNOSIS
- Impaired Gas Exchange related to immature development of the lung and chest wall or insufficient amounts of surfactant.

Expected Outcome:
- The infant will be able to maintain adequate gas exchange as evidenced by blood gas values and pulse oximeter saturations within normal ranges.

Intervention:
- Refer to the section on respiratory distress syndrome.

Evaluation:
- Infant will maintain a normal respiratory rate and be free of any evidence of respiratory distress.
- Infant will maintain normal oxygen saturations on pulse oximetry.

NURSING DIAGNOSIS • Risk for Impaired Skin Integrity related to immature epidermis.

Expected Outcome: • Skin will remain intact without evidence of breakdown.

Intervention	Rationale
1. Assess skin every shift: integrity, color, perfusion, turgor, temperature, and edema.	Early identification of problems will help prevent extensive tissue damage.
2. Extremely premature infants may benefit from a warm mist into the incubator or into a plastic tent covering the infant under a radiant warmer.	Infants < 28 weeks' gestation and less than 7–14 days of age have high insensible water loss through their skin.
3. Minimize use of adhesives. Avoid tape on any infant < 32 weeks' gestation and less than 7 days of age.	Infants < 32 weeks' gestation and less than 7–14 days of age are at the highest risk for skin injury from adhesives because of the weak junction between the epidermis and dermis.
4. Use pectin barriers and karaya base electrodes and change electrodes daily and as needed if poor skin integrity develops. Do not apply over the nipple area to avoid scarring of the tissue.	Nonadhesive products are less likely to tear skin.
5. Remove adhesives slowly with water-soaked cotton balls. Use a pressure gauze dressing, not adhesive bandages, for stasis of bleeding.	The epidermis can be torn from the dermal layer if adhesives are roughly torn from the skin.
6. Clean off povidone-iodine solution with sterile water after procedures and before dressing wounds.	Povidone-iodine solution can irritate the skin, and the preterm skin has increased permeability, placing the infant at risk for systemic absorption of the chemical.
7. Rotate sites for temperature probes daily, or as recommended by the manufacturer, and oximeter probes every 8–12 hours and as needed. Avoid hot packs or heat-retaining plastic.	Poorly perfused tissue is vulnerable to heat injury.
8. Monitor and document IV sites every hour. Check IV patency before administering drugs or blood products.	Excessive IV infiltrates may cause permanent damage to skin, muscle, or nerves.
9. Notify physician of IV infiltrates promptly if the infiltrate warrants treatment with hyaluronidase.	Hyaluronidase, given within 1 hour of an IV infiltrate, can decrease damage to the tissue.
10. Elevate the site of an IV infiltrate to assist in the absorption of fluid. Do not use warm packs on IV infiltrates.	Injured tissue cannot dissipate heat effectively, and warm packs may increase tissue damage.
11. Turn and reposition immobilized infants every 1–2 hours. Avoid pressure points or constriction of blood flow from dressings, tubing, probes, or clothes. Place the infant on a foam egg crate–or sheepskin-type mattress to decrease friction and pressure points.	Neonates cannot communicate their needs to caretakers. Repositioning promotes mobilization of dependent edema.
12. Use less alkaline soaps (e.g., Lowila, Aveeno, Basis, Neutrogena, Purpose, Oilatum) for infant bathing.	The acid pH of the skin has bacteriostatic properties.

Evaluation: • Skin shows no evidence of trauma, fissures, or excoriation.

NURSING DIAGNOSIS • Ineffective Thermoregulation related to prematurity.

Expected Outcome: • A neutral thermal environment will be maintained.

Intervention	Rationale
1. Maintain skin probe when on incubator servocontrol and calibrate the probe every shift.	Proper functioning of the equipment must be ensured.
2. Set skin probe at 36.5°C and adjust it according to the infant's temperature.	
3. Change temperature probe every 24 hours, or as recommended by the manufacturer, and as needed.	Prolonged contact may cause tissue damage, or a loose probe may result in iatrogenic hyperthermia.
4. Monitor for signs and symptoms of temperature instability, check incubator temperature and heater output, and relate findings to axillary temperature and incubator servocontrol probe site.	Wide fluctuations in incubator temperature can be a sign of sepsis or neurologic dysfunction in the infant, or may be indicative of equipment malfunction.
5. Use a neutral thermal environment chart to estimate initial incubator temperature.	Maintenance of the infant in the neutral thermal environment decreases oxygen needs by avoiding metabolism of brown adipose tissue to produce heat and by avoiding increase in basal metabolic rate in response to hyperthermia.
6. Do not bathe an infant until body temperature stabilizes above 36.5°C.	Bathing produces major evaporative heat loss.
7. Plastic wrap may be placed over the bed or around the infant. Caution should be taken with an infant who is not intubated to ensure that the plastic does not fall over the infant's face.	Plastic wrap allows the radiant heat to penetrate through to the infant while decreasing insensible water loss and diminishing the effects of convection and evaporation heat loss.
8. Assess overall circulatory status: capillary refill, skin and mucous membrane color.	Temperature instability affects blood pressure, heart rate, and oxygenation. • Signs and symptoms of hypothermia (<36.5°C) include apnea, bradycardia, tachypnea, poor perfusion, cyanosis, acidosis, feeding intolerance, lethargy irritability, hypoglycemia, and seizures. • Signs and symptoms of hyperthermia (>37.2°C) include apnea, dehydration, sweating, seizures, tachycardia, flushing, hypotension, and carbon dioxide retention.
9. Provide clothing based on environmental temperature and medical status. Do not clothe the infant under a radiant warmer.	Clothing decreases heat loss in an incubator.

Evaluation: • The infant's axillary temperature is maintained between 36.5 and 37.2°C.

NURSING DIAGNOSIS • Ineffective Infant Feeding pattern related to immature reflexes.

Expected Outcomes:
- The neonate will tolerate nipple or gavage feedings without evidence of fatigue, respiratory difficulty, or emesis.
- The infant will receive or ingest adequate calories to support growth.

Intervention	Rationale
1. Assess gestational age, physical condition, and neurologic status.	Asphyxia, sepsis, and intracranial hemorrhage may impair the infant's ability to suck. Immature infants may be unable to coordinate suck and swallow.
2. Maintain strict intake and output measurement. Monitor response to fluid changes. Report abnormal laboratory results.	The premature kidney has limited ability to conserve fluid or excrete excess fluid, placing the infant at high risk for dehydration or fluid retention.
3. Provide supplement nipple enteral feedings with gavage feeding or IV fluids as ordered (see Fig. 21–2).	Supplemental feedings allow the compromised neonate to conserve energy.
4. Provide a calm environment for nippling.	Signs and symptoms of difficulty in handling feedings include tachypnea, coughing, gagging, choking, cyanosis, bradycardia, and crying.
5. Document and use the type of nipple tolerated best by the infant.	Infants with a weak suck may not be able to suck from a hard nipple. Infants with a strong such may choke or aspirate with a soft nipple that has an easy flow.
6. Provide rest periods as needed. Limit nippling to maximum of 20–30 minutes, and supplement with gavage feedings.	The preterm infant may not be able to sustain an effective suck.
7. Give medications at beginning of feedings.	Medication is received even if the infant does not complete the nipple feeding.
8. Use pulse oximeter and cardiac monitor to assist in assessing the tolerance of feeding methods.	Feeding problems may occur as apnea, bradycardia, or oxygen desaturation.
9. Feed as scheduled. Record residuals, emesis, and skill with nippling.	Careful documentation allows caregivers to assess the infant's readiness for feeding advancement.
10. Gavage feedings (Fig. 21–2):	
• If <32–34 weeks' gestation, gavage all feedings unless medical order allows nippling.	Preterm infants < 32–34 weeks' gestation do not have a coordinated suck and swallow reflex.
• Elevate head of bed.	May help decrease severity of gastroesophageal reflux.
• Verify proper tube placement before each feeding.	Improper tube placement can result in pulmonary aspiration of feedings.
• Record any gastric residuals obtained before feeding. Note color and consistency of aspirate. Report abnormal findings.	Residuals can be an early sign of feeding intolerance and necrotizing enterocolitis.
• Use No. 5 French feeding tube if <1000 g.	
• Hold syringe no more than 4 inches above stomach.	Rapid infusion of feedings by gavage may result in emesis.
• Place tube orally.	Neonates are preferential nose breathers, and their nasal passages are small.
• Offer pacifier with feedings..	Pacifier use strengthens infant suck, facilitates digestion, and provides a comfort measure.

A mother giving gavage feeding. This infant has a pacifier ▶ nearby. The pacifier is often used during gavage feeding to strengthen the suck, facilitate digestion, and provide comfort.

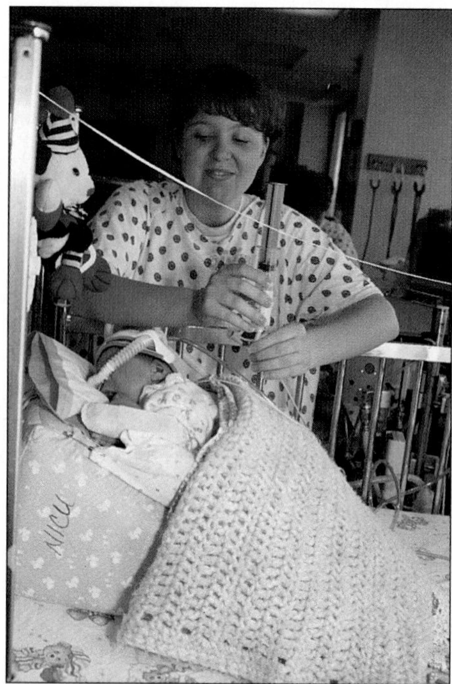

A father bottle feeding an infant in radiant warmer.

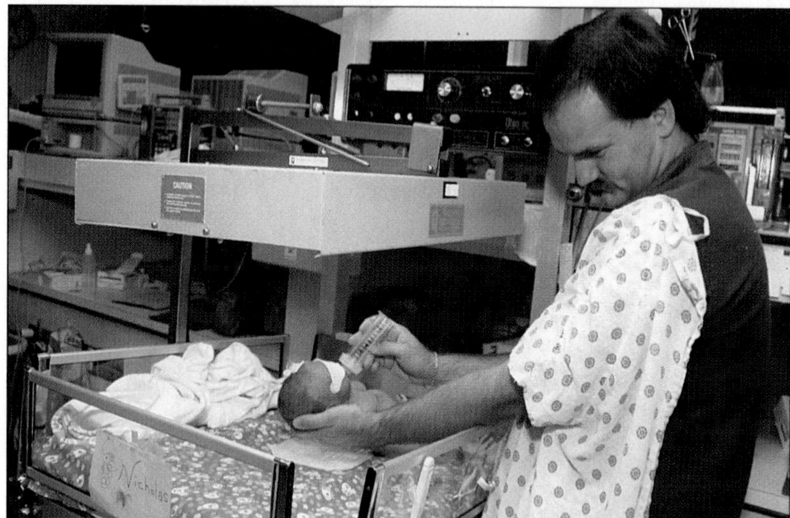

Figure 21–2
Premature infants are usually ineffective feeders because of immature reflexes. Nipple feeding is preferred as long as the infant can tolerate this method and obtain sufficient nourishment. The breast milk or formula is poured into a bottle. A softer nipple is often used because preterm infants may tire easily with the regular nipple. To promote family bonding with the infant, parents are involved as much as possible in the care of their infant. Infants younger than 32–34 weeks' gestation do not usually have their suck and swallow reflexes coordinated well enough to obtain sufficient nourishment by nipple feeding, and must be fed by gavage.

Intervention	Rationale
• Place premature infant on abdomen or right side after feedings.	Gastric emptying improves with right lateral or prone positioning.
11. Teach parents to assess infant's readiness for nipple or breastfeedings as evidenced by ease of respirations, normal muscle tone, and alert state.	Feeding requires high energy input from the infant, and the compromised premature infant may be unable to handle nipple or gavage feedings.
12. Teach parents to avoid other stressors during feedings, such as excessive stimulation, hyperthermia, and hypothermia.	Stressors will increase energy needs.

Evaluation: • The infant demonstrates consistent weight gain along with appropriate head growth and length as documented per growth chart. Infant tolerates feedings without evidence of apnea, bradycardia, or respiratory distress. The infant eventually nipples all feedings within a reasonable time frame without evidence of fatigue or distress.

NURSING DIAGNOSIS • Risk for Infection related to decreased immune function.

Expected Outcome: • The infant remains free of nosocomial infection.

Intervention	Rationale
1. Wash hands between all patient contacts.	Handwashing is the single most effective method of preventing nosocomial infections.
2. Monitor laboratory values, such as CBC and cultures, for indications of infection.	Sepsis in the neonate may have rapid onset, and prompt recognition and treatment is essential.
3. Collect specimens as needed to monitor for infection; collect cultures using aseptic technique.	Sterile technique prevents contamination of the specimen and false-positive results.
4. Monitor vital signs every 4 hours and as needed.	Hypothermia, hyperthermia, hypotension, bradycardia, tachycardia, or apnea can be signs of infection.
5. Document activity level and responsiveness. Assess feeding ability and glucose stability.	Lethargy, poor tone, poor feeding, glucose instability, or extreme irritability can be indicative of sepsis.
6. Provide daily skin care. Identify conditions that increase the risk of infection, such as extreme prematurity, malnutrition, or skin breakdown.	Loss of skin integrity compromises an important barrier against microorganisms.
7. Use aseptic technique for all invasive procedures.	Invasive lines (e.g., umbilical lines, central lines), chest tubes, or endotracheal tubes increase the risk of septicemia in the neonate.
8. Notify visitors of policy: individuals with coughs, cold symptoms, herpes cold sores, or diarrhea should not visit until symptoms clear. Siblings should be screened for recent illness or exposure.	The neonate is immunocompromised and highly susceptible to communicable diseases.

Evaluation: • The infant has normal vital signs, normal perfusion, intact skin, a normal white blood cell count, negative culture findings, and a normal blood glucose level, and will be free of apnea episodes.

NURSING DIAGNOSIS • Altered Growth and Development related to prematurity and prolonged exposure to the hospital environment.

Expected Outcome: • The infant will maintain equilibrium of physiologic status. The infant will maintain restful sleep states for weight gain.

Intervention	Rationale
1. Recognize signs of overstimulation and intervene appropriately. • *Mild stress response:* gaze aversion, yawning, hiccups, grimacing, tongue thrusting, slack jaw, bowel movements, sneezing, and coughing. • *Moderate stress response:* flushing, mottling, sighing, regurgitation, finger splaying, extension of arms and legs, jitteriness, jerky movements, and limpness. • *Severe stress response:* hypoxia, pallor, cyanosis, tachypnea, bradycardia, and arrhythmia.	The neonate attempts to adapt to his environment by modifying body functions and behavioral responses. If he cannot fully adapt to external events, the disruption in the neonate's adaptive mechanisms causes identifiable stress response cues. Infants who cannot adapt to chronic stress may have poor growth patterns.
2. Promote flexed positioning of the infant.	The flexed position promotes self-regulation or coping behavior in the preterm infant.

Intervention	Rationale
3. Decrease overstimulation by: • Dimming lights in room. • Shading eyes or covering the incubator with a blanket. • Coordinating care to minimize disturbance of the infant. • Do not wake infant when in deep sleep. • Provide a quiet environment: close incubator doors quietly, avoid placing equipment on top of incubator. • Hold, touch, or stroke infant to comfort. • Provide pacifier when interested.	The preterm or ill neonate is especially limited in his ability to cope and is easily overwhelmed by the overstimulating NICU environment.

Evaluation: • The infant will rest in a flexed position. The infant will tolerate handling and stimulation with minimal stress responses.

NURSING DIAGNOSIS • Knowledge Deficit (care of the preterm infant) related to lack of exposure to accurate information.

Expected Outcomes:
- The parents will have realistic expectations of their preterm infant.
- The parents will have an adequate knowledge base to care for their infant.

Implementation and Evaluation: • See Care of the Family.

Evaluation: • Verbal statements by parents document their understanding of the infant's status.

NURSING DIAGNOSIS • Risk for Altered Parenting secondary to situational crisis (preterm birth).

Expected Outcomes:
- The parent will exhibit parent–child attachment behavior.
- The parent will develop role identity as a parent.

Implementation and Evaluation: • See Care of the Family.

Evaluation:
- Family members are involved in problem solving directed at appropriate solutions.
- Family assumes caretaking responsibilities.
- Family members contact available resources as needed.

POSTMATURITY

Postmaturity syndrome occurs when placental function is inadequate to supply the nutritional and respiratory demands of the fetus. Fetal growth is affected, and the ability of the fetus to tolerate the stress of labor and delivery may be compromised.

Etiology. The placenta develops completely by the fifth month of gestation and achieves peak function by 36 weeks' gestation. Placental growth continues then at a slow rate, with a decrease noted after 42 weeks' gestation. Contributing etiologies such as maternal systemic disease, uterine anomalies, placenta abnormalities, and fetal factors (i.e., multiple gestation) may alter placental function and thereby cause abnormalities in fetal growth to appear even earlier than 42 weeks' gestation.

Incidence. Approximately 6% of all pregnancies extend beyond 42 weeks' gestation. Approximately one third of these postdate pregnancies, or 2% of all pregnancies, result in an infant with postmaturity syndrome (Thorp & Creasy, 1990).

PATHOPHYSIOLOGY *of Postmaturity*

A postterm pregnancy exceeds 294 days or 42 weeks, as timed from the last menstrual period, or 280 days from the time of ovulation. The fetus is at risk for problems of postmaturity or dysmaturity because of placental dysfunction. Placental dysfunction results in a compromised blood supply to the fetus. The fetus is at risk for nutritional deficiency, hypoxia, or asphyxia. The fetus may show evidence of growth retardation. Skin may be wrinkled because of the loss of subcutaneous fat. The loss of vernix caseosa, which protects the skin, may leave the skin **macerated** (discolored and softened). When oxygen delivery to the smooth muscle of the gastrointestinal tract is inadequate, a fetus under stress relaxes the anal sphincter control and passes meconium (stool) in utero. Nailbeds stain after 4 to 6 hours of exposure to meconium; more than 12 hours of exposure is needed to stain vernix caseosa. Meconium is green, but changes over time to yellow-green or bright yellow as the bilirubin degrades. Clifford (1954) described three stages of progressive changes seen in the newborn with postmaturity syndrome:

Stage I: maceration accompanied by loss of vernix caseosa, with dry and cracking skin that is parchment-like, wrinkled, and peeling. Infant appears malnourished, but alert or apprehensive.

Stage II: all of the findings of Stage I, plus meconium-colored amniotic fluid, meconium on the newborn's skin, and green meconium staining of the umbilical cord.

Stage III: all of the findings of Stages I and II, plus yellow staining of the nails and skin along with a conversion to yellow-green staining of the umbilical cord and placenta.

Clinical Manifestations (see Fig. 21–3)

- Intrauterine growth retardation
- Dehydration
- Dry, cracked, wrinkled, parchment-like skin
- Long, thin arms and legs; decreased subcutaneous tissue, with hanging skinfolds
- Advanced hardness of the skull
- Absence of vernix and lanugo
- Skin maceration, especially in folds
- Meconium (brown-green) staining of the skin
- Appearance of hyperalertness or apprehension

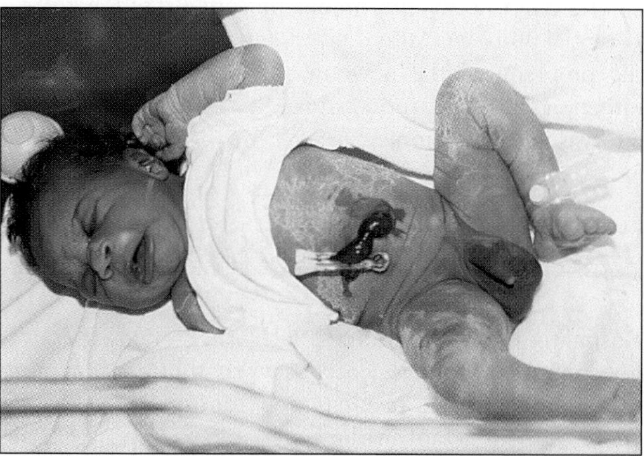

Figure 21–3
This infant exhibits signs of postmaturity. The most obvious sign is the desquamation of his skin because of the loss of protective vernix. The relative deep wrinkles on his thighs and legs suggest that he recently lost subcutaneous fat, also a typical feature of postmaturity. This infant also passed meconium into the amniotic fluid, which increases the risk for respiratory problems. (Courtesy of Parkland Memorial Hospital, Dallas, Texas.)

Physical examination and complete review of the maternal history confirm the diagnosis of postmaturity. If meconium was passed by the fetus before delivery and the neonate shows signs of respiratory distress, evaluation should include a chest x-ray to assess for any evidence of aspiration. An infant who is stressed at the time of delivery is also at high risk for perinatal asphyxia and must be observed closely for any evidence of seizure activity.

Therapeutic Management

Infants with postmaturity syndrome require aggressive management of fluid and nutrition to avoid further weight loss. They are at high risk for hypoglycemia and may require frequent monitoring of their glucose level.

Respiratory support is given as needed and may include oxygen as well as positive pressure ventilation. Calcium levels may be checked to assess for hypocalcemia. A hematocrit evaluation should be done to exclude polycythemia. If polycythemia is present, a partial exchange transfusion may be required, especially if the infant is symptomatic (i.e., cyanosis, hypoglycemia, seizures).

NURSING CARE OF THE POSTMATURE INFANT

Assessment

The gestational age of the infant should be assessed on admission to the newborn nursery. Appropriateness of growth is determined, and physical examination is performed to identify postmature characteristics.

Nursing Diagnosis and Planning

- Altered Growth and Development related to placental insufficiency as evidenced by postmaturity syndrome. ***Expected Outcome:*** *The infant will exhibit no evidence of respiratory distress, hypoglycemia, hypocalcemia, or asphyxia.*
- Risk for Impaired Skin Integrity related to altered nutritional state (postmaturity syndrome). ***Expected Outcome:*** *The infant will exhibit normal skin integrity.*

Implementation

A complete physical examination is performed, with special attention given to respiratory status, serum glucose, and temperature. Because the postmature infant has limited glycogen stores, the infant should be observed for signs and symptoms of hypoglycemia. He should also be observed for signs of symptoms of respiratory distress (see the section on respiratory distress syndrome). The infant's temperature is taken on admission and every hour until stable.

The postmature infant has special skin needs because of the loss of vernix caseosa in utero. The skin is allowed to slough naturally and should be washed with nonalkaline soap or water only.

Evaluation

Is the infant pink in room air? Does the infant exhibit a normal respiratory pattern and normal temperature? Is the infant's skin smooth and intact, without evidence of breakdown?

Meconium Aspiration Syndrome

Meconium aspiration usually occurs only in term or postterm infants, although it may occur in preterm infants who have experienced intrauterine asphyxia. The amniotic fluid is stained with meconium.

Pathophysiology. A chemical pneumonitis can develop and, in some cases, mechanical ventilation is required. Fetal distress and hypoxia may occur. Complete or partial airway obstruction can also occur.

Etiology and Incidence. When asphyxia in utero occurs, there is stimulation of peristalsis and relaxation of the anal sphincter, which releases meconium into the amniotic fluid. Although aspiration of meconium may occur whenever meconium is passed into the amniotic fluid, the likelihood of aspiration increases when the infant experiences severe asphyxia leading to gasping respirations in utero.

Meconium-stained amniotic fluid is seen in 5% to 15% of births, with meconium aspiration pneumonia occurring in 5% of these infants. Mechanical ventilation is required in 30% of cases, and 5% to 10% of cases may be fatal.

Clinical Manifestations

- Mild to severe respiratory distress
- Tachypnea
- Cyanosis
- Retractions
- Nasal flaring
- Grunting
- Yellow-green staining of nailbeds and skin
- Prolonged expiration phase of respirations
- Coarse breath sounds

Diagnostic Evaluation. A chest x-ray shows hyperexpanded areas with areas of atelectasis. Arterial blood gases show respiratory and metabolic acidosis and a low PaO_2, even with 100% oxygen administration.

Therapeutic Management. When meconium is observed, the key to therapeutic management is prevention through suctioning of the mouth and pharynx as soon as the head is delivered and before delivery of the rest of the body. Once the infant is delivered, the vocal cords are visualized with a laryngoscope. If meconium is present below the area of the vocal cords, an endotracheal tube is inserted to facilitate deep suctioning and ventilation, if necessary. Less severely affected infants may require only warmed, humidified oxygen. Extracorporeal membrane oxygenation (ECMO), a form of cardiopulmonary bypass, may be used with infants who do not respond to conventional treatment because of the severity of their disease.

Nursing Care. A nurse who observes meconium during labor should notify the proper personnel that there is a potential problem. After delivery, nursing care is related to the problems of the newborn. The infant is at risk for infection and respiratory distress. See the section on respiratory distress syndrome.

RESPIRATORY DISTRESS SYNDROME

Respiratory distress syndrome (RDS), also known as hyaline membrane disease, occurs when there is immature development of the respiratory system or an inadequate amount of surfactant in the lungs. Infants with RDS are unable to keep their lungs expanded and the alveoli open. RDS is the leading cause of respiratory failure in the preterm infant.

Etiology. RDS occurs in infants with immature lung development or insufficient amounts of surfactant. Predisposing factors include prematurity, asphyxia at birth, cesarean delivery, a diabetic mother (especially <38

PATHOPHYSIOLOGY *of RDS*

In the preterm infant, anatomic immaturity of the chest wall, lung parenchyma, and capillary endothelium contribute to the development of RDS. The immature chest wall anatomy increases the chances of lung collapse at the end of expiration. Immaturity of the lung parenchyma and capillary endothelium result in less surface area for gas exchange. In the preterm as well as the term infant, RDS may be caused by a decreased total amount of pulmonary surfactant and/or a qualitative alteration of the surfactant present. The resulting inability to keep the lungs expanded causes the lung to be relatively noncompliant with changes in intra- and extrathoracic pressure, decreasing air exchange. Lung repair begins after 24–48 hours, even as further cell damage takes place. Hyaline membranes, consisting of debris from necrotic cells enmeshed in a proteinaceous filtrate of serum, are phagocytosed by macrophages. Cuboidal cells replace the damaged alveolar and airway epithelium, and eventually flatten. New capillaries develop and make contact with the regenerating cells of the alveoli. Surfactant synthesis begins and helps the repaired alveoli to remain expanded. Diuresis is usually a sign that the acute phase of RDS has ended and recovery is taking place. The differential diagnosis of RDS should include transient tachypnea of the newborn, pulmonary insufficiency of prematurity, group B streptococci pneumonia, and anatomic malformations.

CONTRIBUTING FACTORS IN THE PATHOPHYSIOLOGY OF RDS

Immature Chest Wall

The ribs and costal cartilages are relatively soft and pliable.

The intercostal muscles have a low total muscle mass and are prone to fatigue, providing inadequate stabilization of the rib cage.

The highly compliant rib cage allows the lower chest wall to collapse when the diaphragm contracts, inadequately expanding the lungs.

The diaphragm is easily fatigued because it has a decreased number of fatigue-resistant muscle fibers.

Immature Lung Tissue

Alveoli are few in number and poorly developed, providing less surface area for gas exchange.

Type 1 epithelial cells lining the alveoli are relatively thick, impeding their ability to exchange gases.

The walls of the capillaries surrounding the alveoli are relatively thick, impeding gas exchange.

Few of the capillaries surrounding the alveoli actually touch the alveoli, making them unavailable for gas exchange.

The lung lymphatic system is poorly developed, resulting in decreased clearance of fetal lung fluid and pulmonary edema.

Decreased Surfactant

In the preterm infant, an insufficient amount of surfactant is produced.

Numerous factors can adversely affect the production and metabolism of surfactant, including acidosis, hypercapnea, hypoxia, shock, pulmonary edema, mechanical ventilation, over- or underinflation of the lungs, and infection.

COMPLICATIONS OF RDS

Pulmonary	Acute: pneumothorax, pneumomediastinum, pulmonary interstitial emphysema Chronic: bronchopulmonary dysplasia
Cardiovascular	Patent ductus arteriosus, hypotension
Renal	Decreased urine output
Metabolic	Acidosis, hyponatremia, hypernatremia, hypocalcemia, hypoglycemia
Hematologic	Anemia, disseminated intravascular coagulation
Neurologic	Seizures, intraventricular hemorrhage
Other	Secondary infection, retinopathy of prematurity, complications of umbilical vessel catheterization

weeks' gestation), acute antepartum hemorrhage, multiple gestation, and a sibling who had RDS. Affected boys outnumber affected girls 2 to 1.

Incidence. Incidence and severity are inversely related to gestational age and birth weight, with as many as 40,000 infants affected each year in the United States (Walfman, 1994). The incidence in infants weighing less than 2500 g at birth may be as high as 16%. The mortality rate is 10% to 20% with most deaths occurring during the acute phase and in infants with birth weight less than 1000 g. About 20% of survivors have bronchopulmonary dysplasia, a prolonged course of respiratory failure lasting months to years and occasionally resulting in death (Chapter 29).

Clinical Manifestations. Symptoms of RDS usually appear at or shortly after birth, worsen over the first 24 to 48 hours, and gradually improve over the next 3 to 5 days. Signs and symptoms include:

- Tachypnea
- Inspiratory retractions (e.g., suprasternal, substernal, intercostal)
- Paradoxic seesaw respirations
- Inspiratory nasal flaring
- Audible expiratory grunt
- Chest x-ray findings showing overall hypoventilation and a reticular granular pattern (i.e., ground glass appearance)
- Apnea, seen with worsening lung function
- Central cyanosis (a late, ominous sign), indicating increased hypoxemia and an advanced stage of deterioration.
- Blood gases initially showing a decrease in the concentration of oxygen in the blood. Carbon dioxide levels in the blood rise as respiratory failure occurs as a result of repeated apnea or poor air exchange because of weak respiratory muscle function. As respiratory failure progresses, there is a slow development of metabolic acidosis and, as the concentration of carbon dioxide in the blood increases, a mixed metabolic and respiratory acidosis develops. Respiratory failure may result in death if supportive management is not timely and appropriate.

Therapeutic Management

Supportive Care. The goals of supportive care are to keep oxygen consumption as low as possible and to maintain adequate nutrition and hydration. Every effort should be made to maintain the infant in a neutral thermal environment. Oxygen consumption increases rapidly above or below the neutral thermal environment. Evaporation is a significant contributor to fluid loss in premature infants. Measures should be taken to minimize fluid loss via evaporation as well as loss of heat. Because handling stimulates movement and oxygen consumption, the infant should be handled as little as possible. Paralyzation or sedation may be needed to prevent movement and asynchronous breathing against the ventilator. A minimum of 60 kcal/kg/day should be provided with sufficient amino acids to prevent catabolism of endogenous proteins and ketoacidosis.

Respiratory Care. Oxygen should be given to maintain pO_2 within the normal range (Table 21–2). Interrupting oxygen administration, even briefly, may cause hypoxemia, pulmonary vasoconstriction, and reduced cardiac output. Mechanical ventilation should be started when the infant's respiratory system requires additional assistance. Low blood oxygen levels, high levels of carbon dioxide in the blood, or increasing respiratory and metabolic acidosis may be indications for mechanical ventilation (see Table 21–2). Apnea with bradycardia that is unresponsive to stimulation, regardless of the blood gas values, is also an indication that mechanical ventilation is needed. With intubation and continuous positive airway pressure or positive pressure ventilation, radiographic changes usually appear less severe. In most infants with RDS, surfactant replacement therapy improves oxygenation and lung mechanics, thereby decreasing the need for supplemental oxygen and high ventilator pressures. The infant should be monitored closely for complications.

TABLE 21–2 *Normal Neonate Blood Gas Parameters*

	CAPILLARY	ARTERIAL
pH	7.30–7.35	7.35–7.45
pCO_2	40–45	35–45
pO_2	40–60	55–65

NURSING CARE OF THE NEWBORN WITH RDS

Assessment

The nurse should identify infants at risk for RDS by reviewing the perinatal history for risk factors. The respiratory system is assessed for signs of respiratory distress, including tachypnea, apnea, retractions, nasal flaring, and grunting (Fig. 21–4). During auscultation of the chest, the nurse assesses the infant's breath sounds, comparing and contrasting the left and right sides and noting the equality of breath sounds, the quality of air entry, and the presence of rhonchi, crackles, and wheezes.

Assessment of the cardiovascular system includes determining the heart rate and noting any murmurs that may indicate a cardiac malformation or patent ductus arteriosus. A shift in the location of the point of maximal impulse may indicate a shift in heart position secondary to a pulmonary air leak.

> Central cyanosis in the newborn usually indicates severe hypoxia.

Peripheral cyanosis may progress to central cyanosis, which may become obscured as the infant's color further deteriorates to pale gray. Initially, extremely ill infants may have a blood pressure that is slightly higher than normal, progressing to hypotension as the infant's condition deteriorates.

The nurse evaluates the results of laboratory tests for abnormal findings. Blood gas abnormalities, acid–base imbalances, disturbances in electrolyte and glucose homeostasis, and early signs of complications such as sepsis

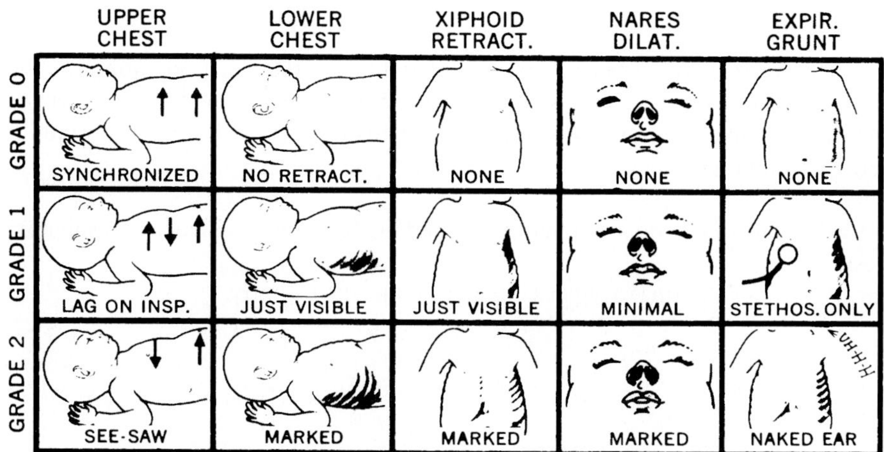

Figure 21–4

Criteria for respiratory distress. Grade 0 for each criterion indicates no respiratory distress; grade 2 for each criterion indicates severe distress. (Courtesy of Mead Johnson & Company, Evansville, IN. Adapted from Silverman, W., & Anderson, D. [1956]. Controlled clinical trial of effects of water mist on obstructive respiratory signs, death rate and necropsy finding among premature babies. Reproduced by permission of *Pediatrics*, Vol. 17, page 1. Copyright 1956.)

require immediate intervention. All indwelling lines as well as the endotracheal tube should be assessed frequently to assure that they are patent and securely in place.

Nursing Diagnoses

- Impaired Gas Exchange related to immaturity of the lungs and chest wall and/or insufficient amounts of surfactant.
- Ineffective Airway Clearance related to obstruction or inappropriate positioning of an endotracheal tube.
- Ineffective Breathing Pattern related to asynchronous breathing between the infant and the ventilator, ventilator malfunction, or inappropriate ventilatory support.
- Risk for altered parenting secondary to situational crisis (sick newborn).
- Potential for injury related to extremes in acid–base balance, oxygen levels, carbon dioxide levels, or barotrauma from mechanical ventilation.

Planning, Implementation, and Evaluation: The Newborn With RDS

NURSING DIAGNOSIS
- Impaired Gas Exchange related to immature development of the lung and chest wall and/or insufficient amounts of surfactant.

Expected Outcome:
- The infant will be able to maintain adequate gas exchange as evidenced by blood gas values and oxygen saturations within normal ranges.

Intervention	Rationale
1. Identify infants at risk.	Anticipating respiratory problems before delivery helps assure that support measures are in place if they are needed.
2. Monitor respiratory status for evidence of respiratory distress (e.g., tachypnea, retractions, grunting, nasal flaring, quality of breath sounds, apnea), and notify physician if deterioration occurs.	Prompt recognition of increasing respiratory distress or impending respiratory failure aids in prompt institution of appropriate support measures.
3. Monitor blood gases, pulse oximetry, and transcutaneous CO_2/O_2, and notify physician of abnormal values.	Abnormal values may indicate a need to modify the infant's management plan.
4. Position the infant to support her respiratory efforts.	Prone positioning supports the relatively flexible chest wall and helps maximize lung expansion during the infant's respiratory efforts. When in the supine position, the infant should have her neck slightly extended and her nose pointed toward the ceiling in a "sniffing" position to prevent narrowing of the airway.

Intervention	Rationale
5. Institute appropriate support measures as needed to help decrease the infant's oxygen consumption: maintain infant in neutral thermal environment, minimize handling, provide sedation or paralyzation if appropriate.	Many actions undertaken by the nurse in caring for the infant's other needs can positively or negatively affect the infant's respiratory status by altering her oxygen requirements.

Evaluation:
- Infant will maintain a normal respiratory rate and be free of any evidence of respiratory distress.
- Infant will maintain normal oxygen saturations on pulse oximetry.

NURSING DIAGNOSIS
- Ineffective Airway Clearance related to obstruction or inappropriate positioning of an endotracheal tube.

Expected Outcome:
- The infant's artificial airway will be correctly positioned and patent as evidenced by equal and adequate breath sounds and chest wall movement.

Intervention	Rationale
1. Assess infant's chest for equal and adequate bilateral breath sounds and expansion during inspiration.	With complete obstruction of the endotracheal tube, no chest movement is noted and the infant's work of breathing markedly increases. Partial obstruction of the endotracheal tube causes diminished breath sounds and chest movement. Inappropriate positioning of the endotracheal tube results in unequal breath sounds between the right and left lungs or between the upper and lower lung lobes on the same side.
2. Reposition or suction the endotracheal tube as needed (see Fig. 21–5). Preoxygenate before suctioning.	Correct positioning of a patent airway is crucial for providing appropriate respiratory assistance. Removing tracheal secretions promptly not only optimizes ventilatory management but also decreases the risk of pneumonia and atelectasis.

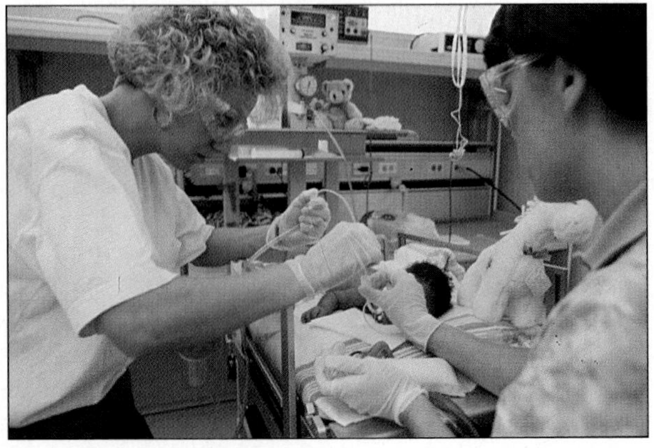

Figure 21–5
Management of respiratory function is a priority in the care of a preterm infant. It involves the nurse, respiratory therapist, and physician. The need to remove secretions must be balanced against the risk of tiring the infant or causing hypoxia with the suctioning procedure. Auscultation of the chest is performed before and after suctioning to determine whether there are accumulated secretions and whether the lungs have equal expansion. (Courtesy of Cook Children's Medical Center, Fort Worth, Texas.)

Evaluation: • The infant's breath sounds and chest wall movements are adequate and equal bilaterally.

NURSING DIAGNOSIS • Ineffective Breathing Pattern related to asynchronous breathing between the infant and the ventilator, ventilator malfunction, or inappropriate ventilatory support.

Expected Outcome: • Ventilatory support will appropriately complement the infant's respiratory efforts as evidenced by blood gas parameters within normal ranges.

Intervention	Rationale
1. In conjunction with the respiratory therapist, administer and monitor the respiratory support ordered by the physician. Monitor serial blood gases to assess response to support measures. Notify physician if values are not within stated parameters.	The respiratory support given the infant should be enough to maintain blood gases within the stated parameters, but not so much that the parameters are consistently exceeded and the potential for iatrogenic respiratory complications is increased.
2. Check ventilator settings hourly, and silence the ventilator alarms only temporarily. Check all ventilator tubings hourly for proper connections and the presence of excessive water.	Malfunctioning of the ventilator can lead to severe complications such as pneumothorax, hypoventilation, hypoxia, and aspiration. Silencing the alarms for long periods may result in failure to recognize a ventilator malfunction.
3. Attempt to ensure synchronous breathing between the infant and the ventilator by promoting an environment conducive to sleep through the judicious use of sedatives and the use of ventilators capable of synchronizing with the infant's respirations.	An asynchronous breathing pattern between the infant and the ventilator decreases the effectiveness of both the infant's efforts and the ventilator's assistance.

Evaluation: • The combination of the infant's spontaneous respiratory effort and ventilator assistance maintains blood gas parameters within normal ranges.

NURSING DIAGNOSIS • Potential for Injury related to extremes in acid–base balance, oxygen levels, carbon dioxide levels, or barotrauma from mechanical ventilation.

Expected Outcome: • The respiratory assistance provided will prevent or promptly treat extremes in blood gas parameters and will minimize potential barotrauma.

Intervention	Rationale
1. Evaluate blood gases for evidence of abnormal or unacceptable values, and notify physician immediately.	Both acidosis and alkalosis, along with both high and low levels of oxygen and carbon dioxide, can have a harmful effect on almost all body systems.
2. Monitor the infant closely for evidence of complications (see Table 21–2).	Promptly identifying complications and immediately undertaking measures to resolve them can decrease the risk of harmful sequelae.

Evaluation: • Action is undertaken in a timely manner whenever blood gas results fall outside of established parameters or whenever effects of barotrauma are noted.

NURSING DIAGNOSIS
- Risk for Altered Parenting secondary to situational crisis (sick newborn).

Expected Outcomes:
- The parent will exhibit parent–child attachment behavior.
- The parent will develop role identity as a parent.

Implementation and Evaluation:
- See Care of the Family.

Evaluation:
- Family members are involved in problem solving directed at appropriate solutions.
- The family assumes caretaking responsibilities.
- Family members contact available resources as needed.

NEONATAL SEPSIS

Neonatal sepsis occurs when bacteria or their poisonous products, known as endotoxins, gain access to the bloodstream, causing systemic signs and symptoms.

PATHOPHYSIOLOGY *of Neonatal Sepsis*

Bacteria can reach the fetus or infant and cause infection in one of four ways: (1) bacteria can pass through the maternal bloodstream through the placenta (e.g., *Listeria monocytogenes, Treponema pallidum, Mycobacterium tuberculosis,* rubella virus, *Toxoplasma,* cytomegalovirus, syphilis); (2) bacteria from the vagina or cervix can enter the uterus (e.g., group B streptococci); (3) the infant may come in contact with bacteria as it passes through the birth canal (gram-negative organisms and group B streptococci); (4) the infant may come in contact with bacteria in its environment after birth (coagulase-positive or -negative staphylococci) (Cole, 1991).

Etiology. The infant is at risk for sepsis because of a number of maternal, neonatal, and environmental factors (see accompanying box). The organisms most often responsible for sepsis in the neonate are group B streptococcus, *Escherichia coli, L. monocytogenes, Pseudomonas, Enterococcus, Staphylococcus aureus, Staphylococcus epidermidis,* and *Candida.*

Incidence. The incidence of bacterial sepsis is inversely proportional to birth weight and gestational age, ranging from 1 per 1000 live births in the term infant to as high as 300 per 1000 live births in the premature infant undergoing prolonged hospitalization. The mortality rate ranges from 10% to 50%, and is higher in premature infants and infants with early-onset sepsis.

Clinical Manifestations. The early signs and symptoms of sepsis may be vague and nonspecific. Often, the mother or nurse first recognizes that something is wrong. The infant may have respiratory or gastrointestinal symptoms. Common clinical manifestations of sepsis include the following:

- Temperature instability: hypothermia or hyperthermia
- Lethargy, irritability, poor feeding, change in muscle tone or activity
- Respiratory distress: grunting, flaring, retractions, tachypnea, or apnea
- Persistent pulmonary hypertension
- Tachycardia, bradycardia, cyanosis, decreased perfusion, pallor, mottling, hypotension, or shock
- Vomiting, increasing gastric residuals, diarrhea, ileus, abdominal distension, or bloody stools
- Jaundice or hepatosplenomegaly
- Jitteriness, bulging fontanelle, decreased response to stimuli, or seizures
- Petechiae, purpura, or rashes
- Hypoglycemia or hyperglycemia
- Metabolic acidosis

Therapeutic Management. Treatment of symptomatic infants is aggressive. Asymptomatic infants who are at high risk for sepsis may also warrant treatment. Treatment begins with obtaining diagnostic tests such as blood, urine, tracheal, and cerebrospinal fluid cultures; CBC with differential and platelet count; and latex agglutination panels on blood and urine. As soon as the cultures have been obtained, antibiotic therapy is started with broad-spectrum agents such as ampicillin and gentamicin. Once positive cultures are obtained, the antimicrobial therapy is modified as needed according to the sensitivities exhibited by the organism. Aminoglycoside levels should be monitored to assure serum levels within the therapeutic range and to avoid toxic levels. The duration of antimicrobial therapy depends on the culture results and the infant's response to treatment.

Supportive measures make up a large part of the treatment of septic infants. The infant should be maintained in a neutral thermal environment. Respiratory support may include supplemental oxygen or even intubation and mechanical ventilation. Serial blood gas determinations can help to assess the adequacy of respiratory interventions. Glucose homeostasis and fluid balance must also be assessed and supported as clinically indicated. Monitoring of blood pressure, centrally if possible, and determination

Risk Factors for Neonatal Sepsis

MATERNAL	NEONATAL	ENVIRONMENTAL
Premature or prolonged rupture of amniotic membranes	Prematurity	Exposure to bacteria from caregivers
Chorioamnionitis	Perinatal asphyxia	Exposure to bacteria from contaminated equipment
Endometritis	Congenital defects causing an opening in the skin or mucosa	Invasive procedures (e.g., the use of venous or arterial catheters, endotracheal tubes)
Peripartum infection or fever	Prolonged hyperalimentation	Surgical procedures
Urinary tract infection	Concurrent neonatal diseases	Resuscitation
Leukocytosis	Male sex	
Uterine tenderness	Low birth weight	
Fetal tachycardia	Developmental or congenital immune defects	
Precipitous delivery	Congenital heart disease	
Prolonged or difficult labor	Intracranial bleeding	
Abruptio placentae	Difficult or traumatic labor or delivery	
Colonization of organisms in genital tract	Meconium staining	
Cardiovascular disease	Prenatal or intrapartal stress	
Poor or no prenatal care	Multiple gestation	
Poor nutrition	Immature immune system	
Low socioeconomic status	Antimicrobial therapies	
Recurrent abortion	Galactosemia	
Substance abuse		
Premature labor		
Foul-smelling amniotic fluid		

of hourly urine output can help to determine whether blood pressure support is needed. The infant's hematocrit level should be maintained at 40% or greater to help assure adequate oxygen-carrying capacity. Serial platelet counts should be monitored to help identify the development of disseminated intravascular coagulation.

Additional interventions are being investigated and used in some areas. These include immunoglobulin administration, exchange transfusion, granulocyte transfusion, and fibronectin transfusion (Kenner & Lott, 1994). The safety and efficacy of these therapeutic interventions have not been established.

NURSING CARE OF THE INFANT WITH NEONATAL SEPSIS

Assessment

The nurse should review the maternal history and the labor and delivery history to identify infants at risk for the development of sepsis. All infants considered at risk should be observed closely for the development of the often subtle signs and symptoms of sepsis. Accurate charting of the infant's behavior during each shift allows nurses to determine whether the behavior they observe is different or abnormal for that infant. The nurse should notify the physician immediately if he observes any change in the infant's respiratory status, muscle tone, or activity; any lack of interest in or intolerance of feedings; or temperature outside of the normal range.

> The infant's condition can deteriorate rapidly from apparently normal to fulminant septic shock and death, especially if the causative agent is group B streptococcus.

Once diagnostic tests are ordered, the nurse should evaluate the results for abnormal values and bring them to the attention of the physician. Monitoring culture results and notifying the physician of any positive results and antibiotic sensitivities can help assure prompt institution of specific therapy.

Nursing Diagnosis and Planning

- Risk for Injury related to effect of sepsis on all body systems. ***Expected Outcome:*** *Harmful effects of sepsis on the infant will be avoided or minimized as evidenced by lack of complications.*
- Ineffective Thermoregulation related to stress of infection and unstable central temperature control. ***Expected Outcome:*** *The infant's temperature will remain within the normal range.*

- Altered Nutrition: Less Than Body Requirements related to lack of interest in nipple feedings or feeding intolerance. ***Expected Outcome:*** *The infant's growth will progress appropriately along established growth curves for postconceptual age.*

Implementation and Evaluation

In most cases, early identification and treatment can prevent the complications of sepsis. Diagnostic tests should be completed before antibiotic therapy is initiated. Antimicrobial therapy cannot be specific for the invading organism until the cultures have grown and antimicrobial sensitivities have been determined.

Infants at risk for sepsis should be observed closely to ensure early recognition and treatment.

> The infant's temperature is monitored closely because both hypothermia and hyperthermia may be signs of sepsis. Hyperthermia is rare.

Extra measures may be necessary to warm or cool the infant to minimize the harmful effects of temperature extremes.

Early in the clinical course of sepsis, the infant may be unable or unwilling to take oral feedings. Adequate fluid and caloric intake should be assured by administering gavage feedings or intravenous fluids as ordered.

Evaluation

- Has the infant been able to maintain body temperature within normal limits without extraordinary nursing intervention?
- Has the infant shown the expected weight gains for his age?
- Have severe complications of sepsis been avoided?
- Were changes in the infant's condition reported to the physician in a timely manner?

NECROTIZING ENTEROCOLITIS

Necrotizing enterocolitis (NEC) is the most commonly acquired gastrointestinal tract disorder in the neonate, and is characterized by necrotic lesions of the mucosa of the small and large intestines, predominately the ileum and proximal colon.

Etiology. Although the etiology of NEC has not been identified, it seems to be multifactorial. Factors that have been postulated to contribute to the development of NEC are listed in the accompanying box. The factors may differ in importance between term and preterm infants.

PATHOPHYSIOLOGY *of NEC*

Although NEC has been the focus of considerable study for many years, the pathogenesis remains in question and may be different in preterm and term infants. In the preterm infant, the immaturity of the gastrointestinal tract may be a crucial factor in the development of NEC. In the term infant, NEC probably begins with an ischemic injury to a portion of the intestinal mucosa. Without adequate blood supply, the mucosal cells are injured, and many die. Without the protective enzymes normally secreted by the mucosal cells, digestive enzymes destroy the mucosal cells. Nonpathogenic bacteria, which normally thrive in the nutrients from formula feedings, can easily invade the damaged intestinal wall, releasing toxins and hydrogen gas and causing necrosis. Normal peristalsis ceases, and intestinal distension occurs as the disease progresses. Perforation of the intestines may occur if the full thickness of the intestinal wall is damaged, resulting in a surgical emergency.

Incidence. It is estimated that NEC will develop in 1% to 15% of all infants admitted to the NICU. The incidence of NEC increases with decreasing gestational age. Between 80% and 90% of affected infants are premature, and 10% to 20% are term. The onset of signs and symptoms usually occurs within the first 14 days of life, but may not occur for several weeks. NEC tends to develop at an earlier age in infants closer to term and with higher birth weight.

Factors Postulated to Contribute to the Development of NEC

Asphyxia
Shock
Hypoxia
Hypothermia
Hypotension
Hypovolemia
Polycythemia
Anemia
Enteral feedings
Exchange transfusion
Infection: bacterial and viral
Patent ductus arteriosus
Respiratory distress syndrome
Hypertonic medications and feedings
Umbilical artery catheterization
Congenital heart disease
Prematurity

Clinical Manifestations

- Apnea and bradycardia
- Temperature instability
- Lethargy
- Abdominal distension, with skin often shiny and discolored
- Bile-stained gastric residual or emesis
- Bloody stools
- Visible, distended bowel loops
- Decreased or absent bowel sounds
- Abdomen tender to palpation
- Hypotension or shock

Diagnostic Evaluation. Radiographic evidence includes dilated bowel loops, thickened bowel walls, air within the intestinal wall (pneumatosis intestinalis), air in the portal vein, or free air in the abdominal cavity (pneumoperitoneum). Laboratory findings include increased or decreased white blood cell count, decreased platelet count, metabolic acidosis, and electrolyte imbalances.

NURSING CARE OF THE INFANT WITH NEC

Assessment

Early signs, such as apnea, bradycardia, temperature instability, and lethargy, mimic those seen in sepsis and should raise the nurse's suspicion.

> Any infant with symptoms similar to those seen with sepsis who then develops feeding intolerance, abdominal distension, bile-stained gastric residuals or bloody stools should be brought to the attention of the physician immediately.

Any deviations from normal in blood pressure or respiratory status may signal the beginning of a rapid deterioration. Prompt recognition and appropriate support measures are needed.

Nursing Diagnosis and Planning

Nursing Diagnosis

- Altered Nutrition: Less than Body Requirements, related to dependence on prolonged parenteral nutrition and loss of intestinal tissue from necrosis.

Expected Outcome

Infant's growth will progress appropriately along established growth curves for postconceptual age.

Nursing Diagnosis

- Risk for Infection related to bacterial invasion of the bowel wall or bowel perforation.

Expected Outcome

The infant will be free of any signs of infection as evidenced by CBC parameters within normal limits and negative blood culture findings.

Nursing Diagnosis

- Fluid Volume Deficit related to extravascular accumulation of fluids in the intestine and abdominal cavity.

Expected Outcome

The infant will maintain normal fluid, electrolyte, and acid–base balance

Nursing Diagnosis

- Ineffective Breathing Pattern related to abdominal distension and apnea

Expected Outcome

The infant will maintain adequate breathing patterns without assistance as evidenced by blood gas values and pulse oximetry readings within normal ranges.

Implementation

During the acute phase of the disease, the infant's vital signs should be assessed and recorded every 1 to 2 hours. Supporting the infant's respirations and blood pressure is essential in helping the infant to survive the acute phase. Positioning the infant to minimize the detrimental effects of the pressure of the abdominal contents against the diaphragm can help optimize the infant's respiratory support. Rarely do these infants tolerate lying on their abdomen. Nasogastric suction is used for abdominal decompression. An environment with minimal stimulation decreases stress on the already compromised infant and helps optimize the overall supportive care. Loud noises and bright lighting should be avoided whenever possible. Tactile stimulation should be kept to a minimum during the acute phase of the illness. Appropriate administration of volume expanders, antibiotics, and hyperalimentation, along with obtaining and assessing laboratory tests, is important throughout the disease process.

Once the infant appears to have recovered and is taking feedings, the nurse must monitor the infant closely for evidence of feeding intolerance, such as abdominal distension, large residuals, and bile-stained emesis. The disease may recur, or scar tissue at the affected site may produce a complete or partial intestinal obstruction. Infants who have recovered from NEC remain at risk for gastrointestinal problems for several weeks.

Evaluation

- Are the infant's biochemical nutritional parameters and growth parameters within acceptable parameters throughout the hospital course?

- Are infants treated appropriately when exhibiting signs and symptoms of sepsis?
- Is there evidence of complications from sepsis or its treatment?
- Was the infant's circulating fluid volume maintained at appropriate levels as evidenced by blood pressure and urine output within acceptable ranges?
- Are the infant's breath sounds and chest wall movements adequate and equal bilaterally?
- Is the combination of the infant's spontaneous respiratory effort and any respiratory assistance able to maintain blood gas parameters within normal ranges?

RETINOPATHY OF PREMATURITY

Retinopathy of prematurity (ROP), formerly called retrolental fibroplasia, is a potential complication of prematurity. High oxygen levels in the blood, along with other factors, lead to changes in the developing retinal vessels that result in scar formation and may cause permanent vision impairment or blindness.

PATHOPHYSIOLOGY *of ROP*

Retinal vascularization occurs in the late weeks of gestation. The fetus at 26 weeks has delicate capillaries covering only half of the retina. The blood vessels are forming, moving in a pattern from the inner, nasal portion of the eye toward the temporal periphery. The retina becomes vascularized from the optic nerve, extending anteriorly toward the ora serrata. Most retinal vascularization is complete by 32 weeks' gestation, but even at term, the temporal periphery of the retina may not be completely vascularized.

In response to hyperoxia or other stresses, the retinal vessels constrict. Necrosis as a result of this constriction is known as vaso-obliteration. Vessels that have not been obliterated attempt to reestablish circulation through neovascularization, the proliferation of new vessels. These new vessels cause the damage (ROP) seen by the ophthalmologist when the eye is examined. ROP occurs at the juncture between the vascularized and avascular retina.

If neovascularization reestablishes the circulation and further vascularization proceeds normally, ROP regresses and excessive vessels are reabsorbed. However, if the vessels continue to extend into the vitreous, fluid leakage and hemorrhage occur, causing retinal scar formation. This scar tissue can place traction on the retina, resulting in retinal detachment and blindness.

Etiology. When this disease process was first described in the 1950s, oxygen administration was believed to be the single etiology. It is now known that the oxygen level in the blood, not the percentage of oxygen administered, is a major factor in the development of ROP.

> ROP is caused in part by varying oxygen concentrations in the blood that result in vasoconstriction and subsequent proliferation and abnormal vascular growth in the retina of the immature infant's eye.
>
> Many other contributing factors are now being linked to ROP. The most important factor is immaturity as determined by gestational age or birth weight. The second major risk factor is the level and duration of oxygen therapy.

Higher oxygen requirements and prolonged oxygen therapy correlate with an increased incidence of severe ROP. Sepsis, intraventricular hemorrhage, and acidosis also have been correlated with an increased incidence of severe ROP (Hunter & Mukai, 1992). Numerous other elements are considered potential risk factors, and research continues to attempt to establish a cause and effect relationship (see accompanying box).

Incidence. Approximately 25% of all premature infants have some form of ROP. Eighty percent of the less severe stages of ROP, regress spontaneously (Hunter & Mukai, 1992).

Clinical Manifestations. ROP is classified into three zones (location) and five stages (severity of disease) and according to the presence or absence of disease.

Diagnostic Evaluation. Screening ophthalmoscopic examinations are recommended for premature neonates who were delivered at less than 35 weeks' gestation or who weighed less than 1800 g and received supplemental oxygen.

Risk Factors Associated with the Development of ROP

Prematurity with very low birth weight (<1500 g)
Hyperoxia
Asphyxia
Sepsis
Hypercapnia or hypocapnia
Blood transfusion
Apnea
Prolonged ventilator support
Nutritional deficiencies

From the Committee for the Classification of Retinopathy and Prematurity. (1984). *Archives of Ophthalmology, 102,* 1131. Copyright 1994, American Medical Association.

Infants delivered at less than 30 weeks' gestation or less than 1300 g should be examined, regardless of oxygen exposure (American Academy of Pediatrics and American College of Obstetricians and Gynecologists, 1992). Initial eye examinations start at 4–6 weeks of age. Repeat examinations are required until vascularization reaches the ora serrata.

When extensive Stage 3+ disease is present in zone I or zone II, the threshold level for surgery is reached. This level indicates that the infant is at significant risk for permanent blindness. Infants at the threshold level may undergo cryotherapy or laser surgery for intervention, with the goal of limiting pathogenic vascular proliferation. Cryotherapy entails freezing the avascular area of the retina to prevent further abnormal neovascularization. Laser photocoagulation is also being used for retinal ablation. Scleral buckling or vitrectomy may be used to treat Stage 4 and Stage 5 ROP in an attempt to reattach the retina (Hunter & Mukai, 1992).

NURSING CARE OF THE INFANT WITH ROP

Assessment

Although the pathogenesis of ROP is still under investigation, there is a known association between oxygen use in the preterm infant and the development of ROP. Assessment should consist of proper usage of oxygen, following unit protocol for its administration and monitoring. Parents must be informed if their infant is at risk for the development of the disease. Parents should be informed of the screening ophthalmology examinations before they occur and be informed promptly of the findings. Education also includes informing parents of the possible side effects of mydriatic drops. Part of the daily assessment of the preterm infant includes assessment of visual attentiveness, including the eventual development of the ability to focus on objects.

Nursing Diagnosis and Planning

- Altered Growth and Development (ROP) related to preterm birth. ***Expected Outcome:*** *The infant's vision will be normal, and ophthalmologic examination finds no evidence of ROP.*
- Knowledge Deficit (ROP) related to lack of exposure to accurate information. ***Expected Outcome:*** *Parents are informed in a timely manner of all medical interventions prescribed for the infant.*
- Ineffective Infant Feeding Pattern related to the effects of mydriatic drug administration. ***Expected Outcome:*** *No side effects of the mydriatic drugs will be noted.*
- Risk for Sensory and Perceptual Alterations related to visual changes secondary to ROP. ***Expected Outcome:*** *If cryotherapy or laser surgery is performed, the infant will experience an uneventful and comfortable recovery from the procedure.*

Implementation. The nurse should verify that the pulse oximeter, used to measure the infant's percutaneous oxygen saturation, is working properly. Alarm limits are set as ordered to assist in identifying the hyperoxic and hypoxia infant. The probe site is changed every 12 hours and as needed because probes can cause skin breakdown and constrict blood flow.

Administer oxygen according to nursery protocol. Verify and document administered oxygen concentration (FiO_2) at least every 1 to 2 hours. Although the pathogenesis of ROP is still under investigation, current information mandates judicious use of oxygen and strict monitoring protocols. Report all abnormal blood gas results to the physician in a timely manner.

Parents should be provided with information about ROP if their infant is at risk. Parents often develop trust in their infant's caretakers if they are kept well informed of all aspects of the infant's health and management plans during the lengthy hospitalization.

Explain to parents the reason for the ophthalmology examinations and the possible side effects for the infant.

Eye drops should be given as ordered, making sure that the drop enters the eye. Request assistance to achieve success because eyes do not dilate properly without correct administration of drops. Uncertainty about the success of drop administration may lead to inadvertent overdose if dosing is repeated.

Feeding intolerance has been reported after the administration of dilating ophthalmologic drops (mydriatic). Monitor for signs of feeding problems after drop administration: abdominal distension, rigid abdomen, spitting, or feeding residuals.

Use a cardiorespiratory monitor as well as a pulse oximeter if an eye examination is to be performed. Oculocardiac reactions have occurred, and resulted in cardiac arrest, with the administration of dilating drops in the preterm infant.

The infant's heart rate and breathing pattern should be monitored. They should remain stable, without apnea or bradycardia.

After administering the drops and after the examination, shield the infant from direct light because pupils may remain dilated for several hours.

If cryotherapy or laser surgery is performed, vital signs and pulse oximetry readings are documented every 15 to 30 minutes until they are stable and then every 1 to 2 hours, according to nursery routine, after the procedure. The infant should be assessed for eye drainage, either purulent or bloody. Ice packs may be ordered for lid edema, and pain medication (e.g., acetaminophen) may be used. A quiet room with dim lights (or a blanket over the incubator) is desirable. Signs of respiratory distress or abdominal distension, as a complication of anesthesia or the eye medication, should be monitored. Initiate enteral feedings slowly when ordered, and monitor the infant for gastric residuals or emesis.

Evaluation

- Are the infant's feeding patterns and respiratory and cardiac status normal for his age?
- Is there drainage from the eye?
- Are the parents asking appropriate questions regarding their infant's condition and treatment?
- Are the parents able to discuss the care of their child?

HYPOGLYCEMIA

Hypoglycemia is an abnormally low level of glucose (sugar) in the blood. It may result from an excessive rate of removal of glucose from the blood or from decreased secretion of glucose into the blood. Hypoglycemia in the neonate is defined as a plasma glucose concentration of less than 40 mg/dl.

Etiology. Hypoglycemia can be caused by decreased availability of glucose or increased use of glucose because of either increased demand or hyperinsulinemia. The accompanying box lists risk factors for hypoglycemia in the neonate (Cowett, 1992).

Incidence. The incidence of hypoglycemia varies with the infant's gestational age at birth and appropriateness of growth.

> Postmature and large for gestational age (LGA) neonates are at higher risk than the AGA term infant, but the neonates who are most likely to experience hypoglycemia are premature infants and infants who are small for gestational age (SGA).

The incidence of hypoglycemia in the preterm SGA infant may be as high as 67% (Cowett, 1992).

Clinical Manifestations

- May be asymptomatic
- Apnea
- Bradycardia
- Cyanosis
- High-pitched cry
- Hypotonia
- Irregular respirations
- Jitteriness
- Lethargy
- Poor feeding
- Seizures
- Tachypnea
- Temperature instability

Diagnostic Evaluation. A blood glucose concentration can be determined by laboratory chemical determination. Although this method is the most accurate, it is lengthy. For this reason, screening tests are used in most nurseries. A drop of blood, which can be obtained by a heelstick, is placed on special filter paper and, after a specified interval, wiped from the strip of paper. Color changes of the filter paper give reasonable estimates of the serum glucose concentration. Severely low readings are often verified by laboratory determinations, but intervention is initiated before the results are available because of the potential for sequelae from prolonged hypoglycemia.

Laboratories use plasma to measure glucose; bedside screening tests use whole blood, which gives a 10% to 15%

PATHOPHYSIOLOGY *of Hypoglycemia*

Glucose is the major source of energy for the fetus and is transported from the mother across the placenta to the fetus. This glucose is used to support the rapid growth taking place. In the last weeks of gestation, excess glucose is stored in the liver and skeletal muscle as glycogen or converted to fatty acids and then stored as triglycerides in fat cells. Insulin is not transported across the placenta, and the fetus must produce his own insulin.

At delivery, this glucose supply ceases, and the infant must depend on his own hepatic glycogen stores and glucoregulatory mechanism to mobilize and use glucose. With its steady source of glucose stopped by the clamping of the umbilical cord, the neonate experiences a decrease in glucose concentration, reaching a nadir (lowest level) at 1–3 hours of postnatal age.

The neonate's requirement for glucose is relatively high because of several factors. High energy needs postnatally result from increased metabolic and motor activity. The larger brain in proportion to body size requires glucose as its fuel source. Access to glucose is limited because of the neonate's immature liver enzyme system, including a decreased response to glucagon, the hormone that promotes the release of glucose from glycogen stores.

Risk Factors for Hypoglycemia in the Neonate

DECREASED GLUCOSE PRODUCTION OR IMPAIRED MOBILIZATION

Adrenal insufficiency
Inborn errors of metabolism
Prematurity
Infant small for gestational age
Maternal propanolol use

INCREASED GLUCOSE USE

Asphyxia
Congenital heart disease
Hypothermia
Hypoxia
Sepsis

INCREASED GLUCOSE USE SECONDARY TO HYPERINSULINISM

Maternal diabetes mellitus (infant of a diabetic mother)
Infant large for gestational age
Rh incompatibility (infant with erythroblastosis fetalis)
Infant undergoing an exchange transfusion
Maternal medications (beta-sympathomimetic tocolytic agents, thiazides)
Beckwith-Wiedemann syndrome
Pancreatic tumor

Data from Cowett, R. M. (1992). Hypoglycemia and hyperglycemia in the newborn. In R. A. Polin & W. W. Fox (Eds.), *Fetal and neonatal physiology*. Philadelphia: W. B. Saunders.

lower glucose reading (Cowett, 1992). Errors in the screening test can result from inaccurate timing, inadequate quantity of blood, improper technique in wiping or washing blood from the filter paper, alcohol contamination of the sample, or improper storage of strips.

Infants who are hypoglycemic but asymptomatic may be given enteral feedings of formula or D_5W. Frequent glucose checks are needed to monitor response.

> Symptomatic infants may require IV fluids, giving a bolus of 200 mg/kg IV glucose (2 ml/kg $D_{10}W$) with concurrent initiation of continuous IV fluids. If IV access is not readily available, intramuscular glucagon can be given to promote the release of glucose stores.

In some cases of intractable hypoglycemia, steroids may be used to stimulate gluconeogenesis from noncarbohydrate sources, or diazoxide may be given to suppress pancreatic insulin secretion.

NURSING CARE OF THE INFANT WITH HYPOGLYCEMIA

Assessment

The assessment begins at the time of birth. Risk factors such as maternal diabetes, sepsis, shock, or perinatal asphyxia alert the caretaker that the infant may be at risk for hypoglycemia. Determination is also made of gestational age and appropriateness of growth. Delays in enteral feedings or in the initiation of IV fluids also place the infant at higher risk. Inappropriate or changes in behavior, including commonly associated clinical signs and symptoms, are monitored.

Nursing Diagnosis and Planning

Nursing Diagnoses

- Risk for Injury related to physiologic damage secondary to hypoglycemia.
- Altered Nutrition, Less than Body Requirements, related to inadequate supply of glucose or increased glucose use in the neonate.

Expected Outcome

- The neonate will show no signs or symptoms of hypoglycemia and will maintain blood glucose levels within normal range for age.

Implementation

Monitor for signs and symptoms of hypoglycemia, but remember that infants may be asymptomatic. Infants at risk should be identified by obtaining a complete perinatal history to identify factors such as maternal hypertension, maternal diabetes, fetal distress, intrauterine growth retardation, or perinatal asphyxia.

Because preterm, LGA, and SGA infants are at increased risk for hypoglycemia, a gestational age assessment should be performed and the infant's weight, length, and head circumference plotted on a growth curve to determine appropriateness of growth.

> The neonate experiences a decrease in glucose concentration that reaches a nadir at 1–3 hours of age.

A blood glucose level should be obtained with a screening strip (e.g., Dextrostix, Chemstrip bG) by 1 hour of age on all neonates or according to nursery policy. Clean the puncture site with povidone-iodine solution, and allow it to dry before the puncture (see Chapter 18). Blood glucose levels of less than 60 mg/dl should be reported.

> Puncture the foot only in the lateral pads of the heel. Neonatal osteomyelitis is an iatrogenic complication of heelsticks performed improperly.

Administer glucose according to the physician's orders or standing orders. Initiate IV fluids or enteral feedings promptly because prolonged hypoglycemia places the infant at risk for severe neurologic sequelae.

Enteral feedings should be provided by nipple or gavage if required. The compromised infant may be unable to safely nipple feed secondary to respiratory distress or lethargy. If $D_{25}W$ is given IV (usually through a central venous line), it should be followed with a continuous infusion of IV fluid. Monitor the infant for rebound hypoglycemia and for the patency of the IV. Monitor IV sites for signs of infiltration, and treat IV infiltrates with hyaluronidase because glucose infiltration can cause severe skin extravasation.

Because hypothermia increases glucose requirements, decrease the risk of hypoglycemia by providing the infant with a neutral thermal environment. If signs and symptoms persist, the physician should be notified according to nursery protocol. Persistent hypoglycemia requires extensive medical evaluation and treatment.

Evaluation

- Have the infant's blood glucose levels remained within normal range for age?
- Has the infant shown clinical manifestations of hypoglycemia?
- If the infant developed hypoglycemia, were appropriate nursing interventions implemented?

HYPOCALCEMIA

Hypocalcemia is the result of inadequate stores of calcium, ineffective calcium homeostasis because of immature hormonal control, the inability to mobilize calcium, or interference with calcium usage. Neonatal hypocalcemia is defined as total serum calcium concentration of less than 7.0 mg/dl.

Etiology. The causes of neonatal hypocalcemia can be divided into three major categories: early onset, late onset, and other (Anast, 1991):

Early (< 48 hours of age)

- Premature
- Infant of a diabetic mother
- Placental insufficiency
- Asphyxia
- Iatrogenic

PATHOPHYSIOLOGY ***of Hypocalcemia***

Calcium and phosphate are actively transported across the placenta to the fetus, and at birth, the serum calcium levels are higher for the fetus than for the mother. Because **parathyroid hormone** (PTH, produced by the parathyroid glands in response to low serum calcium levels) and **calcitonin** (a hormone that inhibits bone resorption or breakdown) do not cross the placenta, the fetus has low PTH and calcitonin levels at birth secondary to the relative hypercalcemia experienced in utero (Anast, 1991).

At birth, the active transport of calcium stops, and the neonate must establish calcium homeostasis. As the serum calcium levels decrease, the calcitonin levels also decrease and there is the stimulus for the production of PTH. This pattern is a normal physiologic process, and the serum calcium concentration stabilizes and begins to rise after 48–72 hours of life. In contrast, the preterm or stressed infant may experience severe or prolonged hypocalcemia. Premature or asphyxiated infants probably experience an increase in calcitonin levels, whereas infants of diabetic mothers have a temporary functional hypoparathyroidism (DeMarini et al., 1993).

Late (after the first week of life)

- Maternal hyperparathyroidism
- Maternal vitamin D deficiency
- High-phosphate formula (cow's milk)
- Intestinal malabsorption
- Hypomagnesemia leading to impaired parathyroid function
- Congenital hypoparathyroidism (DiGeorge sequence)

Other

- Alkalosis (decreased movement of calcium from bone)
- Bicarbonate administration
- Transfusion of citrate-preserved blood
- Furosemide therapy
- Renal disease

Incidence. Thirty percent of infants delivered at 37 weeks' gestation, 35% of infants asphyxiated at birth, 50% of infants of insulin-dependent diabetic mothers, and 90% of very low–birth-weight infants (1500 g) have hypocalcemia in the first days of life (DeMarini et al., 1993).

Clinical Manifestations

- May be asymptomatic
- Tremors, twitching
- Hyperexcitability, irritability

- High-pitched cry, laryngospasm
- Tachycardia
- Apnea
- Electrocardiographic changes
- Seizures (rare)

Diagnostic Evaluation. Either ionized or undissociated serum calcium levels are measured. Norms for blood ionized calcium range from 4.8 to 5.2 mg/dl. Undissociated calcium is bound to protein, and this calcium is measured as total calcium. Total calcium levels are 7.0 to 12.0 mg/dl in the term infant younger than 1 week old and 8.0 to 10.5 mg/dl in the child.

Neonatal hypocalcemia is defined as a total serum calcium concentration of less than 7.0 mg/dl.

Initiation of formula feedings is often the only treatment necessary to correct early hypocalcemia. In infants who are limited in their enteral intake or who have significant hypocalcemia, therapy includes both oral and parenteral calcium administration. Oral supplements are given with enteral feedings. IV supplementation may be given as bolus doses or continuous infusion with IV fluids. Persistent hypocalcemia requires further diagnostic evaluation.

NURSING CARE OF THE INFANT WITH HYPOCALCEMIA

Assessment

The neonatal history is reviewed to identify infants who are at risk for hypocalcemia. Signs and symptoms of hypocalcemia should be reported to the physician. Laboratory tests are performed as ordered and abnormal results reported. Once hypocalcemia is identified, assessment includes identification of the etiology.

Nursing Diagnosis and Planning

Nursing Diagnosis

- Altered Nutrition: Less Than Body Requirements, related to transition to extrauterine life.

Expected Outcome

No signs and symptoms of hypocalcemia will be observed.

Implementation

The infant should be observed for signs or symptoms of hypocalcemia. Identify infants who are at highest risk for hypocalcemia (see *Incidence*), although infants may be asymptomatic. Monitor serum calcium levels as ordered.

Calcium maintains cell membrane permeability and is essential for muscle contraction and nerve transmission. If the total calcium level is less than 7.0 mg/dl, place the infant on a cardiac monitor with an oscilloscope and observe for prolonged Q-T interval or arrhythmias. If oral calcium is ordered, give the medication with enteral feedings because it may cause gastric irritation.

If an IV bolus infusion of calcium is ordered by the physician, monitor the infant's heart rate during administration. Administer slowly according to recommendations given by the drug manufacturer. If bradycardia or arrhythmia occurs, stop administration immediately.

The IV site should be observed for signs of infiltration, and hyaluronidase used to treat infiltrates. Extravasation of calcium-containing fluid can produce necrosis and ulceration. Many medications precipitate with Ca^{++} and should not be mixed together in IV lines. Do not mix calcium with $NaHCO_3$ because this combination also will form a precipitate in IV fluids.

Evaluation

- Was the high-risk infant monitored closely for hypocalcemia?
- Is the infant's nutritional intake normal for his age?
- Were abnormal laboratory values reported promptly to the physician?
- If the child manifested signs of hypocalcemia, were appropriate nursing interventions implemented?

PHENYLKETONURIA

Phenylketonuria (PKU) is a genetic disorder that results in central nervous system (CNS) damage from toxic levels of phenylalanine in the blood. In PKU, there is a deficiency of phenylalanine hydroxylase, the enzyme needed to convert phenylalanine to tyrosine.

Etiology. PKU is an **autosomal recessive** disorder and is manifested only in the **homozygote** (individual who inherited two identical genes for a specific trait).

Incidence. PKU occurs in approximately 1 per 12,000 births (Theorell & Degenhardt, 1993).

Clinical Manifestations

In All Children

- Digestive problems and vomiting
- Myoclonic or grand mal seizures
- Musty or mousy odor of the urine
- Mental retardation

PATHOPHYSIOLOGY *of PKU*

PKU refers to a group of biochemical diseases associated with enzymatic blocks in the conversion of the essential amino acid phenylalanine to tyrosine. Classic PKU consists of the absence of the enzyme phenylalanine hydroxylase. This deficiency results in the toxic accumulation of phenylalanine in the bloodstream after the ingestion of protein containing phenylalanine. Phenylalanine can adversely affect the myelinization process in CNS development. Most of that process takes place during the first decade of life. Mental retardation occurs and will progress if treatment is not implemented.

In Older Children

- Eczema
- Hypertonia
- Hypopigmentation of the hair, skin, and irises
- Hyperactive behavior

Diagnostic Evaluation. Small quantities of blood are collected on special filter paper cards. Screening is done using bacterial inhibition (Guthrie test) or chromatographic or fluorometric assays. A positive result is not diagnostic, but indicates which infants should be further evaluated. PKU is characterized by serum phenylalanine levels greater than 25 mg/dl (normal level is < 2 mg/dl) (Buist & Tuerck, 1992).

All 50 states require routine screening of all newborns for PKU.

With early postpartum discharge, screening is often performed at less than 2 days of age because of the concern that the infant will be lost to follow-up. Because the test is dependent on the accumulation of phenylalanine, screening done before the third day of life has a higher risk of a false-negative outcome. For this reason, testing should be repeated at several days of age.

Therapeutic Management. Infants with PKU are treated with a special diet that restricts phenylalanine intake. Phenylalanine tolerance varies according to the infant and the severity of the enzyme deficiency. The goal of therapy is to limit phenylalanine intake while providing enough to meet the body's requirement of this essential amino acid. Dietary management must be started early in neonatal life because the untreated infant will show evidence of CNS damage by several weeks of age.

Another consideration is women with the disorder who become pregnant.

Maternal PKU has resulted in fetal effects such as mental deficiency, microcephaly, retarded growth, and an increased incidence of structural defects. Affected children are presumably damaged during pregnancy by the elevated phenylalanine level in the mother, with the severity of the effects paralleling the increasing levels of phenylalanine in maternal blood (Jones, 1988).

Adolescent girls require counseling about fetal risks. The goal is to control phenylalanine levels before conception and maintain strict control during the pregnancy.

NURSING CARE OF THE INFANT WITH PKU

Assessment

Although a family history of PKU would alert the caregiver to an infant at risk, most infants with PKU are unidentified at birth. Neonatal symptoms are usually not present. A screening test, part of the newborn screen done in all states, would be the first diagnostic procedure. This newborn screen would include testing for PKU and congenital hypothyroidism as well as any other screening tests mandated by local and state public health departments, such as sickle cell trait, galactosemia, or maple syrup urine disease. A positive screening result requires further diagnostic evaluation to verify the diagnosis.

Treatment should be instituted as soon as the diagnosis is confirmed because the best results are obtained with early treatment. The infant is provided with a diet that eliminates phenylalanine.

With blood levels used as a guide, phenylalanine supplementation is given to provide minimum body requirements.

The growth pattern and neurobehavior of the affected child must be followed.

Termination of diet restrictions results in the recurrence of high phenylalanine levels, but there is less concern about the effects of these high levels once brain development and myelinization are near completion.

Brain development and myelinization occur by 6 to 8 years of age, but attempts may be made to restrict the child's diet until he is older. Affected girls should be encouraged to continue diet restrictions throughout their childbearing years.

Nursing Diagnosis and Planning

Nursing Diagnoses

- Altered Growth and Development secondary to an **inborn error of metabolism** (genetically determined biochemical disorder).
- Altered Nutrition, Less than Body requirements, related to an inborn error of metabolism.
- Knowledge Deficit (PKU) related to special dietary restrictions secondary to PKU.
- Altered Family Processes related to birth of an infant with chronic dietary needs.

Expected Outcomes

- Developmental delays and mental retardation are minimized because of early identification of infants with PKU.
- The family will be able to adapt to the necessary changes in lifestyle or diet.

Implementation

The newborn screen according to hospital protocol should be obtained. Contamination of the filter paper with fingers, body oils, urine, stool, or alcohol can interfere with test results. Umbilical cord blood is not an acceptable source for screening purposes.

Rescreen infants by 14 days of age if the initial screen was done before 24 to 48 hours of age. Provide parental education about the risks and benefits of screening for infants who require a repeat test because of early discharge.

Follow-up is provided for all infants if the initial screening result is abnormal. The nurse assists with referral to a genetic center that is capable of diagnosing and treating the infant. Early diet control must be implemented. Phenylalanine requirements change rapidly in the first months of life. Encourage parental compliance with monitoring requirements for the infant diagnosed with PKU. Rigid regimens for diet control will not be successful unless the family accepts the changes required. Assist the family in dealing with lifestyle changes by initiating referrals as needed (e.g., to social service agencies, registered dietician, and support groups).

Encourage the parents to express their feelings about the infant's diagnosis and the risk of PKU in future children. Assist family members in recognizing the problems caused by the disease, and help them to identify strategies for dealing with the stress of having a child with a chronic illness.

Physical measurements and neurologic and intellectual development should be documented through standardized testing. If good control is established early, normal infant growth and development should occur.

Evaluation

- Was the infant screened for PKU?
- If the infant's initial PKU screening was abnormal, was there follow-up?
- Was early diet therapy implemented for the infant with PKU?
- Has the family adapted to the changes required to care for the infant?

ABO–RH INCOMPATIBILITY

The possibility of blood incompatibility exists whenever the blood type of the fetus is different from the blood type of the mother. The most common difference is between the major blood groups of A, B, and O, but differences in Rh factor also occur and are usually more severe. Both types of incompatibility involve a maternal antibody response to antigens in the fetus's blood. This response leads to destruction of the fetus's red blood cells and results in anemia.

PATHOPHYSIOLOGY AND ETIOLOGY *of ABO–Rh Incompatibility*

The hemolytic process that occurs with both ABO and Rh incompatibilities begins in utero. In ABO incompatibility, the mother's blood type is usually O and the blood type of the infant is either A or B. The serum of type O mothers contains antibodies against blood types A and B. These antibodies can cross the placenta and destroy the red blood cells of the fetus. Although incompatibility can exist if the mother's blood type is A and the fetus's blood type is B, or the reverse, it is rarely seen because antibodies of mothers with blood type A or B rarely cross the placenta.

In Rh incompatibility, the mother is Rh negative and the fetus or newborn is Rh positive. When fetal blood cells enter the mother's circulation, the mother forms antibodies against the Rh factor that she does not have. Once a mother has formed antibodies, subsequent pregnancies are affected because the mother's antibodies cross the placenta and destroy the fetus's red blood cells. In Rh incompatibility, a higher degree of hemolysis occurs, with more serious consequences for the fetus. Because the anti-Rh antibody often recirculates through the reticuloendothelial system, hemolysis and anemia may recur.

Incidence. ABO incompatibility occurs in 12% to 20% of all pregnancies, but only 3% to 4% show evidence of sensitization with a positive direct Coombs' test result. Fewer than 1% of Rh-incompatible pregnancies result in Rh sensitization and symptoms, largely because of the use of Rh_o immune globulin (RhoGAM).

Clinical Manifestations. Signs and symptoms of both ABO and Rh incompatibility are the same and are listed in order of increasing severity of the hemolytic process.

- Jaundice
- Anemia
- Hepatosplenomegaly
- Hydrops fetalis

Diagnostic Evaluation. All mothers should have their blood typed before or during their initial pregnancy. The fetus affected by Rh incompatibility may be diagnosed with hydrops fetalis, a progressive condition related to hemolysis resulting in fetal hypoxia, generalized edema, and eventual circulatory collapse, during prenatal ultrasound testing. This condition may cause death in utero shortly before birth. Routine screening of the infant's blood type and a direct Coombs' test during the first hours after birth help to identify infants with blood group incompatibilities. Assessment of the infant's hematologic indices, such as reticulocyte count, hematocrit level, and red blood cell morphology help to determine the extent of hemolysis. Bilirubin levels can also help to determine the severity of disease. The greater the increase in the bilirubin level from one measurement to the next, the more severe the hemolysis.

Therapeutic Management. Some infants with mild ABO incompatibility may not require treatment. Most infants requiring treatment respond well to good hydration and phototherapy. Rarely does an infant with ABO incompatability have hemolysis severe enough to necessitate an exchange transfusion.

The hemolytic process in Rh incompatibility is almost always severe, and many of these infants require a blood transfusion for anemia at or shortly after birth. Most also require an exchange transfusion to remove antibody-coated red blood cells as well as bilirubin, which may approach toxic levels shortly after birth. Additional red blood cell transfusions for recurrent anemia as well as repeat exchange transfusions may be necessary during the slow resolution phase of Rh incompatibility.

RhoGAM allows destruction of fetal red blood cells in the maternal circulation and prevents maternal production of anti-Rh antibodies. The usual dose is 300 µg intramuscularly, given within 72 hours of delivery or abortion. The widespread use of RhoGAM in mothers who are Rh negative and who give birth to Rh-positive infants has decreased the incidence of Rh incompatibility. Missed abortions or miscarriages of Rh-positive fetuses can sensitize the Rh-negative mother and account for most cases of Rh incompatibility.

NURSING CARE OF THE INFANT WITH ABO–Rh INCOMPATIBILITY

Assessment

Determination of the mother's blood type should be made prenatally or as soon after admission as possible to identify mothers at risk for giving birth to infants with ABO or Rh incompatibilities. Blood typing and direct Coombs' test should be performed on cord blood soon after delivery whenever an infant is identified as being at risk. Obtaining and assessing laboratory values in symptomatic infants can help in the timely institution of appropriate treatment. Noting the rate of change in laboratory test results can help to determine the infant's response to therapy.

If the infant requires an exchange transfusion, the donor blood must be checked carefully to ensure that it is type O; Rh negative; low-titer anti-A, anti-B; and cross-matched with the mother's plasma and red blood cells. During the transfusion, the infant should be monitored for changes in heart rate, blood pressure, oxygen saturation, body temperature, respiratory status, and integrity of indwelling catheters used for the exchange. Both during and after the exchange transfusion, the infant must be monitored for evidence of complications, such as infection, thrombosis, air embolism, arteriospasm affecting the lower extremities, hypoglycemia, acid–base imbalance, hypernatremia, hyperkalemia, hypocalcemia, coagulopathy, necrotizing enterocolitis, cardiac arrthymias, volume overload, and hypothermia.

Nursing Diagnosis and Planning

- Altered Tissue Perfusion (cerebral, cardiopulmonary, renal, gastrointestinal, and peripheral) related to anemia. ***Expected Outcome:*** *The infant will be able to adequately perfuse all tissues.*
- Risk for Injury related to complications of toxic bilirubin levels and exchange transfusion. ***Expected Outcome:*** *Complications from toxic bilirubin levels and exchange transfusion will be avoided or minimized.*

Implementation

Ensure adequate hydration of the infant by administering appropriate fluids in the necessary amounts. Administer phototherapy according to established guidelines (see this chapter, Hyperbilirubinemia, for nursing care). Monitor the infant's blood indices and bilirubin levels, and promptly report deviations from normal or expected values. If an exchange transfusion is performed, the infant's vital signs are assessed every 5 to 15 minutes during the procedure and the infant is monitored closely afterward for evidence of complications.

Evaluation

- Was the infant's hematocrit level maintained within normal ranges?
- Was there perfusion of all tissues as evidenced by blood pressure within normal range and brisk peripheral capillary refill? Were complications either nonexistent or properly identified and appropriately treated?

HYPERBILIRUBINEMIA

Neonatal hyperbilirubinemia, an increase in serum bilirubin levels, is a common occurrence in the neonate. It may or may not be clinically significant. As bilirubin levels rise, some of the excess bilirubin is deposited in body tissues, resulting in a temporary yellow discoloration of the infant's skin and sclera. High bilirubin levels can penetrate and damage brain cells, a condition referred to as kernicterus.

Etiology. The most common causes of hyperbilirubinemia are listed in Table 21–3.

PATHOPHYSIOLOGY *of Hyperbilirubinemia*

Most of the bilirubin produced in the neonate comes from the breakdown of old or abnormal red blood cells by enzymes in the liver and spleen. The hemoglobin in the red blood cells is broken down into iron, protein, and bilirubin. The potentially toxic free bilirubin binds to albumin and is transported to the liver, where it undergoes conjugation, which renders it harmless. In the conjugated form, bilirubin is excreted from the body through the urinary and intestinal tracts. Conjugated bilirubin cannot be reabsorbed by the intestines, but an enzyme present in the intestines of the neonate can convert the bilirubin back to the unconjugated type, which can be reabsorbed into the bloodstream. This process can contribute significantly to the amount of bilirubin the neonate must process.

TABLE 21–3 *Causes of Hyperbilirubinemia*

MECHANISM	RELATED TO	CAUSED BY
Increased bilirubin availability	Overproduction of bilirubin	Polycythemia Decreased red blood cell lifespan Hemolysis (anemias, medication, infection) Extravascular blood (bruises, enclosed hemorrhages)
	Increased reabsorption of bilirubin from intestines	Delayed passage of meconium Increased enzyme activity Delayed enteral feedings Swallowed blood
Decreased bilirubin secretion	Altered liver metabolism of bilirubin	Prematurity indicates immature liver Decreased uptake by liver Inadequate perfusion of liver Decreased enzyme activity (deficiency or inhibition)
	Liver obstruction	Biliary atresia Cystic fibrosis Hyperalimentation Tumor
Combined overproduction and undersecretion of bilirubin	Congenital infection: toxoplasmosis, rubella, herpes, syphilis, hepatitis Asphyxia Infant of diabetic mother	
Uncertain mechanism	Breast milk jaundice Infants of Chinese, Japanese, Korean, Greek, or Native American descent	

Data from Poland, R. L., and Ostrea, E. M., Jr. (1986). Neonatal hyperbilirubinemia. In M. H. Klaus & A. A. Fanaroff (Eds.), *Care of the high-risk neonate* (3rd ed.). Philadelphia: W. B. Saunders. Blackburn, S. T., and Loper, D. L. (1992). *Maternal, fetal, and neonatal physiology.* Philadelphia: W. B. Saunders.

Incidence. Hyperbilirubinemia develops during the first few days of life in 45% to 60% of term infants and as many as 80% of preterm infants.

Clinical Manifestations. The yellow discoloration of the skin that is known as jaundice usually appears when the serum bilirubin level reaches 5 to 7 mg/dl.

> Jaundice is often seen first in the face, especially the nose. It then descends to the torso and then to the extremities.

In the term infant, peak levels are generally reached by the 3rd or 4th day of life, followed by a gradual decrease in bilirubin levels until normal values are reached at about the 10th day of life. In the preterm infant, peak levels are generally reached by the fifth day of life, followed by a slow decline in bilirubin levels until normal values are reached around the end of the first month of life.

Diagnostic Evaluation. Serum bilirubin levels should be obtained whenever clinical jaundice is present or in infants with conditions known to cause hyperbilirubinemia. The direct bilirubin is a measurement of conjugated bilirubin, and the indirect bilirubin is a measurement of unconjugated bilirubin. The total bilirubin level is the direct level plus the indirect level. Any premature infant who is clinically jaundiced and term infants with total bilirubin values of 13 mg/dl or higher should be evaluated to determine the etiology of the jaundice. Total bilirubin levels are generally higher in breastfed infants than in bottle-fed infants and higher in infants of Asian, African, or Native American descent. Other diagnostic tests that may help to determine the etiology include a direct Coombs' test, peripheral blood smear, reticulocyte count, blood type, and Rh status of both mother and infant.

Therapeutic Management. It is difficult to set rules for when to start therapy and which therapy to use. The underlying cause of hyperbilirubinemia as well as the infant's gestational age, chronological age, clinical status, weight, history, and risk factors, and the rate of rise in the bilirubin level must be considered.

Treatment of hyperbilirubinemia usually begins with phototherapy, which consists of exposing the infant to light in the blue part of the spectrum. The light source can be a single quartz-halogen spotlight; a bank of fluorescent bulbs, either blue, cool white, or daybright; or a blanket of white light filaments with a fiberoptic light source. This light causes a chemical reaction in the skin that converts unconjugated bilirubin to a form that can be excreted by the body. Phototherapy is usually given continuously, with short breaks as dictated by other infant care needs.

If phototherapy does not reduce the bilirubin level or if the bilirubin level is dangerously high, the infant may require an exchange transfusion. A double-volume exchange, in which the infant's blood volume is replaced twice, can lower the bilirubin level to approximately one half of the original value. Exchange transfusions should always be performed in the NICU. The infant's blood is removed, and donor blood of the appropriate type is given to the infant in small amounts through an umbilical venous catheter. Phototherapy is almost always used to treat infants requiring an exchange transfusion.

> During phototherapy, special care should be taken to assure that the infant is well hydrated to offset the effects of increased insensible water loss brought on by the phototherapy.

In infants whose bilirubin level responds slowly to phototherapy, phenobarbital is sometimes given to enhance liver enzyme action and increase bilirubin excretion. It may take 3 to 7 days for phenobarbital to begin to significantly improve the bilirubin level. Term infants seem to respond better to phenobarbital therapy than preterm infants.

Breastfed infants may have elevated bilirubin levels that do not seem to decrease with the usual management. Stopping breast milk feedings for 24 to 48 hours usually results in a decrease in the bilirubin level.

NURSING CARE OF THE INFANT WITH HYPERBILIRUBINEMIA

Assessment

The nurse can assess the infant for the presence of jaundice by pressing lightly on the skin with a fingertip. Common assessment sites are the nose and upper chest. Assessment for jaundice should take place in natural light whenever possible. The yellow color of jaundice will be easier to see over the fingerprint area than over the surrounding skin. In infants with dark skin, the first evidence of jaundice may be yellowing of the sclera. The infant should also be assessed for evidence of bruising, petechiae, cephalhematoma, prematurity, pallor, plethora, and enlarged liver or spleen, as well as perinatal risk factors, which can help to identify infants at risk for hyperbilirubinemia.

Nursing Diagnosis and Planning

Nursing Diagnoses

- Risk for Fluid Volume Deficit related to increased insensible water losses from phototherapy.
- Risk for Altered Body Temperature related to heat from phototherapy lights or lack of clothing to expose skin to phototherapy.
- Risk for Injury to Neurologic System related to deposition of bilirubin in brain tissue.

Expected Outcomes

- The infant will be free from jaundice.
- The infant will maintain body temperature within a normal range.
- The infant will maintain a normal fluid balance.
- The infant will not sustain injury to the neurologic system.

Implementation

To maximize the amount of skin exposed, phototherapy is usually administered with the infant completely undressed or wearing only a diaper. While phototherapy is in use, the infant's eyes are covered with an opaque mask that is usually secured in place with a headband or cloth adhesive (Velcro). Several types of eye shields are commercially available.

> The infant's eyes must be protected at all times during phototherapy to prevent retinal damage from the light source.

Care must be taken to ensure that the eye shield does not slip down and cover the infant's nares, compromising normal breathing. Eye patches can be removed when the light source is off (e.g., during feedings) to assess the eyes and allow the infant visual stimulation. The infant's position is changed frequently to ensure maximal skin exposure to the light source. The infant's bilirubin level is monitored one to four times a day to assess the effectiveness of phototherapy. The nurse monitors the infant's temperature every 2 to 4 hours to ensure maintenance within normal limits. The additional heat generated by the phototherapy unit places the infant at risk for hyperthermia. The lack of clothing on the infant increases the possibility of heat loss through convection, conduction, radiation, and evaporation, and may lead to hypothermia. Any signs of feeding intolerance, such as diarrhea or lactose intolerance, are recorded and reported so that appropriate feeding changes can be made. Because infants receiving phototherapy have increased insensible water losses, their intake and output should be closely monitored to ensure adequate hydration.

Evaluation

- Is the infant free of jaundice?
- Has the infant's body temperature remained within normal limits for his age during phototherapy?
- Does the infant remain free of neurologic insults related to hyperbilirubinemia?
- Has the infant maintained fluid and electrolyte balance?

Home Care. Term infants who are otherwise healthy may be treated with phototherapy at home. This practice not only saves health care costs and resources but also allows the family to interact with the infant in a more natural environment. The equipment and care are the same as for the hospitalized infant. Home health nurses make visits once or twice each day during treatment to assess the infant and obtain bilirubin levels.

INTRAVENTRICULAR HEMORRHAGE

Intracranial hemorrhage is bleeding that has occurred somewhere within the brain of the neonate. It is a general descriptive term that includes hemorrhage into and around the ventricles. Periventricular (around the ventricles) hemorrhage is bleeding that occurs in the parenchyma (i.e., within the periventricular white matter of the brain).

PATHOPHYSIOLOGY *of Intraventricular Hemorrhage*

Intracranial hemorrhage usually occurs as a hemorrhage in the germinal matrix that spreads throughout the ventricular system. In premature infants the subependymal area of the germinal matrix, located adjacent to the lateral ventricles, is a highly vascularized, gelatinous area that matures with gestational age. This area is essentially totally involuted by term, but is fragile in the preterm infant. Approximately 15% of infants with intraventricular hemorrhage (IVH) also experience a hemorrhagic infarction in the parenchyma, known as periventricular hemorrhagic **infarction.** This occurrence most likely represents a venous infarction in association with a large IVH.

Etiology. Increases in cerebral blood flow may occur with systemic hypertension, rapid volume expansion, hypercarbia, anemia, and hypoglycemia. Decreased cerebral blood flow is associated with hypotension occurring pre- or postnatally. Even fluctuations in cerebral blood flow, as seen with mechanically ventilated preterm infants with respiratory distress, place the infant at risk. The anatomy of the maturing germinal matrix, the forces of labor and vaginal delivery, asphyxia, or respiratory disturbances in the infant cause an increase in cerebral venous pressure, another risk factor. Other factors that may contribute to the development of IVH include disturbances of platelet–capillary function and coagulation, the tenuous capillary integrity in the vessels of the germinal matrix, and the vulnerability of the matrix capillaries to injury based on the anatomy of its vascular support (Volpe, 1995).

The pathogenesis of IVH is multifactorial. Structural and functional differences in the immature CNS place the premature infant at risk for IVH. Factors that affect the regulation of cerebral blood flow or cerebral venous pressure contribute to the occurrence of germinal matrix–intraventricular hemorrhage.

Incidence. The incidence of IVH is directly correlated with the degree of prematurity. The overall incidence is approximately 20% in premature infants. The first month of life is considered a high-risk period, but most cases of IVH (90%) occur in the first 3 days of life. If the hemorrhage extends, it usually does so within the first 10 days of life (Volpe, 1995).

Clinical Manifestations

- No notable clinical signs (most common)

With mild to moderate intraventricular hemorrhage:

- Altered level of consciousness
- Hypotonia
- Subtle aberrations of eye position or movement

With severe intraventricular hemorrhage, rapidly occurring (least common):

- Stupor, coma
- Apnea, respiratory deterioration
- Seizures
- Pupils fixed, nonreactive to light (difficult to evaluate in the very preterm infant)
- Bulging anterior fontanel
- Flaccid tone
- Metabolic disturbances: metabolic acidosis, glucose abnormalities
- Temperature instability
- Bradycardia
- Hypotension
- Decreasing hematocrit value
- Abnormalities of water homeostasis: inappropriate antidiuretic hormone secretion, diabetes insipidus

Diagnostic Evaluation. IVH is diagnosed by ultrasound scan of the neonatal cranium. A grading of the severity of the hemorrhage is based on the presence and amount of blood noted:

Grade 1: Germinal matrix hemorrhage
Grade 2: IVH
Grade 3: IVH with >50% of ventricular area filled with blood; some dilation of ventricles
Grade 4/Intraparenchymal: Periventricular hemorrhagic infarction or other parenchymal lesion

Computed tomography and magnetic resonance imaging scan of the head are also useful, but less commonly used, diagnostic tools.

Therapeutic Management. Postnatal intervention focuses on maintaining the multisystem stability of the infant, including thermoregulation, correction or support of respiratory problems, normalization of blood pressure and coagulation studies, management of seizures, and limitation of stressful events that may compromise cerebral blood flow or cerebral venous pressure. The mortality rate for infants with severe IVH is approximately 20%.

Management is initially geared to prevention. If the preterm birth of the infant cannot be stopped, plans should be made to deliver the infant at a perinatal center specializing in high-risk deliveries.

Infants with IVH are at risk for post-hemorrhagic ventricular dilation as a result of disturbances of cerebrospinal fluid flow or absorption. Infants must be followed for the development of increased intracranial pressure, rapid head growth, and hydrocephalus, as documented by serial cranial ultrasound examinations. Serial lumbar punctures to remove excessive cerebrospinal fluid and blood may be used to control and treat post-hemorrhagic hydrocephalus. If the hydrocephalus does not respond to this therapy or does not improve over time, a ventriculoperitoneal shunt may be needed.

Long-Term Outcome. Infants with IVH are at increased risk for major neurologic sequelae, including spastic motor deficits and major cognitive deficits. The highest risk occurs when the IVH is associated with an intraparenchymal lesion, such as periventricular hemorrhagic infarction. Families require counseling to help them cope with the diagnosis as well as to provide them with information about the long-term follow-up required by the infant.

NURSING CARE OF THE INFANT WITH IVH

Assessment

Preterm infants delivered at less than 34 weeks' gestation are at increased risk for IVH. Nursing care measures include identifying the infant at risk and limiting activities that might negatively affect the infant.

Fluctuations in cerebral blood flow are associated with mechanical ventilation, restlessness or agitation, hypercarbia, hypovolemia, patent ductus arteriosus, and high inspired oxygen concentrations. Increases in cerebral blood flow or blood pressure may be seen in the preterm infant during rapid eye movement sleep, noxious stimulation, spontaneous motor activity, caretaking activities that require handling of the infant, tracheal suctioning, hypercarbia, hypoglycemia, anemia, rapid volume infusion (i.e., colloid infusions, hyperosmolar solutions, exchange transfusions), pneumothorax, seizures, and surgical ligation of a patent ductus arteriosus. Increased cerebral venous pressure that may contribute to IVH is associated with labor and delivery, asphyxia, and respiratory disturbances, such as pneumothorax and tracheal suctioning. Perinatal asphyxia and systemic hypotension may decrease cerebral blood flow and produce IVH. Disturbances in coagulation may also be a factor (Volpe, 1995).

The family requires assistance in coping with the diagnosis and their concerns for long-term sequelae. The parents must be made aware of the need for long-term follow-up.

Nursing Diagnosis and Planning

Nursing Diagnoses

- Altered Tissue Perfusion, Cerebral.
- Altered Growth and Development related to IVH.
- Knowledge Deficit related to lack of exposure to accurate information regarding potential sequelae of IVH.
- Altered Family Processes related to birth of a potentially handicapped child.

Expected Outcomes

- The infant will have a normal cranial ultrasound.
- The infant will not exhibit any evidence of hydrocephalus or long-term neurologic dysfunction.
- The infant will attain developmental milestones at or near the appropriate time.
- The parents will verbalize an understanding of the long-term prognosis for their infant.

Implementation

Caretaking activities are modified (e.g., attention to how the infant is turned and positioned for diaper changes) to decrease stress whenever possible. Noxious or harmful stimuli are avoided or modified to minimal levels. Care activities are clustered to avoid disturbing the infant, but the infant is allowed to recover from any intervention before another is begun. Recovery is evidenced by normalizing heart rate, respiratory pattern, muscle tone, and oxygen saturation. Episodes that rapidly increase blood pressure, such as seizures or infant agitation, are identified and reported so that treatment can be implemented. Blood products and hyperosmolar solutions are given slowly to prevent rapid changes in intravascular volume. Ventilator settings are monitored and modified in a timely manner to avoid excessive ventilator support and increased risk of pneumothorax. Any sign of prolonged bleeding is identified and reported immediately.

Parents are given simple, but complete explanations about the risk of IVH and the studies needed to diagnose the problem. If the infant has IVH, the parents understand the need to monitor for post-hemorrhagic hydrocephalus and the need for long-term developmental follow-up.

Evaluation

- Is the infant's cranial ultrasound normal?
- Does the infant exhibit any signs of neurologic dysfunction?
- Is the infant attaining developmental milestones at the predicted age?
- Are the parents discussing the infant's present and long-term prognosis?

NEONATAL SEIZURES

A seizure is not a disease process, but rather a symptom of an underlying abnormality. A seizure is defined as a paroxysmal alteration in neurologic function (i.e., behavioral, motor, or autonomic; Volpe, 1989). Although seizures are not life threatening, the underlying pathology may damage the brain. For this reason, seizures should be considered a medical emergency.

PATHOPHYSIOLOGY *of Neonatal Seizures*

Seizures are caused by excessive synchronous electric discharges or depolarizations of neurons. The mechanism of neonatal seizures is not clearly understood. Possible explanations include an excess of excitatory neurotransmitter compared with inhibitory neurotransmitter, altered permeability of the neuronal membrane inhibiting sodium movement, and an imbalance between depolarization and repolarization of the neurons. Because of the overall anatomic and physiologic immaturity of the nervous system in the neonate, well-organized generalized seizures are rare.

Etiology. The most common cause of seizures is perinatal asphyxia leading to hypoxic–ischemic encephalopathy, accounting for as many as 65% of neonatal seizures. Another 15% of cases can be attributed to intracranial hemorrhage. Other causes include metabolic disturbances, meningitis, cerebral infarcts, drug withdrawal, hyperthermia, hypoglycemia, hypocalcemia, sodium and potassium imbalances, congenital anomalies of the CNS, and inherited syndromes.

Incidence. Seizures occur in 0.2% to 1.4% of all live births. As many as 20% of preterm infants and as many as 25% of all NICU admissions are affected.

Clinical Manifestations

- *Subtle seizures.* Sustained eye opening, tonic horizontal deviation of the eyes, blinking or eyelid fluttering, sucking, smacking, drooling, tongue thrusting, pedal-

ing movements of the legs, swimming movements of the arms, and apnea. These manifestations are more common in preterm infants and infants with hypoxic ischemic encephalopathy.
- *Clonic seizures.* Focal: slow, rhythmic, jerking movements involving the face, neck, trunk, or extremities on one side of the body. Infants may be unconscious during and after this type of seizure. Multifocal: jerking movements migrating from one body part to another sequentially. These seizures are more common in term infants and infants with hypocalcemia.
- *Tonic seizures.* Focal: sustained flexion or extension of the leg or arm, or asymmetric posturing of the neck or trunk, or both. Generalized: tonic extension of both arms and both legs (decerebrate posturing), possibly involving tonic flexion of the arms with extension of the legs. These seizures are more common in premature infants.
- *Myoclonic seizures.* Focal: flexing movements of the arm. Multifocal: asynchronous twitching of several body parts. Generalized: bilateral flexing jerks of the arms, occasionally involving the legs as well. These seizures are seen in both premature and term infants.

Diagnostic Evaluation. Appropriate intervention is based on identifying the underlying cause of the seizure. Any evaluation should begin with a detailed patient history, including family history, maternal history during pregnancy, labor and delivery history, and early neonatal history. A detailed physical examination followed by a thorough neurologic evaluation can provide clues to the underlying cause. The history and physical examination help in prioritizing further diagnostic studies. Laboratory tests, such as serum glucose, sodium, potassium, calcium, magnesium, blood urea nitrogen, and blood gas values, are routinely performed when investigating the cause of a seizure. Studies of the cerebrospinal fluid to exclude meningitis are an essential part of the diagnostic work-up. TORCHS* titers to exclude congenital viral infection and amino acid and organic acid studies to exclude inborn errors of metabolism are often included. Cranial ultrasound and computed tomography or magnetic resonance imaging scan of the head are also useful diagnostic tools.

NURSING CARE OF THE INFANT WITH NEONATAL SEIZURES

Assessment

Although seizures are difficult to recognize in the neonate, especially if they are subtle, prompt recognition and treatment of the underlying cause are essential in preventing or minimizing damage to the brain. Jitteriness or tremors may be mistaken for seizures.

> If the movement can be initiated by a stimulus, such as touch, it is probably a tremor. If it cannot be stopped or controlled with gentle restraint or passive flexion, it is probably a seizure.

The nurse can help to minimize the infant's risk for seizures by assessing the routine laboratory studies (see this section on diagnostic evaluation) for abnormalities that might predispose the infant to seizures. If seizure-like activity is noted, the nurse should document the time it began and ended, the body part involved and the type of movement noted, the infant's level of consciousness, the effect on the infant's color and respiratory status, and the infant's condition after the seizure.

Nursing Diagnosis and Planning

- Risk for Neurologic Injury related to the underlying cause of the seizure. ***Expected Outcome:*** *The infant will not exhibit any evidence of long-term neurologic dysfunction.*
- Knowledge Deficit, Parental (seizures), related to the cause of the seizure and the long-term prognosis. ***Expected Outcome:*** *The parents will verbalize an understanding of the causes and treatment of seizures and the long-term prognosis for their infant.*

Implementation

Whenever the nurse sees an infant exhibiting seizure-like behavior, the physician should be notified immediately because seizures can be a sign of a serious disorder or disease. The nurse supports the infant during the seizure by maintaining a patent airway, assessing for adequate respirations, and monitoring the heart rate. To help protect the infant, the nurse does not attempt to restrain the extremities or force anything into the infant's mouth. Once the seizure has stopped, the nurse monitors the infant's vital signs, assures adequate oxygenation and ventilation, and provides comfort and warmth. The nurse plans the infant's care to minimize environmental stimuli. The nurse administers anticonvulsants as ordered, monitoring their effectiveness as well as their effects on other body systems, particularly the respiratory system. The nurse educates the family to help them understand the diagnostic work-up and the underlying cause of the infant's seizures. The nurse teaches the parents to recognize the signs of seizure activity, care for the infant during and after a seizure, administer anticonvulsants, and recognize their side effects. (See the section on seizures in Chapter 40 for further discussion of the care of a child experiencing a seizure.)

*T, Toxoplasmosis; O, other (i.e., hepatitis B, varicella zoster, human parvovirus, coxsackie virus); R, rubella; C, cytomegalovirus infection; H, herpes simplex; S, syphilis.

Evaluation

- Does the infant exhibit signs of neurologic damage?
- Are the parents verbalizing an understanding of the cause of seizures and the long-term care of their child?

INFANTS OF ADDICTED MOTHERS

Infants born to women who abuse drugs during their pregnancy may experience withdrawal symptoms after birth.

> **PATHOPHYSIOLOGY AND ETIOLOGY**
>
> Drugs of low molecular weight readily cross the placenta and become distributed in fetal tissues. Drugs that can cause withdrawal in the infants of mothers who use them include:
>
> | | |
> |---|---|
> | Alcohol | Meperidine |
> | Cocaine | Morphine |
> | Heroin | Pentazocine |
> | Amphetamines | Marijuana |
> | Lysergic acid diethylamide (LSD) | Chlorpromazine |
> | | Diphenhydramine |
> | Phenobarbital | Codeine |
> | Diazepam | Methadone |
> | Lithium | Theophylline |
> | Barbiturates | |
>
> The fetus is repeatedly exposed to the drug and becomes dependent on the drug. Once the umbilical cord is cut, the source of the drug is removed and the infant may experience drug withdrawal. Some drugs also cause congenital anomalies and growth retardation.

Incidence. Chemical dependence is one of the most commonly missed diagnoses in the management of pregnant women. The true incidence of perinatal substance abuse is unknown because self-reporting of use is unreliable and toxicology screens usually detect use over only a short time frame.

Clinical Manifestations. The onset of withdrawal symptoms is variable. Symptoms may be present at birth or may not occur until 4 to 10 days after delivery. Infants born addicted to narcotics may exhibit withdrawal symptoms for 4 to 12 months. Between 70% and 90% of affected infants exhibit signs and symptoms as described below.

W = Wakefulness
I = Irritability
T = Tremulousness, temperature variation, tachypnea
H = Hyperactivity, high-pitched persistent cry, hyperacusia, hyperreflexia, hypertonus
D = Diarrhea, diaphoresis, disorganized suck
R = Respiratory distress, rub marks, rhinorrhea
A = Apnea, autonomic dysfunction
W = Weight loss or failure to gain weight
A = Alkalosis (respiratory)
L = Lacrimation (American Academy of Pediatrics, 1990)

Specific information about cocaine is provided in the accompanying box.

Diagnostic Evaluation. When drug withdrawal has been identified or is suspected, obtaining urine and blood toxicology/drug screens on the mother as well as obtaining urine, blood, and meconium toxicology/drug screens on the infant can help to confirm the diagnosis.

Therapeutic Management. Between 30% and 50% of infants who experience withdrawal respond well to supportive measures. Sensory stimulation can be decreased by swaddling; a quiet, darkened environment; and comfort measures to prevent excessive crying. Frequent, small feedings of high-caloric formula help to supply the additional caloric requirements.

> ***Effects of Cocaine on the Fetus and Neonate***
>
> Of the many substances that can cause drug withdrawal in the neonate, cocaine is one of the most commonly used and has some of the most serious effects.
>
> The rate of cocaine use in pregnant women is increasing (Day et al., 1993). Although cocaine use occurs in all races and ethnic groups and at all socioeconomic levels, cocaine-exposed neonates are particularly prevalent in inner-city hospitals (Bandstra & Burkett, 1991). One such institution reported that 31% of infants tested had positive results for cocaine (Ostrea et al., 1992). The primary route of cocaine administration in pregnant women is smoking of crack cocaine (Bandstra & Burkett, 1991). Cocaine affects the fetus primarily through fetal, placental, and uterine blood flow (Woods et al., 1987). A spectrum of anomalies occur, depending on the extent of diminished blood flow and the time during gestation of exposure. Infants are likely to be born prematurely and with intrauterine growth retardation, and defects in the skeletal, respiratory, cardiovascular, genitourinary, and central nervous system have been reported.
>
> From Plessinger, M. A., & Woods, J. R. (1993). Maternal, placental, and fetal pathophysiology of cocaine exposure during pregnancy. *Clinical Obstetrics and Gynecology, 36*(2), 267–278.

More specific therapy may be required when withdrawal symptoms are severe. Infection, hypoglycemia, hypocalcemia, hypomagnesemia, hyperthyroidism, CNS hemorrhage, and anoxia must be excluded as the etiology of the symptoms. Pharmacologic agents used in the treatment of withdrawal include tincture of paregoric, tincture of opium, morphine, methadone, diazepam (Valium), chlorpromazine (Thorazine), and phenobarbital. Medication doses can be stabilized and then tapered once the infant sleeps well, eats effectively, and gains weight for 3 to 5 days. Failure to taper the dose may result in prolonged hospitalization. Treatment may last a few days or several weeks, depending on the severity of symptoms and the infant's response to treatment. Long-term follow-up of the infant's physical and mental development should be supervised by a physician who is knowledgeable about the symptoms and treatment of addicted infants and willing to communicate effectively with the parents. Social workers are essential in determining the parents' ability to care for the infant after discharge.

NURSING CARE OF THE INFANT WITH AN ADDICTED MOTHER

Assessment

The nurse can help to identify infants who are at risk for withdrawal by obtaining a social history of the parents and a detailed maternal drug history, including prescription and nonprescription drugs. The nurse should assess infants who are at risk for the presence of signs and symptoms of withdrawal. When drug withdrawal has been identified or is suspected, obtaining urine and blood toxicology/drug screens on the mother and urine, blood, and meconium toxicology/drug screens on the infant can help to confirm the diagnosis.

Nursing Diagnosis and Planning

Nursing Diagnoses

- Disorganized Infant Behavior related to altered CNS secondary to withdrawal from addictive substance.
- Altered Nutrition: Less than Body Requirements, related to increased activity, increased metabolic rate, and altered gastrointestinal motility.
- Impaired Skin Integrity related to friction burns on extremities and skin breakdown on the buttocks from diarrhea.
- Altered Parenting related to substance abuse and addiction
- Altered Family Processes related to poor parental self-esteem, addictive personality, and the infant's altered neurologic functioning.

Expected Outcomes

- The infant will maintain vital signs within the normal limits for newborns and will not exhibit signs of increased irritability or seizures.
- The infant will exhibit growth and weight gain at the expected rates for healthy infants.
- The infant will be free of skin breakdown.
- Parents will demonstrate acquaintance and attachment behaviors while interacting appropriately with their infant.
- Parents will demonstrate their ability to provide the appropriate care for their infant.

Implementation

Nursing care is aimed at decreasing environmental stimuli, meeting the infant's nutritional needs, and promoting healthy parent–infant interaction. The infant's care is coordinated to limit the number of times the infant is disturbed. Noise and light levels in the nursery, especially in the infant's immediate vicinity, are maintained at minimal necessary levels. A light blanket can be placed over the top of the isolette to darken the area. Appropriate comfort measures are provided immediately when the infant exhibits irritability. These may include offering a pacifier, swaddling the infant, or rocking. The infant's ability to nipple feed is assessed, and the infant is gavage fed if necessary to provide adequate fluid and caloric intake. Weight gain is monitored daily, and length and head circumferences are monitored weekly to assure that nutritional intake is sufficient for growth. Because these infants are usually irritable, providing their nursing care can be challenging and stressful. Parent–infant interaction is at an especially high risk in these cases, and special effort is made to involve the parents in the infant's care. Contact between parents and social services, such as child protection and community health agencies, is made before discharge in an effort to optimize the functioning of the family unit and the long-term outcome of the child.

Evaluation

- Is the infant able to tolerate normal environmental stimuli?
- Does the infant exhibit behavior within normal limits for his age?
- Is the infant's weight, length, and head circumference increasing along established norms for age and sex?
- Does the infant have healthy, intact skin?
- Are the parents verbalizing their understanding of the infant's condition and needs?
- Are the parents demonstrating their ability to provide for the infant's physical and emotional needs?

FETAL ALCOHOL SYNDROME

Fetal alcohol syndrome (FAS) is the severe form of birth defects experienced by the infant exposed to alcohol in utero. Although more subtle effects are sometimes seen, FAS refers to the classic defects of persistent symmetric growth retardation, malformations of the face and skull, skeletal and cardiac malformation, and CNS functional abnormalities, including mental retardation.

PATHOPHYSIOLOGY *of Fetal Alcohol Syndrome*

Alcohol crosses the placenta rapidly; therefore, the fetus experiences blood levels of alcohol equivalent to the maternal levels. Heavy prenatal alcohol exposure can result in decreased brain cell number, diminished intelligence, and brain malformation (Jones, 1988).

Etiology. Ethanol-induced brain malformations seem to be a result of direct **cytotoxicity** (destruction of certain cells). Ethanol also affects lipid metabolism and membrane function, and alters levels of cyclic adenosine monophosphate) (Dodson, 1992). It is unclear whether any amount of alcohol ingested during pregnancy is safe.

Ethanol is a neuroteratogen in humans, and ethanol or its by-products can cause permanent damage to the fetus.

Incidence. The incidence of FAS varies by country and ethnic group. In the United States, the incidence is one to two per 1000 births (Wright & Catz, 1992).

Clinical Manifestations

- Pre- and postnatal onset of growth deficiency
- Microcephaly
- Short palpebral fissures
- Smooth philtrum (the vertical groove in the median portion of the upper lip), with thin upper lip
- Joint anomalies
- Altered palmar crease patterns
- Short distal phalanges
- Cardiac defects, with ventricular septal defect and auricular septal defect most common
- Mental deficiency with average intelligence quotient of 63
- Tremulousness in the neonatal period
- Irritability in infancy; hyperactivity in childhood
- Other abnormalities, including cervical vertebral malformations, ear anomalies, cleft lip and palate, severe cardiac defects, renal anomalies, strawberry hemangiomata, and genital anomalies (Jones, 1988; Dodson, 1992)

Diagnostic Evaluation. FAS is diagnosed through physical examination and perinatal history, and a referral is often made to a geneticist. The Fetal Alcohol Study Group of the Research Society on Alcoholism proposed three specific criteria for the diagnosis of FAS. To make the diagnosis of FAS, one abnormality from each of the following categories must be present:

1. Prenatal or postnatal growth retardation; failure to thrive, with weight, length, or head circumference at less than the 10th percentile.
2. CNS involvement, including signs of neurologic abnormalities (e.g., irritability in infancy, hyperactivity during childhood), developmental delay, hypotonia, or intellectual impairment (mild to moderate mental retardation).
3. Characteristic facial dysmorphology (at least two of three):
   - Microcephaly (head circumference at less than the third percentile).
   - **Microphthalmia** (abnormally small eyes) or short palpebral fissures.
   - Poorly developed philtrum, thin upper lip (vermilion border), and flattening or absence of the maxilla (Pietrantoni & Knuppel, 1991).

Infants with FAS require early intervention to maximize their developmental potential.

Families require counseling to help them cope with the diagnosis as well as to help them understand the risks involved in future pregnancies if lifestyle changes are not made.

NURSING CARE OF THE INFANT WITH FAS

Assessment

The family requires assistance in coping with the diagnosis as well as the difficulties associated with an irritable infant. Special attention must be given to involving the parents in the care of the infant.

When FAS is suspected, an extensive diagnostic work-up is required. Microcephaly, hypotonia, tremulousness, and irritability can raise levels of suspicion. Feeding difficulties may be encountered as well.

Nursing Diagnosis and Planning

Nursing Diagnoses

- Ineffective Infant Feeding Pattern related to congenital anomaly.
- Altered Growth and Development related to FAS.

- Knowledge Deficit (infant's anomalies and potential sequelae) related to lack of exposure to accurate information.
- Altered Family Processes related to birth of a handicapped child.

Expected Outcomes

- The infant will establish sleep–wake and feeding patterns conducive to appropriate weight gain and growth.
- Parents will recognize FAS and acknowledge the potential for future problems.
- The family's energies will be directed toward caring for their infant.

Implementation

Daily weight gain is monitored, and intake and output are measured and documented. Various feeding strategies (e.g., varying the positioning of the infant; trying smaller, more frequent feedings; using different nipples) should be attempted until the infant is successful with nipple feedings or breastfeedings. Because parents may become frustrated or feel inadequate in dealing with a difficult feeder, it is important to assist the parents with feeding in a supportive manner. Promoting early parent–infant attachment will support the child's well-being. Encourage the family to visit frequently, and involve parents in caretaking activities.

The infant with FAS is likely to have severe permanent neurologic and developmental sequelae. Discuss the infant's recognizable anomalies and the possible sequelae. Allow the parents to verbalize their concerns about their infant's future. Avoid encouraging unrealistic expectations; rather, acknowledge the infant's existing problems and suggest coping strategies.

The family is in a crisis situation, and the mother may experience guilt or may be blamed by other family members for the infant's handicap. Encourage the family to verbalize their feelings. Initiate referrals to appropriate community resources. The needs of the high-risk family are significant and require long-term follow-up.

Evaluation

- Is the infant gaining weight at a rate that is appropriate for his age?
- Are the infant's sleep patterns appropriate for his age?
- Are the parents discussing the cause and prevention of FAS?
- Is the family able to identify its own strengths and weaknesses, coping skills, and support systems?
- Have referrals to community resources been made and implemented?

CARE OF THE FAMILY

Most parents look forward to the birth of an infant with great anticipation, believing that it will be one of the happiest events of their lives. However, this event may be one of the most stressful and depressing times of the parents' lives if the infant is born prematurely, ill, or with a congenital defect. Family dynamics are severely altered, and the family members are in crisis. More so than at any other time, the care of the family cannot be separated from the care of the patient. Nurses caring for infants in the NICU must recognize the needs of the parents and must be prepared to implement appropriate measures to meet those needs (Fig. 21–6). It is important to have a basic understanding of the process of parent–infant attachment as well as the grief process.

Parent–Infant Attachment

As the pregnancy progresses, the parents experience many emotions and begin to reorganize their lives to include the expected infant. Many have strong feelings for the fetus. Plans are made not only for the immediate needs of the infant, but often for each step of the child's life from infancy to adulthood. By the time the pregnancy has reached full term, most parents have accepted the fetus as an individual and are eager to get to know the newest addition to their family. For the first hour or so immedi-

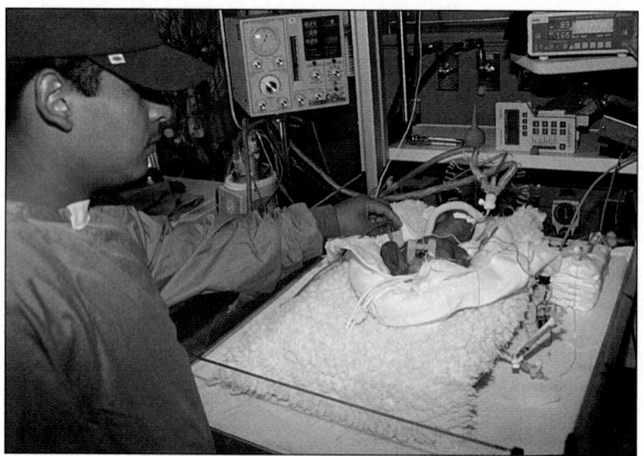

Figure 21–6
Parents of the preterm infant may not have had adequate time to prepare themselves emotionally to accept their infant as a separate individual. They may be tentative in their contact with the baby and afraid to become too strongly attached in case he dies. Parents often grieve because their expectations did not materialize. The staff must include the parents in the child's care to promote the development of emotional ties. (Courtesy of Parkland Memorial Hospital, Dallas, Texas.)

ately after birth, the infant is alert. During this time, the parents become engrossed in their newborn, verifying the infant's sex, the number of fingers and toes, the infant's overall health and well-being, and any resemblance to either parent or other family members. The infant's apparent interest in his parents and surroundings further encourages and enhances this acquaintance process. If the infant meets the parents' expectations as they become acquainted, strong feelings of attachment begin to form, signaling the start of the bonding process. If the acquaintance process does not take place or is interrupted, or if the infant does not meet the expectations of one or both parents, parent–infant attachment may be delayed, placing the future parent–infant relationship at risk.

If the infant is born prematurely, the parents may not have had enough time to prepare themselves emotionally and psychologically for parenthood or to develop strong feelings for the fetus. Before, during, and after a premature delivery, the parents may feel neglected because the primary focus of the health care team seems to be the infant. The experience is not reassuring and is not what the parents had envisioned. Many premature infants have medical complications, some of which are life threatening, necessitating immediate intensive care. Medical personnel, whose faces the parents cannot even see, disappear with their infant, often without saying a word. The parents may feel anger, guilt, inadequacy, blame, and grief because the pregnancy did not reach full term.

Some parents experience a full-term, uncomplicated pregnancy witness the birth of their infant, and realize soon thereafter that their infant is not completely normal. Congenital defects may be evident at birth (e.g., many malformations, some chromosomal disorders). However, some life-threatening problems, such as heart defects and inborn errors of metabolism, may not be evident for several hours or even days after birth. The emotions of parents in these situations may suddenly plummet from euphoria to despair. The parents may perceive the infant's condition as their own inability to conceive a normal child, and they may feel the same anger, guilt, inadequacy, blame, and grief experienced by the parents of premature infants.

Many barriers to parent–infant interaction are present in the NICU. The unfamiliar, high-tech, busy NICU may seem like a harsh, unfriendly environment to the parents. They may feel inadequate as parents because they can do little to protect and care for their infant. Numerous wires, cables, tubings, needles, pumps, and monitors surround the infant and often present a barrier to parent–infant interaction. Most decisions about their infant's care are made by strangers who may not take the time to explain why the therapy is needed, how it will be performed, and what the markers of success or failure are. For these reasons, the parents may feel that their infant does not need them, and they may withdraw.

Withdrawal also may serve as a coping mechanism as parents try not to become attached to their infant in an effort to protect themselves from future emotional pain.

Infants who are premature, critically ill, or malformed often do not behave and respond to their environment and caregivers in the same way as healthy infants. This difference in response may confuse parents and make them feel inadequate as they attempt to interact with and care for their infant. As nurses skillfully meet the infant's needs, the parents may feel that their infant does not really need them and may be better off without them.

Grief

Grief occurs when an individual loses something that was loved and valued. The stages of the grief process are outlined in Chapter 17. Parents of high-risk infants commonly experience grief. Even if the infant does not die, most parents grieve the loss of the anticipated child. People move through the grief process at their own pace, and some never work all the way through it. People may move back and forth between the stages as well. The degree to which parents exhibit grief is not necessarily congruent with the severity of their infant's condition. The parents' experiences with grief as well as cultural and social expectations may influence the expression of grief. Often parents and other family members are at different stages in the grief process and therefore have different needs. It is challenging to meet the diverse needs of two people who are visiting the infant at the same time. Some health professionals have specialized training and skills to assist individuals in dealing with grief and loss, but the nurse, as caretaker of the infant, is usually the one to first come in contact with the parents. By recognizing the steps of the grief process, the nurse may be better prepared to understand the parents' needs and identify actions that will best meet those needs.

NURSING CARE OF THE FAMILY

Assessment

Assessment begins with a determination of how well the parents understand their infant's diagnosis and current condition. Next, it is important to determine how the parents are coping or adapting to their situation. Any support systems being used by the parents should be identified. The stage of the grief process that each parent is experiencing should be noted as well as any apparent movement between the stages. Parental visits to the NICU can be assessed for frequency, length, and the presence of acquaintance or caregiving behaviors.

Nursing Diagnosis and Planning

- Altered Parenting related to inadequate childbirth and parenting preparation, separation from the infant, infant's condition, or NICU environment. ***Expected Outcome:*** *Parents will visit the infant frequently, demonstrating an understanding of the NICU environment as they gradually assume caregiving tasks as their infant's condition allows.*
- Altered Family Processes related to unexpected hospitalization of the infant, isolation from the infant, or the grief process. ***Expected Outcome:*** *Parents will demonstrate an ability to deal constructively with the grief process.*
- Ineffective Family Coping, Compromised, related to the stressful nature of the infant's birth and hospitalization. ***Expected Outcome:*** *Parents will demonstrate the ability to deal appropriately with their infant's hospitalization by using the coping mechanisms available to them.*
- Knowledge Deficit related to lack of understanding of the infant's condition and prognosis. ***Expected Outcome:*** *The parents will verbalize an understanding of their infant's current condition and expected outcomes.*

Implementation

The nurse should attempt to become acquainted with the infant's parents. If time permits, contacting them before delivery and scheduling a tour of the NICU may alleviate some anxiety by helping them to become familiar with the NICU environment and staff. Every effort should be made to encourage parents to visit as often as they like. During visits, the parents should be given a complete, honest report of their infant's current status, his response to therapy, and plans for future interventions. The purpose of the various monitors, pumps, and other equipment should be explained in simple terms. Parents should be encouraged to get as close to the infant as the situation allows. The infant should be referred to by name. Avoiding difficult topics may plant the seeds of distrust and weaken the nurse's effectiveness in dealing with the parents. Parents should be encouraged to express their attitudes, feelings, and emotions, and these should be acknowledged and accepted nonjudgmentally. The nurse should facilitate referrals to support services, such as social workers or counselors. As soon as the infant's condition allows, the parents should be encouraged to touch, hold, talk to, and care for their infant. At all times, the nurse should remember that the infant belongs to the parents, and their concerns, rights, and duties should not be ignored. As the infant nears readiness for discharge, the nurse can initiate referrals to appropriate specialists and agencies in an effort to assure the ongoing care of the infant and family.

Evaluation

- Are parents visiting the infant whenever they are able and are they comfortable in the NICU environment?
- Do the parents understand the grief process and recognize their position within it?
- Are the parents using the coping mechanisms available to them as needed?
- Can the parents explain their infant's current condition and relate the expected outcomes?
- Can parents demonstrate their willingness and ability to assume caregiving tasks as their infant's condition allows?
- Are the parents able to identify the long-term needs of their infant and the resources available to deal with them?

Discharge Planning and Home Care

The survival rate of high-risk neonates continues to increase. Reasons for this increase include advances in technology, both diagnostic and therapeutic; growth of knowledge about fetal and neonatal physiology and pathophysiology; and an increase in scientific management strategies. There has also been an improvement in long-term outcome, but this improvement has not kept pace with the survival rate. As a result, a significant number of neonates with long-term health problems require special attention after discharge and often need readmittance. These problems include neurodevelopmental difficulties in the areas of motor, language, and learning; respiratory difficulties, such as apnea, bronchopulmonary dysplasia (BPD), and an increased incidence of sudden infant death syndrome; gastrointestinal difficulties, such as gastroesophageal reflux and ostomies from gastrointestinal malformations or surgery; vision difficulties related to ROP; and difficulties in growth, such as failure to thrive.

The care of preterm infants who are otherwise healthy and do not have any of these long-term problems may also be challenging for parents. These infants are generally immature neurologically and less socially interactive, providing cues that are difficult for the parents to interpret. Some of the infants' responses to their parents' caregiving may even seem negative (Johnson & Grubbs, 1975).

Current trends in health care aimed at minimizing health care costs have resulted in an increased number of technology-dependent infants being discharged from the hospital. Appropriate discharge planning and coordinated home care are essential for optimizing the long-term outcome of these infants.

Discharge planning begins with the infant's admission to the NICU. Many potential problem areas can be identified during the initial assessment of the infant and review of the mother's chart. Congenital anomalies, extreme prematurity, very low birth weight, and the disease processes that are present on admission can identify infants at risk for long-term complications. Maternal use of alcohol, tobacco, or illicit drugs not only identifies an infant at risk but also may indicate social problems in the home that may affect the infant's long-term outcome. As the infant's hospitalization evolves, some of the initial concerns may be resolved or modified, and new problems may be identified. Nurses in the acute care setting play an integral part in identifying the infant's needs as well as assessing the parents' ability to care for the infant.

At some institutions, the infant's primary nurse has the responsibility for coordinating the discharge process. At others, these duties are undertaken by a full-time discharge coordinator. Regardless of who leads the process, it must be multidisciplinary, including the physician, nurse, respiratory therapist, physical or occupational therapist, social worker, pharmacist, nutritionist, home health care provider, and family members who will provide the infant's care. Professionals from other disciplines are involved as needed. Meetings of the team members should be held to discuss each case at regular intervals during the hospitalization and as needed. Many institutions have weekly discharge planning rounds for all infants.

Several factors must be considered to determine the appropriate time for discharge. First, and most important, the infant must meet the discharge eligibility criteria established by the physician or hospital. A minimum weight requirement, the ability to maintain a normal temperature in an open crib in regular clothing, and the ability to tolerate enteral feedings, usually by nursing or nippling, are common criteria. Next, the readiness of the parents or primary caregivers must be assessed. The parents should be involved in the infant's care as early as possible. Even before the infant can be held or fed by the parents, they can be involved in temperature taking, diaper changing, and education about their infant's special needs. The assessment and caregiving skills of the parents need to be equal to the infant's needs before discharge can be safely undertaken. Having the parents stay with their infant in the hospital for a few nights just before discharge, commonly called rooming-in, can help in this assessment. The home also must be prepared before discharge. All necessary equipment must be in place, working properly, and thoroughly familiar to the parents. The home should have a telephone with emergency numbers clearly posted nearby beside it. Some infants may require the home to be appropriately climate controlled. In addition, any community agencies, home health nursing agencies, or other support services that will be needed must be notified of their role in the infant's discharge plans. Finally, the physician who will be providing the follow-up care for the infant must be apprised of the infant's history and current status, and plans must be made for regular visits. The first visit is usually 7 to 14 days after the infant leaves the hospital. Without careful consideration of each of these factors, the infant's long-term potential cannot be maximized.

KEY CONCEPTS

- Between 5% and 10% of infants born in the United States require special care beyond the level of the normal newborn nursery.
- Nursing care practice in the NICU requires scrupulous assessment skills, meticulous attention to detail, and gentle, hands-on care.
- Problems, both active and anticipated, must be identified, and appropriate intervention instituted in a timely manner.
- The neonate is at risk for a multitude of problems, including respiratory distress, bacterial and viral infection, birth anomalies (e.g., cardiac, gastrointestinal, neurologic), intracranial hemorrhage, birth injuries, seizures, hyperbilirubinemia, hypoglycemia, and hypothermia.
- The NICU environment, as structured by the nurse, should nurture both the infant and the parent to optimize outcome.
- The care often extends beyond the hospitalization, where long-term follow-up is needed to support the physical and developmental growth of the infant.

REFERENCES

American Academy of Pediatrics and American College of Obstetricians and Gynecologists. (1992). *Guidelines for perinatal care* (3rd ed.). Elk Grove Village, IL: Author.

Anast, C. (1991). Disorders of calcium and phosphorus metabolism. In H. W. Taeusch, R. A. Ballard, & M. E. Avery (Eds.), *Diseases of the newborn* (6th ed.). Philadelphia: W. B. Saunders.

Ballard, J. L., Khoury, J. C., Wedig, K., Wang, L., Eilers-Walsman, B. L., & Lipp, R. (1991). New Ballard score, expanded to include extremely premature infants. *Journal of Pediatrics, 119*(3), 417–423.

Bandstra, E. S., & Burkett, G. (1991). Maternal-fetal and neonatal effects of in utero cocaine exposure. *Seminars in Perinatology, 15*(4), 288–301.

Battaglia, F., & Lubchenco, L. (1967). A practical classification of newborn infants by weight and gestational age. *Journal of Pediatrics, 71*(2), 159–163.

Blackburn, S. T., & Loper, D. L. (1992). *Maternal, fetal, and neonatal physiology*, (p. 645). Philadelphia: W. B. Saunders.

Buist, N. R., & Tuerck, J. M. (1992). The practitioner's role in newborn screening. *Pediatric Clinics of North America, 39*(2), 199–211.

Clifford, S. H. (1954). Postmaturity: With placental dysfunction. Clinical syndrome and pathologic findings. *Journal of Pediatrics, 44*, 1.

Cole, F. S. (1991). Bacterial infections in the newborn. In H. W. Taeusch, R. A. Ballard, & M. E. Avery (Eds.), *Diseases of the newborn* (6th ed., p. 351). Philadelphia: W. B. Saunders.

Committee for the Classification of Retinopathy of Prematurity. (1984). An international classification of retinopathy of prematurity. *Archives of Ophthalmology, 102*, 1130–1134.

Cowett, R. M. (1992). Hypoglycemia and hyperglycemia in the newborn. In R. A. Polin & W. W. Fox (Eds.), *Fetal and neonatal physiology*. Philadelphia: W. B. Saunders.

Day, N. L., Cottreau, C. M., & Richardson, G. A. (1993). The epidemiology of alcohol, marijuana, and cocaine use among women of childbearing age and pregnant women. *Clinical Obstetrics and Gynecology, 36*(2), 232–245.

DeMarini, S., Tsang, R., & Rath, L. (1993). Fluids, electrolytes, vitamins, and trace minerals: Basis of ingestion, digestion, elimination and metabolism. In C. Kenner, A. Brueggemeyer, & L. P. Porter (Eds.), *Comprehensive neonatal nursing: A physiologic perspective*. Philadelphia: W. B. Saunders.

Dodson, W. E. (1992). Deleterious effects of intrauterine drug exposure on the nervous system. In R. A. Polin & W. W. Fox (Eds.), *Fetal and neonatal physiology*. Philadelphia: W. B. Saunders.

Hunter, D. G., & Mukai, S. (1992). Retinopathy of prematurity: Pathogenesis, diagnosis, and treatment. *International Ophthalmology Clinics, 32*(1), 163–184.

Johnson, S. H., & Grubbs, J. P. (1975). The premature infant's reflex behaviors: Effect on the maternal–child relationship. *Journal of Obstetric, Gynecological and Neonatal Nursing, 4*(3), 15–21.

Jones, K. L. (1988). *Smith's recognizable patterns of human malformation* (4th ed.). Philadelphia: W. B. Saunders.

Kenner, C., & Lott, J. W. (1994). Experimental therapy. In J. W. Lott (Ed.), *Neonatal infection: Assessment, diagnosis, and management* (pp. 137–149). Petaluma, CA: NICU.

Klaus, M. H., & Fanaroff, A. A. (1993). *Care of the high-risk neonate* (4th ed.). Philadelphia: W. B. Saunders.

Lubchenko, L. O. (1976). *The high risk infant* (p. 6). Philadelphia: W. B. Saunders.

Lubchenko, L. O., Hansman, C., & Blackstrom, L. (1968). In J. H. P. Jonxis, H. K. A. Visser, J. A. Troelstra (Eds.), *Aspects of prematurity and dysmaturity*. Springfield, IL: Charles C Thomas.

Ostrea, E. M., Brady, M., Gause, S., Raymundo, A. L., & Stevens, M. (1992). Drug screening of newborns by meconium analysis: A large-scale, prospective, epidemiologic study. *Pediatrics, 89*(1), 107–113.

Pietrantoni, M., & Knuppel, R. (1991). Alcohol use in pregnancy. *Clinics in Perinatology, 18*(1), 93–111.

Plessinger, M. A., & Woods, J. R. (1993). Maternal, placental, and fetal pathophysiology of cocaine exposure during pregnancy. *Clinical Obstetrics and Gynecology, 36*(2), 267–278.

Poland, R. L., & Ostrea, E. M., Jr. (1986). Neonatal hyperbilirubinemia. In M. H. Klaus & A. A. Fanaroff (Eds.), *Care of the high-risk neonate* (3rd ed., pp. 242–248). Philadelphia: W. B. Saunders.

Silverman, W., & Anderson, D. (1956). Controlled clinical trial of effects of water mist on obstructive respiratory signs, death rate and necropsy findings among premature babies. *Pediatrics, 17*, 1.

Theorell, C. J., & Degenhardt, M. (1993). Assessment and management of metabolic dysfunction. In C. Kenner, A. Brueggemeyer, & L. P. Porter (Eds.), *Comprehensive neonatal nursing: A physiologic perspective*. Philadelphia: W. B. Saunders.

Thorp, J. A., & Creasy, R. K. (1990). Postdate pregnancy. In N. M. Nelson (Ed.), *Current therapy in neonatal-perinatal medicine* (2nd ed.). Toronto: B. C. Decker.

Volpe, J. J. (1989). Neonatal seizures: Current concepts and revised classification. *Pediatrics, 84*(3), 422–428.

Volpe, J. J. (1995). *Neurology of the newborn* (3rd ed.). Philadelphia: W. B. Saunders.

Walfman, B. L. E. (1994). Hyaline membrane disease. In T. L. Gomella (Ed.), *Neonatology* (3rd ed., pp. 421–425). Norwalk, CT: Appleton and Lange.

Woods, J. R., Plessinger, M. A., & Clark, K. E. (1987). Effect of cocaine on uterine blood flow and fetal oxygenation. *Journal of the American Medical Association, 257*(7), 957–961.

Wright, L. L., & Catz, C. S. (1992). Drug distribution during fetal life. In R. A. Polin & W. W. Fox (Eds.), *Fetal and neonatal physiology* (Vol. I.). Philadelphia: W. B. Saunders.

BIBLIOGRAPHY

Avery, G. B., Fletcher, M. A., & MacDonald, M. G. (1994). *Neonatology: Pathophysiology and management of the newborn* (4th ed.). Philadelphia: J. B. Lippincott.

Bakewell-Sachs, S., & Porth, S. (1995). Discharge planning and home care of the technology-dependent infant. *Journal of Obstetric, Gynecologic, and Neonatal Nursing, 24*(1), 77–83.

Bass, L. S. (1991). What do parents need when their infant is a patient in the NICU? *Neonatal Network, 10*(4), 25–33.

Beachy, P., & Deacon, J. (1993). *Core Curriculum for Neonatal Intensive Care Nursing*. Philadelphia: W. B. Saunders.

Bell, G. L., & Lau, K. (1995). Perinatal and neonatal issues of substance abuse. *Pediatric Clinics of North America, 42*(2), 261–281.

Bernes, S. M., & Kaplan, A. M. (1994). Evolution of neonatal seizures. *Pediatric Clinics of North America, 41*(5), 1069–1104.

Best, M. A. (1993). The family in crisis. In P. Beachy & J. Deacon (Eds.), *Core Curriculum for Neonatal Intensive Care Nursing*. Philadelphia: W. B. Saunders.

Blackburn, S. (1992). Alterations of the respiratory system in the neonate: Implications for clinical practice. *Journal of Perinatal and Neonatal Nursing, 6*(2), 46–58.

Blackburn, S. (1995). Problems of preterm infants after discharge. JOGNN, *24*(1), 43–49.

Blackburn, S. T., & Loper, D. L. (1992). *Maternal, fetal, and neonatal physiology*. Philadelphia: W. B. Saunders.

Boeckling, A. C. (1992). Exogenous surfactant therapy for premature infants. *Journal of Perinatal and Neonatal Nursing, 6*(2), 59–66.

Brazelton, T. B. (1995). Working with families: Opportunities for early intervention. *Pediatric Clinics of North America, 42*(1), 1–9.

Chasnoff, I. J. (1991). Chemical dependency and pregnancy. *Clinics in Perinatology, 18*(1), 1–186.

Committee on Substance Abuse, American Academy of Pediatrics. (1990). Drug exposed infants. *Pediatrics, 86*(4).

Denehy, J. A. (1992). Interventions related to parent-infant attachment. *Nursing Clinics of North America, 27*(2), 425–443.

Dietch, J. S. (1993). Periventricular-intraventricular hemorrhage in the very low birth weight infant. *Neonatal Network, 12*(1), 7–16.

Drake, E. (1995). Discharge teaching needs of parents in the NICU. *Neonatal Network, 14*(1), 49–53.

Dubowitz, L., Dubowitz, V., & Goldberg, C. (1970). Clinical assessment of gestational age in the newborn infant. *Journal of Pediatrics, 77*(1), 1–10.

Franck, L., & Vilardi, J. (1995). Assessment and management of opioid withdrawal in ill neonates. *Neonatal Network, 14*(2), 39–48.

Gerdes, J. S. (1991). Clinicopathologic approach to the diagnosis of neonatal sepsis. *Clinics in Perinatology, 18*(2), 361–381.

Gray, B. M., Egan, M. L., & Pritchard, D. G. (1990). The group B streptococci: From natural history to the specificity of antibodies. *Seminars in Perinatology, 14* (suppl. 4), suppl., 10–21.

Griffin, T. (1990). Nurse barriers to parenting in the special care nursery. *Journal of Perinatal and Neonatal Nursing, 4*(2), 56–67.

Harrigan, R., Naber, M. M., Jensen, K. A., & Tse, A. (1993). Perinatal grief: Response to the loss of an infant. *Neonatal Network, 12*(5), 25–31.

Haut, C., & O'Brien, E. (1994). Supporting parental bonding in the NICU: A care plan for nurses. *Neonatal Network, 13*(8), 19–25.

Huffman, D. M., Price, B. K., & Langel, L. (1994). Therapeutic handling techniques for the infant affected by cocaine. *Neonatal Network, 13*(5), 9–14.

Hummel, P. A., & Eastman, D. L. (1991). Do parents of preterm infants suffer chronic sorrow? *Neonatal Network, 10*(4), 59–65.

Kanto, W. P., Hunter, J. E., & Stoll, B. J. (1994). Recognition and medical management of necrotizing enterocolitis. *Clinics in Perinatology, 21*(2), 335–346.

Kenner, C., Brueggemeyer, A., & Porter, L. P. (1993). *Comprehensive neonatal nursing: A physiologic perspective.* Philadelphia: W. B. Saunders.

Kliegman, R. M., Walker, W. A., & Yolken, R. H. (1994). Necrotizing enterocolitis: Research agenda for a disease of unknown etiology and pathogenesis. *Clinics in Perinatology, 21*(2), 437–456.

Korones, S. B., & Bada-Ellzey, H. S. (1993). *Neonatal decision making.* St. Louis: Mosby–Year Book.

Kosloske, A. M., & Musemeche, C. A. (1989). Necrotizing enterocolitis of the neonate. *Clinics in Perinatology, 16*(1), 97–111.

Koszarek K. (1991). Nursing assessment and care for the neonate in acute respiratory distress. In J. Nugent (Ed.), *Acute respiratory care of the neonate.* Petaluma, CA: NICU.

Lott, J. W. (1994). *Neonatal infection: Assessment, diagnosis, and management.* Petaluma, CA: NICU.

MacKendrick, W., & Caplan, M. (1993). Necrotizing enterocolitis: New thoughts about pathogenesis and potential treatments. *Pediatric Clinics of North America, 40*(5), 1047–1060.

Mattson, S., & Smith, J. E. (1993). *Core curriculum for maternal-newborn nursing.* Philadelphia: W. B. Saunders.

Merenstein, G. B., & Gardner, S. L. (1993). *Handbook of neonatal intensive care* (3rd ed.). St. Louis: Mosby–Year Book.

Novotny, E. J. (1993). Neonatal seizures. *Seminars in Perinatology, 17*(5), 351–356.

Nowicki, P. T., & Nankervis, C. A. (1994). The role of the circulation in the pathogenesis of necrotizing enterocolitis. *Clinics in Perinatology, 21*(2), 219–234.

Nugent, J. (1991). *Acute respiratory care of the neonate.* Petaluma, CA: Neonatal Network.

Polin, R. A., & Fox, W. W. (1992). *Fetal and neonatal physiology.* Philadelphia: W. B. Saunders.

Pomerance, J. J., & Richardson, C. J. (1993). *Neonatology for the clinician.* Norwalk, CT: Appleton and Lange.

Pramanik, A. K., Holtzman, R. B., & Merritt, T. A. (1993). Surfactant replacement therapy for pulmonary diseases. *Pediatric Clinics of North America, 40*(5), 913–936.

Remington, J. S., & Klein, J. O. (1990). *Infectious diseases of the fetus and newborn infant.* Philadelphia: W. B. Saunders.

Rushton, C. H. (1990). Necrotizing enterocolitis: Part II. Treatment and nursing care. *American Journal of Maternal Child Nursing, 15*(5), 309–313.

Schwarz, E. H., Trotter, C., & Maurer, B. W. (1990). Neonatal sepsis: Controversial therapies. *ResMedica, 5*(4), 33–40.

Sheldon, R. E., & Venkataraman, P. S. (1990). Tetany. In N. M. Nelson (Ed.), *Current therapy in neonatal-perinatal medicine* (2nd ed.). Toronto: B. C. Decker.

Shellabarger, S. G., & Thompson, T. L. (1993). The critical times: Meeting parental communication needs throughout the NICU experience. *Neonatal Network, 12*(2), 39–45.

Snyderman, S. E. (1990). Phenylketonuria. In N. M. Nelson (Ed.), *Current therapy in neonatal-perinatal medicine* (2nd ed.). Toronto: B. C. Decker.

Stamos, J. K., & Rowley, A. H. (1994). Timely diagnosis of congenital infections. *Pediatric Clinics of North America, 41*(5), 1017–1034.

Stoll, B. J. (1994). Epidemiology of necrotizing enterocolitis. *Clinics in Perinatology, 21*(2), 205–218.

Taeusch, H. W., Ballard, R. A., & Avery, M. E. (1991). *Diseases of the newborn* (6th ed.). Philadelphia: W. B. Saunders.

Tappero, E. P., & Honeyfield, M. E. (1993). *Physical assessment of the newborn.* Petaluma, CA: NICU.

Valaes, T. N., & Harvey-Wilkes, K. (1990). Pharmacologic approaches to the prevention and treatment of neonatal hyperbilirubinemia. *Clinics in Perinatology, 17*(2), 245–273.

Zahr, L. K., & Montijo, J. (1993). The benefits of home care for sick premature infants. *Neonatal Network, 12*(1), 33–37.

Zaichkin, J., & Houston, R. F. (1993). The drug-exposed mother and infant: A regional center experience. *Neonatal Network, 12*(3), 41–49.

22

The Child With an Infectious Disease

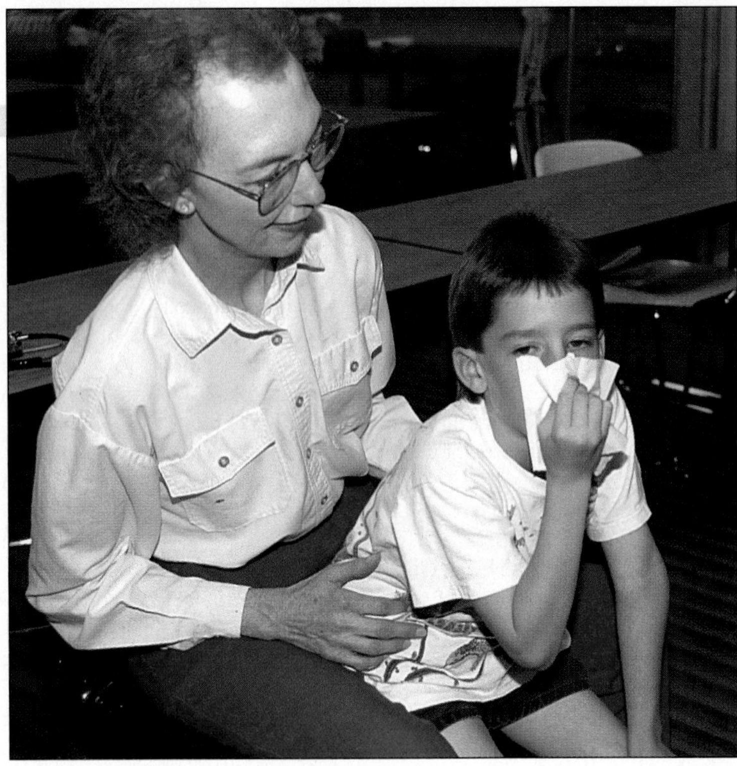

CHAPTER OVERVIEW

LEARNING OBJECTIVES

After studying this chapter, you should be able to:

- Describe the infectious process.
- Describe the modes of transmission for infectious diseases.
- Discuss the types of vaccines.
- Discuss the recommendations for scheduled vaccines.
- Discuss the pathophysiology, clinical manifestations, complications, and nursing management of childhood infectious diseases.
- Discuss the pathophysiology, clinical manifestations, complications, and nursing management of sexually transmitted diseases.
- Use the nursing process to describe the nursing care of a child with an infectious disease.

KEY TERMS

adaptive immune system: a defense system that recognizes foreign invaders, synthesizes and delivers immune products to infection sites, directs action against invaders, and has deactivation mechanisms

antitoxin: a particular kind of antibody produced by the body in response to the presence of a toxin

attenuated vaccine: vaccines derived from microorganisms or viruses whose virulence has been weakened owing to passage through another host

exanthem: an eruption or rash on the skin

immunity: resistance of the body to the effects of a harmful organism or its toxin

inactivated vaccines: vaccines that contain killed microorganisms

infection: invasion of an organism by a pathogenic or nonpathogenic organism, such as bacteria, viruses, protozoa, helminths, or fungi

inflammation: a tissue response to injury or destruction of cells

innate immune system: a host defense system that consists of barriers (skin), phagocytosis, and circulating soluble factors

pathogen: a disease-producing microorganism

prodrome: the initial stage of a disease; symptoms indicative of an approaching disease

toxin: a poison produced by pathogenic microorganisms

vector: a carrier that transfers an infective agent from one host to another

virulence: the ability of an organism to produce its effect

Infectious diseases are a major reason health care is sought for infants and children. Although most infections are not life-threatening, some children develop complications that can be fatal. At increased risk is the infant or child with an immature or compromised immune system. In addition, there is an impact on the family when a child is ill. Absence from work and the accompanying missed income can be devastating, for both single- and two-income families.

Nurses in both community and hospital settings should be able not only to recognize the signs and symptoms of infectious diseases, but also to educate parents about them. In the hospital setting, relatively mild diseases, such as chickenpox, may pose potentially fatal problems to the immunosupressed child. In such cases, the staff nurse must assess and recognize the signs and provide appropriate protection by isolating the infected child. In the community setting, the office or school nurse may be the professional who first recognizes the manifestations of infectious diseases, and must take measures to limit the exposure of other children.

Many infectious diseases present with subtle and common symptoms that may be difficult to identify. Because rashes and fever are common symptoms of many diseases, it is very important to obtain a complete history, including the earliest signs of the developing disease (prodrome), recent exposures, and a description of the rash. Once the causative organism and disease are identified, the focus of care will be to provide comfort measures for symptoms (e.g., fever and itching) and to prevent the spread of the disease. The family and child may also require assistance in adjusting to the isolation necessitated by the disease. Finally, the nurse must educate the child and parents as to the modes of transmission for infectious diseases and the importance of immunizations.

CLINICAL REFERENCE PAGES

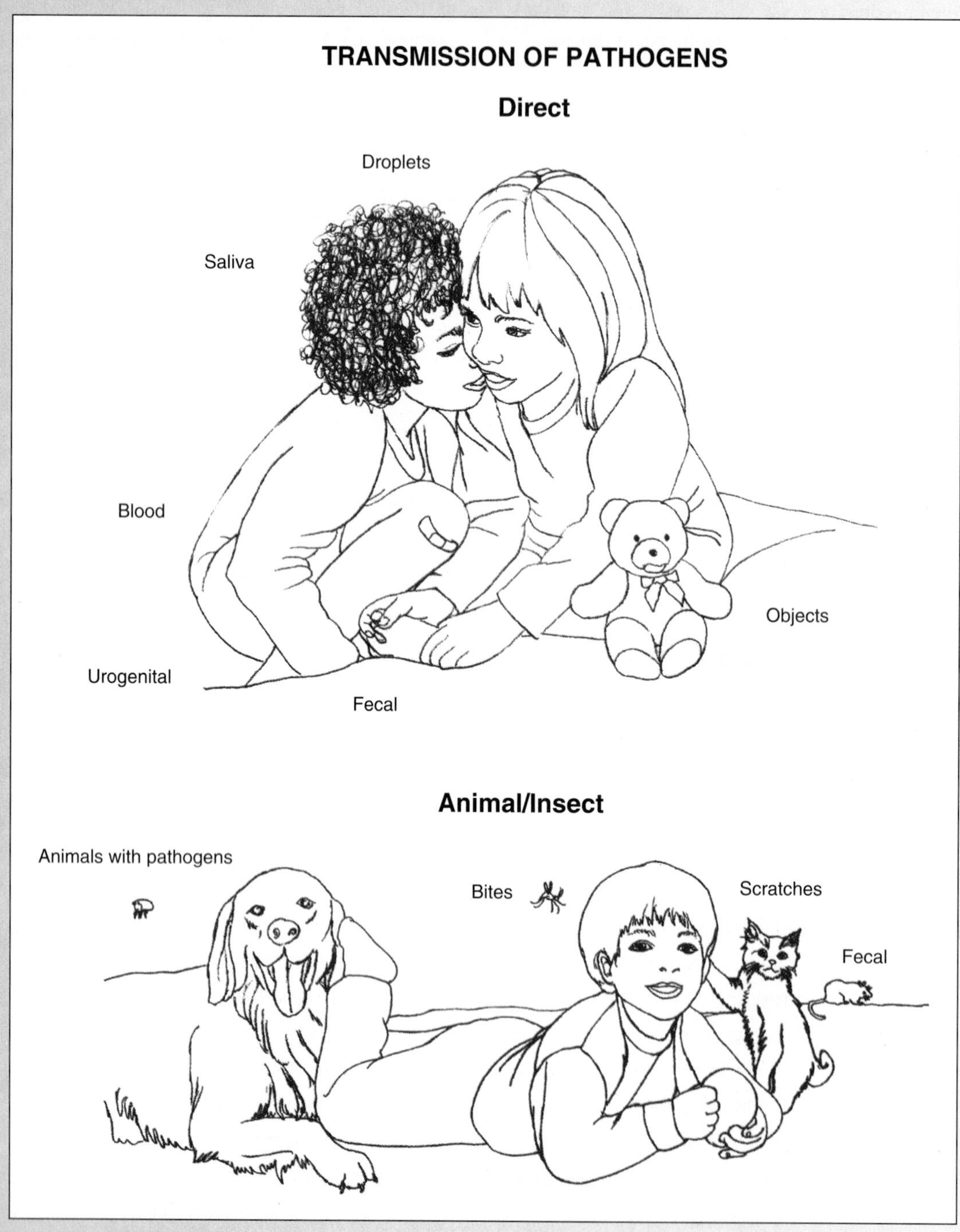

REVIEW OF DISEASE TRANSMISSION

Microorganisms exist throughout both external and internal environments. Most of them are harmless residents—a normal part of human flora. However, an organism that invades body tissue, causing tissue damage and disease, is a **pathogen.** For pathogens to invade a host, they must breach the normal host defenses, either by attaching to or penetrating the host. The power of these pathogens, known as their **virulence,** depends on their ability to overcome the host defense mechanisms. Thus, a highly virulent organism can cause disease with relative ease.

Microorganisms can have one of several relationships with the host: commensalism, mutualism, or parasitism (see accompanying box). Those that cause infectious disease are classified into five types: bacteria, viruses, fungi, protozoa, and helminths. The specific properties of each

Microorganisms and Host Relationships

- *Commensalism:* Host provides shelter and food for the organism; organism retains the ability to exist independently.
- *Mutualism:* Host provides shelter and food for the organism; both benefit.
- *Parasitism:* Host provides shelter and food; the parasite benefits, but the host may be harmed.

are discussed later in the chapter, along with related diseases.

Exogenous pathogens are those that are transmitted from outside the body. They are transmitted by direct contact, animal or insect contact, through contaminated food or water, or by contact with a contaminated object. The organisms are carried by a **vector** from one host to another. The vector may be an insect or an animal. For example, a certain species of mosquito carries the malaria parasite; likewise, certain bats carry the rabies microorganism. Transmission may occur by inhalation, ingestion, injection (insect bites), or direct contact (sexual). During pregnancy, for instance, pathogens from the woman may invade the fetus; thus, a woman whose birth canal is infected can transmit the infectious organisms to her newborn infant. Breast milk may also be the source of the pathogen, if it is infected.

Endogenous transmission of pathogens involves the body's normal flora or microorganisms. Normally, the human flora contain harmless microorganisms. They exist in the skin, nose, mouth, gastrointestinal tract, and urogenital tract. For example, *Staphylococcus epidermidis* inhabits the skin, and *Escherichia coli* is found in the intestines. These microorganisms are beneficial, playing an important role in the body's defenses. They help prevent colonization by virulent pathogens by maintaining an acidic pH environment to discourage pathogen attachment; by taking up epithelial space to prevent growth of pathogens; and by stimulating the immune system. Nevertheless, situations may arise in which these normally benign organisms become virulent, as will be described.

Infection and Host Defenses. The first stage of **infection** begins with *colonization.* Microorganisms invade either by adhering to tissues or invading cells. When replication of the pathogen first begins, it does not cause tissue damage. Thus, colonization can occur without development of a clinical infection. As the host "recognizes" the invasion, the defense system—the immune response—is activated. There are two components of the immune response: (1) the **innate immune system** or nonspecific immune response, and (2) the adaptive immune system, or nonspecific immune response (see Chapter 23).

For a discussion of pediatric differences in the immune system, see the Clinical Reference Pages in Chapter 23.

The first line of defense in the innate immune system is the skin. Generally, the skin serves as a barrier, preventing colonization of most pathogens: The acid secreted in sweat and by sebaceous glands inhibits pathogenic invasion. Mucous membranes trap the organisms, preventing them from adhering to the epithelial walls. Tears, saliva, and urine wash, flush, and protect epithelial cells from invading organisms. Nevertheless, the innate system may be unable to prevent the invasion. Phagocytosis, the process by which phagocytic cells are able to digest and thereby destroy foreign microorganisms, is overwhelmed. Large numbers of pathogens, or their **toxins,** can inhibit phagocytosis. When this occurs, the **adaptive immune system** is activated. This system "recognizes" and responds to pathogens and destroys them. The adaptive immune system "imprints" these pathogens so that if the body again encounters them, the response will be rapid and specific.

Transmission of Pathogens. For a pathogen to maintain its infectious state, it must be transmitted to another host. Exit transmission occurs through several sources (see preceding figure). From the respiratory tract, for example, pathogens are shed through sneezing, coughing, and talking. Because these transmission mechanisms are relatively uncontrollable, infections can easily be spread in crowded conditions; that is, one person can directly spread pathogens to another person's respiratory tract.

Pathogens may also be shed through fecal matter. When personal hygiene is poor and handwashing is not routinely practiced, there are ample opportunities for pathogens to enter through the mouth. Unclean hands may also contaminate food.

In the urogenital tract, pathogenic transmission does not generally occur through infected urine. Rather, sexual activity involving direct mucosal contact is the most common means of transmission of sexually transmitted diseases (STDs). Newborn infants can be infected by direct contact during birth if the mother's birth canal is infected. Saliva is another avenue of transmission, as is direct contact with infected skin. Pathogens can also be present in breast milk and can infect a nursing infant.

A tick or mite can inject pathogens into the skin and blood of the host. Contamination with the blood of the infected host can then occur through transfusions, blood products, and use of contaminated needles. Moreover, a pregnant woman can transmit such pathogens through the placenta.

Immunity. **Immunity** is the resistance of the body to the effects of harmful agents. It occurs as an antigen-antibody reaction that takes place whenever a foreign agent or its toxins enter the bloodstream. Immunity can be either active or passive (see Chapter 23).

IMMUNIZATIONS

Immunizations are effective in decreasing and, in some cases, eliminating childhood infectious diseases. Smallpox has been virtually eliminated, and the incidence of diphtheria, pertussis, tetanus, measles, mumps, rubella, and poliomyelitis has greatly declined in the United States. This success has not been achieved without controversy and change. In the 1970s and 1980s, the safety of the pertussis portion of the diphtherial/tetanus/pertussis (DTP) vaccine was questioned (Cody et al., 1981; Kulenkampff et al., 1974). The reported incidence of children presenting with acute, severe encephalopathy and, in rare instances, permanent brain damage within 1 to 2 days after receiving the DTP vaccine raised many questions (Cherry et al., 1988). In response, controlled studies were conducted that indicated that there was no significant causal relationship between the pertussis vaccine and permanent neurologic illnesses (Griffin et al., 1991; Walker et al., 1988; Howson & Fineberg, 1992; Blumberg et al., 1993). The 1994 report by the National Institute of Medicine concluded that, on rare occasions, acute encephalopathy after DTP vaccination might result in permanent neurologic damage (Chen et al., 1995). However, the risk of permanent damage was determined to be so small that it was found not to outweigh the risk of the disease (Larson, 1994). With the concern over the safety of the pertussis vaccine, some parents elected not to immunize their children, which resulted in an increase in pertussis cases. Medical concern has led to the development of the acellular pertussis vaccine, which has fewer reported side effects (Marcinak et al., 1993; Pichichero et al., 1993). The acellular vaccine is presently licensed only for use as the fourth and fifth dose of DTP (Wexler, 1995c).

Despite the availability of immunizations, some diseases have reemerged. During the 1980s, there was a rising incidence of measles with outbreaks occurring in three major groups: preschoolers, school-age, and college-age. The outbreak of the disease in preschoolers represented a failure to administer the vaccine at the recommended age. In the school-age and college-age populations, however, the disease was identified as not preventable because almost all of those affected had been immunized previously (Markowitz et al., 1989). Those factors identified as contributing to the rising incidence of communicable disease are listed in the accompanying box (American Academy of Pediatrics, 1989; Brunell, 1990).

Major reasons identified for low immunization rates during health care visits include providers who lack knowledge regarding contraindications for giving immunizations and providers who are unwilling to administer multiple vaccines. Other reasons are inadequate access to medical care and the lack of public knowledge regarding immunizations (Hutchins et al, 1989; McConnochie & Roghmann, 1992; Abbotts & Osborn, 1993).

Barriers to Immunization

Complexity of the health care system. Parents delay vaccinating children when they become confused or frustrated with the health care system. Special barriers include:

- Appointment-only clinics
- Excessively long waiting periods
- Inconvenient scheduling
- Inaccessible clinic sites
- The need for formal referral from a primary health care provider
- Language and cultural barriers

Expense of immunization services.

Parental misconceptions about disease severity, vaccine efficiency and safety, complications, and contraindications (see below).

Inaccurate record-keeping by parents and health care workers.

Reluctance by the health care worker to give more than two vaccines during the same visit.

Lack of public awareness of the need for immunizations.

COMMON MISCONCEPTIONS ABOUT ADMINISTRATION AND SAFETY OF VACCINES

The following conditions or circumstances are NOT true contraindications to the administration of vaccines:

- Mild acute illness with low-grade fever or mild diarrhea in an otherwise normal child
- A reaction to a previous dose of DTP vaccine with only soreness, redness, or swelling in the immediate vicinity of the injection site

Factors Contributing to the Rising Incidence of Communicable Disease

- Low immunization rate in inner-city preschool children
- Outbreak of disease in infants too young to be immunized
- Outbreak of disease in previously immunized children
- Failure to respond to immunization in some vaccinated children
- Waning immunity

During the 1990s, many changes have been made in the scheduling of childhood immunizations. Additional changes will likely be made in the coming years with the advent of new vaccines currently being tested. One of the goals of the United States government is to have completed immunization of 90% of children aged 2 years by the year 2000 (U.S. Department of Health and Human Services, 1990). Immunization is a critical component of a child's health care. Knowledge of immunization schedules and an awareness of potential delays will aid the health care provider in the identification of children who have not been fully immunized. Health care providers must provide parents with accurate information regarding immunizations, as they remain the primary and safest means of managing preventable infectious diseases.

Types of Vaccines

Artificially active or artificially passive immunity is produced through the administration of a vaccine. Several preparations of vaccines can accomplish immunity, including the following:

- **Live or Attenuated Vaccines**—Vaccines that have had their virulence (potency) diminished so as to not produce a full-blown clinical illness. In response to vaccination, the body produces antibodies and causes immunity to be established. Examples include measles and hepatitis A vaccines.
- **Killed or Inactivated Vaccines**—Vaccines that contain pathogens made inactive by either chemicals or heat. These vaccines, which are noninfectious, cause the body to produce antibodies. Their disadvantage is that they elicit a limited immune response from the body; therefore, several doses are required. Examples include the Salk polio, rabies, and pertussis vaccines.
- **Toxoids**—Bacterial toxins that have been made inactive by either chemicals or heat. The toxins cause the body to produce antibodies. Examples include diphtheria and tetanus vaccines.
- **Human Immune Globulin**—Obtained from the pooled blood of many people, this type of vaccine provides antibodies to a variety of diseases, such as measles, rubella, and infectious hepatitis. Its disadvantage is that it only offers temporary passive immunity. Some immune globulin can be disease-specific, and is derived from individuals with a specific disease.
- **Animal Serums (Antitoxins)**—Derived from the serum of immunized animals, these vaccines have the disadvantage of being foreign substances, which may cause hypersensitivity reactions. Thus, a history and sensitivity testing should precede vaccine administration. The serums derived from this method are used to stimulate production of antibodies for hepatitis, chickenpox, rabies, diphtheria, smallpox, cytomegalovirus (CMV), botulism, snakebites, and spider bites.

Immunization Schedule

Two agencies make recommendations regarding vaccinations in the United States. They work closely together and generally their recommendations are similar. The Advisory Committee on Immunization Practices (ACIP) is responsible for determining the recommendations for the public sector. The American Academy of Pediatrics (AAP) Committee on Infectious Diseases is responsible for recommendations concerning private pediatric practice. Collectively, these two entities have made recommendations that have resulted in a number of changes over the past few years. Changes in recommendations are published in *Morbidity and Mortality Weekly Reports (MMWR)* for the ACIP and in *Pediatrics* for the AAP.

Please see **Appendix A: Recommended Childhood Immunization Schedule, United States** for the American Academy of Pediatrics' recommendations on immunization. See also Table 22–1.

Recent recommendations incorporate the addition of *Haemophilus influenzae B (Hib)* and hepatitis B vaccines to the vaccination schedule. In addition, a second dose of the measles vaccine and a fourth dose of oral poliovirus vaccine (OPV) have been added. The acellular pertussis vaccine is approved for use as the fourth and fifth doses. The varicella vaccine has been licensed for use in individuals older than 1 year of age who have not had varicella (AAP, 1995). A hepatitis A vaccine was licensed in early 1995 for use in individuals older than 2 years of age. Final recommendations have not been released, but the hepatitis A vaccine has been recommended for high-risk groups, including individuals traveling in countries with a high incidence of hepatitis A; persons in communities with frequent outbreaks of hepatitis A; intravenous drug users; individuals who engage in homosexual activity; and persons with chronic liver disease (Clark, 1996; Wexler, 1995a). Recent recommendations from the Centers for Disease Control and Prevention (CDC) and ACIP may have an effect on the polio vaccine schedule. It has been recommended that the enhanced inactivated polio vaccine be used for the first two doses, followed by two doses of oral polio vaccine. However, it is not expected that this change will be adopted before 1997 (AAP, 1995).

All states require immunizations for children enrolled in licensed child care programs and school. Some states further require immunizations in the upper grades and at the time of college entrance.

A group of children who may be overlooked are those who receive home-schooling. It is of utmost importance, therefore, that immunization records be traced and that vaccinations be given over the course of the fewest number of visits possible.

Text continued on page 594

TABLE 22–1 *Summary of Rules of Childhood Immunization*

VACCINE (STORAGE TEMPERATURE)	AGE USUALLY GIVEN	AGE RULES	FOR PERSONS WHO HAVE FALLEN BEHIND	CONTRAINDICATIONS AND PRECAUTIONS†	RULES OF SIMULTANEOUS ADMINISTRATION	ROUTE
DTP (Consider use of a combined DTP-Hib vaccine.) DTaP (35–46°F)	2 mo, 4 mo, 6 mo, 12–15 mo, 4–6 yr. May start as early as 6 weeks old. May give dose #4 as early as 12 mo old if 6 mo have elapsed since #3. Consider DTaP for doses #4 & #5, but use no earlier than 15 mo.	DTP is not given to children ≥ 7 yr. (Use Td instead.) Consider for doses #4 & #5, at age ≥ 15 mo.	For infant or young child, doses #2 & #3 may be given 4 weeks after previous dose. Dose #4 may be given as soon as 6 months after dose #3. If dose #4 is given before the child's 4th birthday, wait at least 6 months for dose #5. If dose #4 is given after the child's 4th birthday, dose #5 is not needed.	Previous anaphylactic reaction to this vaccine Moderate or severe illness Previous encephalopathy within 7 days after DTP Undiagnosed progressive neurologic problem Previous history of fever ≥ 105°F within 48 hours after dose** Previous continuous crying lasting 3 or more hours** Previous convulsion within 3 days after immunization** Previous pale or limp episode, or collapse** DTaP: Same contraindications and precautions as for DTP	Can give with all others at separate sites	IM
DT (child) (35–46°F)	Only used if child had serious reaction to "P" in DTP, or has an unstable neurologic disorder.	"D" (larger dose of diphtheria toxoid) is not given to children ≥ 7 yr.	Use as you would for DTP but only when there has been a contraindication to the "P" component of the DTP.	Previous anaphylactic reaction to this vaccine Moderate or severe illness	Can give with all others at separate sites	IM
TD (adult) (Store at 35–46°F)	Booster now recommended between ages of 11–16 yr, then every 10 yr.	For unvaccinated children ≥ 7 years & adults, a primary series is needed (childhood DTPs count; see next box).	For those never vaccinated or those who have fallen behind: • #1 • #2 given 1 month later • #3 given 6 months after #2 • Booster given every 10 years for adults.	Previous anaphylactic reaction to this vaccine Moderate or severe illness	Can give with all others at separate sites	IM

OPV (Store at ≤ 7°F)	2 mo, 4 mo, 6 mo, 4–6 yr. May start as early as 6 weeks of age. ACIP, AAFP recommend dose #3 at 6 mo. AAP recommends dose #3 at 6–18 mo.	Not routinely given to anyone 18 years or older. New recommendation of ACIP (11/94) is to give dose #3 at 6 mo *instead of* at 15–18 mo.	ACIP recommends waiting 6 weeks between doses #1, #2, & #3; AAP says 4 weeks is adequate. If dose #3 is given after the child's 4th birthday, no other booster is needed. If dose #3 is given after the child's 4th birthday, ACIP recommends waiting at least 6 weeks between doses #2 and #3.	Previous anaphylactic reaction to this vaccine Moderate or severe illness Cancer, leukemia, lymphoma, immunodeficiency or HIV Taking a drug that lowers resistance to infection (anti-CA, high-dose steroids) Someone in the household with the above problems IPV (inactivated polio vaccine) is available when OPV is contraindicated Consider IPV when an adult in the household or other close contact is not immune to (never vaccinated against) polio In pregnancy, neither OPV nor IPV is recommended, but if immediate protection is needed, use OPV	Can give with all others	PO
MMR (Store at 35–46°F)	Dose #1 at 12–15 mo. Dose #2 is given at 4–6 yr (ACIP, AAFP) or 11–12 yr (AAP). Can be given as early as 6 mo of age in an outbreak, but additional doses should be given as indicated above.	If dose #1 was given before 12 mo, dose #1 should be repeated at 12–15 mo, with a minimum of 1 mo between doses.	Give whenever behind. There should be a minimum spacing of 1 month between dose #1 and dose #2.	Previous anaphylactic reaction to this vaccine Moderate or severe illness Pregnancy or possible pregnancy within next 3 months (use contraception) Anaphylactic allergic response to eggs or neomycin Cancer, leukemia, lymphoma, or immunosuppression HIV positivity is *not* a contraindication Taking large doses of immunosuppressive drugs, including steroids. If blood products or immunoglobulin were recently received, consult ACIP/AAP recommendations regarding delay time.	Can give with all others at separate sites. (Space 1 month from varicella if not given at the same time.)	SC

(continued)

TABLE 22–1 *Summary of Rules of Childhood Immunization (continued)*

VACCINE (STORAGE TEMPERATURE)	AGE USUALLY GIVEN	AGE RULES	FOR PERSONS WHO HAVE FALLEN BEHIND	CONTRAINDICATIONS AND PRECAUTIONS[†]	RULES OF SIMULTANEOUS ADMINISTRATION	ROUTE
HbOC HibTITER or PRP-T ActHib OmniHib or	2 mo, 4 mo, 6 mo, 12–15 mo (4 doses). 2 mo, 4 mo, 6 mo, 12–15 mo (4 doses).	Only one dose of either HbOC, PRP-OMP, or PRP-T is given at 15 mo or older. Not routinely given to children ≥ 5 yr of age. Same as for HbOC.	These rules are for HbOC (HibTITER) and PRP-T (ActHib, OmniHib) only: If dose #1 is given up to 7 mo, give dose #2 & #3 spaced 2 mo after previous dose (1 mo minimum) and booster at 12–15 mo. If dose #1 is given at 7–11 mo (up til 12 mo), only 3 doses are needed; dose #2 is given 2 mo after #1; then a booster is given at 15 mo (minimum spacing of 1 mo between doses). If dose #1 was given at 12–14 mo, give booster at 15–16 mo. No further doses are needed. If the child is 15–60 mo, only one dose is needed.	Previous anaphylactic reaction to this vaccine Previous anaphylactic reaction to diphtheria toxoid if using HbOC (HibTITER). This vaccine contains small amounts of diphtheria toxoid. PRP-OMP (PedvaxHiB) does not. Moderate or severe illness	Can give with all others at separate sites	IM
PRP-OMP PedvaxHiB (Store at 35–46°F)	2 mo, 4 mo, 12–15 mo. (3 doses only).	Same as for HbOC.	These rules are for PRP-OMP (PedvaxHiB) only: If dose #1 is given up to 7 mo, give dose #2 spaced 2 mo later (1 mo minimum) and booster at 12 mo. If dose #1 is given at 7–11 mo, give dose #2 spaced 2 mo later (1 mo minimum) and booster at 12–15 mo. If dose #1 is given at 12–14 mo, give dose #2 spaced 2 mo later.			
Hep B[§] (Store at 35–46°F)	Dose #1 at 0–2 mo, #2 at 2–4 mo, #3 at 6–18 mo. If mother is HBsAg-positive: give at birth, 1–2 mo, 6 mo, plus HBIG at birth. If mother is not a carrier but is from an endemic area, complete the series by 12 mo of age. ACIP recommends vaccinating 11–12 yr olds not already vaccinated. AAP recommends vaccinating all adolescents.	Series can be started at any age; same spacing of doses as routine Strongly consider for all adolescents.	If the child has fallen behind, do not start over; rather, continue the series. Minimum spacing: 1 mo between doses #1 and #2; 2 mo between doses #2 and #3. Commonly used spacing options: 0, 1, 6 months; 0, 2, 4 months; or 0, 1, 4 months.	Previous anaphylactic reaction to this vaccine Hypersensitivity to thimerosal Moderate or severe illness	Can give with all others at separate sites	IM

	ACIP recommends catch-up vaccine for children <11 yr of age whose parents are from endemic areas. Vaccinate children and teens who are in high-risk groups (defined in ACIP statement on hepatitis B or Redbook).					
Varicella vaccine [Store at or below 5°F (−15°C)]	AAP recommends routinely giving at 12–18 mo. ACIP recommendations are expected to agree. AAP recommends vaccinating all children ≥ 12 mo old, adolescents, and young adults who have not had prior infection with chickenpox. ACIP recommendations are expected to agree.	Susceptible children ≤ 12 yr of age receive only one dose. Susceptible children and adults ≥ 13 yr of age receive 2 doses given 4–8 weeks apart.		Anaphylactic allergic response to neomycin. Blood dyscracias, leukemia, lymphomas, or immunosuppression, active tuberculosis, pregnancy.	Can be given with all others, but at separate sites. (Space 1 mo from MMR if not given at same time.)	SC

*For full immunization information, see recent ACIP statements as published in the *MMWR*, or the AAP recommendations as published in the *1994 Redbook*.

†AAFP recommendations agree with the ACIP recommendations.

‡Note: While moderate or severe acute illness is a reason to postpone vaccination, *mild acute illness is not.*

§Dosing of Hepatitis B vaccine: Engerix: 1)10 μg = dose for 0–19 yr olds (including infants of HBsAg-positive mothers). 2) 20 μg = dose for those ≥ 20 yr old. Recombivax-HB: 1) 2.5 μg = dose for infants born to HBsAg-negative mothers and children up to age 11 yr; 2) 5 μg = dose for infants of HBsAg-positive mothers and for children ages 11–19; 3) 10 μg = dose for ages ≥ 20 yrs.

Note: The two hepatitis B vaccines have different packaging and concentrations. Read package insert carefully to determine proper volume of vaccine to administer.

**These are precautions, not contraindications. Generally, when these conditions are present, the vaccine should not be given. However, there are situations when the benefit outweighs the risk and the vaccination should be considered (e.g., during a pertussis outbreak).

Adapted from ACIP, AAP*, and AAFP** by Deborah Wexler, MD, with review by Advisory Board ad hoc team, Immunization Action Coalition, May 1995.

This table was developed to combine the "rules of childhood immunization" onto one page. It was devised especially to assist health care workers in immunization clinics in determining appropriate use and scheduling of vaccines. It can be posted in immunization clinics or clinicians' offices. The table will be revised at least yearly because of the changing nature of national immunization recommendations.

Thank you to Coalition Advisory Board members William Atkinson, MD, MPH, Karl Chun, MD, Joan Foreman, PHN, Neal Halsey, MD, Robert Jacobson, MD, Samuel Katz, MD, Anne Kuettel, PHN, Harold Margolis, MD, James McCord, MD, Carolyn McKay, MD, Margaret Morrison, MD, for their review and comments on this table. Final responsibility for errors or omissions lies with the editor.

Your comments are welcome. Please send them to Deborah Wexler, MD, Immunization Action Coalition, 1573 Selby Ave., Suite 229, St. Paul, MN 55104 or call 612-647-9009, or fax 612-647-9131.

State requirements can be obtained from each state health department. Appendix A and Table 22–1 outline the current recommendations for immunization of healthy children in the United States.

Hepatitis B Vaccine. Recent recommendations include the administration of the hepatitis B vaccine to infants. Hepatitis B has become a major health problem. Previously, high-risk individuals were defined as those who had contact either through blood or sexual activity. Children were considered to be at high risk if they were born to infected mothers, or if they were adolescents engaging in certain high-risk behaviors, such as IV drug use, sexual activity with several partners, or sexual activity with homosexuals. Despite the use of these criteria to identify high-risk individuals, however, the rate continued to increase. As a result, recommendations were made to screen all pregnant mothers and to provide immunization during the perinatal period to those testing positive. Because of the high cost of the hepatitis B vaccine, some providers were reluctant to include this vaccine in the immunization schedule. In 1991, the ACIP recommended that the hepatitis B vaccine be given to all infants, regardless of their mother's status. The scheduling of the vaccine is determined by the degree of exposure. An infant whose mother tests positive receives human B immune globulin (HBIG), along with the first dose of the hepatitis B vaccine, within 12 hours of birth (CDC, 1991). The vaccination schedule for an infant whose mother tests negative consists of a series of three immunizations given at 0 months (birth), 1–2 months of age, and then 4 months after the initial dose. At-risk adolescents also should be identified. Because risk factors are often difficult to identify, adolescents living in communities with a high incidence of drug use, adolescent pregnancy, and/or sexually transmitted diseases should be universally vaccinated.

Pneumococcal Vaccine. Pneumococcal infections commonly cause acute otitis media, pneumonia, meningitis, and sinusitis in children. Pneumococcal infection is the major cause of bacteremia in infants and children 2 years of age or younger. Children with predisposing conditions, such as human immunodeficiency virus (HIV), nephrotic syndrome, and sickle cell disease, and those undergoing splenectomy or organ transplantation are considered to be at high risk for pneumococcal infections. There are 84 pneumococcal serotypes, some of which are prevalent only in children and others of which occur only in adults. Some types are penicillin-resistant. Children who are 2 years of age or older and who are at increased risk for acquiring a pneumococcal infection should be immunized. A 23-valent pneumococcal vaccine is currently available. For children younger than 2 years of age, the vaccine has limited effectiveness and is not, therefore, recommended. Children who are younger than 10 years of age and who remain at high risk should be revaccinated every 3 to 5 years (CID Redbook, 1994).

Meningococcal Vaccine. Meningococcal infections, which are most prevalent in children younger than 5 years of age, can cause meningococcemia, meningitis, and pneumonia. A meningococcal vaccine is recommended for children 2 years of age or older who belong to a high-risk group (those with asplenia, those receiving chemoprophylaxis, and those in semiclosed communities, such as daycare centers with a history of outbreaks). Routine immunization of children with this vaccine is not recommended. The duration of the vaccine's effectiveness is not known, but is likely to be less than 3 years. Children who continue to be at high risk should be considered for revaccination after 2 or 3 years (CID Redbook, 1994).

Children With an Uncertain History of Immunization

When a lapse in immunization occurs, the entire series does not have to be restarted. Rather, DTP, OPV, Hib, or hepatitis B vaccine should be administered at the next available visit. Charts of children should be flagged to remind health care providers of the immunization status of these children. In the case of children who have unknown or uncertain immunization status, appropriate immunization should be administered. Readministration of measles, mumps, and rubella (MMR); Hib vaccine; OPV; or hepatitis B vaccine to someone who is immune has no harmful effects. For children older than 7 years of age, the tetanus-diphtheria (Td) vaccine, rather than the DTP vaccine, should be administered (CID Redbook, 1994).

Refugee children present special difficulties, as their immunization status may vary from complete to incomplete. Relocation from refugee camps can hinder follow-up care. Moreover, refugees are at risk for tuberculosis and hepatitis B. They are tested before entering the United States but may enter the country while receiving treatment. Follow-up care is of utmost importance. Some may enter the United States without screening and should be evaluated for these diseases.

Table 22–2 presents recommendations for immunizing children who were not immunized during infancy.

Administration of Vaccines

The manufacturer's packaging insert for each vaccine includes recommendations for handling, storage, administration site, dosage, and route. Personnel responsible for handling vaccines should be familiar with storage requirements to minimize the risk of vaccine failures. When multidose vials are used, sterile technique should be used to prevent contamination. To ensure safe administration, the vaccines should be given by the recommended route. In children who have not yet developed the gluteal muscle (those younger than 2 years), the preferred site for intra-

TABLE 22-2 *Recommended Immunization Schedules for Children Not Immunized in the First Year of Life*

RECOMMENDED AGE/TIME	IMMUNIZATION
Children Younger than 7 Years	
First visit	DTP, HBV, MMR, OPV, Hib (for those < 5 years of age); tuberculin testing
Interval after first visit 1 month	DTP, HBV, (OPV may be given if accelerated vaccination is indicated)
2 months	DTP, OPV, Hib (for children who received first dose before 15 months of age)
>8 months	DTP, DTaP, HBV, OPV (unless third dose given earlier)
4–6 years (school entry)	DTP or DTaP (unless fourth dose given after 4 years of age); OPV (unless third dose given after 4 years of age)
11–12 years	MMR
10 years later	Td
Children 7 Years and Older	
First visit	HBV, OPV, MMR, Td
Interval after first visit: 2 months	HBV, Td, OPV (may be given 1 month after first visit if accelerated polio vaccination is indicated)
8–14 months	HBV, Td, OPV (not given if third dose was given earlier)
11–12 years	MMR
10 years later	Td

From Committee on Infectious Diseases (Redbook, 1994). *Report of the Committee on Infectious Diseases* (p. 24). Elk Grove, IL: American Academy of Pediatrics.

muscular (IM) injections is the anterolateral aspect of the thigh. The deltoid muscle can be used in children 18 months and older. The ventrogluteal site may be used in older children (see Chapter 19). Vaccines intended for IM administration need to be injected deep into the muscle mass to avoid irritation and possible necrosis. The needle used for IM injections must be long enough to reach the muscle mass. Generally, a needle measuring $\frac{7}{8}$ inch or longer is adequate for a normal 4-month-old infant (CID Redbook, 1994; Hick et al., 1989).

The nurse's responsibilities in administering vaccines are listed in the accompanying box.

The gluteal site is not recommended at any age for the administration of the hepatitis B vaccine. This is because there is diminished immunogenicity in the gluteal site (CID Redbook, 1994).

Nursing Responsibility in Administering Vaccines

- Know the recommended immunization schedule and the recommended alternative schedule for those with lapsed immunizations or unknown immunization history.
- Acquire up-to-date information because recommendations are revised frequently.
- Assess the family's beliefs and values to assist in the education of the family as to the rationale for immunizations, the risks and side effects, and the risks of nonimmunization.
- Take a careful history to determine possible contraindications or precautions, reporting any pertinent information to practitioner. Educate the family as to the rationale for any contraindications.
- "Gloves are not required when administering vaccinations unless the persons who administer the vaccine will come in contact with potentially infectious body fluids or have open lesions" (CID Redbook, 1994).
- Some vaccines come mixed into one syringe (DTP-Hib). Other vaccines should not be mixed. Check manufacturer's recommendations.
- Administer vaccines according to the manufacturer's recommended sites. Improper administration can result in "local irritation, induration, skin discoloration, inflammation, and granuloma formation" (CID Redbook, 1994).
- Aspirate to make sure that the needle has not been placed in a blood vessel.
- Wash hands before vaccine administration and between patients.
- Review with the parents common side effects and the signs of potential severe reactions that warrant contacting the practitioner.
- Administer prophylactic acetaminophen before or shortly after administration of DTP. Instruct the parents to continue age-appropriate dosing every 4 to 6 hours for at least 24 hours.
- For painful or red injection sites, apply cold compresses for the first 24 hours, then use warm or cold compresses as long as needed.
- Give multiple administrations in different sites and document those sites in the medical record.
- Document parental consent in the medical record. Documentation should also include the type of vaccine, date of administration, manufacturer and lot number, expiration date, administration site, any data pertinent to risks and/or side effects, and signature and title of the person administering the immunization.

More than one immunization may be administered at the same age or time. Some vaccines, such as DTP, are given as a multiple vaccine. When more than one injection is to be given, vaccines should be administered using separate syringes, not mixed into one. They should be given at different sites (preferably in different thighs), and the site used for each vaccine should be documented in order to identify possible reactions (Selekman, 1994).

> When giving DTP, Hib, and hepatitis B vaccines simultaneously, it is advisable to administer the most reactive vaccine (DTP) in one leg and to inject the others, which cause less of a reaction, into the other leg.

Precautions and Contraindications

Clearly, the main goal of a vaccine is to achieve immunity with the fewest possible side effects. Most vaccines have no side effects; when side effects do occur, they are usually mild. For example, fever and local irritation often occur in conjunction with the DTP vaccine, whereas fever and rash are frequently associated with the MMR vaccine.

Some severe side effects have been reported, however. These events are usually not predictable. There are reported cases of healthy children developing paralytic polio after administration of OPV. Reactions to the MMR vaccine have included anaphylactic reactions, both in children with and without a history of egg allergy. This has prompted consideration of other possible causative agents. For instance, the MMR vaccine contains neomycin, which may be the cause of the sensitivity. Prior to administration of the MMR vaccine, it is recommended that a thorough history be obtained by the health care provider, including any known history of allergy to eggs, neomycin, or related antibiotics (Kwittken et al., 1993; Levine & Lavi, 1991).

> Live measles vaccine is produced by chick embryo cell culture, so the possibility of anaphylactic hypersensitivity in children with egg allergies should be considered. If there is a question of sensitivity, children should be tested before administration of MMR vaccine. If a child tests positive for sensitivity, the killed measles vaccine may be given as an alternative.

> Any immunization may cause an anaphylactic reaction. All offices and clinics must have epinephrine 1:1000 available.

Immunocompromised Children. Children who are immunologically compromised should not receive live bacterial or viral vaccines in most cases. However, the nature of their immunodeficiency will determine whether some live vaccines may be administered safely. For instance, children who are receiving short-term low doses, or low to moderate long-term doses, of steroids may receive live viral vaccines, but those who are being treated with large amounts of systemic steroids should not receive live viral vaccines. The exception is children with HIV, who may receive the MMR vaccine but not OPV. The rationale for this is that the MMR vaccine does not shed the viruses.

> Siblings and household contacts of immunocompromised children should not receive the OPV, but may be given the inactivated poliovirus vaccine (IPV).

Education

All health care providers who administer immunizations are required by federal law to provide general information about immunizations to the child/parents, preferably in the family's native language. Before administering a vaccine, parents should read the federally required information about that vaccine and have the opportunity to ask questions. The providers must use either the Vaccine Information Pamphlets (VIPs) or a handout that provides all required information (CID Redbook, 1994). Each VIP pamphlet is 8 pages long, therefore, parents may have as many as 24 pages of information to read during a single office visit. It is necessary that the parents feel comfortable with the information, as well as with the answers to any questions. It has been shown that the VIPs do increase the knowledge level of the parents and are beneficial. Providers should consider providing the information prior to scheduled vaccinations so that parents can take the time to read all the information (Clayton et al., 1994). Providers are encouraged to obtain written informed consent for each vaccine administered. If signatures are not obtained, the patient's medical record should document that the vaccine information was reviewed.

> When taking an immunization history, the nurse should avoid asking the question, "Are your child's immunizations up to date?" This question will frequently be answered with a yes, but will fail to give the nurse sufficient information. The nurse may gain more information by asking "Can you tell me when and what was the last shot your child had?"

New Vaccines

Although many changes in immunization practices have already occurred, more will be forthcoming. Vaccines currently being tested are the CMV, herpes simplex, and the Epstein-Barr vaccine.

VIRAL INFECTIONS

Viruses are small parasitic organisms. They have some characteristic that cause them to be very different from other organisms. They contain only one type of nucleic acid—either DNA or RNA. This prevents the organisms from being able to reproduce on their own. Instead, a host cell is needed to allow the virus to replicate.

The virus first attaches itself to a host cell. Some of the viruses are selective as to the cells to which they attach; for example, the HIV virus prefers the T cell. After attachment, they must invade the interior of the cell. Replication of the virus' nucleic material begins after the envelope and capsule (capsid) are shed and the nucleic material of the virus is released into the cell; the host cell then assists in the formation of the necessary nucleic material. New capsules are formed and are released into the host and new host cells. The infected host cell can respond to the viral invasion by cell death (lysis) and destruction. Infected cells can also remain alive and continue to function while new viral particles are slowly released. This type of slow release is what occurs in a symptomless person who is a carrier of the virus.

A virus can invade a host, remaining dormant until a trigger stimulates the virus to begin replicating. Many of the triggering factors are not understood. However, some factors, such as stress, have been identified as triggers in such viral diseases as herpes simplex, which results in the formation of cold sores.

Viral Exanthems. An **exanthem** is defined as an eruption or rash on the skin. Several childhood diseases are characterized by rashes with different characteristics. Indeed, it is possible for rashes to have more than one characteristic (see Chapter 11, Common Skin Lesions, pp. 218–219). Viral exanthems presented in this section include rubeola (measles), rubella (German measles), erythema infectiosum (fifth disease), and roseola infantum.

Rubeola

(Red Measles, Hard Measles, Regular Measles)

Causative agent:	RNA virus
Incubation period:	7 to 14 days
Infectious period:	ranges from 1 to 2 days before onset of symptoms to 4 days after rash appearance
Transmission:	airborne particles or direct contact with infectious droplets
Immunity:	natural disease or live attenuated vaccine at 15 months and 4 to 6 years, or 11 to 12 years of age
Season:	winter/spring

Clinical Manifestations (Fig. 22–1). The measles virus enters the body and slowly spreads. Respiratory symptoms appear after about an average of 10 days. The child will have a profuse runny nose (coryza), cough, and fever. Conjunctivitis may be present, along with photophobia. *Koplik spots* appear approximately 2 days before the appearance of the rash. Koplik spots are small, blue-white spots with a red base found on the buccal mucosa. These spots last approximately 3 days, after which time they slough off. The measles rash usually begins behind the ears, at the hairline, on the forehead, and on the upper part of the neck. It spreads downward to the feet. The rash is red, maculopapular, blanches easily with pressure, and will gradually turn a brownish color. The duration of the rash is about 6–7 days.

A partially immune child, such as an infant younger than 9 months of age who has passively acquired maternal antibodies, or a child given immune gamma globulin, may contract modified measles. The prodromal period is shorter and the symptoms are minimal, with few to no Koplik spots. The rash progression follows the pattern of regular measles.

Atypical measles occurs in those who have received the killed measles vaccine. They present with a sudden onset of fever with a headache; dry, nonproductive cough; chest pain; and, rarely, Koplik spots. The rash, which has a yellow hue, begins on the distal extremities and spreads upward, stopping at the nipple line. There is edema of the extremities and there can be hepatosplenomegaly.

Complications. Owing to the respiratory involvement, secondary bacterial infections, such as pneumonia and otitis media, can occur. These are the most common complications. There may also be complications involving the central nervous system (CNS). Cases of encephalitis, seizures, and subacute sclerosing panencephalitis (SSPE) have been reported. (Levine & Lavi, 1991; Griffin et al., 1991).

Therapeutic Management. The treatment of measles is symptomatic whether the child is hospitalized or remains at home. If hospitalized, the child will require respiratory isolation. During the febrile period, the child should be restricted to quiet activities and bed rest.

The AAP has recommended that vitamin A be considered for the treatment of measles in certain circumstances, including:

- Children ages 6 months to 2 years who are hospitalized with complications (pneumonia, croup, diarrhea)
- Children older than 6 months of age who have the following risks: immunodeficiency, evidence of vitamin A deficiency, impaired intestinal absorption, or moderate to severe malnutrition

In such children, vitamin A has been found to reduce morbidity and mortality. It is believed that vitamin A plays a role in cell integrity and the immunity system (AAP, 1993).

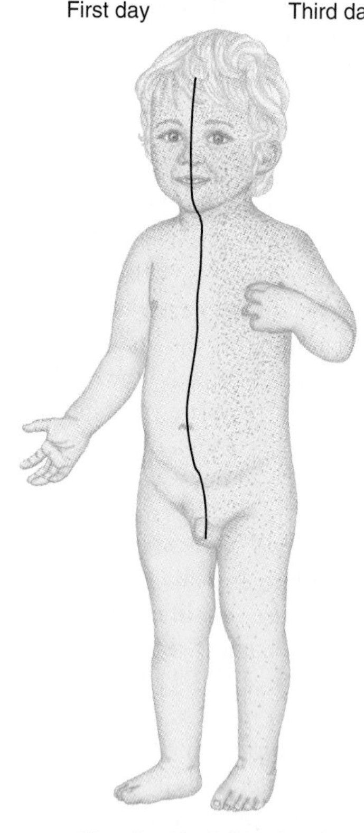

Measles Rash Distribution

- Preceded by Koplik spots on buccal mucosa
- Begins behind ears, at hairline, on upper neck, and spreads downward toward feet
- Red, maculopapular rash that gradually turns brownish
- Duration: 6–7 days

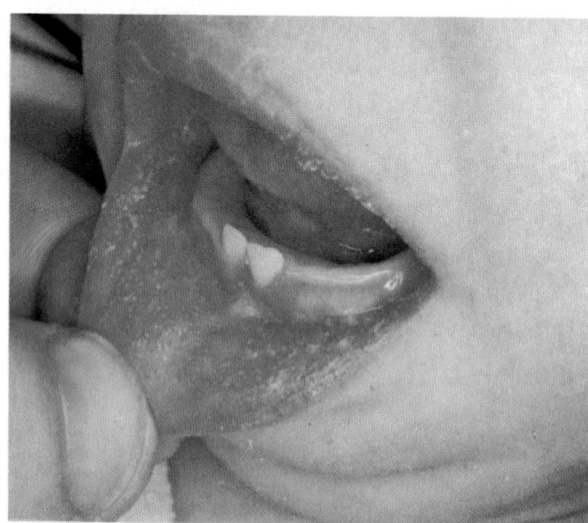

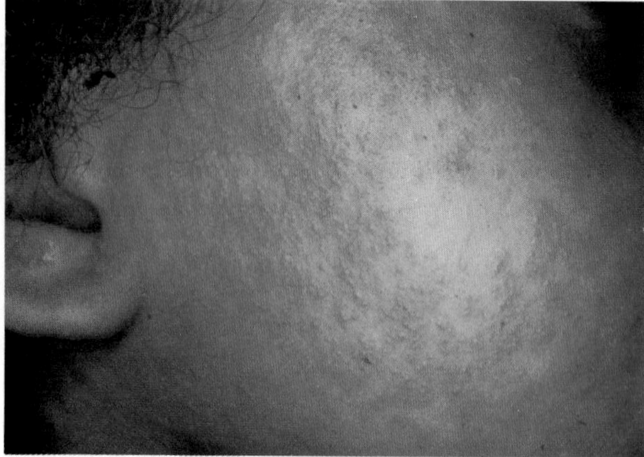

Measles Rash, Dark Skin

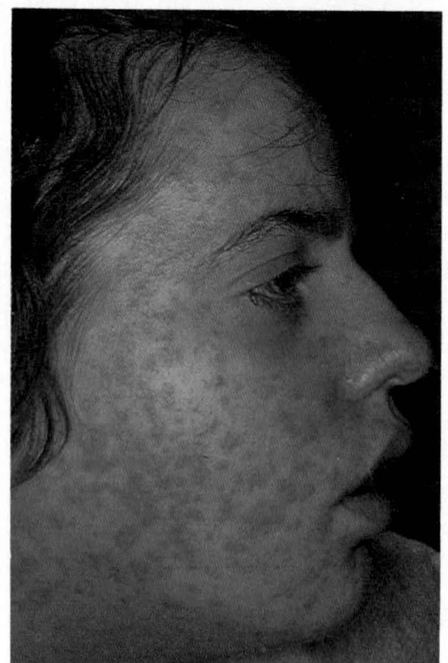

Measles Rash, Light Skin

Figure 22–1

Rubeola (measles) lesions and rash distribution. (Photos from Feigin, R. D., & Cherry, J. D. [Eds.]. [1992]. *Textbook of pediatric infectious diseases* [3rd ed.]. Philadelphia: W. B. Saunders, p. 773, Figs. 81–1 and 81–2; and Hurwitz, S. [1993]. *Clinical pediatric dermatology: A textbook of skin disorders of childhood and adolescence* [2nd ed.]. Philadelphia: W. B. Saunders, p. 350, Fig. 12–5.)

Respiratory isolation for a child with measles requires masks for those in close contact with the child. Gowns and gloves are not indicated. Handwashing is advised after touching the child or contaminated objects and before caring for another child. Articles that are contaminated should be bagged and labeled before reprocessing (CID Redbook, 1994).

Rubella

(3-Day Measles, German Measles)

Causative agent:	RNA virus
Incubation period:	14 to 21 days
Infectious period:	ranges from 10 days before onset of symptoms to 15 days after rash appearance
Transmission:	airborne particles or direct contact with infectious droplets; transplacental
Immunity:	natural disease or live attenuated vaccine at 15 months, 4 to 6 years, or 11 to 12 years of age
Season:	winter/spring

Clinical Manifestations (Fig. 22–2). Rubella is usually a mild disease for children and adults. The virus enters the host, producing a rash after about 14 to 16 days. It is common for young children to be asymptomatic until the appearance of the rash. Older children may complain of profuse nasal drainage, diarrhea, malaise, sore throat, headache, low-grade fever, polyarthritis, eye pain, aches, chills, anorexia, and nausea. In children all ages, there is usually lymphadenopathy involving the posterior cervical and posterior, auricular, and suboccipital nodes.

The rash presents as a pinkish-rose maculopapular exanthem which begins on the face, neck, scalp, and neck. It spreads downward to include the entire body within 1 to 3 days. As the rash spreads to the trunk, the rash on the face begins fading. Petechiae spots, which are reddish and pinpoint, may occur on the soft palate. This is referred to as Forschheimer's sign.

Complications. Rubella has relatively few complications. The most common are arthritis and arthralgia, which occur more often in adult women than in children or adolescents. Mild thrombocytopenia may also occur, but is usually self-limiting and of short duration. A rare complication

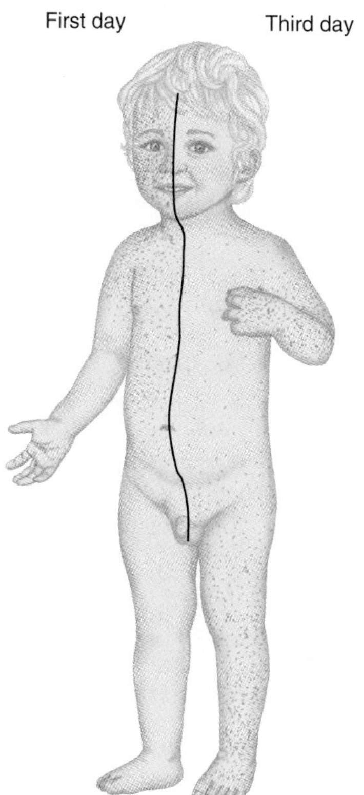

• Begins on face, neck, scalp, and spreads downward to entire body. Fades on face as it spreads to trunk.

• Pinkish, maculopapular

• Reddish, pinpoint petechiae may occur on soft palate (Forscheimer's sign)

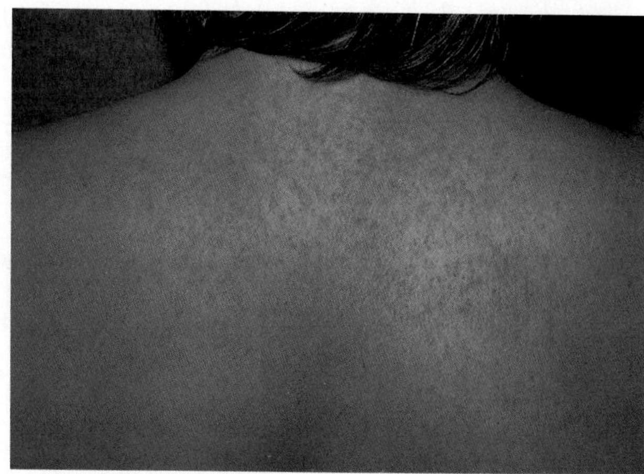

Figure 22–2
Rubella (German measles) lesions and rash distribution. (Photo from Hurwitz, S. [1993]. *Clinical pediatric dermatology: A textbook of skin disorders of childhood and adolescence* [2nd ed.]. Philadelphia: W. B. Saunders, p. 356, Fig. 12–13.)

is encephalitis, which is usually less severe than measles-related encephalitis.

Rubella has serious consequences for a pregnant mother and the fetus.

The most devastating complication of rubella occurs during the first trimester of a pregnancy, with at least one major congenital anomaly occurring in 21% to 54% of exposed fetuses. Infection during later months of pregnancy can also result in fetal damage. Maternal rubella is associated with an increased incidence of fetal death by stillbirths and abortions, an increased rate of premature births, and growth retardation (Bialecki et al., 1989).

Congenital rubella can result in growth retardation, cataracts, retinopathy, and cardiac anomalies. The most common complication is sensorineural deafness. Some of the manifestations may not be present at birth, but may develop at a later time. These late-occurring problems include mental retardation, diabetes mellitus, thyroid disorders, and encephalopathy.

Therapeutic Management. Treatment is generally supportive, and the disease is self-limiting.

Care of a child with rubella involves contact isolation. Infants with congenital rubella also require contact isolation. They should be considered contagious until they are 1 year old or until repeated cultures yield negative results. Some of these children will continue to shed the virus for up to 12 months. Contact isolation requires masks, gowns, and gloves for contact with any infectious material. Contaminated articles must be bagged and labeled before reprocessing (CID Redbook, 1994).

Erythema Infectiosum

(Parvovirus B19, Fifth Disease)

Causative agent:	Parvovirus 19
Incubation period:	4 to 14 days, or up to 20 days
Infectious period:	unknown, but thought to extend from the prodromal period until appearance of the rash
Transmission:	airborne particles, respiratory droplets, blood, blood products, transplacental
Immunity:	natural disease is thought to provide antibodies for immunity
Season:	winter/spring

Erythema infectrosum was first described in 1889. In 1975, parvovirus B19 was recognized as the causative agent, and the disease was classified as the fifth known childhood exanthem. This disease is most common in children ages 5 to 14 years, but may also occur in adults.

Clinical Manifestations (Fig. 22–3). Fifth disease is a relatively mild systemic disease. Typically, the child will be well, but will present with an intense, fiery red, edematous rash on the cheeks, which gives the appearance of the child having been slapped. Prior to the appearance of the rash, many children are asymptomatic or have nonspecific symptoms, such as headache, runny nose, malaise, and mild fever. The appearance of the rash may be aggravated by environmental temperatures. Approximately 1 to 4 days following the facial rash, an erythematous, maculopapular, lacy rash will appear on the trunk and extremities. This rash fades with a central clearing area, giving rise to the lacy appearance. Fifth disease may last for 2 to 39 days and may reappear when aggravated by factors such as exercise, warm baths, rubbing of the skin, and stress.

Complications. Owing to the mildness of the disease, there are usually no reported complications, especially in children. Most reported complications occur in the adult population. There can be mild to severe arthralgia. Children with chronic hemolytic anemia, sickle cell disease, or immunocompromised systems can be at risk. Because this virus attacks the hematopoietic cells of the bone marrow, it produces a decrease in the number of erythrocytes. Normally, this poses no problem except in individuals whose hemoglobin levels are already compromised. These children may experience transient aplastic crisis, which may be treated effectively with blood transfusions. Immunocompromised children respond to the use of IV immunoglobulin.

Pregnant women are at risk for intrauterine infection. Fifth disease has resulted in fetal death, hydrops, and miscarriages. Although the rate of fetal deaths secondary to fifth disease ranges from 9% (Feigin, 1992) to 20% (Waagner, 1993), there does not appear to be any correlation with any specific fetal deformities.

Therapeutic Management. No specific treatment is indicated, but supportive care as needed can be provided. Contact isolation is indicated for hospitalized children with fifth disease. Contact isolation requires gowns and gloves for contact, and bagging and labeling of contaminated materials before reprocessing (CID Redbook, 1994).

Roseola Infantum

(Exanthem Subitum, Sixth Disease, 3-Day Fever)

Causative agent:	human herpesvirus 6 (HHV-6)
Incubation period:	estimated to be 5 to 15 days
Infectious period:	unknown, but is thought to extend from the febrile stage to the time the rash first appears
Transmission:	saliva
Season:	spring and fall

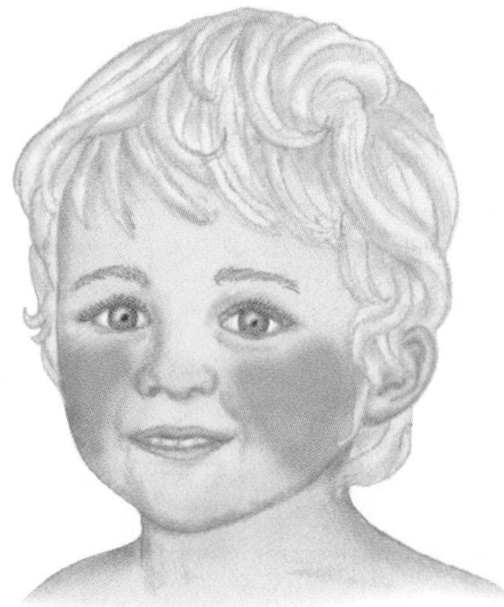

Erythema Infectiosum: "Slapped Cheek" Appearance
• Presents with fiery red edematous rash on cheeks—"slapped cheek" appearance
• Followed in 1–4 days by erythematous maculopapular lacy rash on trunk and extremities

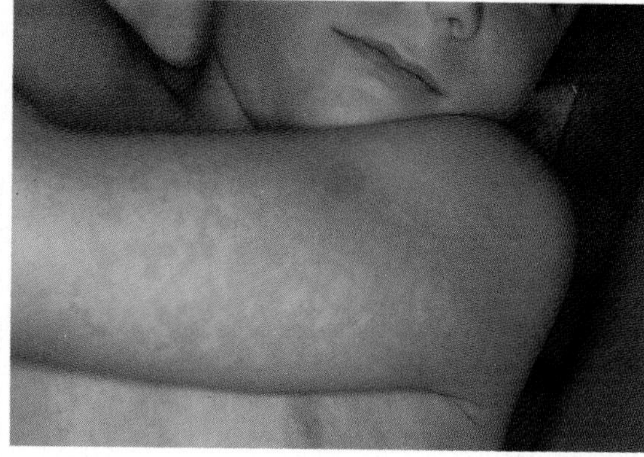

Figure 22–3

Erythema infectiosum lesions and rash distribution. (Photo from Hurwitz, S. [1993]. *Clinical pediatric dermatology: A textbook of skin disorders of childhood and adolescence* [2nd ed.]. Philadelphia: W. B. Saunders, p. 358, Fig. 12–15.)

Clinical Manifestations (Fig. 22–4). Roseola was the sixth childhood exanthem identified. The causative agent was not identified until 1988, and although HHV-6 appears to be the major causative agent, other viruses have been linked to the disease. Most clinical cases of roseola occur in children in the 6- to 18-month-old age group. The disease initially presents with a sudden high fever (103°–106°F), malaise, and irritability. Frequently, the child remains active and alert. An intermittent or constant fever may persist for 3 to 5 days. There may be a mild cough, runny nose, abdominal pain, headache, vomiting, and diarrhea. After 3 to 5 days, the fever subsides, and within several hours to 2 days, a rash appears. The rash consists of rose-pink maculopapules or macules that blanch with pressure. The rash presents predominantly on the neck and trunk and may be surrounded by a whitish ring. Normally, it persists for 24 to 48 hours before fading.

Complications. Complications associated with roseola are uncommon. However, convulsions related to the high fever may occur, and there have been rare cases of encephalitis, hemiplegia, paresis, and mental retardation reported.

Therapeutic Management. The treatment of roseola is supportive.

NURSING CARE OF THE CHILD WITH A VIRAL EXANTHEM

Assessment

It is important to obtain a history of the onset and progression of the rash, as well as any associated symptoms. Recent exposures, the child's immunization history, and any prior history of the disease need to be explored and documented. Additionally, it is important to note any medications taken, any history of upper respiratory infection, and any exposure to known infections. The skin and mucous membranes should be examined, and the distribution and type of rash should be recorded. The eyes, nose, ears, and throat should also be examined for signs of inflammation, swelling, and/or secretions. The temperature of the child should be documented, as should his general state of health. The spleen, liver, and lymph nodes should be examined for any enlargement.

Nursing Diagnosis and Planning

The following nursing diagnoses and expected outcomes may be appropriate following assessment of the child with a viral exanthem.

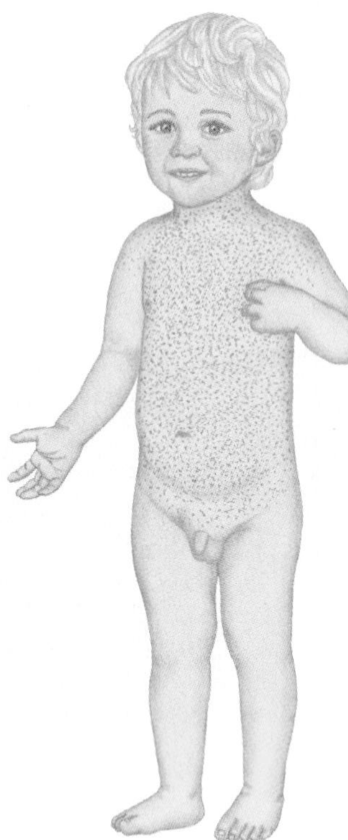

- Rash appears several hours to 2 days after fever subsides
- Erythematous maculopapular or macular; may be surrounded by whitish ring
- Blanches with pressure
- Predominantly on neck and trunk
- Usually persists for 24–48 hours

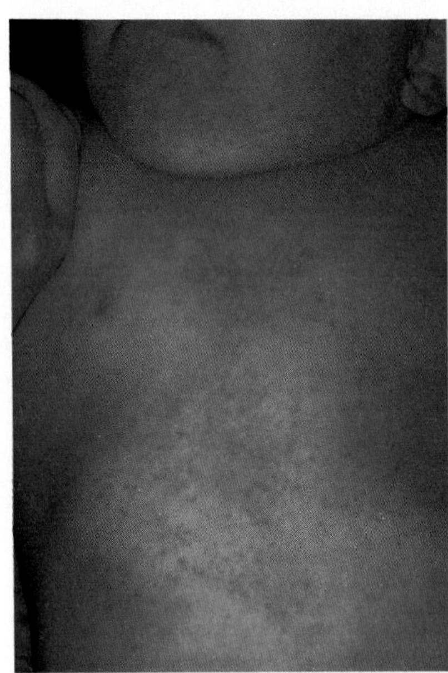

Figure 22–4
Roseola infantum lesions and rash distribution. (Photo from Hurwitz, S. [1993]. *Clinical pediatric dermatology: A textbook of skin disorders of childhood and adolescence* [2nd ed.]. Philadelphia: W. B. Saunders, p. 358, Fig. 12–16.)

Nursing Diagnoses

- Impaired Skin Integrity related to rash/scratching
- Hyperthemia related to infection
- Risk for Infection for Nonimmune Contacts related to the contagious nature of the virus
- Social Isolation related to the isolation requirements
- Knowledge Deficit related to home care needs
- Pain related to malaise/joint discomfort

Expected Outcomes

- The child will have intact skin and mucous membranes.
- The child's body temperature will be within normal limits.
- The infection will be limited to the original source, and no other children will contract the disease.
- The child and family will understand and maintain activity restrictions.
- The parents will demonstrate an understanding of their child's care.
- The child will demonstrate absence of pain/discomfort.

Implementation

Children with typical uncomplicated viral exanthems are usually cared for at home. Hospitalization is indicated when there are complications. Care of the hospitalized child will be determined by the child's specific needs. The hospitalized child will require respiratory or contact isolation. High-risk children and children with an infectious disease should not be cared for by the same nurse.

Home Care Instructions

1. For *elevated temperature*, the child's activity should be restricted to quiet activities and bed rest. As the fever decreases, the activity level can be increased gradually to a normal level. Fever can be controlled with acetaminophen, sponge baths, decreased clothing, decreased environmental temperature, and increased fluid intake. Bed linens may need to be changed frequently during periods of high fevers. Parents should be instructed about the possibility of *febrile seizures*. Seizure precautions should be in effect for any child with a seizure history.
2. The amount of *skin irritation and discomfort* will vary. Lukewarm baths using colloid preparations (Aveeno) or baking soda ($\frac{1}{2}$ cup in tub of water) may help to relieve itching. Creams or emollients may also provide comfort. Soaps should be avoided to prevent drying of irritated skin. Fingernails should be short. If the child continues to scratch, mittens or socks can be applied to the hands. It is essential to maintain the integrity of the skin and prevent any secondary infections. Should secondary infections occur, antibiotic therapy may be necessary.
3. *Coughing* can be managed with cool humidification of the room and antitussives.
4. For *arthralgia*, anti-inflammatory medications may be used. Involvement of weight-bearing joints may warrant bed rest.
5. Some viral exanthems cause *photophobia*. In such cases, keeping the room dimly lighted or providing sunglasses for the patient may be helpful. If the patient has conjunctivitis, secretions or crust should be removed with tepid water and a clean cloth to prevent contamination.
6. *Fluid intake* is important. The parents and child should understand that fluid intake is critical in successfully managing febrile stages of the disease. The child should be encouraged to drink cool liquids frequently. If the child's mucous membranes are involved soft, bland foods may be beneficial.
7. As the child progresses through the stages of illness, it will be necessary to provide *diversional activities* during the period of isolation. Evaluation of the child's favorite activities will provide ideas. The activities chosen should reflect the child's stage of wellness.
8. *Parents' understanding* of the care necessary for their child is important. Parents need to be educated about immunizations and measures to prevent the spread of infectious diseases. They should also be taught to recognize the signs and symptoms of complications so that they can seek medical treatment when warranted. Providing parents with written instructions that they can refer to at home may prove helpful.

Evaluation

- Has the skin remained intact?
- Was isolation of the infectious child maintained?
- Did the child's body temperature remain within normal limits?
- Did the family receive instruction in the care of the child?
- Is the child free of joint discomfort?

Mumps

Causative agent:	paramyxovirus
Incubation period:	usually 16 to 18 days, but may extend to 25 days
Infectious period:	usually 1 to 2 days (7 days prior to swelling to 9 days after onset)
Transmission:	airborne droplets, salivary secretions, possibly urine
Immunity:	natural disease or live attenuated mumps vaccine
Season:	late winter/spring

Clinical Manifestations. Prodromal manifestations may include fever, muscular pain, headache, and malaise. These are often followed by the classic clinical sign of parotid glandular swelling (parotitis), although a substantial number of individuals experience no such swelling. When parotid swelling does occur, it may be accompanied by fever.

Complications. Mumps generally affect the salivary glands, but can involve multiple organs. The most common complication is aseptic meningitis, with the virus being identified in the cerebrospinal fluid (CSF). Common signs include nuchal rigidity, lethargy, and vomiting. These individuals usually recover completely. Meningoencephalomyelitis is another complication that generally has a good prognosis.

The complication that appears to cause most concern among parents is orchitis (inflammation of a testis), which occurs in males. Unilateral orchitis occurs more frequently than bilateral orchitis. About 1 week after the appearance of parotitis, there is an abrupt onset of pain, tenderness, fever, chills, headache, and vomiting. The affected testicle becomes red, swollen, and tender. Atrophy resulting in sterility occurs only in a small number of cases.

Although deafness does not occur frequently, mumps is one of the leading causes of unilateral nerve deafness. The loss can be transient or permanent. Other rare complications include pancreatitis, nephritis, thyroiditis, myocarditis, arthritis, and mastitis.

Therapeutic Management. Uncomplicated mumps may require only symptomatic care. Respiratory isolation is indicated until 9 days after the onset of the parotid swelling. Orchitis requires bed rest, intermittent application of ice packs, and emotional support. Meningoencephalomyelitis, which reflects CNS involvement, presents with fever, headache, nausea, vomiting, nuchal rigidity, and changes in sensorium. The affected child is treated symptomatically and generally has an uneventful recovery.

NURSING CARE OF THE CHILD WITH MUMPS

Assessment

It is important to obtain a history of the onset of symptoms and to examine the patient's ears and throat. The characteristics of the lymph nodes in the neck should be documented, as should the temperature of the child and the general level of wellness. A neurologic evaluation should also be performed. In boys, an examination of the testes should be included in the assessment.

Nursing Diagnosis and Planning

The following nursing diagnoses and expected outcomes may be appropriate following assessment of the child with mumps.

Nursing Diagnoses

- Hyperthermia related to infection
- Pain related to parotid swelling, joint malaise
- Altered Nutrition: Less Than Body Requirements related to pain inflammation
- Risk of Infection related to the contagious nature of the virus
- Social Isolation related to isolation requirements
- Knowledge Deficit related to home care needs

Expected Outcomes

- The child's body temperature will be within normal limits.
- The child will demonstrate or acknowledge absence of pain/discomfort.
- The child will eat 90% of meals and have sufficient caloric intake.
- The infection will be limited to the original source, and no other children will contract the disease.
- The child and family will understand and maintain activity restrictions.
- The parents will demonstrate an understanding of their child's care.

Implementation

Typically, children with mumps are not hospitalized unless there are complications. When a child is hospitalized, he will be placed in isolation according to the facility's policies. Handwashing is of utmost importance. Contaminated articles should be disposed according to the facility's policies. The family, child, and visitors should be instructed on good handwashing. Because the disease is airborne, the child or family should be instructed to cover the child's nose and mouth during sneezing or coughing episodes.

Home Care Instructions

1. Generally, children with mumps are not seriously ill. They will be uncomfortable, however. Antipyretics and analgesics can be given to control fever and malaise.
2. Warm or cold compresses applied to the neck may be of benefit. As intake of food may be painful, soft, bland foods may be preferred. Foods that are acidic or spicy should be avoided.
3. The affected child will need to be isolated while infectious.
4. While in isolation, diversional activities should be planned according to the child's interests. Bed rest may be of benefit during the prodromal period.
5. In boys with orchitis, ice packs, bed rest, and scrotal support may be indicated.
6. Emotional support may be of great importance to the parents. Concern over sterility may be a real source of stress.
7. Parental education regarding the course of the disease and any potential complications may need to be reinforced. Parents often need additional instruction in preventing the spread of infection and maintaining their child's immunizations.

Varicella-Zoster Infections

(Chickenpox, Shingles)

Causative agent:	varicella-zoster virus
Incubation period:	10 to 21 days
Infectious period:	1 to 2 days before the onset of rash to 5 days after the onset of lesions and crusting of the lesions
Transmission:	direct contact, droplet, airborne particles
Immunity:	natural disease with recurrence with zoster
Season:	late winter through early spring

Chickenpox is the result of a primary infection with the varicella-zoster virus. Typically, this is one of the most common childhood diseases seen in children ages 5 to 9 years. Zoster (shingles), which is the reactivation of the latent varicella-zoster virus, occurs most frequently in the elderly. It can also occur in children, however, especially adolescents and young adults. Varicella and zoster in children are not usually life-threatening. However, in children who are immunosupressed, this relatively mild disease can cause serious disease, which may become life-threatening.

Clinical Manifestations (Fig. 22–5)

Varicella. During the 24 to 48 hours prior to the appearance of the rash, symptoms may include a slightly elevated body temperature, malaise, and anorexia. The macular rash generally first appears on the trunk and scalp. The lesions may be in various stages of development, beginning as macular and developing into a red papular rash. The lesions soon become teardrop vesicles with an erythematous base. The vesicles become pustular after which they begin to dry and to develop a crust. The lesions appear in crops, beginning on the trunk and scalp and moving (sparsely) to the extremities. These crops of lesions generally appear in three successive eruptions over a period of 3 to 4 days. The number of lesions will vary from child to child, but children in the household with secondary cases generally have more extensive rashes than the child with the primary case. The lesions may appear on the mucous membranes in the mouth, genital area, and rectum.

The natural disease was initially thought to offer lifelong immunity, but there have been reports of second attacks. These occur usually in immunocompromised chil-

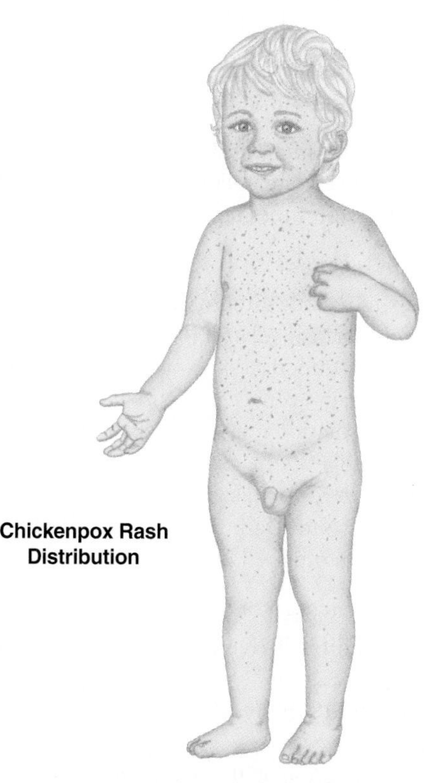

Chickenpox Rash Distribution
• Macular rash 24 to 48 hours following slight fever, malaise, anorexia
• Lesions appear in "crops," first on trunk and scalp, then moving sparsely to extremities. May appear in mucous membranes (mouth, genital area, rectum).
• Generally 3 successive eruptions over 3–4 days
• Lesions begin as a macular rash, develop into a red papular rash, then move quickly into teardrop vesicles with erythematous base. Vesicle becomes pustular, begins drying, and a crust develops.
• Rash varies from child to child

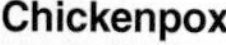

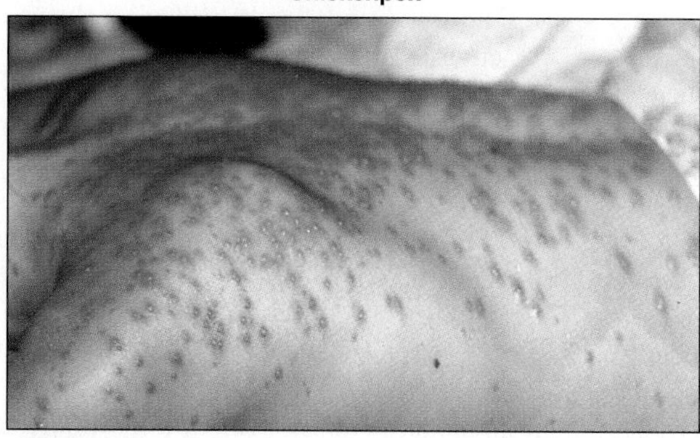

Shingles

Figure 22–5

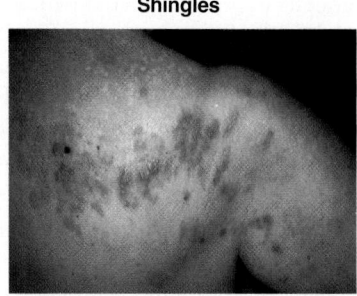

Chickenpox and shingles lesions, and rash distribution. (Shingles photo from Moschella, S. L., & Hurley, H. J. [1992]. *Dermatology* [3rd ed.]. Philadelphia: W. B. Saunders, p. 219, Fig. 8–25*D*.)

dren, those with a subclinical infection, and those who had chickenpox early in infancy (Weller, 1983).

Zoster (Shingles). During the primary infection with varicella, the varicella-zoster virus enters the sensory nerve ending and the dorsal root ganglion and establishes a latent infection. The activation of the infection causes zoster (shingles). It presents with pain and tenderness along the involved nerve and surrounding skin for approximately 2 weeks before the appearance of the rash. The intensity of the pain can range from an unpleasant, abnormal sensitivity to touch to burning, tingling, itching, sharp knife-like prickling, or even deep pain. Unilateral crops of lesions appear along the nerve. These macules and papules progress through the same stages as the varicella. There may be enlargement and tenderness of the lymph nodes in the same region. Zoster is generally thought to be a disease of the elderly, but it can also occur in children, especially those who are immunocompromised, have HIV infection, have had intrauterine exposure, or were infected during the first year of life.

Complications. The most common complication of varicella zoster virus is secondary bacterial infection of the skin lesions. Staphylococci and group A, β-hemolytic streptococci are the usual causative agents. CNS complications have been associated with mild to severe varicella infections. Encephalitis with ataxia, tremor, and nystagmus may occur from the third to the eighth day. The prognosis is generally good unless there is severe CNS involvement, usually manifested by convulsions and coma. Children with these complications may have future CNS difficulties, including seizures, mental retardation, or behavior disorders.

Varicella pneumonia, which is a common complication in adults, rarely occurs in children. Reye's syndrome has been known to occur following varicella infection. Corneal involvement may occur if lesions affect the eye.

Complications of zoster are rare. However, there can be the same difficulties with secondary infections as with varicella.

Therapeutic Management. Treatment is symptomatic and supportive for the healthy child. In the hospital setting, patients with varicella or zoster infections must be placed in strict isolation. For the immunocompromised child, the use of antiviral medications may be indicated. Acyclovir is the drug of choice owing to its minimal toxicity. IV acyclovir should be administered as soon as possible to immunocompromised children who present with active varicella or zoster infections. Presently, the use of acyclovir in otherwise healthy children is not recommended.

For children at high risk for developing severe varicella or zoster, varicella-zoster immune globulin (VZIG) has been proven to be effective in providing passive immunity. It should be administered within 96 hours of exposure. Immunocompromised children, newborn infants of mothers having active varicella infections at time of birth or with siblings at home with active varicella infection and HIV-positive children are considered to be at increased risk. VZIG is not recommended for healthy children.

NURSING CARE OF THE CHILD WITH A VARICELLA-ZOSTER INFECTION

Assessment

A history detailing the onset of symptoms should be obtained, and the lesions should be examined. The appearance, distribution, and stages of lesions should be documented. The child's body temperature and level of general wellness should also be noted.

Nursing Diagnosis and Planning

The following nursing diagnoses and expected outcomes may be appropriate following assessment of a child with varicella-zoster infection.

Nursing Diagnoses

- Impaired Skin Integrity related to lesions/scratching
- Hyperthermia related to infection
- Risk for Infection of Nonimmune Contacts related to the contagious nature of the virus
- Social Isolation related to isolation requirements
- Knowledge Deficit related to home care needs
- Pain related to malaise
- Altered Nutrition: Less Than Body Requirements related to mucosal lesions

Expected Outcomes

- The child will have intact skin and mucous membranes.
- The child's body temperature will be within normal limits.
- The infection will be limited to the original source, and no other children will contract the disease.
- The child and family will understand and maintain activity restrictions.
- The parents will demonstrate an understanding of their child's care.
- The child will demonstrate or acknowledge absence of pain/discomfort.
- The child will eat 90% of meals and have sufficient caloric intake.

Implementation

Hospitalized patients with varicella infections are placed in strict isolation, which requires wearing of a mask, gown, and gloves at all times. All contaminated materials must be bagged and labeled before reprocessing. Handwashing should be done after contact with the patient and before contact with another patient. Patients exposed to varicella should be kept in strict isolation for 8 to 21 days after the onset of rash in the infected individual. At birth, neonates with mothers who have active varicella infections should be placed in strict isolation. Secretion/drainage precautions should be in effect for patients with zoster infections.

Home Care Instructions

1. Most children with varicella-zoster infections are treated at home. They should be isolated from all individuals susceptible to infection (those who are immunocompromised, pregnant, or elderly). Parents should notify the child's school or daycare facility.
2. Fever can be controlled with antipyretics, such as acetaminophen.
3. Pruritis can be managed with antihistamines (diphenhydramine hydrochloride [Benadryl]) and drying lotions (calamine lotion). Baths of colloid preparations (Aveeno), oatmeal, or baking soda may also relieve discomfort. Nails should be kept short and clean to help prevent secondary infections. For small children, mittens may prevent scratching. Clothing that is soft, lightweight, and one piece may provide comfort. Daily bathing and clean linens may help to prevent secondary infections. If secondary infections occur, systemic antibiotics are indicated.
4. For children with mucosal involvement, hydration status must be monitored. Offering liquids that are soothing, such as popsicles and Jell-O, may be beneficial. Acidic, scratchy foods may be irritating to the mouth. The diet should include soft, bland foods.
5. An ophthalmologist should be consulted if the child develops lesions of the cornea.
6. Diversional activities during the infectious period can help the child cope with isolation from activities and peers. The activities selected should reflect the child's level of wellness and interests and should not cause overheating or irritation of the skin.
7. Parents should be educated to recognize signs and symptoms of complications. They should also have a good understanding of the importance of preventing the spread of varicella, especially among individuals who are at high risk for complications from the disease.

Cytomegalovirus

Causative agent:	human CMV
Incubation period:	unknown except for 3 to 12 weeks after blood transfusions and 4 weeks to 4 months after organ transplantation
Transmission:	saliva, urine, blood, semen, cervical secretions, breast milk, organ transplants
Immunity:	none, although CMV immune globulin, used only in seronegative transplant patients, has had moderate effectiveness. A CMV vaccine is currently being tested.

CMV infection is a common cause of congenital infection in infants. A child may become infected with the virus during the prenatal, perinatal, or postnatal period. The manifestations of the disease will depend on the age and the immune status of the child. CMV causes a primary infection, which is followed by a latency period that may persist for life. CMV infection is most devastating for the fetus, the immature neonate, and the immunocompromised.

Clinical Manifestations. Nearly 1% of all neonates are congenitally infected with CMV. The infecting mothers either have a primary infection or a recurrent infection. Of the neonates who acquire CMV in utero, only 10% are symptomatic with jaundice, lethargy, convulsions, hepatosplenomegaly, petechial rash, respiratory distress, microcephaly, and/or intracerebral calcifications. Although 90% of infants with congenital CMV are asymptomatic at birth, they may later develop complications, such as mental retardation, hearing loss, chorioretinitis, and learning disabilities. The newborn infant may become infected while passing through the infected birth canal. Again, these infants are generally asymptomatic, but can continue to shed the virus for up to 5 years.

During the postnatal period, the infant may acquire CMV from a maternal or nonmaternal source. Maternal infection can be transmitted through breast milk. Blood transfusions, which can be numerous in the premature infant, can also be a source of CMV infection.

Children who are not infected congenitally or perinatally often acquire the virus during their toddler or preschool years. It is thought that as many as 80% of toddlers are infected. Children who are in daycare settings have an increased infection rate (Yow, 1990). The teen years may be another period of acquisition owing to sexual activity. These adolescents are generally asymptomatic, but can present with a mononucleosis-like syndrome with fever, hepatosplenomegaly, mild hepatitis, and absence of heterophile antibody. Diagnosis is confirmed when there is a significant increase in the CMV antibody titer and/or a positive immunoglobulin M test result (IgM) with a positive culture of body fluids and symptoms consistent with a CMV infection.

Therapeutic Management. An antiviral drug (ganciclovir) has been successful in treating retinitis in immunocompromised patients. Experience with this drug in the pediatric population has been limited. The risk of exposure associated with blood transmission can be reduced by using CMV-negative donors for neonatal transfusions. At present, there is no safe and effective antiviral drug available to treat CMV. There have been live virus vaccines developed, but they have not been tested sufficiently.

For the hospitalized neonate who is shedding the virus, isolation precautions must be instituted. Controversy persists as to whether strict isolation is required, or whether good handwashing is sufficient to prevent the spread of infection. Because the child who acquires CMV during the neonatal period may continue shedding the virus for months or even years, parental education regarding good hygiene, proper handling of diapers, and good handwashing is indicated.

NURSING CARE OF THE CHILD WITH CYTOMEGALOVIRUS

Assessment

A history of the patient's symptoms and possible exposures must be obtained.

Nursing Diagnosis and Planning

The following nursing diagnosis and expected outcomes may be appropriate following assessment of the child with CMV infection.

Nursing Diagnosis

- Knowledge Deficit related to management, treatment, and prevention of CMV.

Expected Outcomes

- The parents will demonstrate an understanding of their child's care.
- The parents will demonstrate an understanding of the course of the disease and the prognosis.
- The spread of infection will be prevented.

Implementation and Evaluation

In children with congenitally acquired CMV, there may be a wide range of manifestations, so nursing care will vary according to the child's specific needs. When developmental delays, mental retardation, neurologic deficits, or hearing losses occur, the nurse can help coordinate the health care team's efforts to meet the child's needs. Parents will need support and education in caring for a child with developmental deficits. The nurse will play a key role in identifying the need for referral and any resources available in the community, including parental support groups.

Epstein-Barr Virus

(Infectious Mononucleosis)

Causative agent:	Epstein-Barr virus (herpes-like virus)
Incubation period:	4 to 7 weeks
Infectious period:	unknown; commonly, the virus is shed before clinical onset of disease until 6 months or longer after recovery. Asymptomatic carriers are common.
Transmission:	saliva, close intimate contact, blood
Immunity:	none; natural disease with life-long latent infection
Season:	can occur during any season

The primary site of infection is the epithelial cells and the B lymphocytes. The Epstein-Barr virus has been well recognized as the causative agent for infectious mononucleosis. It has also been associated with other diseases, especially in other countries. It has been identified as a cofactor in Burkitt's lymphoma, often seen in Africa, and in the cases of nasopharyngeal carcinoma seen in China and Southeast Asia. The Epstein-Barr virus alone cannot cause the lymphomas or the carcinoma, but it does so in association with other factors.

Clinical Manifestations. Infectious mononucleosis typically occurs in otherwise healthy individuals. It occurs most commonly in older children and young adults. Clinical signs include fever, exudative pharyngitis, lymphadenopathy, and hepatosplenomegaly. The severity of clinical signs can range from asymptomatic and mild to severe and fatal. Some patients develop a maculopapular rash. Children may complain of malaise, headache, fatigue, nausea, and abdominal pain. The acute illness usually continues for 2 to 4 weeks and is followed by a gradual recovery. The prognosis is generally excellent if there are no complications.

Complications. There is risk of splenic rupture associated with Epstein-Barr virus, occurring most frequently during the second week of the illness. The precipitant factor for the rupture is generally related to trauma, which may be as mild as palpitation during examination. The swelling of the pharynx and tonsils can be severe enough to compromise a child's respiratory status. Neurologic complication can include convulsions, ataxia, nuchal rigidity, meningitis, Bell's palsy, transverse myelitis, encephalitis, and Guillain-Barré syndrome. Pneumonia and mycocarditis are common but usually resolve completely. Hepatitis is considered to be part of the disease process. The resulting outcome of these complications will depend on the severity of the virus and the course of the complications.

Therapeutic Management. The illness is generally self-limiting; therefore, treatment is supportive. Complications will require appropriate medical treatment. Steroids may be indicated for tonsillar swelling associated with complications.

NURSING CARE OF THE CHILD WITH EPSTEIN-BARR VIRUS

Assessment

A history should be obtained, including presenting signs and symptoms. Physical examination of the pharynx should be performed, with documentation of any redness or swelling. Any rashes should be noted, including a description of their distribution and appearance. The spleen and liver should be evaluated for enlargement. The child's body temperature should be recorded and her nutrition and hydration status evaluated.

Nursing Diagnosis and Planning

The following nursing diagnoses and expected outcomes may be appropriate following assessment of a child with Epstein-Barr virus.

Nursing Diagnoses

- Hyperthermia related to infection
- Altered Nutrition: Less Than Body Requirements related to tonsillar swelling and pain
- Risk for Fluid Volume Deficit related to tonsillar swelling and pain
- Powerlessness related to bed rest and missing school
- Pain related to the infectious process
- Altered Family Processes related to care of a child with acute illness and long convalescence

Expected Outcomes

- The child's body temperature will be within normal limits.
- The child will eat 90% of meals and have sufficient caloric intake.
- The child's intake will be within an acceptable range, with adequate output (1–2 ml/kg/hr), moist mucous membranes, and appropriate skin turgor.
- The child and family will understand the reason for bed rest and will make arrangements for homebound teaching.
- The child will demonstrate or acknowledge absence of pain.
- The parents will understand the disease process and the appropriate supportive measures in caring for their child.

Implementation

Because Epstein-Barr virus is self-limiting, nursing care is mainly supportive. Most children are cared for at home. Hospitalization for hydration therapy may be necessary if the child is unable to swallow. Care in both settings involves bed rest, hydration, and relief of discomfort.

Home Care Instructions

1. Bed rest is indicated during the acute stage of the illness.
2. Acetaminophen may be useful in controlling discomfort secondary to fever and enlarged tonsils. Corticosteroids have been used in severe cases, but because of the potential for immunosuppression, they are used cautiously. Acyclovir has been used, but has not produced significant results. Penicillin or erythromycin may be given for documented infection of the pharynx.
3. Activity restrictions during the acute and recovery stage, especially contact sports, should be instituted to protect the child's enlarged spleen. With improvement in clinical signs, the child should be allowed to resume normal activities as tolerated.
4. The parents and child need to be prepared for a slow and gradual recovery. It is not unusual for fatigue to continue, necessitating a gradual return to school activities.
5. Hydration should be monitored and encouraged.
6. In children with sore throat, soothing liquids, bland foods, Jell-O, and milk shakes may be better tolerated than a regular diet.
7. Anxiety related to missed school work may be anticipated. Homebound teaching may be arranged if the child will be absent from school for a prolonged period of time.
8. The parents should have an understanding of the disease and the usual course of recovery. They may need support in exploring options for caring for their child, who may require a lengthy recovery period. This may be difficult, especially when both parents work outside the home.

Poliomyelitis

Causative agent:	enterovirus-poliovirus
Incubation period:	3 to 6 days for abortive; 7 to 21 days for paralytic
Infectious period:	shortly before onset of clinical illness; the virus is shed in the pharynx for 1 week after onset and in the feces for several weeks to months
Transmission:	fecal-oral; oral-oral (respiratory)
Immunity:	OPV vaccine
Season:	summer and fall

There are three forms of poliovirus: Brunhilde, Lansing, and Leon. The virus, which enters the body either through ingestion or inhalation, has a preference for the CNS, affecting only certain cells, such as the anterior horn cells of the spinal cord.

Clinical Manifestations. Initial symptoms of poliomyelitis are fever, malaise, anorexia, nausea, headache, sore throat, and generalized abdominal pain. This stage, referred to as abortive poliomyelitis, is generally so mild and brief that it may go unrecognized. The second stage is nonparalytic poliomyelitis. The symptoms are the same as for the abortive stage except that they are more intense, with soreness and stiffness of the trunk, neck, and limbs. If there is no further progression to paralysis, the temperature will fall and the meningeal symptoms will decrease. Recovery can begin within 3 to 10 days. The third stage is the paralytic stage in which flaccid paralysis is the most obvious sign. With paralysis, there is deterioration and atrophy of the muscles. There may be an asymmetric distribution of the symptoms. Generally, the lower extremities and the large muscle groups are affected. There can also be cervical involvement, which is called bulbar polio. This is the most life-threatening form of polio because it affects the respiratory and vasomotor centers. Damage to the respiratory center can result in an inability to sustain respirations.

Therapeutic Management. There is no specific treatment for poliomyelitis. Rather, treatment is specific for each child's needs. For paralytic polio, hospitalization may be necessary. Enteric precautions are indicated, requiring the use of gowns and gloves if soiling or contact with infective material is likely. In patients with respiratory paralysis, mechanical ventilation will be necessary. Physical therapy helps to maintain muscle integrity and prevent contractures.

The prognosis for polio depends on the severity of nerve damage. It may be months before the full extent of damage and the probable degree of recovery can be determined.

NURSING CARE OF THE CHILD WITH POLIOMYELITIS

Assessment

A history of symptoms should be obtained, along with an immunization history. In immunocompromised children, it is also important to obtain a history of contact with anyone who recently received the active polio vaccine. The patient should be observed for neurologic symptoms and respiratory distress, and the body temperature should be documented.

Nursing Diagnosis and Planning

The following nursing diagnoses and expected outcomes may be appropriate following assessment of a child with poliomyelitis.

Nursing Diagnoses

- Pain related to infection/headache/malaise
- Hyperthermia related to the infectious process
- Impaired Physical Mobility related to limited ability to move
- Fear related to prognosis/possible paralysis
- Ineffective Family Coping: Compromised, related to chronic disease, financial considerations, interruption of parental work schedule

Expected Outcomes

- The child will demonstrate or acknowledge absence of pain.
- The child's body temperature will be within normal limits.
- The child will demonstrate maximal ability to move.
- The parents and child will express feelings and demonstrate a minimal amount of fear.
- The parents will demonstrate a knowledge of the child's illness, prognosis, and care and will begin exploring alternatives for caring for the child at home.

Implementation

The primary focus of nursing should be preventive, as the incidence of polio has been drastically reduced by the development and use of the polio vaccine. For the child with paralytic polio, hospitalization may be necessary, and nursing care should focus on prevention of muscle and skeletal deformities. Active and passive range of motion exercises are indicated. Constipation is common, and fluid intake and nutrition should be monitored. If mechanical ventilation is indicated, the nursing care is the same as for any patient receiving ventilator support.

Nursing care of abortive polio is focused on reducing the fear of the parents/child and minimizing muscular deformities. The child can be treated at home with analgesics, sedatives, and bed rest until the fever subsides. Nonparalytic polio can be treated at home.

Home Care Instructions

1. Parents need to be taught to recognize signs of deterioration so that they may seek medical treatment in a timely manner.
2. Muscle tightness and spasms may be controlled with analgesics and the application of hot packs. Hot baths may also provide relief. A firm mattress with a footboard is necessary.
3. Physical therapy should be included as part of the treatment regimen for these children.

Rabies

Causative agent:	rhabdovirus
Incubation period:	5 days to more than 1 year; can extend to 6 years, but the average is 2 months
Infectious period:	10 days (if the animal is still healthy, rabies is unlikely). However, bats may harbor the virus for a longer period of time.
Transmission:	bites with contaminated saliva, scratches from claws of infected animals, airborne transmission in laboratory settings and in bat-infested caves, transplantation of corneas from undiagnosed donors
Immunity:	human diploid cell vaccine (HDCV)
Season:	can occur during any season

Rabies is a virus that can infect any warm-blooded animal. In the United States, the reservoir consists of skunks, bats, raccoons, foxes, squirrels, and woodchucks. Dogs and cats may also be reservoirs but the use of animal vaccines makes them a less common source of infection.

Clinical Manifestations. The rhabdovirus results in a slowly developing infection. The virus travels up the axons of the motor or sensory neurons to the brain. For this reason, bites that occur on the feet or lower extremities result in longer incubation periods than do bites on the face. Incubation periods are shortened in children. When left untreated, the virus will cause vague symptoms. The child may complain of not feeling well. There may be a sore throat, headache, fever, discomfort at the site of the bite, hyperactivity, anxiety, muscle spasms, and/or convulsions. The decreased ability to swallow results in drooling or aspiration, which explains the use of the term hydrophobia in connection with rabies. Once the disease has established itself, it is fatal. Once symptoms appear, the disease generally lasts 5 to 6 days before progressing to death.

Therapeutic Management. The focus of rabies management is preventive. In individuals who are at high risk for contracting rabies, the HDCV is recommended. It can be administered either intradermally or intramuscularly in a three-dose schedule. A booster is recommended when titers fall below acceptable levels.

When a child is bitten by an animal, a determination must be made as to whether or not to treat that child. Factors to be considered include the geographic area, type of animal, circumstances of the bite, and the animal's vaccination record. If the animal is available, it can be observed for 10 days or killed for microscopic examination of the brain.

The bite wound should be cleansed with copious amounts of soap and water. Ethyl alcohol should be flushed into the wound. If the wound is a puncture wound, a catheter should be inserted to irrigate the wound. The child will be given passive immunization (human rabies immune globulin) for protection until the vaccine stimulates the production of antibodies. The immune globulin is given as soon as possible, but should not be given after the eighth day following active immunization. It is given in a split dose, with half given directly into the wound and half given intramuscularly. The vaccine (HDCV) is administered at the same time, but in a different location. The schedule for administering HDCV is on days 3, 7, 14, and 28. Rabies vaccine is the only vaccine that can be given post-exposure and result in successful vaccination.

NURSING CARE OF THE CHILD EXPOSED TO RABIES

Assessment

A complete history of the event should be obtained, including the type of animal involved, identification of the animal as wild or domestic, immunization record of the animal, and the location of animal. This information will determine the course of action. The wound should be examined and a description noted in the child's record.

Nursing Diagnosis and Planning

The following nursing diagnoses and expected outcomes may be appropriate following assessment of a child exposed to rabies.

Nursing Diagnoses

- Anxiety related to the potential diagnosis and treatment
- Fear related to multiple injections
- Anticipatory Grieving related to infection and impending death (for untreated patient)

Expected Outcomes

- The child and family will demonstrate an understanding of the course of treatment.
- The child will demonstrate minimal fear during multiple injections.

Implementation

For the patient who has developed rabies, nursing actions will be supportive. The child will be in strict isolation and standard precautions will be instituted. The family will need support in preparing for the child's inevitable death and in coping with feelings of guilt. The patient will need the supportive care indicated for any dying patient.

For the patient who will undergo a complete series of vaccinations, the nurse may use needle therapy. Allowing the child to administer injections to a doll may help to relieve the anxiety associated with multiple injections. For the older child, an explanation of the injection process and reasons for treatment may be adequate. Allowing the child to choose the injection site may confer some measure of control.

BACTERIAL INFECTIONS

Bacteria are abundant in our environment, yet relatively few cause diseases that have an impact on humans. Bacteria are organisms that contain both DNA and RNA. They lack a nuclear membrane but have a complex cell wall. Outside the cell wall may be capsules, flagella, or pili. The properties of the cell wall determine the bacteria's classification as either gram-positive or gram-negative. Gram-positive bacteria have a thicker wall that helps resist bile activity, drying, and other environmental factors. Gram-positive bacteria can cause chronic inflammation of dermal tissue, fever, and shock. Gram-negative bacteria have a thinner cell wall. Many bacteria have flagella which help propel the bacteria through their environment. They may also have pili, which are rigid projections that assist in attachment to the host cell or other bacteria. The capsules help hide the bacteria's presence from the host and make phagocytosis by the host cell more difficult.

> Bacteria are classified by three characteristics:
> - shape (rods or cocci)
> - reaction of gram stain (positive or negative)
> - ability to grow in the presence of oxygen (aerobic or anaerobic)

Bacteria excrete toxins. Exotoxins are highly poisonous substances that cause cell damage by cell lysis, inhibition of protein synthesis, or interference with passage of nerve impulses. Endotoxins, which are a portion of the gram-negative cell, cause fever, shock, and disseminated intravascular coagulation (DIC).

Diphtheria

Causative agent:	*Corynebacterium diphtheriae* (gram-positive, nonmotile bacillus)
Incubation period:	2 to 5 days
Infectious period:	ranges from 2 weeks or less up to several months in an untreated individual
Transmission:	contact with carrier or disease: droplets
Immunity:	vaccine with boosters; passive immunity from maternal antibodies; natural disease (in which case immunization is necessary)
Season:	fall and winter

Clinical Manifestations

- Nasal: Discharge of foul-smelling mucopurulent material; low-grade fever
- Tonsillar/pharyngeal: low-grade fever; thin, gray membrane on tonsils and pharynx; "bull neck" (neck edema)

Therapeutic Management. Treatment includes the administration of IV diphtheria antitoxin and antibiotics.

Nursing Interventions. Nursing care of the child with diphtheria involves strict isolation, bed rest, and monitoring of the child's respiratory status.

Pertussis
(Whooping Cough)

Causative agent:	*Bordetella pertussis* (gram-negative bacillus)
Incubation period:	6 to 20 days
Infectious period:	catarrhal stage (1–2 weeks) until the fourth week
Transmission:	direct contact or respiratory droplets from coughing
Immunity:	vaccine (provides limited immunity)
Season:	can occur during any season

> Because infants do not receive maternal immunity, they are very susceptible to pertussis. Pertussis is a highly contagious illness and there is a high infant mortality rate associated with it.

Clinical Manifestations. There are three stages of pertussis: catarrhal, paroxysmal, and convalescent (see accompanying box).

Complications. The most common complication of pertussis is pneumonia. There can be varying degrees of other respiratory complications, too, ranging from atelectasis, to interstitial or subcutaneous emphysema, to pneumothorax. Approximately 90% of the deaths attributable to pertussis are related to respiratory complications. Anoxia can lead to CNS involvement. Malnutrition and dehydration may result from extensive vomiting and can be very dangerous, especially for infants. Other complications may include otitis media, ulcers of the frenulum of the tongue, epistaxis, hernia, and rectal prolapse.

Therapeutic Management. Hospitalization and supportive care may be necessary for the infant, whereas older children can usually be managed at home. Infants are placed in respiratory isolation and respiratory status is monitored with a cardiopulmonary monitor and pulse oximeter.

Antimicrobials are effective during the catarrhal stage. However, if the disease has progressed to the paroxysmal stage, antibiotics have little effect. The antibiotic of choice is erythromycin. Corticosteroids and albuterol have been used to reduce paroxysmal coughing.

Stages of Manifestation of Pertussis

Catarrhal
Duration: 1–2 weeks
Symptoms: Symptoms of upper respiratory infection (rhinorrhea, lacrimation, mild cough, low-grade fever)

Paroxysmal
Duration: 2–4 weeks or longer
Symptoms: Increased severity of cough. Repetitive series of coughs during a single expiration, followed by massive inspiration with a whoop. Cyanosis, protrusion of tongue, salivation, distension of neck veins. Coughing spells may be triggered by yawning, sneezing, eating, or drinking, and may induce vomiting.

Convalescent
Duration: 1–2 weeks
Symptoms: Episodes of coughing, whooping, and vomiting which decrease in frequency and severity. Cough may persist for several months.

NURSING CARE OF THE CHILD WITH PERTUSSIS

Assessment

A complete respiratory history is essential. The child's complete immunization history and any known exposures need to be documented. Documentation of parents' description of events prior to admission including coughing, secretions, cyanotic episodes, and child's activity level should be included. Assessment of the child's respiratory, fluid, nutrition, output, and neurologic status is included.

Nursing Diagnosis and Planning

The following nursing diagnoses and expected outcomes may be appropriate following assessment of a child with pertussis.

Nursing Diagnoses

- Ineffective Airway Clearance related to thick secretions
- Impaired Gas Exchange related to apnea and coughing spells
- Fluid Volume Deficit related to poor intake
- Fatigue related to coughing spells
- Anxiety (parent and child) related to frequent coughing paroxysms

Expected Outcomes

- The child's respiratory status will be within normal parameters for rate, depth, and ease.
- The child's coughing episodes will decrease in frequency and duration.
- The child's hydration status will be within normal parameters.
- The child will have periods of uninterrupted rest.
- The parents will maintain a calm, supportive environment.

Implementation

Nursing care of the child with pertussis centers around supportive therapy. The child's respiratory status should be monitored with a cardiopulmonary monitor and pulse oximeter. The limits of the monitor should be checked frequently. Monitors should be explained to parents to help alleviate anxiety associated with beeping monitors. Suction and oxygen equipment should be readily available. Supplemental oxygen may be ordered by the physician. If the child requires oxygen therapy, parents should receive instructions as to the necessity of maintaining the usage of oxygen equipment. Some children will only require additional oxygen during the paroxysmal spells. The nurse should monitor the child's oxygen levels during these episodes.

Because the child's coughing paroxysms may be triggered by noises or episodes of fright, a quiet environment is necessary. The nurse should maintain a quiet, reassuring approach when caring for the infant. Paroxysmal episodes should be monitored and accurately recorded. Parents will need support during the child's coughing spells, as these episodes can be extremely frightening.

The nutritional status of the infant should be closely monitored. Small, frequent feedings may be of benefit if the feeding process becomes exhausting for the infant. Should the child's intake be insufficient, gavage or parenteral nutrition may be instituted. If the child has vomiting episodes, oral care will be necessary.

Nursing care should be clustered to prevent exhaustion of the child. Rest is important for these children. Diversional activities should be age-appropriate. Parental support and education are important. Parents may need emotional support to deal with feelings of guilt, especially if they chose not to immunize their child.

Home Care Instructions

1. The parents should encourage bed rest and activities that foster a decreased activity level (reading, playing Nintendo games, board games, etc.).
2. Fluid intake should be encouraged by offering popscicles, Jell-O, juices, etc.
3. If no humidifier is available, humidification can be provided by periodically placing a child in a bathroom filled with mist from the shower or by making a mist tent using a sheet over the top of a playpen.
4. Small, frequent feedings, with periodic rest periods, are indicated to prevent fatigue and coughing paroxysms.
5. Good handwashing techniques must be instituted to prevent spreading the disease to others.
6. Parents should be instructed to recognize signs and symptoms that indicate the need for medical attention.

Scarlet Fever

(Scarletina)

Causative agent:	group A β-hemolytic streptococci
Incubation period:	1 to 7 days (average of 3 days)
Infectious period:	acute stage until 36 hours after antimicrobial therapy
Transmission:	airborne (inhalation or ingestion); direct contact
Immunity:	none
Season:	late fall/winter/spring

Clinical Manifestations (Fig. 22–6). The onset of scarlet fever can be characterized by abrupt fever, vomiting, headache, abdominal pain, pharyngitis, and chills. The fever reaches a peak by the second day and returns to normal within 5 to 6 days. Within 24 hours, a red, fine, papular rash appears in the axillas, groin, and neck. The rash then spreads peripherally to cover the entire body. The rash will blanch upon pressure except in areas of deep creases (Pastia's sign). Desquamation begins on the face at the end of the first week and flaking proceeds down the trunk. This may con-

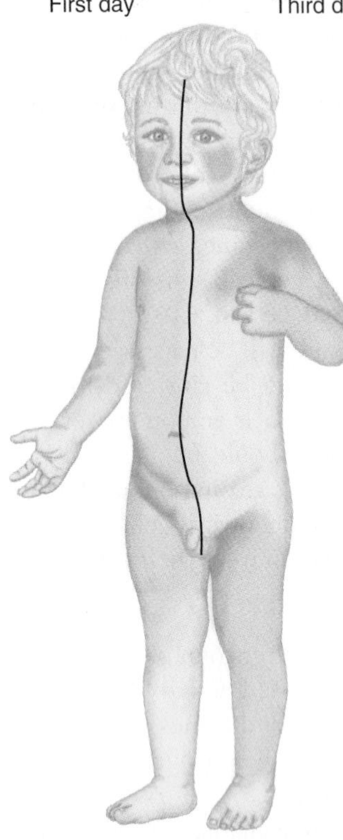

- Red, fine, papular rash appears within 24 hours of fever and other symptoms. In dark skin, the rash is often seen as punctate papular elevations.
- Begins in axillas, groin, and neck, and spreads to cover entire body
- Desquamation begins on face at end of first week and flaking proceeds down trunk. May continue up to 6 weeks.
- Tongue: Initially presents with white, furry coat with red projecting papillae (white strawberry tongue). By the 4th day, the white sloughs off, leaving a red swollen tongue (strawberry tongue).

Scarlet Fever Rash Distribution

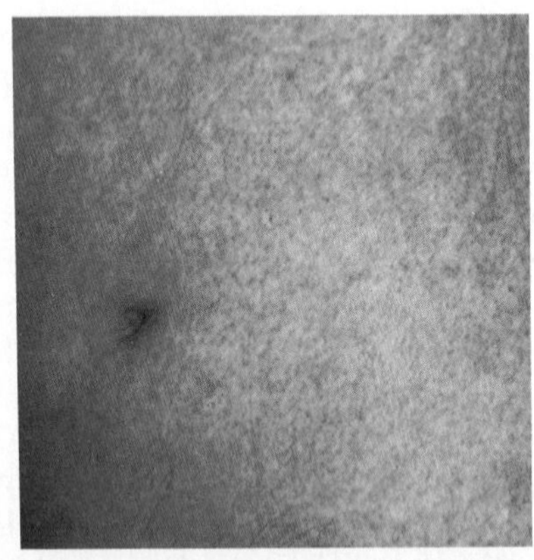

◀ Rash, Light Skin

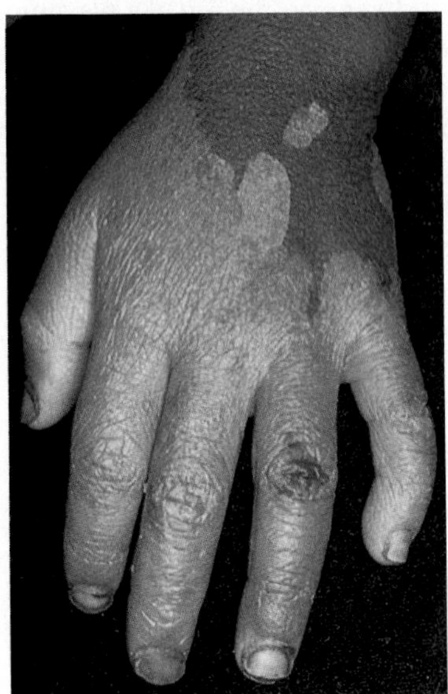

Desquamation, Dark Skin

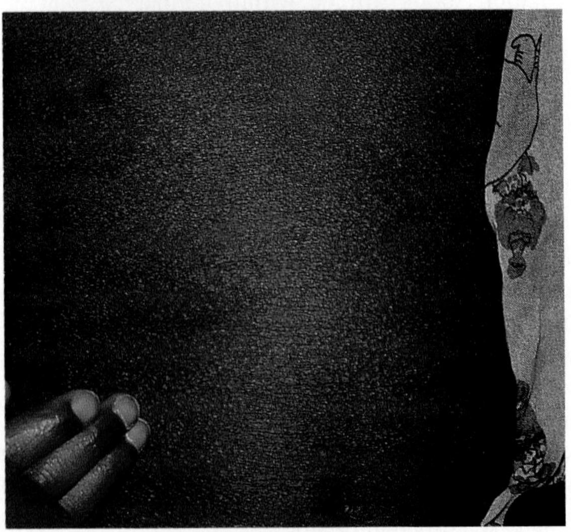

Rash, Dark Skin ▶

Figure 22–6

Scarlet fever rash and distribution. Note the characteristic skin peeling. (Photos from Hurwitz, S. [1993]. *Clinical pediatric dermatology: A textbook of skin disorders of childhood and adolescence* [2nd ed.]. Philadelphia: W. B. Saunders, pp. 353–354, Figs. 12–8, 12–10, 12–11.)

tinue for up to 6 weeks. The tongue is initially coated with a white, furry covering with red projecting papillae (so-called white strawberry tongue). By the fourth day, the white strawberry tongue sloughs off, leaving a red, swollen tongue (so-called strawberry tongue). The tonsils are edematous and may be covered with a gray-white exudate, which may spread to the pharynx. Petechial hemorrhages cover the soft palate.

Complications. Complications generally result from extension of the streptococcal infection. They may include sinusitis, otitis media, mastoiditis, peritonsilar abscess, bronchopneumonia, meningitis, osteomyelitis, rheumatic fever, and glomerulonephritis.

Therapeutic Management. The preferred treatment for any streptococcal infection is penicillin. Erythromycin or cephalosporins can be substituted for patients who are penicillin-sensitive. Supportive care for symptoms is indicated. A throat culture is necessary for accurate identification of the causative agent. Drainage and secretion precautions should be instituted until 24 hours after antimicrobial therapy is started.

NURSING CARE OF THE CHILD WITH SCARLET FEVER

Assessment

A complete history of symptoms should be obtained and documented. The nurse should assess the child's throat, tongue, rash, nutritional and fluid intake, vital signs, and level of general wellness, documenting the findings in the child's chart. Any history of sensitivity to penicillin should be explored and prominently noted.

Nursing Diagnosis and Planning

The following nursing diagnoses and expected outcomes may be appropriate following assessment of a child with scarlet fever.

Nursing Diagnoses

- Pain related to pharyngitis
- Hyperthermia related to infection
- Impaired Skin Integrity related to rash and sloughing of skin
- Altered Nutrition Less Than Body Requirements related to difficulty in swallowing
- Knowledge Deficit related to home care

Expected Outcomes

- The child will exhibit no signs of pain or discomfort.
- The child's body temperature will return to normal parameters.
- Skin and mucous membranes will be intact.
- The child will eat 90% of meals and have sufficient caloric intake.
- The parents will demonstrate a knowledge of the care necessary for their child.

Implementation

Generally, children with scarlet fever are cared for at home. However, children with severe symptoms and complications may require hospitalization and supportive care. In such cases, vital signs should be monitored, especially body temperature. Fluids should be encouraged, especially cool, nonacidic liquids. Medications should be given as ordered. Antipyretics should be used for fever control. The parents should understand the course of treatment and the importance of any medications prescribed. Bed rest and quiet activities may be of benefit during the acute stage.

Home Care Instructions

1. Teaching should be provided to assist parents in identifying signs or symptoms of complications.
2. Parents should be informed of the importance and necessity of taking prescribed medications for the duration of the treatment regimen.
3. Cool drinks and liquid refreshments (popsicles, milkshakes) may be soothing and will help to maintain hydration.
4. Throat lozenges, analgesics, antiseptic throat spray (Chloraseptic), and cool mist may be used to relieve discomfort.
5. Encouraging quiet activities will help to prevent fatigue.
6. In providing oral care, acidic preparations should be avoided. Saline rinses may provide comfort and promote hygiene.
7. A soft, bland diet should be offered.

RICKETTSIAL INFECTIONS

Rickettsia are small, parasitic bacteria that are transmitted to humans by bloodsucking arthropods. A vertebrate is not necessary for the survival of the bacteria, and the host arthropod appears not to be affected adversely by the rickettsia. Replication of the rickettsia in the new host cell causes cell death, which may be accompanied by vasculitis with thrombosis, increased permeability, tissue edema, hemorrhage, circulatory failure, and meningoencephalitis. The disease cannot be transmitted from person to person.

Rocky Mountain Spotted Fever (RMSF)

Causative agent:	*Rickettsia rickettsii*
Reservoir:	wild rodents, dogs
Vector:	tick (wood, dog, Lone Star)
Incubation period:	2 to 14 days (average of 7 days)
Transmission:	bite of infected tick
Season:	April through September

Clinical Manifestations. The onset of RMSF is marked by nonspecific symptoms, such as headache, fever, anorexia, and restlessness. On the third day, a characteristic rash appears. The maculopapular or petechial rash begins on the extremities (palms and soles) and spreads to the rest of the body. As the rash progresses, there can be hemorrhagic and necrotic lesions. Gangrene of the distal parts of the body can result from thrombosis. Edema develops, beginning in the periorbital area and progressing to a generalized edema of the body and extremities. Delayed treatment can lead to a mortality rate of 25%.

Therapeutic Management. With early detection, tetracycline and chloramphenicol have been found to be effective in treating RMSP. These drugs inhibit the growth of the organism; however, if vascular damage has already occurred, the drugs may not alter the course of the disease. Antibiotic therapy is continued until the child has been afebrile for at least 2 to 3 days. The usual duration of therapy is 6 to 10 days.

NURSING CARE OF THE CHILD WITH ROCKY MOUNTAIN SPOTTED FEVER

Assessment

The assessment of children presenting with RMSF should include obtaining a complete history—of skin eruptions, medications taken, exposure to infectious diseases, and recent hiking or other activities in wooded areas. The rash should then be examined, with documentation of its distribution and morphology. The child's vital signs, especially body temperature, should also be assessed and noted.

Nursing Diagnosis and Planning

The following nursing diagnoses and expected outcomes may be appropriate following assessment of a child with Rocky Mountain Spotted Fever.

Nursing Diagnoses

- Impaired Skin Integrity related to rash
- Knowledge Deficit related to prevention of exposure

Expected Outcomes

- The child's skin will be intact.
- The parents will demonstrate an understanding of preventive measures, such as avoidance of tick-infested areas, protective clothing, and proper removal of ticks.

Implementation

The nursing care of the child with RMSF will include the administration of tetracycline. Because tetracycline can cause staining of the teeth, straws should be used and the mouth should be flushed after administration. Hospitalized children will require supportive care for their presenting symptoms.

Education in the prevention of RMSF is necessary. The parents/child should be instructed to avoid tick-infested areas, wear protective clothing, use tick repellent, and inspect themselves frequently for ticks to reduce contact with infected ticks. Removal of ticks should be accomplished using an instrument such as tweezers. The tick should be removed as close to the skin as possible, and touching of the tick with bare hands should be avoided.

Chapter 34 also discusses tick bites.

Evaluation

- Was the child's skin integrity maintained?
- Can the child and family discuss preventive measures related to reducing contact with infected ticks?

BORRELIA INFECTIONS

Borrelia are a genus of spiral bacteria transmitted to humans by arthropods. The diseases caused by Borrelia are relapsing fever and Lyme disease. Relapsing fever is spread from person to person by lice. The bacteria are present in the lice and are introduced into the bite wound when the bite is rubbed. This infection is spread when people fail to wash thoroughly and when clothes are not changed. Lyme disease is spread by tick bites and is the most common vector-borne disease in the United States (Steere, 1993; Gordon, 1994).

Lyme Disease

Lyme disease is a multisystem illness that affects the skin and the musculoskeletal, cardiovascular, and nervous systems.

Causative agent:	*Borrelia burgdorferi* (spirochete)
Incubation period:	3 to 32 days
Vector:	tick
Transmission:	bite of infected tick (person-to-person transmission not possible)
Season:	May to November

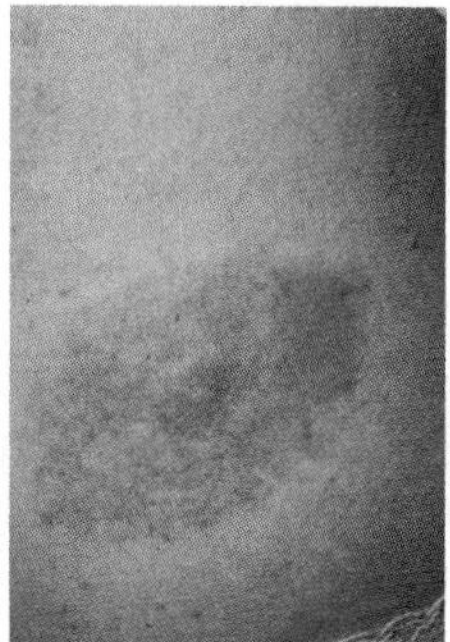

Figure 22–7
Characteristic lesion of Lyme disease. (From Larson, W. G., Adams, R. M., & Maibach, H. I. [1991]. *Color text of contact dermatitis.* Philadelphia: W. B. Saunders, p. 191.)

Clinical Manifestations (Fig. 22–7). An erythematous macular or papular rash forms at the site of the tick bite within 4 to 20 days. This rash can enlarge to 1 cm in diameter, with a clearing in the center. It may itch, prickle, or burn. The rash generally lasts for 3 weeks, during which time it gradually fades. Other manifestations that accompany the rash are malaise, fatigue, headache, stiff neck, arthralgias, vomiting, nausea, and sore throat. There can be general lymphadenopathy. These symptoms may occur from 1 to 4 months after the bite. The symptoms generally resolve over a few days, but many individuals have a recurrence of symptoms. Skin lesions may recur, but are smaller and more diffuse than the initial ones. CNS symptoms may include headache with myelitis, meningitis, Bell's palsy, and cerebral ataxia.

Symptoms that may appear months later include arthritis, recurrent cranial nerve deficits, spastic paraparesis, encephalitis, and dementia.

Therapeutic Management. Presently, treatment involves the use of penicillin and tetracycline. Early detection and treatment appear to affect the course of the disease. Individuals identified in early stages and treated do not progress to later stages of the disease. The difficulty lies in the detection of the spirochete. These bacteria are very difficult to identify, especially in later stages. Presently, there is no reliable diagnostic test for Lyme disease. The diagnosis is based primarily on clinical symptoms, with serologic tests used as an adjunct.

NURSING CARE OF THE CHILD WITH LYME DISEASE

Assessment

Assessment should include a complete history of rash onset and characteristics, medications taken, recent exposures to infectious diseases, and recent hiking, or other activities in wooded areas. The rash should be examined and its distribution and morphology documented.

Nursing Diagnosis and Planning

The following nursing diagnoses and expected outcomes may be appropriate following assessment of a child with Lyme disease.

Nursing Diagnoses

- Impaired Skin Integrity related to rash
- Pain related to rash, headache, and/or joint pain
- Knowledge Deficit related to prevention of exposure

Expected Outcomes

- The child's skin will be intact.
- The child will demonstrate or acknowledge a lack of pain.
- The child/parents will demonstrate a knowledge of preventive measures.

Implementation

Nursing care should focus on the presenting symptoms. Fever, headache, and arthralgia should be treated with antipyretics and analgesics. Antibiotics should be given as

Preventive Measures to Avoid Insect Bites

- Children should wear long pants, long-sleeved shirts, long socks, and a hat when in woods and grassy areas. Pants should be tucked into socks. Paths should be followed and dense areas avoided.
- Insect repellents which contain DEET and permethrines should be used. Clothing and exposed skin should be protected every 4–8 hours. Care should be taken to avoid contact of repellent with the child's eyes or mouth. The repellent should not be applied to the hands so as to avoid contact with the eyes and mouth.
- Repellents should be used with caution in infants because of the risk of encephalopathy.
- Insect repellent should not be applied to wounds or irritated skin.
- The body should periodically be inspected for the presence of ticks, which may resemble small moles or blood blisters.
- Ticks should be removed with tweezers. The tick should be removed as close to the skin as possible.
- Care should be taken to avoid handling the tick with bare hands or crushing the tick's body.
- Ticks may be preserved in alcohol for later identification.
- Pets should be kept free of ticks by dipping and spraying during tick season. The yard should be kept free of brush and undergrowth.

ordered. Parents should have an understanding of the course of treatment. Generally these children will be treated at home, so home care education is important. Education in the prevention of Lyme disease continues to be an important factor (see the accompanying box).

Evaluation

- Was the child's skin integrity maintained?
- Is the child free of pain?
- Can the child and parents verbalize an understanding of prevention of Lyme disease?

HELMINTHS

Helminth is a classification for worms that live as parasites. The three groups that have the greatest impact on humans are tapeworms, flukes, and roundworms (Table 22–3). Children are more commonly infected than adults, primarily as a result of frequent hand-to-mouth activity and the likelihood of fecal contamination. Transmission may occur by oral-fecal ingestion, ingestion of contaminated tissue from another host, skin penetration, or the bite of a bloodsucking insect.

Therapeutic Management. Treatment consists of the administration of oral anthelmintic medications effective against a specific helminth. Treatment is provided to the entire family. Enteric isolation and education of the family regarding personal hygiene and sanitary practices are also necessary.

NURSING CARE OF THE CHILD WITH A HELMINTHIC INFECTION

Assessment

Nursing assessment involves assisting in the collection and evaluation of the parasite. A thorough history, including the child's general wellness, personal hygiene practices, and nutritional intake, should be obtained.

Nursing Diagnosis and Planning

The following nursing diagnoses and expected outcomes may be appropriate following assessment of a child with a helminthic infection.

Nursing Diagnoses

- Risk for Injury related to the physical effects of the helminthic infestation
- Knowledge Deficit related to transmission modes, enteric isolation, personal hygiene practices that will prevent recurrence, medical treatment, and signs and symptoms of complications
- Anxiety related to the social implications of infestation
- Risk for Infection of close contacts related to ease of disease transmission

Expected Outcomes

- The child will demonstrate wellness, without signs or symptoms of abdominal distension, anemia, abdominal cramping/pain, weight loss, malnutrition, or abdominal obstruction.

TABLE 22–3 *Common Helminths*

	TRANSMISSION	MANIFESTATIONS	DIAGNOSIS	TREATMENT
Round worm (Ascaris lumbricoides)	Ingestion of eggs from contaminated soil or food; transfer to mouth from fingers, toys, etc.	Abdominal pain or distension; abdominal obstruction; vomiting with bile staining; pneumonitis	Fecal smear	Mebendazole Pyrantel pamoate
Pin worm (Enterobius vermicularis)	Ingestion or inhalation of eggs; transfer from hands to mouth	Nocturnal anal itching; sleeplessness	Scotch Tape test & microscopic examination	Mebendazole Pyrantel pamoate
Tapeworm (Taenia saginata)	Ingestion from handling or eating infected beef or pork	Asymptomatic; segments of worms seen in stool; abdominal pain; nausea; anorexia, weight loss, insomnia	Fecal smear or microscopic examination	Niclosamide
Hookworm (Necator americanus)	Skin penetration from direct contact with contaminated soil	Dermatitis; anemia; pneumonitis; blood loss; malnutrition	Fecal smear or microscopic examination	Pryantel pamoate

- The parents and child will demonstrate an understanding of the prescribed home care regimen.
- The parents will demonstrate compliance with therapy.
- The parents will demonstrate an understanding of the disease that will reinforce compliance with treatment modalities.
- Infestation will remain with the original source, and no further infestation will occur.

Implementation

Nursing care of children with intestinal parasitic worms includes assisting with the collection of specimens, treatment of infections, and prevention of reinfection. Most parasites are identified in fecal smears obtained from stool specimens. Clear instructions regarding the collection of specimens should be provided to the parents. Sample size and number, as well as proper storage, should be clearly explained.

Stool specimens that have not been contaminated with urine are ideal. However, obtaining urine-free specimens may be difficult, especially in very young children. Older children can be cooperative in obtaining the specimen. At home, clear plastic wrap can be placed over the toilet bowl, or a potty chair can be used. If the child wears diapers, specimens can be collected from the diaper. These specimens do not need to be collected in a sterile manner. The specimen is collected using a clean tongue blade and is placed in the specified container. The container should be marked with the patient's name and the date and time of collection. It should then be refrigerated until it is delivered to the laboratory.

Besides assisting with specimen collection, the nurse provides education regarding the course of treatment. Parents should be informed of the necessity and rationale for evaluating and treating the entire family for infection. They need to clearly understand the various modes of transmissions and the methods that are effective in preventing cross-contamination of family members.

Teaching the family about prevention is the most important responsibility of the nurse. Families need to gain a clear understanding of good hygiene and health habits (see the Home Care Instructions that follow).

Home Care Instructions: Parasitic Infections

1. Handwashing (including under the fingernails) with soap and water should be done before eating or handling of food, as well as after toileting.
2. Placing hands in the mouth and nail biting should be discouraged.
3. Toilets or other appropriate facilities should be used for toileting.
4. Clean bathroom facilities, cleaned with agents containing bleach, should be provided.
5. Scratching of the anal area with bare hands should be discouraged.
6. Dogs and cats should be kept at a distance from play areas and sandboxes, and the latter need to be covered when not in use.
7. Shoes should be worn when outside.
8. All fruits and vegetables should be washed before being eaten.
9. Diapers should be changed frequently and disposed of properly (out of children's reach).
10. Swimming facilities that allow diapered children should be avoided.
11. Only bottled water should be used during camping outings.

FUNGAL INFECTIONS

Fungi are free-living organisms that can be found throughout the environment. Some species of fungi represent part of the normal human flora, especially those in the mouth, intestine, vagina, and skin. A fungus is transmitted through inhalation or penetration of tissue as a result of trauma. Fungi grow very slowly, so clinical symptoms may appear only after a prolonged period of time. They are aerobic, can grow in a wide range of temperatures, and are resistant to most antibiotics. They exist in two forms: *mold* and *yeast.*

Infections caused by fungi are classified into four groups:

1. opportunistic—secondary to a defect in host immunity
2. systemic—involving deep tissues and organs
3. subcutaneous—limited to deep subcutaneous tissue
4. superficial—limited to skin, hair, and nails

Common forms include *Tinea capitis*, *Tinea pedis*, and Candida, which are discussed in greater detail in Chapter 34.

SEXUALLY TRANSMITTED DISEASES

Classic sexually transmitted diseases (STDs), which include syphilis and gonorrhea, were at one time thought to be under control. However, with the increasing sexual activity of adolescents and the microbial-resistant strains of certain organisms, there has been an alarming increase in the incidence of these diseases in the pediatric population. In addition to the classic STDs, newer infections include *Chlamydia trachomatis*, human papillomavirus, and HIV. (HIV is discussed in Chapter 23.) STDs have been identified in neonates, older children, and adolescents. Neonates are at risk for transplacental transmission from an infected mother or from direct contamination during the birthing process. Experimentation with sexual activity places adolescents at significant risk for STDs. As the age of initial intercourse has dropped over the past decade, the incidence of STDs has increased. Often, adolescents lack knowledge of methods for preventing STDs. Moreover, the use of drugs and alcohol makes unsafe, unprotected sex more likely to occur, thereby placing the adolescent at risk for STDs, HIV, and pregnancy.

Children who have not been infected during the neonatal period but who later present with signs and symptoms of an STD should be evaluated for possible sexual abuse. These children may present without the typical genital symptoms, but with a variety of physical or behavioral complaints. Related changes in behavior may include insomnia, eating disorders, bed-wetting, or emotional withdrawal. A careful, complete examination is required. The examination should include inspection of oral, anal, and genital mucosa for any signs of trauma or infection. Because obtaining a complete history may be difficult, children should undergo a complete laboratory evaluation, and all potentially infected areas should be cultured.

Gonorrhea

Causative agent:	*Neisseria gonorrhoeae*
Incubation period:	2 to 7 days
Transmission:	intimate contact, perinatal transmission, sexual abuse, sexual intercourse

Gonorrhea has become the most commonly reported STD. It may be transmitted three different ways:

- *Perinatal transmission* can occur during delivery of a neonate or with premature rupture of the membranes. The neonate can acquire the disease through aspiration of vaginal secretions, which leads to sepsis; direct contact through the conjunctiva; or direct contact through attachment of a fetal scalp monitor.
- A second route of transmission occurs with *sexual abuse.* Any child with a positive culture without a prior history of voluntary sexual behavior should be strongly considered as a potential sexual abuse victim. There has been documentation of transmission through sexual play with children, but this is rare. Studies have shown that almost all children diagnosed with gonorrhea at the age of 1 year or older have had sexual abuse documented.
- The last route of transmission is *voluntary sexual activity.* This route remains the primary route of infection among adolescents. However, sexual abuse should not be excluded as a possibility.

Clinical Manifestations. Ophthalmia neonatorum is the most common type of gonorrheal infection in the infant, presenting 1 to 4 days after birth. A thick, purulent discharge from the eyes may be present and, if not treated promptly, will progress to corneal ulceration, rupture, and blindness. Ophthalmia neonatorum has been controlled through the prophylactic administration of silver nitrate or antimicrobial agents, such as erythromycin or tetracycline given immediately after birth. In older children, ophthalmic infection can be the result of self-inoculation from the genital site.

Girls with gonorrheal infection may present with a purulent vulvovaginitis, whereas boys often have urethritis. A history of purulent discharge with burning during urination is often elicited. Adolescent girls may present with cervicitis, urethritis, perihepatitis, and salpingitis. Approximately 15% of those affected will develop pelvic inflammatory disease (PID), which can lead to infertility (Rawstron, 1993).

Therapeutic Management. Antibiotic-resistant *N. gonorrhea* strains have influenced the choice of therapy. Currently, the drug of choice for gonorrhea is a third-generation cephalosporin, such as ceftriaxone. All patients with gonorrhea should be evaluated for both syphilis and chlamydia owing to the fact that they coexist in up to 45% of cases of gonorrhea. Ceftriaxone is effective in treating syphilis, but not chlamydial infections. It is recommended, therefore, that a course of tetracycline or doxycycline be administered in conjunction with ceftriaxone for those with chlamydial infection. Patients with gonococcal infections should be placed in contact isolation until 24 hours after antibiotic therapy is begun.

Syphilis

Causative agent:	*Treponema pallidum*
Incubation period:	acquired primary—10 to 90 days (average of 21 days)
Transmission:	intimate contact, transplacental, sexual

Congenital syphilis may be transmitted transplacentally by an infected mother at any time during pregnancy or birth. Acquired syphilis is contracted through sexual contact. In children, syphilis that is diagnosed after the neonatal period can almost always be linked to sexual abuse.

Clinical Manifestations. Infants with congenital syphilis may be asymptomatic or may exhibit symptoms within the first 3 months of life. The classic signs are rhinitis, maculopapular rash, and hepatosplenomegaly. Diagnostic x-ray films may show osteochondritis, periosteitis, and/or metaphyseal changes, especially in the long bones of the femur and humerus. Late manifestations are a result of the scarring from the systemic disease process. There is involvement of the bones, teeth, eyes, and eighth cranial nerve. The teeth are notched (Hutchinson's teeth), and hearing loss can occur suddenly around the age of 8 to 10 years.

Acquired syphilis has the same clinical course in children as in adults. Primary syphilis presents with a painless chancre at the site of exposure. It is generally a single, rounded ulcer with a rubbery base and defined margins. The lesion may persist for 3 to 6 weeks before healing. Secondary syphilis may occur 3 to 6 weeks after the appearance of the chancre. The primary lesion may still be present, or it may have healed. Symptoms include local or generalized rash, general adenopathy, malaise, fever, headache, and pharyngitis. As a result of the systemic infection, a positive culture of syphilis may be obtained from CSF. The secondary stage may last from 3 to 12 weeks before resolving.

The latent stage begins with the resolution of the secondary stage. This stage is a result of the chronic **inflammation** of bone, teeth, and the CNS. Signs include Hutchinson's teeth, interstitial keratitis, eighth nerve deafness, bone changes, frontal bossing, and saddle nose (Behrman, 1996).

Therapeutic Management. Syphilis responds well to penicillin. Aqueous crystalline penicillin G or procaine penicillin are effective with congenital syphilis. Acquired syphilis can be treated with benzathine penicillin G. Tetracycline or doxycycline can be used if there is a history of penicillin allergy.

Chlamydial Infection

Causative agent:	*Chlamydia trachomatis, Chlamydia psittaci, Chlamydia pneumoniae*
Incubation period:	3 days up to 5 to 6 weeks with conjunctivitis; 2 to 12 weeks with pneumonia; 5 to 10 days with urethritis
Transmission:	during birthing process with infected mother, sexual activity

Chlamydia has become one of the most prevalent sexually transmitted disease. Infants are infected during the birthing process. Chlamydia can cause morbidity in the infant and is responsible for neonatal eye infections and interstitial pneumonia.

Clinical Manifestations. Neonatal conjunctivitis presents with a watery discharge that becomes purulent. There is eyelid edema, and the conjunctiva may become inflamed. Mucoid rhinorrhea may be associated with the infection. Many infants with conjunctivitis will develop infection of the nasopharynx, which can progress to pneumonia. These infants may have a history of a cough and congestion. Radiographic studies may reveal hyperinflation, infiltrates, and atelectasis. There may be long-term abnormalities of pulmonary function resulting in chronic respiratory problems.

Urethritis with dysuria, urinary frequency, and/or mucopurulent discharge may indicate chlamydial infection. Any identification of this organism in presexual children is indicative of possible child abuse.

Therapeutic Management. In infants with conjunctivitis or pneumonia, a 10- to 14-day course of erythromycin is recommended. In children older than 8 years of age, doxycycline may also be used.

Trichomoniasis

Causative agent:	*Trichomonas vaginalis*
Transmission:	perinatal contact during delivery, sexual activity

Only 25% to 50% of female patients with trichomoniasis will exhibit symptoms. Most male patients are asymptomatic. When symptoms occur, they may include dysuria, vaginal itching and burning (in females), and a foamy, yellowish-green, foul-smelling discharge. Infected mothers can infect their newborn infants during birth. Children having a positive culture for trichomonas should be investigated for possible sexual abuse.

Therapeutic Management. The treatment of choice is a single dose of metronidazole for adolescents and adults. For prepubertal girls, the drug is given in three divided doses. Sexual partners should also be treated. Metronidazole should not be used during the first trimester of pregnancy (CID Redbook, 1994, pp. 475–476).

Human Papillomavirus

Causative agent:	Human papillomavirus (HPV)
Incubation period:	4 weeks to many months
Transmission:	direct sexual contact, perinatal contact during delivery

Human papillomavirus is responsible for the common wart and for venereal warts (condylomata acuminata). These anogenital warts may be contracted through direct sexual contact, or perinatally during the delivery process. Children with anogenital warts should be investigated for sexual abuse. Warts can be obtained through autoinoculation from other body sites. It is necessary for there to be a break in skin integrity for infection to occur.

Anogenital warts begin as small papules that grow into soft, clustered lesions. They are found in moist areas, such as the labia minora, vagina, cervix, anus, rectum, and glans penis. Most warts in children resolve within several years.

Therapeutic Management. Treatment can include cryotherapy, electrotherapy, CO_2 laser therapy, and application of 25% podophyllin. For sexually active individuals, transmission can be decreased by the use of condoms.

NURSING CARE OF THE CHILD WITH A SEXUALLY TRANSMITTED DISEASE

Assessment

The nurse should obtain a complete history of the child's or adolescent's sexual activity. In particular, any discharge from the vagina or penis, itching around the genitals or anus, soreness or swelling in the genital area, pain, body rashes, odors from the genitals, and fever or fatigue should be noted and documented.

Nursing Diagnosis and Planning

The following nursing diagnoses and expected outcomes may be appropriate following assessment of a child with an STD.

Nursing Diagnoses

- Risk for Infection of others related to contagiousness of disease
- Impaired Skin Integrity related to inflammation
- Low Self-Esteem: Situational, related to having a socially unacceptable disease
- Knowledge Deficit related to etiology, treatment, and prevention of STDs

Expected Outcomes

- The infection will remain with original source, with no further disease transmission.
- The skin will be intact.
- The child will demonstrate or acknowledge a lack of pain/discomfort.
- The child will express a positive self-image, as well as actions that reflect that attitude.
- The child and family will demonstrate compliance with the medication protocol and will verbalize a plan of prevention.

Implementation

The nurse plays a key role in the education of young people about STDs. Often, the school nurse is the health care professional adolescents feel they can trust, so they may be the care provider who is in the best position to educate this population. Anyone dealing with adolescents must project a nonjudgmental approach and must offer reassurance of confidentiality. The nurse must be aware of symptoms and assist in identifying those who are at risk for STDs. The nurse may be the one to assume responsibility for helping the adolescent obtain proper medical treatment and gain an understanding of the importance of completing the entire course of medication.

Evaluation

- Was the STD transmitted to another individual?
- Can the child verbalize an understanding of the etiology, treatment, and prevention of STDs?
- Is the child showing either verbal or nonverbal signs of discomfort?
- Does the child express positive feelings about self?
- Is the child/family compliant with the treatment plan?

SUMMARY: NURSING CARE OF THE CHILD WITH AN INFECTIOUS DISEASE

Children from infancy to adolescence may experience an infectious disease. Many of these diseases are self-limiting and rarely produce a devastating illness, yet health care is still indicated. The nursing care involved in caring for a child with an infectious disease is focused mainly on providing symptomatic care and comfort. The nurse must have a knowledge of the course of the disease, its mode(s) of transmission, and appropriate measures for preventing exposure. This knowledge will allow the nurse to intervene and to provide the education and emotional support required by these families.

Nurses can play an important role in the education of adolescents about their sexuality. There has been a rapid increase in the incidence of STD and pregnancy among the adolescent population. The nurse is in a position to develop rapport with individuals in this age group and to provide the necessary counseling for adolescents to deal with these issues.

Assessment

A. History of exposure(s) to infectious diseases
B. History of current symptoms
C. Physical examination
   1. Documentation of type, configuration, and distribution of lesions
   2. Documentation of vital signs (especially body temperature)
   3. Documentation of general wellness
   4. Documentation of other manifestations (arthralgia, malaise, pain, etc.)

Nursing Diagnosis

- Risk for Infection (cross-contamination of self or others) related to infectious disease
- Impaired Skin Integrity related to scratching, lesions, inflammation, and/or infection of lesions
- Altered Body Temperature related to infection
- Fatigue related to fever secondary to infectious disease
- Pain related to joint inflammation
- Social Isolation related to the communicable disease
- Knowledge Deficit related to lack of information or inexperience with infectious diseases

Planning, Implementation, and Evaluation: The Child With an Infectious Disease

NURSING DIAGNOSIS • Risk for Infection (cross-contamination of self or others) related to infectious disease

Expected Outcome:
- No other individuals will contract the infection
- The child will demonstrate absence of infection, as evidenced by vital signs that are within normal parameters for the child; resolving lesions with no evidence of redness or swelling; a white blood cell count that is within acceptable limits for the child; and a lack of irritability/lethargy.

Intervention	Rationale
1. Initiate isolation or infection precautions. Instruct the family as to the requirement for isolation (gowns, gloves, masks) and the underlying rationale. Instruct the family about proper handwashing techniques.	These precautions help prevent transmission of infectious organisms from the patient to others.
2. Instruct the family and child about the underlying concepts and the modes for preventing the spread of infectious disease.	Understanding promotes compliance with isolation techniques.
3. Instruct the family and child about the sources of infection and about the risk of spreading infection.	This promotes an understanding of and cooperation with the treatment protocol and other necessary procedures.
4. Inform the family and child about reporting methods, signs and symptoms of disease, risks of transmission of disease, and potential complications.	Providing information about the disease's causes and treatment, as well as preventive measures, promotes understanding and reduces others' risk of exposure.
5. Instruct the family and child in proper handwashing techniques and medical asepsis.	This helps to prevent the transmission of pathogens to others.
6. Assess the child for fever, malaise, fatigue, lesions, or other signs of disease. Monitor laboratory values.	This information helps to differentiate between various infectious diseases.
7. Administer prescribed medication(s) to control progression of disease or to treat the infection. Instruct the family about the action and side effects of the medication(s) chosen.	Medication is used to prevent or treat infections. Sharing of information promotes compliance with the treatment regimen.
8. Provide written instructions for treatment and care upon discharge. Assess the parents' knowledge of the instructions and, if necessary, have them demonstrate procedures/techniques.	Providing this information will assist parents in maintaining compliance in the home setting.

Evaluation:
- No other individual has contracted the disease.
- The child is free from infection and afebrile.

NURSING DIAGNOSIS • Impaired Skin Integrity related to scratching, lesions, inflammation, and/or infection of lesions

Expected Outcome: • The child will have improved skin integrity as evidenced by healing of existing lesions; absence of lesion extension; decreased scratching; and decreased discomfort.

Intervention	Rationale
1. Keep the child's nails short and clean.	This helps to prevent self-contamination and scarring.
2. Use restraints or mittens on infants if necessary.	This prevents the child from scratching.
3. Bathe or soak the child in cool water (32–38°C). Use oatmeal colloid (Aveeno) or baking soda ($\frac{1}{2}$ cup in bath water), rather than soap, which can be irritating. Use superfatted soaps or soaps for sensitive skin (Dove, Basis, Neutrogena, Aveeno).	Cool baths soothe pruritis and may help to prevent scratching. By contrast, hot water may cause vasodilatation and increase pruritus. These special soaps are less alkaline and thus less drying.
4. Administer antihistamines or antipruritics as prescribed.	Antihistamines counteract the release of histamines, which causes itching. Antipruritics have a sedative effect.
5. Dress the child in lightweight clothing that is not irritating. Avoid wools and scratchy materials.	This type of clothing provides ventilation and minimizes perspiration that otherwise might intensify itching.
6. Apply soothing lotions, such as calamine, to lesions.	The lotions promote drying of lesions and aid in preventing scratching and discomfort. Avoid the use of diphenhydramine-containing calamine, as it can be very sensitizing.
7. Avoid the use of topical corticosteroids unless so ordered by the physician.	Topical steroids can be misused, and they can mask infections. Intermittent rather than continuous use will provide improved results with less risk of side effects.
8. Apply emollient creams (Lubriderm, Moisturel, Curel, or petroleum jelly).	The creams seal in water and hydrate the skin. They can have a soothing effect on the skin.

Evaluation:
• The skin is intact and any previously injured areas are healing.
• The skin lesions show no signs of secondary infection.
• The child is afebrile.
• The child scratches infrequently or not at all.

NURSING DIAGNOSIS • Altered Body Temperature related to infection

Expected Outcome:
• The child will be afebrile as evidenced by a body temperature that is within normal parameters for the child.
• The child will be alert and oriented.

Intervention	Rationale
1. Administer antipyretics as ordered.	These agents reduce the body temperature to normal parameters (37°C).
2. Keep the environment cool (in conjunction with antipyretic administration).	A cool environmental temperature helps to reduce a child's body temperature by promoting evaporation.

Intervention	Rationale
3. Keep clothing and bedding minimal (in conjunction with antipyretic administration).	A cool environmental temperature helps to reduce a child's body temperature by promoting evaporation.
4. Encourage fluid intake (in conjunction with antipyretic administration).	This helps to maintain the child's hydration level. An elevated temperature is associated with increased metabolism and fluid use.
5. Apply a cool, moist compress to the skin (in conjunction with antipyretic administration). Use tepid water to avoid shivering. Do not use alcohol for sponge baths.	This assists in heat dissipation. Shivering, however, increases metabolism and causes heat production. Alcohol produces too rapid a heat loss, is absorbed through the skin, and has a drying effect on the skin.

Evaluation:
- The child maintains a body temperature within normal parameters.
- The child is alert and oriented.

NURSING DIAGNOSIS
- Fatigue related to fever secondary to infectious disease
- Pain related to joint inflammation

Expected Outcome:
- The child will experience an increase in comfort level and energy as evidenced by verbalization of decreased discomfort; a relaxed body posture; decreased crying and irritability; and maintenance of body temperature at baseline parameters for age.

Intervention	Rationale
1. See the measures previously identified to decrease disruptions in the skin and causes for discomfort related to impaired skin integrity.	Relieving the symptoms will decrease the amount of discomfort from impaired skin integrity.
2. Administer antipyretics as ordered.	These agents help to reduce the body temperature to normal parameters (37°C).
3. Keep the environment cool and provide light clothing and bedding. Monitor the child's temperature every 4 hours, or less if indicated.	These measures decrease skin irritation. Monitoring temperatures will direct the necessity of additional nursing measures or the effectiveness of the measures.
4. Administer antihistamines and antipruritics as ordered.	These agents reduce itching and discomfort.
5. Apply lotions and provide soaks or baths using oatmeal colloids or baking soda.	These measures decrease the level of skin irritation discomfort.
6. Encourage bed rest.	Bed rest provides comfort in individuals with joint pain or fever.
7. Provide cool, nonacidic liquids (popsicles, Jell-O).	These liquids provide comfort while encouraging and maintaining adequate intake.
8. Allow the child to gargle.	Saline rinses may soothe irritated lesions. Avoid the use of commercial mouthwashes because they can cause drying and irritation.
9. Provide lozenges to relieve irritation of the mouth and throat.	They provide a soothing effect.

Intervention	Rationale
10. Provide cool mist.	This keeps mucous membranes moist and decreases the irritation caused by drying.
11. Monitor the status of lesions.	This is a measure of the effectiveness of nursing measures.
12. Provide activities that are age-appropriate and energy-appropriate depending on the child's level of wellness.	These activities afford the child suitable diversion.
13. Keep the child's skin clean and change linens and clothing frequently. Wash clothes and linen in mild detergent and double-rinse.	Clean clothing helps to prevent the spread of secondary infections. Double-rinsing reduces the potential irritants in the clothing, thereby minimizing irritation.

Evaluation:
- The skin and mucous membranes are free of signs of irritation.
- The child demonstrates minimal evidence of discomfort.

NURSING DIAGNOSIS
- Social Isolation related to the communicable disease

Expected Outcome:
- The child and family will understand the necessity for isolation and will incorporate this isolation into their home management as evidenced by the child participating in activities, maintaining appropriate interactions with peers, and verbalizing knowledge of the duration of isolation.

Intervention	Rationale
1. Provide activities involving play with masks, gowns, and gloves.	This may help the child adjust to personnel who are required to use these when caring for the child.
2. Encourage parents to stay with the child.	This promotes contact with the family, helping the child adjust to activity limitations, reducing boredom, and providing emotional support.
3. Encourage contact with friends and family via telephone or mail.	Such activities promote social interaction with others and help to prevent boredom.
4. Provide age-appropriate play activities.	This prevents boredom and promotes normal growth and development.
5. Explain to the family and child the purpose for and duration of the isolation.	Such an understanding will promote compliance with the treatment regimen and isolation requirements.

Evaluation:
- The child engages in appropriate activities.

NURSING DIAGNOSIS
- Knowledge Deficit related to lack of information or inexperience with infectious diseases.

Expected Outcome: • Parents will be able to verbalize and/or demonstrate the care necessary to manage their child's health care needs at home, as well as the preventive measures necessary to prevent the spread of the infectious disease.

Intervention	Rationale
1. Instruct parents about the requirements for isolation (gloves, gown, masks).	This information will help to prevent transmission to others.
2. Instruct the parents of measures that can decrease discomfort from lesions and pruritis.	These measures will decrease the child's level of discomfort.
3. Instruct the parents as to the signs and symptoms that would indicate potential complications related to their child's infectious disease.	This knowledge allows parents to identify situations requiring medical attention.
4. Instruct parents in the administration of any ordered medications, and have parents demonstrate administration. Educate parents about the signs and symptoms of adverse reactions to medications.	Understanding the treatment regimen will promote compliance. Parents will then seek medical help when appropriate.
5. Provide parents with information about both the positive and the negative aspects of immunizations. Answer parents' questions about various aspects of immunization.	This information promotes understanding of infectious diseases and their prevention.

Evaluation: • The parents verbalize and/or demonstrate appropriate home care.
• The parents immunize their child(ren).

KEY CONCEPTS

- Microorganisms that cause infectious disease are classified as bacteria, viruses, fungi, protozoa, and helminths.
- The skin is the first line of defense in the innate immune system.
- Modes of transmission for infectious diseases include direct contact, animal contact, insect contact, through contaminated food or water, or by contact with a contaminated object.
- The transmission of pathogens into the host occurs through modes of inhalation, ingestion, injection (insect bites), and direct contact (sexual).
- Vaccines can be live or attenuated, killed or inactivated, toxoids, human immune globulin, or animal serums or antitoxins.
- Personnel administering and handling vaccines must be aware of recommendations for handling, storing, and administering the vaccines. Special attention should be given to the site, dosage, and route.
- The hepatitis B vaccine should not be administered into the gluteal site because of decreased immunogenicity at this site.
- When a lapse in immunization occurs, the entire series does not have to be restarted.
- Children who are immunologically compromised should not receive live bacterial or viral vaccines.
- Assessment of the child with an infectious disease should include documentation of type, configuration and distribution of lesions, temperature, and any other manifestations.
- Children with infectious disease usually can and should be cared for at home.
- Children with STDs who have not been infected during the neonatal period should be evaluated for possible sexual abuse.
- Gonorrhea, the most common STD, can be transmitted during delivery of a neonate or premature rupture of the membranes, through sexual abuse, and through voluntary sexual activity.
- Positive findings associated with STDs include discharge from the vagina or penis, itching around the genitals or anus, soreness or swelling in the genital area, pain, body rashes, odors from the genitals, and fever or fatigue.

REFERENCES

Abbotts, B., & Osborn, L. (1993). Immunizations status and reasons for immunization delay among children using public health immunization clinics. *American Journal of Disease in Children, 147,* 965–968.

American Academy of Pediatrics Committee on Infectious Diseases. (1989). Measles: Reassessment of the current immunization policy. *Pediatrics, 84,* 1110–1113.

American Academy of Pediatrics Committee on Infectious Diseases. (1993). Vitamin A treatment of measles. *Pediatrics, 91*(5), 1014–1015.

American Academy of Pediatrics Committee on Infectious Diseases. (1995). Recommendations for the use of live attenuated varicella vaccine. *Pediatrics, 95,* 791–796.

Behrman, R. E., Kliegman, R., & Arvin, A. (1996). *Nelson's textbook of pediatrics* (pp. 777–781). Philadelphia: W. B. Saunders.

Bialecki, C., Feder, H., & Grant-Kels, J. (1989). The six classic childhood exanthems: A review and update. *Journal of the American Academy of Dermatology, 21*(5), 891–903.

Blumberg, D., Lewis, K., Mink, C., Christenson, P., Chatfield, P., & Cherry, J. (1993). Severe reactions associated with diphtheria-tetanus-pertussis vaccine: Detailed study of children with seizures, hypotonic-hyporesponsive episodes, high fevers, and persistent crying. *Pediatrics, 91,* 1158–1165.

Brunell, P. (1990). Measles one more time. *Pediatrics, 86,* 474–477.

Centers for Disease Control. (1991). Hepatitis B virus: A comprehensive strategy for eliminating transmission in the United States through universal childhood vaccination. *MMWR, 40*(RR-13), 1–19.

Chen, R., Ellenberg, S., Evans, G. (1995). CDC officials help physicians answer DTP-safety questions. *AAP News, 3,* 9–11.

Cherry, J., Brunell, P., Golden, G., & Karzon, D. (1988). Report of the Task Force on Pertussis and Pertussis Immunization. *Pediatrics, 81*(6), 789–914.

Clark, G. (1996). FDA officials license new hepatitis A vaccine. *AAP News, 12*(5), 6.

Clayton, E., Hickson, G., & Miller, C. (1994). Parent's response to vaccine information pamphlets. *Pediatrics, 93,* 369–372.

Cody, C., Baraff, L., Cherry, J., Marcy, S. M., & Manclark, C. (1981). Nature and rates of adverse reactions associated with DTP and DT immunizations in infants and children. *Pediatrics, 68,* 650–660.

Committee on Infectious Diseases (Redbook, 1994). *Report of the Committee on Infectious Diseases.* Elk Grove Village, IL: American Academy of Pediatrics.

Feigin, R. D., & Cherry, J. D. (1992). *Textbook of pediatric infectious diseases* (3rd ed.) (p. 1630). Philadelphia: W. B. Saunders.

Gordon, S. L. (1994). Lyme disease in children. *Pediatric Nursing, 20*(4), 415–418.

Griffin, M., Ray, W., Mortimer, E., Fenichel, G., & Schaffner, W. (1991). Risk of seizures after measles-mumps-rubella immunization. *Pediatrics, 88,* 881–885.

Howson, C., & Fineberg, H. (1992). The ricochet of magic bullets: Summary of the Institute of Medicine Report, adverse effects of pertussis and rubella vaccines. *Pediatrics, 89,* 318–324.

Hutchins, S., Escolan, J., Markowitz, L., Morgan, R., & Orenstein, W. (1989). Measles outbreak among unvaccinated preschool-aged children: Opportunities missed by health care providers to administer measles vaccine. *Pediatrics, 83,* 369–74.

Kulenkampff, M., Schwartzman, J., & Wilson, J. (1974). Neurological complications of pertussis inoculation. *Archives of Diseases in Children, 49,* 46–49.

Kwittken, P. L., Rosen, S., & Sweinberg, S. K. (1993). MMR vaccine and neomycin allergy. *American Journal of Diseases of Children, 147*(2), 128–129.

Larson, L. (1994). Report: Vaccine might trigger reactions. *AAP News, 10*(4), 1–16.

Levine, B., & Lavi, S. (1991). Perils of childhood immunizations against measles, mumps, and rubella. *Pediatric Nursing, 17,* 159–215.

Marcinak, J., Ward, M., Frank, A., Boyer, K., Froeschler, J., & Hosbach, P. (1993). Comparison of the safety and immunogenicity of acellular (BIKEN) and whole-cell pertussis vaccines in 15- to 20-month-old children. *American Journal of Disease in Children, 147,* 290–294.

Markowitz, L., Preblud, S., Orenstein, W., Rovira, E., Adams, N., Hawkins, C., & Hineman, A. (1989). Patterns of transmission in measles outbreaks in the United States, 1985–1986. *New England Journal of Medicine, 320,* 75–81.

McConnochie, K., & Roghmann, K. (1992). Immunization opportunities missed among urban poor children. *Pediatrics, 89,* 1019–1026.

Pichichero, M., Francis, A., Marsocci, S., Green, J., & Disney, F. (1993). Comparison of diphtheria and tetanus toxoids and bicomponent acellular pertussis vaccine in infants. *American Journal of Disease in Children, 147,* 295–300.

Rawstron, S., Bromberg, K., & Hammerschlag, M. (1993). STD in children: Syphilis and gonorrhoea. *Genitourinary Medicine, 69,* 66–75.

Selekman, J. (1994). The guidelines for immunizations have changed . . . again. *Pediatric Nursing, 20*(4), 376–378.

Steere, A. (1993). Current understanding of Lyme disease. *Hospital Practice, 93,* 37–44.

U.S. Department of Health and Human Services. (1990). Healthy people 2000: National health promotion and disease prevention. (Publication No. 91–502/2). Washington, DC: Author.

Waagner, D. C. (1993). Childhood exanthems. In S. L. Kaplan (Ed). *Current Therapy in Pediatric Infectious Disease* (3rd ed.) (pp. 274–278). St. Louis: B. C. Decker.

Walker, S., Jick, H., Perera, D., Knauss, T., & Thompson, R. (1988). Neurological events following diphtheria-tetanus-pertussis immunization. *Pediatrics, 81,* 345–349.

Wexler, D. L. (1995a). Hepatitis A vaccine now licensed. *Needle Tips & the Hepatitis B Coalition News, 5*(1), 1.

Wexler, D. L. (1995b). Summary of rules of childhood immunizations, *Needle Tips and the Hepatitis B Coalition News, 5*(1), 13–14.

Wexler, D. L. (1995c). Ask the experts. *Needle Tips and the Hepatitis B Coalition News,* 5(1), 4.

Weller, T. (1983). Varicella and herpes zoster: Changing concepts of the natural history, control, and importance of a not-so-benign virus. *New England Journal of Medicine, 309,* 1362–1368; 1434–1440.

Yow, M. (1990). CMV infection in young women. *Hospital Practice,* March 30, 1990, 61–79.

BIBLIOGRAPHY

Abramson, J., & Givner, L. (1993). Rickettsial diseases. In S. L. Kaplan (Ed.), *Current Therapy in Pediatric Infectious Disease* (3rd ed.) (pp. 621–622). St. Louis: B. C. Decker.

American Academy of Pediatrics. (1995). Polio vaccine schedule likely to change, but not until 1997. *AAP News, 11*(11), 1.

American Academy of Pediatrics Committee on Adolescence. (1994). Sexually transmitted diseases. *Pediatrics, 94*(4), 568–572.

American Academy of Pediatrics Committee on Infectious Diseases. (1993). Universal hepatitis B immunization. *Pediatrics, 89*(4), 795–800.

American Academy of Pediatrics Committee on Infectious Diseases. (1993). The use of oral acyclovir in otherwise healthy children with varicella. *Pediatrics, 91*(3), 674–676.

Ben-Amitai, D., & Ashkenazi, S. (1993). Common bacterial skin infections. *Pediatric Annals, 22*(4), 225–233.

Bobo, J., Gale, J., Thapa, P., & Wassilak, S. (1993). Risk factors for delayed immunization in a random sample of 1163 children from Oregon and Washington. *Pediatrics, 91*, 308–314.

Brown, H. P. (1989). Recognizing STDs in adolescents. *Contemporary Pediatrics*, 6, 17–36.

Centers for Disease Control. (1992). Pertussis vaccination: Acellular pertussis vaccine for the fourth and fifth doses of the DPT series. Update to supplementary ACIP Statement. *MMWR, 41*(RR-15), 1–5.

Centers for Disease Control. (1992). Pertussis vaccination: Acellular pertussis vaccine for reinforcing and booster use—Supplementary ACIP statement. Recommendations of the Immunization Practices Advisory Committee (ACIP). *MMWR, 41*(RR-1), 1–10.

Centers for Disease Control. (1993). Compendium of animal rabies control. (1993). *MMWR, 42*(RR-3), 1–8.

Centers for Disease Control. (1993). Standards for pediatric immunization practice. *MMWR, 42*(RR-5), 1–10.

Clark, G. (1994). Immigrants challenge U.S. medical practice. *AAP News, 10*(3), 18–20.

Couzens, G. S. (1992). How to detect Lyme disease. *The Physician and Sportmedicine, 20*(4), 140–147.

Cowden, F. M., & Mindel, A. (1992). Sexually transmitted diseases in children: Adolescents. *Genitourinary Medicine, 69*(2), 141–147.

Dennehy, P. H., (1993). Should oral acyclovir be used to treat chickenpox in normal children. *Contemporary Pediatrics, 10*, 31–48.

Englund, J. A. (1993). Varicella-zoster virus infections. In S. L. Kaplans (Ed.), *Current Therapy in Pediatric Infectious Diseases*. (3rd ed.). (pp. 265–269). St. Louis: B. C. Decker.

Feder, H., & Anderson, I. (1989). Fifth disease: A brief review of infections in childhood, in adulthood, and in pregnancy. *Archives of Internal Medicine*, 149, 2176–2178.

Feigin, R. D., & Cherry, J. D. (1992). *Textbook of Pediatric Infectious Diseases* (3rd ed.). Philadelphia: W. B. Saunders.

Friden, I. J., & Resnick, S. D. (1991). Childhood exanthems: Old and new. *Pediatric Clinics of North America, 38*(4), 859–883.

Fulginiti, V. A. (1992). Commentaries: How safe are pertussis and rubella vaccines? *Pediatrics, 89*(2), 334–336.

Gerner, H. M. (1992). Varicella zoster. *Journal of the American Academy of Nurse Practioners, 4*(4), 157–159.

Gershon, A. (1994). Live attenuated varicella vaccine soon to be licensed. *The report on pediatric infectious diseases. 4*(9), 33–34.

Ginsburg, C. M. (1983). Acquired syphilis in prepubertal children. *Pediatric Infectious Disease, 2*(3), 232–234.

Gittes, E. B., & Irwin, C. E. (1993). Sexually transmitted diseases in adolescents. *Pediatrics in Review, 14*(5), 180–189.

Goh, B. T., & Forster, G. E. (1993). STD in children: Chlamydia oculogenital infection. *Genitourinary Medicine, 69*(3), 213–221.

Gordon, S. (1994). Lyme disease in children. *Pediatric Nursing, 20*(4), 415–418.

Grose, C., Meehan, T., & Weiner, C. P. (1992). Prenatal diagnosis of congenital cytomegalovirus infection by virus isolation after amniocentesis. *Pediatric Infectious Disease Journal, 11*(8), 605–607.

Gurevich, I. (1991). Fifth disease and other parvovirus B 19 infections. *Heart and Lung, 20*(4), 342–344.

Halsey, N. A. (1993). Discussion of Immunization Practices Advisory Committee/American Academy of Pediatrics recommendations for universal infant hepatitis B vaccination. *Pediatric Infectious Disease Journal, 12*(5), 446–449.

Halsey, N. A. (1993). Increased mortality after high titer measles vaccines: Too much of a good thing. *Pediatric Infectious Disease Journal, 12*(6), 462–465.

Hess, D. L. (1993). Chlamydia in the neonate. *Neonatal Network, 12*(3), 9–12.

Hick, J., Charboneau, J., Brakke, D., & Goergen, B. (1989). Optimum needle length for diphtheria-tetanus-pertussis inoculation of infants. *Pediatrics, 84*, 136–137.

Jackson, M. A., Burry, V. F., & Loson, L. C. (1992). Complication of varicella requiring hospitalization in previously healthy children. *Pediatric Infectious Disease Journal, 11*(6), 441–445.

Jenny, C. (1992). Sexually transmitted diseases and child abuse. *Pediatric Annals, 21*(8), 497–503.

Koff, R. S. (1993). Hepatitis B today: Clinical and diagnostic overview. *Pediatric Infectious Disease Journal, 12*(5)L, 428–437.

Krugman, S., Katz, S., Gershon, A., & Wilfert, C. (1993). *Infectious diseases of children* (9th ed.). St. Louis: Mosby–Year Book.

Pagano, J. S. (1992). Epstein-Barr virus: Culprit or consort? *New England Journal of Medicine, 327*(24), 1750–1751.

Peter, G., & Halsey, N. (1995). Redbook Committee considers increased IVP use. *AAP News, 11*(10), 13.

Prose, N. S., Abson, K. G., & Berg, D. (1992). Lyme disease in children: Diagnosis, treatment, and prevention. *Seminars in Dermatology, 11*(1), 31–36.

Rawston, S. A., Bromberg, K., & Hammerschlag, M. R. (1993). STD in children: Syphilis and gonorrhoea. *Genitourinary Medicine, 69*, 66–75.

Schmidt, M. J., Olson, J. G., & Krebs, J. W. (1993). Rabies goes wild. *Contemporary Pediatrics, 10*,36–46.

Sexton, D. J., & Corey, G. R. (1992). Rocky Mountain "spotless" and "almost spotless" fever: A wolf in sheep's clothing. *Clinical Infectious Diseases, 15*, 439–48.

Sonnenblick, H. C. (1992). Abstract: Erythema infectiosum. *Pediatrics in Review, 13*(6), 236–237.

Yagupsky, P. (1993). Bacteriologic aspects of skin and soft tissue infections. *Pediatric Annals, 22*(4), 217–224.

Zemel, L. S. (1992). Lyme disease—A pediatric perspective. *Journal of Rheumatology, 19*, 1–13.

23

The Child With Immunologic Alterations

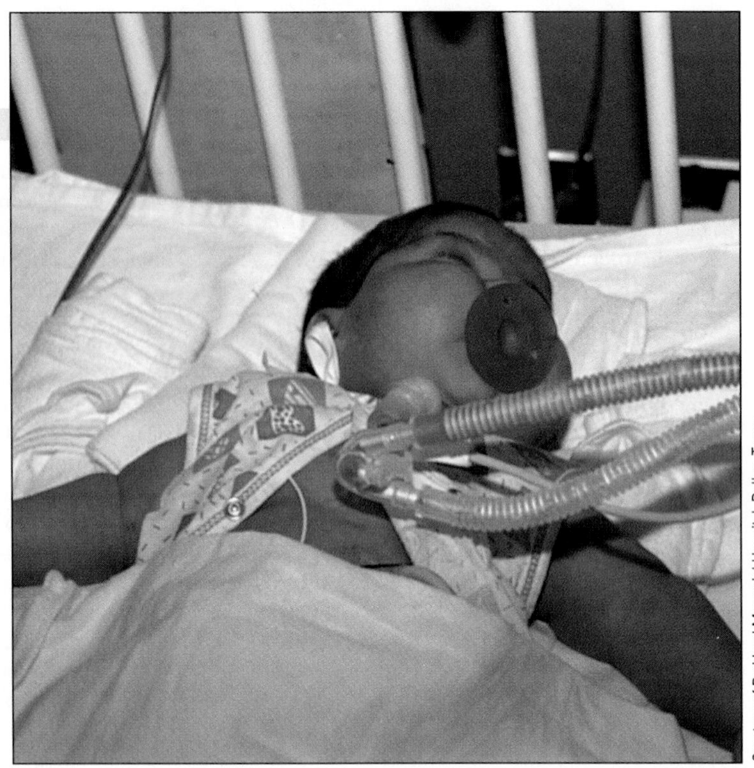

Courtesy of Parkland Memorial Hospital, Dallas, Texas

CHAPTER OVERVIEW

LEARNING OBJECTIVES

After studying this chapter, you will be able to:

- Describe how the immune system attempts to maintain homeostasis of the internal and external environment and what happens when it overfunctions or underfunctions.
- Explain how neonates acquire active and passive immunity.
- Delineate how to prevent the spread of organisms in children with an immunodeficiency.
- Describe how to care for and support HIV-affected children and their families throughout the entire spectrum of illness.

- Outline what to teach and reinforce with families about long-term corticosteroid therapy for systemic lupus erythematous and penicillin therapy for rheumatic fever.
- Describe nursing interventions to help prevent sudden death in an anaphylactic reaction and in Kawasaki disease.

KEY TERMS

active immunity: the protection, which can last months, years, or even a lifetime, that forms in response to exposure to antigens in nature or vaccines

allergy: the immune system's response to an allergen that causes a hypersensitivity reaction in various body systems

antibody: a protein that the immune system produces to bind to specific antigens and eliminate them from the body

antigen: a substance that possesses unique configurations enabling the immune system to recognize it as foreign

autoimmune disease: disease that occurs when the immune system produces antibodies—called autoantibodies—against cells of the body

complement: an accessory system to a humoral response which is composed of serum proteins that facilitate enzyme action and antigen death

immune (lymphoreticular) system: the body's internal defense against foreign substances, such as bacteria, viruses, parasites, and fungi

immunodeficiency: a defect in the immune system leading to increased susceptibility to multiple infections, including repeat infections

leukocytes: white blood cells, whose chief function is to protect the body against foreign substances; there are five types: lymphocytes, monocytes, neutrophils, eosinophils, and basophils

lymphocytes: the primary white blood cells of the immune system (e.g., B lymphocytes or B cells and T lymphocytes or T cells)

nonspecific immune functions: protective barriers, such as chemicals, interferon, inflammation, and phagocytosis, which are activated in the presence of an antigen, but are not specific to that antigen

passive immunity: antibody transfer from a person with active immunity to a person who does not have that antibody

specific immune functions: a humoral (B-cell and antibody production) and cell-mediated (T cell) response that is activated in a highly discriminatory way to antigens that survive in the body

Immunologic alterations typically are chronic, lasting for months to years and interfering with a child's life to some degree. Physical symptoms may range from simple, such as impaired skin integrity, to complex, such as a risk of overwhelming infection. As with other chronic illnesses, there are intervals of wellness, relapses, and sometimes a decline in health; repeated office visits and hospitalizations; disruptions in family routines; altered social interactions; strains on finances; and anxiety about the future.

Initially, the nurse supports the family in dealing with a new and often devastating diagnosis. Care during the acute phase of the illness may be critical in nature, as underlying organisms are diagnosed and treated and high fevers and pain are managed. As a crisis resolves, the nurse prepares the family for discharge by identifying community resources and referrals for ongoing support. The nurse also teaches the family: how to prevent the spread of microorganisms through infection control practices at home; parameters for when to call the physician; and ways to optimize the child's health through maintaining skin integrity, the body's first line of protection against microorganisms, and a diet that includes proteins and calories, which support immune cell growth. Nurses also play a vital role in advocating for children with such stigmatized conditions as HIV infection.

Despite all efforts, rehospitalization is often inevitable. The family is an integral part of the multidisciplinary team, keeping the physicians, nurses, and social workers informed of changes in the child's condition, administering medications, providing respiratory care, and often making difficult decisions about continued treatment and comfort.

Because the science of immunology is still evolving, nurses must remain current about the newest information. This chapter outlines how nurses can support and teach the family and care for the child diagnosed with an immunologic alteration.

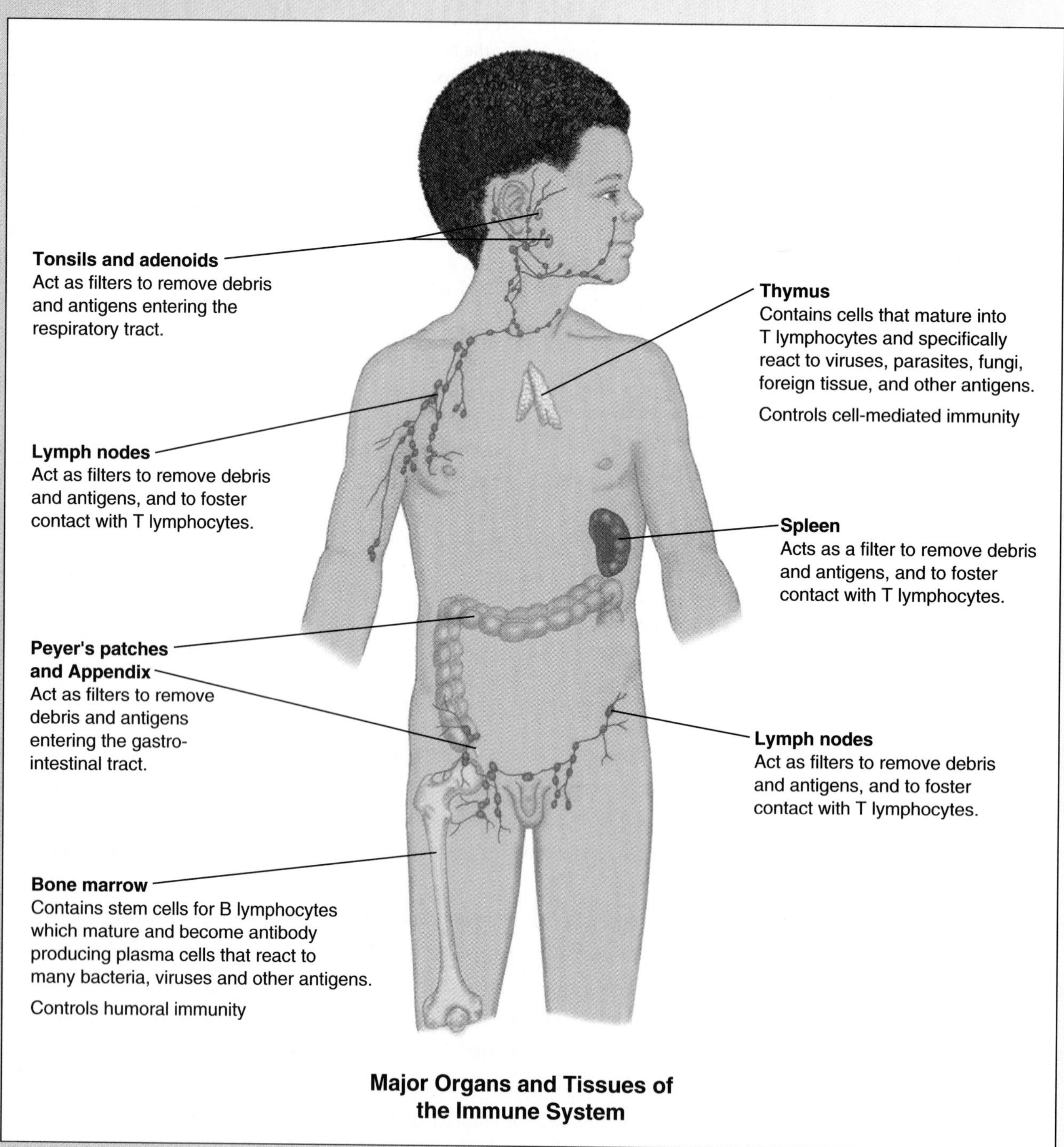
Tonsils and adenoids
Act as filters to remove debris and antigens entering the respiratory tract.
Thymus
Contains cells that mature into T lymphocytes and specifically react to viruses, parasites, fungi, foreign tissue, and other antigens.
Controls cell-mediated immunity
Lymph nodes
Act as filters to remove debris and antigens, and to foster contact with T lymphocytes.
Spleen
Acts as a filter to remove debris and antigens, and to foster contact with T lymphocytes.
Peyer's patches and Appendix
Act as filters to remove debris and antigens entering the gastro-intestinal tract.
Lymph nodes
Act as filters to remove debris and antigens, and to foster contact with T lymphocytes.
Bone marrow
Contains stem cells for B lymphocytes which mature and become antibody producing plasma cells that react to many bacteria, viruses and other antigens.
Controls humoral immunity

Major Organs and Tissues of the Immune System

REVIEW OF THE IMMUNE SYSTEM

The body's network of first-line or external defenses—intact skin and mucous membranes, and such processes as sneezing, coughing, and tearing—help keep it free of disease. When a foreign substance is able to penetrate these first line defenses, the internal defense system—the **immune system**—provides secondary protection through both nonspecific and specific responses. The immune system is able to (1) distinguish the body's own cells, or "self," from foreign substances, or "nonself;" (2) activate a response against "nonself;" (3) detect and destroy foreign substances; (4) suppress a response against "self;" and (5) store information (Schindler, 1988).

Foreign substances or antigens possess unique configurations whereby the immune system recognizes them as foreign. The system responds to the invader by producing proteins called **antibodies.** Each antibody is specific for a particular **antigen,** contains sites that are complimentary, and can combine with the antigen. This combination of antigen and antibody is called the antigen-antibody complex, or immune complex, which then acts to destroy the antigen (Schindler, 1988).

The major organs and tissues of the immune system are the bone marrow, thymus, spleen, lymph nodes, and lymphoid tissue. These organs and tissues are connected to one another by both the circulatory and the lymphatic systems. Cells important to the immune system are listed in the accompanying table.

Nonspecific Immune Functions. The body's innate immune system consists of **nonspecific immune functions,** which are protective barriers activated in the presence of an antigen but not specific to that antigen. Among these nonspecific immune functions are: *chemical barriers,* such as bactericides and fungicides and enzymes in body secretions; *interferon,* a protein produced in response to viruses; *inflammation,* increased capillary permeability, vasodilation, phagocytosis ("cell-eating") and elimination of cell products. *Phagocytosis* may occur itself or as part of the inflammatory response (see figure). The phagocytes ingest the antigen and either survive or die. In dying, the phagocytes release additional chemicals that draw more phagocytes to the area. Increased capillary permeability and vasodilation result in redness and edema. The products of phagocyte-antigen death include toxins that give

CELLS INVOLVED IN THE IMMUNE RESPONSE

	Nonspecific Immune Response
Granulocytes	
Neutrophils	First leukocytes to respond to tissue damage. Ingest and destroy antigens, especially bacteria, by phagocytosis. Increase in number during acute inflammation, bacterial infection, and necrosis. Immature neutrophils are called bands.
Eosinophils	Neutralize histamine. Increase in number during allergic reactions and infestation with parasitic worms.
Basophils	Secrete histamine, heparin, and serotonin in immediate hypersensitivity reactions. Basophils that leave the blood stream are called mast cells.
Agranulocytes	
Monocytes/Macrophages	Monocytes are large phagocytic agranulocytes. In the tissues they are called macrophages. Monocytes ingest and introduce antigens into the circulation. Macrophages engulf bacteria and cellular debris to finish the cleanup process started by the neutrophils.
	Specific Immune Response
B lymphocytes	Noncirculating, short-lived cells responsible for humoral immunity. Produce antibodies to bacteria. First responder to viral infection.
T lymphocytes	Responsible for cellular immunity. Interact with specific antigens on cell surfaces and directly attack invading microorganisms. Respond to viruses, fungi, parasites, and foreign tissue. T-cell regulatory functions mobilize or deactivate the other cells in the immune system.
Helper (CD4) T cells	Recognize antigens that have been processed and presented to them by B cells or macrophages. CD4 cells secrete lymphokines that stimulate B cells to manufacture antibodies.
Suppressor T cells	Inhibit the actions of helper T cells and B cells. Help keep the immune system cells in check.
Killer T cells	Phagocytize target cells; make cells more vulnerable to chemical attack via production of lymphokines.

Material compiled from Applegate, E. J. (1995). *The anatomy and physiology learning system: Textbook* (p. 300). Philadelphia: W. B. Saunders; Copstead, L. E. (1995). *Perspectives on pathophysiology* (p. 191). Philadelphia: W. B. Saunders.

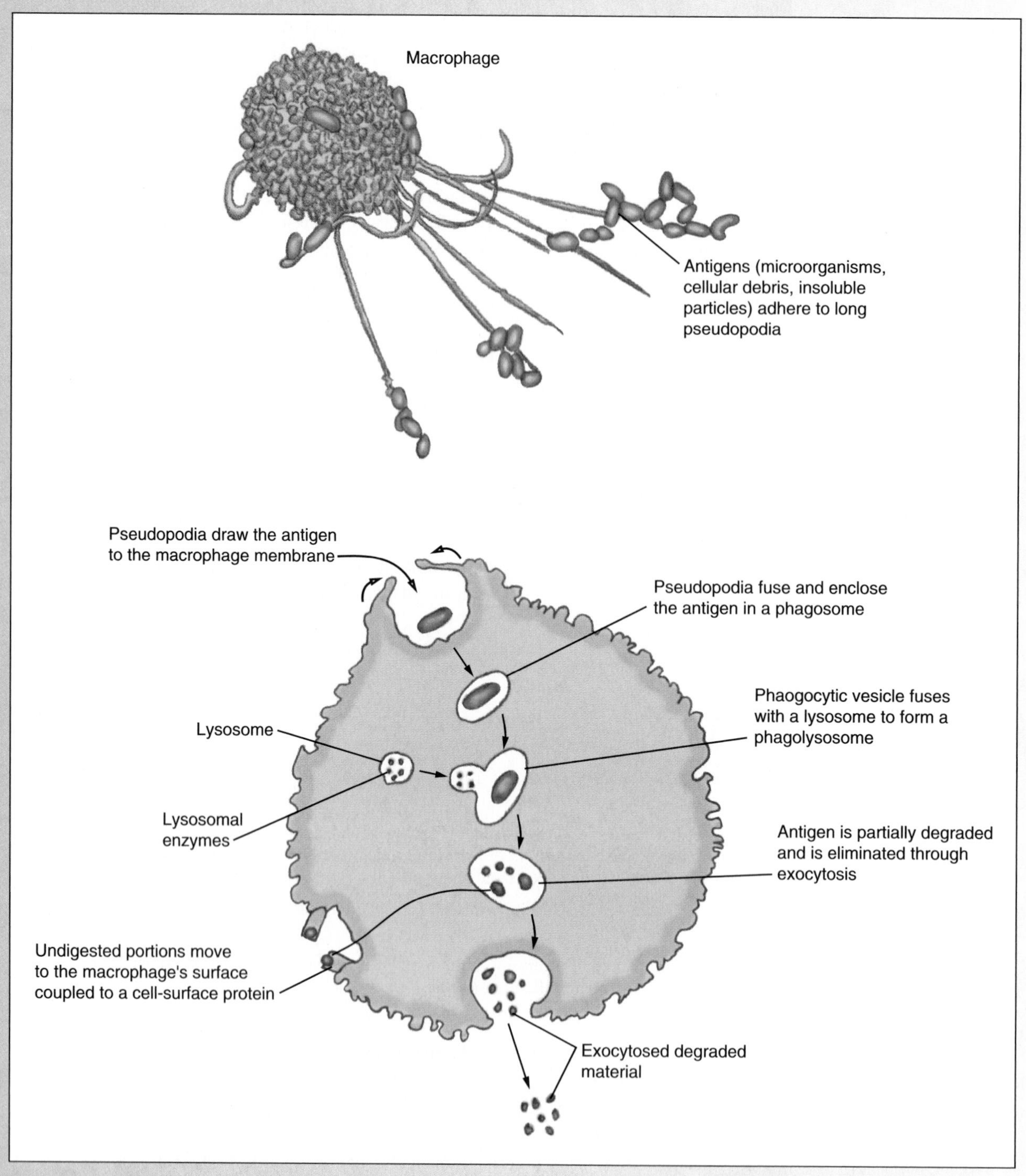

Macrophage
Antigens (microorganisms, cellular debris, insoluble particles) adhere to long pseudopodia
Pseudopodia draw the antigen to the macrophage membrane
Pseudopodia fuse and enclose the antigen in a phagosome
Phaogocytic vesicle fuses with a lysosome to form a phagolysosome
Lysosome
Lysosomal enzymes
Antigen is partially degraded and is eliminated through exocytosis
Undigested portions move to the macrophage's surface coupled to a cell-surface protein
Exocytosed degraded material

rise to fever, pain, and purulence. As the antigens are destroyed, the toxins are cleared from the lymph nodes, which often become enlarged. If the immune response is effective, the inflammation subsides. If it is ineffective, fever follows. In general, bacteria cause a greater febrile response than viruses (Belanti, 1985).

Specific Immune Functions. If the antigen survives within the phagocyte, then there are two types of **specific immune functions** that can recognize and destroy it: humoral and cell-mediated. Although immunologists have traditionally distinguished between humoral and cell-mediated immunity, it has become clear that both responses are closely related (Schindler, 1988). The white blood cells called **lymphocytes** function in both types of immune function. Lymphocytes circulate throughout the blood and the lymphatic system. They make up 53% to 57% of white blood cells in the first year of life, when specific immunity is developing rapidly, but only 25% to 30% after 12 years of age. Two classes of lymphocytes are

IMMUNOGLOBULIN FUNCTION AND PEDIATRIC IMPLICATIONS

IG TYPE	% OF TOTAL IG*	FUNCTION AND PEDIATRIC SIGNIFICANCE	LOCATION
IgG	70–80	Contains most antibodies against bacteria, viruses, and fungi in blood and body spaces. Crosses the placenta; provides maternal antibody protection to infants. Responsible for Rh reactions. IgG response is longer and stronger than that of the other immunoglobulins.	Appears in all internal body fluids; present in majority of B cells.
IgM	5–10	Produced 48–72 hours after an antigen enters the body and remains in the blood. First immunoglobulin produced in response to bacterial and viral infections. Responsible for transfusion reactions in the ABO blood typing system. Does not cross placenta, so values are low in newborns. However, IgM is produced early in life and level increases after 9 months of age. Presence in cord or infant blood may mean infection in utero or newborn period.	Appears mostly in intravascular serum. Attached to B cells; released into plasma during immune response.
IgA	10–15	Prevents infection across mucous membranes—local immunity. Especially important in antiviral protection. Passes to newborn in breast milk. Those having congenital IgA deficiency are prone to autoimmune disease.	Appears in body fluids (nasal and respiratory secretions, saliva, tears, breast milk).
IgE	0.004	Leads to release of histamines producing an allergic response. Elevation may indicate allergy in children. Plays a role in defense against parasites.	Appears in serum. Found on the surface membranes of basophils and mast cells. Produced by plasma cells in mucous membranes and tonsils.
IgD	0.2	Poorly understood. Thought to influence B cell differentiation.	Appears in small amounts in serum. Attached to B cells.

*Normal immunoglobulin values differ for age.

Material compiled from Applegate, E. J. (1995). *The anatomy and physiology learning system: Textbook* (p. 300). Philadelphia: W. B. Saunders; Copstead, L. E. (1995). *Perspectives on pathophysiology* (p. 191). Philadelphia: W. B. Saunders.

involved in the immune response: B lymphocytes (B cells) and T lymphocytes (T cells). B cells, which promote the humoral response, mature in the bone marrow, becoming plasma cells that produce antibodies. Antibodies are classified as immunoglobulins G, M, A, D, and E, often abbreviated IgG, IgM, IgA, IgD, and IgE (see accompanying table, Immunoglobulins). T cells, which are responsible for the cell-mediated response, mature in the thymus and react specifically to viruses, fungi, parasites, foreign tissue, and other antigens. There are three types of T cells: suppressor T cells, natural killer cells, and helper T cells, often referred to as $CD4^+$ cells (Bellanti, 1985; Schindler, 1988).

The Humoral Response. The humoral response chiefly involves B cells, although the cooperation of helper T cells is almost always necessary. Macrophages ingest antigens and introduce them into the circulation, where they contact B cells. The B cells and helper T cells interact. The helper T cells secrete substances that cause B cells to multiply and differentiate into plasma cells, producing vast quantities of antibodies specific to the antigen. The antibodies combine with the antigens and form immune complexes. The antibodies either destroy the antigens or activate an accessory system called **complement,** a series of serum proteins involved in enzyme action and antigen death. Suppressor T cells reduce the production of antibodies after the antigens are eliminated from the body (Schindler, 1988).

The Cell-Mediated Response. A cell-mediated response is also initiated by macrophages presenting antigens. Once activated, helper T cells secrete substances that spur additional T cells to grow. One set of T cells—called natural killer cells—tracks down and kills viruses. Suppressor T cells draw the immune response to a close (Schindler, 1988).

Prenatal Development of Immunity. During fetal development, T cells and B cells are found in the liver. Shortly before birth and for several months after, T cells move to the thymus, where they develop. B cells mature in the bone marrow and lymphoid tissue. A normal fetus can produce IgM by 10.5 weeks, IgG by 12 weeks, and IgA by 30 weeks. Therefore, there may be elevated IgM antibody in cord blood if there has been an intrauterine infection. The normal newborn infant gradually begins its own humoral and cell-mediated response to infections, acquiring immunity both actively and passively (Marlow & Redding, 1988). (See the accompanying box, Pediatric Differences in the Immune System.)

Active Immunity. **Active immunity** means the body has reacted to an antigen through either a humoral or a cell-mediated response, or both. The effect of active immunity is relatively long-lived and is measured in months, years, or even a lifetime. Active immunity may follow exposure

Pediatric Differences in the Immune System

The organs of the immune system mature during infancy and childhood.

- Lymphoid tissue increases in mass during infancy and early childhood. It reaches adult size by 6 weeks of age, grows larger during the prepubertal years, and involutes at puberty.
- The thymus reaches its peak mass before puberty and then involutes.
- The spleen reaches its full size during adulthood.
- The number of Peyer's patches increases until the adult mean is exceeded during adolescence.

Immaturity of the immunologic system places the infant and young child at greater risk for infection.

- The infant has a limited capacity to mount an antibody response. The ability to respond to infections develops gradually as the infant acquires immunity actively and passively.
- Because of the immaturity of the inflammatory response in neonates, the more common signs and symptoms of infection (e.g., fever) are less pronounced, making diagnosis more difficult.
- Neonates' diminished nonspecific immune response allows for more rapid spread of infection, leading potentially to sepsis.
- The term newborn receives an adult level of IgG as a result of transplacental transfer from the mother that persists for 6–9 months. This is followed by a physiological drop in IgG level.
- Premature infants are more susceptible to neonatal infections because of lower levels of transplacental transfer of IgG from the mother and a more severe physiological drop in IgG.
- IgM, IgE, IgD are normally at low levels at birth. IgM, IgE, IgA, IgD do not cross the placenta. The immunoglobulins reach adult levels at different ages (Behrman, 1996):

  IgM: 1 yr
  IgA: 6–7 yr
  IgG: 7–8 yr
  IgE: 10–15 yr
- Absolute lymphocyte counts reach a peak during the first year. Helper T cells reach adult levels by 6 years of age.
- Passive placental transfer of IgG may affect infants' response to active immunization (i.e., pertussis and/or diphtheria).
- Immature or inexperienced immune cells affect the reliability of delayed hypersensitivity skin reactions. For this reason, allergy skin tests are not routinely used with infants.

Disorders of the immune system present differently in children than in adults.

- Primary immunodeficiencies typically present in the first six months of life.
- HIV infection, the major secondary immunodeficiency in children, typically (1) infects an infant through the mother, not sexually; (2) is diagnosed by measuring an aspect of the virus, not antibodies as in adults; and (3) has a shorter latency period in infants with several different AIDS-defining illnesses.

AGE-ADJUSTED CD4⁺ COUNTS

IMMUNOLOGIC CATEGORY	<12 MONTHS	1–5 YEARS	6–12 YEARS
No evidence of suppression	≥1500	≥1000	≥500
Evidence of moderate suppression	750–1499	500–999	200–499
Severe suppression	<750	<500	<200

Modified from Centers for Disease Control. *MMWR, 43* (RR-12), (September 30, 1994). 1–10.

to antigens occurring in nature or in vaccines. Immediately after exposure, there is a latency period when antibody levels are low. During the latency period, the body "recognizes" the antigen as foreign and makes antibodies. The predominant antibodies produced early after exposure to antigens are IgM and, subsequently, IgG. Upon second exposure to an antigen, antibodies appear at a faster rate. The latency period is shortened or nonexistent. Usually after a second exposure, the antibody levels remain high and persist for much longer periods of time. The predominant antibody in a secondary response is IgG (Bellanti, 1985).

Infants receive specific live or attenuated vaccines on a recommended schedule to induce immunity against the antigens in the vaccine (see Appendix A).

Passive Immunity. **Passive immunity** results from antibody transfer from a person with active immunity to one who does not possess that antibody. Transfer of antibodies from a woman to her fetus is an example of passive immunity. The fetus receives maternal IgG antibodies across the placenta with the result that the infant is protected against many infections. Most maternal antibodies dissipate in the infant by 6 to 9 months of age, but some persist for up to 18 months. The duration, however, depends on the level of that particular antibody in the maternal plasma during pregnancy. Protection against measles may last through the second year of life, whereas protection against certain bacterial infections may last only 1 to 2 months. The reason neonates are so susceptible to bacteria, such as *Escherichia coli,* is because these antibodies do not cross the placenta. Breastfed infants have some added protection against infections and allergens that invade by way of the mucous membranes (e.g., gastroenteritis and asthma). This is because colostrum and breast milk contain IgA antibodies (Marlow & Redding, 1988).

COMMON LABORATORY AND DIAGNOSTIC TESTS OF IMMUNE FUNCTION

Function of the immune system is evaluated by a variety of laboratory tests. Laboratory evaluation determines intactness of its major functions, B-cell immunity, T-cell immunity, and phagocytosis (see table, Common Laboratory and Diagnostic Tests of Immune Function). Many values vary significantly with the age of the child, especially during infancy. This is particularly true with regard to the differential in a complete blood count (CBC), the amount of various immunoglobulins, the lymphocyte surface antigen count (e.g., $CD4^+$ count), and the total lymphocyte count. Normal age-related declines in $CD4^+$ counts occur from birth to 6 years of age (see table). An age-adjusted $CD4^+$ lymphocyte count assesses the degree of immunosuppression resulting from HIV infection.

Allergy. Measurement of eosinophilia and IgE levels, along with a radioallergosorbent test (RAST) and skin testing, is helpful in diagnosing allergic reactions (see table, Laboratory and Clinical Tests for Allergy).

LABORATORY AND CLINICAL SCREENING TESTS FOR ALLERGY

TEST	FINDINGS SUGGESTIVE OF ALLERGY
CBC, differential	Excess eosinophils (> 5% of WBCs)
Total eosinophil count	>750 eosinophils
Nasal smear	Excess eosinophils
Serum IgE	Elevated for age
RAST test, antigen-specific IgE	Increase in antigen-specific IgE in the serum
Skin testing	Urticarial wheal appears on skin within ½ hour after administration of selected potential allergens. The reaction can be immediate or delayed and can even include anaphylaxis.

Modified from Centers for Disease Control. (September 30, 1994). *MMWR, 43* (RR-12), 1–10.

COMMON MEDICATIONS FOR IMMUNOLOGIC AND ALLERGIC DISORDERS

DRUG	ACTION	DOSAGE	ADMINISTRATION	SIDE EFFECTS	NURSING CONSIDERATIONS
Acyclovir	Interferes with DNA synthesis and viral replication Treats initial and recurrent mucosal and cutaneous herpes infections and varicella-zoster infections in immunocompromised patients	To treat varicella zoster in children: 500 mg/m^2 q 8 hr; continue for 7 days To treat mucosal or cutaneous herpes simplex in children younger than 12 years of age: 250 mg/m^2 q 8 hr; continue for 7 days	PO, IV, topical	Frequent nausea and vomiting with oral dose; burning or stinging and pruritus with topical therapy	Space doses evenly; use a disposable glove to apply topical ointment.
Aspirin	Produces analgesic, anti-inflammatory effect Decreases elevated body temperature Inhibits platelet aggregation Treats mild to moderate pain, fever, and inflammatory conditions such as rheumatic fever and Kawasaki disease Also used to reduce the risk of myocardial infarction	Usual pediatric dose: 65 mg/kg/24 hr in 4–6 divided doses, not to exceed 3.6 g/day To treat acute rheumatic fever in children: 100mg/kg/day, then decrease to 75 mg/kg/day for 4–6 weeks	PO, rectal	Occasional GI distress: cramping, heartburn, abdominal distension, mild nausea, bruising, bleeding	Do not give to children with chickenpox or flu (increases risk of Reye syndrome) Give with milk or food to decrease gastric symptoms In long-term therapy, monitor plasma salicylic acid concentration and urinary pH Assess skin for bruising. Take temperature 1 hr after administering aspirin and note decrease Evaluate the therapeutic effect on patient's pain.
Beclomethasone dipropionate	Produces local steroidal activity with minimal systemic corticosteroid effects Controls bronchial asthma and relieves allergic rhinitis	Inhalation in children 6–12 years of age: 1–2 inhalations 3–4 times/day; maximum of 10 inhalations/day Intranasal administration in children 6–12 years of age: 1 inhalation 3 times per day	Inhalation, intranasal	Occasional throat irritation, hoarseness, dry mouth, coughing, wheezing, and/or fungal infection with inhalation Occasional local irritation, burning, stinging, dryness, and/or headache with intranasal administration	Do not change dose schedule or discontinue the drug. With inhalation, maintain careful mouth hygiene; rinse mouth with water after inhalation. Contact the physician if the patient develops a sore throat. With intranasal administration, contact the physician if there is no improvement in symptoms, sneezing, or nasal irritation. Use bronchodilators (if ordered) before corticosteroid administration.

Didanosine (ddl)[1]	Inhibits replication of retroviruses, including HIV	90–135 mg/m^2 q 12 hr.	PO	Frequent diarrhea, headache, nausea, vomiting, abdominal pain, skin disorders	
Diphenhydramine hydrochloride (Benadryl)	Competes with histamines, resulting in anticholinergic, antipruritic, antitussive, and antiemetic effects Treatment of allergic reactions Prevents nausea and vomiting, and relieves pruritus and skin irritation	For allergic reactions: 5 mg/kg/24 hr in 4 divided doses in children > 20 lb	PO, IM, IV, topical	Frequent drowsiness, dizziness, muscular weakness, dry mouth/nose/throat/lips Urinary retention Thickening of bronchial secretions with PO, IM, or IV administration	Monitor patient for paradoxical reaction.
Epinephrine	Increases heart rate and vasoconstriction of blood vessels Dilates pupils For bronchial asthma attacks, emphysema, allergic reactions, and anaphylaxis and for management of glaucoma	For anaphylaxis or asthma: 0.01 mg/kg subcutaneously (0.01 ml/kg of 1:1000 concentrate), may repeat in 20-min to 4-hr intervals	Subcutaneously, IV, inhalant, ophthalmic	Frequent restlessness, anxiety, tremors, headache, tachycardia with palpitations, and tissue blanching at injection site	Monitor the rate, depth, rhythm, and type of respirations; quality and rate of pulse; and BP (for elevation) Evaluate the patient for clinical improvement
Hydrocortisone	Has anti-inflammatory properties Prevents/suppresses development of local heat, redness, swelling, and tenderness	Topical use in adults: apply sparingly to affected area 2–4 times/day. Check with physician for current pediatric recommendations.	PO, topical, IM/IV, rectal	With topical use: occasional itching, redness or irritation may occur.	Apply sparingly after shower or bath for best absorption; rub thoroughly into the affected area; do not cover Avoid contact with eyes and exposure of treated area to sunlight.
Intramuscular immune globulin	Provides passive immunity Used after exposure to hepatitis A or B Prevents or modifies symptoms of measles in individuals exposed within previous 6 days Treats idiopathic thrombocytopenic purpura	In immunodeficiency diseases: IM: 1.2 mg/kg initially; then 0.6 mg/kg q 2–4 weeks. Maximum single dose is 20–30 ml in infants and small children	IM, IV	Frequent localized tenderness at injection site Occasional urticaria, angioedema	Give IM injection to a large muscle mass. Monitor vital signs q 15 min × 4 during the first hour of IV infusion, observing for a precipitous fall in BP Keep epinephrine on hand.
Intravenous immune globulin	Prevents bacterial infections associated with B-cell immunodeficiency	Check manufacturer guidelines for current recommendations		Rarely chills, fever, lethargy, chest tightness, nausea, vomiting Anaphylaxis	

(continued)

COMMON MEDICATIONS FOR IMMUNOLOGIC AND ALLERGIC DISORDERS *(continued)*

DRUG	ACTION	DOSAGE	ADMINISTRATION	SIDE EFFECTS	NURSING CONSIDERATIONS
Ketoconazole	Usually fungistatic Treats candidiasis	Mild to moderate infections in children older than 2 years of age: 3.3–6.6 mg/kg/day as a single dose	PO, topical, shampoo	Frequent nausea, vomiting, pruritus	Monitor hepatic function and be alert for the presence of dark urine, pale stools, fatigue, anorexia/nausea/vomiting. Monitor bowel activity, sleep patterns, and skin reactions. Prolonged therapy usually necessary.
Nystatin	Generally fungistatic For treatment of candidiasis	Oral suspension In infants: 100,000–200,000 U 4 times/day In children: 400,000–600,000 U 4 times/day Topical application in adults: apply 2–3 times/day Check with physician for current pediatric recommendations	PO, topical	Occasional nausea, vomiting, diarrhea, GI distress with high doses Rare hypersensitivity reaction, irritation with topical use	Evaluate the patient's food intake. Do not miss a dose. Give oral medication after meals. Clean the patient's mouth before applying; use a swab. Do not give food for 30 minutes. For topical use, keep the area clean and dry; apply a thin layer, wearing a glove.
Penicillin G. See drug references for other forms of penicillin.	Interferes with cell wall replication of susceptible organisms Treats mild to moderate infections of the respiratory tract and skin Used for prophylaxis following rheumatic fever	Children > 27 kg: 600,000–1.2 million U one time. Children < 27 kg and infants: 300,000–600,000 U one time 25,000–90,000 U/day in 3–6 divided doses	IM PO	Frequent GI reaction: nausea, vomiting, and diarrhea Occasional pain, induration at IM injection site May cause hypersensitivity reaction including anaphylaxis	Administer into a large muscle mass or on an empty stomach. Report skin eruptions and respiratory status after administration.

Prednisone	Has anti-inflammatory properties Prevents/suppresses development of local heat, redness, and swelling secondary to inflammation Used as substitution therapy for adrenal insufficiency as well as nonendocrine disorders, such as rheumatic carditis; collagen, intestinal, ocular, renal, and skin diseases; asthma; cerebral edema, malignant conditions	Usual pediatric dose: 0.14–2 mg/kg/day	PO	With long-term therapy: muscle wasting, osteoporosis, spontaneous fracture, amenorrhea, cataracts, glaucoma, peptic ulcer	Give with food. Do not change dose/schedule or discontinue drug. Notify physician of fever, sore throat, muscle aches, weight gain or swelling. Follow the prescribed diet. Maintain hygiene. Do not give any other medications. Assess growth. Monitor follow-up laboratory studies. Inform other physicians and dentists of therapy.
Trimethoprim/sulfamethoxazole (TMP-SMX)[2]: Bactrim, Septra	Bactericidal to susceptible organisms Prevents and treats PCP, as well as chronic urinary tract infections, shigellosis, enteritis, otitis media, chronic bronchitis	For preventing PCP: 150 mg TMP/M^2/day with 750 mg SMX/M^2/day in divided doses, twice a day on consecutive days per week.	PO	Frequent anorexia, nausea, vomiting, rash (7–14 days after therapy begins); urticaria, occasional diarrhea; abdominal pain; pancreatitis	Check for family history of sensitivity. Give on an empty stomach with large glass of water. Monitor renal, hepatic, and hematology reports in long-term use. Observe the patient for skin rashes, bleeding, bruising, fever, and/or sore throat.
Zidovudine[3]	Inhibits replication of HIV by interfering with transcription of RNA and DNA	Infants younger than 2 weeks of age: 2 mg/kg q 6 hr Infants 2–4 weeks of age: 3 mg/kg q 6 hr Children 4 weeks–13 years of age: 180 mg/m^2 q 6 hr	PO	Frequent anemia, neutropenia, nausea, vomiting	Monitor the results of blood studies every 2–4 weeks.

Adapted from Hodgson, B., Kryror, R., & Kingdon, R. (1996). *Nurses' drug handbook 1996.* Philadelphia: W. B. Saunders.

Dosage for #1 and 3 taken from Parrott, R. H., & Rathlev, M. C. (1993). *Access to primary health care for children with HIV: A guide for pediatricians, family physicians and nurse practitioners.* Washington, DC: Childrens National Medical Center.

Dosage for #2 taken from CDC. (April 28, 1995). 1995 revised guidelines for prophylaxis against PCP for children infected or perinatally exposed to HIV. *MMWR 44;* RR–4.

COMMON LABORATORY AND DIAGNOSTIC TESTS OF IMMUNE FUNCTION

TEST	FUNCTION	NURSING CONSIDERATIONS
Serum immunoglobulins (IgG, IgM, IgA and IgE)	Tests humoral immunity Measures levels of immunoglobulins by separating them through immunoelectrophoresis.	Immunization and toxoids received in the last 6 months as well as blood transfusions, tetanus antitoxin, and gamma globulin received in the last 6 weeks can affect results and should be noted on the laboratory requisition. Total immunoglobulins tend to be elevated in early months, then decrease over the first year of life. These also may be unusually high early in HIV infection, then decreaase.
Lymphocyte surface antigen	Determines the types and subtypes of lymphocytes present in blood. Names of lymphocyte surface antigens are based on "clusters of differentiation" (CDs). CD antigens on a leukocyte allows its identification. The two most commonly used surface antigens and the cell types they identify are: CD4: Helper T cells. CD8: Suppressor T cells.	To determine the number of a particular type of cell, a complete blood count (CBC) must also be done.
Serum antibody titer to antigens in vaccines received (e.g., D,T)	Tests humoral immunity.	Tests antibody level to specific antigens.
Skin tests to mumps, tuberculin, tetanus, candida	Tests cell-mediated immunity.	Measures the immune system's ability to develop antibody to foreign substances.
Differential WBC count	Part of the CBC, composed of five types of WBC (leukocytes): neutrophils, eosinophils, basophils, monocytes, and lymphocytes. The differential WBC count is expressed as cubic millimeters (mm^3) and percent of the total number of WBC.	These tests measure if immune cells can ingest and destroy foreign substances.
Allergy skin tests	Upon administration of antigen into the skin to test either immediate or delayed-type hypersensitivity.	Because anaphylactic reactions can occur even in the presence of minimal allergen exposures, emergency equipment and medications should be immediately available.
Radioallergosorbent test (RAST)	Measures the quantity and increase of antigen-specific IgE present in the serum. Exact quantities of antibodies to pollens, foods, etc. can be tested.	More expensive than traditional allergy skin testing, but provides precise information without risk of hypersensitivity reaction.

Refer to appendix for normal values.

Material compiled from: Corbett, J. V. (1992). *Laboratory tests and diagnostic procedures with nursing diagnoses.* East Norwalk, CT: Appleton & Lange; Kee, J. L. (1991). *Laboratory and diagnostic tests with nursing implications.* East Norwalk, CT: Appleton & Lange; Taeusch, H. W., Christiansen, R. O. & Buescher, E. S. (1996). *Pediatric and neonatal tests and procedures.* Philadelphia: W. B. Saunders.

IMMUNODEFICIENCIES

Lack of one or more components of the immune system results in **immunodeficiency** disorders. These can be inherited, acquired through infection or other illness, or produced as a side effect of certain medications. Some children are born with defects of their immune system. Children born with defects in the humoral system are unable or only partially able to produce antibodies, thus making them susceptible to bacterial infections. Other children are born with an abnormal thymus, which affects T cell production. These children are more susceptible to viral and fungal infections, as well as to certain cancers. In very rare cases, children demonstrate a deficiency in both B cells and T cells, which is termed severe combined immunodeficiency disease. The most devastating acquired immunodeficiency is human immunodeficiency virus (HIV) infection, which destroys helper T or $CD4^+$ cells (Schindler, 1988).

A variety of medications may also cause acquired immunodeficiency. For example, antibiotics disrupt normal flora, making the body more susceptible to other microorganisms. Immunosuppressive agents and corticosteroids suppress components of the immune system, resulting in a decrease in the inflammatory response and an increased risk of bacterial invasion. Children who are immunodeficient may present with a variety of clinical features (see accompanying box).

Clinical Findings Associated With Immunodeficiency

FREQUENTLY PRESENT, HIGHLY INDICATIVE SIGNS

- Repeated or persistent respiratory tract infection
- Repeated or persistent otitis or sinusitis
- Severe bacterial infections
- Opportunistic infections, such as *Pneumocystis carinii* pneumonia or cryptosporidiosis
- Poor response to appropriate therapy

FREQUENTLY PRESENT, SOMEWHAT SUGGESTIVE

- Skin lesions
- Failure to thrive or grow
- Chronic diarrhea
- Thrush
- Hepatosplenomegaly
- Anemia, thrombocytopenia, neutropenia
- Small or absent lymph nodes, tonsils, and adenoids

Body Fluids Potentially Infectious With Blood-Borne Pathogens

- Human blood
- Blood products
- Blood components, such as factor
- Semen
- Vaginal secretions
- Cerebrospinal fluid
- Synovial fluid
- Pleural fluid
- Pericardial fluid
- Peritoneal fluid
- Amniotic fluid
- Saliva contaminated with blood
- Body fluids visibly contaminated with blood
- Unfixed tissues or organs
- HIV-containing cell or tissue cultures
- HIV or hepatitis B virus (HBV)–containing culture medium or other solutions

From Occupational Safety and Health Administration. (1992). *Occupational Exposure to Bloodborne Pathogens.* Washington, DC: U.S. Department of Labor.

HIV Infection

HIV infection is an acquired cell-mediated immunodeficiency disorder causing a wide spectrum of illness in children ranging from no symptoms to mild and moderate symptoms to severe symptoms. AIDS represents the most severe illness.

Etiology. HIV in a body fluid (see accompanying box) can enter an uninfected person's body in several ways, including sharing of needles/syringes or engaging in unprotected sexual intercourse with an infected person. Infected women may transmit the virus to an infant across the placenta during pregnancy, at delivery, and through breastfeeding. The chance of such transmission is about 25% (Sullivan, 1993) and may be as low as 8% for women who received Zidovudine during pregnancy and delivery and whose newborns received Zidovudine for 6 weeks after birth (Centers for Disease Control [CDC], 1994).

In the past, some children became infected with HIV through the transfusion of blood and blood products. In addition, approximately 50 cases of HIV infection from sexual abuse have been reported anecdotally (Parrott & Rathlev, 1993).

Incidence. In the United States approximately 6000 children younger than 13 years of age have been diagnosed as having AIDS. Perinatal transmission has been implicated

PATHOPHYSIOLOGY *of HIV Infection*

HIV is a retrovirus composed of a single positive strand of RNA. It contains an enzyme, reverse transcriptase, which plays a key role in viral replication. HIV gains entry into a $CD4^+$ cell by direct fusion of the viral envelope to $CD4^+$ receptors on the cell surface. Within the $CD4^+$ cell, reverse transcriptase causes the synthesis of HIV DNA. This integrates with the $CD4^+$ DNA. HIV then uses the $CD4^+$ cell to make more of itself. The new viruses assemble at the host surface. As they bud through the cell membrane, the viruses mature and can infect other $CD4^+$ cells. The most critical result of HIV entry into the $CD4^+$ cell is cell death. HIV infection leads to gradual destruction of more and more $CD4^+$ cells (McGrath, 1990). Because $CD4^+$ cells control B-cell function, children with HIV infection are deficient in both humoral and cell-mediated immunity. Immunoglobulins become nonfunctional, making the child extremely vulnerable to infections.

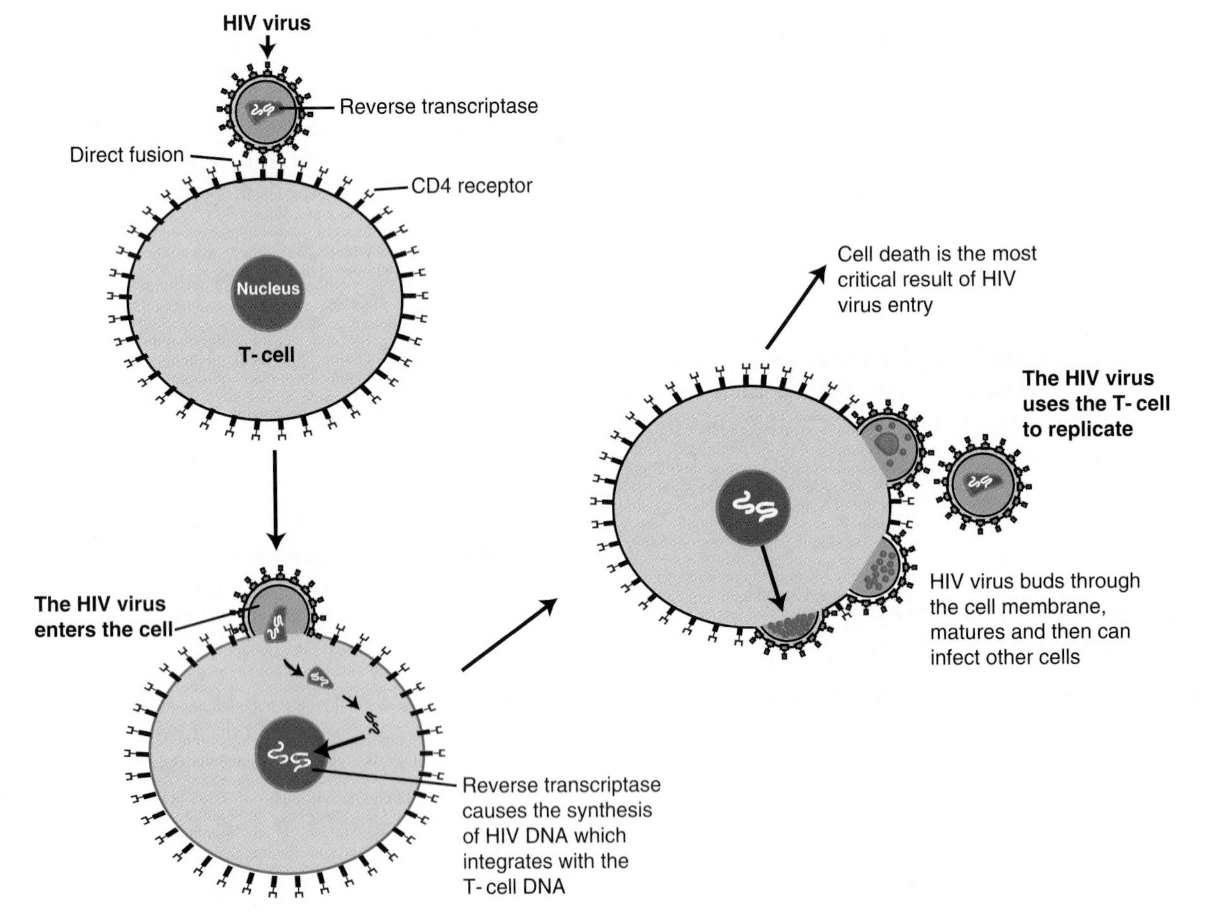

in 89% of the accumulated cases. Although only 2000 teenagers with AIDS have been reported in this country, 10 times that number of 20- to 29-year olds have been diagnosed with the disease. Given that the known median incubation period from the time of acquisition of HIV to the manifestation of AIDS in adults is probably 10 years, it is likely that many of these young adults became infected in their teens (CDC, 1994).

Clinical Manifestations. The time between infection and the diagnosis of AIDS is shorter in infants and young children (average of 4 years) than it is in adolescents or adults (Whinney, 1993). However, only a small number of children experience the onset of severe symptoms by 4 months of age. Most have a longer latency period, with significant illness being manifested by 6 or 7 years of age (Wara, 1992; Whinney, 1993). The occurrence of *Pneumo-*

cystis carinii pneumonia (PCP), an opportunistic infection, significantly reduces survival (Simonds et al., 1993). Among children with perinatally acquired HIV infection, PCP occurs most often in infants 3–6 months of age. PCP in infants is often acute in onset and results in a poor prognosis (CDC, 1995).

The CDC classify the clinical manifestations of HIV infection as mild, moderate, or severe in children younger than 13 years of age. Mild signs of the illness may be nonspecific (CDC, 1994):

- lymphadenopathy
- hepatomegaly
- splenomegaly
- dermatitis
- parotitis
- recurrent or persistent upper respiratory infection, sinusitis or otitis media

In moderate disease, some signs are considered to be important if they persist or recur (CDC, 1994):

- anemia or neutropenia
- diarrhea
- fever
- herpes simplex
- oral candidiasis

Other signs of moderate infection include the following: (CDC, 1994):

- bacterial meningitis, pneumonia, or sepsis (one episode)
- cardiomyopathy
- complicated chickenpox
- hepatitis
- nephropathy
- herpes zoster
- lymphocytic interstitial pneumonia (LIP)

In addition to LIP, the most common AIDS-indicator illnesses in children younger than 13 years of age are as follows (Moye, 1995):

- serious bacterial infections (multiple or recurrent)
- PCP
- cytomegalovirus (CMV)
- encephalopathy
- wasting syndrome

Diagnostic Evaluation. The diagnosis of HIV infection is established by measuring HIV antibody (in children older than 18 months of age) or HIV antigen (in children younger than 18 months of age). HIV antibody testing in an infant younger than 18 months of age indicates only that the child's mother is infected. Therefore, the diagnosis of HIV infection can only be made in young children when the virus or some component of the virus is detected in two different samples of blood drawn at two different times. It has been reported that 95% of perinatally infected children can be diagnosed by 6 months of age (Table 23–1) (Parrott & Rathlev, 1993).

$CD4^+$ counts are used to assess a young child's immune status, risk for disease progression, and need for PCP prophylaxis after 1 year of age. These counts are measured at ages 1 and 3 months; every 3 months until the age of 2 years; and at least every 6 months thereafter. More frequent monitoring of $CD4^+$ counts is indicated when PCP prophylaxis and antiretroviral therapy is recommended (CDC, 1995).

TABLE 23–1 *Testing for the Presence of HIV*

PURPOSE OF TEST	NAME OF TEST	AGE OF CHILD	NURSING CONSIDERATIONS
To detect HIV antibodies	ELISA, EIA for initial test Western blot for confirmatory test	>18 months of age	A positive HIV antibody test result in a child younger than 18 months of age indicates only that the mother is infected, as maternal IgG antibodies persist in infants for 6 to 9 months and, in some cases, as long as 18 months.
To detect HIV antigen	p24 antigen Immune-complex dissociated p24 core antigen	<18 months of age; can be useful at any age	These tests demonstrate the virus or components of the virus; some are more sensitive than others in children younger than 6 months of age. Only a positive result is significant; two or more positive results are diagnostic for HIV infection.
To detect whole HIV	HIV culture		
To detect HIV DNA	Polymerase chain reaction (PCR)		
To detect HIV antibody produced by the infant	IVAP, Elispot HIV IgA, IgM	<18 months of age	These tests are not routinely available or relied upon.

ELISA = enzyme-linked immunosorbent assay; *EIA* = enzyme immunoassay; *IVAP* = in vivo adhesive platelet.

Data from Parrott, R. H., & Rathlev, M. C. (1993). *Access to primary health care for children with HIV: A guide for pediatricians, family physicians and nurse practitioners.* Washington, DC: Children's National Medical Center.

Therapeutic Management. The treatment regimen for children with HIV infection includes a modified immunization schedule to prevent disease; prophylaxis against opportunistic infections, especially PCP; antiretroviral therapy aimed at inhibiting viral replication; and the aggressive use of medications to treat infections.

Children with HIV infection can respond to routine immunizations. In addition to DTP, Hib, MMR, and HB vaccines, the American Academy of Pediatrics (AAP) and the Public Health Service have made additional recommendations for vaccinating children exposed to or infected with HIV (Table 23–2) (AAP, 1994).

New CDC guidelines recommend beginning prophylaxis against PCP at 4 to 6 weeks of age for all children who have been exposed perinatally to HIV; continuing prophylaxis through 12 months of age for children diagnosed with HIV infection; and making decisions regarding prophylaxis for HIV-infected children older than 12 months of age based on $CD4^+$ counts and whether PCP has previously occurred. The first drug of choice is TMP-SMX. Dapsome and Pentamedine may also be used (CDC, 1995).

Several antiretroviral drugs are now in different stages of investigation, and two drugs—zidovudine (Zdv) and didanosine (ddI)—have been approved for use either alone or in combination in children with significant immunodeficiency or symptoms. Many children taking these drugs experience height and weight gains, decreased signs and symptoms associated with HIV infection; improvement in immunologic and neurologic function; and a better short-term survival rate. Protease inhibitors are now approved for combination therapy (in adults) with Zdv and ddI. When used properly, they may result in the decrease of viral load to undetectable levels in the blood (FDA Press Release, 1996; Health & Human Services News, 1995, 1996).

TABLE 23–2 *AAP Recommendations for Routine Active Immunization of Children With HIV Infection*

VACCINE	HIV-AFFECTED CHILDREN
Diphtheria, tetanus, and pertussis (DTP)	Yes
Oral polio vaccine (OPV)	No
Inactivated polio vaccine (IPV)*	Yes
Mumps, measles, and rubella (MMR)	Yes
Influenza*	Consider
Pneumococcal†	Yes
Haemophilus influenzae B (Hib)	Yes
Hepatitis B	Yes

*Including siblings and other family members.

†At or after 2 years of age.

Note: Always check for the most current immunization schedule.

Administer IG after measles exposure, VZIG after chickenpox exposure, and TIG in the management of tetanus-prone wounds.

Data from Parrott, R. H., & Rathlev, M. C. (1993). *Access to primary health care for children with HIV: A guide for pediatricians, family physicians and nurse practitioners.* Washington, DC: Children's National Medical Center; and the American Academy of Pediatrics, Committee on Infectious Diseases. (1994). *Immunizations in special clinical circumstances: HIV infection and AIDS.* In G. Peter (Ed.), *Red Book* (pp. 51–67, 254–270). Elk Grove Village, IL: AAP.

NURSING CARE OF THE CHILD WITH HIV INFECTION

Assessment

Many children with HIV infection experience normal health. However, as the immune system becomes more compromised and symptoms develop, hospitalization eventually becomes necessary. Therapeutic management focuses on the treatment of serious bacterial and opportunistic infections that may affect multiple organs and systems. The nurse must set the stage for engaging the family in a helping relationship. Any biases or judgments on the part of the nurse with regard to mode of transmission must be put aside so that they do not interfere with listening, supporting, and providing care.

The initial assessment should include a determination of whether a diagnosis of HIV infection has been made, as well as what the family understands about the spectrum of illness, including immunologic status (see accompanying box, Teaching Guidelines: The Child Exposed to HIV Infection). It is important that the nurse assess the child's growth and development according to age-appropriate scales and ask the caregivers about any fever, nausea, vomiting, diarrhea, ear pulling, or changes in appetite, sleep pattern, or behavior that may suggest secondary infections.

The physical examination should focus on the following parameters, which may be indicative of an infection:

- Hydration status—assessing the skin for turgor and the mucous membranes for moistness, drying, or cracking; confirming the absence or presence of tears; determining whether the anterior fontanel is palpable and soft; measuring intake, urine output, and specific gravity
- Respiratory status—listening and observing for nasal flaring, retractions, cough, difficult breathing, tachypnea, grunting, wheezing, rhonchi, and decreased breath sounds
- Mouth lesions—observing for white patches on the tongue or inside the cheeks, or blisters on the lips
- Skin lesions (especially in the diaper area)—observing for blotchy, red, flat areas, or blistering or dryness

The nurse should also assess pain by obtaining a self-report from the child, using number or color scales when appropriate; observing the child's speech, facial expressions, body movements and responses; and talking with the family.

Unlike other chronic illnesses, pediatric HIV infection is often an intergenerational health problem. Most fami-

TEACHING GUIDELINES *The Child Exposed to HIV Infection*

Review the following at the time of initial testing and subsequent clinic visits until the diagnosis is established:

TRANSMISSION

HIV can be spread from:
- unprotected sexual intercourse
- sharing of needles
- an infected mother to her baby
- open wounds (if there is blood-to-blood contact)

HIV cannot be spread by:
- sharing of knives, forks, spoons, or cups
- using the same toilet seats, bathtubs, or showers
- coughing or sneezing
- hugging, holding, or touching people

PREVENTION

The best way to prevent the spread of HIV is to:
- abstain from sex and from sharing of needles (or)
- use latex condoms with nonoxynol 9 (and)
- wash needles in a 1:10 bleach solution

The best way to prevent pregnancies is to:
- abstain from sex (or)
- use a condom
- use birth control pills
- undergo tubal ligation

If infected with HIV:
- do not breastfeed
- do not donate blood, sperm, or organs

TESTING

- The most common HIV tests used in older children and adults are the ELISA and the Western blot that measure antibodies to the virus.
- The most common HIV tests used in younger children are the p24 antigen, HIV culture, and PCR that measure the virus or components of the virus.
- CD4 counts indicate how well the immune system is working.

ILLNESS (AIDS)

Children with HIV infection may initially be asymptomatic. Mild and moderate symptoms include:
- persistent upper respiratory and ear infections
- thrush
- skin conditions
- vomiting and diarrhea
- enlarged liver, spleen, lymph nodes, and parotid gland
- growth and development problems
- LIP—a rare lung disease

Some severe symptoms of the illness include:
- opportunistic infections, like PCP and CMV
- recurrent bacterial infections, like sepsis and meningitis
- severe developmental delay
- wasting syndrome

HOME CARE

Offer a high-calorie, high-protein diet:
- Mix formula as directed.
- Do not add extra water or cereal to formula.
- Give supplemental vitamins and minerals as ordered.

Practice basic infection control (see Teaching Guidelines: Basic Infection Control for the Child With Immunodeficiency) and Standard Precautions, including the following practices:
- Avoid touching blood.
- Do not share toothbrushes, pierced earrings, razors, or nail clippers.
- Use a barrier when caring for a cut or bloody nose.
- Cover open sores.
- Leave scabs alone.
- Wipe up blood spills with a paper towel, wash the area with soap and water, rinse with bleach and water, and air-dry.
- Wrap disposable materials soiled with blood in newspaper, tie off in a plastic bag, and throw away in a plastic-lined trash can.
- Wash hands with soap and water if you touch blood.
- Rinse blood-soiled clothing with hydrogen peroxide or cold water and then wash as usual.
- Allow blood to air-dry on "dry clean only" clothing.

Keep the following immunizations up-to-date:
- inactivated polio
- pneumococcal vaccine at 2 years of age
- flu shot each fall
- IG after measles exposure
- VZIG after chickenpox exposure
- TIG for tetanus-prone wounds

Call the doctor if any of the following symptoms occur:
- fever higher than 101° F
- vomiting and diarrhea
- decreased appetite, difficulty swallowing, drooling
- rashes, bumps, lumps, or sores on the skin
- coughing or chest congestion
- ear pain, pulling on the ears, or drainage from the ears
- wounds that will not heal
- exposure to measures or chickenpox

Give prophylaxis against PCP and antiretroviral drugs as ordered.

To answer questions about pediatric HIV infection as well as to obtain educational materials, Call Project CHAMP (Children's HIV/AIDS Model Program), 202–884–5450; The National Pediatric HIV Resource Center, 210–268–8251; The National Cancer Institute Pediatric Branch, 301–402–0696; The CDC National AIDS Hotline, 1–800–342–2437; The Association for the Care of Children's Health, 301–654–6549; or The Child Welfare League of America, 202–638–2952.

lies affected by the disease have limited financial resources (Allbritten, 1990). As a result, the nurse may consult with a social worker to help ensure that basic needs, such as food, housing, and transportation, are met. Other issues, such as disclosure, permanency planning, and "Do Not Resuscitate" (DNR) orders, will need to be explored when the time is right. For example, when trust is established, families may talk about where they are with disclosure. Some choose to share the diagnosis with a trusted friend. For most, however, keeping the secret is a way of life. Although it is stressful and lonely, there are many legitimate reasons for doing so. (Tasker, 1992). The nurse can listen to families as they talk about their reasons and ask what other family members and friends know, including the child.

Because it is currently assumed all women and children with HIV infection will eventually develop AIDS and die, the nurse, at some point, may ask an infected mother what her plans are for her child(ren)'s future. This can include exploring the efficacy of standby guardianship, kinship care, or foster and adoptive placement (Merkel-Holguin, 1994). In addition, families have to make difficult decisions about an infected child's ongoing care. Should aggressive treatment continue, or should the goal of treatment be to make the child comfortable? Most of the time, these decisions are made in consultation with a multidisciplinary team. The nurse can help assess when that time is right.

Nursing Diagnoses

- Risk for Infection related to cell-mediated immunodeficiency
- Altered Nutrition: Less Than Body Requirements related to inadequate caloric intake
- Impaired Gas Exchange related to secondary or opportunistic infections
- Ineffective Airway Clearance related to ineffective cough or fatigue
- Risk for Impaired Skin Integrity related to cell-mediated immunodeficiency
- Altered Growth and Development related to effects of the virus on the neurologic system, chronicity, separation, and hospitalization
- Pain related to physical condition
- (Primary Caregiver) Anxiety related to fear of disclosure
- Ineffective Management of Therapeutic Regimen Noncompliance, related to lack of support systems or denial of the illness
- Anticipatory Grief related to expected loss (refer to care plan in Chapter 17)

Planning, Implementation, and Evaluation: The Child With HIV Infection

NURSING DIAGNOSIS

- Risk for Infection related to cell-mediated immunodeficiency

Expected Outcome:

- The child will be free of secondary and opportunistic infections.
- The child's immunization record will be up-to-date. (See Teaching Guidelines: Basic Infection Control for the Child With Immunodeficiency. Standard Precautions information appears in Appendix G.)

Intervention	Rationale
1. Follow basic infection control and Standard Precautions at all times. (See Teaching Guidelines: Basic Infection Control for the Child With Immunodeficiency, as well as Standard Precautions in Appendix G.)	Children with HIV are susceptible to infections.
2. Administer antimicrobial therapy as ordered; monitor the child for side effects.	Children with HIV mount a poor antibody response. Common pathogens include Salmonella; Shigella; Campylobacter; Yersinia; *Giardia lamblia; Isospora belli;* and Cryptosporidium.
3. Administer antipyretics for fever as ordered; monitor the effects and notify the physician if the fever does not resolve. Offer fluids. Organize care to allow for rest periods.	Children with HIV often have fevers. The increased respiratory rate that accompanies increased activity can lead to further fluid loss.

TEACHING GUIDELINES *Basic Infection Control for the Child With Immunodeficiency*

Review the following basic infection control practices for the child with immunodeficiency:

TO PREVENT CONTACT WITH GERMS

- Keep immunizations up-to-date.
- Keep child home when sick.
- Turn away when someone coughs or sneezes.
- Do not share cups, bottles, plates, utensils, drinks, or pacifiers.
- Do not kiss babies on the mouth.
- Do not use fingers as a pacifier.
- Discard unused refrigerated formula after 24 hours.
- Change diapers—away from food areas—every 2 to 3 hours or sooner if the baby has a stool.
- Dispose of trash daily.

TO CREATE A BARRIER TO GERMS IF CONTACT IS UNAVOIDABLE

- Cover your mouth when coughing or sneezing.
- Use a tissue to wipe nose.
- Cover unused food and formula and refrigerate.
- Keep a bowl close by if feeling nauseated.
- Fold soiled disposable diapers inward and tab.
- Discard dirty diapers and used tissues in a tightly covered, plastic-lined container.
- Cover sand boxes when not in use.

TO KILL GERMS IF CONTACT IS MADE

- Wash hands (using friction) with soap and warm water for 15 seconds before eating and after using the bathroom, wiping noses, changing diapers, cleaning up vomit, or catching a sneeze.
- Provide meticulous skin and mouth care.
- Carefully wash all fruit and vegetables that are to be eaten raw.
- Cook food well, especially meat, fowl, and eggs.
- Wash eating utensils, baby bottles, nipples, and pacifiers with soap and hot water or in the dishwasher.
- Rub the inside of the nipple with salt and rinse well if slimy.
- Clean kitchen and bathroom surfaces, shelves, pails, trash cans, and mops routinely.
- Clean litter boxes, bird cages, and turtle homes frequently and carefully.

Intervention	Rationale
4. Administer intravenous immunoglobulin (IVIG) as ordered; monitor the child for side effects. Notify the physician of any reaction and adjust the rate as ordered.	Administration of IVIG can prevent serious bacterial infections and hospitalizations; however, it does not affect the child's overall survival rate.
5. Reinforce principles of infection control, appropriate immunization schedules, and indications for contacting a physician (See Home Care Guidelines: The Child Exposed to HIV Infection). Teach families how to administer medications and take the child's temperature, as well as when to administer antipyretics at home.	The best way to prevent the spread of organisms at home is through good handwashing. The child with HIV and the siblings receive inactivated polio vaccine. All household members receive the influenza vaccine. If the child with HIV is exposed to the measles or chickenpox, the family must notify the physician immediately.

Evaluation:

- The child does not acquire an infection.
- The child responds to antimicrobial therapy and is free of secondary and opportunistic infections.
- The child is afebrile.
- The child's immunizations are up-to-date.
- The family notifies the physician immediately if the child is exposed to measles or chickenpox.

NURSING DIAGNOSIS • Altered Nutrition: Less Than Body Requirements related to inadequate caloric intake

Expected Outcome:
- The child will eat foods from the recommended food groups.
- The child will take in adequate calories to meet metabolic and growth needs.
- The child will be free of pain when eating.
- The child will have a regular bowel pattern.

Intervention	Rationale
1. Offer foods high in protein and calories; give vitamin and mineral supplements; consult with a nutritionist.	Children with HIV are often small in size and stature. Mouth sores and malabsorption can exacerbate problems with weight gain.
2. Offer milk, juice, or water after meals.	Children can fill up on liquids before eating.
3. Offer licks of a popsicle or ice before meals.	Cold may numb the mouth when sores are present.
4. Allow older children to use a straw.	A straw keeps liquids from touching sore spots.
5. Offer soft, bland, lightly seasoned foods that are nutritious and easy to eat.	Spicy or salty foods can irritate mouth sores. Favorite foods can be mashed, ground, or pureed to facilitate consumption.
6. Serve food at room temperature.	Hot or cold temperatures can aggravate mouth sores.
7. Offer six small meals a day. Increase calories by adding milk, butter, or cheese to potatoes, eggs, casseroles, vegetables, soups, or gravies; by using sauces on rice, noodles, or potatoes; and by offering shakes.	There may be times when children just do not have an appetite. Allow them to eat the food they want, but attempt to increase calories.
8. Offer bland, low fiber, non irritating foods, as ordered, along with Pedialyte, Gatorade or cranberry juice.	Children with HIV often have stomach cramps and diarrhea because of secondary infections.
9. Encourage the family to visit at mealtimes, or assign a consistent person to feed the child at a set time.	There may be psychosocial reasons for a child's inability to gain weight.
10. Weigh the child each A.M., and review caloric intake every 24 hours. Measure specific gravity at every void; compare consistency of stools; and obtain specimens as ordered.	It is important that the child follow his/her own growth curve, even if small for age.
11. Begin tube or parental feedings as ordered.	Alternative feeding techniques are necessary when the child is not gaining weight or is deviating from the established growth curve because of mouth or esophageal lesions, malabsorption, or neurologic findings.
12. Review with the family how to reconstitute formula at home, give vitamins, increase protein and calories and adjust intake based on oral lesions and evidence of malabsorption; teach families how to give alternative feeds as ordered.	Proteins and calories are important to immune cell function. Because some families may add water to formula to make it last longer while others may add cereal to increase calories, it is important to reinforce formula preparation.

Evaluation:
- The child is eating from all recommended food groups.
- The child is growing.
- The child's stools are of normal consistency and frequency for the child.

NURSING DIAGNOSIS

- Impaired Gas Exchange related to secondary or opportunistic infections
- Ineffective Airway Clearance related to ineffective cough or fatigue

Expected Outcome: The child will:

- have clear breath sounds
- have normal pulse and respiratory rates for age
- breathe comfortably with minimal exertion.

Intervention	Rationale
1. Maintain oxygen therapy as ordered and monitor pulse oximetry values.	Changes in the child's pulse oximetry values or clinical condition may indicate a need for a change in oxygen therapy.
2. Administer PCP prophylaxis/treatment, as ordered, with a large glass of water or juice; monitor the child for side effects.	Specific sulfonamides, such as Bactrim and Septra, can help prevent or treat PCP. PCP causes dyspnea, tachypnea, cyanosis, and a nonproductive cough.
3. Administer corticosteroids, as ordered, with food or milk (see the section entitled The Child Receiving Corticosteroid Therapy); monitor the child for side effects.	Corticosteroids are used to treat lymphocytic interstitial pneumonia (LIP). LIP is an insidious condition causing parotid gland enlargement, hypoxia, and digital clubbing.
4. Perform chest physiotherapy (PT) as ordered. Turn and position the child every 2–3 hours; elevate the head of the bed (HOB). Encourage the child who is able to get out of bed to do so frequently. Practice coughing and deep breathing using an incentive spirometer. Obtain a sputum culture as ordered.	Changing position and getting out of bed, even if held upright in someone's arms, allows for lung expansion and helps to prevent atelectasis to dependent lung segments; Improvement in breath sounds on auscultation should be noted.
5. Instruct the parents how to administer Bactrim (and steroids as ordered) at home; teach the family chest PT and techniques for coughing and deep breathing exercises, as well as administration of aerosol treatments at home. Arrange for oxygen tanks and nebulizers as ordered.	PCP prophylaxis is usually taken twice a day, 3 days a week. Nebulizer treatments help to open the airway before chest PT. Nebulizer pieces are cleaned with warm water after each treatment and left to air-dry. They are soaked in white vinegar and water for 30 minutes at the end of the day.

Evaluation:

- The child has improved breath sounds on auscultation.
- The child's pulse oximetry value is greater than 95%.
- The child breathes effortlessly when at rest.
- The child expectorates upper airway secretions.

NURSING DIAGNOSIS

- Risk for Impaired Skin Integrity related to cellular immunodeficiency

Expected Outcome:

- The child's skin will be clean, dry, and intact.
- The child's throat/mouth will be free of sores/inflammation.

Intervention	Rationale
1. Use mild soap; offer liquids throughout the day; apply baby oil to the scalp; avoid tight braids or pony tails; use salve to keep lips moist.	Children with HIV may have very dry skin/scalp/lips.

Intervention	Rationale
2. Clean open sores with warm water; pat or air-dry. Apply antiviral agents as ordered; cover with a nonadherent pad; monitor effectiveness of treatment.	Children with HIV may develop herpes lesions on the skin or in the mouth. Acyclovir is often ordered.
3. Clean the child's teeth 2–3 times a day with a soft brush. For infants, clean the mouth with a cotton swab and plain water.	The skin inside the mouth must be kept clean to prevent infections and dental caries.
4. Using a cotton swab, clean the mouth and apply an oral antifungal agent. Do not offer food or drink for 30 minutes after application. Monitor the effects of treatment.	Children with HIV often develop a fungal infection due to *Candida albicans*, which causes pain with swallowing and can spread down the esophagus. Nystatin is used initially, followed by ketoconazole.
5. Use extra care to keep the diaper area smooth and soft; change diapers as soon as they are wet; clean with mineral oil and warm water; pat or air-dry. Do not use wipes.	Some brands of disposable diapers and wipes may be irritating to the skin; use cloth diapers as needed.
6. Leave the diaper area open to the air; avoid wiping (squeeze a wet cloth over the bottom to wash stool away); pat or air-dry (do not rub); apply a thin layer of antifungal agent as ordered; monitor its effectiveness. Handle the child gently.	Children with HIV often develop fungal infections in the diaper area. Nystatin powder is used if the rash is wet and weepy; nystatin cream allows the skin to breathe; Maalox (applied topically) and colloidal oatmeal baths are effective if skin breakdown is severe.
7. Reinforce techniques to be used at home for meticulous mouth and skin care. Mouth care includes inspecting for white patches, blisters, and sores that recur and persist despite meticulous treatment and care. Skin care of the diaper area is especially important. Teach the family how to administer topical antifungal agents.	Skin and mucous membranes are the body's first line of defense against germs that challenge the immune system.

Evaluation:
- The child does not develop further skin breakdown.
- The child's skin lesions and open sores are healing.

NURSING DIAGNOSIS
- Altered Growth and Development related to the effects of the virus on the neurologic system, chronicity, separation, and hospitalization

Expected Outcome:
- The child's motor, cognitive, and psychosocial development will be within normal limits.

Intervention	Rationale
1. Encourage the family to visit the child as often and as long as possible; supplement family visits with visits from volunteers.	Personal interaction is essential to prevent withdrawal and promote language and motor skills.
2. Administer antiretroviral drugs as ordered; monitor the child for side effects.	HIV can infect brain cells; opportunistic organisms, like CMV and Toxoplasma can cause brain infections; thrombocytopenia can cause internal bleeding. As a result, some children with progressive disease exhibit developmental delay. Many children taking antiretroviral drugs, however, have regained lost developmental milestones and gained weight.

Intervention	Rationale
3. Interact with the child according to his/her developmental age. Provide safe, age-appropriate toys; integrate physical, occupational, and speech therapy techniques into the child's activities of daily living (ADLs) and play. Assess the child each week for changes in any aspect of development.	Children with symptomatic HIV infection can appear developmentally indistinguishable from noninfected family members; motor impairment may become more profound as the disease progresses; impaired children, however, show a level of general comprehension that is not measurable (Glass, 1995).
4. Reinforce physical and occupational therapy techniques, but not to the point of pain. Encourage the family to follow speech therapy instructions, especially those that enhance receptive language skills.	As a child begins to lose motor function, the family continues to feel hopeful when general comprehension persists.
5. Teach the family how to give antiretroviral agents at home, keeping a log and adjusting the schedule to accommodate school schedules.	The antiretroviral regimen may include a combination of 2 or 3 drugs in addition to the other medications a child is taking. A daily log helps families keep track.

Evaluation: • All aspects of the child's development are within normal limits.

NURSING DIAGNOSIS • Pain related to the physical condition

Expected Outcome: The child will:

- be able to communicate where pain is located, if any
- participate in activities to the extent he/she is able
- be comfortable.

Intervention	Rationale
1. Continuously anticipate, assess, recognize, and treat pain appropriately.	Pain management requires multidisciplinary input: the caregiver reports pain to the physician, who may order analgesics.
2. Offer acetaminophens and nonsteroidal anti-inflammatory drugs (NSAIDs) for mild pain; add codeine for moderate pain and morphine or methadone for severe pain.	A "ladder" approach to analgesia has proven effective in managing pain (Oleske, 1995).
3. Plan care so that rest periods are possible and everything that requires touching is done at once. Line the bed with soft blankets or cushions, or a partially inflated mattress. Alternate positions, using the palms of your hands for lifting.	Interventions 3, 4, and 5 are some common-sense, nonpharmacologic interventions for managing pain (Oleske, 1995).
4. Keep the environment calm; speak in gentle tones; play quiet music; dim the lights.	
5. Apply mild heat; offer a warm bath.	
6. Teach deep breathing exercises and use distraction techniques (imagining; singing; watching TV; reading a story) to manage pain.	Giving children an active voice in controlling pain can help lessen it.

Intervention	Rationale
7. Teach the family how to administer analgesics and use nonpharmacologic interventions for managing pain at home. Remind the family to call the doctor if the pain cannot be controlled.	Children should not have to be in pain. There is always something that can be done. Families know their children best and are positioned to assess and manage pain at home with lots of support.

Evaluation:
- The child's pain improves.
- The child participates in age-appropriate activities.

NURSING DIAGNOSIS
- Anxiety (Primary Caregiver) related to fear of disclosure

Expected Outcome: The family will:
- share the diagnosis with health care professionals who need to know
- move through the stages of disclosure and feel comfortable sharing feelings about the diagnosis with one significant person
- answer the child's questions honestly and share the diagnosis when the time is right.

Intervention	Rationale
1. Listen quietly when the family talks about the diagnosis of HIV; note their stage of disclosure (secrecy, exploratory, readiness, or disclosure).	Sharing the diagnosis involves a continuum, with secrecy on one end and full disclosure at the other (Tasker, 1992). Families initially will want to keep their feelings about the diagnosis private. However, there may come a time when they wish to talk; the nurse should develop rapport and gain trust.
2. Encourage the family to share the diagnosis with health care professionals.	Health care professionals who plan and coordinate care need to know the diagnosis.
3. Help the family decide who else needs to know the child's diagnosis; ask them to name one person they wish to share the diagnosis with; encourage peer support groups when ready.	Although many people would like to know the diagnosis, only a handful need to know. Ask families to consider the following when choosing whom to tell: the child's age; clinical condition; health care requirements; the likelihood that bloody injuries will occur; universal precautions.
4. Encourage the family to be honest with the child and to explain the reason for doctors' visits and procedures.	While it is a personal choice when to tell the child the diagnosis, families need to understand that children will worry more if no one talks with them or if they sense dishonesty.
5. Encourage the family to listen to the questions the child is asking and to answer them briefly using words they can understand. Look for readiness cues that indicate the child wants to know more.	It is important for families to understand what their children are asking and to keep responses short and simple.
6. Encourage the family to speak with a health care professional when the child asks questions that are difficult to answer.	Role playing is a useful technique that allows families to practice potential responses to difficult questions. The nurse can offer to accompany them if they decide to share the diagnosis.
7. Promote normal routines at home.	Children with HIV can go to school, church, and parties; play sports and games; and develop or maintain friendships.

Evaluation:

- The family shares the diagnosis with all appropriate health care professionals and at least one significant person.
- The family moves through the stages of disclosure and seeks out support from peers.
- The family answers the child's questions in a developmentally appropriate way.

NURSING DIAGNOSIS

- Ineffective Management of Therapeutic Regimen: Noncompliance related to lack of support systems or denial of the illness

Expected Outcome:

- The mother will keep her health care appointments.
- The family will eventually accept the diagnosis.
- Family members will view themselves as valued members of the health care team.

Intervention	Rationale
1. Use language that shows respect.	HIV-affected families do not want their children called "innocent victims" or "AIDS babies," nor do they wish to be judged as promiscuous or substance abusers. Labels can create barriers, which can result in noncompliance with health care recommendations.
2. Encourage the mother to keep her own doctor's appointments.	HIV-affected women often neglect their own health care needs as they attend to those of their children.
3. Accept the parents' use of denial during periods of emotional respite.	The diagnosis of HIV brings about a series of losses; including the loss of the future and all that the future holds for a child.
4. Maintain realistic hope when possible.	Less than 25% of all seropositive babies develop HIV infection themselves, and most live more than 4 years.
5. Refer the family to the social worker for assistance with finances, transportation, food, housing, clothing, medical care, and respite care, as needed, at home.	Although some women with HIV infection are judged to be uncaring because of missed appointments or because their child fails to gain weight, many simply lack the basic resources for compliance.

Evaluation:

- The mother takes care of herself.
- The parents move from denial to anger to acceptance of the diagnosis.
- The parents are active, participatory, and valued members of the health care team.

The Child Receiving Corticosteroid Therapy

Corticosteroids, given as part of a treatment regimen, act as natural products of the adrenal glands, reducing local and systemic inflammatory symptoms.

Topical steroids are applied to the skin or mucous membranes to reduce edema and redness and to counteract itching. They may be used to treat ophthalmic reactions and skin conditions, such as eczema. An example of a topical steroid is hydrocortisone cream.

Systemic steroids reduce the inflammatory symptoms of generalized allergic reactions (e.g., asthma, hives, and severe contact dermatitis). Systemic steroids are also given increasingly to treat malignant or autoimmune disorders. An example of a systemic steroid is prednisone.

Aerosol steroids produce a very strong, local action and can control symptoms in children with asthma and allergic rhinitis who are corticosteroid-dependent. An example of an aerosol steroid is beclomethasone (see Chapter 29, The Child With Chronic Respiratory Alterations, and Chapter 34, The Child With Integumentary Alterations).

Pathophysiology: Side Effects. Corticosteroids have many different effects, including anti-inflammatory and immunosuppressive properties: inhibition of the process of edema, capillary dilatation, phagocytic activity, and the migration of leukocytes into an inflamed area (Hodgson, Kryror, & Kingdon, 1994).

Incidence of Side Effects. The side effects of steroids vary widely with the child and the medication. Generally, the higher the dose and the longer the medication is taken, the more serious are the side effects. A broader knowledge of reactions and a wider selection of types of steroids and alternatives have significantly reduced untoward reactions in recent years.

Clinicial Manifestations of Corticosteroid Excess. Clinical manifestations of excess topically administered steroids include:

- skin atrophy
- delayed wound healing
- telangiectasis or dilation of the cheek blood vessels
- striae
- excess absorption leading to any of the clinical manifestations of systemic use

Some clinical manifestations of excess steroid administered systemically include:

- edema, particularly in the face
- gastrointestinal irritation, even bleeding
- bruising and delayed wound healing
- susceptibility to infections
- growth limitations
- hypertension
- loss of muscle mass
- increased appetite and weight gain
- amenorrhea
- pancreatitis
- joint pain and osteoporosis
- cataracts

Diagnostic Evaluation of Corticosteroid Excess. The diagnosis of corticosteroid excess is suspected following the occurrence of the described clinical manifestations and is confirmed by administering a bolus of adrenocorticotropic hormone (ACTH) to the child. This challenges the adrenal gland to respond to pituitary stimulation. If serum cortisol levels do not rise after administration of ACTH, adrenal suppression—or cortisone excess—is present.

Therapeutic Management. Every effort is made to prevent corticosteroid excess by observance of the following guidelines:

- Institute short-term, high-dose therapy (for 1 week or less) if there is a strong indication for the use of steroids.
- If long-term use is necessary, alternate-day administration may be prescribed.
- At the time of an acute infection or surgery, supplementary steroids are indicated for children who have received them over a long period of time.

Killed vaccines are substituted for live ones in children receiving high-dose and/or long-term steroids (see previous section on HIV infection).

> For the child receiving corticosteroids, gradual tapering of the dose is essential in both short- and long-term use in order to allow for a gradual return of function in the pituitary-adrenal axis. Failure to do so can result in manifestations of adrenal insufficiency, such as hypoglycemia with seizures, weakness, hyperkalemia and hyponatremia, shock, and vascular collapse.

NURSING CARE OF THE CHILD RECEIVING CORTICOSTEROID THERAPY

Assessment

Assessment of a child receiving long-term steroid therapy should include height and weight measurements, as well as blood pressure at each visit. In addition, the nurse should observe the child for facial puffiness, abdominal pain, increased appetite, blurred vision, and increased thirst or urination. Families may report recent illnesses, bruising, or delayed wound healing.

Nursing Diagnosis and Planning

The following nursing diagnoses and expected outcomes may be appropriate following assessment of a child receiving corticosteroid therapy.

- Ineffective Management of Therapeutic Regimen: Noncompliance related to associated complications. ***Expected Outcome:*** *The child will take all medications as directed.*
- Body Image Disturbance related to changes caused by treatment. ***Expected Outcome:*** *The child will share feelings about any changes in appearance.*
- Risk for Infection related to immunosuppression. ***Expected Outcome:*** *The child will not experience secondary infections.*
- Risk for Injury related to knowledge deficit. ***Expected Outcome:*** *The child will not experience injuries.*

Implementation

The nurse should provide the family with written instructions that specifically state what to do if a dose is missed and when to decrease doses. It is crucial to stress with the family not to discontinue corticosteroid therapy abruptly. In addition, the child should take the medication with foods or milk to minimize the risk of gastrointestinal bleeding. The family must know the benefits of corticosteroids, as well as the fact that changes in appearance, if any, are temporary and reversible. Because the child's appetite may be increased, encouraging low-calorie snacks throughout the day is appropriate. The nurse should remind the family that salt may increase fluid retention. Referral to a nutritionist can be helpful. The nurse can compare changes in appearance and weight gain at each visit and encourage the child to express his feelings about such changes.

Because corticosteroids may mask infections, the nurse should instruct the family to call the doctor in the event of a temperature elevation, cough, runny nose, ear tenderness, decreased appetite, nausea, vomiting, diarrhea, or behavioral change. The family can even call if the child "just doesn't seem right." In addition, the family routinely checks the child's skin for bruising and signs of wound infection, such as redness, and report those lesions that do not resolve as expected. The family should not treat the child with over-the-counter products without first consulting the physician. It is also necessary for the child receiving long-term therapy to avoid others who are sick. The parents must notify the physician of any exposure to a communicable disease, such as measles or chickenpox.

In order to minimize injuries, the nurse should reinforce teaching regarding potential environmental hazards and accident prevention strategies based on the child's developmental age (see Chapter 13, Safety). If the child should get a cut, the parents may hold gentle pressure to the site for 3 to 5 minutes to stop the bleeding and prevent hematoma formation. The child may wear a Medic-Alert bracelet stating the key clinical manifestations of corticosteroid excess or adrenal insufficiency (as described).

Evaluation

- Is the child taking corticosteroids as directed?
- Is the child expressing her feelings about any changes in appearance?
- Is the child free of infections?
- Is the child's skin intact?

AUTOIMMUNE DISORDERS

Sometimes the immune system's ability to differentiate "self" from "nonself" breaks down and the body begins to make antibodies against its own cells, tissues (particularly connective tissue), and organs. Such antibodies are known as autoantibodies. Autoantibodies are common in such conditions as rheumatic fever (RF) and systemic lupus erythematosus (SLE). The response is exacerbated by a malfunction of helper T and suppressor T cells. That is, there are too many helper cells and not enough suppressor cells to turn off the immune response. Frequently, immune complexes develop in **autoimmune diseases** like SLE, whereby the continuous production of autoantibodies overloads the immune complex removal system (Schindler, 1988).

Rheumatic Fever

Rheumatic fever (RF) is an inflammatory autoimmune disease that affects the connective tissue of the heart, joints, subcutaneous tissues, and/or blood vessels of the central nervous system. The most serious complication is rheumatic heart disease, which affects the cardiac valves—most commonly the mitral valves—causing scarring and permanent damage.

PATHOPHYSIOLOGY *of Rheumatic Fever*

The most popular current theory suggests that the colonization of the pharynx with group A beta-hemolytic streptococci triggers an abnormal immunologic response in patients with RF. Sensitized B cells produce antistreptococcal antibody that forms immune complexes. These immune complexes cross-react with cardiac tissue, producing a myocardial and valvular inflammatory response (Wolfe & Wiggins, 1992).

Etiology. RF characteristically presents 2 to 6 weeks following an untreated or partially treated group A beta-hemolytic streptococcal infection of the upper respiratory tract. The initial infection may or may not produce symptoms of pharyngitis (Freund et al., 1993). There may be predisposing genetic factors. Crowding, particularly in the bedroom and classroom, also increases the risk (Grimes & Woolbert, 1990).

Incidence. RF is a disease in transition. Its incidence decreased dramatically in the last two decades, yet there was an unexpected resurgence in the late eighties (Marlow & Redding, 1988; Ayoub, 1992). The average annual incidence is fewer than 1 per 10,000, and the presence of the disease in school-aged children—the most susceptible population—is less than 1 per 1000 (Wolfe & Wiggins, 1992). The disease is slightly more common in girls, and is now more common in African-American children than in caucasians.

Clinical Manifestations. Major manifestations of RF include the following (Fig. 23–1):

- polyarthritis—tender, painful, joints, especially in the elbows, knees, ankles, and wrists
- carditis—inflammation of all parts of the heart, primarily the mitral valves
- chorea—involuntary movements affecting the legs, arms, and face (including speech ability)
- erythema marginatum—red skin lesions that start as flat or slightly raised macules, usually over the trunk, and spread peripherally
- subcutaneous nodules—small, non-tender lumps often located over the joints

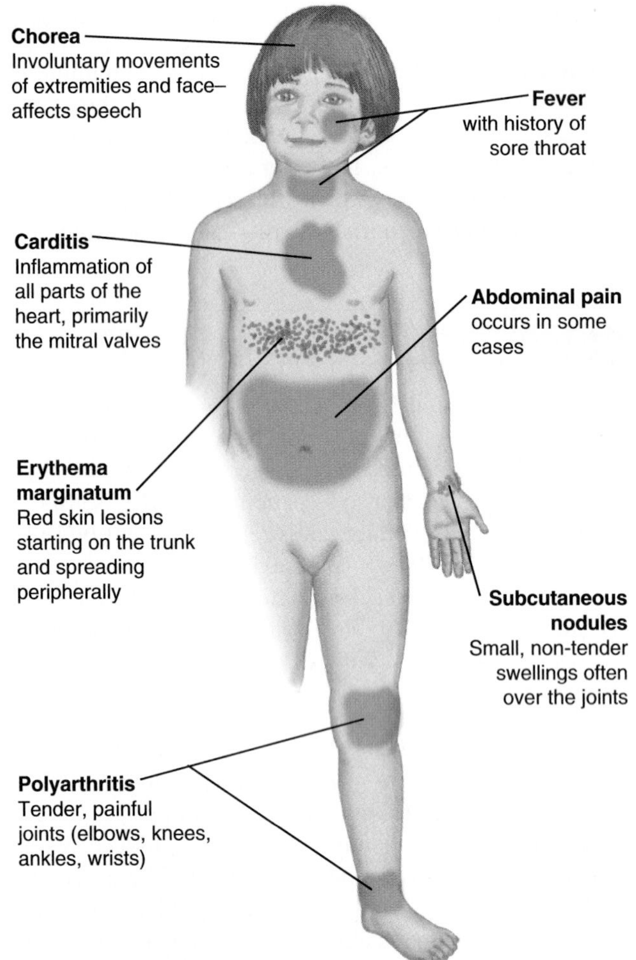
Chorea
Involuntary movements of extremities and face–affects speech
Fever
with history of sore throat
Carditis
Inflammation of all parts of the heart, primarily the mitral valves
Abdominal pain
occurs in some cases
Erythema marginatum
Red skin lesions starting on the trunk and spreading peripherally
Subcutaneous nodules
Small, non-tender swellings often over the joints
Polyarthritis
Tender, painful joints (elbows, knees, ankles, wrists)

Figure 23–1
Clinical manifestations of rheumatic fever.

Diagnosis of Acute Rheumatic Fever by Jones Criteria

MAJOR MANIFESTATIONS

Carditis
Polyarthritis
Chorea
Erythema marginatum
Subcutaneous nodules

MINOR MANIFESTATIONS

Fever
Arthralgia
Previous rheumatic fever or rheumatic heart disease
Elevated erythrocyte sedimentation rate (ESR) or positive C-reactive protein (CRP)
Prolonged P-R interval

Plus supporting evidence of preceding streptococcal infection: history of recent scarlet fever, positive throat culture for group A Streptococcus, increased antistreptolysin-o (ASO) titer, or other streptococcal antibodies.

Modified from Hollister, J. R. (1992). Rheumatic diseases. In W. E. Hathaway, W. W. Hay, J. R. Groothuis, & J. W. Paisley (Eds.), *Current pediatric diagnosis and treatment* (pp. 828–841). East Norwalk, CT: Appleton & Lange.

Although arthritis is the most common manifestation, carditis is by far the most serious, as it is the major cause of morbidity and mortality during the acute as well as the chronic phase (Ayoub, 1992).

Diagnostic Evaluation. A diagnosis of RF is confirmed by the presence of two major manifestations or one major and two minor manifestations from the Jones criteria (see box), plus evidence of a recent streptococcal infection by one of the following positive diagnostic studies:

- anti-streptolysin O titer
- streptozyme
- anti-DNAase B assay

Other test results that may indicate inflammation (Freund et al., 1993) include increased

- C-reactive protein
- antihyaluronidase
- erythrocyte sedimentation rate

In patients with suspected carditis, a chest x-ray study may demonstrate enlargement of the heart. An electrocardiogram will show rhythm abnormalities and evidence of myocarditis and an echocardiogram will demonstrate the size and location of lesions (Freund et al., 1993).

Therapeutic Management. The medical management of RF includes eradication of the streptococcal bacteria and treatment of other symptoms, such as inflammation, congestive heart failure, and chorea. Penicillin is administered orally four times a day for 10 days or as a single intramuscular injection. Prescribed anti-inflammatory agents include aspirin. (Aspirin should not be given to a child who has chickenpox or other viral infection.) The duration of therapy is tailored to meet the needs of the child, but use of aspirin for 2 to 6 weeks, with a reduction in dose toward the end of the treatment regimen, is usually sufficient.

Streptococcal prophylaxis for 5 years, or through adolescence, whichever is greater, is the most important aspect of therapeutic management because damaged valves can become further damaged with repeat infections. Intramuscular penicillin, administered every 28 days, is the drug of choice. Alternatives include oral penicillin taken four times a day or sulfonamides for children who are sensitive to penicillin.

NURSING CARE OF THE CHILD WITH RHEUMATIC FEVER

Assessment

Initially, the nurse determines whether any family members have had a sore throat or unexplained fever within the past 2 months. The child should be monitored throughout the course of hospitalization for any cardiac complications. The nurse should assess temperature, pulse, respiration, and blood pressure and should observe the child for signs of carditis, including shortness of breath, edema of the face, abdomen, or ankles, and precordial pain. Examination of the joints may reveal very tender elbows, knees, ankles, and wrists, with small lumps. The nurse may assess pain using a self-report and the standard number and color scales (see Chapter 20, The Child in Pain). Children with RF may have red skin lesions spreading peripherally from the trunk. When questioned, parents may report the child has had rapid, purposeless, involuntary movements.

Nursing Diagnosis and Planning

The following nursing diagnoses and expected outcomes may be appropriate following assessment of a child with rheumatic fever.

- Knowledge Deficit related to medication and activity restrictions. ***Expected Outcome:*** *The child will comply with the medication regimen and activity restrictions.*
- Ineffective Individual Coping related to confinement. ***Expected Outcome:*** *The child will experience minimal emotional distress.*
- Pain related to polyarthritis. ***Expected Outcome:*** *The child will be comfortable.*
- Risk for Injury related to streptococcal infection. ***Expected Outcome:*** *The child will inform parents at the first sign of a sore throat.*

Implementation

The nurse must administer antibiotics, analgesics, and antipyretics as ordered and report to the physician any fever or pain. In addition to medications, children with RF require modified bed/chair rest with bathroom privileges and meals at the table for 2 to 6 weeks until the elevated erythrocyte sedimentation rate—secondary to the inflammatory autoimmune process—decreases to within normal limits. Children should not return to school while there is clear evidence of rheumatic activity, as described under clinical manifestations. While the child's activities are restricted, the nurse and family should talk about limiting visitors and phone calls and arranging for quiet, yet enjoyable, activities. Family members and friends may purchase board, card, and computer games, movies, puzzles, crafts, models, and riddle books for the school-age child. Such activities will help to minimize activity, as well as cardiac output. The affected child may develop a daily schedule that includes rest periods interspersed with these diversional activities and some limited exercise (e.g., passive range of motion). An art or play therapist can work with the child who is extremely anxious because of confinement. Such anxiety may place undue stress on the heart.

Nursing comfort measures include alternating heat and cold to affected joints; repositioning; massage; and providing distraction using guided imagery and relaxation. Seizure precautions are warranted if the child is experiencing chorea. At home, parents must practice safety measures. For example, the child who cannot control movements may need to sleep on a mattress on the floor and may require assistance going up and down stairs. The child may be embarrassed by his uncontrolled movements, especially in front of peers, and will need reassurance that these symptoms are temporary.

The nurse should encourage the child to tell the parents if anyone in school has "a strep throat" and to take antibiotics as ordered. The family may be allowed to offer an older child a choice of monthly injections versus daily oral administration. If the child chooses the oral route, then the nurse must instruct the family about the required dose, frequency of administration, duration, effects, and side effects, as well as the potential cardiac complications if the regimen is not followed precisely.

Evaluation

- Is the child taking antibiotics as ordered?
- Is the child following modified bed rest guidelines?
- Is the child coping with confinement according to developmental age?
- Is the child free of pain?
- Has the child informed the parents of a sore throat?

Systemic Lupus Erythematosus

SLE is a chronic, multisystem, autoimmune disease characterized by inflammation of the connective tissue. SLE varies in severity and is marked by remissions and exacerbations (Fuller & Hartley, 1991; Legun, 1990; Hollister, 1992).

Etiology. Although the etiology of SLE is not known, genetic, environmental, hormonal, and immune response factors are likely to be responsible. Environmental factors may include exposure to the sun, ultraviolet light, stress, fatigue, viruses, bacteria, certain medications, as well as some food additives. Exacerbations can occur with the cessation of birth control pills, menses, pregnancy, and the postpartum period (Legun, 1990; Marlow & Redding, 1988).

Incidence. The incidence of SLE in the United States ranges from 0.6 in 100,000 to 1 in 1000 persons. In young

PATHOPHYSIOLOGY *of Systemic Lupus Erythematosus*

Many abnormalities in the immune system are associated with SLE. A reduction in the number of suppressor T cells allows for the formation of autoantibodies against proteins that are made by the cell nucleus of the body's collagenous connective tissue. These autoantibodies—referred to as antinuclear antibodies, or ANAs—initiate an abnormal immune complex response, producing inflammation and damaging tissues and organs, including the skin, joints, heart, lungs, kidneys, brain, and circulatory vessels (Legun, 1990; Fuller & Hartley, 1991; Marlow & Redding, 1988).

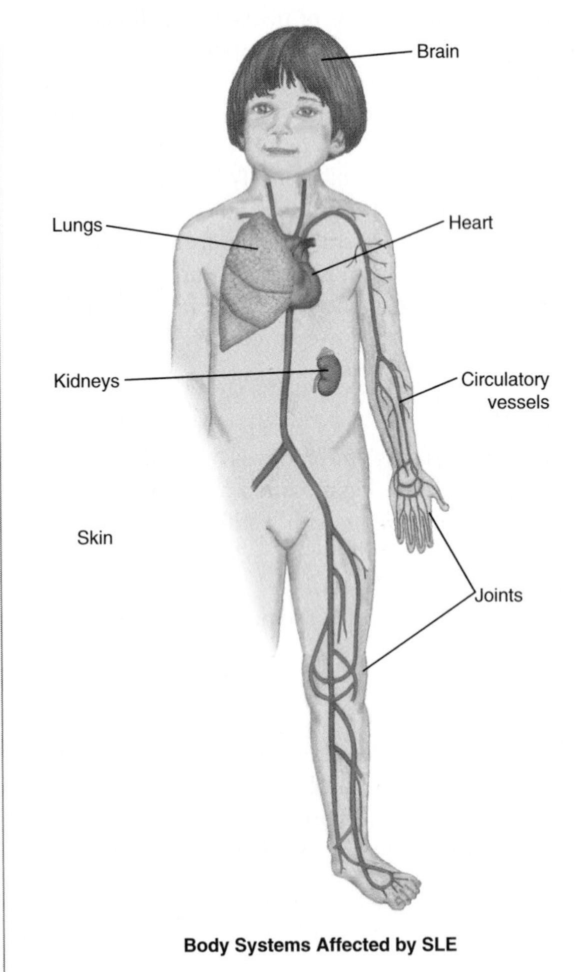

Body Systems Affected by SLE

children, the female-to-male ratio is 3:1; after puberty, this ratio increases to 9:1. Onset is most common in girls between the ages of 9 and 15. More African-American, Latino, and Asian children are affected than caucasian children (Pohlgeers et al., 1990; Fuller & Hartley, 1991; Legun, 1990).

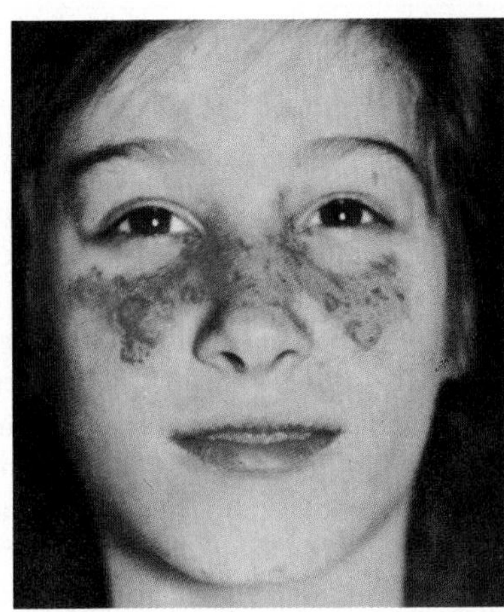

Figure 23–2
The butterfly rash of systemic lupus erythematosus. (From Behrman, R. E., Kliegman, R. M., & Arvin, A. M. [1996]. *Nelson textbook of pediatrics* [15th ed.]. Philadelphia: W. B. Saunders, Color Plate Fig. 150–1.)

Clinical Manifestations. Malaise, arthralgia, and recurrent fever of unknown etiology frequently are among the early manifestations of SLE. The symptoms, however, depend on what organs the immune complexes affect and may include the following:

- malar "butterfly" rash—fixed red, flat, or raised rash over the cheeks and bridge of nose (Fig. 23–2)
- discoid rash—red, round, raised patches that spread
- photosensitivity—skin rash from sun exposure
- oral and nasal ulcers—usually painless lesions
- arthritis—painful, swollen joints with edema
- pleuritis and pericarditis
- renal disorders—protein or red cells in urine
- neurologic disorders—headaches, personality changes, seizures, or psychosis
- hematologic disorders—anemia, leukopenia, lymphoma, or thrombocytopenia
- immunologic disorders and ANA (Legun, 1990)

The most serious complications of SLE include renal disease and neurologic problems.

Diagnostic Evaluation. The presence of four or more of the clinical manifestations listed above, whether or not they occur simultaneously, is diagnostic for SLE (Fuller & Hartley, 1991). In addition, a number of tests can diagnose and monitor the progress of SLE. A positive ANA test is highly suggestive of SLE, but it can also be positive in other autoimmune disorders. Blood urea nitrogen (BUN) levels, gammaglobulin levels, and sedimentation rate may be elevated. Pathologic changes compatible with SLE may be confirmed by electrocardiography, renal function studies, and tissue biopsies demonstrating immune complexes (Fuller & Hartley, 1991; Marlow & Redding, 1988).

Therapeutic Management. The treatment of SLE is tailored to the organ system(s) affected, is symptom-related, and is aimed at preventing exacerbations and complications. Helping the child and family develop long-term coping strategies is important. Corticosteroids are most often given to control the inflammatory response (see the earlier section, The Child Receiving Corticosteroid Therapy). If disease control is inadequate or if the side effects of corticosteroid therapy are intolerable, immunosuppressants, such as cytoxan, may be given. Aspirin and NSAIDs may be used to treat arthritis, serositis, and febrile attacks. Children with renal and neurologic disorders generally receive anticonvulsant and antihypertensive therapy, whereas those with skin lesions and joint problems take antimalarial drugs, such as chloroprine. Killed vaccines, rather than live ones, are used in affected children. A low-salt diet may reduce fluid retention and prevent elevated BUN levels; a low-protein diet helps to preserve renal function (Fuller & Hartley, 1991).

NURSING CARE OF THE CHILD WITH SYSTEMIC LUPUS ERYTHEMATOSUS

Assessment

During a period of disease exacerbation, a child may become acutely ill. The nurse should monitor vital signs, mobility, activity, and pain, and should complete a neurologic examination assessing for decreased sensation, weakness in the extremities, and changes in behavior. Of equal importance is evaluation of the effect of living with a chronic illness on a young girl's self-image and interaction with peers.

Nursing Diagnosis and Planning

The following nursing diagnoses and expected outcomes may be appropriate following assessment of a child with SLE.

- Body Image Disturbance related to changes secondary to the disease process and treatments. ***Expected Outcome:*** *The child will share feelings about appearance.*
- Activity Intolerance related to the disease process. ***Expected Outcome:*** *The child will participate in activities to the extent possible.*
- Pain related to arthritis and numbness of the hands and feet. ***Expected Outcome:*** *The child will be free of pain.*
- Ineffective Management of Therapeutic Regimen: Noncompliance related to associated complications and developmental level. ***Expected Outcome:*** *The child will take all medications as directed.*

Implementation

It is important for the nurse to help the child and family understand the reasons for drug therapy and the need for activity restriction. Another goal is to avoid any triggers that may cause exacerbations (e.g., avoiding exposure to the sun or to people who are sick). For a preteen or adolescent, it is often difficult to achieve a balance between the need to take risks and be accepted by peers and the realities imposed by a chronic illness (see Chapter 17, The Child With a Chronic or Terminal Illness).

It is important for the teenager with a chronic illness to participate, to whatever extent possible, in activities at home, school, church, and within the community. The affected child may gain some control by documenting the level of fatigue three times a day, along with the preceding activities. Together with parents or the nurse, she can then use this information to make sensible decisions about overall participation in sports and extracurricular activities.

The teenager must also understand the importance of taking prescribed medications as ordered (see The Child Receiving Corticosteroid Therapy). The nurse should explain to the child and family the dose, frequency, duration, beneficial effects, and side effects of the drugs prescribed, as well as the ill effects of not following the prescribed treatment regimen. The teenager should be encouraged to plan an appropriate and convenient self-administration schedule.

Children with SLE may feel angry that this could happen to them, and may feel alienated from peers. Wearing makeup can mask rashes and improve appearance. Keeping a diary also helps the child vent anger. An affected peer who is in remission can offer support. The American Lupus Society (310-542-8891) and The Lupus Foundation (301-670-9292 or 800-558-0121) have local chapters in many cities and states.

Evaluation

- Does the child share feelings about his/her appearance?
- Does the child participate in sports and extracurricular activities without becoming overfatigued?
- Is the child free of pain?
- Is the child taking all medications as directed?

IMMUNE COMPLEX DISORDERS

Immune complexes are clusters of interlocking antigens and antibodies. Under normal conditions, immune complexes are removed from the blood. In some circumstances, however, immune complexes continue to circulate. Eventually, they become trapped in the tissues of the kidney, lungs, skin, joints, or blood vessels. There, they set off reactions that lead to tissue inflammation and damage. Immune complexes play a major role in the pathogenesis of Kawasaki disease (KD) (Schindler, 1988; Bellanti, 1985).

Kawasaki Disease

Kawasaki disease, also called mucocutaneous lymph node syndrome, is a febrile generalized vasculitis of unknown etiology. KD is a major cause of acquired heart disease in children in the United States (Dajani et al., 1993).

Etiology. The cause of KD remains unknown. However, an infectious agent is strongly suggested by the disease's predominance among young children who apparently lack immunity and by the existence of outbreaks (Shackelford & Strauss, 1991).

Incidence. In children younger than 5 years of age, the incidence of KD is six to nine per 100,000. It has been estimated that there are at least 2000 cases per year in the United States. The disease occurs year round in this country, with an increased number of cases observed in the winter and spring. Eighty percent of cases occur in chil-

PATHOPHYSIOLOGY *of Kawasaki Disease*

In the acute phase of KD, there are more helper T cells than suppressor T cells, and there are increased numbers of B cells spontaneously secreting IgG and IgM. Antibody-antigen complexes form and are thought to bind to the vascular epithelium, causing inflammation of the vessels and increased platelets, resulting in clot formation. Vascular changes in the myocardium and coronary arteries may lead to aneurysms and myocardial infarction, resulting in death (Levin, Tizard, & Dillon, 1991).

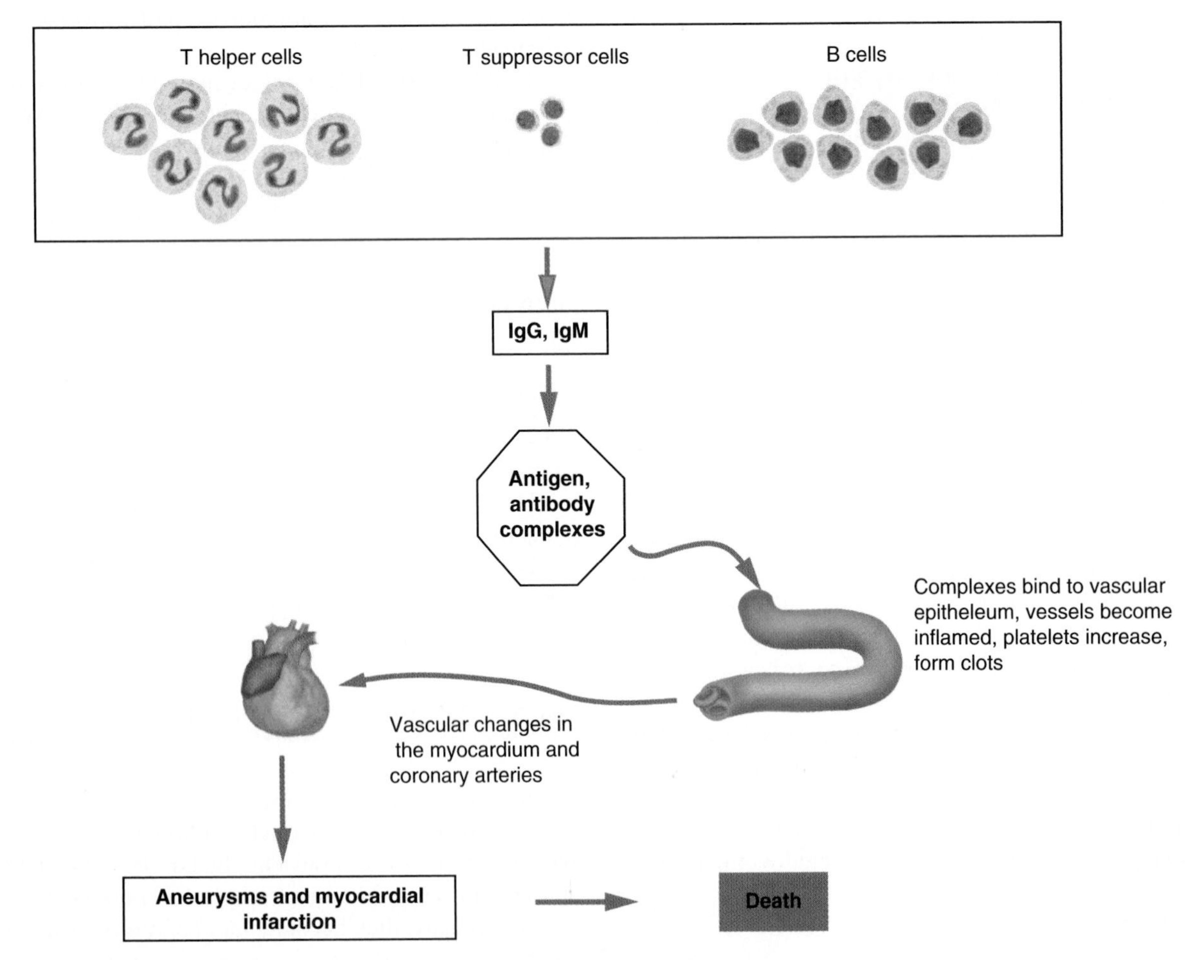

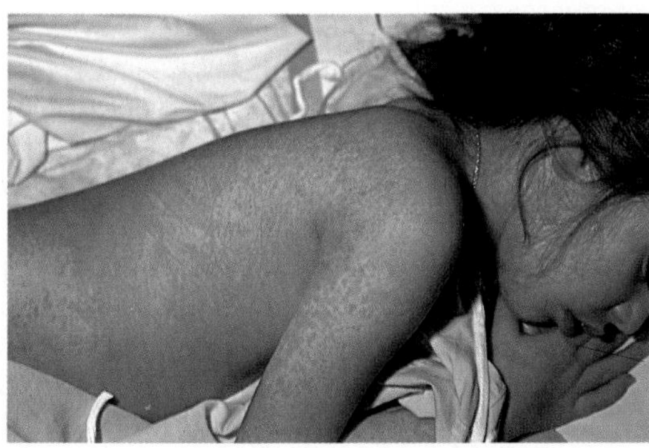

Figure 23–3
Erythematous rash of Kawasaki disease. (From Lookingbill, D. P., Marks, J. G., Jr. [1992]. *Principles of dermatology* [2nd ed.]. Philadelphia: W. B. Saunders, p. 223, Fig. 15–5A.)

dren younger than five years of age, and most are younger than 2 years old. The onset of the disease is rare after 8 years of age (Dajani et al., 1993). KD is more common in boys than in girls. There are striking differences in incidence among different racial groups, with a much higher incidence in Japanese children. The recurrence rate is 0.8% (Lux, 1991).

Clinical Manifestations. KD manifests itself in three phases. The acute stage lasts approximately 10 days and is characterized by an abrupt onset of fever persisting more than 5 days, as well as other clinical symptoms, including:

- bilateral, nonpurulent conjunctivitis
- changes in the mouth (i.e., erythema, fissures, and crusts of the lips; strawberry tongue)
- changes in the peripheral extremities, such as induration of the hands and feet and erythema of the palms and soles
- erythematous rash (Fig. 23–3)
- enlarged cervical lymph nodes

The second or subacute phase begins after 10 days and extends to day 25. The fever disappears and most symptoms resolve. This phase is characterized by the following: (Dajani et al., 1993; Lux, 1991; Marlow & Redding, 1988).

- extreme irritability
- anorexia
- desquamation of the fingers and toes
- arthritis and arthralgia
- cardiovascular manifestations

Coronary aneurysm formation may occur about 11 days after the onset of fever, followed by acute myocardial infarction secondary to thrombosis of these aneurysms (Wolfe & Wiggins, 1992). The final or convalescent stage begins on day 26 and lasts until the sedimentation rate returns to normal and all signs of illness have disappeared. Deep transverse grooves, called bow's lines, may appear on the child's nails owing to the brief arrest in maturation of the cells during the period of high fever (Lux, 1991).

Diagnostic Evaluation. Fever of 5 days' duration, along with four of the five primary clinical findings as described during the acute phase, establishes the diagnosis of KD (Dajani et al., 1993). Cardiac changes may be apparent on electrocardiography. Laboratory data are nonspecific. The white blood cell (WBC) count is elevated during the acute phase, as are the sedimentation rate and C-reactive protein level. Platelets rise excessively during the subacute phase (Marlow & Redding, 1988). Aneurysms are usually detected by echocardiogram (Lux, 1991).

Therapeutic Management. The Committee on Infectious Diseases of the AAP recommends that all children diagnosed with KD within 10 days of onset should receive IVIG and high doses of aspirin to control coronary aneurysm formation and fever (Shackelford & Strauss, 1991). After the fever subsides, the aspirin dose is lowered, but continued, in order to decrease platelet aggregation for at least 3 months and as long as 1 year. Follow-up echocardiographic studies are done at 3 and 8 weeks postdiagnosis and then annually until the aneurysms resolve (Lux, 1991).

NURSING CARE OF THE CHILD WITH KAWASAKI DISEASE

Assessment

The nurse should assess the child's vital signs. Continued fever may affect dietary intake and hydration status. Changes in pulse, respiration, blood pressure, and color, along with shortness of breath, chest pain, and decreased activity, may suggest cardiac complications as well as pain. It is important to examine the child's eyes, mouth, and skin for signs of infection and the joints for redness, swelling, and tenderness. The nurse should determine the parents' anxiety level. They often are frightened by how sick the child is and the threat of a possible devastating sequela. Families appreciate talking about their fears; learning about the course of the illness, the treatment plan, and the prognosis; and participating in the child's care.

Nursing Diagnosis and Planning

The following nursing diagnoses and expected outcomes may be appropriate following assessment of a child with KD.

- Risk for Fluid Volume Deficit related to fever. ***Expected Outcome:*** *The child will maintain fluid and electrolyte balance.*
- Pain related to fever, skin manifestations, and joint inflammation. ***Expected Outcome:*** *The child will rest comfortably.*
- Fear (caregivers') related to changes in the child's behavior and uncertainty about the long-term progno-

sis. ***Expected Outcome:*** *The parents will accept that their previously healthy child has a serious disease with a long recuperative period.*

Implementation

The nurse should administer aspirin with milk or food and IVIG as ordered. Often, a test dose of IVIG is given before initiating an infusion. During the test dose, as well as during the infusion, it is important to monitor the child's vital signs and any adverse reactions to IVIG, including facial flushing, tightness in the chest, chills, dizziness, nausea, vomiting, diaphoresis, and hypotension. The blood pressure is checked every 15 minutes for the first hour and every 30 minutes thereafter until the infusion is complete. A precipitous fall in blood pressure may occur 30 to 60 minutes after the infusion has begun, and is often related to the rate of infusion. The physician will usually lower the prescribed rate of infusion if such a reaction occurs, and may order diphenhydramine (Benadryl) and acetaminophen to control side effects. Epinephrine is given for anaphylactic reactions.

Nursing care focuses on comfort measures and adequate hydration. The nurse and parents must encourage fluid intake by offering frozen popsicles or ice to numb affected mucous membranes; giving liquids that are high in calories and low in acid (while avoiding citrus and sodas) through a straw; and/or applying topical anesthetics 15 to 60 minutes before offering favorite foods that are soft and bland. The nurse or family should provide mouth care following any intake other than water, and should apply salve to soothe cracked, dry lips.

Sponge baths with tepid water often decrease fever and relieve discomfort from skin manifestations. Because desquamation increases the risk of infection, it is important to keep the child's skin clean and dry and to avoid soap irritants. If itching is severe, the physician should be notified.

Toddlers and preschool children fear hospitalization and body changes, often exhibiting regressive behavior and sleeping poorly. Feeding, skin care, and position changes may cause pain. The nurse and family can work together to manage the child's pain by planning care so that everything that requires touching is done at once, and by arranging for rest periods in between. It may help to line the bed with soft blankets from home and to use the palms of the hands when lifting the child. Even in the hospital, it is possible to keep the environment calm by talking in gentle tones, playing soft music, restricting visitors/phone calls, and avoiding bright overhead lights. The nurse should assure the often frightened and anxious family that pain and irritability will eventually resolve, and

TEACHING GUIDELINES *for the Child Discharged With Kawasaki Disease*

Review the following at the time of hospital discharge of a child diagnosed as having Kawasaki disease:

SKIN

- Rinse with water only.
- Avoid soaps and lotions.
- Use salve on the lips.
- Call the physician for severe itching.

TEMPERATURE

- Record the child's temperature in the A.M. and P.M. before giving aspirin.
- Bring the temperature chart to all physician's appointments.

ARTHRITIS

- Look for hot, reddened joints.
- Observe for pain with touch or movement.
- Elevate affected joints.
- Call the physician if the child refuses to walk.

HEART

- Offer a low-cholesterol diet.
- Give aspirin as ordered.
- Call the physician for bleeding or bruising, color changes, shortness of breath, chest pain, or decreased activity level.

PERSONALITY

- Discuss personality changes with household members.
- Provide support and reassurance.
- Encourage quiet activities and rest periods.
- Eliminate stimulation at naptime and bedtime.
- Play soft music and use dim lights.

ANOREXIA

- Offer liquids high in calories but low in acid.
- Avoid citrus juices and sodas.
- Give bland foods initially.
- Prepare favorite dishes.

Adapted from Lux, K. M. (1991). New hope for children with Kawasaki disease. *Journal of Pediatric Nursing, 6,* 159–165.

should praise them for their hard work in keeping the child comfortable. Discharge instructions include provisions for a cardiac follow-up examination (see the accompanying box, Teaching Guidelines for the Child Discharged with Kawasaki Disease).

Evaluation

- Is the child taking adequate amounts of fluid and maintaining electrolyte balance?
- Are the parents able to verbalize the course of the illness and their commitment to follow-up care?

ALLERGIC REACTIONS

Allergy is the immune response to an antigen—called an allergen—that causes a hypersensitive reaction in various body systems. This hypersensitive reaction occurs with a second exposure to an antigen and can be immediate or delayed. One classification of allergic reactions reflects the pathophysiology of each type (Table 23–3). In most children with allergies, there is a genetic link. Common allergic conditions include allergic rhinitis, hives, eczema, asthma, colic, and migraines (Table 23–4). Aller-

TABLE 23–3 *Classification of Allergic Reactions*

TYPE		PATHOPHYSIOLOGY	EXAMPLES
I	Immediate (anaphylactic) hypersensitivity	IgE attaches to mast cells and basophils, causing rupture and release of all contents (i.e., histamines).	Allergic rhinitis, acute anaphylaxis, hives, eczema, asthma
II	Cytotoxic hypersensitivity	An allergen (e.g., a red blood cell) stimulates IgE or IgM to react and mobilize complement to destroy the allergen.	Transfusion reaction after receiving incompatible blood
III	Arthus hypersensitivity (immune complex)	Immune complex is formed and can destroy tissues.	Serum sickness, glomerulonephritis
IV	Delayed cell-mediated hypersensitivity	An allergen reacts with T lymphocytes, and these lead other cells to produce damage.	Contact dermatitis (poison ivy)

TABLE 23–4 *Common Allergic Conditions in Children*

ALLERGENS	MANIFESTATIONS	DIAGNOSIS
Inhalants		
Pollen, dust, mold, dander	Sneezing; red itchy nose, eyes, pharynx, and palate; edematous nasal passages; tongue clicking; runny or congested nose; mouth breathing; chronic cough; dark circles under eyes; nose wrinkling; pale, boggy nasal mucous membranes	Allergic rhinitis
Applicants		
Heat, cold, wool, cosmetics, hair-permanents, sunscreens, plants, grasses	Well-defined red, raised skin or mucosal lesions	Hives
Foods		
Milk, wheat, eggs, strawberries, tomatoes, oranges, chocolate, nuts, shellfish	Intestinal cramping, nausea, vomiting, and diarrhea	Colic
	Bronchospasm	Asthma
	Red patches on cheeks, face, wrists, neck, hands, extremities; swelling; itching; weeping; scales and crust	Eczema
	Well-defined red, raised skin or mucosal lesions	Hives
	Vascular headaches	Migraines
Medicines		
Penicillin, cephalexin, immunizations, allergy immunotherapy, chemotherapy	Redness, swelling, pain	Local inflammation
	Weakness, restlessness, edema, laryngospasm, and cardiovascular collapse	Anaphylaxis
Insects		
Bees, wasps, hornets	Redness, swelling, pain	Local inflammation
	Weakness, restlessness, edema, laryngospasm, and cardiovascular collapse	Anaphylaxis

gic rhinitis is an immediate hypersensitive reaction to allergens trapped by hairs and mucus that line the inside of the nose. (See Chapter 28 for a complete discussion of allergic rhinitis.) Anaphylaxis is a life-threatening allergic response. Allergic reactions are related to the antibody IgE.

Anaphylaxis

Anaphylaxis is a severe immediate hypersensitivity reaction to an excessive release of chemical mediators affecting the entire body.

PATHOPHYSIOLOGY *of Anaphylaxis*

Anaphylaxis occurs when an allergen binds with IgE on the mast cells and basophils, accompanied by a release of histamine and other chemical mediators that affect the magnitude of the response. The reaction is severe and life-threatening and may result in anaphylactic shock. Anaphylaxis may be caused by an allergen that has previously evoked a response, or one that has not.

Etiology. Penicillin is the major cause of anaphylaxis, although other antibiotics and medications may also cause such a reaction. In addition, an anaphylactic response may be caused by foods, such as eggs, nuts, or shellfish; insect stings; immunizations and allergy immunotherapy; and diagnostic contrast media, chemotherapeutic agents, and blood products.

Incidence. Anaphylaxis is rare in infancy and childhood.

Clinical Manifestations. The onset of anaphylaxis is sudden, usually occurring within seconds to minutes after exposure to an allergen. Initial symptoms of impending anaphylaxis include:

- sneezing
- tightness or tingling of the mouth or face
- severe itching of the skin, especially the head and upper trunk
- rapid development of erythema
- a sense of "impending doom"

These may be followed by gastrointestinal and respiratory symptoms, which may include:

- nausea, vomiting, diarrhea, and cramping
- rhinorrhea, stridor, wheezing, and hoarseness

The most serious features of anaphylaxis are:

- laryngospasm
- edema
- cyanosis
- hypotension
- vascular collapse and cardiac arrest

Diagnostic Evaluation. Anaphylaxis occurs suddenly, allowing no time for diagnosis. The etiology is determined later by obtaining the patient's history, and the suspected allergen is confirmed by skin or RAST studies.

Therapeutic Management

Treatment of anaphylaxis must begin immediately, as it is only a matter of minutes before the child will go into shock. Successful management of anaphylaxis also requires anticipating recurrences and reducing risks.

Epinephrine is the first drug of choice in the acute treatment of anaphylaxis. Administration of corticosteroids and antihistamines helps to prevent waves of anaphylaxis several hours later. To manage anaphylactic shock, one must:

- ensure an adequate airway, possibly by endotracheal intubation
- place a tourniquet proximal to the site of injection or insect sting
- administer epinephrine in the uninvolved extremity and in the area of reaction, with repeat dosing within 5 to 10 minutes
- administer oxygen
- start an IV
- administer corticosteroids and antihistamines
- keep the child warm and lying flat or with feet slightly elevated

Children who have experienced insect sting anaphylaxis and demonstrate venom-specific IgE antibodies on skin or RAST studies are candidates for venom immunotherapy (Adamski, 1990).

NURSING CARE OF THE CHILD WITH ANAPHYLAXIS

Assessment

During the acute phase of anaphylaxis, it is essential for the nurse to monitor the child closely for airway obstruction and vascular collapse. Assessment should include noting airway patency, respiratory rate and effort, heart rate, peripheral pulses, capillary refill, oxygen saturation, urine output, and level of consciousness. Following emergency efforts, the nurse can try to determine the cause of the attack by questioning the family about when the symptoms first occurred, what foods were ingested, what medications were administered, and whether there may have been an insect sting.

Nursing Diagnosis and Planning

The following nursing diagnoses and expected outcomes may be appropriate following assessment of a child with anaphylaxis.

TEACHING GUIDELINES ***Preventing Insect Stings***

- Select clothes with whites or khaki colors, not dark or decorative ones.
- Wear fitted clothes with long sleeves, pants, and shoes.
- Use unscented soaps, lotions, and deodorants.
- Apply insect skin protection.
- Avoid orchards, flowers, blooming trees, or shrubs.
- Stay away from picnic areas.
- Keep out of the garden.
- Keep car windows closed while driving.
- Screen all windows.
- Cover all garbage cans.
- Move away slowly from approaching insects.

- Ineffective Breathing Pattern and Decreased Cardiac Output related to an excessive hypersensitive reaction to an allergen. ***Expected Outcome:*** *The child will maintain a patent airway and adequate cardiac output (short-term).*
- Knowledge Deficit related to allergens and prevention through risk reduction. ***Expected Outcome:*** *The child and family will avoid known allergens (long-term).*

Implementation

Initially, the nursing goal is to maintain an adequate airway by administering oxygen and assisting with aerosol treatments and intubation as necessary. A laryngoscope, intubation tray, and tracheostomy kit should be available and the code cart should be nearby. In the case of an insect sting or injected medication, a tourniquet applied to the affected extremity just proximal to the site may help to confine the allergen. It is important to have IV access—with a large-bore needle—in at least one site, preferably two, for medication administration. The nurse will give IV fluids, epinephrine, corticosteroids, and antihistamines as ordered and inform the physician of the patient's improvement or deterioration. Extra fluids (crystalloids or colloids) and plasma expanders should be administered if the child shows signs of vascular collapse.

Because epinephrine causes vasoconstriction and an increase in cardiac output, a child receiving the drug may experience heart palpitations and tachycardia. This is very frightening and is aggravated by the emergency nature of the situation. The nurse should talk to the child and gently offer reassurance. It is important for someone to stay with the family and provide frequent reports about how the child is doing.

Following emergency efforts, the nurse should assure the child and family that it was not their fault that the anaphylactic reaction happened, and should discuss how to prevent recurrences and reduce risks. If the allergen is thought to be food, then the family may monitor and record intake in a diary for later reference. If the allergen is thought to be an insect sting, then the nurse can teach the family about the haunts and habits of insects (see the accompanying box, Teaching Guidelines: Preventing Insect Stings). An insect sting kit should be kept with a child who is not receiving venom immunotherapy. The Epi-Pen Jr. for children delivers 0.15 mg of epinephrine through a spring-loaded injector. The parent must hold the injector against the skin of the upper outer region of the child's thigh for 10 seconds after administering the injection in order to deliver the medication completely. A Medic-Alert bracelet can inform other adults in the child's life as to the allergen (Adamski, 1990).

Evaluation

- Is the child awake and alert with adequate oxygenation and a patent airway?
- Are the child's vital signs within normal limits for age?
- Is the family taking appropriate steps to reduce the risks of another anaphylactic reaction?

KEY CONCEPTS

- The immune system attempts to maintain homeostasis of the internal environment with the external environment through nonspecific functions (inflammation and phagocytosis) and specific functions (humoral and cell-mediated immunity). Any derangement results in an immunologic imbalance whereby the immune system either underfunctions or overfunctions. When it underfunctions, there is an increased susceptibility to infections (immunodeficiency). When the immune system overfunctions, it produces antibodies against cells of the body in autoimmune disease, or against external sensitizing agents, forming the basis for allergies.
- The immune response is produced either actively or passively. Active immunity means the body has reacted to antigens in nature or vaccines that last months to a lifetime. Passive immunity results from antibody transfer from a person with active immunity to a person who does not have that antibody. The effect of passive immunity is transitory.

- Children with acquired or congenital immunodeficiency are vulnerable to bacterial infections. The best way to prevent the spread of organisms is to wash hands routinely and to follow basic infection control practices based on three principles: (1) prevent contact with organisms, (2) create barriers if contact is unavoidable, and (3) kill organisms if contact is made.
- HIV infection is the most well-known acquired immunodeficiency disease. It causes a wide spectrum of illness in children, ranging from no symptoms to mild and moderate symptoms to severe symptoms. AIDS represents the most severe illness. Standard treatments include a modified immunization program, antiretroviral therapy, PCP prophylaxis, and the aggressive use of antibiotics. Nurses have the challenging tasks of promoting normal growth and development preventing infections, providing comfort, and respiratory management. In addition, nurses must support families in dealing with a stigmatizing illness that is ultimately terminal.
- Corticosteroids have immunosuppressive and anti-inflammatory properties. Tapering the dose during both long- and short-term therapy regimens allows for the gradual return of pituitary-adrenal function.
- Prophylaxis with penicillin for 5 years, or through adolescence, whichever period is longer, is the most important aspect of therapeutic management for RF. IM injection is the route of choice. Oral medication is an alternative, if given precisely and faithfully.
- In Kawasaki disease, coronary aneurysms may occur about 11 days after the onset of fever, followed by an acute myocardial infarction secondary to thrombosis of the aneurysms. Nursing management includes administering IVIG and aspirin to reduce the formation of the aneurysms and fever.
- Emergency treatment takes priority in an anaphylactic reaction, as it is only a matter of minutes before the child will go into shock. Initially, the goal is to maintain an adequate airway, sometimes necessitating endotracheal intubation. This is followed by the administration of epinephrine.

REFERENCES

Adamski, D. B. (1990). Assessment and treatment of allergic response to stinging insects. *Journal of Emergency Nursing, 16*(2), 77–82.

Allbritten, D. J. (1990). *Children With HIV/AIDS: A sourcebook for caring: A guide for establishing programs for children.* Alexandria, VA: National Association of Children's Hospitals and Related Institutions (NACHRI).

American Academy of Pediatrics, Committee on Infectious Diseases. (1994). Immunizations in special clinical circumstances; HIV infection and AIDS. In G. Peter (Ed.), *Red Book* (pp. 51–67, 254–270). Elk Grove Village, IL: AAP.

Ayoub, E. M. (1992). Resurgence of rheumatic fever in the United States: The changing picture of a preventable illness. *Postgraduate Medicine, 92,* 133–142.

Bellanti, J. (1985). *Immunology: Basic processes (2nd ed.).* Philadelphia: W. B. Saunders.

Centers for Disease Control and Prevention (CDC). (April 28, 1995). 1995 revised guidelines for prophylaxis against PCP for children infected with or perinatally exposed to HIV. *MMWR, 44,* RR–4.

Centers for Disease Control and Prevention (CDC). (1994). Recommendations for the use of zidovudine to reduce perinatal transmission of HIV. *MMWR, 43*(11), 285–287.

Centers for Disease Control and Prevention. (1994, November). *HIV/AIDS surveillance report* (mid-year ed.). Atlanta, GA: Author.

Corbett, J. V. (1992). *Laboratory tests and diagnostic procedures with nursing diagnoses.* E. Norwalk, CT: Appleton & Lange.

Dajani, A. S., Taubert, K. A., Gerber, M. A., Shulman, S. T., & Ferrieri, P. (1993). Diagnosis and therapy of Kawasaki syndrome in children. *Circulation, 87,* 1776–1780.

FDA Press Release. (1996, March). FDA grant accelerates the approval to third protease inhibitor to treat HIV.

Freund, B. D., Scacco-Neuman, A., Pisanelli, A. S., & Benchot, R. (1993). Acute rheumatic fever revisited. *Journal of Pediatric Nursing 8*(3), 167–176.

Fuller, C., & Hartley, B. (1991). Systemic lupus erythematosus in adolescents. *Journal of Pediatric Nursing, 6,* 251–257.

Glass, P. (1995, June). Neurodevelopmental aspects of HIV+. Workshop co-sponsored by the National Pediatric and Family HIV Resource Center. Greenbelt, MD.

Grimes, D. E., & Woolbert, L. F. (1990). Facts and fallacies about streptococcal infection and rheumatic fever. *Journal of Pediatric Health Care, 4,* 186–192.

Health and Human Services News. (1996, March). FDA approves second protease inhibitor to treat HIV.

Health and Human Services News. (1995, December). FDA approves first protease inhibitor for treatment of HIV.

Hodgson, B., Kryror, R., & Kingdon, R. (1994). *Nurses' drug handbook 1994.* Philadelphia: W. B. Saunders.

Hollister, J. R. (1992). Rheumatic diseases. In W. E. Hathaway, W. W. Hay, J. R. Groothuis, & J. W. Paisley (Eds.), *Current pediatric diagnosis and treatment* (pp. 768–776). East Norwalk, CT: Appleton & Lange.

Kee, J. L. (1991). *Laboratory and diagnostic tests with nursing implications.* East Norwalk, CT: Appleton & Lange.

Legun, L. A. (1990). Systemic lupus erythematosus during pregnancy. *Journal of Obstetrics and Gynecology, 19,* 304–310.

Levin, M., Tizard, E. J., & Dillon, M. J. (1991). Kawasaki syndrome: recent advances. *Archives of Diseases in Childhood, 66,* 1369–1372.

Lux, K. M. (1991). New hope for children with Kawasaki disease. *Journal of Pediatric Nursing, 6,* 159–165.

Marlow, D. R., & Redding, B. A. (1988). *Textbook of pediatric nursing.* Philadelphia: W. B. Saunders.

McGrath, M. S. (1990). Immunology of AIDS: Overview. In P. T. Cohen, M. A. Sande, & P. A. Volberding (Eds.), *The AIDS knowledge base* (1st ed.), 3.2.1. Waltham, MA: The Medical Publishing Group.

Merkel-Holguin, L. A. (1994). *Because you love them: A parent's planning guide.* Washington, DC: The Child Welfare League of America.

Moye, J. (1995, June). Update: Prophylaxis of opportunistic infections in pediatric HIV disease. Workshop co-sponsored by the National Pediatric and Family HIV Resource Center. Greenbelt, MD.

Occupational Safety and Health Administration. (1992). *Occupational exposure to bloodborne pathogens.* Washington, DC: U.S. Department of Labor.

Oleske, J. (1995, June). Pain in pediatric HIV disease: Meeting the challenge. Plenary session co-sponsored by the National Pediatric and Family HIV Resource Center. Greenbelt, MD.

Parrott, R. H., & Rathlev, M. C. (1993). *Access to primary health care for children with HIV: A guide for pediatricians, family physicians and nurse practitioners.* Washington, DC: Children's National Medical Center.

Pohlgeers, A. P., Eid, N. S., Schikler, K. N., & Shearer, L. T. (1990). Systemic lupus erythematosus: Pulmonary presentation in childhood. *Southern Medical Journal, 83,* 712–714.

Schindler, L. (1988). *Understanding the immune system.* Washington, DC: U.S. Department of Health and Human Resources, Public Health Service, National Institutes of Health.

Shackelford, P. G., & Strauss, A. W. (1991). Kawasaki syndrome. *New England Journal of Medicine, 324,* 1664–1666.

Simonds, R. H., Oxtoby, M. J., Caldwell, B., Gwinn, M. L., & Rogers, M. F. (1993). *Pneumocystis carinii* pneumonia among U.S. children with perinatally acquired HIV infection. *Journal of the American Medical Association, 270,* 470–478.

Sullivan, J. (1993). Mechanisms of maternal-fetal HIV transmission. *Clinical Immunological Spectrum, 4,* 5.

Taeusch, H. W., Christiansen, R. O., & Buescher, E. S. (1996). *Pediatric and neonatal tests and procedures.* Philadelphia: W. B. Saunders.

Tasker, M. (1992). *How can I tell you?* Bethesda, MD: Association for the Care of Children's Health.

Ward-Wimmer, D., & Riley, M. W. (1991). *Caring at home: A guide for families.* Washington, DC: The Child Welfare League of America.

Wara, D. W. (October, 1992). Address at the Annual Meeting of the American Academy of Pediatrics. San Francisco, CA.

Whinney, S. M., Pagano, M., & Thomas, P. (October, 1993). Age at AIDS diagnosis for children with perinatally acquired HIV. *Journal of Acquired Immune Deficiency Syndrome, 6*(10), 1139–1144.

Wolfe, R. R., & Wiggins, J. W. (1992). Cardiovascular diseases. In W. E. Hathaway, W. W. Hay, J. R. Groothuis, J. W. Paisley (Eds.), *Current pediatric diagnosis and treatment* (pp. 517–575). East Norwalk, CT: Appleton & Lange.

BIBILIOGRAPHY

American Academy of Pediatrics, Task Force on Pediatric AIDS. (1992). Guidelines for human immunodeficiency virus (HIV)–infected children and their foster families. *Pediatrics, 89,* 681–683.

American Academy of Pediatrics, Task Force on Pediatric AIDS. (1991). Education of children with HIV infection. *Pediatrics, 88,* 645–648.

Boxer, M. B. (1993). Anaphylaxis without cause. *Emergency Medicine, 25*(1), 21–30.

Cohen, F. L., & Durham, J. D. (1993). *Women, children and HIV/AIDS.* New York: Springer.

Copstead, L. (1995). *Perspectives on pathophysiology.* Philadelphia: W. B. Saunders.

Cunha, B. A. (1992). Kawasaki disease. *Emergency Medicine, 24*(12), 209–213.

Greenberg, P. (1992). Immunopathogenesis of HIV infection. *Hospital Practice, 27*(2), 109–124.

Hong, R. (1992). Diseases due to immunologic deficiency disorders. In R. E. Behrman (Ed.), *Nelson textbook of pediatrics* (14th ed., pp. 550–557). Philadelphia: W. B. Saunders.

Iseki, M., & Heiner, D. C. (1993). Immunodeficiency disorders. *Pediatrics in Review, 14,* 226–236.

Jones, E. M., & Callen, J. P. (1991). Collagen vascular diseases of childhood. *Pediatric Clinics of North America, 38,* 1019–1039.

Melish, M. E. (1992). Kawasaki syndrome: A 1992 update. *Pediatric Dermatology, 9,* 335–337.

Mofenson, L. M., Moye, J., Jr., & Bethel, J. (1992). Prophylactic intravenous immunoglobulin in HIV-infected children with CD4+ counts of 0.20×10^9 or more. *Journal of the American Medical Association, 268,* 483–488.

Newburger, J. W., Takahashi, M., Beiser, A., Burns, J., Bastian, J., Chung, K., et al. (1991). A single intravenous infusion of gamma globulin as compared with four infusions in the treatment of acute Kawasaki syndrome. *New England Journal of Medicine, 324,* 1633–1638.

Pizzo, P. (1990). Pediatric AIDS: Problems within problems. *Journal of Infectious Disease, 161,* 316–325.

Reisman, R. E. (1992). Natural history of insect sting allergy: Relationship of severity of symptoms of initial sting anaphylaxis to re-sting reactions. *Journal of Allergy and Clinical Immunology, 90,* 335–339.

Selekman, J. (1990). The multiple faces of immune deficiency in children. *Pediatric Nursing, 16*(4), 351–361.

Simonds, R. J., & Chauock, S. (1993). Medical issues related to caring for HIV-infected children in and out of home. *Pediatric Infectious Disease Journal, 12*(10), 845–851.

Stafford, C. T., Moffitt, J. E, & Yates, A. B. (August 15, 1992). Insect sting anaphylaxis: Referral is imperative. *Emergency Medicine, 24*(11), 230–232.

Taubert, K. A., Rowley, A. H., & Shulman, S. T. (1991). Nationwide survey of Kawasaki disease and acute rheumatic fever. *Journal of Pediatrics, 119(2),* 279–282.

Working Group on Antiretroviral Therapy. (1993). Antiretroviral therapy and medical management of the HIV-infected child. *Pediatric Infectious Disease Journal, 12,* 513–522.

24

The Child With Fluid and Electrolyte Alterations

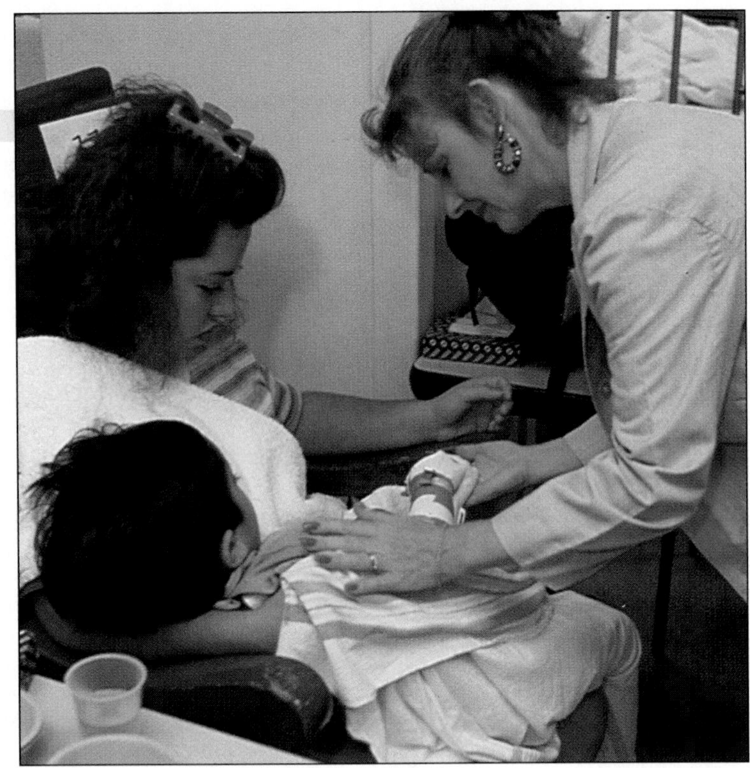

CHAPTER OVERVIEW

LEARNING OBJECTIVES

After studying this chapter, you should be able to:

- Identify the regulatory mechanisms that maintain fluid and electrolyte balance in the body.
- Describe the differences in body fluid and electrolyte composition and regulation in infants and children compared with those of adults that make them especially vulnerable to imbalances.
- Describe the processes of dehydration and acid-base imbalance.
- Differentiate between the various types of acid-base disturbances.
- Examine the processes of diarrhea and vomiting.
- Integrate assessment findings with nursing implementation to determine the success of therapy.
- Describe nursing interventions to prevent fluid and electrolyte imbalances.

KEY TERMS

acidosis: abnormal accumulation of acid or loss of base from the body, with pH equal to or less than 7.35

alkalosis: abnormal accumulation of bicarbonate or loss of acid in the body, with pH equal to or greater than 7.45

anuria: severe diminution of urine formation, less than 0.5 ml/kg/hr, usually indicative of kidney failure; may be secondary to severe dehydration

ECF: extracellular fluid found outside the cell, comprising approximately one third of the body's fluid in older children and about half of the fluid in infants

hypertonic (hypernatremic) dehydration: state in which the solute concentration is above that of normal body fluids (i.e., sodium > 145 mEq/L)

hypotonic (hyponatremic) dehydration: state in which the solute concentration is below that of normal body fluids (i.e., sodium < 135 mEq/L)

ICF: intracellular fluid found within the cells, comprising approximately two thirds of the body's fluid in older children and about half of the fluid in infants

interstitial fluid: fluid surrounding the cell, including lymph fluid

intravascular fluid: fluid contained with the blood vessel (e.g., plasma)

isotonic (isonatremic) dehydration: state in which the solute concentration is practically identical to that of body fluids (i.e., sodium between 135 and 145 mEq/L)

oliguria: diminished amounts of urine output

Infants and young children are at a greater risk than adults for disturbances in fluid and electrolyte balance due to differences in body composition, higher metabolic rate, and immaturity of physiologic regulating systems. These differences are especially significant in the infant, whose proportion of total body water and basal metabolic rate are greater than in adults and older children. Any source of fluid loss from the body—such as diarrhea, vomiting, hemorrhage, shock, ostomy drainage, fluid loss from burns—can result in a fluid or electrolyte imbalance. Diarrhea alone has been associated with 9% of all hospitalizations for children under age 5 years (Kleinman, Sack, & Dale, 1994).

Nurses, as well as parents, need to be able to quickly recognize the signs and symptoms of fluid and electrolyte loss. The condition of infants and young children can change rapidly when fluid and electrolyte imbalances occur. Most cases of dehydration can be cared for at home with the use of oral rehydration solutions. Some children, however, will not respond and will require intravenous management in the hospital setting.

This chapter includes a review of the basic principles of fluid and electrolyte balance and acid-base balance. The pathophysiology and clinical manifestations of dehydration, diarrhea, and vomiting are discussed, as well as the treatment and nursing care for these common childhood disorders.

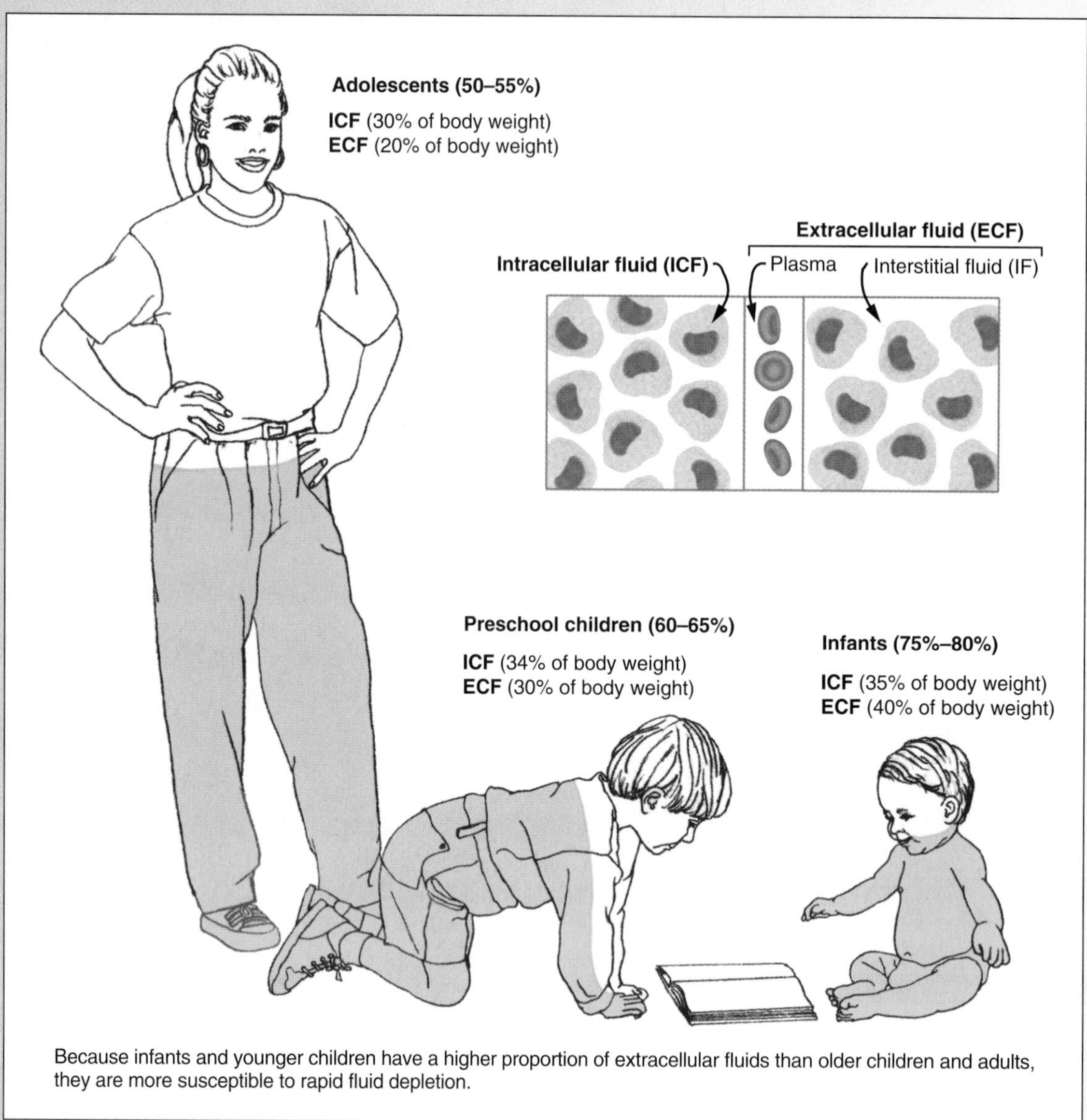

Because infants and younger children have a higher proportion of extracellular fluids than older children and adults, they are more susceptible to rapid fluid depletion.

FLUID AND ELECTROLYTE IMBALANCES IN CHILDREN

Unique characteristics of children affect fluid and electrolyte balance. Infants and young children are more vulnerable than adults to changes in fluid and electrolyte balance (see accompanying box, Pediatric Differences Related to Fluid and Electrolyte Balance). Under normal conditions, the amount of fluid ingested during a day should equal the amount of fluid lost through sensible water loss (such as urine output) and insensible water loss (via the respiratory tract and skin). Insensible water loss per unit of body weight is significantly higher in infants and children. The faster respiratory rates of infants and young children also result in higher evaporative water losses. Any condition that prevents normal oral fluid intake (such as vomiting) or results in fluid losses (such as diarrhea, hyperventilation, burns, or hemorrhage) is especially significant because it depletes the body's store of water and electrolytes much more rapidly in infants and young children than in adults.

It is essential that parents know and understand all medications their child is on in order to prevent drug interactions that might cause electrolyte imbalances or interference with therapy.

Pediatric Differences Related to Fluid and Electrolyte Balance

INFANTS

- Can lose fluids equal to their ECF within 2–3 days due to the higher percentage of water in the ECF.
- Have a decreased ability to concentrate urine, due to immature renal function.
- Have a higher rate of peristalsis.
- Have an immature lower esophageal sphincter, which makes them more prone to gastroesophageal reflux, which can lead to dehydration and electrolyte disturbances.
- Have a harder time compensating for acidosis due to decreased ability to acidify urine.

INFANTS AND YOUNG CHILDREN

- Have a higher metabolic turnover of water due to a higher metabolic rate (if losses are not replaced rapidly, imbalance occurs).
- Are unable to verbalize or communicate thirst.

INFANTS AND CHILDREN

- Have a proportionately greater body surface area in relation to body mass, resulting in greater potential for fluid loss via the skin and GI tract.
- Have a higher proportionate water content (premature infants have 90%, full-term infants, 75%–80%, preschool-age children 60%–65%, and adolescents and adults approximately 55%), with a larger proportion of fluid in the extracellular space.
- Have a lower functioning immune system, with more tendencies to infectious diseases, fever, food intolerances and allergies, gastroenteritis, and respiratory infections, all of which can result in fluid and electrolyte disturbances and fluid volume deficit.

Body water is located in two major compartments: within the cell (intracellular) and outside of the cell (extracellular). These two compartments are separated by the cell membrane, across which body fluid is continually exchanged. Extracellular fluid **(ECF)** is located in several places: interstitial spaces (surrounding the cells, such as lymph fluid); **intravascular** (fluid within the blood vessels or plasma); and transcellular (such as cerebrospinal fluid, pericardial, pleural, synovial, sweat, and digestive secretions). Because the ECF interacts with the outside environment, a child is more likely to lose ECF than intracellular fluid **(ICF).** ECF is lost first when fluid loss occurs (i.e., through illness, trauma, or fever). The intracellular compartment is more difficult to dehydrate. In the neonate, approximately 40% of body water is located in the extracellular compartment, compared with 20% in the adolescent and adult. Because approximately 50% of this ECF is exchanged daily in an infant, dehydration can occur very suddenly and rapidly if there is inadequate fluid intake or excessive fluid losses. Because of the infant's higher metabolic rate, the rate of water turnover is rapid. In the infant, half of the ECF may be exchanged compared with an adult exchange of one sixth of the ECF in a similar time. Depletion of ECF, often caused by gastroenteritis, is one of the most common problems among infants and young children. In adults and older children, because a greater proportion of fluids is located in the intracellular compartment, severe fluid depletion does not occur as rapidly. Maturity in terms of body space distribution is usually reached around age 3 years.

Body fluids are basically composed of two elements: water and solutes. *Water* is the primary constituent, with the infant's weight being approximately 75% water to the adult's 60%. As a rule of thumb, the volume of total body water decreases with increasing age. There is an inverse relationship between total body water and total body fat. Neonates, and particularly premature infants, have a lower proportion of fat compared with adults. *Solutes* are composed of both electrolytes and nonelectrolytes. The majority of the body's solutes are electrolytes, primarily sodium (Na), potassium (K), chloride (Cl), and calcium (Ca). The primary electrolyte of the ECF is sodium; potassium is the primary electrolyte in the ICF. The extracellular compartment contains more sodium and chloride during infancy, causing increased vulnerability of infants to electrolyte imbalances. Changes in concentration of these electrolytes may result in cellular dysfunction and illness. Problems of fluid and electrolyte balance always involve both water and electrolytes; thus treatment includes replacement of both, calculated according to serum electrolyte laboratory values. The major electrolyte disturbances are outlined in the accompanying table, Overview of Fluid and Electrolyte Disorders. A discussion of diarrhea and vomiting, common causes of fluid and electrolyte disturbances in children, is presented later in this chapter.

The table Assessment of Fluid and Electrolyte Disturbances lists clinical manifestations and the possible disturbances that could cause them.

Medications commonly used in fluid and electrolyte disorders and common laboratory and diagnostic tests are listed in the accompanying tables.

ALTERATIONS IN ACID–BASE BALANCE IN CHILDREN

Alterations in acid-base balance can affect cellular metabolism as well as enzymatic processes, and the ability of the body to regulate this status is crucial. Children can experience acid-base imbalance as a result of many pathologic conditions. The pH, or measure of acidity or alkalinity of

OVERVIEW OF FLUID AND ELECTROLYTE DISORDERS

	PRECIPITATING EVENTS	CLINICAL MANIFESTATIONS
Hyponatremia (sodium < 135 mEq/L)	Fever Increased water intake without electrolytes Decreased sodium intake Diabetic ketoacidosis Burns and wounds SIADH Malnutrition Cystic fibrosis Renal disease Vomiting, diarrhea, nasogastric suction	Neurologic: • Usually do not show signs until sodium reaches 125 mEq/L • Behavioral changes, irritability, lethargy, headache, dizziness, apprehension Cardiovascular • Increased heart rate • Decreased blood pressure • Cold, clammy skin Muscle cramps (especially abdominal) Nausea
Hypernatremia (sodium > 145 mEq/L)	Water loss or deprivation High sodium intake Diabetes insipidus Diarrhea Fever Hyperglycemia Renal disease	Intense thirst Oliguria Agitation, restlessness Flushed skin Peripheral and pulmonary edema Dry, sticky mucous membranes Nausea and vomiting Serum Na ≥ 150 mEq/L: disorientation, seizures, hyperirritability when at rest
Hypokalemia (potassium < 3.5 mEq/L)	Stress Starvation Malabsorption Excessive loss of GI fluids through vomiting, diarrhea, sweat, nasogastric tube Administration of diuretics (especially furosemide, ethacrynic acid, and thiazide diuretics) IV fluids without added potassium Administration of corticosteroids Diabetic ketoacidosis	Muscle weakness, paralysis Leg cramps Decreased bowel sounds Weak and irregular pulse, tachycardia or bradycardia, cardiac arrhythmias Hypotension Ileus Irritability, fatigue
Hyperkalemia (potassium > 5.0 mEq/L)	Increased intake of potassium (e.g., salt substitutes) Decreased urine excretion Kidney failure Metabolic acidosis Hyperglycemia Potassium-sparing diuretics Dehydration (severe) Too rapid administration of IV potassium Burns	Irritability, anxiety Twitching, hyperreflexia Weakness, flaccid paralysis Nausea/diarrhea Bradycardia Cardiac arrest (concern if potassium > 8.5 mEq/L) Apnea, respiratory arrest
Hypocalcemia (calcium < 8.5 mg/dl; ionized calcium < 4.5 mg/dl)	Inadequate intake of calcium Vitamin D deficiency Renal insufficiency Calcium losses (e.g., infection, burn, loop diuretics) Alkalosis Administration of diuretics Hypoparathyroidism	Numbness and tingling of fingers, toes, nose, ears, and circumoral area Hyperactive reflexes, seizures Muscle cramps/tetany Laryngospasm Lethargy and poor feeding in the newborn Positive Trousseau's and Chvostek's signs Hypotension Cardiac arrest
Hypercalcemia (calcium > 10.5 mg/dl; ionized calcium > 5.5 mg/dl)	"Milk alkali" syndrome (chronic ingestion of calcium carbonate antacids or milk) Excessive IV or oral calcium administration Acidosis Prolonged immobilization Hypoproteinemia Renal disease Hyperparathyroidism Hyperthyroidism	Lethargy, weakness, anorexia Thirst Itching Behavioral changes: confusion, personality change, stupor Nausea, vomiting, constipation Bradycardia, cardiac arrest

ASSESSMENT OF FLUID AND ELECTROLYTE DISTURBANCES

	CLINICAL MANIFESTATION	POSSIBLE FLUID AND/OR ELECTROLYTE DISTURBANCE
Heart Rate	Rapid, weak, thready	Fluid volume deficit
	Rapid, bounding	Fluid volume excess
	Weak, irregular, slowing	Severe hyperkalemia
	Weak, irregular, rapid	Severe hypokalemia
Respirations	Rapid, deep	Metabolic acidosis
	Slow, shallow	Respiratory alkalosis
Blood Pressure	Increased	Fluid volume excess
	Decreased	Late stages of shock; fluid volume deficit; hypokalemia or hyperkalemia, hyponatremia
Skin	Poor elasticity	Fluid volume deficit
	Pallor	Fluid volume deficit
	Cool to touch	Fluid volume deficit; increased or decreased sodium
	Poor capillary refill	Fluid volume deficit
Edema		Fluid volume excess (usually)
Dry Mucous Membranes		Fluid volume deficit
Decreased Salivation and/or Tearing		Fluid volume deficit
Behavioral Changes	Lethargy	Fluid volume deficit
	Irritability	Fluid volume deficit
	Increased restlessness	Hyperkalemia
	Comatose	Markedly increased acidosis or alkalosis
Sensory Changes	Thirst	Fluid volume deficit, increased sodium and/or calcium
	Tingling in extremities	Hypocalcemia, alkalosis
	Abdominal cramps	Hyponatremia, hyperkalemia
	Muscular cramps	Hypocalcemia, hypokalemia
	Light-headedness or dizziness	Respiratory alkalosis
	Nausea	Hypercalcemia, hypokalemia or hyperkalemia
Neurologic Changes	Hypotonia	Hypokalemia, hypercalcemia
	Weakness	Metabolic acidosis
	Hypertonia:	
	Positive Chvostek's sign	Hypocalcemia
	Tremors, cramps, tetany	Hypocalcemia, alkalosis

Data from Finberg, L., Kravath, R., & Hellerstein, S. (1993). *Water and electrolytes in pediatrics* (pp. 135–138). Philadelphia: W. B. Saunders; and Horne, M., Heitz, U., & Swearingen, P. (1991). *Fluid electrolyte and acid-base balance: A case study approach* (Chaps. 8, 9, 10). St. Louis: Mosby–Year Book.

COMMON LABORATORY AND DIAGNOSTIC TESTS FOR FLUID AND ELECTROLYTE IMBALANCE

	DESCRIPTION	INDICATIONS	NORMAL FINDINGS	NURSING CONSIDERATIONS
Urine Osmolality	24 hr urine collection or random test	Altered fluid status	300–900 mOsm/kg	No preparation Done by nurse
Urine Sodium	24 hr urine collection or random urine specimen	Altered fluid status, hyponatremia	50–130 mEq/L	No preparation Done by nurse
Urine Specific Gravity	Random urine specimen	Altered fluid status	1.002–1.030	No preparation Done by nurse
Urea Nitrogen	Random urine specimen	Altered fluid status Renal function	5–18 mg/dl	No preparation Sample collected by nurse
Serum Osmolality	Random urine specimen	Altered fluid status Measures solute concentration of blood	275–295 mOsm/kg	No preparation Draw blood needed for sample

MEDICATIONS COMMONLY USED FOR FLUID AND ELECTROLYTE DISORDERS

DRUG AND INDICATION	DOSAGE	SIDE EFFECTS	NURSING CONSIDERATIONS
Antidiarrheals			
Diphenoxylate hydrochloride with atropine sulfate (Lomotil, Lonox, others)	*PO:* 0.3–0.4 mg/kg/day in three or four divided doses Not indicated for children less than age 2 years	CNS: lethargy, confusion, drowsiness, headache CV: tachycardia GI: nausea/vomiting, abdominal cramps, distension	Do *not* administer if child is dehydrated. May be crushed and given with food or fluid. Monitor stool patterns. Monitor fluid status.
Kaolin and pectin (Kaopectate, others) • For mild to moderate diarrhea • Not established for children <3 years of age	*PO:* 3–6 yr: 15–30 ml 6–12 yr: 30–60 ml Give after each loose stool; not to exceed eight times/day	Constipation (usually mild and transient)	Shake before giving. Advise patient not to use for longer than 48 hours or if fever develops. Could reduce absorption of other concurrently administered medications.
Loperamide hydrochloride (Immodium, Pepto Diarrhea Control) • For acute, nonspecific diarrhea • Not indicated for children < age 2 years	*PO:* 2–5 yr: 1 tsp after first loose stool, then 1 tsp after each, not to exceed 3 tsp/day 6–8 yr: 2 tsp or 1 caplet after first loose stool, then 1 tsp or ½ caplet after each, not to exceed 4 tsp or 2 caplets per day	Nausea, vomiting Constipation, cramps, dry mouth	If acute diarrhea does *not* improve in 48 hours, discontinue. Do not use if fever increases. May be given by either liquid or tablets. Monitor stool pattern. Monitor fluid status. May cause drowsiness.
Bismuth subsalicylate (Pepto-Bismol) • Usually used for "traveler's" diarrhea • Not established for use in children < age 3 years	*PO:* 3–6 yr: 1 tsp or 1/3 tablet 6–9 yr: 2 tsp or 2/3 tablet 9–12 yr: 1 tbsp or 1 tablet every 30–60 minutes up to eight times per day	Temporary darkening of stools With high doses: constipation, bismuth toxicity, bluish gum line, tinnitus, bleeding disorders	Chew tablets. Beware of salicylates. Educate child/family that a blackish discoloration of the tongue and stool may occur.
Antiemetics			
Trimethobenzamide hydrochloride (Tigan, Tegamide, others)	15–40 kg: *PO:* 100–200 mg/dose, tid or qid *Rectal:* 100 mg/dose, tid or qid <15 kg: *Rectal:* 100–200 mg/dose, tid or qid	CNS: extrapyramidal reactions, drowsiness, confusion, dizziness, headache, blurred vision Hypotension	Avoid use in children with hepatotoxicity, acute vomiting, or allergic reactions. May be given PO, IM, PR (IM not usually used in children). Oral capsules may be taken apart and mixed with food. Do not give with aminoglycosides or other ototoxic drugs.
Prochlorperazine (Compazine)	>10 kg or > 2 yr *PO:* 0.4 mg/kg/day divided into three or four doses *IM:* 0.13 mg/kg	CNS: extrapyramidal reactions, lowered seizure threshold, drowsiness Jaundice, agranulocytosis Hypotension ECG changes: prolonged PR interval, flattened T waves	Monitor blood pressure closely. Do *not* give IV for children <10 kg or <2 yr. Use only to manage vomiting of known etiology.
Ondansetron hydrochloride (Zofran) • Prevention of nausea and vomiting associated with chemotherapy	*IV:* 0.15 mg/kg prior to chemotherapy, then 0.15 mg/kg 4 and 8 hours after first dose	Constipation Rare cases of rash, tachycardia, hypotension Transient blurred vision	IV only. Usually for patients receiving chemotherapy or those not tolerating other antiemetics.
Promethazine (Phenergan, Provigan)	*IM, PO, rectal, IV:* 0.25–0.5 mg/kg q 4–6 hr	CNS: similar to prochlorperazine Hypotension Nausea, vomiting, constipation Nasal stuffiness	Oral form may be given with food or fluid (to decrease gastric upset; tablet may be crushed or mixed). Avoid heavy exercise after administration. Only for prolonged vomiting of known etiology.

body fluids, is regulated within a narrow range (normal blood pH is 7.35 to 7.45). Maintenance of serum pH within normal limits is crucial to maintaining cellular function, enzyme activity, and neuromuscular membrane potentials. Chemical buffers, the respiratory system, and the kidneys work together to keep the blood pH within normal range. Acid is constantly produced as a by-product of metabolism. The body attempts to maintain blood pH within normal limits by reducing the buildup of acid. Chemical and cellular buffer systems minimize the effect of alterations in blood pH by neutralizing excess acids and bases that accumulate in body fluids. Two of the most significant buffers are bicarbonate and proteins. Bicarbonate, the most important buffer for plasma and **interstitial fluids,** is responsible for the majority of ECF buffering and can exert its effects relatively quickly (within minutes).

When alterations in pH become too much for the buffer systems to handle, compensatory mechanisms in the renal and respiratory systems are activated. The lungs remove carbon dioxide from the blood, reducing the amount of carbonic acid and raising the blood pH. The respiratory system works rapidly to compensate for acid-base disturbances. If the blood pH drops below normal **(acidosis),** respiratory rate and depth will increase, removing CO_2 and raising blood pH. Conversely, in the presence of **alkalosis,** respiratory rate and depth will decrease, thus lowering blood pH.

Kidneys regulate bicarbonate and remove hydrogen ions from the blood. If the blood is too alkaline, the kidneys conserve hydrogen ions, thus lowering blood pH. In the presence of acidosis the kidneys excrete hydrogen ions and conserve bicarbonate, raising blood pH. Renal compensatory processes work more slowly than respiratory mechanisms, usually within 1 to 2 days. If compensatory mechanisms are ineffective, acid-base imbalances occur. When a dysfunction results in decreased hydrogen ion concentration in the blood, the arterial pH increases (alkalosis). When a dysfunction results in an increase in hydrogen ions, the arterial pH decreases (acidosis).

The four types of acid-base imbalances, involving either respiratory or metabolic mechanisms, are summarized in the accompanying tables.

> Treatment of metabolic acid-base disturbance is oriented toward correcting the underlying problem; treatment of respiratory imbalance is directed toward re-establishing alveolar ventilation.

MECHANISMS OF ACID-BASE DISTURBANCES

	PRIMARY DISTURBANCE	PRINCIPLE COMPENSATORY RESPONSE*
Metabolic Acidosis	Decreasing HCO_3	Hyperventilation causes decreased $PaCO_2$
Metabolic Alkalosis	Increasing HCO_3	Hypoventilation causes increased $PaCO_2$
Respiratory Acidosis	Increasing $PaCO_2$	Release of HCO_3 and increased renal reabsorption of HCO_3
Respiratory Alkalosis	Decreasing $PaCO_2$	Decreased renal reabsorption of HCO_3

*Important items to remember when acid-base compensation occurs:

- Normal values from which to interpret blood gases:
  $PaCO_2$ = 40–45 mmHg
  pH = 7.35–7.45
  Bicarbonate = 22–26 mEq/L
- When metabolic compensation occurs, assume respiratory alteration in origin
- When respiratory compensation and release of tissue buffers occurs, assume metabolic in origin

Data from American Academy of Pediatrics. (1990). *Textbook of pediatric advanced life support* (pp. 49–52). American Heart Association; and Horne, M., Heitz, U., & Swearingen, P. (1991). *Fluid, electrolyte and acid-base balance: A case study approach* (pp. 404–405). St. Louis: Mosby–Year Book.

SELECTED LABORATORY VALUES FOR ACID-BASE DISTURBANCES

TEST	METABOLIC ACIDOSIS	METABOLIC ALKALOSIS	RESPIRATORY ACIDOSIS	RESPIRATORY ALKALOSIS
ABG: pH	<7.35	>7.45	<7.35	>7.45
$PaCO_2$ (mmHg)	<40	>45	>45	<35
PaO_2 (mmHg)	WNL or slightly decreased	Decreased	Decreased	Decreased
HCO_3 (mEq/L)	<22	>26	WNL or slightly increased	Decreased
K^+ (mEq/L)	>4.0	Decreased	WNL	Slightly decreased
Na^+ (mEq/L)	Varies according to condition	Decreased	WNL	Slightly decreased
Cl^- (mEq/L)	Usually increased	Decreased	WNL	Slightly increased

ACID-BASE DISTURBANCES: PRINCIPLE CAUSES, CLINICAL MANIFESTATIONS, AND TREATMENT

CONDITION	PRINCIPLE CAUSES	CLINICAL MANIFESTATIONS	PRINCIPAL TREATMENT METHODS
Metabolic Acidosis	Ketoacidosis (DKA, alcohol-induced ketoacidosis) Increasing metabolic rates from fever, RDS, seizures Interferences with normal metabolism: ketosis, tissue hypoxia Loss of bicarbonate from diarrhea, ileostomy or fistula drainage Acute and chronic renal failure ECF expansion and decreasing HCO_3 concentration	Increasing heart rate, arrhythmias (fibrillation) Cold, clammy skin (mild to moderate acidosis) Warm, dry skin (severe acidosis) Level of consciousness changes from fatigue and confusion to stupor and coma	Identify and treat underlying disorder. Provide $NaHCO_3$, K^+ replacement and mechanical ventilation as indicated.
Metabolic Alkalosis	Volume depletion related to various conditions such as vomiting, pyloric stenosis, gastric drainage, and diuretics Increased alkali intake Medical conditions such as cystic fibrosis	Arrhythmias (atrial-ventricular with prolonged QT interval) Increasing heart rate Level of consciousness changes from apathy and confusion to stupor Muscular weakness	Will depend on the underlying cause; mild to moderate alkalosis usually does not require treatment. Use of fluids with NaCl and KCl, along with isotonic saline, histamine H_2 receptor antagonist (such as cimetidine) to decrease gastric hydrochloric acid, acidifying agents, and potassium-sparing diuretics (e.g., aldactone or mannitol).
Respiratory Acidosis	Pulmonary disease (BPD, hyaline membrane disease, croup) Airway obstruction Chest conditions such as flail chest, pneumothorax Acute and chronic respiratory failure Neuromuscular abnormalities such as Guillain-Barré syndrome, toxins, drugs, paralysis CNS depression from sedative overdose, trauma, anesthesia	Increasing heart rate Arrhythmias with hypotension Increasing rate/depth of respirations, forceful use of accessory muscles with retraction and cyanosis Increasing intracranial pressure	Correction of ventilation problem: use of oxygen, intubation, mechanical ventilation, $NaHCO_3$.
Respiratory Alkalosis	Hyperventilation from CNS stimulation such as emotions, fear, hysteria, pain, salicylate poisoning Decreased lung compliance and hypoxemia from conditions such as pulmonary edema, CHF, pneumonia, asthma, pulmonary emboli Pregnancy Compensation from metabolic acidosis Sepsis	Dizziness, paresthesias, lightheadedness, diaphoresis Increasing rate/depth of respirations Arrhythmias (changes in ST-T wave)	Mild to moderate usually does not require specific treatment. For hyperventilation-induced conditions: oxygen, rebreathing oxygen masks, psychological reassurance; mechanical ventilation if severe condition. Sedatives/tranquilizers for anxiety-induced, acetazolamide to prevent motion sickness.

DKA, diabetic ketoacidosis; RDS, respiratory distress syndrome; ECF, extracellular fluid; BPD, bronchopulmonary dysplasia; CNS, central nervous system; CHF, congestive heart failure.

DEHYDRATION

Dehydration, or fluid loss in excess of fluid intake, is a common condition affecting infants and children. Dehydration is classified as isotonic, hypotonic, or hypertonic (Table 24–1). **Isotonic dehydration,** the most common type occurring in children, results when water and electrolytes are lost in approximately the same proportion as they exist in the body, and serum sodium levels remain within the acceptable normal range (135 to 145 mEq/L). **Hypotonic dehydration** occurs when the loss of electrolytes is greater than loss of water, resulting in a serum sodium level less than 130 mEq/L. **Hypertonic dehydration** occurs when the loss of water is greater than the loss of electrolytes and the serum sodium level is greater than 150 mEq/L.

TABLE 24–1 *Types of Dehydration: Etiology, Clinical Manifestations, and Laboratory Values*

	ISOTONIC DEHYDRATION	HYPOTONIC DEHYDRATION	HYPERTONIC DEHYDRATION
Etiology	Most common type of dehydration in children Vomiting, diarrhea Insensible fluid loss via respiratory and integumentary Decreased PO intake with increased activity	*Renal losses:* Diuretics, hyperglycemia, nephritis, adrenal insufficiency *Extrarenal losses:* Vomiting, diarrhea, third-space burns, tube drainage *Other:* CHF, SIADH, nephrosis; administration of large amounts of electrolyte-free solutions (plain water) during illness or postoperatively	*Renal losses:* Diuretics, diabetes insipidus, adrenal insufficiency *Extrarenal losses:* Vomiting, diarrhea *Other:* Fever, increased sodium in formula, diet, or tube feeding; administration of hypertonic sodium IV fluids
Clinical Manifestations	Mild thirst Skin turgor poor Dry skin and mucous membranes Decreased urine output Skin temperature cold Body temperature afebrile ↔ febrile Lethargic	Increased thirst Skin turgor very poor Skin usually clammy Decreased urine output Mucous membranes dry to slightly moist Skin temperature cold Body temperature afebrile ↔ febrile Very lethargic; concern about seizures	Thirst very increased Skin turgor fair Skin texture thickened or "doughy" Decreased urine output Mucous membranes parched Skin temperature cold ↔ hot Body temperature afebrile ↔ febrile Lethargic; hyperirritable with stimulation
Laboratory Values	Serum sodium: 130–150 mEq/L *Urine:* Sodium usually WNL Specific gravity slightly elevated Osmolality usually WNL Volume usually WNL or slightly decreased	*Renal losses:* Serum sodium < 130 mEq/L Urine sodium increased Urine specific gravity decreased Urine osmolality decreased Urine volume increased *Extrarenal losses:* Serum sodium < 130 mEq/L Urine sodium decreased Urine specific gravity increased Urine osmolality increased Urine volume decreased *Other:* Serum sodium < 130 mEq/L Urine sodium decreased Urine specific gravity increased Urine osmolality increased Urine volume decreased	*Renal losses:* Serum sodium > 150 mEq/L Urine sodium increased Urine specific gravity decreased Urine osmolality decreased Urine volume increased *Extrarenal losses:* Serum sodium > 150 mEq/L Urine sodium decreased Urine specific gravity increased Urine osmolality increased Urine volume decreased *Other:* Serum sodium > 150 mEq/L Urine sodium decreased Urine specific gravity increased Urine osmolality increased Urine volume decreased

Data from Behrman, R. E., Kliegman, R. M., & Arvin, A. M. (1996). *Nelson textbook of pediatrics* (15th ed.). Philadelphia: W. B. Saunders.

PATHOPHYSIOLOGY *of Dehydration*

In the early phases of dehydration, fluids, with some electrolytes, are lost from the ECF. If the fluid loss continues, loss of ICF can occur.

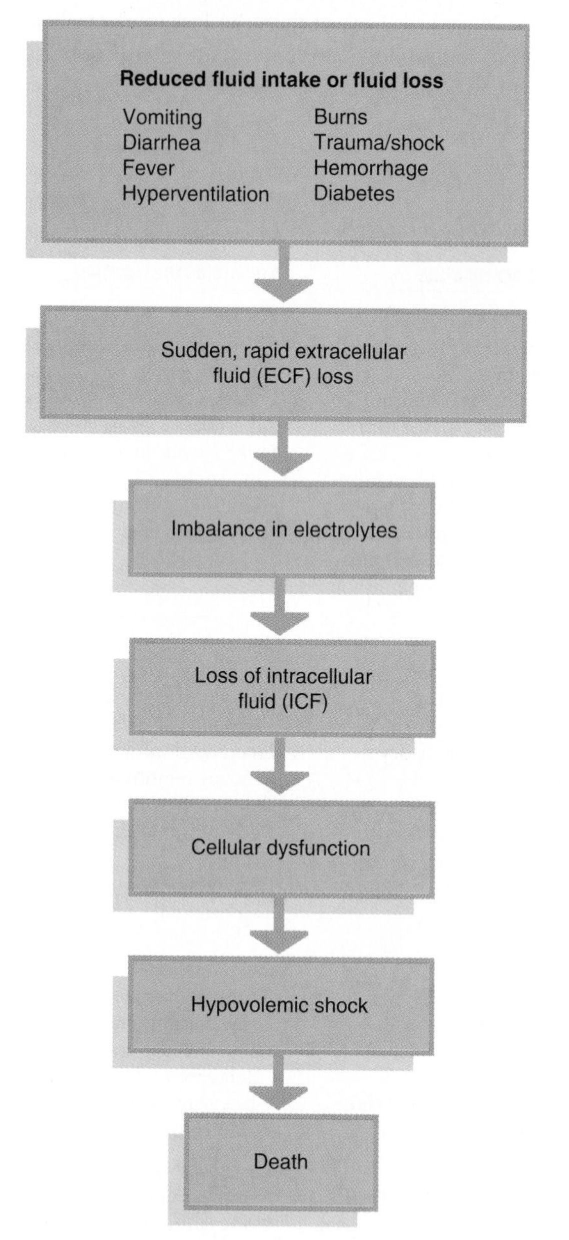

Dehydration can lead to shock.

Etiology. There are many varied causes of dehydration. Common alterations that may lead to dehydration are due to disturbances in the following systems:

- Gastrointestinal tract: vomiting, diarrhea, pyloric stenosis, malabsorption
- Endocrine system: fever, diabetes mellitus, cystic fibrosis
- Skin: burns
- Lungs: tachypnea
- Kidneys: renal failure
- Heart: congestive heart failure

Incidence. Any age-group can be affected, but neonates and infants are especially vulnerable to the effects of dehydration due to the factors discussed in the Clinical Reference Pages.

Clinical Manifestations. For infants and young children with isotonic dehydration, the fluid deficit is described as 5% (mild), 10% (moderate), or 15% (severe) dehydration, describing the percentage of body weight lost. Approximately 1 g of body weight is the equivalent of 1 ml of body fluid. A weight loss or gain of 1 kg (2.2 lb) in 24 hours represents a 1-liter fluid loss or gain.

- *Mild dehydration:* 3% to 5% loss of body weight; fluid volume loss of <50 ml/kg.
- *Moderate dehydration:* 6% to 9% loss of body weight; fluid volume loss of 50–90 ml/kg.
- *Severe dehydration:* 10% or more loss of body weight; fluid volume loss of ≥100 ml/kg.

Because total body water and ECF volume compose a smaller percentage of body weight in older children and adolescents than in infants, any percentage of body weight lost from dehydration represents a more severe fluid depletion. Therefore isotonic dehydration in the older child is classified as mild if 3% body weight is lost, moderate if 6% body weight is lost, and severe if 9% body weight is lost.

The signs and symptoms associated with isotonic dehydration are listed in Table 24–2. As with impending shock, the most essential manifestations include changes in heart rate, behavior/sensorium, urine output, skin qualities, and, in infants, fontanels.

Changes in heart rate, sensorium, and skin color are earlier indicators of impending shock than blood pressure due to a child's ability to compensate and maintain an adequate cardiac output.

Diagnostic Evaluation. The key parameters in attempting to determine the type and degree of severity of dehydration include:

- a history of acute or chronic fluid loss
- serum electrolyte laboratory values
- clinical manifestations
- weight of the child

Therapeutic Management. Management is directed at correcting the fluid and electrolyte imbalance and then proceeding to treat the causative factors. If the child is awake and alert and able to take fluids by mouth, oral rehydration therapy (ORT), such as Pedialyte, Infalyte, or the World Health Organization's solution, is given. Pedialyte or Infalyte for neonates and infants and electrolyte drinks (such as

TABLE 24–2 *Clinical Signs and Symptoms Associated With Severity of Isotonic Dehydration*

	MILD DEHYDRATION	MODERATE DEHYDRATION	SEVERE DEHYDRATION
Loss of Body Weight	<5%	5%–10%	10%
Skin Color	Pale	Dusky	Mottled
Skin Turgor	Decreased	Moderately decreased	Markedly decreased
Urine Output	Decreased	Oliguria	Marked oliguria and azotemia
Thirst	Slight	Moderate	Intense
Tears	Present	Decreased	Absent
Mucous Membranes	Dry	Very dry	Parched
Blood Pressure	Normal	Normal or slightly above or below normal	Low
Pulse	Normal or tachycardia	Tachycardia	Increased tachycardia and thready pulse
Anterior Fontanels	Level or flat	Slightly sunken	Sunken

From Betz, C. L., Hunsberger, M. M., & Wright, S. (1994). *Family-centered nursing care of children* (2nd ed., p. 921). Philadelphia: W. B. Saunders; Straughn, A., & English B. (1996). Oral rehydration therapy. *Maternal Child Nursing, 21,* 144–147.

Gatorade or Exceed) for older children may be attempted (see Table 24–4). This regimen usually involves quick rehydration within 4 to 6 hours. If the child is unable to take fluids by mouth, and there is a need to replace ongoing fluid losses, then parenteral fluid and electrolyte therapy is initiated. Isotonic intravenous fluids (dextrose 5% in lactated Ringer's solution or dextrose 5% in 0.9% sodium chloride solution) are given. If necessary, potassium is added to the intravenous solution once urine output is adequate. The accompanying box presents guidelines for maintenance fluid requirements and minimum urine output by age and weight.

Rate of administration of replacement fluids is determined by the type of dehydration. For the child with isotonic or hypotonic dehydration, lost fluids are replaced over 24 hours (in addition to the child's maintenance fluid requirements). Half the amount of estimated fluids are replaced over the first 8 hours; the remaining half, over the next 16 hours. With hypertonic dehydration, lost fluids are replaced more slowly (over 48 hours) to prevent a sudden decrease in serum sodium level. Potassium losses must also be replaced; this process should proceed slowly to avoid hyperkalemia. Potassium replacement should be begun only after urine output is adequate.

Potassium should never be added to an intravenous solution in the presence of oliguria or anuria (i.e., urine output less than 0.5 ml/kg/hr).

Potassium replacement should be administered with extreme caution. Some guidelines to use for the administration of potassium chloride are listed below.

- *Never* give by IV push.
- Give no more than 40 mEq/L, no faster than 1 mEq/kg/hr.
- Always check the dose and dosage calculations of potassium chloride. (Incorrect placement of a decimal point can result in a lethal dose for a child.)
- Do not administer potassium chloride if urine output is less than 1–2 ml/kg/hr (depending on child's age and hydration status.)
- Add potassium chloride to IV fluids with the plastic IV bag in the upright (noninfusion) position rather than in the down (infusion) position to avoid the risk of inadequate mixing. (Inadequate mixing could result in the child receiving an excessive amount of potassium chloride in the first few minutes.)

Maintenance Fluid Requirements and Minimum Urine Output

Fluid Requirements by Body Weight

Up to 10 kg:	100 ml/kg/day
10–20 kg:	1000 ml/kg/day + 50 ml/kg/day for each additional kg between 10 and 20 kg
20+ kg:	1500 ml/kg/day + 20 ml/kg/day for each additional kg over 20 kg

Minimum Urine Output by Age-Group

Infants and toddlers:	>2–3 ml/kg/hr
Preschoolers and young school-age:	>1–2 ml/kg/hr
School-age and adolescents:	0.5–1 ml/kg/hr

NURSING CARE OF THE CHILD EXPERIENCING DEHYDRATION

Assessment

Because dehydration can develop very quickly in infants and young children, the nurse must be alert for early signs of dehydration in children with conditions in which fluid losses are likely to occur, such as diarrhea, vomiting, burns, diabetes, trauma, and fever.

The general appearance of the child should be assessed, as well as specific parameters:

Intake and output: Measure all fluid intake and losses accurately (including vomitus, urine, stools, nasogastric drainage, sweat, wound drainage).

Urine output and specific gravity: Output of less than 1–2 ml/kg/hr or specific gravity above 1.020 may indicate dehydration. However, glucose, large amounts of protein, and radiographic dyes elevate the specific gravity and may interfere with accuracy of this parameter.

Weight: Weight is a crucial indicator of fluid status. Accurate measurement of the weight of the unclothed child is essential. Changes in weight related to changes in IV lines or dressings should be identified by documenting "with IV." Weight gain during illness may indicate fluid retention or pulmonary or generalized edema. The weight should be rechecked, and the child should be assessed for pulmonary crackles and periorbital edema.

Stools, vomitus: Frequency, type, and consistency should be assessed and documented.

Sweating: Estimate from dampness of clothing and linen.

Serum electrolytes: See Overview of Fluid and Electrolyte Disturbances table in Clinical Reference Pages.

Skin: Assess color, temperature, turgor (Fig. 24–1), moisture, and capillary refill.

Mucous membranes and presence of tears: Dry or sticky mucous membranes and absence of tears indicate dehydration.

Anterior fontanel: Sunken or depressed fontanel in infants indicates dehydration. Suture lines may also become prominent with dehydration.

Vital signs: Fever increases metabolic rate and fluid requirements. Pulse is rapid, weak, and thready with dehydration. Metabolic acidosis, which often accompanies dehydration, is compensated for by an increased respiratory rate. Blood pressure is decreased in moderate and severe dehydration.

Behavior: Irritability, lethargy, confusion, or seizures may be present. Cry may be high pitched and weak.

Nursing Diagnosis and Planning

The following nursing diagnoses and expected outcomes are examples that may be appropriate in the treatment of dehydration in the child.

Nursing Diagnosis

- Fluid Volume Deficit related to fluid volume loss in gastrointestinal contents, hemorrhage, burns, other illness, or failure of regulatory mechanisms

Expected Outcome

The infant/child will display adequate fluid volume as evidenced by:

- age-appropriate urine output (1–2 ml/kg/hr)
- age-appropriate urine specific gravity
- elastic skin turgor and moist mucous membranes
- serum pH and electrolyte levels within normal limits
- return to pre-illness weight.

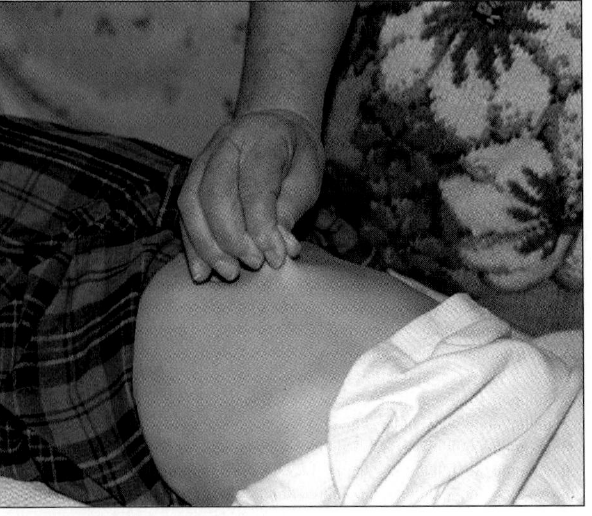

Figure 24–1

Testing skin turgor. *Turgor* refers to the elasticity of the skin, which is affected by the extent of hydration. The nurse tests turgor by gently grasping the skin. When the skin is released, it should instantly spring back into place; if it does not, tissue turgor is considered poor. (Courtesy of the University of Texas at Arlington School of Nursing, Arlington, Texas)

TEACHING GUIDELINES *for Dehydration*

SIGNS AND SYMPTOMS OF DEHYDRATION

Parents should be taught to watch for the following signs and symptoms of dehydration:

- Fewer wet diapers
- No tears when crying
- Irritability, high-pitched cry
- Difficult to awaken
- Increased respiratory rate or difficulty in breathing
- Sunken fontanel, sunken eyes with dark circles
- Vomiting or many loose stools
- Abnormal skin color, temperature, or dryness

Parents of infants younger than age 6 months should seek professional assistance early, because their child's condition may worsen more rapidly than the older child's.

ORAL REHYDRATION THERAPY

It is important for parents to understand that giving plain water alone or in large amounts can be extremely dangerous. Instead, commercially available oral rehydration solutions, such as Infalyte or Pedialyte for infants, and sports drinks such as Gatorade, Exceed, or 10-K for older children, should be used.

Implementation

The nurse plays an important role during treatment of conditions that predispose children to dehydration. Discussions of nursing care of the child with vomiting and diarrhea follow in this chapter. One of the nurse's responsibilities is to teach parents how to prevent dehydration. Parents should be taught to give infants and young children extra fluids during hot weather and to avoid overdressing. During minor illness, taking the child's temperature and providing additional fluids in the presence of fever may prevent the child from developing more serious problems. Parents should be taught how to identify the early signs and symptoms of dehydration and to seek professional help if they occur. (See Teaching Guidelines box.)

Parents should also be taught how to replace fluids when their child is mildly dehydrated.

> It is important for parents to understand that giving plain water alone or in large amounts can be extremely dangerous.

Undiluted skim milk should not be given because of its high solute content. Electrolyte solutions such as Infalyte, Pedialyte, or Gatorade contain the appropriate concentration of electrolytes and should be used when fluid is the child's only intake for a prolonged period of time.

When caring for the hospitalized child with fluid and electrolyte imbalance, the nurse assumes the responsibility of continuously monitoring the child's condition and administering oral and IV fluids safely. (See Chapter 19 for IV therapy.) When caring for children with conditions such as fever, burns, diarrhea, vomiting, or trauma, the nurse must continuously assess for signs of dehydration. For interventions, see discussion of specific disorders.

Evaluation

- Is urine output appropriate for age (1 to 2 ml/kg/hr) with specific gravity of 1.005 to 1.020?
- Is skin elastic and soft?
- Are mucous membranes moist?
- Is the child taking an age-appropriate amount of fluid?
- Are vital signs within age-appropriate limits?
- Are serum pH and electrolyte levels within normal limits?
- Do parents verbalize home care required?

DIARRHEA

Diarrhea, one of the most common disorders in childhood, is defined as an increase in the frequency, fluidity, and volume of stools. Diarrhea accompanies many childhood disorders. Diarrhea in children may be acute or chronic, inflammatory or noninflammatory. Diarrhea caused by viral infection is usually called gastroenteritis. Viral gastroenteritis is the most common cause of diarrhea in children over age 1 year.

If not treated, acute diarrhea can lead to dehydration, electrolyte imbalance, and hypovolemic shock. Acute diarrhea can be life-threatening in infants and small children if gastrointestinal fluid losses are not adequately replaced.

Etiology. There are many and varied causes of both acute and chronic diarrhea, listed in Table 24–3.

Incidence. Diarrhea, and ensuing dehydration, is the number one killer of children worldwide and is a major cause of morbidity, as well as a primary symptom of many other conditions. Within the United States, diarrhea accounts for

PATHOPHYSIOLOGY *of Diarrhea*

Increased motility and rapid emptying of the intestines results in impaired absorption of nutrients and water, as well as electrolyte imbalance. Water, sodium, potassium, and bicarbonate are drawn from the extracellular space into the stool, resulting in dehydration, electrolyte depletion, and metabolic acidosis.

Diarrhea occurs when there is excess fluid in the small intestine. This can result from a number of processes:

- Bacterial toxins stimulate active transport of electrolytes into the small intestine. Cells in the mucosal lining of the intestines are irritated and secrete increased amounts of water and electrolytes.
- Organisms invade and destroy intestinal mucosal cells, decreasing intestinal surface area and impairing the intestine's capacity to absorb fluids and electrolytes.
- Inflammation decreases the intestine's ability to absorb fluid, electrolytes, and nutrients. This occurs in malabsorption syndromes.
- Increased intestinal motility results in impaired intestinal absorption.

TABLE 24–3 *Causes and Manifestations of Diarrhea in Infants and Children*

CAUSES OF DIARRHEA	MANIFESTATIONS
Intestinal infection: • Bacterial: *Campylobacter jejuni,* Salmonella,* E. coli* • Viral: Rotavirus* (acuse of over 50% of cases of acute diarrhea in children, enteric adenovirus) • Parasitic: *Giardia lamblia,* Cryptosporidium** (high incidence of both in daycare centers) • Fungal overgrowth	Watery stools containing mucus and possibly blood. Pain, cramps, nausea, vomiting, and fever (over 101.6°F [38.5°C] with bacterial infection). Risk of dehydration, electrolyte imbalances, and shock
Food intolerance (lactose intolerance, overfeeding, introduction of new foods)	Diarrhea, increased mucus in stools, flatus, and pain after ingestion of lactose or offending food
Malabsorption (cystic fibrosis, dissaccharide deficiencies, celiac disease)	Diarrhea, cramps, distension, steatorrhea occur after meals May experience anorexia, weight loss, and fatigue
Medications (antibiotics, iron)	Diarrhea after administration of medications
Colon disease (ulcerative colitis, Crohn's disease, enterocolitis)	Inflammation and ulceration of intestinal walls, increased motility May have 10–20 stools a day Abdominal pain, fever, chills, anorexia, and weight loss
Irritable bowel syndrome	Diarrhea alternating with constipation or normal bowel function Pain, distension, and nausea may be present
Intestinal obstruction	Partial obstruction may result in diarrhea caused by increased intestinal motility. Pain, nausea, and sometimes bloody stools
Emotional stress (anxiety, fatigue)	Increased motility
Infectious disease (otitis media, upper respiratory infection, urinary tract infection)	Diarrhea frequently accompanies other infections.

*Most common causative organisms.

approximately 10% of all acute care visits by children under age 2 years (Cohen & Ballistreri, 1989). It can either be a short- or long-term condition; in infants and young children, however, diarrhea can be life-threatening if the losses are not replaced.

Clinical Manifestations. Diarrhea may manifest either quickly or insidiously, and includes the following systems manifestations:

Integumentary

- Dry, hot skin
- Changes in skin texture and turgor
- Dry mucous membranes

GI: small intestine:

- Cramps, nausea, vomiting
- Large volume of stools, light in color
- Stools tend to be soupy, greasy, foul-smelling

GI: large intestine:

- Urge to defecate but often insignificant stool present
- Mushy, jelly-like, or even bloody fecal matter
- Stool usually dark in color
- Stool rarely foul-smelling

Other manifestations of diarrhea include:

- Increased heart and respiratory rates
- Decreased tearing
- Fever

Diagnostic Evaluation. Because there are many causes of diarrhea, the diagnostic workup is frequently geared toward ruling out infectious agents as well as anatomic and physiologic reasons, such as allergies, food intolerances, and bowel problems. Tests to be performed after an initial history has assessed for food intolerances, stress, or school/work problems include the following:

Stool: cultures (for bacteria, ova, parasites, rotavirus), pH, red blood cells, leukocytes, glucose (use of Clinitest), blood (use of guaiac or Hemoccult)

Breath hydrogen test: checking for carbohydrate malabsorption

Blood tests: especially electrolytes, blood urea nitrogen, glucose, as well as blood cultures (especially if an infectious agent is suspected)

X-rays: to check for possible bowel abnormalities

History: food/formula intolerance and/or allergies

Therapeutic Management. Treatment of diarrhea is aimed at restoring fluid and electrolyte balance and returning the bowel to normal function. Preventing spread of infection to others is an important component of care. Mild cases of diarrhea can usually be treated at home (AAP, 1996; O'Loughlin et al., 1995). Parents must be informed of specific fluid intake requirements and signs of dehydration, which would signal a worsening of the child's condition. Treatment includes the replacement of fluids, early feedings, and close monitoring and observation for the treatment of diarrhea and prevention of dehydration. Early reintroduction of feeding can prevent dehydration, reduce stool frequency and volume, and hasten recovery. Research indicates that healing is facilitated by early reintroduction of nutrients back into the intestinal tract (Halpern, 1991; Pizarro, 1991). Early reintroduction of oral fluids represents a change from the more traditional approach of "resting the bowel"; i.e., placing the child NPO, using intravenous therapy for fluid replacement, and a more gradual introduction of food (Meyers, 1995; Gremse, 1995). Oral rehydration therapy (ORT) is begun within the first 24 hours of illness, with initial feedings including breast milk, electrolyte solutions such as Infalyte or Pedialyte, or dilute formula for infants and electrolyte solutions such as Gatorade for older children. Research has indicated that rice cereal–based products, such as Infalyte, are better at decreasing stool output and increasing fluid absorption because of the molecular structure of the rice and should be considered initially for the dehydrated child with diarrhea (Barclay et al., 1995; Fayad et al., 1993; Pizarro, 1991).

The ORT solutions have changed from the days of homemade recipes (mixtures of water, salt, sugar, and cereals) to today's commercially available, lower osmolality fluids. The high carbohydrate contents of fluids such as

TABLE 24–4 *Comparison of Clear Liquids and Oral Rehydration Solutions*

PRODUCT	SUGARS (g/L)	NA (mmol/L)	K (mmol/L)	OSMOLALITY (mOsm/L)
Apple juice	100–150	3	28	700
Cola	50–100	2	0.1	550
Ginger ale	50–100	3	1.0	540
Chicken broth	0	250	8	450
Gatorade	46	20	3	330
WHO Solution	20	90	20	310
Pedialyte	25	45	20	250
Infalyte	30 g/L of rice syrup solids	50	25	200

Data from Snyder, J. (1987). Cereal-based oral rehydration therapy: Theory and practice. Symposium Proceedings, February 17, 1987, pp. 33–36.

apple juice or colas may further aggravate diarrhea and cause additional fluid loss due to their osmotic effect (see Table 24–4). Infants may advance from clear liquids to a lactose hydrolyzed milk or soy formula after 24 hours and toddlers to a bland milk-free diet. The reintroduction of cow's milk may cause diarrhea to begin again because of possible lactase deficiency. For this reason, diluted formula may be given, gradually advancing to full strength. In some instances, it may be necessary to give the infant a soy formula until the deficiency resolves. The child is gradually advanced to a more solid diet. Common foods that are especially well tolerated during diarrhea are bland foods consisting primarily of starch, including rice, maize, wheat, and potatoes.

For infants with mild to moderate diarrhea who have not become dehydrated, ORT is started at home. If an infant or child has become mildly to moderately dehydrated and requires a visit to a clinic or emergency department, ORT solution is still recommended (Johnson, 1994). Feeding of solids or formula is started as soon as the child is rehydrated. For a child with severe dehydration and ongoing losses, ORT is not recommended. Such children are usually admitted to a hospital for observation and intravenous therapy.

If the diarrhea is caused by a bacteria, parasite, or fungus, other types of medication along with antibiotics may be ordered. The use of antidiarrheal medication is not recommended in children under age 2 years due to the binding nature of these products and the potential for toxicity. Antidiarrheal medications have not been found to shorten the course of the diarrhea.

> Diarrhea caused by pathogens occurs as the body attempts to rid itself of the organism, and the use of antidiarrheal medications may in fact increase fluid and electrolyte losses by allowing the pathogen to remain in the body longer.

Prognosis. Most children experiencing diarrhea and subsequent dehydration usually have a relatively quick recovery, provided the cause of the diarrhea is determined and therapy is started as soon as possible.

NURSING CARE OF THE CHILD WITH DIARRHEA

Assessment

The child's condition and hydration status should be the first area of assessment; as discussed above, the concern about dehydration is the potential for shock. The child/family should be questioned about possible food allergies, intolerance to foods, food eaten over the past 24 hours, and outbreaks of diarrhea in the nuclear or extended family. If diarrhea is present, stools should be assessed using the acronym ACCT (amount, color, consistency, time) and odor. When assessing and monitoring for ACCT, the nurse should note the quantity and quality of the stool; description of the stool's color (i.e., green, brown, black, clear, blood-tinged); consistency (watery, loose, runny); presence of mucus; and the length of time the stool consistency has changed.

Other ongoing assessments include monitoring of intake and output; assessing the current weight and then comparing with the last known weight; assessing for thirst, along with skin turgor and texture and mucous membranes; and monitoring the child's level of activity.

Nursing Diagnosis

- Fluid Volume Deficit related to increased stool output
- Impaired Skin Integrity related to exposure to stool
- Risk for Infection (in others) related to lack of knowledge about transmission prevention
- Altered Nutrition: Less Than Body Requirements related to decreased intake and inability of body to absorb fluid
- Knowledge Deficit related to home care

Planning, Implementation, and Evaluation: The Child With Diarrhea

NURSING DIAGNOSIS • Fluid Volume Deficit related to increased stool output

Expected Outcome: • The child will maintain fluid balance within normal limits as evidenced by age-appropriate urine output, capillary refill < 2 seconds, elastic skin turgor, moist mucous membranes, and maintenance of pre-illness weight.

Intervention	Rationale
1. Weigh child carefully on admission and daily on the same scale and at the same time each day.	Weight is a useful indicator of fluid status.

Intervention	Rationale
2. Monitor and document intake and output hourly. Monitor urine color every 4 hours and specific gravity when appropriate. Weigh diapers after each voiding and stool. (Each gram of diaper weight is equivalent to 1 ml of urine.) Notify physician of signs of dehydration.	Urine output should be at least 2 ml/kg/hr for infants and toddlers, and 1 ml/kg/hr for school-age children.
3. Monitor vital signs at least every 4 hours or more frequently as indicated. Temperature should not be taken rectally. Report abnormalities to physician.	Dehydration can quickly lead to shock in infants and small children. Use of a rectal thermometer can stimulate peristalsis and cause more diarrhea.
4. Assess for signs of dehydration (dry mucous membranes, decreased tearing, and sunken fontanel) frequently. Assess and document amount, frequency, color, and consistency of stools.	Such signs are often the first signs of dehydration.
5. Administer PO and IV fluids as ordered. Check IV for patency/infiltration every hour. Check restraints for pressure and position frequently.	Excessive output without replacement leads to fluid deficit and electrolyte imbalances.
6. Administer medications as ordered (antidiarrheals, antibiotics, antiprotozoals).	Medications may be administered to treat the cause of the diarrhea as well as to assist in minimizing possible sequelae.
7. Maintain NPO status if ordered.	During acute stage of diarrhea, oral intake may increase peristalsis.
8. Send stools to laboratory for culture and other ordered tests. Perform tests for guaiac, pH, and reducing substance. Monitor laboratory reports (electrolytes, pH, hematocrit, serum albumin, urine specific gravity). Notify physician of abnormal laboratory values or increased frequency of stooling.	Laboratory reports are monitored to evaluate response to therapy.
9. Implement measures to reduce fever (antipyretics as ordered). (See Chapter 18 for discussion of care of the child with fever.)	

Evaluation: The infant/child is well hydrated as evidenced by moist mucous membranes, flat fontanel, age-appropriate urine output (1 to 2 ml/kg/hr), and specific gravity of 1.005–1.020. Stools are formed and the child has fewer than four per day.

NURSING DIAGNOSIS • Impaired Skin Integrity related to exposure to stool

Expected Outcome:
- The child will have no sign of skin breakdown, as evidenced by intact perineal and perianal skin.
- The child will exhibit signs of healing on affected or excoriated areas.

Intervention	Rationale
1. Assess the extent of skin breakdown (color, texture, lesions, drainage).	Skin breakdown greatly increases potential for infection.

Intervention	Rationale
2. Attempt to reduce peristalsis and avoid solutions/foods irritating to mucosal lining.	Reduces external stimuli that aggravates the condition.
3. Wash diaper area with water and mild soap after each stool and dry thoroughly. Commercial cleaning wipes often contain alcohol and may cause irritation and pain. Apply medicated ointment or cream as ordered. Do not use plastic pants if hydrocortisone cream is used, because plastic can increase absorption of medication.	Thorough and consistent skin care routine decreases the risk of skin breakdown.
4. Expose affected area to air as much as possible (not with explosive diarrhea). Keep clothing and linen clean and dry.	Exposure of skin to air decreases irritation and promotes healing.
5. Use protective moisture barriers, such as creams or ointments.	Barrier creams are useful for protection from diarrheal stools.

TEACHING GUIDELINES *for the Child With Diarrhea*

DIET

Diet depends on the age of the child and the severity of the diarrhea.

Mild diarrhea (mushy stools) in children younger than age 2 years: Extra fluids are needed and may be given by adding 1 to 2 ounces of extra water to each bottle of formula or juice. If the infant is taking solids, give a soft diet consisting of the ABCs (applesauce, strained bananas, and strained carrots), rice, potatoes, and other bland foods without dairy products.

Moderate diarrhea (watery or frequent stools) in children younger than age 1 year: Clear fluids (oral electrolyte solutions) for 24 hours. Infalyte, Pedialyte, Rehydralyte (or other generic products with compositions identical to Pedialyte) are ideal. Half-strength Gatorade or other sports drinks may be substituted until Pedialyte or a similar electrolyte solution is obtained. Jell-O water, Kool-Aid, or soda pop should not be used as the only intake because they contain little or no salt. Avoid using red Jell-O because it can look like blood in the stools. Boiled skim milk, chicken or beef broth, or other concentrated solutions can cause serious complications because they contain too much salt. The infant should be given as much liquid as he wants to drink.

After the infant has been on clear liquids for 6 to 24 hours, regular formula can be resumed. If the diarrhea was severe or if the diarrhea does not improve after 3 days on regular formula, the infant should be given soy formula (Isomil, ProSobee) instead of cow's milk formula. The formula should be diluted with 1 or 2 ounces of extra water per bottle until the stools are no longer watery. Diluted formula should not be used for more than 24 hours. Soy formula should be continued until the diarrhea is gone for 3 days.

Solids may be given after liquids are fully tolerated. Appropriate foods include the ABCs (applesauce, bananas, strained carrots), mashed potatoes, rice cereal mixed with water, and other bland foods without dairy products.

Breast feeding should not be discontinued because of mild to moderate diarrhea. Extra water should be offered between breast feedings.

Moderate diarrhea (watery or frequent stools) in children age 1 to 2 years:

- *Day 1:* Clear liquids (Infalyte, Pedialyte, Gatorade). Avoid fruit juices. As with younger infants, Kool-Aid, popsicles, and water should not be used as the only intake because they contain little or no salt.
- *Day 2:* Saltine crackers, toast with honey, rice, mashed potatoes, applesauce, bland soups, or other bland foods without dairy products.
- *Day 3:* Lean meats, soft-boiled eggs, noodles, soft cooked fruits and vegetables, and active culture yogurt. Avoid cheese, which contains 80% of the lactose found in milk.
- *Day 6:* Regular diet without milk.
- *Day 8:* Milk and milk products can gradually be added.

Intervention	Rationale
6. Perform axillary or otic temperatures only; *no* rectal temperatures.	Rectal temperature stimulates peristalsis.
7. Turn child every 2 hours and protect reddened bony prominences. Use prophylactic pressure-relieving devices in bed and chairs.	Decreasing pressure on irritated skin promotes healing.
8. Teach parents skin care routines (see Teaching Guidelines for the Child With Diarrhea).	Parents need to be involved in care of the child.

Evaluation: The child is free from alterations in skin integrity, as evidenced by absence of irritation, excoriation, redness, blisters, pruritus, and signs of infection.

Mild or moderate diarrhea in children over age 2 years:

- Give foods high in starch (breads, crackers, rice, mashed potatoes, and noodles) because these are easily absorbed during diarrhea.
- Give clear liquids. Reduce or eliminate milk and milk products, except active-culture yogurt, which is digested by the *Lactobacillus* organism. Avoid raw fruits and vegetables, beans, spices, and any other foods that cause loose stools.
- Resume normal diet 1 day after the diarrhea is gone, which is usually in 3 or 4 days.

PREVENTING SPREAD OF INFECTION

Diarrhea is very contagious. Thorough handwashing after diaper changing or using the toilet is crucial to prevent others in the household from getting diarrhea. All family members should be taught the importance of thorough and frequent handwashing. Diapers should be changed on a surface designated for that purpose and *not* on the kitchen counter where food is prepared. Changing areas should be cleaned with disinfectant after each diaper change.

SKIN CARE

To prevent breakdown of the sensitive skin in the diaper area, diarrhea stools should be completely washed off with mild soap and water after each bowel movement. (Washing the child under running water in the bathtub makes the job easier. The tub should be cleaned with disinfectant before anyone else uses it.) The skin should be dried gently and a layer of zinc oxide or other protective ointment applied. Changing diapers immediately after bowel movements is important to prevent skin breakdown. The use of commercial baby wipes should be avoided, because they may sting excoriated skin.

To prevent overflow of diarrhea from the diaper, diapers should be applied snugly. A cotton washcloth can be placed inside the diaper to trap some of the more watery stool. Superabsorbent diapers and diapers with elastic leg bands also cut down on cleanup time.

WHEN TO CALL THE DOCTOR

Call the doctor immediately if:

- The child does not urinate for longer than 6 hours
- Crying produces no tears or the mouth becomes dry
- The infant's fontanel appears sunken
- Blood appears in the diarrhea or the diarrhea becomes severe (e.g., a bowel movement every hour for more than 8 hours or more than 10 watery bowel movements in one day)
- Severe abdominal cramps occur
- The child becomes dizzy when standing
- The child starts acting very sick
- Fever over 100°F (37.8°C) has been present for more than 72 hours
- Mild diarrhea lasts more than 1 week

Adapted with permission from Schmitt, B.D. (1992). *Instructions for pediatric patients* (pp. 61–62). Philadelphia: W. B. Saunders.

NURSING DIAGNOSIS: • Risk for infection (in others) related to lack of knowledge about transmission prevention

Expected Outcome:
- Child shows no signs of diarrhea
- Family members show no signs of infection and demonstrate correct isolation technique. (See Chapter 18 and Appendix G for further discussion of isolation technique.)

Intervention	Rationale
1. Practice careful handwashing. Wear gloves when caring for child. Isolate child according to institution policy.	Good handwashing and adherence to isolation guidelines help prevent nosocomial infection.
2. Instruct family and visitors in proper handwashing and observe return demonstration. Assess parents' understanding of the need for isolation. Discuss importance of maintaining isolation and explain isolation technique. Teach how to contain organisms and demonstrate techniques to prevent spread. Offer explanations using simple, accurate terminology appropriate to the parents' level of understanding.	If isolation measures are not maintained, infection may spread to family and others.
3. Dispose of linen and other soiled items correctly.	Proper disposal of contaminated articles decreases risk of spread of infection.

NURSING DIAGNOSIS: • Altered Nutrition: Less Than Body Requirements related to decreased intake and inability of body to absorb fluid

Expected Outcome:
- The child will tolerate diet, as evidenced by weight gain and no recurrence of diarrhea.

Intervention	Rationale
1. Assess child's weight on admission and daily.	See above.
2. Monitor intake and output.	See above.
3. Assess serum electrolytes, calcium, vitamins B_{12} and K, folic acid, and zinc levels if ordered.	Laboratory values are assessed to determine actual or potential deficiencies.
4. Assess and document bowel sounds and abdominal distension.	Peristalsis (as evidenced by bowel sounds) is necessary in order to tolerate PO/NG feedings. Hyperactive bowel sounds may indicate excessive peristalsis.
5. When ordered, begin clear liquids, such as noncarbonated electrolyte drinks for older children and oral rehydration solutions (Pedialyte, Infalyte) for infants and younger children. Discourage the use of Popsicles and other sugary drinks.	Fluids high in sugar lack necessary electrolytes and can create a higher osmotic environment, actually causing more dehydration.
6. Offer ORT solution in small, frequent feedings (beginning with 5 to 15 ml by spoon every 20 minutes; if tolerated, volume can be gradually increased, waiting longer periods between feedings to decrease stimulation of peristalsis).	Fluids should be offered in small amounts at first to prevent gastric distension.

Intervention	Rationale
7. Give liquids at room temperature.	Cold liquids stimulate peristalsis.
8. Limit apple juice, or omit in early stages.	High osmolality of apple juice can cause loose stools.
9. Encourage easily digestible, bland foods when child can tolerate solid food.	Once rehydration has been achieved, a regular diet as tolerated provides necessary nutrients.
10. Discourage use of foods with high fat or sugar content; add milk products last. Soy formula (ProSobee, Isomil, Nursoy) may be substituted for cow's milk formula.	Temporary lactose intolerance (for 4 to 6 weeks) is common following diarrhea; cow's milk may aggravate diarrhea.
11. Keep room as odor-free as possible. Provide oral hygiene.	Minimizing unpleasant stimuli increases intake and feelings of well-being.

Evaluation: The child retains food and fluids and resumes normal bowel elimination patterns.

Home Care

Because diarrhea is often treated at home, parents need clear, specific instructions on how to care for their sick child (see Teaching Guidelines box). The main goal is to prevent dehydration by giving enough oral fluids to keep up with the fluids lost in diarrhea. A common myth is that the bowel should be "put to rest" by restricting food and fluids. Limiting fluids can be dangerous, especially in infants and small children. Severe dehydration can develop quickly in a fluid-restricted infant with diarrhea (Schmitt, 1992).

VOMITING

Vomiting is the forcible ejection of stomach contents through the mouth, involving a complex reflex that is associated with sweating, salivation, and often tachycardia (all symptoms of autonomic nervous stimulation). Other terms that may be used to further describe vomiting include spitting up (or chalasia, which is a normal process during infancy), regurgitation (associated with gastroesophageal reflux or overfeeding), and, if severe, projectile vomiting (usually indicative of obstruction, tumor, pyloric stenosis, or increasing intracranial pressure). Isolated incidents of vomiting are usually of little concern. However, consequences can be serious if vomiting is persistent and prolonged.

Etiology. There are many possible causes of vomiting, which are listed in the accompanying box.

PATHOPHYSIOLOGY *of Vomiting*

The process of vomiting is controlled through the emetic center located in the reticular core of the medulla (in the brain stem), which receives stimuli from one of three sources:

1. Stimulation of vagal and sympathetic afferent nerves, such as from irritation, distension, or obstruction, or inflammation
2. Chemical stimulation from drugs (e.g., ipecac and other opioids), cerebral hypoxia, inner ear disturbances, and increased intracranial pressure
3. Higher cortical centers, with stimuli such as sights, odors, and fright/fear

The mechanism of vomiting occurs in the presence of several complex reflexes:

1. Autonomic nervous system discharge, which causes salivation, sweating, pallor, and increased heart rate
2. Contraction of the stomach antrum and duodenum
3. Relaxation of the remainder of the stomach, esophagus, and sphincters
4. Closure of the glottis and soft palate
5. Contraction of the diaphragm and abdominal muscles, which increases intra-abdominal pressure and compresses abdominal contents, thus propelling them into the esophagus and out the mouth.

Possible Causes of Vomiting

Infectious: Pancreatitis, gastritis, appendicitis, hepatitis, inner ear conditions, food poisoning
Obstructive: Pyloric stenosis, small bowel obstruction (intussception, Hirschsprung's disease), tumors, appendicitis
Allergic: Allergies to foods, formulas, or medications; chemotherapy; lactose intolerance
Metabolic: Diabetic ketoacidosis, toxic ingestion, increased intracranial pressure, tumors, gastroesophageal reflux, tracheoesophageal fistula
Psychologic: Emotional stress, fear, anxiety, control issues, bulemia
In association with diarrhea: Gastroenteritis
Sudden onset in healthy child: Infection
Present in other family members: Food poisoning, infection
In association with fever, abdominal pain, and tenderness: Appendicitis, infection
After ingestion of toxic plants or liquids: Poisoning
After feeding in infants: Obstruction, gastric reflux, gastric distension, poor feeding techniques, air swallowing
Other: Overeating, motion sickness, pregnancy

Incidence. Vomiting, which occurs very frequently during childhood, is usually a symptom of some other underlying problem or disease. Vomiting and ensuing emesis can also result from allergic reactions, side effects of medications (such as chemotherapy), toxic effects of medications or ingested substances, and certain eating disorders.

Clinical Manifestations

- Sour milk curds without green or brownish color or undigested food from stomach
- Greenish emesis: usually indicates presence of bile and possible intestinal obstruction below ampulla of Vater
- Fecal odor: indicates lower intestinal obstruction or peritonitis
- Blood-tinged, bright red or coffee ground: bright red blood indicates that the blood has not been in contact with gastric juices; therefore, bleeding must be occurring at or above the cardia or in the stomach

Force of Vomiting

- Regurgitation: could be due to overfeeding
- Forceful: could indicate some obstruction
- Projectile: may indicate either obstruction, tumor, or increased intracranial pressure

Diagnostic Evaluation. Vomiting is usually of short duration and is not severe. However, if vomiting continues and the child is starting to appear deficient in fluid and/or electrolytes, the following tests may be indicated:

- Complete blood count and electrolyte studies (blood urea nitrogen, and glucose levels) and urine tests
- Radiographic studies (if an obstructive process is suspected)
- Blood cultures (if infectious disease is suspected)
- Arterial blood gases

Therapeutic Management. The primary focus of managing vomiting is detection and treatment of the cause, with the secondary intent to prevent complications. ORT, as indicated for treatment of diarrhea, is also appropriate for the vomiting child and may be given in small, frequent amounts every 10 to 20 minutes (volume dependent on child's weight and age). As the vomiting decreases in frequency, the amount and interval between feeding can increase. If the vomiting is severe or prolonged in neonates and young infants, however, IV therapy is initiated. Most children will respond well to the above, but some will require antiemetics such as trimethobenzamide hydrochloride (Tigan) or promethazine (Phenergan), especially if the cause is unknown and vomiting is predictable and of limited duration.

Once the vomiting has ceased, it is important to reintroduce liquids/foods gradually as tolerated. Finally, having the child wash his mouth or brush his teeth after vomiting is important in ridding the mouth of the hydrochloric acid as well as freshening the mouth.

The vomiting child should be placed in an upright or sidelying position to prevent aspiration.

NURSING CARE OF THE VOMITING CHILD

Assessment

It is important to determine and describe the type and force of vomiting (i.e., "spitting up" as opposed to regurgitation, forceful, or projectile vomiting), as well as the character, or ACCT, of the occurrence. Because vomiting is often associated with gastric distension, the relationship, if any, with infant feeding should be assessed (e.g., poor feeding techniques, failure to bubble/burp, improper positioning).

Nursing Diagnosis and Planning

The following nursing diagnoses and expected outcomes may be appropriate in the treatment of the vomiting child.

Nursing Diagnoses

- Fluid Volume Deficit related to increased loss of GI contents
- Altered Nutrition: Less Than Body Requirements related to inability of body to retain gastric contents.

Expected Outcomes

The child will

- Maintain fluid balance within normal limits as evidenced by age-appropriate fluid intake
- Have appropriate urine output (1 to 2 ml/kg/hr), capillary refill less than 2 seconds, elastic skin turgor, and moist mucous membranes
- Maintain electrolyte balance within normal limits as evidenced by serum sodium and potassium levels within normal limits, normal level of activity and alertness
- Tolerate diet as evidenced by no recurrence of vomiting.

Implementation

Because vomiting is often the primary symptom of many different conditions, it is very important to assess and record its occurrence, as well as any other associated manifestations. Nursing interventions are frequently determined by the cause of the vomiting and therefore may be very specific. For example, if the vomiting is found to be due to incorrect feeding techniques and/or solutions, the nurse's role is to educate the family regarding appropriate feeding techniques (e.g., adequate bubbling and burping as well as positioning after the feeding) and preparation of formulas.

Major concerns with vomiting are dehydration and fluid and electrolyte imbalance; therefore, it is essential that hydration status be carefully assessed, including accurate monitoring of intake and output, weight, fontanels in infants, skin turgor, eyes, skin, and heart and respiratory rates. Once the cause of vomiting is determined, nursing interventions are directed toward measures to ensure a continued reduction in the vomiting. If gastroesophageal reflux is suspected, correct positioning during and after feeding, in addition to increasing frequency, decreasing volume, and increasing thickness of feedings, is important.

In reintroducing oral fluids and feedings for the child who is vomiting, it is important to start with an appropriate electrolyte-containing solution. It is best to offer ORT solution in small, frequent feedings to avoid gastric distension (5 to 15 ml every 20 minutes). If tolerated, the volume can be gradually increased, waiting longer between feedings. If the child has repeated vomiting or vomits large volumes, the physician should be notified so IV therapy may be initiated (Tucker & Sussman-Karten, 1987). If oral fluids are well tolerated, solid foods may be gradually added. Another important consideration is education for the child and/or family about avoidance of certain foods (such as fatty, acidified, or seasoned foods), as well as minimizing stimuli such as stress, anxiety, or unfavorable-smelling foods, which might lead to nausea and subsequent vomiting. Antiemetic medications, decreased stimuli, and avoidance of food or activities that might tend to upset the stomach either directly or by association may be helpful in decreasing nausea and vomiting. It is also necessary to remember that vomiting is also often linked with eating disorders (especially in adolescents) or control issues (all ages), which would require further followup (see Chapter 41).

Nursing care of the vomiting child is directed toward:

- Observation and reporting of vomiting
- Assessing for associated symptoms, such as dehydration
- Implementing measures to reduce the vomiting
- Recording accurate intake and output
- Evaluating the effectiveness of therapy
- Preventing aspiration

Evaluation

- Is the child taking age-appropriate amounts of fluid without vomiting?
- Is the child's urine output 1 to 2 ml/kg/hr?
- Is the child's skin turgor elastic, with capillary refill 2 seconds or less?
- Does the child have moist mucous membranes?
- Is the fontanel flat and soft, but not depressed?
- Do the parents verbalize home care required?

KEY CONCEPTS

- Infants and children are at a much greater risk than adults for fluid and electrolyte disturbances.
- The three mechanisms by which acid-base balance is maintained are chemical buffering, respiratory control of carbon dioxide, and renal regulation of bicarbonate and secretion of hydrogen ions.
- The two major forms of acid-base disturbance are acidosis and alkalosis, either of which may be respiratory or metabolic in nature.
- Treatment of metabolic disturbances is directed toward correcting the underlying problem; interventions for respiratory alterations are implemented toward reestablishing alveolar ventilation.

- Dehydration may be classified as isotonic (most common), hypotonic, or hypertonic.
- Monitoring of intake and output, vital signs, and level of activity (or sensorium) are crucial in appropriately assessing the child with a fluid and/or electrolyte disturbance.
- Diarrhea can lead to loss of bicarbonate (and subsequent acidosis); vomiting will cause the loss of hydrochloric acid (and subsequent alkalosis).
- Oral rehydration therapy is indicated for the child with diarrhea, mild/moderate/severe dehydration, and vomiting.

REFERENCES

American Academy of Pediatrics (1990). *Textbook of pediatric advanced life support* (pp. 49–52). American Heart Association.

Anonymous. (1996). Practice parameter: The management of acute gastroenteritis in young children. American Academy of Pediatrics, Provisional Committee on Quality Improvement, Subcommittee on Acute Gastroenteritis. *Pediatrics, 97*(3), 424–435.

Behrman, R., & Kleigman, R. (1994). *Nelson's essentials of pediatrics* (2nd ed.). Philadelphia: W. B. Saunders.

Bertz, C. L., Hunsberger, M. M., & Wright, S. (1994). *Family centered nursing care of children* (2nd ed.). Philadelphia: W. B. Saunders.

Cohen, M. B., & Balistreri, G. F. (1989). Infant diarrhea. *Contemporary Pediatrics, 3*, 89–114.

Fayad, I. M., Hashem, M., Duggan, C., Refat, M., Bakir, M., Fontaine, O., & Santosham, M. (1993). Comparative efficacy of rice-based and glucose-based oral rehydration salts plus early reintroduction of food. *Lancet, 342*(8874), 772–775.

Finberg, L., Kravath, R., & Hellerstein, S. (1993). *Water and electrolytes in pediatrics* (2nd ed.). Philadelphia: W. B. Saunders.

Gremse, D. A. Effectiveness of nasogastric rehydration in hospitalized children with acute diarrhea. *Journal of Pediatric Gastroenterology and Nutrition, 21*(2), 145–148.

Halpern, J. (1991). Oral rehydration therapy: the best response to diarrheal dehydration. *Journal of Emergency Nursing, 17*(2), 99–101.

Horne, M., Heitz, U., & Swearingen, P. (1991). *Fluid, electrolyte and acid-base balance: A case study approach.* St. Louis: Mosby–Year Book.

Johnson, K. (Ed.). (1994). *The Harriet Lane handbook.* St. Louis: Mosby–Year Book.

Kleinman, R., Sack, D., & Dale, C. (1994). Diarrhea management with oral rehydration therapy. *Pediatric Basics, 67*, 10–16.

Meyers, A. (1995). Modern management of acute diarrhea and dehydration in children. *American Family Physician, 51*(5), 1103–1118.

O'Loughlin, E. V., Notaras, E., McCullough, C., Halliday, J., & Henry, R. L. (1995). Home-based management of children hospitalized with acute gastroenteritis. *Journal of Pediatrics and Child Health, 31*(3), 189–191.

Pizarro, D., et al. (1991). Rice-based oral electrolyte solutions. *New England Journal of Medicine, 324*(8), 517–521.

Schmitt, B. D. (1992). *Instructions for pediatric patients.* Philadelphia: W. B. Saunders.

Snyder, J. (1987). Cereal based oral rehydration therapy: Theory and practice. Symposium Proceeding. 2/17/87. pp. 33–36.

Straughn, A., & English, B. (1996). Oral rehydration therapy: A neglected treatment for pediatric diarrhea. *Maternal Child Nursing, 21*, 144–147.

Tucker, J. A., & Sussman-Karten, K. S. (1987). Treating acute diarrhea and dehydration with an oral rehydration solution. *Pediatric Nursing, 13*(3), 169–174.

BIBLIOGRAPHY

Balisteri, W. (1990). Oral rehydration in acute infantile diarrhea. *The American Journal of Medicine, 88* (Suppl 6A), 30S–33S.

Barclay, D. V., Gil-Ramos, J., Mora, J. O., & Dirren, H. (1995). A packaged rice-based oral rehydration solution for acute diarrhea. *Journal of Pediatric Gastroenterology and Nutrition, 20*(4), 408–416.

Binder, H. (1990). Pathophysiology of acute diarrhea. *The American Journal of Medicine, 88* (Suppl 6A), 2S–4S.

Boynton, R., et al. (1988). *Manual of ambulatory pediatrics.* (2nd ed.). Glenview, IL: Scott, Foresman.

Buzby, M. (1992). Infectious gastroenteritis in infants and children. *Gastroenterology Nursing, 14*(6), 302–306.

Candy, C. (1987). Recent advances in the care of children with acute diarrhea. *Journal of Advanced Nursing, 12*(1), 95–99.

Casteel, H., & Fiedorek, S. (1990). Oral rehydration therapy. *Pediatric Clinics of North America, 37*(2), 295–311.

Cusson, R. (1992). Rice-based oral rehydration fluid in the treatment of infant diarrhea. *Journal of Pediatric Nursing, 7*(6), 414–415.

Duggan, C., Glass, R., & Santosham, M. (1993). Oral rehydration therapy in children. *Patient Care, 27*(8), 59–62.

Dukes, G. (1990). Over-the-counter antidiarrheal medications. *The American Journal of Medicine, 88* (Suppl 6A), 6A–26S.

Ellett, M. L., Fitzgerald, J. F., & Winchester, M. (1993). Dietary management of chronic diarrhea in children. *Gastroenterology Nursing, 15*(4), 170–177.

Figueroa, D., et al. (1993). A controlled trial of bismuth subsalicylate in infants with acute watery diarrheal disease. *New England Journal of Medicine, 328*(23), 1653–1658.

Grisanti, K., & Jaffe, D. (1991). Dehydration syndromes. Oral rehydration and fluid replacement. *Emergency Medicine Clinics of North America, 9*(3), 565–588.

Hazinski, M. (1988). Understanding fluid balance in the seriously ill child. *Pediatric Nursing, 14*(3), 231–236.

Hedman, D. (1991). Stabilization of the infant and child. *Journal of Post Anesthesia Nursing, 6*(3), 165–169.

Issenman, R. M., & Leung, A. K. (1993). Oral and intravenous rehydration of children. *Canadian Family Physician, 39,* 2129–2136.

Keller, V. E. (1995). Management of nausea and vomiting in children. *Journal of Pediatric Nursing: Nursing Care of Children and Families, 10*(5), 280–286.

Maldonado, Y., & Yolken, R. (1990). Rotavirus. *Clinical Gastroenterology, 4*(3), 609–624.

Meyers, A. (1994). Fluid and electrolyte therapy for children. *Current Opinion in Pediatrics, 6*(3), 303–309.

Reis, E. C., Goepp, J. G., Katz, S., & Santosham, M. (1994). Barriers to use of oral rehydration therapy. *Pediatrics, 93*(5), 708–711.

Snyder, J. (1991a). Use and misuse of oral therapy for diarrhea. Comparison of US practices with American Academy of Pediatrics recommendations. *Pediatrics, 87*(1), 28–33.

Snyder, J. (1991b). Oral therapy for diarrhea. *Hospital Practice, 26*(5A), 86–88.

25

The Child With Upper Gastrointestinal Alterations

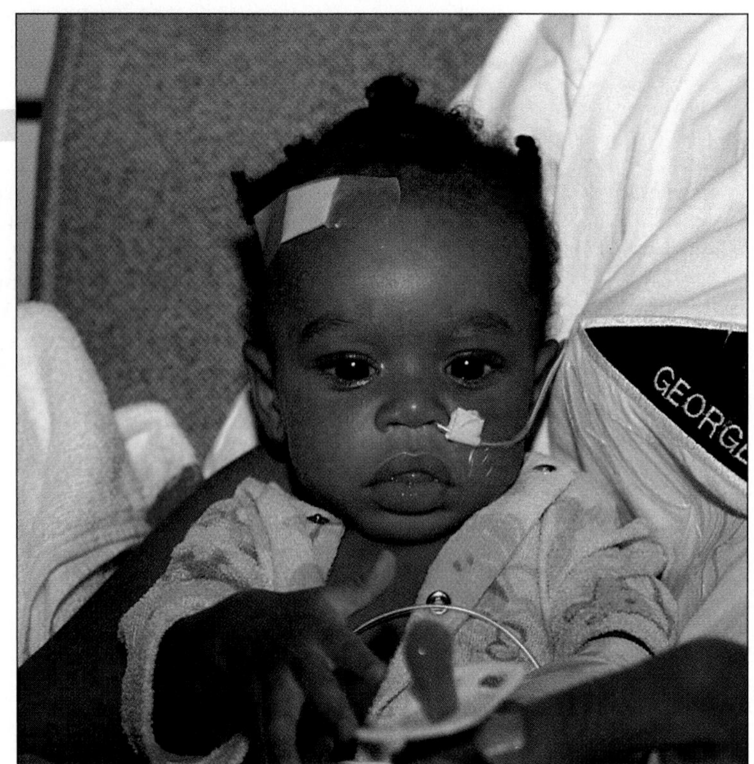

CHAPTER OVERVIEW

LEARNING OBJECTIVES

After completing this chapter, you should be able to:

- Describe the development of the upper gastrointestinal (GI) system and its relationship to selected congenital defects.
- Describe the anatomy and physiology of the upper GI system in the infant and child.
- Describe the common diagnostic and screening tests used for alterations in upper GI function.
- Identify the nursing implications of common medications used in the treatment of upper GI alterations.
- Discuss and display an understanding of the pathophysiology, etiology, clinical manifestations, diagnostic evaluation, and therapeutic management of cleft lip and palate, esophageal atresia, tracheoesophageal fistula, diaphragmatic and hiatal hernias, gastroesophageal reflux, pyloric stenosis, and ulcers.
- State expected nursing diagnoses for upper GI alterations.
- Use the nursing process to develop nursing care plans and teaching guidelines for the child with upper GI alterations.
- Develop guidelines for home care for the child with upper GI alterations.

KEY TERMS

achalasia: failure of smooth muscle fibers of the GI tract to relax, resulting in a functional obstruction and difficulty in passage of food and chyme along the GI tract

atresia: absence or abnormal closure of a normal body orifice or passage

dysphagia: inability or difficulty in swallowing

fistula: an abnormal passage or communication between two organs or tissues

fundoplication: a 270° to 360° wrap of the stomach fundus around the distal esophagus to tighten the lower esophageal sphincter and prevent gastric reflux

hematemesis: vomiting of bright red blood or of denatured blood that looks like "coffee grounds"; usually represents a bleeding source proximal to the jejunum

melena: rectal passage of black, tarry stools, indicating denatured blood from the upper GI tract

occult bleeding: bleeding in such minute quantity that it can only be recognized by microscopic or chemical means

peristalsis: progressive, wave-like movements caused by contraction and relaxation of the longitudinal and circular muscles of the GI tract; propels a bolus of food or fluid forward

projectile vomiting: vomiting that is projected with force, perhaps 2 to 4 feet away from the mouth; may be preceded by deep gastric left to right peristaltic waves; characteristic of pyloric stenosis

pylorus: the distal opening of the stomach where the stomach contents pass into the duodenum; surrounded by muscle bands

The child with an upper gastrointestinal (GI) alteration and his family have many special needs. Some problems—such as tracheoesophageal fistula or diaphragmatic hernia—begin at birth, with life-threatening consequences. Or, the parent may have difficulty accepting the appearance of a child with cleft lip and palate. Other problems—such as gastroesophageal reflux and ulcers—develop after birth and provide long-term challenges in management and treatment. Sudden, unexpected surgery may occur, as in pyloric stenosis. As a result of these alterations, nutrition, elimination, respiratory status, skin integrity, body image, family processes, growth and development, and educational needs may be affected.

The nurse provides a vital link in the care of these children. Acute care at birth, education about prenatal development, preoperative and postoperative care, home care, and teaching are essential nursing activities. Coordinating care with other specialties and national support groups can be useful as well. To perform these functions the nurse must have an understanding of normal anatomy and physiology, differences in GI function in children and adolescents, common diagnostic tests, and medications. In addition, the specific nursing care of common alterations in GI function should be understood.

CLINICAL REFERENCE PAGES

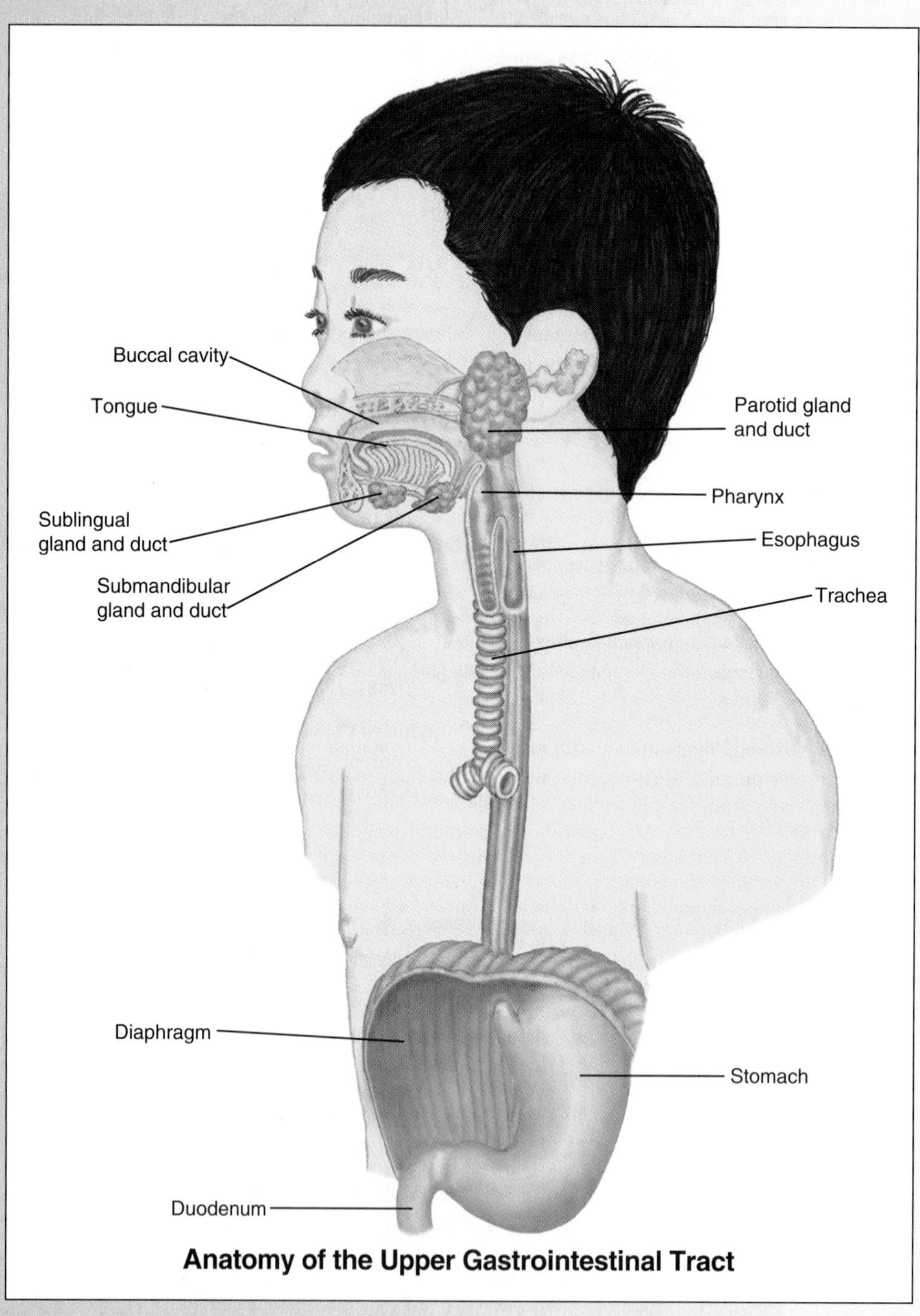

Anatomy of the Upper Gastrointestinal Tract

REVIEW OF THE UPPER GASTROINTESTINAL SYSTEM

The upper GI system includes the *mouth, esophagus,* and *stomach*. Its primary functions are to take in food and fluids, begin the digestive process, and propel food into the intestines, where nutrients are absorbed. To understand alterations, it is first necessary to understand normal structure and function.

The *mouth,* or buccal cavity, is the entrance to the GI tract. Here, food is broken up and mixed with saliva. This process starts the digestion of carbohydrates. The submandibular, parotid, and sublingual glands secrete saliva in response to the smell, taste, or thought of food. The tongue contains taste buds that distinguish salt, sweet, sour, and bitter sensations, and is essential for swallowing.

At birth, the *esophagus* measures approximately 10 cm in length; it lengthens to 18 to 25 cm by adulthood. The upper third of the esophagus consists of striated voluntary muscle; the lower two thirds consists of smooth muscle. The upper esophageal sphincter prevents the reflux of esophageal contents into the pharynx and lungs, and prevents esophageal distension during respiration; the lower esophageal sphincter (LES) prevents the reflux of gastric contents into the lower esophagus.

Swallowing is under both voluntary and involuntary control. As food is chewed, it forms a small bolus, or mass; the tongue propels the bolus toward the oropharynx. The presence of this mass in the oropharynx stimulates the medulla, causing the soft palate to rise. The nasal passages close, the pharyngeal muscles contract, the larynx closes and respiration is inhibited. As a result of these processes, food is propelled to the esophagus. Through **peristalsis,** the bolus moves on to the LES, the muscle relaxes, and the bolus enters the stomach.

The *stomach* lies in the epigastric, umbilical, and left hypochondrial regions of the abdomen. It is a muscular pouch, shaped somewhat like a gourd, where the bolus is received. As the LES and the **pylorus** contract, the stomach muscles churn the contents. The contents mix with the digestive juices to form chyme. The chyme moves on to the pylorus and thence to the duodenum. (See the gastric enzyme table in the Chapter 26 Clinical Reference Pages.)

A mucus–bicarbonate barrier in the stomach provides a thick layer of mucus and a buffer zone to neutralize acid. Stomach acids diffuse slowly through this layer toward the gastric wall; they are neutralized by bicarbonate ions from the surface epithelial cells. Thus, a neutral pH is maintained at the gastric epithelial surface.

Prenatal Development. The primitive gut is formed from the endoderm in the first 4 weeks of embryologic development. The primitive gut then gives rise to three sections of the GI tract, each having an individual blood supply and rate of development:

Foregut: from pharynx to duodenum, including the liver, pancreas, and biliary tract
Midgut: from duodenum to transverse colon
Hindgut: descending colon, rectum, and anal canal

Problems in the development of each of these three sections give rise to specific malformations and disease states. Anatomically, development is complete at birth, but physiologically the GI tract is immature.

Fetal swallowing, intestinal motility, and defecation are detectable in the second trimester, but the most rapid and extensive development of the GI system occurs in the third trimester. The newborn must be able to adapt from total parenteral nutrition to total enteral nutrition because the placenta no longer performs nutrient exchange and waste removal.

Pediatric differences in the upper GI system are listed in the accompanying box.

Pediatric Differences in the Upper Gastrointestinal System

- Infants have minimal saliva.
- Swallowing not under voluntary control until 6 weeks.
- Infants and children have less stomach capacity.

AGE	STOMACH CAPACITY (ML)
Newborn	10–20
1 week	30–90
2–3 weeks	75–100
1 month	90–150
3 months	150–200
1 year	210–360
2 years	500
10 years	750–900
16 years	1500
Adult	2000–3000

- Stomach lies transversely, is horizontal in abdomen of infants.
- Stomach is round in infant and toddler periods.
- Peristaltic waves may reverse in infancy, causing spitting up and vomiting.
- Secretory cells don't reach adult levels until 2–3 years.
- Low HCl concentration is seen until school age.
- Peristalsis is faster; food remains in the stomach for a shorter period of time.
- Fever increases rate of propulsion.

COMMON LABORATORY AND DIAGNOSTIC TESTS FOR UPPER GI DISORDERS

	DESCRIPTION	NORMAL FINDINGS	INDICATIONS	PREPARATION AND NURSING IMPLICATIONS
			Stool	
Occult Blood (Guaiac, Hematest)	Stool smeared on filter paper and prepared with solution	Negative	Inflammatory conditions, bowel necrosis Ulcers, severe (GER)	Done by nurse Blue is positive
			Endoscopy	
Fiberoptic Upper GI Endoscopy	Direct visualization of the lining to the esophagus, stomach, and proximal duodenum; also creates mechanism for biopsies, cultures	Normal mucosa	Persistent abdominal pain, vomiting, failure to thrive, hematemesis, **achalasia.** Used to rule out esophagitis, GER, ulcers, esophageal atresia	NPO at least 6 hours prior to exam Conscious sedation Monitoring of respiratory function during sedation
Gastric Biopsy	Small biopsy samples are obtained during endoscopy	Normal tissues	Identifies changes in mucosa and helps determine severity of damage Ulcers, GER	Same as endoscopy Watch for GI bleeding Hematest stools
			Radiologic Exams	
Flat Plate, Abdomen	Anterior and posterior X-rays	Normal gas patterns, no masses	Identifies stool and gas patterns, excludes obstruction or perforation Pyloric stenosis, tracheoesophageal (TE) fistula, esophageal atresia, diaphragmatic hernias	Usually no preparation Teaching
Barium Swallow	Radiopaque contrast media and/or air swallowed	Normal swallowing, no anatomic defects	Esophageal abnormalities, swallowing difficulties, LES function Esophageal atresia, TE fistula, GER	NPO for 2–4 hours before exam Adequate fluids essential after exam to prevent barium impaction
Upper GI Exam	Radiopaque contrast material swallowed or inserted per NG tube; outlines stomach, pyloric canal.	Normal gastric emptying, no abnormalities	Determines gastric emptying time TE fistula, pyloric stenosis, ulcers, strictures, achalasia	NPO for 4 hours before exam Adequate fluids essential after exam to prevent barium impaction
Ultrasound	Noninvasive use of sound waves to identify anatomy and inflammation	Normal anatomy	Identifies anatomic abnormalities and inflammatory conditions Pyloric stenosis, abdominal pain	No preparation, though a full bladder may be needed to provide a window to view pelvic organs
Gastroesophageal Scintigraphy	Radioisotope injected or put in formula; nuclear scan	Normal gastric emptying time, no reflux	Most accurate method to identify GER	NPO at least 4 hours prior to exam Patient teaching
Ambulatory pH Studies	Small catheter with pH probe positioned in distal esophagus Number of reflux events recorded and correlated with episodes of vomiting, apnea, bradycardia, cyanosis	No drop in pH indicating reflux	Clarifies relationship between reflux episodes and clinical symptoms GER	NPO at least 4 hours before probe placement Protocols vary among institutions Patient teaching Requires 18–24 hours
Esophageal Manometry	Catheter measures the pressures of the LES, esophageal body, and upper esophageal sphincter	Normal pressure for age	Evaluates swallowing disorders, esophageal motility GER, TE fistula	NPO at least 4 hours prior to probe placement Used less frequently in children

MEDICATIONS COMMONLY USED FOR UPPER GI DISORDERS

	INDICATIONS	DOSE	COMMON SIDE EFFECTS	NURSING IMPLICATIONS
		Antacids		
Maalox, Amphojel (available OTC)	Decreases pH and activity of pepsins. Used for palliative relief of GER, and as initial treatment for ulcers. Used only to decrease discomfort from reflux and ulcers; do not cure the problem.	Infants: 2–5 ml Children: 5–15 ml PO per dose, usually 1 and 3 hr after meals and h.s. May be given for up to 6 wk.	*Aluminum:* Constipation, bowel obstruction, toxic serum levels of aluminum *Magnesium:* Diarrhea *Calcium:* Renal damage	Provide teaching to prevent overuse. Compliance may be a problem. Interfere with absorption of several drugs, including digoxin, penicillin, sulfonamides, and cimetidine. Maintain fluid intake for age. Observe constipation.
		Gastric Secretion Inhibitors: H_2 Receptor Antagonists		
Tagamet (cimetidine)	Used to decrease acid, gastrin, and pepsin secretion at the gastric mucosa for GER, and gastric ulcers	20–40 mg/kg/day PO or IV QID usually 30 min before meals and h.s.	Diarrhea, myalgias, neutropenia, gynecomastia, vomiting headaches, fatigue	Numerous drug interactions, including theophylline and phenytoin. Antacids decrease absorption. Avoid smoking.
Zantac (ranitidine)	Same as Tagamet	1–4 mg/kg/day PO divided into 2 doses every 12 hr or 1–4 mg/kg/day in divided doses q 6–8 hr	Fewer side effects than cimetidine; headache, GI disturbance, malaise, irritability, rash, sedation	More potent than cimetidine. Used for GER.
Pepcid (famotidine)	Same as Tagamet	Available OTC in lower doses.		Newest—being tested on children.
		Mucosal Protective Agents		
Carafate (sucralfate)	Provides adherent gel barrier that covers the ulcer site. Also stimulates prostaglandin release to strengthen the mucosal barrier.	Now available in liquid form. 1 g PO QID 1 hr before meals and h.s.	Constipation, dry mouth, skin rashes	Not approved for use in children under 12 yr. Often used with H_2-receptor antagonists. Tablets are large and difficult to swallow.
		Prokinetic Agents		
Urecholine (bethanechol)	Used to increase LES pressure and to accelerate gastric emptying time and peristalsis in GER	0.4–0.6 mg/kg/24 hr PO. Given 30–60 min before meals and h.s.	Hypotension, nausea, bronchospasm, wheezing, salivation, flushing, blurred vision	**Do not give IV or IM.** Antidote is atropine. Contraindicated in ulcer disease, asthma.
Reglan (metoclopramide)	Same as Urecholine	0.1 mg/kg/dose IV or PO. Given 30 min before meals and h.s. 1–2 mg/kg/dose IV 2–6 hr as an antiemetic.	Multisystem extrapyramidal side effects, fatigue, irritability, restlessness, rarely irreversible tardive dyskinesias	Use with Benadryl as an antiemetic.
Propulsid (cisapride)	Same as Urecholine	0.15–0.3 mg/kg/dose, 3 times a day	No CNS disturbances; may cause diarrhea, abdominal cramps but are dose-related	Newest drug but very promising. May take several days to achieve maximum relief.

Data from Greene, M. G. (1991). *The Harriet Lane handbook: A manual for pediatric house officers* (12th ed.). St. Louis: C. V. Mosby; Hubbard, P. (1994). Medication review: Cisapride, *ANNA Journal, 21*(6), 374–380; Andrews, C. (1994). Ulcer-healing drugs and their actions and side effects. *Nursing Times, 90*(33), 38–40; and Sterling C., et al. (1991). Nursing responsibility in the diagnosis, care, and treatment of the child with gastroesophageal reflux. *Journal of Pediatric Nursing, 6*(5), 331–336.

DISORDERS OF PRENATAL DEVELOPMENT

Cleft lip and palate, esophageal atresia, tracheoesophageal fistula, and diaphragmatic hernias are all the result of abnormal fetal development that may have drastic consequences on the early life of a child.

Cleft Lip and Palate

Cleft lip (CL), cleft palate (CP), and cleft lip and palate (CL/P) are separate anomalies that are closely related in etiology, pathophysiology, and nursing care, so they will be discussed together. These distinct problems are all abnormal openings in the lip or palate. The defects may occur unilaterally on either side or bilaterally.

Incidence. Incidence ranges from 1:1000 births for CL/P to 1:2500 births for CL. There is a male dominance in CL, and a female dominance in CP. The incidence is higher in Asians, and lowest in blacks (Behrman, Kliegman, & Arvin, 1995). Cleft lip and palate accounts for 35% to 40% of these facial malformations.

PATHOPHYSIOLOGY AND ETIOLOGY *of Cleft Lip and Palate*

Cleft lip and/or palate are the result of embryologic failures in development due to multiple genetic and environmental factors. They result in an abnormal opening in the lip, palate, and sometimes nose. Cleft lip results when the medial nasal and maxillary processes fail to join at 6 to 8 weeks of gestation. Cleft palate is a failure of the primary palatal shelves or processes to fuse at 7 to 12 weeks of gestation. Each of these abnormalities appear as distinct malformations but may also appear together.

Achieving suction during feedings may be impossible, and fluids may enter the nose, putting the child at risk for aspiration, feeding difficulties, and respiratory distress.

Clinical Manifestations (Fig. 25–1)

Cleft Lip

- Notched vermilion border
- Variable sized clefts that involve the alveolar ridge
- Dental anomalies (deformed, supernumerary, or absent teeth)

Cleft Palate

- Nasal distortion
- Midline or bilateral cleft with variable extension from uvula and soft and hard palates
- Exposed nasal cavities

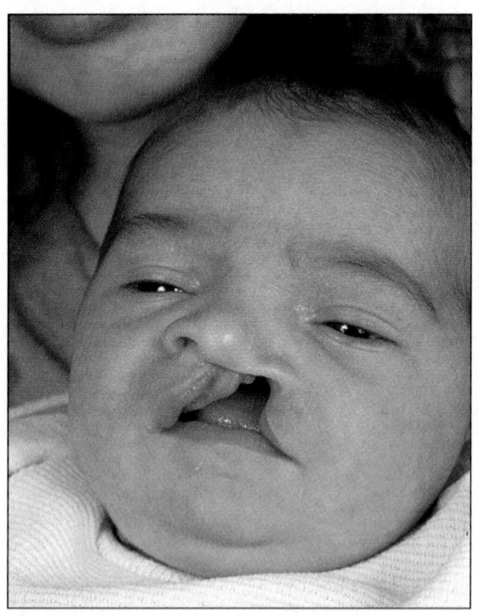

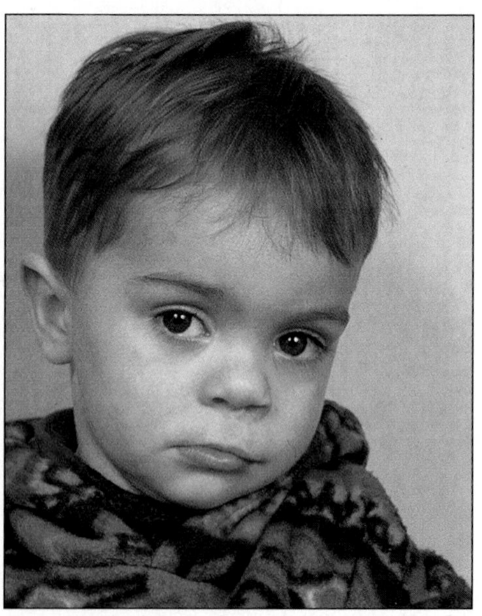

Figure 25–1
Child born with a cleft lip and palate, before (A) and after (B) repair. Repair of facial clefts usually requires multiple surgeries at different stages in the child's growth. Early repair of a cleft lip facilitates parent–infant bonding and improves feeding. Results are generally quite good with today's surgical, orthodontic, and speech therapy techniques. (Courtesy of Children's Medical Center, Dallas, Texas)

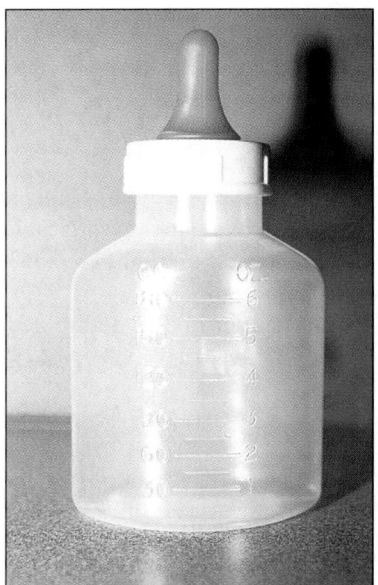

◀ A feeder with compressible plastic sides allows the person feeding the baby to gently squeeze the sides of the bottle to help eject the breast milk or formula. A slightly longer nipple allows the milk to be swallowed with less chance of entering the nasopharynx, and yet is not so long that it stimulates the gag reflex.

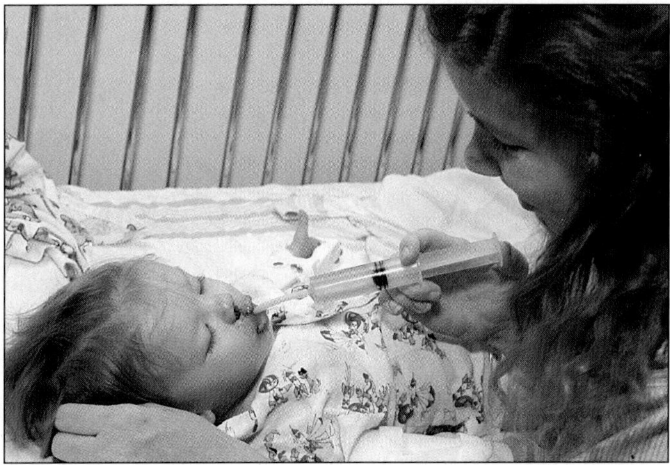

After repair, a syringe with a rubber tip is used ▶ for feeding to prevent trauma to the incision.

Figure 25–2

Before and after repair of a cleft lip or palate, special feeding techniques are essential for adequate nutrition.

Diagnostic Evaluation. Diagnosis is based on observation at birth and complete examination in the neonatal period. Cleft lip is diagnosed through visual inspection of the lip. The first sign of CP may be formula coming from the nose. A gloved finger placed in the mouth to feel the defect or visualization with a flashlight will confirm diagnosis.

Therapeutic Management. Management of the child is based on the severity of the defect. A number of professionals are involved in this process, including surgeons, nurses, geneticists, psychiatrists, ENT specialists, audiologists, and occupational and speech therapists. Orthodontists and plastic surgeons become involved in the lengthy management. Pediatricians will provide ongoing child health care.

The first intervention involves modifying feeding techniques as needed to allow adequate growth. Use of specialized feeding techniques, obturators, and unique nipples and feeders can usually accomplish this goal and provide for early discharge home with parents (Fig. 25–2).

Cleft lip repair is usually performed by age 4 weeks and at some centers in the first 2 to 3 days of life (Richard, 1994a). Early repair may improve bonding and makes feeding much easier. The surgical technique involves the use of a staggered suture line to minimize scarring. Some cosmetic modifications may be needed again at age 4 to 5 years.

Cleft palate repair is individualized and based on degree of deformity and size of child. Closure is completed between ages 6 months and 2 years. Most teams recommend repair by age 1 year. Earlier closure facilitates speech development (Richard, 1994a).

Concurrent treatment of altered dentition, recurring otitis media, speech dysfunction, emotional issues, and cosmetic concerns complete the ongoing therapy. Children with CP are at high risk for developing chronic otitis media. Parents should be aware of this so that otitis media is diagnosed early to decrease the chance of long-term scarring and hearing loss (Resnick & Zarem, 1996).

NURSING CARE OF THE CHILD WITH A CLEFT LIP OR PALATE

Assessment

Cleft lip and palate are readily apparent at birth and the degree of involvement should be documented. Ability to suck, swallow, and breathe without distress and handle normal secretions must be evaluated. Because the appearance of cleft lip and palate is usually unexpected and frightening to parents and families, assessment of their reactions is equally important. This assessment should include documentation of the parents' interactions with the neonate and their feelings about the situation.

Parents of an infant with a cleft lip or palate may need help to resolve the fact that their infant has a malformation that affects his appearance. The parents must deal with many questions from family members, stares from strangers, and feelings of pity from other new parents. Nursing interventions and information are critical here. Providing information about the etiology of the defect and showing them pictures of other children both before and after surgical repair can give them some relief from these fears and concerns. In addition, modeling and encouraging bonding efforts of touching, holding, and examining their newborn can be very reassuring.

Nursing Diagnoses

- Altered Nutrition: Less Than Body Requirements related to inability to suck and/or to surgical repair
- Knowledge Deficit related to special feeding techniques and surgery
- Altered Family Processes related to visible birth defect
- Impaired Skin Integrity related to surgical repair
- Risk for Infection related to surgical repair
- Pain related to surgical incisions
- Altered Health Maintenance related to need for long-term care

Planning, Implementation, and Evaluation: The Child With a Cleft Lip or Palate

NURSING DIAGNOSIS

- Altered Nutrition: Less Than Body Requirements related to inability to suck and to surgical repair
- Knowledge Deficit related to special feeding techniques and surgery

Expected Outcome: The child will:

- complete feeding desired within 30 minutes.
- follow the normal growth curve, and be content during and after feedings.

The parents will:

- express satisfaction with progress of feedings.
- understand expected preoperative and postoperative care.

Intervention	Rationale
1. Assess degree of cleft and impairment of sucking.	Infants with cleft lip alone or simple cleft dental arch may be successful with breast or bottle feeding without modification.
2. Teach ESSR method (see Teaching Guidelines for the Child With Cleft Lip and Palate).	Infants who are fed using this method have a better growth rate than children who use other methods (Richard, 1994b).

TEACHING GUIDELINES *for the Child With Cleft Lip or Palate*

A. Teach ESSR method:
   1. ENLARGE nipple by cross-cutting hole so that food is delivered to the back of the throat without sucking.
   2. STIMULATE sucking by rubbing the nipple on the lower lip.
   3. SWALLOW.
   4. REST to allow the child to finish swallowing what has been placed in his mouth. Refer to Richard (1991, 1994b) for further information.

B. Evaluate feeding at each visit by observing parents giving feeding because this is a major area of concern for families of children with cleft lip and palate.

C. To reduce anxiety and aid bonding, provide before and after pictures and written information such as that available from the Cleft Palate Foundation.

D. Teach care for the child in elbow restraints:
   1. Do not apply too tightly. They should be loose but still prohibit flexion of the elbow.
   2. Remove restraints at least every 2 hours for 10–15 minutes and play games with the child that encourage flexion. Assess skin integrity and range of motion during this time.
   3. Remove only one at a time with parent or nurse in constant attendance.

Intervention	Rationale
3. Keep care and teaching as simple as possible.	Nutrition, parent–infant relationship, and compliance may be improved if "normal" techniques can be utilized.
4. Provide alternative assistive feeding devices as needed and ordered.	Techniques and equipment vary among institutions. Use what is available and effective for each child.
5. Burp frequently and hold child in more upright position.	Minimizes air swallowing and GI gas
6. Document feeding program in written form for parents to be able to use at home, and provide to other health professionals.	Provides consistency at home and when in contact with numerous medical personnel required for treatment of the child
7. Provide emotional support to parents as they learn to feed their child.	Self-care and bonding are improved when parents can assume total care.
8. Keep accurate record of growth using growth chart.	Identifies growth changes early when intervention can be most effective
9. Explain preoperative and postoperative procedures: NPO for 6 hours, IV, use of arm restraints, appearance of repair in immediate postoperative period.	Decreases parental anxiety and encourages involvement
10. Postoperatively:	
a. Keep straws, pacifiers, spoons, or fingers away from mouth for 7–10 days. No oral temperatures.	Reduces stress on surgical repair and prevents accidental tearing of very fine sutures
b. Advance diet as ordered and tolerated from clear liquids to normal *soft* diet within 48 hours.	Minimizes nutritional deficits and stress on child No foods that can tear sutures are offered.
c. For CL repair, resume preoperative feeding techniques.	Little evidence exists that sucking causes excess suture stress (Richard, 1994a).
d. For CP repair, provide short nipples that don't rest on palatal sutures; give baby food, or baby food mixed with water (Richard, 1994a).	Recent studies indicate that nipples may be used postoperatively without stressing sutures (Richard, 1994a).

Evaluation:

- Is the child following appropriate growth curve?
- Is the child happy and content during and after feedings?
- Is parent satisfied with feeding technique being used and time to complete a feeding?
- Can parent explain expected preoperative and postoperative care?

NURSING DIAGNOSIS

- Altered Family Processes related to visible birth defect

Expected Outcome:

- Parents will bond with child, as evidenced by desire to hold and care for child, ability to identify positive aspects of the child, and assumption of home care responsibilities.

Intervention	Rationale
1. Encourage parents to discuss their fears, concerns, and negative emotions.	Grief, anxiety, confusion, guilt, denial, and anger are not uncommon and should be expressed.
2. Encourage touching and holding.	Encourages bonding and prevents a delayed attachment

Intervention	Rationale
3. Make appropriate referral to a cleft lip/palate team of nurses, physicians, and other specialists as soon as possible.	They can provide accurate information and begin to outline a plan of action.
4. Express acceptance of the baby by modeling feeding and close physical contact.	Aids adaptation process
5. Refer to community resources and parent groups. See Resource list at end of book (Appendix H).	Acceptance and adaptation are aided by sharing with others in similar situations.
6. Encourage parents to share concerns about long-term care and stresses it places on family emotionally and financially.	This is a long-term concern that requires extensive follow-up and can strain many family's resources. Identifying concerns early can increase problem-solving options.

Evaluation:
- Can parents identify positive aspects of their child?
- Do parents hold, cuddle, and make eye contact with child?
- Have parents sought community or national support?

NURSING DIAGNOSIS
- Impaired Skin Integrity related to surgical repair
- Risk for Infection related to surgical repair

Expected Outcome:
- The repair site will heal without complications, as evidenced by incision that is clean, free from exudate or redness.

Intervention	Rationale
1. Clean lip repair site with sterile water using a cotton swab or saline, after feeding and as ordered. Use a rolling motion from the suture line out. Have parents demonstrate this cleaning technique.	Decreases medium for bacterial growth, decreases crusting, and minimizes scarring
2. Apply anti-infective ointment as ordered.	Prevents infection, crusting, and scarring
3. Use elbow restraints to keep child from touching the repair site. Continue for 6–8 days. Remove q 2 hr for 10–15 minutes. Remove only one at a time with parent or nurse in constant attendance.	Prevents accidental rupture or tear of sutures Promotes contact with child, decreases anxiety, and allows nurse to assess skin integrity and circulation
4. Do not brush the child's teeth for 1–2 weeks.	Prevents accidental tear of palatal sutures
5. Keep child in supine position or on side lateral to repair.	Prevents contact of suture lines with bed linens
6. Observe for redness, swelling, excessive bleeding, drainage, or fever.	Signs of infection must be identified early because additional inflammation can increase scarring.
7. Rinse mouth with water after feedings to clean palate repair.	Rinses food and residual sugars from suture lines, reducing risk of infection
8. Encourage parents to hold and cuddle as desired by child.	Crying puts additional stress on suture line.

Intervention	Rationale
9. Maintain lip protective devices.	Prevents separating lip suture lines

Evaluation:
- Is the suture site clean, dry, and without redness, heat, or drainage?
- Is the suture site intact and healing without crusting or excessive scarring?
- Are arms and hands free of skin breakdown, or limited range of motion?

NURSING DIAGNOSES
- Pain related to surgical incisions

Expected Outcome:
- The child will be free from pain, as evidenced by resumption of normal activities, ease of comforting, and parental perception of no pain.

Intervention	Rationale
1. Assess pain using appropriate tools (see Chapter 20).	Infants and young children do not react to pain in typical adult ways, and alternative methods of assessment are needed to validate assessment findings.
2. Provide comfort measures, especially holding, rocking, and parental voices.	Increases parent involvement, relieves discomfort, and reduces stress on sutures caused by crying
3. Provide analgesics and sedatives on a regular basis as ordered. Pain should decrease significantly after 24–48 hours.	Prevents peaks of pain that cannot be managed appropriately
4. Report pain not managed by usual means.	May be an indication of hematoma formation or other complications of repair.

Evaluation:
- Does the child participate in age-appropriate activities?
- Is the child receiving pain medications?
- Does the child appear relaxed and content at rest?
- Does the parent think the child is in pain?

NURSING DIAGNOSIS
- Altered Health Maintenance related to need for long-term care

Expected Outcome:
- Parents will seek continued follow-up to evaluate and manage long-term complications.

Intervention	Rationale
1. Make appropriate and early referrals for any problems with speech impairment or language-based learning disabilities.	These are common complications of CL/P. Early intervention minimizes harm.
2. Monitor for recurrent or chronic otitis media. Schedule frequent hearing tests.	Due to craniofacial deformities, these can be very common and must be treated to prevent language and learning problems.
3. Encourage early speech attempts. Arrange speech therapy as needed.	CP can make speech difficult to understand and child may feel self-conscious about "errors" she makes. Practice improves development.

Intervention	Rationale
4. Encourage good dental care.	Abnormalities of teeth and alveolar ridge make malocclusion and dental caries a major concern.

Evaluation:
- Do the parents continue to seek follow-up care (ENT, speech therapy, dentist)?
- Does the child have age-appropriate speech?
- Does the child have normal hearing?
- Does the child have normal dentition?

Esophageal Atresia With Tracheoesophageal Fistula

Esophageal **atresia** and tracheoesophageal **fistula** (TEF) are congenital malformations in which the esophagus terminates before it reaches the stomach and/or a fistula is present that forms an unnatural connection with the trachea. Figure 25–3 reviews types of TEF.

PATHOPHYSIOLOGY *of Esophageal Atresia and TEF*

TEF is the result of an embryonal failure to differentiate the foregut into the trachea and esophagus and the incomplete fusion of them into distinct organs. The failure occurs between the fourth and fifth week of pregnancy and is manifested in several ways (see Fig. 25–3).

The presence of a fistula between the esophagus and trachea causes oral intake to enter the lungs or large amounts of air to enter the stomach. Coughing, choking, and severe abdominal distension can occur. Eventually, aspiration pneumonia and severe respiratory distress will develop in the untreated child, and death may occur without surgical intervention. Esophageal atresia occurring by itself causes respiratory distress secondary to aspiration of saliva and any oral fluids that may be given before diagnosis.

Etiology and Incidence. The cause of TEF and esophageal atresia is unknown. Esophageal atresia with or without TEF occurs in 1 in 2,000 to 4,500 births with no difference in the sexes. From 30% to 50% have other associated anomalies of the cardiac, GI, and central nervous systems. Prematurity and low birth weight are frequent concomitant problems that have a significant impact on long-term prognosis. See Figure 25–3 for further discussion of their incidence.

Clinical Manifestations

Any child who exhibits the "3 Cs" of **coughing, choking** with feedings, and **cyanosis** should be suspected of TEF.

- Failure to pass suction catheter, nasogastric (NG) tube at birth
- Excessive oral secretions
- Vomiting
- Abdominal distension
- Airless, scaphoid abdomen (atresia without fistula)

Diagnostic Evaluation. A history of maternal polyhydramnios is a significant prenatal clue. If TEF is suspected prenatally, diagnosis can be made at the ideal time, in the delivery room. Atresia should be suspected if an NG tube can't be passed 10 to 11 cm beyond the gum line. This suspicion is confirmed with an abdominal X-ray that will identify a proximal esophagus dilated with air (atresia) or abdominal distention (fistula). The specific type of defect can be identified by the radiologist after instilling less than 1 ml of a water-soluble contrast medium into the NG tube and documenting its movement into the tracheal tree and the proximal pouch. This is then withdrawn from the pouch to minimize the risk of aspiration. Bronchoscopy and endoscopy are also used to identify and assess fistulas.

Therapeutic Management

Esophageal atresia and TEF represent a critical neonatal surgical emergency. While the baby is awaiting transfer to a neonatal unit and surgery, management centers on prevention of aspiration.

Keeping the infant supine or prone with the head of the bed elevated decreases the chance of gastric secretions entering the lungs. An NG tube must be in place and aspirated every 5 to 10 minutes to keep the proximal pouch clear of secretions. IV fluids are essential. Normal newborn care is appropriate with special attention to keeping the baby warm and oxygenated.

Surgical repair is the mainstay of treatment. Initial repair includes the ligation of the fistula and end-to-side anastomosis of the atresia to decrease the severity of stricture formation. If the gap between the two parts of the esophagus is too large, a staged repair is necessary and a gastrostomy tube (G-tube) and cervical esophagostomy are placed. Later anastomosis, colon interposition, and dilation can be expected. Evaluation and treatment of esophageal motility dysfunction, gastroesophageal reflux, strictures, bronchitis, and pneumonia may occur as the child grows.

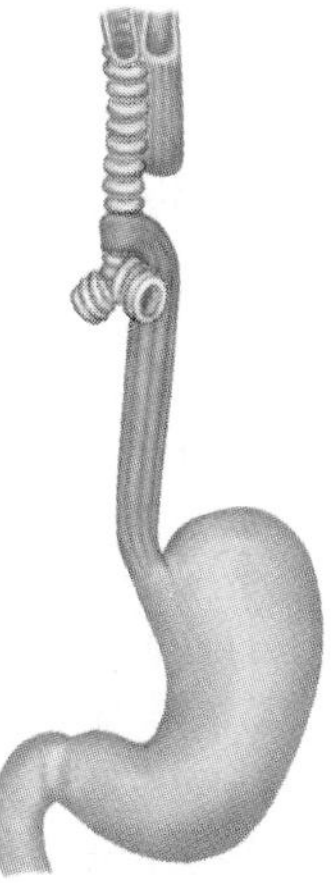

Esophageal Atresia with Distal TEF

Incidence: 85%–88%
Clinical Manifestations: Feeding causes regurgitation and coughing. Constant flow of saliva. Gastric distention.
Diagnostic Findings: Contrast reveals blind pouch. Air on abdominal x–ray.
Surgical Treatment: One-stage surgical repair to ligate fistula and anastomose esophagus.

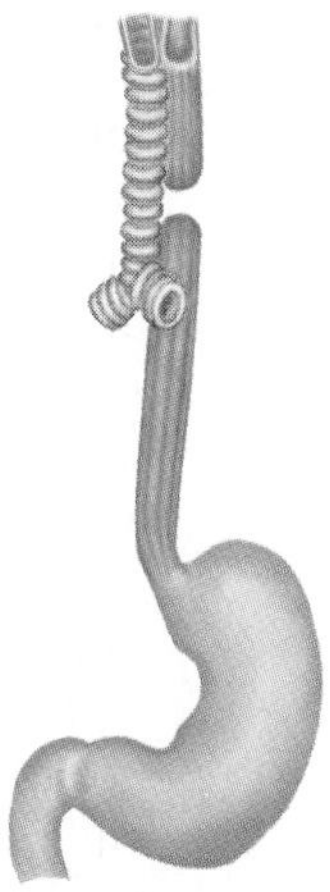

Esophageal Atresia Without Fistula

Incidence: 6%–8%
Clinical Manifestations: Excess oral secretions. Regurgitation of feedings.
Diagnostic Findings: Blind pouch. No air in abdomen.
Surgical Treatment: Two–stage repair 1) Gastrostomy and cervical esophagostomy. 2) Colon interposition to create patent esophagus.

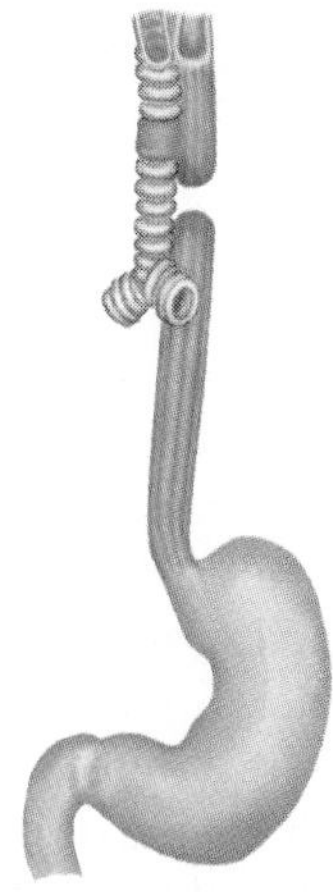

Proximal Esophageal Fistula with Trachea; Distal Segment Has No Communication

Incidence: 1%
Clinical Manifestations: Excessive oral secretions. Immediate respiratory distress with oral intake.
Diagnostic Findings: PO contrast outlines tracheal tree. No air in abdomen.
Surgical Treatment: One or two-stage repair depending on length of separation.

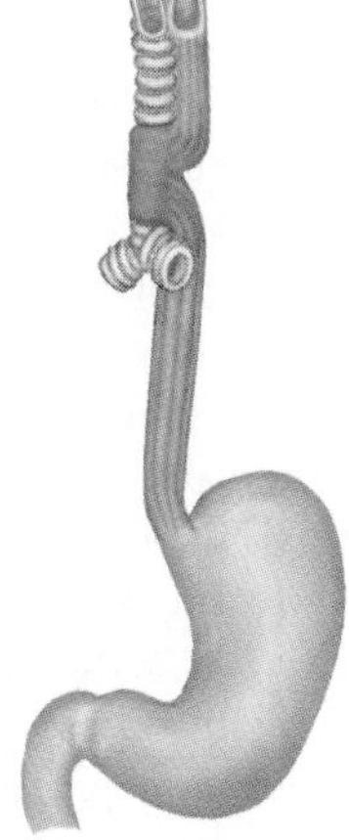

Proximal and Distal Esophageal Fistulas with Trachea

Incidence: 1%
Clinical Manifestations: Excessive secretions. Respiratory distress with feedings.
Diagnostic Findings: PO contrast outlines tracheal tree. Air in abdomen.
Surgical Treatment: Ligation of fistulas and anastomosis of esophagus.

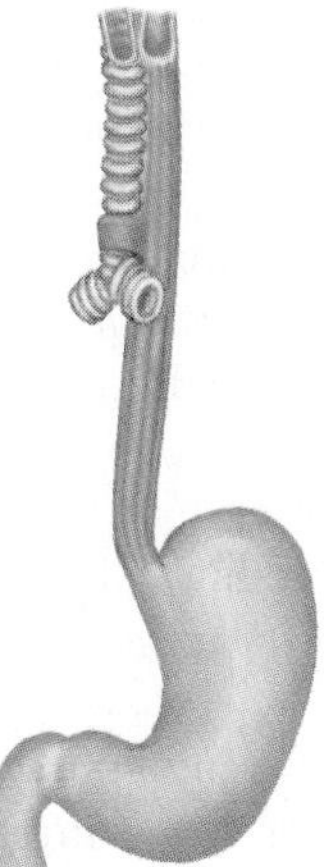

TEF Without Atresia (Also called "H Type")

Incidence: 4%
Clinical Manifestations: Minimal symptoms unless regurgitation occurs. Choking, coughing. Abdominal distention.
Diagnostic Findings: Bronchoscopy demonstrates fistula.
Surgical Treatment: Ligation of fistula

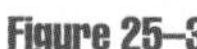

Figure 25–3

Types of esophageal atresia and tracheoesophageal fistulas.

NURSING CARE OF THE INFANT WITH TEF

Assessment

The infant with TEF is at constant risk for aspiration. Assessment for respiratory distress in the immediate period after birth is essential. The nurse must examine the infant for excessive oral secretions, choking, and cyanosis. Difficulty swallowing, regurgitation, vomiting, and unexplained cyanosis after an initial feeding in the infant who is not diagnosed at birth are important assessment findings that must be reported to the physician immediately. Abdominal distention should be measured and the infant continually assessed for distress (vital signs, respiratory effort, nasal flaring, retractions, cyanosis). A newborn assessment should be completed with special attention to identifying any concomitant congenital defects.

Family assessment of anxiety levels, fears, concerns, and knowledge level will provide important information for planning nursing care and teaching.

Nursing Diagnosis and Planning

The following nursing diagnoses and expected outcomes are appropriate following assessment of the infant with TEF:

- Risk for Aspiration related to TEF. ***Expected Outcome:*** *The infant will not aspirate, as evidenced by control of oral secretions without coughing, cyanosis, or adventitious breath sounds.*
- Altered Nutrition: Less Than Body Requirements related to possible feeding difficulties. ***Expected Outcome:*** *The infant will gain weight and follow growth chart at appropriate level.*
- Risk for Impaired Skin Integrity related to G-tube and esophagostomy. ***Expected Outcome:*** *The infant will maintain skin integrity as evidenced by intact skin around G-tube and esophagostomy.*
- Risk for Infection related to surgical repair. ***Expected Outcome:*** *The infant will have surgical site, G-tube site, and esophagostomy free from infection, as evidenced by clean, intact skin without drainage, exudate, or redness.*
- Pain related to surgical repair. ***Expected Outcome:*** *The infant will be free from pain, as evidenced by resumption of normal activities, ease of comforting, and relaxed facial features.*
- Anxiety (Parental) related to neonatal surgical emergency. ***Expected Outcome:*** *The parents will express feelings and concerns.*
- Knowledge Deficit related to home care needs and follow-up care. ***Expected Outcome:*** *The parents will demonstrate safe G-tube feedings and esophagostomy care.*

Implementation

Nursing interventions are different in the preoperative and postoperative periods. In the immediate period after birth, placement in a radiant warmer and administration of humidified oxygen are essential to relieve respiratory distress. The child is prepared for surgery, remains NPO, and is hydrated with IV fluids. Maintaining thermoregulation and fluid balance are essential, so monitoring temperature and other vital signs, using radiant warmers, and keeping accurate intake and output records are important.

It is essential to minimize the risk of aspiration. Using a chalasia board that helps keep the child at a 30° angle while supine can be useful to decrease reflux. However, a prone position is preferred (see Fig. 25–5). See Teaching Guidelines for the Child With GER (p. 716). Placing a suction catheter in the proximal pouch and mouth will keep secretions to a minimum. Maintaining constant assessment of respiratory status is essential. Even after surgical repair, these children are prone to gastroesophageal reflux.

> Directing teaching toward the parents is important at this time if they are emotionally ready to listen. Their anxieties must be addressed by careful listening, supporting, sharing emotions, and encouraging their bonding with the infant.

In the immediate postoperative period monitoring respiratory status, supporting fluid balance and nutrition, maintaining thermoregulation, providing pain relief, monitoring for infection, and promoting bonding with parents take priority. The child will likely have a chest tube in place. Patency must be maintained, suction monitored, and output documented. Respiratory rate, effort, and the presence of abnormal breath sounds should be documented. Thermoregulation can significantly affect respiratory status in the newborn, so monitoring and maintaining temperature with a radiant warmer may be needed.

IV fluid, antibiotics, and parenteral nutrition may be ordered. The nurse must maintain patency of the IV, monitor intake and output, assess for dehydration, sunken fontanel, decreased urine specific gravity, and possible fluid overload. Daily weights and measurement of head circumference can aid in assessing growth. Pain medications must be administered as needed based on objective assessment measures used in each institution.

If a cervical esophagostomy has been performed as the first stage of a surgical repair, keep it covered with gauze to absorb saliva and provide skin care. Frequent cleaning with half-strength hydrogen peroxide and assessing for redness, breakdown, or exudate is essential because this wet area can become easily macerated and infected. Referral to an enterostomal therapist can be helpful in teaching parents its care. See Teaching Guidelines for the Child With Transesophageal Fistula.

TEACHING GUIDELINES *for the Child With Transesophageal Fistula*

A. Teach care of esophagostomy (cover with clean gauze).
   1. Change gauze frequently to prevent constant wetness.
   2. Clean with half-strength hydrogen peroxide once daily.
   3. Use skin barriers to prevent breakdown.
   4. Assess for redness, exudate, yeast infections, swelling, and pain.
   5. Consult with enterostomal therapist for support in skin care.

B. Provide oral stimulation with use of pacifier or small amounts of fluid per bottle to allow practice in swallowing.

C. Teach care of gastrostomy tube (care will vary with type used).
   1. For new gastrostomy, clean insertion site daily with half-strength hydrogen peroxide, rinse with water, and apply antimicrobial ointment. Rotate tube daily.
   2. After 1–2 weeks, soap and water and tub baths may be used to clean site. Stomahesive powder may be used to decrease moisture.
   3. Keep tube open to air in postoperative period.
   4. While site is healing, stabilize the tube at 90° angle to prevent excessive movement using Hollister Tube Drainage Attachment, nipple with gauze at base, or Silicone retention disks.
   5. Well-healed site can be secured with tape or Op-Site.
   6. Use skin barriers (SkinPrep) to prevent breakdown.
   7. Report exudate, heat, or leakage of formula.
   8. Use nystatin for monilia, antimicrobial ointment for redness, and enterostomal therapy products for skin breakdown.
   9. Utilize support of enterostomal therapist to individualize care for each type of tube available.

In the immediate postoperative period, the gastrostomy tube is elevated, allowing gastric contents to pass to the small intestine and air to escape, which promotes comfort and decreases risk of leakage at the anastomosis. Sucking a pacifier satisfies sucking needs, provides early training in swallowing, makes feeding easier later, and provides comfort through distraction. Pacifiers should not be offered until the child can tolerate oral secretions.

Numerous G-tubes are available for placement during surgery or percutaneously. These include the use of traditional gastrostomy tubes and Foley catheters that use air or saline balloons to anchor them. The Medical Innovation Corporation (MIC) tube is a silicone tube with an anchoring device and a sliding ring that prevents inward or outward migration of the tube (Huddleston et al., 1989). The percutaneous endoscopic gastrostomy (PEG) tube uses internal and external crossbars to stabilize it perpendicularly in the fistula created for insertion (Neal & Slayton, 1992). The gastrostomy feeding Button™ (Fig. 25–4) can be used in any well-established gastrostomy site and eliminates the extension of a tube beyond the surface of the abdomen (Huth & O'Brien, 1987). The button is a mushroom-shaped silicone device that has "wings" to anchor it and has the advantages of a cosmetically pleasing appearance, decreased skin breakdown, increased comfort, and full immersibility in water. Tube selection is usually made by the physician, but long-term successful care and use of the tube is a nursing and parental responsibility.

Parents should be taught the techniques of G-tube feeding and care. (See Teaching Guidelines for the Child With TEF and Chapter 18, Application of Nursing Principles to Pediatrics.) Skin care at the site may include cleaning with half-strength hydrogen peroxide, rotating the tube, and using Skin Prep and other ostomy skin care products. Redness, exudate, pus, heat, or leakage of formula should be reported.

Parent education and support are critical components. This should include discussing feelings and anxieties, providing information about home care, practicing with special techniques, providing stimulation, and using appropriate resources such as enterostomal therapy and dietitians.

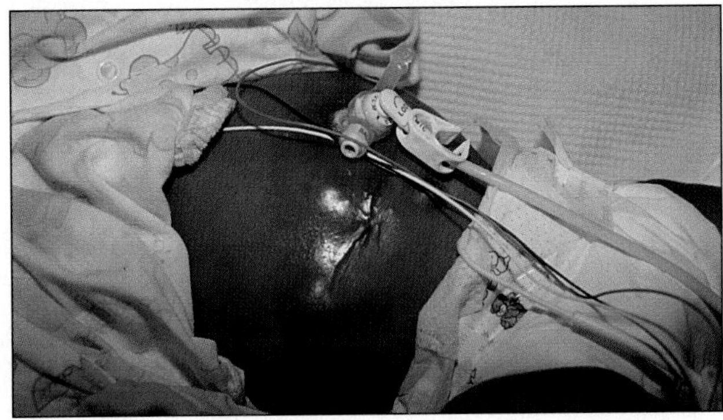

Figure 25–4
The skin level gastrostomy button is good for children who require long-term gastrostomy feeding. It is relatively flat, reduces skin breakdown, increases comfort, and is fully immersible in water. (Courtesy of Parkland Memorial Hospital, Dallas, Texas)

TABLE 25–1 *Upper Gastrointestinal Hernias*

DESCRIPTION	CLINICAL MANIFESTATIONS	THERAPEUTIC MANAGEMENT	NURSING MANAGEMENT
Hiatal Hernia Protrusion of a portion of the stomach through the esophageal hiatus of the diaphragm	Similar to GER: • Vomiting • Coughing, wheezing, short periods of apnea • Failure to thrive	Medical management similar to GER Surgical repair of defect	Monitor intake and output, document vomiting, observe for respiratory distress, routine postoperative care for GI surgery Parent teaching about surgery, medical treatment of reflux (See Teaching Guidelines for the child with GER)
Congenital Diaphragmatic Hernia (CDH) Opening in the diaphragm through which abdominal contents herniate into the thoracic cavity during prenatal development *and* some degree of pulmonary hypoplasia determined by the timing and size of the herniation Mortality: 50%–80% Degree of pulmonary hypoplasia determines outcome Incidence: 1 in 2,200–5,000	Clinical findings dependent on severity of defect • Fetal ultrasound shows abdominal organs in chest • Diminished or absent breath sounds on affected side • Bowel sounds may be heard over chest • Cardiac sounds may be heard on right side of chest • Respiratory distress developing soon after birth: dyspnea, cyanosis, nasal flaring, tachypnea, retractions • Scaphoid abdomen	If diagnosed prenatally, move mother to tertiary care center. Neonatal emergency! Nasogastric intubation with suction Ventilate with high frequency ventilaton, manage acidosis with bicarbonate and ventilation ECMO Manage pulmonary hypertension Surgical reduction of hernia after physiologically stable May wait 6–18 hours after birth Respiratory support, ECMO until lungs functioning after surgery	Identify clinical findings and report immediately Semi-Fowler's position on affected side with head of bed elevated Maintain patency of NG tube Monitor IV fluids Maintain mechanical ventilation, ECMO, chest tubes, assess oxygenation Provide minimal stimulation Routine postoperative care Monitor for signs of infection, respiratory distress, and feeding difficulties, and report to physician Support family mourning loss of perfect child Provide clear, truthful information Encourage parent to see and touch infant Provide referral with support groups Discharge teaching Feeding techniques

Evaluation

- Can the child coordinate sucking and swallowing?
- Is the child tolerating oral feedings without choking, coughing, or cyanosis?
- Is the child growing according to growth chart?
- Is the surgical site clean, dry, intact, and free of redness, drainage, or exudate?
- Is the skin intact without breakdown around G-tube and esophagostomy?
- Is the child resting contentedly without pain medication?
- Can the parents explain need for surgical procedure?
- Do parents demonstrate appropriate care of G-tube or esophagostomy?
- Have parents assumed all care responsibilities?

Upper Gastrointestinal Hernia

A hernia is an abnormal protrusion of part of an organ or tissue through the structures that normally contain it. Hernias can be either congenital or acquired. Some hernias are able to be reduced, whereas others become incarcerated and cannot be returned by manipulation. A medical emergency occurs when a hernia becomes strangulated and blood supply is cut off. This condition can occur suddenly and requires immediate treatment. The most common hernias of the upper GI tract are discussed in Table 25–1.

DISORDERS OF FUNCTION

Gastroesophageal reflux, pyloric stenosis, and ulcers may develop in children and can have important nursing implications for nutritional support, fluid balance, respiratory function, and parental education.

Gastroesophageal Reflux

Gastroesophageal reflux (GER) is regurgitation of gastric contents back into the esophagus. GER is a normal physiologic phenomenon; all adults and infants reflux periodically, especially after meals. Reflux can be divided into three types: physiologic, functional, and pathologic (see box on following page).

Etiology. Many factors contribute to the development of GER. Neurologic impairment such as cerebral palsy, Down syndrome, and head injury may affect the transmission of neural signals to the LES. Delayed gastric emptying of a liquid meal due to distension may also contribute. LES relaxations can also be triggered by partial or incomplete swallowing dysfunctions, or drugs such as theophylline or caffeine. Increased intra-abdominal pressure incurred while straining, crying, coughing, or slumping tend to promote increased episodes of GER. These postural effects are most likely large factors in infants. Obesity and hiatal hernias also promote GER. Finally, during the first 6 months of life the LES pressure undergoes maturational development. Because infants have a short abdominal LES, this predisposes them to increased instances of GER. As the infant grows the LES matures and the reflux improves.

PATHOPHYSIOLOGY *of GER*

The LES, a zone of tonically contracted smooth muscle surrounding the distal esophagus, is innervated by vagal nerves and receives signals from multiple organs. A defect in this neural control may result in a dysfunctional LES with periods of transitory spontaneous relaxation. This allows gastric contents to reflux back into the esophagus.

In addition, the esophagus traverses both the abdominal and thoracic cavity, with the LES positioned strategically between the two. Most of the LES is abdominal. The greater the length of intra-abdominal esophagus, the more competent this valve becomes. Any condition that shortens the abdominal segment of the LES will increase the likelihood of reflux.

Incidence. Pathologic GER occurs in about 3% of all newborns (Sterling et al., 1991). Boys are affected three times more than girls, and premature infants more than full-term infants. Almost all infants with GER will have symptoms by age 6 weeks. In the absence of therapy, 2% to 5% will die of respiratory complications, and 3% to 5% will develop significant esophageal scarring that will require medical and surgical management.

Clinical Manifestations

All Types of GER

- Vomiting or spitting up after a meal
- Hiccuping
- Recurrent otitis media related to pooled secretions in the nasopharynx during sleep

Pathologic GER

- Weight loss, failure to thrive
- Irritability, discomfort, abdominal pain
- Heartburn, **dysphagia**
- **Hematemesis, melena**
- Anemia
- Respiratory problems: coughing, choking, wheezing, pneumonia, apnea, bradycardia

Diagnostic Evaluation. A variety of chronic and acute illness have been associated with GER. It is necessary to confirm the presence of GER only after other major conditions have been ruled out. Diagnostic tests include barium swallow, upper GI study, fiberoptic endoscopy, esophageal manometry, ambulatory pH studies, and gastroesophageal

Types of Gastroesophageal Reflux

Physiologic
- Infrequent emesis
- Parents may not be concerned or think it is normal

Functional
- Painless, frequent emesis after meals
- No failure to thrive
- 40% asymptomatic by 3 months
- 70% asymptomatic by 18 months
- Medical management very effective

Pathologic
- Failure to thrive
- Aspiration pneumonia
- Apnea
- Frequent emesis, amount varies
- Often requires surgery

Data from Shannon, R. (1993). Gastroesophageal reflux in infancy. Review and update. *Journal of Pediatric Health Care, 7*(2), 71–75.

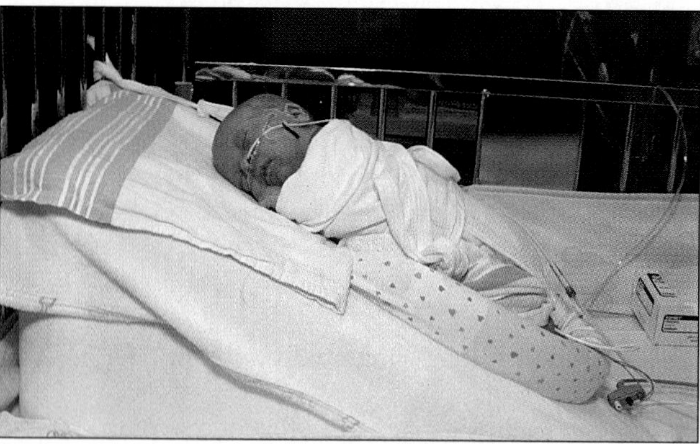

Figure 25–5
The infant having gastroesophageal reflux may be positioned prone on a wedge that provides a head-up tilt of 30 degrees. A harness around the torso keeps the baby positioned properly. This child also had liver failure, which caused increased intra-abdominal pressure and accounts for the jaundice.

scintography. See the table on common laboratory and diagnostic tests in the Clinical Reference Pages for a complete discussion of these tests.

Therapeutic Management. Therapy for GER is based on the severity of symptoms and includes diet, position, medications, and surgery. Many infants suspected of functional GER are treated conservatively without the benefit of diagnostic testing that can be time consuming and costly.

Diet. Small, frequent feedings of predigested formulas such as Nutramigen or Pregestimil will reduce the amount of formula in the stomach, decrease distension, and minimize reflux. These smaller, more frequent feedings with frequent burping are often tried as the first line of treatment. Feedings thickened with rice cereal may reduce episodes of emesis but do not affect reflux time (Orenstein, 1992). Some preliminary studies indicate thickened feedings actually may increase the risk of GER by delaying gastric emptying time (Orenstein, 1992). Formulas may need to be concentrated and NG tube feedings supplemented for the child with failure to thrive. Caffeine and fatty foods decrease LES pressure and should be eliminated.

Positioning. Much attention has been given to the best positioning for GER. It is generally suggested that a 30° head elevated prone position (Fig. 25–5) results in fewer and shorter episodes of GER (Orenstein, 1990). A simple prone position may be equally effective (Orenstein, 1992). The American Academy of Pediatrics Task Force on Infant Positioning and SIDS has noted that infants with GER or other conditions may be placed in the prone position (AAP, 1992).

Medications. Though most medications used in the treatment of GER have not been FDA approved for children, their use is quite common. Antacids for symptom relief, H_2-receptor antagonists to decrease acid secretion, and prokinetic agents to accelerate gastric emptying may be used. See the table on common medications in the Clinical Reference Pages.

Treatment of Acute Bleeding. Bleeding is a complication of longstanding GER and esophagitis. Washing out of the stomach with lavage via an NG tube is commonly performed for the evacuation of blood and blood clots during an episode of upper GI bleeding. The use of iced saline lavage to stop bleeding is no longer advocated. Radiologic procedures or surgery to coagulate bleeding vessels may be needed.

Surgery. Up to 15% of infants with GER will require **fundoplication**. A 270° to 360° wrap to the stomach fundus is made around the distal esophagus. This tightens the LES and prevents gastric reflux. The child may develop a gas bloat syndrome because of the inability to burp and may require a gastrostomy tube as a temporary mechanism for gastric decompression.

NURSING CARE OF THE INFANT WITH GER

Assessment

Nursing assessment begins with a thorough history, including the amount and frequency of feedings, changes in formula, and positioning during feedings. The frequency and pattern of emesis, including documentation of whether it is projectile, painful, or contains blood, should be made. A medical history of frequent respiratory problems of pneumonia, apnea, choking, or cyanosis should be gathered.

Observation of the child during a feeding can provide critical information about choking, gagging, coughing, color change, and comfort during feeding.

The child's length, weight, and head circumference should be plotted on a growth chart. The infant should be assessed for Sandifer movements, unusual postural habits that may be observed in infants with severe reflux-induced esophagitis. These typically irritable infants may demonstrate head-cocking, arching, and thrashing of the arms. It has been suggested that drawing the head to one side may relieve pain by keeping gastric secretions from entering the esophagus or mouth. If a history of respiratory symptoms is present, the infant is assessed for abnormal breath sounds or retractions.

Family assessment should not be overlooked and should include observations of parent–child interactions, feeding styles, and discussion of feelings and concerns about the child who vomits frequently, is difficult to feed, and may have failure to thrive.

Nursing Diagnosis and Planning

The following nursing diagnoses and expected outcomes are appropriate following assessment of the child with GER:

- Risk for Aspiration related to GER. ***Expected Outcome:*** *The infant will maintain a patent airway, without signs of aspiration or respiratory distress.*
- Fluid Volume Deficit related to vomiting. ***Expected Outcome:*** *The infant will retain feedings, with regurgitation of less than 10 ml.*
- Altered Nutrition: Less than Body Requirements related to anorexia, vomiting, and dysphagia. ***Expected Outcome:*** *The infant will maintain and gain weight according to growth chart.*
- Pain related to esophagitis. ***Expected Outcome:*** *The infant will remain free from discomfort of esophageal irritation.*
- Impaired Swallowing related to esophagitis. ***Expected Outcome:*** *The infant will swallow effectively without choking, coughing, or cyanosis.*
- Risk for Infection related to surgical repair. ***Expected Outcome:*** *The infant will have a surgical site that is clean, dry, and free from redness or exudate.*
- Knowledge Deficit related to disease process and home care. ***Expected Outcome:*** *The parents will learn infant cardiopulmonary resuscitation (CPR); explain GER and the reasons for diagnostic tests, medications, dietary changes, and/or surgery.*
- Impaired Home Maintenance Management related to complex, long-term care. ***Expected Outcome:*** *The parents will demonstrate effective coping mechanisms for dealing with the long-term consequences of GER.*

Implementation

Nursing care requires a thorough understanding of the therapeutic management as well as postoperative care. It involves dietary modifications, positioning, medication administration, respiratory support, and perioperative care. See Teaching Guidelines for the Child with GER.

Dietary Modifications. Formulas and feeding routines are frequently changed to promote optimal gastric emptying. Parents need to understand the reasons for these changes and may require assistance with developing new feeding techniques or schedules. If thickened formula is used, 1 to 3 tsp of rice cereal per ounce of formula is most commonly used and may require cross-cutting the nipple. Parents may need assistance in this area. Thickened formula is fed only to infants who are not on solid foods. Toddlers are fed their solids first, followed by liquids. Chocolate and caffeine should be eliminated from the diets of older children, but be prepared to offer alternative "treats." A good rule of thumb for all children is to never take something away without first providing something in its place.

Positioning. Proper positioning is one of the mainstays of reflux management. Ideally, the goal is to maintain the infant in an upright angle 24 hours a day, at a 60° angle when supine, and at a 30° angle when prone. This positioning is maintained until the infant remains asymptomatic for 6 weeks. The use of slings, harnesses, achalasia boards, wedges, and towel rolls are essential and are available for home use in a variety of sizes. Because all infant care must be done in this position, changing tables, cribs, and car seats must all be modified and require extensive home teaching from the nurse.

Providing developmental stimulation is essential for the child who may have more limited mobility. Using mobiles, activity boxes, mirrors, and musical toys can be useful, as can moving the child's crib into areas of activity.

Medications. The nurse will administer GER medications as ordered but must be aware of the many drug interactions and side effects associated with the sometimes complicated and long-term regimen. Medications must be scheduled around mealtimes, so the nurse should determine the feeding schedule of the child and assist the family in adjusting their schedule if necessary. See the table of common medications in the Clinical Reference Pages for a discussion of nursing implications for these drugs.

Respiratory Support. The varying respiratory alterations presents many challenges. Parents of infants with GER may feel overwhelmed with doubt and anxiety about their ability to adequately care for their child.

TEACHING GUIDELINES *for the Child With GER*

Explain feeding alterations:
- Small frequent feedings.
- Thicken with 1–3 tsp rice cereal per ounce of formula.
- Cross-cut nipple or try different nipples.
- Consult pediatric dietitian for assistance and support.

Modify posture of infant:
- Keep upright at 30–45° angle at all times.
- Use wedge, folded or rolled blankets and towels, slings, and specially made boards in crib.
- Avoid infant seats because they increase gastric pressure and decrease LES tone.
- Contact home health resources for follow-up and education.

Teach parents about medications:
- Teach important side effects.
- Use charts to keep track of numerous medications.
- Provide written information on all medications.
- Notify physician about any motor dysfunction, extreme irritability, or skin rashes.
- Reinforce proper scheduling of medications.
- Caution about drug interactions: Don't mix antacids with other drugs, don't add any other drug without physician approval because numerous drug interactions are possible with cimetidine.

Provide respiratory support:
- Teach infant CPR to all caregivers.
- Provide monitoring education and support.

Explain GER:
- Explain and provide written information about the disease process and its possible complications of bleeding, apnea, choking, cough, and esophagitis.

Provide emotional support:
- Encourage discussion of fears, concerns, and frustrations.
- Contact community resources and national support groups for information and support.
- Arrange respite care if needed.

Repeated instructions, written materials, home health nurse visits, emotional support, and support groups can be very important. Infants experiencing apnea, bradycardia, or color change will need continuous cardiac/apnea monitoring. This requires extensive parental training and follow-up. The ability of *all* caretakers to perform infant CPR must be determined and training offered.

Surgical Care. Because surgery is considered the last resort in the treatment of GER, sufficient preoperative preparation time is available to answer questions, prepare the parent for IVs, NG tube, and possible gastrostomy. See the discussion of preoperative and postoperative care for the child with TEF for a discussion of specific nursing interventions. Frequently a gastrostomy tube will be placed at the time of fundoplication. This provides relief from gastric distension and provides a mechanism for enteral tube feedings. The ability to burp or vomit will eventually return after a fundoplication. Postoperative problems of retching and difficulty in swallowing should be discussed with parents. In addition, parents need to understand about the possibility of the development of dumping syndrome. Dumping syndrome begins within 30 minutes after a feeding and may include diaphoresis, palpitations, weakness, syncope, abdominal fullness, nausea, or diarrhea. This will improve with age.

Home Care. Supporting the parents and modifications in positioning, diet, and administering medications are essential nursing interventions. Continued follow-up and support by a nurse are of paramount importance. The nurse should be prepared to teach about diet, positioning, medications, and respiratory support by demonstrating specific techniques, providing appropriate equipment, and leaving written schedules and information. Because the plan of care is usually continued for at least 6 weeks after symptoms improve, long-term relationships with the family may develop and provide essential support for all family members.

Evaluation

- Is the child's airway patent without choking, coughing, cyanosis, or retractions?
- Is the child growing according to the growth chart?
- Can the child retain feedings with regurgitations of less than 10 ml?
- Does the child take medications as prescribed at correct time and dosages?
- Is the child content and comfortable during feedings?
- Have the parents and all caregivers demonstrated infant CPR?
- Can the parents explain GER and the reasons for positioning and dietary modifications?
- Can parents verbalize side effects that require physician notification?
- Can the parents explain need for surgical procedure?
- Do parents demonstrate appropriate care of G-tube?
- Have parents assumed all care responsibilities?

Hypertrophic Pyloric Stenosis

Pyloric stenosis results when the circular areas of muscle surrounding the pylorus hypertrophies and blocks gastric emptying. This is one of the most common surgical disorders of early infancy.

Etiology. The exact cause of pyloric stenosis remains unknown, but muscular hypertrophy is not present at birth. Pyloric stenosis may be associated with other GI anomalies such as malrotation, short gut syndrome, esophageal and duodenal atresia, anorectal anomalies, hiatal hernia, and GER. Heredity and family predisposition seem to increase the risk of pyloric stenosis.

Incidence. The incidence of pyloric stenosis is 1 in 500 births. First-born children and offspring of affected children are at highest risk. Males are affected five times more often than females, and full-term infants more than premature infants. There is also a higher incidence found in white infants than black or Asian infants (Borkowski, 1994).

PATHOPHYSIOLOGY *of Hypertrophic Pyloric Stenosis*

Pyloric spasms cause milk curds to be propelled against a narrowed pyloric channel and subsequently irritate its sensitive mucosal lining. Edema of the pyloric mucosa results. This edema further reduces the size of the pyloric canal and creates resistance to the flow of milk. To promote gastric emptying and compensate for this resistance the pylorus contracts with more force and gradually enlarges in size. This enlarged pyloric muscle slowly begins to constrict the pyloric channel and when the mucosal edema subsides, the resistance to flow still remains. A vicious cycle develops that progresses to a high-level obstruction of the pyloric canal.

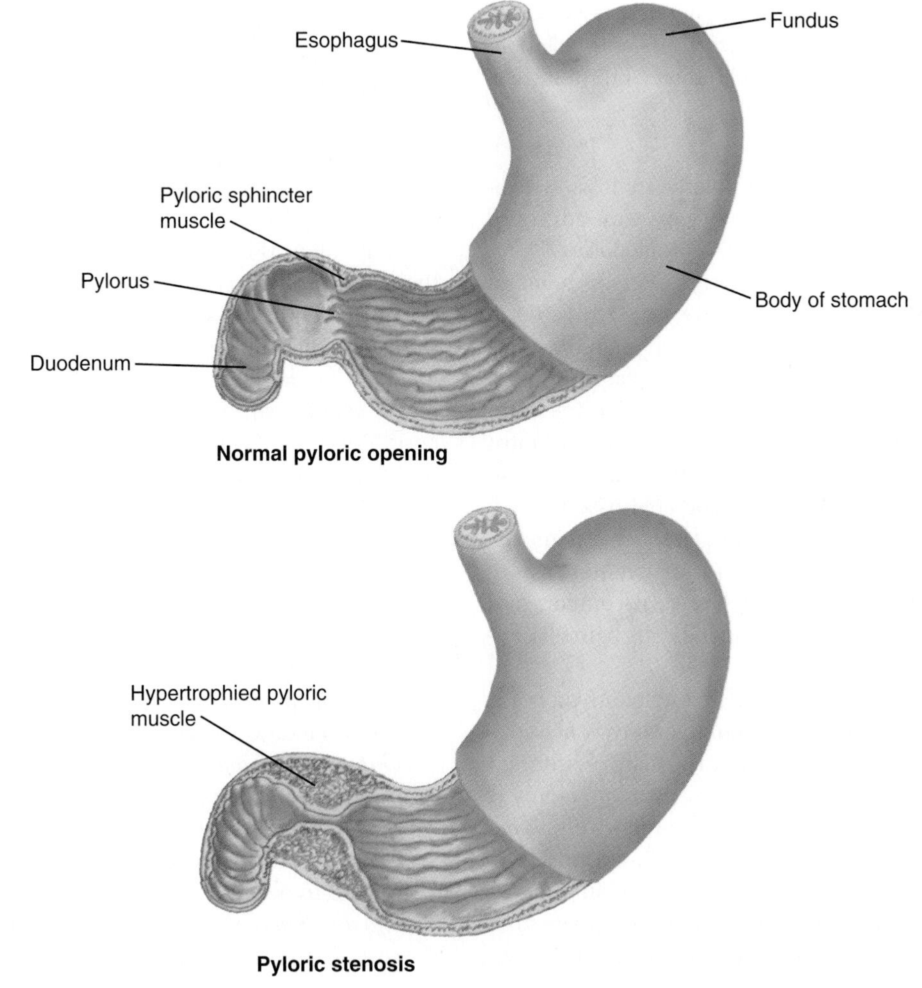

Clinical Manifestations

- Previously healthy infant with progressive, **projectile, nonbilious vomiting**
- Movable, palpable, firm, olive-shaped mass in right upper quadrant
- Visible deep gastric peristaltic waves from left upper quadrant to right upper quadrant immediately before vomiting
- Irritability, hunger, crying
- Sunken fontanel, poor skin turgor, dry mucous membranes, decreased urine output
- Metabolic alkalosis
- Jaundice
- Constipation

Diagnostic Evaluation. Diagnosis is based on a history of vomiting, visible peristaltic waves, and a palpable pyloric mass. When the mass can't be palpated, radiology and ultrasound studies are helpful. A flat plate of the abdomen will show a narrow pylorus with a dilated stomach and absent gas distal to the pylorus. Ultrasound can confirm the presence of a pyloric mass. A barium swallow will outline the long narrow pyloric canal and identify delayed gastric emptying. Laboratory findings may indicate metabolic alkalosis due to vomiting, including decreased serum potassium and sodium levels, increased pH and bicarbonate, and decreased chloride level. Indirect bilirubin may be elevated.

Therapeutic Management. Because pyloric stenosis is usually diagnosed early, few infants are seen with advanced states of dehydration, malnutrition, and alkalosis. If present, they must be corrected before surgery. An infant who is slightly dehydrated with a CO_2 of 25 mEq/L or less, or an infant who is moderately dehydrated with a CO_2 of 26 to 35 mEq/L is managed with replacement parenteral fluids and electrolytes, and an NG tube for stomach decompression. Once the stomach is empty, most infants will stop vomiting. Surgery is usually delayed 24 to 48 hours until fluid and electrolyte and acid-base balance is corrected. Infants severely dehydrated and malnourished with CO_2 levels about 35 mEq/L may require a 3- to 5-day course of IV fluids, electrolyte replacement, and infusions of plasma or packed red blood cells before surgical repair.

There is universal agreement that a pyloromyotomy is the definitive treatment. The pyloromyotomy is not considered an emergency procedure but is usually performed without delay on well-hydrated infants. Pyloromyotomy is performed through a right transverse incision well above the liver edge. The enlarged circular pyloric muscle is incised longitudinally without puncturing the submucosa or lumen. This releases the obstruction and allows free passage of fluid from the stomach to the duodenum.

NURSING CARE OF THE CHILD WITH HYPERTROPHIC PYLORIC STENOSIS

Assessment

Hypertrophic pyloric stenosis is suspected in infants who present with a history of projectile vomiting, especially after meals. A thorough nursing history is obtained that includes the infant's feeding schedule with type, amount, and frequency of formula taken. The relationship of feedings to vomiting is determined and documented. Vomiting is assessed for frequency, amount, color, and consistency, as well as projection.

GATHERING INFORMATION FROM PARENTS Gathering a history about the amount and characteristics of vomiting can be difficult since descriptive terms are nonspecific and estimation of amounts is very inconsistent. Useful questions might include:

Could you wipe it off the child with a diaper or rag?
Did it require a change of clothes for the infant or caregiver?
If it was on a bed or sheet, how big a circle did it make?
If it was on the floor, how big a circle did it make?
Does it happen after every feeding?
Does it look like what he just ate or is it curdled?
What color is it?
Does it appear to be under force and project away from the child?

Encouraging the parents to keep a written record of these answers can provide essential assessment information.

The infant is checked for signs of dehydration such as the absence of tears, weak cry, depressed fontanel, poor skin turgor, and dry mucous membranes. Signs of potassium, sodium, and chloride depletion should be noted. The abdomen is checked for distension, tenderness, bowel sounds, the presence of a pyloric mass, or gastric peristaltic waves. The family is assessed for their understanding of the disorder, the presence of a viable support system, and their ability to participate in their child's care.

Nursing Diagnosis and Planning

The following nursing diagnoses and expected outcomes are appropriate following assessment of the child with hypertrophic pyloric stenosis:

- Fluid Volume Deficit related to vomiting. ***Expected Outcome:*** *The infant will have a balanced intake and output; be free of signs of dehydration; have urine output of greater than 1–2 ml/kg/hr.*
- Altered Nutrition: Less Than Body Requirements related to persistent vomiting. ***Expected Outcome:*** *The infant will tolerate regular feedings; continue to show growth according to growth chart.*

- Impaired Skin Integrity related to surgical incision. ***Expected Outcome:*** *The infant will have a clean, dry, intact incision without redness or exudate.*
- Risk for Infection related to surgical incision. ***Expected Outcome:*** *The infant will have a clean, dry, intact incision without redness or exudate.*
- Knowledge Deficit related to need for surgery or pyloric stenosis. ***Expected Outcome:*** *The parents will describe pyloric stenosis; verbalize an understanding of expected preoperative and postoperative care; assume total care of the infant before discharge.*

Implementation

Preoperatively the infant is NPO and is stabilized with IV fluids and electrolytes. Vital signs, daily weights, and monitoring of laboratory values and intake and output are essential nursing interventions. Intake and output should include all IV and PO fluids, blood products, emesis, urine output, stools, and NG drainage. The dehydrated infant should be kept warm and quiet. Oral care and skin massage with lotions and oils may be provided because skin and membranes are more susceptible to breakdown in their dehydrated state. The head of the bed is elevated and the infant placed prone to reduce the risk of aspiration. The NG tube should be patent, properly positioned, and the amount, color, and type of drainage recorded. Respiratory distress should be assessed.

Postoperatively, the care varies with each surgeon. Most surgeons remove the NG tube immediately and begin feeding within the first 4 to 6 hours after surgery if bowel sounds are normal. Because gastric peristalsis is normally depressed for 12 to 18 hours after the pyloromyotomy, others delay feedings for 24 hours and leave the NG tube in place.

Feeding is started with small amounts of an oral electrolyte solution such as Pedialyte and the amount is slowly increased. Formula is offered in half-strength concentrations and advanced to full strength within 48 hours after surgery. If the child is receiving breast milk, dilution is not necessary. Feedings are not advanced until the child can tolerate the previous amount without vomiting. Intravenous fluids are continued until the infant is taking and retaining sufficient amounts of formula.

> Approximately one third of all infants experience some vomiting during the early postoperative periods, but vomiting is usually temporary and without complications.

Postoperative nursing care follows the same guidelines as preoperative care with accurate monitoring of all vital signs, laboratory values, respiratory problems, and hydration. In addition, the small surgical incision should be assessed for redness, swelling, or drainage. Parents should be encouraged to participate as much as possible in their child's care, but they may need emotional support in the unfamiliar environment of the hospital setting.

Home Care. Because symptoms normally abate in the immediate postoperative period, parents may find taking care of their infant much easier than it had been before repair. However, they need to be instructed to report any excessive vomiting, abdominal tenderness, fever, incisional redness, or drainage. If the child is discharged before the diet has been fully advanced to full strength, written instructions about how the diet should be advanced are essential.

Evaluation

- Are intake and output balanced?
- Does the child have a flat fontanel, good skin turgor, moist mucous membranes, urine specific gravity ≤ 1.025, and sodium level within normal limits?
- Is the child tolerating previous oral feedings without vomiting?
- Has weight returned to pre-illness level?
- Is surgical site clean, dry, intact, and without drainage or redness?
- Can parents explain need for surgery and routine preoperative and postoperative care?
- Have parents assumed all care responsibilities?

Ulcers

A peptic ulcer is an area of sharply circumscribed loss of the mucosa, submucosa, or muscular tissue occurring in areas of the digestive tract exposed to acid and pepsin. Peptic ulcers can be either primary or secondary, gastric or duodenal. Primary or idiopathic ulcers occur in the absence of underlying systemic disease. Secondary or stress ulcers are acute and are found in conjunction with other illnesses such as shock, respiratory failure, sepsis, hypoglycemia, severe burns, or intracranial lesions.

Gastric ulcers occur in the stomach, particularly the gastric antrum, and are uncommon in childhood. Duodenal ulcers occur in the pylorus or duodenum, are often chronic in nature, frequently lead to complications, and are the most commonly encountered ulcers in children.

Etiology. Known factors that can alter the mucus–bicarbonate barrier in children include the following:

Bile salts: Bile breaks down adherent mucous structure of the gastric-duodenal lining and exposes the mucosa to acid.

Lack of prostaglandins: Prostaglandins augment both the mucus gel lining and bicarbonate secretion. Deficiencies of mucosal prostaglandins may cause impairment of the mucus–bicarbonate barrier.

Genetic factors: There may be a familial tendency for duodenal ulcers. This together with environmental factors may predispose children to ulcer formation. An association between ulcer activity and blood type O is also noted.

Bacteria: *Helicobacter pylori (H. pylori)* is a gram-negative spiral bacteria that has been identified in the gastric antrum of children with duodenal ulcer. It infects the majority of adults with ulcer disease. It acts by weakening the gastric mucosal barrier and allowing acid and peptic digestion of the susceptible mucosa.

Psychological factors: Importance of psychological factors is questionable. They likely influence exacerbations or complications but not initial ulcer activity.

Stress: Stress accounts for at least 80% of secondary ulcers encountered during infancy and early childhood. They tend to be acute and occur in seriously ill children.

Diet: Diet does not seem to influence the development of ulcer disease in children. Although certain foods may cause indigestion, there is no convincing data that dietary factors cause, perpetuate, or reactivate ulcers, especially duodenal. However, colas, teas, and chocolate do increase acid secretions and may play a factor.

Medications: Many medications such as aspirin, nonsteroidal anti-inflammatory agents, indomethacin, tobacco, and alcohol are known to adversely affect the gastroduodenal mucosa in adults but appear to have little importance in pediatric ulcer disease.

PATHOPHYSIOLOGY *of Ulcers*

The stomach and duodenum are lined by a thick mucus–bicarbonate barrier, a layer of mucus that provides a buffer zone for acid neutralization. Stomach acids diffuse slowly through this layer toward the gastric wall, but are encountered and neutralized by slowly diffusing bicarbonate ions liberated from surface epithelial cells. The establishment of a neutral pH at the gastric epithelial surface provides protection from the combined effects of acid and pepsin. Ulcers result when any imbalance in the process occurs and erosions develop on the surface of the gastric or duodenal mucosa.

Incidence. The true incidence of peptic ulcer disease in children is unknown because ulcers often spontaneously heal before a diagnosis is made. The average age for ulcer activity is 11 to 12 years, with boys affected 2 to 3 times more than girls. Duodenal ulcers occur more frequently in children over age 6 years; children under age 6 frequently develop gastric ulceration. Stress ulcers account for 80% of ulcers occurring during infancy and early childhood, affect both sexes, and are equally distributed between the stomach and duodenum.

Clinical Manifestations

- Burning, cramping pain when stomach is empty
- Awakening during the night or early morning hours complaining of abdominal discomfort
- Vomiting in children under age 6 years
- Hematemesis and melena common in infants and young children
- Anorexia

Diagnostic Evaluation. Fiberoptic upper endoscopy is the diagnostic tool of choice for all children, including neonates. Endoscopy not only provides direct visualization of the lining of the esophagus, stomach, and proximal duodenum, but also creates a mechanism for biopsies or cultures. Other tests include ultrasound to rule out gallstones, tumors, or mechanical obstruction. Fecal **occult blood** samples may be done to check for GI bleeding.

Therapeutic Management. Medical management is the most common treatment for ulcer disease in children. Factors that are considered for ulcer treatment include drug safety, symptom relief, patient and parent compliance, and the prevention of complications or ulcer recurrence. A bland diet with milk and small frequent feedings was long felt to be the mainstay of ulcer therapy. It has been shown, however, that the protein and calcium in milk actually stimulate more acid secretions than they buffer. A regular diet low in caffeine is now generally prescribed because caffeine is a potent stimulant of acid secretion and exacerbates GER. A diet high in fiber and polyunsaturated oils may also play a role in ulcer prevention (Andrews, 1994).

Medications now are considered the first line of treatment. They include antacids, H_2-receptor antagonists, mucosal protective agents, and prokinetic agents. See the Commonly Used Medications table in the Clinical Reference Pages for a discussion of their actions, dosage, side effects, and nursing implications.

Surgery is indicated for management of ulcer complications such as hemorrhage, perforation, or obstruction. Vagotomy, pyloroplasty, ligation of a bleeding vessel, or closure of a perforation may be performed.

If the child is actively bleeding, an NG tube is inserted to remove blood, decompress the stomach, and estimate blood loss. Intravenous fluids, oxygen, blood replacement, and vasoactive drugs like Pitressin (vasopressin) may be given. Balloon tamponade with a Sengstaken-Blakemore tube may be indicated. Blood or clots are removed with room temperature gastric lavage. The use of iced saline lavage to stop GI bleeding is no longer advocated because it increases bleeding and clotting times and prolongs the prothrombin time. It also imposes a risk of hypothermia on an already compromised child.

Long-term prognosis for peptic ulcer disease diagnosed in children remains controversial; however, marked improvement in symptoms is noted with the use of H_2-blockers and other medications. Without adequate treatment, peptic ulcer disease frequently persists into adult life.

NURSING CARE OF THE CHILD WITH ULCERS

Assessment

Nursing assessment of the child with peptic ulcer disease begins with a thorough history, including family history of ulcer disease, past episodes of abdominal pain, or recent stressful events in the home, school, or community. A complete assessment of pain includes the nature of pain and its location; its relationship to meals, defecation, or voiding; episodes of nocturnal pain; and medications being used to effectively relieve the pain. The child is examined for the presence of epigastric tenderness, nausea, vomiting, abdominal distension, hematemesis, melena, or recent changes in appetite or eating habits. All stools and emesis should be checked for the presence of blood. Bowel sounds are auscultated for 5 minutes. If vomiting is present the child is assessed for signs of dehydration. If bleeding is observed, the child is monitored for changes in vital signs, and the physician is notified immediately. Finally, the family is assessed for their understanding of the disease, the presence of a viable support system, and their ability to participate in their child's care.

Nursing Diagnosis and Planning

The following nursing diagnoses and expected outcomes are appropriate following assessment of the child with ulcers:

- Altered Nutrition: Less Than Body Requirements related to vomiting, anorexia, and pain. ***Expected Outcome:*** *The child will tolerate normal diet without vomiting and will continue to grow according to growth chart.*
- Fluid Volume Deficit related to vomiting or hemorrhage. ***Expected Outcome:*** *The child will have moist mucous membranes, good skin turgor, and urine output of at least 1–2 ml/kg/hr.*
- Pain related to gastritis or duodenal ulceration. ***Expected Outcome:*** *The child will remain free from abdominal pain; be free of complications of bleeding and perforation.*
- Risk for Noncompliance related to unpalatable prolonged medical therapy. ***Expected Outcome:*** *The child will take medication as prescribed.*
- Knowledge Deficit related to disease, diagnosis, and treatment regimen. ***Expected Outcome:*** *The child/parents will identify events that may be contributing to stress and anxiety; verbalize an understanding of ulcer development and the rationale for diagnostic tests, medications, and surgery; describe signs and symptoms of complications and side effects of medications; assume responsibility for all home care.*

Implementation

One of the first nursing interventions is preparing the child for diagnostic tests. Because fiberoptic endoscopy is often used, the child must be prepared for conscious sedation. Keeping the child NPO for at least 6 hours, maintaining an IV, and monitoring vital signs and respiratory function during the procedure are nursing responsibilities. Upper GI examinations and ultrasound may also be used.

The major focus of nursing interventions is teaching. Please see Teaching Guidelines for the Child with an Ulcer for a discussion of medication information, dietary restrictions, and complications that must be understood by the parents and child. See also the table of common medications in the Clinical Reference Pages.

Home Care. Ulcers are managed almost exclusively in the home environment so teaching, follow-up, and home health referral are essential. Correct use of medications and dietary modifications are parental responsibilities that may require educational materials, emotional support, help with time organization, and encouragement to continue even when symptoms are relieved. See Teaching Guidelines for the Child With Ulcers.

Evaluation

- Is child tolerating his regular diet without vomiting?
- Has weight returned to pre-illness level?
- Is child well hydrated with moist mucous membranes, good skin turgor, urine specific gravity $\leq$ 1.025, and balanced intake and output?
- Is child free from complaints of abdominal pain?
- Is child taking and tolerating all medications?
- Can parents and child (if age-appropriate) explain the disease process, the diagnostic tests, dietary restriction, and medications?
- Are medications being administered correctly?
- Can parents explain warning signs that require immediate physician notification?

TEACHING GUIDELINES *for the Child With an Ulcer*

Explain the pathophysiology of ulcer development, its causes, diagnosis, and therapeutic management.
- Emphasize its relationship to acute illness.
- Help the older child identify sources of excess stress in his life that can be modified.
- Teach stress reduction activities such as relaxation, exercise, and support groups.

Prepare parents for medication administration.
- See Clinical Reference Pages for complete discussion of common ulcer drugs.
- Do not administer antacids within 1 hour of other antiulcer medications.
- Do not stop when symptoms improve; continue for full 6–8 weeks.
- Do not use aspirin or other nonsteroidal anti-inflammatory drugs as they may cause bleeding.
- Do not use over-the-counter relief without physician knowledge.
- Do not add other drugs without physician knowledge since metabolism and absorption may be altered by ulcer medications.

Help parents make changes in diet as prescribed.
- Provide well-balanced diet with many choices for the child who is anorexic.
- Seek assistance from dietary services as needed.
- Provide meals and snacks every 2–3 hours.
- Avoid coffee, chocolate, and caffeine.
- Avoid foods that cause the child discomfort.

Teach parents complications and side effects. Give parents a list of complications that should be reported including:
- Coffee ground emesis
- Weight loss
- Tarry stools
- Increased pain
- Diarrhea
- Vomiting
- Any CNS changes, especially dyskinesias.

KEY CONCEPTS

- The GI system is formed in the first 4 weeks of embryologic development, so congenital defects can be traced to this period.
- Development is anatomically complete at birth but physiologically immature, affecting enzyme secretion, capacity, and sphincter tone.
- Assessment of GI distress is very difficult in small children and must include a thorough history, physical assessment, and general appraisal of the child's distress, as well as the parent's perception of the child's pain.
- Fluid balance is very quickly affected if the child is experiencing vomiting, diarrhea, or anorexia so the nurse must assess changes quickly and completely.
- Gastroesophageal alterations often put the child at risk for respiratory distress secondary to aspiration and compression of the abdomen into the pulmonary spaces. Assessment of respiratory function and maintaining the airway are critical interventions.
- Medications play a crucial role in management of some upper GI alterations so the nurse must be aware of dosages, indications, side effects, and teaching needs.
- Emotional needs of parents need to be addressed quickly if the child has a congenital condition.
- Home care and teaching have a high priority because parents manage many of these alterations at home or after surgical repair.
- Community and home health resources are a critical part of nursing care for the child with these alterations.

REFERENCES

American Academy of Pediatrics Task Force on Infant Position and SIDS. (1992). Positioning and SIDS. *Pediatrics, 89,* 1120–1126.

Andrews, C. (1994). Ulcer-healing drugs and their actions and side effects. *Nursing Times, 90*(33), 38–40.

Barone, M. (1996). *The Harriet Lane handbook: A manual for pediatric house officers* (12 ed.). St. Louis: C. V. Mosby.

Behrman, R. E., Kliegman, R. M., & Arvin, A. M. (1995). *Nelson textbook of pediatrics* (15th ed.). Philadelphia: W. B. Saunders.

Borkowski, S. (1994). Common pediatric surgical problems. *Nursing Clinics of North America, 29*(4), 551–562.

Hubbard, P. (1994). Medication review: Cisapride. *ANNA Journal, 21*(6), 374–380.

Huddleston, K., Vitarelli, R., Goodmundson, J., & Kok, S. (1989). MIC or Foley: Comparing gastrostomy tubes. *Maternal Child Nursing, 14*(1), 20–26.

Huth, M., & O'Brien, M. (1987). The gastrostomy feeding button. *Pediatric Nursing, 13*(4), 241–245.

Neal, J., & Slayton, D. (1992). Neonatal and pediatric PEG tubes. *Maternal Child Nursing, 17*(4), 184–191.

Orenstein, S. R. (1990). Prone position in infant GE reflux: Is elevation of the head worth the trouble? *Journal of Pediatrics, 117*(2), 184–187.

Orenstein, S. R. (1992). GE reflux. *Pediatric Review, 13*(5), 174–182.

Resnick, J., & Zarem, H. (1996). Diseases and injuries of the oral region. In F. D. Burg, J. R. Ingelfinger, W. R. Wald, & R. A. Polin (Eds.), *Gellis and Kagan's current pediatric therapy 15.* Philadelphia: W. B. Saunders.

Richard, M. (1994a). Common pediatric craniofacial reconstructions. *Nursing Clinics of North America, 29*(4), 791–799.

Richard, M. (1994b). Weight comparisons of infants with complete cleft lip and palate. *Pediatric Nursing,* (2), 191–196.

Richard, M. (1991). Feeding the newborn with cleft lip and/or palate: The enlargement, stimulate, swallow, and rest (ESSR) method. *Journal of Pediatric Nursing, 6*(5), 317–321.

Shannon, R. (1993). Gastroesophageal reflux in infancy: Review and update. *Journal of Pediatric Health Care, 7*(2), 71–75.

Sterling, C., Jolley, S., Besser, A., & Matteson-Kane, M. (1991). Nursing responsibility in the diagnosis, care, and treatment of the child with gastroesophageal reflux. *Journal of Pediatric Nursing, 6*(5), 331–336.

BIBLIOGRAPHY

Berube, M., & Parrish, R. (1994). Home care of the infant with gastroesophageal reflux and respiratory disease. *Journal of Pediatric Health Care, 8*(4), 173–180.

Bockus, H. L. (1985). *Gastroenterology.* Philadelphia: W. B. Saunders.

Bockus, S. (1991). Troubleshooting your tube feedings. *American Journal of Nursing, 91*(5), 24–30.

Composto, R., & Eichelberger, C. (1992). Congenital diaphragmatic hernia: Pathophysiology and nursing care. *Neonatal Network, 11*(6), 57–61.

Curtin, G. (1990). The infant with cleft lip or palate: More than a surgical problem. *Journal of Perinatal/Neonatal Nursing, 3*(3), 80–89.

Eisenberg, R. (1990). *Gastrointestinal radiology: A pattern approach.* Philadelphia: J. B. Lippincott.

Eliason, M. (1991). Cleft lip and palate: Developmental effects. *Journal of Pediatric Nursing, 6*(2), 107–113.

Fishbach, F. (1988). *A manual of laboratory diagnostic tests* (3rd ed.). Philadelphia: J. B. Lippincott.

Haas-Beckert, B., & Heyman, M. (1993). Comparison of two skin-level gastrostomy feeding tubes for infants and children. *Pediatric Nursing, 19*(4), 351–354.

Hagelgans, N., & Janusz, B. (1994). Pediatric skin care issues for the home care nurse: Part 2. *Pediatric Nursing, 20*(1), 69–76.

Kenner, C., Brueggermeyer, A., & Gunderson, L. (1993). *Comprehensive neonatal nursing: A physiologic perspective.* Philadelphia: W. B. Saunders.

Kent, P., & Curley, M. (1992). Challenges in nursing: Infants with congenital diaphragmatic hernia. *Heart and Lung, 21*(4), 381–389.

Kirks, D. (1984). *Practical pediatric imaging: Diagnostic radiology of infants and children.* Boston: Little, Brown.

Litwack-Saleh, K. (1993). Practical points in the care of the patient post-cleft lip and palate repair. *Journal of Post Anesthesia Nursing, 8*(1), 35–37.

McCance, K., & Huether, S. (1994). *Pathophysiology: The biologic basis for disease in adults and children.* St. Louis: C. V. Mosby.

Moreno, C., & Iovanne, B. (1993a). Congenital diaphragmatic hernia: Part I. *Neonatal Network, 12*(1), 19–27.

Moreno, C., & Iovanne, B. (1993b). Congenital diaphragmatic hernia: Part II. *Neonatal Network, 12*(2), 21–27.

Purtilo, D., & Purtilo, R. (1989). *A survey of human diseases.* Boston: Little, Brown.

Roberts, A. (1991). Systems of life: The digestive system Part 1. *Nursing Times, 87*(11), 45–48.

Roberts, A. (1991). Systems of life: The digestive system Part 2. *Nursing Times, 87*(15), 65–68.

Sleisenger, M., & Fordtran, J. (1993). *GI diseases: Pathophysiology, diagnosis and management.* Philadelphia: W. B. Saunders.

Smith, J. (1988). Big differences in little people. *AJN, 88*(4), 459–462.

Sterling, C., Schaffer, S., & Jolley, S. (1993). Home management related to medical treatment for childhood gastroesophageal reflux. *Pediatric Nursing, 19*(2), 167–173.

Wellman, C., & Coughlin, S. (1991). Preoperative and postoperative nutritional management of the infant with cleft palate. *Journal of Pediatric Nursing, 6*(3), 154–158.

Yeo, H. (1992). Surgical intervention of esophageal atresia with tracheoesophageal fistula. *Professional Nurse, 8*(1), 50–53.

Yetter, J. F. (1992). Cleft lip and cleft palate. *American Family Physician, 46*(4), 1211–1221.

Young, R., & Murray, N. (1991). Adapting intravenous pumps for enteral feeding. *Maternal Child Nursing, 16*(4), 212–216.

26

The Child With Lower Gastrointestinal Alterations

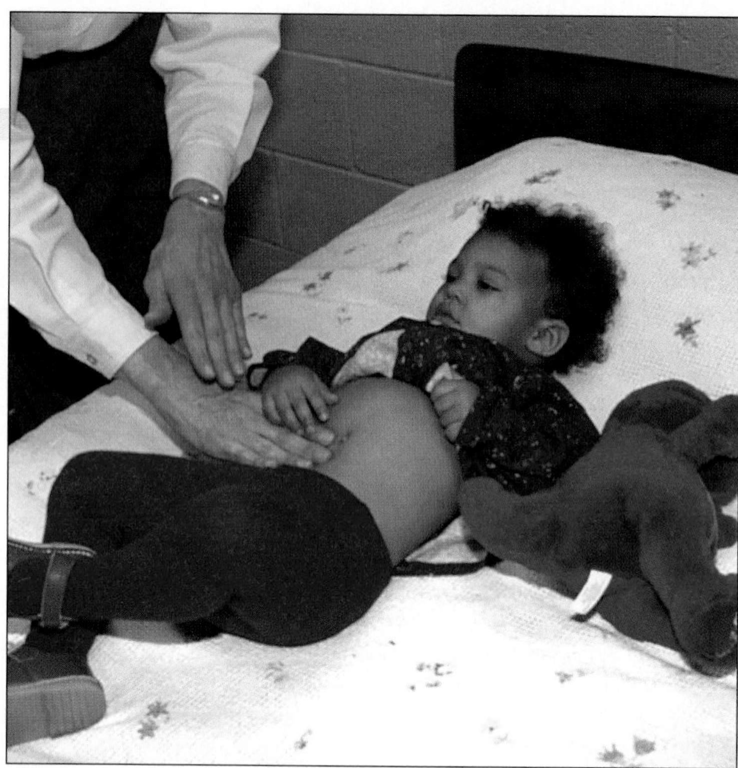

CHAPTER OVERVIEW

LEARNING OBJECTIVES

After studying this chapter, you should be able to:

- Describe the development of the lower gastrointestinal (GI) system and its relationship to selected congenital defects.
- Describe the anatomy and physiology of the GI system in the infant and child.
- Describe the normal physiology of the liver and its functions.
- Describe the common diagnostic and screening tests used with alterations in lower GI function.
- Identify the nursing implications of common medications used in the treatment of lower GI alterations.
- Discuss and display an understanding of the pathophysiology, etiology, clinical manifestations, diagnostic evaluation, and therapeutic management of the following disorders: lactose intolerance, celiac disease, Hirschsprung's disease, abdominal wall defects, constipation, irritable bowel syndrome, imperforate anus, intussusception, Crohn's disease, ulcerative colitis, appendicitis, infectious gastroenteritis, biliary atresia, hepatitis, and cirrhosis.
- State expected nursing diagnoses for lower GI alterations.
- Use the nursing process to develop nursing care plans and teaching guidelines for the child with lower GI alterations.
- Develop guidelines for home care for the child with lower GI alterations.

KEY TERMS

acholic: free from bile

atresia: congenital absence or closure of a body orifice; obliteration of a tubular organ

encopresis: fecal incontinence after age 4 years

fistula: abnormal communication between two organs or from one organ to the outside of the body

ganglion: a cluster of nerve cells outside the central nervous system; responsible for intestinal peristalsis

ileocecal valve: the ringlike mucous membrane at the junction of the terminal ileum and cecum

levator ani muscle: part of pelvic diaphragm, responsible for elevating anus into correct area in embryologic development

McBurney's point: one-half to 2 inches from the right anterior superior iliac spine, a point of special tenderness in appendicitis

meconium: first stool passed by neonate; greenish-black, sticky substance that results from bile, epithelial cells, and amniotic fluid in the GI tract

portoenterostomy: a connection created from the portal system to the GI system, specifically diverting bile from liver tracts to jejunum

tenesmus: ineffective, painful, or continuous urge to defecate

transmural: through all layers of the wall of a cavity

villi: small finger-like projections in the mucosa of the intestine; responsible for absorption

The child with a lower gastrointestinal (GI) alteration has many special needs. Because of the regular necessity of eating and elimination, lower GI problems affect many aspects of daily life. Medications, surgery, diet alterations, and special elimination needs become a way of life for many children. Activity level, growth and development, and even lifespan can be affected.

The nurse plays a vital role with these children. Providing care during surgical and acute care of the illness is only the beginning. Because of the chronic nature of some of these conditions, the nurse must coordinate care with other specialties and arrange long-term follow-up for children and their families. Community and home-based care are essential components of care, and the nurse's role must include teaching, nutritional support, emotional support, stomal management, and integration with all health care professionals involved in the child's care.

CLINICAL REFERENCE PAGES

Pediatric Differences in the Lower GI System

- Because the neonate's delicate tissues are unable to secrete adequate amounts of enzymes and fluids, infection and trauma can develop. Vomiting and diarrhea often result.
- The immature neonatal liver is not yet efficient in its detoxifying ability, which causes diminished vitamin and mineral breakdown.
- In the neonate, the large intestine is relatively short, with less epithelial lining to absorb water from a fecal mass. As a result, stools have a soft consistency, with more rapid peristalsis.

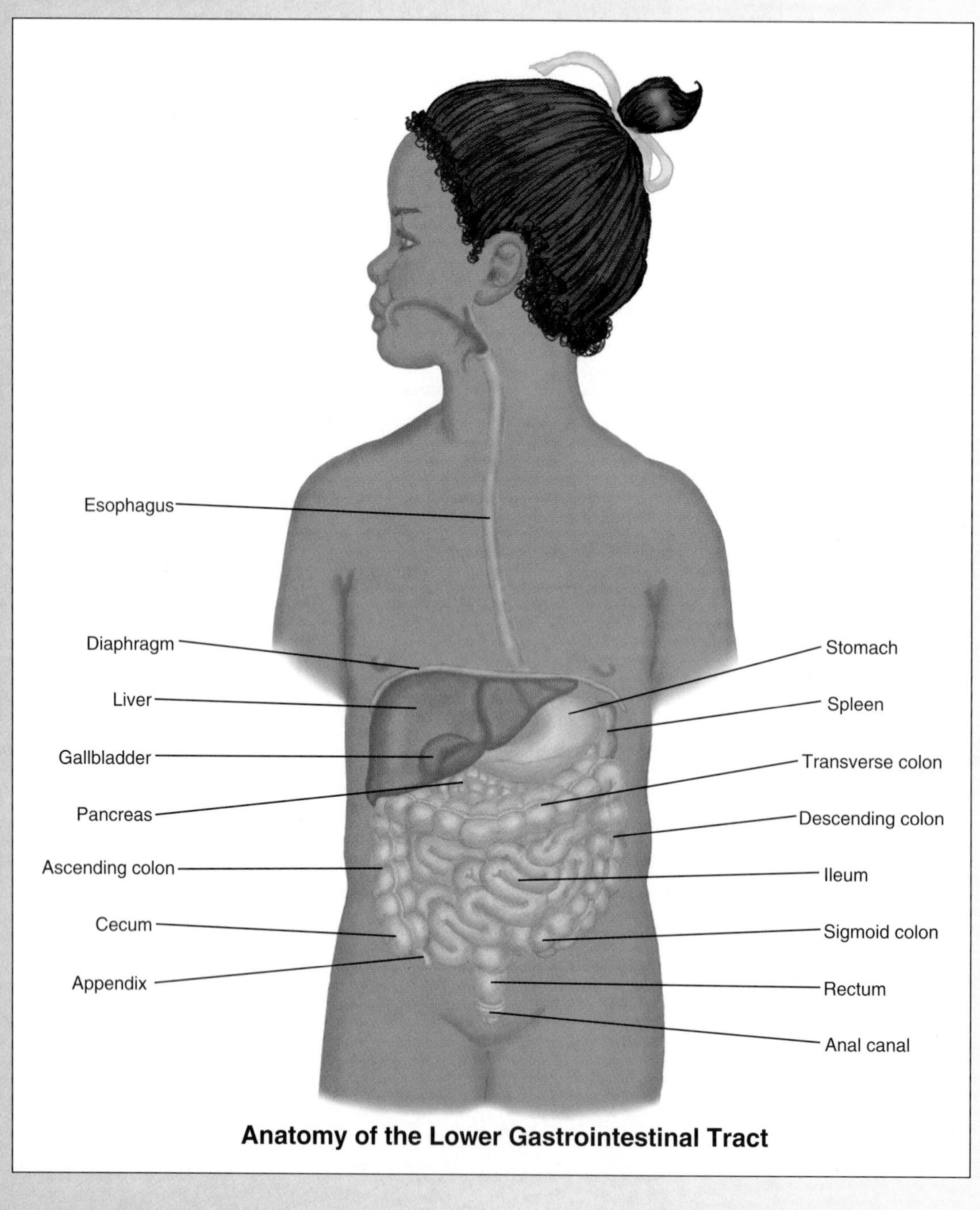

Anatomy of the Lower Gastrointestinal Tract

ANATOMY AND PHYSIOLOGY REVIEW

The lower GI system includes the duodenum, liver, gallbladder, pancreas, jejunum, ileum, cecum, appendix, ascending colon, transverse colon, descending colon, sigmoid colon, rectum, and anus. The primary functions of the lower GI tract are to digest and absorb nutrients, to detoxify and excrete unwanted waste, and to aid in fluid and electrolyte balance.

The *duodenum* is the first part of the small intestine, extending from the pylorus to the jejunum. Partially digested chyme from the stomach enters the duodenum, where pancreatic enzymes and bile are excreted to further break down fats, carbohydrates, and proteins.

The *pancreas* is an oblong gland lying behind the stomach that secretes enzymes to digest food and glucagon and insulin to control motility and absorption.

The *liver,* the largest organ in the body, is located under the right diaphragm. The liver lies predominantly in the right upper quadrant, with the left lobe extending into the left upper quadrant. It is divided into two lobes separated by the falciform ligament. Within each lobe are numerous lobules, which form the functional units of the liver. It is unique in that it is supplied with blood from two sources: (1) the hepatic artery supplies oxygenated blood, and (2) the hepatic portal vein supplies deoxygenated blood with absorbed nutrients from the GI tract. The liver has numerous functions, including phagocytosis, bile production, detoxification, glycogen storage and breakdown, and vitamin storage. The production of bile is essential for the absorption of fat and excretion of the end products of blood cell breakdown.

The primary function of the *gallbladder,* a sac-like structure attached to the underside of the right lobe of the liver, is to store bile for secretion into the duodenum when stimulated by the presence of fat in its lumen.

The *jejunum* and *ileum* form the remainder of the small intestine. Absorption of all nutrients and vitamins occurs here through the *villi* and microvilli by the processes of diffusion and active transport. Absorption of vitamin B_{12} occurs only in the terminal ileum.

The large intestine starts with the *cecum.* This blind pouch, 2 to 3 inches long, begins at the **ileocecal valve,** which prevents reverse peristalsis into the small intestine. Attached to it is the *appendix,* a worm-like tube about 3 inches long. The open end of the cecum attaches to the remainder of the colon, which is divided into four sections: the *ascending, transverse, descending,* and *sigmoid colon.* One major function of the large intestine is water reabsorption, which occurs mostly in the cecum and ascending colon. Intestinal bacteria ferment the remaining CHO and aid in the synthesis of B vitamins and vitamin K. Final breakdown of bile occurs here. Mucus secretion and peristalsis of wastes are also important functions.

The *rectum* is the last 7 to 8 inches of the intestine, and the *anal canal* refers to the last 1 to 2 inches. Stool is stored in the rectum until distension of the rectal walls initiates the defecation reflex, the final stage of the GI processes.

Major Digestive Enzymes. See table.

Prenatal Development. The GI system is formed from the endoderm in the first 4 weeks of embryologic development. The primitive gut then gives rise to three separate sections of the GI tract, each with its own blood supply and own rate of development:

- Foregut: from pharynx to duodenum including the liver, pancreas, biliary tract
- Midgut: from duodenum to transverse colon
- Hindgut: descending colon, rectum, anal canal

Problems in the development of each of these three sections give rise to different malformations and disease states. Anatomically, the development is complete at birth, but physiologically, the GI tract is immature.

MAJOR DIGESTIVE ENZYMES

	ENZYME	FUNCTION
Mouth	Amylase	Complex carbohydrate to simple carbohydrate
Stomach	Pepsin	Proteins to proteoses
Small Intestine	Enterokinase Peptidases Sucrase, maltase, lactase	Activates trypsin Peptides to amino acids Disaccharides to monosaccharides
Pancreas	Trypsin Lipase Amylase	Peptides to amino acids Fat to fatty acids and glycerol Carbohydrates to disaccharides
Liver, Gallbladder	Bile	Emulsifies fat, allowing lipase to function Increases fat and fat-soluble vitamin absorption

COMMON LABORATORY AND DIAGNOSTIC TESTS

	DESCRIPTION	NORMAL FINDINGS	INDICATIONS	PREPARATION AND NURSING IMPLICATIONS
		Stool		
Culture and Sensitivity	Organisms from a small sample of stool are grown in culture media	Normal GI flora	To identify organisms and determine their antibiotic sensitivity (e.g., infectious diarrhea)	• No preparation • Deliver to laboratory immediately. • Keep free from contamination.
Reducing Substances (Clinitest)	Stool diluted with water and then tested for undigested carbohydrates using Clinitest tablets	Negative	Malabsorption syndromes (e.g., lactose intolerance, sprue, chronic diarrhea)	• No preparation • Done by nurse • Check for color change in solution.
Occult Blood (Guaiac, Hematest)	Stool smeared on filter paper and prepared with solution	Negative	Inflammatory conditions, bowel necrosis (e.g., inflammatory bowel disease, *Shigella*, intussusception)	• No preparation • Done by nurse • Blue is positive.
Leukocytes	Stool smeared on slide and examined microscopically for PMNs	Negative	Inflammatory conditions, gastroenteritis (e.g., *Shigella*)	• No preparation • Send stool sample or rectal swab to laboratory.
		Urine		
Urobilinogen	Dipstick or lab analysis to determine bile by-products in urine	Negative	Hepatic dysfunction and obstruction (e.g., hepatitis, biliary atresia, cirrhosis)	• No preparation • Done by nurse
		Blood		
Liver Function Tests	Serum levels measured to give indication of liver function	LDH: 150–300 U/L AST: 0–34 IU/L ALT: 1–37 IU/L Total bilirubin: 0.2–1.0 mg/dl Ammonia: 15–45 U/dl	Suspected liver problems (e.g., biliary atresia, hepatitis, cirrhosis)	• No preparation • Venipuncture
Breath Hydrogen Test	Carbohydrate solution given PO and exhaled breath samples collected over 3 hours	Less than 20 ppm above baseline	Maldigestion/malabsorption syndromes (e.g., lactose intolerance, celiac disease). Inadequately digested carbohydrate produces hydrogen when acted on by GI flora.	• Child prepares by fasting for 4–12 hours. • Noninvasive • May require face mask to collect expired air • Nurse provides teaching about procedure.

Colonoscopy	Direct viewing of colon using fiberoptic scope and camera inserted per rectum	Normal mucosa, patent bowel	Identifies mucosal changes and abnormalities in the lumen of the colon (e.g., celiac disease, inflammatory bowel disease)	Preparation includes • NPO • teaching • bowel cleansing • sedation
Biopsy (Jejunal, Rectal, Liver)	Small piece of tissue is removed for analysis	No abnormal tissue	Determines amount of mucosal inflammation and the absence of ganglion cells (e.g., Hirschsprung's disease, hepatitis, biliary atresia, celiac disease, cirrhosis)	Preparation includes • teaching • bowel cleansing • sedation or anesthesia if percutaneous (liver)
		Radiologic Examinations		
Abdominal Flat Plate	Anterior and posterior X-rays		Identifies stool and gas patterns, inflammation, patency of GI tract (e.g., abdominal pain, imperforate anus, intussusception, appendicitis)	• Usually no preparation other than teaching
Barium Enema, Air Contrast Barium Enema	Radiopaque contrast media and/or air placed in large intestine via rectum		Identifies abnormalities in the surface of the bowel lumen and determines patency of bowel. Provides hydrostatic reduction of intussception (e.g., inflammatory bowel disease, Hirschsprung's disease, imperforate anus)	Preparation includes • NPO • teaching • bowel cleansing Adequate fluids essential after exam to prevent barium impaction.
Ultrasound	Noninvasive use of sound waves to identify anatomy and inflammation		Identifies anatomic abnormalities and inflammatory conditions (e.g., appendicitis, imperforate anus)	• Teaching • For pelvic ultrasound, full bladder needed to improve visualization of pelvic organs.

MEDICATIONS COMMONLY USED FOR LOWER GI DISORDERS

	INDICATIONS	DOSE OR ROUTE	COMMON SIDE EFFECTS	NURSING IMPLICATIONS
Lactase Preparations (Lact-aid, Dairy-Ease, Lac-Dose)	Lactose intolerance	Follow over-the-counter directions (varies with product)	Distension	• Available over the counter. • Provide teaching to prevent overuse. • Only useful when taken before or immediately after consumption of dairy products.
GoLYTELY	Bowel cleansing before diagnostic procedures	25–60 ml/kg/hr	Nausea, vomiting, bloating	• Must be given at correct rate until clear fluid passes per rectum. • May need NG tube to ensure this rate in young children.
Mineral Oil	Chronic constipation to decrease pain of defecation	30–75 ml BID	Leakage of oil per rectum; fat-soluble vitamin deficiencies with prolonged use	• Must be continued until passage of stool no longer painful. • Supplement fat-soluble vitamins. • Tasteless and odorless if cold. • May be mixed with juice to increase palatability.
Colace (Docusate Sodium)	To soften stool when treating chronic constipation and encopresis	Age 3–6 yr: 20–60 mg Age 6–12 yr: 40–120 mg per day	Abdominal cramping (rare)	• Increase fluid intake. • Not recommended for extended use. • Available in syrup.
Imodium (Loperamide)	To decrease forward propulsion of stool and increase water reabsorption in diarrhea and irritable bowel syndrome	4–8 mg/day	Constipation, distension, drowsiness	• Discontinue use after 48 hr except in irritable bowel syndrome. • Available over-the-counter.
Lomotil (Diphenoxylate HCl and Atropine Sulfate)	Same as Imodium	0.3–0.4 mg/kg/day in divided doses	May prolong infectious diarrhea by delaying removal of colon toxins; nausea, vomiting, dry mouth, flushing, severe drowsiness, blurred vision.	• Increase fluid intake. • Monitor fluid balance.
			Inflammatory Bowel Disease	
Corticosteroids *Prednisone*	Active flare-ups and initial disease	PO, IM, IV	Related to dose and length of treatment: growth retardation, tendency for infection, Cushingoid changes	• Doses must be tapered when acute disease is contained, and never abruptly discontinued. • High initial dose may be needed. • If PO, give with food.
Cortenema, Proctofoam	Tenesmus, anogenital lesions	Enema	May produce some systemic effects with prolonged use	• Retain for 30 minutes or overnight.
Antibacterial, Anti-inflammatory (Sulfasalazine [Azulfidine])	Chronic management of colonic disease: ulcerative colitis, Crohn's lower bowel	PO, enema	Nausea, vomiting, anorexia, skin rash, headache, anemia	• Start with low doses and increase. • Used with steroids in acute disease. • Give folate supplement.
Antibiotics (Flagyl)	Fistulas in Crohn's	PO, IV	Neurotoxicity, GI complaints	• May not be therapeutic for 2–3 weeks. • Doses high and may cause neurotoxicity.
Antidiarrheals (Lomotil, Imodium)	Crohn's symptom relief	PO	Constipation, drowsiness, blurred vision	• Used sparingly. • Controversial.

Inflammatory bowel disease section adapted with permission from the article "Inflammatory Bowel Disease: Primary Health Care Management of Ulcerative Colitis and Crohn's Disease," from the August, 1991 issue of *The Nurse Practitioner*, © Springhouse Corporation.

DISORDERS OF ABSORPTION AND DIGESTION

Digestive and absorptive disorders are the direct result of an inability of the body to break down or absorb specific nutrients. The two most common in children are celiac disease and lactose intolerance.

Lactose Intolerance

The inability to tolerate lactose, the sugar found in dairy products, is the result of an absence or deficiency of lactase, an enzyme found in the secretions of the small intestine required for the digestion of lactose. There are two types of lactose intolerance: congenital and developmental. Congenital lactose intolerance, which is very rare, appears at birth, with a complete absence of lactase. Developmental lactose intolerance, which is more commonly seen, is a deficiency of lactase that appears in early to late childhood.

> **PATHOPHYSIOLOGY** *of Lactose Intolerance*
>
> An absence or deficiency of lactase leads to an inability to digest lactose and the subsequent accumulation of lactose in the lumen of the small intestine. As a result, water is drawn into the colon, resulting in watery osmotic diarrhea containing undigested lactose. In addition, GI bacteria break down lactose and release hydrogen, which causes excess gas production, bloating, and abdominal pain.

Etiology. Most cases of lactose intolerance are the result of inadequate levels of lactase. The exact reason for this deficiency is unknown. The disease is likely to be more severe during and after other illnesses affecting the GI mucosa, such as viral gastroenteritis or food poisoning.

Incidence. The disease appears to have a racial association, with higher incidence in Asians, Arabs, Jews, African Americans, and southern Europeans.

Clinical Manifestations

- Diarrhea, frothy but not fatty
- Abdominal distension
- Crampy abdominal pain
- Excessive flatus

The symptoms are not usually seen until lactase activity begins to decrease after age 3 years or during other GI insults. If the child has congenital lactose intolerance, symptoms will be immediate and may be severe.

Diagnostic Evaluation. A history of improvement after implementing a lactose-free diet provides a presumptive diagnosis. This can be supported by the finding of 1+ or greater sugars during Clinitest examination of the stool. Breath hydrogen testing may give an indication of the amount of lactase available by indirectly measuring the amount of undigested carbohydrate. (See the table Common Laboratory and Diagnostic Tests in the Clinical Reference Pages.)

Therapeutic Management. The treatment for lactose intolerance is removal of lactose from the diet. In most cases, total elimination is unnecessary. Removing milk as the beverage of choice can provide enough relief from symptoms. Additional dietary changes may be required to provide adequate sources of calcium and, in the infant, protein and calories. Formulas that do not contain lactose (Isomil, Nursoy, Nutramigen, ProSobee, and other soy-based formulas) may be given to the infant suspected of having lactose intolerance.

These dietary changes can be supplemented with the use of commercial lactase preparations (Lact-Aid, Dairy-Ease, Lac-Dose) that can be taken with lactose-containing food to provide adequate lactase levels and variable relief from symptoms.

NURSING CARE OF THE CHILD WITH LACTOSE INTOLERANCE

Assessment

Assessment will reveal a healthy-looking child with episodic abdominal pain and occasional diarrhea without any nutritional deficiencies or other health problems. If the problem is congenital and thus likely to be more severe, diarrhea may be a major concern. The neonate or infant may appear extremely dehydrated, with severe diarrhea and weight loss. The child and family may or may not be able to correlate symptoms with food intake.

Nursing Diagnosis and Planning

The following nursing diagnoses and expected outcomes may be appropriate in the treatment of lactose intolerance in the child.

- Pain related to bloating and flatus. ***Expected Outcomes:*** *The child will be free from abdominal pain, as evidenced by age-appropriate play and activity; have normal bowel sounds with a soft abdomen that is not painful during palpation.*
- Diarrhea related to maldigestion. ***Expected Outcome:*** *The child will have soft, formed stools without evidence of fat.*
- Knowledge Deficit related to dietary changes. ***Expected Outcomes:*** *The child will take in a minimum of 800 mg calcium per day as reported by dietary history. The family will state foods to be avoided or provided in small amounts;*

TEACHING GUIDELINES *for the Child With Lactose Intolerance*

- Provide information about high-lactose foods (i.e., milk, ice cream).
- Help parents eliminate all sources of lactose until symptoms subside.
- Assist parents to find soy-based, lactose-free formulas as needed for infants (Isomil, Nursoy, Nutramigen, ProSobee).
- Encourage breast-feeding mother to limit dairy products.
- Provide information about alternative calcium sources (e.g., egg yolk, green leafy vegetables, dried beans, cauliflower, molasses, supplements).
- Gradually add yogurt, hard cheeses, and small amounts of milk to assess tolerance.
- Teach proper use of lactase products (see table Medications Commonly Used for Lower GI Disorders in the Clinical Reference Pages).
- Refer parents to dietary resources for assistance, ideas, and/or recipes.

provide adequate calcium sources in diet; select appropriate lactase products.

Implementation

The chief nursing intervention is teaching. (See Teaching Guidelines for the Child With Lactose Intolerance.) Symptoms are often relieved after a lactose-free diet is followed for a short time. Foods containing small amounts of lactose may be added gradually after this time to assess the child's reaction. If small amounts of milk are tolerated, it is useful to offer food or lactase preparations simultaneously with milk. These simple changes can offer instant relief.

After diagnosis and initial management, this condition is often perceived to be only a minor nuisance. However, emotional support for the family may be needed. Referring the family to self-help and information groups and encouraging them to share successes and concerns are important nursing interventions.

Evaluation

Is the child happy, content, and free of excess gas and bloating?

Does the child show adequate growth according to a growth chart?

Does food diary indicate intake of at least 800 mg calcium daily for a child age 1 to 10 years?

Has parent sought outside information about dietary changes from dietitian or support group?

Does parent express satisfaction with control of child's condition?

Celiac Disease

Celiac disease, also known as gluten enteropathy or tropical sprue, results from the inability to fully digest the gliadin or protein part of wheat, barley, rye, and oats. This is a lifelong deficiency requiring dietary modification to prevent chronic maldigestion and malabsorption.

Etiology. Celiac disease is considered to be genetic. From 80% to 90% of children with celiac disease have the genetic marker HLA-B8, a human leukocyte antigen complex located on chromosome 6. This chromosomal variation results in the inability to digest gliadin, causing severe GI mucosal changes that continue on exposure to gluten.

Incidence. The incidence of celiac disease varies in different regions. In the United States incidence is about 1:10,000 live births (Behrman, 1996). There is a much higher incidence in Europe. Siblings and children of affected patients have the highest risk of the disease (Auricchio, Greco, & Troncone, 1988).

Clinical Manifestations

- Diarrhea
- Growth failure is present; the child is usually less than 25th percentile on growth charts
- Abdominal distension
- Vomiting
- Anemia
- Irritability and anorexia
- Muscle wasting and edema
- Celiac crisis produces profuse, watery diarrhea, and vomiting

The symptoms are not seen until 3 to 6 months after the introduction of grains to the diet, usually at age 9 to 12 months.

Diagnostic Evaluation. The measurement of serum antigliadin antibody (AGA) is a reliable diagnostic test and allows for continued assessment and evaluation of dietary changes. In the past, this test required specialized laboratory equipment. However, a newer method, the strip AGA test, requires a single drop of blood and results can be determined quickly for approximately $5. Its ease of use makes the diagnosis of celiac disease simpler and more cost effective. The test is also effective in evaluating the adequacy of dietary changes.

Jejunal biopsy will unequivocally identify the presence of ulcerations in the GI tract. The diagnosis is supported by monitoring the reaction to a gluten-free diet.

PATHOPHYSIOLOGY *of Celiac Disease*

Gluten—the protein found in rye, oats, barley, and wheat—breaks down into gliadin and other by-products. Celiac disease results from an inability to digest gliadin. This results in the accumulation of glutamine in the intestine, which has a toxic effect on the mucosal cells. This leads to atrophy of the villi and a marked decrease in the absorptive surface. Malabsorption of fats, carbohydrates, and vitamins develops. *Celiac crisis* is a result of sudden accumulation of glutamine and the subsequent destruction of the mucosal cells causing severe diarrhea and dehydration.

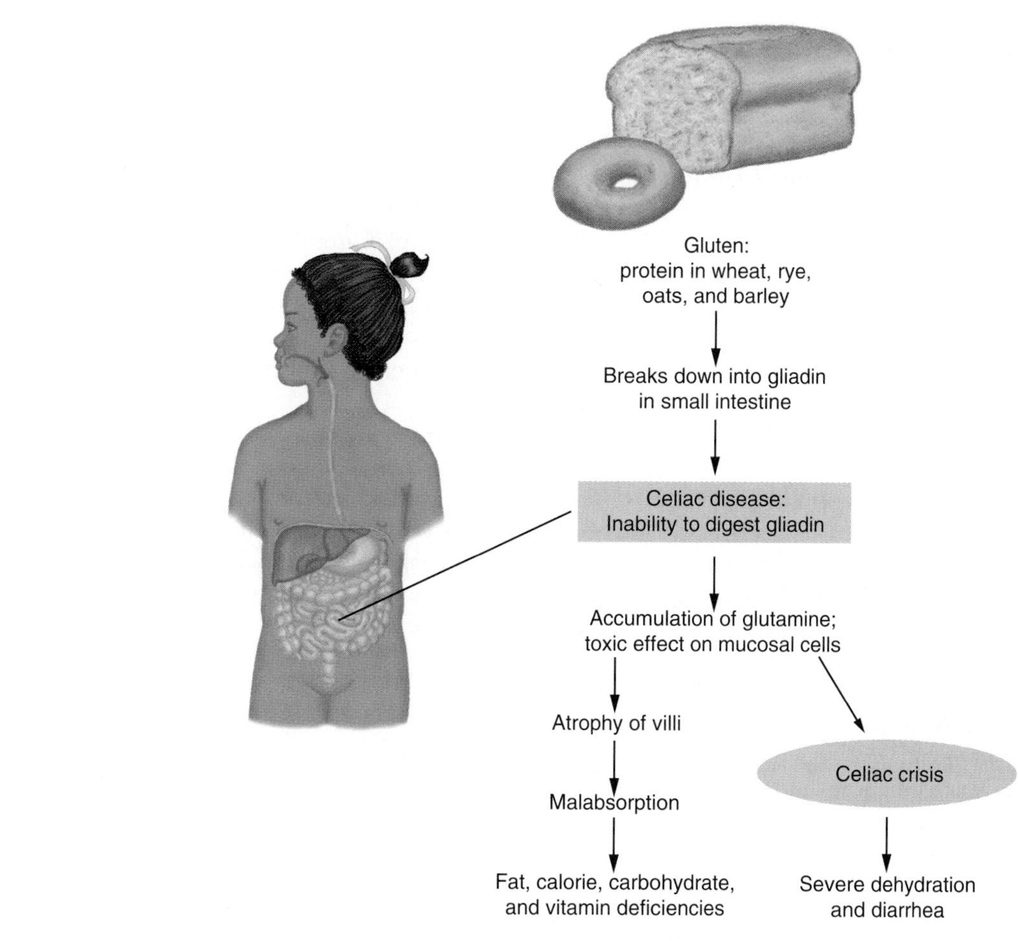

Symptoms are often relieved in one week by removal of gluten from the diet.

Further diagnostic testing can be done using the breath hydrogen excretion test to identify the amount of carbohydrate malabsorption occurring. This test is not specific for sprue. D-Xylose testing indicates the amount of mucosal damage; the remaining absorptive surface can be estimated. (See the table Common Laboratory and Diagnostic Tests in the Clinical Reference Pages.)

Therapeutic Management. Dietary management is the mainstay of treatment. All wheat, rye, barley, and oats should be eliminated from the diet and replaced with corn and rice. Vitamin supplements, especially of fat-soluble vitamins and folate, may be needed in the early period of treatment to correct deficiencies. These restrictions are likely to be lifelong, although small amounts of grains may be tolerated after the ulcerations have healed. Support from dietary services is essential for maintenance.

Occasionally, the child is first seen by a health care provider because of celiac crisis. Celiac crisis causes profuse, watery diarrhea and vomiting and can lead to severe dehydration and metabolic acidosis very quickly. The cause of the crisis—usually infection or hidden sources of gluten—must be identified. The child is given intravenous (IV) fluids to correct fluid and acid-base imbalance, albumin to treat shock, and corticosteroids to decrease severe mucosal inflammation.

NURSING CARE OF THE CHILD WITH CELIAC DISEASE

Assessment

Assessment of the infant with celiac diseases usually reveals an irritable, malnourished, failure-to-thrive infant aged 9 to 12 months. Any child with diarrhea, especially one with foul-smelling, fatty stools and significant growth delays, should be suspected of having this disorder. A noticeable decline in the child's rate of growth as charted on the growth curve, associated with the addition of grains to the diet, is essential supportive evidence.

Abdominal assessment will reveal distension and ascites with an increasing girth; observation will identify other signs of malnutrition such as thin edematous extremities, pallor, and muscle wasting. Anemia is a common finding.

The child who presents with severe diarrhea, foul-smelling stools, vomiting, poor perfusion, edema, or changes in vital signs (shock or metabolic acidosis) should be referred for emergency care of celiac crisis.

Nursing Diagnoses and Planning

The following nursing diagnoses and expected outcomes may be appropriate in the treatment of celiac disease in the infant or child.

- Altered Nutrition: Less Than Body Requirements related to malabsorption. ***Expected Outcome:*** *The infant/child will have soft, formed stools without diarrhea.*
- Pain related to abdominal distension. ***Expected Outcome:*** *The infant/child will be free from abdominal pain, as evidenced by age-appropriate play and activity.*
- Altered Growth and Development related to malnutrition. ***Expected Outcome:*** *The infant/child will return to and follow normal growth pattern on growth chart.*
- Knowledge Deficit related to dietary changes. ***Expected Outcomes:*** *The family will offer appropriate foods to infant/child as evidenced by food diary; state need for lifelong dietary changes; seek emotional and educational support as needed.*
- Fluid Volume Deficit related to celiac crisis. ***Expected Outcome:*** *The infant/child will be adequately hydrated, as evidenced by moist mucous membranes and good skin turgor.*

Implementation

Celiac disease is a lifelong condition that requires significant dietary and lifestyle changes. Continued support is needed for these families.

The chief nursing intervention is teaching parents how to modify their child's diet. (See Teaching Guidelines for the Child With Celiac Disease.) Pain will likely be relieved quickly by elimination of gluten in the diet. Involvement of dietitians and nutritionists in teaching and follow-up is helpful. Careful and consistent follow-up will be necessary to make sure that the infant is able to resume a normal growth and development pattern as soon as possible. When the child has normal stools without diarrhea and resumes her normal growth pattern, teaching will have been effective.

Because this is a lifelong condition, support groups can be useful in managing the problem. The American Celiac Society is an excellent source for information and support (see Appendix H). Referral to this group and other family support organizations is essential. Encourage the parents to share their fears and concerns about the chronic nature of the disease and its impact on their family life.

Evaluation

Does the child have soft, formed stools without diarrhea?

Is the child free of abdominal pain?

Has the child resumed normal growth pattern per growth chart?

Does food diary indicate an intake of approximately 100 kcal/kg for infant through 3-year-old child?

Do parents use available support and education groups?

TEACHING GUIDELINES *for the Child With Celiac Disease*

- Home care by the parent and family is the mainstay of treatment.
- All wheat, rye, barley, oats, and hydrolyzed vegetable protein must be eliminated from the diet.
- Provide information about the use of corn, rice, or millet as substitute grain foods.
- Encourage use of vitamin supplements, especially folate and fat-soluble vitamins.
- Refer to national support groups and dietary resources.
- Read all labels on food and medications carefully to avoid any unknown additives.
- Provide anticipatory guidance to parents of adolescent about adolescents' need to experiment with foods and "go along with the crowd."
- Provide additional counseling and information for the school-age child and adolescent who is becoming independent in food choices.

Do parents express satisfaction with the way they are coping with dietary changes?

ALTERATIONS IN MOTILITY AND DISORDERS OF OBSTRUCTION

Disorders of obstruction and alterations in motility result from blockages in the patency of the GI tract or in its ability to produce normal peristalsis without diarrhea or constipation.

Hirschsprung's Disease

Also known as congenital aganglionosis or megacolon, Hirschsprung's disease is the result of an absence of **ganglion** cells in the rectum and to varying degrees upward in the colon. About 80% of cases affect the rectosigmoid region, 15% progress to the right colon, and 5% involve the entire colon (Hatch, 1988).

Etiology. The disease is a result of an embryologic failure of migration of the hindgut ganglion cells to the most caudal portion of the GI tract, the rectum. The initiating factor in this failure is unknown.

Incidence. Hirschsprung's disease occurs in 1 in 500 live births with a 4:1 male to female ratio (Hatch, 1988). It has a strong hereditary component and a higher incidence in children with Down syndrome.

Clinical Manifestations

- Delayed passage or absence of **meconium** stool in the neonatal period *is the cardinal sign.*
- Chronic constipation beginning in the first month of life results in pellet-like or ribbon stools that are foul-smelling.

PATHOPHYSIOLOGY *of Hirschsprung's Disease*

Ganglions provide parasympathetic innervation of the colon. In Hirschsprung's disease, ganglions are absent from a variable length of colon extending proximally from the anus. Adequate peristalsis cannot occur in the affected colon, leading to a tonic contraction of the lumen. This produces a functional bowel obstruction, chronic constipation, and the passage of ribbon stools. It can lead to a complete bowel obstruction. Because of the constriction of the lumen, huge amounts of feces and gas collect proximal to the aganglionic portion, resulting in a gross enlargement of this segment. The enlarged segment of colon is actually normal in function.

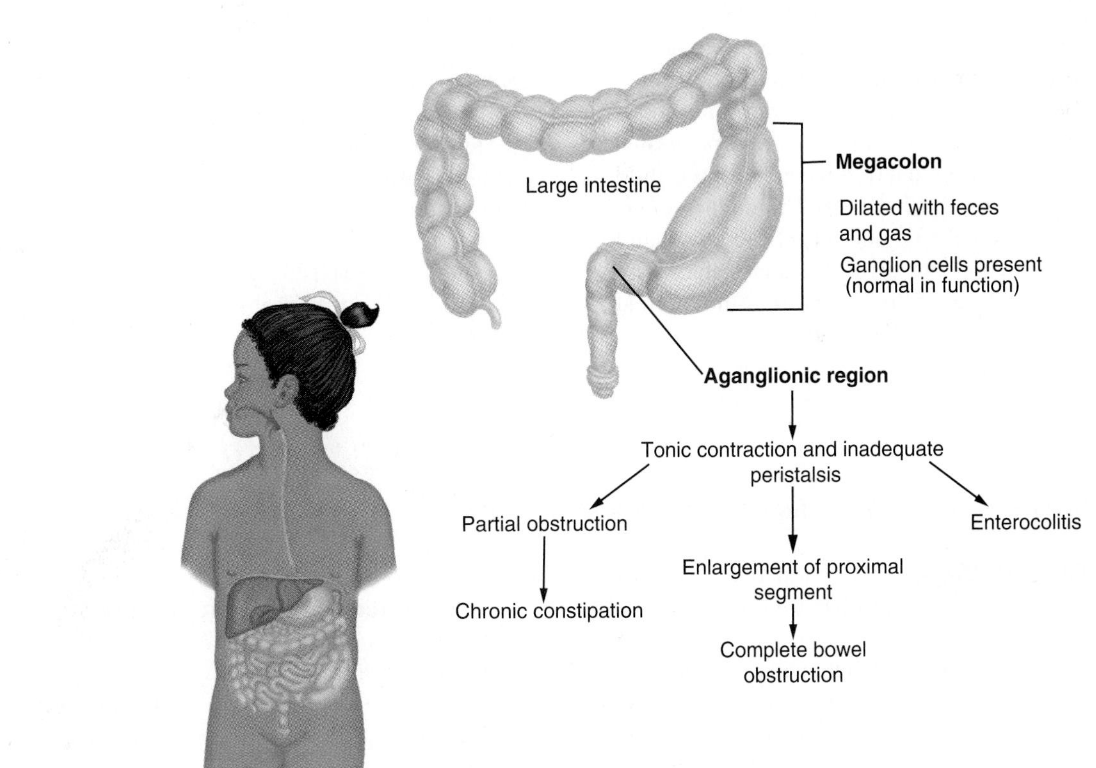

- Bowel obstruction, especially in the neonatal period.
- Abdominal pain and distension
- Failure to thrive

Diagnostic Evaluation

> Any child who fails to pass meconium within the first 24 hours and who is prone to constipation or stool infrequency in the first month after birth is suspected of having Hirschsprung's disease.

Rectal exam will reveal the absence of stool followed by an often explosive release of gas and feces related to the sudden but transient increase in rectal size.

Barium enema will demonstrate an abrupt change in the size of the colon from a very distended ganglionic proximal portion to the contracted, saw-toothed appearance in the aganglionic distal portion, with a "transitional zone" of tapered bowel between them. Significantly, the child will fail to evacuate barium after the examination. The definitive diagnosis is made by rectal biopsy. During biopsy, a small core, or "punch sample," which contains all layers of the bowel mucosa, is removed. Absence of ganglionic cells in the sample confirms the diagnosis of Hirschsprung's disease.

Therapeutic Management. Treatment for mild to moderate Hirschsprung's disease is based on relieving the chronic constipation with stool softeners and rectal irrigations. See the discussion of dietary changes and constipation under Nursing Care, below.

Treatment for moderate to severe Hirschsprung's disease involves removing the aganglionic portion of the intestine in a two-step surgical intervention. In the neonatal period, the obstruction is relieved by performing a temporary colostomy with the most distal section of normal bowel. A complete surgical repair is delayed until the child weighs 8 to 10 kg, at which time a "pull-through" is performed to excise all aganglionic portions of the bowel and reanastomose the normal bowel to the anal canal. The colostomy is closed during this procedure, and normal bowel function returns shortly thereafter.

NURSING CARE OF THE CHILD WITH HIRSCHSPRUNG'S DISEASE

Assessment

The child with Hirschsprung's disease will have constipation that has been present since the neonatal period and frequent passage of foul-smelling ribbon-like or pellet stools. Nutritional status should be assessed because malnutrition can develop secondary to extreme distension or enterocolitis. Thin extremities, abdominal distension, and a history of poor feeding should be noted.

If the child is acutely ill on presentation, enterocolitis must be suspected. Evaluation of bowel sounds and abdominal distension, frequency of vomiting and diarrhea, and changes in abdominal circumference should be documented. Temperature should be assessed by a route other than rectal.

It is important to assess the family's concerns and their methods of dealing with the problem. This disease can drain family and financial resources during the diagnosis and surgical treatment. In a mild form of the disease, diagnosis may not be made until the child is older. Assessing the older child's feelings about chronic constipation and its treatment is important.

Nursing Diagnoses

- Constipation related to aganglionic bowel
- Risk for Fluid Volume Deficit or Excess related to surgical preparation
- Impaired Skin Integrity related to colostomy and surgical repair
- Risk for Infection related to surgical repair
- Altered Nutrition: Less Than Body Requirements related to GI surgery
- Pain related to surgical incisions
- Knowledge Deficit related to need for surgery, irrigation, and/or care of ostomy
- Body Image Disturbance related to colostomy and irrigations

Planning, Implementation, and Evaluation: The Child With Hirschsprung's Disease

NURSING DIAGNOSES

- Constipation related to aganglionic bowel
- Risk for Fluid Volume Deficit or Excess related to surgical preparation

Expected Outcome:

- The child will pass soft, formed stools without retention.
- The child will be free from fluid or electrolyte disturbance related to bowel cleansing as evidenced by moist mucous membranes, urine specific gravity of 1.005 to 1.025, and normal serum sodium, potassium, and bicarbonate levels.

Intervention	Rationale
1. Assess child's bowel function and characteristics of stool.	Essential for accurate diagnosis of problem.
2. Prepare child for pull-through surgery or placement of temporary colostomy:	The only cure for this problem is to remove the aganglionic portion of the bowel to assure a return to normal peristalsis.
a. Administer isotonic saline enemas until return is clear. (See Chapter 18 for discussion of administering enemas to children.)	Saline is used to prevent fluid and electrolyte disturbance related to the use of tap water or hypertonic solutions.
b. Hold buttocks together for a short time.	Infants are unable to retain enema.
c. Monitor input and output of each enema.	Significant retention may occur related to obstruction and impaction.
OR	
a. Use a polyethylene glycol-electrolyte lavage solution (GoLYTELY) PO or through nasogastric (NG) tube until clear fluid is passed through rectum. It must be given at 25 to 60 ml/kg/hr to achieve appropriate effect. Use only in children over age 5.	GoLYTELY cleanses the bowel in less than 6 hours without absorption or fluid/electrolyte disturbance or the use of extended dietary limitations and enemas (Konings, 1989).
b. Monitor for nausea or vomiting.	High quantities of fluid are required for successful use of GoLYTELY and the infant or small child may have difficulty with gastric emptying.
3. After bowel cleansing:	
a. Keep child NPO until surgery.	Any intake will eliminate clean bowel required for safe and successful surgery.
b. Provide IV fluids as needed.	Adequate hydration is essential for surgery.
c. Maintain strict intake and output records.	Prevents and identifies fluid imbalances.

Evaluation:
- Has the child tolerated bowel cleansing enemas as evidenced by moist mucous membranes, urine specific gravity of 1.002 to 1.030, and serum sodium of 139 to 145 mmol/L?
- Has child remained NPO?
- Does child demonstrate balanced intake and output?
- Does the child pass soft, formed stools without retention following completion of surgical correction?

NURSING DIAGNOSES
- Impaired Skin Integrity related to colostomy and surgical repair
- Risk for Infection related to surgical repair

Expected Outcome:
- The surgical sites are clean and free from exudate, redness, or drainage.
- The colostomy site is intact without bleeding or skin irritation.
- The child is afebrile.

Intervention	Rationale
1. Administer neomycin 1.0% solution per rectum or stoma as ordered.	Sterilizes bowel for surgery by acting locally to reduce bacterial buildup without systemic absorption of medications.

Intervention	Rationale
2. Administer PO or IV antibiotics as ordered.	Further sterilizes the bowel and/or prevents infection at the surgical incision. Antibiotics that act directly on GI flora (neomycin) may be given by PO route even if child is NPO.
3. a. Monitor vital signs using tympanic or axillary temperature.	Fever is a sign of infection. Rectal mucosa may be traumatized by thermometer.
b. Include abdominal circumference with each vital sign measurement.	Abdominal circumference is important in identifying ileus or obstruction.
4. a. Assess surgical site for redness, swelling, and drainage.	Early signs of infection must be reported immediately.
b. Assess stoma for bleeding and skin breakdown around the area.	Because of the sensitive nature of children's skin, breakdown can occur very quickly and must be identified and treated early.
c. Assess anal area after pull-through procedure for patency of any appliance that may be in place, presence of stool, redness, or discharge.	Infection is common in this area if meticulous hygiene is not practiced.
5. Provide meticulous skin care to abdominal, perineal, and ostomy sites by changing dressings and appliances as needed.	Prevents skin breakdown and infection.
6. Use appropriate size, hypoallergenic ostomy supplies (e.g., Little Ones Ostomy products).	Prevents skin breakdown.
7. Report any fever, unusual drainage, redness, or odor to physician.	These are signs of infection.
Long-Term Care	
8. Encourage parent and/or child to begin ostomy care as soon as possible. (See Chapter 18 for discussion of ostomy care for children.)	Supervised practice increases self-care, decreases anxiety about ostomy care.

Evaluation:
- Is child afebrile?
- Are surgical sites free from redness, purulent drainage, excess heat, and dehiscence?
- Is colostomy free from bleeding and skin breakdown?

NURSING DIAGNOSIS
- Altered Nutrition: Less Than Body Requirements related to GI surgery

Expected Outcome:
- The child has normal bowel sounds, is passing stool, and tolerates regular diet.
- The child is free from signs of dehydration or electrolyte disturbance, as evidenced by moist mucous membranes, good skin turgor, urine specific gravity within age range, and normal serum sodium, potassium, and bicarbonate levels.

Intervention	Rationale
1. Keep child NPO until bowel sounds return or flatus is passed.	Evidence of return of peristalsis is needed before resuming PO intake.
2. Set NG tube to intermittent suction until peristalsis returns.	Provides decompression and decreases vomiting.

Intervention	Rationale
3. Administer IV therapy as ordered until child tolerates appropriate PO intake.	Provides fluid, glucose, and electrolytes during NPO period.
4. Assess for dehydration and overload, including urine specific gravity, intake and output, skin turgor, mucous membranes, daily weight, and vital signs.	Accurate assessment will aid in managing fluid volume needs.
5. Begin with clear liquids and advance to regular diet as tolerated.	Slow reintroduction aids tolerance to foods and prevents vomiting or diarrhea.

Evaluation:
- Are bowel sounds active and present in all four quadrants?
- Does child have good skin turgor and moist mucous membranes?
- Does child demonstrate balanced intake and output?
- Is presurgical weight maintained within 5%?
- Is child tolerating age-appropriate diet without vomiting or diarrhea?

NURSING DIAGNOSIS
- Pain related to surgical incisions

Expected Outcome:
- The child will be free from pain as evidenced by resumption of age-appropriate activities, sleeping without interruption, and interacting with caretakers.

Intervention	Rationale
1. Assess pain using appropriate tools (see Chapter 20).	Infants and young children do not react to pain in typical adult ways. Alternative methods of assessment are needed to validate assessment findings.
2. Provide comfort measures and involve parents (repositioning, back rubs, music, holding, rocking, massage, parental voices).	Increases parent involvement and relieves discomfort.
3. a. Provide pain medications on a regular basis as ordered.	Prevents peaks of pain that cannot be managed appropriately.
b. Assess for respiratory depression.	Narcotics can cause respiratory depression.
c. Provide patient-controlled analgesia (PCA) where appropriate.	School-age children may be capable of controlling their own pain using PCA devices. (See Chapter 20.)
4. Report pain not managed by usual means.	May be an indication of bowel obstruction, infection, or other complication.

Evaluation:
- Is child sleeping without fitfulness?
- Is child participating in age-appropriate play activities when awake?
- Does parent feel that child's pain is under control?
- Are pain medications being given?

NURSING DIAGNOSIS
- Knowledge Deficit related to need for irrigation, surgery, and/or care of ostomy
- Body Image Disturbance related to colostomy and irrigations

Expected Outcome:
- The parent will state necessity of rectal irrigations and/or surgical intervention.
- The parent and/or child will assume responsibility for care of ostomy.
- The child and family will express feelings about irrigations and ostomy care.

TEACHING GUIDELINES *for the Child With Hirschsprung's Disease*

- Teach parents and child about the need for bowel cleansing before surgery because this can be stressful and time consuming.
- Explain surgical procedure, including the possible need for a temporary colostomy and any anal device used to maintain the pull-through.
- Provide tour of operating room and recovery room for parents and child, if desired, to reduce anxiety.
- Encourage parents to participate in care as much as possible to promote self-care and control and decrease anxiety.
- Teach colostomy care (see Chapter 18), including the use of appropriate size, hypoallergenic equipment available for care of children's colostomies.
- Arrange support services from enterostomal therapist; such assistance in education and emotional support is essential.

Intervention	Rationale
1. Teach parents how to complete rectal irrigations.	This is the first method of disease management that is tried. It may be successful in mild cases.
2. Teach parents how to assess for distension and obstruction.	As parents manage irrigations at home, they must be able to identify problems early and notify physicians appropriately.
3. Encourage parents to share feelings, anxieties, and concerns about the need for irrigations.	This can be stressful and invasive for the child and family. Recognizing concerns and encouraging parents to share them will relieve some anxieties.
4. Explain surgical repair and recovery process (see Teaching Guidelines for the Child With Hirschsprung's Disease).	Information decreases anxiety.
5. Encourage preschoolers and early school-age children to draw pictures, use dolls, and play to express concerns about bodily appearance, irrigations, and colostomy.	These methods can give nurse valuable assessment data that cannot be gathered verbally from small children.
6. Teach ostomy care in the immediate postoperative period. Encourage parents to participate and learn while in a supervised setting.	Decreases anxiety; increases competency and self-control.
7. Encourage child to assume care as soon as possible if ostomy occurs in the older child. (See Chapter 18 for discussion of ostomy care for children.)	Promotes self-care and positive body image.
8. Refer to support groups for children with ostomies (see Appendix).	Provides information, support, reassurance, and assistance in caring for child.

Home Care: Many of the nursing interventions discussed above will be carried over to home care. In mild cases, and in more severe cases before surgery, home care is the essential intervention. Parents must be taught rectal irrigations, assessment of bowel functioning, high-fiber nutrition, and even colostomy care. Helping parents and children identify signs of bowel obstruction is essential. Dietitians and enterostomal therapists can assist in some teaching and care.

After surgery, assessing all surgical incision sites for redness, drainage, or exudate is important. Minor dressing changes may be needed and can be taught to parents or older children.

Evaluation:
- Can parent explain the need for irrigations, surgery, and colostomy?
- Can parent identify distension, vomiting, and failure to pass stool as symptoms of obstruction?
- Does parent and/or child perform all irrigations and colostomy care without assistance?
- Does parent share concerns and anxieties about invasive nature of care?

Abdominal Wall Defects

Gastroschisis, omphalocele, and umbilical hernia are disorders of fetal gut development that can have a devastating impact on the infant. Table 26–1 presents an overview of these disorders, and outlines the nursing care.

Constipation and Encopresis

Constipation is the infrequent and difficult passage of dry, hard stools. One of the major concerns regarding constipation is the development of **encopresis,** or fecal incontinence. With encopresis, children often complain that soiling is involuntary and occurs without warning. Parents find the situation frustrating, and soiling often becomes a major issue between parent and child (Seth & Heyman, 1994). Often encopresis causes the child to feel ashamed or embarrassed, and he may avoid situations in which embarrassment might be heightened, such as spending the night with a friend, or even going to school. If the condition persists over a long period of time, it usually affects the child's self-esteem and may impair social relations. Often, the parents experience guilt and shame or revulsion, disgust, or anger, and may project these feelings onto the child.

Etiology. Constipation can have many causes, such as changes in diet, dehydration, lack of exercise, emotional stress, certain drugs, pain from anal fissure, or excessive milk intake. If the child has no neurologic or anatomic disorders, encopresis is usually the result of recurrent fecal impaction and enlarged rectum caused by chronic constipation. Predisposing factors for encopresis include inadequate or inconsistent toilet training or some type of psychological stress, such as starting school or the birth of a sibling.

Incidence. Constipation can affect any child at any time, though it peaks at age 2 to 3 years (Hatch, 1988). Encopresis generally affects preschool and school-age children, with 1.5% to 3% of the population being affected. There are more boys than girls affected. There is a higher incidence of encopresis in lower socioeconomic classes and among children with learning disabilities.

PATHOPHYSIOLOGY *of Constipation and Encopresis*

When stool passes into the rectum, distension of the walls stimulates mass peristaltic movements in the bowel. This is called the defecation reflex. If defecation is not desired, the external sphincter contracts and voluntary retention of stool occurs. As the stool remains in the rectum, the rectum relaxes and the defecation reflex wanes. Water reabsorption from the colon continues, resulting in hard, dry, stool that is difficult to pass. The eventual passage of that stool may result in pain or anal fissures. If retention of stool continues, more fissures may develop or become worse, so that eventually even soft stool may produce pain. A cycle of pain develops whereby the stool is retained to avoid pain but the retention leads to even more difficult defecation.

Over time, the rectum becomes enlarged. This can produce a failure to control the external sphincter, resulting in encopresis.

Clinical Manifestations

Constipation

- Abdominal pain and cramping without distension
- Palpable, movable fecal masses with large amount of stool inside an enlarged rectum
- Diarrhea; overflow may be chief complaint
- Normal or decreased bowel sounds
- Malaise, anorexia, headache
- Nausea and vomiting
- Anal fissure

Encopresis

- Evidence of soiling clothing
- Scratching or rubbing anal area, due to irritation
- Fecal odor without apparent awareness by the child
- Social withdrawal and avoidance of extended contact with others (such as overnight stays, camp)

TABLE 26–1 *Abdominal Wall Defects*

	GASTROSCHISIS	OMPHALOCELE	UMBILICAL HERNIA
Pathophysiology/Etiology/ Clinical Manifestations	Embryonal weakness in abdominal wall causes herniation of gut on one side of umbilical cord during early development. Most commonly right side Viscera outside of abdominal cavity and not covered with sac	Large herniation of gut into umbilical cord Viscera outside of abdominal cavity but inside translucent sac covered with peritoneum and amniotic membrane	Imperfect closure of umbilical ring allows gut to push outward at umbilicus during straining and crying. Viscera inside abdominal cavity and under skin Usually 1–3 cm, easily reduced
Incidence	1 in 20,000 live births More common in males	1 in 5000–10,000 live births	Most common in low–birth-weight or black infants
Associated Anomalies	Malrotation of intestines Decreased abdominal capacity **Atresia,** stenosis rare Higher incidence of Meckel's diverticulum Other anomalies rare	Malrotation of intestines Decreased abdominal capacity Atresia, stenosis common Higher incidence of Meckel's diverticulum One-third to one-half of cases have cardiac, genitourinary, or chromosomal anomalies Associated with Beckwith syndrome (hypoglycemia, macrosomia, macroglossia)	Commonly occurs in children with Down syndrome, hypothyroidism, Hurler syndrome
Morbidity and Mortality	Mortality 10%–15%	Mortality 20%–30% Common complications include sepsis and intestinal obstruction	Minimal
Therapeutic Management	Immediate IV, NG tube placement Total parenteral nutrition Synthetic material (Silastic) is used to cover the gut in a sac (if sac has ruptured or omphalocele is large). The sac is suspended over the child's abdomen, and gravity is used to slowly return gut to the abdominal cavity over 2–8 days or longer if defect is large. Defect is closed surgically after all contents have been returned to the abdominal cavity. Even if defect is small, immediate surgical repair may be done in several stages. If diagnosed prenatally, surgical delivery is recommended. Necrotic bowel may need to be removed surgically.		Most disappear spontaneously by 1 year of age. No surgical repair unless it causes symptoms, persists past age 5 years, becomes strangulated, or continues to grow

Diagnostic Evaluation. Abdominal X-rays may demonstrate an enlarged rectum with large amounts of stool and gas. The definitive diagnostic procedure is a rectal examination. This is rarely performed because of its emotional impact on the child and the possibility of pain from anal fissure. A thorough history is usually sufficient for diagnosis.

Therapeutic Management. The best form of treatment is prevention of the chronic problem using appropriate diet, exercise, and establishing regular toileting habits. Education about "normal" bowel function can prevent a psychogenic component to the problem.

> The focus of management is to remove the impaction, "retrain" the rectum to be aware of when it is full, and help the child overcome the pain-retention cycle.

Treatment usually involves three approaches (Ellett, 1990):

1. Overcoming withholding
   a. Enemas until impaction is cleared
   b. Stool softener or laxative
   c. Mineral oil 30 to 75 ml BID to decrease pain of defecation

TABLE 26–1 *Abdominal Wall Defects (continued)*

	GASTROSCHISIS	OMPHALOCELE	UMBILICAL HERNIA
Nursing Care	Thermoregulation critical because significant heat loss can occur through exposed intestines. Use warmers, monitor temperature. Use sterile technique in dealing with defect. Immediately cover with warm, moist, sterile gauze and wrap with plastic to keep moist. Minimize movement of infant and handling of intestines. Assess for circulatory compromise, obstruction, and sepsis: monitor temperature, pulses, capillary refill, skin color, changes in respiratory patterns, and heart rate. Observe for respiratory distress secondary to high intra-abdominal pressure as gut returns to peritoneal cavity. Fluid volume management is crucial nursing responsibility: monitor intake and output and daily weights, assess fontanels, monitor electrolytes, and maintain IV line. Postoperatively, monitor and manage ileus, which commonly lasts for 2–4 weeks: maintain NG tube for decompression, monitor bowel sounds and stools, and measure abdominal girth. Maintain parenteral nutrition to sustain growth. Offer pacifier to meet sucking needs Provide emotional support for parents as they deal with the "loss of the perfect child" Encourage parents to provide care as they are able, talk to and touch infant and hold him when appropriate.		Binding is not effective in reducing or minimizing bulge. Monitor for changes in size of hernia. Assess for increased bowel sounds, and irreducible mass, which may indicate strangulation.
Teaching and Home Care	Encourage parents to hold, cuddle, and bond with infants as soon as possible. Provide developmental stimulation for long-term hospitalization. Assist parents in dealing with feelings of guilt and disappointment. Use pictures to help parents understand nature of defect. Contact national support groups and community resources. Teach parents signs of bowel obstruction: vomiting, pain, irritability, anorexia, and firm abdomen. Provide follow-up from nutritional support personnel as needed.		Teach parents signs of strangulation: vomiting, pain, irreducible mass at umbilicus. Contact physician immediately if strangulation is suspected.

2. Dietary changes
   a. Limiting milk intake
   b. Increasing water intake
   c. Increasing residue in diet
3. Changing the retention habit
   a. Sitting on the commode for 5 to 10 minutes approximately 20 to 30 minutes after meals

The goal is to pass two to three soft stools per day without pain within the first month. Medications are weaned slowly over 3 to 6 months after fear of pain has been lost.

NURSING CARE OF THE CHILD WITH CONSTIPATION/ENCOPRESIS

Assessment

The nurse should obtain a thorough history of the soiling events, including frequency, intensity, and duration. It is often helpful to interview the parents and child separately to reduce the child's embarrassment, since parent–child relationships are often strained. The nurse can explain to parents that a medical history and examination will be performed to rule out organic causes of the chronic constipation such as Hirschsprung's disease or spina bifida occulta.

Nursing Diagnosis and Planning

The following nursing diagnoses and expected outcomes may be appropriate in the treatment of constipation or encopresis in the child.

- Constipation or Bowel Incontinence related to inconsistent patterns of elimination, anxiety, or pain during elimination. ***Expected Outcome:*** *The child will have normal bowel function as evidenced by the passage of soft stools without pain or incontinence.*
- Ineffective Family Coping related to persistent stress, guilt, and embarrassment about child's elimination difficulty. ***Expected Outcomes:*** *The family will function effectively as a unit; openly discuss their problems; develop a plan to achieve control over incontinence.*
- Social Isolation related to embarrassment, peer teasing, and odor from bowel incontinence. ***Expected Outcomes:*** *The child will verbalize positive, realistic feelings about self; verbalize appropriate ways to achieve control over bowel incontinence.*
- Impaired Skin Integrity related to poor hygiene in anal area, bowel incontinence, and lack of knowledge. ***Expected Outcome:*** *The child will maintain skin integrity as evidenced by clean, intact skin.*

Implementation

Because constipation and encopresis really represent a continuum of the same problem, this nursing care plan presents options that can be tried as needed to deal with the problem. Simple constipation may resolve using only dietary changes or helping change a habit of retention, severe encopresis may require all interventions to be continued over a period of 3 to 6 months.

Overcoming Withholding. Before bowel retraining can begin, the child's bowel must be evacuated of all hard stool and impactions. This is best accomplished with the use of appropriate size Fleet or isotonic enemas every 12 hours until the impaction is cleared, usually within 48 hours. Parents should be taught to administer enemas at home, or they may be performed by the nurse.

During this time, the child should be monitored for hypernatremia or hyperphosphatemia, which could result from repeated use of Fleet enemas. (See Chapter 18 for discussion of enema administration.) After cleansing has been achieved, the child is started on mineral oil 30 to 75 ml (1 Tbsp/10 kg) BID (Ellett, 1990). This may be continued in lower doses for 1 to 2 months after initial cleansing. This is best tolerated when it is given chilled or mixed with cold drinks. Mixing the oil with chocolate milk, blending it with ice cubes and fruit juice, or chilling it help to disguise the taste. It is not unusual for the child to leak oil when doses are high, and parents and children need to be aware that this does not constitute encopresis. At the end of this intervention, the child should be passing soft stool without pain or incontinence.

Dietary Changes. Dietary modifications are used as a part of the treatment. Increasing water and fiber intake by offering granola bars, dried fruits, whole grain cereals, and fresh vegetables with low-fat dip can increase the bulk in stool and make it easier to pass. Decreasing sugar and milk intake will also help keep stools soft. Fat-soluble vitamins should be supplemented during the use of mineral oil because the oil can interfere with vitamin absorption in the small intestine.

Changing the Retention Habit. To help reestablish a normal bowel habit, it is recommended that the child be required to sit on the toilet for 5 to 10 minutes after breakfast and dinner. This will allow the normal gastrocolic reflex to assist with defecation and will eliminate the need to be involved with retraining during school hours. Star charts and small prizes are helpful in rewarding success.

These interventions are continued for at least 3 to 6 months, during which time the rectum will resume its normal size and the child will relearn to attend to the defecation reflex. If fecal impaction occurs at any time, enemas are again administered and the dosage of mineral oil adjusted.

Emotional Support. As these interventions are being carried out, it is essential to allow the child and parents to express their feelings of success and failure with the program. To minimize the damage to the child's self-esteem, self-care should be encouraged as much as possible. To decrease embarrassment, it is helpful for school-age children to have a complete change of pants and underwear at school, should leakage or an accident occur. Age-appropriate support groups may be available in a center with a large population or encopresis clinic.

> **PARENT–CHILD COMMUNICATION** Teaching is a major intervention with this problem. However, encouraging the child and parents to share feelings of shame and embarrassment are equally important. Allow the child to verbalize any concerns he may have and provide age-appropriate anatomic information to help him understand the etiology of the problem. Using drawings and books may be an effective way to begin this sharing of feelings and information. Relieving the child of the shame and embarrassment may improve his cooperation with the plan of care.

Home Care. Because this is an outpatient, home-treated condition, teaching parents is the critical intervention. The parents need to understand the correct way to administer enemas (see Chapter 18). They also need support in implementing and documenting the successes and setbacks since the plan is implemented over a 3- to 6-month period. The child and parents need encouragement to continue even when only small successes are being made. This is a problem that develops over time and takes time, patience, and perseverance to resolve.

Evaluation

For constipation and encopresis:

Is child passing soft stool without pain?

Does food diary indicate foods from all food groups with high fiber being consumed?

For encopresis:

Is child experiencing any incontinence?

Are mineral oil, enemas, or laxatives still needed?

Are fat-soluble vitamin supplements being taken during first phase of treatment?

Is child experiencing success with control of bowels?

Irritable Bowel Syndrome

Irritable bowel syndrome is the result of increased motility that can lead to spasm and pain. It includes diarrhea or recurrent abdominal pain.

PATHOPHYSIOLOGY *of Irritable Bowel Syndrome*

The precipitating factors in irritable bowel syndrome are unknown but result in two distinct problems. The first is disorganized contractility, which causes spasmodic peristaltic rushes and lulls. This disorganization causes an alternating diarrhea and constipation and intermittent abdominal pain. The second component is excess mucus production in the lumen of the bowel. This produces maldigestion and the passage of incompletely digested food and nutrients.

Etiology. Stress and emotional factors are thought to be the most common cause of this disorder. There is supposition that an abnormality in the autonomic nervous system accounts for the changes in motility and secretion, but this has not been adequately documented (Milla, 1988). In infants, it may be related to a lactase deficiency. It is not associated with any psychopathology.

Incidence. Irritable bowel syndrome is most common from ages 16 to 20 months, and again in school-age children and adolescents, with girls outnumbering boys 3:1. It tends to occur in families with a positive history for other bowel disturbances or infantile colic. From 10% to 15% of school-age children experience these "attacks" (Behrman, Kliegman, & Arvin, 1996). The disease tends to resolve by age 20 but may recur as a "spastic colon" in adulthood (Behrman, Kliegman, & Arvin, 1996).

Clinical Manifestations

- Diffuse abdominal pain unrelated to meals or activity
- Alternating constipation and diarrhea, with the presence of undigested food and mucus in stool
- Normal growth

Diagnostic Evaluation. The diagnosis is based on the elimination of major GI pathology, including Crohn's disease, giardiasis, lactose intolerance, or genitourinary abnormalities. Abdominal ultrasound, stool cultures, abdominal X-ray, and complete gynecologic assessment are often ordered.

Therapeutic Management. There is no definitive treatment for this poorly understood functional bowel problem. Management is aimed at decreasing symptoms. The primary intervention should be reassurance that it is a self-limiting, intermittent problem. Unless lactose intolerance is suspected, no dietary modifications are required other than the maintenance of a healthy, well-balanced, moderate fiber diet. If the disease continues, a fear-pain cycle may develop that can have a significant impact on the daily activity of the child. Psychiatric support in this area may be helpful (Berk, 1985).

NURSING CARE OF THE CHILD WITH IRRITABLE BOWEL SYNDROME

Assessment

Assessment will reveal a healthy-looking toddler or school-age child with episodic abdominal pain and intermittent mucoid diarrhea. Growth and activity will be normal. The pain may be worse during stressful family or school situations, though the child is unlikely to make that association. Monitoring growth rate, assessing diet, and keeping a log of episodes will provide useful assessment information.

Family and psychosocial assessment may reveal a family that is worried about a serious life-threatening disease and is very focused on the bowel habits of the child. They may not be reassured by the normal findings on a physical and developmental examination.

Nursing Diagnosis and Planning

The following nursing diagnoses and expected outcomes may be appropriate in the treatment of irritable bowel syndrome in the child.

- Pain related to hyperperistalsis. ***Expected Outcomes:*** *The child will be free of abdominal pain, as evidenced by age-appropriate play and activity; not exhibit guarding during palpation.*
- Diarrhea related to maldigestion. ***Expected Outcome:*** *The child will have soft, formed stools without evidence of mucus.*

- Anxiety related to emotional aspects of disease. ***Expected Outcome:*** *The parent/child will verbalize the self-limited nature of the disease.*

Implementation

The chief nursing interventions are teaching and reassurance. Health promotion activities such as exercise, balanced nutritional diet, and school activities have the best influence on the disease. Antispasmodics and pain medications are not likely to have an effect. If the child develops fecal masses, laxatives and enemas may be needed to return the intestine to a more physiologic state.

Because of the associated psychosocial component, referral to mental health and family counseling services can be effective in cases that are unresponsive to other measures. The child and family will express feelings and concerns that will assist in evaluating the interventions.

Home Care. Providing support for the family and child as they deal with this self-limited disease is an essential nursing intervention. Teaching the child and family about the Food Guide Pyramid and the need for many servings in the lower portion of the pyramid may help improve fiber intake. Encourage the parents and child to keep track of servings in each group as a way to evaluate nutritional practices. Exercise should be encouraged through the use of family walks and outings, bicycling, and playing ball with friends and family. Healthy lifestyle changes that can improve symptoms in the child may also improve overall health for the family. Allowing the child and family to express frustration and fears about pain and diarrhea that can't be "cured" will provide important psychosocial assistance.

Evaluation

Does child complain of abdominal pain?
Does infant guard abdomen during palpation?
Are stools soft, formed, and free of mucus?
Does child participate in age-appropriate activity and play?
Does family express satisfaction with control of problem?

Imperforate Anus

Imperforate anus (anal *atresia,* anal agenesis) is the incomplete development or absence of the anus in its normal position in the perineum. There are two major types: (1) high, in which the blind pouch is above the **levator ani muscle,** and (2) low, in which the pouch is below the levator ani muscle (Table 26–2). Anal membrane atresia, a minor anorectal malformation, is the presence of a thin membrane over the anal opening.

PATHOPHYSIOLOGY ***and Etiology of Imperforate Anus***

Anal agenesis is the direct result of an embryologic failure of migration and development of the hindgut during the 7th to 10th week of development. The exact time this migration failure occurs determines the severity of the lesions. The failure may also result in sacral agenesis and abnormalities in the urethra and vagina.

Incidence. Imperforate anus occurs in varying severity in from 1 in 500 to 1 in 5000 births (Behrman, Kliegman, & Arvin, 1996). It has a high incidence of associated anomalies, including genitourinary, sacral, and additional GI anomalies.

Clinical Manifestations

- Failure to pass meconium stool
- Absence or stenosis of the anorectal canal
- Anal membrane
- External fistula to the perineum

Diagnostic Evaluation. An initial examination of the perineum as part of the neonatal examination is an essential first step. This should include determining the patency of the rectum with a small finger or rectal tube if a lesion is suspected. X-ray examination, ultrasound and computed tomography scan can be useful in determining the level of the lesion and the amount of muscle involved in the defect.

Determining patency of the anus in the neonatal period is essential for early detection and treatment.

Therapeutic Management. Anal stenosis is easily treated with repeated and staged dilatation. All other forms of atresia require surgical intervention. A low defect can be successfully treated by opening the perineum with anoplasty followed by serial dilatations. High defects are best treated using a two-stage correction with a transverse colostomy and a later "pull-through" procedure requiring a more extensive surgical intervention. The goal of treatment for anal stenosis, anal membrane atresia, and the low type of imperforate anus is to achieve continence. In the higher defects, complete continence may be impossible but some degree of control is attainable.

NURSING CARE OF THE CHILD WITH AN IMPERFORATE ANUS

Assessment

During the neonatal assessment the defect should be easily identified on sight. However, a rectal thermometer or

TABLE 26-2 *Imperforate Anus: Types and Treatments*

TYPE	DESCRIPTION	TREATMENT
	Low Anomalies	
Anal Stenosis 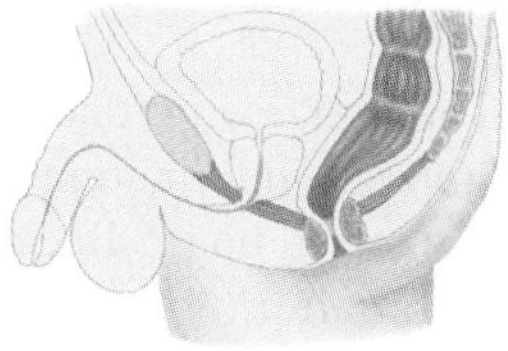	Congenital anal stenosis is a narrowing of the anorectal canal that may occur at any point or extend its entire length. Diagnosis can be established by digital and endoscopic examination.	Can often be corrected by manual dilations.
Imperforate Anal Membrane 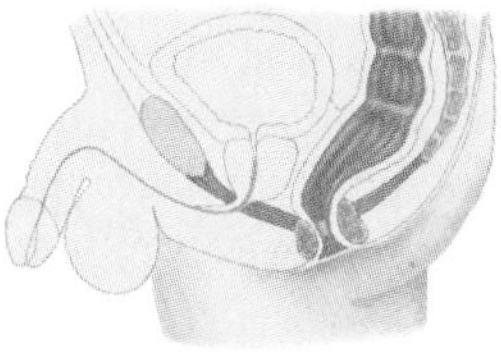	A thin cutaneous membrane persists across the anal opening. Meconium fills the rectum and can frequently be seen as a discoloration of the membrane.	Incision or excision of the membrane followed by anal dilatations until bowel function is normal.
Anal Agenesis (Low) 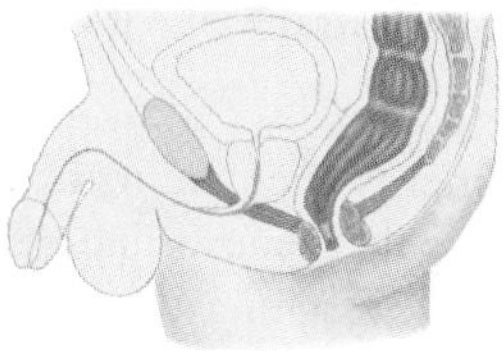	The rectum ends in a blind pouch below the levator ani muscle.	Surgery, varying with the type of lesion and fistula.
	High Anomalies	
Anal Agenesis (High) 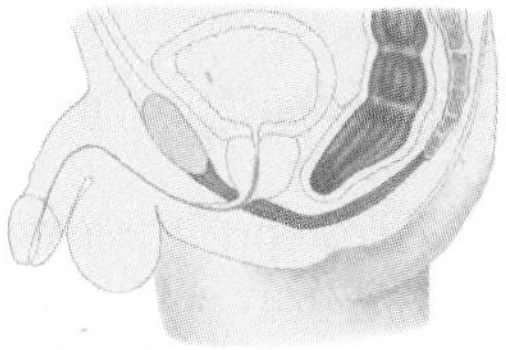	The rectum ends in a blind pouch above the levator ani muscle. Anal agenesis (low and high) accounts for 80% of anorectal malformations. Most infants with anal agenesis have associated **fistulas** of various types (rectovaginal, rectoperitoneal, rectourethral).	Surgery, varying with the type of lesion and fistula.
Rectal Atresia 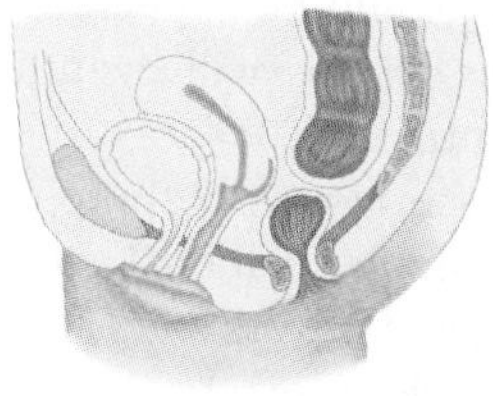	In this rare anomaly, the anus is normal but the rectal canal is not continuous. Lower rectal pouch can be identified by careful examination with the little finger; usually a complete block is encountered.	Surgery: Anastomosis through an abdominoperineal approach.

tube may be necessary to determine patency if meconium is not passed in the first 24 hours after birth. The presence of stool in the urine, vagina, or in a skin dimple should be reported immediately as an indication of abnormal anorectal development. If anorectal malformations are confirmed, nursing assessment should be continued to identify any other GI problems (tracheoesophageal fistulas, esophageal atresia) or urogenital malformations (fistulas), which commonly occur.

Assessment should include the parent's feelings of loss or guilt about the birth defect. It is not unusual to find them distraught and feeling "somehow responsible" for the problem with their neonate.

Nursing Diagnosis and Planning

The following nursing diagnoses and expected outcomes may be appropriate in the treatment of imperforate anus in the neonate.

- Bowel Incontinence related to incomplete formation of anus. ***Expected Outcome:*** *The infant will pass soft, formed stools without pain or bleeding.*
- Risk for Impaired Skin Integrity related to colostomy. ***Expected Outcomes:*** *The infant will maintain skin integrity at the incision site as evidenced by lack of redness, drainage, or swelling at the incision site; maintain pink, dry skin that is free from breakdown around the colostomy.*
- Knowledge Deficit related to home care needs and surgery. ***Expected Outcomes:*** *The parents will verbalize an understanding of the need for immediate intervention; demonstrate ability to perform anal dilatations; demonstrate ability to care for temporary colostomy.*

Implementation

Once diagnosis is made, immediate plans are made for surgical intervention. For a low lesion, this will necessitate a perineal surgical incision. Skin care at the anoplasty site is a primary intervention and includes keeping the area clean and observing for signs of infection. A side-lying position with the legs flexed or a prone position to keep the hips elevated can reduce edema and pressure on the surgical site. The anal surgical site should be clean, dry, and without redness, swelling, or drainage.

If the lesion is a high type, the first surgery usually includes a temporary colostomy. Colostomy care in the neonate can be difficult because of the sensitive nature of the neonate's skin. Hypoallergenic supplies of an appropriate size are necessary, and parent teaching needs to be a major focus. Because this involves an abdominal surgical site, the child will be NPO, will have an NG tube in place, and will require IV fluid management until GI motility returns. (See Hirschsprung's Disease and Chapter 18.) The colostomy site should be pink, without evidence of drainage, swelling, or skin breakdown. A fresh colostomy stoma will be red and edematous, but this should decrease with time.

Anal dilatations are often begun soon after surgery; the parents will need to be taught how to perform these. The goal of this therapy is a functionally sized anus that is able to pass stool of a normal caliber.

Parental Support and Education. The nurse can decrease parental anxiety by offering appropriate information and providing time for parents and infant to bond. Because the surgical repair is done very soon after birth, parents must be provided with time alone with the infant so that an initial relationship can be developed. In addition, parents should be allowed and encouraged to share their feelings about the birth defect and express emotions about the outcomes of the surgery. If these interventions are successful, the parent will have face-to-face communication, close physical contact, and verbal interaction with their infant and will share their feelings with the nursing staff.

Education should include a description of the pathophysiology of imperforate anus, skin and colostomy care, and the expected recovery for their child, including the need for IV fluids, NG suction, and frequent vital signs and assessments.

Home Care. Anal dilatation at home by the parents is necessary to achieve and maintain bowel patency. Therefore, an important part of nursing care is teaching the parents how to perform them. Parents should be instructed to

- Use only dilators supplied by their physician
- Use a water-soluble lubricant
- Insert the dilator no more than 1 to 2 cm into the anus to prevent damage to mucosa

After instruction, ask the parents to demonstrate, and correct their technique if necessary.

If their infant has a temporary colostomy, the parents must also be instructed in colostomy care and maintenance. (See discussion of colostomy care in Chapter 18.)

Because achieving bowel continence can vary with the severity of the lesion, parental education must be individualized. Delayed bowel training should be expected, but over 80% of children with these lesions will eventually achieve an acceptable level of continence.

It may be advisable to refer the family to appropriate resources for counseling and support. National support groups such as the Pull-Through Network can also be helpful to the families of these children (see Appendix H).

Evaluation

Are surgical sites clean, dry, and free from redness, breakdown, or purulent drainage?

Is colostomy functioning without redness, purulent drainage, or skin breakdown?

Can parents explain need for immediate surgery?
Do parents perform anal dilatations using appropriate size dilator, lubricant, and insertion depth of 1 to 2 cm into anus?
Are parents caring for colostomy without problems or concerns?
Are parents satisfied with their understanding and management of the condition?

Intussusception

Intussusception is an invagination of a section of the intestine into the distal bowel, which results in bowel obstruction. In children, this most often occurs as a section of terminal ileum telescopes into the ascending colon through the ileocecal valve. It is the most common cause of bowel obstruction in children age 3 months to 6 years (Behrman, Kliegman, & Arvin, 1996). Though relatively rare, it does represent a pediatric emergency with "classic" assessment findings.

Etiology. In young children, the cause of intussusception is unknown. There is evidence that hypertrophy of mesenteric lymphoid tissue secondary to a viral infection is a contributing factor (Kirks, 1984). Pathology within the colon, such as a mass or anatomic defect, is the most likely cause in children older than age 6 years.

Incidence. This problem generally affects infants, with 75% occurring before age 2 and 40% in infants age 3 to 9 months. It occurs in 1 to 4 per 1000 births, has a 3:1 male to female ratio, and has a higher incidence in children with celiac disease and cystic fibrosis (Behrman, Kliegman, & Arvin, 1996; Kirks, 1984). Recurrence risk is 3% to 10% and usually occurs within the first 48 hours (Kirks, 1984; Ladebauche, 1992).

Clinical Manifestations

- Well-nourished with no history of GI problems
- Paroxysms of pain subside and recur during the first several hours, then progress to a more constant severe pain.
- Vomiting

PATHOPHYSIOLOGY *of Intussusception*

As the bowel telescopes inside itself, obstruction develops. In addition, the mesenteric vessels become trapped between the walls of the two layers and ischemia occurs. This pressure on the bowel leads to bleeding and "currant jelly" stools. Mesenteric ischemia also causes edema and possible strangulation or infarction of the bowel, which can progress to perforation, peritonitis, sepsis, shock, and death.

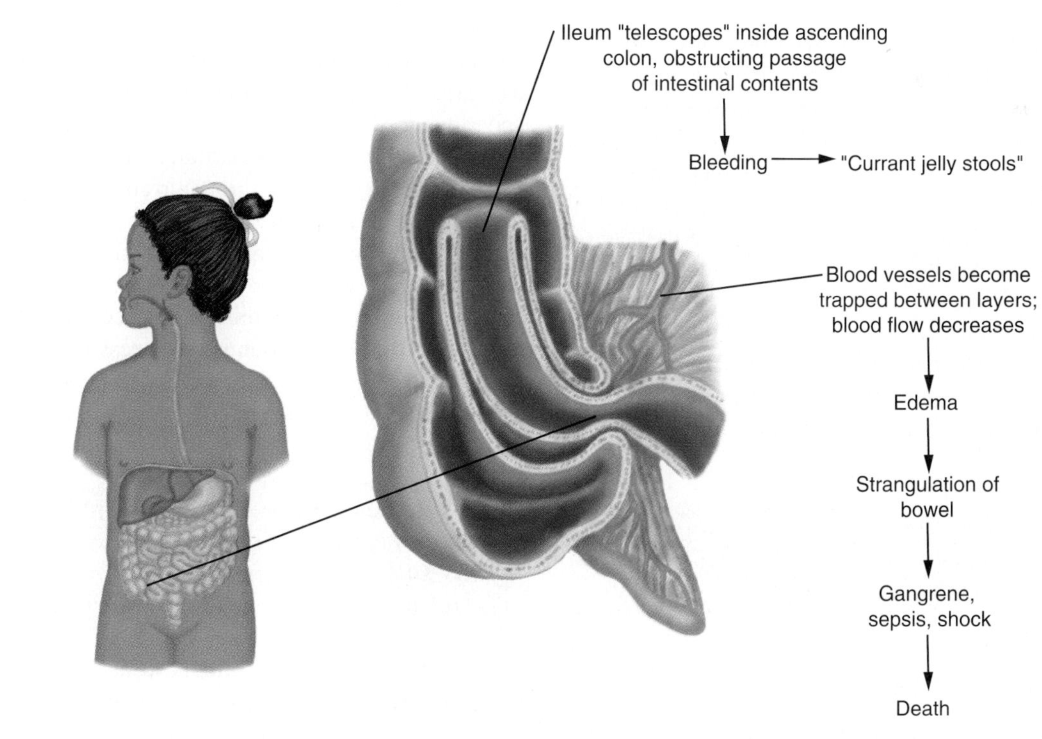

- Passage of bloody mucus stool ("currant jelly"), diarrhea; this may not occur until postoperative period.
- Sausage-shaped abdominal mass
- Symptoms of shock and sepsis are present if obstruction has been present for greater than 12 to 24 hours.
- Lethargy, listlessness

Diagnostic Evaluation. Abdominal X-rays may indicate abnormal gas patterns related to the bowel obstruction or a soft tissue mass. Ultrasound is useful in identifying the location of the intussusception and the amount of edema in the area. Definitive diagnosis and treatment can be obtained simultaneously with the use of barium enema or air enema.

Therapeutic Management. The goal of treatment is to restore the bowel to its normal position and function as quickly as possible. In children who do not show symptoms of shock or sepsis, attempts at hydrostatic reduction are made with barium or air enema until free flow of barium into the terminal ileum is evident. This can be done in 70% to 85% of cases. If reduction fails or findings indicate damage to the bowel, immediate surgery is performed. If the intussusception is detected and reduced within 24 hours, morbidity is minimal. However, overall mortality remains 5% to 10% (Behrman, Kliegman, & Arvin, 1996).

NURSING CARE OF THE CHILD WITH INTUSSUSCEPTION

Assessment

The nursing history typically reveals a previously healthy infant who suddenly begins crying and drawing up his legs in severe pain. This may resolve only to recur a short time later and become more constant in nature. The child should be assessed for signs of bowel obstruction: vomiting, nausea, distension, and hypoactive or hyperactive bowel sounds. A palpable abdominal mass and passage of currant jelly stools will help confirm the diagnosis. Hydration status, including urine output, specific gravity, skin turgor, and mucous membranes, is assessed on admission. Fever, increased heart rate, changes in level of consciousness or blood pressure, and respiratory distress should be reported immediately as possible indications of sepsis or peritonitis.

> The presence of colicky abdominal pain, vomiting, or passage of currant jelly stools should alert the nurse to the probability of intussusception.

Nursing Diagnosis and Planning

The following nursing diagnoses and expected outcomes may be appropriate in the treatment of intussusception in the child.

- Altered Tissue Perfusion (GI) related to ischemia of bowel. ***Expected Outcome:*** *The child will have a patent bowel as evidenced by passage of soft, formed, Hematest-negative stools.*
- Pain related to bowel obstruction. ***Expected Outcomes:*** *The child will be free from abdominal pain, as evidenced by age-appropriate play and activity; not exhibit guarding during palpation.*
- Fluid Volume Deficit related to vomiting/diarrhea. ***Expected Outcomes:*** *The child will tolerate age-appropriate food and fluids without vomiting or recurrence of symptoms; be free from fluid and electrolyte disturbances, as evidenced by return to normal weight, moist mucous membranes, good skin turgor, and normal serum sodium level and hematocrit.*
- Knowledge Deficit related to possibility of surgery and need for immediate intervention. ***Expected Outcomes:*** *The parents will verbalize an understanding of the need for immediate intervention; explain the mechanisms of intussusception and hydrostatic reduction.*
- Sleep Pattern Disturbance related to colicky abdominal pain. ***Expected Outcome:*** *The child will return to normal sleep patterns.*

Implementation

Once diagnosis is made, immediate plans are made to admit the child to the hospital for hydrostatic reduction. Prompt assessment for dehydration, shock, or sepsis is essential, including documenting mental status, capillary perfusion, and urine output. The child is given IV fluids and an NG tube is inserted if distension is present. During reduction, pain medications or sedation may be needed to decrease spasm. After reduction, clear liquids are started and advanced gradually as tolerated. The nurse must observe for the passage of barium and note the characteristics of stool. In addition, the recurrence of previous symptoms of bowel obstruction should be noted; risk of recurrence following nonsurgical reduction is about 10%. Resumption of a normal diet, activity, and the passage of stool without blood will indicate a successful outcome.

If hydrostatic reduction is unsuccessful, the child must be prepared for abdominal surgery. (See Chapter 18 and the discussion of nursing care under Hirschsprung's disease.)

> If hydrostatic reduction is unsuccessful, continue to monitor for the return of normal bowel function (normal stool), because spontaneous resolution could occur, eliminating the need for surgery.

Postoperatively, the child is kept NPO until bowel function returns. Nasogastric suction and IV therapy, pain medications, maintenance of respiratory function, frequent assessment, and meeting developmental needs remain the nurse's roles. (See Chapter 15.)

During this difficult time for parents, it is essential to relieve their anxiety by providing appropriate information. This should include a description of the pathophysiology of intussusception, the usefulness of hydrostatic reduction, and the expected recovery for their child, including the need for IV fluids, NG suction, and frequent vital signs and assessments. In addition, emotional support can be provided by encouraging them to participate in their child's care, listening to their concerns, and encouraging expression of their feelings during this stressful time.

VISUALIZING INTUSSUSCEPTION A rubber glove or balloon can be a useful teaching tool for parents. As you press one finger (representing the terminal ileum) into the inflated glove (the distal colon) and cause it to go inside itself, the telescoping can be visualized. The balloon can also demonstrate how hydrostatic reduction works. As you press on the distal portion (the glove) with your hand, you can feel how the telescoped portion (the finger) is pushed back to its normal position. Give parents their own balloon to help them better understand the mechanisms.

Evaluation

- In preoperative period, does child achieve moist mucous membranes, good skin turgor, urine specific gravity less than 1.025, and return to pre-illness weight?
- Is child passing soft, formed, Hematest-negative stool?
- Does infant guard abdomen when palpated?
- Is child demonstrating age-appropriate activity levels and play?
- Is child tolerating age-appropriate food and fluids without vomiting or recurrence of symptoms?
- Can parents explain rationale for hydrostatic reduction?
- Are all questions from the parents answered to their satisfaction?

INFLAMMATORY AND INFECTIOUS DISORDERS

Disorders that result from infection or chronic inflammatory changes in the lower GI tract are included in this section. These disorders are of major concern because of their effects on growth and development. Though some are easily resolved, like appendicitis, others, such as inflammatory bowel disease, can cause lifelong alterations in nutrition and elimination. Nursing care of these disorders includes nutritional support, assistance with elimination, skin care issues, infection control concerns, risk for repeated surgeries, and emotional support for families and can provide quite a challenge for nurses.

Inflammatory Bowel Disease

Inflammatory bowel disease is a chronic inflammatory condition of the small or large intestine. It includes two distinct conditions: ulcerative colitis and Crohn's disease. Ulcerative colitis affects only the colon and involves both the mucosal and submucosal layers of the intestine. Crohn's disease can occur anywhere in the GI tract from mouth to anus and is **transmural,** involving all layers of the intestine. Table 26–3 outlines the differences between ulcerative colitis and Crohn's disease.

Etiology. The exact cause of inflammatory bowel disease is not known. Several "triggers" have been identified, including viral and other infectious agents, food allergies, vasculitis, increased intestinal permeability, immunologic dysfunction, and genetic factors. The supposed psychogenic relationship has been under recent investigation and is now thought to be a result of the debilitating chronic infection instead of a direct cause (Cooke, 1991).

Incidence, Clinical Manifestations, and Diagnostic Evaluation. See Table 26–3.

Therapeutic Management. Management for inflammatory bowel disease is multidimensional and includes medication, dietary and nutritional support, and symptomatic treatment. Pharmacologic treatment includes anti-inflammatory, antibacterial, antibiotic, and immunosuppressive drugs. See Medications Commonly Used for GI Disorders in Clinical Reference Pages at the beginning of this chapter.

For ulcerative colitis, avoidance of milk products and the use of a low-fiber, low-residue, high-protein diet can be useful. Parenteral nutrition (TPN) may be needed during acute flare-ups or surgery to maintain nutritional support. Total colectomy is the only true cure.

Crohn's disease is best managed before permanent structural changes have developed. Malnutrition is a common problem and can involve protein, fat, carbohydrate, and vitamin deficiencies. Nutritional support and teaching are essential. Surgery is not curative but may be necessary for treatment of abscesses, fistulas, or chronic recurrent obstruction. Bowel resection is the usual procedure.

NURSING CARE OF THE CHILD WITH AN INFLAMMATORY BOWEL DISEASE

Assessment

Recurrent or chronic diarrhea is the primary finding of the nursing history with inflammatory bowel disease. The major assessment findings are a result of this diarrhea and the associated malabsorption that occurs. Weight loss, dehydration, anorexia, growth failure, vitamin deficiencies, and anemia are common. The severity of the GI symp-

TABLE 26–3 *Crohn's Disease and Ulcerative Colitis*

	CROHN'S DISEASE	ULCERATIVE COLITIS
Pathophysiology	Affects entire GI tract Transmural involvement Cobblestone appearance of mucosa Fistulas common Remissions and exacerbations	Involves only colon, starting at the rectum and moving upward Mucosa/submucosa only Mucosa lacking in most cases Fistulas rare Remissions uncommon
Diagnostic Evaluation *Colonoscopy* *Rectoscopy* *Barium enema*	"Skip" lesions with deep fissures and granulomas Normal	Continuous spreading with superficial ulceration No normal mucous membrane
Incidence	5 per 100,000 and increasing Equal sex distribution Not seen in infants Peaks in teens, early 20s Clusters in families Associated with higher standard of living	5 per 100,000 Equal sex distribution Peaks between age 15–40 years Clusters in families Affects whites more than other races
Clinical Manifestations	Abdominal pain Diarrhea, nonbloody Fever Palpable abdominal mass Anorexia and severe weight loss Significant growth impairment Perianal and anal lesions Fistulas and obstructions Extraintestinal symptoms (arthralgia and arthritis)	Abdominal pain unusual Diarrhea, occasionally with hemorrhage and anemia No masses Moderate weight loss Mild growth impairment Rare Fistulas and obstructions rare Risk of toxic megacolon
Morbidity and Mortality	Life expectancy not reduced 50%–70% will eventually require surgery for obstruction or fistula	12%–15% mortality 10% chance of cancer after 10 years

toms and the amount and length of steroid use will have a significant influence on a child's growth rate. Remissions and exacerbations of symptoms are common. Frank blood is possible in ulcerative colitis. Intermittent cramping discomfort that is exacerbated by eating is common in Crohn's disease. The child with Crohn's disease may complain of oral lesions and perianal skin breakdown.

Inflammatory changes can also occur outside of the GI system. Arthralgia and arthritis, especially of the lower extremities, can cause discomfort and mobility problems.

Depression, anxiety, fears about social interactions, and low self-esteem are found and are most likely related to the need to have quick access to restrooms at all times and be "close to home" should an accident occur. The chronic nature of this condition and its unknown prognosis can lead to family stress and tax the family financial resources and family support systems. Assessment should include questions about family and peer support, resources, and knowledge about the disease.

Nursing Diagnosis and Planning

The following nursing diagnoses and expected outcomes may be appropriate in the treatment of inflammatory bowel disease in the child.

- Altered Nutrition: Less Than Body Requirements related to chronic malabsorption. ***Expected Outcomes:*** *The child will have acceptable bowel patterns as evidenced by passing no more than four stools a day and being free from nocturnal diarrhea; receive adequate nutrition, as evidenced by normal hemoglobin and growth that follows the growth curve.*
- Pain related to cramping. ***Expected Outcome:*** *The child will be free from abdominal pain, as evidenced by resumption of normal activity and no complaints of pain.*
- Self-Esteem Disturbance related to chronic diarrhea and colostomy. ***Expected Outcome:*** *The child will have a positive self-concept as evidenced by leading an active lifestyle without depression.*

PATHOPHYSIOLOGY *of Inflammatory Bowel Disease*

The triggering factor, be it viral, allergic, or immunologic, causes the bowel to "respond" as if to an injury and results in capillary vasoconstriction and histamine release within the bowel. The histamine has two effects on the bowel. The first is vasodilation, which results in swelling that can cause malabsorption by distorting the surface area of the villi. Swelling then produces cell death and ulceration, which can progress to the development of fissures, strictures, fistulas, adhesions, and bowel obstruction. The second effect of histamine release is increased capillary permeability, which results in increased fluid in the intestine and subsequent diarrhea. Crohn's disease affects all the layers of the bowel, and ulcerative colitis affects the mucosa and submucosa only.

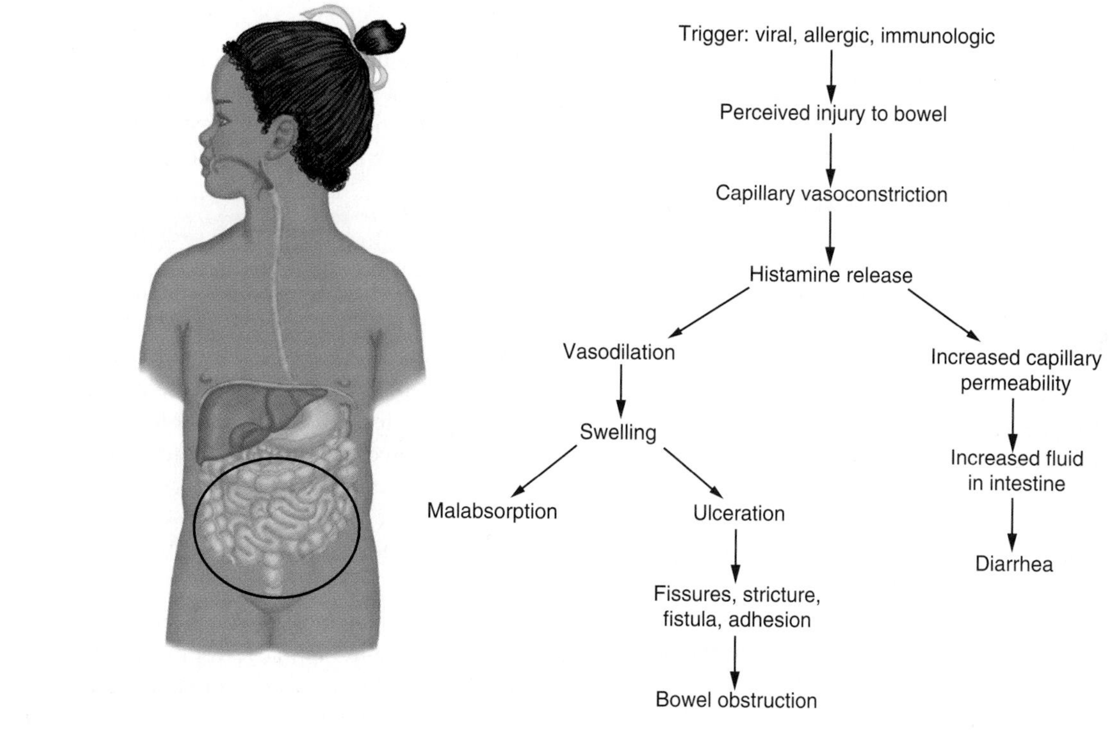

- Altered Growth and Development related to malnutrition, chronic illness, and steroid use. ***Expected Outcome:*** *The child will meet normal developmental milestones as evidenced by progress on standard developmental screenings.*
- Body Image Disturbance related to weight loss and water retention from steroid therapy. ***Expected Outcome:*** *The child will state reasons for changes in body appearance, and share concerns about changes with family and support personnel.*

Implementation

Nursing care centers on maintaining pharmacologic interventions, developing long-term nutritional management, educating, and providing emotional support.

Medications. Teaching appropriate administration of medications is an important nursing role. Enemas are used before critical diagnostic tests and as a method of medication administration. Any child who will be taking steroids needs to understand the importance of regular administration. They should be given with food or antacids if GI distress becomes a problem. The steroids, though beneficial in symptom suppression, may actually exacerbate the growth delays associated with inflammatory bowel disease. See the Clinical Reference Pages for a discussion of medications used to control inflammatory bowel disease.

Nutritional Management. Nutritional support varies with the disease and the patient's tolerance to changes. In general, maintaining a low-fiber, low-residue, milk-free diet provides some relief, though strict restrictions do not alleviate symptoms. A balanced nutritious diet is recommended as are vitamin, iron, and folate supplements. During periods of acute flare-up or surgery, TPN and lipids may be needed to restore a seriously malnourished child. These will not change the course of the inflammation in the bowel but will provide essential nutritional support. Elemental diets, which can be absorbed without significant digestion, may be used during acute episodes of Crohn's disease to allow for bowel rest. NG or gastrostomy tube feedings during the night may be necessary during puberty to prevent further growth impairment. Continued assessment of nutritional status, growth patterns, and development are important parts of nursing care for this chronic problem. Assessing of the number of stools, nutritional status, weight, developmental milestones, and pain will help in evaluating response to treatment.

Family Education and Support. Education and support can be provided by appropriate community resources. The Crohn's Colitis Foundation of America will supply educational materials and give the child and family information on local resources and support groups (see Appendix H). Long-term nursing care can be improved by providing consistent caregivers and encouraging relationships to form. Self-care and management should be major goals in working with children with inflammatory bowel disease and other chronic diseases (see Chapter 17). The parents and child will be assuming responsibility for home care.

Because this is a long-term health problem with numerous medical, pharmacologic, and surgical interventions required, family support and financial resources can be strained to the limit. National and local support groups may be able to give essential support to the family in these areas. In addition, emotional support of caregivers becomes very important.

Home Care. Home care is a mainstay of treatment. Teaching parents how to administer steroids, including providing information on their inherent side effects and the importance of not discontinuing their use abruptly, should be a high priority. The techniques of enema administration and skin care of perianal lesions should also be learned by the caregivers. Keeping nutrition diaries can also provide useful information. TPN may be administered at home, and parents need complete instructions.

In addition, helping children and parents know when to seek care is important. Sudden exacerbations of symptoms, weight loss, blood loss, and severe abdominal pain should be reported to health care professionals.

Evaluation

Does child take all medications as ordered?
Can child and parent explain actions, side effects, and correct administration of all medications?
Is child free from nocturnal diarrhea?
Is child passing more than four stools per day?
Does child and family seek help when exacerbations occur?
Is child gaining weight appropriately and following the growth chart?
Is child's hemoglobin between 11 and 16?
Does child complain of abdominal pain?
Does child participate in age-appropriate activities without evidence of depression?
Has child or family sought external support through appropriate referral groups?

Appendicitis

Appendicitis is the inflammation and infection of the vermiform appendix, a small lymphoid, tubular, blind sac at the end of the cecum. It is the most common cause of emergency surgery in children and adolescents.

PATHOPHYSIOLOGY *of Appendicitis*

Obstruction of the appendix allows normal mucus secretions to accumulate in the appendix, producing distension. Distension eventually causes occlusion of the capillaries and engorgement of the walls of the appendix. Microabscesses form, and can progress to abscess and fistulas. Perforation occurs as a result of tissue breakdown and swelling. Bowel contents then contaminate the mesenteric bed and peritoneum, leading to peritonitis and sepsis.

Etiology. Common causes of obstruction and subsequent appendicitis include lymphoid swelling related to viral infection, impacted fecal material, foreign bodies, and parasites. In most cases, no definitive cause can be identified at time of surgery.

Incidence. Appendicitis occurs with equal frequency in both sexes, with most cases occurring during adolescence and early adulthood. There are approximately 4 appendectomies per 1000 children under age 14 years (Behrman, Kliegman, & Arvin, 1996). Appendicitis is uncommon under age 4 years, but in those cases, it has a very high frequency of perforation, most likely related to the difficulty in diagnosis.

Clinical Manifestations

- Pain progressing in intensity and localizing to the right lower quadrant at **McBurney's point** (Fig. 26–1)
- Nausea and vomiting
- Anorexia
- Diarrhea or constipation
- Fever and chills

Appendicitis may be *very* difficult to assess in young children.

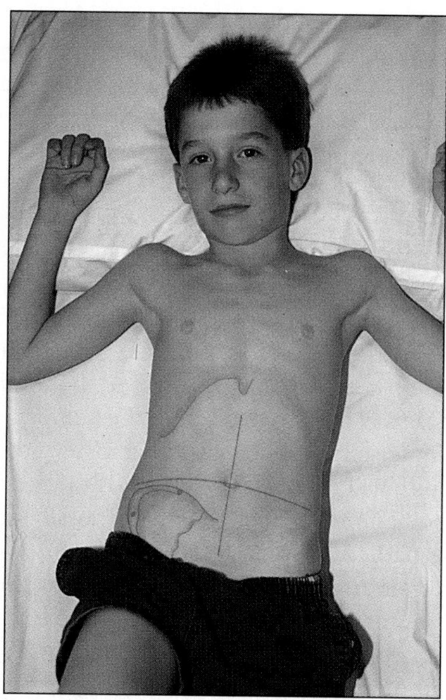

Figure 26–1
McBurney's point is midway between the right anterior superior iliac crest and the umbilicus. It is usually the location of greatest pain in the child with appendicitis. (Photo courtesy of University of Texas at Arlington School of Nursing)

Diagnostic Evaluation. Diagnosis is usually based on the classic abdominal findings of pain at McBurney's point: guarding, rebound tenderness, nausea, vomiting, and fever. The presence of a white blood cell count of 15,000 to 20,000 cells/μl can support the clinical findings. A quick, safe, and accurate diagnosis can usually be made with ultrasound, which indicates an enlarged, incompressible appendix that may be fluid filled and locally inflamed.

Therapeutic Management. The definitive treatment for appendicitis and suspected appendicitis is appendectomy. Preoperatively the child is managed with fluid therapy, immobilization to control pain, NPO, and antibiotics. The procedure may be done laparoscopically or with an open abdominal approach if perforation is suspected.

NURSING CARE OF THE CHILD WITH APPENDICITIS

Assessment

Nursing assessment will reveal a history of vomiting, pain, fever, and diarrhea or constipation. Physical examination will find abdominal tenderness and guarding. The child may assume a supine position with the right leg flexed to decrease tension on the abdominal wall. The nurse must be keenly aware of the symptoms of perforation, including a sudden relief from pain followed by an increase in pain, rigid abdomen, and early shock symptoms. Behavioral changes and refusal to eat are important indicators in infants.

It is important to assess anxiety in the child and family who are most likely facing surgery. The child may be combative toward abdominal assessment because of the pain. The parents may have financial concerns related to the unplanned surgery.

Nursing Diagnosis and Planning

The following nursing diagnoses and expected outcomes may be appropriate in the treatment of appendicitis in the child.

- Pain related to abdominal inflammation and surgical incision. ***Expected Outcome:*** *The child will be free from pain, as evidenced by resumption of normal activity and movement, with no complaints of pain.*
- Risk for Infection related to rupture and surgery. ***Expected Outcomes:*** *The child will have a clean, dry surgical incision that is free from redness, heat, or exudate; be afebrile with a WBC count of 5,000 to 15,000 cells/μl.*
- Fluid Volume Deficit related to vomiting and/or diarrhea. ***Expected Outcome:*** *The child will be well-hydrated, as evidenced by moist mucous membranes, good skin turgor, and urine output of at least 2 ml/kg/hr.*
- Anxiety related to unplanned surgery. ***Expected Outcomes:*** *The parent/child will express feelings about surgery; verbalize necessity for emergency hospitalization.*

Implementation

On admission, vital signs should be assessed for signs of sepsis or shock. Comfort measures may be instituted, including topical cold, pain medications, and encouraging positions of comfort. Enemas or laxatives should not be administered. No heat should be applied to the abdomen because this may increase the chance of perforation secondary to vasodilation. IV fluid therapy should be instituted to prepare the child for surgery and correct any existing acid-base disturbance related to vomiting and diarrhea.

If the procedure is performed laparoscopically, discharge should be expected within 24 hours. Open surgical removal may require several days of recovery in the hospital. After either surgery, the child will be NPO until bowel function has returned. For the child with a perforation, IV antibiotics are continued for a longer period of time and hospitalization may be 5 to 14 days. During this time the diet should be advanced gradually as tolerated so that the child can tolerate a normal diet without vomiting or diarrhea.

Ruptured Appendix. The child with a ruptured appendix requires special care. If perforation is suspected, the child should be prepared for insertion of an NG tube for decompression and the possibility of an external drainage device after surgery. IV antibiotics may be started. Postoperatively, this child will have had more major surgery, requiring a larger incision, possibly lavage, and the placement of drains. These drains may be attached to suction, and asepsis and patency must be maintained at all times. The amount of drainage should be carefully recorded. The wound may be left open and treated with sterile wet-to-dry (saline-soaked gauze) dressings and wound irrigations with antibacterial solutions. Pain from the incision and from frequent dressing changes should be managed with analgesics, especially opioids, given around the clock (see Chapter 20, The Child in Pain). Continued assessment of abdominal pain is essential in evaluating the presence of abscess or fistula. Vital signs including temperature should be monitored every 2 to 4 hours. Nasogastric suction will likely be continued postoperatively until normal bowel sounds return. Positioning the child to facilitate drainage and minimize the spread of infection into the upper abdomen should be done by elevating the head of the bed or having the child lie on the operative side.

Home Care. After surgery and discharge parents must be prepared to assume responsibility for the child's care. The surgical incision and any drain sites must be assessed for redness, drainage, dehiscence, or suture infections and any problems reported to the physician. The diet should be advanced slowly. Parents should begin with liquids and soft foods and progress to the child's normal diet if it can be tolerated without nausea or vomiting. Parents should be taught to watch for vomiting, abdominal pain, or distension as possible signs of bowel obstruction or peritoneal infection.

Evaluation

Does child complain of pain?
Does child demonstrate guarding on abdominal palpation?
Has child returned to normal activity level?
Does the child have normal bowel sounds?
Is surgical incision clean, dry, and free from redness, heat, purulent drainage, or dehiscence?
Is child afebrile with WBC count of 5,000 to 15,000 cells/µl?
Is child tolerating age-appropriate regular diet without vomiting, diarrhea, or increased abdominal pain?

Infectious Gastroenteritis

Infectious gastroenteritis is caused by a group of viruses, bacteria, and parasites that are capable of causing serious communicable diarrhea, massive fluid and electrolyte loss, sepsis, and death. For further discussion, see Chapter 24.

Etiology. Ingestion of contaminated food or water and person-to-person contamination are the most likely causes of infectious gastroenteritis in the United States. High-risk groups include children in day-care centers, preschools, and chronic care facilities and those infected with the human immunodeficiency virus. *Giardia* is the most common pathogen in toddlers, and rotavirus is most common in infants (Cheney & Wong, 1993). In most incidences the pathogen is not identified. See Table 26–4.

PATHOPHYSIOLOGY ***of Infectious Gastroenteritis***

As the pathogen adheres to the mucosa of the intestine, it is no longer affected by peristaltic waves and is not removed from the site. Epithelial invasion occurs, causing an inflammatory response and epithelial cell death. This leads to ulcerations, pseudomembranes, bleeding, and possibly sepsis. As the pathogens multiply, they may produce toxins. Enterotoxins (e.g., cholera, *Shigella*) cause fluid and electrolyte shifts that result in increased secretion into the intestine and simultaneous decrease in absorption secondary to edema. This results in massive diarrhea and dehydration. Cytotoxins (e.g., *Salmonella*) produce local edema, malabsorption, and dehydration. Some pathogens are also capable of producing neurotoxins (e.g., *Shigella*) that act outside of the GI tract.

Incidence. Gastroenteritis is one of the most common outpatient infectious diseases. In children under age 5 years, 2 to 2.5 cases per year can be expected. Infections peak in the summer and have an equal sex distribution. Despite the usually self-limiting nature of the condition, mortality is estimated to be 0.25 deaths per 1000 live births in the first year of life (Cheney & Wong, 1993).

Clinical Manifestations. Gastroenteritis will likely present with some degree of the following.

- Diarrhea of varying amount and consistency
- Tenesmus
- Abdominal pain
- Fever
- Vomiting
- Dehydration
- History of travel to other regions of the world or country

See Table 26–4 for findings specific to each causative organism.

Diagnostic Evaluation. Definitive diagnosis can be made by rectal or stool culture that is positive for a pathogen, but these cultures are expensive and result in many false negatives. Ova and parasites are more reliably found. Only children who appear toxic or have bloody stools, abdominal pain, or *tenesmus* usually receive a diagnostic workup. The presence of fecal WBCs and blood can support the presumptive diagnosis based on clinical findings. Blood

TABLE 26–4 *Characteristics of Infectious Diarrhea*

INFECTIOUS AGENT	CHARACTERISTICS	CLINICAL MANIFESTATIONS	DIAGNOSTIC FINDINGS	TREATMENT
Shigella (Enteroinvasive With Cytotoxin)	Incubation 1–7 days Most common in summer Fecal-oral spread Remains communicable for 1–3 weeks	Symptoms last 5–10 days Diarrhea begins as watery, progresses to small, bloody, mucus Severe abdominal pain High fever Neurologic symptoms (headache, nuchal rigidity, convulsions) Risk for sepsis, hemolytic uremic syndrome, rectal prolapse, DIC	Blood, mucus, WBCs in stool Positive culture in some cases	Bactrim 8–10 mg/kg/day × 5 days OR Ampicillin 50–100 mg/kg/day × 5 days Enteric precautions Identify source if possible
Salmonella (Enteroinvasive)	Incubation 6 hours–3 days Most common in summer, fall Usually food-borne Infectious for duration of illness and variable period afterward	Symptoms last 2–5 days Rapid onset Secretory diarrhea Abdominal pain, nausea, vomiting common	+blood, PMNs in stool	For infants younger than age 12 weeks, same as *Shigella* Enteric precautions Identify source if possible
E. coli (Enteroinvasive With Enterotoxin)	Variable incubation Most common in summer Food-borne most common	Green, watery, secretory diarrhea May cause hemorrhagic colitis Fever	+blood, PMNs	Same as *Shigella* Enteric precautions
Campylobacter	Incubation 1–8 days Most common in infants and adolescents	History of consumption of contaminated shellfish Severe abdominal pain Foul-smelling, watery diarrhea	+blood, PMNs	Possibly treated with erythromycin × 7 days Enteric precautions
Giardia Lamblia	Most common cause of parasitic diarrhea Spread in water	Afebrile Abdominal distension, flatulence Variable diarrhea	–blood, –PMNs, +ova and parasites Parasite found on duodenal biopsy	Flagyl × 7 days Enteric precautions Treat all unknown water sources with chlorine/iodine before drinking
Rotavirus	Incubation 1–3 days Common in winter months Accounts for 50% of cases of acute diarrhea in children	Symptoms usually last 2–6 days History of preceding or concurrent respiratory illness Fever for 24–48 hours	–blood, –PMNs, ova and parasites	No pharmacologic treatment Enteric precautions Immunization under development
C. Difficile	Antibiotic-associated Most common nosocomial diarrhea	Diarrhea develops after antibiotic treatment	+blood, PMNs	Cholestyramine used to enhance mucosal recovery and decrease length of diarrhea Possibly treated with Vancomycin or Flagyl × 10 days

cultures may also be needed in the acutely ill infant and young child. An unprepared sigmoidoscopy can be useful in the diagnosis of the amount of mucosal involvement and in obtaining more reliable cultures and may be useful in diagnosis. See Table 26–4.

Therapeutic Management. The priority therapy is to replace water and correct acid-base or fluid and electrolyte disturbances with IV fluids or PO electrolyte replacement liquids. The rate of replacement may be as high as 50 to 100 ml/kg over 4 to 6 hours (one to two and a half times maintenance) (Cheney & Wong, 1993). Because diarrhea is high in sodium, potassium, and bicarbonate, oral rehydration solutions (e.g., WHO formula, Pedialyte) should be used to match losses. Hospitalization for treatment is not uncommon, especially in the infant or small child, to allow for continued assessment and management of symptoms or sepsis. Antimicrobial therapy is useful in *Shigella* and *Giardia*, and some cases of *Salmonella*, *Clostridium difficile*, and *Escherichia coli*, but not rotavirus.

Antimotility drugs (Lomotil, Imodium) are occasionally used for severe diarrhea but may in fact delay the clearance of the pathogen and increase the extent of the invasion. They should not be used for longer than 48 hours. Large doses of Pepto-Bismol can cause salicylate poisoning in children and should not be used. Adsorbent drugs (cholestyramine) are useful in *C. difficile* diarrhea because of their ability to bind the toxin that is present.

See Chapter 24 for further discussion.

NURSING CARE OF THE CHILD WITH INFECTIOUS GASTROENTERITIS

Assessment

Obtain an adequate history of the event, including the length of symptoms, frequency and consistency of stools, and the presence of blood or mucus in stools. Noting the amount, color, consistency, and time (ACCT) of each stool is a consistent way to document findings. The concurrent appearance of symptoms in other members of the family can also be helpful in diagnosis. Any travel to other countries or wilderness areas should also be documented. Evaluating formula and food preparation at home and in day-care facilities as well as examining sanitation and hygiene in these places can provide valuable information.

The child may appear moderately to severely dehydrated with hyperactive bowel sounds and severe diarrhea, often bloody in nature. Blood in the stool usually appears after the maximum fluid loss has occurred and can be useful in determining the stage of illness. The presence of abdominal pain, vomiting, tenesmus, and fever should be assessed. Complaints of headache, nuchal rigidity, irritability, and seizures are important to note as symptoms of the neurotoxic effects of *Shigella*.

Assessment of hydration status is critical. Poor urine output, high urine specific gravity, poor skin turgor, dry mucous membranes, crying without producing tears, a sunken/depressed fontanel in infants, and skin tenting can occur quickly with the large amount of fluid lost through diarrhea. Loss of bicarbonate from severe diarrhea and dehydration make metabolic acidosis a major concern. The compensatory mechanisms of increased respiratory rate and effort are important to document.

Nursing Diagnosis and Planning

The following nursing diagnoses and expected outcomes may be appropriate in the treatment of infectious gastroenteritis in the child.

- Fluid Volume Deficit related to severe diarrhea. ***Expected Outcomes:*** *The child will be adequately hydrated without electrolyte disturbance, as evidenced by moist mucous membranes, good skin turgor, return to normal weight, and normal serum sodium, potassium, and bicarbonate levels; have soft, formed stools without diarrhea, blood, or mucus.*
- Risk for Infection related to exposure of family members and others to infectious agents. ***Expected Outcome:*** *The child will not transmit pathogens to others.*
- Pain related to abdominal cramping. ***Expected Outcome:*** *The child will be free from abdominal pain, as evidenced by return to normal activity and no complaints of pain.*
- Knowledge Deficit related to disease and its control. ***Expected Outcome:*** *The parents will demonstrate an understanding of the communicability of the condition, as evidenced by use of enteric precautions when handling child's secretions.*
- Altered Nutrition: Less Than Body Requirements related to malabsorption. ***Expected Outcomes:*** *The child will resume normal diet; regain weight lost during acute phase within 1 week after symptoms abate.*
- Risk for Impaired Skin Integrity related to skin contact with feces and necessity for frequent cleansing. ***Expected Outcome:*** *The child will maintain skin integrity as evidenced by clean, dry intact skin without redness, drainage, or breakdown.*

Implementation

Critical nursing interventions are related to the fluid volume deficit. IV fluids with electrolyte corrections and bicarbonate are essential to establish homeostasis. Accurate intake and output measurements and weights are important. Monitoring skin turgor, urine output, and serum electrolyte levels will provide evaluation criteria in this area. See Chapter 24 for further discussion.

Providing safety, assessing neurologic symptoms, and monitoring for seizures are also priorities for the child with *Shigella*.

Prevention of the spread of infection remains a critical nursing intervention. Thorough handwashing is a must. Isolation techniques must be strictly enforced for all staff and family members to minimize the risk of infection. These must be maintained at home for up to 2 weeks, or less if antibiotics are given.

Pain and fever may be treated with acetaminophen, but symptomatic treatment with antidiarrheals is not recommended without physician prescription because it tends to increase the length of symptoms. Symptomatic care of the febrile child includes tepid sponging and light dressing.

Parents and children will require teaching about these interventions and the disease process during this period. (See Teaching Guidelines for the Child With Infectious Diarrhea.) Because this is a public health concern, dietary recalls can be important in establishing the causation and minimizing the risk of spread to the public.

Home Care. The most important intervention that can be implemented at home is proper rehydration to prevent the need for hospitalization and IV therapy. See Chapter 24 for a discussion of oral rehydration fluids and an extensive nursing care plan about caring for the child with diarrhea. After rehydration has been successful and symptoms have subsided, feeding should resume. Clear liquids for 24 hours after symptoms have subsided is recommended. After that time, the normal diet is slowly resumed. Isomil DF, a lactose-free formula with added fiber, is a good start for the formula-fed infant. Older children and toddlers can gradually resume a soft diet of easily digestible foods such as cereals, cooked vegetables, and lean meats.

The prevention of spread of infection is also essential for home care. Handwashing; disinfection of contaminated linens, clothes, and diapers; and the use of surface disinfectant sprays are important.

Evaluation

Has child returned to preinfection weight?
Does child have good skin turgor, moist mucous membranes, and urine specific gravity of less than 1.025?
Does child have serum sodium of 139 to 145-mmol/L and serum potassium of 4.1 to 5.2 mmol/L?
Is child passing soft, formed stools without diarrhea, blood, or mucus?
Can child tolerate age-appropriate regular diet?
Are other family members free from infectious diarrhea?
Is child complaining of abdominal pain?
Does child guard abdomen to palpation?
Is day-care facility practicing appropriate infection control procedures, if appropriate?

HEPATIC DISORDERS

Disorders that involve the liver and biliary tract may be the result of congenital malformations or acquired infection. Because of the importance of the liver in metabolism, alterations in its function can affect many body systems, including the cardiovascular, skin, renal, neurologic, hematologic, and immunologic systems. These disorders can also have significant effects on growth and development. Nursing care may involve nutritional support, infection control, developmental stimulation, family support, and intensive physiologic care during a period of crisis and/or transplant.

Biliary Atresia

Biliary atresia refers to the obstruction or absence of the extrahepatic bile ducts. At birth, the liver structure itself is normal without inflammation, but the structural problem leads to significant cellular damage and eventual liver failure and death.

Etiology. The cause of biliary atresia is unknown. Because the problem originates during the prenatal period, viruses, toxins, and chemicals cannot be ruled out. It is unlikely to recur within the same family.

Incidence. Extrahepatic biliary atresia occurs in 1 in 10,000 to 20,000 births, with a slightly higher incidence in females (MacDonald, 1991).

TEACHING GUIDELINES *for the Child With Infectious Diarrhea*

- Teach parents adequate handwashing.
- Encourage day-care providers to use gloves when changing diapers, clothing, and linens.
- Allow child to use a separate bathroom if available.
- Administer PO fluids using appropriate rehydration solutions (WHO, Pedialyte, Rehydralyte) in small, frequent amounts (every 30 minutes).
- Document progress of diarrhea using ACCT method.
- Bacterial gastroenteritis may be communicable for several weeks after symptoms abate so enteric precautions need to be continued.
- When PO intake resumes, avoid foods containing lactose. Use special formulas (Isomil DF) and introduce milk products gradually.
- Keep day-care providers aware of dietary changes, and provide supervision in food or formula preparation as needed.

PATHOPHYSIOLOGY *of Biliary Atresia*

Obstruction of the extrahepatic bile ducts causes obstruction of the normal flow of bile out of the liver and into the gallbladder and small intestine. As a result bile plugs form and cause bile to back up in the liver. This causes inflammation, edema, and hepatic degeneration. Eventually the liver becomes fibrotic, and cirrhosis and portal hypertension develop, leading to liver failure. The gradual degeneration of the liver causes jaundice, icterus, and hepatomegaly. Because bile is not present in the intestine, fat and fat-soluble vitamins cannot be absorbed. This leads to malnutrition, deficiencies of fat-soluble vitamins, and growth failure.

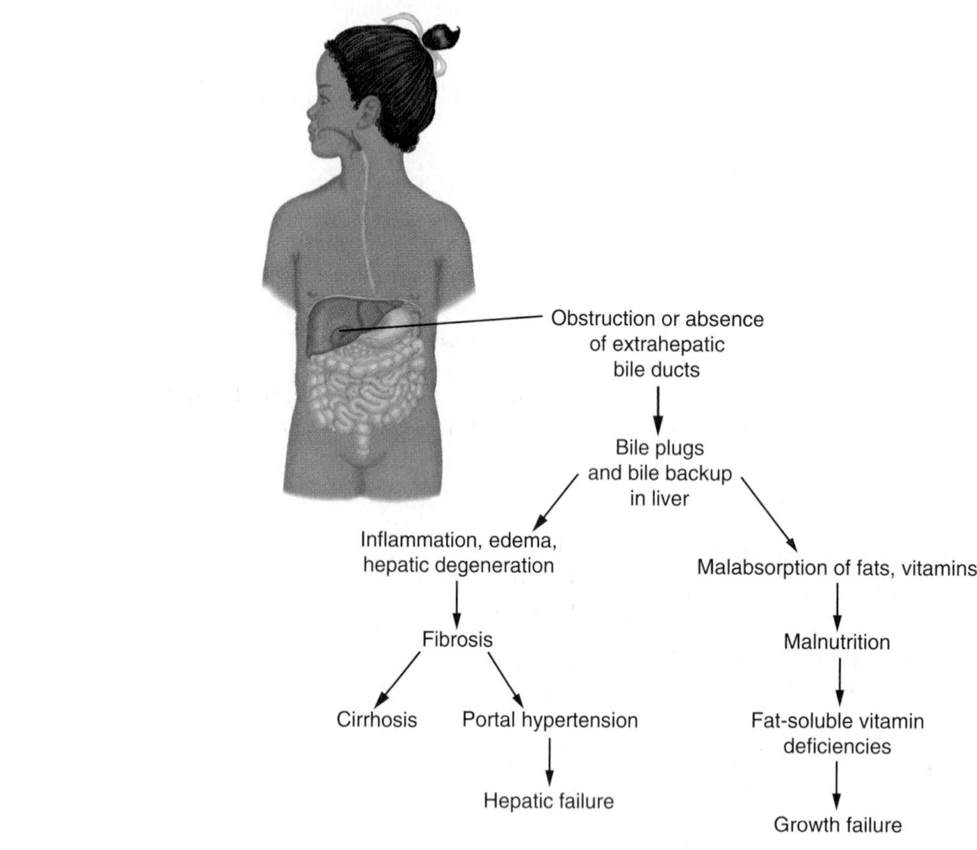

Clinical Manifestations

- Child is apparently healthy at birth.
- Jaundice occurs within 2 weeks to 2 months.
- **Acholic** (light in color, due to absence of bile pigment) stools
- Bile-stained urine
- Hepatomegaly

Diagnostic Evaluation. Investigations of liver function (bilirubin, aminotransferases [ALT, AST]) and clotting studies (prothrombin time, partial thromboplastin time) are useful screening tools. Metabolic screens are essential in these patients in order to rule out inborn errors of metabolism such as galactosemia and alpha-1 antitrypsin deficiency, which can produce similar initial findings. Hepatitis and other viral titers are also necessary to eliminate neonatal hepatitis as the source of dysfunction. Urine and stool should be examined and urobilinogen levels determined as an indication of the degree of obstruction.

Liver biopsy can provide a definitive diagnosis if bile plugs, edema, and fibrosis are found in the presence of normal hepatic lobular structure (Behrman, Kliegman, & Arvin, 1996). Cholangiography may be used to determine the extent of atresia.

Therapeutic Management. During and after exploratory laparotomy, the size of the lesion can be identified and drainage can be attempted. If no correctable lesion is found, a hepatic **portoenterostomy** (Kasai procedure) will be performed to allow for drainage of bile from the liver. This procedure allows bile to flow directly into the intestine through an anastomosis of the jejunum to the porta hepatis, the point at which the hepatic ducts join to form the common bile duct. The Kasai procedure does provide some long-term benefits; however, hepatic dysfunction will persist. The main goal of this procedure is to allow growth and development of the child until such time as a liver transplant can be performed.

The medical management of the child involves the management of malnutrition and symptom relief. Medium chain triglyceride (MCT) oil or TPN provides essential nutrition. Vitamin malabsorption must be treated to prevent night blindness (vitamin A), neuromuscular degeneration (vitamin E), rickets (vitamin D), and hypoprothrombinemia (vitamin K) (Behrman, Kliegman, & Arvin, 1996). Assessment for and treatment of portal hypertension with its concomitant problems of ascites and variceal bleeding must be instituted. Controlling bleeding, restricting salt, and using diuretics are important in managing portal hypertension.

NURSING CARE OF THE CHILD WITH BILIARY ATRESIA

Assessment

During the early phase of disease, in the first months of life, the infant with biliary atresia will appear jaundiced, with mild hepatosplenomegaly and increased abdominal girth. As the disease progresses, the child may appear thin, with failure to thrive, marked jaundice, and evidence of rickets secondary to chronic vitamin D deficiency.

Pruritus becomes a major problem; the child may develop skin infections or xanthoma (lipid deposits in the skin) secondary to retention of cholesterol in the skin.

After the Kasai procedure, the child needs to be assessed for evidence of portal hypertension, which may include the development of ascites and GI bleeding. Even after repair, it would not be unusual to find *acholic* stools and bile-stained urine.

Psychosocial and family assessment should have a high priority. This is a life-threatening, chronic problem that requires surgical intervention, contacts with numerous health care personnel, repeated hospitalization, and eventually an extended wait for a transplant. Information about family and financial resources, emotional support, and the feelings of the child and family about progress and management of the disease should be gathered. For more information see Chapters 16 and 17.

Nursing Diagnosis and Planning

The following nursing diagnoses and expected outcomes may be appropriate in caring for the infant with biliary atresia.

- Altered Nutrition: Less Than Body Requirements related to malabsorption. ***Expected Outcome:*** *The infant will receive adequate nutrition, as evidenced by following the growth curve and being free of vitamin deficiency conditions.*
- Risk for Infection related to pruritus and surgical site. ***Expected Outcome:*** *The infant will have intact skin without breakdown or purulent drainage.*
- Altered Growth and Development related to chronic malnutrition. ***Expected Outcome:*** *The child will meet normal developmental milestones as evidenced by progress on standard developmental screening tests.*
- Sensory/Perceptual Alterations related to increased blood toxins. ***Expected Outcome:*** *The infant will be alert and will interact with the environment.*
- Ineffective Family Coping: Compromised related to life-threatening illness. ***Expected Outcomes:*** *The parents will demonstrate knowledge of the disease process and prognosis during discussions with health care personnel; deal with grief, as evidenced by expressing feelings about the "loss of the perfect child," and seeking family, community, and national support.*

Implementation

Nursing interventions are centered on six major areas: nutritional support, skin care, developmental stimulation, continued assessment, education, and emotional support.

Nutritional Support. Providing adequate calories, aiding in vitamin supply and absorption, and preventing hepatic encephalopathy are important goals. Calorie counts, daily weights, and abdominal girths are important assessments and will provide the data necessary to improve nutritional support. Concentrating calories with the use of Polycose and providing MCT supplements that do not require the presence of bile salts to digest will significantly change the nutritional status of the child. NG tube feeding or TPN may become necessary at times. Supplements of vitamins A, D, E, and K as well as calcium, phosphate, and zinc are essential for adequate nutrition. Protein may need to be limited to avoid the development of hepatic encephalopathy. Using growth charts and weighing on a monthly basis will provide evaluation criteria.

Skin Care. Bile acid binders such as cholestyramine and phenobarbital aid in the excretion of bile salts and decrease pruritus and the development of xanthomas (Behrman, Kliegman, & Arvin, 1996). Colloidal oatmeal baths (Aveeno) can be comforting for severe itching. Prevention of skin breakdown due to severe scratching is essential. Gloves during sleep, soothing lotions, and creams for dry skin may prevent infection.

Developmental Stimulation. Teaching parents activities to provide developmental stimulation and using resources available through physical and occupational therapy are essential. As the child awaits transplant, efforts should be made to facilitate as much development as possible by providing stimulation for gross and fine motor skills and social and emotional growth. Routine screening tests can document developmental growth and help evaluate interventions.

Continued Assessment. Continued assessment for the development of portal hypertension cannot be overlooked. The parents must be taught to watch for GI bleeding and the development of severe edema and ascites. Should this occur, sodium restriction, diuretics, IV albumin, and hospitalization may become necessary.

Family Education and Support. The family has many educational needs, and the nurse needs to be involved in helping them understand the disease process, deal with nutritional changes, manage skin care, assess for danger signs, and enhance development. See Chapter 17. National resources are available to help these families. The Children's Liver Foundation is able to provide programs, educational materials, and referral to support groups as needed (see Appendix H).

> The nurse who can listen to parental concerns, provide resources and support, and encourage participation and involvement is a critical member of the health care team. The nurse should provide information about daily care and focus attention to the future liver transplant and its long-term care and treatment. Because this usually occurs within the first 2 years of life, age-appropriate explanations for the toddler are also indicated.

The child and family should be prepared for the eventual need for a liver transplant and the possible death of their child. This is a life-threatening condition that requires numerous hospitalizations and many diagnostic tests and produces immense stress on families. Arranging the educational and emotional support needed by the family so that they can manage their child until liver transplantation becomes possible is a critical nursing intervention.

Home Care. The parents must be able to assume all home care responsibilities. This includes being able to monitor growth and nutritional intake, mix special formulas, manage NG feedings, provide skin care, and give medications. Their ability to assess for GI bleeding, ascites, edema, and skin infections is critical so that treatment can begin as soon as possible.

Evaluation

- Is child's growth following growth chart?
- Is child showing symptoms of protein malnutrition or vitamin deficiencies?
- Is child's skin free from breakdown or purulent drainage?
- Are developmental milestones being met?
- Is child alert and interacting with his environment?
- Do parents report severe edema, ascites, infections, or GI bleeding?
- Are parents involved in support groups or utilizing information networks?
- Can parents explain rationale and procedures in obtaining a liver transplant?

Viral Hepatitis

Hepatitis is an acute or chronic inflammation of the liver caused by several different viruses and some toxins or disease states. Though each type of hepatitis is unique, there are many similarities in assessment findings and treatment.

Etiology. The most common causes of viral hepatitis are discussed in Table 26–5. Rubella, cytomegalovirus (CMV), herpes simplex, and Epstein-Barr virus may also occasionally produce hepatitis in children.

The most common mode of transmission of *hepatitis A (HAV)* is person to person, by the fecal-oral route. Hepatitis A virus is highly contagious and spreads readily in households and day-care centers. Epidemics of HAV have been caused by eating shellfish contaminated by human sewage. HAV infection can also be acquired by swimming in contaminated water.

Hepatitis B virus (HBV) is primarily transmitted parenterally or by sexual contact. Sharing or reusing contaminated needles or syringes, exposure to infected blood or bloody fluids, and sexual activity are the most common modes of HBV transmission (American Academy of Pediatrics, 1994). The most important modes of transmission for HBV infection in children are perinatal transmission from an HBV-infected mother to her infant and exposure to infected drugs or blood products (Ramos-Soriano & Schwarz, 1994). HBV infection transmitted by blood transfusions has decreased in recent years as a result of improved blood product screening procedures. Contaminated body fluids splashed into the mouth or eyes can cause HBV infection. HBV can survive in the dried state for 1 week or longer, and percutaneous contact with contaminated objects can transmit infection. Hepatitis B is not spread by the fecal-oral route.

Incidence. There are over 60,000 cases of hepatitis reported each year. A large number of hepatitis A outbreaks can be traced to day-care centers. The risk of an outbreak of HAV occurring in a day-care center increases with the number of children enrolled who are younger than age 2 years and who wear diapers (AAP, 1994). Because the virus may be excreted for 2 to 3 weeks before the appearance of clinical signs and for 2 to 3 weeks afterward, outbreaks are common wherever good handwashing is not practiced.

In the United States and other western industrialized countries hepatitis B infection occurs most often in adoles-

PATHOPHYSIOLOGY *of Viral Hepatitis*

Hepatitis viruses cause necrosis of the parenchymal cells of the liver. The inflammatory response causes swelling and blockage of the drainage system in the liver. Biliary stasis and further destruction of the hepatic cells occurs. Because bile cannot be excreted by the liver into the intestine, it appears in the blood (hyperbilirubinemia), urine (urobilinogen), and skin (hepatocellular jaundice).

Hepatitis infection may result in asymptomatic or mild illness, in which complete regeneration of liver cells occurs within 2 to 3 months. More severe forms of hepatitis include *fulminant hepatitis,* in which hepatic necrosis and death can occur within 1 to 2 weeks, and *subacute or chronic hepatitis,* which can result in permanent scarring of the liver and impaired liver function. Chronically infected persons are carriers of the disease and are at increased risk for developing chronic liver disease (cirrhosis, chronic persistent hepatitis) or liver carcinoma later in life.

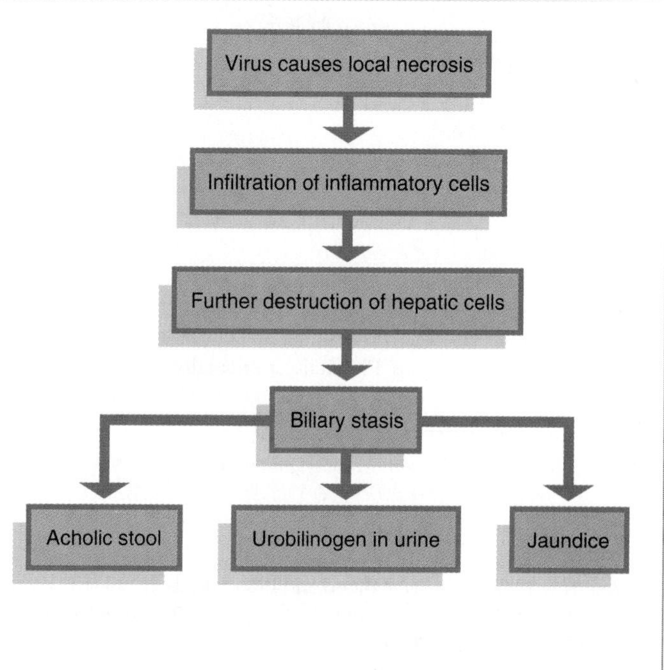

cents and adults. From 5% to 8% of the U.S. population has been infected with HBV, and 0.2% to 0.9% are chronically infected. In developing countries where sanitation is poor, HBV occurs most often in infants and children younger than age 5 years. From 70% to 90% of the adult population of these areas has been infected, and 8% to 15% are chronically infected. Infection with hepatitis B is the leading cause of acute and chronic liver disease worldwide (Katkov, 1995).

Clinical Manifestations. In infants and preschool-age children, hepatitis A is usually either asymptomatic or causes mild, nonspecific symptoms such as anorexia, malaise, and easy fatigability. The disease causes more severe symptoms of nausea, jaundice, and malaise in adults.

> Because most children with hepatitis A are asymptomatic or have mild, nonspecific symptoms the disease may not be diagnosed until an outbreak of hepatitis occurs. Thus, spread of HAV infection in a day-care center often occurs before the initial case is identified.

Hepatitis B may cause a wide range of clinical manifestations, ranging from asymptomatic infection to fatal acute fulminant hepatitis.

Symptomatic acute hepatitis occurs in two stages:

Anicteric (Absence of Jaundice) Phase (Lasts Approximately 5 to 7 Days)

- Anorexia, nausea and vomiting
- RUQ or epigastric pain
- Fever
- Malaise; child feels ill
- Fatigue, depression, irritability

Icteric (Jaundice) Phase (Lasts 4 Weeks or Less)

- Jaundice, urticaria
- Dark urine and light-colored stools
- Child begins to feel better as jaundice becomes more apparent.
- Acute fulminating hepatitis is marked by bleeding problems, encephalopathy, ascites, and acute hepatic failure. Fulminant hepatitis is due primarily to hepatitis B and hepatitis C.

The symptoms and clinical changes should return to normal within 3 months of onset. If not, a chronic state should be suspected. Infection with hepatitis B, hepatitis D, and hepatitis C can result in chronic hepatitis and cirrhosis. Chronic HBV infection can also cause hepatic carcinoma.

Diagnostic Evaluation. A history of exposure to jaundiced children, confirmed outbreaks in day-care centers, or percutaneous exposure to blood or body fluids should raise suspicion of hepatitis. Although there is no liver function test specific for hepatitis, tests of liver function, especially AST, ALT, and bilirubin levels and sedimentation rate can be indications of liver damage caused by hepatitis. Serum bilirubin levels peak 5–10 days after jaundice appears. History and course of the disease are essential in making the appropriate diagnosis.

Hepatitis is diagnosed by identification of the antigens (HBsAg, HBeAg) responsible for the disease or the anti-

TABLE 26–5 *Differentiation of Viral Hepatitis*

TYPE/ETIOLOGY	TRANSMISSION	INCUBATION	CLINICAL MANIFESTATIONS	RECOVERY PROGNOSIS
Hepatitis A Virus (HAV), Previously Called Infectious Hepatitis	Fecal-oral	15–50 days (average 28 days) Most contagious 1–2 weeks before symptoms Onset at 25–30 days	Mild, flulike symptoms or asymptomatic, no jaundice in children Adolescents: fever, malaise, anorexia, nausea, jaundice	Good prognosis. Chronic infections, carriers don't occur. Recovery provides lifelong immunity.
Hepatitis B Virus (HBV), Previously Called Serum Hepatitis	Blood and blood products Secretions Prenatally, perinatally Sexual contact	50– 180 days (average 60–90 days) Onset at 4 months	Same as HAV Severity ranges from asymptomatic to fatal fulminant infection. Anicteric or asymptomatic most common in children 90% of neonates will develop chronic carrier state.	Good prognosis. Generally a full recovery except in chronic carriers. 20% of adults develop chronic carrier state and are predisposed to cirrhosis and hepatocellular cancer.
Hepatitis C (HCV) Non-A, Non-B Hepatitis	Blood and blood products	14–180 days (average 40–60 days)	Same as HAV	50% progress to chronic hepatitis and cirrhosis or cancer.
Hepatitis Delta Virus (HDV) Occurs only in patients with acute or chronic HBV infection	Blood and blood products More common in Mediterranean countries, and among IV drug users and hemophiliacs	21–90 days	Occurs with HBV and causes it to be more severe.	More likely to develop fulminating hepatitis than other strains.
Hepatitis E Virus (HEV) Enterically Transmitted Non-A, Non-B Hepatitis	Fecal-oral More common in adults	15–60 days (average 26–42 days)	Epidemic with characteristics of HAV Uncommon in developed countries	High incidence of mortality in pregnant women.

Data from Balisteri (1988) and Aach et al. (1992).

bodies (anti-HAV, anti-HBc, anti-HBe, anti HBs, or anti-HCV) that develop as a result. IgM anti-HAV antibodies are present at the onset of illness and usually disappear within 4 months, but may persist for 6 months or longer. IgG anti-HAV antibodies develop shortly after IgM anti-HAV antibodies. The presence of IgG without IgM anti-HAV antibodies indicates past infection (AAP, 1994). HCV serologic assays are used mainly for detection of chronic hepatitis C because they remain negative for at least 1–3 months after onset of the illness (Behrman, Kliegman, & Arvin, 1966)

Liver biopsy may be needed to evaluate the chronic active forms of the disease and to determine the extent of damage in advanced or fulminant cases.

Therapeutic Management. There is no specific treatment for acute viral hepatitis. In uncomplicated viral hepatitis, treatment is mainly supportive because the disease is self-limiting. Treatment is aimed at maintaining comfort and adequate nutritional balance. A low-fat, balanced diet can be helpful if the child is bothered by nausea and anorexia. Hospitalization is rarely needed.

In fulminant hepatitis, intensive care may be required to provide hemostasis, nutritional and fluid support, neurologic assessment, and management until the liver has had a chance to recover.

Hepatitis A. Control of further spread is essential. Because HAV may survive on contaminated objects for weeks, good handwashing and thorough disinfection of diaper-changing surfaces are imperative. Children and adults who have had direct contact with a person infected with HAV should receive immune globulin (IG) (0.02 ml/kg) as soon as possible after exposure. A vaccine has been developed to prevent HAV infection, and immunization is recommended for child day-care center workers, homosexually active males, military personnel, and travelers to areas of high endemicity. Cases of hepatitis should be promptly reported to local public health officials. Test-

Persons Who Should Receive Hepatitis B Immunization

- All infants; infants of HBsAg-positive mothers require postexposure prophylaxis with HBIG and vaccine
- Infants and children at risk for acquiring HBV should be immunized by age 6–9 months
- Adolescents, particularly those at high risk
- IV drug users
- Sexually active heterosexual persons with more than one sex partner and sexually active homosexual males
- Health care workers at risk for exposure to blood or body fluids
- Residents and staff of institutions for developmentally disabled persons
- Hemodialysis patients
- Patients with bleeding disorders who receive certain blood products
- Household contacts and sexual partners of HBV carriers
- International travellers to areas where HBV is endemic
- Inmates of correctional facilities

Used with permission of the American Academy of Pediatrics. *Report of the Committee on Infectious Disease, 1994 Red Book.* 23rd edition, Elk Grove Village, IL, 1994.

ing for IgM anti-HAV antibody should be done on suspect cases of day-care center employees and household contacts of infected persons (AAP, 1994).

Hepatitis B. Children with acute or chronic HBV should be cared for with scrupulous standard precautions. The most effective means of preventing HBV infection is immunization with hepatitis B vaccine. Hepatitis B vaccination is recommended for all newborns as part of the routine childhood immunization schedule (AAP, 1994). (See Table 22–2 in Chapter 22.) Other persons who should receive hepatitis B immunization are listed in the accompanying box. Hepatitis B immune globulin (HBIG) is effective in preventing HBV infection if given within 2 weeks after exposure (AAP, 1994). It is possible to prevent hepatitis D by preventing hepatitis B.

NURSING CARE OF THE CHILD WITH VIRAL HEPATITIS

Assessment

Nursing history may identify a source of infection. In children, flulike symptoms of fever, malaise, anorexia, fatigue, and nausea may be the *only* symptoms of viral hepatitis. Abdominal assessment may find RUQ tenderness and hepatomegaly. Stools will be pale and clay-colored, and urine may be dark and "frothy." Jaundice, if present, is best assessed in sclera, nailbeds, and mucous membranes and usually follows a cephalocaudal progression. In HBV, arthralgias may be the presenting complaint.

Fulminant hepatitis will likely present with acute hepatic failure with associated encephalopathy, bleeding, fluid retention, ascites, and icteric appearance.

Nursing Diagnosis and Planning

The following nursing diagnoses and expected outcomes may be appropriate in the treatment of hepatitis in the child.

- Altered Nutrition: Less Than Body Requirements related to anorexia. ***Expected Outcomes:*** *The child will tolerate age-appropriate diet without weight loss, vomiting, or abdominal pain; return to normal activity level.*
- Risk for Infection related to exposure of family members to infectious agents. ***Expected Outcomes:*** *The family will practice good handwashing and other necessary isolation procedures; remain free from infection.*
- Risk for Injury related to fulminant hepatitis. ***Expected Outcome:*** *The child will return to preillness weight and activity level.*
- Knowledge Deficit related to home care and long-term prognosis. ***Expected Outcome:*** *The parents will verbalize a basic understanding of hepatitis and the importance of treatment.*

Implementation

Unless fulminant hepatitis develops, children are usually treated at home, so parental education is crucial. Teaching parents about the importance of a nutritious low-fat diet as tolerated by the child, rest, and general supportive care are important. The child with hepatitis is often anorexic. Several small meals and snacks throughout the day are better tolerated than regular portions at mealtimes. Fatigue and malaise can last for several weeks. Adequate rest and sleep are important for recovery. Because hepatitis A is not infectious within a week after the onset of jaundice, the child may return to school at that time if he feels well enough. The parents should be taught the danger signals that could indicate a worsening of the child's condition, specifically changes in neurologic status, bleeding, and fluid retention. Jaundice may appear to get worse before it resolves, and parents should be prepared for this possibility. Parents should be taught not to give their child any over-the-counter medications, because impaired liver function may result in inadequate metabolism and excretion of the medication. Adolescents should be cautioned not to drink alcohol during the illness or recovery period.

Prevention of spread of infection is an essential intervention for HAV. This should include enteric precautions for at least 1 week after the onset of jaundice and excellent handwashing. (See Chapter 18 for a discussion of isolation procedures.) Handwashing is the most important preventive measure. Family members must be taught how to institute appropriate precautions and to clean exposed household surfaces with bleach, $\frac{1}{4}$ cup to each gallon of water (Belkengren & Sapala, 1989). Diapers should not be changed on or near surfaces used for preparing or serving food. The nurse should explain to family members the ways in which HAV (fecal-oral route) and HBV (parenteral route) are spread to others. Education about the new recommendations concerning hepatitis A and hepatitis B vaccination should be provided (see Chapter 22 and Appendix A).

If the child has HBV, especially neonatal HBV, the parents should be prepared for the possibility of a chronic carrier state and the development of cirrhosis and hepatocellular cancer in later years. If the child with HBV has a history of illicit IV drug use, the nurse has the responsibility of teaching about the dangers of such behaviors, including the risk of transmission of hepatitis and other infections. The child should be assisted in obtaining counseling through a drug program.

Home Care. Children with hepatitis are almost always managed at home. Nursing interventions include teaching parents handwashing skills, use of gloves, disinfection of contaminated surfaces and articles, monitoring for complications, providing a well-balanced, low-fat diet, and monitoring other family members for infection. All children should be immunized for hepatitis.

Evaluation

Has the child maintained preillness weight within 5%?
Is the child free of vomiting?
Have the stools returned to brown color and is urine pale yellow?
Is child participating in age-appropriate activities and play?
Do family members practice good handwashing and adhere to isolation procedures?
Has hepatitis spread to other family members?
Have all family members obtained immunization as appropriate?
Can parents explain symptoms to watch for in other family members?

Cirrhosis

Cirrhosis is a chronic, degenerative condition of the liver that results in the development of bands of fibrous tissue, firm nodules, and connections between the central and portal areas of the liver. This scarring causes irreversible damage to the liver.

Etilogy. Cirrhosis in children usually results from chronic liver disease such as hepatitis B infection or biliary atresia. Sickle cell disease, inborn errors in metabolism such as alpha-1 antitrypsin deficiency and disturbances in copper metabolism, cystic fibrosis, and Wilson's disease are also possible causes in children.

Incidence. Cirrhosis is uncommon in children but as the lifespan of children with chronic disease continues to rise, it will become more common. Children with biliary atresia, chronic hepatitis, cystic fibrosis, or sickle cell disease are at risk.

Clinical Manifestations. The symptoms are often nonspecific, vague, and slow to develop. They result from either liver cell failure or portal hypertension.

Results of Liver Cell Failure

- Jaundice
- Intense pruritus
- Steatorrhea
- Distension
- Edema
- Anemia, bleeding tendencies
- Anorexia
- Frequent infections
- Poor growth

Result of Portal Hypertension

- Splenomegaly
- Varices, GI bleeding

Result of Both

- Ascites

Diagnostic Evaluation. Because the most likely cause of cirrhosis in children is chronic biliary obstruction, evaluation is based on the history of pre-existing conditions, including biliary atresia and hepatitis. The presence of clinical manifestations of chronic liver disease and the history of one of these conditions is used for a presumptive diagnosis. Liver function tests such as bilirubin, aminotransferases, ammonia, albumin, cholesterol, and prothrombin time, support the diagnosis. Definitive diagnosis is a liver biopsy, which will identify fibrous scarring and changes of hepatic vasculature.

Therapeutic Management. Because there is no effective treatment to halt the progression of cirrhosis, management is aimed at relieving the cause if possible. Any infectious agents should be treated and obstructive causes repaired. Supportive care, including rest, nutritional support, fluid management, and relief of symptoms are included. Management of life-threatening complications, especially bleeding varices, ascites, and hepatic encephalopathy, take priority in medical management. Monitoring liver

PATHOPHYSIOLOGY *of Cirrhosis*

Stasis of bile causes inflammation and hepatomegaly. If this continues, destruction of the liver begins. As the liver attempts to heal itself, fibrotic regeneration and nodules develop, and function is impaired. This scarring can cause altered hepatic blood flow and decreased liver cell function. Changes in hepatic blood flow can cause scarring and collapse of the hepatic vasculature, increased vascular resistance, and eventually portal hypertension. As the liver cells decrease in function, more die and the liver can't produce necessary proteins or bile, causing malabsorption and malnutrition. As liver cells continue to die, the cycle is repeated.

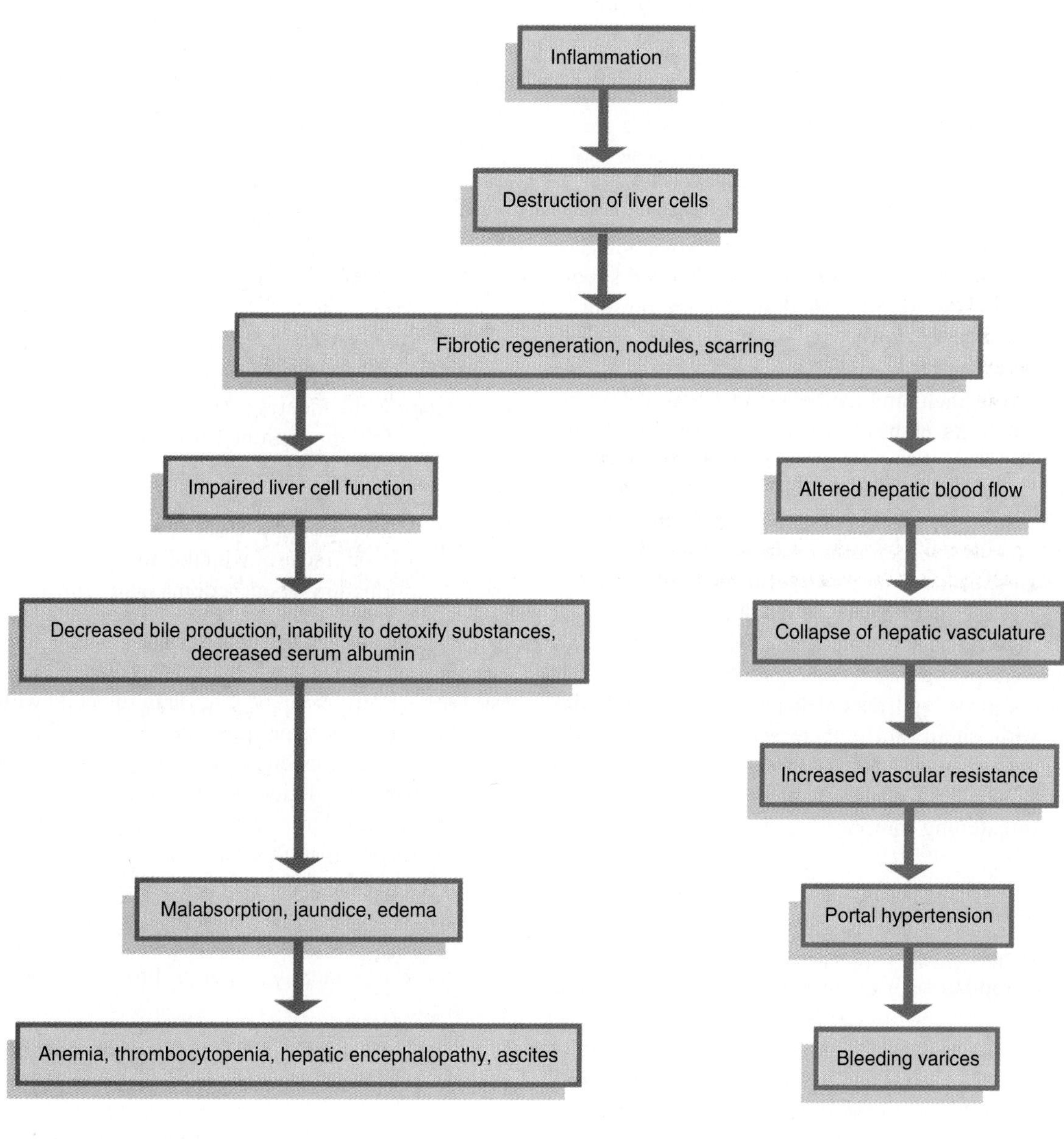

function is important in order to evaluate the child for eventual liver transplantation.

Definitive therapy is a liver transplant.

NURSING CARE OF THE CHILD WITH CIRRHOSIS

Assessment

History and general appraisal will likely reveal a child with a history of failure to thrive and of chronic biliary obstruction or hepatitis B infection. The child may present in varying degrees of distress and discomfort. Many children will present with vague complaints or be asymptomatic. The earliest findings are likely to be anorexia, nausea, indigestion, fatigue, and RUQ pain or fullness. Monitoring height and weight using a growth chart, gathering information on a typical day's food intake, and assessing sleep habits and activity levels can help identify these more general problems and provide essential supportive evidence.

Abdominal palpation will likely reveal splenomegaly and RUQ tenderness or hepatomegaly. Distended superficial veins; tight, shiny skin; and edema may be present.

Jaundice and pruritus may be detected, especially if the cirrhosis is the result of biliary obstruction. A complete skin assessment, including nailbeds and sclera, will identify jaundice at its earliest stages. The skin should be examined for breakdown or infection caused by intense scratching. The amount and location of edema should also be noted. This skin assessment may also reveal bruises related to thrombocytopenia and pale color related to anemia. A stool specimen may be useful in identifying the degree of bile obstruction and malabsorption.

The most critical assessment needs to be centered on detecting signs of the three major complications of cirrhosis: ascites, varices, and encephalopathy. The child who presents with significantly increased abdominal girth, edema, vomiting blood, or changes in level of consciousness should be referred for emergency medical care of these life-threatening complications.

Nursing Diagnosis and Planning

The following nursing diagnoses and expected outcomes may be appropriate in the treatment of cirrhosis in the child.

- Altered Nutrition: Less Than Body Requirements related to malabsorption and anorexia. ***Expected Outcome:*** *The child will return to preillness weight, eat an age-appropriate balanced diet, and intake adequate fluids.*
- Risk for Impaired Skin Integrity related to pruritus. ***Expected Outcome:*** *The child will maintain skin integrity as evidenced by intact skin without breakdown or infection.*
- Risk for Fluid Volume Excess related to ascites and edema. ***Expected Outcome:*** *The child will be free from ascites and edema.*
- Risk for Injury related to thrombocytopenia and varices. ***Expected Outcome:*** *The child will be free from bleeding.*
- Knowledge Deficit related to long-term prognosis. ***Expected Outcomes:*** *The parents will verbalize symptoms of ascites, bleeding varices, and encephalopathy that should be reported immediately; explain prognosis; seek support from community resources.*

Implementation

The goal of nursing care is to sustain the child in optimum condition until a liver transplant can be achieved. The care can be divided into four areas: nutritional support, skin care, prevention of complications, and developmental and parental support.

Nutritional Support. Providing optimum nutrition for the child to grow and develop is a major nursing intervention. The diet needs to be high carbohydrate, high calorie, normal protein, and low fat. Protein may need to be limited in case encephalopathy develops. Because anorexia can be a problem, creative food options, NG tube feedings, and TPN may be needed. These changes put minimal stress on the liver while meeting the growth requirements of the child. In addition, sodium restriction can help prevent edema. Multivitamins with vitamin A, D, E, and K supplements are essential. Vitamin K injections may be needed. Monitoring the child's weight on a daily and weekly basis and recording intake and output can provide critical information about edema and growth. Support from dietary personnel can be valuable when working with and teaching these families.

Skin Care. Pruritus can be intense in the child with cirrhosis. Continued assessment for open lesions, scratch marks, and bleeding are essential. Colloidal oatmeal baths and topical antipruritic lotions such as Calamine may provide temporary relief. Drugs are not usually an option for itch relief because impaired liver function affects metabolism of drugs. Use of sedatives, opioids, Tylenol, and alcohol is strictly avoided. Keeping the nails trimmed short or wearing cotton gloves during sleep can minimize damage to the skin from scratching. Ease of bruising should also be noted.

Prevention of Complications. These are critical interventions.

Infection: Prevent exposure to infection. Monitor for fever and report immediately.

Ascites: Monitor for edema, give diuretics as ordered, maintain low-sodium diet, give albumin as ordered.

Child will likely have to be hospitalized for treatment; monitoring intake and output and weight, maintaining fluid balance, and monitoring abdominal girth and distension are nursing concerns.

Bleeding: Administer stool guaiac tests, avoid injections, give vitamin K as ordered, and protect from injury. Identify bleeding as soon as possible. While child is hospitalized nursing care involves transfusing blood or blood products safely, maintaining fluid balance, monitoring pulse and blood pressure, administering oxygen therapy, and assisting with endoscopic sclerotherapy or the placement of a Sengstaken-Blakemore tube for compression of bleeding esophageal varices.

Encephalopathy: This results from a buildup of ammonia in the blood from the incomplete breakdown of protein. Limiting protein in the diet, giving lactulose as ordered to decrease the GI bacteria that produce ammonia, administering antibiotics as ordered, and monitoring changes in behavior and level of consciousness are nursing responsibilities.

Developmental and Parental Support. Children with cirrhosis are chronically ill and require much time and effort to maintain optimum health. Providing developmental stimulation on a daily basis is essential, and parents need education and support services to achieve this. In addition, parents need to be educated about the disease, its prognosis, the feasibility of a liver transplant, and the risk of complications. As the parents cope with the potential loss of their child, community resources and national support groups such as The Children's Liver Foundation are helpful.

Home Care. The focus of home care is in teaching. Because the child will be cared for at home unless a serious complication arises or the child is hospitalized for a liver transplant, parents need much information. Helping the parents develop meals and snacks that meet special nutritional needs on a day-to-day basis can be difficult, and dietary personnel can provide invaluable information. Preventing infection is something parents can control somewhat by sheltering the children from infected individuals as much as possible. The most critical intervention is helping parents identify when they should seek help, specifically if the child develops GI bleeding, changes in level of consciousness, or severe edema. The healthier the child can remain, the better the child and family can focus on developmental skills and preparation for liver transplant.

Evaluation

Is the child growing appropriately according to growth chart?
Is skin intact, clean, and free of lesions or infection?
Is abdomen soft and nondistended without edema?
Is the child free from infection?
Is the child free from GI bleeding?
Is child alert, oriented, and participating in age-appropriate activities?
Can the parent verbalize prognosis and daily care?
Does the parent report complications immediately?

KEY CONCEPTS

- The GI system is formed in the first 4 weeks of embryologic development, so congenital defects can be traced to this period.
- Development of the GI system is anatomically complete at birth but physiologically immature, affecting enzymes, sphincter tone, permeability, secretion, and reabsorption.
- Some GI disorders (lactose intolerance, celiac sprue) are managed by simple dietary changes.
- Passage of the first meconium is a critical nursing observation that can assist with diagnosis of Hirschsprung's disease and imperforate anus.
- GI surgery to repair congenital defects and inflammatory conditions requires nursing care similar to that for an adult but with special emphasis on nutrition, fluid status, pain control, parental involvement, and developmental level of the child.
- Assessment of GI distress is very difficult in small children and must include a thorough history, physical assessment, and general appraisal of the child's distress.
- Using appropriate isolation precautions is essential to prevent spread of infection in GI disorders.
- Home care and teaching have a high priority because parents must have the necessary information to care for their child during the management of GI alterations.

REFERENCES

Aach, R., Hirschman, S., & Holland, P. (1992). The ABCs of viral hepatitis. *Patient Care, 26*(13), 34–38.

American Academy of Pediatrics. (1994). *Report of the Committee on Infectious Diseases,* 1994 Red Book. (23rd ed.). Elk Grove Village, IL: AAP.

Auricchio, S., Greco, L., & Troncone, R. (1988). Gluten-sensitive enteropathy of childhood. *Pediatric Clinics of North America, 35*(1), 157–187.

Balistreri, W. (1988). Viral hepatitis. *Pediatric Clinics of North America, 35*(3), 375–407.

Behrman, R., Kliegman, R. M., & Arvin, A. M. (1996). *Nelson textbook of pediatrics.* (15th ed.). Philadelphia: W. B. Saunders.

Belkengren, R., & Sapala, S. (1989). Pediatric management problems: Hepatitis. *Pediatric Nursing, 15*(6), 638–639.

Berk, J. E. (Ed). (1985). *Bockus gastroenterology.* Philadelphia: W. B. Saunders.

Cheney, C., & Wong, R. (1993). Acute infectious diarrhea. *Medical Clinics of North America, 77*(5), 1169–1196.

Cooke, D. (1991). Inflammatory bowel disease: Primary health care management of ulcerative colitis and Crohn's disease. *Nurse Practitioner, 16*(8), 27–39.

Ellett, M. (1990). Constipation/encopresis: A nursing perspective. *Journal of Pediatric Health Care, 4*(3), 141–146.

Hatch, T. (1988). Encopresis and constipation in children. *Pediatric Clinics of North America, 35*(2), 257–280.

Katkov, W. N. (1995). Hepatitis vaccines. *Gastroenterology Clinics of North America, 24*(1), 147–159.

Kirks, D. R. (1984). *Practical pediatric imaging: Diagnostic radiology of infants and children.* Boston: Little, Brown.

Konings, K. (1989). Preop use of GoLYTELY in pediatrics. *Pediatric Nursing, 15*(5), 473–474.

Ladebauche, P. (1992). Intussusception in pediatric patients. *Journal of Emergency Nursing, 18*(3), 275–279.

MacDonald, C. (1991). Biliary atresia. *Journal of Pediatric Nursing, 6*(6), 374–383.

Milla, P. J. (1988). Gastrointestinal motility disorders in children. *Pediatric Clinics of North America, 35*(2), 311–330.

Ramos-Soriano, A. G., & Schwarz, K. B. (1994). Recent advances in hepatitides (Part I). *Gastroenterology Clinics of North America, 23*(4), 753–767.

Seth, R., & Heyman, M. B. (1994). Management of constipation and encopresis in infants and children. *Gastroenterology Clinics of North America, 23*(4), 621–636.

BIBLIOGRAPHY

Barone, M. (1996). *The Harriet Lane handbook: A manual for pediatric house officers* (14th ed.). St. Louis: Mosby-Year Book.

Bishop, W., & Ulshen, M. (1988). Bacterial gastroenteritis. *Pediatric Clinics of North America, 35*(1), 69–87.

Evans, K. (1990). Pediatric management problems: Constipation. *Pediatric Nursing, 16*(6), 590–591.

Fischbach, F. (1988). *A manual of laboratory diagnostic tests* (3rd ed.). Philadelphia: J. B. Lippincott.

Frost, G. (1992). Hirschsprung's disease in infants and children. *Gastroenterology Nursing, 15*(1), 45–48.

Griffiths, A., Nguyen, P., Smith, C., MacMillan, J., & Sherman, P. (1993). Growth and clinical course of children with Crohn's disease. *Gut, 34*(7), 939–943.

Heitlinger, L., & Lebenthal, E. (1988). Disorders of carbohydrate digestion and absorption. *Pediatric Clinics of North America, 35*(2), 239–256.

Katzman, E. (1989). What's the most common helminth infection in the US? *MCN, 14*(3), 193–195.

Keating, P. (1990). Constipation. *Community Outlook,* December, *4,* 9–10.

Kirschner, B. (1988). Inflammatory bowel disease in children. *Pediatric Clinics of North America, 35*(1), 189–207.

Kirsner, J. B., & Shorter, R. G. (1988). *Inflammatory bowel disease.* Philadelphia: Lea and Febiger.

McCance, K., & Huether, S. (1994). *Pathophysiology: The biologic basis for disease in adults and children.* St. Louis: Mosby.

MacDonald, T. (1993). Etiology of Crohn's disease. *Gut, 34*(2suppl), 939–943.

Martin, S. (1992). The ABCs of pediatric LFTs. *Pediatric Nursing, 18*(5), 445–449.

Not, T., Ventura, A., Peticarari, S., Basile, S., Torre, G., & Dragovic, D. (1993). A new, rapid, noninvasive screening test for celiac disease. *The Journal of Pediatrics, 123*(3), 425–427.

Pappas, S. C. (1995). Fulminant viral hepatitis. *Gastroenterology Clinics of North America, 24*(1), 161–173.

Perucca, R. (1992). Understanding Crohn's disease. *Journal of Intravenous Nursing, 15*(3), 164–169.

Riddlesberger, M. (1988). Evaluation of the gastrointestinal tract in the child: CT, MRI and isotopic studies. *Pediatric Clinics of North America, 35*(2), 281–310.

Roberts, A. (1991). Systems of life: The digestive system Part 1. *Nursing Times, 87*(11), 45–48.

Roberts, A. (1991). Systems of life: The digestive system Part 2. *Nursing Times, 87*(15), 65–68.

Roberts, A. (1991). Systems of life: The digestive system Part 3. *Nursing Times, 87*(19), 61–64.

Roberts, A. (1991). Systems of life: The digestive system Part 4. *Nursing Times, 87*(24), 61–64.

Rushton, C. (1988). The surgical neonate: Principles of nursing management. *Pediatric Nursing, 14*(2), 141–151.

Sivit, C. (1993). Diagnosis of acute appendicitis in children: Spectrum of sonographic findings. *American Journal of Radiology, 161*(7), 147–152.

Smith, J. (1988). Big differences in little people. *American Journal of Nursing, 88*(4), 459–462.

Stroh, S., Stern, P., & McCarthy, S. (1989). Fecal incontinence in children: A clinical update. *MCN: The American Journal of Maternal-Child Nursing, 14*(4), 252–254.

Vegunta, R., Cooney, D., & Cooney, D. R. (1993). Surgical management of abdominal wall defects in infants. *AORN Journal, 58*(1), 53–63.

27

The Child With Genitourinary Alterations

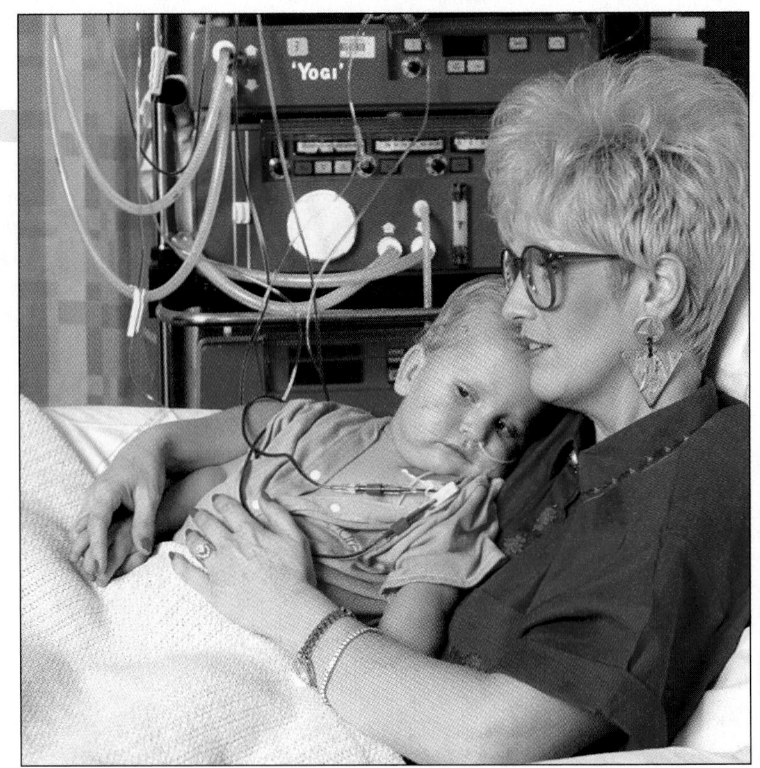

Courtesy of Children's Medical Center, Dallas, Texas

CHAPTER OVERVIEW

LEARNING OBJECTIVES

After studying this chapter, you should be able to:

- Describe the anatomy and physiology of the urinary tract system of the infant and child.
- Describe the most common diagnostic and screening tests associated with alteration in genitourinary function.
- Identify nursing implications of common medications used in the treatment of urinary tract alterations.
- Discuss and display an understanding of common alterations in the urinary tract system.
- State expected nursing diagnoses for children with alterations in the urinary tract system.
- Use the nursing process to discuss nursing care of children with common alterations of the urinary tract system.
- Develop guidelines for home care for the child with an alteration of the urinary tract system.

KEY TERMS

arteriovenous fistula: a connection between an artery and vein, usually for the purpose of hemodialysis

arteriovenous graft: a U-shaped plastic tube inserted between an artery and a vein, usually for the purpose of hemodialysis

dysuria: pain on urination

edema: presence of abnormally large amounts of fluid in the intercellular tissue spaces of the body

frequency: urination at short time intervals

hypercalciuria: excessive calcium in the urine

hyperlipidemia: high cholesterol and triglyceride levels in the blood

hypoalbuminemia: low albumin levels in the blood

proteinuria: protein in the urine

renal scarring: area of nonfunction in the kidney

urgency: sudden urge to urinate

Genitourinary alterations in children encompass a wide range of illnesses. An older child with a urinary tract infection may have a single acute illness, whereas a child with end-stage renal disease has a chronic illness that will involve periodic hospitalizations and interfere with daily functioning. The effects of the illness on the child and family depend on the nature of the illness, age at onset, severity and prognosis, family functioning, and economic burden (Hamburg, 1983).

Nurses care for children with genitourinary disorders in a variety of settings. In the hospital, the nurse may care for a child in an acute phase of nephrotic syndrome. In the home, the nurse may teach administration of an intravenous antibiotic or peritoneal dialysis, or may monitor compliance with a treatment plan. In the community setting, the nurse may assist in the care of a child with genitourinary alterations in a local physician's office or public health setting and collaborate with the pediatric nephrologist or dialysis or transplant center.

CLINICAL REFERENCE PAGES

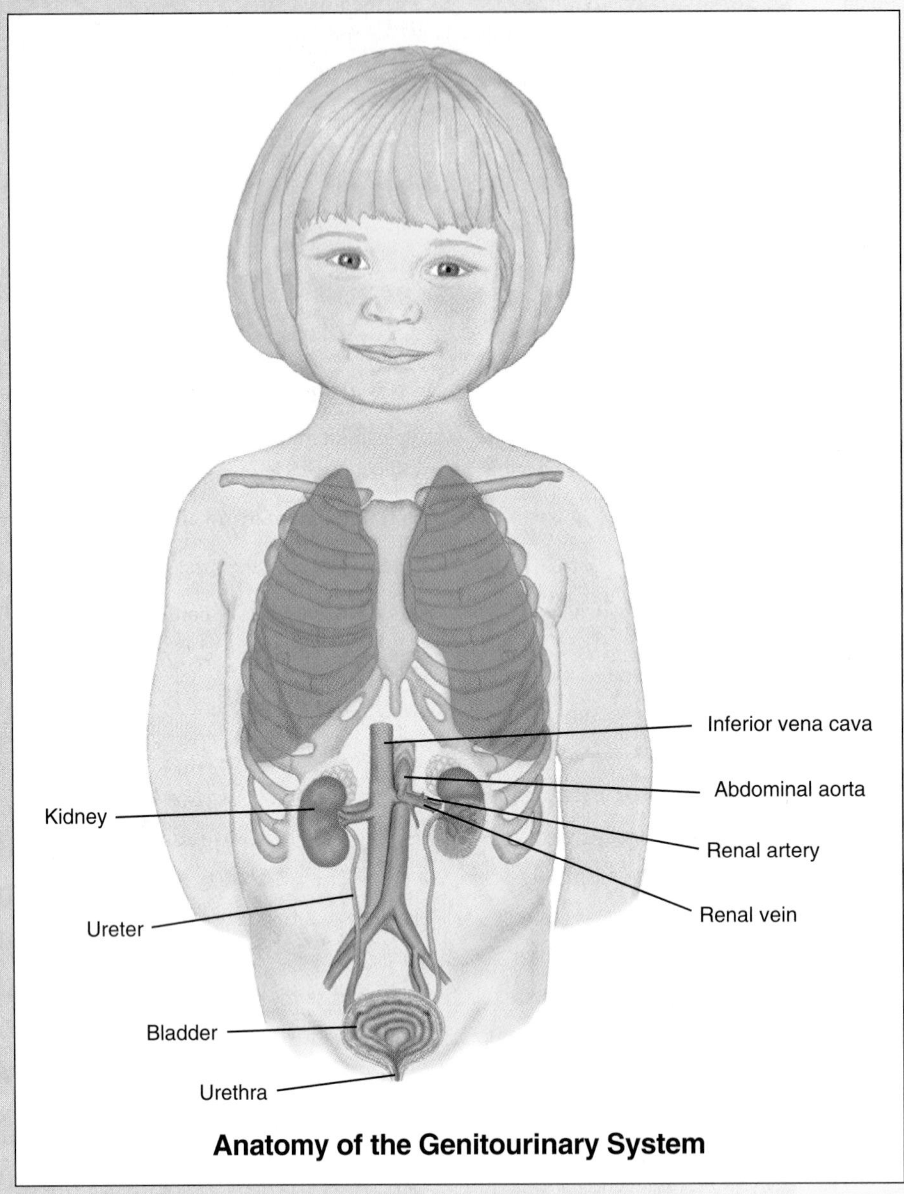

Anatomy of the Genitourinary System

Pediatric Differences in the Genitourinary System

- In a healthy infant the kidneys operate at a functional level appropriate for the size of the body. However, the functional reserves are reduced when the infant is under stress.
- By age 6 to 12 months, kidney function is nearly like that of the adult.
- In premature infants (under 34 weeks' gestation) the reabsorption of glucose, sodium, bicarbonate, and phosphate is reduced.
- The kidneys of young infants cannot concentrate urine as efficiently as those of older children and adults. After the first few weeks of life, the kidneys' acidifying ability reaches the adult level. But with acidosis, there is only a small increase in acid secretion, and susceptibility to acidemia rises.
- Most children with acute renal failure regain normal function.

REVIEW OF THE GENITOURINARY SYSTEM

The urinary system consists of the kidneys, ureters, bladder, and urethra (see figure). The urinary system upper tract includes the kidneys and ureters; the lower tract includes the bladder and urethra. Pediatric differences in the genitourinary system are listed in the box below.

The bean-shaped *kidneys* lie one on each side of the spinal column. In an adolescent or adult, the kidney is about the size of a fist; in an infant, the kidney is proportionally larger. The upper portion of the left kidney lies at about the twelfth rib, with the right kidney slightly lower than the left kidney. The hilum, the indentation in the kidney, is the area where the blood vessels, lymphatics, nerves and ureter enter the kidney. The kidney is encased by a thin fibrous capsule. The outer region of the kidney is the cortex, the inner region is the medulla; both can be observed with the kidney dissected longitudinally. The cortex contains the glomeruli and tubules, and the medulla contains the renal pyramids. The renal pelvis, located in the area of the hilum, is an extension of the upper end of the ureter.

The *nephron* is the kidney's functional unit (see figure). The nephron does the work of the kidney. It consists of Bowman's capsule, glomerulus, proximal tubule, loop of Henle, distal tubule, and collecting duct. Each kidney contains about a million nephrons.

Blood enters the kidney through the renal arteries, which branch off the abdominal aorta. The renal artery divides and subdivides, eventually culminating in the afferent arterioles, which feed into the glomerular capillaries. The glomerular capillaries empty into the efferent arterioles. Peritubular capillaries surround the proximal tubule, the loop of Henle, and the distal tubules. The capillaries drain into the venous system. Blood returns to the body through the renal vein, which enters the inferior vena cava.

Kidney Function. The kidneys maintain fluid and chemical balance through glomerular filtration, tubular reabsorption, and secretion. The kidney has important hormonal functions:

Produces renin, which helps with the regulation of blood pressure. Release of renin is primarily stimulated by decreased pressure in the afferent arterioles of the glomerulus.

Produces erythropoietin, which stimulates red blood cell production by the bone marrow.

Metabolized vitamin D to its active form, which is important in calcium metabolism.

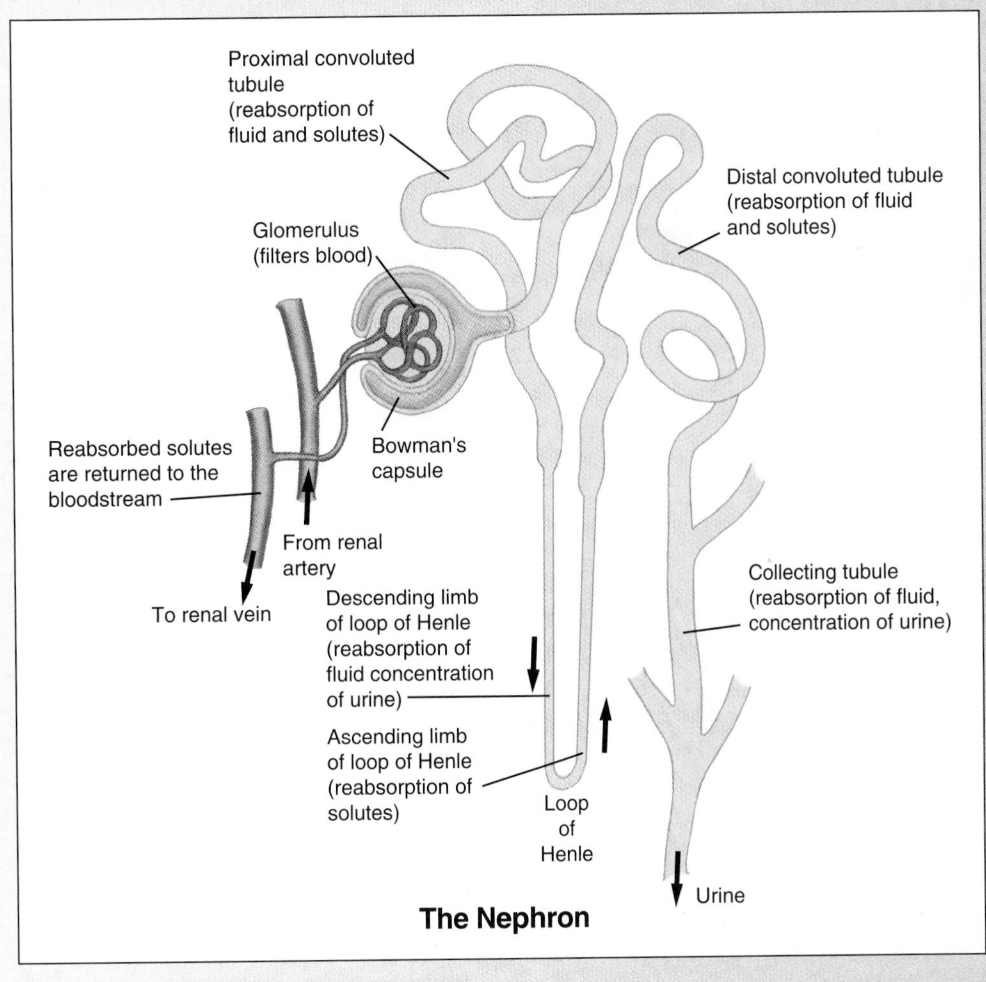

The Nephron

MEDICATIONS COMMONLY USED IN THE TREATMENT OF GENITOURINARY DISORDERS

	ACTION/USE	DOSAGE AND ADMINISTRATION	SIDE EFFECTS	NURSING IMPLICATIONS
Chlorambucil (Leukeran)	Inhibits DNA and RNA synthesis. Can cause bone marrow suppression. Used for some forms of leukemia and lymphoma. Can be used in nephrotic syndrome in combination with corticosteroids for those patients who are steroid dependent or have frequent relapses.	0.2 mg/kg/day PO for 8–10 weeks	*Occasional:* Bone marrow depression. *Rare:* Nausea, vomiting, or abdominal discomfort. High dose may result in problems with decreased fertility	Baseline CBC should be done before initiation of therapy and weekly during course of treatment. Patients have increased risk of infection. Should be advised to report any febrile illness or exposure to chickenpox. Live vaccines should not be administered to children receiving this medication.
Chlorothiazide Sodium (Diuril)	Produces diuresis. Blocks reabsorption of sodium, potassium, and chloride by the distal convoluted tubule. Decreases renal calcium excretion. Helps reduce plasma and extracellular fluid volume. Used for edema associated with renal dysfunction, hypertension, and hypercalciuria.	10–20 mg/kg/day PO in 2 divided doses	*Frequent:* Hypokalemia *Occasional:* Hypotension, gastrointestinal (GF) disturbance	Obtain baseline electrolyte values. Monitor vital signs and intake/output, as well as electrolytes, during therapy. Instruct parents to offer foods high in potassium while their child is on this medication (i.e., bananas, orange juice, potatoes). Educate parents regarding signs and symptoms of dehydration.
Nifedipine (Procardia)	Calcium channel blocker that is a potent peripheral vasodilator. Used for hypertension in children.	*Hypertension:* 30 mg BID PO *Hypertensive emergency:* 5–10 mg PO (sublingual) q 30 min as needed	*Frequent:* Dizziness, flushing, headache, peripheral edema *Occasional:* Cough, mood changes, sore throat, nasal congestion, gingival hyperplasia	For hypertensive emergency, capsule should be punctured and contents squeezed under tongue. Capsule can also be bitten, chewed, and swallowed. Patients should monitor blood pressure closely and practice good *daily* oral hygiene.
Imipramine Hydrochloride (Tofranil)	Tricyclic antidepressant. Blocks reuptake of norepinephrine and serotonin by presynaptic neurons, which increases their availability in the CNS. Exhibits anticholinergic effects, which makes it useful in the treatment of nocturnal enuresis.	25 mg h.s. PO for children older than 6 years (when used for treatment of nocturnal enuresis)	*Frequent:* Drowsiness, dry mouth, urine retention, postural hypotension *Occasional:* GI disturbance *Adverse effect:* Overdosage may result in potentially fatal arrhythmias	Caution about possibility of postural hypotension. This is usually not problematic with bedtime dosing. Parents *must* be instructed on effects of overdosage and that safe keeping of the drug is essential.
Furosemide (Lasix)	Inhibits renal reabsorption of sodium and chloride and promotes excretion of potassium. Used to treat edema associated with renal disease, congestive heart failure, and acute pulmonary edema.	*PO:* 1–2 mg/kg q 6–8 hr; may be increased to maximum of 6 mg/kg *IV:* 1–2 mg/kg q 2 hr; maximum 6 mg/kg	*Frequent:* Hypokalemia, GI upset *Occasional:* Dizziness, postural hypotension, rash, photosensitivity	Baseline electrolyte values should be documented and levels rechecked on a regular basis. Instruct parents on foods with high potassium values. Structure dosing to avoid nighttime diuresis. Assess patient's hydration status and educate parents on same (i.e., weights, intake and output pattern). Avoid overexposure to sunlight.

Cyclosporine (Sandimmune)	Inhibits T-cell activity, thus decreasing immune response. Used in conjunction with corticosteroids to prevent rejection of transplanted organs.	*PO: Initially*, 14–18 mg/kg per day in 2 divided doses. Then 5–10 mg/kg/day as maintenance. Available in capsule or solution form. Must be stored at room temperature and solution must be administered with proper syringe to ensure adequate dosing. *IV:* 5–6 mg/kg/day until patient able to take PO. Dosage may be altered to achieve desired serum levels.	*Frequent:* Hypertension, hirsutism, gingival hyperplasia, hand tremors *Occasional:* Headache, GI upset, hyperkalemia. *Rare:* Seizures, allergic reaction. *Adverse effects:* Nephrotoxicity (will see increased serum creatinine), especially with high serum levels	Most pediatric patients receive cyclosporine via the oral route. It is important that the family is instructed to give the medication at the same time each day to maintain adequate serum levels. Patients need to maintain good daily oral hygiene and may use over-the-counter hair removal preparations if needed. Nurses should instruct the families on the importance of keeping clinic and lab appointments. It is also essential that the patient's blood pressure is measured regularly. Family must consult the nephrologist before the child takes *any* other medication because many medications interfere with cyclosporine metabolism.
Epoeitin Alfa (Epogen, Procrit)	A glycoprotein produced in the kidneys that stimulates RBC production. Used for the treatment of anemia associated with chronic renal failure or ESRD. May also be used for anemia related to chemotherapy.	*Initially* 50–100 U/kg IV (subcutaneous) 3 times a week. Will decrease when desired hematocritis reached.	*Frequent:* Pain when given subcutaneously *Occasional:* Hypertension, headache, iron deficiency. *Rare:* Nausea/diarrhea, urticaria, seizures, thrombus formation (due to increased viscosity of blood).	Iron stores should be evaluated before therapy. Iron supplementation given if stores inadequate. Patient's blood pressure should be well controlled before beginning therapy and monitored regularly. CBC with differential and platelets should be done on a regular basis. Parents should understand that their child's activity/energy level will *increase* with successful therapy. Compliance may become a problem if child perceives the subcutaneous route as too painful.
Oxybutynin Chloride (Ditropan)	Exerts direct antispasmodic effects on smooth muscle. Is used to relieve symptoms associated with uninhibited bladder contractions.	2.5–5 mg b.i.d. PO	*Frequent:* Dry mouth. *Occasional:* Facial flushing, constipation, urine retention, blurred vision, heat intolerance.	Exposure to warm/hot environments should be limited. Teachers should know about "dry mouth" effect so that those children can have an access to water as needed.

Data from Hodgson, B., et al. (1996). *Nurses drug handbook 1996*. Philadelphia: W. B. Saunders; Shanno, M., et al. (1995). *Govoni and Hayes: Drugs and Nursing Implications*. Norwalk, CT: Appleton and Lange.

COMMON LABORATORY AND DIAGNOSTIC TESTS FOR GENITOURINARY DISORDERS

	DESCRIPTION	NORMAL FINDINGS	INDICATIONS	NURSING CONSIDERATIONS
Blood Urea Nitrogen (BUN)	End product of protein metabolism	0 to 6 mo, 4–15 mg/dl 6 to 24 mo, 5–15 mg/dl 2 yr to adult, 5–25 mg/dl	Gross indicator of renal function	Increases in renal insufficiency
Computed Tomography (CT Scan)	Computerized calculations revealing a pattern of shades	Normal appearance	Renal tumors	Sedation may be required; child lies on back, and should be still; oral contrast material may be administered; child is usually NPO due to sedation and/or oral contrast material
Cystoscopy	Bladder and urethra are examined with cystoscope, a tubular lighted telescopic lens	Normal appearance	Examination of bladder and lower tract; visualization of tumor and stones; removal of small stones; biopsy of bladder or tumors; fulguration of bladder tumors and posterior urethral valves	Usually performed under general anesthesia; little pain involved; encourage fluids; assess ability to void postprocedure
Intravenous Pyelogram (IVP)	Intravenous injection of contrast material concentrates in urine and is seen in kidneys and urine; serial X-ray studies are done; a postvoid film is done after child has emptied the bladder	Normal appearance; activity in kidneys by 2–5 min; no residual urine on postvoid film	Determines bladder's ability to empty completely; provides information about kidneys, ureters, and bladder anatomy; identifies masses that compress urinary system	Child should be NPO for a period of time in preparation for receiving contrast material; assess child for hypersensitivity to contrast material; contraindications include decreased renal function
KUB (Kidney, Ureter, Bladder), Flat Plate Scout Film	Abdominal X-ray film	Normal abdominal structures	Diagnoses renal stones; done before renal studies	No discomfort
Renal Arteriogram (Angiogram)	Contrast material is injected by catheter inserted into femoral artery, then into abdominal aorta and renal artery; visualizes vascular structures of kidney	Normal renal vasculature	Assesses for renal artery stenosis and preparation for renal transplant donor surgery	Direct pressure exerted on puncture site; child is usually on complete bed rest for a period of time postprocedure
Renal Biopsy	Removal and examination of kidney tissue	Normal tissue	Diagnosis and prognosis of renal disease	Sedation usually required; child lies on abdomen; for renal transplantation child lies on back; biopsy usually NPO due to sedation
Renal Scan (Radioisotope Renogram)	Injection of radioactive agent to allow visualization of kidney structures and function; serial films are taken	Prompt uptake and excretion of radioactive agent	Evaluate blood flow and renal function; assess renal scarring; identify pyelonephritis	Minimal radiation exposure; child must remain still for procedure
Renal Ultrasound	Noninvasive; high frequency sound waves are directed at kidneys, ureters, and bladder	Normal size, shape, position, function of kidneys	Assess position, size, and contour of kidneys, ureters, and bladder; detect obstruction and stones; localize for renal biopsy	Child lies on abdomen; if for transplantation child lies on back

Retrograde Pyelogram	Contrast dye is injected through a catheter into renal pelvis	Normal contour and size of ureters and kidneys	Identification of disease of ureters and renal pelvis and obstructive disease	Renal impairment does not influence visualization; procedure is done in X-ray department or surgery; child should be NPO for sedation or general anesthesia
Serum Creatinine (Cr)	By product of muscle metabolism; production is constant as long as muscle mass remains constant	0 to 2 wk, 0.2–0.8 mg/dl 2 wk to 2 yr, 0.2–0.6 mg/dl 2 to 4 yr, 0.3–0.6 mg/dl 4 to 6 yr, 0.4–0.8 mg/dl 6 to 10 yr, 0.4–0.8 mg/dl 10 to 12 yr, 0.5–1.0 mg/dl female: 12 yr to adult, 0.5–1.0 mg/dl male: 12 yr to adult, 0.5–1.3 mg/dl	Increases in renal insufficiency	Should be assessed before giving nephrotoxic chemotherapeutic agents
Serum Osmolality	Measurement of concentration of blood, determined by solute in blood	275–295 mOsm/kg	Indication of fluid and electrolyte balance	Helpful in evaluating hydration status, liver disease, and antidiuretic hormone function
		Urinalysis (UA)		
Specific Gravity	Measurement of concentration of urine	1.002–1.030	Provides information regarding hydration and renal concentration ability	Specific gravity will be higher if protein or glucose is present
pH	Determines acidity	4.6–8.0	Increases in urinary infections	Effected by diet
Protein	Detection of protein in urine	Negative	May be first indication of renal disease	Early-morning specimens are preferable because they are more concentrated
Glucose	Detection of glucose in urine	Negative	Screen or confirm diabetes and monitor effectiveness of diabetes control; may be present in child with weight loss, dehydration, infection, and renal disease	Nonspecific, needs further evaluation
Ketones	Formed in liver and completely metabolized; alteration in carbohydrate metabolism leads to excessive ketone production	Negative	Mainly associated with diabetes; may be present with fever, anorexia, diarrhea, fasting, starvation, prolonged vomiting	Children are more prone to develop ketonuria
Leukocyte Esterase	Enzyme released during WBC breakdown	Negative	May be present when WBC in urine	Indicates possible urinary tract infection
Nitrites	Produced by bacteria	Negative	May be present when bacteria in urine	In infant and child, bacteria may not be present in bladder long enough to produce sufficient nitrites to yield positive results

(continued)

COMMON LABORATORY AND DIAGNOSTIC TESTS FOR GENITOURINARY DISORDERS *(continued)*

	DESCRIPTION	NORMAL FINDINGS	INDICATIONS	NURSING CONSIDERATIONS
White Blood Cells (WBC)	Microscopic finding of WBCs in urine	0–2/HPF	Seen with infection	Urine culture is indicated
Red Blood Cells (RBC)	Microscopic finding of RBCs in urine	0–2/HPF	Trauma, stones, infection, glomerulonephritis	Normal in menstruating females
Bacteria	Microscopic presence of bacteria in urine	None	Urinary tract infection	Urine culture is indicated
Casts	White cell casts and red cell casts originate in kidney tubules	None	Pyelonephritis, glomerulonephritis, renal infarction, collagen disease, and interstitial inflammation of kidney	Helps in diagnosis
Urine Culture and Sensitivity	Presence of bacteria and/or other pathogens	Negative or < 100,000 colonies/ml urine from clean catch or sterile bag specimen	Isolation and identification of pathogens in urinary tract; identification of antibiotic sensitivity	See Chapter 27 for specimen collection guidelines
		Urodynamics		
	Invasive test involving urethral and rectal catheters and perineal surface electrodes; measures urine flow, bladder capacity, sensation, sphincter function, and bladder pressures; measures voluntary and involuntary contractions	Normal bladder function	Voiding dysfunction, abnormal urinary tract	Inform child and family of procedure; provide support for child throughout procedure; provide diversionary activities
		Voiding Cystourethrogram (VCUG)		
	Contrast dye instilled in bladder; child or infant voids after bladder is full; serial films taken	Negative for reflux and dilatation of posterior urethra, complete bladder emptying	Detects reflux of urine into ureters and its severity; detects bladder emptying problems; detects urethral problems	Can be done in nuclear medicine department to decrease radiation exposure; procedure is invasive; provide support and diversionary activities for child

URINARY TRACT INFECTIONS

Urinary tract infections (UTIs) are common in children. Urinary tract infections are characterized by the presence of bacteria in urine and an inflammatory response. These infections can have long-term complications that include high blood pressure, decreased renal function, and, rarely, end-stage renal disease (ESRD).

PATHOPHYSIOLOGY *of Urinary Tract Infections*

Cystitis is an infection in the bladder. Pyelonephritis is an infection in the kidney. The diagnosis of chronic pyelonephritis refers to damage to the kidney from previous infections. An abnormal urinary tract system can predispose an infant or child to UTIs. **Renal scarring,** associated with UTIs, is the result of inflammation and **edema** in the kidney. Scarring usually occurs in the first 3 to 5 years of life.

Etiology. Urinary tract infections, except in newborn infants, are caused by bacteria ascending from the area around the outside of the urethra. Urinary tract infections in newborn infants may be caused by bacteria in their blood, which seeds in the kidney.

Fecal organisms are the most common infecting organisms due to the proximity of the rectum to the urethra. *Escherichia coli* is the most common bacteria in acute UTIs of children (Gonzalez, 1996). Other bacteria known to cause UTIs are group B streptococci, *Klebsiella pneumoniae, Proteus* species, *Enterobacter* species, *Enterococcus* species, and *Staphylococcus* species. Viruses and fungi, specifically *Candida* species, can also cause infections.

Incidence. Infections in the neonatal period are more common in boys than girls. In infants and children, UTIs are more common in girls due to the shorter length of the urethra in females. Symptomatic UTIs occur in about 1.4 per 1000 newborn infants. Urinary tract infections occur in 1.2% to 1.9% of school-age females and are most common in the 7 to 11 year age-group. Sexually active females are at increased risk for cystitis (Behrman, Kliegman, & Arvin, 1996).

Clinical Manifestations. The clinical manifestations of UTI vary widely. Some of the factors that influence clinical manifestations are patient age, gender, underlying anatomic or neurologic abnormalities, and frequency of recurrence. Symptoms in the young child and infant are more vague and nonspecific.

Infants

- Nonspecific
- Fever or hypothermia in neonate
- Irritability
- Poor feeding
- Vomiting
- **Dysuria** as evidenced by crying when voiding
- Change in urine odor or color

Children

- Abdominal or suprapubic pain
- Voiding **frequency**
- Voiding **urgency**
- Dysuria
- New or increased incidence of enuresis

Children With Pyelonephritis

- Same symptoms as children with UTI
- Fever
- Back pain
- Costovertebral angle tenderness
- Nausea and vomiting
- Appear sick

Diagnostic Evaluation. A UTI is diagnosed by the presence of bacteria in the urine. A urinalysis and urine culture must be obtained before the diagnosis of UTI can be made. A urine catheter obtained by clean catch or sterile bags which yield a single organism $>10^5$ is accurate in determining bacteria. The collection technique should match the desired goal. When accurate determination of bacteria is the goal, bladder catheterization or suprapubic aspiration is the collection of choice. Unfortunately, both methods are intrusive. If catheterization or suprapubic aspiration is used to obtain a urine culture, the growth of almost any bacteria indicates infection.

Radiographic studies are indicated for children who are likely to have renal damage associated with structural abnormalities:

- Children less than age 5 years
- All boys
- Girls with pyelonephritis or a secondary infection
- Children with suprapubic mass
- Children with abnormal urinary stream
- Children with increased blood urea nitrogen (BUN) or serum creatinine level
- Children with elevated blood pressure

The radiologic studies may include renal ultrasound, renal scan, voiding cystourethrogram (VCUG), or intravenous pyelogram. A renal scan may be used to differentiate pyelonephritis from cystitis and identify renal scarring.

The specimen can be collected in a variety of methods, depending on the developmental level of the child and clinic procedures. A midstream clean catch urine specimen can be obtained from a child who can void on demand. In girls, the labia majora are spread apart and cleaned. In uncircumcised boys, the foreskin is gently retracted and the glans penis and meatus is cleaned. After the urinary stream has started, urine is collected in a sterile container. In infants and non–toilet-trained children, a urine specimen may be collected by attaching a bag to the perineum. The perineal area must be meticulously cleaned and the specimen collected within 30 minutes. If the child or infant does not void within 30 minutes, the bag is changed (see Chapter 18). Urine can be collected by urethral catheterization into the bladder. Careful attention to cleaning and aseptic technique are necessary to avoid introducing bacteria into the bladder.

In infants, urine can be collected by a physician performing a suprapubic aspiration. The area above the pubis is cleaned with an antiseptic solution, a needle attached to a syringe is inserted into the bladder, and urine is aspirated.

Therapeutic Management. Antibiotics are used in the treatment of UTIs. Oral antibiotics are used for children with cystitis. The antibiotic chosen should be sensitive to the specific bacteria, easily administered, and have minimal adverse effects. A urine culture should be repeated 2 to 3 days before treatment completion. Antibiotic therapy is usually 7 to 10 days in length. For children with pyelonephritis and all infants, intravenous antibiotic therapy is necessary until their condition improves, they are able to take oral antibiotics, and they have negative urine culture.

In addition, when anatomic abnormalities are detected therapeutic management may include prophylactic antibiotic therapy. Serial radiographic studies and possibly surgical intervention may be indicated. These children should be followed by a pediatric nephrologist or urologist.

NURSING CARE OF THE CHILD WITH URINARY TRACT INFECTION

Assessment

A history of signs and symptoms of UTI should be obtained from the child and family. Signs and symptoms vary according to age. The younger the child, the more vague and nonspecific the history may be (see Clinical Manifestations above).

Physical assessment should include temperature, blood pressure, abdominal examination for masses, examination for costovertebral angle tenderness, and genital examination for abnormalities. A urinalysis and urine culture should be obtained before initiation of antibiotics.

Nursing Diagnosis and Planning

The following nursing diagnoses and expected outcomes may be appropriate following assessment of the child with UTI:

- Risk for Injury related to complications of infectious process leading to kidney disease. ***Expected Outcome:*** *The child will be free of recurrent UTIs that could lead to progressive renal damage.*
- Fluid Volume Deficit related to decreased intake and increased fluid loss. ***Expected Outcome:*** *The child will maintain adequate intake of fluids and electrolytes for age.*
- Knowledge Deficit related to disease process, diagnostic tests, antibiotic administration, and preventive measures for UTI. ***Expected Outcome:*** *The parent/child will verbalize an understanding of disease process, diagnostic tests, and preventive measures for UTIs. The child will receive follow-up care including antibiotic administration.*

Implementation and Evaluation

Nursing care includes administration of antibiotics, promotion of comfort, maintaining good hydration, preparing the child and parents for diagnostic procedures, and monitoring for response to treatment and complications.

The child and family should be given information on the prevention of UTIs. The child and parents should be taught good perineal hygiene. Females should be taught to wipe from front to back after urination and/or a bowel movement to avoid moving bacteria from the anus to the urethra. Fluid intake including water should be encouraged. The child should be encouraged to avoid "holding" urine and to urinate at least four times a day. The bladder should be emptied with each void to avoid residual urine. Bubble baths should be avoided secondary to possible urethral irritation. Cotton underwear, which breathes, is preferred over nylon, which tends to hold moisture-promoting bacterial growth. Prophylactic antibiotics may be prescribed to be taken daily. For older children, antibiotics are best administered at bedtime due to urinary stasis during the night.

Good hydration is important, especially if the child has been nauseated, vomiting, or feeding poorly. Oral fluid should be encouraged if possible. Intravenous hydration may be required. The child should be observed for signs of dehydration: poor skin turgor, dry mucous membranes, a sunken fontanel, decreased output, and decreased perfusion. Daily weights, intake and output, and urine specific gravity are indicators of hydration. Acute renal infection can impair the kidney's ability to concentrate urine, leading to falsely low specific gravity readings (Reynolds & Hoberman, 1995).

The importance of follow-up appointments, radiologic studies, urinalysis, and cultures should be stressed secondary to the risk of renal damage. Explanation of diagnostic tests should be given to the parent. The most common manifestations of renal damage are elevated blood pressure, decreased renal function, and, rarely, end-stage renal disease. Prevention of subsequent UTIs is a measure of the success of preventive teaching. Compliance with the treatment plan also is part of the evaluation of nursing care.

GLOMERULONEPHRITIS

The term *glomerulonephritis* refers to a group of kidney disorders in which the main focus of injury is the glomerulus (see Clinical Reference Pages). Glomerulonephritis is characterized by inflammation of the capillaries contained in the glomerulus.

This inflammation can result from several different causes, such as infection, a systemic disease process, or a primary defect in the glomerulus itself. The majority of disorders are termed "acute" glomerulonephritis and usually occur following a bacterial or viral infection. Acute post-streptococcal glomerulonephritis is the most common type and is characterized by hematuria, **proteinuria,** edema, and renal insufficiency.

Etiology/Incidence. Acute post-streptococcal glomerulonephritis occurs as an immune reaction to streptococcal infection of the throat or skin. This disorder most commonly occurs in school-age children, with a slightly higher incidence in males. Clinical symptoms of acute glomerulonephritis usually appear 1 to 3 weeks after a streptococcal infection (Brouhard, 1992).

Clinical Manifestations

The presence of hematuria is essential for the diagnosis of acute post-streptococcal glomerulonephritis.

- Hematuria may range in severity from microscopic to gross, as evidenced by "smoky" or "tea-colored" urine.
- Edema may be noted, especially in the eyelids and ankles.
- Decreased urine output may be experienced.
- Hypertension may be present.
- Fever may or may not be present.
- Fatigue is experienced by many children.

PATHOPHYSIOLOGY *of Acute Post-streptococcal Glomerulonephritis*

Acute glomerulonephritis following an infection with streptococci is thought to occur as a result of an immunologic response. The body responds to the *Streptococcus* bacteria by forming antibodies, which combine with the bacterial antigens to form immune complexes. As these antigen–antibody complexes travel through the circulation, they become "trapped" in the glomerulus and activate an inflammatory response, which results in injury to the capillary walls. As a result of the inflammation, the size of the capillary lumen is smaller, which decreases the glomerular filtration rate and leads to renal insufficiency. Additionally, injury to the capillary walls interferes with their permeability so that "larger" molecules such as proteins can pass through into the urine.

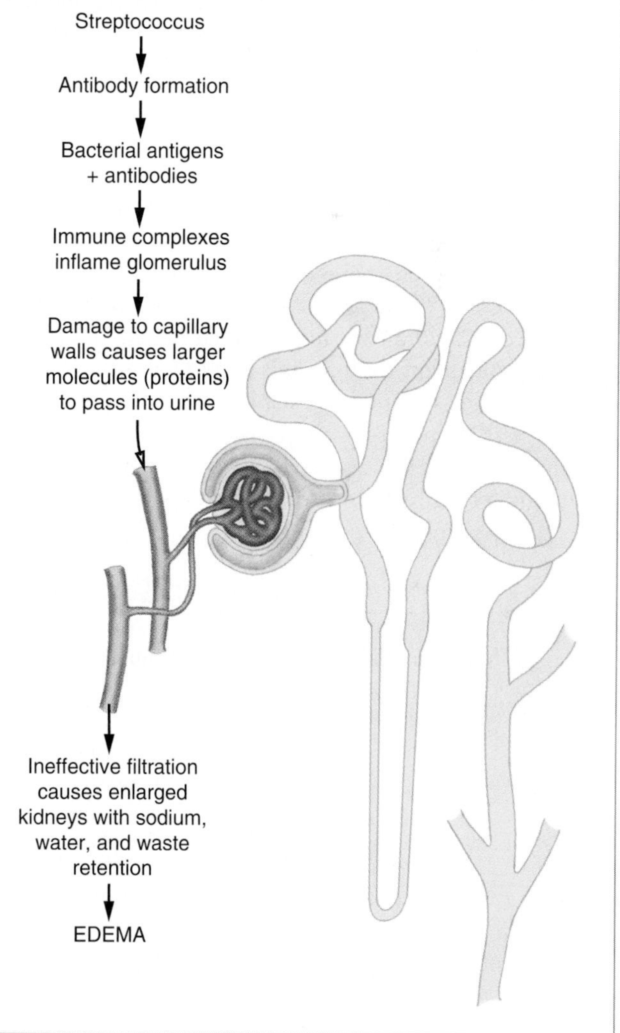
Streptococcus
Antibody formation
Bacterial antigens + antibodies
Immune complexes inflame glomerulus
Damage to capillary walls causes larger molecules (proteins) to pass into urine
Ineffective filtration causes enlarged kidneys with sodium, water, and waste retention
EDEMA

Diagnostic Evaluation. The diagnosis of acute post-streptococcal glomerulonephritis can be made by the history, presenting symptoms, and laboratory results. (See Table 27–1, p. 789.) A urinalysis will reveal hematuria with red cell casts. The presence of these casts indicates glomerular injury. Proteinuria is also present but typically is not as severe as in nephrotic syndrome. Blood chemistry values are usually within the normal range. However, if the renal insufficiency is severe, BUN and creatinine levels will be elevated. Electrolyte disturbances such as high serum potassium and low serum bicarbonate may be present due to inadequate glomerular filtration. A complete blood count is done. The white blood cell (WBC) count is usually within normal limits and mild anemia is common. The lower hemoglobin and hematocrit values are reflective of the "dilutional" effect of the extra fluid in the blood as a result of decreased glomerular filtration. Immunologic studies are important in diagnosing acute post-streptococcal glomerulonephritis. Serum complement (C_3) may be low due to the fixation of complement in the immune complexes. Streptozyme, which indicates the presence of antibodies to streptococcal bacteria, is high if the child has not received antibiotics. Culture of the throat or skin lesion (if present) may be helpful for isolating the bacteria. Again, this is only useful if the infection is recent and the child has not received antibiotics. A renal biopsy may be indicated for two reasons. First, for those children whose signs and symptoms are not characteristic of acute post-streptococcal glomerular nephritis, and second, for those children whose symptoms don't improve as expected.

Therapeutic Management. There is no specific therapy for acute post-streptococcal glomerulonephritis. Medical management is aimed at the associated signs and symptoms and is guided by the degree of renal dysfunction the child experiences. Children with acute renal failure should be hospitalized to allow for fluid and electrolyte management until their renal function has stabilized. Antihypertensive therapy may be necessary. This can be accomplished by limiting sodium and water intake or by the administration of diuretics or antihypertensive medication. The prognosis for children with acute post-streptococcal glomerulonephritis is excellent. The acute clinical episode is usually self-limiting, and laboratory values normally return to baseline in 6 to 12 weeks. Most children enjoy a complete recovery.

NURSING CARE OF THE CHILD WITH ACUTE POST-STREPTOCOCCAL GLOMERULONEPHRITIS

Assessment

The child should be evaluated for symptoms of fluid overload. The respiratory system should be assessed for presence of any respiratory difficulty such as cough, increased respiratory rate, or increased work of breathing. Auscultate the breath sounds for crackles. Assess the child for presence of edema, especially in lower extremities. Obtain vital signs and weight. Monitor laboratory values.

> Be sure that blood pressure is obtained with an appropriately sized cuff. Using too small a cuff can give a falsely high reading, and a cuff that is slightly too big is unlikely to mask high blood pressure readings (see Chapter 18, Table 18–1).

Determine the child's and family's understanding of the illness and reason for hospitalization.

Nursing Diagnosis

- Fluid Volume Excess related to decreased urine output
- Risk for Activity Intolerance related to fatigue
- Risk for Impaired Skin Integrity related to edema and decreased activity
- Altered Nutrition: Less Than Body Requirements related to fluid and diet restrictions
- Anxiety related to knowledge deficit regarding disease process or hospitalization

Planning, Implementation, and Evaluation: The Child With Acute Post-Streptococcal Glomerulonephritis

NURSING DIAGNOSIS • Fluid Volume Excess related to decreased urine output

Expected Outcome: • The child will maintain normal fluid status, as evidenced by urine output of at least 1–2 ml/kg/hr, normal blood pressure, no increase in weight, and no symptoms of respiratory distress.

Intervention	Rationale
1. Measure and record fluid intake, including oral intake and intravenous fluids, and urine output each shift. Report output of urine less than 1–2 ml/kg/hr.	Frequent, accurate assessment of intake and output is essential for evaluating fluid status. Children with severe renal impairment may require measurement of intake and output every 2 to 4 hours. Urine output of less than 1–2 ml/kg/hr represents renal failure.

Intervention	Rationale
2. Obtain daily weights. Remember to weigh the patient on the same scale at about the same time each day. Young children should be weighed without diapers, and older children should wear only gowns.	Accurate daily weights are important for determining fluctuation in fluid status. Weight measurements can vary from scale to scale. Children's clothing and presence of a wet diaper can also affect the weight. The time of day a child is weighed is important because a child will weigh more after consuming meals and fluids than he will upon awakening in the early morning.
3. Measure blood pressure with appropriately sized cuff every shift and document. Report increasing values. More frequent readings may be required if the child has significant hypertension or receives antihypertensive medication.	Hypertension may result from fluid overload. The child should be calm and cooperative while the blood pressure is obtained. An elevated measurement in a child who is upset or combative is not reliable.
4. Assess respiratory effort and auscultate breath sounds every shift. Report rapid respirations, retractions, nasal flaring, or crackles.	Children with fluid excess may develop pulmonary edema.
5. Limit fluid intake as ordered. Inform parents, visitors, and hospital staff of need to limit fluids.	Fluid intake may be restricted to match urine output in an attempt to maintain fluid balance. Children may "sneak" drinks or obtain drinks from people who are unaware of the restrictions.
6. Ensure low-sodium diet is followed if ordered. Inform parents and visitors of diet restrictions.	Excessive sodium will increase fluid retention. Parents and visitors frequently bring food and treats from outside the hospital.

Evaluation: The child has

- adequate urine output for weight
- no weight gain during the hospitalization
- normal blood pressure for age
- nonlabored respirations.

NURSING DIAGNOSIS

- Risk for Activity Intolerance related to fatigue

Expected Outcome:

- The child will be rested, as evidenced by the ability to tolerate daily care and play activities.

Intervention	Rationale
1. Arrange daily care so that child has some uninterrupted time for sleep and naps.	It is important that the child has an opportunity to rest.
2. Encourage parents to bring favorite sleep toy or blanket for child.	Rest is promoted by helping the child to feel comfortable.
3. Allow for nap time and bed time to coincide with child's home schedule as much as possible. Try to follow home rituals.	Rest is promoted by helping the child to feel comfortable.
4. Limit play time to short periods and extend as child's condition improves.	Child may tire easily when first hospitalized.

Evaluation:

- The child is able to tolerate usual activities for age.

NURSING DIAGNOSIS • Risk for Impaired Skin Integrity related to edema and decreased activity

Expected Outcome: • The child will exhibit no signs of skin breakdown, as evidenced by skin that is intact, normal color for race, and nontender to touch.

Intervention	Rationale
1. Have child change position at least q 2 hr during the day.	Frequent change of position decreases pressure on the skin, especially over bony prominences. Position change also helps to decrease edema in dependent areas such as the ankles and eyelids.
2. Elevate lower extremities with pillows when child is sitting or lying in bed. If child has peripheral intravenous (IV) line, elevate the extremity.	Because edema is largely dependent, elevation will help decrease severity. Placement of IV line decreases use of an extremity, increasing potential for edema.
3. Maintan good hygiene by giving daily baths and cleaning skin well after bowel movements and diaper changes. Use lotion to prevent dry skin. Change linen daily.	Presence of dirt and excrement is irritating to the skin. Dry skin is more prone to breakdown, and massaging skin with lotion also promotes circulation.
4. Promote activity as child improves. Ask for child's participation in daily care. Encourage child to visit playroom or engage in play activities in his room.	Activity increases circulation and promotes reabsorption of fluid in edematous areas.

Evaluation: • The child has healthy skin, as evidenced by intact skin surface, appropriate skin color for race, and skin that is nontender to touch.

NURSING DIAGNOSIS • Altered Nutrition: Less Than Body Requirements related to fluid and diet restrictions

Expected Outcome: • The child will have adequate hydration and nutrition, as evidenced by moist mucous membranes and maintenance of weight at "pre-illness" level.

Intervention	Rationale
1. Assess for signs of dehydration (dry mucous membranes, listlessness, poor skin turgor, tachycardia) and report.	Dehydration could occur due to fluid restriction and effects of diuretics.
2. Monitor daily weights. Obtain "pre-illness" weight from parents.	Small fluctuation in weight can indicate fluid loss or gain. Weight below pre-illness level may indicate dehydration or weight loss from decreased food intake.
3. Consult with dietary department about palatable low-sodium food and drinks. Allow parents to bring "favorite" foods from home if these foods comply with dietary orders.	Low-sodium foods taste different, and children may refuse to eat them. Offering the child foods that are different from those available in the hospital may encourage him to eat.

Evaluation: • Child has moist mucous membranes and maintains "pre-illness" weight.

NURSING DIAGNOSIS • Anxiety (child/parent) related to knowledge deficit regarding disease process or hospitalization

Expected Outcome: • Anxiety will be decreased in the child, as evidenced by cooperation with daily care and interest in developmentally appropriate play. Parents will verbalize understanding of disease process.

Intervention	Rationale
1. Allow parents and child to voice concerns.	Provides support and a basis for assessing their understanding of disease process.
2. Explain all procedures to the child and parents. Tell them what will happen, why it will happen, when it will happen, and how it will feel.	Information enables the child and parents to understand procedures and anticipate these events. Children fear the unknown. Knowing what to expect helps decrease anxiety.
3. Allow parents to participate in the child's care as appropriate.	Parents are familiar people and can provide comfort to the child.
4. Provide age-appropriate play activities.	Play is diversional and therapeutic.
5. Allow for emotional support.	A favorite blanket or sleep toy may be very comforting to a child. Also, if the child is a thumbsucker, ensure that the favorite thumb or fingers are accessible by choosing an IV site that allows them to be free of tape or restraints.

Evaluation:
- The child experiences minimal anxiety as evidenced by cooperation with care activities and interest in play.
- The parents participate in their child's care as appropriate, provide comfort to the child, and verbalize an understanding of the disease process.

Home Care: If the child has been hypertensive or is to be discharged on antihypertensive medications, before going home the parents should be provided with a blood pressure cuff and stethoscope and instructed how to measure blood pressure. The child's blood pressure should be assessed before medication is given. The parameters for when to hold medication should be clear to the family, as should the parameters for when to call the physician because of high readings. The parents should be instructed to monitor intake and output and provided with parameters appropriate for their child.

NEPHROTIC SYNDROME

The term nephrotic syndrome refers to a kidney disorder characterized by proteinuria, **hypoalbuminemia,** and edema. Nephrotic syndrome may be classified as primary or secondary. Primary nephrotic syndrome results from a disorder within the glomerulus of the kidney. A child may develop nephrotic syndrome secondary to a systemic disease such as hepatitis, systemic lupus erythematosus, heavy metal poisoning, or cancer. The most common type of nephrotic syndrome in children is primary.

Etiology/Incidence. The cause of primary nephrotic syndrome is not fully understood. Success in controlling the disease by the use of immunosuppressive drugs suggests the possibility of an immunologic component. Primary nephrotic syndrome can arise from one of four types of renal lesions. In the majority of children, minimal alterations of the glomerulus are seen on histologic examination. Accordingly, the most common disorder is termed minimal change nephrotic syndrome (MCNS). Minimal change disease accounts for almost 80% of childhood nephrotic syndrome (Barrett, 1993). The remainder of children develop nephrosis as a result of focal segmental

PATHOPHYSIOLOGY *of Nephrotic Syndrome*

Primary nephrotic syndrome occurs from an alteration in the glomerulus. Loss of plasma proteins through the glomerulus gives rise to the following symptoms.

Proteinuria occurs when protein is lost into the urine due to the increased permeability of the glomerular basement membrane. The majority of urinary protein is albumin; however, other proteins may be present. Proteinuria is essential for the diagnosis of nephrotic syndrome. Blood albumin values will be low (hypoalbuminemia) as a result of the loss of albumin through the defective glomerulus. Decreased levels of albumin reduce the plasma oncotic pressure so that the intravascular fluid moves into the interstitial spaces. This shifting of fluid reduces the intravascular volume, which decreases the amount of renal blood flow due to hypovolemia.

In an effort to increase blood volume, the kidney stimulates renin production. Renin causes increased excretion of aldosterone, resulting in renal tubular reabsorption of sodium, which in turn causes water retention. The net effect of this phenomenon is edema. In addition, the serum values of cholesterol and triglycerides will be elevated. This is thought to occur from increased stimulation of lipoprotein production due to the decrease in oncotic pressure. Loss of immunoglobulins into the urine is common in nephrotic syndrome. Most notably, levels of IgG are decreased, which makes these children more susceptible to infection. Before the use of antibiotics, infection was a frequent cause of death in these patients.

Children with nephrotic syndrome are in a hypercoagulable state, predisposing them to venous thrombosis. This tendency occurs as a result of several factors. Decreased intravascular volume (hypovolemia) causes increased concentration of red blood cells and platelets and slowing of circulation. Urinary loss of proteins that inhibit coagulation also contributes to the risk of thrombus formation.

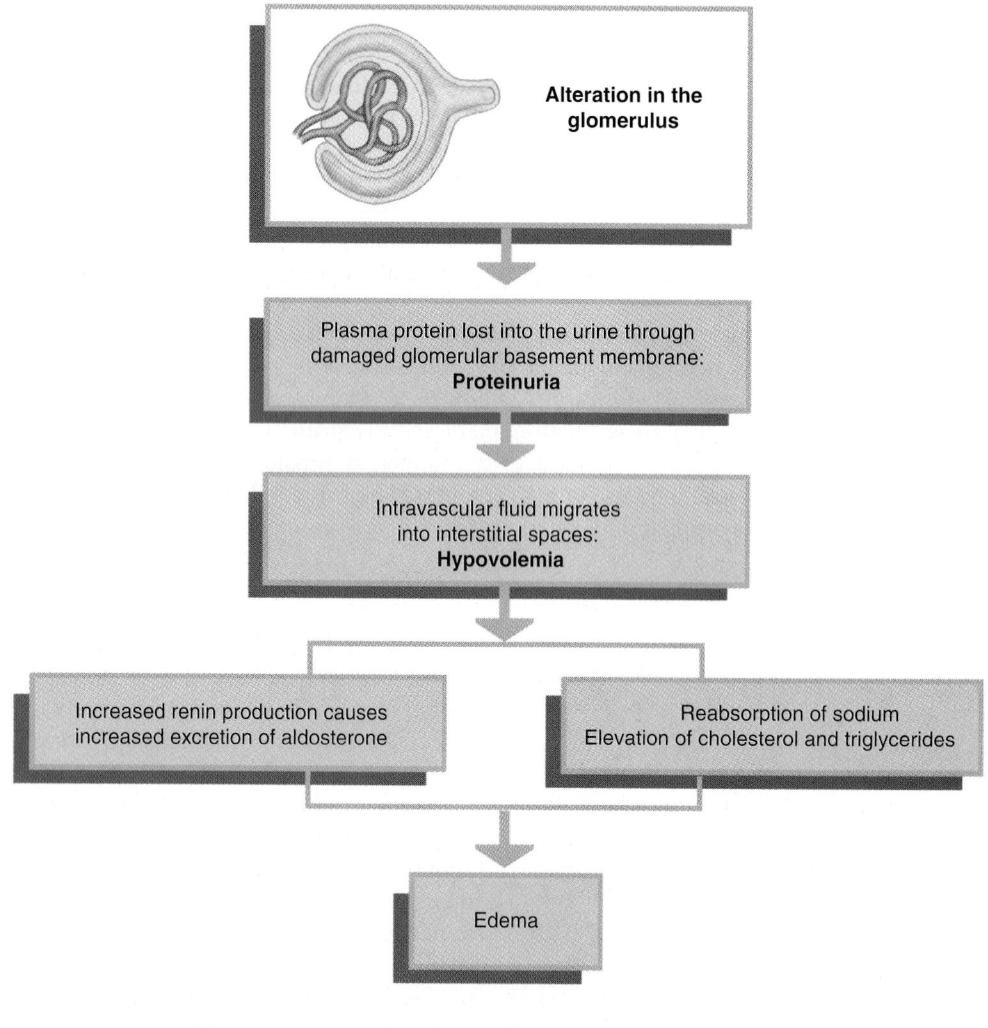
Alteration in the glomerulus
Plasma protein lost into the urine through damaged glomerular basement membrane: Proteinuria
Intravascular fluid migrates into interstitial spaces: Hypovolemia
Increased renin production causes increased excretion of aldosterone
Reabsorption of sodium
Elevation of cholesterol and triglycerides
Edema

glomerulosclerosis. More rarely, the disorder will arise due to membranoproliferative glomerulonephritis or mesangial proliferation.

Primary nephrotic syndrome most frequently occurs in children between ages 2 and 6 years. There is a slightly higher incidence in males. The prognosis for children with MCNS is very good. Manifestations of the disease usually decrease with age so that relapses are rare in adolescence. Unfortunately, the diagnosis of focal segmental glomerulosclerosis carries a worse prognosis. This disease is progressive and often results in end-stage renal disease.

Clinical Manifestations

- Edema is usually first noted in the periorbital spaces and dependent areas of the body. The edema is "pitting" in nature, and is most noticeable over the bony prominences of the lower extremities.

> Children with nephrotic syndrome often awaken with only facial edema and, as the day progresses, become noticeably edematous in their abdomen, genital area, and lower extremities.

- Anorexia
- Fatigue
- Abdominal pain may occur from the presence of extra fluid in the peritoneal area. Edema of the bowel may cause decreased absorption of nutrients and diarrhea.
- Recent upper respiratory infection is common. Many children are misdiagnosed with "allergies" due to periorbital edema and respiratory symptoms.
- Increased weight
- Normal blood pressure

Diagnostic Evaluation. The diagnosis of nephrotic syndrome can be made based on the clinical presentation, age of the child, and laboratory results (Table 27–1). Serologic tests for hepatitis, human immunodeficiency virus, or syphilis, or ANA titers are done to rule out systemic disease as a cause for nephrotic syndrome.

A kidney biopsy may be done if a lesion other than MCNS is suspected. This would occur if the child had a nontypical presentation, as evidenced by being older than 10 years or having gross hematuria or hypertension. A biopsy is also indicated for the child who does not respond as expected to pharmacologic treatment.

Therapeutic Management. It is not unusual for the child with primary nephrotic syndrome to be hospitalized briefly during the initial onset of the disease to provide palliative treatment for the edema, perform necessary diagnostic testing, and initiate therapy. It is during this time that the parents are educated about the disease process and necessary home care.

The edematous child should be placed on a no added salt diet. The caregiver should not use salt when cooking, the child should not be permitted to use the salt shaker, and the caregiver should avoid serving high-sodium foods such as pickles, salted chips, and cured meats. If edema is severe, or if the child is hypertensive, sodium intake may be further restricted. Some children can develop respiratory complications from being edematous. Increased fluid in the abdomen can interfere with expansion of the lungs. Excessive fluid in the lung tissue can cause pulmonary edema.

When proteinuria is massive and the child is edematous, oral penicillin is commonly given to reduce the likelihood of developing an infection.

> Peritonitis may be a problem in these patients due to abdominal edema. This excess fluid is an excellent culture medium for bacteria. The organism most likely to cause an infection is *Streptococcus pneumoniae.*

Severe edema in the lower extremities can give rise to cellulitis due to fluid stasis and poor circulation.

TABLE 27–1 *Nephrotic Syndrome Versus Acute Post-Streptococcal Glomerulonephritis: Comparison of Diagnostic Findings*

	NEPHROTIC SYNDROME	ACUTE POST-STREPTOCOCCAL GLOMERULONEPHRITIS
Urinalysis	3–4+ proteinuria per Albustix Protein excretion greater than 40 mg/m^2/hr in a timed urine collection Microscopic hematuria *may* be present	0–2+ proteinuria per Albustix Hematuria present and may range from microscopic to grossly visible
Laboratory Findings	Low serum albumin (<2.5 g/dl) Elevated serum cholesterol and triglycerides Elevated hemoglobin, hematocrit, and platelet count Normal electrolytes Normal complement levels Negative ASO titer and streptozyme	Serum albumin normal Normal values for cholesterol and triglycerides Hemoglobin and hematocrit are normal or low Serum potassium may be elevated, sodium may be low BUN and creatinine may be elevated Complement levels are low ASO titer and streptozyme are positive
Physical Findings	Normotensive or hypotensive	Frequently hypertensive

The child is usually placed on diuretic therapy until urinary protein loss is controlled. If the edema is marked and causes the child to have decreased mobility, poor oral intake, or decreased urine output, salt-poor albumin may be given intravenously. The administration of albumin helps restore normal plasma osmotic pressure and promotes the movement of interstitial fluid back into the intravascular compartments. Furosemide is given intravenously after the albumin infusion to enhance diuresis and decrease the chance of fluid overload.

Therapy for remission is usually instituted with prednisone at a dose of 2 mg/kg/day (maximum 60 mg) divided into two or three doses. This regimen is continued until the child is in remission.

> Remission is achieved when the urine is 0–trace for protein for Albustix for 5 to 7 consecutive days.

During Initial Therapy. During initial therapy, steroids are generally continued at the same daily dose for a total of 4 to 6 weeks, then switched to an alternate-day schedule and slowly tapered.

In the event of a relapse, steroid therapy is less prolonged. Once remission is achieved, dosing decreases to alternate days and is tapered more quickly. This is done to minimize prednisone side effects (see Common Medications table in Clinical Reference Pages).

Some children respond to steroids quickly and achieve remission in 5 to 7 days, whereas others may not respond for 4 weeks. If proteinuria continues beyond 6 weeks of daily steroid therapy, the child is said to be steroid-resistant and a kidney biopsy is done to determine the exact nature of the disease.

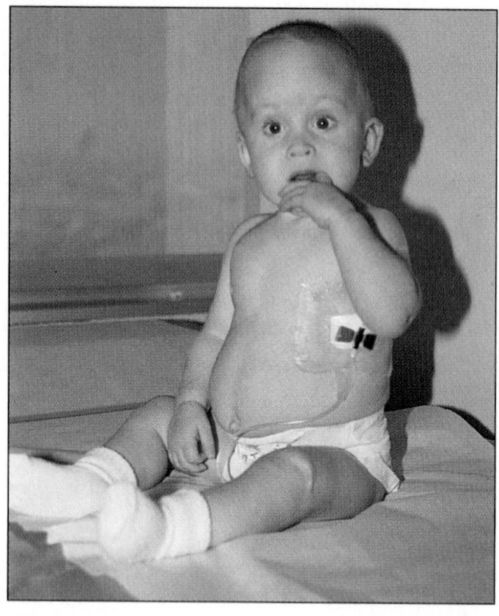

Figure 27–1
This child has nephrotic syndrome that is presently in remission. She previously received steroid therapy, and is now receiving cyclosporine chemotherapy to control the process. During the acute phase of the nephrotic syndrome, the child may have massive edema because blood proteins are lost in the urine. Skin pallor is also common. (Courtesy of Children's Medical Center, Dallas, Texas)

Children who initially respond to steroid therapy but have relapses while on a tapering schedule or shortly after stopping steroids are said to be steroid-dependent. These children may benefit from a course of an alkylating agent such as cyclophosphamide or chlorambucil. The risks and benefits of this therapy must be carefully considered, and the parents should be informed of all possible side effects (see Common Medications table). A kidney biopsy is usually done before starting therapy. Recently, the use of cyclosporine in those children who remain steroid-dependent despite a course of an alkylating agent has proven to be effective in maintaining remission (Fig. 27–1).

When the child is in remission a pneumococcal vaccine should be given to help protect him from pneumococcal infection in the event of a relapse. It may also be beneficial for the child with nephrotic syndrome to receive a flu vaccine each year, since there can be an exacerbation of the disease following an infection.

NURSING CARE OF THE CHILD WITH NEPHROTIC SYNDROME

The nurse should monitor the child's vital signs as ordered to detect any changes that may be early signs of infection or hypovolemia. Careful documentation of the child's fluid intake and urine output should be done as well as obtaining accurate daily weights. This is essential in determining fluid status. Nursing care should include assessment of the amount of edema present in the child each shift, specifically in the periorbital areas, abdomen, genitalia, and lower extremities. The laboratory results are monitored and the urine checked daily with Albustix for protein. The nursing history should include the child's immunization status and known recent exposures to communicable diseases. Assessment of the family's understanding of the disease process and treatment is important so that the nurse can make appropriate referrals and provide the parents with information.

Nursing Diagnoses

- Risk for Impaired Skin Integrity related to edema and decreased circulation
- Risk for Infection related to urinary loss of gammaglobulins and immunosuppressive therapy
- Risk for Fluid Volume Deficit (intravascular) related to proteinuria, edema, and effects of diuretics
- Fluid Volume Excess related to decreased excretion of sodium and water retention
- Anxiety (parental) related to hospitalization of child and caring for a child with chronic disease

Planning, Implementation, and Evaluation: The Child With Nephrotic Syndrome

NURSING DIAGNOSIS • Risk for Impaired Skin Integrity related to edema and decreased circulation

Expected Outcome: • The child will exhibit no signs of skin breakdown, as evidenced by the absence of redness, tenderness to touch, and ulceration.

Intervention	Rationale
1. Ensure that the child changes position q 2 hr.	Frequent position change decreases pressure on body parts and helps relieve edema in dependent areas.
2. Maintain good hygiene by giving daily baths and changing linen daily. Use lotion for dry skin.	Body secretions and debris on linens can irritate the skin. Gentle massage when bathing and applying lotion help increase circulation.
3. Support or elevate edematous body parts with pillows while child is in bed or sitting in a chair.	Edema is gravity dependent. Elevation will help decrease edema.
4. Promote physical activity as child is able to tolerate by providing developmentally appropriate play activities.	Increased activity helps promote circulation.

Evaluation: • The child's skin is intact with no redness or tenderness.

NURSING DIAGNOSIS • Risk for Infection related to urinary loss of gamma-globulins and immunosuppressive therapy

Expected Outcome: • The child will have no evidence of an infection, as evidenced by normal WBC count, normal body temperature, and absence of abdominal pain and cough.

Intervention	Rationale
1. Screen visitors for signs of infection such as upper respiratory symptoms, sore throats, or exposure to communicable diseases.	Avoid exposure to people with an active infectious process. Communicable diseases, especially varicella, pose a serious threat because the child on immunosuppressive therapy is not able to respond appropriately to infection.
2. Administer antibiotics as ordered.	Antibiotics are usually given for peritonitis prophylaxis during the edematous phase.
3. Use good handwashing techniques, and instruct family to do the same.	Helps decrease transmission of germs.
4. Monitor child for fever, cough, sore throat, or complaints of abdominal pain each shift. Monitor laboratory values.	Frequent assessment ensures early detection of infectious process. Abdominal pain may be an indication of peritonitis.

Evaluation: • The child maintains normal body temperature and laboratory values, and has no complaints of pain or cough.

NURSING DIAGNOSIS

- Risk for Fluid Volume Deficit (intravascular) related to proteinuria, edema, and effects of diuretics

Expected Outcome:

- Child has no evidence of hypovolemia, as evidenced by blood pressure measurement within normal limits, adequate urine output, and hemoglobin and hematocrit values within normal range.

Intervention	Rationale
1. Monitor vital signs, including blood pressure and pulse, every shift. Report variance from baseline.	Low blood pressure and increased heart rate are signs of hypovolemia. Blood pressure may also be elevated due to renin release.
2. Monitor intake and output every shift. Report if child has output of less than 1–2 ml/kg/hr of urine.	Accurate intake and output measurement is essential for evaluating fluid status.
3. Monitor laboratory values.	Increasing values of hemoglobin, hematocrit, and platelets may indicate hemoconcentration or low intravascular volume.
4. Assess for signs of dehydration such as appearance of mucous membranes, capillary refill, and level of activity. (Capillary refill may be altered due to edema; assess in nonedematous area.) Report positive findings.	The pathophysiology of nephrotic syndrome may predispose the child to decreased intravascular volume. This is compounded by the use of diuretics.

Evaluation:

- The child's vital signs remain within normal limits and urine output is adequate. The child has moist mucous membranes and remains interactive.

NURSING DIAGNOSIS

- Fluid Volume Excess related to decreased excretion of sodium and water retention

Expected Outcome:

- The child will not demonstrate fluid overload, as evidenced by stable daily weights and no respiratory difficulty.

Intervention	Rationale
1. Monitor intake and output each shift.	Accurate intake and output is essential for evaluating fluid status.
2. Obtain accurate daily weights. Weigh child on same scales, at same time each day, in gown only.	Daily weights are necessary to detect changes in fluid status. Clothing or presence of wet diaper can alter weight. Readings of weight can vary from scale to scale and time of day.
3. Adhere to dietary sodium restriction.	Excessive sodium intake increases amount of water retention.
4. Measure and record abdominal girth each day. Ensure accuracy by measuring in same area each time.	Edema commonly occurs in the abdomen.
5. Monitor blood pressure at least once each shift.	Increased total body fluid volume and concurrent steroid therapy can result in increased blood pressure.
6. Administer diuretics as ordered.	Diuretics may aid in the elimination of excessive fluid.

Intervention	Rationale
7. Assess pulmonary status by listening to breath sounds for crackles, observing for signs of increased work of breathing and presence of cough.	Fluid overload can result in pulmonary edema.

Evaluation: • Child's weight does not increase and the child experiences no cough, increased respiratory rate, or retractions.

NURSING DIAGNOSIS • Anxiety (parental) related to hospitalization of child and caring for a child with chronic disease

Expected Outcome: • Parents will demonstrate a more relaxed state, as evidenced by participating in the care of their child and verbalizing an understanding of the disease process.

Intervention	Rationale
1. Allow parents to verbalize frustration and fears. Encourage them to ask questions and provide them with information about nephrotic syndrome and its treatment.	Verbalization of fears is often therapeutic in itself. Information helps decrease anxiety because people often fear the unknown.
2. Incorporate the parents' help in the daily care of the child. Have them practice using Albustix, taking blood pressures, and assessing edema.	Nephrotic syndrome can be a chronic condition and is usually managed at home. It is important for the parents to feel comfortable with caring for their child.
3. Arrange for a dietary consult.	Steroid therapy stimulates appetite. Patients should be informed about low-calorie snacks and portion size. The child will also need to be on sodium restriction during the edematous phase of disease.

Evaluation: • The parents verbalize understanding of their child's condition and required treatment. The parents actively participate in the child's care.

Home Care: Preparing the family for discharge is an essential element of nursing care. The caregivers should be proficient in reading Albustix and should be sent home with a full container and a prescription for refills. It is best if they keep a daily calendar of Albustix readings. The need to check the urine daily may continue for an indefinite time because a positive reading for protein in the urine may be the only symptom of relapse.

In addition to daily Albustix readings, the child should have daily weights and blood pressure measurements. His weight may fluctuate not only from fluid status changes, but also from rapid weight gain from increased appetite while on steroids. The child may also be hypertensive from steroid therapy as well. The parents should be educated about all medications their child will be taking. It is very important that they check with the nephrologist before giving their child any over-the-counter cold medication, because many of these preparations contain ephedrine, which can aggravate hypertension.

Parents should be instructed to report exposure to chickenpox or development of fever immediately. Children on steroids are not able to respond appropriately to viral or bacterial infections and may require additional treatment. Finally, these children should not receive live vaccinations during steroid therapy due to their impaired immune response.

ENURESIS

Enuresis refers to a condition in which the child is unable to control bladder function although he has reached an age at which control of voiding is expected. Nocturnal enuresis, or bed wetting, is common in children. Children who have never been dry at night for prolonged periods are said to have primary nocturnal enuresis. Secondary, or "acquired" enuresis, refers to the child who starts having problems with wetting when previously he has been dry. A child with a history of daytime wetting along with complaints of urgency or frequency may have a more complex problem.

PATHOPHYSIOLOGY *and Etiology of Enuresis*

Control of urination is related to the maturity of the central nervous system. By age 5 years, most children are aware of bladder fullness and are able to control voiding. Children generally achieve daytime urinary control first, with nighttime dryness occurring later. Girls seem to master this earlier than boys. Children who have primary nocturnal enuresis may have delayed maturation of this portion of the central nervous system. They are not able to "sense" bladder fullness and do not awaken to void.

A child with secondary enuresis or with problems of daytime control and complaints of dysuria, urgency, or frequency should be evaluated for other conditions. Bladder infections can give rise to such symptoms. Excessive calcium loss in the urine—**hypercalciuria**—can be associated with complaints of painful urination, urgency, frequency, or wetting. These symptoms occur because the presence of calcium crystals in the urine is irritating to the bladder. Hypercalciuria can result from increased absorption of calcium in the gastrointestinal tract or from ineffective reabsorption of calcium in the renal tubules.

Children with a strong history of daytime urinary urgency and inability to "hold" their urine may suffer from uninhibited bladder contractions. In these children, their bladders are very sensitive to urine volume. Moderate to large amounts of urine in the bladder give rise to strong contractions of the bladder muscle. Many of these children will squat and sit on their foot or cross their legs when they feel the urge to void in an attempt to obtain bladder control. Rarely, children with these symptoms may suffer from an anatomic abnormality.

Incidence. Primary nocturnal enuresis is common, affecting about 20% of children at age 5 years (Behrman, Kliegman, & Arvin, 1995). It occurs more frequently in boys and in children with a family history of bed wetting. Most children will eventually outgrow bed wetting without therapeutic intervention. Only 10% of children having nighttime wetting also have associated symptoms and problems during the day (Meadow, 1992).

Clinical Manifestations

- History of bed wetting with no prolonged period of dryness in a child older than age 5 years
- Normal daytime voiding pattern

Diagnostic Evaluation. The diagnosis of primary nocturnal enuresis is based on the history and presenting clinical symptoms. Urinalysis and urine culture should be done to rule out possibility of infection. Additionally, the child's urine should be checked for the presence of excessive calcium. (See Laboratory and Diagnostic Tests table in the Clinical Reference Pages.)

Therapeutic Management. Several approaches can be used to treat the child with primary nocturnal enuresis. First, the family and child can try some general interventions. The child should participate in the care of the wet sheets. This is not done as punishment but rather to help the child take ownership of the problem (Warady, Alon, & Hellerstein, 1991). Participation can range from having the young child strip the bed and/or take the soiled linen to the laundry room to the older child actually doing the laundry. Some children have benefited by limiting their fluid intake at night and voiding just before going to bed. The child can be assisted to "think" about what a full bladder feels like and picture waking up and going to the bathroom. This imagery is done as the child lies in bed before drifting off to sleep. Reward systems have also been helpful for the child with primary nocturnal enuresis. The child can be given a calendar and a roll of favorite stickers. For each dry night the child places a sticker on the calendar. The family will decide on a special reward or outing when the child has achieved a certain number of stickers or consecutive dry nights.

Behavioral conditioning through the use of alarms has been successful in the older child with nocturnal enuresis. A device worn on the child's pajamas contains a moisture-sensitive alarm. As the child starts to void, the alarm goes off, awakening the child so that he can go to the bathroom. The alarm system must be used consistently and given a minimum trial of several months in order to evaluate its effectiveness.

Several medications have been used for the treatment of nocturnal enuresis. Imipramine hydrochloride, a tricyclic antidepressant, has been effective, although the mechanism of action is not known. The parents should be cautioned regarding safe storage of this medication due to potential side effects of overdosage. DDAVP, or desmopressin acetate, has also been helpful because of its antidiuretic property (see Common Medications table).

Hypercalciuria can be managed by two approaches. First, a 3-day diet history is evaluated by a dietician for sodium and calcium intake. If the diet is found to be excessive in these elements, appropriate diet restrictions are made. If the diet history reveals an acceptable amount of sodium and calcium, medication may be prescribed. Most often, a thiazide diuretic is used, which works by increasing the reabsorption of calcium in the renal tubules.

Children who are affected by uninhibited bladder contractions may benefit from voiding on a frequent basis to keep urine volume in the bladder to a minimum. The use of an anticholinergic such as oxybutynin chloride, which relaxes the smooth muscle of the bladder, may be helpful.

NURSING CARE OF THE CHILD WITH ENURESIS

Assessment

The nurse should obtain a full set of vital signs. The child and parents should be assessed for their understanding of enuresis and for what types of interventions they have already tried. The nurse should also ask if the child participates in social activities with peers, such as sleepovers, and if the child is concerned with the problem of wetting. Therapy is much more successful for the older child who really wants to be dry than for the younger child who is not bothered by bed wetting. The nurse should assist the child in obtaining a urine specimen.

Nursing Diagnosis and Planning

The following nursing diagnoses and expected outcomes may be appropriate following assessment of the child with enuresis:

- Situational Low Self-Esteem related to bed wetting or urinary incontinence. ***Expected Outcome:*** *The child will demonstrate positive self-image, as evidenced by increased interest in peer activities and positive self-statements.*
- Impaired Social Interaction related to bed wetting or urinary incontinence. ***Expected Outcome:*** *The child will participate in age-appropriate activities such as sleepovers and overnight camp.*
- Ineffective Family Coping: Compromised related to negative social stigma and increased laundry load. ***Expected Outcome:*** *The child will demonstrate effective coping, as evidenced by harmonious family interactions and verbalization of decreased stress related to enuresis.*
- Risk for Impaired Skin Integrity related to prolonged contact with urine. ***Expected Outcome:*** *The child will have no rashes or redness in the perineal area.*

Implementation

Enuresis can be a frustrating problem for both the child and his family. The nurse can help by providing them with correct information about the reason for enuresis and the different therapeutic modalities. It is important that the family chooses the treatment that will best meet their needs. Follow-up to determine the effectiveness of treatment is essential, because becoming dry can be a long process and the nurse is instrumental in providing support to the child and family.

Evaluation

- Is the child verbalizing a decrease in stress within the family related to the enuresis?
- Is the child showing an increased interest in peer activities?
- Is the child experiencing increased dry nights?

VESICOURETERAL REFLUX

Vesicoureteral reflux (VUR) is defined as the backflow or reflux of urine from the bladder into the ureters and possibly the kidneys. The urine returns to the bladder after voiding. Vesicoureteral reflux is associated with UTIs.

Incidence. The incidence of VUR is unknown. A familial tendency exists. One-third of the siblings of a patient with VUR have VUR (Noe, 1992). Seventy percent of children with VUR have spontaneous resolution (Sherbotie & Cornfield, 1991).

Clinical Manifestations. Urinary tract infection is the most common clinical manifestation. Vesicoureteral reflux is diagnosed as part of UTI evaluation.

Diagnostic Evaluation. Voiding cystourethrogram (VCUG) or nuclear medicine cystogram is the standard radiologic evaluation for the detection and grading of reflux. The International Classification of Reflux identifies the grades of reflux on a scale of I to V (see Pathophysiology box). Grade I describes reflux into the ureter only and no dilation. Grade V, the most severe, describes gross dilation and reflux involving the kidney. The child should receive at least one VCUG to examine the lower tract. Subsequent examination can include nuclear medicine cystogram, thus minimizing radiation exposure (Belman, 1995).

Renal scan is used to assess renal scarring and function.

Urodynamic studies are helpful when voiding dysfunction (frequency, urgency, or incontinence) is present.

Therapeutic Management. Medical management includes the administration of low-dose prophylactic antibiotic therapy attempting to prevent an UTI. Antibiotics are continued until the reflux is resolved as documented by cystogram. The child with grade I or II reflux is most likely to resolve spontaneously. In addition to antibiotics,

PATHOPHYSIOLOGY *of Vesicoureteral Reflux*

In normal urinary tract functioning, there is a valve-like mechanism at the junction of the ureter and bladder that prevents urine from refluxing into the ureters. As urine fills the bladder or the bladder contracts during voiding, pressure in the bladder occludes the opening to the ureter. When a defect occurs at the vesicoureteral junction, VUR occurs. The defect at the vesicoureteral junction is considered a congenital abnormality.

In VUR urine returns to the bladder as residual, which increases the risk of infection. Bacteria in the urine may be carried up to the kidney, causing pyelonephritis and renal damage. Kidney damage may occur from the pressure of urine in the kidney and repeated UTIs. Reflux is associated with hypertension.

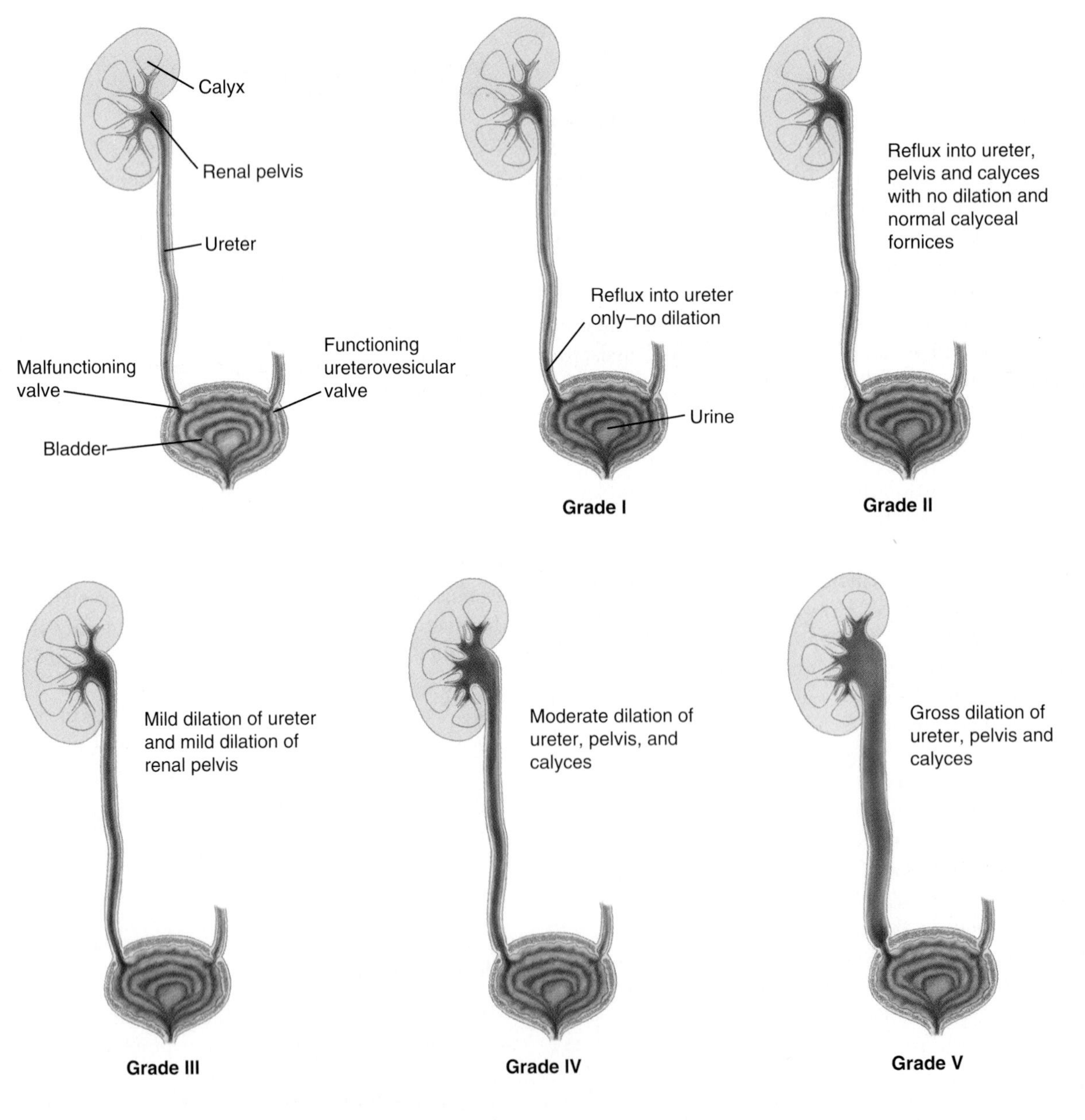

serial urine cultures and cystograms are necessary. Blood studies may be done to monitor BUN and serum creatinine secondary to the risk of kidney damage associated with VUR. Blood pressure should be monitored secondary to the risk of high blood pressure associated with VUR.

The surgical intervention is reimplantation of the ureter into the bladder. Surgical intervention is indicated when UTIs occur despite prophylactic antibiotic therapy and when the patient or family is noncompliant with medical regimen leading to UTIs. Follow-up care should include prophylactic antibiotic therapy, serial urine cultures, cystograms, kidney function tests (BUN and serum creatinine), and blood pressure monitoring.

NURSING CARE OF THE CHILD WITH VESICOURETERAL REFLUX

Assessment

Urinary tract infection is the most common clinical manifestation. The nurse should be aware of the clinical manifestations of UTIs. See Urinary Tract Infection section for nursing assessment of VUR.

Nursing Diagnosis and Planning

The following nursing diagnoses and expected outcomes may be appropriate following assessment of the child with vesicoureteral reflux:

- Risk for Injury related to possibility of kidney damage. ***Expected Outcomes:*** *The child will demonstrate resolution of vesicoureteral reflux; be free of recurrent UTIs, as evidenced by negative urine cultures.*
- Knowledge Deficit related to disease process, diagnostic tests for VUR and prevention measures for UTIs. ***Expected Outcome:*** *The parents will verbalize an understanding of disease process, diagnostic tests, and preventive measures for UTIs. The child will receive follow-up care, including antibiotic administration.*

Implementation

Nursing care includes the treatment and prevention of UTIs. See Urinary Tract Infection section of this chapter.

Questions and concerns of the family should be answered. The parents and the child, in a simple age-appropriate manner, should be educated regarding the treatment plan, medical, or surgical management. If medical management is elected, parents and the child should understand that the treatment may be for years and compliance is important. Follow-up will include antibiotic therapy, urine cultures, renal function tests (BUN and serum creatinine), blood pressure monitoring, and nuclear cystograms.

If surgical treatment is required, parents and child should be given information regarding the surgical procedure and preoperative and postoperative care. They should understand that an inpatient hospitalization will be required. Medications will be given for pain and bladder spasms, which frequently occur after surgery. Follow-up care will involve prophylactic antibiotics until a postsurgery cystogram supports that the VUR has been corrected.

Evaluation

- Is the child free of recurrent UTIs?
- Has the child incurred kidney damage?
- Has the child received follow-up diagnostic testing and antibiotic therapy?

CRYPTORCHIDISM

Cryptorchidism (undescended or "hidden" testes) occurs when one or both testes fail to descend through the inguinal canal into the scrotal sac.

PATHOPHYSIOLOGY *of Cryptorchidism*

In normal fetal development, the testes descend from the abdomen during the seventh to ninth month of gestation (Sugar, 1995). The exact reason for failure of the testes to descend is not known. It is thought to be a result of an abnormality of the testis itself or because of insufficient hormonal stimulation for the normal process of descent. Sperm production is decreased in the undescended testis, and there is increased risk of developing a malignancy when the child reaches adulthood. Inguinal hernias are commonly associated with cryptorchidism.

Incidence. Cryptorchidism is a common urologic problem. Premature infants have a higher incidence of undescended testes due to the relatively late developmental descent during intrauterine life. From 4% to 5% of normal healthy males will have undescended testes at birth (Mitchell & Ganesan, 1990). Most infants will have spontaneous descent of their testes during the first year of life.

Clinical Manifestation

- Testes not palpable or easily guided into the scrotum

Testes can retract into the inguinal canal if the infant is upset or cold. Examination of the male genitalia should take place in a warm room with the infant calm. It is also helpful for examiners to warm their hands before palpating the scrotum.

Diagnostic Evaluation. One or both testes may be undescended. If the testis is not palpable, its location can be determined by ultrasound. The "missing" testis may be found at any point along the process vaginalis, or it may be located in the abdomen. Location of an intra-abdominal testis may have to be done by surgical exploration. When neither testis can be palpated, the child is evaluated for their presence by hormonal stimulation and measurement of testosterone response. True absence of both testes is rare.

Therapeutic Management. Initially, the infant with undescended testes is managed by observation, because he may have spontaneous descent of the testes during the first 12 months of life. After age 1 year, medical or surgical treatment may be instituted. Human chorionic gonadotropin (HCG) may be used to correct cryptorchidism. HCG is the pituitary hormone that stimulates the production of testosterone and has resulted with limited success in helping to bring the testis down. The treatment of choice is surgical correction, or orchiopexy. The most common complications from this surgery are bleeding and infection. The purpose of therapy is to preserve testicular function, provide a normal-appearing scrotum, and enable the child to perform self-testicular exams as he matures to screen for malignancy.

NURSING CARE OF THE CHILD WITH CRYPTORCHIDISM

Assessment

A physical examination should be performed, with careful attention given to examination of the genitalia. Assess the parents' knowledge of undescended testes and the importance of treatment.

Nursing Diagnosis and Planning

The following nursing diagnoses and expected outcomes may be appropriate following assessment of the child with cryptorchidism:

- Knowledge Deficit (parental) related to cause and management of cryptorchidism. ***Expected Outcome:*** *The parents will verbalize an understanding of cryptorchidism.*
- Anxiety related to possible decreased fertility and increased risk of testicular malignancy. ***Expected Outcomes:*** *The child will receive appropriate referrals for fertility testing when appropriate; perform regular testicular self-examination during adolescence.*

Implementation

Nursing care should be directed at educating parents and providing them with information and resources. If the child has bilateral undescended testes or absence of testes, referrals to a counselor, psychologist, or subspecialist may be appropriate.

Evaluation

- Have the parents verbalized an understanding of the cryptorchidism and its management?
- Do the parents understand their responsibilities to guide their child when he is an adolescent to perform regular testicular self-examination?

HYPOSPADIAS

Hypospadias is a congenital anomaly in which the actual opening of the urethral meatus is "below" the normal placement on the glans of the penis (Fig. 27–2). The

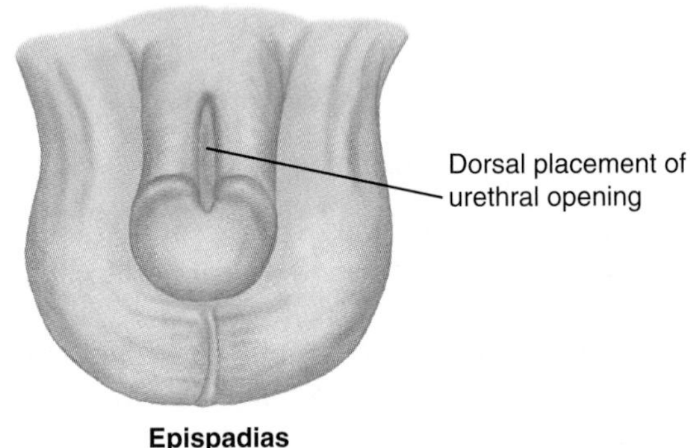

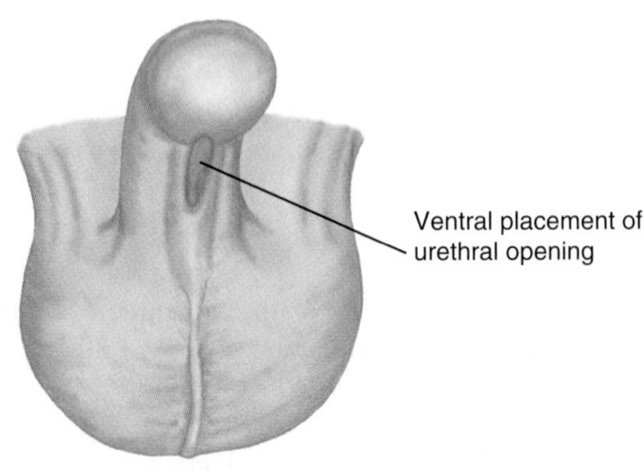

Figure 27–2
Epispadias and hypospadias are congenital anomalies in which the urethral opening is "above" or "below" its normal location on the glans of the penis. Stenosis of the opening could occur, possibly leading to urinary tract infections or hydronephrosis. Hypospadias might interfere with fertility if left uncorrected.

degree of "misplacement" of the urethral opening may vary. The urethra may open only slightly ventral to the glans or as far back as the penoscrotal junction. Hypospadias may be accompanied by chordee, or downward curvature of the penile shaft. Associated anomalies may include undescended testes and inguinal hernias. Dorsal placement of the urethral opening, epispadias (Fig. 27–2), may also occur but is less common.

PATHOPHYSIOLOGY *of Hypospadias*

Hypospadias occurs from incomplete development of the urethra in utero. The exact cause of the defect is not known but is thought to be related to genetic, environmental, and hormonal influences (Sugar, 1995).

The displacement of the urethral meatus does not usually interfere with urinary continence. However, stenosis of the opening can occur, which would give rise to partial obstruction of outflowing urine. This might result in UTIs or hydronephrosis (Kumor, 1992). Furthermore, ventral placement of the urethral opening might interfere with fertility in the mature male, if left uncorrected.

Etiology and Incidence. Hypospadias, including minor degrees, occurs in 1 of every 500 male children (Gonzalez, 1996). There is increased risk if either the father or a sibling has the anomaly. Testes are undescended in 10% of affected males, and there is an increased risk for inguinal hernias.

Clinical Manifestations

- Ventral placement of the urethral opening

Diagnostic Evaluation. Diagnosis is based on physical examination.

Therapeutic Management. Correction of hypospadias is accomplished by surgical intervention. The surgical procedure should be done before the age of toilet training as the location of the meatus may make it difficult for the child to urinate standing up. Surgery is usually done when the child is less than age 18 months. Children with hypospadias should not be circumcised because the foreskin may be used in the surgical reconstruction. Postoperatively, the child will have some type of urinary diversion to allow for healing of the meatus. Indwelling urinary catheters or urethral stints are commonly used. Additionally, the child's activity must be restricted for several days. These treatments are better tolerated by the younger child.

The goal of surgery is to make urinary and sexual function as normal as possible and to improve the cosmetic appearance of the penis.

NURSING CARE OF THE CHILD WITH HYPOSPADIAS

Assessment

A general physical examination should be done with special attention to the genitalia. Palpate the abdomen for a distended bladder or enlarged kidneys. Assess urinary function by questioning the parents about UTIs, quality of urinary stream (whether it is steady or intermittent), dribbling, or family history of genitourinary problems. Evaluate the parents' understanding of hypospadias and the surgical procedure necessary for corrections.

Nursing Diagnosis and Planning

The following nursing diagnoses and expected outcomes may be appropriate following assessment of the child with hypospadias:

- Knowledge Deficit (parental) related to diagnosis of hypospadias, surgical procedure, and postoperative care. ***Expected Outcomes:*** *The parents will verbalize an understanding of hypospadias and the reason for surgical correction; actively participate in the postoperative care.*
- Risk for Infection related to indwelling catheter. ***Expected Outcome:*** *The child will remain free of urinary tract infection, as evidenced by normal urinalysis and absence of fever.*
- Impaired Physical Mobility related to surgical procedure on the penis. ***Expected Outcome:*** *The child will tolerate activity restriction, as evidenced by participating in developmentally appropriate bedside play, infrequent episodes of crying, and normal sleep patterns.*

Implementation

Parents should receive detailed preoperative teaching and be encouraged to participate in the postoperative care of their child. The parents should be able to demonstrate proper care of the catheter or stint before discharge.

Encourage the child to drink frequently. High fluid intake is necessary to maintain hydration and free flow of urine. Monitor vital signs each shift and report above-normal temperatures. Observe urine for cloudiness or foul smell. Provide the child with a variety of diversional activities and administer pain medication as ordered. Allow child to be "mobile" by transporting him in a wagon or cart. Encourage parents to bring favorite sleep toys or music to help the child feel less anxious.

Evaluation

- Can the parents explain the surgical procedure and postoperative care of their child?
- Are the parents participating in the care of their child?
- Is the child comfortable and participating in age-appropriate play?

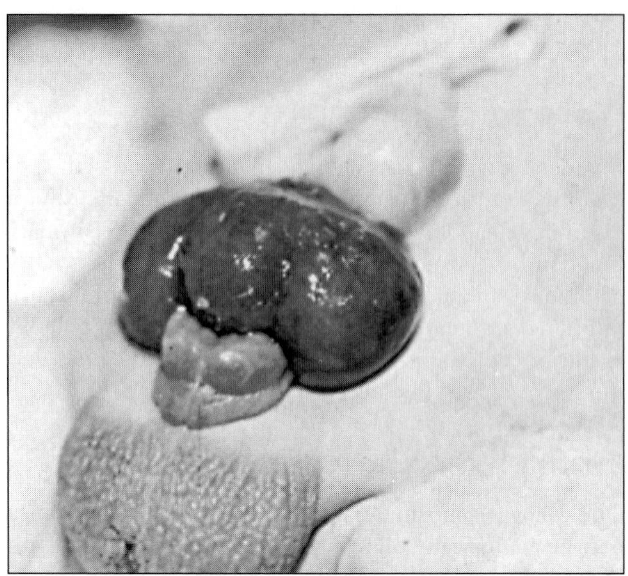

Figure 27–3
Classic bladder exstrophy. The bladder is exposed in the midline; the umbilical cord is displaced caudally; the penis is epispadiac, and the scrotum is broad. (From Behrman, R. E., Kliegman, R. M., & Arvin, A. M. [1996]. *Nelson textbook of pediatrics* [15th ed.]. Philadelphia: W. B. Saunders, p. 1542)

PATHOPHYSIOLOGY *of Bladder Exstrophy*

Bladder exstrophy occurs as the result of inappropriate growth of the cloacal membrane, mesoderm, and lower abdominal wall during embryonic development (Gearhart & Jeffs, 1990). There are variations in the severity of exstrophy ranging from isolated epispadias to extrusion of fused bladder and intestinal mucosa. The degree of deformity depends on when the disruption occurs during fetal development. The earlier in gestation, the more severe the defect. If exstrophy of the bladder is left untreated, the child will suffer from complete urinary incontinence and sexual dysfunction, and be at increased risk for developing cancer of the bladder mucosa due to constant exposure and irritation. Most infants born with bladder exstrophy have normal kidneys, but may be at risk for kidney damage due to VUR and bladder dysfunction, which can occur after reconstructive surgery.

BLADDER EXSTROPHY

Bladder exstrophy is a congenital anomaly characterized by the extrusion of the urinary bladder to the outside of the body through a defect in the lower abdominal wall (Fig. 27–3). Exstrophy of the bladder may be associated with genital abnormalities as well as defects of the anus. Infants born with exstrophy also have widening of the symphysis pubis, but rarely suffer serious orthopedic problems as a result.

Etiology and Incidence. The cause of bladder exstrophy is not known. This anomaly occurs in about 1 in 30,000 births, with a higher incidence seen in male infants (Bowers et al., 1995).

Clinical Manifestations

- Exposed bladder mucosa
- Displaced anal opening
- Widened symphysis pubis
- Defects of external genitalia (more severe in males)

Diagnostic Evaluation. Bladder exstrophy is diagnosed by physical examination. Generally, these children are otherwise healthy, full-term infants. In some cases additional radiologic studies may be indicated to define the severity of the defect.

Therapeutic Management. At birth, care should be taken to protect the exposed bladder tissue from drying while allowing drainage of urine. This is best accomplished by covering the bladder with a nonadhering plastic wrap, such as the commercial kind used for food storage. The use of petroleum jelly gauze should be avoided because this type of dressing can dry out, adhere to the mucosa, and damage the delicate tissue when removed. Treatment of bladder exstrophy requires surgical management and occurs in a series of staged reconstructions. Ideally, the initial surgery for closure of the abdominal defect should occur within the first few days of life. The goal of subsequent surgeries is to reconstruct the bladder and genitalia and enable the child to achieve urinary continence. These infants have a high incidence of VUR. Commonly, they receive prophylactic antibiotic therapy. Urinary tract infection should be ruled out in the event of a febrile illness.

NURSING CARE OF THE CHILD WITH BLADDER EXSTROPHY

Assessment

The nurse should determine the parents' understanding of their child's condition. A physical examination of the newborn should be made with special attention to the patency of the anus, adequacy of urine output, and condition of exposed bladder mucosa. The older child should be assessed for urinary continence and history of UTIs. Also, the child's self-perception and social interaction should be evaluated.

Nursing Diagnosis and Planning

The following nursing diagnoses and expected outcomes may be appropriate following assessment of the infant with bladder exstrophy:

- Impaired Tissue Integrity related to exposed bladder mucosa. ***Expected Outcome:*** *The infant will maintain integrity of bladder mucosa, as evidenced by tissue that is smooth, moist, red, and intact.*
- Knowledge Deficit (parental) related to diagnosis and treatment of anomaly. ***Expected Outcome:*** *The parents will understand their child's diagnosis and surgical management, as evidenced by verbalization, asking appropriate questions, participating in the child's care, keeping follow-up appointments, and following prescribed medical regimen.*
- Risk for Infection related to anatomical defect, surgical procedures, and probable abnormal bladder function. ***Expected Outcomes:*** *The infant will maintain body temperature that is within normal limits; demonstrate no complications of UTIs, as evidenced by normal kidney function.*
- Body Image Disturbance related to physical appearance of lower abdomen and genitalia. ***Expected Outcome:*** *The child will develop positive body image, as evidenced by participating in age-appropriate activities, demonstrating good hygiene, and verbalizing positive self-statements.*

Implementation

Nursing care of the newborn with bladder exstrophy is focused on maintaining the integrity of the bladder until surgical closure is performed. Providing emotional support for the parents and family is important. Often, they are overwhelmed by the appearance of their new baby and information regarding treatment for the anomaly. The nurse should encourage them to verbalize their fears and concerns and supply them with appropriate information. Nursing care of the older child with bladder exstrophy should include evaluation of psychosocial development. If problems are noted, appropriate referrals should be made. The nurse should also monitor laboratory values and urinalysis to assess for renal function.

Home Care. Parents should be informed of the signs and symptoms of UTI and instructed to report these to their physician. If the child is on antibiotics, the family should be educated about importance of taking the medicine as prescribed and possible side effects that could occur.

Evaluation

- Has the infant remained free of infection?
- Does the infant have normal kidney function?
- Are the parents participating in the child's care, including keeping follow-up appointments and following the prescribed care of the child?

MISCELLANEOUS DISORDERS AND ANOMALIES OF THE GENITOURINARY TRACT

Other disorders and anomalies associated with the genitourinary tract are described in Table 27–2. Most of them require surgical correction as noted. For both psychological and mechanical reasons, these defects are usually corrected at a young age; some may require more than one surgery.

ACUTE RENAL FAILURE

Acute renal failure is defined as the sudden, severe loss of kidney function. In acute renal failure, the kidneys can no longer filter waste products, regulate fluid volume, nor maintain chemical balance. Most children with acute renal failure regain renal function.

PATHOPHYSIOLOGY *and Etiology of Acute Renal Failure*

Acute renal failure is categorized as prerenal, intrarenal, or postrenal.

Prerenal acute renal failure is the result of decreased perfusion of the kidney. The kidney must have adequate blood flow for effective functioning. The decreased blood flow and subsequent ischemia cause cell swelling, cell injury, and possible cell death. Possible causes are dehydration, perinatal asphyxia, hypotension, septic shock, hemorrhagic shock, and renal artery obstruction.

Intrarenal acute renal failure is the result of actual damage to kidney tissue. Possible causes include nephrotoxins such as aminoglycosides and contrast dye, ureterovesical obstruction, hemolytic-uremic syndrome, glomerulonephritis, and pyelonephritis.

Postrenal acute renal failure is the result of obstruction of urine outflow. The obstruction increases pressure within the kidney, which decreases renal function. Possible causes include ureteropelvic obstruction, ureterovesical obstruction, posterior urethral valves, neurogenic bladder, and outlet obstruction by stones, tumor, or edema.

Incidence. Acute renal failure in the pediatric patient is uncommon.

Clinical Manifestations

- Electrolyte imbalances
- Fluid imbalances

TABLE 27–2 *Miscellaneous Disorders and Anomalies of the Genitourinary Tract*

DISORDER/ANOMALY	THERAPEUTIC MANAGEMENT
Hydrocele: Painless swelling of the scrotum caused by a collection of fluid	Some experts recommend repairing by age 1 year if not resolved. Others indicate repairing if, in the absence of a hernia, it is readily reducible by examination, progressively enlarging, or persisting as years pass.
Phimosis: Inability to retract the prepubice at an age when it should be retractable (usually age 3 years)	Accumulation of secretion of sebaceous glands and mild cases can be corrected through cleaning and manual retraction. More severe cases require surgical enlargement of the phimotic ring or circumcision.
Chordee: Ventral curvature of penis associated with hypospadias. Chordee with hypospadias may create potential problems with sexual function	Release of fibrous band through surgery
***Epispadias* (Fig. 27–2):** Urethral opening located on the dorsum of the penis	Surgical correction directed at bladder neck reconstruction, if necessary, and penile and urethral lengthening as needed
Ambiguous Genitalia: Female pseudohermaphroditism: Normal internal structures; is potentially fertile Male pseudohermaphroditism: Fetal testis does not receive stimulation to produce testosterone. The sex of rearing must be feminine in such a child True hermaphroditism: Infant has both ovarian and testicular tissues, with abnormal internal and external genital structure Anatomic disruption of normal female or male structures: The mechanism is neither hormonal nor chromosomal	Sex assignment is dictated by the external genital appearance and the sexual potential of the child as an adult. Reconstructive surgery, if necessary, should be performed before age 3 years. Genetic workup may be indicated because many of these conditions are inherited or autosomal recessive or X-linked traits. Psychological support should also be provided.

- Increased BUN and serum creatinine
- Acid-base imbalances
- Nonspecific manifestations (poor feeding or decreased appetite, vomiting, lethargy, seizures, pallor)

Diagnostic Evaluations. Determining the underlying cause of acute renal failure is very important. If the underlying cause can be reversed, renal function usually returns to normal. Evaluation includes the following.

History. The history will often give an indication of the underlying cause of the acute renal failure. A history of vomiting, diarrhea, and fever may indicate dehydration and prerenal acute renal failure.

Accurate Intake and Output. Acute renal failure is usually associated with oliguria (urine output <1 ml/kg/hr). Urine output may be normal or increased.

Laboratory Data. Serum creatinine and BUN levels are increased. BUN, an end product of protein catabolism, may reflect the nutritional status of the child. Metabolic acidosis may occur, as indicated by a low serum bicarbonate. Serum potassium may be increased. Serum sodium may be increased or decreased.

Physical Examination. The child may be hypertensive. Edema secondary to decreased urine output and fluid overload may be present. The child may be in respiratory distress secondary to fluid overload.

Urethral Catheterization. Catheterization can help in diagnosing urethral and bladder neck obstruction.

Renal Ultrasound. Renal ultrasound may help with diagnosis of obstruction and postrenal acute renal failure.

Renal Scan. Renal scan may be helpful in the diagnosis of the cause of renal failure. It can assess blood flow, function, and obstruction.

Therapeutic Management Without Dialysis

Fluid Imbalances. Fluid balance is an important component of the management of a child with acute renal failure. If the child is dehydrated, fluid replacement is essential. Fluid restriction is necessary in a child who has decreased or absent urine output and is adequately hydrated or fluid overloaded.

Electrolyte Imbalances

Potassium. Most children with acute renal failure have a high potassium level, requiring intervention when the serum potassium level is >6.0 mEq/L. Medications can be given orally, rectally, and intravenously to maintain a normal potassium level. Potassium is restricted from the diet and IV fluids.

Sodium. The sodium level may be elevated or decreased. It is more common for the level to be decreased due to water overload. The sodium administered is adjusted to maintain a normal sodium level.

Acid-Base Imbalances. Children with acute renal failure are unable to excrete hydrogen ions and ammonia through the kidney and develop metabolic acidosis (low serum bicarbonate). Additional sodium bicarbonate can be administered orally or intravenously.

Therapeutic Management With Dialysis

INDICATIONS FOR DIALYSIS

- Severe fluid overload
- Pulmonary edema or congestive heart failure secondary to fluid overload
- Severe hypertension
- Metabolic acidosis not responsive to medications
- Hyperkalemia not responsive to medications
- BUN greater than 120 mg/dl

Dialysis is a process of removing waste products and excess body fluid, and regulating electrolytes and minerals. There are two types of dialysis: hemodialysis and peritoneal dialysis (see box on p. 804).

NURSING CARE OF THE CHILD WITH ACUTE RENAL FAILURE

Assessment

The child's history can assist in determining the cause of acute renal failure. A history of dehydration, blood loss, perinatal asphyxia, aminoglycoside administration, or abnormal voiding is important to obtain.

Physical examination should include blood pressure, temperature, heart rate, and pulse. The child's weight should be obtained. Assessment for fluid overload is needed. Examine for edema in areas such as legs, back, and face. Breath sounds should be assessed for pulmonary edema.

Laboratory data should be monitored. The most reliable indication of acute renal failure is an elevated creatinine level. Electrolyte levels, including sodium, potassium, and bicarbonate, are needed.

Nursing Diagnosis and Planning

The following nursing diagnoses and expected outcomes may be appropriate following assessment of the child with acute renal failure:

- Fluid Volume Excess related to kidney dysfunction. ***Expected Outcome:*** *The child will exhibit no signs of fluid deficit or excess, as evidenced by pre-illness weight, absence of edema, and clear breath sounds.*
- Risk for Infection related to invasive procedures and fluid overload. ***Expected Outcome:*** *The child will be free of infection, as evidenced by normal WBC count and absence of fever.*
- Altered Family Processes related to child hospitalized with a serious disorder. ***Expected Outcome:*** *The child/family will exhibit positive coping strategies, as exhibited by performing activities of daily living and prescribed treatment for the child.*
- Altered Nutrition: Less Than Body Requirements related to anorexia and decreased intake due to restrictions. ***Expected Outcome:*** *The child will maintain pre-illness weight and express a desire for selected nutritious foods.*
- Knowledge Deficit related to disease process, its therapy, and prognosis. ***Expected Outcome:*** *The child/parents will demonstrate an understanding of the disease process, its therapy, and prognosis.*

Implementation

The nurse caring for a child with acute renal failure must monitor and assess fluid balance. Accurate intake and output measurements are very important. Limiting fluid intake may be necessary and may be easier if small, frequent amounts are taken. Older children can participate in determining the fluids that are given. Peritoneal dialysis or hemodialysis may allow for more liberal fluid restrictions. Fluid status is assessed by weight, blood pressure, heart rate, and assessment for edema, skin turgor, mucous membranes, and fontanel.

When performing procedures such as drawing blood, IV catheter placement, or dialysis on these infants and children, it is important to use aseptic technique due to the risk of infection (see the box on p. 804). Monitoring sites of invasive procedures for redness, warmth, and drainage can detect infection early. Body temperature and WBC counts are indicators of infection. The nurse may administer antibiotics as ordered by the physician.

The child and family will require support and reassurance. They need opportunities to verbalize concerns and feelings and ask questions. The family should be allowed to participate in the care of their child as much as possible.

The child and family need to be kept informed of the child's status. They need to be given explanations tailored to the individual family. The family and child should be allowed to guide the nurse in the amount of information they need. This is a very stressful time for the child and family, and information may need to be repeated.

Evaluation

- Has the child maintained fluid balance?
- Is the child free of infection?
- Is the family exhibiting positive coping skills?
- Has the child maintained his pre-illness weight?
- Can the parents/child verbalize an understanding of the disease and its treatment?

Dialysis

Dialysis is a process of removing waste products and excess body fluids, and regulating electrolytes and minerals. It is sometimes necessary in acute renal failure. When chronic renal failure progresses to end-stage renal disease, dialysis or kidney transplantation is required.

There are two types of dialysis: hemodialysis and peritoneal dialysis.

HEMODIALYSIS

Hemodialysis cleanses the blood by circulating it through a special filter referred to as an artificial kidney. Blood is pumped through the artificial kidney and returned to the body. Hemodialysis occurs through a vascular access such as a double lumen central line or an **arteriovenous fistula** or shunt. The access is surgically placed. Children who receive chronic dialysis usually receive treatments three times per week for 3–4 hours each time.

The major complications of hemodialysis include access infection and access obstruction. In addition, there is a disruption of school, peer, and family life due to the treatment schedule. However, children treated with hemodialysis in a specialized pediatric unit can thrive. In infants and small children, hemodialysis is technically more difficult and fluid and electrolyte shifts more pronounced.

Hemodialysis is more efficient and requires less time than peritoneal dialysis. In addition, there is less responsibility for the family.

PERITONEAL DIALYSIS

In peritoneal dialysis, fluid enters the peritoneal cavity through a catheter, which may be placed at the bedside or surgically placed. The dialysis fluid is allowed to dwell, during which time waste products, chemicals, and fluid pass through the peritoneal membrane into the fluid. The fluid is then drained and the process is repeated.

In children receiving chronic dialysis, the exchanges can be performed overnight with an automated cycler, or manually four to five times per day. The treatments generally are performed at home.

Peritoneal dialysis is technically easier than hemodialysis. Advantages over hemodialysis include more independence for the child and family, and a more steady physiologic state due to the more frequent dialysis. The disadvantages include the risk of infections (peritonitis and catheter exit site), and family and child fatigue from treatment demands.

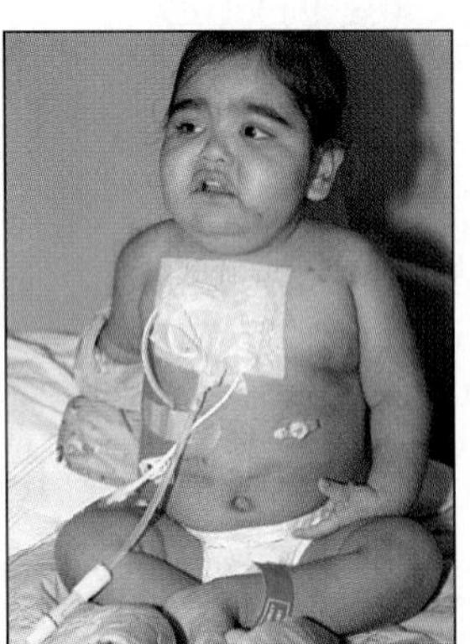

◀ Peritoneal dialysis. Implanted lines allow instillation of the dialyzing fluid into this child's peritoneal cavity. This child has rejected a transplanted kidney and receives peritoneal dialysis until another transplant will be attempted. She was previously on steroids in an attempt to control rejection, which accounts for the characteristics typical of Cushing's syndrome.

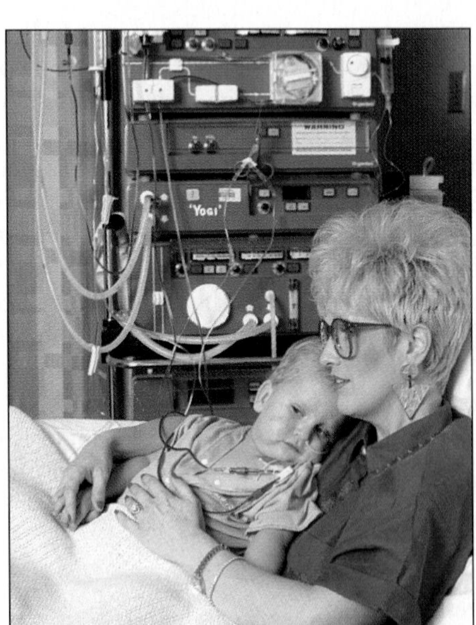

Child receiving hemodialysis. Family members should participate in the child's care as much as possible.

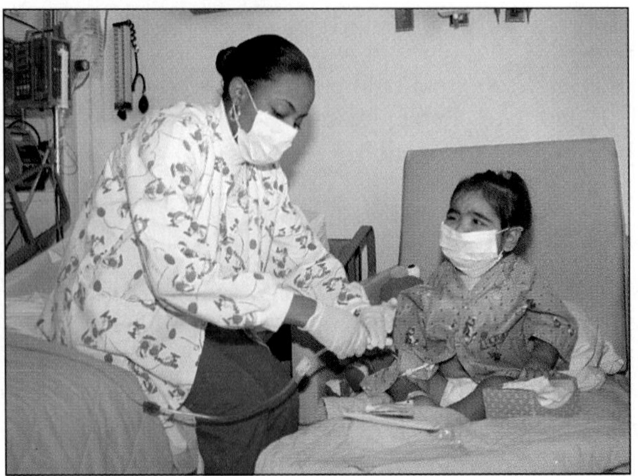

Infection of the peritoneal cavity is the chief hazard of peritoneal dialysis. When the lines are open to begin or end the dialyzing cycle, both adult and child wear masks.

Photos courtesy of Children's Medical Center, Dallas, Texas.

CHRONIC RENAL FAILURE AND END-STAGE RENAL DISEASE

Chronic renal failure is an irreversible loss of kidney function which occurs over months to years. It can be managed conservatively with medications and diet restrictions. Chronic renal failure progresses to end-stage renal disease (ESRD), which is defined as the permanent irreversible loss of kidney function, that can no longer be managed conservatively to maintain life and health. Dialysis or transplantation is required to treat ESRD. This usually occurs when only 5% to 10% of kidney function remains.

Pathophysiology. Regardless of the cause of kidney damage, chronic renal failure progresses to ESRD. The exact mechanisms are unclear. The factors that may contribute negatively are ongoing immunologic injury, hyperfiltration (the overwork of the remaining nephrons), high dietary protein and phosphorus intake, persistent proteinuria, and hypertension.

Etiology. The causes of chronic renal failure in children are different from those in adults. The most common cause, especially in younger children, is congenital anomalies such as obstruction, VUR, and renal dysplasia. Children can develop chronic renal failure from diseases such as glomerulonephritis, pyelonephritis, and hemolytic-uremic syndrome. Generally secondary causes of ESRD such as diabetes and high blood pressure are not seen in children. As adults, approximately 35% of people with insulin-dependent diabetes will develop ESRD (Foster, 1994).

Incidence. The incidence of chronic renal failure among children younger than age 16 years varies between 1.5 and 3.0 per million (Fogo & Kon, 1994).

Clinical Manifestations

- Electrolyte imbalance
- Fluid imbalance (dehydration or fluid overload)
- Acid-base imbalance
- Renal bone disease (osteodystrophy)
- Anemia
- Poor growth
- Hypertension
- Fatigue
- Decreased appetite, poor feeder
- Nausea and vomiting

Diagnostic Evaluation. Chronic renal failure may present itself nonspecifically. Physical examination may reveal short stature and failure to thrive. The child may have high blood pressure. Blood work may reveal electrolyte abnormalities, calcium and phosphorus abnormalities, and/or anemia. Bone X-rays may reveal renal osteodystrophy. The child may have normal fluid volume, be dehydrated, or be fluid overloaded.

The history may or may not include known renal disease. Fatigue, poor concentration, increased sleeping, poor feeding or decreased appetite, nausea, and vomiting are common complaints.

Diagnostic tests may be performed to determine etiology and prognosis. These may include VCUG, renal ultrasound, renal scan, and renal biopsy.

Therapeutic Management

Chronic Renal Failure. The diet of a child with chronic renal failure is modified secondary to the decreased ability of the kidney to regulate fluids, electrolytes, minerals, and waste products. Salt and fluid may be restricted to prevent fluid overload and hypertension. Protein intake is restricted due to the kidney's inability to remove waste products. Phosphorus is restricted to help prevent bone disease. Potassium may be restricted due to the kidney's inability to remove it.

In addition to diet modifications, medications are given. Diuretics may be helpful in fluid balance and blood pressure control. Antihypertensive medication may be required for blood pressure control. Sodium bicarbonate may also be necessary to maintain acid-base balance. Vitamin D and phosphorus binding medications may be helpful in preventing bone disease.

New advances in the treatment of infants and children with chronic renal failure such as recombinant erythropoietin and recombinant growth hormone have improved the quality of life of these children. Recombinant erythropoietin is used to treat anemia, thus avoiding repeated blood transfusions and improving the energy level. The use of recombinant growth hormone has allowed significant improvement in the growth of children with chronic renal failure.

End-Stage Renal Disease. Once a child reaches ESRD, dialysis or transplantation is required for health and life. The diagnosis of ESRD is made by monitoring serum creatinine, glomerular filtration rate (GFR), and the quality of life of the child. Generally, ESRD is diagnosed when the GFR reaches around 10%.

Dialysis. See box, p. 804.

Kidney Transplantation. Transplantation is the goal for most children with ESRD. Kidney transplantation offers the best opportunity to have a normal lifestyle. Unfortunately, transplantation is not a cure. Children who have been transplanted must continue to take immunosuppressive medication, have blood tests, and keep clinic appointments.

Kidneys come from two types of donors: living donors and cadaveric donors. A living donor is someone in the child's family such as a parent or grandparent. A person who donates must be in good health and have healthy kidneys. A cadaveric donor kidney is from someone who is brain dead. A cadaveric donor must have a consent from their family and have healthy kidneys. The blood types of the donor and recipient need to be compatible. Transplants using kidneys from a relative have been more successful in children than those using cadaveric kidneys.

The most common complication of kidney transplantation is rejection. Immunosuppressive medications, taken to help prevent rejection, include cyclosporine, azathioprine, and prednisone. Newer immunosuppressive drugs include tacrolimus (Prograf), mycophenolate mofetil, and a new form of cyclosporine (Neoral).

As with all medications, immunosuppressive medications have side effects. When the immune system is suppressed, there is an increased risk of infection related to the body's decreased ability to fight infection. Children with renal transplants should be monitored for infection and may take anti-infective medications routinely.

High blood pressure is a complication of transplantation. High blood pressure may be caused by the underlying renal disease, the transplanted kidney, or a side effect of the immunosuppressive medications.

NURSING CARE OF THE CHILD WITH CHRONIC RENAL FAILURE OR END-STAGE RENAL DISEASE

Assessment

The assessment of the child with chronic renal failure or ESRD is directed toward clinical manifestations of the renal failure and its possible complications.

Blood work is monitored for abnormalities and response to interventions. Assessment for potential anemia is made by monitoring the hemoglobin and hematocrit. In addition, response to therapy is assessed in the child receiving recombinant erythropoietin.

Serum calcium and phosphorus, alkaline phosphatase, parathyroid hormone level, and bone X-rays are obtained to monitor for renal osteodystrophy.

Fluid status should be assessed for fluid overload and dehydration. Fluid status is evaluated by weight, blood pressure, heart rate, edema, skin turgor, mucous membranes, and fontanel.

Growth and development are evaluated. Accurate weight and height should be obtained. Dietary intake, as well as any vomiting, should be obtained to evaluate caloric intake. Information regarding attainment of development tasks, school performance, and peer relationships are helpful.

Nursing Diagnosis and Planning

The following nursing diagnoses and expected outcomes may be appropriate following assessment of the child with chronic renal failure or end-stage renal disease:

- Altered Nutrition: Less Than Body Requirements related to decreased appetite and dietary restrictions. ***Expected Outcome:*** *The child will receive adequate nutrition for growth and health as measured by appropriate growth for age.*
- Knowledge Deficit related to disease process, treatment, and/or diet restrictions. ***Expected Outcome:*** *The child/parents will understand the disease process, its treatment, and dietary restrictions.*
- Fluid Volume Excess/Deficit related to fluid and electrolyte imbalances secondary to renal dysfunction. ***Expected Outcome:*** *The child will exhibit no signs of fluid overload or deficit as measured by weight, blood pressure, and absence of edema or signs of dehydration.*
- Altered Growth and Development related to restricted diet, chronic illness, and anemia. ***Expected Outcome:*** *The child will attain maximum growth and development.*
- Altered Family Processes related to having a child with chronic and potentially life-threatening disease. ***Expected Outcome:*** *The child and family will achieve successful coping strategies, as measured by their ability to care for child.*
- Risk for Impaired Skin Integrity related to edema and poor nutrition. ***Expected Outcome:*** *The child's skin will not show signs of break in skin integrity (redness, irritation, breaks).*

Implementation

The care of the child with chronic renal failure or ESRD is complex and requires a multidisciplinary team.

Adequate nutritional intake should occur according to the dietary restriction parameters. The diet of the child with chronic renal failure should be individualized and should include foods the child likes. Small, frequent meals may be helpful. Diet supplements may be necessary to meet caloric needs. Recombinant growth hormone may allow the child to have adequate growth.

Information needs of children with chronic renal failure and their families are multifaceted. The parents need information regarding diet, medications, potential effects of the renal failure, and its treatment. They need to be informed regarding treatment options such as hemodialysis, peritoneal dialysis, and transplantation.

The child should receive appropriate fluid intake. Ongoing assessment of hydration status should occur. The child and family should be instructed in fluid restriction and hydration assessment such as weight, blood pressure, and appearance of edema.

The child should be encouraged to participate in appropriate activities such as school attendance for the school-age child and peer activities for the adolescent. Parents may need encouragement to treat their children age appropriately.

The child with chronic renal failure and the family need support. They need opportunities to ask questions, verbalize feelings, and express concerns. Involving the child in her own care and decisions regarding treatment is beneficial. The family should be assessed for prior successful coping strategies and encouraged to use those. Additional help from social service, psychology, or psychiatry may be helpful.

Evaluation

- Has the child shown normal growth patterns for age?
- Can the parents and the child discuss diet restrictions?
- Is the child free of edema?
- Is the family involved in the care of the child?
- Has the integrity of the child's skin been maintained?
- Has the child verbalized anxiety related to disease?

CHILDHOOD HEMOLYTIC-UREMIC SYNDROME

Hemolytic-uremic syndrome (HUS) is an acute disorder characterized by anemia, thrombocytopenia, and acute renal failure.

PATHOPHYSIOLOGY *of Hemolytic-Uremic Syndrome*

Most affected children have an associated prodrome of gastrointestinal symptoms, which suggests that an infectious agent may be the cause of HUS. Studies have shown a strong association between the syndrome and an enteric infection with *Escherichia coli* 0157:H7 (Ashkenazi & Pickering, 1990). Two important characteristics of *Escherichia coli* 0157:H7 contribute to the development of HUS. First, because this bacteria attaches itself to the intestinal mucosa, its clearance through normal intestinal peristalsis is decreased, allowing the bacteria to grow and multiply. Secondly, the bacteria produces a toxin that damages the endothelial cells of capillary walls, and the subsequent inflammatory response results in occlusion of capillaries. This is especially significant in the renal glomeruli. The occlusion of glomerular vessels decreases filtration and results in acute renal failure. However, it is important to understand that the vascular process seen in HUS can affect *any* organ. Anemia results from fragmentation of red blood cells, which are damaged as they try to pass through the occluded vessels and are removed from circulation by the spleen. Thrombocytopenia occurs because the platelets get trapped within the small vessels.

Etiology and Incidence. Hemolytic-uremic syndrome is the most common cause of acute renal failure in children, usually affecting children younger than age 4 years (Rowe et al., 1991). The peak incidence of the syndrome is spring and summer, although HUS can occur at any time.

Escherichia coli 0157:H7 has been isolated from various domestic animals. Outbreaks of gastrointestinal symptoms have been associated with recent consumption of undercooked meat.

Clinical Manifestations

- Gastrointestinal illness characterized by abdominal pain, fever, vomiting, and bloody diarrhea may be present or child may have recent history of these symptoms.
- Pallor
- Irritability
- Lethargy
- Decreased urine output

Diagnostic Evaluation. Physical examination may reveal dehydration, petechiae, edema, and hepatosplenomegaly. Laboratory evaluation will reveal low hematocrit, hemoglobin, and platelet counts. Coagulation studies, prothrombin time, and partial thromboplastin time will be normal. Serum creatinine and BUN will be elevated. If renal failure is severe, the child may have serum electrolyte abnormalities and fluid overload, which would give rise to hypertension and possibly congestive heart failure.

The child may have central nervous system involvement. Symptoms such as lethargy, seizures, or coma may result from vascular damage in the brain.

Therapeutic Management. Treatment of HUS is supportive and mainly addresses the problems resulting from anemia, thrombocytopenia, and renal insufficiency. Transfusion of packed red blood cells is given to diminish the effects of severe anemia. Although the patient may have a low platelet count, platelet transfusions are not routinely given unless the patient has problems with uncontrolled bleeding or needs a surgical procedure. Dialysis may be instituted to maintain balance of fluid and electrolytes. Dialysis also allows for adequate nutrition even in the patient with no urine output.

Although most children recover without long-term problems, there is potential for these patients to develop chronic renal insufficiency or ESRD.

NURSING CARE OF THE CHILD WITH HEMOLYTIC-UREMIC SYNDROME

Assessment

The nurse should obtain a full set of vital signs and weight. Auscultate the breath sounds for crackles and the heart tones for clarity. Assess the child's level of consciousness. Examine the extremities and abdomen for presence of edema. Palpate the abdomen for tenderness and auscultate for bowel sounds. Record intake and output and monitor laboratory values. Observe the child for petechiae, bleeding, or bruising.

Nursing Diagnosis and Planning

The following nursing diagnoses and expected outcomes may be appropriate following assessment of the child with HUS:

- Fluid Volume Excess related to decreased urine output. ***Expected Outcome:*** *The child will demonstrate fluid volume balance, as evidenced by absence of respiratory difficulty or severe hypertension.*
- Risk for Injury related to low platelet count. ***Expected Outcome:*** *The child will demonstrate no bruises or active bleeding.*
- Activity Intolerance related to anemia. ***Expected Outcome:*** *The child will experience frequent rest periods.*
- Altered Nutrition: Less Than Body Requirements related to fluid volume restrictions and decreased absorption. ***Expected Outcome:*** *The child will maintain adequate nutrition, as evidenced by moist mucous membranes and appropriate daily caloric intake.*
- Anxiety (parental) related to severity of illness and therapeutic measures (transfusions and dialysis). ***Expected Outcome:*** *The parents will demonstrate decreased anxiety, as evidenced by providing comfort to their child, participating in daily care as appropriate, and verbalizing understanding of illness.*

Implementation

Ensure that dietary and/or fluid restrictions are followed. Report symptoms of fluid overload such as respiratory difficulty, hypertension, or increase in weight. If the platelet count is very low, protect the child from injury by padding bed rails and assisting with ambulation. Remove sharp objects and inform play specialists and parents about precautions. Structure nursing care activities so that the child is able to have uninterrupted naps and sleep time. Assess child's hydration status every shift. If the child is able to tolerate oral feedings, offer small, frequent meals. Provide the parents with correct information about HUS and treatment modalities. Parents may be fearful of HIV transmission from blood transfusions. They may also believe that if their child starts dialysis she will become "dependent" on it. They need to know that this is usually a temporary measure to allow the kidneys to "get well." Allow the parents to participate in the care of their child according to their comfort level.

Evaluation

- Has the child maintained fluid balance?
- Is the child free of bruising or bleeding?
- Is the child well hydrated?
- Are the parents able to verbalize their fears regarding their child's illness?

KEY CONCEPTS

- The kidney reaches near-adult function at age 6 to 12 months.
- Infants cannot concentrate urine as efficiently as older children and adults.
- The clinical manifestations of urinary tract infections vary according to the child's age, underlying anatomic or neurologic abnormalities, and frequency of recurrence.
- Nursing care of the child with a urinary tract infection includes giving information to the parents and child on prevention through perineal hygiene, increased fluid intake, emptying of bladder, and the wearing of cotton underwear.
- Children with glomerulonephritis should be assessed for the presence of any respiratory difficulty such as cough, increased respiratory rate, and difficulty breathing, which may indicate fluid overload.
- Children at risk for fluid volume excess due to decreased urine output should be weighed daily on the same scale, at the same time, wearing only gowns. Infants should have their diapers removed.
- Children with edema should have their position changed at least every 2 hours and their lower extremities elevated when they are sitting or lying in bed.
- Edema related to nephrotic syndrome is first noted in the periorbital spaces and dependent areas of the body. The child may awaken with facial edema; as the day progresses, edema becomes more noticeable.
- Most children will eventually outgrow enuresis with therapeutic intervention.
- Urinary tract infection is the most common clinical manifestation of vesicoureteral reflux. Medical management includes low-dose prophylactic antibiotic therapy.
- Most infants with cryptorchidism will have spontaneous descent of their testes during the first year of life.
- The goal of surgery to correct hypospadias is to make urinary and sexual function as normal as possible and to improve the cosmetic appearance of the penis.
- Most children with acute renal failure regain renal function.

REFERENCES

Ashkenazi, S., & Pickering, L. K. (1990). *E. coli* 0157:H7—A new GI pathogen to contend with.

Behrman, R., Kliegman, R. M., & Arvin, A. M. (1996). *Nelson textbook of pediatrics* (15th ed.). Philadelphia: W. B. Saunders.

Bowers, V., Hawnigan, K., & Kushner, K. (1995). Bladder extrophy and epispadias. In K. Karlowicz (Ed.), *Urologic nursing: principals and practice* (pp. 565–592). Philadelphia: W. B. Saunders.

Brouhard, B., & Travis, L. (1992). Acute postinfectious glomeralonephritis. In C. M. Edelmann (Ed.), *Pediatric kidney disease* (2nd ed., pp. 1195–1215). Boston: Little, Brown.

Clark, G., & Barratt, T. (1993). Minimal change nephrotic syndrome and focal segmental glomerulosclerosis. In M. Holliday, T. Barratt, & E. Avener, (Eds.), *Pediatric nephrology* (3rd ed., pp. 767–783). Baltimore: Williams & Wilkins.

Duckett, J. W. (1989). Hypospadias. *Pediatrics in Review, 11,* 37–42.

Fogo, A., & Kon, V. (1994). Pathophysiology of progressive renal disease. In M. A. Holliday, T. M. Barratt, & E. D. Avner (Eds.), *Pediatric nephrology* (pp. 1228–1240). Baltimore: Williams & Wilkins.

Foster, D. W. (1994). Diabetes mellitus. In K. J. Isselbacher, E. Braunwald, J. D. Wilson, J. B. Martin, A. S. Fauci, & D. L. Kasper (Eds.), *Harrison's principles of internal medicine* (pp. 1979–2000). New York: McGraw-Hill.

Gearhart, J. P., & Jeffs, R. D. (1989). State of the art reconstructive surgery for bladder exstrophy at the Johns Hopkins Hospital. *American Journal of Diseases in Children, 143,* 1475–1478.

Gearhart, J., & Jeffs, R. (1990). Management and treatment of classic bladder exstrophy. In K. Ashcroft (Ed.), *Pediatric urology* (pp. 269–300). Philadelphia: W. B. Saunders.

Gonzalez, R. (1996). Urologic disorders in infants and children. In R. Behrman, R. Kliegman, & A. Arvin (Eds.), *Nelson textbook of pediatrics* (15th ed., pp. 1546–1548) Philadelphia: W. B. Saunders.

Kumor, V., Cotran, R., & Robbins, S. (1992). *Basic pathology* (pp. 437–470). Philadelphia: W. B. Saunders.

Meadow, S. R. (1992). Enuresis. In C. M. Edelmann (Ed.), *Pediatric kidney disease* (2nd ed., pp. 2015–2021). Boston: Little, Brown.

Mitchell, M., & Ganesan, G. (1990). The undescended testis. In M. Green & R. Haggerty (Eds.), *Ambulatory pediatrics* (pp. 423–426). Philadelphia: W. B. Saunders.

Reynolds, R. E., & Hoberman, A. (1995). Diagnosis and management of pyelonephritis in infants. *Maternal/Child Nursing, 20,* 78–100.

Rowe, P. C., Orribine, E., Wells, G. A., & McLaine, P. N. (1991). Epidemiology of hemolytic-uremic syndrome in Canadian children from 1986 to 1988. *Journal of Pediatrics, 119,* 218–223.

Sherbotie, J. R., & Cornfield, D. (1991). Management of urinary tract infections in children. *Medical Clinics of North America, 75,* 327–338.

Shortlife, 1995.

Sugar, E. & Huyler-Grant, C. (1995). Disorders of the external genitalia in children. In K. Karlowicz (Ed.), *Urologic nursing: Principals and Practice* (pp. 498–595). Philadelphia: W. B. Saunders.

Warady, B. A., Alon, U., & Hellerstein, S. (1991). Primary nocturnal enuresis: Current concepts about an old problem. *Pediatric Annals, 20,* 246–255.

BIBLIOGRAPHY

Barkin, R., & Rosen, P. (1993). *Emergency pediatrics: A guide to ambulatory care* (3d ed.). St. Louis: C. V. Mosby.

Bergstein, J. M. (1992). The urinary system and pediatric gynecology. In R. E. Behrman (Ed.), *Nelson Textbook of pediatrics* (14th ed., pp. 1323–1328). Philadelphia: W. B. Saunders.

Borkowski, S. (1991). Vesicoureteral reflux. *Journal of Pediatric Health Care, 5,* 315–320.

Brouhard, B., & Travis, L. (1992). Pediatric infectious glomerulonephritis. In C. M. Edelmann, et al. (Eds.), *Pediatric kidney disease* (2nd ed., pp. 1199–1215). Boston: Little, Brown.

Clark, G., & Barratt, T. M. (1993). Minimal change nephrotic syndrome and focal segmental glomeruloscerosis. In M. A. Holiday, T. M. Barratt, & E. D. Avner (Eds.), *Pediatric nephrology* (pp. 767–787). Baltimore: Williams & Wilkins.

Cole, B., & Salinas-Madrigal, L. (1993). Acute proliferative glomerulonephritis and crescentic glomerulonephritis. In M. A. Holiday, T. M. Barratt, & E. D. Avner (Eds.), *Pediatric nephrology* (pp. 697–718). Baltimore: Williams & Wilkins.

Dwyer, J. (1993). Vegetarian diets for treating nephrotic syndrome. *Nutrition Reviews, 51,* 44–46.

Goldbloom, R. B. (1992). *Pediatric clinical skills.* New York: Churchill Livingstone.

Gulanick, M., Puzas, M., & Wilson, C. R. (1992). *Nursing care plans for newborns and children: Acute and critical care.* St. Louis: C. V. Mosby.

Hendrix, W. (1992). Dialysis therapies in critically ill children. *Clinical Issues in Critical Care Nursing, 3*(3), 605–613.

Jones, C. L., Walker, R., & Powell, H. R. (1992). Management of the nephrotic child. *Journal of Paediatric Child Health, 28,* 201–203.

Kelsch, R. C., & Seduran, A. B. (1993). Nephrotic syndrome. *Pediatrics in Review, 14,* 30–37.

Montagnino, B., Welch, V., & Hoyler-Grant, C. (1995). Congenital anomalies that affect the kidney, ureter, and bladder. In K. Karlowicz (Ed.), *Urologic nursery: Principles and practice* (pp. 567–592). Philadelphia: W. B. Saunders.

Seigler, R. L., Milligan, M. K., Burningham, T. H., Christofferson, R. D., Chang, S. Y., & Jorde, L. E. (1991). Long term outcome and prognostic indicators in the hemolytic-uremic syndrome. *Journal of Pediatrics, 118,* 195–200.

Sugar, E., & Hayler-Grant, C. (1995). Disorders of the external genitalia in children. In K. Karlowiez (Ed.), *Urologic nursing: Principles and practice* (pp. 498–518). Philadelphia: W. B. Saunders.

Wilson, L. M. (1992). Diagnostic procedures in renal disease. In S. A. Price & L. M. Wilson (Eds.), *Physiology of disease processes* (pp. 634–646). St. Louis: Mosby-Year Book.

28

The Child With an Acute Respiratory Disorder

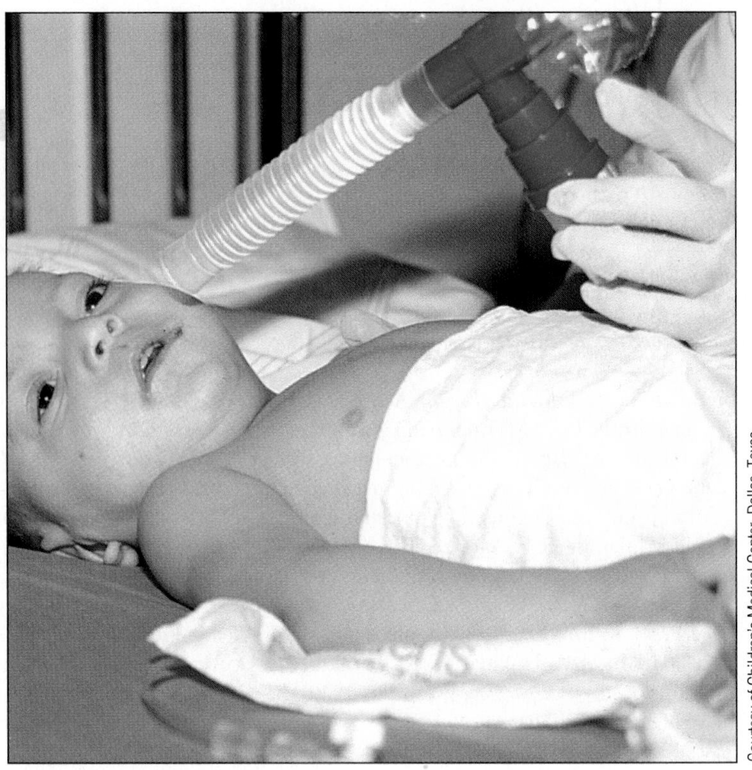

CHAPTER OVERVIEW

LEARNING OBJECTIVES

After studying this chapter, you should be able to:

- Describe the differences in the anatomy and physiology of the respiratory system of the infant/child.
- Explain how the structure and function of the infant's or child's respiratory system increases the risk for respiratory disease.
- Outline nursing care for a child with allergies.
- Discuss and display an understanding of the pathophysiology, clinical manifestations, and therapeutic management of common acute respiratory alterations.
- Identify the nursing care needs of infants and children with acute respiratory alterations.
- Outline a care plan for a child with croup and bronchitis.
- Develop guidelines for home care for a child with an acute respiratory alteration.

KEY TERMS

atelectasis: collapsed or airless state of the lung (may involve all or part of the lung)

crackle: abnormal discontinuous nonmusical sound heard on auscultation, primarily during inhalation; also called rale

grunting: sound similar to a "grunting" noise that can be heard with or without a stethoscope

nasal flaring: serious sign of air hunger; widening of nares to enable infant to take in more oxygen

orthopnea: ability to breathe easily only in upright position

retractions: abnormal movement of the chest walls during inspiration; may occur intercostally and substernally

rhonchi: adventitious breath sounds caused by the passage of air through an airway obstructed by thick secretions; do not clear with coughing

stridor: a shrill, harsh sound that can be heard during inspiration or expiration, or both; produced by the flow of air through a narrowed segment of the respiratory tract

wheezing: high-pitched, musical whistles heard with or without a stethoscope

Alteration of the respiratory system is the most common cause of illness in the infant and the child. Infants and children under age 3 years are at increased risk to develop respiratory infections due to their immature immune system, smaller upper and lower airways, and underdeveloped supporting cartilage. Although most respiratory infections are self-limiting, infants and young children can quickly experience respiratory distress as mucus and edema obstruct their small airways.

Parents should be taught preventive measures, which include adequate rest, good nutrition, and good hygiene with emphasis on handwashing. Even with the most careful hygiene and preventive measures, most children will experience some type of respiratory infection each year. School nurses often first see these children in the school health office and may be the primary health caregivers of these children.

Most children can be cared for at home by their parents and will not require hospitalization. Those children who are hospitalized are being discharged from the hospital earlier in their recovery than in the past. The current health care environment underlines the need for nurses to teach parents home care of their child, including observations that might indicate the need to enter the health care system. Parents, especially first-time parents, are often frightened by the sudden onset of respiratory symptoms, which may or may not indicate a severe problem. This chapter will provide the foundation for the nurse to assess and respond to common acute respiratory alterations.

CLINICAL REFERENCE PAGES

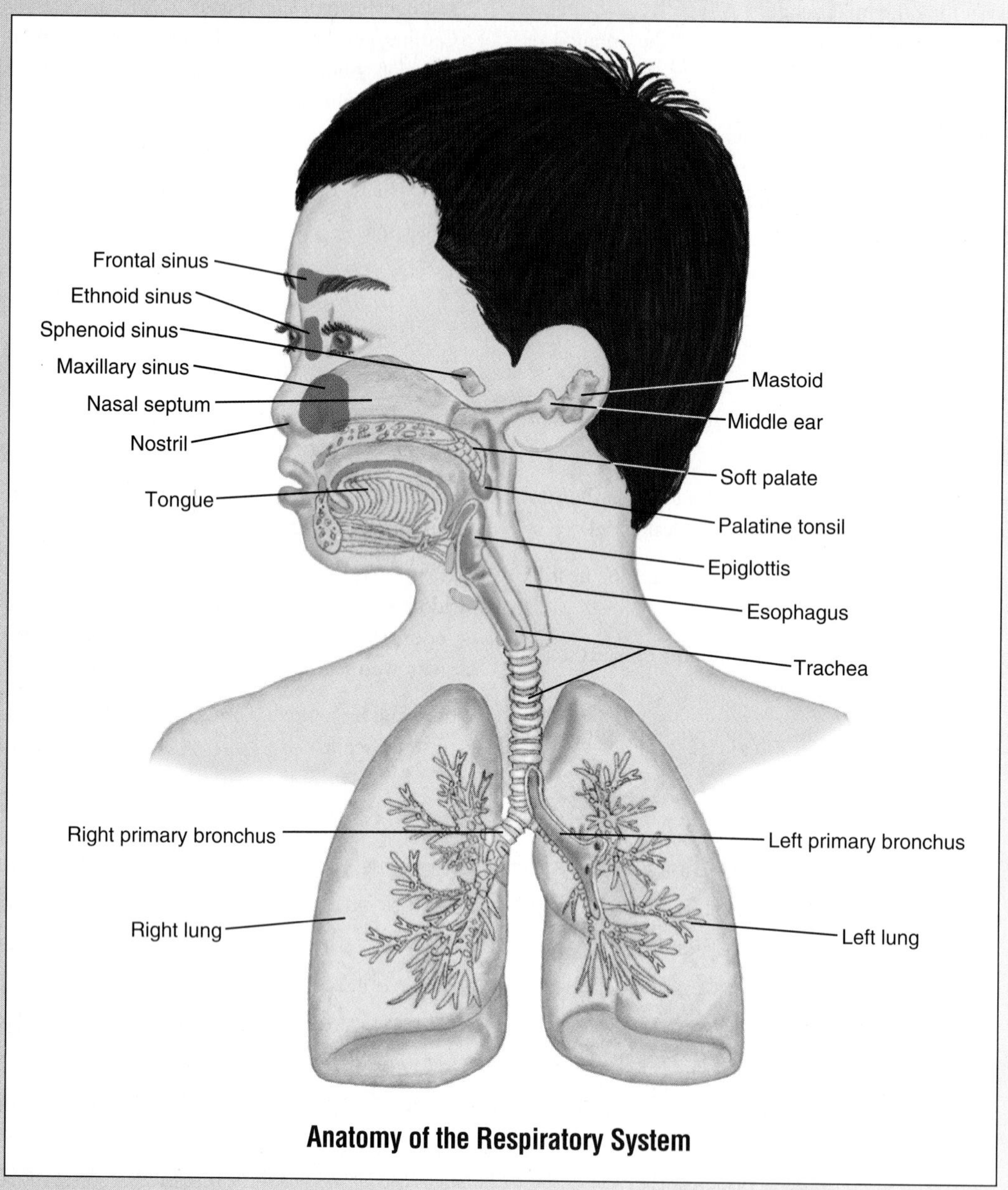

Anatomy of the Respiratory System

REVIEW OF THE RESPIRATORY SYSTEM

The respiratory system consists of the *nose, pharynx, trachea, bronchi,* and *lungs.* It is further divided into the *upper respiratory tract* (nose, pharynx, larynx) and the *lower respiratory tract* (trachea, bronchi, and lungs) (see the accompanying figure).

The Upper Airway. Air enters the body through the nares, or nostrils, two nasal cavities lined with mucous membrane. Air is prepared for entry into the lungs through filtration, humidification, and warmth.

The pharynx, or throat, carries air into the respiratory tract and food and liquids into the digestive system. The *nasopharynx* is located immediately behind the nasal cavity, the *oropharynx* behind the mouth. The *laryngeal pharynx* lies below the oropharynx and opens into the larynx toward the front and the esophagus toward the back.

The *larynx* is located between the pharynx and the trachea. The vocal cords are at the upper end of the larynx. The *epiglottis* covers the larynx during swallowing and helps keep food out of the lower respiratory tract. Ciliated mucous membranes line the larynx and trap dust and

Pediatric Differences in the Respiratory System

- Lack of surfactant in premature infants. Increased risk of respiratory distress syndrome prior to 34 weeks' gestation.
- Smaller lower airways and supporting cartilage that is underdeveloped and predisposes the child to an increased risk of obstruction by mucus, edema, and foreign bodies.
- Lung size is proportional to body height. Therefore, lung volumes and capacities do not vary from age to age. Neonate's airway is 50% smaller than that of adults.
- Infant is obligatory nose-breather and therefore has difficulty breathing through the mouth.
- Diaphragm is neonate's major respiratory muscle. Intercostal muscles are not well developed. Retractions are more common in the infant than in older children and adults.
- Brief periods of apnea (10–15 sec) are common in the neonate. The respiratory pattern may be irregular.
- Respiratory rate is higher than that of adults.
- Increased metabolic rate raises oxygen needs.
- Alveoli develop from approximately 20 million to 200 million by age 3 years. There is a gradual decrease of alveoli after age 3 years, few develop after age 8 years.
- Lung surface increases until 5–8 years.
- Eustachian tubes are relatively horizontal, which increases the risk for bacteria to enter the middle ear.
- Actual lung growth continues into the adolescent years.
- Trachea size approximately triples by adulthood.
- Tonsillar tissue is normally enlarged in early school-age children.
- Infants and children use abdominal muscles to inhale until about age 5–6 years.
- Flexible larynx is more susceptible to spasm.

other particles. The particles are then carried to the pharynx to be removed by sneezing, blowing, or coughing.

Cilia are hairlike processes that move mucus and fluid. Damage to cilia interferes with the removal of mucus from the respiratory tract.

There are three types of tonsils: the oval *palatine tonsils* are located on either side of the pharynx, the *lingual tonsils* below the palatine tonsils at the base of the tongue, and the *pharyngeal tonsils*, or *adenoids*, at the nasopharyngeal border. The tonsils are composed mainly of lymphoid tissue and help filter the circulating lymph of bacteria and other foreign material that enters the body, especially through the mouth and nose.

The Lower Airway. The *trachea* conducts air between the larynx and the lungs. It divides into right and left main *bronchi* at its lower end, the *carina*. The right main bronchus is shorter and wider than the left. The main bronchi divide into *lobar bronchi*, *segmental bronchi*, and *bronchioles* and terminate in *alveoli*. Mucus-secreting goblet cells line the bronchi and protect the lungs from dust and bacteria.

The *lungs* are two conical structures within the thoracic cavity. In the right lung are three *lobes* (upper, middle, lower); in the left, two lobes (upper, lower) (see Fig. 11–17). The *pleura* consists of two layers, the *parietal pleura* and the *visceral pleura;* the parietal pleura lines the entire thoracic cavity and the *visceral pleura* encases each lung. The pleura aids in maintaining lung stability. Separation of the lungs from the thorax is prevented through the negative pressure within the intrapleural space. *Diffusion* of gases takes place in the lungs. Terminal bronchioles lack mucus-secreting goblet cells and cilia, and gas exchange does not take place here.

Distal to the terminal bronchioles are the alveoli, where most gas exchange occurs. Thinness of the alveolar walls aids in gas exchange. Within the alveolar walls there is an almost solid sheet of capillaries, so that the alveolar gases are in close proximity to the capillary blood.

Prenatal Respiratory Development. The respiratory system must be developed prior to birth in order for the neonate to survive. The placenta performs oxygenation in utero, but the neonate must be able to inflate the lungs, establish continuous breathing, and have the ability to transfer the gases needed to meet metabolic needs.

Postnatal Respiratory Changes. Postnatal changes in the respiratory system are listed in the accompanying box.

> Adaptation to extrauterine life is mainly dependent on the lungs. At birth the infant must inflate the lungs, establish continuous breathing, and possess a mature enough system to facilitate the gas transfer needed to meet metabolic needs.

Gas Exchange and Transport. Two-way diffusion takes place between the walls of the alveoli. In diffusion, there is movement of molecules from an area of greater concentration to one of lesser concentration. Blood entering the lung capillaries is somewhat low in oxygen. Oxygen will diffuse from the alveoli, where its concentration is higher, into the blood. Similarly, carbon dioxide moves out of the blood and into the alveoli. Most oxygen that diffuses into

Postnatal Changes in the Respiratory System

- Compression of thorax during delivery forces out some fetal lung fluid.
- Respirations are stimulated by hypoxemia, hypercarbia, cold, tactile stimulation, and a possible decrease in the concentration of prostaglandin E_2.
- Inflation of the normal lung is complete within a few breaths, and most alveoli are expanded within first hour of life.
- Premature infant has a more compliant chest wall and weaker muscles than a term infant.
- Surfactant in the lung liquid lowers surface tension and facilitates lung expansion.
- Pulmonary blood flow increases.
- Closure of foramen ovale and the ductus arteriosus establishes separate pulmonary and circulatory systems.

the capillary blood in the lungs is bound to the hemoglobin of red blood cells. A small percentage is dissolved in plasma. For oxygen to enter the cells, it must separate from hemoglobin. The uptake and delivery of gases by the blood is a continuous process (see the accompanying figure).

Carbon dioxide diffuses into the blood from the tissues and is transported to the lungs by the blood. In this activity hemoglobin acts as a buffer that enables blood to take up carbon dioxide without altering the pH significantly. Ventilation occurs through *inspiration* and *expiration.* In inspiration the diaphragm contracts and flattens, expanding the vertical dimension of the chest; the lung volume increases. In expiration the diaphragm and chest wall relax, decreasing thoracic volume. Intrathoracic pressure increases and gas flows out of the lungs, taking with it carbon dioxide that was delivered to the lungs by the blood. Ventilation of the lungs is intermittent. Inspired air is 21% oxygen; end-expired air is 16% oxygen and 35% carbon dioxide.

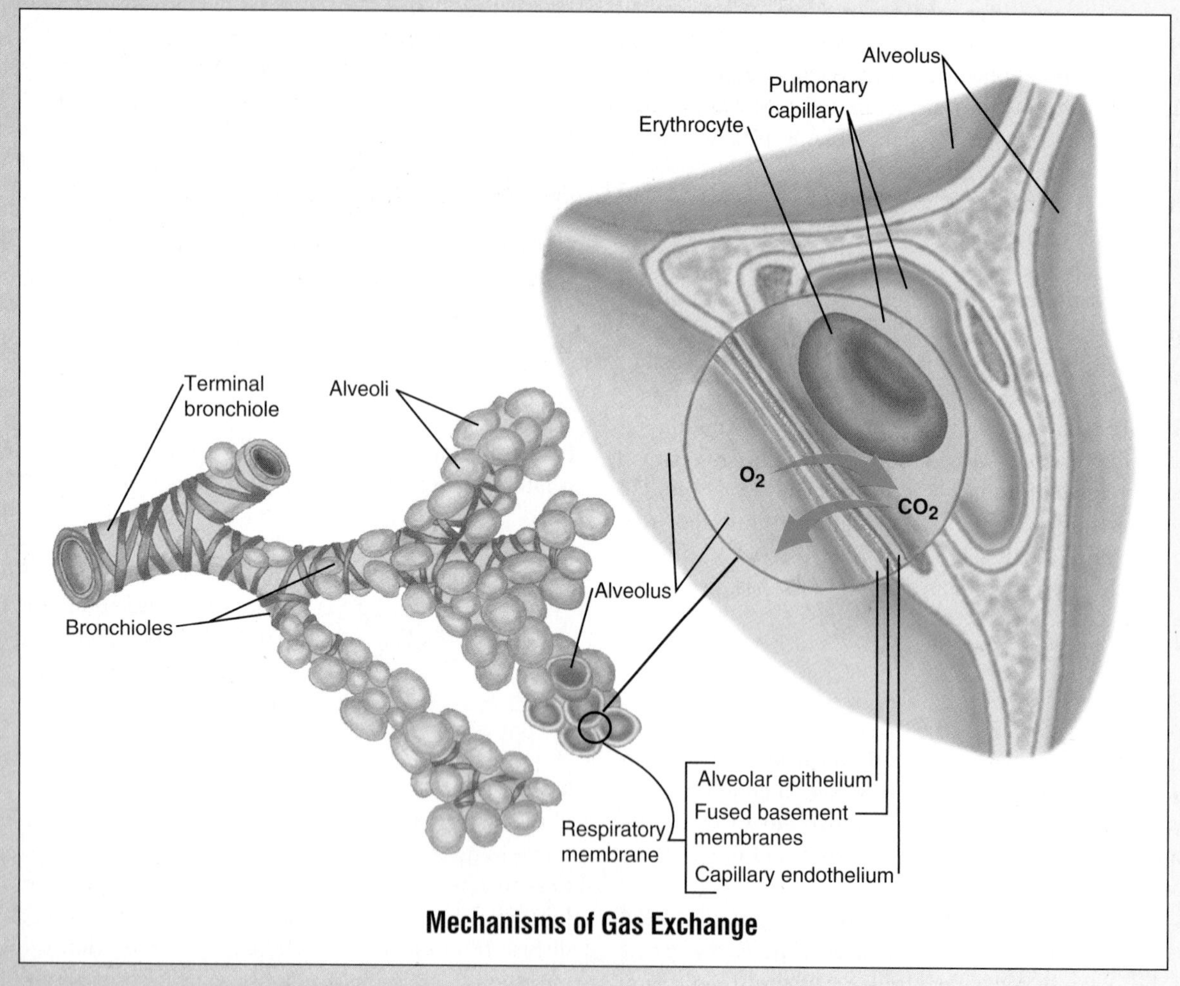

Mechanisms of Gas Exchange

DIAGNOSTIC TESTS

In most cases, respiratory tract diseases are diagnosed based on the results of a physical examination and the clinical manifestations. However, sometimes specific diagnostic tests are called for (see the accompanying table).

Blood Gas Analysis. Arterial blood gas (ABG) analysis plays an important role in the investigation of pulmonary function. ABGs most frequently include values for PaO_2, $PaCO_2$, pH, and HCO_3^-. Samples of arterial blood for these readings are more reliable than capillary or venous blood, especially in patients with poor peripheral perfusion.

COMMON LABORATORY AND DIAGNOSTIC TESTS FOR RESPIRATORY DISORDERS

TEST	DESCRIPTION	NORMAL FINDINGS	INDICATIONS	NURSING CONSIDERATIONS
Postero-anterior and lateral chest X-rays	Visualizes airways, lungs, heart, great vessels	Normal appearance of internal structures of chest	Respiratory disease of lungs	Assist in holding child
Computed tomography (CT scan)	Defines lesions located within chest wall, pleural space, mediastium, and lung parenchyma	Normal cross section of lung tissue	Tumors or masses To evaluate response to therapy aimed at defined lesions	Sedation and immobilization Withhold feedings 3–4 hr pretest because of frequent use of contrast medium
Bronchoscopy	Visualize tracheobronchial tree through a scope	Normal appearance of tracheobronchial tree or successful removal of foreign body or mucus plugs	Visualization, biopsy of lesions, cultures To remove a foreign body or mucus plugs	Rigid bronchoscopy is usually performed under general anesthesia Fiberoptic flexible bronchoscopy can be performed while child is awake or sedated Child should be closely observed for signs of airway obstruction Mist may be given to decrease swelling and edema
Laryngoscopy	Direct visualization of larynx with a scope	Normal appearance of larynx	Stridor and local abnormalities	Mirror (indirect) laryngoscopy can be performed on children age 4–5 yr or older; in infants and younger children, direct laryngoscopy or transnasal laryngoscopy with flexible bronchoscope will give much better results General anesthesia usually required Topical anesthesia and mild sedation given with fiberoptic exam Fluids and foods withheld until effects of local anesthetic have worn off and gag reflex has returned
Lung biopsy	Open thoracotomy to remove pulmonary tissue	Normal lung tissue	Histology and culture of tissue and inspection of lung	General anesthesia and chest tube postoperatively
Percutaneous lung puncture	Needle aspiration through intercostal space	No culture growth	Used only in critically ill child with interstitial pneumonia who has not responded to treatment	No preparation Observe for manifestations of pneumothorax
Cultures	Throat, blood, nasopharyngeal, sputum	No culture growth, normal flora	Isolate and identify pathogens	See Chapter 18 for procedures

ABGs should be used primarily to determine acid-base balance and not for oxygen saturation. See Chapter 18 for information regarding obtaining arterial blood samples.

Pulmonary Function Tests. Probably the most useful tests of ventilatory function are *vital capacity* and *expiratory flow rates,* both measured by spirometry. These tests can be performed in most children by age 6 years. Accurate measurements are difficult to obtain in younger children and infants because they are unable to follow commands. Pulmonary function tests assess the degree of pulmonary disease, response to therapy, and presence of restrictive or obstructive disease. They are also done to test the child's response to bronchodilators should pulmonary function be affected.

The child to be tested must receive instruction and practice in blowing, pushing, and holding respirations. The child should become familiar with the mouthpiece and the nose clip in order to feel comfortable with their use.

Noninvasive Monitoring of Oxygen

Pulse Oximetry. *Pulse oximetry* is a simple, noninvasive, continuous method for measuring oxygen saturation for the purpose of determining the need for or response to oxygen therapy. It is fully described in Chapter 18.

Transcutaneous Monitoring. *Transcutaneous monitoring* continuously monitors oxygen and carbon dioxide concentrations in the body through the use of an electrode. Electrode sites must be changed every 3 to 4 hours to prevent burning of the skin, and the machine must be recalibrated each time electrodes are changed. The readings may not be accurate if the tissue perfusion is poor.

COMMON RESPIRATORY MEDICATIONS

Medications for treating respiratory illness are described in the accompanying table. See also the Common Medications table in Chapter 29.

MEDICATIONS COMMONLY USED FOR ACUTE RESPIRATORY DISORDERS

DRUG	ACTION AND USES	DOSAGE	ADMINISTRATION	SIDE EFFECTS	NURSING CONSIDERATIONS
Ribavirin (Virazole)	Virustatic through disruption of RNA and DNA synthesis, interfering with viral replication Used for severe lower respiratory tract infections due to RSV in selected high-risk infants and children	Deliver mist containing 20 mg/ml; continue for 12–18 hr/day for 3–7 days	Aerosolized or inhaled	Can precipitate in respiratory devices; therefore can interfere with effective respiratory support of infants undergoing mechanical ventilation. Rash, conjunctivitis.	Respiratory tract secretions for nasal washings should be obtained before first dose or at least during first 24 hr of therapy. Obtain baseline respiratory reading. Monitor intake and output, fluid balance. Assess skin for rash. Monitor blood pressure (BP); assess lung sounds, respirations. Warn pregnant personnel and visitors of the possible teratogenic risks associated with exposure to ribavirin. Precipitation of the drug on contact lenses has been associated with conjunctivitis.
Amantadine hydrochloride (Symadine, Symmetrel)	Antiviral against influenza Prevents penetration of influenza A virus into host cells and can inhibit viral coating	1–9 yr: 4.4–8.8 mg/kg/day, 2–3 divided doses, up to 150 mg per day 9–12 yr: 100 mg b.i.d.	Oral (capsules and syrup)	Nausea, dizziness, difficulty concentrating, insomnia, orthostatic hypotension, anorexia, constipation.	Obtain specimens for viral diagnostic test before giving first dose. Monitor BP, intake and output, food tolerance, neurologic effects, and any skin rashes. Doses should be evenly spaced and the nighttime dose should be taken several hours before sleep to avoid insomnia.

UPPER AIRWAY DISORDERS

Sinusitis

Sinusitis, although not itself a serious disorder, may lead to life-threatening complications. Inflammation and infection of the sinuses can be acute or chronic.

Etiology. Acute sinusitis often follows a viral upper respiratory tract infection. Children with chronic sinusitis often have allergic rhinitis or acute otitis media with effusion. Hypertrophied adenoids, immune deficiencies, and foreign body obstruction in the nose also predispose children to sinusitis. Children with cystic fibrosis have a high incidence of sinusitis because of highly viscous mucous secretions and nasal polyps.

The most common causative organisms are *Streptococcus pneumoniae, Hemophilus influenzae, Branhamella catarrhalis,* and *Staphylococcus aureus.*

Incidence. Infections of the sinuses can occur in infancy as well as in childhood, but they are most common during the school-age period.

Clinical Manifestations

Acute

- Signs and symptoms of a "cold" that do not improve after 14 days
- Low-grade fever
- Purulent nasal discharge
- Nasal congestion
- Headache, tenderness, and a feeling of fullness over affected sinuses (irritability in younger children)
- Edema over the affected sinuses (occasional)
- Halitosis
- Cough (usually increases when child is lying down)

Chronic

- Low-grade fever (intermittent)
- Purulent nasal discharge, postnasal drip
- Chronic cough
- Recurrent headache
- Sneezing
- Impaired senses of taste and smell
- Halitosis
- Malaise, anorexia

Diagnostic Evaluation. Sinus X-rays show mucosal thickening, opacification, and air-fluid levels in children over age 1 year. Sinus X-rays are of no value in younger children because of their small sinuses. A computed tomography (CT) scan provides detailed anatomic information. Because of the thick bone of the maxilla in the anterior face and the small size of the sinus, transillumination of the sinuses is not useful.

PATHOPHYSIOLOGY *of Sinusitis*

Acute sinusitis occurs when the sinus cavity is invaded by bacteria, causing mucosal inflammation and edema that block narrow sinus channels. Increased volumes of secretions are produced, and the affected sinuses fill with purulent material. Inflammation and infection interfere with the protective cleansing action of the cilia covering the sinus mucous membranes. Impaired mucociliary transport leads to stagnation of secretions within the sinuses and provides a medium for bacterial growth.

Chronic sinusitis is usually a complication of acute sinusitis. Prolonged or repeated infections result in irreversible changes in the mucosal lining of the sinus. Nasal polyps, deviated septum, and enlarged adenoids inhibit sinus drainage and can also lead to infections. The frontal and sphenoid sinuses are most often involved in children.

Infection from sinusitis may spread to the middle ear, causing otitis media. Serious complications occur when infection spreads either directly through the bone or along the venous channels of the skull into adjacent structures, such as the orbit or the central nervous system.

Therapeutic Management. Antibiotics are the mainstay of treatment. In addition to antibiotics, treatment includes analgesics, hydration, the application of moist heat, and topical decongestants. The use of decongestants and antihistamines in the treatment of sinusitis is controversial. Antihistamines may be used to treat allergy symptoms associated with chronic sinusitis, but they tend to impair sinus drainage by thickening secretions. Steroid nasal sprays may be used to reduce inflammation while avoiding the rebound effect of decongestant nosedrops.

Obstructive deformities such as enlarged adenoids or polyps are surgically corrected. If orbital cellulitis develops, the child should be hospitalized immediately and parenteral antibiotic therapy begun.

NURSING CARE OF THE CHILD WITH SINUSITIS

Assessment

The child should be questioned and examined to determine the location of pain or fullness. Pain may occur in the forehead, over the cheekbones or upper teeth, or may radiate to the top of the head. The face should be inspected and palpated for edema. Temperature should be assessed and the nose and throat inspected for the presence of purulent discharge. The nasal mucous membranes are inspected for erythema and edema.

Nursing Diagnosis and Planning

The following nursing diagnoses and expected outcomes may be appropriate in the treatment of sinusitis in the child.

- Ineffective Airway Clearance (upper airway) related to increased secretions. ***Expected Outcome:*** *The child will have decreased inflammation and edema.*
- Pain related to edema and inflammation of sinus mucous membranes. ***Expected Outcome:*** *The child will verbalize decreased pain.*
- Knowledge Deficit related to home care. ***Expected Outcome:*** *The parents/child will verbalize and demonstrate an understanding of home care measures for sinusitis.*

Implementation

Nursing care consists of administering antibiotics, promoting drainage of purulent secretions, promoting comfort, monitoring for response to treatment, and observing for complications. The child and parents must be taught the importance of taking the antibiotics as prescribed. Sinus drainage is facilitated by generous oral fluid intake. Hydration is accomplished through increased clear fluid intake and a bedside humidifier.

Warm moist compresses applied two to three times daily help decrease swelling and pain. Periorbital edema should be carefully watched and any increase in swelling or drainage from the eyes reported to the physician. Breathing warm mist in a hot shower or through hot, moist towels can help liquefy and mobilize nasal mucus and exudate, as can saline nosedrops. Nosedrops should be administered after gently cleaning the nasal passages. Acetaminophen is given for fever and discomfort. The amount, color, and consistency of nasal drainage should be noted and evaluated to determine if the child is responding to treatment.

The child's response to treatment and the development of complications should be evaluated carefully. Parents should be taught to contact the physician promptly if symptoms become worse or the child does not seem to be feeling better after 3 or 4 days.

Evaluation

- Has the amount of inflammation and edema decreased?
- Is the child resting comfortably?
- Are the parents able to provide comfort measures and other care for their child at home?

Allergic Rhinitis

Allergic rhinitis is an inflammatory disorder of the nasal mucosa, it has a pattern of seasonality, is recurrent, and has specific triggers. It is sometimes referred to as *seasonal allergic rhinitis, seasonal pollinosis,* and *hay fever.* Some children have symptoms year-round (*perennial allergic rhinitis*).

PATHOPHYSIOLOGY *of Allergic Rhinitis*

Allergens (pollens, mold, spores, dust mites, animal dander) are deposited on the nasal mucosa. Inflammation of the area causes permeability of the nasal mucosa. Local IgE is produced and sensitization of the respiratory tissues occurs. Mast cell mediators are released, producing vasodilation, mucosal edema, mucus secretions, stimulation of itch receptors, and reduction of the threshold for sneezing.

Etiology. Common causative agents are *dust mites, feathers, danders of household pets, mold spores, pollen of trees, grasses,* and *weeds.* There is usually a family history similar to that seen in atopic dermatitis and asthma. Unlike atopic dermatitis, allergic rhinitis does not predispose the child to the development of asthma.

Incidence and Prognosis. The onset of allergic rhinitis usually occurs after about age 5 years and before age 20. It is estimated that 5% to 9% of children have this type of allergic response (Behrman, 1995).

Allergic rhinitis can be improved and sometimes cured by avoidance of known allergens or by immunotherapy. A child will sometimes develop a tolerance to a particular antihistamine. Changing to a different medication is usually effective. Over time, the child can usually return to the original medication.

Clinical Manifestations

- Watery rhinorrhea
- Paroxysmal sneezing
- Itching of nose, eyes, ears, and palate
- Allergic salute: upward rubbing of the nose, which can leave a crease below the bridge (Fig. 28–1)
- Allergic shiners (dark circles under the eyes from congestion and edema) (Fig. 28–1)
- Dry lips from mouth breathing
- Pale, boggy nasal mucous membranes (eosinophilia)
- Nasal obstruction

Diagnostic Evaluation. A thorough personal and family history should be taken with a review of the presenting signs and symptoms. A nasal smear for eosinophils is done. Skin testing is done if signs and symptoms continue after treatment with medication. The radioallergosorbent test

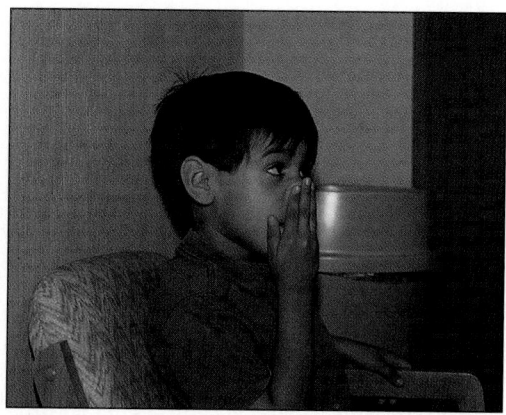

Figure 28–1
Children with allergic rhinitis often have dark circles under their eyes ("allergic shiners"). They are often seen rubbing their noses upward with the palm—an allergic salute. (Courtesy of Dallas County Hospital District Community Oriented Primary Care Clinic, Dallas, Texas.)

(RAST) is used only when skin testing is difficult due to generalized dermatitis, when the child is very young, and when the child is too ill for skin testing.

Therapeutic Management. The treatment of choice is to eliminate the allergen from the child's environment (see Teaching Guidelines box). When this is impossible, as in the case of pollen in the air, medications may be prescribed. Finally immunotherapy may be implemented. For a discussion of environmental control and immunotherapy see the section on asthma in Chapter 29.

Antihistamines and bronchodilators are given to relieve symptoms. Antihistamines are most effective when given before or very early in an allergic episode. A decongestant may be given in conjunction with an antihistamine if nasal congestion is a problem. Topical intranasal corticosteroids (for example, beclomethosone) are quite effective in children who do not respond to antihistamines and decongestants (see medications table in the Clinical Reference Pages in Chapter 29). Systemic side effects are absent. It usually takes several days of treatment before the effects of topical corticosteroids are felt by the child. Children with severe symptoms who do not respond to treatment may be given systemic corticosteroids. Relief is usually attained within 24 hours.

NURSING CARE OF THE CHILD WITH ALLERGIC RHINITIS

Assessment

The child is assessed for symptoms of allergic rhinitis: watery rhinorrhea, paroxysmal sneezing, and itching of nose, eyes, ears, and palate. Nasal obstruction may also be present. Children taking medication for rhinitis should be assessed for side effects of the medication, including drowsiness, excitability, and dry mucous membranes. The child is also observed for manifestations of sinusitis, a common complication of allergic rhinitis.

Nursing Diagnosis and Planning

The following nursing diagnoses and expected outcomes may be appropriate in the treatment of allergic rhinitis in the child.

- Ineffective Airway Clearance (upper airway) related to nasal congestion secondary to an allergic process. ***Expected Outcome:*** *The child will have clear upper airway passages, as evidenced by ability to breathe through the nose.*
- Knowledge Deficit related to disease process. ***Expected Outcome:*** *The parents/child will verbalize an understanding of the cause and treatments of the disease.*

Implementation

Nursing care is focused on early identification of signs and symptoms of allergic rhinitis and support of the therapeutic management of the disease. After the identification of the allergens, it is often necessary to counsel parents regarding environmental control, administration of medications, and immunotherapy if it is implemented.

Drowsiness is the most common side effect of antihistamines, which can usually be eliminated if the child takes a combination antihistamine and decongestant. Some children experience dry mucous membranes and excitability. Other drug therapy was discussed under therapeutic management.

When specific allergens have been identified, those things should be eliminated or controlled. During pollen season the child should stay indoors as much as possible and the windows should be kept closed if the house is air-conditioned. After being outdoors the child should shower and wash hair to remove pollens from the body. Animals who have been outside may also be a source of contamination. See Teaching Guidelines for Allergy-Proofing the Home for further instructions for parents.

Receiving immunotherapy can be a traumatic experience. It is often difficult for children to understand how getting an injection is going to help them.

> Children should be closely supervised for 20 to 30 minutes after an injection in case anaphylaxis develops.

Warm water or saline irrigations of the nasal passages can be used to soften crusted secretions and wash out irritants. Saline can be mixed by adding $\frac{1}{4}$ teaspoon of salt to a

TEACHING GUIDELINES *for Allergy-Proofing the Home*

Suggest the following to decrease the child's exposure to allergens:

POLLEN AND DUST

- Wash sheets and blankets in hot water.
- Avoid wool and down blankets.
- Encase pillows and mattresses in dust-proof covers.
- Replace carpet with wood, tile, slate, or vinyl.
- Replace drapes and blinds with curtains and shades.
- Replace upholstered furniture with wood or plastic.
- Keep closet doors shut.
- Cover hot air vents with filters.
- Install air cleaners.
- Use multi-layer vacuum bags.
- Clean with a towel treated to attract dust.
- Run air conditioners.
- Keep humidity at 40%–50%.

MOLD

- Clean with a mold inhibitor.
- Dry shoes thoroughly.
- Use a moisture remover in closets.
- Stay out of the basement.
- Replace foam rubber mattresses with springs.
- Run an air conditioner.
- Keep the humidity below 35%.
- Run a dehumidifier.
- Ventilate the house.
- Store firewood outside.
- Limit the number of indoor plants.

DANDER

- Keep pets outside if possible.
- Ventilate the house.
- Install air cleaners.
- Encase mattresses and pillows in dust-proof covers.
- Wash cats with water.

cup of warm water. Saline nosedrops are also available over the counter.

Evaluation

- Is the child able to breathe through his nose?
- Have the parents made changes in the home, if necessary, to reduce the child's exposure to environmental allergies?
- If the child is receiving immunotherapy, are the parents bringing the child for scheduled injections?

Otitis Media

Otitis media is one of the most common illnesses of childhood. The term otitis media refers to infection or blockage of the middle ear. Based on duration, otitis media can be classified as *acute*—up to 3 weeks' duration, *subacute*—from 3 weeks' to 3 months' duration, or *chronic*—more than 3 months' duration.

Otitis media is generally described as acute otitis media or otitis media with effusion. Descriptions of the types of otitis media can be found in the accompanying box.

Etiology. The most common bacterial pathogens causing acute otitis media are *Streptococcus pneumoniae*, *Haemophilus influenzae*, and *Moraxella catarrhalis*. Although viruses do

Types of Otitis Media

Acute Otitis Media

- Also called acute purulent otitis media, acute suppurative otitis media
- Infection of the middle ear with sudden onset and short duration

Otitis Media With Effusion

- Also called secretory otitis media, chronic otitis media with effusion, serous otitis media, "glue ear," nonsuppurative otitis media
- Presence of fluid (effusion) behind the tympanic membrane with no signs of infection
- Effusions can be serous (thin and watery), mucoid (mucous-like), or purulent (pus-like)

Otitis Media Without Effusion (myringitis)

- Inflammation of the tympanic membrane

Chronic Otitis Media

- Also called chronic suppurative otitis media
- Chronic disease of the middle ear with or without ear drainage
- May or may not have effusion (Goyocoolea & Hueb, 1991)

PATHOPHYSIOLOGY *of Otitis Media*

The immature anatomy of the child's middle ear and eustachian tube predisposes infants and toddlers to otitis media (see the figure below). When the eustachian tube is obstructed, as frequently occurs with enlarged adenoids or mucosal edema from an upper respiratory infection, effective drainage and ventilation of the middle ear cannot occur. Air that is normally present in the middle ear is absorbed by the blood, resulting in a "vacuum" or negative pressure in the middle ear. Fluid (effusion) accumulates within the middle ear space, creating a medium for bacterial growth. If the eustachian tube remains nonfunctional for a prolonged period, the fluid within the middle ear becomes thick and dark in color ("glue ear"). Mild temporary conductive hearing loss often occurs in otitis media with effusion due to decreased mobility of the ossicles and the tympanic membrane. Permanent conductive hearing loss can result from repeated episodes of otitis media and may interfere with the development of language and cognitive skills. Chronic otitis media with effusion is the most common cause of hearing loss in children.

Infection (acute otitis media), most often is the result of pathogens traveling from the nasopharynx, often following an upper respiratory infection. In the presence of effusion, negative pressure in the middle ear draws mucus through the eustachian tube from the pharynx whenever the child cries, yawns, or sucks forcefully on a nipple. Purulent fluid accumulates in the middle ear space, causing pressure and pain. Otitis media with effusion may precede or follow acute otitis media.

Complications of otitis media include conductive hearing loss and sensorineural hearing loss. The infection of acute otitis media can spread to surrounding tissues, causing mastoiditis or intracranial complications such as meningitis or brain abscess. Inflammation and pressure from otitis media may result in tympanosclerosis (scarring of the tympanic membrane), perforation of the tympanic membrane, and cholesteatoma (pus and debris in the middle ear).

See also Figure 11–6.

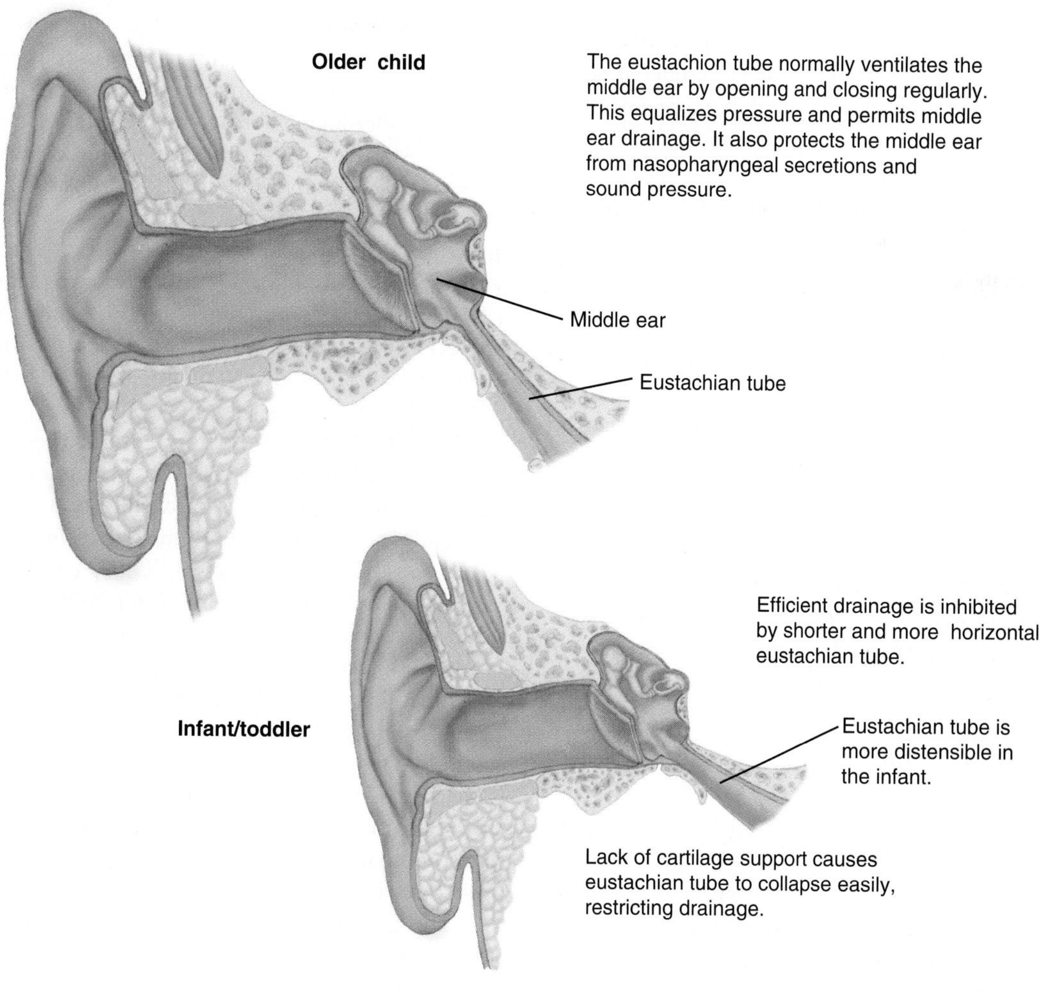
Older child
The eustachion tube normally ventilates the middle ear by opening and closing regularly. This equalizes pressure and permits middle ear drainage. It also protects the middle ear from nasopharyngeal secretions and sound pressure.
Middle ear
Eustachian tube
Infant/toddler
Efficient drainage is inhibited by shorter and more horizontal eustachian tube.
Eustachian tube is more distensible in the infant.
Lack of cartilage support causes eustachian tube to collapse easily, restricting drainage.

not cause otitis media, they are thought to predispose the child to ear infection by altering host defenses and contributing to eustachian tube dysfunction. Allergies are also thought to precipitate otitis media.

Factors that increase the risk of otitis media include exposure to illness in other children in daycare centers, household smoking, bottle-feeding, and congenital conditions such as Down syndrome and cleft palate (Marchant, 1990). The use of a pacifier beyond age 6 months has also been identified as a risk factor (Niemelä, Uhari, & Möttönen, 1995).

Bottle-feeding contributes to ear infection because of the position of the infant during feeding. Reflux of formula up the eustachian tube from the nasopharynx occurs when the infant swallows while supine. Breast-feeding offers some protection from ear infection by providing maternal antibodies and by decreasing allergy incidence as well as from the more upright position of the infant while nursing.

Incidence. The peak incidence of otitis media occurs between ages 6 and 36 months, with a smaller peak occurring in the 4- to 7-year age-group. Most initial episodes of otitis media occur about age 6 months, when there is a decline in maternal antibodies. The onset of otitis media in the first year of life increases the risk of recurrent disease (Behrman, 1995).

By the end of the third year of life, 50% to 70% of all children have experienced at least one episode of acute otitis media. Most children under age 5 have two to three episodes of otitis media each year. Boys have a slightly higher incidence of otitis media than girls.

The incidence of otitis media is highest in winter and spring and lowest in the summer months.

Clinical Manifestations

Acute Otitis Media

- Otalgia (earache). Infants may pull their ears or roll their heads.
- Irritability, sleep disturbances, persistent crying in infants
- Fever
- Vomiting, anorexia, diarrhea (infants especially)
- Tympanic membrane appears bulging, opaque, usually red, with decreased mobility. Light reflex diffuse. Landmarks obscured.
- Drainage, usually yellowish-green, purulent, and foul smelling (indicates perforation of the tympanic membrane)

Otitis Media With Effusion

- Tinnitus, popping sounds
- Hearing loss, (usually conductive) up to 35 decibels. Delays in speech development may result from prolonged hearing loss. In the older child, hearing loss may manifest as behavior problems, poor school performance, disturbed sleep, irritability, and decreased responsiveness.
- Mild balance disturbances. May result in delays in motor skills.
- Tympanic membrane appears retracted, dull gray or yellow; air-fluid level or air bubbles may be visible through tympanic membrane; mobility is decreased, landmarks distorted (see Fig. 28–2).
- Tympanogram shows a flattened tracing and negative pressure.

Diagnostic Evaluation. Diagnosis of otitis media is based on history findings and direct visualization of the tympanic membrane (otoscopy). In *acute otitis media*, the tympanic membrane is opaque rather than shiny and translucent. The membrane appears full or bulging and the landmarks are obscured (see Fig. 28–2). The color is sometimes, but not always, red. Pneumatic otoscopy shows decreased mobility. *Otitis media with effusion* is characterized by clear fluid behind a dull gray or yellow transparent membrane (see Fig. 28–2). In otitis media with effusion, mobility of the tympanic membrane is also decreased and the landmarks are obscured. Pneumatic otoscopy should be used, rather than otoscopy alone, to diagnose otitis media with effusion. In addition, tympanometry can be used to confirm what was seen with the eye (American Academy of Pediatrics, 1994b).

Therapeutic Management. Acute otitis media is treated with oral antibiotics. Amoxicillin is usually used initially. Amoxicillin/clavulanate (Augmentin) is effective against beta-lactamase-producing organisms resistant to amoxicillin alone. Alternative antibiotics such as erythromycin/sulfisoxazole (Pediazole), trimethoprim/sulfamethoxazole (Bactrim, Septra), cefaclor (Ceclor), or cefixime (Suprax) may be prescribed for penicillin-resistant organisms or in cases of penicillin allergy. Antibiotics are given for a total of 10 to 14 days. The child should be examined again at the end of the course of antibiotic therapy (after 10 to 14 days) to assess for persistent infection or for middle ear effusion.

The child who suffers frequent, recurrent otitis media or middle ear effusion may be placed on prophylactic antibiotic treatment with amoxicillin or a sulfonamide in one daily dose at bedtime. Prophylactic antibiotics may be given for as long as 6 months. These children should be examined monthly to monitor for middle ear effusion. Hearing should be assessed with audiometry.

Some practitioners believe that, due to the prevalence of infection related to multiple-drug resistant bacteria, antimicrobial treatment of otitis media should be modified by individualized treatment based on risk factors, substantially curtailing antimicrobial treatment for otitis media with effusion and looking again at the practice of antimicrobial prophylaxis to prevent acute otitis media recurrences (Paradise, 1995). More research is needed in this area.

The usefulness of decongestants or antihistamines in the prevention and treatment of otitis media is controversial. Although these medications are widely prescribed,

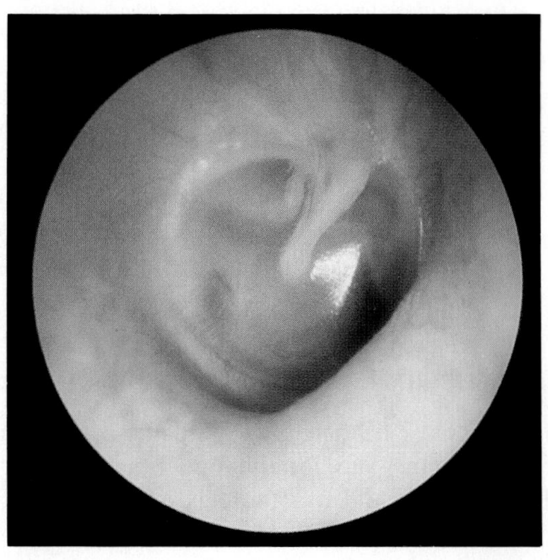

◀ Normal right tympanic membrane and middle ear

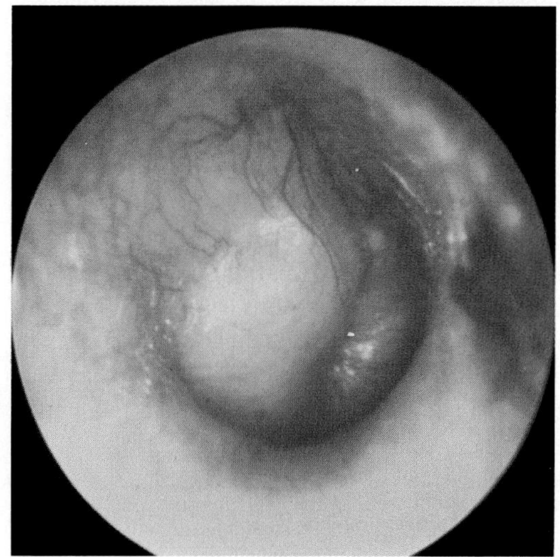

Acute otitis media: Bulging right tympanic membrane ▶

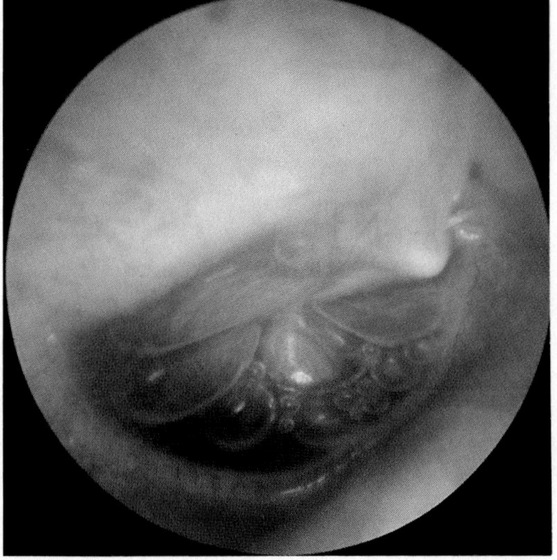

◀ Otitis media with effusion: Air-fluid level and bubbles visible through right retracted, translucent tympanic membrane

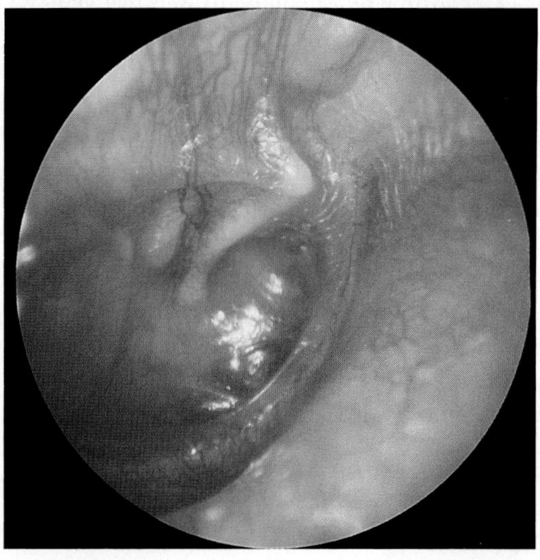

Otitis media with effusion: Severely retracted, opaque right tympanic membrane ▶

Figure 28–2

Appearance of tympanic membrane in otitis media as compared with normal tympanic membrane. (From Bluestone, C.D., & Klein, J.O. [1995]. *Otitis media in infants and children.* [2nd ed.]. Philadelphia: W. B. Saunders, Color Plate Figs. 1 through 4.)

most research does not support their use except to control nasal drainage or congestion. Acetaminophen is given to help relieve pain and fever of acute otitis media.

Initial treatment of otitis media with effusion may include observation or antibiotic therapy. Parents should be encouraged to control environmental risk factors. The American Academy of Pediatrics (AAP) has recommended that antihistamines, steroids, adenoidectomy (in the absence of adenoid pathology), and tonsillectomy **not be used** in the treatment of otitis media with effusion in children ages 1 through 3 years (American Academy of Pediatrics, 1994b).

In cases of persistent ear infection despite antibiotic therapy or otitis media with effusion that persists for over

3 months, *myringotomy* with insertion of *tympanostomy tubes* may be performed. During this surgery mucoid material is removed from the middle ear and a tympanostomy tube is inserted through the tympanic membrane. A tympanostomy tube is a small polyethylene tube inserted into the middle ear to equalize the pressure on both sides of the tympanic membrane and to keep the ear aerated. Negative pressure in the middle ear is thus relieved, allowing the middle ear mucosa to return to normal and growth of the eustachian tube to occur. The tube usually falls out spontaneously in 6 to 12 months. This may provide enough time for the effusion process to resolve, but some children require repeated insertions of tympanostomy tubes because of persistent eustachian tube dysfunction. Adenoidectomy may be performed at the same time as tube insertion. Tympanostomy tubes are inserted under general anesthesia, usually in a day surgery setting.

NURSING CARE OF THE CHILD WITH OTITIS MEDIA

Assessment

The parent should be asked if the child has had a recent upper respiratory tract infection or previous ear infections. The child is assessed for fever and pain. Because signs of ear infection may be subtle in infants, the nurse should assess not only for obvious signs of ear pain such as head rolling and pulling at the ear, but also for nonspecific findings like irritability, diarrhea, or refusal of feedings. Older children may complain of pain or a feeling of fullness in the affected ear. The ear is examined with an otoscope, noting the color, mobility, and translucency of the tympanic membrane as well as the appearance of the external canal. The tympanic membrane should be inspected carefully for signs of perforation. Any drainage from the ear should be cultured and the color, consistency, and odor noted. Hearing and language development should be assessed.

Nursing Diagnosis and Planning

The following nursing diagnoses and expected outcomes may be appropriate in the treatment of otitis media in the infant or child.

- Pain related to inflammation and pressure in the middle ear. ***Expected Outcomes:*** *The child will be free of pain, as evidenced by sleeping through the night, not pulling at the ears, and crying less; have tympanic membranes that appear shiny, pearly gray, with normal landmarks, visible light reflex, and normal mobility on tympanogram.*
- Knowledge Deficit related to disease process and treatment regimen. ***Expected Outcomes:*** *The parents will demonstrate methods of feeding the infant that decrease the risk of otitis media; keep child's ears dry if tympanostomy tubes are in place; follow treatment regimen.*
- Risk for Altered Body Temperature related to inflammation. ***Expected Outcome:*** *The child will display a normal body temperature.*
- Risk for Fluid Volume Deficit related to elevated temperature and decreased intake. ***Expected Outcome:*** *The child will have moist mucous membranes, good skin turgor, and appropriate intake for age.*

Implementation

Parents must be taught the importance of giving antibiotics on time and for the prescribed number of days. Because the child usually feels much better after a few days of medication, it is common for parents to feel that the antibiotics are no longer necessary and to stop giving them. Compliance may be increased by giving written as well as oral instructions for administering medications. Providing a medication record form on which to record doses taken and a calibrated measuring device for liquid medications is also helpful.

> Compliance may be increased through specific teaching regarding administration of antibiotics. "After a few days, your child may seem to be well and show no signs of otitis media. If you stop giving the antibiotic at that time some of the pathogens or 'bugs' that caused the otitis media may still be alive and your child can experience a relapse."

Acetaminophen can be given to relieve discomfort. The child's fluid intake should be increased if fever is present. The parents should be told to notify the physician if the child has not improved after 48 hours of antibiotic treatment or if there is drainage from the affected ear. The importance of follow-up visits to ensure that the ear is free of infection and effusion and that the child's hearing is normal should be emphasized.

If the child is undergoing myringotomy with insertion of tympanostomy tubes, the nurse should prepare the child and parents as for any outpatient surgical procedure. The procedure should be explained in clear terms and questions answered simply and honestly. Postoperatively, the child is monitored for ear drainage. A small amount of reddish drainage is normal for the first few days after surgery. However, the parents should report any heavier bleeding or bleeding that occurs after 3 days. The parents should also be instructed to report any fever or increased pain. The child should not blow his nose for 7 to 10 days. Most physicians prefer that the child's ears be kept dry if tubes are in place, but some feel that a small amount of water in the ears is not harmful. Bath and lake water are potential sources of bacterial contamination, however, and chlorinated swimming pool water can be irritating to tympanic membranes with tubes. The usual recommendation is to place ear plugs or cotton balls covered with petroleum jelly in the ears during baths and shampoos. Swimming is allowed only with ear plugs and with the physician's approval. Diving and swimming deeply under water are prohibited. The size and appearance of the tympanostomy tubes should be described to the parents, and they should be reassured that if the tubes fall out it is not an emergency but that the physician should be notified.

Otitis media is usually a chronic problem, with frequent recurrences of infection and effusion. The parents should be taught the early signs of ear infection and the importance of seeking care if they occur. Because hearing impairment from middle ear effusion can be very difficult for parents to detect, the child with chronic otitis media should have periodic hearing evaluations.

The nurse should teach parents methods to decrease the risk of recurrent otitis media, such as encouraging breast-feeding during infancy, discontinuing bottle-feeding as soon as possible, feeding the infant in an upright position, and never giving the infant a bottle in bed. Parents should be told not to smoke in the child's presence because passive smoking increases the incidence of otitis media.

Evaluation

- Did the parents complete the treatment regimen by giving the entire dose of the prescribed antibiotic?
- Were follow-up appointments to determine the resolution of the otitis media kept?
- Is the child sleeping an appropriate amount of time for his age?
- Is the child afebrile?

Laryngomalacia (Congenital Laryngeal Stridor)

Laryngomalacia is caused by flaccidity of the epiglottis and supraglottic aperture and weakness of airway walls. It is the most common cause of **stridor** in the neonatal period.

Pathophysiology. Congenital laryngeal stridor is related to a delay in development of neuromuscular control. The epiglottis and supraglottic aperture are flaccid. The epiglottis is sucked into the airway during inspiration.

Etiology and Incidence. The embryologic origin of the defect is unknown. Some children have a degree of inspiratory obstruction even after apparent clinical resolution. Some may develop stridor with respiratory infection, exertion, or crying throughout childhood (Behrman, 1995).

Laryngomalacia is the most common congenital laryngeal defect. It occurs more frequently in males.

Clinical Manifestations

- Noisy, crowing, inspiratory respiratory sounds (stridor) are present.
- **Retractions** may or may not be present.
- Stridor is usually present at birth (may begin as late as age 2 months).
- Symptoms increase when infant is in supine position.

Diagnostic Evaluation. Diagnosis is based on a good history and direct laryngoscopy.

Therapeutic Management. Symptoms usually resolve without treatment by age 18 to 24 months. In rare instances, endotracheal intubation or tracheostomy may be required.

NURSING CARE OF THE INFANT WITH LARYNGOMALACIA

Assessment

The neonate is observed for stridor, retractions, and dyspnea. The nurse notes any signs of acute respiratory distress. Because some infants have feeding problems, the infant should be observed for feeding difficulties.

Nursing Diagnosis and Planning

The following nursing diagnoses and expected outcomes may be appropriate in the treatment of laryngomalacia in the infant.

- Ineffective Breathing Pattern related to partial obstruction of airway. ***Expected Outcome:*** *The infant will have a decrease in stridor.*
- Ineffective Airway Clearance related to congenital weakness of supraglottic structures. ***Expected Outcome:*** *The infant will have no signs of respiratory distress, such as dyspnea, retractions, or restlessness.*
- Anxiety (parental) related to infant's respiratory distress. ***Expected Outcomes:*** *The parents will verbalize an understanding of the child's malformation; verbalize and demonstrate comfort and ease when caring for the infant.*

Implementation

Assessment and documentation of the infant's respiratory status is carried out every 2 hours and as needed. Obstruction increases during crying with respiratory infections, and stridor increases in the supine position when the neck is flexed. The prone position with the neck hyperextended improves the child's breathing. A respiratory tract infection might put undue stress on the infant's system.

As part of discharge teaching, parents are taught the signs of respiratory distress in order to monitor any changes that might indicate infection in the respiratory tract. The ability of the parents to return-demonstrate the teaching should be part of the evaluation of the effectiveness of teaching.

If the child has feeding difficulties, a smaller nipple may be tried. Smaller, more frequent feedings are sometimes better tolerated by infants with respiratory difficulties. The ability of parents to comfortably care for their child indicates effectiveness in the discharge teaching.

Evaluation

- Has the infant's stridor decreased?
- Has the infant's respiratory distress decreased?
- Are the parents able to care for the infant?

Pharyngitis

Pharyngitis, inflammation of the pharynx and surrounding lymphoid tissue, may be viral or bacterial in origin. Although pharyngitis is self-limiting and is a relatively minor disorder, streptococcal infections can have serious complications, such as rheumatic fever and acute glomerular nephritis.

Pathophysiology. The most common organisms causing pharyngitis are viruses and Group A beta-hemolytic streptococci. Pharyngitis often accompanies the common cold. Tonsillitis is usually present with pharyngitis.

Etiology. Viral pharyngitis may be caused by adenovirus, parainfluenza virus, influenza virus, coxsackievirus, and respiratory syncytial virus. Streptococci account for approximately 15% of pharyngitis cases. Streptococcal pharyngitis is rare before age 3 years. Streptococci are spread by close droplet transmission.

Incidence. The most common age for pharyngitis is between 4 and 7 years, when most children begin preschool and school and have increased exposure to microorganisms. Group A beta-hemolytic streptococci infection occurs most frequently in the winter.

Clinical Manifestations. Signs and symptoms differ somewhat between viral and bacterial pharyngitis.

> The only reliable means of determining if pharyngitis is viral or bacterial is with a throat culture.

Not all children with pharyngitis complain of a sore throat, particularly if they are preschool age. Instead the child may complain of a "stomachache" or simply refuse to eat. Table 28–1 compares viral and bacterial pharyngitis.

Diagnostic Evaluation. A throat culture is the most reliable means of distinguishing between viral and bacterial pharyngitis. Because it takes 1 to 2 days to obtain results from a throat culture, more rapid screening tests are often used. If a rapid strep test is negative, a throat culture may be taken. Rapid strep tests have approximately 20% incidence of false-negative results. Because approximately 10% of children carry Group A streptococci in their throats, a positive throat culture is not proof of active infection.

Therapeutic Management. During the acute phase of pharyngitis, the child is kept quiet and given acetaminophen or ibuprofen for pain. Older children may find gargling with warm saline solution comforting. Cool, bland liquids are best tolerated because of the discomfort caused by swallowing solids or irritating liquids.

The use of antibiotics should be restricted to those children who test positive to antigen detection tests or cultures. Streptococcal pharnygitis is best treated orally with penicillin or penicillin V for 10 days. Erythromycin may be used in children who are allergic to pencillin. Children placed on penicillin therapy are noninfectious to others 24 hours after being placed on therapy.

NURSING CARE OF THE CHILD WITH PHARYNGITIS

Assessment

Assessment of the child with pharyngitis includes inspection of the pharynx for the presence of erythema, exudate,

TABLE 28–1 *Comparison of Viral and Bacterial Pharyngitis*

VIRAL PHARYNGITIS	BACTERIAL PHARYNGITIS
Gradual onset	Abrupt onset (may be gradual in children < age 2 years)
Sore throat (reaches a peak on the second or third day)	Sore throat (usually severe)
Erythema and inflammation of the pharynx and tonsils (may be slight), vesicles or ulcers on tonsils	Erythema and inflammation of the pharynx and tonsils
Fever (usually low grade, but may be high)	Fever (usually high, 103–104°F [39.4°–40°C], but may be moderate); begins early in illness and usually lasts 1–4 days
Hoarseness, cough, rhinitis, conjunctivitis, malaise, anorexia (early)	Abdominal pain, vomiting, headache
Cervical lymph nodes may be enlarged and tender	Cervical lymph nodes may be enlarged and tender
Usually lasts 3 to 4 days	Usually lasts 3 to 5 days

or petechiae. The skin should be inspected for rash and color changes. The child is questioned about onset and location of throat, ear, or abdominal pain. In the preverbal child, the parent may report that the child refuses to eat or begins to cry during feedings. The child's temperature and respiratory status are assessed. The child or parent should be asked about onset of symptoms and any known contact with strep in the school or family. The parent should be asked if the child has been taking any antibiotics at home, because this will interfere with the results of the throat culture.

Nursing Diagnosis and Planning

The following nursing diagnoses and expected outcomes may be appropriate in the treatment of pharyngitis in the child.

- Pain related to inflammation. ***Expected Outcome:*** *The child will experience minimal pain, as evidenced by engaging in age-appropriate play.*
- Fluid Volume Deficit related to elevated temperature and difficulty swallowing. ***Expected Outcome:*** *The child will maintain proper fluid balance, as evidenced by adequate urine output for age and moist mucous membranes.*
- Altered Nutrition: Less Than Body Requirements related to difficulty swallowing. ***Expected Outcome:*** *The child will take bland liquids and foods such as ginger ale, jello, puddings, and flavored ice pops.*

Implementation

Comfort measures for the relief of throat discomfort include administration of acetaminophen, warm salt water gargles ($\frac{1}{4}$ tsp salt per 8 oz glass of water), and warm or cool compresses to the throat. The child should not be forced to eat. Cool, bland liquids should be encouraged to prevent dehydration. Soft foods such as gelatin, soup, mashed potatoes, puddings, cream of wheat, and flavored ice pops are tolerated best. Rest in bed is advisable while the child has fever.

Moist mucous membranes and adequate urine output are signs of proper fluid balance. At the end of treatment the child should be free of signs of infection and show no signs of complications of the disease. Instructions for parents are discussed in the Teaching Guidelines box.

Evaluation

- Is the child resting comfortably?
- Is the child well hydrated?
- Is the child eating and drinking bland foods and liquids?

Acute Nasopharyngitis

Acute nasopharyngitis, or the common cold, is a viral infection of the upper respiratory tract. The severity of the infection varies with the age of the child, nutritional and immunologic status, general health, and presence of allergy and stress. Nasopharyngitis is usually self-limiting but can spread to surrounding structures such as the middle ear and the lower respiratory tract.

Pathophysiology. Nasopharyngitis occurs when viruses invade the mucous membranes lining the nose and throat, causing edema, vasodilation, and production of large amounts of mucus.

Etiology. Nasopharyngitis is caused by a variety of viruses. The infection is spread by droplet inhalation or from placing fingers in the mouth or nose after touching contaminated objects. The incubation period is about 2 to 4 days.

Incidence. Nasopharyngitis is the most frequent infectious disease of infants and children. Most children suffer from between six to nine colds each year. Peak times of occurrence are September (at the beginning of school) and in the spring. Crowding, low socioeconomic class, siblings, daycare centers, and exposure to passive smoking are factors that increase risk for upper respiratory infections.

TEACHING GUIDELINES *for Pharyngitis*

- Antibiotics should be taken for entire prescribed course even if the child is feeling better and is free of symptoms.
- Older child may gargle with saline.
- Offer bland, soft foods such as gelatin, soup, puddings, flavored ice pops.
- Apply warm or cool compresses to throat.
- Leftover antibiotics from siblings or friends should not be used.
- The health care provider should be called if the child has difficulty breathing, increased difficulty swallowing, or if fever lasts more than 3 days.
- If any family members develop fever, sore throat, rhinorrhea, or headache, they should have a throat culture.
- A follow-up with repeat throat culture should be done 3 to 5 days after completing the course of antibiotics.

Clinical Manifestations

- Nasal congestion, sneezing
- Nasal discharge (rhinorrhea), at first clear and watery. Secretions may become thick and purulent if a secondary infection develops.
- Low-grade fever in children (fever of 102°F to 104°F [38.8°C to 40°C] in infants, no fever in neonates)
- Cough caused by secretions draining into the throat, especially at night
- Sore throat
- Irritability and restlessness
- Muscular aches and a chilly sensation
- Cervical lymph nodes may be enlarged.
- Infants may become anorexic or refuse feedings because of difficulty sucking and breathing at the same time. Dehydration may result.
- Sometimes vomiting and diarrhea, particularly in infants
- Symptoms usually last about a week and then gradually subside.

Diagnostic Evaluation. Diagnosis is based on history and clinical symptoms. Allergic rhinitis and early manifestations of measles and pertussis have similar symptoms and should be ruled out. Drug abuse, especially of cocaine and marijuana, also cause similar symptoms and may need to be considered in older children and adolescents.

Therapeutic Management. Treatment is directed at relieving symptoms and preventing complications. There are no medications currently available that will cure or shorten the duration of the common cold. Antibiotics are of no value because nasopharyngitis is a viral infection.

The child should rest in bed as long as fever is present. Acetaminophen may be given for fever and discomfort. Aspirin is not recommended because of the risk of Reye syndrome. Liquids are encouraged to prevent dehydration. Sterile normal saline nosedrops may be helpful in relieving nasal congestion. Oral decongestants such as pseudoephedrine (Sudafed) may be used for relief of nasal obstruction for children over age 6 years.

NURSING CARE OF THE CHILD WITH ACUTE NASOPHARYNGITIS

Assessment

The child is observed for the signs and symptoms outlined above. Respirations should be assessed for ease, rate, and depth. The chest should be auscultated for adventitious breath sounds. Special attention is given to hydration status, particularly in infants, because nasal obstruction makes it difficult for infants to suck and breathe at the same time. Fever that persists longer than 72 hours, earache, stiff neck, extreme irritability, or increased respiratory effort should be reported to the physician because these may be indicators of a secondary bacterial infection.

Nursing Diagnosis and Planning

The following nursing diagnoses and expected outcomes may be appropriate in the treatment of acute nasopharygitis in the child.

- Ineffective Airway Clearance related to increased nasal secretions. ***Expected Outcome:*** *The child will breathe through nose and not experience difficult breathing.*
- Sleep Pattern Disturbance related to inability to breathe through the nose. ***Expected Outcome:*** *The child will experience minimal discomfort related to difficulty breathing, as evidenced by ability to rest comfortably.*
- Knowledge Deficit related to misconceptions about the common cold. ***Expected Outcomes:*** *The child/parents will verbalize knowledge of the disease process; demonstrate behaviors that prevent the spread of infection.*

Implementation

Comfort measures are important in caring for the child with nasopharyngitis. A stuffy nose and copious secretions can be relieved with prescribed nosedrops and decongestants. Nosedrops are most helpful when administered 15 minutes before feedings and at bedtime. When administering nosedrops, effectiveness is increased by instilling 2 drops and then waiting 5 minutes before instilling 2 more drops. This causes vasodilation of the posterior as well as the anterior nasal mucous membranes. Parents should be cautioned against using vasoconstrictive decongestant nosedrops for more than 3 days because of the risk of rebound congestion. Bottles of nosedrops and nasal sprays should be used by only one person to prevent spread of infection. A cool mist humidifier at the bedside while the child sleeps may help relieve dryness of the mucous membranes. Cough suppressants are not recommended because they impair removal of secretions, thus increasing the risk of secondary infection.

Fever can be controlled with acetaminophen and increased fluids. Parents may need to be taught how to take the child's temperature and how to measure the correct dose of medication. The child should rest on the bed or sofa until she is afebrile.

Offering the child's favorite fluids or ice pops at frequent intervals may increase fluid intake. The anorexic child should be given small servings of soup, gelatin, or other soft foods, but she should not be forced to eat. Parents may be reassured that this short period of decreased food intake will not harm the child. To make eating easier for the infant, nasal secretions can be removed with a bulb syringe and normal saline nosedrops administered before each feeding. Providing quiet activities that the child enjoys makes compliance with activity restrictions easier.

Parents and children should be taught methods of preventing the spread of infection such as careful handwashing, proper disposal of tissues, covering mouth and nose while sneezing, and other basic hygiene measures.

Evaluation

- Is the child able to breathe through her nose?
- Is the child able to breathe more easily at night and sleep without waking?
- Can the family verbalize both care and prevention of nasopharyngitis?

Influenza

Influenza or *flu* are terms used to describe a viral infection that causes an illness with a broad spectrum of clinical responses and significant morbidity and mortality in children.

Pathophysiology. The main area of involvement in children is the mucous membrane of the respiratory tract, which shows extensive destruction of its ciliated epithelium. There may be marked desquamation of the tracheal epithelium near the onset of symptoms. Although the main pathology is in the respiratory system, the heart, brain, or lymphoid tissues are occasionally involved in fatal cases.

Etiology. Influenza is caused by the orthomyxovirus family. There are three influenza virus types: A, B, and C.

Respiratory secretions of infected children contain large amounts of the virus; the infection is transmitted directly from person to person by the airborne route or by fomites.

Incidence. Influenza morbidity is highest in school-age children. Infants are also a high-risk group. Pandemic influenza occurs every 10 to 40 years, epidemics of lesser severity occur every 2 to 3 years.

Clinical Manifestations

- Chills and fever
- Flushed face
- Myalgia
- Cough
- Headache
- Sore throat, usually associated with pharyngitis
- Nasal stuffiness
- Photophobia
- Conjunctivitis (mild)
- Rhinitis

Younger children may present with manifestations of other respiratory viruses (parainfluenza virus, respiratory syncytial virus, rhinovirus, and adenovirus), making it difficult to identify the causative organisms. See the descriptions of the manifestations of each of these conditions in this chapter.

Diagnostic Evaluation. Diagnosis is based on clinical manifestations and throat cultures.

Therapeutic Management. Amantadine hydrochloride (Symmetrel) is used in the treatment of influenza A viruses and can be effective when given early in the course of the disease. Ribavirin (Virazole) is active against both influenza A and B viruses.

An inactivated influenza vaccine can be given to children older than 6 months of age in chronic care facilities or those that have other chronic diseases. The American Committee on Immunization Practices publishes specific guidelines for its use.

Bed rest is encouraged and physical activities are restricted. Fluids are encouraged and nonsalicylate antipyretics given for excessive fever. Prophylactic administration of antibiotics is discouraged.

NURSING CARE OF THE CHILD WITH INFLUENZA

The nursing care of the child with influenza includes the measures found in the sections on pharyngitis, nasopharyngitis, and bronchiolitis.

Tonsillitis

Tonsillitis is the term commonly used to describe inflammation and infection of the two palatine tonsils. *Adenoiditis* refers to infection and inflammation of the pharyngeal tonsils, or adenoids, which are located above the palatine tonsils on the posterior wall of the nasopharynx. The purpose of these lymphoid tissues is to filter and protect the respiratory and digestive tracts from invasion by pathogens, but often the tonsils become a site for infection.

Pathophysiology. Infection and inflammation of the tonsils cause them to enlarge. The palatine tonsils may meet in the midline ("kissing tonsils") and cause difficulty swallowing and breathing. If adenoids enlarge they can obstruct the eustachian tubes, resulting in otitis media and hearing impairment. Hypertrophy of the adenoids can also block the passageway between the nose and the throat, causing mouth breathing or obstructive sleep apnea.

Etiology. The cause of tonsillitis, like pharyngitis, may be bacterial or viral. The most common bacterial agents are Group A beta-hemolytic streptococci.

Incidence. Tonsillitis is very common among preschool and young school-age children. Incidence of tonsillitis decreases during middle childhood with normal shrinkage of lymphoid tissue.

Clinical Manifestations. (See also clinical manifestations of pharyngitis.)

- Sore throat; may be persistent or recurrent
- Tonsils enlarged, bright red; may be covered with white exudate or cryptic plugs
- Difficulty swallowing
- Mouth breathing and unpleasant mouth odor
- Fever
- Cough
- *Enlarged adenoids* may cause nasal quality of speech, mouth breathing, hearing difficulty, otitis media, snoring, or obstructive sleep apnea.

Diagnostic Evaluation. The causative agent is identified by a throat culture. A complete blood count with differential, bleeding and clotting profiles, and urinalysis are ordered prior to surgery.

Therapeutic Management. Tonsillitis may be treated medically or surgically. Medical treatment is the same as for pharyngitis and consists of comfort measures and antibiotics for bacterial tonsillitis.

Surgical removal of the tonsils, or tonsillectomy, is controversial. Although some physicians think that a tonsillectomy is warranted in cases of recurrent tonsillitis, the prevailing attitude is more conservative, reserving the procedure for cases of upper airway obstruction, peritonsillar abscess, obstructive sleep apnea, or other serious problems. Tonsillectomy is generally not performed in children younger than age 3 years because of the tendency for remaining tonsillar tissues to hypertrophy. Contraindications to tonsillectomy include active infection and cleft palate. Surgical removal of the tonsils while they are infected may result in spread of the infecting organism and sepsis. In children with cleft palate the tonsils help prevent air escape during speech. Adenoidectomy alone may be performed in cases of recurrent otitis media secondary to eustachian tube obstruction or for persistent nasal or airway obstruction.

Many parents believe that a tonsillectomy will solve their child's problems of frequent sore throats, mouth breathing, and poor weight gain. There is no evidence that a tonsillectomy reduces the incidence of recurrent pharyngitis. The nurse should be prepared to discuss the current treatment philosophy with parents and address their concerns. If tonsillectomy is chosen as the method of treatment, the procedure is often done in a day surgery setting.

PREOPERATIVE NURSING CARE OF THE CHILD UNDERGOING TONSILLECTOMY

Assessment

A complete history is taken and special attention is given to allergy symptoms, difficulty swallowing, or airway obstruction. The child is assessed for signs of active infection (fever, elevated white blood cell [WBC] count) and redness and exudate of the throat. The child should be questioned about the presence of pain in the throat or ears. Because the tonsillar area is so vascular, any bleeding history must be documented and communicated to the primary physician.

Laboratory results (prothrombin time, partial thromboplastin time, platelet count, hemoglobin, hematocrit, urinalysis) are reviewed and the child should be observed for loose teeth to decrease risk of aspiration during surgery.

Nursing Diagnosis and Planning

The following nursing diagnoses and expected outcomes may be appropriate in the treatment of the child undergoing a tonsillectomy.

- Anxiety related to surgery. ***Expected Outcome:*** *The child/parents will exhibit a decreased level of anxiety, as evidenced by relaxed body posture and involvement in play activities.*
- Knowledge Deficit related to surgery and procedures. ***Expected Outcome:*** *The child/parents will verbalize understanding of preoperative teaching.*

Implementation

The child should be reassured that he will still be able to talk after surgery. It should also be explained that although the child's throat will be sore after surgery, he will need to drink liquids. (See also Preoperative Care, Chapter 15.)

POSTOPERATIVE NURSING CARE OF THE CHILD UNDERGOING TONSILLECTOMY

Assessment

Immediately after surgery the child should be assessed for bleeding and for ability to swallow secretions. If bleeding occurs, the child is returned to surgery for recauterization.

Nursing Diagnosis and Planning

The following nursing diagnoses and expected outcomes may be appropriate in the treatment of the child who has undergone a tonsillectomy.

- Risk for Injury (hemorrhage) related to surgery. ***Expected Outcome:*** *The child will experience minimal postoperative bleeding.*
- Ineffective Airway Clearance related to throat discomfort. ***Expected Outcome:*** *The child will maintain a clear airway.*
- Pain related to surgical removal of tonsils. ***Expected Outcome:*** *The child will be comfortable and be able to rest.*
- Risk for Fluid Volume Deficit related to difficulty swallowing and NPO status before surgery. ***Expected***

Outcome: *The child will have adequate fluid intake for age and will experience minimal fluid loss.*

- Knowledge Deficit related to home care. ***Expected Outcome:*** *The parents will verbalize an understanding of the care of their child at home.*

Implementation

The child should be placed in a prone or side-lying position to facilitate drainage. The rate and quality of respirations and breath sounds should be assessed. Vital signs, including blood pressure, should be monitored frequently. (A common protocol is every 15 minutes for the first hour, hourly for 4 hours, and then every 2 to 4 hours for the next 24 hours). Suction equipment should be available, but do not suction unless there is airway obstruction. Although not all clinicians are in agreement, straws and forks may be withheld to prevent trauma to the surgical site.

The child is assessed for bleeding (frequent swallowing; restlessness; fast, thready pulse; vomiting bright red blood). Carefully using a tongue blade, inspect the pharynx with a good light source for clots or bleeding. If bleeding occurs, the child is turned to the side, and the physician notified.

Vomiting of old blood (coffee ground emesis) is common. Antiemetics are given as ordered to decrease throat pain caused by retching. If vomiting occurs, keep the child NPO for 30 minutes and then resume clear liquids.

Nonaspirin analgesics (e.g., acetaminophen) are given as ordered. Adequate analgesia increases fluid intake. Some centers give the analgesic every 4 hours for the first 24 hours because throat discomfort is expected. An ice collar can be applied for comfort.

Provide clear, cool liquids when the child is fully awake. Avoid citrus, carbonated, and extremely hot or cold liquids because they may irritate the throat. Milk and milk products (puddings, ice cream) are avoided initially until the child is tolerating clear liquids well. This is done because milk products can coat the throat and cause the child to clear his throat, thus increasing the risk of bleeding. Adequate fluid intake promotes healing and maintains hydration. See Teaching Guidelines for information regarding home care.

Evaluation

- Does the child have minimal bleeding, nausea, and vomiting?
- Is the child's intake and urine output normal for age?
- Are the child's complaints of pain and/or level of irritability minimal?
- Are vital signs within normal limits?

Croup

Croup is a term used to describe a group of conditions characterized by inspiratory stridor, a harsh (brassy or croupy) cough, hoarseness, and varying degrees of respiratory distress. The major types of croup include acute spasmodic croup, laryngotracheobronchitis (LTB), bacterial tracheitis, and epiglottitis. Although epiglottitis is a type of croup, it is discussed separately because it is a bacterial infection with unique symptoms and treatment. (Table 28–2 compares types of croup.)

TEACHING GUIDELINES ***Following Tonsillectomy***

- Quiet activities for a week after surgery.
- Encourage abundant liquid intake. Avoid citrus juices, which irritate the throat, for 10 days.
- Avoid red liquids, which will give the appearance of blood if the child vomits.
- Add full liquids (cream soups, gelatin, puddings, soups) on the second day and soft foods (mashed potatoes, soft cereals, eggs) as the child tolerates them. Avoid rough or scratchy foods (bacon, chips, popcorn), citrus foods, or spicy foods for 3 weeks.
- The child should be encouraged to chew and swallow, because this exercises pharyngeal muscles and promotes healing.
- Do not give the child any straws, forks, or sharp pointed toys that could be put in the mouth.
- Use acetaminophen; the child may have a prescription for acetaminophen with codeine for sore throat. Do not use aspirin or any medicine containing aspirin, which may affect the clotting time of the blood.
- Pain should not persist past the first week. Notify physician if this occurs.
- Discourage the child from coughing, clearing the throat, or gargling.
- Bad mouth odor is normal and may be relieved by drinking more liquids.
- Earache and slight fever are common.
- Call the physician for any bleeding, persistent earache, or fever over 101°F (38.5°C).
- Bleeding or pain may occur in 7–10 days after surgery. Such bleeding requires immediate medical attention. The risk for bleeding is due to tissue sloughing during the healing process.
- Keep the child away from crowds or places where he may catch a cold for 2 weeks.
- The child may return to school when directed by the physician. This is usually in about 10 days.
- Bring the child for a follow-up appointment in 1–2 weeks.

PATHOPHYSIOLOGY *of Croup*

Croup is a viral infection of the upper airway. Although the entire upper, or nonreactive, airway is involved to some extent in all forms of croup, each type is named according to the anatomic area most severely involved. For example, LTB affects the larynx, trachea, and bronchi. In acute spasmodic croup, the larynx is the area of most severe inflammation.

In all forms of croup, mucosal inflammation and edema cause narrowing of the airway. This narrowing is more dangerous in infants and young children than in adults because of their small airway diameter and flexible larynx, which is more susceptible to spasm.

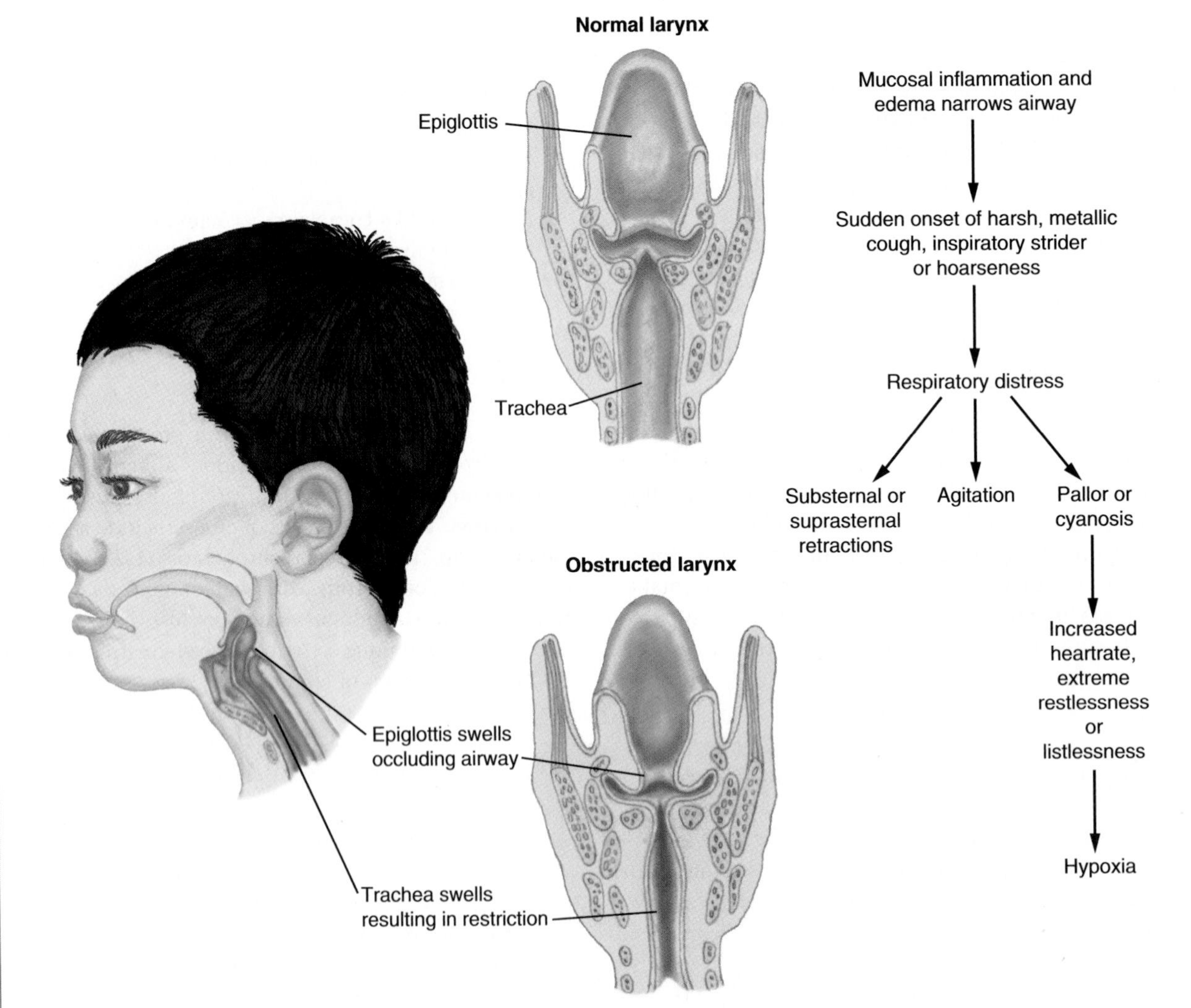

Etiology and Incidence. Parainfluenza viruses cause the majority of cases of viral croup. The cause of acute spasmodic croup is unknown.

Laryngotracheobronchitis, the most frequent form, usually affects infants and toddlers. LTB is the most common cause of airway obstruction in children age 6 months to 6 years. Males have a higher incidence of croup. The disease occurs more often during the winter.

Acute spasmodic croup occurs most often in children age 1 to 3 years. Spasmodic croup occurs more often in anxious and excitable children. There seems to be hereditary predisposition to spasmodic croup.

Bacterial tracheitis is less common than LTB and acute spasmodic croup. It progresses from an upper respiratory infection and may be confused with LTB because of the similarity of manifestations. The child does not respond to treatment for LTB if he has bacterial tracheitis.

The following discussion will focus on LTB, the most common type of croup requiring hospitalization, and acute spasmodic croup. See Table 28–2 for other types of croup.

TABLE 28–2 *Comparison of Types of Croup*

	ACUTE SPASMODIC LARYNGITIS (SPASMODIC CROUP)	ACUTE LARYNGOTRACHEO-BRONCHITIS (LTB)	ACUTE EPIGLOTTITIS	ACUTE BACTERIAL TRACHEITIS
Age Usually Affected	1 to 3 years	3 months to 3 years	3 to 8 years	1 month to 6 years
Location of Swelling and Inflammation	Subglottic (below the vocal cords)	Vocal cords, subglottic, and tissue below vocal cords, including bronchi	Supraglottic (above the vocal cords)	Mucosa of the upper trachea
Cause	Viral, emotional, or genetic predisposition	Usually viral, but may be bacterial	Bacterial (usually *H. influenzae*, type B)	*Staphylococcus* (most common)
Assessment	Sudden onset, usually at night Child awakens with harsh cough, inspiratory stridor, dyspnea, and hoarseness	Gradual onset, usually at night Child awakens with harsh cough and inspiratory stridor	Sudden onset, which may rapidly progress to complete airway obstruction and death Sore throat, dyspnea	Progresses from upper respiratory infection (1–2 days) High fever Stridor Croupy cough Purulent secretions
Treatment	Humidity Increased fluids May treat at home	Humidity Racemic epinephrine IV fluids during respiratory distress Hospitalization may be necessary	IV antibiotics Artificial airway IV fluids Emergency hospitalization	Humidified oxygen Antipyretics IV antibiotics May require intubation

Clinical Manifestations

- Often begins at night and may be preceded by several days of upper respiratory infection symptoms
- Sudden onset of harsh, metallic cough; sore throat; inspiratory stridor and hoarseness
- Use of accessory muscles (substernal, intercostal, suprasternal retractions)
- Frightened appearance
- Agitation
- Usually low-grade fever; occasionally fever as high as 104°F (40°C)
- Symptoms usually worse at night and better in the day; may recur for several nights
- Cyanosis

Diagnostic Evaluation. Diagnosis is made mainly from observation of clinical symptoms. Differentiation between viral croup and bacterial epiglottitis is very important, as treatment varies between the two. However, the use of the *H. influenzae* b (Hib) vaccine has reduced the incidence of epiglottitis. A croup score is often used to describe severity of respiratory distress. ABGs and/or pulse oximetry may be monitored to detect decreased Po_2 levels.

Therapeutic Management. The goal of treatment is to maintain a patent airway. Children with acute spasmodic croup can usually be cared for at home. Treatment for acute spasmodic croup includes mist and increased oral fluid intake. Steam from hot running water in a closed bathroom and cool mist from a bedside humidifier are effective in decreasing mucosal edema. Cool mist humidifiers are recommended over steam vaporizers, which present a danger of scald burns. Taking the child out into the cool, humid night air may also relieve mucosal swelling. Crying aggravates the airway obstruction. If the child develops stridor at rest, cyanosis, severe agitation/fatigue, or moderate to severe retractions, or is unable to take oral fluids, he should be seen in the emergency department.

Children with LTB, usually a more severe type of croup, are hospitalized more often than those with acute spasmodic croup. Nebulized racemic epinephrine may be given to decrease laryngeal edema and bronchospasm. The child must be closely observed for changes in respiratory status and should not be treated with epinephrine on an outpatient basis because the effects of epinephrine are temporary. Children who receive epinephrine should be observed in the emergency department for 2 to 3 hours after treatment and should not be discharged if stridor or retractions are present. Corticosteroid therapy may be used in hospitalized children with croup to reduce inflammatory edema and prevent destruction of ciliated epithelium. Antibiotics are not indicated unless a bacterial infection is present. Acetaminophen is given to reduce fever.

A mist hood may be used for an infant; a mist tent for older children. However, if this distresses the child, cool mist in the room may be more effective. Intravenous fluids may be given until respiratory distress subsides and the child can take adequate fluids by mouth. Sedatives are contraindicated because they depress respirations and could mask restlessness, an early sign of hypoxia.

If signs of moderate or severe hypoxia develop, the child is intubated immediately. Usually the tube remains in place from 3 to 5 days and is removed when the child can breathe around the tube.

NURSING CARE OF THE CHILD WITH CROUP

Assessment

A nursing history typically reveals a recent upper respiratory infection. The child should be assessed for inspiratory stridor, barking cough, and hoarseness. Heart rate and respiratory rate should be assessed. Signs of respiratory distress such as use of accessory muscles; substernal, intercostal, and suprasternal retractions; **nasal flaring;** restlessness and irritability; and pallor or cyanosis should be noted. Cyanosis, increased heart and respiratory rate, extreme restlessness, or evidence of fatigue or listlessness may be signs of hypoxia and should be reported immediately. Breath sounds should be auscultated for adventitious sounds or areas of decreased breath sounds. Temperature and hydration status should also be assessed.

Nursing Diagnoses

- Ineffective Airway Clearance related to mucosal swelling and obstruction of the upper respiratory tract
- Risk for Fluid Volume Deficit related to inadequate oral intake and tachypnea
- Fear related to dyspnea and hospitalization
- Knowledge Deficit related to course of croup and home care

Planning, Implementation, and Evaluation: The Child With Croup

NURSING DIAGNOSIS
- Ineffective Airway Clearance related to mucosal swelling and obstruction of the upper respiratory tract

Expected Outcome:
- The child will breathe without difficulty.
- The child will have heart and respiratory rates within normal limits for age.

Intervention	Rationale
1. Assess child's breathing continuously for signs and symptoms of increased respiratory distress (increased respiratory rate, stridor at rest, nasal flaring, retractions, cyanosis, changes in level of consciousness or increased irritability, decreased or adventitious breath sounds, tachypnea). a. *Never* leave a child with respiratory distress alone. b. Monitor vital signs hourly and as necessary. c. Monitor ABGs or pulse oximetry. d. Notify physician of increased respiratory distress.	The child must be monitored closely to detect early signs of worsening obstruction. Extreme restlessness, listlessness, cyanosis, or a rapid, increasing respiratory rate with an increased heart rate are signs of hypoxia. Increased stridor may be a sign of increasing inflammation. However, decreased stridor may also be an ominous sign, because with severe obstruction not enough air may be able to pass through the larynx to cause loud stridor.
e. If epiglottitis is suspected, call a physician and do not visualize the throat	Visualization may result in laryngospasm and airway obstruction.
2. Provide high humidity as ordered via mist tent or hood. Provide cool, not cold, mist.	High humidity helps liquefy secretions and decreases mucosal edema. Cool mist is also effective in reducing fever. Cold mist may precipitate bronchospasm.
3. Administer O_2 at ordered flow rate. Monitor O_2 concentration (FiO_2) in tent every 2 hours. Monitor ABGs or transcutaneous oxygen concentration frequently.	Oxygen may be ordered to alleviate hypoxia and restlessness. The child's condition must be monitored closely because oxygen use may mask early signs of hypoxia and increasing obstruction.
4. Have emergency intubation equipment (e.g., intubation tray, oxygen, suction, manual resuscitation bag, valve, and mask) closely available.	The child's condition can change rapidly, and respiratory arrest from airway obstruction can occur.

Intervention	Rationale
5. Administer aerosolized racemic epinephrine, as ordered. Assess response to medication. Monitor for tachycardia.	Racemic epinephrine decreases layngeal edema. Tachycardia is a side effect of adrenergic medications. The effect of racemic epinephrine lasts less than 2 hours. Children should be observed for rebound obstruction, which may occur within a few hours after administration of racemic epinephrine.
6. Keep child as quiet as possible. Encourage parent to stay nearby or even to climb inside the mist tent with the child if the child is frightened and refuses to stay inside the tent. If the use of a tent or hood is causing distress, treatment may be more effective if the child is held by a parent and cool mist is directed toward the child's face. Maintain a calm, quiet environment. Provide a security object for the child. Observe the child closely but disturb as little as possible.	Crying aggravates laryngospasm and increases hypoxia. The parent's presence is an effective supportive measure for frightened, agitated infants and children. Anxiety and crying increase the airway obstruction of croup.
7. Support child in an upright position with the head of the bed elevated or with the child being held by the parent.	An upright position facilitates respirations by decreasing pressure from abdominal contents on the diaphragm.

Evaluation: The child will have respiratory and heart rates within normal limits for age, pink mucous membranes and nailbeds, and clear breath sounds with effective air movement.

NURSING DIAGNOSIS • Risk for Fluid Volume Deficit related to inadequate oral intake and tachypnea

Expected Outcome: • The child will drink adequate fluid for age and weight.

Intervention	Rationale
1. Monitor hydration status with intake and output measurements and urine specific gravity. Check mucous membranes, skin turgor, and presence of tears. Weigh daily on same scale and at same time of day.	Increased respiratory rate causes insensible water loss and difficulty swallowing leads to decreased intake.
2. Offer clear liquids as tolerated.	Fluids are encouraged to decrease edema and to decrease viscosity of secretions. Fluids may be given orally if stridor is mild and the child is not tachypneic. Increased oral fluids and a regular diet are offered as soon as the child's condition improves.
3. Give liquids at room temperature.	Cold liquids may increase respiratory distress.
4. Assess child's ability to swallow, observing for respiratory distress.	Tachypnea and laryngospasm often cause dysphagia.
5. Administer IV fluids at ordered rate. Use IV tubing with graduated fluid control chamber to guard against accidental infusion of large volumes of fluid.	Intravenous fluids may be ordered during the acute phase of croup to prevent dehydration. Oral fluids are contraindicated in the presence of severe respiratory distress because of the risk of aspiration and the increased stress put on the systems of the body.

Intervention	Rationale
6. Administer acetaminophen for fever as ordered. Monitor temperature every 4 hours.	Fever increases insensible water loss by increasing metabolic rate.

Evaluation:
- The child will have urine output appropriate for age.
- The child will have urine specific gravity of 1.002 to 1.030.
- The child will have moist mucous membranes.

NURSING DIAGNOSIS
- Fear related to dyspnea and hospitalization

Expected Outcome:
- The child will be less anxious, as evidenced by resting quietly in the mist tent, crying less, and cooperating with nursing care as appropriate for age.
- The parents' anxiety will be decreased, as evidenced by their ability to assist the child to deal with stressors of hospitalization and illness.

Intervention	Rationale
1. Maintain a calm, restful environment. Organize nursing care so as to disturb child as little as possible. Postpone unnecessary procedures until the child is in less distress. Allow for periods of uninterrupted rest.	Anxiety and crying increase oxygen consumption and respiratory distress.
2. Encourage parents to touch and cuddle the child. Toddlers and infants like to be held when they are ill. Parents should be told it is acceptable to sit inside the mist tent with their child. Children who are not in tents can be held in their parents' arms while mist is directed toward their faces.	Parental presence is important in reducing anxiety in infants and young children.
3. Encourage parents' participation in care. Explain ways that they can make their child more comfortable and tell them that their presence is important.	Parents' feelings of helplessness and anxiety are decreased when they are allowed to comfort and care for their child. Participation in the child's care also helps prepare the parents for discharge and home care.
4. Provide parents with breaks as needed and assure them that their child will be cared for in their absence.	Caring for a child in the hospital is exhausting to parents. Fatigue magnifies feelings of anxiety and helplessness.
5. Allow favorite toy or blanket in mist tent.	Familiar objects provide a sense of security for small children in the strange hospital environment.
6. Explain all treatments, equipment, and procedures to child and parents.	Anxiety and fear related to lack of knowledge can be minimized by providing clear and timely explanations.
7. Allow child and parents to ask questions and to discuss fears and concerns.	Cooperation is increased with understanding of the purpose of treatments. Parents are often very anxious because of the sudden onset and frightening nature of croup symptoms. Parents sometimes feel guilty for not having brought the child in for treatment sooner.
8. Use developmentally appropriate communication techniques (e.g., play, puppets, etc.).	A calm, empathetic, and caring approach is helpful in providing emotional support to the child and parents.

Evaluation:
- The child will remain in the mist tent without signs of agitation or being upset (less crying) and will allow nursing staff to touch, hold, and interact with him.
- The child will demonstrate adequate rest/sleep patterns by not waking up during the night and show no signs of fatigue or irritability.
- The child will engage in age-appropriate play.
- The parent will comfort the child.

NURSING DIAGNOSIS
- Knowledge Deficit related to course of croup and home care

Expected Outcome:
- Parents will have accurate knowledge of croup symptoms, be comfortable in home management of croup, and will seek assistance appropriately if symptoms become severe.

Intervention	Rationale
1. Assess parents' level of understanding of croup and previous experiences in coping with the illness. Teach parents that once a child has had an attack, croup tends to reoccur. Teach that maintaining stable environmental temperature and humidity and keeping the child well hydrated may be helpful in decreasing severity of attacks. Teach that croup is a viral infection, and avoiding large groups of people and practicing good health habits to prevent infection may decrease recurrence of croup.	Croup symptoms tend to occur at night, clearing in the morning and then recurring for several nights. Croup usually clears within a few days with no complications. Croup often follows an upper respiratory infection in the croup-prone child.
2. Teach parents the signs and symptoms of respiratory distress. Parents should be taught how to count respirations and how to assess for retractions and cyanosis. a. The child should be closely observed at all times for worsening of his condition, which can occur rapidly. b. Parents should call the doctor if the following occur: • the child has increased difficulty breathing or seems to be getting worse • the child has retractions (tugging in of the skin between, above, or below the ribs) • the child's lips turn bluish or dusky • breathing cool or warm mist does not improve symptoms in 20 minutes • the child has not been able to drink much in the past 24 hours • the child drools or has difficulty swallowing • the child has fever (over 103°F [39.4°C]) • the child seems exhausted, listless, or very agitated.	Parents should be taught appropriate treatment of the child with croup and when to seek medical attention.
3. Explain the importance of providing a humidified environment in treating croup symptoms. Ways to provide humidity include the following: a. Hold and cuddle the child in a steamy bathroom for at least 10 minutes or until symptoms are relieved. Run all the hot water faucets full force with the door closed.	High humidity helps thin secretions and decrease swelling.

Intervention	Rationale
b. Place a humidifier beside the child's bed. A cool mist humidifier, rather than a steam vaporizer, is recommended because of the danger of the child pulling the machine over and burning himself. c. Take the child outside into the cool, moist night air. Opening the freezer door can also be effective.	
4. Explain the importance of adequate hydration and nutrition. The child needs to drink 2 to 4 glasses (500 to 1,000 ml) of fluids daily. Sips of warm fluids during a croup attack help relax the vocal cords and thin mucus.	Adequate hydration is important in thinning secretions. Adequate caloric intake helps replace calories expended fighting the infection.
5. Give acetaminophen for fever. Do *not* give cough syrup or cold medicines.	Acetaminophen is effective in reducing fever and will help the child feel more comfortable. Cough syrups and cold medicines may dry and thicken secretions.
6. After warm mist therapy and some clear liquids, if the child can go back to sleep, run a humidifier at the bedside and check on the child periodically throughout the night. Call the physician immediately if the child seems worse of if he does not seem better in 48 hours.	Close observation is essential to detect worsening of croup symptoms. Worsening of symptoms will not necessarily awaken the child.

Evaluation: Parents are able to explain appropriate treatment of croup and when medical attention is needed.

Epiglottitis (Supraglottitis)

Epiglottitis, acute inflammation and swelling of the epiglottis and surrounding tissue, is a life-threatening, rapidly progressing condition that may cause complete airway obstruction within a few hours of onset.

Etiology and Incidence. Epiglottitis is almost always caused by *Haemophilus influenzae.* Other organisms, such as *Staphylococcus aureus, Haemophilus parainfluenzae, Streptococcus pneumoniae,* and beta-hemolytic streptococci, cause the infection less frequently. Viral epiglottitis is rare.

Epiglottitis occurs most often in children aged 3 to 7 years. Incidence is equal between males and females. The incidence has decreased because of the use of the Hib vaccine.

Clinical Manifestations

- Abrupt onset, rapid progression of symptoms. Often parents report that the child was put to bed well and awakened with a severe sore throat and difficulty swallowing.
- High fever (102.2° to 104°F [39° to 40°C]). Child appears toxic and very ill.
- Sore throat (can progress from a mild sore throat to acute respiratory distress in a few hours)

FOUR Ds OF EPIGLOTTITIS

- Drooling
- Dysphagia (difficulty swallowing)
- Dysphonia (difficulty talking)
- Distressed inspiratory efforts (Nemes, Schmidt, & Kelly, 1988)

- Child appears anxious and frightened; may be irritable or lethargic
- Child insists on sitting upright, often in a tripod position (leaning forward supported by arms, chin thrust out, mouth open).
- Nasal flaring
- Suprasternal, substernal, and intercostal retractions
- Tachycardia
- Pale skin color to cyanosis (depending on degree of airway obstruction)
- Edematous, cherry-red epiglottis
- Elevated WBC count (20,000 to 30,000 mm^3)

Diagnostic Evaluation. The most reliable diagnostic sign of epiglottitis is an edematous, cherry-red epiglottis. However, examination and visualization of the epiglottis is contraindicated until emergency intubation equipment and

PATHOPHYSIOLOGY *of Epiglottitis*

Epiglottitis is a bacterial form of croup. The epiglottis and surrounding structures become inflamed as bacterial infection invades the soft tissue. The epiglottis becomes edematous and cherry red, and may become so swollen that it completely covers the glottis and obstructs the airway. Secretions pool in the hypopharynx and larynx. As the disease rapidly progresses, swelling becomes so severe that the child is unable to swallow and begins to drool. The child's voice is muffled and the throat is very sore. Inspiratory stridor, cough, and irritability are present. Complete airway obstruction can occur rapidly, resulting in hypoxia, acidosis, and death.

Onset of epiglottitis is usually sudden. The child may have had symptoms of a mild upper respiratory infection for a few days before symptoms began. Children with epiglottitis can progress from wellness to complete airway obstruction within 2 to 6 hours.

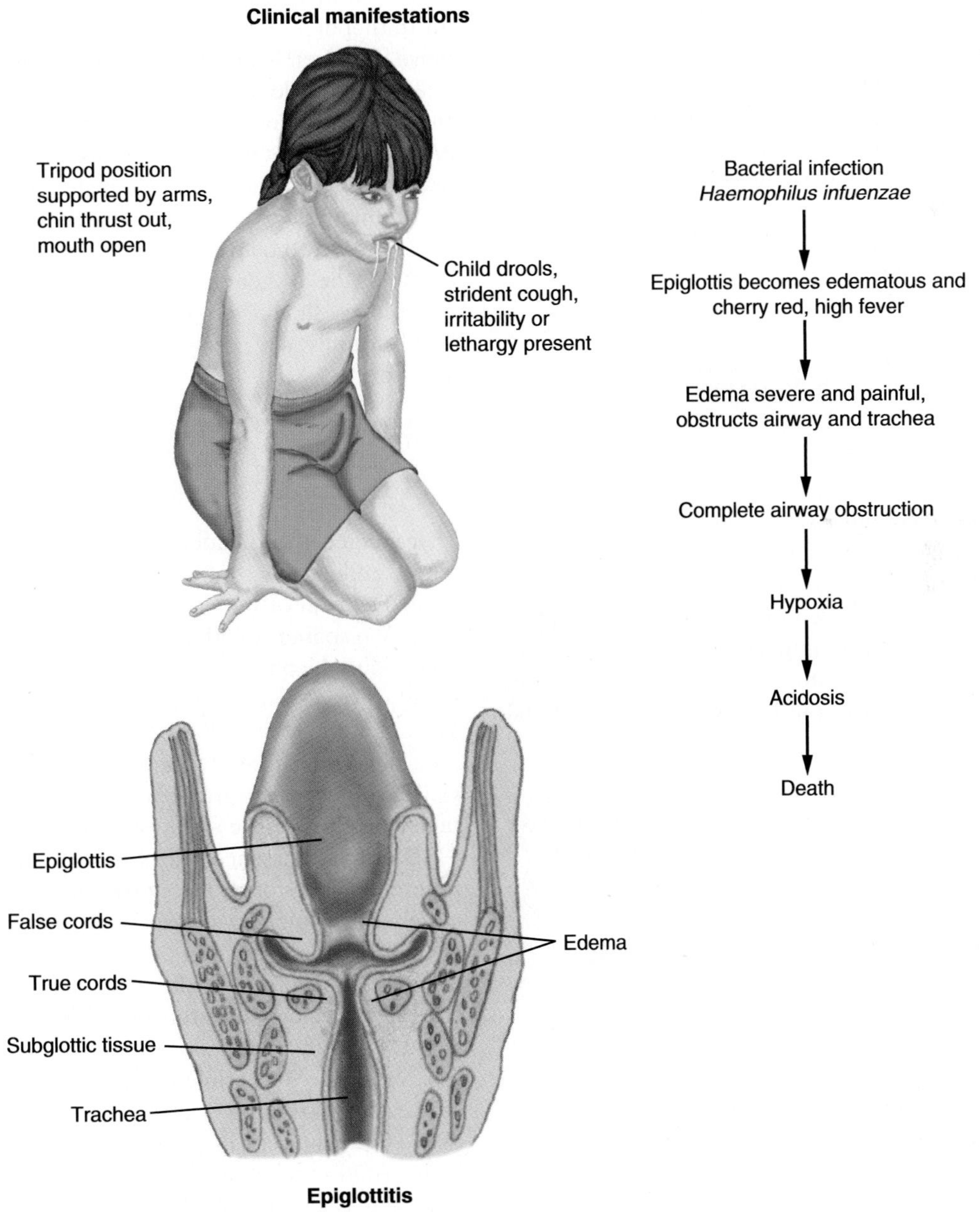

Epiglottitis

qualified personnel are available to support the child in case of laryngospasm and airway obstruction.

Therapeutic Management. The main objective of treatment for epiglottitis is to achieve a patent airway as quickly as possible. The child with epiglottitis has an edematous epiglottis which may completely obstruct the airway at any time. X-rays are best taken at the bedside, where the child can be constantly monitored and emergency equipment is readily available. The danger of airway obstruction is so great that usually all invasive procedures such as venipuncture are postponed until the child is intubated. Once the airway is secured the child is transferred to the intensive care unit. Oxygenation status is closely monitored with ABGs or pulse oximetry, and humidified oxygen is administered. Mechanical ventilation is sometimes used.

Antibiotics are administered for 7 to 10 days. Throat and blood cultures are taken after the child is intubated. Antipyretics are given for fever.

Usually the child improves dramatically after 48 hours of antibiotic therapy and can be extubated at this time. Discharge is in about 3 to 7 days and the child is sent home on oral antibiotics.

NURSING CARE OF THE CHILD WITH EPIGLOTTITIS

Assessment

The nurse should continuously assess for signs of respiratory distress (stridor, nasal flaring, tachypnea, tachycardia, retractions, drooling, changes in level of consciousness, cyanosis). A sudden decrease in respiratory efforts may be a sign of exhaustion and impending respiratory arrest. ABGs and pulse oximetry are monitored. Pulse oximetry should remain ≥95%, with the PaO_2 between 80 and 100 mmHg.

> The throat of a child with suspected epiglottitis should not be examined or cultured, because any stimulation with a tongue depressor or culture swab could cause laryngospasm and complete airway obstruction.

Nursing Diagnosis and Planning

The following nursing diagnoses and expected outcomes may be appropriate in the treatment of epiglottitis in the child.

- Ineffective Breathing Pattern related to edema of the epiglottis. ***Expected Outcomes:*** *The child will have respiratory rate and rhythm within normal limits; breathe without difficulty.*
- Ineffective Airway Clearance related to placement of artificial airway. ***Expected Outcomes:*** *The child will have respiratory effort within normal limits; maintain skin color within normal limits.*
- Fear related to respiratory distress. ***Expected Outcome:*** *The child will demonstrate relaxed body posture and have adequate rest and sleep.*

Implementation

The primary aim of nursing care is to maintain a patent airway. It is essential that the nurse keep the child as calm and quiet as possible. If temperature is taken, it should be by the axillary and not the oral route. The child should be supported in a position of comfort, usually sitting straight up (orthopnic). The child should never be forced to lie down. Children who are anxious and are in respiratory distress are often less fearful on their parents' laps. Parents should be encouraged to hug and comfort their child. Parents' anxiety level must be assessed and controlled because their anxiety is easily transferred to the child.

Humidified oxygen is delivered in high concentrations. Oxygen therapy is usually less upsetting if the parent holds the oxygen tubing in front of the child's face. All procedures should be explained to parent and child clearly, calmly, and according to the child's level of understanding.

> The child with suspected epiglottitis must never be left unattended.

Emergency intubation equipment (oxygen, laryngoscope, endotracheal tube, suction equipment) should be immediately available in case of complete airway obstruction. Worsening of the child's condition should be reported to the physician immediately.

Antipyretics are given for fever. Because of the risk of aspiration, the child is kept NPO and fluids are given IV. The nurse must closely monitor the ordered IV rate as well as urine specific gravity and other indicators of hydration. IV antibiotics are administered as ordered.

If the child has an artificial airway, either endotracheal tube or tracheostomy, the nurse must observe the child closely for respiratory distress and suction the airway as needed. The endotracheal tube must be securely taped to decrease movement of the tube and to minimize the chance of accidental extubation. The child, once intubated, must be restrained to prevent accidental extubation. It may be impossible to reintubate the child because of the severe swelling of the epiglottis. The endotracheal tube is usually kept in place for approximately 24 to 36 hours. After extubation, the child must be watched carefully and is usually placed in a mist tent for 24 hours before being transferred to a pediatric unit. Normal respiratory rate and rhythm and normal color serve as evaluation criteria.

Because epiglottitis progresses rapidly and acute respiratory distress is frightening, both parents and child have high anxiety levels. The nurse should care for the child calmly and efficiently and offer the family much-needed support during hospitalization. Upon discharge the parents need to be instructed how to administer the child's oral antibiotics. They should be reassured that recurrence of epiglottitis is rare. The child should be free of respiratory difficulty, resting well, and show no other distress.

Evaluation

- Is the child breathing without difficulty?
- Are the child's mucous membranes and nailbeds pink?
- Is the child resting quietly and getting an adequate amount of rest and sleep?

LOWER AIRWAY DISORDERS

Bronchitis

Bronchitis is a disease that rarely exists by itself but occurs together with other conditions of the upper and lower respiratory tract. It can be confused with asthma. A cough is the major sign and it usually resolves without therapy in approximately 2 weeks.

PATHOPHYSIOLOGY ***of Bronchitis***

Inflammation of the trachea and major bronchi is present in bronchitis. Mucus production is increased and the mucosa is congested. Due to nonspecific leukocytic migration, purulent secretions can occur even in the absence of a bacterial infection.

Acute bronchitis is a self-limiting disease. Chronic bronchitis in children has been shown to be a factor in the persistence of lung dysfunction and chronic respiratory symptoms (Loughlin, 1990).

Etiology and Incidence. Acute bronchitis is usually viral. Rhinovirus is the most common organism. Other viruses thought to cause bronchitis include respiratory syncytial, influenza virus, parainfluenza virus, and adenovirus. Most bacterial infections occur secondary to a primary viral infection or some other airway problem. They may also occur secondary to foreign body aspiration. Air pollution has also been implicated in the disease.

The disorder is more common in young children and males. It can occur anytime but is more common during the winter months.

Clinical Manifestations

- Gradual onset with rhinitis
- Cough (initially nonproductive but may change to loose cough with increased mucus)
- Coarse and fine moist crackles and **rhonchi** (high-pitched, resembling wheezing of asthma)
- Malaise
- Afebrile or low-grade fever
- Increased mucus, which may be purulent

Diagnostic Evaluation. Chest X-rays are usually normal. Diagnosis is based on the clinical picture.

Therapeutic Management. Treatment is mainly palliative and includes rest, humidification, and increased fluid intake. Exposure to cigarette smoke should be avoided. Cough suppressants are not recommended unless the child is unable to rest due to the coughing. Antihistamines should be avoided because of their drying effect on secretions. Antibiotics should only be given if a bacterial infection is proved through culture or the clinical picture supports the diagnosis.

NURSING CARE OF THE CHILD WITH BRONCHITIS

Assessment

The nurse should assess temperature, appearance of secretions, and respiratory effort every 2 to 4 hours. The child's intake should also be monitored as well as signs of sleep deprivation related to the persistent cough.

Nursing Diagnosis and Planning

The following nursing diagnoses and expected outcomes may be appropriate in the treatment of bronchitis in the child.

- Ineffective Airway Clearance related to increased mucus production. ***Expected Outcome:*** *The child will demonstrate resolution of inflammation, as evidenced by decreased mucous production and decreased coughing.*
- Sleep Pattern Disturbance related to persistent coughing. ***Expected Outcome:*** *The child will experience age-appropriate amounts of uninterrupted sleep.*
- Fluid Volume Deficit related to insufficient intake secondary to malaise. ***Expected Outcomes:*** *The child will ingest appropriate amount of fluid for age and weight; have moist mucous membranes and good skin turgor; maintain weight.*
- Risk for Altered Comfort related to hyperthermia and malaise. ***Expected Outcomes:*** *The child will maintain body temperature within normal limits; show an interest in age-appropriate activities, books, toys, significant others.*

Implementation

Fluids are encouraged by frequently offering small amounts of the child's favorite liquids. Humidification is provided. The child is assessed for signs of dehydration, including daily weights. Acetaminophen is administered for elevated temperature (usually over 101°F [38.3°C]). Quiet activities should be provided for diversion.

Evaluation

- Is the child exhibiting decreased coughing and mucus production?
- Does the child have periods of rest and sleep?
- Is the child's intake adequate for age?
- Has the child maintained a normal body temperature?

Bronchiolitis

Bronchiolitis, an inflammation of the bronchioles, is one of the major causes of hospitalization in infants under age 1 year. Respiratory syncytial virus (RSV) is the causative agent in more than 50% of the cases.

Etiology and Incidence. Children usually acquire the disease from an older child or adult who has a minor respiratory disease. Common contacts are family members or other frequent contacts (e.g., daycare). Those with RSV may be infected through contact with contaminated hands due to high communicability of the virus. Nosocomial outbreaks in pediatric hospitals are a common concern.

> RSV can live on paper or skin for up to 1 hour, and on cribs and other nonporous surfaces for up to 6 hours. Although it is not airborne, it is highly communicable. It is usually transferred by the hands. Meticulous handwashing decreases spread of organisms.

In addition to RSV, other causative organisms include mycoplasma, parainfluenza virus, and some adenoviruses. RSV occurs in annual epidemics during winter and early spring. By age 2 years nearly 100% of children will have had RSV (Nederhand et al., 1989). Immunity is not acquired, but the incidence and severity decrease with age.

Bronchiolitis occurs during the first 2 years of life, with a peak incidence at age 6 months. It is most common during spring and winter. It can occur in epidemic numbers, and in some parts of the country it is the most common cause of hospitalization of infants.

Clinical Manifestations

- Mild upper respiratory tract infection usually precedes development of bronchiolitis.
- Serous nasal drainage, sneezing, low-grade fever, and anorexia are present for several days, followed by the onset of acute respiratory distress.
- Tachypnea present, with respiratory rates of 60 to 80 breaths/min.
- Auscultation of the lungs may reveal **wheezing,** crackles, or rhonchi.
- Intercostal and subcostal retractions are present.
- Cyanosis may or may not be present.
- Nasal flaring may be present.
- Difficulty feeding is due to increased respirations, which interfere with sucking and swallowing.
- Body temperature varies from hypothermic to as high as 105.8°F (41°C).

Diagnostic Evaluation. Diagnosis can be made by clinical presentation and the age of the child. Rapid viral identification can be performed on respiratory secretions obtained by nasopharyngeal washing (see Chapter 18). The diagnostic test is ELISA (enzyme-linked immunofluorescent assay).

Chest X-rays show hyperinflation of the lungs and increased anteroposterior diameter on lateral view. There are scattered areas of consolidation in some patients, which is attributed to atelectasis secondary to obstruction or inflammation of the alveoli. Some infants have normal X-rays.

Therapeutic Management. Mild bronchiolitis can be treated at home with fluids, humidification, and rest. Infants with respiratory distress are hospitalized. Treatment is supportive. Cool, humidified oxygen is delivered to relieve dyspnea, hypoxemia, and insensible water loss from tachypnea.

Parenteral fluids may be necessary for acutely ill infants who are dehydrated due to tachypnea and/or poor intake. The infant should be positioned with the head and chest at a 30- to 40-degree angle with the neck slightly extended to maintain an open airway and decrease pressure on the diaphragm.

Antibiotics are not given unless there is a secondary bacterial infection. The use of antibiotics in children with RSV has been shown to actually increase the probability of the child developing a bacterial infection (Hall et al., 1988).

Ribavirin (Virazole) is an antiviral respiratory drug that appears to interfere with RNA and DNA synthesis, inhibiting viral replication. It is used mainly in hospitalized children with severe RSV and in high-risk children (those with heart disease, chronic respiratory disease, prematurity, immunodeficiency). Administration is via hood, face mask, or oxygen tent over 12 to 18 hours for a minimum of 3 and maximum of 7 days (Fig. 28–3). The drug is most effective if administered within the first 3 days of the disease. It is very expensive and has proven to be teratogenic in some animal studies. Some caregivers experience headaches, burning nasal passages and eyes, and crystallized soft contact lenses (see Common Medications Table in Clinical Reference Pages). There are currently questions related to the efficacy of ribavirin and more research is needed (American Academy of Pediatrics, 1996).

PATHOPHYSIOLOGY *of Bronchiolitis*

In bronchiolitis, edema and accumulation of mucus and cellular debris cause obstruction of the bronchioles. Infants' bronchioles are very small and can quickly become obstructed. Airway resistance is increased during inspiratory and expiratory phases of respiration due to the small air passages. Hyperinflation of the lungs results from air trapping because bronchioles constrict during expiration. **Atelectasis** may occur if obstruction becomes complete and trapped air is absorbed. Normal exchange of gases is impaired and the infant is hypoxic. Some infants develop mild respiratory alkalosis; more frequently metabolic acidosis is observed (see Chapter 24).

The child with bronchiolitis is most acutely ill the first 48 to 72 hours after the onset of the disease. Improvement usually occurs in a few days. Mortality is less than 1%. Some infants' lung function studies remain abnormal for months.

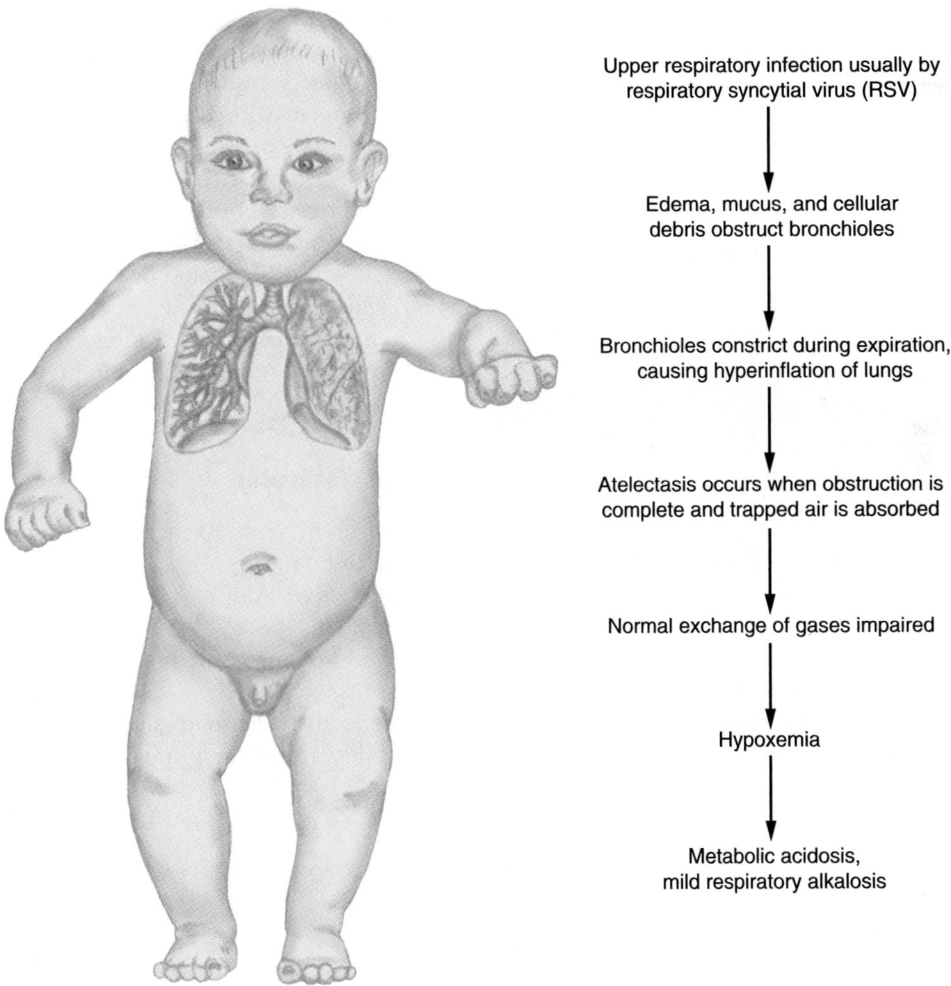
Upper respiratory infection usually by respiratory syncytial virus (RSV)
Edema, mucus, and cellular debris obstruct bronchioles
Bronchioles constrict during expiration, causing hyperinflation of lungs
Atelectasis occurs when obstruction is complete and trapped air is absorbed
Normal exchange of gases impaired
Hypoxemia
Metabolic acidosis, mild respiratory alkalosis

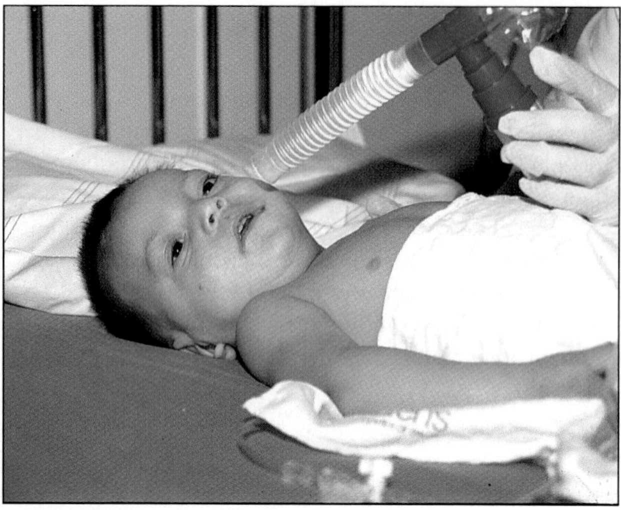

Figure 28–3

Respiratory syncytial virus (RSV) causes many cases of lower respiratory infections, such as bronchiolitis and pneumonia. Personnel who care for these children should maintain contact isolation, including the wearing of gloves and gowns and, of course, by practicing good handwashing. Women who are pregnant or trying to conceive should not care for these children if ribavirin is being administered because of some evidence of possible teratogenic effects of the drug. (Courtesy of Children's Medical Center, Dallas, Texas.)

> Because of the research indicating the possibility of teratogenic effects, health care workers and visitors who are pregnant or are planning pregnancy should not be in the room where ribavarin is being delivered.

NURSING CARE OF THE CHILD WITH BRONCHIOLITIS

Assessment

The respiratory system is assessed for signs of respiratory distress (tachypnea, dyspnea, retractions, cyanosis, and nasal flaring). Breath sounds are auscultated. Respiratory assessment should be ongoing with documentation every 2 hours during the acute phase and as needed if changes occur. Apnea monitoring is indicated in acute disease. The nurse should ascertain that the alarms are set and document any periods of apnea.

The infant is assessed for signs of dehydration (dry mucous membranes, decreased urine output, sunken fontanel, weight loss). Body temperature is monitored closely. The temperature in oxygen tents should be monitored as well as the moisture in the tent, tubing, and on the bedding and/or infant. The infant should be placed close to the nurses' station for easy observation.

> Body weight is the most reliable method of measurement of body fluid loss or gain. One kilogram of weight change represents one liter of fluid loss or gain.

The family's understanding of the disease and their level of anxiety is assessed. The infant is observed for signs of anxiety, restlessness, and/or irritability.

The infant with RSV is isolated in a single room or placed in a room with other RSV patients. Good handwashing is imperative. Nurses caring for these infants should not care for other high-risk patients. The current recommendation is that during peak RSV season, children infected with RSV should be managed with contact isolation, which should include strict attention to good handwashing practices and wearing gowns when soiling of clothing may occur (AAP Committee on Infectious Diseases, 1994).

Nursing Diagnoses

- Impaired Gas Exchange related to edema and increased mucus
- Ineffective Airway Clearance related to increased secretions
- Fluid Volume Deficit related to decreased intake and insensible loss
- Ineffective Thermoregulation related to illness
- Anxiety related to hospitalization, dyspnea

Planning, Implementation, and Evaluation: The Child With Bronchiolitis

NURSING DIAGNOSES

- Impaired Gas Exchange related to edema and increased mucus
- Ineffective Airway Clearance related to increased secretions

Expected Outcome:

- The child will have increased gas exchange, as evidenced by clear breath sounds and the absence of use of accessory muscles.
- The child's airway will clear as evidenced by normal respiratory rate and rhythm and vital signs for age.

Intervention	Rationale
1. Assess respirations: observe and document rate, quality, depth, use of accessory muscles, and flaring of nostrils q 2–4 hr and prn.	Ensures early identification of changes that might indicate impending respiratory distress. Assesses quality of aeration.
2. Auscultate breath sounds q 2–4 hr and prn.	Provides important clues to the condition of the lungs and possible changes taking place (increasing obstruction).
3. Monitor vital signs q 2–4 hr and prn.	Hypoxia causes an increase in pulse, respirations, and blood pressure. A drop in blood pressure and decreasing respirations may be a sign of impending respiratory arrest.
4. Administer humidified oxygen as ordered.	Oxygen decreases hypoxia, and the humidification liquefies mucus and decreases bronchiole edema.
5. Position head at 30–40 degrees with neck slightly extended.	Maintains an open airway and eases respirations by decreasing pressure on the diaphragm.
6. Use continuous pulse oximetry.	Provides continuous monitoring of oxygen saturation.
7. Use cardiorespiratory monitor.	Alarms if infant has period of apnea longer than 15–20 sec.
8. Do not place toys that will cause friction in mist tent if O_2 is being added. Stuffed animals and other cloth toys should also be kept out of the tent.	Friction may cause a spark that, added to the increased O_2, can cause a fire. Cloth toys will become wet from the mist.
9. Schedule care and alter the environment to allow for periods of rest.	Oxygen needs decrease during periods of inactivity.
10. Perform chest physiotherapy as ordered (may involve coordination with respiratory therapy department to schedule treatments before meals or at least 1 hour after meals).	Loosens and eases the removal of mucus that may be obstructing the airways. Scheduling before meals or 1 hour after meals decreases risk of aspiration. This treatment is controversial because it can stress infants and increase respiratory distress.
11. Administer antiviral agents as ordered.	Ribavirin is the drug of choice in high-risk RSV-positive infants.
12. Monitor IV fluids and encourage oral intake as tolerated (Pedialyte, Ricelyte, $\frac{1}{2}$ strength apple juice).	Aids in liquefication of secretions and prevents dehydration from decreased intake of fluids.
13. Instill saline nosedrops (1–2 drops in each nostril) before feeding and prn. Follow with suctioning with bulb syringe.	Dried secretions block nasal passages, and the infant cannot suck and breathe at the same time.

Evaluation:

- The child has clear breath sounds and normal respiratory and heart rate.
- The child is breathing without the use of accessory muscles.

NURSING DIAGNOSIS

- Fluid Volume Deficit related to decreased intake and increased insensible loss

Expected Outcome:

- Adequate fluid volume will be maintained, as evidenced by moist mucous membranes, maintenance of weight, and normal urine output for age.

Intervention	Rationale
1. Monitor intake and output.	Composition of body fluids and electrolytes is influenced by fluid loss and intake. Measurement assists in assessment of hydration and replacement needs.
2. Monitor daily weights.	Short-term weight changes are the most reliable measurement of fluid loss or gain.
3. Offer frequent, varied liquids (frozen juices, ice pops, Pedialyte, Ricelyte). Making a game out of the task is also sometimes helpful.	Replaces normal and insensible loss of fluid and aids in liquefying secretions. Offering favorite liquids increases cooperation.
4. Administer IV fluids as ordered.	Intravenous fluids may be necessary because of feeding difficulties secondary to respiratory distress.
5. Monitor serum electrolytes and report abnormal results.	Indicates electrolyte imbalance and serves as guide in replacement therapy.
6. Assess for signs and symptoms of dehydration (weight loss, poor skin turgor, dry mucous membranes, sunken fontanel).	Indicates infant has a fluid deficit.
7. Observe for decrease in urine output; <2 ml/kg/hr for infant and <1 ml/kg/hr for children over age 2 years is abnormal. Check urine specific gravity. Report levels above 1.030.	Concentrated urine denotes fluid deficit. Increased urine specific gravity can indicate dehydration.

Evaluation:
- The child is hydrated, as evidenced by moist mucous membranes, flat fontanel, and adequate urine output for age.
- The child maintains admission weight.

NURSING DIAGNOSIS
- Ineffective Thermoregulation related to illness

Expected Outcome:
- The child will be afebrile as evidenced by a temperature that is within normal limits for age.

Intervention	Rationale
1. Monitor child's temperature q 2–4 hr and prn.	Establishes a baseline in order to monitor changes.
2. Control environmental temperature by maintaining the room temperature between 72° and 75°F and provide light clothing and covers.	Removal of heat sources enables the body to release heat and lower its temperature.
3. Administer antipyretics, as ordered.	Acetaminophen is the preferred drug for fever reduction. Aspirin should not be given to children with viral disease due to its association with Reye syndrome. Ibuprofen may be used in young children who do not respond to acetaminophen.

Intervention	Rationale
4. Administer tepid bath for temperature > 40°C (104°F) that does not respond to antipyretics.	Cools the body through conduction. Too rapid cooling produces chilling, which further elevates body temperature.
5. Encourage fluid intake as tolerated.	Fever results in fluid loss via the skin and lungs.

Evaluation:
- The child maintains body temperature within normal limits for age.

NURSING DIAGNOSIS
- Anxiety related to hospitalization, dyspnea

Expected Outcome:
- The infant's anxiety will be decreased, as evidenced by less crying, increased rest periods, and decrease in pulse rate.
- The parents will verbalize understanding of the disease, have relaxed body appearance, and be able to demonstrate comforting behaviors toward the infant.

Intervention	Rationale
1. Encourage parents to stay with infant when possible (parents may have other children to care for, may be unable to miss work, may lack transportation, etc.).	Presence of a significant other will provide the child with a familiar person he can trust.
2. If the child's anxiety is increased by being placed in a mist tent, the parent may hold the child while the mist is blown on the child's face.	Crying and anxiety put increased stress on the respiratory system and can decrease the effects of the treatment.
3. Explain hospital routines and all procedures and treatments. Repeat until understanding is verbalized and demonstrated.	Fear of the unknown increases anxiety. Anxiety decreases ability to integrate information and problem solve.
4. Maintain a calm environment. Explain to parents that child may reflect their anxiety.	Anxiety can be transferred to the child by the healthcare provider as well as by the parents.
5. Acknowledge awareness of parents' and/or child's anxiety.	Validates feelings and builds trust through acceptance and understanding of the behavior.
6. Involve parents in care of infant. The mist tent can become a special playhouse for the child. Parents may get in tent with child and play and read with him.	Gives the parents a sense of control. The infant is also given the security of the presence of a familiar person.

Evaluation:
- The parents verbalize an understanding of the care of their child, and verbalize increased feelings of security and trust in the healthcare system.
- The parents comfort and nurture their infant. (See Teaching Guidelines box.)
- The infant experiences age-appropriate amounts of sleep and rest.
- The infant has a pulse that is normal for age.
- The infant does not cry excessively.
- The parents and child demonstrate relaxed body posture.

TEACHING GUIDELINES *for Bronchiolitis*

Teach the parent:

- Recognition of signs and symptoms of respiratory distress: tachypnea (rapid breathing), retractions (drawing in of chest when breathing), and cyanosis (bluish discoloration of skin and mucous membranes).
- Air can be humidified through the use of a humidifier in the child's bedroom.
- Avoid steam vaporizers because of the danger of burns. Warm mist can be provided by filling a humidifier with warm (not hot) water and having the child breath in the mist.
- Mucus can be suctioned from the nose by using a bulb syringe. Secretions can be loosened by using 3 drops of warm saline in each nostril and waiting about a minute before attempting to use the bulb syringe.
- Fluids should be encouraged. Small, frequent feedings of formula or breast milk should be offered if the infant tires when feeding. If coughing produces vomiting, the infant should be refed. Parents can be shown methods of increasing fluid intake through the use of play, e.g., tea parties with small cups and teapots, offering parents 10-ml and 20-ml needleless syringes so child can draw up flavored fluids in syringe and pretend he is a nurse.
- Smoking should be avoided in the presence of a child with respiratory disease.

Pneumonia

Pneumonia is an inflammation of the parenchyma of the lung and may occur as a primary or secondary disease. Pneumonias may be classified by anatomic distribution or by the agents that cause them. Environment, immunity, and the age of the child are all etiologic factors in the pathogenesis of the disease (Table 28–3). The two most common types of pneumonia are viral and bacterial. Children with bacterial pneumonia tend to be more toxic than those with viral disease.

Clinical differentiation between viral and bacterial pneumonia is very difficult. Viruses are the most common causative agents. Pneumonias can be classified as bacterial, viral, mycotic, aspiration, hypostatic, drug/radiation, hypersensitivity pneumonitis, Loeffler syndrome, and "other" (Behrman, 1995). Children with chronic and acute conditions such as acquired immunodeficiency syndrome, cystic fibrosis, congenital defects, and foreign body aspiration are at increased risk to develop pneumonia. Opportunistic infections (*Pneumocystis carinii* pneumonia) may be associated with acquired immunodeficiency syndrome (see Chapter 23).

Viral Pneumonia

Pathophysiology. Invasion of the terminal airways and the alveoli occurs. The infiltrates are usually patchy and affect multiple lobes. Cell destruction is present, with sloughing of cellular debris into the lumen. Multiple organisms can be the causative agents (see Table 28–3).

Etiology and Incidence. The most common causative organisms are shown in Table 28–3. RSV causes a more serious disease in the infant than in an older child.

From 80% to 85% of pediatric pneumonias are caused by viruses. Males are affected slightly more often than females. Children are most commonly affected between ages 2 and 3 years. The incidence diminishes after age 3 years. Environmental conditions (overcrowding) and season of the year are also predisposing factors.

TABLE 28–3 *Common Causes of Pneumonia at Different Ages*

AGE	BACTERIAL	VIRAL	OTHERS
Neonate	Group B streptococci, coliform bacteria	CMV, herpes virus	*Mycoplasma hominis, Ureaplasma urealyticum*
4–16 wk	*S. aureus, H. influenzae, S. pneumoniae*	CMV, RSV	*Chlamydia trachomatis, Ureaplasm urealyticum*
Up to 5 yr	*S. pneumoniae, S. aureus*	RSV, adenovirus, influenza virus A, B	
Over 5 yr	*S. pneumoniae*	Influenza virus A, B	*Mycoplasma pneumoniae*

From Behrman, R., and Kliegman, R. (1994). *Nelson essentials of pediatrics* (2nd ed.). Philadelphia: W. B. Saunders.

Clinical Manifestations. Onset may be acute or insidious. Pneumonia caused by the influenza virus tends to have a more abrupt onset than that caused by some of the other viruses. Temperature tends to be lower than in bacterial pneumonia. The disease usually lasts 5 to 7 days.

- Low-grade to high fever
- Cough
- Crackles
- Wheezing (more common in pneumonia caused by RSV)
- Headache, malaise, myalgia (older children)
- Abdominal pain

Diagnostic Evaluation. The diagnosis is made by chest X-ray, which reveals diffuse infiltrates. The WBC count is usually below 20,000/mm^3.

Therapeutic Management. Treatment is supportive. Antibiotics are not given. More severely ill children may be hospitalized and given oxygen, chest physiotherapy, and IV fluids.

Bacterial Pneumonia

Pathophysiology. The alveoli are filled with fluid and cells. A small segment or the entire lung may be involved. Bacteria can reach the bloodstream via the pulmonary lymphatics. Vital capacity and lung compliance decrease as consolidation increases. There may be plural effusion or empyema.

Etiology. The organisms causing bacterial pneumonia are age-related (see Table 28–3). The child often has a history of a viral infection.

Clinical Manifestations

Pneumococcal Pneumonia

Infants:

- Preceded by mild upper respiratory infection for several days
- Abrupt onset of fever, restlessness, apprehension, respiratory distress
- Grunting respirations
- Nasal flaring
- Supraclavicular, intercostal, and subcostal retractions
- Tachypnea

Children and Adolescents:

- Preceded by brief, mild, upper respiratory infection
- High fever
- Chills
- Cough
- Chest pain
- Restlessness/anxiety
- Rapid respirations

Streptococcal Pneumonia

- Similar to pneumococcal pneumonia with sudden onset
- High fever
- Chills
- Respiratory distress

Staphylococcal Pneumonia

Prior upper respiratory infection with abrupt onset of:

- High fever
- Cough
- Tachypnea
- Grunting respirations
- Sternal and subcostal retractions
- Nasal flaring
- Cyanosis
- Anxiety

Hemophilus Influenza

- Similar to pneumococcal pneumonia with an insidious onset
- Cough
- Fever
- Nasal flaring
- Retractions

Therapeutic Management. Bacterial pneumonias are treated with antibiotic therapy. Some children may need oxygen support. Chest tube drainage of fluid or pus from the pleural cavity may be done in staphylococcal pneumonia.

NURSING CARE OF THE CHILD WITH PNEUMONIA

Assessment

The child with pneumonia should be assessed for signs of respiratory distress, including dyspnea, tachypnea, cyanosis, use of accessory muscles, diminished breath sounds, and crackles. Fever, tachycardia, malaise, anorexia, restlessness, and changes in condition should also be noted.

Nursing Diagnosis and Planning

The following nursing diagnoses and expected outcomes may be appropriate in the treatment of the child with pneumonia:

- Ineffective Airway Clearance related to bronchial obstruction. ***Expected Outcome:*** *The child will have clear airways, as evidenced by the absence of abnormal breath sounds and dyspnea.*
- Ineffective Breathing Pattern related to increased mucus production. ***Expected Outcome:*** *The child will*

demonstrate effective breathing, as evidenced by regular respiratory rate and rhythm within normal limits for age and absence of use of accessory muscles for breathing.

- Impaired Gas Exchange related to increased mucus and accumulation of exudate. ***Expected Outcome:*** *The child will maintain adequate gas exchange, as evidenced by decreased restlessness and improved mucous membrane and nailbed color.*
- Fluid Volume Deficit related to fever, decreased intake, and tachypnea. ***Expected Outcomes:*** *The child will maintain fluid balance, as evidenced by moist mucous membranes, good skin turgor, urine output appropriate for age, and maintenance of age-appropriate weight.*
- Knowledge Deficit related to disease process and home care. ***Expected Outcome:*** *The parents will verbalize an understanding of the process and care of the child.*
- Anxiety (parental) related to infant's dyspnea and hospitalization. ***Expected Outcomes:*** *The parents will show a decrease in anxiety, as evidenced by decreased irritability and increased periods of rest; verbalize and demonstrate comfort and ease when caring for the child.*
- Pain related to coughing and difficulty breathing secondary to disease process. ***Expected Outcome:*** *The child will have decreased pain as evidenced by less irritability, verbalization of decreased discomfort (if age-appropriate), and a relaxed body posture.*

Implementation

Nursing care of the child with pneumonia is directed by the severity of illness and the cause of the disease. Some children will be managed at home and others hospitalized on a general pediatric unit or special care area.

The child's breath sounds, respiratory rate and rhythm, use of accessory muscles, color, vital signs, and degree of restlessness are assessed every 2 hours. Chest physiotherapy should be scheduled before meals and bedtime. Elevating the head of the bed and changing position every 2 hours assist respiratory effort and promote pulmonary drainage. Older children may assume a position of comfort, but still must change their position every 2 hours. The use of infant seats should be avoided because pressure may be placed on the diaphragm, thus actually decreasing lung expansion. The older child is assisted with coughing and deep breathing, and splinting as necessary to ease discomfort. Oxygen should be humidified and monitored. Pulse oximetry aids in the monitoring of oxygen saturation. A cardiorespiratory monitor is used when available.

Oral and/or IV fluids are given as ordered. IV fluids may be indicated when oral intake increases the stress put on an already-compromised body. Intake and output are monitored, and the child is assessed for signs of dehydration (oliguria, poor skin turgor, dry mucous membranes, sunken fontanels, weight loss). Weight should be measured daily. Specific gravity of urine is also checked.

Nursing care is planned to provide for periods of rest. Diversional activities should be designed to conserve energy (books, puzzles, videos, board games). A quiet and cool environment should be maintained and visitors limited. Visiting by anyone with an infection should be restricted.

The nurse should assess for fever and discomfort, and administer antipyretics (acetaminophen), antibiotics, and analgesics as ordered. Normal breathing may cause discomfort. If an analgesic is not ordered, the physician should be notified. Splinting of the affected side by lying on that side may decrease discomfort. Diversional activities and manipulation of the environment are often effective in pain relief.

The family and child (if age-appropriate) need to be provided with information concerning disease and treatment. All procedures and treatments should be explained. The parents are encouraged to stay with their child and participate in the care of the child. Empathy when feelings and concerns are expressed needs to be conveyed. See the Teaching Guidelines box for a discussion of home care.

Pulmonary Noninfectious Irritation

Although we think of foreign body aspiration as the most common type of pulmonary noninfectious irritation in children, other forms of irritation may cause respiratory difficulties. Three of the most common types are adult respiratory distress syndrome (ARDS), passive smoking, and smoke inhalation.

TEACHING GUIDELINES *for Pneumonia*

- Provide rest.
- Increase fluid intake to $1\frac{1}{2}$ times the daily requirement. (The box on page 681 lists fluid requirements.)
- Administer acetaminophen for fever and discomfort.
- Use cool mist humidifier.
- Assess parents' ability to take the child's temperature. Provide needed instruction.
- Administer antibiotics as ordered and give correct dose with entire prescribed amount.
- Give warm liquids (lemonade, apple juice, Pedialyte, Ricelyte) to loosen secretions.
- Avoid exposure to smoking.

Common Items of Aspiration

Nuts	Grapes	Parts of toys
Pins	Bones	Hard candy
Screws	Earrings	Balloons
Coins	Small toys	Popcorn
Seeds	Chunks of food	

Foreign Body Aspiration

The aspiration of a foreign body is most common between ages 6 months and 5 years. Children who put objects in their mouths while they are playing, running, or laughing are at risk to aspirate the object. Certain items have increased incidence of aspiration by infants and children (see accompanying box).

Pathophysiology. Most foreign bodies become lodged in the bronchi. The right main bronchus is a more common site because of its anatomic development (see the discussion of anatomy and physiology in the Clinical Reference Pages). Objects lodged in the larynx cause edema and inflammation. Obstruction in the bronchus is demonstrated by obstructive emphysema or atelectasis. Failure to remove obstructive foreign objects is almost always fatal. Most can be removed mechanically without complications. Delay in treatment can lead to aspiration pneumonia and airway trauma.

Etiology and Incidence. Foreign body aspiration is usually due to the curiosity of children, their oral needs, and/or lack of supervision. Infants and children love to explore and to investigate objects. This often includes putting objects into their mouths. Children also have the uncanny ability to remove small parts from toys and to find other objects that have been put "out of their reach." Adults may give infants and small children foods that they are not developmentally prepared to ingest (hard candy, popcorn, uncooked carrots, hot dogs).

Childhood aspiration can occur at any age but most incidents occur in males before age 5, with a peak age of 1 to 3 years. In a study by Steen and Zimmerman (1990), nuts accounted for the highest incidence of aspiration (68%), followed by fruit and vegetable foreign bodies (e.g., apples, carrots) (14%).

Clinical Manifestations

Immediate Signs and Symptoms

- Sudden, violent coughing
- Gagging
- Wheezing
- Vomiting
- Brief episode of apnea
- Cyanosis

After the above signs and symptoms, the child may be asymptomatic for hours or weeks. If not treated they may develop signs and symptoms related to edema and increased irritation and obstruction:

Laryngeal and Tracheal Obstruction

- Hoarseness
- Croupy cough
- Stridor
- Cyanosis and dyspnea with wheezing (may occur)

Bronchial Obstruction

- Cough
- Wheezing
- Unilateral decreased breath sounds
- Pneumonitis
- Hoarseness
- Stridor
- Respiratory arrest if obstruction and inflammation cause complete obstruction

Diagnostic Evaluation. Diagnosis is based on a good history and the clinical manifestations. Fluoroscopy and chest X-ray are used to reveal the presence of a foreign object in the respiratory tract. X-ray will reveal an opaque foreign body, and laryngoscopy or bronchoscopy confirms the diagnosis and provides an avenue for removal of the object.

Therapeutic Management. Removal of foreign bodies from the respiratory tract is done by direct laryngoscopy or bronchoscopy. After the procedure the child should remain hospitalized for observation of laryngeal edema and respiratory distress. Cool mist is provided and antibiotic therapy is ordered if appropriate.

NURSING CARE OF THE CHILD WHO HAS ASPIRATED A FOREIGN BODY

Assessment

The degree of obstruction should be assessed to determine the appropriate action to take. If the child is aphonic (not speaking) and not breathing, the nurse should follow the guidelines for managing an obstructed airway (see Chapter 14, Table 14–3). Children who are partially obstructed are observed for signs of increasing airway obstruction.

After the object has been removed, the child is observed for signs of obstruction caused by laryngeal edema and soft tissue swelling (restlessness, dyspnea). The parents' knowledge of respiratory distress is also evaluated before discharge.

Parental anxiety and guilt are often observed after an aspiration. In addition to supporting the parents, the nurse also assesses their knowledge of safety.

Nursing Diagnosis and Planning

The following nursing diagnoses and expected outcomes may be appropriate in the treatment of the child who has aspirated a foreign body.

- Ineffective Airway Clearance related to airway obstruction secondary to aspiration of a foreign body. ***Expected Outcome:*** *The child will have normal breath sounds and respiratory rate and rhythm within normal limits for age.*
- Anxiety related to difficulty breathing secondary to aspiration of a foreign body. ***Expected Outcome:*** *The child will display decreased anxiety, as evidenced by a relaxed body posture and participation in age-appropriate play.*
- Altered Family Processes related to feelings of guilt. ***Expected Outcome:*** *The parents will discuss feelings regarding the child's aspiration.*
- Knowledge Deficit related to safety in the care of children. ***Expected Outcome:*** *The parents will verbalize an understanding of safety precautions associated with children.*

Implementation

After removal of the object the nurse observes and documents the child's respiratory status. The child should be placed on a cardiorespiratory monitor.

Liquids are withheld until the child's gag reflex returns postanesthesia. Oral fluids should be started slowly and increased as the child tolerates the intake. Intake and output should be documented. If the child refuses to drink because of a sore throat or is unable to take oral fluids, the physician should be notified so that IV fluids may be started.

Parents are encouraged to verbalize their feelings concerning the child's aspiration episode. Using a developmentally appropriate approach, the nurse should discuss infant and child safety in relationship to aspiration. Parents are encouraged to remove toys with small parts that could be put into the child's mouth. A review of age-appropriate foods is also helpful based on the child's developmental abilities. See Chapter 13 for discussion of specific preventive measures and safety risks.

Evaluation

- Does the child have clear breath sounds and normal respiratory rate and rhythm for age?
- Can the family relate an understanding of safety measures for their child?
- Has the family verbalized their feelings concerning accidents related to aspiration?

Adult Respiratory Distress Syndrome

Although there is not uniform agreement as to what constitutes ARDS, it is generally agreed that ARDS represents severe diffuse lung injury precipitated by a variety of illnesses. The mechanism of lung injury in children is similar to that of adults and usually occurs from 8 to 48 hours after the initial illness, which may be, but is not limited to, aspiration, trauma, drug ingestion, shock, and massive transfusions.

Pathophysiology. The mechanism that initiates and perpetuates the lung injury is not understood. There is a breakdown in the alveolar–capillary barrier with fluid accumulation in the interstitium and alveoli. There are acute and chronic stages of the syndrome. Initially there is capillary congestion and pulmonary edema. Children who do not recover from the acute stage develop fibrosis of the lungs.

Table 28–4 discusses clinical manifestations, therapeutic management, nursing care, and prognosis.

Passive Smoking

Increased attention has been paid to the role of passive smoking in the development of respiratory disease in children. Children with a history of exposure to cigarette smoke have more episodes of airway obstruction, more frequent hospitalizations for respiratory complaints, onset of asthma at an earlier age, and more frequent episodes of otitis media than nonexposed children (O'Sullivan, 1994). Recent studies have supported the hypothesis that environmental tobacco smoke has a role in the development of bronchial hyperresponsiveness in children (Agudo et al., 1994). Preexisting abnormalities of respiratory function associated with in utero exposure to tobacco smoke products and familial predisposition to wheezing are important determinants of wheezing and lower respiratory disease in the first year of life (Tager et al., 1993).

Pathophysiology. Smoke is an irritant that can cause increased airway reactivity and inflammation.

For a discussion of clinical manifestations, therapeutic management, nursing care, and prognosis see Table 28–4.

Smoke Inhalation

As many as 50% of all fire-related deaths are caused by smoke injuries. The severity of lung injury is related to the nature of the material inhaled, the products of incomplete combustion that are generated, and the child's confinement in a closed space. Besides the noxious gases, fine particles of soot may also be inhaled, which may have toxic gases adsorbed on them or which may cause thermal burns.

Pathophysiology. Because the upper airway has a built-in cooling system, most thermal airway injury is limited to the areas above the larynx. Steam inhalation injury is an exception. Combustion of the materials involved causes a wide variety of noxious gases. These include, but are not limited to, oxides of sulfur and nitrogen, acetaldehydes,

TABLE 28–4 *Pulmonary Noninfectious Irritants*

	ADULT RESPIRATORY DISTRESS	PASSIVE SMOKING	SMOKE INHALATION
Clinical Manifestations	Acute, subacute, and chronic phases Pulmonary manifestations may be minimal during acute phase but will move toward respiratory distress (dyspnea, tachypnea, retractions, grunting, cyanosis) May develop severe hypoxemia and, occasionally, hypercapnia It should be noted that there is a primary disease and manifestations of that disease process will also be present	Increased respiratory infections An effect on respiratory function and growth in infants and a small but significant reduction in airway function in older children Possible negative effect on the linear growth of children with cystic fibrosis (Kovesi, Corey, & Levison, 1993)	Singed nasal hair Cough Hoarseness Hemoptysis Soot in sputum Cyanosis Wheezing Carbon monoxide: mild—headaches, mild dyspnea, visual changes, confusion moderate—irritability, diminished judgment, dim vision, nausea severe—hallucinations, confusion, ataxia, collapse, coma
Therapeutic Management	Need to be treated in an ICU Treatment of underlying cause Oxygen/mechanical ventilation Pulse oximetry Maintain cardiac function Stabilize hematocrit Prevention of infection	Awareness of problem and preventive teaching Effective programs to prevent smoking in parents and minors	100% oxygen by mask Arterial blood gases Intubation and tracheostomy equipment available Aerosolized bronchodilators Balance fluid therapy between the need for a large volume of fluid and the need to limit fluid to decrease pulmonary edema Prophylactic antimicrobial therapy is controversial
Nursing Care	Monitor respiratory status Monitor blood gas analysis Psychological support of child and parents Monitor urine output, capillary filling, and perfusion	Involvement in community projects to designate "no smoking" ordinances in public places School-based prevention programs Education of parents as part of anticipatory guidance of the dangers of smoking, both active and passive Role modeling no smoking	Respiratory assessment Support of pulmonary therapy Psychological support of the child and family due to the fear of the trauma of the fire or insult that caused the injury Children who have lost a family member will need long-term psychological support
Prognosis	High mortality, usually more than 50% Those who survive have a good chance of full recovery	Increased numbers of studies have shown the correlation between smoking and respiratory disease. More studies will be needed to show the long-term effects	Most will return to near-normal pulmonary function and few will suffer long-term problems associated with the injury

hydrocyanic acid, and carbon monoxide. Exposure to these gases can cause mucosal edema, activation of irritant receptors, necrosis, sloughing of airway mucosa, inspissation (thickening or drying) of sooty debris, and airway obstruction leading to further hypoxemia, atelectasis, and reduced bacterial clearance (McCoy, 1993).

Carbon monoxide poisoning is a complication of smoke inhalation caused when CO combines with hemoglobin to form carboxyhemoglobin, causing severe hypoxia.

For a discussion of clinical manifestations, therapeutic management, nursing care, and prognosis see Table 28–4.

Apnea

Apnea is defined as the cessation of breathing for 20 seconds or longer or a shorter pause that is accompanied by bradycardia or cyanosis. Premature infants may have periodic breathing, in which there is a shift from regular rhythmic breathing to brief episodes of apnea. This type of breathing pattern consists of three or more respiratory pauses of greater than 3 seconds with less than 20 seconds of respiration between pauses. Rarely, it is associated with changes in heart rate or color. Periodic breathing is very common in premature infants and decreases as the infant's gestational age increases. The cause is unknown and it can be a normal event.

Apparent life-threatening events (ALTEs) refer to a sudden episode characterized by apnea, color change, change in muscle tone, choking, or gagging in an infant who appears otherwise healthy (Brouillette, Weese-Mayer, & Hunt, 1990). In the past, this type of occurrence was referred to as a "near miss sudden infant death syndrome." This was misleading. ALTEs most often occur in infants ≥ 37 weeks' gestational age while they are sleeping, feeding, or awake. Infants who have experienced an ALTE are usually hospitalized for observation and testing.

Apnea of Prematurity

Apnea of prematurity is increased in neonates of 24 to 32 weeks' gestational age. It is the most common type of apnea.

PATHOPHYSIOLOGY *of Apnea of Prematurity*

The pathophysiology of apnea of prematurity varies among infants. There may be immaturity of the respiratory center in the medulla oblongata. Some infants may have an abnormal response to CO_2. As hypoxia increases, the ventilatory response decreases (Stark, 1991). Upper airway obstruction can lead to apnea when there is continued respiratory effort without nasal airflow due to lack of coordination of the diaphragm and intercostal muscles. There may be an abnormal response to stimulation of laryngeal chemoreceptors by liquids such as water or milk, which would explain apnea occurring during feeding and suctioning (Stark, 1991).

Etiology and Incidence. Apnea of prematurity occurs in healthy infants and may be due to upper airway obstruction, immaturity of central control mechanisms, compliant chest wall, and/or abnormal response during rapid eye movement (REM) sleep, which may be related to loss of muscle tone.

Incidence increases as gestational age decreases and usually resolves by 38 weeks. The onset is usually after the first day of life and within, but not limited to, the first week of life.

Clinical Manifestations

- Cessation of breathing for more than 15 to 20 seconds
- Bradycardia

Therapeutic Management. Infants at risk for apnea (<32 weeks' gestation or <1500 grams) should be placed on a cardiorespiratory monitor with alarms set. Gentle cutaneous stimulation (massaging the feet) may be adequate to stimulate breathing. If apnea persists, mask-bag ventilation is required. Oxygen is administered to treat hypoxia.

Continuous positive airway pressure (CPAP) can be used to treat apnea. CPAP prevents obstruction by splinting the upper airway (Stark, 1991).

Drug therapy of caffeine, oral theophylline, or intravenous aminophylline is given to increase central respiratory drive and improve CO_2 sensitivity. Infants who are unresponsive to theophylline and caffeine may respond to doxapram, which stimulates both the respiratory center and peripheral chemoreceptors.

Infant Apnea

It is not abnormal for term infants to have brief periods of periodic breathing during sleep. Apnea of infancy refers to infants greater than 37 weeks' gestation who experience a respiratory pause that lasts > 20 seconds or a shorter pause associated with bradycardia, cyanosis, pallor, and/or marked hypotonia.

PATHOPHYSIOLOGY *of Infant Apnea*

There are three types of apnea associated with infant apnea:

- *Central* (absence of respiratory effort and air movement)
- *Obstructive* (apparent respiratory efforts without air movement or sound)
- *Mixed* (absence of respiratory effort and nasal air movement followed by resumption of respiratory effort without air movement)

Short episodes of apnea are usually central and apnea episodes that last 15 seconds or more are usually mixed.

Etiology. Before making a diagnosis of apnea of infancy, other conditions must be ruled out. The infant who has apnea together with seizures, hypoglycemia, or gastroesophageal reflux should have further testing to determine the etiology of those disorders (Spitzer, 1996). In about 50% of cases, no cause is determined and a diagnosis of apnea of infancy is made.

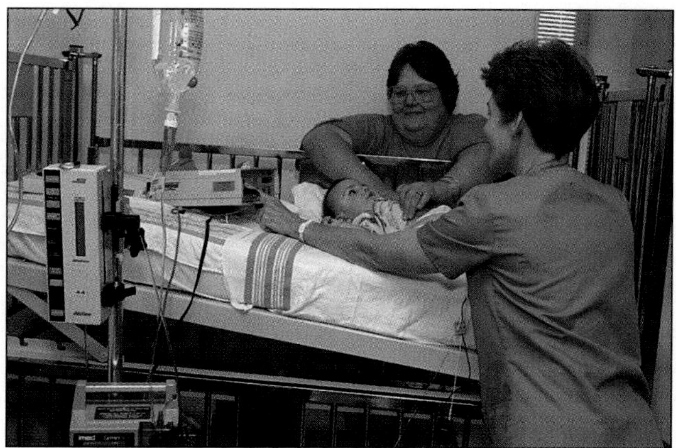

Figure 28–4
Teaching the family about using an apnea monitor and how to respond to alarms is an important element in caring for the child with infant apnea. The nurse must assess the parents' ability to tolerate the stressors of living with a child who is prone to apnea and support them as they deal with these stressors.

Clinical Manifestations

- Cessation of breathing >20 seconds
- Bradycardia
- Color changes (cyanosis, pallor, or erythema)
- Hypotonia

Diagnostic Evaluation. Testing is dependent on the clinical indications and the disease that is being ruled out. Cardiorespiratory and neurophysiologic studies should be done. Included in these studies are chest X-ray, blood chemistry, electrocardiography, and electroencephalography. The pneumocardiogram specifically tests for apnea by recording the heart rate and chest wall movements. It is important to note that the reliability of the test to predict apnea has not been well established.

Therapeutic Management. If a cause cannot be discovered and eliminated, the infant is placed on a home monitoring cardiorespiratory system (Fig. 28–4). A respiratory stimulant (caffeine, theophylline) may be ordered.

NURSING CARE OF THE INFANT WITH APNEA

Assessment

The infant's heart rate and respirations are monitored continuously. The nurse should check to be sure that the alarms on the cardiorespiratory monitor are set. Resuscitative equipment should be available.

If an apneic episode is observed, the nurse should note the time and duration of the episode. Color change, bradycardia, and oxygen saturation should also be noted and documented. The nurse should also document what the infant was doing before the episode and any actions the nurse took to stimulate breathing.

> When a monitor alarm is triggered, the nurse should immediately assess the infant rather than focus on the machine.

Nursing Diagnosis and Planning

The following nursing diagnoses and expected outcomes may be appropriate in the treatment of apnea in the infant.

- Ineffective Breathing Pattern related to apnea secondary to prematurity of respiratory control mechanisms (premature infant)
- Ineffective Breathing Pattern related to apnea of known or unknown etiology (term infant).
  Expected Outcome: *The infant will have regular breathing patterns, as evidenced by respiratory rate and rhythm within normal limits for age.*
- Anxiety (parental) related to fear of infant's death. ***Expected Outcome:*** *The parents will verbalize feelings concerning the infant's periods of apnea.*
- Knowledge Deficit related to apnea monitoring equipment and cardiopulmonary resuscitation (CPR). ***Expected Outcome:*** *The parents will demonstrate ability to perform infant CPR and operate apnea monitor.*

Implementation

The infant with apnea is monitored continuously on a cardiorespiratory monitor. The parameters for heart rate are set according to the infant's age, and the respiratory pause is set at greater than 15 seconds. Resuscitative equipment should be available, and the nurse should be proficient in using it.

The apneic infant can be stimulated by gently tapping the infant's foot or trunk and/or turning the infant over. The infant should not be shaken vigorously. If he does not resume breathing, bag and mask ventilation should be instituted.

A neutral thermal environment should be maintained and suctioning should be avoided when possible. Several studies have shown that feeding affects ventilation. Therefore, infants should be monitored closely when being fed.

If home apnea monitoring is ordered, the family should be instructed in the use of the monitor and in CPR (Fig. 28–4). There are several indications for home apnea monitoring (see accompanying box).

Evaluation

- Have the parents verbalized their fears associated with the infant's apnea?
- Have the parents demonstrated the ability to operate monitoring equipment and to perform CPR?

Indications for Home Apnea Monitoring

- The infant is a survivor of ALTE.
- The infant is a newborn sibling of two or more SIDS infants.
- The infant is premature and has symptoms of idiopathic apnea of prematurity but is otherwise ready for hospital discharge.
- The infant has a tracheostomy.
- The infant has a sleep apnea syndrome caused by a neurologic disorder, periodic breathing, upper airway abnormality, or idiopathic syndromes.

Adapted from Hanly, P. (1992). Mechanisms and management of central sleeping apnea. *Lung, 170,* 1017. Reprinted by permission of Springer-Verlag.

Sudden Infant Death Syndrome

Sudden infant death syndrome (SIDS) is defined as the sudden death of an infant under age 1 year that remains unexplained after a thorough case investigation, including performance of a complete autopsy, examination of the death scene, and review of the clinical history (Willinger & Catz, 1991). It is sometimes referred to as "crib death" by the public. SIDS usually occurs during sleep.

PATHOPHYSIOLOGY *of SIDS*

There have been a wide variety of findings on infants who have died of SIDS. Nonspecific findings such as mild pulmonary edema, vascular congestion, or pulmonary inflammation are commonly found. Other consistent findings include retarded postnatal growth, increased pulmonary arterial smooth muscle, retention of brown fat, brain stem gliosis, and intrathoracic petechiae. The increase in smooth muscle in the larger pulmonary arteries extending to smaller blood vessels close to the alveoli suggests that infants with SIDS have been subjected to chronic hypoxia (Behrman, 1995). However, researchers have not been able to find sufficient evidence to prove this theory. No single organism has been consistently found in SIDS victims.

Etiology and Incidence. There are numerous theories as to the etiology of SIDS. However, the cause is currently unknown. Some of the proposed hypotheses are prematurity, brain stem defects, severe infant botulism, infections, reactions to immunizations, and hypersensitivity to cow's milk. Some studies have suggested a connection with lower socioeconomic status, cultural influences, lack of prenatal care, smoking, sibling with SIDS, and the season of the year (winter).

Numerous reports from countries other than the United States have found a significant association with infants sleeping in the prone position and SIDS. Based on this information the AAP has endorsed a recommendation that healthy infants be placed for sleep on their sides or backs, rather than being placed prone (AAP, 1992). There has been an increase in infants being put to sleep in the supine and side-lying position since 1992. However, in one study conducted of 852 caregivers, 54% of the study infants were still being put to sleep prone (Chessare, Hunt, & Bourguignon, 1995). In a smaller, later study conducted by the National Institute of Child Health and Human Development, 70% of 1,000 caretakers responded that they placed infants younger than 7 months on their sides or backs (AAP, 1996). There is a need for increased education in this area because countries who have had significant decreases in the prone sleeping position are reporting significant decreases in SIDS and the United States has had less than a 2% decrease since 1992 (Chessare, Hunt, & Bourguignon, 1995). There is also a risk factor associated with putting infants to sleep on soft bedding. Infants may suffocate by rebreathing CO_2-laden expired air when sleeping face down on soft bedding (Gilbert-Barnes and Barnes, 1995; Kemp, Nelson, & Thach, 1994).

In a recent survey of pediatricians conducted by the National Institute of Child Health and Human Development, 81% said they recommended placing infants to sleep on their backs (AAP, 1996). Nurses should encourage parents to place healthy infants on their sides or backs for sleep and they should provide the rationale for the parents to increase compliance.

SIDS occurs most frequently between the second and fourth months of life, with 95% of cases occurring by age 6 months. It is more common in boys, low–birth-weight infants, and infants from lower socioeconomic groups. It occurs more often during the winter months. The highest incidence is in Native Americans, followed by blacks.

Clinical Manifestations

- Silent death
- May be found in any position
- May be clutching bedding

Diagnostic Evaluation. Diagnosis is confirmed through autopsy. A medical history of the infant and family should be taken. The infant is examined for signs of illness or trauma. The death scene is also investigated.

NURSING CARE FOR THE FAMILY OF THE INFANT WITH SIDS

Assessment

When a child is brought into the emergency department with suspected SIDS, there is often confusion for the family. If resuscitation was begun at home, they may assume that it was effective and that their child is alive. Assessment of the family's understanding of the situation should be done to plan for teaching and support. The family's emotional status should be assessed. Coping strategies should be evaluated.

The family is interviewed in a calm, slow, and nonthreatening manner. Questions should not imply negligence or any involvement in the death. Parents need to be given time to think before they answer questions. Parents should be told that SIDS is the apparent cause of death and that nothing they or anyone else could have done would have prevented the death.

Nursing Diagnosis and Planning

The following nursing diagnoses and expected outcomes may be appropriate following assessment of the family of the infant with SIDS.

- Altered Family Processes related to death of a child. ***Expected Outcomes:*** *The parents/family will verbalize feelings related to the death of the infant; provide support for one another.*
- Ineffective Family Coping: Compromised related to death of a child. ***Expected Outcome:*** *The parents/family will identify strengths and accept support of other family members, friends, and professionals.*
- Knowledge Deficit related to cause of death. ***Expected Outcome:*** *The parents will verbalize an understanding of their child's death.*

Implementation

The guiding force for the nurse working with a family who has had a child die of SIDS is to provide calm support. The parents are confused about the death and are trying to cope with all of the emotions they are feeling. Most parents will experience a combination of guilt, anger, and emotional pain.

A quiet room should be provided for the family, and someone should remain with them. The family should be assisted with calling family, friends, and/or clergy. The nurse should accompany the physician when the parents are told their child is dead. At this time the parents should also be told that the apparent cause of death is SIDS and that nothing could have been done to prevent the death. By doing this, the stage is set to work to minimize feelings of guilt.

The parents will be interviewed. This interview should be conducted in a slow, nonthreatening manner that in no way reflects guilt or suspicion on the parents. Because the parents will be overwhelmed, questions may need to be repeated for clarity.

Parents should be given the opportunity to say good-bye to their child. A quiet room should be provided with a rocking chair and dim lighting. The parents may not think to ask to see their child. It should be the role of the nurse to provide this opportunity. Parents who are not given the opportunity to hold their child and say good-bye often regret it later. The nurse should accept either decision the parents make in this matter. Each parent will have his or her own way of coping.

After the death of an infant, the nurse might say, "Would you like to have some time alone with your baby? We will bring him to you and you can take as long as you would like to hold him." The infant should be cleaned and wrapped in a blanket and brought to the parents.

The wishes of parents who do not want time alone with their baby should be respected.

The need for an autopsy should be explained. The autopsy will verify the cause of death and confirm for the parents that they did not cause the death.

Prior to the parents leaving the hospital, arrangements for follow-up care should be made. Many hospitals have a team consisting of a social worker, chaplain, and nurse who are called when a suspected SIDS death occurs. Variations of this team may be present or it may be the nurse's role to initiate home care of the family.

The family should be referred to a local SIDS program for information, support, and counseling. Nurses who are involved in home visiting encourage the family to communicate their feelings. Siblings should not be overlooked. Parents may be so overwhelmed with their own grief that they forget the other children. Another reaction might be to overprotect their other children. The nurse should guide the family in identifying the various responses of the family members and in treating them at their correct developmental level. Children in the family who perhaps resented the new baby may have tremendous guilt feelings. The loss of a sibling may be especially traumatic to a toddler who does not understand the changes that are taking place in the family. Routines and rituals which are important to the toddler may be disrupted.

Evaluation

- Has the family joined a support group?
- Is the family able to verbalize feelings associated with the death of their child?
- Is the family using effective coping skills to work toward an understanding of their child's death?
- Has the extended family mobilized to support the family?

KEY CONCEPTS

- Infants and children under age 3 years are at increased risk to develop respiratory infections due to their immature immune system, smaller airways, and underdeveloped supporting cartilage.
- At birth the neonate must inflate the lungs, establish continuous breathing, and transfer gas needed to meet metabolic needs.
- The severity of allergic rhinitis can be decreased through the early identification and treatment of manifestations.
- Warm saline irrigations of the nasal passages can soften crusted secretions and wash out irritants. Saline solution can be made by mixing $\frac{1}{4}$ tsp of salt with 1 cup of water.
- Respiratory obstruction increases during crying and stridor increases in the supine position when the neck is flexed. The prone position with the neck hyperextended improves breathing.
- The only reliable means of determining if pharyngitis is viral or bacterial is with a throat culture.
- Children with nasopharyngitis should be seen by a physician if they have a fever lasting longer than 72 hours, earache, stiff neck, extreme irritability, and/or increased respiratory rate.
- Manifestations of bleeding after a tonsillectomy include frequent swallowing, restlessness, fast thready pulse, and vomiting bright red blood.
- The mucosal edema associated with croup can sometimes be decreased by steam from hot running water in a closed bathroom or a cool humidifier or by taking the child out into the cool, humid night air.
- Children with croup who develop stridor at rest, cyanosis, severe agitation/fatigue, or moderate to severe retractions or who are unable to take oral fluids should be seen in the emergency department.
- The four Ds of epiglottitis are drooling, dysphagia, dysphoria, and distressed inspiratory efforts.
- Examination and visualization of the epiglottis is contraindicated if epiglottitis is suspected because it can cause laryngospasm and airway obstruction.
- Because RSV is highly communicable, during RSV season infected children should be placed in contact isolation. Good handwashing should be emphasized and gowns worn when there is a chance clothing might be soiled.
- Oxygen needs can be decreased in the child in respiratory distress by scheduling nursing care to allow for periods of rest.
- Steam vaporizers should be avoided because of the danger of burns.
- Chest physiotherapy should be scheduled before meals and bedtime.
- If a child is aphonic and not breathing, the guidelines for management of an obstructed airway should be followed.
- During an apneic episode the time and duration, color change, bradycardia, oxygen saturation, what the infant was doing prior to the apneic period, and any actions that stimulated breathing should be documented.
- Healthy infants should be placed on their sides or backs for sleeping.
- When interviewing parents of an infant suspected of dying of SIDS, the nurse should avoid any implication of guilt on the part of the parents.

REFERENCES

Agudo, A., Bardagi, S., Romer, P., & Gonzalez, C. (1994). Exercise-induced airways narrowing and exposure to environmental tobacco smoke in schoolchildren. *American Journal of Epidemiology, 140,* 409–417.

American Academy of Pediatrics (1992). *AAP task force on infant positioning and SIDS.* Elk Grove Village, IL: AAP.

American Academy of Pediatrics (1994a). AAP reaffirms nonprone sleeping position endorsement. *AAP News, 10,* 2.

American Academy of Pediatrics (1994b). New otitis media guidelines released. *AAP News, 10,* 7.

American Academy of Pediatrics (1994c). *Report of the Committee on Infectious Diseases* (23rd ed.). Elk Grove Village, IL: AAP.

American Academy of Pediatrics (1996). SIDS decline linked to parents' actions. *AAP News, 12,* 1.

Anas, N., & Perkin, R. (1984). The pathophysiology of apnea of infancy. *Perinatology–Neonatology, 8,* 65–70.

Behrman, R., Kliegman, R., & Arvin, A. (1996). *Nelson textbook of pediatrics* (15th ed., p. 626). Philadelphia: W. B. Saunders.

Behrman, R., & Kliegman, R. (1994). *Nelson essentials of pediatrics* (2nd ed.). Philadelphia: W. B. Saunders.

Bluestone, C., & Klein, J. (1983). Otitis media with effusion, atelectasis, and eustachian tube dysfunction. In C. Bluestone & S. Stool (Eds.), *Pediatric otolaryngology.* Philadelphia: W. B. Saunders.

Brouillette, R., Weese-Mayer, D., & Hunt, C. (1990). Breathing control disorders in infants and children. *Hospital Practice, 8,* 82.

Chessare, J., Hunt, C., & Bourguignon, C. (1995). A community-based survey of infant sleep position. *Pediatrics, 96*(5), 893–896.

Gilbert-Barnes, E., & Barnes, L. (1995). Sudden infant death: A reappraisal. *Contemporary Pediatrics, 12*(4), 88–107.

Goyocoolea, M., & Hueb, M. (1991). Definitions and terminology. *Otolaryngology Clinics of North America, 24*(4), 757–761.

Hall, C., et al. (1988). Risk of secondary bacterial infection in infants hospitalized with respiratory syncytial viral infection. *New England Journal of Medicine, 113,* 266.

Hanley, P. (1992). Mechanisms and management of central sleeping apnea. *Lung, 170,* 1017.

Kemp, J., Nelson, V., & Thach, B. (1994). Physical properties of bedding that may increase risk of sudden infant death syndrome in prone-sleeping infants. *Pediatric Resident, 36,* 7–11.

Kovesi, T., Corey, M., & Levison, H. (1993). Passive smoking and lung function in cystic fibrosis. *American Review of Respiratory Disease, 148,* 1266–1271.

Loughlin, G. (1990). Bronchitis. In V. Chernick (Ed.), *Kendig's disorders of the respiratory tract in children* (p. 357). Philadelphia: W. B. Saunders.

Marchant, C. (1990). Otitis media today. *Pediatric Consultant, 8,* 1.

McCoy, K. (1993). Pediatric parenchymal diseases. In P. Koff, D. Eitzman, & J. Neu (Eds.), *Neonatal and pediatric respiratory care* (pp. 97–98). Philadelphia: W. B. Saunders.

Nederland, K., et al. (1989). Respiratory syncytial virus: A nursing perspective. *Pediatric Nursing, 15*(4), 342–345.

Nemes, J., Schmidt, E., & Kelly, L. (1988). Epiglottitis: ED nursing management. *Journal of Emergency Nursing, 14,* 70–75.

Niemelä, M., Uhari, M., & Möttönen, M. (1995). A pacifier increases the risk of recurrent acute otitis media in children in day care centers. *Pediatrics, 96*(5), 884–888.

O'Sullivan, B. (1994). Respiratory injury after hydrocarbon poisoning. In D. Schidlow & D. Smith (Eds.), *A practical guide to pediatric respiratory diseases.* Philadelphia: Hanley & Belfus.

Paradise, J. (1995). Managing otitis media: A time for change. *Pediatrics, 96*(4), 712–715.

Spitzer, A. (1996). SIDS and recurring apnea. In F. Burg, J. Ingelfinger, E. Wald, & R. Polin (Eds.), *Gellis and Kagans current pediatric therapy* (pp. 161–162). Philadelphia: W. B. Saunders.

Stark, A. (1991). Disorders of respiratory control in infants. *Respiratory Care, 36*(7), 673.

Steen, K., & Zimmerman, T. (1990). Tracheobronchial aspiration of foreign bodies in children: A study of 94 cases. *Laryngoscope, 100,* 525.

Tager, I., et al. (1993). Lung function, pre- and post-natal smoke exposure, and wheezing in the first year of life. *American Review of Respiratory Disease, 147,* 811–817.

BIBLIOGRAPHY

Adrian, G., Stutman, H., & Marks, M. (1991). Bacterial pneumonias. In V. Chernick (Ed.), *Kendig's disorders of the respiratory tract in children* (p. 371). Philadelphia: W. B. Saunders.

Burton, G., Hodgkin, J., & Ward, J. (Eds.). (1990). *Respiratory care* (3d ed.). Philadelphia: J. B. Lippincott.

Carlson, J. (1993). The psychologic effects of sudden infant death syndrome on parents. *Journal of Pediatric Health Care, 7,* 77–81.

Carson, L. (1992). Triage decisions: An 11-month-old with unexplained respiratory distress. *Journal of Emergency Nursing, 11*(1), 82.

Chernick, V., & Kendig, E. (1990). *Kendig's disorders of the respiratory tract in children.* Philadelphia: W. B. Saunders.

Chiocca, E. (1994). RSV and the high-risk infant. *Pediatric Nursing, 20*(6), 565–568.

Cohen, B., & Brady, M. (1992). Practices surrounding ribavirin administration. *Pediatric Nursing, 18*(3), 253–257.

Crawford, F., et al. (1994). Biomarkers of environmental tobacco smoke in preschool children and their mothers. *Journal of the National Cancer Institute, 86,* 1398–1402.

Gibson, E., Cullen, J., Spinner, S., Rankin, K., & Spitzer, A. (1995). Infant sleep position following new AAP guidelines. *Pediatrics, 96*(1), 69–72.

Gomberg, S. (1990). Mistaken identity—Is it epiglottitis or croup? *Pediatric Nursing, 16*(6), 567–570.

Grisemer, A. (1990). Apnea of prematurity: Current management and nursing implications. *Pediatric Nursing, 16*(6), 606.

Guntheroth, W., Lohmann, R., & Spiers, P. (1990). Risk of sudden infant death syndrome in subsequent siblings. *Journal of Pediatrics, 116,* 520.

Hall, C. B. (1993). Respiratory syncytial virus: What we know now. *Contemporary Pediatrics, 11,* 92–110.

Harris, J., et al. (1992). Respiratory syncytial virus: A pediatric nursing plan of care. *Journal of Pediatric Nursing, 7*(2), 128.

Koff, P., Eitzman, D., & Neu, J. (1993). *Neonatal and pediatric respiratory care.* St. Louis: Mosby–Year Book.

Loughlin, G., & Eigen, H. (1994). *Respiratory disease in children.* Baltimore: Williams & Wilkins.

Ruddy, R. (1993). Croup—Has management changed? *Contemporary Pediatrics, 12*(10), 21–32.

Ryan, C., Yacoub, W., Paton, T., & Avard, D. (1990). Childhood deaths from toy balloons. *American Journal of Disabled Children, 144,* 1221.

Schidlow, D., & Smith, D. (1994). *A practical guide to pediatric respiratory diseases.* Philadelphia: Hanley & Belfus.

Schmidt, B. (1992). *Instructions for pediatric patients.* Philadelphia: W. B. Saunders.

Spiers, P., & Guntheroth, W. (1994). Recommendations to avoid the prone sleeping position and recent statistics for sudden infant death syndrome in the United States. *Archives of Pediatric Adolescent Medicine, 149,* 141–146.

Spurzem, J. (1993). Acute bronchitis: Diagnosis and management. *Hospital Medicine, 12,* 26–32.

Steinschneider, A., & Santos, V. (1991). Parental reports of apnea and bradycardia: Temporal characteristics and accuracy. *Pediatrics, 88*(6), 1100.

Stretton, M., & Newth, C. (1990). Croup and epiglottitis: The critical early diagnosis. *Journal of Respiratory Disease, 11*(12), 1087–1100.

Wagner, T., & Hindi, A. (1984). Hazards of baby powder? *Pediatric Nursing, 10*(2), 124–125.

Waring, W. (1990). Diagnostic and therapeutic procedures. In V. Chernick (Ed.), *Kendig's disorders of the respiratory tract in children* (p. 81). Philadelphia: W. B. Saunders.

Willers, S., et al. (1992). Exposure to environmental tobacco smoke in the household and urinary cotinine excretion, heavy metals retention, and lung function. *Archives of Environmental Health, 47,* 357–363.

Willinger, M., Hoffman, H., & Hartford, R. (1994). Infant sleep position risk for sudden infant death syndrome. *Pediatrics, 93*(5), 814–819.

Youngkins, J. (1991). The impact of one staff nurse's research. *Maternal/Child Nursing, 16,* 133.

29

The Child With Chronic Respiratory Alterations

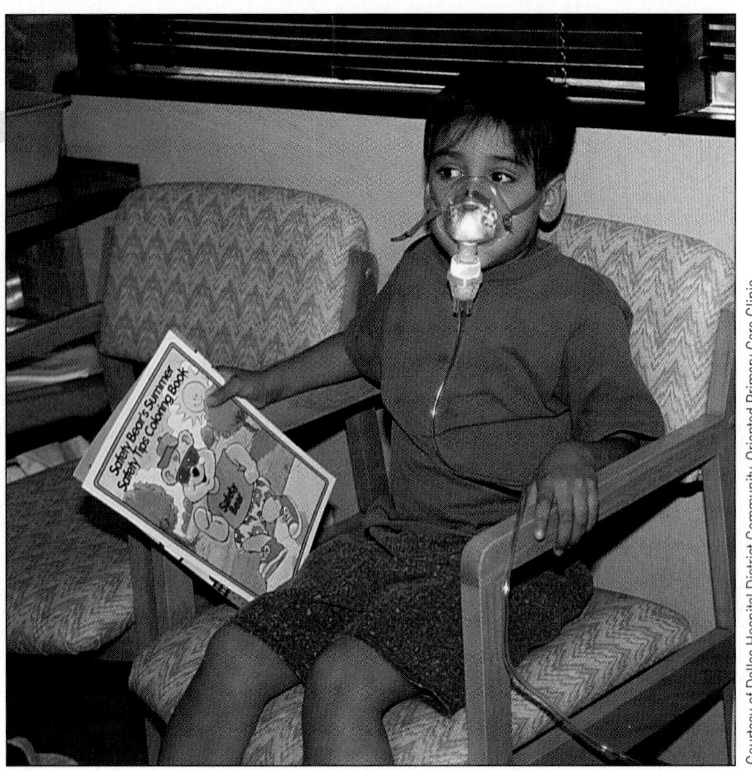

Courtesy of Dallas Hospital District Community-Oriented Primary Care Clinic

CHAPTER OVERVIEW

LEARNING OBJECTIVES

After studying this chapter, you should be able to:

- Discuss and display an understanding of the pathophysiology, therapeutic management, and nursing care of children with chronic respiratory conditions.
- Discuss common medications used in the treatment of chronic respiratory conditions in children and the nursing implications associated with these medications.
- Identify common triggers of asthma symptoms and measures that can be taken to prevent and treat asthma episodes.
- Identify teaching needs associated with asthma.
- Describe the nursing care of the child with cystic fibrosis.
- Discuss measures to maintain adequate oxygenation and provide appropriate developmental stimulation for the child with bronchopulmonary dysplasia.
- Describe the correct method of administering and evaluating tuberculosis skin tests.
- Identify ways to prevent the transmission of tuberculosis and explain the importance of administering antituberculosis medications as prescribed.

KEY TERMS

anergy: impaired or absent ability to react to specific antigens

dyspnea: difficulty breathing

hypercapnia: increased levels of carbon dioxide in the blood, as indicated by an elevated Pco_2 determined by blood gas analysis

hypocapnia: decreased levels of carbon dioxide in the blood

hypoxemia: decreased oxygen level in the blood

hypoxia: decreased oxygenation of cells and tissues

orthopnea: difficulty breathing except in an upright position

tachypnea: increased respiratory rate

wheezing: high-pitched, musical whistles, heard with or without a stethoscope, which may be inspiratory or expiratory and which are caused by bronchial constriction or obstruction of the airway; commonly occurs in asthma

Children with chronic conditions have many special needs (see Chapter 17). The child with a chronic respiratory disease is no different. Medications and treatments become a way of life for many of these children. Their activity level is often altered, and some may have a shortened lifespan.

The nurse plays a very important role in the care of the child with a chronic respiratory disease. Beyond giving acute care to the hospitalized child, the nurse must coordinate and facilitate the child's long-term care. Because of the advances being made in the treatment of chronic pediatric respiratory conditions, the treatment and care of children affected by these disorders is constantly changing and improving. This places an added responsibility on the nurse to stay current in these areas.

CLINICAL REFERENCE PAGES

See the Clinical Reference Pages in Chapter 28 for a review of the respiratory system, including a discussion of pediatric differences.

COMMON LABORATORY AND DIAGNOSTIC TESTS FOR CHRONIC RESPIRATORY DISORDERS

TEST/DESCRIPTION	SIGNIFICANCE OF FINDINGS	INDICATIONS	NURSING CONSIDERATIONS
Radioallergosorbent Test for IgE (RAST) Measures quantity of IgE antibodies in serum after exposure to specific antigens	If the child is not allergic to the antigen, IgE antibody is not detected. A test result is positive in relation to a specific antigen if it is >400% of control.	• Identification of specific allergens • Onset of asthma, hay fever, dermatitis • Systemic reaction to insect venom, drugs, chemicals • Monitoring response to desensitization procedures	Prepare for a peripheral blood sample. Determine whether the child has undergone any radioisotope tests within the past week, as such tests may alter the results.
Pilocarpine Iontophoresis (Sweat Test) Measures sweat electrolyte concentration for diagnosis of cystic fibrosis (CF) Sweating is stimulated on the child's forearm with a small electrical current and pilocarpine; a sweat sample is then collected on preweighed, dry, sterile gauze or filter paper and the amount of sweat sodium and chloride are measured.	*Normal:* ≤ 40 mEq/L *Suggestive of CF:* 40 mEq/L *Positive for CF:* ≥ 60 mEq/L	• Diagnosis of cystic fibrosis	No physical preparation is needed. Offer the parents and child support as they face the implications of a positive diagnosis. Inform the child/parents that the test is painless and that it is usually performed twice to ensure accurate results. Because an adequate amount of sweat is difficult to obtain from infants, the sweat test is usually unreliable in infants < 4 weeks of age.
Chorionic Villus Biopsy (CVB) Detects fetal abnormalities secondary to various genetic disorders Tissue samples obtained via CVB are cultured in media and are examined microscopically and assessed for chromosomal abnormalities.	*Normal findings:* no chromosomal abnormalities detected	• Detection of genetic defects • Family history of genetic disorders or diseases (e.g., CF, sickle cell anemia, Tay-Sachs disease • Prenatal sex determination when the mother is a known carrier of a sex-linked disorder (e.g., hemophilia)	Samples are best obtained between the 8th and 10th weeks of pregnancy. Explain the procedure and purpose of the study to the client. The test takes about 15 minutes. Ask the client to void before the procedure. Ask the client to remove clothing from the waist down; provide a gown. The embryo is localized by ultrasonography. Obtain and record baseline vital signs. Position the client on the examination table and offer support as the vaginal speculum is inserted. Instruct the client to report immediately any abdominal cramping or vaginal bleeding after the procedure.

COMMON LABORATORY AND DIAGNOSTIC TESTS FOR CHRONIC RESPIRATORY DISORDERS *(continued)*

TEST/DESCRIPTION	SIGNIFICANCE OF FINDINGS	INDICATIONS	NURSING CONSIDERATIONS
Aminiotic Fluid Analysis Assessment of fetal health and maturity, and detection of genetic disorders, diseases, and inborn errors of metabolism	Normal findings: clear amniotic fluid, no chromosomal or neural tube abnormalities.	• In utero diagnosis of disorders, such as CF and diabetes mellitus • Detection of genetic and neural tube defects • Test for hemolytic disease in the neonate • Determination of fetal maturity • Prenatal sex determination	The test may be performed from 14 weeks' gestation. Explain the procedure and purpose to the client. The test requires approximately 20–30 minutes. If ultrasonography is performed immediately prior to the procedure, hydrate the client to ensure a full bladder. After the ultrasound examination, ask the client to empty her bladder to prevent perforation during amniocentesis. Record maternal vital signs and fetal heart rate before the procedure and every 15 minutes after the procedure for 1 hour. Assess the client for contractions, pain, and vaginal bleeding every 15 minutes after the procedure. Observe the puncture site for signs of bleeding or drainage.
Mantoux Test Skin test for tuberculosis Purified protein derivative (PPD), 5 TB units (0.1 ml) is injected intradermally into the volar surface of the forearm with a short 26 to 27-gauge needle, beveled side up. A wheal that is 6–10 mm in diameter should appear during the injection. The site is checked in 48–72 hr by a health care professional. Results are recorded in mm (not simply as "positive" or "negative"). The reading is based on induration (hardness), not redness.	*Positive result:* An area of induration ≥ 15 mm (in children of all ages) An area of induration ≥ 10 mm in children younger than 4 years of age or at high risk for exposure An area of induration ≥ 5 mm in the highest risk groups *Negative result:* The Mantoux test cannot rule out the presence of TB, particularly in young infants	• Screening and testing of individuals suspected of having or of having been exposed to TB	More reliable than the tine test, but more difficult to administer. When administering the Mantoux test, withdrawal of the needle should be delayed for 2–3 seconds after injection to minimize leakage of PPD at the puncture site. In most children, skin testing will show a positive reaction 3 to 6 weeks after initial infection. Steroids and immunosuppressants given within 4–6 weeks can cause false-negative skin test results. Positive tuberculin reactivity usually continues for the person's lifetime, even with treatment.
Tine Test Multiple puncture skin test (MPT) for TB (other MPTs include the Aplitest and Heaf tests.) A disposable plastic unit with four stainless steel blades (tines) predipped in OT is applied to the forearm after the skin has been cleansed with alcohol. The site should be circled with a pen to facilitate later interpretation.	*Positive result:* appearance of vesicles with one or more papules measuring at least 2 mm in diameter Patients with positive or doubtful reactions must undergo the Mantoux test.	• Screening test for TB	MPTs are not as accurate as Mantoux test (Behrman, Kliegman, & Arvin, 1996). Problems with MPTs limit their usefulness (AAP, 1994b): • Lack of standardization of antigen dose • High rate of false-negative and false-positive readings • Variability in application of prongs • Lack of standardized test reading (often done by untrained persons, such as parents)

MEDICATIONS COMMONLY USED IN THE TREATMENT OF CHRONIC RESPIRATORY CONDITIONS

NAME AND ACTION	DOSAGE/ROUTE	SIDE EFFECTS	NURSING IMPLICATIONS
Beta$_2$-Adrenergic Agonist Medications			
Albuterol (Proventil, Ventolin, Airet, Volmax): Reduces bronchospasm; rapid-acting Prevents exercise-induced bronchospasm Effective for 4–6 hr	*Oral:* 2–6 yr: initial 0.1 mg/kg daily; maximum 12 mg/daily. 6–14 yr: 2 mg t.i.d., maximum 24 mg/day. Over 14 yr: 2–4 mg t.i.d. *Nebulizer:* ≥5 yr: 2.5–5 mg q 4–6 hr; ≥12 yr: 2.5 mg 3–4 times a day *Metered dose inhaler (MDI):* 1–2 puffs q 4–6 hr while awake, as needed, up to 4 times a day	Nervousness, tremor, tachycardia, palpitations, throat irritation, hypertension, nausea, cramps, dizziness, headache, insomnia	When used to prevent exercise-induced bronchospasm, the inhaler should be used at least 15 minutes before exercise. Correct inhaler technique is important. With aerosol therapy, nebulization with oxygen prevents hypoxemia related to the treatment.
Terbutaline (Brethine, Brethaire, Bricanyl): Reduces bronchospasm Effective for 4–7 hours Relaxes bronchial smooth muscle, relieves bronchospasm	*Oral:* 2.5 mg q 6 hr, maximum 7.5 mg/day *MDI:* 1–2 puffs q 4–6 hr *Nebulizer:* 0.5–1.5 mg q 4–6 hr *Subcutaneous:* <12 yr: 3.5–5 μg/kg/dose given once. >12 yr: 0.25 mg/dose repeated in 15–30 min prn × 1 dose only. Total maximum dose of 0.5 mg within a 4-hr period.	Tachycardia, headache, nausea, tremors, nervousness, insomnia	Prevents exercise-induced asthma and should be given before onset of symptoms.
Metaproterenol (Alupent, Metaprel, Prometa): Reduces bronchospasm; rapid-acting Effective for 3–4 hr	*Oral:* 10–20 mg tablet q 4–6 hr, maximum of 20 mg/dose *MDI:* 1 to 3 puffs q 3–4 hr for children older than 12 years of age; maximum of 12 puffs/day *Nebulizer—over 12 yr:* 50 mg/ml 0.25–0.50 mg/kg in 2 ml of NS q 4–6 hr, max 15 mg	Tachycardia, palpitations, hypertension, nervousness, weakness, headache, nausea, vomiting, bad taste in the mouth	Store in an airtight container that is protected from light.
Epinephrine (adrenalin)	*Subcutaneous:* 0.01 ml/kg of of 1:1000 (1 mg/ml) preparation	Pallor, tremor, anxiety, tachycardia, palpitations, headache	May repeat dose once or twice at 20-minute intervals.
Other Bronchodilators			
Theophylline *Oral:* Dose varies according to age and other factors. Aerosol administration is ineffective. Long-acting theophylline (Slo-bid, Quibron T/Or, Theo-Dur sprinkle, Somophyllin-CRT, Somophylline-GC) Short-acting theophylline (Elixophyllin, Slo-Phyllin, Somophyllin) Reduces bronchospasm; improves mucociliary clearance Duration of effect varies with the preparation used.	*IV infusion:* Dosage is individualized, depending upon the agent used, the route of administration, age, weight, and other factors affecting theophylline clearance. *Oral:* 6 mo–9 yr: 4 mg/kg q 6 hr. 9–16 yr: 3 mg/kg q 6 hr	Tachycardia, hypotension, nausea, vomiting, abdominal discomfort, diarrhea, anorexia, weight loss, jitteriness, irritability, insomnia, headache, learning difficulties, seizures	*Oral:* Give with food to avoid GI distress. Therapeutic serum theophylline levels range from 10–20 μg/ml. Toxicity occurs at levels > 20 mg/ml. Absorption varies between different brands of theophylline, so generic substitutes should not be accepted for prescribed medication. Serum theophylline levels should be monitored closely.
Theophylline ethylenediamine (Aminophylline)	*IV infusion:* Patients not currently receiving theophylline may receive a loading dose of 6 mg/kg, followed by maintenance dosages (IV): 6 mo–9 yr: 1 mg/kg/hr 9–12 yr: 0.9 mg/kg/hr 12–16 yr: 0.6 mg/kg/hr	Gastrointestinal (GI) irritation and central nervous system (CNS) stimulation, palpitations, tachycardia Symptoms of toxicity: frequent vomiting, severe thirst, slight fever, tinnitus, palpitations, possible seizures	To minimize adverse effects, administer IV aminophylline slowly, at a rate ≤ 25 mg/min; loading doses are usually given over a period of 20–30 min. Dilute the solution at least to 250 mg/20 ml. IV push is not recommended.

MEDICATIONS COMMONLY USED IN THE TREATMENT OF CHRONIC RESPIRATORY CONDITIONS *(continued)*

NAME AND ACTION	DOSAGE/ROUTE	SIDE EFFECTS	NURSING IMPLICATIONS
Theophylline ethylenediamine (Aminophylline) (cont.)			Steroids may increase the drug's pharmacologic effect. Do not exceed IV flow rate of 1 ml/min (25 mg/min). Use infusion pump to regulate IV administration. Do NOT administer this drug IM, as it causes severe pain.
Anti-Inflammatory Medications			
Cromolyn (Intal): Reduces airway reactivity Prevents symptoms of exercise-induced asthma.	*MDI:* 2 puffs 2–4 times/day *Nebulizer:* children older than 2 years: 20 mg 6–8 hr	Virtually no side effects May cause coughing or slight pharyngeal irritation with inhalation	This drug has no effect once asthma symptoms start (i.e., it must be taken prophylactically)
Nedrocromal sodium (Tilade): Nonsteroidal anti-inflammatory agent used for preventive management of asthma	*MDI:* children 12 years of age and older: 2 puffs 4 times/day	Mildly unpleasant taste, nausea, headache, throat irritation, cough	No bronchodilating action Useful only for the prevention of asthma symptoms
Corticosteroids			
Inhaled preparations Beclomethasone dipropionate (Beclovent, Vanceril) Triamcinolone acetonide (Azmacort) Flunisolide (Aerobid)	*MDI:* Beclomethasone and triamcinolone: 1–2 puffs q 6–8 hr Flunisolide: 2 puffs q 12 hr	*Inhaled:* Oropharyngeal candidiasis, dysphonia, dry throat, nasal irritation, sneezing	*Inhaled:* Proper inhalation technique and use of a spacer device may help decrease local adverse effects. Rinsing the mouth after each inhalation may help prevent oral candidiasis.
Oral preparations Prednisone Prednisolone Methylprednisolone Reduces airway inflammation; decreases mucus secretion and airway edema; reduces airway hyperresponsiveness	*Oral:* 0.14–2 mg/kg The dose varies with drug used and patient's age and condition. Lowest possible dose should be used. To minimize suppression of the hypothalamic-pituitary-adrenal axis, the drug should be taken between 2 a.m. and 8 a.m. when the adrenal cortex is most active.	*Oral:* Depends on dose frequency and duration of effect Mood changes, increased appetite, fluid retention, infection, weight gain, gastrointestinal distress, impaired growth, decreased bone formation	*Oral:* Do not stop drug abruptly. Take with food or milk to minimize gastric irritation. Alternate-day administration may cause fewer side effects. Chickenpox and measles may lead to fatal complications in children receiving immunosuppressant drugs. Care should be taken to avoid exposure.
Mucolytic agents			
N-Acetylcysteine (Mucomyst): Aerosolized mucolytic agent used in combination with chest physiotherapy for patients with CF. Reduces viscosity of mucus secretions	3–5 ml of 20% solution with an equal volume of NS or 10 ml of 10% solution 3–4 times/day	Stomatitis, nausea, vomiting, hemoptysis, severe rhinorrhea	Unpleasant, pungent odor may cause nausea
Recombinant human DNase (Pulmozyme): Reduces viscosity of sputum in patients with CF.	2.5 mg delivered by nebulizer 1–2 times/day using recommended nebulizer system	Minimal adverse effects Hoarseness, pharyngitis, rash, chest pain	Safety has not been demonstrated in children younger than 5 years of age. The drug should be refrigerated and should not be exposed to room temperatures for > 24 hr.

MEDICATIONS COMMONLY USED IN THE TREATMENT OF TUBERCULOSIS (TB)

NAME AND ACTION	DOSAGE/ROUTE	SIDE EFFECTS*	NURSING IMPLICATIONS
First-Line Drugs			
Isoniazid (INH): Antitubercular bactericidal agent that interferes with cell wall synthesis	Oral/IM *Daily:* 10–15 mg/kg/day *2/week:* 20–30 mg/kg Available in an oral liquid form	Peripheral neuritis, pyridoxine (vitamin B_6) deficiency, hepatotoxicity, glossitis, gastrointestinal disturbance, hypersensitivity, fever	Administer pyridoxine if the patient's diet is deficient in meat and milk. Monitor the patient's liver function.
Rifampin (RIF) (Rifadin): Antitubercular bactericidal agent that inhibits RNA synthesis	Oral/IV *Daily:* 10–20 mg/kg *2/week:* 10–20 mg/kg Available in an oral liquid form	Hepatotoxicity, gastrointestinal disturbance, hypersensitivity, rash, fever, thrombocytopenia, many drug interactions	Instruct the patient to expect orange discoloration of urine, feces, saliva, sputum, sweat, and/or tears. Contact lenses may also stain orange. This drug may render oral contraceptives ineffective.
Ethambutol (EMB) (Myambutol): Antitubercular bacteriostatic agent that inhibits protein synthesis	*Daily:* 15–25 mg/kg *2/week:* 50 mg/kg *3/week:* 25–30 mg/kg	Optic neuritis (decreased acuity and loss of red-green color discrimination), gout; skin rash	Test the patient's vision monthly. Monitor serum uric acid levels. Not recommended in young children.
Streptomycin: Antitubercular bacteriostatic and bactericidal action (inhibits protein synthesis)	IM *Daily:* 20 mg/kg daily 2 or 3/week: 25–40 mg/kg. Maximum 1 g/day	Auditory and renal toxicity, hypokalemia, hypomagnesemia	Monitor the patient's auditory and kidney function. Streptomycin must be given IM. Contraindicated in pregnant women.
Pyrazinamide: May be bacteriostatic or bacteriocidal depending on its concentration at infection site.	15–30 mg/kg/day, maximum 1.5 g/day 2/week: 40–60 mg/kg	Gastrointestinal upset, hepatotoxicity, hyperuricemia, arthralgias	In doses of $\leq$ 30 mg/kg/day this drug is seldom hepatotoxic.
Second-Line Drugs Used for multidrug-resistant *M. tuberculosis* infection			
Capreomycin (Capastat) Kanamycin (Kantrex) Cycloserine (Seromycin) Ethionamide (ETH) (Trecator-SC)	15–30 mg/kg/day 15 mg/kg/day 10–15 mg/kg/day 15–20 mg/kgday	Auditory, vestibular, and renal toxicity; hypokalemia; hypomagnesemia; eosinophilia Seizures, headache, depression, rash, gastrointestinal upset, hepatotoxicity, metallic taste	Administer vitamin B_6 with cycloserine.

*Adverse reactions to TB medications occur must less frequently in children than in adults. It is not necessary to monitor liver function unless the child exhibits signs suggesting hepatitis (abdominal pain, jaundice, vomiting).

ASTHMA

Asthma, or reactive airway disease (RAD), is a leading cause of acute and chronic illness in children and is the most frequent admitting diagnosis in children's hospitals. (Behrman, Kliegman, & Arvin, 1996). Asthma affects two to five million children in the United States. Despite advances in medical treatment, the incidence and death rate from asthma have increased in recent years.

Etiology. The reason some children's airways are more reactive than others is unclear. However, it is known that heredity plays a role. A child who has one parent with asthma has a 25% chance of developing the disease, whereas a child whose parents are both asthmatic has a 50% chance of developing asthma (Behrman, Kliegman, & Arvin, 1996).

An asthma episode may be triggered by a variety of stimuli, such as cold air, smoke, fumes, viral infection, stress, exercise, odors, or drugs (particularly aspirin and NSAIDs). A child does not have to "have allergies" to suffer from asthma, but allergies do play a major role in triggering an episode in many children. The most common allergens causing asthma are inhalants (house dust, dust mites, mold, animal dander), airborne pollens (trees, grasses, weeds), and outdoor seasonal molds. Foods occasionally cause problems, especially in infants, but less commonly in older children.

The immature anatomy of infants and small children predisposes them to increased distress from asthma. Children's smaller, narrower airways and decreased elastic lung recoil make them more prone to airway obstruction. The child's flexible rib cage and underdeveloped chest muscles and diaphragm lead to exhaustion with increased respiratory effort. Although asthma is not actually "outgrown," the severity of asthma attacks often decreases as the child gets older owing to increased airway size, improved diaphragmatic support, and better mucus clearing. However, asthma is considered a lifelong condition and may become increasingly severe after a period of remission.

Incidence. Since the early 1980s, the incidence of asthma has risen in the United States and in other parts of the world (Rachelefsky, 1995). Asthma affects an estimated 12.4 million Americans, nearly double the 6.8 million reported in 1980 (Altman, 1994). Asthma affects 1 in 12 school-age children in the United States and is the leading cause of school absences, causing more than 30% of all school absences due to illness. Although asthma may first appear at any age, the highest incidence of asthma is in the first few years of life. About 50% of new cases of asthma occur in children younger than 1 year of age. Asthma is more common among boys than girls until puberty, when the incidence between the sexes becomes equal (Behrman, Kliegman, & Arvin, 1996). Research has shown that the younger the child is when the asthma first appears, the more likely it is that the asthma will persist into the adult years. Most children with asthma improve by adolescence, but only 20% are symptom-free by early adulthood.

Clinical Manifestations. The manifestations of asthma may vary. A child experiencing an asthma episode may have only a dry cough. Others, however, may exhibit one or more of the following:

- Wheezing
- Dyspnea with prolonged expiration and use of accessory muscles of respiration; may also display retractions, nasal flaring, or stridor.
- Nonproductive cough (with or without wheezing); later becomes productive
- Tachypnea, **orthopnea**
- Restlessness, apprehension, diaphoresis
- Abdominal pain secondary to the strain placed on the abdominal muscles during labored breathing
- A "hunched over" sitting position with arms braced
- Fatigue, as evidenced by difficulty performing simple tasks, such as eating, walking, or even talking, owing to shortness of breath
- Sudden or insidious onset of asthma
- A feeling of chest tightness prior to the onset of more objective signs, followed by dry cough, wheezing, and **dyspnea.**
- Worsening of symptoms after going to bed owing to increased narrowing of the airways at night and pooling of secretions.

At the beginning of the asthma episode, **wheezing** may be heard only with a stethoscope. As the severity of the episode increases, wheezing may be audible to the unaided ear. Children who have severe respiratory distress may not demonstrate wheezing owing to decreased air movement. With treatment, increased wheezing may actually signal that the child's condition is improving.

> Decreased wheezing in a child who otherwise is not improving clinically may incorrectly be interpreted as a positive sign when, in fact, it may signal an inability to move air. A "silent chest" is an ominous sign during as asthma episode.

Diagnostic Evaluation. Wheezing is the classic symptom of asthma, but other symptoms may be present, including shortness of breath, cough, or dyspnea, on exertion. A new case of asthma may begin as a cough without wheezing. The child may have had recurrent bouts of pneumonia or sinusitis. A family history of asthma or allergy is a frequent finding.

Physical examination may be normal if the child is not having an asthma episode at the time of the examination. During an acute episode, auscultation will reveal wheez-

PATHOPHYSIOLOGY *of Asthma*

Asthma is a reversible obstructive airway disease characterized by:

Bronchospasm resulting from constriction of bronchial smooth muscle
Inflammation and edema of the mucous membranes lining the small airways and accumulation of thick secretions in the airways
Increased airway responsiveness to a variety of stimuli

Children with asthma have hyperreactive airways. Normal airways react to irritants and other stimuli by narrowing. The asthmatic child's airways, however, narrow in response to stimuli that do not affect nonasthmatic individuals (see accompanying figure). When exposed to an irritant—whether allergic or nonallergic—the asthmatic child's bronchial smooth muscles go into spasm. Upon exposure to an allergen, antibodies (immunoglobulin E [IgE]) are synthesized and attach to receptors on airway mast cells. Upon reexposure to the antigen, IgE receptors are triggered to activate the mast cells, causing release of mediators (histamine and other substances). These mediators stimulate both immediate and delayed inflammatory responses which cause asthma symptoms. The *immediate phase* is characterized by bronchoconstriction that resolves within 1 to 2 hours. In the *delayed phase,* bronchoconstriction may recur in 4 to 6 hours, and may persist for 2 to 5 hours or longer. An additional *late response* may also occur; this is inflammatory in nature and causes hyperresponsiveness of the airways that lasts several weeks or months. Late asthmatic responses can also occur without a previous early (immediate) response. When asthma is precipitated by nonallergic stimuli (exercise, cold air), bronchospasm usually lasts less than 1 hour and is not followed by a late response.

During an asthma episode, the mucous membranes lining the bronchioles become edematous and secrete large amounts of thick mucus. As a result, the airways narrow, leading to increased airway resistance and respiratory distress. Because small airways are normally wider on inspiration than expiration, the child is able to inhale, but has difficulty exhaling through the narrowed bronchioles. **Wheezing** can be heard as air is forced through the narrow passages during expiration. Air becomes trapped, causing hyperinflation of the alveoli. The child is forced to breathe at increasingly higher lung volumes (Bechler-Karsch, 1994).

Airway obstruction is more severe in some parts of the lungs than in others, and air flows more easily into areas with the least resistance. The blood that flows to the less ventilated portions of the lungs is inadequately saturated with oxygen. Thus, a mismatch between ventilation and perfusion in poorly ventilated areas of the lung occurs, resulting in incompletely saturated blood entering the systemic circulation. Decreased Po_2 levels **(hypoxia)** results. As the child struggles to get enough air, his breathing rate increases **(tachypnea).** Tachypnea lowers carbon dioxide levels in the blood **(hypocapnia).** As the child tires from the increased work of breathing, hypoventilation occurs, and carbon dioxide levels increase. Increased levels of carbon dioxide in the blood **(hypercapnia)** during an asthma episode may be a sign of severe airway obstruction and impending respiratory failure.

ing, tachypnea, and a prolonged expiratory phase. Examination of the chest may show increased anteroposterior diameter (so-called barrel chest). Chest X-ray studies are usually normal except in cases of severe asthma, in which hyperinflation of the airways may be seen. Pulmonary function tests reveal a decreased expiratory flow rate and air trapping.

Rhinitis, sinusitis, and nasal polyps are often present in children with asthma. Eosinophilia is present in both the blood and the sputum. Skin tests are often performed to identify specific allergens. The radioallergosorbent test (RAST) may be used to identify specific antigens. Arterial blood gas measurements may be ordered in patients having a severe asthma episode. Pulse oximetry values are usually monitored in patients who are hospitalized for asthma.

Therapeutic Management of an Acute Asthma Episode

An acute asthma episode can be a frightening experience for both the child and his parents. Often, the child and parents try to treat the episode at home with prescribed medications and breathing treatments. If home measures fail to control an asthma episode, the family often seeks treatment at a hospital emergency department.

First, a bronchodilator (usually albuterol) is administered via a powered nebulizer. In the past, acute asthma episodes were treated with subcutaneous epinephrine, but this practice has largely been replaced by the use of inhaled beta-adrenergic medications (see Medications Commonly Used in the Treatment of Chronic Respiratory Conditions in the Clinical Reference Pages at the begin-

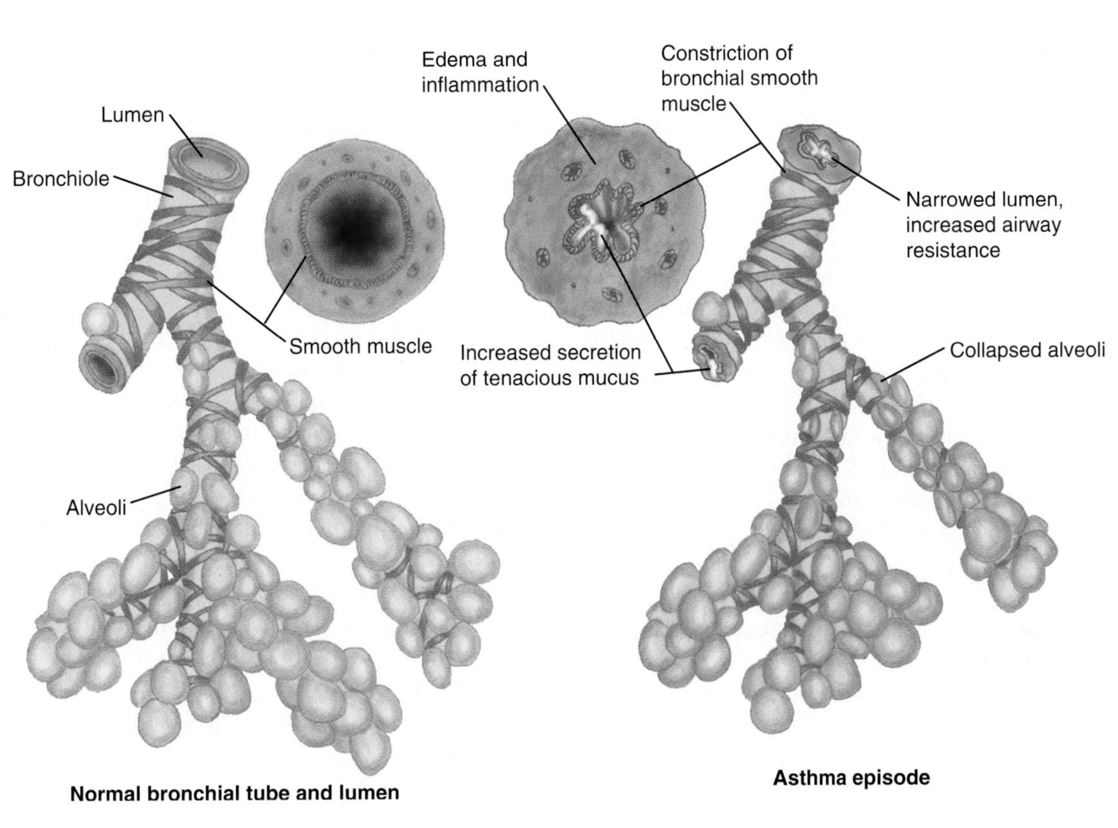

ning of this chapter). If there is cyanosis or marked respiratory distress, humidified oxygen is administered, either by nasal prongs or face mask. An IV line is started to provide fluids as well as venous access for parenteral medications. IV bronchodilators may be ordered. Corticosteroids may be prescribed to decrease inflammation in the airways. Assessment of the degree of airway obstruction and the response to bronchodilator treatment is then performed. Auscultation of breath sounds may not reveal wheezing in the severe phase of an asthma episode because the bronchioles may be "too tight to wheeze." Increased wheezing may be heard after treatment with bronchodilators, signaling increased air movement. Chest X-ray films, arterial blood gas determinations, and/or pulse oximetry values may be obtained to further evaluate the patient's oxygenation status.

Increasingly severe asthma that is unresponsive to vigorous treatment measures is termed *status asthmaticus*. Status asthmaticus is a medical emergency that can result in respiratory failure and death. Hospitalization, usually in an intensive care unit, is indicated. The child is placed on a cardiac-respiratory monitor, and continuous pulse oximetry measurements are initiated. Blood gases and serum electrolytes are monitored. Humidified oxygen is administered via tent nasal cannula or face mask. An IV line is started for administration of fluids and medications. The child is given nothing by mouth except liquids if tolerated. A variety of medications, including nebulized albuterol (either intermittent or continuous) and oral or parenteral corticosteroids, and methylxanthines (aminophylline and theophylline), are administered. If the child does not respond to these medications, subcutaneous epinephrine

(1:1000) at a dose of 0.01 ml/kg with a maximum dose of 0.3 ml or subcutaneous terbutaline may be administered. Endotracheal intubation with mechanical ventilation may be necessary. Acidosis is corrected with IV administration of sodium bicarbonate. Antibiotics may also be administered to treat concurrent infection (such as pneumonia).

Long-Term Management of Asthma

The goals of long-term asthma treatment are to minimize symptoms, prevent acute asthma episodes, avoid side effects of therapy, and help the child maintain a normal lifestyle. Self-management is important in achieving these goals. Children with asthma and their parents need to be taught about asthma and how to control it. Treatment focuses on environmental control, immunotherapy, education about asthma, and medications.

Common Asthma Triggers

Children with asthma and their parents can decrease the frequency and severity of asthma episodes by recognizing and controlling the triggers that precipitate symptoms.

> Common asthma triggers include allergens and irritants in the child's environment, respiratory infections, exercise, and emotions.

Environmental Factors. Because environmental factors frequently trigger asthma episodes, a careful assessment of potential triggers in the child's environment should be made. Common irritants include cigarette smoke, smoke from wood-burning stoves and fireplaces, fumes, deodorants, over-humidified air, and perfume. Allergenic triggers, such as animal dander, seasonal pollens, and molds, often cause problems. House dust can be both an irritant and an allergen.

The extent of environmental control needed depends upon the severity of the child's asthma problem. For the child with mild asthma, merely prohibiting smoking in the house and controlling dust with frequent house cleaning may be adequate. Keeping the humidity in the house below 50% helps to control dust mites. If the child continues to have problems after such measures have been implemented, additional steps to minimize environmental triggers are indicated (see Teaching Guidelines: Allergy-Proofing the Home in Chapter 28).

Allergy. Although allergy is not the cause of asthma in every case, it does play a role in precipitating asthma symptoms in some children, particularly those older than 2 years of age. In children with "extrinsic" or "allergic" asthma, an episode may be precipitated by exposure to allergens, such as dust, pollens, or animal dander. The most effective way to decrease allergy-induced asthma symptoms is for the child to avoid the offending allergen. Skin testing may be performed to identify specific allergic triggers. Increased serum IgE levels may also be found. Specific IgE antibodies may be identified by performing a serologic RAST. Immunotherapy ("allergy shots") may be helpful in decreasing asthma symptoms caused by specific allergens that cannot be avoided. Immunotherapy has been shown to decrease sensitivity to pollens, dander, house dust, and mite antigens. Immunotherapy is used in conjunction with, not in place of, other asthma therapies (Smith, 1993).

Exercise. Exercise is a trigger of asthma in some children. Eighty percent of asthmatics develop some degree of chest tightness, cough, or wheeze with exercise (Plaut, 1988). Exercise-induced asthma (EIA) is thought to be triggered by rapid breathing of large volumes of cool, dry air (as with mouth breathing during exercise). The symptoms of EIA usually begin after 5 to 10 minutes of exercise and often last from 30 minutes to 1 hour.

Measures to prevent EIA include:

- Warming the air by breathing through the nose and/or covering the mouth and nose with a scarf when exercising in cold weather.
- Using an inhaled $beta_2$-agonist or cromolyn before exercise.
- Practicing techniques to decrease hyperventilation (e.g., progressive muscle relaxation, diaphragmatic breathing).

Children with asthma should not be restricted from physical activity. Athletics and active play are important parts of a child's life. Exercise not only increases physical fitness but also enhances self-esteem and offers valuable opportunities for socialization. With adequate treatment, a child with asthma can participate in most physical activities. Swimming is frequently recommended as an ideal sport for children with asthma because the air is humidified and exhaling underwater prolongs exhalation and increased end-expiratory pressure. Other sports that do not require sustained exertion, such as gymnastics, baseball, and weight lifting, are also well tolerated. However, if asthma is well controlled, the child can usually participate in any type of sport.

Infection. Viral respiratory infections are the most frequent triggers of pediatric asthma. Viruses cause chemical mediators (histamine, leukotrienes, and others) to be released from mast cells in the airway, resulting in bronchial inflammation, edema, and increased production of mucus. Viruses are also thought to hinder the effectiveness of some asthma medications by decreasing the sensitivity of beta-adrenergic agonist receptor sites in the airways.

It is advisable for children with frequent or severe asthma to avoid exposure to individuals with a viral respiratory infection. These children also benefit from administration of influenza vaccine.

Emotions. Asthma is not caused by psychosocial problems. However, although emotional upset does not cause asthma, it can exacerbate asthma symptoms. Laughing, crying, or shouting can act as mechanical triggers of bronchoconstriction. Also, a child with asthma may become angry or frustrated with his condition and refuse to take his medication, thus making his symptoms worse. Moreover, anxiety during an episode may cause the child to hyperventilate, aggravating asthma symptoms.

Monitoring Symptoms

Asthma symptoms can best be treated if they are detected early. Children should be taught how to recognize the subtle early symptoms of an asthma episode (itchy chest or chin, cough, irritability or tired feeling, increased breathing rate, dry mouth, unusually dark circles under eyes).

A useful device for monitoring breathing capacity is the peak flowmeter. A peak flowmeter measures the flow of air in a forced exhalation in liters/minute. Peak flow monitoring can help identify the start of an asthma episode, often before the child is aware of symptoms. Peak flow zones divide the peak flowmeter into the colors of a traffic light and can help children and health professionals make decisions about asthma management (see accompanying box) (National Jewish Center for Immunology and Respiratory Medicine, 1995).

Home monitoring of peak expiratory flow rate may be performed several times a day. The results can be compared to the child's normal predicted level and to the results obtained during the past several days, providing an objective assessment of respiratory status. Changes in peak flow rate are helpful in determining the need for treatment modification, as well as in early detection of asthma symptoms.

Medications

Generally, asthma is treated with a combination of medications from two categories: bronchodilators and anti-inflammatory agents (see Medications Commonly Used in the Treatment of Chronic Respiratory Conditions in the Clinical Reference Pages at the beginning of this chapter).

Bronchodilators

Beta$_2$-Adrenergic Agonists. The most commonly prescribed drugs in this category are albuterol (Proventil,

Monitoring Breathing Capacity Using a Peak Flowmeter

The peak flowmeter is a device used to monitor breathing capacity in the child with asthma. It measures the flow of air in a forced exhalation in liters per minute. Peak flow monitoring can help identify the start of an asthma episode, often before symptoms are evident. To help children monitor their asthma, a zone system can be explained as a traffic light, making it easier for them to identify and understand differences in peak flow values.

Peak Flow Zones

Personal best: ______________________

Green: All clear—no asthma symptoms are present (80%–100% of personal best)

Yellow: Caution—acute episode may be present (50%–80% of personal best). A temporary increase in medication may be indicated. Asthma may not be under control. Medication may need to be increased.

Red: Medical alert (below 50% of personal best). An immediate bronchodilator should be taken. Practitioner should be notified if measurements do not return immediately to and stay in yellow or green zones.

HOW TO USE A PEAK FLOWMETER

1. Remove gum or food from the mouth and stand up.
2. Move the pointer on the meter to zero.
3. Hold the meter horizontally, being sure to keep your fingers away from vent holes and the marker.
4. Relax and take a few moderately slow, deep breaths. Slowly take the deepest breath possible with your mouth wide open.
5. Hold your breath while placing the mouthpiece on your tongue. Seal your lips tightly around the mouthpiece.
6. Blow out as hard and fast as possible. Give a short, sharp blast, not a slow blow. (The meter records the fastest huff, not the longest.) Note the number by the marker on the numbered scale.
7. Repeat three times. Wait at least 10 seconds between attempts. (Be sure to move the pointer to zero after each try.)
8. Record the highest of the three readings.
9. Ideally, peak flow values are obtained a minimum of once a day, preferably in the morning. Peak flow measurements should be done before and after administration of an inhaled bronchodilator. The number of measurements should be increased during a flare-up.

Adapted from National Heart, Lung, and Blood Institute (June 1991). *Executive summary: Guidelines for the diagnosis and management of asthma.* Washington, DC: US Department of Health and Human Services.

Ventolin), metaproterenol (Alupent), and terbutaline (Brethine, Bricanyl). These drugs cause relaxation of bronchial smooth muscle and inhibit the release of mediators from mast cells. Results can be achieved most quickly and with smaller doses via inhalation than by other routes because absorption is more efficient. Because the inhaled dose in small, adverse effects of the drug are minimized. Inhaled medications can be delivered by a compressor-driven nebulizer or by a metered dose inhaler (MDI) (see accompanying boxes). If a child has difficulty coordinating inhalation with activation of the MDI, or cannot inhale all of the medication with one breath, a spacer device or holding chamber may be useful. Bronchodilators may be administered together by inhalation and parenterally for additional bronchodilation. Such combined therapy also decreases undesirable side effects, as a smaller dose of each drug is required.

The proper home use of adrenergic drugs by inhalation is particularly important for maintaining control of asthma symptoms. However, parents need to be made aware of the danger of overreliance on these treatment aids. Parents need to know the importance of keeping track of the number of inhaled doses used by their children. Excessive use of the inhaler has been associated with increased mortality from asthma (Howell, Flaim, & Lung, 1992). Overreliance on MDIs has caused delay in seeking medical attention in the presence of worsening asthma (Barnhart & Czervinske, 1995).

Theophylline. One of the oldest medications for asthma still in use today, theophylline relaxes bronchial smooth muscle, decreases airway reactivity, and inhibits mast cell degranulation. Theophylline is effective for longer periods of time than $beta_2$-agonists, and so is useful for the treatment of nighttime symptoms (Weinberger, 1993). Theophylline can be given orally or parenterally. Aerosol administration of theophylline is ineffective. Theophylline is most therapeutic at serum concentrations of 10 to 20 μg/ml. Because rates of theophylline metabolism are extremely variable among children, and because the margin between therapeutic and toxic levels is narrow, serum theophylline levels are monitored closely. Theophylline toxicity occurs at serum levels exceeding 20 μg/ml. Manifestations of toxicity include restlessness, nausea, vomiting, irritability, headache, abdominal pain, diarrhea, fever, cardiac arrythmias, and seizures. Irreversible brain damage or death can result at concentrations of 30 μg/ml. Serum theophylline concentrations vary among children and are not related to the dose alone. Theo-

Tips on Using a Nebulizer

1. Use clean hands and a clean area.
2. Take slow, deep breaths through pursed lips to maximize deposition of aerosolized medication in the lungs.
3. Use all the medication in the nebulizer during one treatment. Do not store medication in the nebulizer for later use.
4. The length of the treatment is usually 10 to 15 minutes if the equipment is working properly and the correct amount of medication and diluent are used. If the length of treatments is prolonged, check the nebulizer or the compressor for defects.
5. Rinse the nebulizer in clean water after each treatment. Allow it to air-dry after loosely covering it with a clean paper towel. Once daily, wash the nebulizer in warm, soapy water; then rinse and soak it for 30 minutes in a disinfecting solution or a solution containing one part white vinegar and four parts water. Never store the nebulizer in a closed plastic bag until it is completely dry. Storing wet equipment promotes the growth of mold and bacteria.

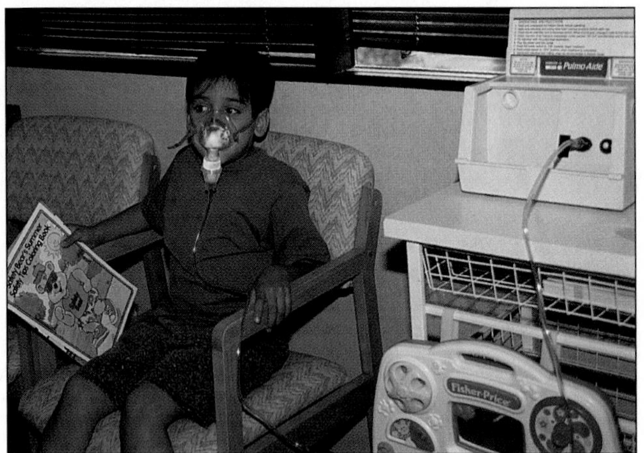

The powered nebulizer delivers a bronchodilator to the child who is having an acute asthma episode. This boy has a viral respiratory infection, which is a common trigger of acute asthma episodes in the pediatric population. (Courtesy of Dallas County Hospital District Community-Oriented Primary Care Clinic)

Adapted from Brim, S. A quick guide for home use of inhalant medications. (1989, January–February). *Pediatric Nursing, 15*(1), 87–94. With permission from Janetti Publications, Inc.

How to Use a Metered Dose Inhaler

1. Stand up. Shake the inhaler well. Remove the cap.
2. Hold the inhaler upright. Hold the mouthpiece 1 to 2 inches from the lips and open your mouth wide.
3. Tilt your head back slightly and breathe out fully.
4. Place your lips tightly around the mouthpiece, press down on the inhaler, and start to breathe in slowly.
5. Breathe in slowly (3–5 seconds), as this allows deeper penetration of the medication.
6. Hold your breath for as long as possible, up to 10 seconds.
7. Remove the inhaler and breathe out slowly through the nose.
8. Wait at least 2 minutes and shake the inhaler again before repeating the dose.
9. Visible mist escaping from the open mouth indicates improper technique. Do not count that try. Relax and repeat.
10. Rinse your mouth with water if desired.
11. Do not use p.r.n. treatments any more frequently than the interval ordered. The use of aerosolized treatments and metered dose inhalers containing the same medication (either prescribed or over-the-counter) is dangerous (Brim, 1989).
12. Report severe side effects to the physician immediately.

phylline is metabolized in the liver. Many factors affect clearance of theophylline, thus affecting the serum levels of the drug (see accompanying box).

Theophylline is used for the treatment of asthma episodes, as well as for preventive treatment. There are many preparations of this drug (see common respiratory medications table in Clinical Reference Pages). Short- and long-acting preparations of different strengths are available. IV theophylline is used in the treatment of acute asthma episodes. When IV theophylline is indicated, aminophylline is usually given. It is important to determine whether the child has recently taken a theophylline preparation before the loading dose is given. If an oral medication containing theophylline has been taken prior to admission, a blood theophylline level is drawn in order to determine the loading dose. The child is observed closely for signs of theophylline toxicity, and serum theophylline levels are drawn at intervals (usually within 6 hours of dosing and again 12 to 24 hours later). As theophylline levels approach 20 μg/ml, the risk of adverse effects increases. The nurse should observe the child carefully for theophylline side effects (gastrointestinal distress, nervousness, insomnia, irritability, headache, tremor, tachycardia, hypotension, diuresis, flushing, fever).

Factors Affecting Theophylline Clearance

Decreased Clearance (Increased Serum Level)

Age < 12 months
Viral respiratory infection
Erythromycin, Tegretol
Oral contraceptives
Influenza trivalent vaccine
High-carbohydrate, low-protein diet
Caffeine
Liver failure, heart failure

Increased Clearance (Decreased Serum Level)

Age between 12 months and 12 years
Smoking
Phenobarbitol
Phenytoin (Dilantin)
Charcoal-broiled beef
High-protein, low-carbohydrate diet

Anti-Inflammatory Agents

Cromolyn Sodium. Cromolyn sodium (Intal) is an inhaled nonsteroidal anti-inflammatory medication that prevents asthma symptoms by blocking the release of mast cell mediators. (See preceding box, How to Use a Metered Dose Inhaler.) Cromolyn has no effect on asthma symptoms once they have begun because this drug has no bronchodilating effect. Rather, cromolyn is primarily used for maintenance therapy in patients with chronic asthma. It may also be used before exercise or exposure to a known allergen to prevent symptoms. Cromolyn is available as a dry powder inhalation, as an MDI preparation, and as a nebulized solution. This medication is most effective against allergen-induced asthma when taken 30 minutes before exposure to the allergen. EIA is best prevented when cromolyn is inhaled a few minutes before exercise. Because cromolyn works best when the bronchioles are as open as possible, an adrenergic drug may be prescribed to be inhaled just before administration of cromolyn.

Cromolyn is one of the safest drugs used in the treatment of asthma and is virtually free of adverse effects. Occasionally, inhalation of cromolyn will irritate the airways, causing a mild cough. Drinking a few sips of water before and after inhalation usually prevents this problem and minimizes the bad taste of this medication. The patient should be aware that cromolyn is a preventive medication and is not effective for the relief of asthma symptoms. A newer anti-inflammatory asthma medication, nedrocromil sodium (Tilade) is available for use in children 12 years and older.

Corticosteroids. Corticosteroids relieve asthma symptoms by decreasing inflammation in the airways. They also potentiate the effect of adrenergic medications. Because of the importance of airway inflammation in the pathogenesis of asthma, inhaled steroids are increasingly being prescribed for the daily management of asthma. Inhalation therapy allows the topical administration of potent anti-inflammatory agents directly at the site of action in the airways. Administration directly at the site of action helps decrease the adverse effects seen with systemic corticosteroid therapy (Barnhart & Czervinske, 1995). Moreover, the use of inhaled steroids sometimes allows a reduction in the dose of systemic steroids.

Corticosteroids can be lifesaving in cases of severe asthma, but because of the potentially severe side effects of systemically administered corticosteroids, oral steroids are used for long-term treatment of chronic asthma only when other measures have failed. Adverse side effects of oral steroids are related to the dose, frequency, duration, and timing of the medication. Treatment for less than 2 weeks may cause only an increased appetite and a feeling of well-being which changes to moodiness when the steroid is stopped. More severe effects of continuous long-term corticosteroid therapy include a cushingoid appearance, growth suppression, osteoporosis, glaucoma, cataracts, peptic ulcer, hyperglycemia, and decreased resistance to infection. To minimize these side effects, steroids may be administered on an every-other-day regimen or in short-term therapeutic "bursts" which are gradually tapered.

NURSING CARE OF THE CHILD WITH ASTHMA

Assessment

Nursing assessment of the child with asthma should begin with a thorough history, which should include any family history of asthma or allergy and any past episodes of asthma, allergy, or other respiratory problems. Asking parents what treatment has been effective in previous asthma episodes may also be helpful. The family's knowledge of asthma (the disease and its management) should be assessed.

Assessment during an acute asthma episode should include vital signs and a careful evaluation of respiratory and oxygenation status. The nurse should note respiratory rate and effort, presence or absence of retractions, use of accessory muscles, nasal flaring, and pulse oximetry values. Level of consciousness is an important indicator of oxygenation and should be assessed carefully. Breath sounds should be carefully auscultated, noting any adventitious sounds or areas of diminished breath sounds. The child should be assessed for neurologic signs of impending respiratory failure (changes in consciousness, increased fatigue, somnolence). As infants and children become more hypoxic, they may not recognize or interact appropriately with their parents. Failure to resist or to cry during painful procedures is an ominous sign (Bechler-Karsch, 1994).

Because tachypnea and decreased intake of oral fluids may cause dehydration, hydration status should also be assessed (urine output, status of mucous membranes, presence of tears, skin turgor, weight).

Included in the psychosocial history should be a record of the child's routines and habits. Previous hospitalizations should be documented, as a past experience may affect the child's perception of the current illness. An assessment of the family's knowledge of the disease, degree of compliance, and growth and development provides the basis for future teaching.

Nursing Diagnoses

Nursing diagnoses that may apply to the child with asthma include:

- Risk for Suffocation related to bronchospasm and mucosal edema
- Ineffective Airway Clearance related to bronchospasm and mucosal edema
- Fatigue related to hypoxia and increased work of breathing
- Anxiety related to hospitalization and respiratory distress
- Altered Family Processes related to chronic disease
- Risk for Fluid Volume Deficit related to increased respiratory rate and decreased oral intake
- Knowledge Deficit related to disease process and treatment

Planning, Implementation, and Evaluation: The Child With Asthma

NURSING DIAGNOSIS

- Risk for Suffocation related to bronchospasm and mucosal edema
- Ineffective Airway Clearance related to bronchospasm and mucosal edema

Expected Outcome:

- The child will have improved gas exchange as evidenced by clear breath sounds, a pulse oximetry value of greater than 95% on room air, no use of accessory muscles, pink mucous membranes and nailbeds, and a capillary refill time of less than 2 seconds.
- The child will be able to clear the airway as evidenced by a respiratory rate and rhythm appropriate for the child's age, the ability to expectorate mucus, and normal vital signs for age.

Intervention	Rationale
Acute Care	
1. Monitor respiratory rate, heart rate, and blood pressure every 15 to 30 minutes. Auscultate breath sounds, assess respiratory rate and effort, and observe color every 15 minutes to 4 hours as the patient's condition indicates. Monitor arterial blood gas (ABG) values, pulse oximetry values, and pulmonary function test results. Notify the physician of any significant change (increased respiratory rate and effort, changes in wheezing, retractions, nasal flaring, severe cough, decreased alertness, cyanosis, increased dyspnea or apprehension). Obtain ABG and other blood studies as ordered.	Subtle changes in the child's condition may serve as an early warning of increased airway obstruction.
2. Administer humidified oxygen at the ordered flow rate. If child has chronic CO_2 retention, do not exceed 2 L/min.	Supplemental oxygen decreases hypoxia secondary to airway edema, mucus, and bronchospasm. Administration of oxygen to a child with chronic CO_2 retention may lead to respiratory depression by decreasing the stimulus to breathe.
3. Help the child assume an upright position or position of comfort. The older child may be most comfortable leaning forward on a pillow or overbed table.	An upright position aids in expansion of the lungs and decreases pressure on the diaphragm.
4. Maintain a patent endotracheal or tracheal airway if the child has been intubated for severe respiratory distress. Suction the airway as needed.	Artificial airways can become obstructed with tenacious mucus.
5. Administer medications as ordered. Assess whether medications are effectively relieving the patient's symptoms. Monitor the patient for side effects. Monitor the serum theophylline level (desired therapeutic level: 10–20 μg/ml). Notify the physician of signs of toxicity.	Refer to the earlier section in the text on medications (pp. 871–874) and the preceding table entitled Medications Commonly Used in the Treatment of Chronic Respiratory Conditions.
6. Provide increased fluid intake (IV and/or oral). Correct dehydration gradually.	Increased fluid intake helps to liquefy secretions and replaces fluid lost through increased respirations. Overhydration can cause obstruction of small airways from accumulation of interstitial fluid.
7. Keep the child NPO during periods of respiratory distress, as ordered by the physician.	Oral fluids are contraindicated in the presence of respiratory distress because of the risk of aspiration.
8. Maintain an IV line.	IV access is necessary for administering medications and fluids.
9. Check that respiratory treatments are given as ordered. Assess the child's breath sounds before and after treatments. Encourage the child to cough and deep breathe, especially after treatments. Suction as needed.	Breathing treatments help to loosen/eliminate secretions and re-expand lung tissue. Mucus plugs can cause atelectasis and alveolar collapse.
10. Ensure that emergency equipment is available (e.g., appropriate-size ventilation bag, endotracheal tubes, laryngoscope, emergency medication).	The child's condition can deteriorate rapidly. Immediate resuscitation may be necessary in the event of severe respiratory distress.

Intervention	Rationale
11. Keep the child as calm as possible. Offer support during periods of respiratory distress.	Anxiety increases bronchospasm.
Long-Term Care	
12. Teach the proper administration of prescribed medications.	See the earlier section on medications (pages 871–874).
13. Assess the patient's compliance with the prescribed treatment regimen.	Compliance is often related to the family's understanding of the disease and treatment.
14. Teach the child/family to recognize early warning signs of an acute episode.	Early treatment of mild asthma symptoms may prevent a severe episode.
15. Prevent infections. (Protect the child from respiratory infections, keep the equipment clean, and use good handwashing techniques.)	Respiratory infections frequently trigger asthma episodes.
16. Assess the family's ability to afford medications. Evaluate the family's need for support services.	Compliance is often affected by economic factors.

Evaluation: The child:

- maintains a patent airway,
- has a respiratory rate that is within normal limits for her age and expends minimal respiratory effort,
- has clear breath sounds with free movement of air.

NURSING DIAGNOSIS

- Fatigue related to hypoxia and increased work of breathing

Expected Outcome:

- The child will exhibit decreased fatigue as evidenced by less irritability and restlessness, uninterrupted sleep periods, and ability to perform usual activities.

Intervention	Rationale
Acute Care	
1. Assess the child for signs and symptoms of hypoxia, including restlessness, fatigue, irritability, increased heart rate, and increased respiratory rate.	Irritability and agitation may be early signs of hypoxia. Prompt treatment of hypoxia decreases fatigue.
2. Organize nursing care to provide periods of uninterrupted rest and sleep.	Periods of quiet decrease stress and promote rest.
3. Encourage the parents' presence, particularly when the patient is a young child.	Parents' presence decreases fear and anxiety.
4. Provide for the patient's physical comfort. Encourage quiet, age-appropriate play activities as the child's condition improves.	Physical and emotional comfort confer a sense of well-being and promote rest.
5. Implement measures to relieve respiratory distress. Monitor the frequency of nebulized medications and serum theophylline levels. Assess the patient's breath sounds after treatments and at appropriate intervals.	Theophylline levels in excess of 20 μg/ml are toxic. The side effects of restlessness and agitation are increased when serum drug levels are too high.

Intervention	Rationale
Long-Term Care	
6. Encourage adequate rest and 8 to 10 hours of sleep each night.	Adequate rest and sleep prevent fatigue and increase the patient's resistance to infection.
7. Teach stress management techniques.	Bronchospasm may be triggered by emotional upset and stress.
8. Encourage regular, appropriate exercise.	Appropriate exercise improves ventilation.

Evaluation:
- The child is able to perform usual activities without undue fatigue.

NURSING DIAGNOSIS
- Anxiety related to hospitalization and respiratory distress

Expected Outcome:
- The child will exhibit reduced anxiety as evidenced by a relaxed body position and a decrease in negative behaviors when the health care worker approaches him.
- Parents will demonstrate reduced anxiety by verbalizing an accurate knowledge of asthma and by participating in the child's care in a calm manner.

Intervention	Rationale
Acute Care	
1. Teach the child techniques to control panic/anxiety and to slow breathing rate (e.g., slow drinking of liquids, visually imagining staying calm, breathing exercises, pursed lip breathing, "belly breathing," etc.).	Concentration on such activities during an asthma episode calms the child and decreases fear of suffocation.
2. Maintain a calm, quiet environment and a reassuring manner. Stay with the child. Give care efficiently and calmly.	The ability to remain calm decreases the patient's oxygen demand and work of breathing.
3. Reassure the child that there is someone nearby to assist if breathing difficulties develop. Tell the child that he will be watched closely at night to allay any fears about going to sleep. Make the call light available for older children.	Calm reassurance by the nurse can decrease the patient's fear of suffocation and facilitate rest.
4. Utilize play therapy.	Therapeutic play allows the child to work through fears in a nonthreatening manner.
5. Encourage the parent(s) to stay with the child. Praise the parents for rooming-in and supporting the child.	The presence of a familiar person can decrease fear and anxiety.
6. Keep parents informed of treatments, routines, and the child's condition.	Reassuring the parents can help calm the child, as the parents' anxiety level is quickly transferred to the child. Frequent and accurate updating of the child's condition reassures parents and decreases fear of the unknown.
7. Encourage expression of feelings by child and parents.	
8. Avoid use of sedatives.	Sedatives may depress respirations.

Intervention	Rationale
9. Explain all procedures in an age-appropriate manner. Facilitate trust by being truthful and acknowledging discomfort of procedures.	Procedures and unfamiliar hospital setting may produce anxiety. Explanation decreases fear of the unknown. Honesty fosters trust.

Evaluation:
- The child cooperates with and participates in treatment and appears relaxed.
- The child obtains adequate rest and sleep.
- The parents verbalize decreased anxiety about hospitalization and disease process.

NURSING DIAGNOSIS
- Altered Family Processes related to chronic disease

Expected Outcome:
- The family will cope with the child's illness and will comply with management of the disease while providing for normal growth and development of the child.

Intervention	Rationale
1. Provide opportunities for the family to express feelings. Recognize and accept negative feelings about the child and the illness.	This nonjudgmental approach helps the family to work through fear, guilt, anxiety, and economic problems.
2. Explore previous coping mechanisms used in times of stress.	Identification and review of previously successful coping skills can assist the family in dealing with the present crisis.
3. Explain all procedures and treatments.	A thorough explanation decreases fear of the unknown and anxiety.
4. Keep parents informed of the child's condition.	Knowledge gives parents a sense of control.
5. Arrange for the family to meet with others affected by asthma. Identify available community resources (see Appendix H).	Meeting others with asthma can assist with problem solving and provide support.

Evaluation:
- The family functions well while providing necessary care for the child using available resources.

NURSING DIAGNOSIS
- Risk for Fluid Volume Deficit related to increased respiratory rate, diaphoresis, and decreased oral intake

Expected Outcome:
- The child will drink adequate fluid for his age and weight, as evidenced by maintenance of body weight prior to illness, moist mucous membranes, and urine output appropriate for age.

Intervention	Rationale
Acute Care	
1. Monitor intake and output, status of mucous membranes, body weight, tearing, and urine specific gravity. Maintain urine specific gravity at 1.003 to 1.020. Monitor electrolytes. Assess skin turgor. Assess the patient's sputum for color, tenacity, and amount.	Rapid respiratory rate, diaphoresis, and increased pulmonary secretions may cause dehydration and increased viscosity of secretions.

Intervention	Rationale
2. Maintain IV infusion at the ordered flow rate. Avoid excessive amounts of fluid.	Adequate hydration enhances liquefaction of secretions, and thinner secretions are more easily expectorated. Excessive fluids may lead to pulmonary edema.
3. Encourage oral fluids when tolerated, with the amount consumed being determined by the calculated needs of the child. Offer favorite fluids. Provide liquids at bedside.	Oral fluids are contraindicated during acute respiratory distress so as to minimize the risk of aspiration. Children are most likely to drink fluids if they are offered fluids they like.
4. Offer liquids at room temperature. Avoid milk and milk products.	Cold liquids may aggravate bronchospasm. Milk sometimes causes increased coughing and production of mucus.
5. Provide a humidified atmosphere.	Humidification helps to liquefy secretions and promotes hydration.
Long-Term Care	
6. Encourage the child to drink at least 3 to 8 glasses (750 to 2000 ml) of fluid per day, depending on age and weight.	Increased fluid intake decreases the viscosity of secretions.

Evaluation: The child
- ingests adequate fluid for age/weight,
- maintains a urine specific gravity of 1.003 to 1.020,
- maintains her pre-illness weight,
- has moist mucous membranes.

NURSING DIAGNOSIS
- Knowledge Deficit related to disease process and treatment

Expected Outcome:
- The child will tolerate normal activities of daily living (exercise, play, school attendance).

Intervention	Rationale
Acute Care	
1. Assess the child's and parents' understanding of asthma. Explain unfamiliar procedures and equipment at the child's level of understanding. Teach the family about the disease, its triggers, and prescribed medications/treatments.	Understanding increases compliance with treatment.
2. Help the family identify precipitating factors (e.g., exercise, infections, allergens, weather changes).	An awareness of triggers may decrease future asthma episodes.
3. Explain the role of emotions and stress in the development of asthma symptoms.	
4. Teach the child and family about the importance of taking medications as prescribed.	Knowledge of medications increases compliance with the therapeutic regimen. This helps to maintain serum drug levels within a therapeutic range.

Intervention	Rationale
Provide written information and instructions about medications (names, side effects, dosages, and times of administration). Teach the family to recognize signs and symptoms that warrant notification of the physician. Reinforce the need to keep follow-up appointments.	
Long-Term Care	
5. Assist in developing an exercise program for the child. Medication may be needed prior to exercise. Teach the importance of a healthy lifestyle (regular exercise, adequate fluids and nutrition, rest, and prevention of infection).	Exercise promotes pulmonary and cardiovascular health and assists the child in leading a normal life.
6. Refer the family to a support group.	Meeting with other children and families affected by asthma provides an avenue for expressing feelings and sharing information. Knowledge of asthma decreases anxiety during acute episodes. The frequency and severity of episodes will be minimized if the child knows the appropriate actions for controlling symptoms.
7. Teach self-management of asthma (see accompanying box entitled Age-Appropriate Self-Management Responsibilities for Children With Asthma. Help the child to identify triggers of asthma symptoms). Teach the necessary skills for home care. Encourage the child to "take charge" of her asthma. The child should know what triggers to avoid, early warning signs of an episode, the correct use of treatment aids (MDI, peak flowmeter), as well as proper administration of medications and techniques for stress reduction and relaxation. Encourage the child/family to participate in programs designed to develop effective self-management and decision-making skills. Some of these programs are listed in the resource appendix at the end of the book.	Helping the child with asthma to learn about her condition can help decrease anxiety during episodes and increase her ability to take appropriate action to control symptoms. Frequency and severity of asthma episodes will be minimized if the child knows what triggers to avoid, early warning signs of an episode, and the correct treatment of symptoms.
8. Teach deep breathing exercises.	
9. Teach importance of follow-up care and of routine health maintenance (keeping immunizations up-to-date, etc.).	Prevention of infection and healthy living habits help to decrease asthma triggers.

Evaluation:
- The child/family verbalize an accurate knowledge of asthma and its treatment.
- The child/family keep follow-up appointments.
- The child returns to normal daily activities.

Home Care

Children with asthma should be encouraged to learn about their condition and to "take charge" of their asthma. Teaching developmentally appropriate self-management skills to children and families has been shown to be an effective tool for improving control over asthma (Howell, Flaim, & Lung, 1992). Asthma self-management programs have been set up in emergency departments, clinics, inpatient hospital units, physician's offices, and schools, as well as at camps for children with asthma.

Teaching the necessary skills to control and manage asthma symptoms can decrease a child's anxiety during

Age-Appropriate Self-Management Responsibilities for Children With Asthma

PRESCHOOL—COOPERATION

Cooperates with medicines and treatments
Begins to learn to identify symptoms and tells an adult helper
Begins to use correct technique when using peak flowmeter
Begins to respond to adult guidance for avoidance of triggers

SCHOOL AGE—LEARNING

Learns the action of medications, and the appropriate dose and time
Asks for daytime medications and treatments at routine times
Uses correct technique when using peak flowmeter
With the aid of an adult helper, reads and records peak flowmeter results
Identifies symptoms and tells adult helper
Discusses treatment of symptoms with adult helper
Identifies factors that make asthma worse
Begins to avoid or control factors that make asthma worse, without reminders

ADOLESCENT—DECISION MAKING

Plans and takes routine medications and treatments
Learns and recognizes medication side effects
Uses techniques to remember medications and treatments
Determines and tells an adult helper when prescriptions for medications need to be refilled by the pharmacy
Uses a peak flowmeter correctly and records measurements
Assesses the severity of symptoms and identifies symptoms early
Treats symptoms appropriately
Recognizes when to contact the health care provider and discusses this with adult helper
Meets with an adult helper on a routine basis to monitor for trends in peak flow numbers and symptom recognition
Avoids and controls factors that make asthma worse, both at home and at school

Reprinted with permission from the National Jewish Center for Immunology and Respiratory Medicine, 1400 Jackson Street, Denver, CO 80206.

episodes and enable the child and family to take appropriate action to control the symptoms of the disease. The frequency and severity of asthma episodes will be minimized if the child knows:

- what triggers to avoid and other prevention measures
- the early warning signs of an asthma episode
- the correct use of treatment aids (nebulizer, MDI, peak flowmeter, symptom diary). (See previous boxes entitled How to Use a Metered Dose Inhaler and How to Use a Peak Flowmeter.)
- the proper administration of medications and their names, prescribed dose, expected effects, side effects, and frequency of use
- the guidelines included in a written crisis plan (when to increase therapy, when to call the physician, when to go to the emergency department)

EMERGENCY ASTHMA MANAGEMENT The following are some symptoms that indicate the need for emergency treatment of asthma:

- Worsening wheeze, cough, or shortness of breath
- A peak flow rate that decreases, or does not change (even after use of an inhaled beta$_2$-agonist), or that is less than 30% to 50% of the child's predicted baseline level or personal best
- Difficult breathing (as evidenced by the child's chest and neck being pulled or sucked in with each breath, or the child hunching over or struggling to breathe)
- Trouble with walking or talking
- Discontinuation of play without the ability to resume activity
- Listlessness and weak cry in an infant; refusal to suck bottle or breast
- Gray or blue lips or fingernails (in which case the child needs emergency treatment *immediately!*)

Adapted with permission from Rachelefsky, G. S. (1995). Asthma update: New approaches and partnerships. *Journal of Pediatric Health Care*, 9, 12–21.

- strategies to control fear and panic during asthma episodes
- the importance of rest and exercise in preventing asthma symptoms

Parents should be assisted in developing a plan for home care that includes a well-balanced diet, regular and adequate sleep/rest, and appropriate activities. Prevention of infection—by keeping immunizations up-to-date and protecting the child from exposure to contagious disease—is important. Parents should be provided with phone numbers and the names of contact persons if they have questions, and a follow-up appointment should be made. See Appendix H for the names, addresses, and phone numbers of asthma resource organizations.

BRONCHOPULMONARY DYSPLASIA

Bronchopulmonary dysplasia (BPD) is a chronic obstructive pulmonary disease that occurs in some infants who have required increased levels of oxygen and mechanical ventilation. BPD usually occurs in premature infants who have survived respiratory distress syndrome (RDS), but it is occasionally seen in term infants who require supplemental oxygen and mechanical ventilation. An infant who requires supplemental oxygen at 1 week of age and is still oxygen-dependent at 28 days is described as having BPD.

PATHOPHYSIOLOGY *of Bronchopulmonary Dysplasia*

Pressures of mechanical ventilation damage bronchial epithelium. The airways are then invaded by macrophages and polymorphonuclear cells, causing airway edema. Alveolar walls become thickened and fibrotic changes occur in the airways and alveoli. The continued use of oxygen affects the growth and development of lung structures, reducing the number of developing alveoli by one third to one half the number within a normal lung (Conte, 1992).

Cystic and atelectatic areas develop in the lungs, predisposing the infant to pulmonary hypertension. There also may be loss of cilia which decreases the lungs' ability to remove mucus, leading to mucus plugs, atelectasis, and pneumonia (Motoyama et al., 1987).

Etiology. BPD is a complication seen in infants who have been exposed to high oxygen concentrations and positive pressure ventilation for prolonged periods of time. Lung immaturity seems to be the key factor in the development of RDS and, ultimately, BPD (Truog et al., 1985). Because lung development varies among infants, gestational age cannot always predict the development of BPD. Term infants with serious respiratory problems, such as meconium aspiration, pulmonary hypertension, and neonatal pneumonia, have also developed BPD after prolonged assisted ventilation (Avery, et al., 1987). It has also been suggested that there may be a genetic predisposition to the condition. White males have been found to be at increased risk (Avery et al., 1987).

Incidence. BPD is the leading cause of morbidity and mortality among infants who have survived RDS. It is the most common chronic lung disease in infants. The overall incidence of BPD in infants who weigh less than 1500 g and who require mechanical ventilation is between 15% and 38% (Northway et al., 1990). Infants with low birth weights are at increased risk for developing BPD. The current high survival rates of low-birth-weight, preterm infants have resulted in an increase in the disorder.

Clinical Manifestations. The clinical manifestations of BPD include the following:

- Tachycardia and tachypnea related to decreased oxygenation
- Increased work of breathing, retractions, and prolonged exhalation with increased use of abdominal and accessory muscles
- Pallor associated with chronic hypoxia
- Cyanosis and activity intolerance (feeding and handling)
- Weight loss or poor weight gain related to increased metabolic workload, hypoxia, and poor feeding
- Restlessness and irritability related to hypoxia
- Wheezing (intermittent or chronic)
- Puckering or pursing of the mouth with flaring of the nares (early signs of impending respiratory distress)

Diagnostic Evaluation. Diagnosis is based on clinical manifestations and radiographic abnormalities. Infants with respiratory symptoms that persist beyond 28 days of life, who are oxygen-dependent beyond 28 days, and who require mechanical ventilation during the first week of life are suspected of having BPD.

Therapeutic Management. The goal of treatment of BPD is to maintain adequate oxygenation in order to promote growth and development, to prevent further lung disease, and to promote healing of the damaged lungs. Treatment consists of oxygen therapy, drug therapy, and nutritional support.

Positive-pressure ventilation should be discontinued as soon as possible. If mechanical ventilation is necessary to maintain life, then the lowest possible inflation pressures should be used, together with expiratory times that allow the lung to empty completely. Weaning from the ventilator may be a slow, tedious process, sometimes requiring many months to complete and often interrupted by infections and other problems (Barnhart & Czervinske, 1995).

Ten percent of infants with BPD will require oxygen therapy for longer than 1 year (Hazinski, 1990). Oxygen can be given through a hood, tent, face mask, or nasal cannula. Oxygen saturation rates should be monitored closely. Children may be discharged from the hospital while still oxygen-dependent.

Diuretics and fluid restriction are often used to treat pulmonary interstitial edema. Furosemide is the most common diuretic used. Because infants with BPD often experience fluid overload and edema, fluid and electrolyte status should be monitored closely. Supplemental calcium, potassium, and chloride may be indicated (Rush et al., 1990). Bronchodilators (theophylline, metaproterenol, cromolyn disodium), when given in the early stages of BPD, can lessen airway resistance and decrease the possibility of lung damage. The corticosteroid dexamethasone is often administered while weaning the infant from mechanical ventilation. Careful monitoring during this process is needed as dexamethasone increases lung compliance, placing the infant at risk for pulmonary barotrauma.

Infants with BPD experience frequent infections owing to increased susceptibility and exposure to invasive treatments and procedures. After the initial stages of BPD, the risk of infection is probably the greatest risk to survival for these infants (Barnhart & Czervinske, 1995). Antibiotics are often needed. Ribavirin may be given to infants with respiratory syncytial virus.

Because of an increased resting metabolic rate, frequent respiratory exacerbations, and feeding problems, the infant with BPD has increased nutritional needs. A realistic feeding goal in these infants is 110 to 150 kcal/kg/day to produce a weight gain of 15 to 20 g/day (Hazinski, 1990). The use of formulas containing 24 cal/oz is appropriate in meeting this requirement, especially in infants in whom fluids are restricted. Formulas may be fortified with vegetable oil, triglycerides, or glucose polymers to increase the calories per ounce (Bernbaum et al., 1989).

Infants with BPD are usually not discharged home until they have reached a gestational age of at least 40 weeks, are able to feed adequately to support growth, and can maintain an acceptable transcutaneous oxygen concentration during routine activities, such as feeding, bathing, and crying (Conte, 1992). Infants who require oxygen therapy at home must be monitored for hypoxia at frequent intervals. Some infants, such as those receiving prolonged ventilation therapy, require a tracheostomy (Fanoroff, Martin, & Hack, 1991).

Prognosis. Most infants with BPD do improve. Mortality ranges from 10% to 25%. Of the infants with BPD, 40% to 50% will require ongoing therapy at home, and some will develop respiratory disease that will continue into adulthood.

Infants with resolved or resolving disease may have chronic bronchial hyperactivity which, in some cases, progresses to bronchial asthma. More than 40% will require rehospitalization during the first year of life because of acute viral respiratory tract infections (Cunningham, McMillan, & Gross, 1991). A significant number of deaths occur after discharge from the hospital (Hagedorn & Gardner, 1989). Infants may show a developmental delay for the first 24 to 36 months of life (Meisels et al., 1986). Morbidity varies depending on the severity of the BPD and the infant's level of prematurity.

NURSING CARE OF THE INFANT WITH BPD

Assessment

The care of the infant with BPD is as varied as the disease itself. The nurse may be caring for an infant who is dependent on mechanical ventilation or one who is receiving oxygen via a cannula, nasal catheter, or hood. Oxygen saturation measurements, determined by pulse oximetry, should be monitored and changes should be documented in relation to hypoxia. Chest X-ray films and blood gas results should be checked and significant changes should be reported. Respiratory rate and effort, color, and vital signs should be assessed every 2 hours and p.r.n. during the acute stage of the disease. Breath sounds should also be auscultated every 2 hours and p.r.n.

Intake and output and daily weights should be obtained and recorded, and infants should be observed for signs of fluid overload. Assessment of fluid status should include an evaluation of the quality and characteristics of breath sounds, presence or absence of edema, vital signs, and respiratory effort. Electrolyte levels should be monitored, and the physician should be notified of abnormal results. The child should also be assessed for signs of infection, such as fever, tachycardia, tachypnea, lethargy, changes in color, and consistency of tracheal secretions.

Growth and development should also be assessed, as infants with BPD are frequently developmentally delayed (Goldson, 1990). The family's response to the child's illness should also be noted. Stressors impacting the family and coping strategies which have been effectively used by the family in the past should be identified. Prior to the child's discharge, the family's ability to cope with a child with a chronic illness should be assessed. This assessment should include physical as well as psychological strengths and weaknesses.

Nursing Diagnosis and Planning

The following nursing diagnoses and expected outcomes are examples that may be appropriate following assessment of the infant with BPD.

- Impaired Gas Exchange related to alveolar damage secondary to high oxygen concentrations and mechanical ventilation. ***Expected Outcome:*** *The infant will maintain adequate gas exchange as evidenced by blood gas values that are within normal range. (See blood gases table in the Clinical Reference Pages of Chapter 28).*
- Ineffective Airway Clearance related to fatigue associated with hypoxia. ***Expected Outcome:*** *The infant will be able to clear the airway as evidenced by a respiratory rate and rhythm and vital signs that are within the normal range for the infant's age. (See Chapter 3 box, Vital Signs for Newborns, p. 55.)*
- Risk for Infection related to lung pathology. ***Expected Outcome:*** *The infant will remain free from infection as evidenced by absence of the following: fever, increased or copious sputum, tachycardia, tachypnea.*
- Altered Nutrition Less Than Body Requirements, related to feeding difficulties secondary to dyspnea and increased metabolic rate. ***Expected Outcome:*** *The infant will exhibit normal growth as evidenced by appropriate increases recorded on a growth chart.*

- Fluid Volume Excess related to interstitial fluid edema. ***Expected Outcome:*** *The infant will show no signs of fluid overload as evidenced by the absence of edema and crackles.*
- Altered Growth and Development related to hypoxia and prolonged hospitalization. ***Expected Outcome:*** *The infant will exhibit optimal growth and development patterns as evidenced by the ability to perform developmental tasks or milestones that are appropriate for the infant's age.*
- Ineffective Family Coping Compromised, related to having a child with a chronic disease who requires frequent hospitalization. ***Expected Outcome:*** *Family members will verbalize an understanding of the care of the child and identify their strengths and weaknesses.*

Implementation

Infants requiring mechanical ventilation are cared for in special care areas. Nurses in these units work with the physician to provide ventilatory assistance at the lowest possible setting. Care should be taken with procedures that can interfere with the endotracheal tube (ETT) (e.g., suctioning, turning, and weighing the infant) so that undue pressure or trauma is not placed on the airway. Sedation may be ordered to minimize trauma to the airway caused by the infant "fighting" the ventilator (Barnhart & Czervinske, 1995). Some infants respond well to gentle touch, positioning, and music, whereas others do better if they are left alone (Barnhart & Czervinske, 1995). When suctioning, special care should be taken to maintain oxygen saturations (see section on Suctioning in Chapter 18). The infant should be assessed for tachypnea, retractions, nasal flaring, pallor, diminished or unequal breath sounds, and restlessness every 2 hours and p.r.n. Changes associated with alterations in blood gas analysis results should always be reported.

Although chest physiotherapy (CPT) is often done by a respiratory therapist, it is the nurse's responsibility to monitor the infant's response to therapy. Pulse oximetry changes related to hypoxia should be observed and documented. Positioning for CPT and other procedures must be done carefully, as the risk for aspiration is high (Barnhart & Czervinske, 1995).

The infant should not be exposed to staff or visitors with respiratory infections. Thorough handwashing is imperative. Sterile technique should be used when suctioning. Mucous secretions should be observed for signs of infection (increased amount, change in color or consistency). Vital signs should be monitored every 2 hours. The infant's position should be gently changed from side to side and from front to back to improve drainage and prevent infection. Infants with BPD should receive all standard immunizations at the normal chronologic age.

Infants with BPD have increased metabolic needs caused by the inflammatory process in the lungs. Premature infants have little caloric reserve to meet the increased caloric needs required to promote lung healing and development. The nutritional needs of the infant may be met through feedings via total parenteral nutrition (TPN), nasogastric tube, gavage, bottle, or breastfeeding. These infants are often poor feeders because of prematurity, hypoxia, and deprivation of oral feeding experiences (Conte, 1992). A gastrostomy tube may need to be placed in infants with severe BPD and feeding problems. The severely ill infant may start with TPN and progress to bottle feeding. Special high-calorie formulas (24 cal/oz) containing medium-chain triglycerides or the addition of polycose to the formula may be useful in meeting the increased caloric needs of these infants. A schedule of small, frequent feedings helps to prevent undue fatigue in the infant. Because oxygen consumption increases during oral feeding, pulse oximetry values, respiratory rate, and work of breathing should be carefully assessed. Studies have shown that infants with BPD have more **hypoxemia** before, during, and after feedings than do low-birth-weight infants without BPD (Singer et al., 1992). Repeated episodes of hypoxia are suspected to play a role in the increased risk for sudden, unexpected death and in later intellectual deficits in children who have had BPD (Garg et al., 1988). The nurse should remain nearby to monitor the infant's condition when the parent first holds and feeds the baby. The infant may expend more calories and oxygen than he gains from such feedings. A nutritional consult should be obtained.

Because infants with BPD often do not tolerate fluids well, they are at risk for fluid imbalance. Strict intake and output parameters are maintained, and the infant is weighed daily. Increased respiratory rate, crackles, edema, decreased breath sounds, cyanosis, or tachycardia may be signs of possible pulmonary edema and should be reported. There is a risk of giving too much fluid in the attempt to provide adequate calories.

Nursing care should be given in a quiet, gentle manner. Stimulation should be based on the infant's ability to tolerate increased sensory input. Appropriate stimulation should be incorporated into care activities and scheduled judiciously in order to avoid overstimulating or exhausting the infant. Nurses can provide ongoing stimulation when giving care by touching, holding, and talking to the infant. By doing this, they also serve as role models for the parents of these children. As the infant improves, areas of need should be identified and a program of infant stimulation should be implemented.

The family should be encouraged to express their feelings and thoughts regarding the care of a child with a long-term disease. Past coping strategies can be identified and discussed. The disease, its treatment, and related procedures should be explained, together with the rationale for intervention. Families are more likely to comply with the prescribed treatment regimen if they understand the reason for the interventions. The family should be kept informed of the infant's condition and any changes that take place. The family should be involved in the care of the child. A social service consult is very important.

Home Care Home care of the infant with BPD decreases the risk of hospital-acquired infection and reduces health care costs. Care at home also improves social development by encouraging interaction between the child and family. Over time, infants who are cared for in a home environment with supportive parents are most likely to do well (Damato, 1991; Northway et al., 1990; Parker, Lindstrom, & Cotton, 1992). Infants are usually able to be discharged home if they (1) are able to feed adequately to gain weight, (2) require only low concentrations of oxygen (less than 1 L/min), and (3) can maintain an acceptable transcutaneous oxygen concentration during routine activities, such as feeding, bathing, and crying (Conte, 1992). Some infants are discharged while still ventilator-dependent.

Preparation for discharge and home care requires a great deal of education and reassurance. Education of the family with a chronically ill or technology-dependent child must begin early. The goal is to teach the family that they can provide care for their child. Education must begin with basic care—i.e., feeding, bathing, holding, and playing. When parents feel comfortable with basic care, they can be taught the medical, nursing, and respiratory procedures that will be necessary at home (Barnhart & Czervinske, 1995). Because infants with BPD are susceptible to respiratory problems, parents must be taught how to prevent infection, such as by using good handwashing technique and by keeping the infant away from adults and children who have upper respiratory infections or communicable diseases. In these infants, relatively minor respiratory infections can rapidly progress to more serious problems, such as pneumonia or bronchiolitis. Parents need to know how to assess their child's respiratory status, as well as how to recognize the early warning signs of illness (see accompanying box). It is important for parents to report these signs to the pediatrician early so as to avoid serious illness and rehospitalization (Barnhart & Czervinske, 1995). Parents also must be given information about the medications their child is to receive at home. Parents should be given the opportunity to practice administering the medications before the child is discharged. A written schedule and checklist for administration, including effects and side effects, should be given to the parents. Specific information on what to do if the infant misses a dose or vomits after a dose should be provided.

The infant may continue to require oxygen at home and may have a tracheostomy. Some infants are discharged while they are still ventilator-dependent. Children with tracheostomy tubes require continuous observation. Older infants and toddlers who require oxygen or mechanical ventilation require close supervision to prevent them from manipulating dials on the ventilator or wandering beyond the length of the tubing. Parents must be vigilant to keep the toddler from placing small toys into the ventilator tubing or artificial airway. Parents of the infant with a tracheostomy are taught tracheostomy care, suctioning, and CPT (see Chapter 18, pp. 473–480), as well as signs of complications (e.g., infection of the tracheostomy, obstruction by secretions, or accidental decannulation) and appropriate actions. Families must be taught the necessary precautions for safe use of oxygen in the home (see Teaching Guidelines). Compliance with these safety measures should be evaluated during home visits (Conte, 1992). Apnea-bradycardia monitors are often sent home with the infant, and parents must be taught cardiopulmonary resuscitation and other emergency measures. Before hospital discharge, contact with emergency services, utility companies, and the telephone company should be made, notifying them that a technology-dependent child will be living in their area (Fig. 29–1). Required actions in case of emergency should be reviewed with the family. Children requiring mechanical ventilation often have the support of nursing care during the day. Children who do not require technologic support may not qualify for supportive care through insurance. This may present a problem for families with limited financial resources who cannot afford in-home babysitters (Conte, 1992). The nurse should review family and other support systems available prior to discharge.

Infants with BPD are often developmentally delayed. A program of appropriate stimulation to foster growth and development should be planned and implemented as early as possible. Home care is best directed and monitored by a multidisciplinary team. Ongoing support by the team, as well as frequent evaluation of the infant's condition and the family's ability to continue to maintain home

Early Warning Signs of Illness in Infants With Bronchopulmonary Displaysia

FINDINGS ON PHYSICAL EXAMINATION

- Changes in pulse, respiration rate, color
- Increased adventitious breath sounds
- Increased intensity of retractions
- Increased cough, thickness and color of secretions
- Fever

ILLNESS WARNING SIGNS

- Change in activity level (irritability, decreased playfulness)
- Change in sleep pattern
- Change in eating or feeding

Adapted with permission from Barnhart, S. L., & Czervinske, M. P. (1995). *Perinatal and pediatric respiratory care* (p. 661). Philadelphia: W. B. Saunders.

TEACHING GUIDELINES *for Safe Use of Oxygen at Home*

SAFETY GUIDELINES	RATIONALE
• Secure the oxygen tank in an upright position.	• Oxygen tanks are highly explosive; if a horizontally positioned tank explodes, the rapid release of oxygen can catapult it through both animate (human bodies) and inanimate objects (walls).
• Keep oxygen tanks at least 5 feet from heat sources and electrical devices (e.g., space heaters, heating vents, fireplaces, radios, vaporizers). • Ensure that no one smokes in the room or in the area of the oxygen tank.	• Smoking increases the risk of fire, which could cause the tank to explode; escaped oxygen would feed the fire.
• Avoid using alcohol-based substances or oil to relieve dryness around the child's mouth (e.g., petroleum jelly, vitamin A & D ointment, baby oil).	• Both alcohol and oil are flammable and increase the risk of fire.
• Keep a fire extinguisher readily available.	• A fire extinguisher may be needed to put out a fire immediately.
• Turn off both the volume regulator and the flow regulator when oxygen is not in use.	• If the volume regulator is on when the oxygen is turned on, the child might receive a rapid, forceful flow of oxygen in the face that could be frightening and uncomfortable. Oxygen leakage, which might not be detected because oxygen is odorless, can cause fire.

Adapted with permission from Hagedorn, M. I., & Gardner, S. L. (1989). Physiologic sequelae of prematurity: The nurse practitioner's role. Part I. Respiratory issues. *Journal of Pediatric Health Care, 3,* 288–297.

ELECTRIC COMPANY
REQUEST FOR SPECIAL CONSIDERATION

Date: ______________________

Name: ______________________
Address: ______________________
____

Phone: ______________________
Account Number: ______________

Attention: Customer Service

Our infant/child, ______________________, is under the care of Dr. ________________ at ______________________ for ________________. This condition(s) requires the use of a cardiorespiratory monitor and/or other life support equipment, specifically:
____

The necessary equipment selected for home care is equipped with a battery backup system that will power the equipment in the event of a power failure for a **limited period of time.** If a power failure occurs, it is imperative to restore service to this home as soon as possible. Please place this home on a priority list for restoration of electric service. If you have advance warning of a temporary interruption in electric service, please notify the parents so alternative arrangements can be made. If you have questions regarding the specifications of the equipment provided, please contact our equipment provider, Pediatric Home Care Associates.

Thank you for your cooperation.

Sincerely yours,

OUR EQUIPMENT PROVIDER IS:

Figure 29–1
Example of a letter that can be used to notify the local public service company that a technology-dependent child is living in their service area. (Courtesy of Pediatric Home Care Associates, Garfield, NJ. From Barnhart, S. L., & Czervinske, M. P. [1995]. *Perinatal and pediatric respiratory care* [p. 662]. Philadelphia: W. B. Saunders)

care, is necessary. Prior to discharge, the family's ability to cope with the needs of a child with BPD should be evaluated. (See Chapter 17 for further discussion of the care of a child with a chronic illness.)

Evaluation

- Are the infant's blood gas values within normal range?
- Is the infant free of signs of infection?
- Can the infant perform developmentally appropriate tasks?

CYSTIC FIBROSIS

Cystic fibrosis (CF), the most common lethal genetic disease in whites, is a chronic multisystem disorder affecting the exocrine glands. The mucus produced by the exocrine glands (particularly those of the bronchioles, small intestine, and the pancreatic and bile ducts) is abnormally thick, causing obstruction of the small passageways of these organs. Although cystic fibrosis is incurable, the life expectancy of affected children has increased dramatically. The median survival age is 30 years, making CF a disease not only of children, but also of young adults. The recent discovery of the CF gene has brought hope for improved treatment and the possibility of eventually developing a cure for the disease.

Etiology. CF is transmitted as an autosomal recessive trait, which means that both parents must carry the gene for the child to be affected. Statistically, for each pregnancy, if both parents carry the CF gene, there is a 25% chance that a child will inherit one CF gene from each parent and have CF, a 50% chance that a child will inherit only one CF gene from either parent and be a carrier, and a 25% chance that the child will inherit only normal genes and be completely free of CF.

The CF gene has been localized to the long arm of chromosome 7. Research continues.

Incidence. CF is the most common lethal genetic disease among caucasians, with an incidence of 1 in 2000 live births. The occurrence of CF among blacks is 1 in 17,000 live births. The disease very rarely affects Hispanics or Orientals. It is estimated that 1 in 20 white Americans carry the gene for CF.

Although most CF cases are diagnosed in infancy and early childhood, 8% to 10% of cases are not detected until adolescence.

Clinical Manifestations. Signs and symptoms of CF vary widely among affected children. The severity of involvement of specific organ systems varies among patients, as does the age at which symptoms begin. Symptoms gradually worsen as the disease progresses, and the outcome is always fatal.

Respiratory System

- Wheezing and a dry, nonproductive cough (earliest pulmonary manifestations)
- Repeated bouts of pneumonia and bronchitis
- Purulent and copious sputum accompanying chronic bacterial infections. The cough at this stage is wet and paroxysmal and may be followed by vomiting.

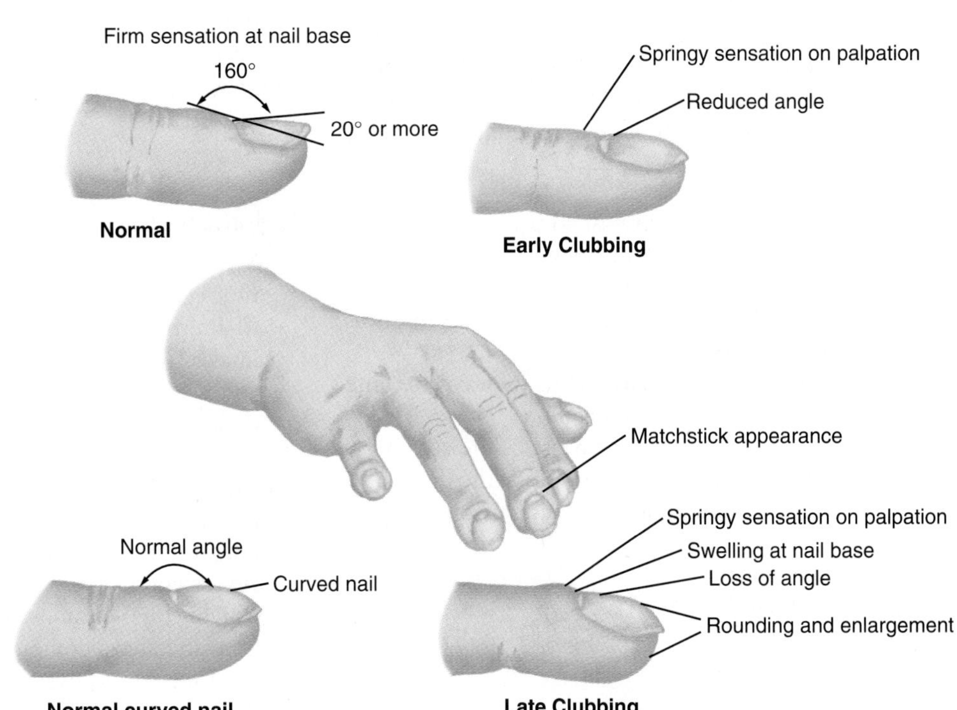

Figure 29–2
Digital clubbing may be an indication of hypoxia, which often occurs in cystic fibrosis and other respiratory disorders.

PATHOPHYSIOLOGY *of Cystic Fibrosis*

CF affects the exocrine glands throughout the body. Abnormally thick mucus obstructs organ passages and leads to respiratory, digestive, integumentary, and reproductive dysfunction and damage.

RESPIRATORY SYSTEM

Abnormally thick, sticky secretions cause obstruction of both the small and large airways. Stasis of secretions from bronchial obstruction provides a medium for bacterial growth. Chronic infection causes the release of toxic chemicals that damage lung tissues and alter host defenses within the airways, thus exacerbating the infection and inflammation. Inflammation may also cause bronchospasm, worsening airway blockage. Because airways dilate on inspiration and constrict on exhalation, air trapping occurs in the peripheral airways narrowed by mucous secretions. Hyperinflation is one of the first findings on chest X-ray studies of a child with CF. Chronic infection leads to atelectasis and eventual fibrosis and destruction of pulmonary tissue. As the disease progresses, the lungs of almost all patients with CF eventually become colonized with *Pseudomonas aeruginosa,* an organism which can never be completely eradicated from the respiratory tract, but which can be controlled with vigorous antibiotic therapy.

With chronic respiratory infection, impaired oxygen and carbon dioxide exchange causes varying degrees of hypoxia, hypercapnia, and acidosis. Fibrotic lung changes occur as the disease worsens and hypoxia increases. Alveolar hypoxia leads to pulmonary vasoconstriction, increasing pulmonary vascular resistance. Increased pulmonary vascular resistance causes the right side of the heart to work harder to pump blood into the lungs. Enlargement of the right ventricle in response to increased pulmonary resistance (cor pulmonale) results. Congestive heart failure may develop. Pulmonary complications include sinusitis, spontaneous pneumothorax, and hemoptysis. Death in patients with CF is almost always the result of respiratory failure.

DIGESTIVE SYSTEM

Eighty-five percent of patients with CF have pancreatic involvement. The pancreatic ducts, blocked by thick mucus, are unable to secrete trypsin, amylase, and lipase into the small intestine. Without these digestive enzymes, proteins, carbohydrates, and fats are poorly absorbed. Bowel obstruction from thickened intestinal mucus and pancreatic insufficiency may be present at birth (meconium ileus).

The islets of Langerhans in the pancreas are normal in patients with CF, but they may decrease in number as the disease progresses and the pancreas undergoes fibrotic changes. Older children with CF sometimes develop insulin-dependent diabetes. Abnormalities of the gallbladder are common.

INTEGUMENTARY SYSTEM

The sweat glands of patients with CF secrete normal amounts of sweat. However, the levels of sodium and chloride in the sweat are two to five times the normal range.

REPRODUCTIVE SYSTEM

Ninety-eight percent of male patients with CF are sterile owing to obstruction of the deferent ducts and seminal vesicles. Female patients have reduced fertility because of abnormally thick cervical mucus, which impedes sperm penetration of the cervical canal.

- Crackles, wheezes, and diminished breath sounds
- Accessory muscle use, retractions, hypoxia, and cyanosis
- Increased cough, dyspnea, tachypnea, and cyanosis as the disease progresses
- Emphysema and atelectasis as the airways become increasingly obstructed with secretions
- Cor pulmonale and congestive heart failure secondary to fibrotic lung changes in later stages of the disease
- Spontaneous pneumothorax or hemoptysis in later stages
- Nasal polyps, sinusitis
- Digital clubbing (Fig. 29–2)
- Barrel chest (increased antero-posterior diameter of chest)

Digestive System

- Steatorrhea (frothy, foul-smelling stools that are 2 to 3 times greater in bulk than normal), flatus
- Malnutrition and growth failure despite normal caloric intake; deficiencies of fat-soluble vitamins A, D, E, and K because of an inability to absorb fats. Vitamin A deficiency may lead to xerophthalmia, and vitamin K deficiency may result in bleeding, especially in infants.
- Children with CF are usually thin and underweight, but with adequate treatment, most attain normal height. Of the children diagnosed as having CF, 50% are assigned less than the 10th percentile for height or weight (FitzSimmons, 1993).
- Protruberant abdomen, barrel chest, wasted buttocks, and thin extremities

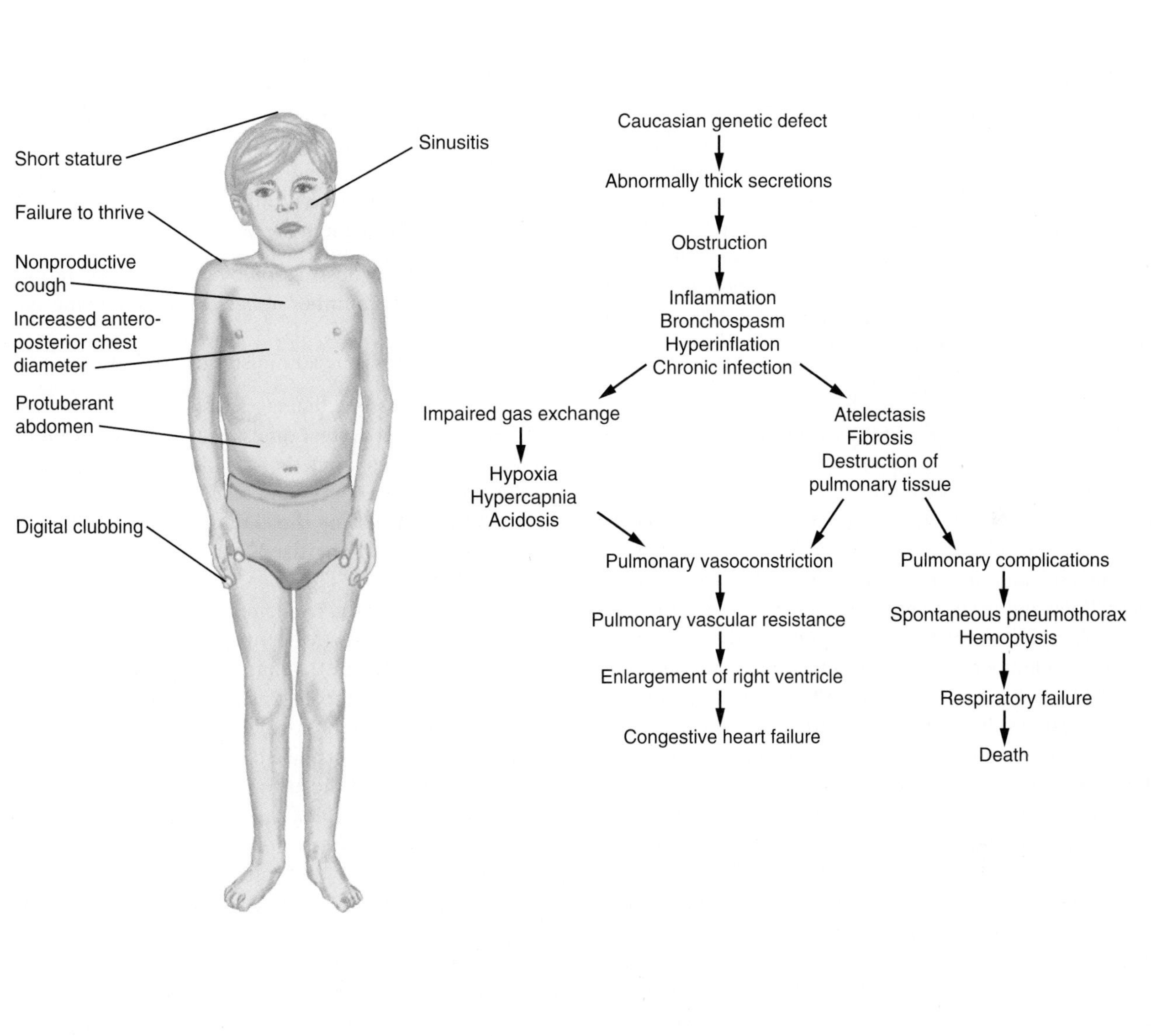

- Meconium ileus in the neonate (earliest manifestation of CF). Intestinal obstruction later in life, called meconium ileus equivalent, may occur and is the result of impacted feces at the ileocecal junction.
- Rectal prolapse and intussusception
- Biliary cirrhosis, portal hypertension, and esophageal varices, secondary to obstruction of the bile ducts, in 2% to 4% of patients
- Increased incidence of insulin-dependent diabetes in older patients with CF

Integumentary System

- Abnormally high concentrations of sodium and chloride in sweat (Mothers often report that their infants "taste salty" when kissed.)
- Risk for electrolyte imbalances during hot weather. Infants are especially prone to developing hyponatremia and hypochloremia.
- Dry mouth and increased susceptibility to infection.

Reproductive System

- An average of 2 years' delay in development of secondary sex characteristics
- Difficulty becoming pregnant because of thick cervical mucus which acts as a barrier to sperm (although this impairment of fertility should not be relied upon as a birth control method)
- Increased incidence of fetal loss and preterm birth, as well as increased neonatal mortality, in pregnant women with CF (although those with mild CF can

carry a pregnancy to term with conscientious prenatal care)
- Sterility secondary to aspermia in approximately 95% of male patients with CF; otherwise normal sexual function

Diagnostic Evaluation. CF has been called the "great imitator," as signs of failure to thrive and chronic respiratory infection or are symptoms of many other childhood conditions. Some infants with CF present at birth with symptoms of severe bowel obstruction (meconium ileus) caused by intestinal plugging by thick, tenacious secretions. More commonly, children with CF are diagnosed during infancy or toddlerhood with poor growth; bulky, greasy stools; and frequent colds or bouts of pneumonia (Barnhart & Czervinske, 1995; Fulginiti, 1993). Early diagnosis and treatment of CF make a difference in the quality and length of life for these children.

The diagnosis of CF requires a positive sweat test, as well as either a positive family history of CF or clinical symptoms consistent with CF. The sweat test is simple, painless, and reliable. It is usually performed twice to ensure accuracy. The sweat test, *pilocarpine iontophoresis*, measures the amount of sodium and chloride in a person's sweat. Sweating is stimulated on the child's forearm with pilocarpine, the sample is collected on absorbent material, and the amount of sodium and chloride is measured. A chloride level greater than 60 mEq/L is considered to be a positive test result; a level of 40 mEq/L is suggestive of CF and requires a repeat test. A sample of at least 50 mg of sweat is required for accurate results. Because this amount is difficult to obtain from small infants, the sweat test is usually not reliable in infants younger than 4 weeks of age.

In addition to the sweat test the following studies are also performed: 72-hour fecal fat determination, liver function tests (ALT, AST), fasting blood glucose test, chest X-ray film, sputum culture (for identification of infective organisms), and pulmonary function tests.

Prenatal diagnosis can be made by DNA analysis of chorionic villi samples or by testing of amniotic fluid. DNA analysis requires blood samples from each parent and an affected child in order to track the CF-affected chromosome. Then, to determine if the fetus is affected by CF, DNA is obtained from chorionic villi at 8 to 10 weeks' gestation. Results can be reported the same day. DNA analysis can also determine whether siblings of the affected child are carriers. (Once the diagnosis of CF is established, siblings should be tested.) Another method for obtaining prenatal diagnosis is by amniotic fluid analysis, whereby samples of amniotic fluid are taken during the second trimester. The results are based on the fact that intestinal alkaline phosphatase in amniotic fluid is reduced when a fetus is affected with CF. Results are usually available in 2 to 4 weeks. Genetic counseling is an important aspect of CF care.

Therapeutic Management. Because the severity and rate of progression of symptoms is different for each child, treatment must be individualized. Therapy is aimed at preventing and treating pulmonary infections, maintaining optimal nutritional status, and promoting psychological adjustment. Children with CF are cared for at home most of the time. They are hospitalized during acute pulmonary infections, end-stage disease, and periodically for IV antibiotic treatment and vigorous CPT.

Respiratory Problems. Because chronic respiratory infection is a major cause of lung damage in patients with CF, the goals of treatment are as follows:

1. to relieve airway obstruction by mobilizing secretions
2. to decrease the number of bacteria by removing secretions
3. to treat infections by administering antibiotics

Segmental postural drainage with inhalation therapy or CPT is performed several times a day to loosen secretions and to move them from the peripheral airways into the central airways where they can be coughed out. Secretions are mobilized by placing the child in various positions and percussing and vibrating the chest (see Chapter 18, Figs. 18–14 and 18–15). CPT over each lung segment, followed by breathing exercises, facilitates drainage and expectoration. Mucolytic agents (Mucomyst, Gelsolin, recombinant DNase or Pulmozyme), bronchodilators (Isuprel, Bronkosol, anti-inflammatory agents, proteolytic agents), and hydrating agents (Amiloride, UTP), are often used with postural drainage to decrease the viscosity of secretions or to increase the size of the airways. (Aitkin, 1992; Behrman, Kliegman, & Arvin, 1996; Light, 1994; Hubbard et al., 1992). A common schedule for pulmonary hygiene is postural drainage for 5 to 10 minutes, followed by nebulization with a prescribed solution, followed by another 10 to 20 minutes of postural drainage. This procedure is repeated twice a day when the child is feeling well, and more often as needed during periods of acute illness.

Exercise is an important part of pulmonary treatment. Some researchers suggest that aerobic exercise, such as jogging or swimming, may be as effective as traditional CPT in relieving pulmonary obstruction (Loutzenhiser & Clark, 1993). Most patients are treated with a combination of exercise and CPT. Patients with CF who exercise regularly have fewer pulmonary exacerbations and generally feel better than those who do not.

Antibiotics have played a major role in increasing the life expectancy of children with CF. Some physicians prescribe antibiotics prophylactically, whereas others use them only during periods of active infection. IV antibiotics are the usual treatment of choice during acute pulmonary exacerbations. Children with CF frequently require higher than usual doses of antibiotics because of their rapid metabolism of these drugs. IV antibiotics are usually administered during hospitalization, but home IV therapy is becoming more widely used, offering substantial savings and minimizing disruption of daily activities. A variety of techniques may be used to achieve stable venous access for IV therapy, such as peripheral catheters attached to heparin locks, peripherally inserted central catheters (PICC), Hickman and Broviac catheters, and implantable central venous catheters (see Chapter 18). Oral or aerosolized antibiotics may be used instead of IV therapy.

Steroids are sometimes prescribed when pulmonary symptoms are unresponsive to antibiotics and increased CPT. However, steroids are used with caution because of the concern that they could worsen *Pseudomonas* infections. Oxygen therapy is used with caution as many children with CF have chronic carbon dioxide retention and are at risk for oxygen-induced carbon dioxide narcosis.

> It is essential that patients with CF be adequately protected from communicable diseases by immunization. In addition to the recommended basic series of immunizations, children with CF should also receive yearly influenza vaccinations.

Digestive Problems. Early in the course of CF, the child will usually have a huge appetite but will be unable to gain weight. Chronic pulmonary infections, increased work of breathing, and malabsorption place an increased caloric and protein demand on the child with CF, raising caloric requirements to approximately 150% of the normal recommended daily allowance (RDA). Children with CF are managed with a high-calorie, high-protein diet, pancreatic enzyme replacement therapy, fat-soluble vitamin supplements, and, if nutritional problems are severe, nighttime gastrostomy feedings or TPN. Fats are not restricted unless steatorrhea cannot be controlled by increased pancreatic enzymes. Infants are usually given a predigested formula (Pregestimil or Nutramigen), which is more easily absorbed. Formulas may also be concentrated to provide increased calories. For the older child, caloric intake may be increased with food supplements or enteral tube feedings (usually at night, either by nasogastric tube or by gastrostomy/jejunostomy).

> Do not mix pancreatic enzyme powder with hot foods or foods containing tapioca or other starches. Enzyme powder should be mixed with nonfat, nonprotein foods, such as applesauce.

Enteric-coated microencapsulated pancreatic enzyme preparations (Cotazym-S, Pancreatin, Pancrease) are administered with every meal and snack. Enzyme dosage is adjusted according to stool formation: less enzyme with constipation, more enzyme with loose, fatty stools. In recent studies (Kuhn & Horn, 1994), bowel obstruction has been reported in association with high-dose enzyme replacement (lipase, >6000 U/kg/meal). Therefore, enzyme dosage should be individualized for each patient and kept as low as possible while still maintaining the child's nutritional status (Behrman, Kliegman, & Arvin, 1996). Extra salt is added to the diet in extremely hot weather.

NURSING CARE OF THE CHILD WITH CYSTIC FIBROSIS

Assessment

The child with CF should be assessed for signs and symptoms in each of the systems usually affected by the disease, as well as for psychosocial adaptation to this chronic condition.

Respiratory Assessment. The child may have had frequent episodes of pneumonia or bronchitis. The chest should be auscultated to detect any crackles, wheezes, areas of diminished breath sounds, or prolonged expiratory phase of respiration. The child should be examined for signs of long-standing respiratory difficulty, such as barrel chest and/or digital clubbing. Respiratory status is assessed by noting the rate, depth, and ease of respirations, as well as the color of the nailbeds and mucous membranes, and by determining pulse oximetry values (Fig. 29–3). The characteristics of the child's cough and the color, amount, and quality of sputum should be noted. Fever, if present, should be documented. Exercise tolerance and the child's ability to sleep lying down at night should also be assessed.

Digestive Assessment. The child should be weighed and measured and height and weight plotted on a stan-

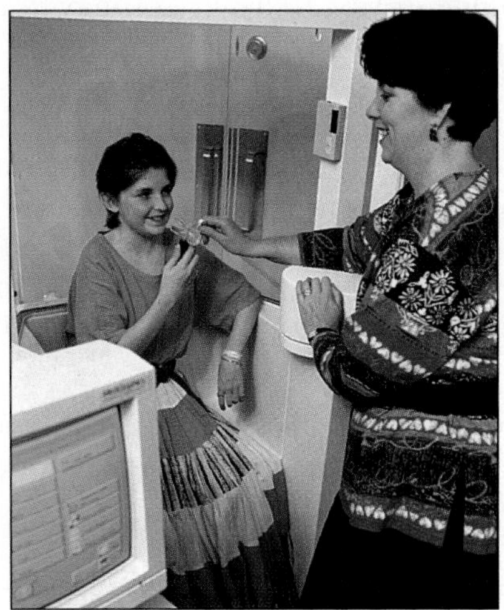

Figure 29–3
Tests of lung capacity and pulmonary function are commonly performed in children and adults with cystic fibrosis. These tests help to evaluate the progression of the disorder and determine whether more vigorous treatment is needed. (Courtesy of Cook Children's Medical Center, Fort Worth, Texas)

dardized growth chart to assess adequacy of growth. Other signs of malabsorption, such as steatorrhea, frequent infections, fatigue, and protruberant abdomen with thin extremities, should be noted. A diet history is useful in assessing the child's caloric intake. The use of vitamins and dietary supplements should be documented. Adequacy of intestinal enzyme replacement can be assessed by determining the number and consistency of stools. Because ulcers and intestinal obstruction often accompany CF, complaints of abdominal pain, blood in the stools, and constipation should be noted. Use of antacids, H_2 blockers, or antireflux medications should also be assessed.

Reproductive Assessment. Girls should be assessed for vaginal itching or drainage, which may indicate vaginal infections. Contraception should be discussed with adolescents.

Integumentary Assessment. The skin should be inspected for cyanosis and for clubbing of the fingers and toes (see Fig. 29–2). The results of pilocarpine iontophoresis should be reviewed.

Nursing Diagnoses

- Ineffective Airway Clearance related to increased pulmonary secretions
- Impaired Gas Exchange related to air trapping within the alveoli secondary to obstruction of the airways by thick mucus
- Risk for Infection related to tenacious secretions and altered body defenses
- Alteration in Nutrition: Less Than Body Requirements, related to poor intestinal absorption of nutrients
- Activity Intolerance related to pulmonary congestion and poor absorption of nutrients
- Self-Esteem Disturbance related to physical changes from chronic illness
- Ineffective Individual/Family Coping: Compromised, related to chronic illness
- Anticipatory Grieving related to potentially fatal diagnosis

Planning, Implementation, and Evaluation: The Child With Cystic Fibrosis

NURSING DIAGNOSIS

- Ineffective Airway Clearance related to increased pulmonary secretions
- Impaired Gas Exchange related to increased pulmonary secretions

Expected Outcome:

- The child will be able to remove secretions from the airway as evidenced by decreased respiratory distress, cyanosis, and coughing.
- The child will maintain an oxygen saturation level of greater than 94%.

Intervention	Rationale
1. Assess the child's respiratory status q 4 hr, or more often if indicated. Observe for increased respiratory distress during activity, feeding, respiratory treatments, or interruption of oxygen therapy.	Frequent respiratory assessment is necessary to detect early changes in oxygenation status.
2. Perform chest percussion and postural drainage q 4 hr and as needed (see Chapter 18, Figs. 18–14 and 18–15). These procedures may be needed as often as q 2 hr during periods of pulmonary infection. Perform treatments at least 1 hour prior to meals or 2 hours after meals to prevent vomiting, as well as before bedtime to clear airways and facilitate rest.	CPT helps mobilize secretions and improves oxygenation.
Auscultate breath sounds before and after treatments. Observe the child's response to and tolerance of procedures.	Assessing breath sounds is helpful in monitoring the effectiveness of treatments.
3. Encourage coughing and deep breathing, and activities that require deep breathing (as tolerated).	Deep breathing facilitates lung expansion and helps mobilize secretions.
Teach child the "huff" maneuver (forced expiratory technique) to mobilize secretions. The child is taught to cough with an open glottis by taking a deep breath, then exhaling rapidly whispering the word "huff."	"Huffing," or forced expiratory technique, reduces the likelihood of bronchial collapse, which occurs with explosive coughing, and improves secretion removal.

Intervention	Rationale
4. Administer expectorants and bronchodilators as ordered.	These medications facilitate thinning and mobilization of secretions.
Teach the parents NOT to give the child cough suppressant preparations.	Cough suppressants inhibit expectoration of secretions and promote infection.
5. Administer humidified, low-flow (≤2 L/min) oxygen carefully as needed and as ordered.	Oxygen must be administered with caution to children with chronic hypoxia because it may depress respirations by causing oxygen narcosis. Humidity loosens and thins secretions.
6. Elevate the head of the bed or support the child in an upright position with pillows if he is dyspneic. Stay with the child during coughing episodes.	An upright position facilitates chest expansion by decreasing pressure on the diaphragm.
7. Administer IV or p.o. fluids as needed and as ordered.	Adequate fluid intake decreases the viscosity of secretions and aids in expectoration.

Evaluation: The child exhibits:

- improved breath sounds
- the ability to participate in usual activities
- a pulse oximetry value of >94% on room air.

The parent:

- demonstrates CPT, inhalation therapy, breathing exercises, and other treatments that will be performed at home.

NURSING DIAGNOSIS

- Risk for Infection related to tenacious secretions and altered body defenses

Expected Outcome:

- The child will have no signs of infection as evidenced by normal body temperature, nonpurulent sputum, and decreased respiratory distress.

Intervention	Rationale
1. Promote optimal nutrition and hydration.	Adequate protein/caloric intake improves the child's defenses against infection.
2. Practice and teach patient and family hygiene measures (thorough handwashing technique, personal cleanliness).	Careful hygiene measures decrease the child's exposure to pathogens.
3. Assess the child's vital signs, noting fever, increased respiratory rate, and/or dyspnea. Assess the patient for malaise or chills. Monitor the child for increased white blood cell count. Observe the color, amount, and consistency of secretions.	These findings will help to determine whether or not the child has an infection.
4. Protect the child from exposure to pathogens by restricting visitors with infections.	Children with CF are susceptible to respiratory infections and should be protected from unnecessary exposure to infecting organisms.

Intervention	Rationale
5. Make sure the child's immunizations are up-to-date. Immunize yearly against influenza.	Children with CF should receive all routine immunizations at the ages recommended by the American Academy of Pediatrics (see Appendix A). An annual influenza vaccine is also appropriate based on the recommendations of the Centers for Disease Control (CDC).
6. Administer antibiotics as ordered.	Antibiotics may be ordered to help fight infection.

Evaluation:
- The child demonstrates a decreased amount of sputum and secretions that are not purulent.
- The child has normal body temperature and a white blood cell count that is normal for age.

NURSING DIAGNOSIS
- Alteration in Nutrition: Less Than Body Requirements related to poor intestinal absorption of nutrients

Expected Outcome:
- The child will have improved nutritional status as evidenced by increased height and weight along the normal growth curve and by adequate intake (eating over 80%) of meals.
- The child will have stools of normal consistency, frequency, and color.

Intervention	Rationale
1. Provide a well-balanced diet that is high in calories, protein, and carbohydrates. Include the child's favorite foods in the diet, particularly when appetite is decreased. Increase caloric intake with oral high-calorie supplements, nocturnal gastrostomy feedings, or parenteral feedings via a central venous catheter, as ordered.	Insufficiency of the pancreatic enzymes lipase, trypsin, and amylase results in malabsorption of fats, protein, and carbohydrates. Because of malabsorption and the stress of chronic illness, the child with CF needs approximately 150% of the normal protein and caloric requirements to maintain growth.
Give infants a partially digested formula, such as Portagen or Pregestimil. Breastfeeding should be encouraged in conjunction with enzyme supplementation.	Nutrients from predigested infant formulas are more readily absorbed.
2. Administer pancreatic enzymes, as ordered, within 30 minutes of eating meals and snacks. Do not mix enzymes with hot or starchy foods. Mix with a small amount of nonfat, nonprotein food such as applesauce.	Pancreatic enzymes must be administered at the time food is eaten in order to be effective. They are inactivated by heat and are partially degraded by gastric acids.
Older children may take enteric-coated pancreatic enzyme capsules. Enzyme beads must not be crushed or chewed.	Enteric coating prevents gastric inactivation. Chewing or crushing the beads destroys the enteric coating, causing inactivation of the enzymes and excoriation of the oral mucosa. Extra enzymes should be added when high-fat foods are eaten.
Wipe off any powder that remains on child's lips. Pancreatic enzymes are not given if the child is NPO.	Prolonged contact with enzyme powder may cause excoriation of oral mucosa.
3. Note the color, consistency, and frequency of stools.	Excess pancreatic enzyme supplements may cause constipation, diarrhea and gastrointestinal bleeding; insufficient enzymes result in malabsorption of fats and proteins, producing steatorrhea.

Intervention	Rationale
4. Administer multivitamins, water-miscible, fat-soluble vitamins; and iron supplements as ordered.	Deficiency of pancreatic enzymes interferes with absorption of fat-soluble vitamins. Pancreatic enzyme replacements interfere with absorption of iron.
5. Supplement the child's diet with salt during extremely hot weather or when the child has a fever. Instruct parents to report promptly any muscle cramping, lethargy, or changes in the child's level of consciousness.	Excessive losses of sodium chloride in the sweat may lead to electrolyte imbalances.
6. Administer CPT before meals.	Performing CPT before meals decreases the chance of vomiting during a treatment.
7. Provide frequent mouth care, particularly before meals and snacks.	Copious, tenacious sputum produces a foul taste and decreases appetite.
8. Assess the child's appetite and food intake.	Early in the disease process, children with CF have a voracious appetite. Poor appetite and anorexia are associated with acute infections and advanced CF.

Evaluation:
- The child maintains weight or gains 1 lb/week if malnourished.
- The parent demonstrates the skills necessary to maintain an alternative feeding method (e.g., gastrostomy, TPN) prior to the child's discharge from the hospital.
- The parent adjusts the pancreatic enzyme dosage appropriately.

NURSING DIAGNOSIS
- Activity Intolerance related to pulmonary congestion and poor absorption of nutrients

Expected Outcome:
- The child will rest comfortably and engage in age-appropriate activities as his energy level allows.

Intervention	Rationale
1. Support the child in a comfortable, upright position.	An upright position facilitates maximum lung expansion.
2. Provide rest periods between treatments. Organize nursing care to provide periods of uninterrupted rest. Keep the child comfortable.	During periods of pulmonary infection, the child's energy reserves are depleted. Children with CF are vulnerable to fatigue because of increased basal metabolic rate, nighttime coughing, and poor oxygenation status.
3. Explain all procedures according to the child's level of understanding. Reassure the child that she will not be left alone when she is having difficulty breathing.	Decreased anxiety facilitates rest.
4. Increase the child's level of activity as tolerated. Provide age-appropriate activities geared to the child's energy level.	Quiet activity decreases boredom.
5. When the child is feeling well, encourage active play and activities, such as swimming and gymnastics.	Exercise loosens secretions and promotes feelings of well-being and self-confidence.

Evaluation:
- The child engages in physical activity as his condition allows.
- The child is able to rest and has decreased episodes of coughing.

NURSING DIAGNOSIS
- Self-Esteem Disturbance related to alteration in appearance and activity intolerance (see Chapter 17)

Expected Outcome:
- The child with CF will have a positive self-concept and feelings of independence.
- The child will engage in age-appropriate activities and participate in self-care.

Intervention	Rationale
1. Encourage the child to express feelings about the chronic illness and its affect on feelings of self-worth.	Physical changes, such as short stature, delayed puberty, clubbing of fingers, and a barrel chest, may cause the child to feel "different." Exercise intolerance and embarrassment about coughing up large amounts of sputum may discourage the child from participating in activities with peers.
2. Assist the child to identify personal strengths and areas of accomplishment.	Recognition of and pride in unique attributes increases self-esteem.
3. Encourage the child to take responsibility for her own care as much as possible.	Children are more likely to adhere to the treatment plan if they are allowed to take control of parts of their illness management. Active participation in decision making promotes autonomy.
4. Teach parents the importance of fostering independence in their child.	Parents of chronically ill children may become overprotective, undermining the self-confidence of the child.
5. Encourage discussion of areas of concern, such as dating, sexuality, and peer acceptance.	Pubertal delays are usually present.
6. Discuss the child's condition with school personnel. Provide printed educational material for teachers. (One excellent resource is *A Teacher's Guide to CF*, available from the CF Foundation, 6931 Arlington Rd., Bethesda, MD 20814, 1–800–FIGHT CF.)	Teachers often have questions about the child's exercise tolerance, diet, medications, and toileting needs. The child's school performance may be affected by fatigue and frequent bouts of respiratory infection. Absenteeism secondary to hospitalization requires coordination with school personnel.

Evaluation:
- The child develops age-appropriate cognitive and social skills.
- The child demonstrates an attitude of acceptance of self and of the illness.

NURSING DIAGNOSIS
- Ineffective Individual/Family Coping: Compromised, related to chronic illness

Expected Outcome:
- The child/family will comply with the treatment regimen.
- The child/family will verbalize feelings about the impact of the illness on their lives.
- The child/family will utilize available support systems and community resources.

Intervention	Rationale
1. Teach the family the importance of carrying out treatments, administering medications, and following the therapeutic plan as outlined by health care providers.	Conscientious compliance with the treatment regimen decreases the frequency of respiratory infections and improves the health and longevity of the child with CF.
Teach parents the skills required to administer nebulizer treatments and medications and to guide or perform breathing exercises, chest percussion, and postural drainage.	Education helps the family feel they have some control in making informed decisions regarding their child's health care.

Intervention	Rationale
Provide written instructions on all aspects of care. (Many excellent materials are available from the CF Foundation, 6931 Arlington Rd., Bethesda, MD 20814, 1–800–FIGHT CF.)	
2. Listen to and encourage the child and family to verbalize their feelings and express their concerns regarding CF. Answer questions honestly and openly.	Identifying concerns and clarifying misconceptions will help the family cope with the stress of chronic illness.
3. Introduce the family to other families affected by CF.	Families of other children with CF can offer suggestions and strategies for dealing with problems.
4. Provide information about available community resources, such as those provided by the Cystic Fibrosis Foundation, Crippled Children's Programs, and the American Lung Association.	These organizations provide information, equipment, and financial support. The financial and emotional burden of CF can be overwhelming.
5. Assist the family in obtaining home care equipment (oxygen and aerosol therapy supplies). Provide parents with the phone numbers of persons to contact if they have questions or problems with equipment or medications.	Parents need support and specific information in order to care for a chronically ill child at home. Availability of resources decreases parents' feelings of frustration and helplessness.
6. Obtain social service consults and home health referrals as needed.	

Evaluation:
- The child/family comply with the treatment plan.
- The child/family utilize available resources.

NURSING DIAGNOSIS
- Anticipatory Grieving related to potentially fatal diagnosis

Expected Outcome:
- The child and family will discuss their feelings about anticipated death and will make realistic plans for the future.

Intervention	Rationale
1. Provide honest information about the disease and its prognosis.	Although tremendous progress has been made in treatment, CF remains a chronic disease with no cure. The median survival age is 30 years. Honesty promotes trust. Families need accurate information in order to make decisions.
2. Listen to the child and family as they discuss feelings about the disease, death, and the future.	Diagnosis of an eventually fatal disease provokes an acute anticipatory mourning reaction among family members. Counseling should begin at the time of diagnosis and continue throughout the course of the disease.
3. Identify additional sources of emotional support and counseling (pastor, mental health services, etc.).	Having several support systems available helps the family cope with the stresses of a chronic, progressive illness.

Evaluation:
- The child/family express feelings of anger, sadness, and fear without guilt.
- The child/family set realistic goals for themselves.

Home Care. Preparation for home care involves teaching family members how to carry out CPT, how to provide breathing treatments, and how to give medications at home. Written instructions should be provided on all aspects of care. The Cystic Fibrosis Foundation (1–800–FIGHT CF) has excellent material available for patients with CF and their families. Families need assistance in obtaining home care equipment. Instructions and practice using the equipment, as well as a phone number to call in case problems arise, should be provided.

Nutrition is an important aspect of home care. Parents should be instructed how to provide a high-calorie, high-protein diet with tolerated fat. Parents often have questions about the appropriate dosage for enzyme supplements. The amount of enzyme is regulated by the child's needs, and the dosage is adjusted until the stool pattern is acceptable (e.g., one to two stools daily in older children; more often in infancy). Enzymes should be taken within 30 minutes of eating. Extra enzymes should be added when high-fat foods are eaten. Extra salt and fluids should be provided during hot weather. Oral hygiene is important because of interference with salivation and excessive mucus production.

TUBERCULOSIS

Tuberculosis (TB) is a reportable contagious disease with a high morbidity and mortality throughout the world. Its incidence had declined until 1985, when it again began to rise. The World Health Organization has declared TB a global crisis (Ott, Horn, & McLaughlin, 1995).

Etiology. *Mycobacterium tuberculosis,* an acid-fast bacillus, causes TB. The principle route of contamination is through inhalation of droplets from a person with active TB. Droplets produced by coughing and sneezing remain suspended in the air. When they are inhaled, they can reach the bronchioles and alveoli.

The risk of infection by the organism is thought to be dependent upon several factors (see the accompanying box). Most children are infected by a family member or babysitter or other person with whom they have frequent contact.

Incidence. After decades of decline in the incidence of TB, the number of cases of TB has risen dramatically in the past decide. Almost 1.3 million cases and 450,000

PATHOPHYSIOLOGY *of Tuberculosis*

TB is most often transmitted by inhalation of contaminated droplets coughed up and expelled from an adult or adolescent with infectious pulmonary TB. The most common site of organism implantation is the respiratory tract. The bacillus multiplies in lung tissue, alveoli, and regional lymph nodes. After an incubation period of 2 to 10 weeks, hypersensitivity develops; at that time, the infected child will test positive on skin tests. Most infected children are asymptomatic at the time of the initial positive skin test result (American Academy of Pediatrics [AAP], 1994b).

The *disease* of TB is differentiated from TB *infection* by the presence of clinical manifestations. The risk of developing TB disease is approximately 5% to 10% over an entire lifetime, and is highest in the first 2 years after infection. Months to years may ensue between a TB infection and development of the disease. Usually, untreated infections become dormant and never progress to clinical disease in the healthy host (AAP, 1994b). The immunologic response of most people is usually strong enough to keep the bacteria from multiplying and spreading. If the host response is adequate, the organism is walled off and the tubercle becomes a healed calcified mass. TB bacilli can remain dormant and cause active disease at a later time if the child's resistance is lowered. If the lesion does not heal and is not walled off, it may continue to enlarge and spread into nearby tissues, or it may enter the blood and spread to other sites (middle ear, brain, kidney, bones, joints, and skin).

TB disease destroys host tissue. When tubercle bacilli multiply, they may damage tissue so badly that the center of the infected area turns to liquid pus. When this liquid escapes through an airway, it is coughed up as sputum, leaving a tiny hole (cavitation) in the lung. This bacteria-laden sputum is infectious. Only rarely do children develop active pulmonary TB with cavitation, and only in such instances is the child infectious to others (Ott, Horn, & McLaughlin, 1995). Children with primary pulmonary TB usually are not contagious because their lesions are small and cough is minimal or absent (AAP, 1994a). The duration of infectivity of treated adults and adolescents depends upon the drug susceptibility of the infecting organism and cough frequency. Although infectivity usually lasts only a few weeks after treatment is begun, it may last longer if the person fails to take the prescribed medication or is infected with a resistant strain.

Risk Factors for Development of Tuberculosis (TB)

1. Contact with adults with infectious TB
2. Chronic illness, immunosuppression, HIV infection
3. Malnutrition
4. Age (infancy and adolescence)
5. Nonwhite racial and ethnic groups; immigrants from areas with a high incidence of TB
6. Urban, low-income living conditions
7. Incarcerated adolescents
8. Children in close contact with any of the following groups of adults: HIV-infected persons, users of IV or other street drugs, poor or medically indigent city dwellers, residents of nursing homes, migrant farm workers

deaths occur among children each year. Homeless persons, especially those living in shelters, have a TB case rate 40 times higher than that of the general population (Starke et al., 1992). More than two-thirds of the reported cases in the United States now occur in urban, low-income areas, and in nonwhite racial and ethnic groups (AAP, 1994a). In the pediatric population, TB occurs most commonly in infants and adolescents and in children with immunosuppressive conditions. Of particular concern is the increase in multidrug-resistant (MDR) TB which develops primarily in persons who do not take medications as prescribed (Ott, Horn, & McLaughlin, 1995).

Clinical Manifestations

- Children ages 3 to 15 years are usually asymptomatic, have normal chest X-ray studies, and can be identified only through a positive skin test.
- Some children develop malaise, fever, slight cough, weight loss, anorexia, lymphadenopathy, or more specific symptoms related to the site of infection (e.g., kidneys, brain, bone, lungs).

Diagnostic Evaluation. Skin testing is the initial method of screening and testing in persons suspected of having TB. In most children, skin testing will produce a positive reaction 3 to 6 weeks after the initial infection, and occasionally as long as 3 months after infection. Positive tuberculin reactivity usually continues for the person's lifetime, even with treatment.

There are two types of antigen preparations used for testing: old tuberculin (OT) and purified protein derivative (PPD). These preparations must be kept refrigerated in a dark place to preserve their potency. Skin testing can be done via an intradermal Mantoux test or a multiple-puncture test (MPT) (e.g., tine test) (see the table entitled Common Laboratory and Diagnostic Tests).

> The test should be read by a health care professional, not by the patient or parent. The reading is based on induration (hardness), not erythema (redness). Results should be recorded in millimeters and not simply as "positive" or "negative" (even if there is no induration). Repeated Mantoux PPD skin testing will not "sensitize" an uninfected person to PPD and will not cause future PPD tests to be positive.

Interpretation of the Mantoux Test Results. Current guidelines developed by the CDC and AAP state that an area of induration of 15 mm or greater is considered to be a positive sign in all children, including those with no risk factors. Induration measuring 10 mm or greater is considered to be a positive result in children younger than 4 years of age and in those with chronic illness or high risk for environmental exposure to tuberculosis. A reaction of 5 mm or greater is considered to be a positive result for the highest-risk groups (see the box entitled Definition of a Positive Mantoux Skin Test in Children). The fact that a child has a negative tuberculin skin test does not rule out the presence of TB, particularly in young infants. Therefore, all positive and doubtful reactions to a tine test must be followed by the Mantoux test.

Children with positive skin test results undergo follow-up examinations, which include periodic chest X-ray films and sputum cultures and smears. Because children often swallow sputum rather than expectorate it, gastric washings to obtain swallowed sputum are sometimes done. A thorough history should be obtained, and all contacts of the affected child should be tested for the disease.

Therapeutic Management. Treatment of TB involves the eradication of TB organisms with medication (multi-drug; see the table in the Clinical Reference Pages entitled Medications Commonly Used in the Treatment of Chronic Respiratory Conditions), provision of optimal nutrition, and prevention of exposure to infection, which could further compromise the child's already challenged immune system. Hospitalization of children with TB may be indicated depending on the severity of the disease, the age of the child, the need for more extensive testing, and/or the child's family and social environment. Unless the child is acutely ill, bedrest is not required.

Preventive Medication Therapy. Isoniazid (INH) is given to prevent TB infection from progressing to active disease. A chest X-ray film is obtained prior to initiation of preventive therapy. In infants and children, the recommended duration of INH therapy is 9 months. For children with HIV infection, a minimum of 12 months of treatment is recommended. Isoniazid is given daily at a dosage of 10 mg/kg. For children with INH-resistant TB infection, rifampin (10 mg/kg in a single daily dose) is administered for 9 months (AAP, 1994b).

Definition of a Positive Mantoux Skin Test in Children

AREA OF INDURATION ≥ 5 mm

- Children in close contact with persons who have known or suspected infectious cases of tuberculosis (TB)
- Children suspected of having TB disease (based on positive chest X-ray findings or clinical manifestations of TB)
- Children with immunosuppressive conditions or HIV infection

AREA OF INDURATION ≥ 10 mm

- Children younger than 4 years of age
- Children with chronic illness (malignant disease, diabetes mellitus, chronic renal failure, malnutrition)
- Children known to have environmental exposure (those born, [or with parents born] in regions of the world where TB is highly prevalent; those in close contact with adults who are HIV-infected, homeless, IV drug users, migrant farm workers, nursing home residents, or incarcerated/institutionalized persons)

INDURATION ≥ 15 mm

- Children older than 4 years of age without any risk factors

Modified from American Academy of Pediatrics, Committee on Infectious Diseases. (1994). *1994 Redbook: Report of the Committee on Infectious Diseases.* (23rd ed., p. 485.) Elk Grove Village, IL: Author. Used with permission of the American Academy of Pediatrics.

If there is doubt that the child will comply with the once-daily dosing regimen of anti-TB medication, twice-weekly therapy, administered by a health care professional, must be provided. Administration of medication must be directly observed by a health care worker or other responsible, mutually agreed upon individual (AAP, 1994b).

Treatment of Active Disease. The major problem in treating active TB is poor compliance in taking medications. Treatment is also complicated by the tendency of mycobacteria to mutate into drug-resistant strains. Drug resistance is an increasing problem. Poor patient adherence to treatment can lead to the development of drug-resistant tuberculosis (Behrman, Kliegman, & Arvin, 1996). In some areas, the incidence of resistance to INH has been as high as 30% (AAP, 1994a). The slow growth of TB organisms makes them particularly persistent.

Isoniazid (INH) is the drug of choice in the treatment of TB in children and is included in all treatment regimens (except INH-resistant cases). Combining INH with rifampin is the most effective treatment of TB in children. Ethambutol can be used as an alternative to rifampin, especially when longer treatment is required. Streptomycin is used for treatment of severe systemic TB (miliary or meningeal disease). Usually, treatment is administered for 6 to 9 months using isoniazid (INH) and rifampin, and is supplemented by pyrazinamide for the first 2 months (AAP, 1994a; Inselman & Kendig, 1990). In cases of INH-resistant TB, 12 to 18 months of therapy with an effective drug (streptomycin, ethambutol, rifampin, or pyrazinamide) is usually necessary to effect a cure (AAP, 1994a).

If multiple resistance to drug therapy develops and treatment is ineffective, surgical resection may be an option.

Bacillus Calmette-Guérin vaccine (BCG) is the only vaccine available for use in the prevention of TB. Unfortunately, BCG varies in the immunity it provides and has resulted in serious reactions. In the United States, it is used mainly for children with negative chest X-ray and skin test results who have had repeated exposures to TB and for asymptomatic HIV-infected children who are at increased risk for developing TB.

NURSING CARE OF THE CHILD WITH TUBERCULOSIS

Assessment

The child is assessed for a positive skin test, malaise, fever, lymphopathy, cough, weight loss, and anorexia. Assessment includes a thorough history of the child and family, including close outside family contacts. Reporting of cases of TB is required by law in all states in the United States. Nurses should assist in searching for the source case and others infected by the source case.

Nursing Diagnosis and Planning

The following nursing diagnoses and expected outcomes are examples that may be appropriate following assessment of the child with tuberculosis.

- Ineffective Gas Exchange related to obstruction of the bronchus secondary to an inflammatory process. ***Expected Outcome:*** *The child will have improved gas exchange as evidenced by clear breath sounds.*
- Ineffective Breathing Patterns related to obstruction of airways. ***Expected Outcome:*** *The child will expectorate mucus.*
- Knowledge Deficit related to disease process and treatment. ***Expected Outcome:*** *The child and family will verbalize an understanding of the disease process and its treatment.*

- Altered Family Processes related to caring for a child with a long-term disease. ***Expected Outcome:*** *The family will be able to meet the increased needs of the child.*
- Risk for Noncompliance related to long-term treatment of TB. ***Expected Outcome:*** *The child, with the help of the family, will adhere to the treatment plan.*
- Altered Nutrition: Less Than Body Requirements, related to anorexia. ***Expected Outcome:*** *The child will have an adequate intake for age as evidenced by weight maintenance and regaining of lost weight.*
- Fatigue related to impaired oxygen transport secondary to the disease process. ***Expected Outcome:*** *The child will exhibit decreased fatigue as evidenced by participation in the activities of daily living and playing with age-appropriate toys.*

Implementation

Evaluation of the child's respiratory status is ongoing and is documented every 2 to 4 hours depending on the severity of the disease. If the child has a cough, its characteristics should be described. The quantity and appearance of any expectorated mucus should also be described and documented. Younger children will swallow, rather than expectorate mucus. Because mucus acts as an emetic, it may cause vomiting. The child's color, activity level, and breath sounds should also be assessed and documented.

Because children with TB are rarely contagious, they are seldom isolated. However, in some areas of high prevalence, where children have a high incidence of exposure and are hospitalized only when they are very ill, they may be placed in isolation to prevent nosocomial TB (American Health Consultants, 1990). Children and adolescents with infectious pulmonary TB whose sputum cultures show acid-fast bacilli (AFB) should be subject to isolation precautions until effective medication therapy has been started and their sputum cultures show a diminishing number of organisms (AAP, 1994a). Children with TB infection or disease can attend school or a child care center if they are receiving TB medication (Jackson, 1993).

Persons exposed to infectious TB, especially those with impaired immunity or children younger than 4 years of age, should receive medical attention. Such individuals will undergo tuberculin skin testing, have a chest X-ray film, and undergo INH preventive therapy. Infected persons may have a negative reaction to skin testing, either because they have not yet developed cellular reactivity or because of anergy (decreased ability to react to antigen).

A well-balanced, age-appropriate diet (see Chapter 12) should be provided. Because the child may be anorexic, a dietary consult and the selection of favorite, nutritious foods are warranted. Frequent, small meals may increase intake. Intake and output should be documented.

Care should be planned to allow for uninterrupted rest peiods. Quiet activities (books, board games, video games, puzzles) provide diversion and decrease anxiety.

The family should be taught the cause and prevention of TB (see the accompanying box, Teaching Guidelines for the Child With Tuberculosis). The importance of nutrition, rest, and avoidance of exposure to other infectious processes should be explained. The side effects of the medications and the importance of adherence to the treatment regimen should also be discussed. Promoting compliance with drug therapy is one of the nurse's most important roles. Families should understand that, even though the child may be asymptomatic, the organism can lie dormant. They also need to understand the consequences of incomplete treatment (reinfection and, possibly, increasingly severe disease). Involvement of social services and the public health department may help the family in meeting the child's needs.

Prevention. Case finding is the most important factor in preventing transmission of TB in children (Gaffney, 1994). Because most children are infected by a family member, the best way to stop transmission of the disease

TEACHING GUIDELINES *for the Child With Tuberculosis (TB)*

Teaching of the child and family should include the following:

- Importance of adequate rest and a nutritionally adequate diet
- Proper administration of anti-TB medications as ordered and the importance of completing the prescribed course of medications
- Ways to prevent transmission of TB bacilli to others:
- Cover mouth and nose with tissue when sneezing, coughing, or laughing.
- Burn contaminated tissues.
- Carefully wash hands or wear gloves when handling sputum-contaminated articles.
- Use disposable articles or disinfect contaminated articles by boiling for 5 minutes or exposing them to bright, direct sunlight for 1 to 2 hours.

is to identify those who are infected and to provide TB therapy (Ott et al., 1995).

Prevention also includes (1) the isolation of adults with active disease, (2) administration of isoniazid to household contacts of patients with TB, and (3) administration of BCG to high-risk populations.

Early detection of the disease is accomplished by routine screening of children. Children at high risk for TB (see the earlier box entitled Risk Factors for Development of Tuberculosis) should be tested annually, using Mantoux tests. Routine annual skin testing of children with no risk factors in low-prevalence areas is not indicated (AAP, 1994b). A test should also be administered when the child has had contact with a person with TB. If the test is negative, it should be repeated 10 weeks after removal of the TB contact. If the child remains in contact with the infected person (parent, grandparent), the child should be retested every 3 months (Inselman & Kendig, 1990).

Evaluation

- Does the child have clear breath sounds and minimal or no cough?
- Does the child take the prescribed medication daily?
- Does the child receive a well-balanced diet and adequate rest?
- Have close contacts of the infected person been identified?
- Have family members and other close contacts obtained medical attention, and are they compliant with the treatment regimen?

KEY CONCEPTS

- Asthma is the most common chronic disease of childhood. Asthma is characterized by bronchospasm, edema of the bronchiolar mucous membranes, and increased secretion of mucus in the airways.
- Asthmatic symptoms signaling spasm of the smooth muscle of the bronchi and bronchioles may be triggered by a variety of stimuli, including allergens, cold air, weather changes, infection, exercise, fatigue, and emotional distress.
- Status asthmaticus—continued severe respiratory distress despite medical treatment—places the child in imminent danger of respiratory arrest and requires immediate hospitalization.
- Nursing care of the child with a severe asthma episode includes administration of inhaled and/or IV bronchodilators or corticosteroids, as ordered; oxygen therapy; IV fluids; and assistance with intubation and mechanical ventilation.
- Nursing care of the child with chronic asthma includes administration of prescribed medications and treatments and education of the child and family about medications, how to avoid triggers of asthma symptoms, how to recognize early warning signs of an asthma episode, and measures that can be taken to prevent severe asthma episodes.
- Cystic fibrosis (CF) is an inherited (autosomal recessive), multisystem disorder characterized by widespread dysfunction of the exocrine glands. Abnormal secretion of thick, tenacious mucus causes obstruction and dysfunction of the pancreas, lungs, salivary glands, sweat glands, and reproductive organs.
- Nursing care of the child with CF includes maintaining a patent airway by administering bronchodilators and performing or supervising respiratory treatments, administering antibiotics and pancreatic enzymes, and teaching the child and family about CF and its treatment.
- Bronchopulmonary dysplasia (BPD) is a chronic obstructive pulmonary disease characterized by thickening of the alveolar walls and bronchiolar epithelium. BPD occurs primarily in premature and low-birth-weight infants who have been mechanically ventilated with high concentrations of oxygen for prolonged periods of time.
- Nursing care of the infant with BPD includes supportive intervention to maintain adequate oxygenation and provision of appropriate stimulation to promote normal growth and development.
- Nursing care of the child with tuberculosis (TB) includes administering and evaluating TB skin tests and administering anti-TB medications as ordered. The nurse also instructs the child and family about the importance of adequate rest, a nutritionally adequate diet, and compliance with the medication regimen, as well as ways to prevent the transmission of TB infection.

REFERENCES

Aitkin, M. (1992). Recombinant DNase inhalation in normal and cystic fibrosis subjects. A phase study. *Journal of the American Medical Association, 267*(14), 1947–1981.

Altman, L. K. (1994, January 4). Childhood asthma seldom outgrown. *New York Times.*

American Academy of Pediatrics. (1992). Chemotherapy for T.B. in infants and children. *Pediatrics, 89,* 161–165.

American Academy of Pediatrics Committee on Infectious Diseases. (1994a). *1994 Redbook: Report of the committee on infectious diseases* (23rd ed.). Elk Grove Village, IL: Author.

American Academy of Pediatrics Committee on Infectious Diseases. (1994b). Screening for tuberculosis in infants and children. *Pediatrics, 93*(1), 131–134.

Avery, M., Tooley, W., Keller, M., et al. (1987). Is chronic lung disease in low birth weight infants preventable? A survey of ten centers. *Pediatrics, 79,* 26.

Barnhart, S. L., & Czervinske, M. P. (1995). *Perinatal and pediatric respiratory care* (468–479). Philadelphia: W. B. Saunders.

Bechler-Karsch, A. B. (1994). Assessment and management of status asthmaticus. *Pediatric Nursing, 20*(3), 217–223.

Behrman, R. E., Kliegman, R. M., & Arvin, A. M. (Eds.). (1996). *Nelson textbook of pediatrics* (15th ed.). Philadelphia: W. B. Saunders.

Bernbaum, J. E., Friedman, S., Hoffman-Williamson, M., et al. (1989). Preterm infant care after hospital discharge, *Pediatric Review, 10,* 195–208.

Brim, S. (1989). A quick guide for home use of inhalant medications. *Pediatric Nursing, 15*(1), 87–94.

Conte, V. H. (1992). Bronchopulmonary dysplasia. In P. L. Jackson & J. A. Vessey (Eds.), *Primary care of the child with a chronic condition.* St. Louis: C. V. Mosby.

Cunningham, C. K., McMillan, J. A., & Gross, S. J. (1991). Rehospitalization for respiratory illness in infants of less than 32 weeks' gestation. *Pediatrics, 88,* 527–532.

Damato, E. (1991). Bronchopulmonary dysplasia: Then and now. *Archives of Disease in Childhood, 65*(10sn), 1076–1081.

Fanaroff A., Martin, M., & Hack, M. (1991). Long-term outcome of respiratory distress in infants. *Respiratory Care, 36,* 707.

FitzSimmons, S. C. (1993). The changing epidemiology of cystic fibrosis. *Journal of Pediatrics, 122*(1), 1–9.

Fulginiti, V., & Lewy, J. (1993). Pediatrics: Update on cystic fibrosis. *Journal of the American Medical Association, 210*(2), 246–248.

Gaffney, K. F., et al. (1994). Think TB: New focus for family assessment. *Pediatric Nursing, 20,* 36–38.

Garg, M., Kurzner, L. I., Bautista, D. B., & Keens, T. G. (1988). Clinically unsuspected hypoxia during sleep and feeding in infants with bronchopulmonary dysplasia. *Pediatrics, 81,* 635–642.

Goldson, E. (1990). Bronchopulmonary dysplasia. *Pediatric Annals, 19*(1), 13–18.

Hagedorn, M. I., & Gardner, S. L. (1989). Physiologic sequelae of prematurity: The nurse practitioner's role. Part I. Respiratory issues. *Journal of Pediatric Health Care, 3,* 288–297.

Hazinski, T. (1990). Bronchopulmonary dysplasia. In V. Chernick (Ed.), *Kendig's disorders of the respiratory tract in children* (p. 311). Philadelphia: W. B. Saunders.

Howell, J. H., Flaim, T. F., & Lung, C. L. (1992). Asthma: Patient education. *Pediatric Clinics of North America, 39*(6), 1343–1359.

Hubbard, R. C., McElvaney, N. G., Birer, P., et al. (1992). A preliminary study of aerosolized recombinant human deoxyribonuclease I in the treatment of cystic fibrosis. *New England Journal of Medicine, 326,* 812–815.

Inselman, L., & Kendig, E. (1990). Tuberculosis. In V. Chernick (Ed.), *Kendig's disorders of the respiratory tract in children.* Philadelphia: W. B. Saunders.

Jackson, M. (1993). Tuberculosis in infants, children, and adolescents: New dilemmas with an old disease. *Pediatric Nursing, 19*(5), 437–442.

Light, M. J. (1994). rhDNase and cystic fibrosis: The penultimate step. *RT Journal of Respiratory Care Practitioners, 7,* 45–48.

Loutzenhiser, J. K., & Clark, R. (1993). Physical activity and exercise in children with cystic fibrosis. *Journal of Pediatric Nursing, 8*(2), 112–119.

Meisels, S., Plunkett, J., Roloff, D., et al. (1986). Growth and development of preterm infants with respiratory distress syndrome and bronchopulmonary dysplasia. *Pediatrics, 77,* 345.

Motoyama, E. K., Fort, M. D., Klesh, K. W., et al. (1987). Early onset of airway reactivity in premature infants with BPD. *American Review of Respiratory Disease, 136,* 50.

National Jewish Center for Immunology and Respiratory Medicine. (1995). *Patient education material.* Denver, CO: Author.

Northway, W. H., Moss, R. B., Carlisle, K. B., et al. (1990). Late pulmonary sequelae of bronchopulmonary dysplasia. *New England Journal of Medicine, 323,* 1793.

Ott, M. J., Horn, M., & McLaughlin, D. (1995). Pediatric TB in the 1990s. *Maternal & Child Nursing 20*(1), 16–20.

Parker, R. A., Lindstrom, D. P., Cotton, R. B. (1992). Improved survival accounts for most, but not all, of the increase in bronchopulmonary dysplasia. *Pediatrics, 90,* 663–668.

Plaut, T. F. (1988). *Children with asthma* (2nd ed.). Amherst, MA: Pedipress.

Rachelefsky, G. S. (1995). Asthma update: New approaches and partnerships. *Journal of Pediatric Health Care, 9,* 12–21.

Rush, M.G., Engelhardt, B., Parker, R. A., et al. (1990). Double blind, placebo-controlled trial of alternate day furosemide therapy in infants with BPD. *Journal of Pediatrics, 117,* 112.

Singer, L., Martin, R. J., Hawkins, S. W., et al. (1992). Oxygen desaturation complicates feeding in infants with BPD after discharge. *Pediatrics, 90,* 3, 380–383.

Smith, L. (1993). Childhood asthma: Diagnosis and treatment. *Current Problems in Pediatrics, 23,* 271–305.

Starke, J. R., Jacobs, R. F., & Jereb, L. (1992). Resurgence of tuberculosis in children. *Journal of Pediatrics, 120*(6), 839–853.

Truog, W., Jackson, J., Badura, R., et al. (1985). Bronchopulmonary dysplasia and pulmonary insufficiency of prematurity. *American Journal of Diseases in Childhood,* 139–351.

Weinberger, M. (1993). Theophylline: When should it be used? *Journal of Pediatrics, 122*(3), 403–405.

BIBLIOGRAPHY

Abmann, E., & Lipsi, K. (1991). Early intervention for technology-dependent infants and young children. *Infants and Young Children, 3*(4), 67–77.

Adriano, G., Stutman, H., & Marks, M. (1991). Bacterial pneumonias. In V. Chernick (Ed.), *Kernig's disorders of the respiratory tract in children* (p. 371). Philadelphia: W. B. Saunders.

American Academy of Pediatrics Committee on Infectious Diseases. (1993). Use of ribavirin in the treatment of RSV. *Pediatrics, 92*(3): 501–504.

American Health Consultants. (1990). Isolation, lab tests considered for infants, children in TB areas. *Hospital Infection Control.*

Barnes, L. P. (1993). Tuberculosis: Implications for patient teaching. *Maternal Child Nursing, 18,* 224.

Bartels, L. A., & Farrington, E. (1994). Nedocromil sodium (Tilade). *Pediatric Nursing, 20*(4), 395–399.

Behrman, R. (1994). *Nelson textbook of pediatrics* (14th ed.) (p. 1077). Philadelphia: W. B. Saunders.

Burton, G. G., Hodgkin, J. E., & Ward, J. J. (Eds). (1991). *Respiratory Care* (3rd ed.). Philadelphia: J. B. Lippincott.

Bye, M. R., Ewig, J. M., & Quittell, B. E. (1994). Cystic fibrosis. *Lung, 172,* 251–270.

Canny, G. J., & Levison, H. (1990). Childhood asthma: A rational approach to treatment. *Annals of Allergy, 64,* 406–418.

Capen, C. L., Dedlow, E. R., Robillard, R. H., Fuller, B. M., & Fuller, C. P. (1994). The team approach to pediatric asthma education. *Pediatric Nursing, 20*(3), 231–237.

Carter, E., Maurice, C., Chesrown, S., Shieh, G., Reilly, K., & Hendeles, L. (1993). Efficacy of intravenously administered theophylline in children hospitalized with severe asthma. *Journal of Pediatrics, 122,* 470–476.

Centers for Disease Control. (1993). Outbreak of Multidrug-resistant tuberculosis at a hospital. *Morbidity and Mortality Weekly Report, 42,* 427–434.

Crescioli, S., Spinazzi, A., & Plebani, M., et al. (1991). Theophylline inhibits early and late asthmatic reactions induced by allergens in asthmatic subjects. *Annals of Allergy, 66,* 245–251.

Cystic fibrosis Foundation.
Guide to Diagnosis and Management of Cystic Fibrosis
Guide to Drug Therapy in Patients With Cystic Fibrosis
Parents' Handbook: Your Child and Cystic Fibrosis
Living with Cystic Fibrosis: A Guide for Adolescents
Teachers' Guide: A Child With CF Is in Your Class
(Available from Cystic Fibrosis Foundation, 6000 Executive Blvd, Suite 309, Rockville, MD 20852).

Davidson, P. (1991). Tuberculosis. Current Opinion. *Infectious Disease, 4,* 134.

Dibble, S. L., & Savedra, M. C. (1988). Cystic fibrosis in adolescents: A new challenge. *Pediatric Nursing, 14*(4), 299–303.

George, R. B., & Owens, M. W. (1991, March). Bronchial asthma. *Disease-a-Month,* 149–196.

Goldberg, R., & Bancalari, E. (1991). Therapeutic approaches to the infant with bronchopulmonary dysplasia. *Respiratory Care, 36*(6), 613–621.

Goldenhersh, M. J., & Rachelefsky, G. S. (1990). Childhood asthma: Management. *Patient Care, 24*(7), 76–80.

Gray, P. H., & Rogers, Y. (1994). Are infants with bronchopulmonary dysplasia at risk for sudden infant death syndrome? *Pediatrics, 93*(5), 774–777.

Greenberger, P. A. (1992). Corticosteroids in asthma: Rationale, use and problems. *Chest: The Cardiopulmonary Journal-Supplement, 101*(6), 418S–421S.

Hammond, L. J., Caldwell, S., & Campbell, P. W. (1991). Cystic fibrosis, intravenous antibiotics and home therapy. *Journal of Pediatric Health Care, 5*(3), 24–30.

Janson-Bjerklie, S. (1990, September). Status asthmaticus. *American Journal of Nursing, xx,* 52–55.

Kazzi, N., Yves, W., & Poland, R. (1990). Dexamethasone effects on the hospital course of infants with bronchopulmonary dysplasia who are dependent on artificial ventilation. *Pediatrics, 88,* 5.

Kelly, H. W., & Hill, M. R. (1992). Asthma. In Dipiro, J. T., Talbert, R. L., Hayes, P. E., et al. (Eds.), *Pharmacotherapy: A pathophysiologic approach.* New York: Elsevier, 408–448.

Kempthorne, J., & Giebink, G. S. (1991, August). Pediatriac approach to the diagnosis and management of otitis media. *Otolaryngologic Clinics of North America, 24*(4), 905–929.

Klein-Berndt, S. (1991). Bronchopulmonary dysplasia in the family: A longitudinal case study. *Pediatric Nursing, 17*(6), 607–611.

Kuitert, L. M., & Kletchko, S. L. (1991). Intravenous magnesium sulfate in acute, life-threatening asthma. *Annals of Emergency Medicine, 20*(11), 1243–1245.

Kuhn, R. J., & Horn, L. (1994). Pancreatic enzyme therapy in patients with cystic fibrosis: The high dose lipase issue. *Pediatric Nursing, 20*(8), 623–624.

Lehne, R. A. (1994). *Pharmacology for Nursing Care* (2nd ed.). Philadelphia: W. B. Saunders.

Mazer, B., Figueroa-Rosario, M. S., & Bender, B. (1990, August). The effect of albuterol aerosol on fine-motor performance in children with chronic asthma. *Journal of Allergy and Clinical Immunology, 86*(2), 243–248.

McMullen, S. (1992). Respiratory distress syndrome and bronchopulmonary dysplasia. *Pediatrics,* 77, 345.

Nemes, J., Schmidt, E., & Kelly, L. (1988). Epiglottitis: ED nursing management. *Journal of Emergency Nursing, 14,* 70–75.

Rhodes, A. M. (1993). TB: Public health statutes. *Maternal Child Nursing, 18,* 225.

Richardson V., Zickler C., & Wheat, L. (1991). Tuberculosis screening and treatment in children. *Journal of Pediatric Health Care, 5*(1), 11–17.

Robertson, C. M. T., Etches, P. C., Goldson, E., & Kyle, J. M. (1992). Eight-year school performance, neurodevelopmental, and growth outcome of neonates with bronchopulmonary dysplasia: A comparative study. *Pediatrics 8*(3), 365–372.

Ryan-Wenger, N. M., & Walsh, M. (1994). Children's perspective on coping with asthma. *Pediatric Nursing, 20*(3), 224–228.

Schmidt, B. D. (1992). *Instructions for pediatric patients.* Philadelphia: W. B. Saunders.

Sinkin, R., Cox, C., & Phelps, D. (1990). Predicting risk for bronchopulmonary dysplasia: Selection criteria for clinical trials. *Pediatrics, 86*(5), 728; *88*(6), 1100.

Sly, R. M. (1991). Aerosol therapy in children. *Respiratory Care, 36*(9), 994–1005.

Snider, D., Reider, H., Combs, D., et al. (1988). Tuberculosis in children. *Pediatric Infectious Disease, 7,* 271–278.

Starke, J. R. (1992). Resurgence of TB in children. *Journal of Pediatrics, 120,* 839–855.

Traver, G. A., & Martinez, M. (1988). Asthma update. Part I. Mechanisms, pathophysiology, and diagnosis. *Journal of Pediatric Health Care, 2*(5), 221, 226.

Traver, G. A., & Martinez, M. (1988). Asthma update. Part II. Treatment. *Journal of Pediatric Health Care, 2*(5), 227–233.

Waring, W. (1990). Diagnostic and therapeutic procedures. In V. Chernick (Ed.), *Kendig's disorders of the respiratory tract in children.* (p. 81). Philadelphia: W. B. Saunders.

Weinberger, M. (1990). *Managing Asthma.* Baltimore, MD: Williams and Wilkins.

Weitzman, M., Gortmaker, S. L., Sobol, A. M., & Perrin, J. M. (1992). Recent trends in the prevalence and severity of childhood asthma. *Journal of the American Medical Association, 268,* 2673–2677.

Wolthers, O. C., & Pedersen, S. (1992). Controlled study of linear growth in asthmatic children during treatment with inhaled glucocorticosteroids. *Pediatrics, 89,* 839–842.

Zahr, L. K., Connolly, M., & Page, D. R. (1989). Assessment and management of the child with asthma. *Pediatric Nursing, 15*(2), 109–114.

30

The Child With Congenital Cardiac Defects

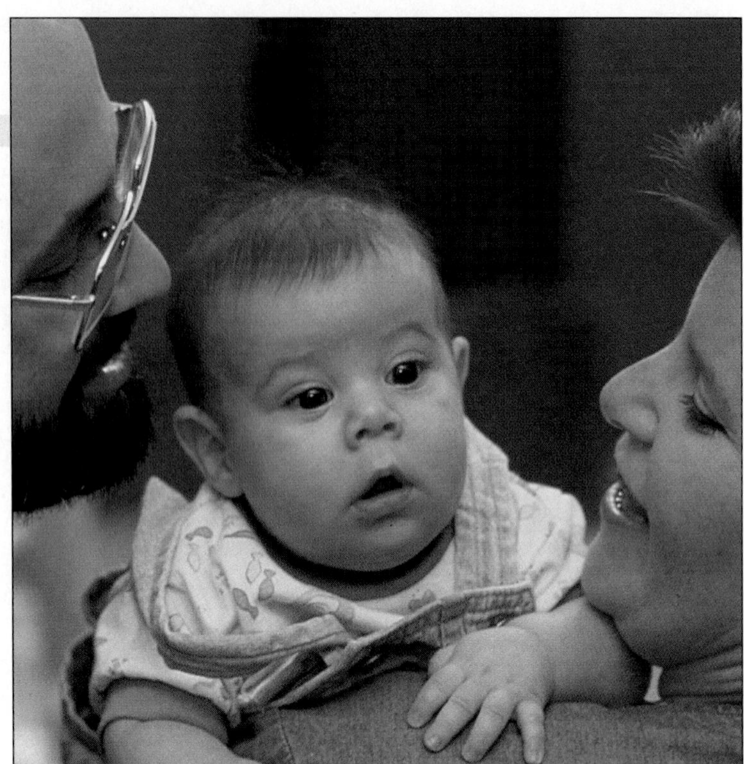

CHAPTER OVERVIEW

LEARNING OBJECTIVES

After studying this chapter, you should be able to:

- Describe the circulatory changes that occur during and after the birth process.
- Describe the anatomy and physiology of the normally functioning heart.
- Discuss the physiology of increased pulmonary blood flow in lesions causing left-to-right shunts.
- Implement the nursing diagnoses specific to caring for infants and children with left-to-right shunts.
- Discuss the physiology of lesions causing right-to-left shunts (i.e., cyanotic lesions).
- Implement the nursing diagnoses specific to caring for infants and children with cyanotic heart disease.
- Discuss the unique presentation behaviors of infants and children with stenotic lesions.
- Discuss the nursing implications of common cardiac medications used in children with cardiac disease.
- Discuss nursing interventions as they relate to specific nursing diagnoses commonly implemented when caring for a child with congenital heart disease.

KEY TERMS

angioplasty: vessel dilation

arrhythmia: an abnormal rhythm of the heart

artery: a vessel that carries blood away from the heart

atresia: the absence of a normal opening or vessel

cardiac catheterization: the process of examining the heart by introducing a thin tube (i.e., catheter) into a vein or artery and passing it into the heart to sample oxygen, measure pressure, and X-ray the area

cardiomegaly: an enlarged heart on chest X-ray

dilatation: to make larger using artificial means (such as a balloon catheter)

echocardiogram: a graphic record of the walls, valves, and vessels of the heart that is produced by reflected sound (ultrasound), of which there are several different types

gradient: a pressure difference

hypertrophy: thickening of the wall

murmur: a sound in the cardiac cycle caused by turbulent blood flow

regurgitation: the abnormal backward flow of blood through a heart valve

shunt: abnormal blood flow from one side of the heart to the other

stenosis: the narrowing or constriction of an opening (such as a heart valve)

valve: an opening, covered by membranous flaps, between two chambers of the heart or between a chamber of the heart and a blood vessel; when closed, no blood normally passes through

valvuloplasty: opening of a valve using mechanical means

Congenital heart disease refers to structural or functional defects within the heart that are present in the developing fetus or at birth. It occurs in 8 of every 1000 live births, or 1% of all live births (Hoffman, 1990). Defects may range from one as simple as an atrial septal defect to one as complex as truncus arteriosus. Other congenital defects may be present as well. Cardiac defects and the attempts to repair them may result in physiologic as well as psychological sequelae to the child.

The precise etiology of congenital heart disease is not yet known. Investigations into environmental and genetic causes are in progress. The genetic component of congenital heart disease has been investigated more thoroughly than the environmental aspect.

This chapter will present an overview of normal cardiac anatomy and physiology, beginning with fetal circulation and extending through the postnatal changes that occur. Commonly used diagnostic tests and medications for children with cardiac disease will also be discussed. The specific congenital lesions will be discussed according to the categories under which they fall: left-to-right shunts, right-to-left shunts, and stenotic lesions. The discussion of all congenital cardiac defects is beyond the scope of this chapter, as there are many different defects.

CLINICAL REFERENCE PAGES

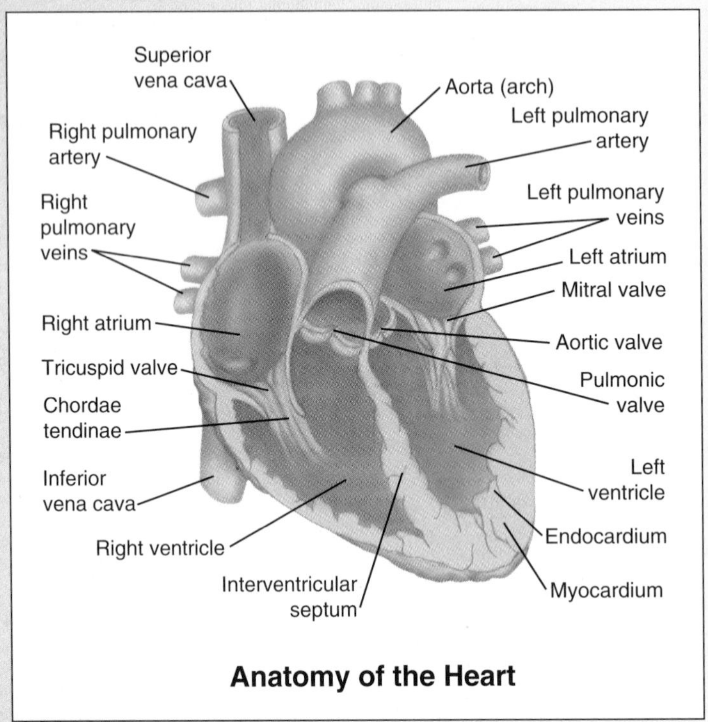

Anatomy of the Heart

REVIEW OF THE HEART AND CIRCULATION

Normal Cardiac Anatomy and Physiology. The heart is a muscular pump divided into four chambers. The two upper chambers are the atria, and the two lower chambers are the ventricles. The chambers are connected by **valves,** veins, and **arteries;** they provide for the oxygenation of blood in the lungs and subsequent distribution of the blood to the body tissues.

Electricity is required for the heart's pumping mechanism to work. This electricity is initiated by a group of cells called the sinus node. The electrical impulse thus initiated sends a message to the relay station, the atrioventricular node, which then carries the impulse to the ventricles through the His bundle, bundle branch system, and finally, the Purkinje fibers.

Each cardiac cycle consists of this electrical activity, which produces depolarization and subsequent repolarization of the cardiac muscle—more simply, a heartbeat. During each cycle, unoxygenated blood returns to the heart via the vena caval system. It enters the right atrium, travels through the tricuspid valve, and into the right ventricle. The blood is then pumped through the pulmonary valve into the pulmonary artery, then travels through the pulmonary system (the lungs) for the removal of carbon dioxide and the addition of oxygen. The blood leaves the lungs via the pulmonary veins and travels through the left atrium by way of the mitral valve, and into the left ventricle. The left ventricle pushes the blood into the aorta, which then delivers blood to the rest of the body. The pressures in the left side of the heart are four to five times higher than those in the right side. A malformation or anomaly in any of the heart's structures may affect blood flow and subsequent hemodynamic stability.

Pediatric differences in the heart and circulation are listed in the accompanying box.

Fetal Circulation. The major difference between fetal and neonatal circulation is the process of gas exchange (Alyn & Baker, 1992). In the fetus, this process occurs in the pla-

Pediatric Differences in the Heart and Circulation

- The heart and the great vessels develop during the first few weeks of gestation. The fetus is most vulnerable to cardiac malformations during this period.
- Annually about 40,000 neonates are found to suffer from congenital heart disease; as a consequence, most of those alterations are due to defects that were present at birth.
- Heart sounds in the neonate are at higher pitch and of greater intensity than in the adult, and the pulse rate is higher. Many variations in these parameters are both possible and normal.
- The chest wall of infants and young children is thin because of the relative lack of subcutaneous and muscle tissue. Innocuous murmurs can be auscultated in structurally normal hearts because of the wall thinness.
- In a very sick child the cardiac output should be evaluated as either adequate or inadequate to meet metabolic demands. Shock may be present even when the cardiac output is normal or high.
- Increased pulmonary vascular resistance in the newborn increases pressure on the right side of the heart. This may delay detection of left-to-right shunts in the newborn period because increased right-sided pressure decreases the left-to-right shunting.

centa. The fetal lungs have a very high resistance to flow because they contain no air. Therefore, there is no transfer of oxygen and carbon dioxide.

The three major shunts that allow blood flow in the developing fetus are the foramen ovale, the ductus arteriosus, and the ductus venosus (see figure on p. 910). These shunts allow oxygen-rich blood returning from the placenta via the venous circulation to reach the systemic arterial circulation. They also return unoxygenated blood from the fetus to the placenta for removal of carbon dioxide and oxygenation. In fetal circulation, the pressures in the left and right sides of the heart are equal.

Transitional and Neonatal Circulation. At birth major changes in the circulatory system occur. With the neonate's first breath, gas exchange is transferred from the placenta to the lungs.

In the normal neonate, the fetal shunts (ductus venosus, ductus arteriosus, foramen ovale) close and resistance to flow in the pulmonary system decreases as systemic resistance increases. Pulmonary vascular resistance decreases and a marked increase in pulmonary blood flow follows. Closure of the ductus arteriosus, along with the increased pulmonary blood flow, enhances left ventricular output. The increase in systemic arterial pressure due to placental closure increases the workload of the left ventricle, and the neonatal heart now functions on its own. The neonatal circulation is now normal. In some neonates it may take several days for the fetal shunts to close.

DIAGNOSTIC TESTS

Remarkable technological advances in the understanding of the cardiovascular system's function and needs have brought refinements in the tools and techniques for detecting and diagnosing congenital heart defects. Invasive procedures are required only in the most extreme cases and those in which treatment is necessary. Nevertheless, no tool or technique replaces good history taking—of both patient and parent or caregiver—and physical examination. Parents know their own children best; they may pick up subtle clues that may not be noted by the practitioner. The physical examination should be thorough. Height and weight should be plotted on the appropriate growth chart. The patient's color should be noted, with specific attention to cyanosis and/or pallor. The fingers (i.e., nailbeds) should be inspected for clubbing and the respiratory status assessed.

> Poor weight gain and failure to thrive are often associated with congenital cardiac disease.

Auscultation is very important when assessing the child with possible congenital cardiac disease (McNamara, 1990). The presence of heart murmurs can be noted at this time, and other heart sounds may be noted that may assist in defining certain defects. Finally, palpation of peripheral pulses and of the liver can give clues to the presence of cardiac disease (Malinowski & Yablonski, 1986).

> Blood pressure measurements in all four extremities should be performed in all patients with suspected heart disease to determine if discrepancies exist between the upper and lower extremities (Park, Lee, & Johnson, 1993).

The most commonly used diagnostic tests in pediatric cardiology are described in the table on page 911.

Common cardiac medications are detailed in the table on pages 912–913.

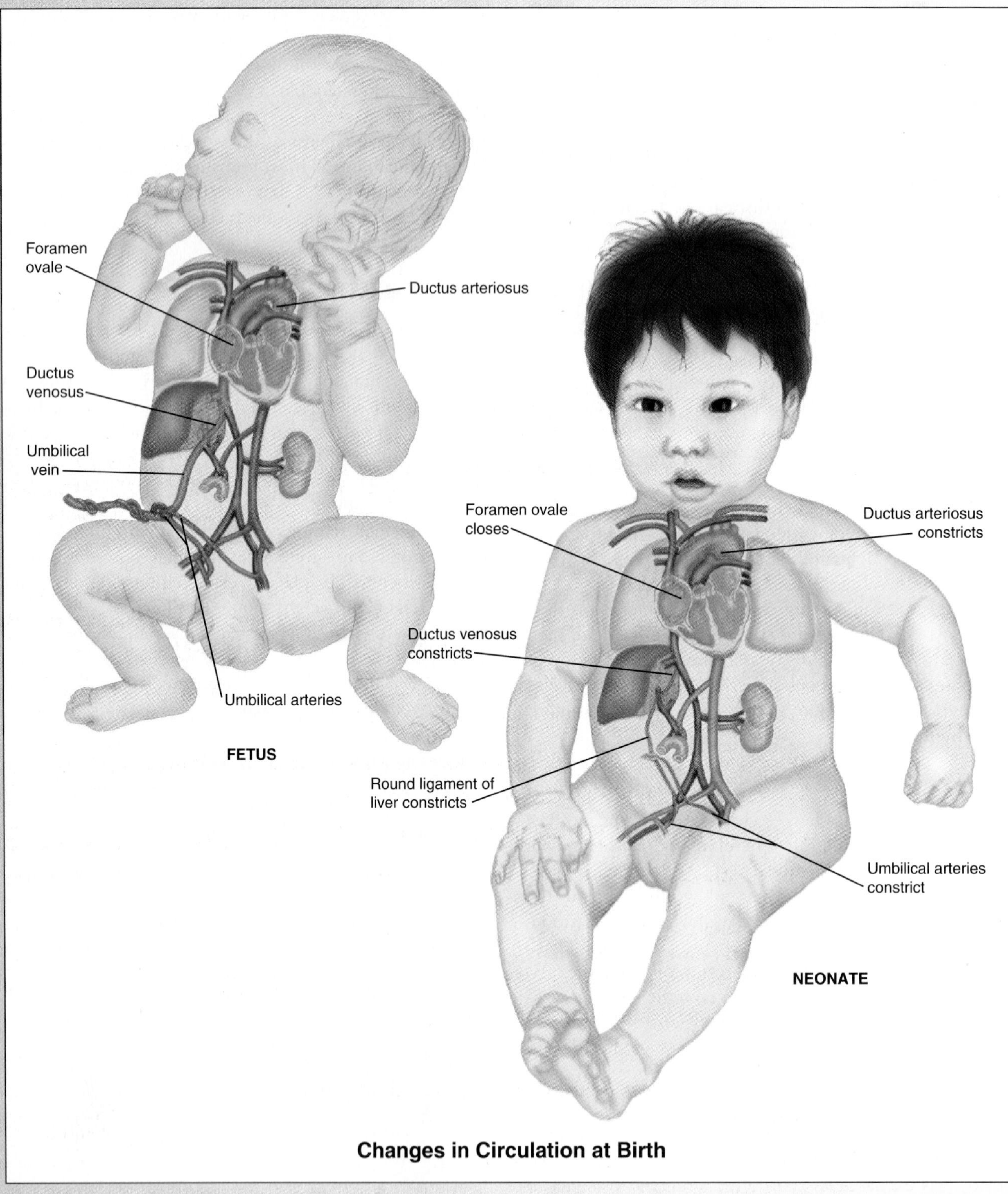

Changes in Circulation at Birth

COMMON DIAGNOSTIC TESTS FOR CARDIAC DISORDERS

TEST	DESCRIPTION	PREPARATION AND NURSING CONSIDERATIONS	COMMENTS
Cardiac auscultation	Placement of stethoscope over various areas of chest to detect normal and abnormal heart sounds	Best done when child is quiet Upper torso clothing should be removed and open front gown placed on older child	"Innocent murmurs" are not associated with congenital heart disease
Electrocardiography (ECG)	Recording of heart's electrical activity from outside surface of body; electrodes are placed in various positions, attached to lead wires; lead wires attached to a machine that records and prints electrical activity	Best done when child is quiet and cooperative Skin should be free of lotions and oils	Detects chamber enlargement and deviations in axis that may be caused by heart defects Determines heart rate and rhythm
Chest radiography (CXR)	X-ray picture of heart and associated organs/structures in chest cavity	No specific preparation Encourage parent/family member to accompany child to X-ray department	Can provide information about heart size and, in some cases, blood flow to lungs
Echocardiography	High-frequency sound waves (ultrasound) that generate an image of heart and associated structures; measures size of cardiac chambers, location and motion of valves, and size of septal defects	Must be done when child is quiet and cooperative If not cooperative, sedation may become necessary	Types of **echocardiograms:** M mode Two-dimensional Doppler Transesophageal Fetal
Magnetic resonance imaging (MRI)	Strong magnetic field surrounds patient; field promotes rotation of nuclei (that normally spin) at predictable speed, allowing visualization of soft tissue, tumors, shunts, myocardial thickness, structure, and valve function	Patient teaching NPO at least 4 hr before procedure if requiring sedation	Patient must be able to lie still for 1 to 2 hr or will require sedation
Cardiac catheterization	Invasive procedure in which catheters are introduced into heart through veins and arteries: performed under fluoroscopy, allows blood samples to be taken from various areas of the heart for oxygen saturation measurements; angiography, involves dye (or contrast agent) injection through a catheter to record blood flow through heart	Patient teaching Sedation Monitoring NPO at least 6 hr before procedure	Assesses pressure readings and/or changes, and hemodynamic function before and after heart surgery Therapeutic interventions, such as balloon dilatation of valves, balloon/blade septostomy for shunt creation, and device closure of certain defects (Smith, 1986; Sondheimer, 1990; Hellenbrand & Mullins, 1989)

CARDIAC MEDICATIONS COMMONLY USED IN CHILDREN

MEDICATION	MECHANISM OF ACTION	DOSAGE	ADMINISTRATION	ADVERSE EFFECTS	NURSING CONSIDERATIONS
Digoxin (Lanoxin)	Increases cardiac contractility by making more calcium available to contractile proteins in heart Causes heart to pump blood more forcefully Decreases heart rate	*PO:* *Loading doses:* Premature infant: 20 μg/kg Term neonate: 30 μg/kg Infants (up to age 2 yr): 40–50 μg/kg Child (age 2 yr and older): 30–40 μg/kg First three doses (loading dose) given over 16–24 hr Maximum digitalizing dose: 1 mg *Maintenance dose:* Premature infant: $\frac{1}{5}-\frac{1}{3}$ loading dose daily Neonates, infants, children: $\frac{1}{5}-\frac{1}{3}$ daily 10 years or older: 125–500 μg/day	May be given IV or PO Elixir prepared to yield 50 μg/ml Therapeutic serum concentration is 0.5 ng/ml to 2.0 ng/ml	Nausea, vomiting, atrioventricular (AV) block, other cardiac arrhythmias, anorexia, vision disturbances, diarrhea, drowsiness	Measure apical pulse before giving. The practitioner will set limits for withholding the dose. Instruct parents to administer with dropper packaged with elixir Instruct parents that excessive vomiting can be a sign of too much digoxin in the blood Do not repeat dose if child vomits. Contact caregiver. Do not mix with formula or food. Give between feedings to decrease chance of spitting up. Encourage parents to administer the drug around the same time every day A potentially dangerous medication Use IV only when necessary
Furosemide (Lasix)	Diuretic that reduces preload by decreasing reabsorption of sodium and chloride in the loop of Henle Activates renal prostaglandins, leads to renal dilatation, and decreases systemic and pulmonary vascular resistance	*PO:* Dose: 1–2 mg/kg/day, up to maximum of 6 mg/kg/day *IV/IM:* Dose: 1–2 mg/kg; should not exceed 4 mg/min when administering.	May be given IV, IM, PO Oral liquid preparation yields 10 mg/ml	Volume depletion, electrolyte (Na^+, K^+, Cl, Ca^{2+}, and Mg^{2+}) depletion, muscle cramps, weakness, nausea, fatigue, diarrhea	Patient may require potassium supplement Encourage potassium-rich foods: citrus fruits, tomatoes, bananas, dates, apricots Refrigerate oral solution Encourage parents to alert school system that school-age child may need to urinate more frequently than other children while taking diuretic
Propranolol (Inderal)	Beta-blocking agent that reduces cardiac oxygen demands by blocking catecholamine-induced increases in heart rate, blood pressure, and force of myocardial contraction	*PO:* 2–4 mg/kg/day divided q 6 hr *IV:* Not used any longer because shorter acting IV beta-blocking agents now available	PO liquid preparation available: 20 mg/5 ml	Hypotension, bradycardia, decreased myocardial function, bronchospasm, fatigue, lethargy, depression, attention deficit disorder, hypoglycemia	Contraindicated in asthma because of bronchoconstriction effects Instruct parents that drug can affect school performance and to contact cardiologist if decreased performance for no other apparent reason

					Can cause hypoglycemia in presence of GI upset (vomiting) or NPO status Instruct parents to give medication at even intervals throughout waking hours Tablets can be chewed or crushed and sprinkled on a small amount of soft food (ice cream, pudding, applesauce) Instruct parents to call about episodes of dizziness, limpness, tiredness, or fainting (possible symptoms of hypotension)
Enalapril (Vasotec)	Afterload reducer that causes dilation of arterial and venous blood vessels Relaxes blood vessels to allow heart to pump blood into vessels more easily Similar to captopril, with longer half-life	*PO:* 0.08 mg/kg/dose q 12–24 hr	Can be given in oral liquid form, which must be used within $\frac{1}{2}$ hour IV form available	Hypotension, cough, rare neutropenia	Instruct patient/family members that patient should rise slowly to sitting or standing position to minimize drop in blood pressure Instruct patient/family to notify physician about light-headedness, dizziness, fainting while taking medication
Captopril (Capoten)	Afterload reducer that causes dilation of arterial and venous blood vessels Relaxes blood vessels to allow heart to pump blood into vessels more easily	*PO:* Neonate: 0.1–0.5 mg/kg/dose q 8–12 hr; maximum of 4 mg/kg/day Infant or older child: 0.1–2 mg/kg/dose q 6–12 hr; maximum of 6 mg/kg/day Adolescent: 6.25–12.5 mg/dose q 8–12 hr; maximum of 50–75 mg/day	PO only	Hypotension (especially in presence of volume depletion), neutropenia, proteinuria, cough, impaired taste, skin rashes	Hypotension common with initial dose Monitor blood pressure 30 min after administration, then every 15 min ×4, then hourly ×3; notify physician of 20% decrease from baseline blood pressure Administer 1 hr before or 2 hr after meals to increase absorption Can cause 15%–30% increase in serum digoxin concentrations; observe for adverse effects of digoxin while administering both agents

From Artman and Graham, 1987; Baker and Alyn, 1992; Delgizzi and Ueda, 1990; Opie, 1995, Skidmore, 1994.

LEFT-TO-RIGHT SHUNTS

An intracardiac **shunt** occurs when the blood flow is forced by a higher pressure to go through an opening that is not normally present. In the case of left-to-right shunts, blood is shunted to the right side of the heart because the left side is normally functioning under a higher pressure than the right side. This shunting allows oxygenated and unoxygenated blood to mix. This results in increased pulmonary blood flow because the abnormal communication or opening sends more blood to the right side of the heart (through the opening) than normal. The four common lesions that result in left-to-right shunts—atrial septal defect (ASD), ventricular septal defect (VSD), patent ductus arteriosus (PDA), and atrioventricular canal defect (AVC)—are described and illustrated in Table 30–1.

NURSING CARE OF THE CHILD WITH A LEFT-TO-RIGHT SHUNT

Assessment

The diagnosis of the child with a left-to-right shunt is not always readily apparent at birth (Moynihan & King, 1989). Many of these children will remain asymptomatic, others may exhibit the signs and symptoms of congestive heart failure (CHF). The older infant may exhibit failure to thrive. Because the diagnosis of a heart defect in the neonatal or infant period is shocking to the parents, a complete assessment of the family unit is important. This assessment should include documentation of their feelings about the diagnosis as well as their interactions with the child. The nursing diagnoses below are not inclusive of all children with left-to-right shunts. They may not all apply to each patient. The nursing diagnoses and subsequent plan of care must be individualized for each patient (Krenner & Hern, 1988; Carter, 1992; Wesorick, 1990; Doengos & Moorhouse, 1991).

Nursing Diagnoses

- Activity Intolerance related to altered cardiac output, as manifested by congestive heart failure
- Knowledge Deficit related to disease process, treatments/interventions, and home care
- Anxiety related to disease process, treatments/interventions, and home care
- Altered Family Processes related to child with heart defect
- Altered Growth and Development related to congenital heart defect
- Risk for Infection related to surgical repair
- Pain related to surgical repair
- Altered Health Maintenance related to long-term needs of child

Planning, Implementation, and Evaluation: The Child With a Left-to-Right Shunt

NURSING DIAGNOSIS
- Activity Intolerance related to altered cardiac output, as manifested by congestive heart failure

Expected Outcome:
- The child will remain free of the signs and symptoms of congestive heart failure.

Intervention	Rationale
1. Assess respiratory rate and rhythm, presence/absence of nasal flaring, use of accessory muscles, and crackles/rhonchi.	Infants with CHF will experience changes in their breathing patterns due to increased at-rest fluid retention in the lungs, liver, and other areas of the body.
2. Assess for other signs of CHF, such as fluid retention noted in the area of the eyes, mouth, hands, feet, and chest, and diaphoresis at rest.	Fluid retention is usually noted in hands and feet because of decreased venous return. Diaphoresis is the body's way of trying to get rid of excess fluid.
3. Assess urine output (1–2 ml/kg/hr). Weigh diapers.	Due to fluid retention, children with CHF may urinate less, thus exhibiting decreased urine output.

Intervention	Rationale
4. Assess caloric intake.	Because the child must use so much energy to breathe, the appetite is decreased.
5. Plan nursing interventions to allow maximum rest for the child.	Organizing nursing activities decreases the child's stress and fatigue.

Evaluation:
- The child exhibits a decrease in the physiologic signs of activity intolerance related to congestive heart failure.

NURSING DIAGNOSIS
- Knowledge Deficit (parental) related to disease process, treatments/interventions, and home care

Expected Outcome:
- Parent will verbalize knowledge of disease process, treatments/interventions, and home care.

Intervention	Rationale
1. Assess parents' readiness to learn and need to know.	A baseline assessment of prior knowledge should be taken into consideration before developing any teaching plan. If parent is not ready, learning will not occur.
2. Provide brief, factual explanations of child's defect or any treatments/interventions, and do so frequently (Runton, 1988).	Simple, repetitive explanations are most likely to be retained by parents.
3. Provide parents with information regarding medications and care techniques that they will be responsible for at home. Do so as soon as these interventions/treatments are implemented.	Informed parents will better ensure continuity of care once the child is discharged. By getting an early start (i.e., when interventions are first initiated), parents have more time to learn.
4. Provide parents with written information when available (Clare, 1985; O'Brien & Boisvert, 1989).	This will provide an adjunct to individual teaching. Provides a reference to the caregiver at home. Written information can be referred to during less stressful times when it may be more likely to be retained.
5. Assess parents' understanding of instructions through return demonstration and repeating information.	Validates that learning has occurred and parent is competent to provide care.
6. Allow parents to ask questions and verbalize concerns and anxieties.	Promotes comfort level with techniques.
7. Assess need for and initiate appropriate referrals to support services, if required.	Provides adequate resources when needed.

Evaluation:
- Parent will verbalize adequate knowledge of disease process, treatments/interventions, and home care, including medications and any other care techniques.

TABLE 30–1 *Common Lesions Resulting in Left-to-Right Shunts*

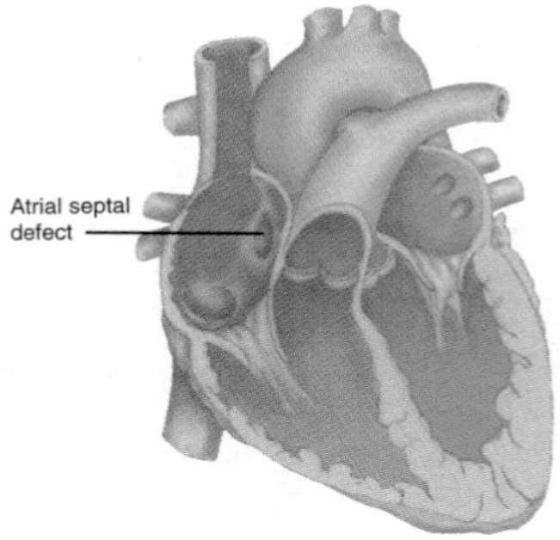

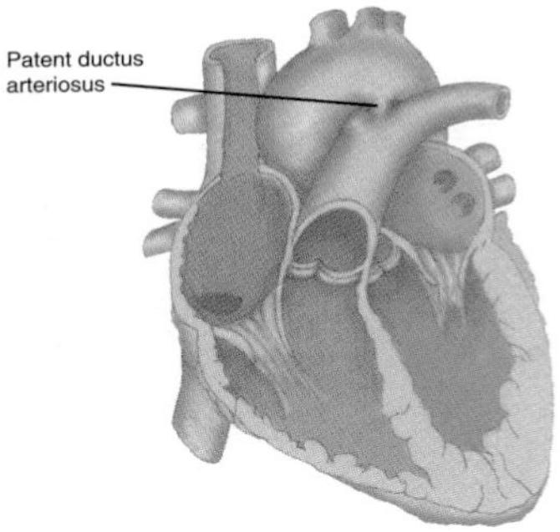

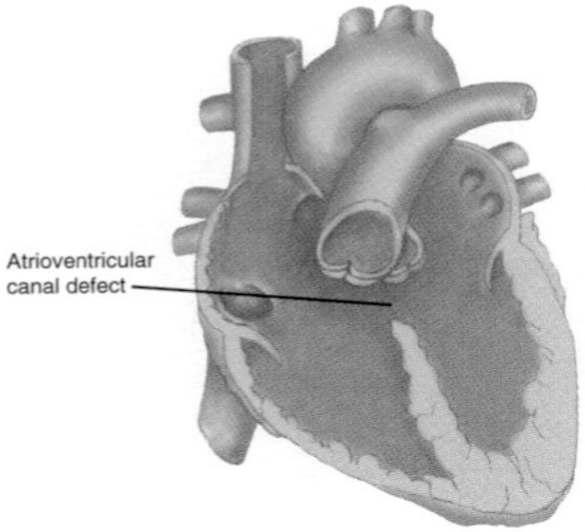

	ATRIAL SEPTAL DEFECT	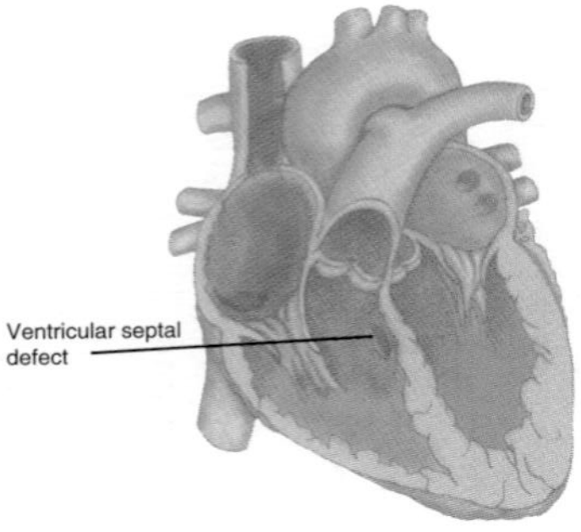 VENTRICULAR SEPTAL DEFECT	PATENT DUCTUS ARTERIOSUS	ATRIOVENTRICULAR CANAL DEFECT
	Atrial septal defect	Ventricular septal defect	Patent ductus arteriosus	Atrioventricular canal defect
Pathophysiology	An opening between the two atria, allowing oxygenated blood and unoxygenated blood to mix. Left-to-right shunting of blood due to the higher pressure on the left side of the heart.	An opening between the two ventricles, allowing oxygenated and unoxygenated blood to mix. Shunting of blood due to the higher pressure on the left side of the heart. VSDs are classified according to location in the septum, i.e., membranous or muscular.	An artery that connects the aorta and the pulmonary artery during fetal life. It generally closes spontaneously within a few hours to several days after birth. Allows abnormal blood flow from the high-pressure aorta to the low-pressure pulmonary artery, resulting in a left-to-right shunt.	Inappropriate fetal development of endocardial cushions. This may produce abnormalities in the atrial septum, ventricular septum, and the atrioventricular valves. A wide variety of defects including an ostium primum ASD, VSD, or atrioventricular valve anomalies. These lesions allow oxygenated and unoxygenated blood to mix, resulting in increased pulmonary blood flow. There are several classifications of atrioventricular canal defects.
Incidence	ASDs account for 12% of all congenital cardiac defects and are more common in females than males (2:1) (Feldt et al., 1989).	VSDs account for approximately one third of all cases of congenital heart disease. Most common cardiac defect; often associated with other lesions, such as pulmonary stenosis and transposition of the great arteries.	PDA accounts for 12% of all congenital cardiac defects; this incidence increases in premature and very low–birth-weight neonates.	Five percent of all congenital heart defects; most common defect in children with Down syndrome.

Clinical Manifestations	Growth retardation Diaphoresis Poor eating Mild fatigue (older child) Dyspnea (older child) Many patients are asymptomatic.	Growth retardation Failure to thrive Diaphoresis Poor eating Tachypnea CHF (see Chapter 31) Some patients are asymptomatic.	CHF Apnea (in premature infants) Tachypnea Retractions Nasal flaring Hypoxemia Bounding peripheral pulses (large PDA) Widened pulse pressure (large PDA) Many patients are asymptomatic.	Clinical manifestations depend on the type of defect. A child with a complete atrioventricular canal defect will show: Exertional cyanosis (especially when crying or feeding) Moderate to severe CHF in infancy.
Complications	CHF and arrhythmias may develop in late adulthood. Changes in pulmonary vasculature occur in early to middle adulthood if defect is not repaired.	CHF and failure to thrive could be the presenting symptoms. Untreated VSD may result in pulmonary hypertension in later years. Surgical complications include residual VSD, conduction system abnormalities, and aortic or tricuspid insufficiency.	CHF, endocarditis. Pulmonary vascular obstructive disease in later life.	Mitral valve regurgitation, heart block, arryhythmias, CHF, and pulmonary hypertension.
Management	Surgical closure at age 4–5 years. All defects are closed in females due to the possibility of clot formation during the child-bearing years. Small ASDs are left open in males, but moderate to large ones are repaired. Open-heart surgery is used, although transcatheter closures have shown much promise.	Some may close spontaneously; if spontaneous closure does not occur, moderate or large defects require surgical closure before school age. If pulmonary hypertension is present, closure necessary by age 1 year. Open-heart surgery is used for closure.	Some produce no symptoms and close spontaneously. Measures to reduce symptomatology of CHF must be undertaken. Can be closed nonsurgically (Callow, 1994) or surgically. Surgical closure done via left thoracotomy and without cardiopulmonary bypass. Indomethacin is sometimes used to promote ductal closure in premature infants.	Surgical patch closure of septal defects, possible mitral valve replacement (severe defect), and recontruction of AV valve tissue.
Prognosis	Mortality after surgery is very low. Complications, which are usually transient, include atrial tachyarrhythmias, sinus node dysfunction, and CHF.	Mortality after surgery is as high as 5% with single defect. Mortality increases in presence of CHF, pulmonary hypertension, and other defects.	Mortality after closure is less than 1%.	Mortality rate of surgery is approximately 10%.

NURSING DIAGNOSIS • Anxiety related to disease process, treatments/interventions, and home care

Expected Outcome: • The parents will experience a reduction in anxiety, as evidenced by verbalization of fears and concerns, participation in their child's care, and knowledge of the child's heart disease.

Intervention	Rationale
1. Describe the nature of the child's disease and symptoms at parents' level of understanding.	Basic explanation will assist parents in understanding why various treatments and interventions are necessary.
2. Explain to parents and child treatments/interventions that may be performed, including what the child will experience and the associated care.	Prior knowledge of events and occurrences can ease anxiety on both the child and parents' part.
3. Allow parents/child to verbalize feelings and concerns related to hospitalization.	Hospitalization is a frightening experience. By allowing verbalization of feelings and concerns related to the experience, nurses can provide assistance in allaying fears and addressing concerns.
4. Allow parents to spend as much time as possible with child while hospitalized, and let them know it's okay to leave the child for periods of rest, shower, etc.	This allows the parent to "parent" and provide support for the child. Giving reassurance that it's okay to leave will promote parental self-care.
5. Encourage participation in child's care.	Eases the sense of loss of control.
6. Assess parents for signs of increased anxiety (i.e., insomnia, facial tension, fatigue).	Parents may need assistance in identifying their anxiety and in developing methods to relieve stress.
7. Provide ancillary services as required (i.e., chaplaincy, social services, financial counseling).	Other services may be needed, such as spiritual support, transportation, and financial assistance.

Evaluation: • Parental anxiety is reduced, as evidenced by their ability to assume normal care, ask appropriate questions about their child's care, and be active participants in decisions regarding their child's care.

NURSING DIAGNOSIS • Altered Family Processes related to heart defect

Expected Outcome: • Parents will verbalize understanding of child's illness and will express feelings about changes brought about by the disease process in an appropriate manner.

Intervention	Rationale
1. Assess child/family for causative/contributory factors of altered family process.	A baseline assessment must occur before developing the plan of care.
2. Support and emphasize strengths of family.	Helps family not to focus on weaknesses.
3. Provide both verbal and written information to family as needed.	Allows review at a later time when things are less stressful.

Intervention	Rationale
4. Provide feedback and praise for compliance with treatment regimen.	Promotes compliance and lets them know they are doing a good job.
5. Assist family in dealing with situational crises by:	
a. suggesting items to be brought from home to help child cope	To make the environment more "comfortable"
b. ascertaining need for financial support of family	To promote wellness among the family
c. referring to support groups/clergy/counseling, if necessary	To help with change in parental role and change in family dynamics, and to receive support from others
d. encouraging parents to leave child for short periods to be with other family members.	To promote wellness among the family

Evaluation: • The parents will express positive feelings for their child and will be able to assume normal care. They will indicate a level of comfort with the defect and seek support as needed.

NURSING DIAGNOSIS • Altered Growth and Development related to congestive heart failure secondary to congenital heart defect

Expected Outcome: • The child will perform motor, social, and/or expressive skills typical of age-group within scope of present capabilities; and perform self-care and self-control activities appropriate for age. The parents will verbalize understanding of developmental delay/deviation and plan(s) for intervention.

Intervention	Rationale
1. Assess causative/contributing factors, such as existing condition that may be contributory, nature of parenting activities, and significant stressful events.	Limited intellectual capacity, physical handicaps, and chronic illness can hinder growth and development. Lack of stimulation and inadequate caretaking, as well as other stressful life events, may be contributing factors.
2. Assess degrees of deviation from developmental norms by identifying developmental age/stage, reviewing expected skills/activities, and noting individual deviations.	Chronological age and developmental age are not always the same. Begin assessment at chronological age and adapt assessment accordingly. All interventions must be individual and specific to this assessment.
3. Assist child/parents to prevent, minimize, or overcome developmental delays or regression by encouraging parental recognition of deviations and objectively discussing contributing factors.	Parents may not always be aware of developmental delays and may need assistance in identifying them. It is best to avoid blame when discussing contributing factors.
4. Plot height and weight on growth chart.	To assess patient's status in relation to growth curve (i.e., to assess for growth retardation).

Evaluation: • The child performs age-appropriate skills and engages in self-care. The parents verbalize understanding of developmental delays/deviations and can identify plan(s) for intervention.

NURSING DIAGNOSIS • Risk for Infection related to surgical repair

Expected Outcome: • The child will remain free of signs of infection, as evidenced by body temperature of <100.5°F, wounds without exudate, and white blood cell (WBC) count within normal limits.

Intervention	Rationale
1. Monitor temperature as ordered (every 1 to 4 hours) and notify physician about fever.	Fever is often the first sign of infection.
2. Monitor for fever, chills, diaphoresis, lethargy, and/or altered level of consciousness.	These are common signs and symptoms of sepsis.
3. Monitor and maintain awareness of how long lines/tubes/catheters have been in place; remove promptly when no longer needed.	The longer the lines/tubes/catheters are in place, the more the patient is at risk for infection. Discontinuing nonnecessary lines/tubes/catheters allows one less avenue for infection.
4. Maintain aseptic technique when changing dressings and handling IV equipment.	To prevent nosocomial infections.
5. Administer antibiotics as prescribed, ensuring correct dosage, route of administration, and patient's response (i.e., adverse effects).	Antibiotics are given prophylactically in most patients undergoing repair of congenital heart disease.
6. Administer antipyretics as ordered, ensuring correct dosage, route of administration, and patient's response (i.e., effectiveness).	To decrease elevated temperature.

Evaluation: • Child maintains body temperature <100.5°F. The wound and other associated sites are dry and intact and free of drainage, and the WBC count is within normal limits.

NURSING DIAGNOSIS • Pain related to surgical repair

Expected Outcome: • The child will be free of discomfort, as evidenced by normal affect/disposition, appropriate vital signs for age and baseline, and restful sleep.

Intervention	Rationale
1. Assess child for signs of discomfort: irritability; changes in heart rate, respiratory rate, and blood pressure; short, shallow respirations; and inability to sleep.	Children exhibit their discomfort by irritability, fast breathing, tachycardia, and inability to sleep.
2. Administer pain medication as ordered, ensuring correct dosage, route of administration, and patient response (effectiveness).	Pain relief is important in the postoperative patient in order to promote ambulation, coughing, and deep breathing.
3. If pain medication is ineffective, notify physician to discuss inadequacy of present regimen.	The nurse is the patient's advocate, and the dosage and/or type of pain medication may be inadequate for individual patient.

Intervention	Rationale
4. Encourage rest periods, incision splinting, and pain medication before the pain becomes unbearable.	To prevent fatigue, which increases pain intensity. Splinting will lessen sternal pain during coughing. Requesting pain medications early prevents unnecessary escalation of pain.
5. Facilitate parent–child contact as soon as possible after procedures or painful interventions.	To promote comfort and safety for the child.

Evaluation: • The child will be free of pain, or pain will be minimized, as evidenced by vital signs within normal limits for age and baseline, restful sleep, and normal affect.

NURSING DIAGNOSIS • Altered Health Maintenance related to long-term needs of child

Expected Outcome: • Parents state need for continued follow-up care to evaluate status and long-term complications.

Intervention	Rationale
1. Teach parents how to administer all necessary cardiac medications and their associated actions and potential adverse effects.	Family members should be taught how to administer all cardiac medications well before discharge. This allows for questions and answers and evaluation of their home care techniques.
2. Reinforce dietary changes/instructions, if applicable.	Patient may be on a reduced salt diet to prevent edema.
3. Discuss cardiac risk factors and importance of exercise, discipline, and so on.	Heart-healthy living is important in all patients, especially those with already compromised function.
4. Teach patient/parents about subacute bacterial endocarditis (SBE) prophylaxis, and provide information card.	Bacterial endocarditis is costly, painful, and occasionally deadly. It can be prevented in most cases with antibiotic prophylaxis (see Recommendations for Bacterial Endocarditis Prophylaxis box).
5. Assess need for outside assistance (financial, emotional, psychological).	Consistency of care can be maintained by initiating community assistance at the time of discharge.
6. Encourage questions and solicit verbalization of all instructions and return demonstration (if applicable) of all home care needs.	To evaluate teaching and to allow any discrepancies to be corrected before discharge.
7. Ensure that patient/family has appropriate follow-up appointment.	Accurate and timely follow-up is pivotal in children with heart disease.
8. Encourge good dental hygiene and care.	Poor dental hygiene can lead to the development of endocarditis.
9. Provide written material when available (i.e., American Heart Association booklet entitled "If your child has a congenital heart defect"). (See Teaching Guidelines box.)	Written information can be referred to during less stressful times, thus increasing retention and understanding.

Evaluation: • The child/parents will state the need for follow-up care to monitor status and avoid long-term complications of congenital heart disease.

TEACHING GUIDELINES *Home Care After Heart Surgery*

ACTIVITY

- Resume regular nap and sleep schedules and play activities (infants).
- Omit play outside for several weeks, allowing inside play as tolerated.
- Avoid activities where the child could fall (like riding tricycles, bicycles, swinging, or sliding) for 2 to 4 weeks after hospital discharge.
- Resume regular bedtime (children).
- Avoid large crowds of people for 1 week after discharge (including daycare and church).

DIET

- Resume regular formula/milk and baby foods (infant).
- Do not give any "new" foods until after the first checkup (infant).
- If baby eats table foods, follow a no-added-salt diet (infant).
- Follow a no-added-salt diet until checkup (children).
- Appetite should pick up at home.

INCISION

- Bathe infant/child with soap and water in the usual way. Do not use a bandage.
- No creams, lotions, or powders on incision until it is completely healed and without scabs.

SCHOOL

- Child may return to school the third week after hospital discharge.
- The child should go to school for half days for the first few days.
- No physical education until 2 months after the operation.

WHEN TO CALL THE DOCTOR

- Faster, harder breathing than normal when child is at rest
- New, frequent coughing
- Turning blue or bluer than normal
- Frequent vomiting or diarrhea
- Pain seems worse instead of better.
- Appetite worse than at time of discharge
- Any new swelling, redness, or drainage of the incision
- Fever >100.5°F

CHECKUP

- An appointment should be made for a 2-week follow-up at the time of discharge.
- Instructions should be given as to the date, time, and location of all follow-up appointments.
- The child will have a chest X-ray, electrocardiogram, and blood test at this visit.
- The checkup will take 2 hours.

DEVELOPMENT

If the child has recently learned how to do something at home before the operation (like drink from a cup, begin to walk, or use the toilet), this skill will probably have to be relearned when the child gets home. This is a common reaction. Young children do not understand the reasons for being in the hospital the way an adult does. The child will need extra love and attention from parents and family members at this time. After some time passes and the child goes home to familiar people and routines, he will become his old self again.

DISCIPLINE

Treat the child normally, the same as other children in the family. Children need to learn right from wrong, how to behave in different situations, and how to cope with everyday problems. If the child is doing something not approved of, he needs to be told. Crying will not hurt the child's heart. If the child does something good, use praise/rewards. Children need their parents' help to learn.

DENTAL CARE

The child should be checked by a dentist every 6 months after age 3 years. Always tell the dentist of the child's heart problem so antibiotics can be given before dental procedures if needed.

GENERAL INFORMATION

- Delay immunizations, circumcision, ear piercing, and dental work until 2 months after surgery.
- Nightmares are a normal reaction for children after hospitalization. Comfort and reassurance that all is back to normal will help. It is best for the child to remain in his own bed during this time.
- Visitors should be limited to two a day for less than half an hour. As the child's activity increases, the number and length of visits can be increased. All visitors should be well. No one with colds, sore throat, flu, or other infections should be allowed to visit.
- Antibiotics should be prescribed before invasive procedures such as ear piercing, dental work, etc.

Recommendations for Bacterial Endocarditis Prophylaxis

DEFECTS REQUIRING PROPHYLAXIS

- Prosthetic cardiac valves
- Previous SBE, even without heart disease
- Most congenital heart malformations
- Acquired valve abnormalities due to surgery, heart disease, or rheumatic fever
- Hypertrophic cardiomyopathy
- Mitral valve prolapse with regurgitation
- Persistent VSD despite surgery
- First 6 months after congenital heart disease repair

DEFECTS NOT REQUIRING PROPHYLAXIS

- Isolated ostium secundum ASD
- Beyond first 6 months after ASD, VSD, or PDA repair
- Mitral valve prolapse *without* regurgitation
- Normal/functional heart murmurs
- Previous Kawasaki disease *without* valvular dysfunction
- Previous rheumatic fever *without* valvular dysfunction
- Pacemakers and implanted defibrillators

PROCEDURES REQUIRING PROPHYLAXIS

- All dental procedures likely to induce gingival or mucosal bleeding, including professional teeth cleaning (not simple adjustment of orthodontic appliances or shedding of deciduous teeth)
- Tonsillectomy and/or adenoidectomy
- Surgical procedures or biopsy involving respiratory or intestinal mucosa
- Bronchoscopy with a rigid bronchoscope
- Incision and drainage of infected tissue
- Genitourinary and gastrointestinal procedures, including most diagnostic and therapeutic procedures that are invasive (sclerotherapy for esophageal varices, esophageal dilation, cystoscopy, urethral dilation, urethral catheterization or surgery if urinary tract infection is present, prostatic surgery, vaginal hysterectomy, and vaginal delivery in presence of infection)

Adapted from Dajani, A. S., et al. (1990). Prevention of bacterial endocarditis: Recommendations by the American Heart Association, *JAMA 264*(22), 2919–2922. Copyright 1990, American Medical Association.

RIGHT-TO-LEFT SHUNTS

Right-to-left shunts occur when blood is shunted to the left side of the heart because one of the right heart chambers has a higher pressure. In defects in which there is a right-to-left shunt, the child is cyanotic because oxygenated blood mixes with unoxygenated blood.

There are at least six congenital heart defects in which there is a right-to-left shunt. These defects—tetralogy of Fallot, transposition of the great arteries, truncus arteriosus, pulmonary **atresia,** tricuspid atresia, and hypoplastic left heart syndrome—are described and illustrated in Table 30–2.

NURSING CARE OF THE CHILD WITH A RIGHT-TO-LEFT SHUNT

Assessment

The child with a right-to-left shunt will be considerably sicker than the child with a left-to-right shunt. Many of these children will present with symptoms in the first week of life. The most common assessment finding in these children is cyanosis (Driscoll, 1990). The child may also become dyspneic after feeding, crying, and other exertional activities. Children with tetralogy of Fallot or with physiology similar to that seen with tetralogy of Fallot may experience hypercyanotic episodes, or "tet spells." These episodes are characterized by increased respiratory rate and depth of respiration and increased hypoxemia. The diagnosis of a heart defect in the neonatal or infant period is shocking to parents; a complete family assessment is important. All of the nursing diagnoses used for children with left-to-right shunts can be applied to the child with a right-to-left shunt. The nursing diagnoses and subsequent plan of care must be individualized for each patient.

Nursing Diagnoses

See nursing diagnoses listed under Nursing Care of the Child With a Left-to-Right Shunt.

Additional Defect-Specific Nursing Diagnoses

- Altered Tissue Perfusion related to hypercyanotic episodes
- Risk for Impaired Gas Exchange related to inadequate ventilatory support, pulmonary hypertension, atelectasis, and congestive heart failure
- Risk for Decreased Cardiac Output related to congestive heart failure

Text continued on page 928

TABLE 30-2 *Common Lesions Resulting in Right-to-Left Shunts*

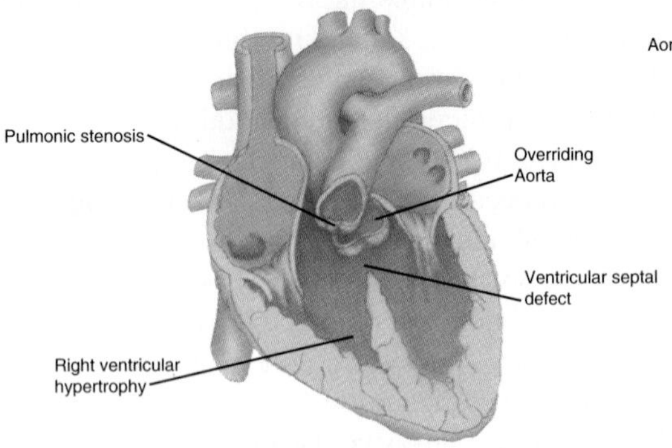

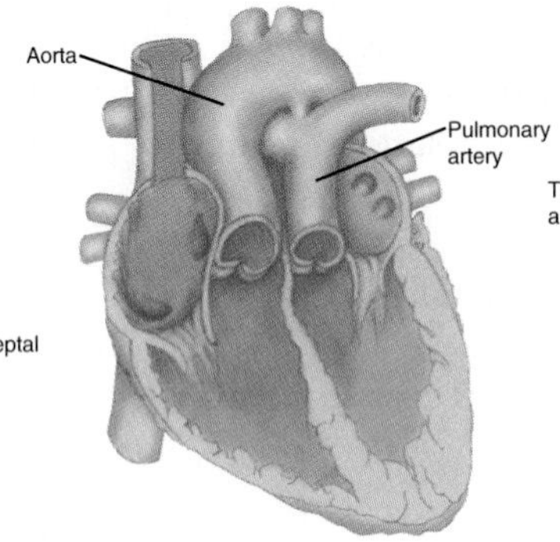

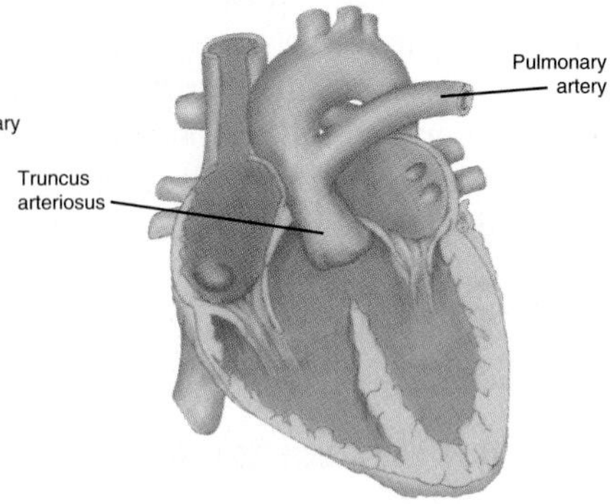

	TETRALOGY OF FALLOT	TRANSPOSITION OF THE GREAT ARTERIES	TRUNCUS ARTERIOSUS
Pathophysiology	Four cardiac anomalies make up tetralogy of Fallot: a ventricular septal defect, pulmonary stenosis, an overriding aorta, and right ventricular **hypertrophy.** There are other associated defects in certain cases. Pulmonary stenosis results in reduction of pulmonary blood flow; the VSD allows mixing of oxygenated and unoxygenated blood (Pinsky & Arciniegas, 1990).	The aorta and the pulmonary artery are reversed; i.e., the aorta rises from the right instead of the left ventricle, and the pulmonary artery arises from the left instead of the right ventricle. Systemic venous blood (unoxygenated blood) returns to the right side of the heart to pass through the aorta back to the body without being oxygenated because of bypassing the lungs. The pulmonary venous blood (oxygenated blood) enters the left side of the heart, returning to the lungs via the pulmonary artery. The systemic (unoxygenated) and pulmonary (oxygenated) circulations are totally separate. There must be some opening (i.e., PDA or septal defect) to allow blood to mix.	A single large vessel arises from the ventricles to give off the systemic, pulmonary, and coronary circulations. The pulmonary artery and aorta are one vessel that overrides both ventricles. There are 3 variations. Most commonly, blood is received from both ventricles, which mixes in the common great artery, causing desaturation. The ventricles have a common outflow tract, allowing systemic and pulmonary blood to mix.
Incidence	The classic form occurs in 9% of children with congenital heart disease.	Responsible for approximately 9% of all congenital heart disease and 10% of all children with cyanotic heart disease. (Van Praagh, 1991; Neches, Park, & Ettedgui, 1990).	Occurs in 2% of all congenital cardiac defects and is often associated with other congenital cardiac lesions (Mair et al., 1989).
Clinical Manifestations	Cyanosis Hypercyanotic episodes or "tet spells" Polycythemia CHF (see Chapter 31) Respiratory distress Clubbing of digits (in respiratory chapter) Squatting episodes Poor growth	Cyanosis Tachypnea Hypoxemia CHF	Cyanosis CHF moderate to severe Bounding pulses Widened pulse pressure Poor growth Activity intolerance

PULMONARY ATRESIA	TRICUSPID ATRESIA	HYPOPLASTIC LEFT HEART SYNDROME
Patent ductus arteriosus Atrial septal defect Pulmonary atresia Small right ventrical	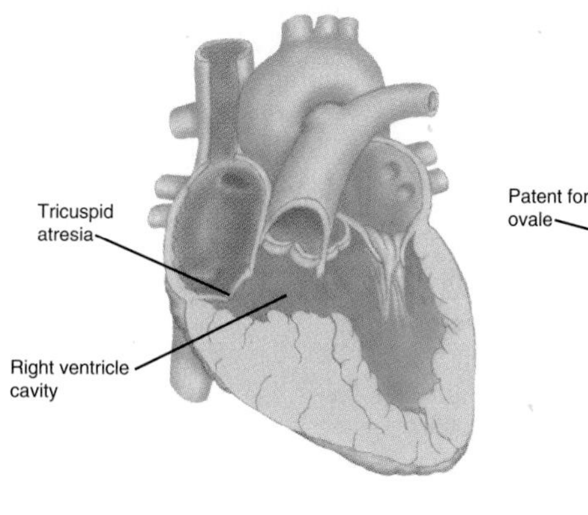 	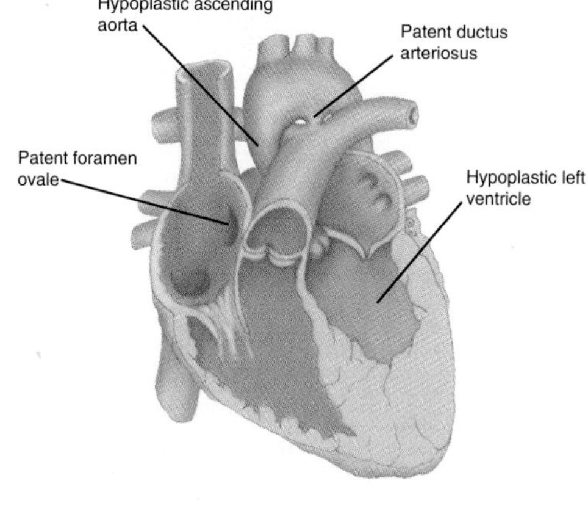
Absence of the pulmonary valve. If no VSD, called pulmonary atresia with intact ventricular septum. No blood flow from the right ventricle to the pulmonary artery. Blood travels to the left side of the heart through a patent foramen ovale. Mixing of systemic and pulmonary circulation occurs. The tricuspid valve cannot perform properly, resulting in right atrial dilation.	Absence of the tricuspid valve, allowing no blood flow between the right atrium and the right ventricle. It is the result of the complete lack of formation of the tricuspid valve during fetal cardiac development. There is no blood flow from the right atrium to the right ventricle and in most cases the right ventricle is underdeveloped and very small. The only way for blood to leave the right atrium is through some form of intra-atrial communication such as a patent foramen ovale or an ASD. There is a complete mixing of unoxygenated and oxygenated blood in the left side of the heart. This mixing results in systemic desaturation and varying amounts of pulmonary obstruction, leading to decreased pulmonary blood flow.	A defect in which there is essentially no left ventricle. There is valvular stenosis or atresia of the aortic and/or mitral valves, normal great vessels, and an intact ventricular septum. The extremely small to absent left ventricle and valvular stenosis or atresia results in inadequate systemic perfusion. There is major resistance to aortic flow. Without a PDA to allow blood flow from the pulmonary artery into the aorta and coronary circulation the neonate will die. This defect occurs due to underdevelopment of the left ventricle and affected valves during fetal cardiac development.
Accounts for 3% of all congenital cardiac defects.	Approximately 2% of all congenital heart defects.	Approximately 2% of all congenital heart defects.
Cyanosis Decreased peripheral pulses Periorbital edema Hepatomegaly Sudden death	Cyanosis (severe in some cases) Clubbing Polycythemia Hypercyanotic episodes Tachycardia Dyspnea	The following are seen after ductal closure: Cyanosis Pallor Decreased peripheral pulses Respiratory distress Pulmonary edema CHF

(continued)

TABLE 30–2 *Common Lesions Resulting in Right-to-Left Shunts (continued)*

	TETRALOGY OF FALLOT	TRANSPOSITION OF THE GREAT ARTERIES	TRUNCUS ARTERIOSUS
Complications	Palliative surgery complications include bleeding, respiratory complications, shunt occlusion, CHF, and paralysis of the diaphragm. Corrective surgery complications include CHF, low cardiac output, bleeding, arrhythmias, and neurologic sequelae. Long-term complications can include heart block, ventricular arrhythmias, severe right ventricular dysfunction, and/or sudden death, although these complications are less with improved surgical techniques.	Death, if not promptly diagnosed and treated. Corrective surgery is now usually performed in the first weeks of life (Koster & Schlosser, 1991; Jensen, 1992). Complications include coronary artery occlusion, stenosis of the switched arteries, and leakage of the new aortic valve.	Early, postoperative complications include low cardiac output, CHF, bleeding, arrhythmias, and neurologic sequelae. Late mortality rate is approximately 12%, usually associated with conduit failure/obstruction, persistent CHF, worsening pulmonary vascular disease, and reoperation (Mair et al., 1989).
Management	Includes medical management, palliation, and surgical corrections. Hypercyanotic episodes must be treated immediately. Prostaglandin E_1 may be required for ductal dependent lesions. A systemic-to-pulmonary shunt may be used palliatively. Corrections include VSD closure, pulmonary valvotomy, and enlargement of right ventricular outflow tract using a patch. Corrective surgery should be done by age 1 year to prevent long-term complications.	Mixing of the two separate circulations must occur. If a PDA is present, medications (i.e., Prostaglandin E_1) are given to keep it patent. The choice of surgical procedure must be made. Balloon atrial septostomy can be used for palliation. Surgical correction includes the arterial switch procedure which establishes normal circulation. This procedure is performed in the first few weeks of life. Other surgical procedures include the Senning procedure, and the Mustard procedure, which create an intra-atrial baffle to direct venous blood to the mitral valve and pulmonary venous blood to the tricuspid valve. The Rastelli procedure involves closure of the VSD with a baffle directing left ventricular blood through the VSD into the aorta.	Involves both medical and surgical therapy. Medical management involves treatment of CHF with various anticongestants and, occasionally, vasodilators. Surgical correction involves separation of pulmonary artery (arteries) from the trunk with patch closure of any aortic openings. The VSD is closed through the right ventricle, and a conduit (tube) is placed between the right ventricle and pulmonary arteries.
Prognosis	Surgical mortality is around 5%.	Postoperative mortality of arterial switch is 8%. Some patients will have sudden cardiac death (Castaneda et al., 1989; Kirklin et al., 1990).	Without surgical intervention, many of the children will die within 1 year. Surgical mortality is as high as 15%; late mortality is approximately 12%.

PULMONARY ATRESIA	TRICUSPID ATRESIA	HYPOPLASTIC LEFT HEART SYNDROME
The complications of shunting procedures include right ventricular dysfunction, chronic decreased cardiac output, and/or ventricular arrhythmias. For total repair, the postoperative complications include low cardiac output, prolonged ventilation, CHF, pleural effusion, chylothorax, bleeding, arrhythmias, neurologic sequelae, and in some cases, protein-losing enteropathy or death. Long-term complications include chronic low cardiac output, bradyarrhythmias and tachyarrhythmias, and sudden death.	Extreme cyanosis or pulmonary edema if associated with transposition of the great arteries; right heart failure if ASD is small. Postoperative complications include low cardiac output, prolonged ventilation, CHF, pleural effusion, chylothorax, bleeding, arrythmias, and neurologic sequelae (Callow, 1987; O'Brien, 1994).	Complications of staged surgical correction include bleeding, low cardiac output, CHF, arrythmias, effusions, and ventricular dysfunction. Complications of cardiac transplantation include rejection, infection, and long-term immunosuppression.
Prostaglandin E_1 is the initial management priority. Balloon atrial septostomy may improve oxygen saturations. A systemic-to-pulmonary shunt can be performed, but has a high (20%) mortality rate. Total repair via several different methods can be performed but may result in major postoperative and long-term complications (Foker et al., 1986).	The treatments and procedures are mostly palliative and problems can exist long after the child reaches adulthood (Sade & Fyfe, 1990). Palliative surgical procedures include a systemic-to-pulmonary shunt or pulmonary artery banding in the child with severe CHF or increased pulmonary blood flow. Corrective surgery may be the *hemi-Fontan* procedure in which the superior vena cava and the right pulmonary artery are joined. This is usually done in children with severe cyanotic heart disease who are too young for the Fontan procedure. The Fontan procedure may be performed partially depending on the child's hemodynamic response. This procedure results in the separation of systemic and pulmonary venous blood within the heart with systemic venous blood now diverted to the pulmonary circulation.	Options for neonates include no treatment, staged surgical correction, or cardiac transplantation (Johnson & Davis, 1991). These children should be maintained on prostaglandin E_1 until a decision regarding treatment is made. Stage 1, performed during the first weeks of life, is known as the *Norwood procedure.* It attempts to make the heart function similar to children born with single ventricles and truncus arteriosus. (The pulmonary artery is anastomosed to the aorta to create a new aorta, a shunt is created to provide pulmonary blood flow, and a large ASD is created.) The final stage is the *Fontan procedure.* Transplantation should be undertaken in a center that specializes in neonatal transplantation. Complications of staged correction include bleeding, low cardiac output, CHF arrhythmias, effusions, and ventricular dysfunction. Complications of cardiac transplantation include rejection, infection, and long-term immunosuppression.
Surgical palliation has a mortality rate as high as 20%.	The surgical mortality is as high as 20%. Postoperative complications include low cardiac output, prolonged ventilation, CHF, pleural effusion, arrhythmias, neurologic sequilae, and protein-losing enteropathy. Long-term complications depend on the repair and can include low cardiac output, arrhythmias, and tachyarrhythmias.	Staged surgical correction and cardiac transplantation are greater than 25%. Without intervention, death is imminent.

Planning, Implementation, and Evaluation: The Child With a Right-to-Left Shunt

NURSING DIAGNOSIS • Altered Tissue Perfusion related to hypercyanotic episodes

Expected Outcome: • The child will remain free of signs of decreased tissue perfusion, as evidenced by absence of profound cyanosis, normal activity level/affect for child, and normal respiratory status and oxygen saturation for child.

Intervention	Rationale
1. Keep child as stress-free as possible by anticipating and meeting the infant's feeding and comfort needs promptly.	Crying and/or agitation may precipitate hypercyanotic episodes.
2. Monitor for signs of hypercyanosis and notify physician if noted.	Severe hypercyanotic episodes can result in metabolic acidosis and can terminate in limpness, syncope, seizures, cerebrovascular accidents, and death.
3. Administer propranolol as ordered, ensuring correct dosage.	Propranolol, a beta blocker, is used for palliative treatment of hypercyanotic episodes. (See the medication table in the Clinical Reference Pages.)
4. Monitor glucose level every 4 to 6 hours if child is NPO and receiving propranolol. Notify physician if glucose level < 60 mg/dl.	Propranolol can cause hypoglycemia if given when patient is NPO or hypovolemic.
5. If hypercyanotic episode occurs, place child in knee-chest position and notify physician.	Knee-chest position is thought to increase pulmonary blood flow by increasing systemic vascular resistance and to improve systemic arterial oxygen saturation by decreasing venous return so that smaller amounts of highly saturated blood reach the heart. Toddlers and older children with unrepaired tetralogy of Fallot, may squat to obtain this position and relieve chronic hypoxia. However, most defects are corrected by this age.
6. Administer other therapies as ordered, such as oxygen and medication, ensuring correct dosage, route, and effectiveness.	Oxygen is used to improve oxygenation and prevent profound hypoxemia. Morphine may be used as a calming agent, and sodium bicarbonate may be used to correct metabolic acidosis.
7. Place child in safe environment (with parent).	Decreases stress and prevents further deterioration due to stress.
8. Instruct patient/family on the signs/symptoms of hypercyanotic episodes.	These episodes may occur at home, and parents need to be able to recognize them and have a plan of action should they occur.

Evaluation: • The child maintains adequate tissue perfusion, as evidenced by absence of profound cyanosis, normal activity level/affect for child, and normal respiratory status and oxygen saturation for child.

NURSING DIAGNOSIS • Risk for Impaired Gas Exchange related to inadequate ventilatory support, pulmonary hypertension, atelectasis, and congestive heart failure

Expected Outcome: • The child maintains adequate gas exchange, as evidenced by normal respiratory status and oxygen saturation for child.

Intervention	Rationale
1. Monitor respiratory status every 1 to 2 hours, assessing respiratory rate, breath sounds, chest expansion, use of accessory muscles, nasal flaring, and retractions. Notify physician of significant changes.	Early signs of inadequate gas exchange are exhibited by respiratory difficulty (i.e., an increase in breaths/minute, nasal flaring, retractions, and use of accessory muscles).
2. Assess/verify ventilator settings every shift and as needed with changes in the child's condition.	To ensure that settings are as ordered and that ventilator adjustments are made with changes in respiratory status.
3. Ensure endotracheal tube security.	To avoid inadvertent dislodgement of the tube.
4. Restrain hands of intubated children.	To avoid inadvertent dislodgement/removal of tube.
5. Verify endotracheal tube position by chest auscultation every 1 to 2 hours or by chest X-ray, as needed.	Proper ventilatory support is dependent on correct tube placement.
6. Suction endotracheal tube every 2 to 4 hours, as required.	To ensure patency and remove unwanted secretions.
7. Administer sedation/paralytics, as ordered, ensuring correct dosage and effectiveness.	Medications are often necessary with children receiving mechanical ventilation. Sedatives can ease pain and anxiety; paralytics will prevent movement.

Evaluation:

- The child maintains adequate gas exchange, as evidenced by normal respiratory status and oxygen saturation for child.

NURSING DIAGNOSIS

- Risk for Decreased Cardiac Output related to congestive heart failure

Expected Outcome:

- The child maintains adequate cardiac output, as evidenced by absence of sinus tachycardia and diaphoresis, warm extremities free of mottling, urine output > 1–2 ml/kg/hr, normal respiratory status and oxygen saturation for child, absence of jaundice, and nonpalpable liver.

Intervention	Rationale
1. Obtain vital sign parameters for each child and set monitor limits accordingly. Vital signs that may be "normal" for children without cardiac disease may not be "normal" for the child with cardiac disease.	Children with CHF will experience changes in their breathing patterns and other vital signs due to increased at-rest fluid retention. Baseline vital signs with appropriate monitoring parameters will assist in determining if patient status improves or deteriorates. Normals for these children may fall outside the range of expected normals.
2. Obtain vital signs every 1 to 4 hours, as ordered, and document. Notify physician if outside prescribed parameters.	Same as above.
3. Assess for signs and symptoms of increasing heart failure every 2 to 8 hours. Note any edema in extremities, trunk, head, and neck.	Congestive heart failure can progress fairly rapidly, so subtle changes are important. Because of decreased venous return, fluid pools in the lower extremities.

Intervention	Rationale
4. Obtain body weight every 12 to 24 hours using same scale at approximately same time of day, and alert physician if excessive weight gain (>50 g/day in infants, >200 g/day in children).	Fluid retention may not always be evident by visual inspection. Weight changes may indicate the body's inability to get rid of excess fluid. Weighing at approximately the same time of day ensures consistency.
5. Maintain accurate intake and output records. Notify physician if urine output is < 1 ml/kg/hr for 4 to 8 hours or if blood is present in urine. Obtain urine specific gravity once or twice a shift and document.	Children with CHF will not wet as many diapers or will urinate less due to fluid retention. An imbalance between the fluid intake and output is important because it gives clues as to how much fluid is being retained.
6. Administer diuretics/afterload reducers, as ordered, ensuring correct dosage and effectiveness.	Diuretics will help to get the fluid out of the body. The response to diuretic administration is very important.
7. Assess respiratory effort every 2 to 4 hours. Notify physician if retracting, flaring, or grunting is a new finding or has increased in severity.	Noting subtle changes in respiratory status may assist in preventing severe CHF. The earlier the assessment findings are noted, the earlier interventions can be implemented.
8. Auscultate breath sounds every 2 to 4 hours. Notify physician if breath sounds decrease or crackles are present.	Pulmonary edema can develop very rapidly and, in fragile infants, can be manifested by decreased breath sounds rather than crackles; crackles indicate fluid in the alveoli.
9. If respiratory effort is increased, place child in reverse Trendelenburg position (elevate head and upper body) to facilitate respiratory effort and decrease work of breathing.	Elevation of the head and upper trunk promotes fluid shifting from the lungs. The less fluid in the lungs, the less respiratory effort is required.
10. Administer humidified O_2, as ordered and during times of exertion and stress, ensuring effectiveness by oxygen saturation measurements.	An increase in the oxygen level in the blood helps to decrease the body's requirements for cardiac output.
11. Palpate liver every 4 to 12 hours. If palpable, document how many centimeters below right costal margin. Notify physician of any new developments.	An increase in liver size is an indication of right-sided heart failure. This size increase makes the liver more palpable below the rib cage.

Evaluation:

- The child maintains adequate cardiac output, as evidenced by absence of sinus tachycardia and diaphoresis, warm extremities free of mottling, urine output > 1–2 ml/kg/hr, normal respiratory status and oxygen saturation for child, absence of jaundice, and nonpalpable liver.

STENOTIC LESIONS

Stenosis is the narrowing or constriction of an opening. Stenosis can occur in a valve or a vessel. The narrowing or constriction results in obstruction of blood flow through this area. The stenotic lesions discussed and illustrated in Table 30–3 are pulmonary stenosis, aortic stenosis, and coarctation of the aorta.

NURSING CARE OF THE CHILD WITH A STENOTIC LESION

Assessment

The child with a stenotic lesion will have varying symptoms, depending on the type and degree of the stenotic lesion. Most of them will have **murmurs** when first seen in the health care setting. Some of these children will remain asymptomatic whereas others may exhibit the signs and symptoms of CHF. Newborns may exhibit tachycardia, tachypnea, dyspnea, pallor, and decreased peripheral pulses. There may be a recent history of vomiting and decreased urine output. Infants with critical valvular aortic stenosis, a life-threatening condition, may exhibit severe CHF, poor peripheral perfusion, **cardiomegaly,** and progressive metabolic acidosis. Older children may exhibit shortness of breath, chest pain, exertional dyspnea, and/or syncope. The nursing assessment should include an overall systems assessment with a focus on the hemodynamic effects of left ventricular outflow tract obstruction. The nursing diagnoses and subsequent plan of care must be individualized for each patient with the assessment findings taken into consideration.

Nursing Diagnoses

See nursing diagnoses listed under Nursing Care of the Child With a Left-to-Right Shunt.

Additional Defect-Specific Nursing Diagnoses

- Altered Tissue Perfusion related to ventricular overload
- Decreased Cardiac Output related to ventricular overload
- Fluid Volume Excess related to left and right ventricular overload and ineffective pumping

Planning, Implementation, and Evaluation: The Child With a Stenotic Lesion

NURSING DIAGNOSIS

- Altered Tissue Perfusion related to ventricular overload
- Decreased Cardiac Output related to ventricular overload

Expected Outcome:

- The infant will maintain adequate tissue perfusion and optimal cardiac output as evidenced by absence of profound cyanosis and limb mottling, normal respiratory status and oxygen saturation for the child, and stable pressure gradient between upper and lower extremity blood pressures.

Intervention	Rationale
1. Assess peripheral perfusion by palpating peripheral pulses, noting any color changes and capillary refill.	Poor peripheral perfusion is usually noted by decreased or absent pulses or blood pressure in the extremities; also, there may be color changes, (i.e., cyanosis, coolness, and mottling) of all extremities. Prolonged capillary refill is an additional sign of poor perfusion.
2. Measure blood pressure in all four extremities.	Depending on the location and degree of stenosis, blood pressure measurements may be different. For example, in a child with coarctation of the aorta, the upper extremities have a higher blood pressure than the lower extremities due to decreased blood flow as a result of the stenosis.
3. Administer oxygen and cardiac medication as ordered, ensuring correct dosage, route, and effectiveness.	Oxygen is used to improve oxygenation and prevent profound hypoxemia. Diuretics are used to relieve congestion.

Evaluation:

- The infant maintains adequate tissue perfusion and optimal cardiac output, as evidenced by absence of profound cyanosis and limb mottling, normal respiratory status and oxygen saturation for child, and stable pressure gradient between upper and lower extremity blood pressures.

TABLE 30–3 *Common Stenotic Lesions*

	PULMONARY STENOSIS	AORTIC STENOSIS	COARCTATION OF THE AORTA
	Stenotic pulmonic valve	Stenotic aortic valve	Coarctation of the aorta
Pathophysiology	The pulmonary valve leaflets are thickened and fused, causing obstruction of blood flow from the right ventricle to the entrance of the pulmonary artery. Pulmonary blood flow is decreased. The narrowing reduces the valve radius, causing increased resistance to blood flow through the valve. This, in turn, causes the right ventricle to pump at a higher pressure, resulting in hypertrophy (enlargement). There are varying degrees and varying severities.	A narrowing of the aortic valve, where blood leaves the left ventricle to enter the aorta and systemic circulation; occurs when valve leaflets, left ventricular outflow tract, or aorta are abnormally formed, resulting in three different forms of aortic stenosis. This obstruction causes the left ventricle to pump at a greater pressure; the resistance to blood flow in the left ventricle can result in decreased cardiac output, left ventricular hypertrophy, and pulmonary vascular congestion.	A narrowing in the aortic arch. In most cases, the narrowing is located distal to the left subclavian artery. The narrowing causes increased resistance to blood flow from the proximal to distal aorta, resulting in *increased pressure in proximal area* and *decreased pressure in distal area* (Gersony, 1989).
Incidence	Accounts for 9% of all congenital cardiac defects, and is commonly associated with other cardiac malformations.	Occurs in approximately 8% of patients with congenital heart disease and is commonly associated with other defects. In females with the disease, it is likely to result in offspring with the same defect.	Accounts for 12% of congenital heart disease, and is frequently associated with other cardiac defects.
Clinical Manifestations	Cyanosis CHF (see Chapter 31) Syncope Many children are asymptomatic.	Dyspnea Exercise intolerance Fatigability CHF Angina (chest pain) Syncope Decreased cardiac output Hypotension Tachycardia Poor feeding Some patients are asymptomatic.	CHF (in presence of VSD) Unequal intensity of pulses in upper and lower extremities Dyspnea Exercise intolerance Claudication in upper extremities in older children previously asymptomatic Some children are asymptomatic. The signs and symptoms depend on degree of narrowing and presence/absence of associated defects.

TABLE 30-3 *Common Stenotic Lesions (continued)*

	PULMONARY STENOSIS	AORTIC STENOSIS	COARCTATION OF THE AORTA
Complications	Postprocedural (i.e., balloon dilation and surgery) complications include valve incompetency, decreased cardiac output, CHF, and restenosis.	Aortic insufficiency is a major complication of catheter or surgical intervention (Ohler, Feagle & Lee, 1989). The surgical complications include CHF, decreased cardiac output, arrhythmias, and/or sudden death. The complications of valve replacement include insufficiency, infection, clot formation, and death.	Surgical complications include CHF, bleeding, hypertension, and paralysis. Restenosis is common. In older children: Dizziness Headaches Syncope
Management	Balloon angioplasty and/or surgical valvotomy (Brock procedure). Balloon angioplasts done in the cardiac catheterization lab dialate the valve.	Nonsurgical treatment: balloon angioplasty to dilate valve. Surgical treatment: commissurotomy to open the valve. Valve replacement may be required later for restenosis.	Aggressive CHF management. Best if repaired by age 2 years. Surgery involves removal of stenotic area with reanastomosis (reattachment) of the two ends or enlargement of the constricted area using a graft. Depends on severity.
Prognosis	Less than 2% mortality for both balloon dilation and surgical valvotomy. May experience restenosis or valve incompetence during chronic phase. Pulmonary valvuloplasty (balloon dilation or stretching of the valve) has <1% mortality for symptomatic patients.	Surgical mortality ranges from less than 2% (subvalvular) to 10%–20% (valvotomy in the critically ill). About 10%–25% of patients will experience restenosis and require additional surgery later on.	Surgical mortality is less than 5%, but increases in infants with associated defects.

NURSING DIAGNOSIS

- Fluid Volume Excess related to left and right ventricular overload and ineffective pumping

Expected Outcome:

- Infant/child exhibits evidence of fluid loss (i.e., frequent urination, weight loss, adequate balance between intake and output).

Intervention	Rationale
1. Administer diuretics as prescribed, ensuring correct dosage, route, and effectiveness.	Diuretics will help body get rid of excess fluid. Effectiveness is evaluated by urine output, either by measuring amount of urine or by weighing diapers.
2. Maintain accurate intake and output.	The fluid intake and output should be about the same. If the intake grossly exceeds the output, the diuretics may not be effective and/or the patient may require fluid restriction.
3. Maintain fluid restriction, if ordered.	The restriction of fluid will help decrease pulmonary and liver edema.

Intervention	Rationale
4. Weigh daily at approximately the same time every day using the same scales, and notify physician of excessive weight gain (> 50 g/day infants; > 200 g/day children).	Excess fluid volume may not always be overtly visible. Weight changes may indicate fluid retention. Weighing the infant or child on the same scales at the same time each day ensures consistency.
5. Change position frequently to prevent skin breakdown associated with edema.	Edematous areas are extremely prone to skin breakdown due to stretching and opacity. Frequent position changes will prevent undesirable pooling of fluid in certain areas.
6. Provide skin care for children with edema.	Same as above.
7. Assess for evidence of increased or decreased edema.	Changes in the amount of edema can indicate the effectiveness or ineffectiveness of therapies, interventions, and nursing care.

Evaluation:
- The child maintains adequate fluid volume and fluid loss as evidenced by frequent urination, weight loss, and adequate balance between intake and output.

EBSTEIN'S ANOMALY

Ebstein's anomaly is a congenital anomaly of the tricuspid valve. It is a rare defect in which the tricuspid valve leaflets fail to develop normally during fetal cardiac development.

Clinical Manifestations. Clinical manifestations vary according to the severity of the defect. The more displaced (downward) the valve, the more tricuspid **regurgitation/stenosis** is noted. Many children are asymptomatic. In children with a large right to left shunt, cyanosis may be present in the first days of life. Signs and symptoms of CHF may be present.

Complications. **Arrhythmias,** cardiac enlargement, CHF, pulmonary stenosis, and tricuspid regurgitation are all potential complications of Ebstein's anomaly.

Therapeutic Management. Medical management requires treatment of CHF and management of tachyarrhythmias. Prostaglandin E_1 may be used in the neonate dependent on a patent ductus arteriosus. Prostaglandin E_1 causes vasodilation and smooth relaxation, which increases dilation and patency of the ductus arteriosus.

Surgical intervention can include systemic to pulmonary shunts, a variation of the Fontan procedure (see p. 927), and plication (shortening) of the atrialized portion of the right ventricle and tricuspid valve repair. If abnormal electrical circuits are present, catheter ablation (removal) should be undertaken before surgical repair to decrease pump time, optimize hemodynamics, thus decreasing the duration of the surgical procedure. Surgical treatment is generally only palliative. Children with Ebstein's anomaly may be referred for cardiac transplantation.

PATHOPHYSIOLOGY *of Ebstein's Anomaly*

The tricuspid valve is displaced downward into the right ventricle. The anterior cusp of the valve has some attachment to the valve ring, but the other leaflets are adherent to the wall of the right ventricle. The leaflets are dysplastic (abnormally developed), and the medial and posterior leaflets are displaced inferiorly, adhering to the right ventricular wall. The function of the tricuspid valve varies depending on the degree of displacement. Tricuspid insufficiency and/or stenosis may be present.

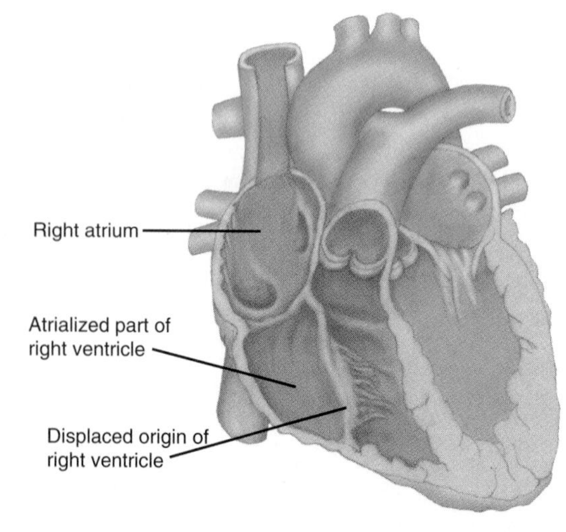

Prognosis. Prognosis is variable. It is usually poor if diagnosed at birth, but surgical palliation may improve neonatal prognosis. The prognosis is excellent if the child is asymptomatic until adolescence. The presence and degree of arrhythmias may determine the late prognosis.

NURSING CARE OF THE CHILD WITH EBSTEIN'S ANOMALY

Assessment

The child should be assessed for cyanosis. Any "spells" that could be attributed to a tachyarrhythmia should also be noted. Assessment for signs and symptoms of CHF failure as well as dehydration are ongoing.

> If large amounts of air enter the intravenous line, in children with intracardiac shunts, a stroke could ensue.

Nursing Diagnosis and Planning

The following nursing diagnoses and expected outcomes are examples that may be appropriate in the treatment of Ebstein's anomaly in the child.

- Decreased Cardiac Output related to congestive heart failure and/or tachyarrhythmias. ***Expected Outcome:*** *The child will remain free of signs and symptoms of congestive heart failure.*
- Altered Tissue Perfusion related to decreased oxygenation. ***Expected Outcome:*** *The child will be adequately perfused.*
- Knowledge Deficit related to disease process, treatments, interventions, home care, and prognosis. ***Expected Outcome:*** *The parents will indicate an understanding of the disease process and the care of their child.*
- Anxiety related to disease process, treatments, interventions, home care, and prognosis. ***Expected Outcome:*** *The parents will verbalize feelings concerning their child and will seek support as needed.*

Implementation and Evaluation

Refer to care plans in this chapter for nursing care related to the above diagnoses. It should be stressed to the parents that their child will be less tolerant of viral illness (with vomiting and diarrhea) than children without the defect. Refer to Chapter 31 for a discussion of the child with congestive heart failure.

KEY CONCEPTS

- With the neonate's first breath, gas exchange is transferred from the placenta to the lungs. The fetal shunts (ductus venosus, ductus arteriosus, foramen ovale) close and resistance to flow in the pulmonary system decreases as systemic resistance increases. Pulmonary vascular resistance decreases and a marked increase in pulmonary blood flow follows.
- Poor weight gain with failure to thrive are common signs of congenital cardiac disease (Norris & Hill, 1994).
- In left-to-right shunts, blood is shunted to the right side of the heart because the pressure is higher on the left side. Oxygenated and unoxygenated blood mixes.
- Common nursing diagnoses associated with infants with congenital heart defects, and their parents, include activity intolerance, knowledge deficit, anxiety, altered family processes, risk for infection, pain, and risk for altered health maintenance.
- In right-to-left shunts, the child is cyanotic because oxygenated blood mixes with unoxygenated blood. These children will be more ill than the child with a left-to-right shunt.
- Hypercyanotic episodes, or "tet spells," are characterized by increased respiratory rate and depth of respiration and increased hypoxemia.
- Stenosis can occur in a valve or a vessel and result in obstruction of blood flow through the area.
- Assessment of the family of a child with a congenital cardiac defect should begin at diagnosis and follow throughout the care of the child.

REFERENCES

Alyn, I. B., & Baker, L. K. (1992). Cardiovascular anatomy and physiology of the fetus, neonate, infant, child, and adolescent. *Journal of Cardiovascular Nursing, 6,* 1–11.

Artman, M., & Graham, T. P. (1987). Guidelines for vasodilator therapy of congestive heart failure in infants and children. *American Heart Journal, 113,* 994–1005.

Baker, L. K., & Alyn, I. B. (1992). Pharmacologic manipulation of preload, afterload, and contractility in the young. *Journal of Cardiovascular Nursing, 6,* 12–29.

Callow, L. (1987). Postoperative nursing care of the patient who has undergone the Fontan procedure. *Focus on Critical Care, 14,* 24–31.

Callow, L., (1994). Nursing implications of interventional device placement in pediatric cardiology and pediatric cardiac surgery. *Critical Care Nursing Clinics of North America, 6,* 133–151.

Carter, V. L. (1992). *Cardiovascular nursing care management at Medical University of South Carolina* (2nd ed.). Charleston, SC: Medical University Press.

Castaneda, A. R., Mayer, J. E., Jr., Jones, R. A., Wernovsky, G., & di Donato, R. (1989). Transposition of the great arteries: The arterial switch operation. *Cardiology Clinics, 7,* 369–376.

Clare, M. D. (1985). Home care of infants and children with cardiac disease. *Heart & Lung, 14,* 218–222.

Dajani, A. S., Bisno, A. L., Chung, K. J. et al. (1990). Prevention of bacterial endocarditis: Recommendations by the American Heart Association. *JAMA, 264,* 2919–2922.

Delgizzi, L. J., & Ueda, J. N. (1990). Using inotropic and vasodilating agents in pediatric patients with cardiac disease. AACN Clinical Issues. *Critical Care Nursing, 1,* 131–147.

Doenges, M. E., & Moorhouse, M. F. (1991). *Nurses pocket guide: Nursing diagnoses with interventions* (3rd ed.). Philadelphia: F. A. Davis.

Driscoll, D. J. (1990). Evaluation of the cyanotic newborn. *Pediatriate Clinics of North America, 37,* 1–23.

Feldt, R. H., Porter, C. J., Edwards, W. D., et al. (1989). Defects of the atrial septum and the atrioventricular canal. In F. H. Adams, G. C. Emmanouilides, & T. A. Riemenschneider (Eds.), *Moss' heart disease in infants, children, and adolescents* (4th ed., pp. 170–188). Baltimore: Williams & Wilkins.

Gersony, W. M. (1989a). Coarctation of the aorta. In F. H. Adams, G. C. Emmanouilides, & T. A. Riemenschneider (Eds.), *Moss' heart disease in infants, children, and adolescents.* (4th ed., pp. 243–255). Baltimore: Williams & Wilkins.

Hellenbrand, W. E., & Mullins, C. E. (1989). Catheter closure of congenital cardiac defects. *Cardiology Clinics, 7,* 351–368.

Hoffman, J. I. E. (1990). Congenital heart disease: Incidence and inheritance. *Pediatric Clinics of North America, 37,* 25–44.

Jensen, C. A. (1992). Nursing care of a child following an arterial switch procedure for transposition of the great arteries. *Critical Care Nurse, 12,* 51–57.

Johnson, A. B., & Davis, J. S. (1991). Treatment options for the neonate with hypoplastic left heart syndrome. *The Journal of Perinatology and Neonatal Nursing, 5,* 84–92.

Kirklin, J. W., Colvin, E. V., McConnell, M. E., et al. (1990). Complete transposition of the great arteries: Treatment in the current era. *Pediatric Clinics of North America, 37,* 171–177.

Koster, N. K., & Schlosser, P. (1991). Nursing management of the neonate undergoing the arterial switch operation. In C. Marvoudis & C. L. Backer (Eds.), *Cardiac surgery: The arterial switch operation.* State of the Art Reviews (5, pp. 177–190). Philadelphia: Hanley & Belfus.

Krenner, C., & Hern, M. J. (1988). Writing a nursing diagnosis for a complex client: The infant with a congenital heart defect. *Journal of Pediatric Nursing, 3,* 256–264.

Mair, D. D., et al. (1989). Truncus arteriosus. In G. H. Adams, G. C. Emmanouilides, & T. A. Riemenschneider (Eds.), *Moss' heart disease in infants, children, and adolescents* (4th ed., pp. 504–515). Baltimore: Williams & Wilkins.

Malinowski, P., & Yablonski, C. (1986). Congenital heart disease in infants: Nursing assessment. *Critical Care Nursing Quarterly, 9,* 6–23.

McNamara, D. G. (1990). Value and limitations auscultation in the management of congenital heart disease. *Pediatric Clinics of North America, 37,* 93–113.

Moynihan, P. J., & King, R. (1989). Caring for patients with lesions increasing pulmonary blood flow. *Critical Care Nursing Clinics of North America, 1,* 195–213.

Neches, W. H., Park, S. C., & Ettedgui, J. A. (1990). Transposition of the great arteries. In A. Garson, Jr, J. T. Bricker, & D. G. McNamara (Eds.), *The science and practice of pediatric cardiology* (pp. 1175–1212). Philadelphia: Lea & Febiger.

Norris, M. K. G., & Hill, C. S. (1994). Nutritional issues in infants and children with congenital heart disease. *Critical Care Nursing Clinics of North America, 6,* 153–163.

O'Brien, P., & Boisvert, J. T. (1989). Discharge planning for children with heart disease. *Critical Care Nursing Clinics of North America, 1,* 297–305.

O'Brien, P., & Smith, P. A. (1994). Chronic hypoxemia in children with cyanotic heart disease. *Critical Care Nursing Clinics of North America, 6,* 215–226.

Ohler, L., Feagle, D. J., & Lee, B. I. (1989). Aortic valvuloplasty: Medical and critical care nursing perspectives. *Focus on Critical Care, 16,* 275–287.

Opie, L. H. (1995). *Drugs for the heart* (4th ed.). Philadelphia: W. B. Saunders.

Park, M. K., Lee, D., & Johnson, G. A. (1993). Oscillometric blood pressures in the arm, thigh and calf in healthy children and those with aortic coarctation. *Pediatrics, 91,* 761–765.

Pinsky, W. W., & Arciniegas, E. (1990). Tetralogy of Fallot. *Pediatric Clinics of North America, 37,* 179–191.

Runton, N. (1988). Congenital cardiac anomalies: A reference guide for nurses. *Journal of Cardiovascular Nursing, 17,* 90–98.

Sade, R. M., & Fyfe, D. A. (1990). Tricuspid atresia: Current concepts in diagnosis and treatment. *Pediatric Clinics of North America, 37,* 151–169.

Skidmore, R. L. *Mosby's 1995 nursing drug reference.* St. Louis: C. V. Mosby.

Smith, P. A. (1986). Current diagnostic and therapeutic catheterization techniques. *Critical Care Nursing Quarterly, 9,* 24–39.

Sondheimer, H. M. (1990). Cardiac catheterization—a new role in the 90s. *Contemporary Pediatrics, 7,* 91–106.

Van Praagh, R. (1991). Transposition of the great arteries: History, pathologic anatomy, embryology, etiology, and surgical considerations. In C. Marvoudis & S. L. Backer (Eds.), *Cardiac surgery: The arterial switch operation.* State of the Art Reviews (5, pp. 7–82). Philadelphia: Hanley & Belfus.

Wesorick, B. (1990). *Standards of nursing care. A model for clinical practice.* Philadelphia: J. B. Lippincott.

BIBLIOGRAPHY

Beekman, R. H., Rocchini, A. P., & Rosenthal, A. (1989). Therapeutic cardiac catheterization for pulmonary valve and pulmonary artery stenosis. *Cardiology Clinics, 7,* 331–340.

Carey, B. E. (1982). Prostaglandin E_1 treatment for neonatal heart defects. *Dimensions of Critical Care Nursing, 1,* 275–283.

Foker, J. E., Braunlin, E. A., St. Cyr, J. A., et al. (1986). Management of pulmonary atresia with intact ventricular septum. *Journal of Thoracic and Cardiovascular Surgery, 92,* 706–715.

Gerraughty, A. B. (1989). Caring for patients with lesions obstructing systemic blood flow. *Critical Care Nursing Clinics of North America, 1,* 231–244.

Gersony, W. M. (1989b). Coarctation of the aorta and ventricular septal defect in infancy: Left ventricular volume and management issues. (Editorial comment). *Journal of the American College of Cardiology, 14,* 1553.

Givens, L., & Ricks, J. (1985). Assessment of clinical manifestations of cyanotic and a cyanotic heart disease and children. *Heart & Lung 14,* 200–204.

Kirklin, J. W., & Barratt-Boyes, B. G. (1986). *Cardiac surgery: Morphology, diagnostic criteria, natural history, techniques, results, and indications.* New York: John Wiley & Sons.

Lock, J. E., Cockerhan, J. T., Keane, J. F., et al. (1987). Transcatheter umbrella closure of congenital heart defects. *Circulation, 75,* 593–599.

Paul, M. H. (1989). Complete transposition of the great arteries. In F. H. Adams, G. C. Emmanouilides, & T. A. Riemenschneider (Eds.), *Moss' heart disease in infants, children, and adolescents* (4th ed., pp. 371–423). Baltimore: Williams & Wilkins.

Radtke, W., & Lock, J. (1990). Balloon dilation. *Pediatric Clinics of North America, 37,* 193–213.

Roberson, D. A., & Silverman, N. H. (1989). Ebstein's anomaly: Echocardiographic and clinical features in the fetus and neonate. *Journal of the American College of Cardiology, 14,* 1308–1311.

Warsaw, M. P., & Winn, C. W. (1988). Pulmonary valvuloplasty as an alternative to surgery in the pediatric patient: Implications for nursing. *Heart & Lung 17,* 521–527.

Whittemore, R., Hobbins, J. C., & Engle, M. A. (1982). Pregnancy and its outcome in women with and without surgical treatment of congenital heart disease. *American Journal of Cardiology, 50,* 641–651.

31

The Child With Cardiovascular Alterations

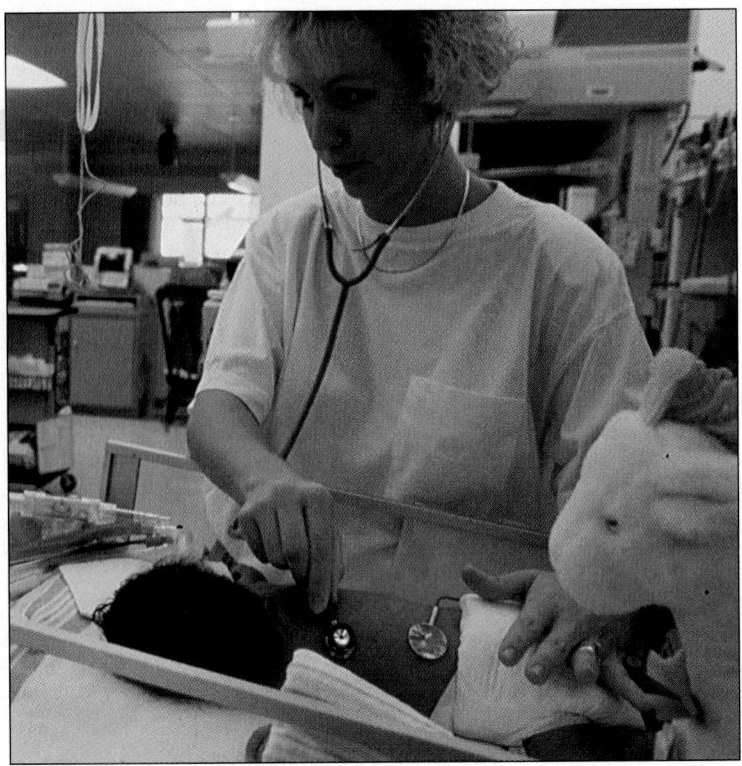

CHAPTER OVERVIEW

LEARNING OBJECTIVES

After studying this chapter, you should be able to:

- Describe the three types of shock in children, and the associated therapeutic management and nursing care appropriate for each.
- Identify nursing interventions that support the management of primary and secondary hypertension.
- Utilize appropriate screening tools and identify diagnostic aids in determining the etiology of hypertension.
- Differentiate symptoms of right-sided and left-sided heart failure.
- Identify nursing interventions that decrease workload on the myocardium in children with heart failure.
- Identify the nurse's role in discharge planning for the child with congestive heart failure and the family.

KEY TERMS

afterload: the amount of resistance against which the heart pumps

bradycardia: slow heart rate for age

cardiac output: the factor of the amount of blood pumped from the heart (stroke volume) and the heart rate

cardiomegaly: enlarged heart

central venous pressure: pressure measured in the right atrium; helpful in determining the amount of circulating blood volume

compensation: maintenance of an adequate blood flow without distressing symptoms, accomplished by cardiac and circulatory adjustments such as tachycardia, cardiac hypertrophy, and increased blood volume from sodium and water retention

decompensation: inability of the heart to maintain adequate circulation, marked by dyspnea, venous engorgement, cyanosis, and edema

ischemia: deficiency of blood supply to an organ

myocardial contractility: the property by which myocardial cells and tissues shorten in response to an appropriate stimulus; force of contraction of the myocardium

oxygen saturation: a measure of the degree to which oxygen is bound to hemoglobin

palpitations: sensation of rapid or irregular heart beat

preload: amount of stretch of the myocardial fibers before contraction; most easily measured by determining central venous pressure (CVP)

pulmonary edema: collection of excessive fluid in the alveoli of the lungs

pulmonary hypertension: increased pressure in the pulmonary arteries and arterioles

pulmonary vascular resistance: the amount of resistance in the pulmonary arteries against which the right heart must pump

pulmonary venous congestion: increased pulmonary pressure leading to the accumulation of excessive fluid and blood in the pulmonary veins

systemic vascular resistance: the amount of resistance in the systemic arteries against which the left heart must pump

systemic venous congestion: increased systemic venous pressure leading to the accumulation of excessive fluid in the systemic veins

tachycardia: increased heart rate compared to norms for age

tissue perfusion: the amount of blood flow distributed to an area

The most common cardiac problems in children result from congenital heart defects (see Chapter 30). This chapter focuses on other disease processes that affect the function of the heart and cardiovascular system; however, in some instances, the etiology may not be directly caused by dysfunction of the heart. For example, a child in septic shock secondary to bacteremia may have severe cardiovascular instability.

The nurse's role is very important in the astute and vigilant monitoring of a child with potential cardiovascular alterations. The degree of change in acuity and rapidity of decompensation are much greater in infants and children than in any other age group. Thus, the skill required of the pediatric nurse in assessing, monitoring, and delivering prompt treatment is an unparalleled nursing challenge.

Parents of children with cardiovascular disease may be anxious and overprotective of their children. Knowing this, the nurse has a responsibility to educate parents about their child's disease and to stress the importance of the child interacting with the environment as normally as possible. The disease must be put into the context of the family's life for effective planning and provision of care to be achieved.

CLINICAL REFERENCE PAGES

Refer to Chapter 30 for a review of the anatomy and physiology of the cardiovascular system and for diagnostic tests.

The medications used in the treatment of cardiac alterations in children include vasopressors, antihypertensives, and antiarrhythmics. Some of the most common of these medications are listed in the accompanying table.

MEDICATIONS COMMONLY USED FOR CARDIOVASCULAR DISORDERS

DRUG/DOSAGE	ACTION	NURSING IMPLICATIONS	SIDE EFFECTS
Potent Vasopressors			
Dopamine: 2–20 μg/kg/min IV drip	Increases blood pressure, cardiac output, heart rate, and renal and peripheral perfusion	Administer via central line. Monitor the patient closely for signs of infiltration or adverse side effects. The drug should not be infused with alkaline solutions.	Cardiac arrhythmias Vasoconstriction
Dobutamine: 2–10 μg/kg/min IV drip	Increases cardiac contractility; moderately increases heart rate	Same nursing implications as for dopamine.	Tachyarrhythmias
Epinephrine: 0.01 μg/kg IV push of 1:10,000 solution; 0.05–0.5 μg/kg/min IV drip	Increases blood pressure and heart rate; acts as vasoconstrictor and bronchodilator	Monitor the patient for signs of infiltration, as a chemical burn may result. Agent should not be infused with alkaline solutions. Monitor the patient closely for adverse side effects.	Tachyarrhythmias Severe vasoconstriction
Isoproterenol: 0.1–1.0 μg/kg/min IV drip	Increases heart rate and cardiac output; decreases peripheral vascular resistance	Close monitoring of the patient's vital signs is imperative.	Sinus tachycardia Arrhythmias Palpitations
Amrinone: 0.75 mg/kg bolus, then 5–10 μg/kg/min IV drip	Used for short-term management of CHF that is refractory to conventional treatment, as well as for low cardiac output following cardiac surgery	Close monitoring of the patient's vital signs and hemodynamic status is imperative. Ensure adequate central venous pressure. Be prepared to administer IV fluids via bolus.	Hypotension Thrombocytopenia Ventricular tachycardia
Antihypertensives			
BETA-ADRENERGICS			
Propranolol: 1–4 mg/kg/day q 6 hr	Inhibits catecholamines and beta-receptor effects on kidneys and heart	Monitor the patient for hypotension, bradycardia, or circulatory collapse.	Cardiac failure Bradycardia Bronchospasm (avoid use in asthmatics)
DIURETICS			
Hydrochlorothiazide: 1–2 mg/kg/day	Depletes extracellular fluid volume by inhibiting sodium transport in the early distal tubule	Monitor K^+ levels.	Hypokalemia
Furosemide (Lasix): 1–2 mg/kg/day up to a maximum of 6 kg/mg/day	Inhibits NaCL reabsorption in the loop of Henle	Monitor the patient for hypotension, excessive diuresis, and transient deafness.	Hypokalemia Ototoxicity Volume depletion
Spironalactone: 1–3 mg/kg/day	Acts as a competitive antagonist of aldosterone	Anticipate that a K^+ supplement will not be needed. Watch for signs of edema and reduced diuresis.	Hyperkalemia Gynecomastia Menstrual irregularities

MEDICATIONS COMMONLY USED FOR CARDIOVASCULAR DISORDERS *(continued)*

DRUG/DOSAGE	ACTION	NURSING IMPLICATIONS	SIDE EFFECTS
VASODILATORS			
Hydralazine: 0.75–1 mg/kg/day	Dilates arterioles and has a direct inotropic effect	Caution the patient about possible dizziness and/or headache, and about the need to change from a standing to a sitting position slowly.	Flushing, headache, tachycardia, palpatations, increased cardiac output, salt and water retention
Sodium nitroprusside: 0.5–8.0 μg/kg/min IV drip	Acts as a potent vasodilator	Monitor the patient's blood pressure very closely. An arterial line should be in place for continuous monitoring of blood pressure.	Sudden severe hypotension Headache Nausea and vomiting Sweating
CALCIUM-CHANNEL BLOCKERS			
Nifedipine: 0.2–0.5 mg/kg sublingual or p.o.; maximum of 30 mg	Interferes with the inward flux of calcium ions through slow channel of active cell membrane	Monitor the patient for hypotension, decreased cardiac function, flushing, nausea, and headache.	Headache Flushing Tachycardia Nausea
ANGIOTENSIN-CONVERTING ENZYME (ACE) INHIBITORS			
Captopril: 0.1–0.3 mg/kg/dose q 6–12 hr; maximum of 2 mg/kg/day	Inhibits conversion of angiotensin I to II, resulting in decreased peripheral vascular resistance	Monitor the patient for hypotension, rashes, facial edema, and blood cell count.	Neutropenia, agranulocytosis, rashes, angioedema of the face, persistent cough
Antiarrhythmics			
Class IA—Quinidine: 15–60 mg/kg/day	Used to treat SVT and atrial/ventricular arrhythmias Slows induction Increases refractory period and action potential duration	Observe the patient for prolonged PR intervals, absence of P waves, hypotension, and tachycardia.	Hypotension, headache, nausea, rash, diarrhea, tinnitus
Class 1B—Lidocaine: 1 mg/kg q 5–10 min; maximum total dose 5 mg/kg	Used to treat ventricular arrhythmias Slows conduction Increases refractory period and increases the action potential	Observe the patient for twitching and tremors, as well as respiratory depression. Administer slowly to prevent vertigo.	Vertigo, paresthesia, seizures
Class II—Propranolol: 1–4 mg/kg/day	Used to treat SVT, refractory VT, and Wolff-Parkinson-White syndrome Prolongs AV conductive beta adrenergic blockers	Observe the patient for untoward reactions involving the gastrointestinal, integumentary system, circulatory, or central nervous system.	Hypotension Bradycardia Decreased myocardial contractility Bronchospasm
Class III—Amiodarone: 5–10 mg/kg/day	Used to treat refractory SVT and to prevent VT Increases the action potential duration and increases the QRS duration Slows conduction	Monitor the patient for heart block, hypotension, and thyroid dysfunction. Serious side effects are common. Used only when other drugs are ineffective.	Bradycardia, hypotension, nausea, nightmares, rash
Class IV—Verapamil: 4–8 mg/kg/day	Used to treat SVT in children older than 1 year of age Slows conduction at the AV node by calcium channel blockade	Use of this agent is contraindicated in infants. Monitor the patient for hypotension and heart failure.	Hypotension Bradycardia Asystole Decreased myocardial contractility
Class V—Digoxin: 0.01–0.02 mg/kg/day	Used to treat SVT and atrial arrhythmias Prolongs AV nodal conduction in both fast (B) and slow (A) pathways	Monitor digoxin levels. Check the dosage with another nurse before administering. Monitor the patient for side effects. Monitor the heart rate before drug administration.	Digoxin toxicity: anorexia, vomiting, bradycardia, lethargy, visual changes
Class VI—Adenosine: 50–300 μg/kg IV bolus	Used to treat SVT Slows AV nodal conduction Suppresses automaticity of atrial and Purkinje tissues	Monitor the patient closely for bradycardia and hypotension.	Transient bradycardia and asystole, flushing, nausea, headache

SHOCK

Shock is defined as an acute, complex pathophysiologic state in which there is failure of the organs to deliver sufficient amounts of oxygen and other nutrients to satisfy the requirements of the tissue beds (Perkin & Levin, 1982). Shock can be more specifically identified according to the etiology underlying this compromised state. The three forms of shock discussed in this chapter are hypovolemic, cardiogenic, and septic.

Etiology

Hypovolemic Shock. Hypovolemic shock can occur as a result of a number of factors. The fluid that is lost may be blood from trauma or surgery, or fluids and plasma from vomiting and diarrhea. Water constitutes a much greater portion of the body weight of an infant and child than of an adult. The bulk of fluid volume is primarily located in the extracellular tissue spaces. Because infants have a large body surface area and increased metabolic rate, there is an increased insensible fluid loss, thus compounding an increased risk of hypovolemia when circulating blood volume decreases (Hazinski, 1990).

Cardiogenic Shock. Cardiogenic shock occurs when myocardial function is impaired and unable to produce a cardiac output that is sufficient to meet the metabolic demands of the body. The causes of cardiogenic shock include structural abnormalities related to congenital heart disease, infectious and noninfectious cardiomyopathies, trauma, ischemia, metabolic abnormalities, drug intoxication, and impaired cardiac function following intracardiac surgical repair. Cardiogenic shock is a late manifestation of all types of shock (Perkin & Levin, 1982).

Septic Shock. Septic shock occurs when microbial toxins (bacteria, virus, fungus, rickettsia) are present in the blood. This can lead to a host response, resulting in a cascade of metabolic, hemodynamic, and clinical changes (Wetzel & Tobin, 1992). Infants and children who have debilitating illnesses, patients who are cared for in the intensive care unit for prolonged periods of time with many invasive lines, and those who are immunosuppressed are at greatest risk for developing septic shock.

Incidence. In the United States, hypovolemic shock is the most common type of shock affecting children, predominantly resulting from hemorrhagic blood loss secondary to trauma (Kallen & Lonergan, 1990). Cardiogenic shock occurs most commonly as a result of myocardial dysfunction in the early postoperative period (Wetzel & Tobin, 1992). The incidence of septic shock is 25% to 35% in patients with bacteremia; however, most of these patients have an underlying chronic illness, so the bacteremia may be a result of a nosocomial infection (Zimmerman & Dietrich, 1987).

PATHOPHYSIOLOGY *of Shock*

HYPOVOLEMIC SHOCK

Hypovolemic shock results from an abnormal decrease in the volume of plasma in the body. When intravascular volume is reduced, the body initially compensates by increasing heart rate and redistributing the blood flow to the vital organs (the brain and heart). There is also uneven or maldistributed blood flow in the microcirculation (arterioles, capillaries, and venules) (Perkin & Levin, 1982). Decompensation occurs when the total blood and fluid volume is reduced by 20% to 25%. If fluid resuscitation is not initiated within an appropriate time frame, decreased oxygen delivery and cellular **ischemia** and necrosis result.

CARDIOGENIC SHOCK

Cardiogenic shock is characterized by low cardiac output and hypotension, which results in inadequate tissue perfusion (circulation of blood through the vascular bed of tissue). Unlike hypovolemic shock, the compensatory mechanisms that occur in a child with cardiogenic shock may cause further myocardial dysfunction. As the blood flow is redistributed away from skin, splenic, and mesenteric circulation, arteriolar and venous resistance increases, helping to maintain the circulation to the vital organs, the heart and brain. The increased **systemic vascular resistance** produces a greater workload on the left ventricle **(afterload).** The increased workload causes increased oxygen demands of the myocardium in response to a depleted oxygen supply. This leads to myocardial ischemia, which further depresses cardiac function, thereby establishing a vicious cycle (Hazinski, 1990).

SEPTIC SHOCK

Septic shock occurs when an invading organism infects a susceptible host. Sepsis is the presence in the blood or other tissues of pathogenic microorganisms or other toxins that results in a spectrum of responses. The responses produce endocrine, metabolic, and immunologic reactions. Endotoxins produced by lysis of bacteria cause a metabolic response that affects the cardiovascular system (Schumer, 1992). During the early phase, there is adequate **tissue perfusion** and even increased cardiac output. The late phase of septic shock is marked by decreased **cardiac output,** increased systemic vascular resistance, and decreased peripheral tissue perfusion. The consequent effects are anaerobic metabolism, acidosis, and increased protein catabolism (Schumer, 1992).

Clinical Manifestations. The clinical manifestations of shock are different for each of the described types of shock (see the list that follows). Infants and children with septic shock demonstrate early signs that indicate a compensated state and then late signs that indicate a decompensated state of shock.

Hypovolemic Shock

- Dry mucous membranes
- Depressed fontanel
- Cold, clammy skin
- Oliguria
- Poor skin turgor
- Reduced capillary refill

Cardiogenic Shock

- Hepatomegaly
- Cardiomegaly
- Increased central venous pressure
- Periorbital edema
- Crackles
- Diaphoresis
- Oliguria
- Reduced capillary refill
- Reduced peripheral pulses

Septic Shock: Early

- Vasodilatation
- Extremities that are warm to the touch
- Purpuric skin lesions
- Tachypnea

Septic Shock: Late

- Rapid, thready pulse
- Cyanosis
- Cold, clammy skin
- Narrow pulse pressure
- Oliguria/anuria

Table 31–1 presents the general appearance of a child in shock.

Hypotension is a late sign of shock. The lower limits for systolic blood pressure in children are as follows.

- Infants younger than 1 month of age: 60
- Infants 1–12 months of age: 70
- Children older than 1 year of age: 70 + (2 × the child's age in years).

Diagnostic Evaluation. The diagnosis of shock in infants and children is established chiefly on the basis of clinical manifestations and medical history. A chest x-ray may help to differentiate cardiogenic shock from hypovolemic and septic shock. In cardiogenic shock, the heart is usually enlarged (**cardiomegaly**) and may show signs of **pulmonary edema.** In hypovolemic or septic shock, the chest x-ray is usually normal, and heart size is smaller than normal. In septic shock, chest x-ray studies may indicate pneumonia, which may be the source of the infection.

Laboratory studies used in the diagnosis of septic shock include blood cultures and cultures of other sites that may be the source of infection (i.e., urine, sputum, wound drainage, indwelling lines). Other laboratory tests for all types of shock include arterial blood gas values, glucose levels, electrolytes, blood urea nitrogen (BUN), creatinine levels, complete blood count (CBC), and coagulation studies.

Therapeutic Management. The therapeutic management of the child in any type of shock includes the steps of basic life support (see Chapter 14).

Monitoring with pulse oximetry and increasing ambient oxygen are indicated in most cases of shock. If vascular access cannot be obtained, an intraosseous line can be

TABLE 31–1 *Assessing a Child's General Appearance: "Looks Good" Versus "Looks Bad"*

	"LOOKS GOOD"	"LOOKS BAD"
Color	Pink mucous membranes Consistent color over the trunk and extremities	Mottled color
Skin Perfusion	Warm Brisk capillary refill (<2 seconds)	Cold (peripheral to proximal cooling) Sluggish capillary refill (>2 seconds)
Activity	Age-appropriate (may be frightened, unhappy, unwilling to be separated from parents) Will engage in play	Fretful, then lethargic
Responsiveness	Age-appropriate	Irritable (early), then lethargic Decreased response to painful stimulus is worrisome
Infant Feeding	Eats well	Weak suck Tires during feeding May develop respiratory distress during feedings

Adapted from Hazinski, M. F. (1990). Shock in the pediatric patient. *Critical Care Nursing Clinics of North America, 2*(2), 313.

used until the child is resuscitated, at which time the temporary intraosseous line can be replaced with an intravenous line. Central access (femoral, subclavian, internal jugular veins) is indicated for rapid administration of large volumes of fluids, the administration of some vasoactive drugs, and the assessment of intravascular filling pressure (Behrman et al., 1996).

> Ensuring a patent airway, effective breathing, and maintaining circulation are always the first steps of management in a critically ill child with shock. These steps may be referred to as ventilation, infusion, and perfusion (VIP).

Hypovolemic Shock. Once the airway, breathing, and circulation (ABCs) are established, the next most important aspect of treatment in an infant or child with hypovolemic shock is adequate vascular access. A crystalloid infusion of normal saline (NS) or lactated Ringer's (LR) solution should be initiated promptly. If the hypovolemic shock is attributable to hemorrhage, whole blood should be administered to replace losses after the child has received 40 ml/kg of crystalloid (Kallen & Lonergan, 1990).

Colloids (albumin) are protein-containing fluids that may be used in volume resuscitation after the initial treatment with crystalloids. Colloids are primarily used for dehydration or body fluid losses other than blood.

Cardiogenic Shock. The initial management of an infant or child with cardiogenic shock includes adequate oxygenation by maintaining the airway and proper ventilation. Cardiogenic shock is most commonly seen postoperatively in patients undergoing cardiac surgery (Hazinski & Barkin, 1992). Invasive monitoring of **central venous pressure,** arterial blood pressure, and pulmonary artery pressure helps to identify hemodynamic changes in the postoperative period and allows early recognition of signs of cardiogenic shock. However, vigilant monitoring and recognition of the subtle clinical signs and symptoms of decreased cardiac output (e.g., cyanosis, decreased skin temperature, and delayed capillary refill) also can detect the early stages of shock, allowing the state of uncompensated cardiac failure to be avoided.

If there is an excess of intravascular fluid volume, diuretics may be prescribed. Usually, furosemide (Lasix), 1 mg/kg, provides effective diuresis. If diuresis is marginal, there may be inadequate kidney perfusion and peritoneal dialysis may be ordered (Nixon & O'Donnell, 1992).

The heart rate must be in the normal range or higher than normal to improve the cardiac output. Children, especially infants younger than 6 months of age, have a decreased ability to increase stroke volume, and thus are much more dependent upon an increased heart rate to improve cardiac output. In the postoperative cardiac patient, heart block or other arrhythmias may occur. A temporary pacemaker in children with arrhythmias is indicated to achieve the desirable heart rate.

Pharmacologic Therapy. Pharmacologic therapy is the mainstay of medical treatment in children with cardiogenic shock. Frequently, a combination of pharmacologic therapy is necessary to stabilize the child (see the table entitled Medications Commonly Used for Cardiovascular Disorders in the Clinical Reference Pages).

Sodium nitroprusside (Nipride) (see Common Medications table) is a valuable pharmacologic agent used in combination with the vasopressor drugs. Nipride reduces systemic and **pulmonary vascular resistance,** thereby decreasing the afterload or the workload on the ventricle. As a precipitous drop in arterial blood pressure may occur with the infusion of Nipride, titration of the medication is necessary to achieve the optimal tissue perfusion.

Extracorporeal Membrane Oxygenation (ECMO). ECMO is a means of mechanical circulatory and pulmonary support for infants and children in severe end-stage cardiogenic shock. ECMO requires venous and arterial cannulation, usually of the right internal jugular vein and right common carotid artery. In the early postoperative period in patients who have undergone cardiac surgery, transthoracic cannulation may be performed, involving the right atrium and ascending aorta (Rogers et al., 1989).

ECMO is used with great success in neonates with respiratory distress syndrome, persistent fetal circulation, and meconium aspiration pneumonia. In the pediatric population, ECMO is used primarily to treat children with persistently low cardiac output or severe, reversible pulmonary hypertension following surgical repair of congenital heart defects (Klein et al., 1990).

Septic Shock. The therapeutic management of septic shock involves restoring hemodynamic status with fluid resuscitation and promptly treating infection using antibiotics. Surgery may also be indicated to eliminate the source of the infection. Inotropic medications are used to manage the cardiovascular instability. Vasoconstrictors may be used to increase vascular tone and counteract the effects of toxins in the vasculature. Maintaining a secure, patent airway may be necessary if significant respiratory distress occurs.

Patients with abscesses, gastrointestinal obstruction, or other sources of continued microorganism production may need prompt surgical intervention. Even though the child may seem very ill and unable to tolerate an operation, surgery may offer the only hope for survival (Zimmerman & Deitrich, 1987).

NURSING CARE OF THE CHILD WITH SHOCK

Assessment

Nursing assessment of a child with shock should be thorough, with attention focused on the cardiopulmonary system. Early identification of shock in infants and children is crucial to decreasing morbidity and mortality (see the previous section entitled Clinical Manifestations).

An assessment of airway, breathing, and circulation is the primary focus in caring for a child in shock. Ensuring a patent airway and monitoring the child's respiratory effort to confirm adequate air exchange with good chest expansion are the initial concerns. The central circulation is assessed by checking a brachial, carotid, or femoral pulse.

Hypovolemic Shock. A child with hypovolemic shock may have a history of vomiting and diarrhea, or anorexia. The parent may report a decrease in "wet diapers," or that the child has not voided recently. If the history is consistent with a traumatic event, there may be obvious signs of injury or bleeding.

The child in hypovolemic shock will require frequent assessment of vital signs, including blood pressure (every 15 minutes to every 1 hour). Skin color, turgor, and temperature should be monitored very closely. The anterior fontanel (if present) should be assessed to determine whether it is depressed or full. A depressed fontanel may be a manifestation of dehydration, whereas a full or level fontanel usually suggests that fluid volume is adequate.

Additionally, the neurologic status of the child must be assessed and monitored closely. A depressed or deteriorating level of consciousness should be reported promptly. The heart and lungs should be auscultated, and the peripheral pulses palpated. Capillary refill time, moistness of mucous membranes, and general muscle tone/strength should be assessed. Urine output must also be monitored closely. In very young children, diapers should be weighed to quantify urine output. Moreover, if the child has diarrhea, a urine bag or Foley catheter should be placed. The abdomen should be palpated and auscultated for the presence of bowel sounds. Abdominal injury must be ruled out, especially if the abdominal girth appears to be increasing, with evidence of abdominal distension. Any abnormal bruising or obvious trauma must be recognized quickly.

Cardiogenic Shock. A child with cardiogenic shock requires close monitoring of the heart and lungs for adventitious sounds. The liver should be palpated and its size measured. The child's respiratory effort must also be assessed. Retractions, grunting, and nasal flaring may be apparent. Periorbital and peripheral edema may be present. Close monitoring of the peripheral pulses and capillary refill is extremely important.

Septic Shock. The early signs of septic shock include hyperthermia or hypothermia. The temperature should be monitored every 1 to 2 hours. The skin may be warm and flushed in early septic shock (hyperdynamic phase) or ashen and cold in late shock (hypodynamic phase). Indeed, shock of any etiology may cause microcirculatory dysfunction, leading to abnormal coagulation factors and platelet dysfunction. Therefore, the skin should be observed closely for signs of petechiae, oozing of blood from invasive lines, or purpuric lesions. The presence of petechiae that are spread diffusely over the body may indicate severe sepsis. It is important to remember that hypotension is a late sign of all types of shock in pediatric patients.

Nursing Diagnosis

The following nursing diagnoses and expected outcomes are examples that may be appropriate following assessment of the child with shock.

- Altered Tissue Perfusion (cardiopulmonary, cerebral, and peripheral) related to decreased cardiac contractility (cardiogenic shock), decreased body fluid volume (hypovolemic shock), abnormal distribution of blood flow, and/or metabolic acidosis (septic shock)
- Impaired Gas Exchange related to possible decreased pulmonary blood flow, increased interstitial fluid in alveoli, and inflammatory response of alveoli
- Risk for Infection related to invasive venous and arterial lines, indwelling catheter(s), presence of endotracheal tube, and possible incisional wounds
- Anxiety and Fear related to the care of a critically ill child with a possibly grave prognosis

Planning, Implementation, and Evaluation: The Child With Shock

NURSING DIAGNOSIS

- Altered Tissue Perfusion (cardiopulmonary, cerebral, and peripheral) related to decreased cardiac contractility (cardiogenic shock), decreased body fluid volume (hypovolemic shock), abnormal distribution of blood flow, and/or metabolic acidosis (septic shock)

Expected Outcome:

- The child will have adequate tissue perfusion as evidenced by strong peripheral pulses, normal capillary refill time, vital signs within normal limits for age, pink mucous membranes and nail beds, and no evidence of dyspnea.

Intervention	Rationale
1. Assess systemic perfusion and vital signs every 1–2 hours.	Astute monitoring can identify the early signs of shock.

Intervention	Rationale
2. Measure intake and output (I & O) accurately. Report urine outputs of <1 ml/kg/hr or >5 ml/kg hr. Also report major discrepancies between I & O.	Decreased urine output indicates decreased renal perfusion.
3. Establish IV access quickly. Deliver an initial fluid bolus with an infusion pump or by IV push for a period of 10–15 minutes in children with hypovolemic or septic shock. Repeat fluid boluses as ordered.	Children with hypovolemic or septic shock require rapid fluid resuscitation.
4. Check blood glucose levels every 2–4 hours.	Neonates and infants have high glucose requirements and low glycogen stores. Hypoglycemia and hyperglycemia may occur during stress.
5. Administer vasopressors using an IV controller or infusion pump to ensure accurate delivery of medication. It is preferable to administer such agents through a central line.	Dopamine, dobutamine, and epinephrine can cause tissue necrosis if infiltration occurs in peripheral tissues. An arterial line and an intensive care setting are indicated for continuous blood pressure monitoring.
6. Administer vasodilators cautiously, using an IV controller or infusion pump to ensure accurate delivery of medication. Monitor the patient's blood pressure closely after initiation of Nipride therapy.	Nipride may cause a precipitous drop in systolic blood pressure. Confirm an adequate circulating blood volume before initiating Nipride therapy.
7. Weigh the patient daily on the same scale. Report any rapid weight gain to the physician.	In cardiogenic shock, there may be a significant weight gain within a short period of time owing to systemic or **pulmonary venous congestion.**
8. Administer diuretics as ordered. Note the degree of diuresis. Monitor electrolyte levels.	Diuretics are indicated for patients with pulmonary edema and **systemic venous congestion.** Potassium is lost through the urine with diuretic therapy.
9. Administer antibiotics promptly, as ordered, for children with septic shock.	Treatment of the underlying infection is the primary concern in caring for children with septic shock.

Evaluation:

- The child has adequate tissue perfusion as evidenced by pink color, brisk capillary refill, alertness and responsiveness, and normal vital signs for age.
- The child does not progress to uncompensated shock nor does irreversible tissue necrosis occur.

NURSING DIAGNOSIS

- Impaired Gas Exchange related to possible decreased pulmonary blood flow, increased interstitial fluid in alveoli, and inflammatory response of alveoli

Expected Outcome:

- The child will have adequate oxygen and carbon dioxide exchange as evidenced by an **oxygen saturation** level ≥ 95%–100%, arterial blood gas values that are within normal limits, pink mucous membranes and nail beds, and no evidence of dyspnea.

Intervention	Rationale
1. Assess respiratory rate and effort, color, chest expansion and aeration. Note signs of respiratory distress and report them to the physician promptly.	Children usually develop respiratory arrest before cardiac arrest. Prompt recognition of related symptoms allows early treatment and intervention.

Intervention	Rationale
2. Administer oxygen as ordered. Make sure the mode of delivery is appropriate for the age of the patient.	The size and age of the child may determine the mode of oxygen delivery that will be best tolerated. Forced inspired oxygen increases the partial pressure of oxygenation, leading to improved tissue oxygenation.
3. Have available the appropriate equipment for endotracheal intubation (laryngoscope, blades, tubes, tape, face mask, Ambubag, and suction).	Children with uncompensated states of shock develop respiratory distress and failure quickly. Endotracheal intubation and positive pressure ventilation is often necessary.
4. Monitor arterial blood gas values, oxygen saturation, and hemoglobin levels.	These parameters indicate the amount of oxygen delivered to tissue beds.
5. Maintain a patent airway. Suction nasopharyngeal or endotracheal secretions as needed. Hyperventilate the patient with 100% oxygen before suctioning. Reposition the child to enhance postural drainage.	Children with shock may have a decreased level of consciousness, impaired cough reflex, and increased secretions. If pneumonia is present, secretions may be thick and copious.

Evaluation:
- The child has an oxygen saturation > 95% on room air, blood gas values that are within normal limits, pink mucous membranes and nailbeds, and a normal breathing rate and pattern.

NURSING DIAGNOSIS
- Risk for Infection related to invasive venous and arterial lines, indwelling catheter(s), presence of an endotracheal tube, and possible incisional wounds

Expected Outcome:
- The child will not develop a nosocomial infection.

Intervention	Rationale
1. Maintain strict aseptic technique when handling IV lines, invasive tubes, and incisional or puncture sites.	Contamination of invasive lines, which allows bacteria to enter the blood, or of open wounds may lead to sepsis. A child in a compromised state and with poor nutritional status is at high risk for infection.
2. Monitor the child's temperature closely. Notify the physician of rectal temperatures >38.5°C or 101.0°F. Observe secretions/body fluids, incisions, and puncture sites for evidence of erythema, edema, or purulence. Report positive blood culture results and elevated white blood cell counts promptly.	A septic work-up may be indicated. CBC and blood, urine, sputum, and wound cultures may be ordered.
3. Administer antipyretics as ordered. Avoid the use of aspirin in children.	Reye syndrome has been associated with the use of aspirin in children.
4. Ensure adequate caloric intake. If the child is unable to tolerate oral or nasogastric feedings, discuss alternative methods of feeding with the physician.	Febrile and septic children have increased metabolic demands and require increased caloric intake.

Evaluation:
- The child does not develop a nosocomial infection.
- The child is afebrile, and culture results are negative.

NURSING DIAGNOSIS
- Anxiety and Fear related to the care of a critically ill child with a possibly grave prognosis

Expected Outcome:
- The child/parent expresses feelings, verbalizes an understanding of the condition, and demonstrates coping skills.

Intervention	Rationale
1. Provide concise, accurate information to parents. Assess the child's developmental level and level of comprehension. Provide simple explanations of procedures before initiating them. Provide information in a calm, relaxed, and concerned manner. Answer all questions honestly. Be empathetic.	Providing accurate information to the family will allay fear of the unknown and will promote feelings of control. It may be necessary to repeat information several times in order for the parents to fully comprehend it.
2. Allow the child/parents to vent their feelings, concerns, and anxieties.	Decreasing anxiety will decrease the child's oxygen requirements and the level of parental distress.
3. Encourage the parents to participate in the child's care as appropriate (bathing, combing hair, etc.).	Allowing parents/guardians to participate in the child's care promotes a sense of control and a feeling of usefulness, rather than helplessness.
4. Be nonjudgmental in response to parents' actions. Utilize available resources (e.g., a social worker, chaplain, or other family members) to help calm parents who are exhibiting uncontrolled feelings.	Inappropriate and irrational behaviors may be demonstrated during high periods of stress. It is important that the individuals not feel embarrassed or ashamed, and that they be allowed to vent feelings of anger.
5. Assess the parents' perceptions of the event and provide reassurance or clarify any misconceptions. Determine the availability of support systems and encourage their utilization. Help the parents to identify coping mechanisms that have been effective in the past, and encourage the parents to determine whether these mechanisms may be effective during the current crisis.	The balancing factors that are critical to crisis resolution include the perception of the event, the available support systems and coping mechanisms. Maximizing these balancing factors helps the family to manage the crisis and provides much needed support.

Evaluation:
- The parents/child are able to vent their feelings to staff or significant others.
- The family demonstrates a decreased level of anxiety and utilizes available resources and effective coping mechanisms.

CONGESTIVE HEART FAILURE

Congestive heart failure (CHF) is a clinical syndrome that reflects the heart's inability to pump sufficiently in order to meet the metabolic demands of the body. The heart becomes overloaded and is unable to deliver adequate cardiac output. In infants and children, inadequate cardiac output is most commonly caused by congenital heart defects that produce an excessive volume or pressure load on the myocardium.

Etiology. Conditions that cause heart failure in the pediatric population include congenital heart disease, endocardial fibroelastosis, open-heart repair for congenital heart defects, and conditions that cause severe hypoxia in the myocardium and pulmonary and systemic vasculature. A variety of acquired conditions may cause CHF in the pediatric population. The most common conditions are rheumatic heart disease, endocarditis and myocarditis, cardiomyopathies, and severe dysrhythmias (Talner, 1989).

Incidence. In infants, congestive heart failure occurs most often in association with a diagnosis of congenital heart disease. After the first 3 months of life, endocardial fibroelastosis is the most frequent cause of heart failure; after 1 year of age, a variety of conditions, many of which are acquired, may cause heart failure (Talner, 1989).

PATHOPHYSIOLOGY *of Congestive Heart Failure*

In children, a combination of both left-sided and right-sided heart failure is usually present. In left-sided failure, the left ventricle is unable to pump blood out to the systemic circulation. The blood then backs up into the left atrium and pulmonary veins, causing increased left atrial and pulmonary venous pressure. The lungs become congested with blood, which leads to **pulmonary edema.**

In right-sided failure, the right ventricle is unable to pump blood adequately to the pulmonary arteries and the pulmonary vasculature. This causes less blood to be oxygenated and increases the right atrial and systemic venous pressures. The end result is that when the heart is overloaded, it is unable to deliver adequate cardiac output.

Clinical Manifestations. The clinical manifestations of CHF include the following:

Right-Sided Heart Failure

- Periorbital and facial edema
- Hepatomegaly
- Splenomegaly
- Ascites
- Wheezing
- Neck vein distension (children)

Left-Sided Heart Failure

- Tachypnea
- Dyspnea
- Crackles
- Intercostal muscle and sternal retractions
- Wheezing

Right- and Left-Sided Heart Failure

- Tachycardia
- Cardiomegaly
- Gallop heart rhythm
- Decreased peripheral perfusion
- Excessive diaphoresis
- Sudden, prodigious weight gain
- Decreased urine output
- Cyanosis and/or pallor

Diagnostic Evaluation. The diagnosis of CHF is established on the basis of clinical signs and symptoms, a chest x-ray, ECG, and echocardiogram. Laboratory studies that may be indicated to determine the presence of heart failure in children include arterial blood gas values, serum electrolyte levels, CBC, sedimentation rate, serum glucose and calcium levels, and urinalysis.

Therapeutic Management. Therapeutic management of the infant/child with CHF depends on the etiology of the heart failure and the severity of the condition. If the etiology is a congenital heart defect and the defect can be treated surgically, then surgery is indicated. Children with dilated cardiomyopathy and certain complex congenital heart defects may be candidates for a cardiac transplant. Infection, rejection, and development of accelerated coronary artery disease are serious complications that limit long-term survival in cardiac transplant patients. Therefore, the decision for transplantation is made only after careful selection of potential recipients (Muirhead, 1992).

In heart failure that is caused by hypoxia and dysrhythmias, treatment centers on correcting the underlying condition, improving ventilation, and providing antidysrhythmic medication. When heart failure is not responding to surgical intervention, or when surgical intervention may be the cause of heart failure, pharmacologic medical management is required.

The most common agents used in the management of CHF include oxygen, positive inotropic agents, vasodilators, and diuretics. Digoxin and furosemide are the initial drugs utilized in a child with heart failure. Captopril may be added if signs of heart failure persist (Kaplan, 1990). (See the previous table entitled Medications Commonly Used for Cardiovascular Disorders.)

Children with acute heart failure occurring in the neonatal or postoperative period are treated with oxygen and mechanical ventilation; catecholamines, such as epinephrine, dopamine, and dobutamine; IV diuretics; and vasodilators, such as sodium nitroprusside and nitroglycerin. Additionally, prostaglandin E_1 (PGE_1) may be administered in the neonatal period for ductal-dependent congenital heart defects with cardiovascular collapse to maintain patency of the ductus arteriosus prior to surgical therapy (Kaplan, 1990).

NURSING CARE OF THE CHILD WITH CONGESTIVE HEART FAILURE

Assessment

Assessment of the child with congestive heart failure includes close monitoring of vital signs and a thorough cardiovascular examination as described in the earlier section in this chapter entitled Shock. Recognition of the early signs of congestive heart failure will expedite early treatment and prevent decompensation to a more severe state. The early symptoms of tachypnea, poor feeding, and diaphoresis during feeding should be noted and the physician alerted as soon as possible.

Nursing Diagnosis and Planning

The following nursing diagnoses and expected outcomes may be appropriate following assessment of the child with congestive heart failure.

- Altered Tissue Perfusion (cardiopulmonary and peripheral) related to increased workload of the heart. ***Expected Outcome:*** *The child will have adequate tissue perfusion as evidenced by pink mucous membranes and nail beds, a capillary refill of <2 seconds, good peripheral pulses, and an activity level that is within normal limits.*
- Altered Nutrition, Less Than Body Requirements related to increased energy expenditure. ***Expected Outcome:*** *The child will demonstrate appropriate weight gain and no significant loss of weight over a short period of time.*
- Knowledge Deficit related to special care requirements at home. ***Expected Outcome:*** *The parents will demonstrate appropriate care of the child and verbalize a readiness to assume care of the child with special needs at home.*

Implementation

Plan nursing care in such a way as to provide undisturbed rest periods for the child. Elevate the head of the bed to decrease the workload of breathing. Oxygen administration may be ordered for stressful periods, especially during bouts of crying or invasive procedures.

Administer medications as ordered. Digoxin is commonly ordered to increase **myocardial contractility.** (See the section of this chapter entitled Dysrhythmias for nursing implications.) Monitor the effectiveness of diuretic therapy. Accurate intake and output and daily weight measurements should be obtained to detect fluid retention. All diapers should be weighed and the urine output recorded and assessed in relation to the diuretics administered.

Monitor electrolyte levels and report any abnormalities, especially hypokalemia, to the physician immediately. If vasodilators or angiotensin-converting enzyme (ACE) inhibitors (captopril) are ordered, the patient's blood pressure should be monitored and hypotension should be reported and evaluated before administering the dose.

> Feed the infant or child in a relaxed environment. The infant with CHF tends to tire easily during feedings. Frequent, small feedings may be less tiring. If the child is unable to consume an appropriate amount during that time period, nasogastric feedings should be considered.

Nutrition and Weight Gain. For breastfeeding infants, accurate weight measurements before and after each feeding may be indicated to determine whether the child's intake is adequate. A concentrated formula containing 24 to 28 calories per ounce may need to be introduced if weight gain is inadequate. With moderate to severe CHF, the infant/child may require bolus or continuous nasogastric feedings. Weekly or biweekly weight measurements should be obtained once the child is discharged to document adequate weight gain.

A weight gain of more than 50 g/day may indicate fluid overload. Assess urine output, evaluate the child for evidence of facial or peripheral edema, auscultate lung sounds, and report the weight gain to the physician.

Parent Teaching. Education of the parents should begin when the child is diagnosed with CHF. The term *congestive heart failure* should be explained carefully to the parents to allay any fear that the child's heart is going to stop. The nurse should explain that there are varying degrees of heart failure ranging from mild to severe, and should inform the parents about the signs and symptoms the child may exhibit, as well as when to call the physician. All medications should be explained thoroughly to the parents, and they should be given the opportunity to administer the medications to the child before hospital discharge. The parents should also be taught infant/child cardiopulmonary resuscitation (CPR). However, a home cardiorespiratory monitor is usually not indicated. If the child requires a nasogastric tube, the parents should be thoroughly trained in the proper method for inserting the tube, checking its placement, and administering the formula or pumped breast milk. A referral to visiting nurses or other community resources may be indicated if the parental resources are insufficient. Home care of the child with CHF can be frightening for the parent/family, and respite care may prove to be a valuable resource in reducing the stress in the family.

Evaluation

In evaluating the child with CHF, the following should be determined:

- Has the heart failure improved with surgical or medical treatment?
- Is the child experiencing adequate weight gain and normal growth and development?
- Have the parents begun to overcome their fears and to learn to monitor symptoms, administer medications, and support the child nutritionally?

HYPERTENSION

Hypertension is defined as an average systolic and/or average diastolic blood pressure that exceeds or is equal to the 95th percentile for age and sex, based on measurements obtained on at least three occasions. Normal blood pressure is defined as a systolic and/or diastolic blood pressure that is less than the 90th percentile for age and sex (Table 31–2).

The two major categories of hypertension are essential (primary or idiopathic) and secondary (symptom of underlying disease).

Etiology. Essential hypertension is considered to be an inherited disorder. However, with essential hypertension, the manifestations of the elevated blood pressure may be a response to an environmental stimuli. In both adults and children, there tends to be an exaggerated blood pressure response to physical and emotional stresses as compared to normotensive individuals. Some individuals with essential hypertension have an increased blood pressure in response to increased levels of sodium; this finding is most consistent in the African-American population. There is also evidence to believe that there may be a basic defect in the sodium ion transport mechanism in patients with essential hypertension (Hiner & Falkner, 1992).

Additional determinants of blood pressure in children are height and weight. Children with elevated blood pressure are usually taller and heavier than their age-matched peers. Obesity is a common concurrent condition in children with hypertension (Hiner & Falkner, 1992).

The causes of secondary hypertension in the pediatric population include coarctation of the aorta, endocrine disorders, bronchopulmonary dysplasia, and various renal and renovascular diseases. Coarctation of the aorta is the most common cardiovascular cause of hypertension (see Chapter 30). Renal arterial disease in the neonate is usually caused by renal artery thrombosis secondary to umbilical artery catheters or polycythemia. Renal parenchymal disease is a common cause of hypertension in all age groups. Hypertension caused by endocrine disorders is unusual, and is usually treatable (Mendoza, 1990).

TABLE 31–2 *90th Percentiles for Blood Pressure Measurement in Boys and Girls: Newborn to 18 Years of Age*

AGE	BOYS	GIRLS
Newborn	87/68	76/68
6 months	105/66	106/66
1 year	105/69	105/67
2 years	106/68	105/69
4 years	108/69	107/69
6 years	111/70	111/70
8 years	114/73	114/72
10 years	117/75	117/75
12 years	121/77	122/78
14 years	126/78	125/81
16 years	131/81	128/81
18 years	136/84	127/80

Data from the Report of the Second Task Force on Blood Pressure Control in Children, National Heart, Lung and Blood Institute (NHLBI), 1987.

PATHOPHYSIOLOGY *of Hypertension*

The arterial blood pressure provides information about the systolic and diastolic arterial measurements. The systolic pressure reflects the stroke volume of the heart, the rate of the blood ejected, and the elasticity of the aorta. The diastolic pressure reflects the resting pressure of the arterial system. This is affected by the peripheral vascular resistance or the diameter of the arteries and the heart rate. An increase in the heart rate decreases the diastolic or ventricular filling time.

Hypertension, or increased arterial blood pressure over time, may produce cardiac enlargement and subsequent cardiac failure, cerebrovascular disease, renal disease and failure, retinal disease, and accelerated atherosclerosis and coronary heart disease. These effects are predominantly seen with primary or essential hypertension (Berenson et al., 1989).

Incidence. There have been few documented studies in the pediatric population to determine the incidence of hypertension. In a study of high-school children (O'Quin et al., 1992), the reported incidence of hypertension ranged from 2% to 6%. The study demonstrated a higher incidence of hypertension in boys than in girls. The incidence of hypertension in junior-high-school students has been reported to be 1.1%. There was no significant difference in blood pressure according to racial group in children, which is a different finding than in the adult population (Sinaiko et al., 1989).

Clinical Manifestations. Children with primary hypertension rarely have clinical evidence of disease, and the elevated blood pressure is usually detected during a routine physical examination. However, high elevations of blood pressure can lead to the following manifestations:

Essential or Primary Hypertension

- Dizziness
- Headaches (severe, occipital)
- Epistaxis
- Visual disturbances
- Neurologic deficits (late sign)
- Extremity weakness
- Cerebrovascular accident

Secondary Hypertension

Renal:

- Weight loss or failure to gain weight
- Facial or pretibial edema
- Pale mucous membranes
- Unilateral or bilateral abdominal mass

Cardiovascular:

- Absent or decreased femoral pulses
- Decreased blood pressure in the lower extremities compared to the upper extremities
- Cardiomegaly
- Murmur
- Signs/symptoms of CHF (see page 949).

Diagnostic Evaluation. The differentiation of primary or essential hypertension from secondary hypertension requires a comprehensive physical examination and a complete medical history. Blood pressure measurements are done on all four extremities and repeated twice if elevated. Blood tests (a complete blood count, urinalysis, BUN, creatinine, uric acid and electrolyte), an echocardiogram, an ultrasonogram of the kidneys, and an arteriogram may be performed to rule out any diseases that may be causing secondary hypertension.

The diagnosis of primary or essential hypertension is established primarily by exclusion of an underlying disease. A family history of hypertension, a diagnosis established in the pre-adolescent or adolescent period, and the racial group (African American) are factors that suggest an increased likelihood of primary hypertension (Kaplan et al., 1992).

Therapeutic Management

Primary Hypertension

Nonpharmacologic Therapy. Nonpharmacologic treatment may include weight reduction, physical conditioning, dietary modifications, and stress modification. If the nonpharmacologic treatments are maximized, the need for pharmacologic therapy in children with hypertension should be less than 1% (Second Task Force on Blood Pressure Control in Children, 1987).

Weight Reduction. There is a direct relationship between obesity and hypertension in children and adolescents. Even a modest weight reduction has been shown to decrease blood pressure by 40% to 80%. Weight loss in children is often difficult to accomplish, however. A consistent gradual weight loss plan should be initiated (Daniels, 1992).

Physical Conditioning. An exercise program should be initiated in conjunction with the dietary weight reduction plan. Not only does exercise facilitate weight loss, it also has the effect of lowering blood pressure, an effect which is independent of weight loss. It has been found that 30 minutes of aerobic exercise three times per week may result in a consistently lower resting blood pressure. In adolescents, weight lifting may also have a lowering effect on blood pressure. Any weight lifting or aerobic exercise program should be initiated under the supervision of a physician. Power lifting and body building should be discouraged in children or adolescents with hypertension (Daniels, 1992).

Dietary Modifications. Moderate sodium restriction is recommended in hypertensive children and adolescents. The degree of sodium restriction necessary to decrease blood pressure effectively has not been established, but it is recommended that the dietary intake should be not greater than 5 to 6 g/day (Second Task Force on Blood Pressure Control in Children, 1987).

There is sufficient evidence showing an association between alcohol and hypertension. The mechanism for this association is currently being studied, but it is believed to be related to the role of the renin-angiotensin system and neurotransmitters. Smoking has also been shown to produce an aldosterone-like hypertension in young people. Therefore, avoidance of alcohol and tobacco is recommended (Ingelfinger, 1989).

Relaxation Techniques. Relaxation techniques and biofeedback have resulted in modest reductions in blood pressure in the adult population. Information on the efficacy of these techniques in children is not yet available. However, according to the Second Task Force on Blood Pressure Control in Children (1987), reducing undue environmental stress and providing support for coping with family and school difficulties may be effective strategies for blood pressure control.

Pharmacologic Treatment. Pharmacologic treatment of primary hypertension may be indicated if there is significant diastolic hypertension, evidence of target organ injury, and clinical signs and symptoms related to blood pressure elevation. The primary drugs used are (1) alpha- and beta-adrenergic receptor blockers; (2) diuretics; (3) vasodilators, including calcium-channel blockers; and (4) ACE inhibitors. (See previous table entitled Medications Commonly Used for Cardiovascular Disorders.)

> It is very important to infuse IV antihypertensive medications very slowly and to have an arterial line in place for monitoring. Sudden hypotension may result after initiation of these medications.

Secondary Hypertension

Treatment of the underlying disease process is the focus of therapy in secondary hypertension. If the secondary disease is coarctation of the aorta or is renovascular in nature, surgery may be indicated. The emphasis of therapy in patients with renal parenchymal or endocrine pathology is on the disease process; effective treatment will result in secondary control of blood pressure.

NURSING CARE OF THE CHILD WITH HYPERTENSION

Assessment

Blood Pressure Screening. Blood pressure screening should be initiated when a child is 3 years old and should continue through adolescence. The blood pressure should be checked at least yearly. The environment should be as quiet as possible when auscultating the blood pressure, and the patient's arm should be supported at the heart level. If the child is found to have an elevated blood pressure, the measurement should be repeated two more times, allowing a 2- to 3-minute interval between blood pressure checks.

Physical Assessment. The assessment of a child with hypertension should include inspection of the skin to detect any evidence of edema, to ascertain the color of the mucous membranes, and to document the presence or absence of café au lait spots or moon face. Any of these findings may indicate an underlying disease that may be the cause of the hypertension. The pulses should be palpated for symmetry and strength. A child with coarctation of the aorta may have bounding upper extremity pulses and diminished or absent femoral and pedal pulses. The heart is auscultated to determine the heart rate, as well as any sign of heart murmur or gallop. The abdomen is auscultated for evidence of bruit. A neurologic examination is indicated in children with acute, severe hypertension to detect signs of a possible cerebrovascular accident.

Nursing Diagnosis and Planning

The following nursing diagnoses and expected outcomes may be appropriate following assessment of the child with hypertension.

- Altered Tissue Perfusion (peripheral and cardiovascular) related to elevation in systolic and/or diastolic arterial blood pressure. ***Expected Outcome:*** *The child will maintain normal tissue perfusion with blood pressure at a controlled level (< 95th percentile for age).*
- Ineffective Management of Therapeutic Regimen, Noncompliance related to restrictions on diet, motivation for physical conditioning, and possible medication regimen. ***Expected Outcome:*** *The child will adhere to dietary, physical conditioning, and medication therapy.*
- Altered Tissue Perfusion (cerebral) related to prolonged or acute hypertensive episodes. ***Expected Outcome:*** *The child will not demonstrate neurologic insult or damage.*

Implementation

Nursing implementation focuses on education and support of the family in adhering to the treatment regimen. The nurse may consult a dietician and collaboratively develop a teaching plan regarding a low-sodium and weight-reduction diet, if ordered. When counseling the family/child about dietary modifications, it is important to include the whole family in making the necessary dietary changes. Motivation and compliance will be much improved if the change in diet is supported by all family members.

If a physical conditioning program is prescribed, the nurse should ascertain what physical activities the child enjoys so that these activities can be incorporated into the conditioning plan. Other family members or friends should be encouraged to join the child in the exercise program. Give praise and encouragement for progress in weight loss and increased endurance. Encourage the child to vent feelings about any possible problems related to home or school situations. Discuss methods for facilitating relaxation that may be helpful during periods of stress.

The child who is hospitalized with acute, severe hypertension may require medications (see previous table entitled Medications Commonly Used for Cardiovascular Disorders). Once the child is stabilized after an acute hypertensive crisis, oral antihypertensive medication will likely be prescribed. It is important to reinforce the importance of compliance with the medication regimen and of periodic, follow-up evaluations during discharge planning.

Evaluation

Has the child:

- Been evaluated by the primary physician?
- Maintained a blood pressure that does not exceed the 95th percentile for age?
- Maintained weight loss?
- Adhered to a low-sodium diet?
- Complied with the medication regimen?

DYSRHYTHMIAS

The identification of dysrhythmias in the pediatric population is similar to that in the adult population. The electrocardiographic findings are the same in the pediatric population as in the adult population, with a few variations. The heart rate is usually faster in both normal and abnormal rhythms, and increases from birth to about 2 months of age and then gradually begins to decrease with age. The QRS and PR intervals are usually shorter and increase with age (Hanisch & Perron, 1992).

PATHOPHYSIOLOGY *of Dysrhythmias*

Supraventricular **tachycardia** (SVT) and ventricular tachycardia (VT) usually occur as a result of reentry phenomenon or as an autonomic ectopic focus.

Bradydysrhythmias most commonly are related to hypoxia as a result of respiratory arrest. Insufficiency or atrioventricular (AV) block occurs when there is a defect, either in the conduction system along the AV node or in the bundle of His, which prevents the conduction of the impulse from the atria to the ventricle.

Etiology. Many cardiac dysrhythmias in childhood are associated with underlying cardiac disease. Dysrhythmias may occur in the preoperative period in children with congenital heart disease, or they may occur in the early or late postoperative period. Other underlying conditions that may produce dysrhythmias include myocarditis or myocardial ischemia, cardiomyopathy, certain drugs, hypoxia, metabolic disturbance, increased intracranial pressure, and adverse effects of antidysrhythmic drug therapy (Strasburger, 1991).

Children may also have dysrhythmias without any evidence of underlying cardiac disease. The etiology may be congenital, idiopathic, genetic, or a result of increased vagal tone (Hanish & Perron, 1992).

Incidence. Dysrhythmias in the pediatric population are relatively common; however, most are not life-threatening. For example, premature atrial contractions and sinus arrhythmias occur in about 50% of children, but are not life-threatening (Klitzner, 1991). The most common, potentially serious dysrhythmias seen in children are SVT, VT, and bradydysrhythmias. SVT is the most common serious dysrhythmia, occurring in about 1% of the population and primarily affecting children younger than 1 year of age (Strasburger, 1991).

Clinical Manifestations. The clinical manifestations of dysrhythmias may include the following:

Infant/Toddler

- Poor feeding
- Tachypnea
- Lethargy or irritability
- Symptoms of congestive heart failure and low cardiac output (see the Clinical Manifestations section for Congestive Heart Failure and Table 31–1).

School-Age Child/Adolescent

- Palpitations
- Dizziness
- Syncope
- Exercise intolerance

Diagnostic Evaluation. The primary tool used for diagnosing pediatric dysrhythmias is the 12-lead ECG.

Therapeutic Management

Supraventricular Tachycardia. Children who are asymptomatic and without hemodynamic decompensation should be treated conservatively. The use of vagal maneuvers is controversial and frequently is unsuccessful in children (Binder et al., 1991; Till et al., 1989). Adenosine is an effective antiarrhythmic because of its ability to directly slow electrical conduction through the AV node (see the previous table entitled Medications Commonly Used for Cardiovascular Disorders). If the child with SVT is hemodynamically unstable and demonstrates signs of cardiogenic shock, synchronized cardioversion is the treatment of choice (American Heart Association and American Academy of Pediatrics [AHA & AAP], 1994).

Ventricular Tachycardia. The treatment of VT involves synchronized cardioversion. Lidocaine, 1 mg/kg, may be administered before the cardioversion. (See the table at the beginning of this chapter entitled Medications Commonly Used for Cardiovascular Disorders).

Bradydysrhythmias. Bradydysrhythmias are treated with adequate ventilation, oxygen, and chest compression. Epinephrine and atropine may be used when adequate ventilation and oxygenation are assured, but heart rhythm has not improved (AHA & AAP, 1994). In children with complete heart block, placement of a temporary or permanent pacemaker may be necessary.

NURSING CARE OF THE CHILD WITH DYSRHYTHMIAS

Assessment

Children with dysrhythmias require a thorough cardiovascular assessment (previously described in the earlier section entitled Shock), as they are prone to developing cardiogenic shock. In a stable or compensated child with dysrhythmias, it is important to obtain a comprehensive and accurate history of activity tolerance. Older children may have unexplained episodes of dizziness, **palpitations,** or syncope.

Nursing Diagnosis and Planning

The following nursing diagnoses and expected outcomes are examples that may be appropriate following assessment of the child with dysrhythmias.

Nursing Diagnoses

- Altered Tissue Perfusion related to decreased ventricular filling or decreased rate of heart contraction, leading to inadequate cardiac output
- Risk for Injury related to syncopal episodes
- Decreased Cardiac Output related to fatal arrhythmias (VT)

Expected Outcomes

The child will:

- Convert to normal rhythm or will be in a compensated hemodynamic state as evidenced by pink mucous membranes and nail beds, brisk capillary refill, and good-quality pulses
- Remain free of syncopal episodes and injury
- Not succumb to sudden death as a result of dysrhythmias

Implementation

Nursing implementation involves immediate care of the child who is experiencing the dysrhythmia, as well as education of the child/family. The child/family will require information regarding: (1) monitoring for future signs and symptoms of dysrhythmias; (2) administering medications

TEACHING GUIDELINES *Home Care Instructions for Digoxin Administration*

- Instruct family members to administer digoxin every 12 hours as ordered.
- Check the dosage of the medication twice, and with another family member.
- If a dosage is missed, and is not identified until 4 or more hours later, do not administer that dose.
- If the child vomits after digoxin is administered, do not repeat dose.
- If more than one consecutive dose is skipped, notify the physician.
- Do not mix with formula or food.
- Keep out of reach of children.
- Measure pulse before administering.

as ordered; and (3) appropriate emergency measures to initiate, including CPR, once the child has been discharged from the hospital.

The nurse should consult the physician immediately if a child experiences sustained SVT, VT, or bradyarrhythmias. The child should be monitored in an intensive care unit until the dysrhythmia has resolved and the child is hemodynamically stable.

It is imperative that the dosage for digoxin be checked twice by two professional nurses before administration. The therapeutic range for digoxin is narrow, which means that drug toxicity can easily occur. An overdose of digoxin can be fatal to the child.

As one of the first signs of digoxin toxicity may be **bradycardia,** the heart rate should be auscultated before administering the drug. If the heart rate is abnormally low for the child's age, the physician should be notified before the next dose is given.

Parameters should be set by the prescribing physician indicating the pulse reading below which digoxin should be withheld. The physician should be notified of the pulse rate and of the fact that the medication has been withheld.

Other signs and symptoms of digoxin toxicity include heart block, premature ventricular contractions, and ventricular fibrillation. Less specific signs include lethargy, nausea, vomiting, anorexia, and diarrhea. Digoxin is frequently prescribed orally and is usually administered every 12 hours on a home schedule (See the accompanying box entitled Home Care Instructions for Digoxin).

Ventricular fibrillation is rare in the pediatric population. If it occurs, defibrillation and CPR should be initiated as soon as possible.

Education of the child and family is imperative for those patients with life-threatening dysrhythmias. The child should be taught to identify the signs and symptoms of dysrhythmia, including palpitations, dizziness, and fatigue. These symptoms should be reported to the parent or teacher as soon as possible and medical attention should be pursued. Children who take antiarrhythmics at home need to adhere to the prescribed medication schedule closely and must be careful not to skip any doses. Parents and teachers also need to be aware of signs/symptoms that may indicate early dysrhythmia, and all caretakers should complete a formal course in CPR.

Evaluation

When evaluating the child with dysrhythmias, it is important to determine:

- Are the dysrhythmias controlled with medication?
- Have the child, parents, and other caregivers received instruction about medications, activity limitations, and the possibility of a life-threatening event?

BACTERIAL ENDOCARDITIS

Bacterial endocarditis is an inflammation resulting in an infection of the valves, endothelium, and endocardium. It is caused by a bacterial or fungal agent.

PATHOPHYSIOLOGY *of Bacterial Endocarditis*

In patients with congenital heart defects, there is a pressure gradient within the structures of the heart. The pressure gradient causes turbulence, which may result in damage or disruption of the endocardium or endothelium. Deposition of fibrin and entrapment of platelets may occur at these sites of disruption, and a fibrin clot may form. In the presence of bacteria, this clot can then entrap circulating microorganisms, causing a vegetation to form. With further proliferation of the microorganisms and fibrin and platelet formation, the vegetation may increase in size, becoming entrapped within a fibrin protective sheath. The bacteria contained within can quickly destroy the surrounding tissue and valve structures (Kaplan, 1992).

Etiology. Bacterial endocarditis most commonly occurs in children with congenital heart disease, with the exception of children with repaired atrial septal defects or repaired patent ductus arteriosus. Other children at risk for endocarditis include those with rheumatic heart disease (see Chapter 23), prosthetic heart valves, "calcific" aortic valve disease, hypertrophic cardiomyopathy, mitral valve prolapse with insufficiency, and previous bacterial endocarditis (Kaplan, 1992). The bacterial organisms most commonly responsible are gram-positive organisms, including *Staphylococcus aureus, Streptococcus viridans,* and *Staphylococcus epidermidis* (Kaplan & Shulman, 1989; Doerr & Starke, 1996).

Incidence. The incidence of bacterial endocarditis in neonates has increased over the last decade. This is probably attributable to the increased survival of neonates and the use of indwelling vascular catheters (Doerr & Starke, 1996). Endocarditis is still a cause of morbidity and mortality, despite the use of prophylactic antibiotics, owing to several factors (Behrman et al., 1996):

- The infecting agents have changed
- Some physicians and dentists remain unaware of the threat of the disease and the preventive measures available
- Diagnosis may be difficult when delayed
- Several groups have emerged who are at increased risk, including IV drug users, survivors of cardiac surgery, and children/infants with lowered resistance who require intravascular catheters

Clinical Manifestations. The clinical manifestations of bacterial endocarditis include the following:

- Heart murmur
- Fever, malaise, or sweating
- Signs and symptoms of heart failure
- Anemia
- Increased sedimentation rate
- Myalgias and arthralgias
- Headache
- Anorexia

Diagnostic Evaluation. The diagnosis of bacterial endocarditis is primarily established on the basis of a positive blood culture of the causative organism and visualization of a vegetation on echocardiographic studies. Other laboratory tests that may help to confirm the diagnosis are an elevated sedimentation rate and C-reactive protein level. An ECG is usually not helpful in the diagnosis of bacterial endocarditis (Kaplan & Shulman, 1989).

Therapeutic Management. Prevention is the most important means of therapeutic management for bacterial endocarditis. Children at risk should establish and maintain a good oral hygiene routine to reduce the incidence of periodontal infections.

> Children at risk for bacterial endocarditis who are undergoing surgical interventions or procedures involving the respiratory tract, genitourinary tract, or gastrointestinal tract will require prophylactic antibiotics before and after the procedure.

Bacterial endocarditis prophylaxis is also recommended when any dental procedures are planned that may induce gingival or mucosal bleeding, or that involve incision and drainage of infected tissue (American Heart Association, 1990).

The treatment for bacterial endocarditis includes parenteral antibiotics for 2 to 6 weeks, depending on the pathogen involved and the clinical circumstances. The prolonged course of antibiotics is necessary because the bacteria within the vegetations are protected from phagocytic and other host defense mechanisms, and the density of bacteria is very high at these sites (Kaplan & Shulman, 1989).

Surgical interventions, such as excision of the vegetation, and, in some circumstances, removal of an infected valve and other structures, may be indicated. The child should be evaluated for circulatory compromise, and surgical intervention should be addressed before there is significant deterioration in the child's condition (Citak et al., 1992).

NURSING CARE OF THE CHILD WITH BACTERIAL ENDOCARDITIS

Assessment

Assessment of the child with bacterial endocarditis requires close monitoring of temperature elevations and vital signs. Vital signs should be monitored every 2 to 4 hours, along with a thorough cardiovascular assessment. There may or may not be a murmur; if there is, any change in the murmur should be reported.

Nursing Diagnosis and Planning

The following nursing diagnoses and expected outcomes may be appropriate following assessment of the child with bacterial endocarditis.

- Altered Tissue Perfusion (peripheral) related to hemodynamic instability as a result of impaired valvular or myocardial function. ***Expected Outcome:*** *The child will have adequate tissue perfusion as evidenced by pink mucous membranes and nail beds, a capillary refill time of less than 2 seconds, strong peripheral pulses, vital signs that are within normal limits, and a level of consciousness that is within normal limits.*

- Hyperthermia related to bacterial infection. ***Expected Outcome:*** *The child will maintain a body temperature that is within normal limits.*
- Pain (headaches, arthralgias, myalgias) related to hyperthermia. ***Expected Outcome:*** *The pain associated with headaches, arthralgias, and myalgias will be reduced or eliminated.*
- Knowledge Deficit (parental) related to home care of child with bacterial endocarditis. ***Expected Outcome:*** *The parents will be able to administer medications and monitor the conditions of their child.*

Implementation

The child will require vigilant monitoring of vital signs, peripheral perfusion, and hemodynamic stability. Any change in heart murmur or tissue perfusion should be reported immediately. The child's activity level may be diminished, necessitating assistance with activities of daily living. Opportunities for quiet activities such as reading, watching videos, drawing, and doing puzzles should be provided.

The child's temperature should be monitored every 2 to 4 hours and plotted on a graph. If the child is receiving an aminoglycoside antibiotic, serum peak and trough levels should be monitored. The nurse should be sure to administer the antibiotics at the appropriate time, with trough levels drawn 15 minutes before the dose and peak levels drawn 1 hour after the dose is administered. Acetaminophen is administered p.r.n. for fever, as ordered by the physician, once the initial blood cultures are drawn. Acetaminophen may also be administered for persistent headaches, arthralgias, and myalgias. The nurse should reassure the child/parents that the aches and malaise will resolve eventually.

The child may go home on parenteral antibiotic therapy. Make sure that the parents have access to adequate community resources and confirm that they have undergone formal instruction in the use of the IV mode selected (e.g., Heparin lock, Port-a-cath, Hickman catheter, or percutaneous line) and the proper administration of antibiotics. Provide reassurance and support to the family and child regarding the extensive and lengthy therapy required for treatment.

Evaluation

When evaluating a child with bacterial endocarditis, the following should be determined:

- Are the child's vital signs improved?
- Are the blood culture results negative?
- Is there evidence of vegetation on echocardiography?
- Have symptoms of malaise, arthralgia, myalgia, and fever subsided?

KEY CONCEPTS

- There are three types of shock in children: cardiogenic, hypovolemic, and septic. The most common is hypovolemic shock.
- Children have a greater body surface area and increased metabolic rate, which predispose them to loss of circulating blood volume and dehydration at an increased rate.
- Hypotension is a late sign of shock. Decreased level of consciousness, poor peripheral perfusion, and decreased urine output are indicators of impending shock.
- Maintaining a patent airway, supporting breathing, and maintaining circulation are the essential aspects of treatment for shock.
- The initial management of children with primary hypertension includes diet modification, reduction of weight (when needed), physical conditioning, and relaxation techniques.
- An appropriate-size blood pressure cuff, two repeat blood pressure readings on all four extremities, and a careful medical history are essential in the diagnosis of hypertension.
- Signs of right-sided heart failure include ascites, liver and spleen enlargement, edema, and neck vein distension. Signs of left-sided heart failure include dyspnea, rales, tachypnea, intercostal muscle and sternal retractions, and wheezing. Signs of both left- and right-sided heart failure are tachycardia, cardiomegaly, gallop rhythm, decreased peripheral perfusion, excessive diaphoresis, and weight gain.
- Measures to decrease the workload on the heart include limiting the time the child is allowed to bottle-feed or nurse, elevating the head of the bed, allowing for uninterrupted rest periods, and providing oxygen during stressful periods.
- Education of parents regarding medications, monitoring for signs and symptoms of congestive heart failure, and decreasing stress in the environment are imperative in home discharge planning for infants/children with congestive heart failure.

REFERENCES

American Heart Association. (1990). Committee on the Prevention of Rheumatic Fever, Bacterial Endocarditis, and Kawasaki Disease of the American Heart Association. Prevention of bacterial endocarditis. *Journal of the American Medical Association, 264*(22), 2919–2922.

American Heart Association and American Academy of Pediatrics. (1994). Chameides, L., & Hozenski, M. F. (Eds.). *Textbook of pediatric advanced life support.* Dallas: Author.

Behrman, R., Kleigman, R., & Alvin, A. (1996). *Nelson textbook of pediatrics* (15th ed.). Philadelphia: W. B. Saunders.

Berenson, G. S., Lawrence, M., & Soto, L. (1989). The heart and hypertension in childhood. *Seminars in Nephrology, 9*(3), 236–246.

Binder, L. S., Boeche, R., & Atkinson, D. (1991). Evaluation and management of supraventricular tachycardia in children. *Annals of Emergency Medicine, 20*(1), 51–54.

Citak, M., Rees, A., & Mavroudis, C. (1992). Surgical management of infective endocarditis in children. *Annals of Thoracic Surgery, 54*(4), 755–760.

Daniels, S. R. (1992). Primary hypertension in childhood and adolescence. *Pediatric Annals, 21*(4), 224–234.

Doerr, C., & Starke, J. (1996). Infective endocarditis. In J. Ingelfinger, E. Wald, & R. Polon (Eds.), *Gellis & Kagen's current pediatric therapy*. Philadelphia: W. B. Saunders.

Hanisch, D. G., & Perron, L. (1992). Complex dysrhythmias in infants and children. *American Association of Critical Care Nurses—Clinical Issues, 3*(1), 255–267.

Hazinski, M. F. (1990). Shock in the pediatric patient. *Critical Care Nursing Clinics of North America, 2*(2), 309–324.

Hazinski, M. F., & Barkin, R. M. (1992). Shock. In R. M. Barkin (Ed.), *Pediatric emergency medicine—concepts and clinical practice* (pp. 84–118). St. Louis: Mosby.

Hiner, L., & Falkner, B. (1992). Essential hypertension in childhood and adolescence. *Child Nephrology Urology, 12*, 119–123.

Ingelfinger, J. R. (1989). Nutritional aspects of pediatric hypertension. *Bulletin of New York Academy of Medicine, 65*(10), 1109–1120.

Kallen, R. J., & Lonergan, J. M. (1990). Fluid resuscitation of acute hypovolemic hypoperfusion states in pediatrics. *Pediatric Clinics of North America, 37*(2), 287–294.

Kaplan, E. L. (1992). Bacterial endocarditis prophylaxis. *Pediatric Annals, 21*(4), 249–255.

Kaplan, E. L., & Shulman, S. T. (1989). Endocarditis. In F. H. Adams, G. C. Emmanouilides, and T. A. Riemenschneider (Eds.), *Moss' heart disease in infants, children, and adolescents* (4th ed., pp. 718–729). Baltimore: Williams & Wilkins.

Kaplan, R. A., Hellerstein, S., & Alon, U. (1992). Evaluation of the hypertensive child. *Child Nephrology Urology, 12*, 106–112.

Kaplan, S. (1990). New drug approaches to the treatment of heart failure in infants and children. *Drugs, 39*(3), 388–393.

Klein, M. D., Shaheen, K. W., Whittlesey, G. C., Pinsky, W. W., & Arciniegas, E. (1990). Extracorporeal membrane oxygenation for the circulatory support of children after repair of congenital heart disease. *Journal of Cardiovascular Surgery, 100*, 498–505.

Klitzner, T. S. (1991). Arrhythmias in the general pediatric population: An overview. *Pediatric Annals, 20*(7), 347–349.

Mendoza, S. (1990). Hypertension in infants and children. *Nephron, 54*, 289–295.

Muirhead, J. (1992). Heart transplantation in children: Indications, complications, and management considerations. *Journal of Cardiovascular Nursing, 6*(3), 44–55.

Nixon, H., & O'Donnell, B. (1992). The surgery of congenital heart disease. *Essentials of Pediatric Surgery* (4th ed., pp. 283–292). Stoneham, MA: Butterworth-Heineman.

O'Quin, M., Sharma, B. B., Miller, K. A., & Tomsovic, J. (1992). Adolescent blood pressure survey: Tulsa, OK 1987–1989. *Southern Medical Journal, 85*(5), 487–490.

Perkin, R. M., & Levin, D. L. (1982). Shock in the pediatric patient: Part I. *The Journal of Pediatrics, 101*(2), 163–169.

Rogers, A. J., Trento, A., Siewers, R. D., Griffith, B. P., Hardesty, R. L., Pahl, E., Beerman, L. B., Fricker, F. J., & Fischer, D. R. (1989). Extracorporeal membrane oxygenation for postcardiotomy cardiogenic shock in children. *Annals of Thoracic Surgery, 47*, 903–906.

Schumer, W. (1992). Primary cellular injury. In D. E. Fry (Ed.), *Multiple system organ failure* (pp. 17–24). St. Louis: Mosby.

Second Task Force on Blood Pressure Control in Children. Report of the Second Task Force on Blood Pressure Control in Children: National Heart, Lung, and Blood Institute—1987. *Pediatrics, 79*(1), 1–25.

Sinaiko, A. R., Gomez-Marin, O., & Prineas, R. J. (1989). Prevalence of "significant" hypertension in junior high school-aged children: The children and adolescent blood pressure program. Part 1. *The Journal of Pediatrics, 114*(4), 664–669.

Strasburger, J. F. (1991). Cardiac arrhythmias in childhood. *Drugs, 42*(6), 974–983.

Talner, N. S. (1989). Heart failure. In F. H. Adams, G. C. Emmanouilides, T. A. Riemenschneider (Eds.), *Moss' heart disease in infants, children, and adolescents* (pp. 890–911). Baltimore: Williams & Wilkins.

Till, J., Shinebourne, E. A., Rigby, M. L., Clarke, B., Ward, D. E., & Rowland, E. (1989). Efficacy and safety of adenosine in the treatment of supraventricular tachycardia in infants and children. *British Heart Journal, 62*, 204–211.

Wetzel, R. C., & Tobin, J. R. (1992). Shock. In M. C. Rogers (Ed.), *Textbook of pediatric intensive care*, Vol. 1 (2nd ed., pp. 563–613). Baltimore: Williams & Wilkins.

Zimmerman, J. J., and Dietrich, K. A. (1987). Current perspectives on septic shock. *Pediatric Clinics of North America, 34*(1), 131–163.

BIBLIOGRAPHY

Akagi, T., Benson, L. N., Lightfoot, N. E., Chin, K., Wilson, G., & Freedom, R. M. (1991). Natural history of dilated cardiomyopathy in children. *American Heart Journal, 121*(5), 1502–1506.

Awadallah, S. M., Kavey, R. W., Byrum, C. J., Smith, F. C., Kveselis, D. A., & Blackman, M. S. (1991). The changing pattern of infective endocarditis in childhood. *The American Journal of Cardiology, 68,* 90–94.

Berenson, G. S., Shear, C. L., Chiang, Y. K., Webber, L. S., & Voors, A. W. (1990). Combined low-dose medication and primary intervention over a 30-month period for sustained high blood pressure in childhood. *The American Journal of the Medical Sciences, 299*(2), 79–86.

Carcillo, J. A., Pollack, M. M., Ruttimann, U. E., & Fields, A. I. (1989). Sequential physiologic interactions in pediatric cardiogenic and septic shock. *Critical Care Medicine, 17*(1), 12–16.

Chadwick, E. G., & Shulman, S. T. (1986). Prevention of infective endocarditis. *Modern Concepts of Cardiovascular Disease, 55*(3), 11–15.

Coody, D., Yetman, R., & Portman, R. (1995). Hypertension in children. *Journal of Pediatric Health Care, 9,* 3–11.

Corbett, J. (1994). Update on mitrial pharmocological treatment for hypertension. *Maternal-Child Nursing, 19,* 184.

Crawford, F. A., Gillette, P. C., Case, C. L., and Zeigler, V. (1992). Surgical management of dysrhythmias in infants and small children. *Annals of Surgery, 216*(3), 318–326.

Daberkow, E. (1992). Permanent pacemakers in children. *Journal of Cardiovascular Nursing, 6*(3), 56–64.

Deal, J. E., Snell, M. F., Barratt, T. M., & Dillon, M. J. (1992). Renovascular disease in childhood. *Journal of Pediatrics, 121,* 378–384.

Delgizzi, L. J., & Ueda, J. N. (1990). Using inotropic and vasodilating agents in pediatric patients with cardiac disease. *AACN Clinical Issues in Critical Care Nursing, 1*(1), 131–147.

Delius, R. E., Zwischenberger, J. B., Cilley, R., Behrendt, D. M., Bove, E. L., Deeb, M., Heidelberger, K. P., & Bartlett, R. H. (1990). Prolonged extracorporeal life support of pediatric and adolescent cardiac transplant patients. *Annals of Thoracic Surgery, 50,* 791–795.

Farine, M., & Arbus, G. S. (1989). Management of hypertensive emergencies in children. *Pediatric Emergency Care, 5*(1), 51–55.

Franklin, C. D. (1992). The etiology, epidemiology, pathogenesis and changing pattern of infective endocarditis, with a note on prophylaxis. *British Dental Journal, 172*(10), 369–373.

Gillette, P. C., Case, C. L., Oslizlok, P. C., Zeigler, V. L., & O'Connor, A. W. (1992). Pediatric cardiac pacing. *Cardiology Clinics, 10*(4), 749–754.

Hagedorn, M. I., & Gardner, S. L. (1990). Physiologic sequelae of prematurity: The nurse practitioner's role. Part III. Congestive heart failure. *Journal of Pediatric Health Care, 4,* 229–236.

Higgins, S. S., Hardy, C. E., & Higashino, S. (1989). Should parents of children with congenital heart disease and life-threatening dysrhythmias be taught cardiopulmonary resuscitation? *Pediatrics, 84*(6), 1102–1104.

Houtman, P. N., & Dillon, M. J. (1991). Screening for hypertension in fit children. *Journal of Human Hypertension, 5,* 345–348.

Houtman, P. N., & Dillon, M. J. (1992). Medical management of hypertension in childhood. *Child Nephrology Urology, 12,* 154–161.

Howard, J., et al. (1991). Cardiovascular risk factors in children. A bloomsday research report. *Journal of Pediatric Nursing, 6*(4), 222–227.

Ingelfinger, J. R. (1989). Noninvasive evaluation of pediatric hypertension. *Pediatric Annals, 18*(9), 551–560.

Ko Kon, J., Deal, B. J., Strasburger, J. F., & Benson, D. W. (1992). Supraventricular tachycardia mechanisms and their age distribution in pediatric patients. *The American Journal of Cardiology, 69,* 1028–1032.

McGarvey, S. T., & Zinner, S. H. (1989). Blood pressure in infancy. *Seminars in Nephrology, 9*(3), 260–266.

Schieken, R. M. (1992). Effects of childhood hypertension on the heart. *Child Nephrology Urology, 12,* 128–132.

Stanley, J. C. (1992). Surgical intervention in pediatric renovascular hypertension. *Child Nephrology Urology, 12,* 167–174.

Strong, W. B., Deckelbaum, R. J., Gidding, S. S., Kavey, R. W., Washington, R., Wilmore, J. H., & Perry, C. L. (1992). AHA Medical/Scientific Statement—Special Report: Integrated cardiovascular health promotion in childhood. *Circulation, 85*(4), 1638–1650.

Suddaby, E. C., & Riker, S. L. (1991). Defibrillation and cardioversion in children. *Pediatric Nursing, 17*(5), 477–481.

Trippel, Maj. D. L., Wiest, D. B., & Gillette, P. C. (1991). Cardiovascular and antiarrhythmic effects of esmolol in children. *Journal of Pediatrics, 119,* 142–147.

32

The Child With Hematologic Alterations

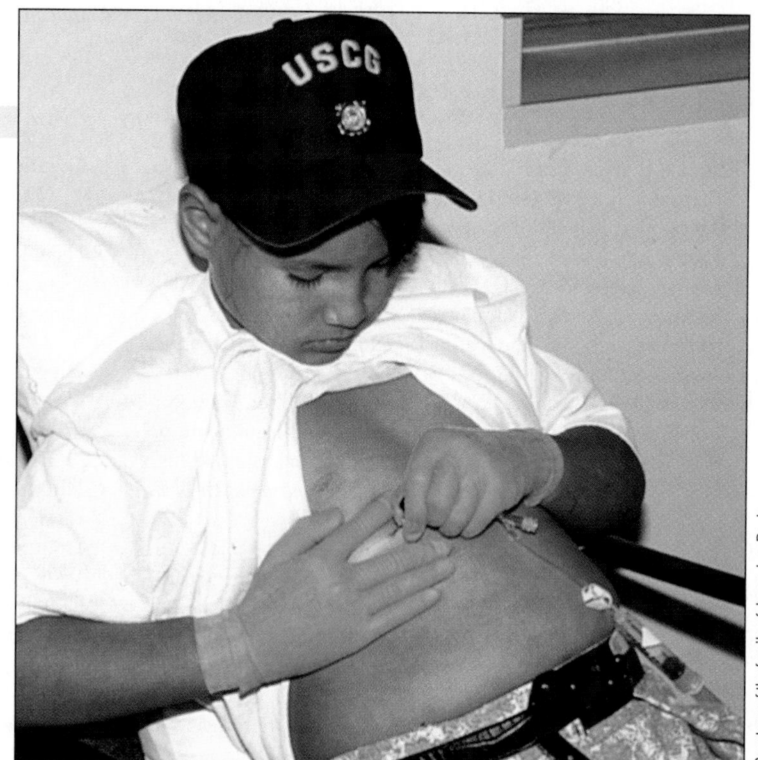

Courtesy of the family of Jason Lee Davis

CHAPTER OVERVIEW

LEARNING OBJECTIVES

After studying this chapter, you should be able to:

- Describe the anatomy and physiology of blood.
- Discuss the pediatric differences related to blood.
- Discuss the role of the nurse in the prevention of iron deficiency anemia.
- Describe common factors in the care of a child with anemia.
- Demonstrate an understanding of the pathology and therapeutic management of common hematologic alterations.
- List nursing diagnoses for children with hematologic alterations.
- Describe nursing care for children with hematologic alterations.

KEY TERMS

autoimmune disorder: a disorder in which the body launches an immunologic response against itself

chelation: binding of a metallic ion with a structure so that the ion is inactivated

erythropoiesis: production of erythrocytes

extramedullary: outside the bone marrow

granulocytes: polymorphonuclear leukocytes (neutrophils, eosinophils, or basophils)

hematopoiesis: production of blood cells; normally occurs in the bone marrow, but may occur in extramedullary sites

hemolysis: breakdown of red blood cells

hemosiderosis: focal or general increase in tissue iron stores without associated tissue damage

pancytopenia: a reduction in all types of blood cells

reticulocyte: immature red blood cells; normal value for children is 1%

reticuloendothelial system: the collection of cells, throughout the body, which are capable of phagocytosis

When caring for infants and children with blood disorders, the nurse is challenged in the areas of preventive, acute, and chronic care. Depending on the disorder and the condition of the child, care may be given in the home, in an outpatient setting, or in the hospital. It is not unusual for a child to be seen in an outpatient setting (clinic, school), referred to a hospital for diagnosis and stabilization, and returned to the home for maintenance. Genetic counseling may be indicated for patients/families with certain types of blood disorders.

Almost all medications can be given at home, including desferoxamine mesylate (Desferal), IV immune globulin (IVIG), IV antibiotics, factor products, and even blood transfusions. Parents are learning to manage infusion therapy to some degree, particularly monitoring and discontinuing infusions when appropriate. Children with chronic diseases are monitored in outpatient facilities.

CLINICAL REFERENCE PAGES

ANATOMY AND PHYSIOLOGY REVIEW

Hematology is the study of the blood and blood-forming tissues. In fetal life, red blood cells (RBCs) are produced by various tissues, but after birth, their production is exclusively controlled by the bone marrow, primarily in the long bones. With age, RBC production is assumed by the more membranous bones of the vertebrae, sternum, and ribs. The number of RBCs is affected by age, gender, and the altitude at which a person lives.

Normally, RBCs are biconcave discs that are capable of changing shape as they flow through the microvasculature of the body. They have a fairly uniform size that is determined mainly by the amount of cellular content of substances, primarily hemoglobin. Their function is to transport oxygen to tissues.

Essential to this ability to carry oxygen is an appropriate amount of hemoglobin, whose production is dependent on sufficient amounts of circulating iron. Iron is absorbed from dietary intake by the intestines and stored by the liver in both soluble and insoluble forms, to be used when necessary.

The stimulus for production of RBCs is a decrease in circulating oxygen which, in turn, stimulates the kidneys to produce a hormone called erythropoietin. Erythropoietin stimulates the production of RBC precursors and causes them to mature rapidly. Disorders of the kidney can affect the individual's ability to produce this hormone, and, thus, can affect RBC production by the bone marrow.

Polycythemia, an increase in the number of RBCs, is a less common symptom than anemia, which is a decrease in the number of RBCs or their hemoglobin content. Anemia results from one of three problems: blood loss, decreased production of RBCs or hemoglobin, or increased destruction of RBCs.

White blood cells (WBCs), or leukocytes, are formed in the bone marrow and in lymphatic tissue. They fight foreign substances in the body by destroying cells through phagocytosis and by forming antibodies which, in turn, destroy unwanted tissue. WBC disorders result from decreased production of WBCs or a disruption in the function of the cells (see accompanying box).

Platelets are the cells that are partially responsible for blood clotting. They are manufactured in the bone marrow and circulate in the blood for about 10 days before they die. Platelet disorders occur because the bone marrow is not producing enough to meet the demands of the body.

Types and Functions of White Blood Cells

Granulocytes: Phagocytic cells found in bone marrow
- **Neutrophils:** Fight bacteria
- **Eosinophils:** Fight parasites and respond to allergens
- **Basophils:** Secrete heparin and speed fat removal

Monocytes: Phagocytize large cells, including necrotic tissue; they are, therefore, important in fighting chronic infection

Lymphocytes: Found in bone marrow, spleen, thymus, and other lymph glands and tissue
- **T cells:** Made in the thymus and responsible for cell-mediated immunity
- **B cells:** Responsible for humoral immunity

Characteristics of the Pediatric Hematologic System

- The life span of RBCs in neonates is shortened.
- By 2 months of age, erythropoiesis increases, leading to increased reticulocytes in the blood and a rise in hemoglobin.
- RBCs are produced in the marrow of all bones. After 5 years of age, RBC production in the shafts of the long bones (tibia, femur) is reduced, and production ceases entirely at the age of 20 years. Hematopoiesis primarily takes place in the marrow of the ribs, sternum, vertebrae, pelvis, skull, clavicle, and scapulas.
- The number of RBCs varies according to age. The increased need for oxygen in utero accounts for the higher RBC and hemoglobin level of infants.

MEDICATIONS

Caring for infants and children with blood disorders requires a knowledge of a wide variety of drugs and blood products. The accompanying table presents the medications that are commonly used in the management of blood disorders in children (see p. 964).

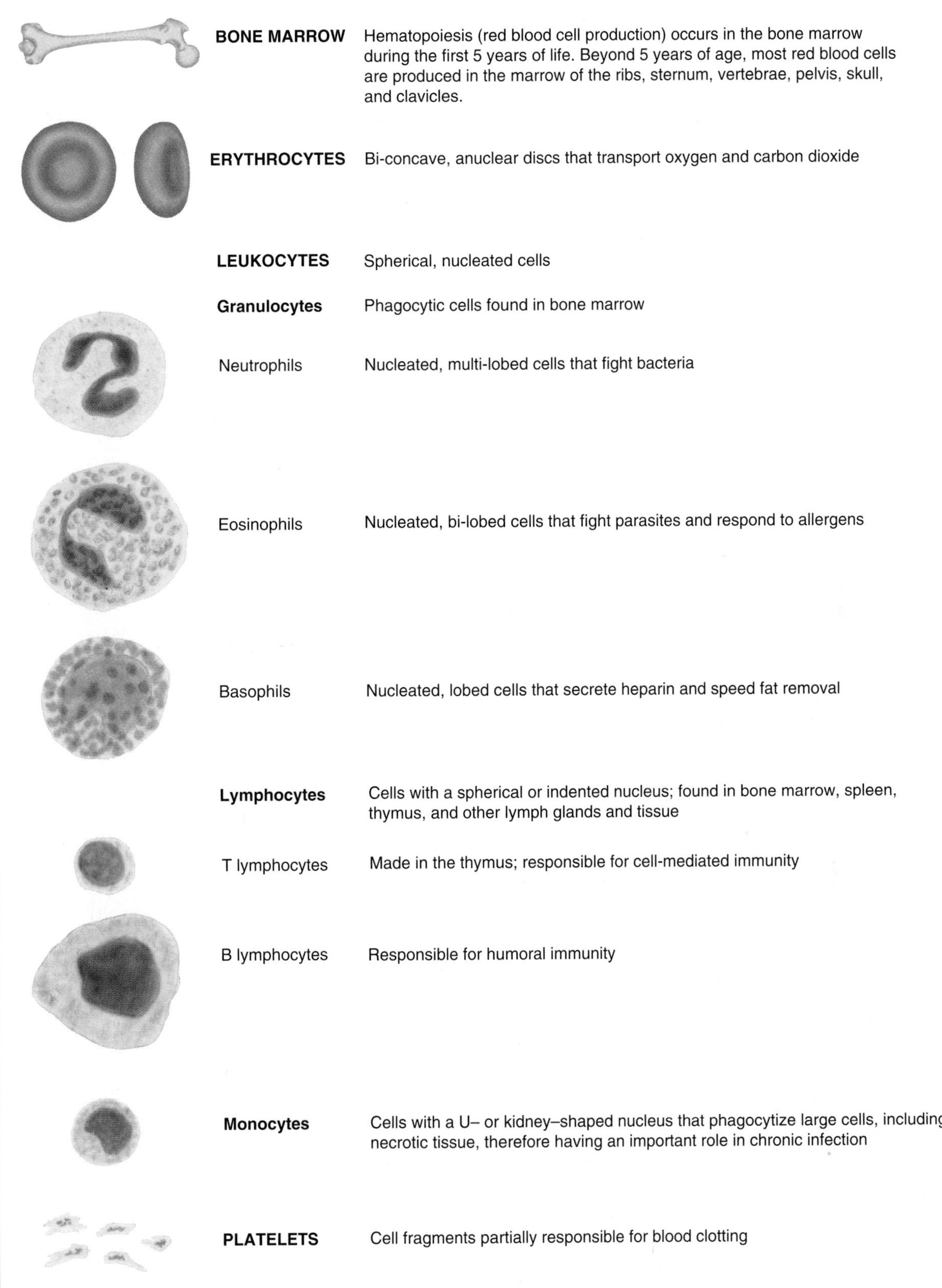

BONE MARROW
Hematopoiesis (red blood cell production) occurs in the bone marrow during the first 5 years of life. Beyond 5 years of age, most red blood cells are produced in the marrow of the ribs, sternum, vertebrae, pelvis, skull, and clavicles.
ERYTHROCYTES
Bi-concave, anuclear discs that transport oxygen and carbon dioxide
LEUKOCYTES
Spherical, nucleated cells
Granulocytes
Phagocytic cells found in bone marrow
Neutrophils
Nucleated, multi-lobed cells that fight bacteria
Eosinophils
Nucleated, bi-lobed cells that fight parasites and respond to allergens
Basophils
Nucleated, lobed cells that secrete heparin and speed fat removal
Lymphocytes
Cells with a spherical or indented nucleus; found in bone marrow, spleen, thymus, and other lymph glands and tissue
T lymphocytes
Made in the thymus; responsible for cell-mediated immunity
B lymphocytes
Responsible for humoral immunity
Monocytes
Cells with a U– or kidney–shaped nucleus that phagocytize large cells, including necrotic tissue, therefore having an important role in chronic infection
PLATELETS
Cell fragments partially responsible for blood clotting

Review of the Hematologic System

MEDICATIONS COMMONLY USED FOR HEMATOLOGIC DISORDERS

DRUG	ACTION	DOSAGE	ROUTE OF ADMINISTRATION	SIDE EFFECTS
Iron (Fe) *Ferrous Fumarate* *Ferrous Gluconate* *Ferrous Sulfate*	Essential element in the formation of hemoglobin	*Iron deficiency anemia (IDA):* 2–3 mg/kg/24 hr, given in 3–4 divided doses *Term infants and children:* 1–2 mg/kg/24 hr, given in 3–4 divided doses	Oral; better absorbed if given with vitamin C and between meals	Gastrointestinal irritation Black, tarry stools
Desmopressin Acetate (DDAVP)	Promotes endothelial release of factor	*Hemophilia and von Willebrand disease (VWD):* Intranasal: 2–4 µg/kg/dose IV: 0.2–0.4 µg/kg/dose over 15–30 minutes	Intranasal IV	Headache Nausea Nasal congestion Flushing Abdominal cramps
Deferoxamine Mesylate (Desferal)	Binds with free iron and is then excreted in the urine	*Severe, acute iron poisoning:* IM or IV: 1 g followed 4–8 hr later with 0.5 g *Less severe cases:* Sub Q: 20–40 mg/kg over 8–24 hr Total dose should not exceed 6.0 g IM or IV.	SC IM IV, at a rate not to exceed 15 mg/kg/hr IM administration	Flushing Urticaria Hypotension Pain at injection site
Immune Globulin	Supplements immune status Sometimes given to suppress the body's autoimmune response	*Idiopathic thrombocytopenic purpura (ITP):* 400 mg/kg/dose, IV, qd × 5 days	IM IV	Low-grade fever Rare hypertensive reaction Tenderness at injection site
Factor VIII *Factor IX*	Supplements inadequate factor in hemophiliacs	Dosage varies with individual patients	IV Must be reconstituted just before administration	Very rare reactions
Cyclosporin (Sandimmune)	Antirejection drug used in transplants	**Initial:* 14–18 mg/kg/dose p.o. qd *Post-transplant:* dose decreases incrementally	Oral; dilute with milk or juice and drink promptly IV dose, given over 2–6 hr Monitor renal function closely	Elevated blood urea nitrogen (BUN) and creatinine levels Elevated bilirubin and liver enzymes Hypertension Acne Nausea and vomiting Headache
EMLA	See Chapter 20, The Child in Pain			

Abbreviations: IV, intravenous; SC, subcutaneous; IM, intramuscular

Data from Benitz, W. E., & Tatro, D. S. (1988). *The pediatric drug handbook.* Chicago: Year Book Medical Publishers; and Nathan, D. G., & Oski, F. A. (Eds.). (1993). *Hematology of infancy and childhood* (4th ed.). Philadelphia: W. B. Saunders.

IRON DEFICIENCY ANEMIA

Iron deficiency is the most common cause of anemia in children. Iron deficiency anemia (IDA) may be characterized by mild or marked anemia.

Etiology. Several factors can contribute to IDA, including growth rate, lack of absorption of iron, blood loss, and diet.

Incidence. Anemia related to inadequate dietary iron is unusual before 4 to 6 months of age, and occurs most often in children between the ages of 9 to 24 months. It is usually related to the intake of large amounts of milk and foods that do not contain supplemental iron (Behrman et al., 1996). The incidence has dropped in recent years owing to education about and availability of iron-fortified formula. IDA may also occur in the adolescent population when a proper diet is not followed, or when adolescent girls experience menarche, but the condition rarely comes to the attention of a specialist.

Clinical Manifestations. The clinical manifestations of IDA vary with the degree of anemia, but may include:

- Extreme pallor with porcelain-like skin
- Tachycardia
- Lethargy
- Irritability

Diagnostic Evaluation. Any child presenting with anemia should first have a complete history taken, with particular emphasis placed on assessing nutritional intake. The results of a complete blood count (CBC) in patients with IDA will show low hemoglobin levels and microcytic, hypochromic RBCs. The **reticulocyte** count is usually normal or slightly elevated. Serum ferritin levels and serum iron/iron binding capacity should be determined.

Therapeutic Management. Long-term therapy is directed at increasing the dietary intake of iron and reducing the consumption of cow's milk. The absorption of dietary iron-rich foods is unreliable and will not rapidly provide the body with enough iron to correct the anemia. Therefore, affected children are given a daily oral iron preparation of ferrous sulfate. Iron therapy is continued for 3 months after the hemoglobin and hematocrit levels return to normal. Follow-up monitoring should include a CBC and reticulocyte count. An increase in the reticulocyte count should be noted within 72–96 hours of the initiation of iron therapy. An increase in the hemoglobin level can be expected in 4–30 days. Because the response to iron therapy is so rapid, blood transfusions are rarely indicated, unless the cardiovascular compromise caused by the anemia is severe.

NURSING CARE OF THE CHILD WITH IRON DEFICIENCY ANEMIA

Assessment

Parents may state that their child is more quiet than usual, with an increased desire to be held. In cases of extreme anemia, the mother may state that she felt her child's heart racing when holding him or her. More often than

PATHOPHYSIOLOGY ***of Iron Deficiency Anemia***

The element iron is a necessary component for the manufacture of hemoglobin in RBCs. Without an adequate amount of iron, the bone marrow continues to manufacture RBCs, but their content of hemoglobin is decreased, making these RBCs inefficient to carry oxygen to vital tissue. Too little oxygen decreases peripheral vascular resistance, which increases the workload of the heart, producing the symptoms seen in an anemic state. The normal neonate is born with enough stored iron to produce adequate amounts of hemoglobin for 4 to 6 months (Chow et al., 1984). The average life of an RBC is about 120 days. Thus, it follows that IDA is usually not seen in children before the age of 9 months. As RBCs undergo **hemolysis,** intracellular iron is released into the circulation for use by the body. Adults are able to use this breakdown of RBCs as their primary source of iron. Children grow very rapidly and increase their circulating blood volume at the same time. Because the breakdown of RBCs in children is not as rapid as their need to make new ones, children must have increased dietary consumption of iron. Various factors can contribute to a lack of absorption of iron by the gastrointestional tract. When cow's milk is introduced into the diet before the age of 1 year, infants do not get the iron they need from iron-fortified formula. Large amounts of cow's milk may take the place of iron-fortified cereals and iron-rich baby food. Additionally, breast milk is a poor source of iron, and dietary supplements must be introduced to augment the nutrients in the breast milk. Blood loss from an infant's intestine occurs very slowly and has several causes. The immature intestine may be unable to tolerate the protein in cow's milk. Irritation of the bowel results in hemorrhages of the microvasculature, resulting in blood loss in the stool. Although unusual, parasitic infections can also irritate the intestinal lining, causing slow blood loss. The storage of iron in the fetus takes place during the third trimester of gestation. Premature neonates who are born before about 32 weeks' gestation require supplemental iron sooner, as they have inadequate iron storage.

not, there is a history of introduction to cow's milk before the age of 12 months, as well as a history of increased consumption of milk, to the exclusion of solid foods.

> Parents may not readily or accurately report their child's dietary intake without being asked specific questions. Ask the parent to begin the dietary history at the time the child awoke yesterday, describing the child's activities and exactly what the child ate. Correlating activity with diet may enable you to obtain a better history, and may alert you to feeding patterns for which counseling may be indicated.

The physical examination reveals a pale, tired-appearing child with mild to severe tachycardia. If the anemia is severe, a heart murmur may be heard that will disappear as the anemic state is reversed.

Nursing Diagnosis

The following nursing diagnoses may be appropriate following assessment of the child with IDA.

- Altered Tissue Perfusion related to anemia
- Altered Nutrition: Less Than Body Requirements related to parental knowledge deficit of age-appropriate nutritional needs
- Knowledge Deficit related to age-appropriate nutritional intake

Planning, Implementation, and Evaluation: The Child With Iron Deficiency Anemia

NURSING DIAGNOSIS • Altered Tissue Perfusion related to anemia

Expected Outcome: • The child will have adequate or optimal tissue perfusion as evidenced by oxygen saturation values greater than 95%, a normal level of consciousness for age, and a urine output of at least 1–2 ml/kg/hour.

Intervention	Rationale
1. Examine the child for signs of decreased tissue perfusion by assessing vital signs, activity level, capillary refill time, mucous membrane color, oxygen saturation level, and urine output. Document and report any abnormalities to the physician.	Visible deterioration in tissue perfusion is an early warning sign that vital organs are in danger of not receiving enough oxygen.
2. Administer packed RBCs as ordered for transfusion.	Packed RBCs are used for transfusions in children to deliver needed cells without the risk of volume overload associated with whole blood transfusion.

Evaluation:
- The child maintains an oxygen saturation level of greater than 95%.
- The child experiences no deterioration in activity level, urine output, or cardiac output.

NURSING DIAGNOSIS • Altered Nutrition: Less Than Body Requirements related to parental knowledge deficit of age-appropriate nutritional needs

Expected Outcome: • The child will have normal iron, hemoglobin, and hematocrit levels within 6 weeks after initiation of therapy.

Intervention	Rationale
1. Assess the child's past and current nutritional history.	Therapy is based on the child's history.

Intervention	Rationale
2. Instruct the caregiver to continue to give the infant iron-fortified formula until the infant is 12 months of age. If the child is older than 12 months, milk intake should be decreased to $\leq$ 24 oz/day.	Cow's milk is poorly digested by the gastrointestinal tract and is not rich in iron. The American Academy of Pediatrics (AAP) recommends continuing iron-fortified formula until the child is 12 months of age. Decreasing milk intake will encourage consumption of other iron-rich foods.
3. Begin the child on iron-fortified formula, and, if old enough, iron-rich foods. Depending on the child's age, suggest intake of liver, dried beans, cream of wheat, iron-fortified cereal, apricots, prunes, egg yolks, and dark, leafy green vegetables.	Iron-fortified formula and food will establish healthier eating habits.
4. Administer vitamin C as ordered, along with foods rich in vitamin C.	Vitamin C increases the absorption of iron by the body.
5. Administer oral iron supplements as ordered by the physician. Iron is usually given in 3 divided doses between meals. It may be given with a citrus fruit or juice.	The immediate need is to increase iron intake beyond that absorbed from formula or food.
6. Administer iron through a straw or medicine dropper placed at the back of the mouth. Brush or wipe teeth after administration.	Iron will temporarily stain the teeth.
7. Keep medication out of reach of children.	Iron poisoning is possible with overdose.
8. Monitor the child's laboratory values, including reticulocyte count and hemoglobin level.	The reticulocyte count should peak in 5–7 days. It also serves as an objective test for determining the parents' degree of compliance with therapy. The hemoglobin level should increase in 4–30 days (Behrman et al., 1996).
9. Parents should be instructed to expect dark, black stools, and the nurse should inquire about their presence.	Absence of tarry stools may indicate lack of compliance with therapy.
10. Obtain a social service consult for enrollment in the WIC program, if warranted (see Chapter 12).	Poor nutritional habits may be attributable to a lack of resources.

Evaluation:
- The child experiences no recurrence of IDA.
- The child has normal iron, hemoglobin, and hematocrit levels and the child and family demonstrate a change in eating habits.

NURSING DIAGNOSIS
- Knowledge Deficit related to age-appropriate nutritional intake

Expected Outcome:
- The parent will effectively administer iron and will demonstrate or confirm an appropriate change in the child's diet.

Intervention	Rationale
1. Explain the need for iron in the manufacture of RBCs in the body, the effect of iron therapy on laboratory test results, the potential outcome with no intervention, the lack of iron in cow's milk, and its effect on the body.	Explanations of the rationale for therapy to help ensure compliance with therapy.

TEACHING GUIDELINES *for Home Care of the Child With Iron Deficiency Anemia*

DIETARY CHANGES

- Provide iron-fortified formula if the child is < 12 months of age.
- If the child is > 12 months of age, limit cow's milk to ≤ 24 oz/day.
- Increase the child's intake of iron-rich foods, with selections based on the age of the child: liver, dried beans, cream of wheat, iron-fortified cereal, apricots, prunes, egg yolks, dark, leafy green vegetables.

ADMINISTRATION OF IRON

- Administer iron in three divided doses between meals.
- Give with vitamin C–rich fluids.
- Administer iron through a straw or medicine dropper placed at the back of the mouth, away from the teeth. Brush or wipe off teeth.
- Iron supplementation causes black, tarry stools.

FOLLOW-UP CARE

- Keep appointments for follow-up evaluations.
- Expect blood work to be done at follow-up visits.

Intervention	Rationale
2. Obtain a nutritional consult.	The nutritionist will reinforce the principles taught by the nurse. Prevention of iron-deficiency anemia is the goal of nursing care.
3. Teach the parent the appropriate method for administering iron. (See Teaching Guidelines for Home Care of the Child With Iron Deficiency Anemia.)	Do not assume the parent is able to administer iron effectively.

Evaluation: • The child and/or family demonstrates compliance with the prescribed therapy, and verbalizes appropriate questions.

SICKLE CELL DISEASE

Sickle cell disease (SCD) refers to a group of genetic disorders characterized by the production of sickle hemoglobin (HbS), chronic hemolytic anemia, and ischemic tissue injury. The more common forms of sickle cell disease include homozygous HbSS disease (sickle cell anemia), HbSC disease (sickle C disease), and the sickle beta-thalassemic syndromes. SCD is an inherited, lifelong disease that primarily affects African Americans, but can also occur in Mediterranean and Middle Eastern populations. Morbidity and mortality from the severe forms of the disease has decreased as a result of newborn screening for the disease, routine prophylactic penicillin, and pneumococcal and *Haemophilus influenzae* vaccines (Bray et al., 1994).

Etiology. SCD is an autosomal recessive disease (see Chapter 2, Fig. 2–2). If one parent has the HbS trait and the other parent is normal, there is a 50% chance that each offspring will inherit the trait. Children with the HbS trait are not symptomatic. If each parent carries the trait, there is a 25% chance that their offspring will be normal, a 50% chance that the child will carry the trait, and a 25% chance that each child will have the disease.

Incidence. Approximately 8% of African Americans carry the sickle cell trait. Among African-American infants, 1 in 375 is affected with sickle cell disease (Selekman, 1993).

Diagnostic Evaluation. In the past, many infants died from complications of SCD before being diagnosed. Newborn screening for SCD, however, has dramatically decreased the mortality from this disease. A laboratory diagnosis is established on the basis of a CBC, examination for sickled RBCs on the peripheral smear, and hemoglobin electrophoresis. These children will have elevated reticulocyte counts because the lifespan of their sickled RBCs is shortened.

Clinical Manifestations and Therapeutic Management. All the clinical manifestations of SCD are a result of the sickled cells being unable to flow easily through the microvasculature and, consequently, their clumping, which obstructs blood flow. Large amounts of fetal hemoglobin (HgF) present in the first few months of life obscure the presence of sickle cell hemoglobin, so symptoms of the disease usually do not appear until 4 to 6 months of age (Bray et al., 1994).

Most of the organ systems, including the eye, liver, kidney, skin, and lungs, are affected by the disease. Delayed puberty and growth are common; the child usu-

PATHOPHYSIOLOGY *of Sickle Cell Disease*

The normal RBC is a biconcave disc that is capable of changing shapes to enable the cells to flow easily through the microvasculature of the body. Under conditions of low oxygen concentration, acidosis, and dehydration, the RBCs in a child with SCD change shape, assuming a sickle shape, that prevents them from flowing easily through the smallest blood vessels. These sickled cells clump together, causing occlusions in the small vessels. With reoxygenation, most of the sickled RBCs resume their normal shape. However, after repeated sickling and unsickling, the cells become irreversibly sickled and their lifespan is reduced from 120 days to 12 days.

Sickled cells cause microvascular occlusion, leading to tissue ischemia, infarcts, and organ damage. The lungs, spleen, and brain are the organs most seriously affected by the complications of SCD. The normal spleen functions to filter bacteria in the blood. The spleen of a child with SCD does not function properly much past the age of 5 years. Precautions must be taken to protect the child from those bacteria that the spleen normally filters. The large vessels are also affected, leading to strokes and other vaso-occlusive events.

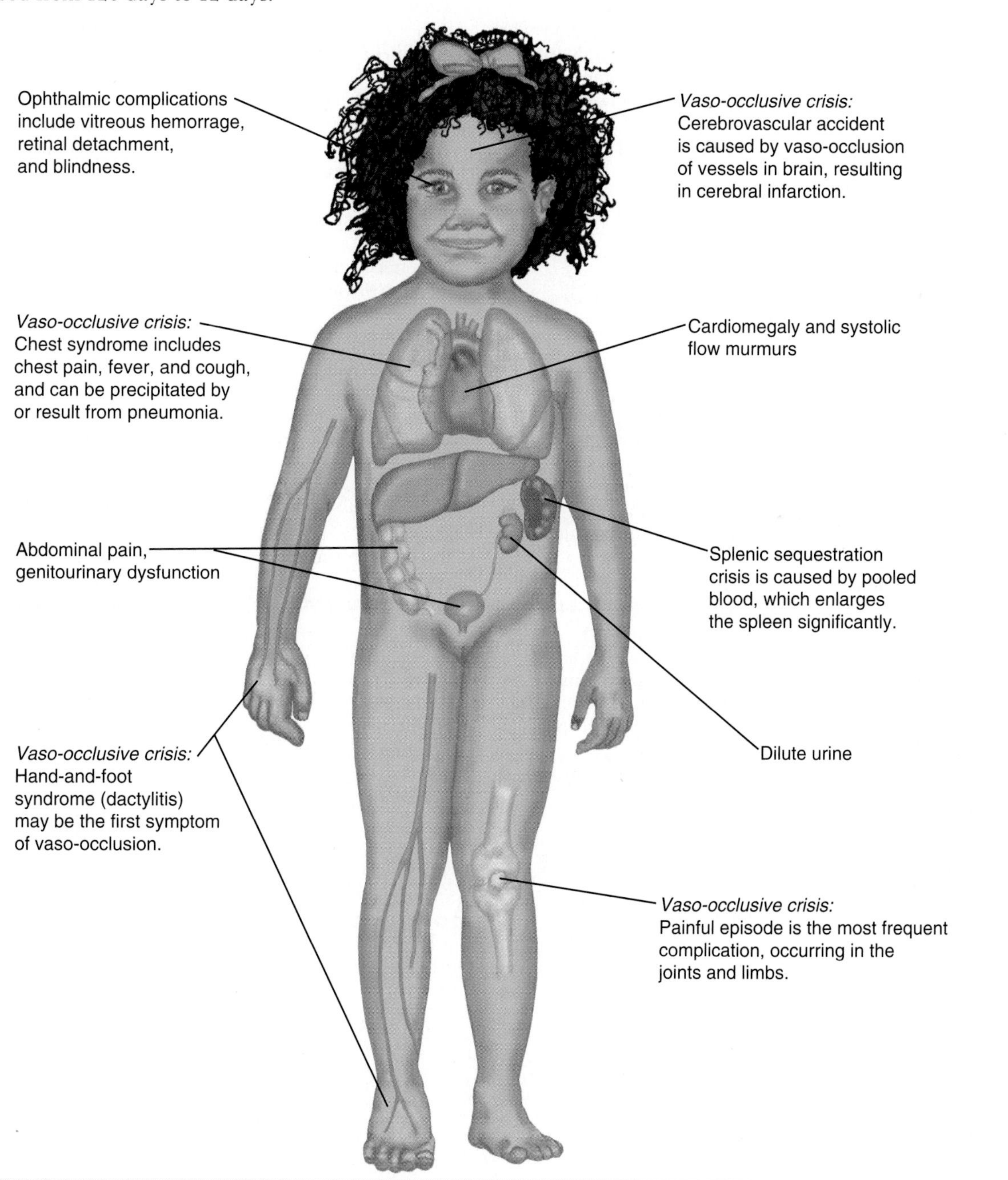
Ophthalmic complications include vitreous hemorrage, retinal detachment, and blindness.
Vaso-occlusive crisis: Cerebrovascular accident is caused by vaso-occlusion of vessels in brain, resulting in cerebral infarction.
Vaso-occlusive crisis: Chest syndrome includes chest pain, fever, and cough, and can be precipitated by or result from pneumonia.
Cardiomegaly and systolic flow murmurs
Abdominal pain, genitourinary dysfunction
Splenic sequestration crisis is caused by pooled blood, which enlarges the spleen significantly.
Vaso-occlusive crisis: Hand-and-foot syndrome (dactylitis) may be the first symptom of vaso-occlusion.
Dilute urine
Vaso-occlusive crisis: Painful episode is the most frequent complication, occurring in the joints and limbs.

TABLE 32–1 *Clinical Manifestations and Therapeutic Management of Sickle Cell Disease*

COMPLICATIONS	CHARACTERISTICS	SYMPTOMS	TREATMENT
Vaso-occlusive Crisis			
Painful episode	Most common type of crisis Typically produces bone or joint pain, but pain can occur anywhere Pain may come and go Frequency of pain is individualized	*Mild:* joint or bone pain lasting for a few hours *Severe:* joint or bone pain lasting for days	Oral analgesics IV narcotics (usually, morphine), which may be given by continuous infusion IV fluids at $1\frac{1}{2}$–2 times the maintenance dose
Acute chest syndrome	Common cause of hospitalization Sometimes confused with pneumonia Can recur	Chest pain Fever Cough	IV fluids Antibiotics Oxygen Respiratory treatments Blood transfusion
Dactylitis ("hand and foot syndrome")	Occurs in children ages 6 mo to 4 yr of age Unknown cause, but may be cold- or stress-induced Self-limiting complication	Swelling of hands and/or feet Pain Warmth of affected area	Oral analgesics Hydration (p.o. or IV) Warm compresses applied to the affected area Rest
Cerebrovascular accident	Without therapy, stroke will recur in 50% of patients (Vichinsky, 1991)	Change in level of consciousness Vomiting Vision changes Ataxic gait Spasms of extremities Seizures Extremity numbness Inability to move joint or extremity Slurred speech Unrelenting headache	Long-term blood transfusion, therapy for indefinite period and possibly chelation therapy May require extensive rehabilitation
Acute Splenic Sequestration	Blood volume pooling in the spleen, causing splenic enlargement Life-threatening condition (hypovolemic shock) Usually occurs in children ages 6 mo to 4 yr One episode increases risk of future occurrences	Decreased hemoglobin level Acutely ill-looking child Pallor Irritability Tachycardia Priapism Impressively enlarged spleen Hypovolemic shock	Blood transfusions to restore circulating blood volume Eventual splenectomy in cases of persistent recurrence Partial splenectomies may be considered to eliminate further sequestration but preserve some splenic function
Acute Anemia Secondary to Erythroblastopenia	Caused by parvovirus, which ceases blood cell production by the bone marrow Usually lasts for 5–10 days Rarely recurs	Pallor Lethargy Headache Fainting History of upper respiratory infection	Blood transfusions and treatment of symptoms

ally has small stature throughout adolescence but will attain normal growth in the early 20s.

Parents should be taught to assess the size of the spleen in order to monitor the child closely.

The symptoms that result from having sickled RBCs are referred to as "painful episodes." A painful episode may be precipitated by infection, dehydration, hypoxia, trauma, or general stress. Repeated vaso-occlusive crises as well as a virtually continual state of anemia, are the factors that produce long-term problems later in the life of the patient with SCD. Table 32–1 presents the Clinical Manifestations and Therapeutic Management of SCD.

Meperidine (Demerol) is no longer recommended for long-term pain management owing to its side effects. Morphine is the current drug of choice.

Because the spleen of people with SCD is not functioning properly or because they have had their spleen surgically removed owing to complications, children and adults with SCD are considered to be immunocompromised. Bacterial septicemia is the major cause of death in children with SCD between the ages of 1 to 3 years, the period of highest mortality (West, West, & Ohene-Frempeng, 1994). The bacteria *Streptococcus pneumoniae* and *Haemophilus influenzae* are normally destroyed by the reticuloendothelial system of the spleen (Vichinsky, 1991), but as children with SCD do not have a properly functioning spleen, they are considered to be more susceptible to infection with these bacteria. For this reason, daily penicillin therapy is begun at the time of diagnosis for many children with HbSS disease but not those with HbSC disease because HbSC is not as serious as HbSS. Research is being done to determine the feasibility of discontinuing penicillin as the child reaches school age. The pneumococcal vaccine should be given at the ages of 1, 2, and 5 years. The *H. influenzae* vaccine is recommended at 2 months of age. The hepatitis B series should be given due to the number of transfusions these children receive. Moreover, they should receive the influenza vaccine annually (Vichinsky, 1991).

The severity of sickle cell disease can be decreased by increasing fetal hemoglobin (HbF). In some centers antineoplastics (azacitidine and hydroxyurea) and food additives (butynate compounds) may be used for this purpose. However, there are unknown consequences of long-term use, especially on growth and development. Side effects of anti-neoplastics include the reduction of bone marrow function. Treatment is also directed at ending painful episodes quickly. High-dose methylprednisolone is sometimes given with analgesics for this purpose.

Cure of Disease. Bone marrow transplant with a matched donor has been successful with a small percentage of children, but the risk of transplantation must be weighed against the risk of having the disease. Research also continues in the area of gene therapy.

NURSING CARE OF THE CHILD WITH SICKLE CELL DISEASE

Assessment

Upon initial diagnosis, the subjective data usually include parental concern that the child is in pain. The parents may have noticed swelling of the joints or the child's refusal to move an extremity, or the child crying out when a joint is moved or touched. Fever and irritability may accompany the pain. Parents of a child already diagnosed with SCD who have been educated about the signs of complications will give a much more detailed history of the present illness. Nurses who are familiar with a child and his or her individual presentation of painful episodes become very adept at assessing the severity of that child's condition.

Just because a child has SCD does not mean that one should assume that the child's pain does not have another serious etiology.

Despite their ability to verbalize symptoms, assessment of adolescents who are experiencing pain presents a unique challenge. During the developmental time in their life when they most want to fit in with their peer group, teenagers with SCD are different. After the initial pain of an episode has subsided, the teen may seek attention from health care providers in an attempt to avoid their peer group, verbalizing continued symptoms that would make them unable to return to their normal activities. Objective data will vary according to the type of painful episodes.

Refer to the section on Clinical Manifestations and Therapeutic Management for data on physical assessment.

Nursing Diagnosis

The following nursing diagnoses may be appropriate following assessment of the child with SCD.

- Impaired Tissue Perfusion related to vaso-occlusion and anemia
- Pain related to vaso-occlusion
- Risk for Infection related to chronic immunosuppressed state
- Ineffective Family/Individual Coping related to chronic illness
- Anticipatory Grieving related to potentially fatal diagnosis

Planning, Implementation, and Evaluation: The Child With Sickle Cell Disease

NURSING DIAGNOSIS
- Impaired Tissue Perfusion related to vaso-occlusion and anemia

Expected Outcome:
- The child's oxygen saturation level will be maintained at a level greater than or equal to 95%.
- There will be no long-term complications from a lack of oxygen.

Intervention	Rationale
1. Assess the child's respiratory status q 4 hr and p.r.n.	Respirations are assessed frequently to detect changes in respiratory status quickly. The child's level of consciousness is an early indicator of decreasing oxygen perfusion to the brain.
2. Pulse oximetry.	O_2 saturation levels can be monitored through pulse oximetry.
3. Administer oxygen as ordered to keep saturation levels ≥ 95%.	Delivering oxygen helps to ease the child's work of breathing. Oxygen does not reverse the sickling process, but may prevent more sickling. Oxygen is not typically used during a painful episode unless hypoxia is present. Long-term administration can depress bone marrow activity and actually increase the anemia.
4. Elevate the head of the bed to a comfortable level.	Raising the HOB facilitates chest expansion by decreasing pressure on the diaphragm.
5. Encourage deep breathing.	Children with chest syndrome breathe shallowly and with guarding. Deep breathing facilitates lung expansion.
6. Administer packed RBCs as ordered.	Transfusions of normal RBCs will increase the oxygen-carrying capacity of the blood.

Evaluation:
- The child is able to resume usual activities.
- The child maintains an oxygen saturation level ≥ 95%.

NURSING DIAGNOSIS
- Pain related to vaso-occlusion

Expected Outcome:
- The child will have decreased pain as evidenced by a lowered score on the pain assessment tool selected.

Intervention	Rationale
1. Assess pain q 1–2 h and p.r.n. using a pain assessment tool appropriate for the child's age.	Pain can be very severe in vaso-occlusive crisis and is relieved for only short periods of time. Use of an assessment tool is more objective than individual nurse's or parents' assessments of pain.
2. Administer analgesics as ordered.	Analgesics may be administered q 2 hr to begin with, or a patient-controlled analgesic pump or continuous infusion may be required.
3. Administer IV fluids at a rate that is $1\frac{1}{2}$ to 2 times the maintenance rate.	Increased fluid volume helps reduce the viscosity of the blood, thus alleviating sites of vascular occlusion.

Intervention	Rationale
4. Administer packed RBCs as ordered.	This increases circulating blood, carrying oxygen to help alleviate the painful episodes.
5. Use nonpharmacologic pain control measures.	Comfort measures often help distract the patient from the discomfort (see Chapter 20).

Evaluation:
- The child expresses decreasing pain.
- The child is able to resume usual activities quickly.

NURSING DIAGNOSIS
- Risk for infection related to chronic immunocompromised state

Expected Outcome:
- The child will have no signs of infection (e.g., no elevated temperature or respiratory rate, redness or swelling of skin or tissue, adventitious breath sounds).
- The child will receive prompt treatment for signs of infection.

Intervention	Rationale
1. Monitor vital signs q 4 hr and p.r.n. Report any elevations in temperature to the physician.	Elevated temperature and increased respiratory rate may be signs of infection.
2. Administer antipyretics and antibiotics as ordered.	Antibiotics may be given prophylactically due to a high risk for infection.
3. Administer penicillin daily as ordered. Give Pneumovax and *Haemophilus influenzae* type b vaccines.	Patients are at a high risk for pneumococcal infections and should receive penicillin daily every 12 hours. The Pneumovax and *Haemophilus influenzae* type b vaccines should be given to prevent sepsis.
4. Teach the parents signs of infection to watch for, as well as the proper way to obtain the child's temperature. Confirm that the parent has a thermometer.	Do not assume that the parent has a thermometer or knows how to accurately obtain a temperature reading.

Evaluation:
- The child/parent demonstrates a prompt response to any signs of infection. (Prompt recognition of these signs, together with administration of antibiotics, will bring vital signs to normal for age, and will prevent the further spread of infection or worsening of symptoms.)

NURSING DIAGNOSIS
- Ineffective Family/Individual Coping related to chronic illness

Expected Outcome:
- The child and family will comply with the treatment plan and follow-up visits.
- The child and family will verbalize feelings about the impact of the illness on their lives.
- The child and family will utilize available support systems and community resources.

Intervention	Rationale
1. Teach the family the necessity of and rationale for following the treatment plan as outlined by the health care team.	Conscientious adherence to the treatment regimen decreases the frequency of hospitalization and improves the child's health and longevity.

TEACHING GUIDELINES *for Home Care of the Child With Sickle Cell Disease*

- Encourage fluid intake ($1\frac{1}{2}$ to 2 times the daily requirement).
- Expect frequent urination.
- Provide for adequate rest periods.
- Avoid cold and heat stress.
- Avoid known sources of infection.
- Avoid prolonged exposure to the sun.
- Monitor the child's body temperature.
- Know the proper use of a thermometer.
- Administer penicillin daily.
- Call the primary caregiver if symptoms of infection are evident.
- Know the physician's telephone number.

Intervention	Rationale
2. Provide written instructions on all aspects of care and on complications. Provide the address and phone number of the local Sickle Cell Foundation (see Teaching Guidelines for Home Care of the Child With Sickle Cell Disease).	Education helps the family gain a sense of control by allowing them to make informed decisions regarding their child's health. Written instructions can be referred to later when the parent is less stressed and able to comprehend.
3. Listen and encourage the child and family to verbalize their feelings and express their concerns regarding SCD. Answer questions honestly and openly.	Identifying concerns and clarifying misconceptions will help the family cope with the stress of chronic illness.
4. Introduce the family to other families of children with SCD.	Families of other children with SCD can offer support, suggestions, and strategies for dealing with problems.
5. Provide parents with phone numbers of persons to contact if they have questions or problems. The Sickle Cell Foundation has information on the disease and on support groups in the area.	Availability of resources decreases parents' feelings of frustration and helplessness.

Evaluation: The child/family:

- Complies with the treatment plan.
- Utilizes available resources.
- Demonstrates increased positive coping mechanisms.

NURSING DIAGNOSIS

- Anticipatory Grieving related to potentially fatal diagnosis

Expected Outcome:

- The child and family will discuss their feelings about anticipated death and will make realistic plans for the future.

Intervention	Rationale
1. Provide honest information about the disease and its progress.	Although tremendous progress has been made in treatment, SCD remains a chronic disease with no cure. Honesty promotes trust. Families need accurate information to make decisions.
2. Listen to the child and family as they discuss their feelings about the disease, death, and the future.	Diagnosis of an eventually fatal disease provokes an acute anticipatory mourning reaction among family members. Counseling should begin at the time of diagnosis.
3. Identify additional sources of emotional support and counseling such as the Sickle Cell Foundation (see Appendix H).	Having several support systems available helps the family cope with stresses of chronic, progressive illness.

Evaluation: The child/family:

- Is able to express feelings of anger, sadness, and fear without guilt.
- Sets realistic goals for themselves.

β-THALASSEMIA

β-Thalassemia major, or Cooley's anemia, is the most severe form of thalassemia, a group of disorders characterized by reduced production of one of the globin chains in the synthesis of hemoglobin. These disorders are found primarily in people of Mediterranean descent, although the disease has been reported in the Asian and African population, as well.

Etiology/Incidence. Inheritance is by an autosomal recessive pattern. If the child inherits only one gene for β-thalassemia, he or she may have only a mild anemia, hence the term "thalassemia minor." β-Thalassemia affects about 1400 people in the United States (Martin & Butler, 1993).

Clinical Manifestations. The clinical manifestations of β-thalassemia include the following:

- Pallor
- Small size for age
- Severe anemia (hemoglobin < 6 mg/dl)
- Microcytic, hypochromic RBCs

Diagnostic Evaluation. A child presenting with severe anemia should undergo a bone marrow aspiration to rule out the presence of other disorders. In addition to a CBC, testing should include quantification of reticulocyte count, serum iron level, total iron-binding capacity, hemoglobin electrophoresis, and HbA and HbF levels to confirm the diagnosis.

Therapeutic Management. Chronic transfusion therapy has been the treatment of choice for these children. In order to prevent the severe side effects and bony changes associated with the disease, the hemoglobin is maintained at 9 to 10 mg/dl.

The major complication of chronic transfusion therapy is hemosiderosis. In order to prevent organ damage from too much iron in the body, **chelation** therapy with a drug called deferoxamine (Desferal) is used. The drug is most effective when given by SC or an IV route. In order to avoid hospitalizing affected children, the drug is often given at home by continuous subcutaneous injection via pump infusion over a 12-hour period at night. If the child has an implantable infusion device, a continuous IV infusion over a 72-hour period once a week may be used. These approaches preserve some degree of normalcy in lifestyle for the family. Therapy is continued until the iron level returns to an acceptable level. This can be accomplished within months of initiating chelation therapy.

PATHOPHYSIOLOGY *of β-Thalassemia*

Normal hemoglobin (HbA) is composed of two α- and two β-polypeptide chains. In thalassemia, a hereditary anemia, there is a genetically determined reduction or absence in either the α or β chain, causing abnormal synthesis of hemoglobin, which impairs the RBCs' ability to carry oxygen. In β-thalassemia, the problem is too little β and too much α.

Classified as minor, intermediate, or major, the severity of the disease is based on the degree of imbalance in the globin chain. β-thalassemia is classified as thalassemia major; thus, its complications are severe.

Typically, during the second 6 months of life, a severe anemia develops. RBCs are hemolyzed as they are produced. Because the body's natural response to a reduction in circulating hemoglobin is to try to produce more erythrocytes (RBCs), the bone marrow begins massive production. Progressive disease constantly stimulates the bone marrow. The body perceives this as an inability to keep up with the need for RBCs. As a result, **extramedullary** (outside the bone marrow) sites of production of RBCs begin **erythropoiesis.** The result is a chronic state of production and destruction of RBCs with a resulting inadequate amount of normal circulating hemoglobin.

Iron is necessary for the production of hemoglobin and is a by-product of the hemolysis of RBCs. Normally, the intestines absorb small amounts of iron. In this disorder, however, the body increases the absorption of iron for some reason. Combined with the increase in iron from the breakdown of RBCs, as well as the increased amounts of iron introduced into circulation by the transfusions necessary to treat thalassemia, **hemosiderosis** occurs, usually during the second decade of life.

The results of this excessive erythropoiesis and hemolysis are considerable. The bones become thin and fragile from excessive erythropoiesis. Hepatosplenomegaly occurs as a result of extramedullary erythropoiesis and hemosiderosis. Impaired growth and delayed puberty occur. Without proper management, multisystem organ dysfunction ensues.

Once a patient requires 200 to 250 ml of packed RBCs/kg/year, a splenectomy is considered. Usually, the transfusion requirements drop by 50% following the procedure (Martin & Butler, 1993).

Although the procedure is not as widely used in the United States, as in other countries, the disease is treated by performing bone marrow transplantations for children with a matched sibling. The success of this procedure in children younger than 16 years of age with no hepatitis or portal fibrosis is approximately 85% with transplantation (Johnstone, 1996).

NURSING CARE OF THE CHILD WITH β-THALASSEMIA

Assessment

Subjective data may include the parents' observation that their child is not as active as other children the same age. The child may sleep more than other children, or want to be held often.

These children have a pale appearance and a microcytic, hypochromic anemia, usually less than 6 mg/dl. Symptoms are related to the degree of anemia.

An older child with the disease or a child who has not received adequate treatment will likely have characteristic facial deformities, including maxillary hyperplasia and malocclusion (see accompanying box). Hepatosplenomegaly is usually seen at this time, but is not a symptom in infancy.

Characteristic Features of a Child With β-Thalassemia

Features develop as a consequence of inadequate treatment.

- Frontal bossing (prominent and protruding forehead)
- Maxillary prominence
- Wide-set eyes with a flattened nose
- Hepatosplenomegaly
- Greenish-yellow skin tone
- Osteoporosis, as a chronic consequence

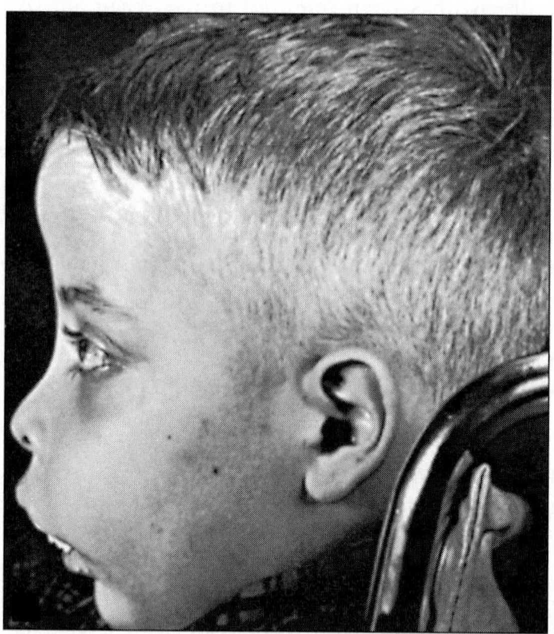

Massive expansion of the marrow of the face and skull produces characteristic facies. (Photo from Behrman, R. E., Kliegman, R. M., & Arvin, A. M. [Eds.]. [1996]. *Nelson textbook of pediatrics* [15th ed., p. 1402]. Philadelphia: W. B. Saunders.)

Nursing Diagnosis and Planning

The following nursing diagnoses and expected outcomes may be appropriate following assessment of the child with β-thalassemia.

- Inadequate Tissue Perfusion related to anemia. ***Expected Outcome:*** *The child will experience prompt resolution of severe anemia.*
- Body Image Disturbance related to altered appearance and the perception of having a chronic disease. ***Expected Outcome:*** *The child/family will verbalize feelings related to changes in appearance and the limitations imposed by the disease process.*
- Family Anxiety related to the diagnosis. ***Expected Outcome:*** *The child and/or family will express feelings about the disorder, lifestyle disruptions as a result of treatment, and possible genetic transmission of the disease.*
- Knowledge Deficit related to the disorder. ***Expected Outcome:*** *The child/family will verbalize an understanding of the disorder.*

Implementation

The nurse can expect to begin transfusions immediately in affected children while assessing for cardiovascular compromise from the anemia. Preparing the child and family for diagnostic procedures will help alleviate fears. Once the diagnosis is made, education should begin. Parents need to understand the importance of proper and ongoing follow-up. If bone marrow transplantation is offered as an option, parents will need support from the nursing staff as they make this decision. The family needs much support as they begin chelation therapy, which is very time-consuming and interferes with family routines (see Teaching Guidelines box). The nurse should routinely monitor the family's compliance with therapy.

If parents are considering having another child, genetic counseling should be offered to them. If both parents carry the defective gene, with each pregnancy, there is a 1 in 4 chance of having another child with the disease. Genetic counseling should also be made available to the affected child once he or she has reached maturity. If the child marries someone who carries the thalassemia gene,

TEACHING GUIDELINES *for Home Chelation Therapy*

SUBCUTANEOUS ROUTE VIA PORTABLE INFUSION PUMP

- Check needle security and placement.
- Check pump for proper infusion rate.
- Call the physician if the site becomes inflamed or painful.
- Check needle security throughout the day, especially when the child wakes from sleep.
- Call the physician/clinic/home health nurse if the infusion site becomes puffy, red, or painful.
- Call the physician/clinic/home health nurse if pump alarms cannot readily be reset.

INTRAVENOUS ROUTE: IMPLANTABLE INFUSION DEVICE*

- Teach the parent(s) to operate the intravenous pump.

*Assuming the infusion is begun in the clinic.

with each pregnancy there is a 1 in 4 chance of producing a child with β-thalassemia.

Referral should be made to the Cooley's Anemia Foundation (see Appendix H).

Evaluation

When evaluating a child with β-thalassemia, the following should be determined:

- Is the family compliant with the treatment plan?
- Is the child able to verbalize feelings associated with the treatment and/or the psychosocial implications of the disease?
- Has the family sought genetic counseling?
- Does the family readily verbalize feelings about having a child with β-thalassemia?
- Has the family sought information and support from the Cooley's Anemia Foundation?

HEMOPHILIA

Hemophilia is a lifelong, hereditary blood disorder with no cure. Until recently, the transfusion of replacement blood factors to prevent or stop episodes of bleeding was associated with the risk of contracting hepatitis or human immunodeficiency virus (HIV) because the blood factors were manufactured from pooled human plasma (Hilgartner et al., 1993). Advances in drug therapy preparations have now eliminated that risk.

Etiology and Incidence. Hemophilia is a sex-linked hereditary disorder carried on a gene on the X chromosome (see Chapter 2, Fig. 2–2). Male offspring inheriting the affected X chromosome are afflicted with the disorder. The gene may be silently carried for generations by women who never produce an affected male child, but typically, there is a history of hemophilia in the family. Rarely, female offspring are born with the disorder, but only if they inherit an affected gene from their mother and are the offspring of a father with hemophilia.

PATHOPHYSIOLOGY *of Hemophilia*

There are more than 10 factors in the blood that work in a sequence to produce blood clotting. Factor VIII, or antihemophiliac factor, and Factor IX, or plasma thromboplastin component, are the two missing or defective constituents in the blood that cause hemophilia A, or classic hemophilia, and hemophilia B, or Christmas disease. When these factors are missing or defective, blood does not clot as it should. The two disorders are inherited in the same way and have similar symptoms, and thus will be discussed as one disorder. Normal levels of Factor VIII and IX are 50–150%. The severity of the disease is classified as:

Severe	<1% factor activity
Moderate	1–5% factor activity
Mild	6–50% factor activity

Clinical Manifestations

- Disease severity that is individual, but tends to be familial
- Bleeding after surgery or serious trauma in all individuals with this disease
- Bleeding after tissue trauma in individuals with moderate and severe disease
- Bleeding for no apparent reason in individuals with severe disease
- Most commonly, bleeding in the muscles and joints, especially the knees for moderate and severe disease (Fig. 32–1)
- Commonly, recurrent bleeding in the same joint for severely affected patients
- Swelling, pain, and stiffness (bleeding symptoms)
- May have persistent bleeding only after surgery or trauma if mild form of disease

Children with hemophilia do not bleed greater or faster than normal people, they bleed longer.

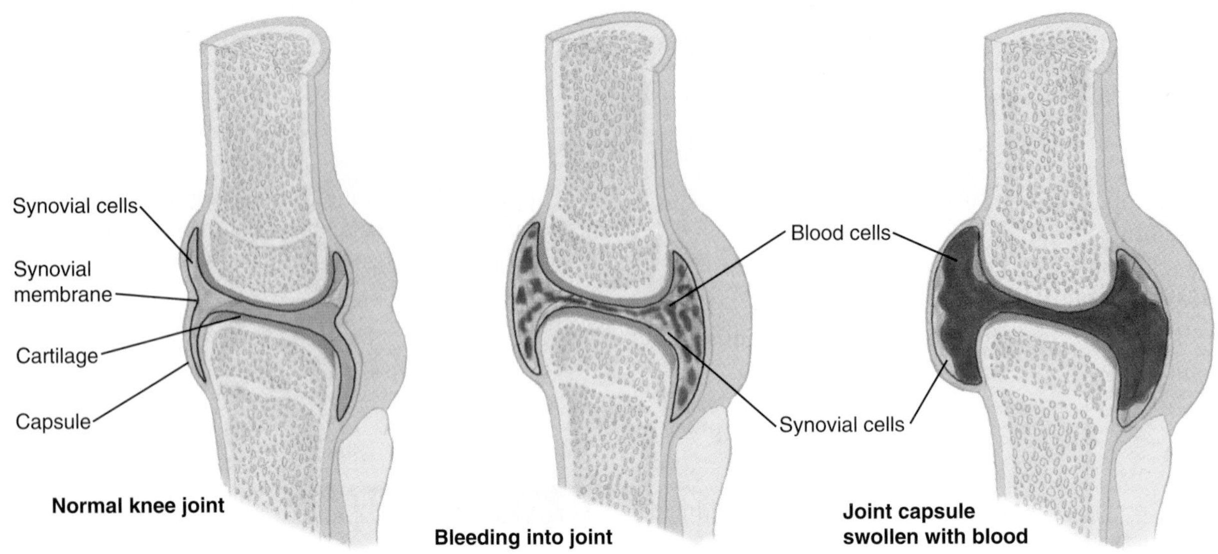

Figure 32–1
Hemarthrosis and joint destruction characteristic of hemophilia.

Diagnostic Evaluation. Hemophilia is sometimes, but not always, diagnosed following circumcision, at which time prolonged bleeding may be observed. Because the most common sites of bleeding are in the muscles and joints, diagnosis may be delayed until the toddler years, when the child becomes more active and the disease has an opportunity to manifest itself. A diagnostic work-up for the child suspected of having hemophilia includes a prothrombin test (PT), partial thromboplastin time (PTT), bleeding time, fibrinogen level, platelet count, quantitative immunoelectrophoretic assay, and factor VIII and factor IX assays.

Therapeutic Management. The management of hemophilia is very individual and depends on the severity of the illness. The purpose of therapy is to prevent excessive bleeding and tissue damage by supplying the body with the missing or ineffective factors (VIII or IX).

Previously, treatment involved transfusions of blood products or administration of freeze-dried products manufactured from blood products. One of the major risks associated with this factor replacement therapy was contracting hepatitis or acquired immunodeficiency syndrome (AIDS). Because of this risk, manufacturers began to heat-treat the blood factor to reduce the risk of viral transmission. Monoclonal products were then developed, and were found to be even safer than the heat-treated products. The most recent development in the treatment of hemophilia is the availability of recombinant antihemophiliac factor, which is derived not from human plasma, but is produced synthetically, from isolation of the gene. Recombinant factor eliminates the risk of transmission of viruses. The freeze-dried product is supplied with sterile water and must be reconstituted before being given IV.

Prophylactic therapy is now being started in infants and young children with severe hemophilia to prevent joint problems. Children ages 1 to 2 years receive factor replacement on a regular schedule if they develop clinical symptoms. Children with mild hemophilia A may be able to utilize desmopressin acetate (DDAVP) intranasal spray to stop bleeding. Children with hemophilia A and B can be given aminocaproic acid (Amicar) or tranexamic acid (Cyclokapron), oral medications that stabilize oral clots and can also sometimes stop nosebleeds.

> Acetylsalicylic (ASA) should not be given to children with factor disorders because it inhibits platelet function.

Aside from administration of factor, children with hemophilia must try to avoid activities that induce bleeding. For mild hemophilia, special precautions can be taken to protect joints, thereby allowing the patient to lead a more normal life. Prophylactic replacement therapy should also be given prior to surgery and some dental procedures. Bleeding is treated with rest, ice, elevation of the affected part, and compression.

NURSING CARE OF THE CHILD WITH HEMOPHILIA

Assessment

Neonatal nurses should frequently observe the circumcision site for prolonged bleeding. The physician should be notified if prolonged bleeding is observed.

Subjective data gathered on a child known to have hemophilia should include information about recent trauma and initial measures to stop bleeding, including how long pressure needed to be applied before the bleeding subsided. Other questions to ask include whether the swelling increased after the surface bleeding stopped, and whether swelling and stiffness occurred without apparent trauma.

Nurses should be alert to the possibility of hemophilia when the parents of a child just learning to crawl or walk express concern that their child bruises easily upon tumbling or falling down. Questions should be asked about previous cuts and scrapes to determine whether the child seemed to require more than the usual amount of pressure application or time for the bleeding to subside.

Nursing Diagnosis

The following nursing diagnoses may be appropriate following assessment of the child with hemophilia.

- Risk for Injury related to prolonged bleeding
- Knowledge Deficit related to diagnosis
- Ineffective Family/Individual Coping related to chronic illness and/or guilt

Planning, Implementation, and Evaluation: The Child With Hemophilia

NURSING DIAGNOSIS
- Risk for Injury related to prolonged bleeding

Expected Outcome:
- Bleeding resulting from injury will be recognized and controlled promptly to prevent permanent damage to tissue.

Intervention	Rationale
1. Assess the area of injury frequently for bleeding over a 24-hour period.	Bleeding may be prolonged and, especially in the case of head trauma, may not be manifested immediately.
2. Measure the injured joint for any change in size.	Joint measurement provides objective, rather than subjective, data for future comparisons.
3. In the case of head trauma, assess the child's level of consciousness and note any behavioral changes.	A decreased level of consciousness and unusual behaviors are early indicators of increased intracranial pressure secondary to hemorrhage.
4. Apply pressure to small superficial wounds and assess the area for subcutaneous bleeding.	Small wounds may ooze blood into the subcutaneous tissue.
5. Administer factor replacement as ordered by the physician.	Factor must be reconstituted just before infusion. It may be given prophylactically if the patient is at great risk for bleeding, as in head trauma, even if no bleeding is apparent.
6. Monitor factor levels as ordered.	With serious injuries warranting hospitalization, factor levels aid physicians in prescribing dosages and in establishing individual thresholds for a particular patient.
7. If a muscle or joint injury occurs, immobilize, elevate, and apply ice to the affected part, as ordered by the physician.	Initial immobilization will help prevent further injury until the bleeding resolves.
8. Offer suggestions for establishing a safe home environment for the child (see Teaching Guidelines for Home Care of the Child With Hemophilia).	A safe home environment will help prevent injuries.

Intervention	Rationale
9. Do not obtain temperature readings rectally.	Rectal thermometers may cause bleeding secondary to tissue trauma.
10. Provide for and expect behaviors consistent with normal growth and development for the child's age.	Parents may tend to overprotect or provide "special" treatment of their child. This unnecessarily limits the child's opportunities for normal psychosocial development and causes decreased self-esteem.

Evaluation: The child or parent:

- Experiences no serious bleeding from injury.
- Complies with the treatment regimen to prevent further injuries.
- Experiences no long-term complications from injury.
- Learns to balance the limitations imposed by the disease and a normal childhood.

NURSING DIAGNOSIS

- Knowledge Deficit related to diagnosis

Expected Outcome:

- The child/family will verbalize an understanding of the diagnosis and demonstrate compliance with the home care regimen.

Intervention	Rationale
1. Assess the child's/family's readiness for learning. Create an environment for learning.	Upon initial diagnosis, the family may need time to adjust to the diagnosis before they are ready to be educated. The appropriate setting for an educational session may be away from the child, so that parents will be able to focus on the information.
2. Upon initial diagnosis and with subsequent follow-up visits, spend time with the family explaining the diagnosis, its sequelae, and treatment. Offer written literature and/or educational tapes.	Education is ongoing and will need to be reinforced with stressed parents. Explaining the rationale for treatment and the disease's sequelae will better ensure compliance with therapy. Written or taped information can be reviewed later, when comprehension is likely to be improved.
3. Offer encouragement and praise for prompt parental recognition and response to bleeds.	Praise will reinforce behavior. Parents want to know they are doing the right things for their child.
4. Teach techniques for reconstitution and infusion of factor at home when the child is old enough for IV access to be established by the parents.	Ease of establishing IV access will depend on the child. Some parents will be able to establish IV access in their child. Many centers are using implantable infusion devices to ensure prompt IV access. Parents are taught techniques for accessing the port, infusing the factor, and heparinizing the port.
5. Topical anesthetics, such as EMLA, can be used when accessing infusion ports or peripheral sites.	The use of topical anesthetics decreases pain, thus causing less trauma.

Evaluation: The child/family:

- Promptly recognizes and reacts to bleeding.
- Safely administers factor replacement at home.

TEACHING GUIDELINES *for Home Care of the Child With Hemophilia*

- Apply prolonged pressure to superficial wounds until the bleeding has stopped.
- Call the physician in the event of blunt trauma, especially trauma involving the joints.
- Establish an age-appropriate, safe environment:
  - Pad table corners.
  - Pad crib rails.
  - Provide extra "joint" padding on clothes.
  - Remove items that can tip over or be pulled down on the child.
  - Do not leave a crawling or toddling child unattended.
- Instruct older children to avoid contact sports and to take precautions with other sports.
  - Pad knees and elbows for physical education class.
  - Use bicycle helmets for any sport in which head injury could occur.
- Call the physician if any head injury occurs.
- When parents are ready:
  - Teach IV line insertion.
  - Teach reconstitution and administration of factor.
- If the child has an implantable infusion device, teach the parents:
  - Site preparation.
  - Sterile technique for insertion of Huber needle.
  - Technique for verification of needle placement.
  - Administration of factor by IV push.
  - Saline and heparin flush.
  - Removal and proper disposal of needle.
- Stress the importance of immunizations, dental hygiene, and routine well-child care.
- Encourage the parents to allow the child to set his own limits of safety when possible.
- Provide for normal growth and development opportunities (safe activities, time with other children, limit-setting, independence).

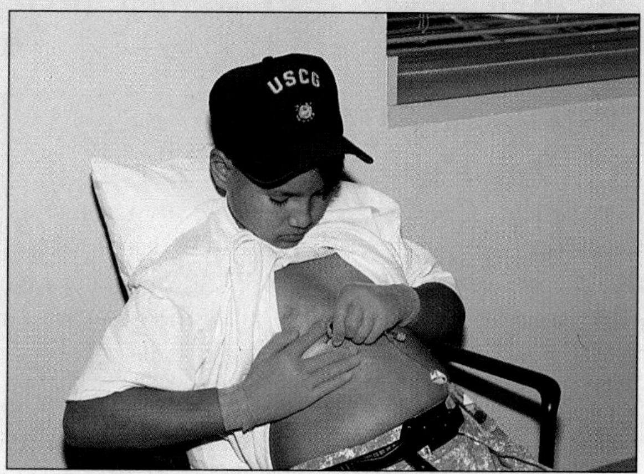

Control of deficient blood clotting in hemophilia requires injection of the missing clotting factors. This young man is injecting his factor into an implanted central venous access port. Sterile technique is essential. (Courtesy of the family of Jason Lee Davis)

NURSING DIAGNOSIS • Ineffective Family/Individual Coping related to chronic illness and guilt

Expected Outcome:
- The child will comply with the treatment plan.
- The family will verbalize concerns about the impact of the illness on their family.
- The child/family will utilize available support systems and community resources.

Intervention	Rationale
1. Teach the family the necessity of taking safety precautions, reacting cautiously to injury, administering medications properly, and following the treatment plan as outlined by health care providers. (See Teaching Guidelines for Home Care for the Child With Hemophilia.)	Conscientious adherence to the treatment regimen decreases the potential for long-term complications.
2. Listen and encourage the child and family to verbalize their feelings and express their concerns regarding hemophilia. Answer questions honestly and openly. Be particularly aware of feelings of guilt expressed by the mother.	Identifying concerns and clarifying misconceptions helps families to cope with the stress of chronic illness.

Intervention	Rationale
3. Introduce the family to other families of children with hemophilia.	Families of other children with hemophilia can offer support, suggestions, and strategies for dealing with problems.
4. Provide the family with the following address: National Hemophilia Foundation, The SoHo Bldg., 110 Greene St., Suite 406, New York, NY 10012.	Access to information and assistance can help the family deal with the sometimes overwhelming financial and emotional burdens of caring for a child with hemophilia, especially if complications occur.

Evaluation: The child/family will:

- Comply with the treatment plan.
- Utilize available resources.
- Balance increased limitations and normal childhood.

VON WILLEBRAND'S DISEASE

Von Willebrand's disease (VWD) is the most commonly inherited bleeding disorder. Because this disorder is less severe than hemophilia, it is less well known. There are at least three major varieties of VWD, classified on the basis of genetic and laboratory studies: type I, type IIA, and type IIB.

Pathophysiology. People with VWD have either underproduction of or dysfunction of von Willebrand protein. This protein carries factor VIII and binds platelets to damaged tissue. Depending upon the severity of the disorder, therapy may be required for increased bleeding.

Etiology. This is an autosomal, usually dominant, inherited disorder.

Clinical Manifestations. The clinical manifestations of VWD include the following:

- History of epistaxis
- Bleeding from the gums
- Prolonged bleeding from cuts
- Excessive bleeding following surgery or trauma
- Menorrhagia in females

Diagnostic Evaluation. A thorough history will ascertain whether the episode of bruising is compatible with the degree of trauma. A family history of bleeding disorders is important.

Laboratory tests may include a bleeding time and PTT, the results of which may be normal. The most clinically useful laboratory test for diagnosing this disorder is the quantitative immunoelectrophoretic assay, which in the presence of the disease, will reveal a discrepancy in the quantity and function of von Willebrand factor in the plasma.

Therapeutic Management. Therapy is aimed at replacing the missing or dysfunctional factor in the blood. In the past, cryoprecipitate or fresh-frozen plasma were given prior to surgery or following trauma with excessive bleeding. Presently, this treatment is only recommended if the cryoprecipitate is donated from a well-screened, unaffected family member or a repeat individual donor. The treatment of choice is DDAVP, which is administered intravenously or intranasally. The DDAVP products are given for type I and type IIA VWD only. In type IIB disease, DDAVP cannot be used, but high-purity (not monoclonal or recombinant) factor VIII products such as KOATE HP or Humate P can be administered (LaFon, 1995).

NURSING CARE OF THE CHILD WITH VON WILLEBRAND DISEASE

Assessment

A careful history detailing episodes of bruising and bleeding is essential. Possible causes of any previous episodes of bleeding, if any can be identified, should also be discussed. The nurse should ask how many times the child has experienced a nosebleed, how long the child bleeds from "normal" trauma, and whether there is a history of prolonged bleeding associated with surgery or trauma associated with prolonged bleeding.

Physical examination usually reveals a normal child except for evidence of bruising that is more excessive than expected for the degree of trauma experienced. If the child is being seen following a major bleeding episode, signs of hemorrhage and/or decreased hemoglobin level will be seen.

Nursing Diagnosis and Planning

The following nursing diagnoses and expected outcomes may be appropriate following assessment of the child with VWD.

- Risk for Injury (Hemorrhage) related to platelet adhesion dysfunction. ***Expected Outcome:*** *The child will experience no life-threatening episodes of hemorrhage.*

- Knowledge Deficit: related to disorder. ***Expected Outcome:*** *The child and/or family will verbalize an understanding of the disorder; accept the presence of a chronic disorder.*

Implementation

Education of the family is aimed at acquiring an understanding of the precautions to take with the child, as well as a knowledge of when prophylactic therapy should be given prior to elective procedures. The child should wear a Medic Alert tag at all times. The family should be referred to the Hemophilia Foundation for support services (see Appendix H.)

The degree of activity limitation will depend on the severity of the disorder. The child's limitations may include avoidance of contact sports, especially football.

Evaluation

When evaluating a child with VWD, the following should be determined:

- Are episodes of bleeding minimal and controlled?
- Is the family able to administer medications when necessary?
- Is the child able to participate in most childhood activities?

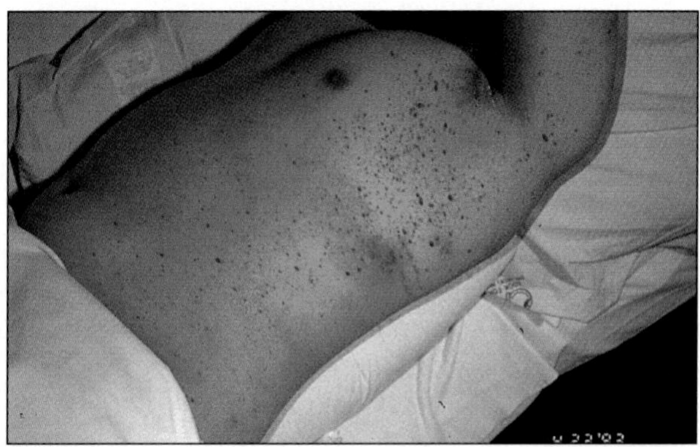

Figure 32–2
Multiple petechiae are characteristic of idiopathic thrombocytopenic purpura. This disorder results in the destruction of circulating platelets and decreased bone marrow production of new platelets. (Courtesy of Cook Children's Medical Center, Hematology-Oncology Clinic)

IDIOPATHIC THROMBOCYTOPENIC PURPURA

Idiopathic thrombocytopenic purpura (ITP) is a hematologic disorder resulting in a reduction in and destruction of platelets. This disorder may be seen by nurses in both inpatient and outpatient settings, depending on the severity of the illness.

Pathophysiology. ITP is an autoimmune disorder resulting in both a destruction of circulating platelets and a decreased production of platelets by the bone marrow. ITP may be acute and self-limiting, or it may be chronic, requiring therapy.

Etiology/Incidence. The cause of ITP is unknown, but it typically occurs 1 to 3 weeks after a febrile, viral illness. The peak age for ITP is 2 to 4 years, and it occurs with equal frequency in male and female patients (Nathan & Oski, 1993).

Clinical Manifestations. The clinical manifestations of ITP include the following:

- Excessive bruising
- Petechiae, especially involving the mucous membranes and sclera (Fig. 32–2)

Diagnostic Evaluation. The initial diagnostic evaluation should include a thorough history and a CBC. The history should include information about any medications the child has taken that could cause thrombocytopenia, and any incidence of illness, especially febrile illness, in the past month. In an affected child, the initial CBC will reveal a low platelet count, often less than 50,000, but the results will otherwise be normal.

If any data in the history or CBC suggest ITP, the physician may order a bone marrow aspirate to rule out an oncologic disorder, and to determine whether megakaryocytes, which are precursors of platelets, are present.

Physical examination of the affected child reveals bruising and petechiae, the severity of which depends on how low the platelet count is and the tolerance of the child to the low platelet count. The spleen and liver are generally normal in size. The greatest risk of a low platelet count is intracranial hemorrhage, so a neurologic assessment is important.

Therapeutic Management. The goal of treatment is to prevent excessive bleeding, especially intracranial bleeding. Therefore, the treatment plan is dependent upon the severity of the thrombocytopenia. Most cases are self-limiting, with a normal platelet count returning within 6 months with no therapy (Gerritsma et al., 1994). However, some physicians prefer to initiate treatment at the time of diagnosis.

Depending on whether the child is an inpatient or outpatient, IV or p.o. steroids may be administered over a 2- to 4-week period. For unknown reasons, the steroids block the autoimmune destruction of platelets. The other drug that may be used to treat ITP is IVIG, which is given once a day for 3 to 5 days. Often, after the first dose of IVIG, the next morning's platelet count is dramatically increased.

ITP is considered to be "acute" if recovery of a normal platelet count is seen within 6 months. The condition becomes chronic if it lasts longer than 6 months (Gerritsma et al., 1994). Children with chronic ITP may initially respond to steroids with an increase in platelet count, but it will not reach normal levels. These children may go for long periods without experiencing problems with excessive bleeding or a low platelet count; the count will then begin to decline again, at which time steroid therapy should be resumed.

When steroids and IVIG do not control the thrombocytopenia in a child with chronic ITP, a splenectomy may be indicated. Splenectomy will cure most children with chronic ITP because the spleen synthesizes the antiplatelet antibody that results in the destruction of circulating platelets. The risk associated with removal of the spleen is sepsis from those organisms that the spleen's **reticuloendothelial system** fights. Without the spleen, the body's ability to fight *Streptococcus pneumoniae, Haemophilus influenzae,* and *Neisseria meningitidis* is limited. This limitation is greater in children younger than 5 years of age, so ITP is managed without splenectomy, if possible, until age 5. Platelet transfusions are given only in children with very low platelet counts, or when active, uncontrolled bleeding occurs.

NURSING CARE OF THE CHILD WITH IDIOPATHIC THROMBOCYTOPENIC PURPURA

Assessment

Parents usually bring their child to the doctor because they have noticed excessive bruising or a "red rash" in the child's mouth or on the child's body. Although this "rash" may look remarkable to a nurse, it often evolves so gradually that it escapes the immediate notice of the parent who sees the child every day. As a result, health care may not be sought until very significant bruising and petechiae, even hematomas, are present. Affected children usually demonstrate normal activity levels for their age, as they do not "feel bad." Assessment should include observation for signs of any further bruising or bleeding, including epistaxis, hematuria, or blood in the stools, as well as for signs of a decreasing level of consciousness, which could indicate intracranial hemorrhage.

Nursing Diagnosis and Planning

The following nursing diagnoses and expected outcomes may be appropriate following assessment of the child with ITP.

- Risk for Injury (Hemorrhage) related to low platelet count. ***Expected Outcome:*** *The child will exhibit no signs of active bleeding or intracranial hemorrhage.*
- Knowledge Deficit related to the disorder and its therapeutic management. ***Expected Outcome:*** *The child/family will verbalize an understanding of ITP and the treatment plan.*
- Risk for Infection related to chronic use of steroids and/or splenectomy. ***Expected Outcome:*** *The child will respond rapidly to treatment for infections.*

Implementation

The implementation of nursing care centers around carrying out physician-ordered treatments, restricting activities which could result in increased bleeding, and educating the family about ITP and home care.

Usually, an IV line is established for the purpose of administering IV steroids or IVIG. Children with ITP can be among the most challenging in terms of establishing IV access because merely puncturing the skin may result in a hematoma, which may be confused with "blowing" the vein. Careful flushing of the IV catheter with normal saline will confirm proper placement of the catheter.

> In children with low platelet counts, ASA should not be given, rectal temperatures should be avoided, and invasive procedures should be performed with extreme caution.

Restricting the activity of a toddler can be a real challenge. Physicians may hospitalize these children just for

TEACHING GUIDELINES *for Home Care of the Child With Idiopathic Thrombocytopenic Purpura*

- Eliminate participation in contact sports, bicycle riding, roller skating, and diving if the child's platelet count is low.
- Use a soft-bristle toothbrush if the platelet count is less than 20,000/mm^3.
- Establish an age-appropriate, safe home environment.
- Pad table corners.
- Pad crib rails.
- Offer extra "joint" padding on clothes.
- Do not leave a crawling or toddling child unattended.

that purpose. Soft-bristled toothbrushes or toothettes should be used on all children whose platelet count is less than 20,000/mm^3. Until the platelet count returns to normal, activities such as bicycle riding, contact sports, diving, and roller skating, should be curtailed.

Education includes teaching the family about the disease process of ITP; the side effects of steroids and IVIG, if used; the necessity of restricting the child's activity; and the importance of proper follow-up evaluations, which usually include weekly platelet counts. Parents should be made aware of the signs and symptoms of infection, as steroids may mask a fever. (See also Teaching Guidelines for Home Care of the Child With Idiopathic Thrombocytopenic Purpura.)

If the child has had a splenectomy, pneumococcus vaccine and/or daily penicillin should be administered. Any signs and symptoms of infection should be reported immediately to the physician so that proper therapy can be initiated before the infection becomes life-threatening.

Very few patients have thrombocytopenia that does not respond to any of the treatments just discussed. Those patients who do not respond to treatment will require additional diagnostic testing and second-line therapeutic regimens.

Evaluation

When evaluating a child with ITP, the nurse should determine the following:

- Have areas of ecchymosis and petechiae been decreased?
- Does the family verbalize and implement a plan of care that decreases the risk of the child incurring an injury that is likely to cause hemorrhage?
- Does the family respond quickly to early signs of infection by notifying the primary health care provider?

DISSEMINATED INTRAVASCULAR COAGULATION

Disseminated intravascular coagulation (DIC) is the abnormal activation of the normal clotting mechanisms in the body. In children, DIC occurs without the overwhelming mortality that is seen in adults. The key to recovery is identification and treatment of the cause of the DIC.

Etiology. DIC is triggered by any factor that causes endothelial damage, liberation of tissue thromboplastin, circulating endotoxins, or immune complexes. In children, some of the most common causes are trauma, hypoxia, necrotizing enterocolitis, shock, liver disease, viral or bacterial infections, and acute promyelocytic leukemia.

PATHOPHYSIOLOGY *of Disseminated Intravascular Coagulation*

The pathophysiology of DIC is very complicated and often is not easily understood as both excessive bleeding and excessive clotting are occurring at the same time. The syndrome of DIC leads to the depletion of platelets and clotting proteins and deposition of platelet and fibrin plugs in the vasculature.

The process of blood clotting follows either an intrinsic or extrinsic pathway (O'Brian & Woods, 1978). Either pathway leads ultimately to prothrombin forming thrombin, which, in the presence of fibrogen, forms fibrin. Fibrinolysis, or clot destruction, requires the presence of thrombin. During this process, the enzyme plasmin lyses fibrin into fragments called fibrin degradation products (FDPs) which interfere with the ability of platelets to adhere to one another. In DIC, initiation of the clotting process is stimulated by endothelial damage or some kind of tissue injury. Platelets and clotting factors are depleted. As clotting is stimulated, the body perceives the need to produce substances to dissolve those clots, and there is an increase in the end-result of clot lysis, FDPs. The overstimulation of both of these normal processes has three major effects on the body: (1) increased, uncontrolled bleeding resulting from the depletion of platelets and clotting factors and overstimulation of the fibrinolytic process, (2) anemia caused by the excessive bleeding and the mechanical fragmentation of RBCs, and (3) organ damage secondary to the formation of emboli.

Although the severity of DIC cannot be predicted, most authorities believe that DIC occurs, to some degree, in all seriously ill infants and children.

Clinical Manifestations. The clinical manifestations of DIC are as follows:

At the Onset of Disease

- Insidious onset corresponding to platelet count and fibrinogen levels
- Excessive bruising
- Oozing from skin puncture sites
- Oozing from sites of mild tissue trauma (e.g., insertion of a nasogastric tube)
- Mild gastrointestinal bleeding

Upon Disease Progression

- Purpural rash
- Worsening of bleeding

Confirmatory Laboratory Findings in the Diagnosis of Disseminated Intravascular Coagulation

- Low platelet count noted on CBC
- RBC fragments on the smear
- Decreased RBCs count
- Prolonged prothrombin time
- Prolonged partial thromboplastin time
- Decreased fibrinogen level
- Elevated levels of fibrin degradation products
- Elevated levels of D-dimer

- Hemoptysis
- Hypoxemia
- Oliguria progressing to renal failure
- Intracranial hemorrhage
- Progressive organ failure

Diagnostic Evaluation. The diagnosis of DIC is confirmed by laboratory testing (see accompanying box).

Therapeutic Management. In order to control DIC, the underlying cause of the condition must first be treated. Treatment then becomes symptomatic. The depleted factors are replaced. Fresh frozen plasma (FFP) is given to normalize the PTT by replacing fibrinogen, prothrombin, and clotting factors. Washed, packed RBCs replace the cells lost in hemorrhage. Exchange transfusions may be used in neonates because they cannot tolerate the excessive fluid volume required to ensure replacement of the platelets, clotting factors, and RBCs by replacement products. Vitamin K is given to normalize the PT. The most familiar drug used to dissolve clots is heparin. However, heparin therapy is almost never used to treat DIC in children except in DIC associated with acute promyelocytic leukemia.

NURSING CARE OF THE CHILD WITH DISSEMINATED INTRAVASCULAR COAGULATION

Assessment

DIC typically develops in a child who is already hospitalized. The subjective and objective data assessed will depend entirely on the initial illness. The nurse must be cognizant of the patient who is at risk for DIC. Any evidence of bleeding at any site of interruption in integument and at every orifice should be assessed. The nurse should also note any changes in the pattern of vital signs. Adequate tissue perfusion should be confirmed, as normal function of an organ is the end result of sufficient oxygenation of that organ. Children with full clinical manifestations of DIC are typically cared for in an intensive care unit.

Nursing Diagnosis and Planning

The following nursing diagnoses and expected outcomes may be appropriate following assessment of the child with DIC.

- Risk for Injury (Hemorrhage) related to depletion of clotting factors and platelets and increased circulating FDPs. ***Expected Outcome:*** *The child will receive prompt treatment for bleeding.*
- Risk for Injury (Organ Damage) related to emboli formation obstructing adequate blood flow. ***Expected Outcome:*** *The child will continue to have proper organ function.*
- Anxiety (Family) related to illness. ***Expected Outcome:*** *The family will demonstrate positive coping mechanisms.*

Implementation

Any areas of active bleeding should be located promptly and pressure applied, if possible. Care should be taken to avoid any unnecessary contact with tissue. IV lines and tubes should be protected to eliminate the additional trauma caused by their reinsertion. Frequent monitoring of vital signs is necessary in order to identify changing patterns. Laboratory results are also monitored carefully. Physician orders are followed with regard to medicines and treatments. Because hypoxemia and acidosis may actually cause DIC, care is taken to provide adequate ventilation in patients with compromised respiration. The morbidity and mortality of children with DIC depend on the underlying causative condition. With prompt recognition of both the cause of DIC and its diagnosis, and with proper management of both, these children usually have favorable outcomes.

Evaluation

When evaluating a child with DIC, the following questions should be asked by the nurse caring for the child at the time of diagnosis:

- Were early signs of DIC identified and the child transferred to an intensive care unit for specialized care?
- Was the family supported and kept informed of the child's condition?
- Are the child's organs functioning?

APLASTIC ANEMIA

Aplastic anemia, or aplastic **pancytopenia,** is a condition affecting both children and adults in which the bone marrow ceases production of the cells it normally manufactures. The result is peripheral **pancytopenia.**

Etiology/Incidence. Aplastic anemia can be either congenital, acquired, or idiopathic. Several rare, inheritable disor-

PATHOPHYSIOLOGY *of Aplastic Anemia*

Aplastic anemia is characterized by cessation of **hematopoiesis** by the bone marrow of **granulocytes,** erythrocytes, and platelets. The disease may be classified as mild, moderate, or severe depending on how low the values are for absolute neutrophil count, platelet count, and absolute reticulocyte count. There are no specific criteria by which to differentiate mild from moderate disease. Even the distinction between moderate and severe disease has been subject to differing definitions in the literature (Khatib et al., 1994).

ders are characterized by aplastic anemia, the most common of which is Fanconi's anemia. Aplastic anemia can also be acquired and a number of agents and conditions have been implicated. These most often include drugs or chemicals and less often radiation exposure, viruses, and immune diseases. Most pediatric cases of aplastic anemia are idiopathic. If the disease is acquired, the causative agent damages the bone marrow, preventing the development of granulocytes, RBCs, and platelets. Aside from antineoplastic agents, the drug used in pediatrics that most commonly causes aplastic anemia is chloramphenicol. Acquired aplastic anemia has a poorer prognosis with a more rapid progression than the primary types.

Annually, in the United States and Europe, the incidence of aplastic anemia is 2 to 6 cases/million. Leukemia, by comparison, has an incidence of 50 cases/million/year (Nathan & Oski, 1993).

Clinical Manifestations. The clinical manifestations of aplastic anemia include the following:

- Petechiae
- Bruising
- Pallor
- Fatigue
- Tachycardia
- Decreased RBC, granulocyte, and platelet counts
- Infection
- Less commonly, major bleeding

Diagnostic Evaluation. Although the diagnosis of aplastic anemia may be suspected from the child's history and the results of a CBC, a bone marrow biopsy must be performed to confirm the diagnosis. Biopsy results should reveal the presence or absence of precursors for the mature cells found in a peripheral blood sample. In aplastic anemia, these precursors are notably absent from the marrow sample. Therefore, the marrow is hypocellular and contains a predominance of lymphocytes.

Therapeutic Management. If the aplastic anemia is determined by history to be acquired, exposure to the causative agent is discontinued immediately. Treatment then is based on symptoms. Platelet and RBC transfusions may be ordered. Granulocyte transfusions are not used owing to their short life span in the circulation. If symptoms of infection are present, antibiotics are administered after appropriate cultures are obtained.

Drugs used to treat aplastic anemia include steroids, cyclosporin, and antithymocyte globulin (ATG) and antilymphocyte globulin (ALG), to which patients can have serious reactions. Some patients are treated with colony-stimulating factors.

Although the drugs just mentioned are usually tried first, allogeneic bone marrow transplantation remains the treatment of choice for patients with severe aplastic anemia for whom a suitable donor has been identified (Khatib, Wilimas, & Wang, 1994). See Chapter 33 for a discussion of bone marrow transplantation.

NURSING CARE OF THE CHILD WITH APLASTIC ANEMIA

Assessment

Subjective assessment usually reveals parents' observations of bruising immediately after an event that would not normally result in a bruise. An observant parent may have noticed petechiae in the child's mouth while assisting the child to brush his teeth. Information should be elicited about drugs recently taken or recent exposures to environmental substances outside the child's usual realm in an effort to determine possible drug- or chemical-related causes for the pancytopenia.

Petechiae, bruising, pallor, lethargy, and tachycardia are the usual abnormal findings, and these are directly related to the degree of pancytopenia. Otherwise, the results of the physical assessment are usually normal.

Nursing Diagnosis and Planning

The following nursing diagnoses and expected outcomes may be appropriate following assessment of the child with aplastic anemia.

- Risk for Infection related to granulocytopenia. ***Expected Outcome:*** *The child will remain free of infection.*
- Risk for Injury (Bleeding) related to thrombocytopenia. ***Expected Outcome:*** *The child will not experience episodes of major bleeding.*
- Impaired Tissue Perfusion related to anemia. ***Expected Outcome:*** *The child's demand for oxygen will be balanced with the body's supply.*
- Knowledge Deficit related to the disease process. ***Expected Outcome:*** *The child and/or family will verbalize an understanding of the disease process and its potential complications.*

Implementation

Nursing care is initially focused on preventing any serious physiologic sequelae of pancytopenia. Because of the increased risk of bacterial infection, affected patients should be assigned to private rooms; depending on the severity of the granulocytopenia, reverse isolation may be warranted. Precautionary measures should be taken, as for any patient with a low platelet count, including no injections, no rectal temperatures, use of a soft-bristled toothbrush or toothette, abstinence from any contact sports or activity, and periodic assessment for increased bleeding.

Physicians' orders should be followed with regard to transfusions, cultures, and antibiotics. Usually, the platelet count will be maintained at a level greater than 20,000/mm^3 to prevent intracranial hemorrhage. The hemoglobin is typically maintained at a level greater than 7 g/dl. If any symptoms of infection are present, a blood culture should be drawn. The need for cultures of other sites will depend on the patient's symptoms.

> Patients with a low WBC count will not produce pus, which is a usual sign of infection.

Antibiotics should be administered immediately in a febrile patient with granulocytopenia owing to the risk for rapid, overwhelming sepsis. Children who are hospitalized, febrile, and granulocytopenic should be assessed frequently for signs of septic shock, including quality of peripheral pulses compared to central pulses, extremity temperature, capillary refill, and vital signs.

Education of the family and patient should include information about the disease process and the complications that should be reported promptly to the physician. If the decision is made to transplant the patient, intense pretransplant education is indicated.

Follow-up studies should include frequent CBCs and physical examinations, at least weekly, whether the patient is discharged from the hospital after spontaneous recovery or following a bone marrow transplant.

Evaluation

In evaluating the child with aplastic anemia, the nurse should ask the following questions:

- Has the family received instruction regarding the disease and home care?
- Has the child remained free from infection?

KEY CONCEPTS

- Caring for children with blood disorders requires an understanding of the anatomy and physiology of blood and blood-forming tissues, of genetics; and of the care of children with a chronic disease.
- In order for RBCs to carry oxygen, there must be an adequate amount of hemoglobin, the level of which is dependent upon sufficient circulating iron.
- Anemia results from blood loss, decreased production of RBCs or hemoglobin, or increased destruction of RBCs.
- The number of RBCs varies according to age, gender, and the altitude at which a person lives.
- Iron deficiency anemia can largely be prevented by teaching parents the importance of providing iron-fortified formula to children until the age of 12 months.
- Morphine is the drug of choice for children with pain secondary to a "painful episode" associated with sickle cell disease.
- Complications associated with sickle cell anemia can be reduced through early screening, parent/child education, routine immunizations, pneumococcal and influenza immunizations, penicillin prophylaxis, and early diagnosis and management of complications.
- Children with decreased platelets and factor disorders should not receive ASA or have their temperature taken rectally. Invasive procedures should be done only when necessary, and then only with extreme caution to avoid hemorrhage.
- Factor prophylaxis is warranted in infants and young children with hemophilia who are at risk for developing joint problems secondary to bleeding.
- Educating the family of a child with ITP about the need to restrict activity and to provide protection is a major nursing challenge.
- Bleeding associated with hemophilia is treated with rest, ice, elevation, compression, and factor replacement as necessary.
- Education of the family about home care for the child with hemophilia should include information on the management of bleeding episodes, environmental safety, administration of medications, health promotion, and normal growth and development.

REFERENCES

Behrman, R. E., Kliegman, R. M., & Arvin, A. (Eds.). (1996). *Nelson textbook of pediatrics* (15th ed). Philadelphia: W. B. Saunders.

Benitz, W. E., & Tatro, D. S. (1988). *The pediatric drug handbook.* Chicago: Year Book Medical Publishers.

Bray, G. L., Muenz, L., Makis, N., & Lessin, L. S. (1994). Assessing clinical severity in children with sickle cell disease. *American Journal of Pediatric Hematology/Oncology, 16*(1), 50–54.

Chow, M. P., Durand, B. A., Feldman, M. N., & Mills, M. A. (1984). *Handbook of pediatric primary care.* New York: John Wiley and Sons.

Gerritsma, H., Schmid, A., Luethy, A. R., Leibundgut, K., Gugler, E., Wagner, H. P., & Hirt, A. (1994). Megakaryocyte growth in vitro predicts outcome in idiopathic thrombocytopenic purpura. *American Journal of Pediatric Hematology/Oncology, 16*(3), 194–199.

Hilgartner, M. W., Donfield, S. M., Willoughby, A., Contant, C. F., Evatt, B. L., Gomperts, E. D., Hoots, W. K., Jason, J., Loveland, K. A., McKinlay, S. M., & Stehbens, J. A. (1993). Hemophilia growth and development study. *American Journal of Pediatric Hematology/Oncology, 15*(2), 208–218.

Johnstone, H. (1996). Thalassemia. In Burg, F., Ingelfinger, J., Wald, E, & Polin, R. (Eds.), *Gellis and Kagan's current pediatric therapy* (pp. 282–283), Philadelphia: W. B. Saunders.

Khatib, Z., Wilimas, J., & Wang, W. (1994). Outcome of moderate aplastic anemia in children. *American Journal of Pediatric Hematology/Oncology, 16*(1), 80–85.

LaFon, J. (1995). *Exploring von Willebrand disease* (pp. 8–11). New York: The National Hemophilia Association.

Martin, M. B., & Butler, R. B. (1993). Understanding the basics of α-thalassemia major. *Pediatric Nursing, 19*(2), 143–145.

Nathan, D. G., & Oski, F. A. (Eds). (1993). *Hematology of infancy and childhood* (4th ed.). Philadelphia: W. B. Saunders.

O'Brian, B. S., & Woods, S. (1978). The paradox of DIC. *American Journal of Nursing, 78*(11), 1878–1880.

Selekman, J. (1993). Update: New guidelines for the treatment of infants with sickle cell disease. *Pediatric Nursing, 19*(6), 600–605.

Vichinsky, E. P. (1991). Comprehensive care in sickle cell disease: Its impact on morbidity and mortality. *Seminars in Hematology, 28*(2), 220–226.

West, T. B., West, D. W., & Ohene-Frempong, K. (1994). The presentation, frequency, and outcome of bacteremia among children with sickle cell disease and fever. *Pediatric Emergency Care, 10*(3), 141–143.

BIBLIOGRAPHY

Bailes, B. K. (1992). Disseminated intravascular coagulation. *AORN Journal, 55*(2), 517–528.

Brewin-Wilson, D. A. (1989). Transient erythroblastopenia of childhood: Implications for nurse practitioners. *Journal of Pediatric Health Care, 3*(4), 200–203.

Buchanan, G. R. (1993). Sickle cell disease: Recent advances. *Current Problems in Pediatrics, 23*(6), 219–229.

Day, S., Dancy, R., Kelly, K., & Wang, W. (1993). Iron overload? In sickle cell disease? *Maternal-Child Nursing, 18,* 330–335.

Drotar, D. O., Agle, D. P., Eckl, C. L., & Thompson, P. A. (1995). Psychological response to HIV positivity in hemophilia. *Pediatrics, 96*(6), 1062–1069.

Ehlers, K. H., Giardina, O. J., Lesser, M. L., Engle, M. A., & Hilgartner, M. W. (1991). Prolonged survival in patients with beta-thalassemia major treated with deferoxamine. *The Journal of Pediatrics, 118*(4), 540–545.

Hilgartner, M. W., & Pochedly, C. (Eds.). (1989). *Hemophilia in the child and adult.* New York: Raven Press.

Jones, P. K., & Ratnoff, O. D. (1991). The changing prognosis of classic hemophilia (factor VIII "deficiency"). *Annals of Internal Medicine, 114*(8), 641–648.

Loupe, D. E. (1989). Breaking the sickle cycle. *Science News, 136,* 360–362.

Lucarelli, G., Galimberti, M., Polchi, P., Angelucci, E., Baronciani, D., Giardini, C., Politi, P., Durazzi, S., Muretto, P., & Albertini, F. (1990). Bone marrow transplantation patients with thalassemia. *New England Journal of Medicine, 322*(7), 417–421.

Miller, C. (1992). *Inheritance of hemophilia.* New York: National Hemophilia Foundation.

Miller, R., & Berman, B. (1994). Transient erythroblastopenia of childhood in infants less than 6 months of age. *American Journal of Pediatric Hematology/Oncology, 16*(3), 246–248.

Morrison, R. A., & Vedro, D. A. (1989). Pain management in the child with sickle cell disease. *Pediatric Nursing, 15*(6), 595–599.

National Hemophilia Foundation. (1990). Your child and hemophilia. New York: Author.

National Hemophilia Foundation. (1991). What you should know about hemophilia. New York: Author.

Samuels, X., & Reid, J. (1994). Common problems in sickle cell disease. *American Family Physician, 49*(6), 1477–1486.

Sporrer, K. A., Jackson, S. M., Agner, S., Laver, J., & Abboud, M. R. (1994). Pain in children and adolescents with sickle cell anemia: A prospective study utilizing self-reporting. *American Journal of Pediatric Hematology/Oncology, 16*(3), 219–224.

Tamary, H., Kaplinsky, C., Shuartzmayer, S., Umiel, T., Pecht, M., Levin, S., & Zaizov, R. (1993). Transient erythroblastopenia of childhood. *American Journal of Pediatric Hematology/Oncology, 15*(4), 386–391.

U.S. Department of Health and Human Services, The Agency for Health Care Policy & Research. (1993). Sickle cell disease: Screening, diagnosis, management, and counseling in newborns and infants. Rockville, MD: Author.

Zappa, S. (1994/1995, Winter). A topical anesthetic and hemophilia care. *Nursing Network/Psychosocial News,* 5,6.

Zipursky, A., Chachula, D. M., & Brown, E. J. (1993). The reversibly sickled cell. *American Journal of Pediatric Hematology/Oncology, 15*(2), 219–225.

33

The Child With Cancer

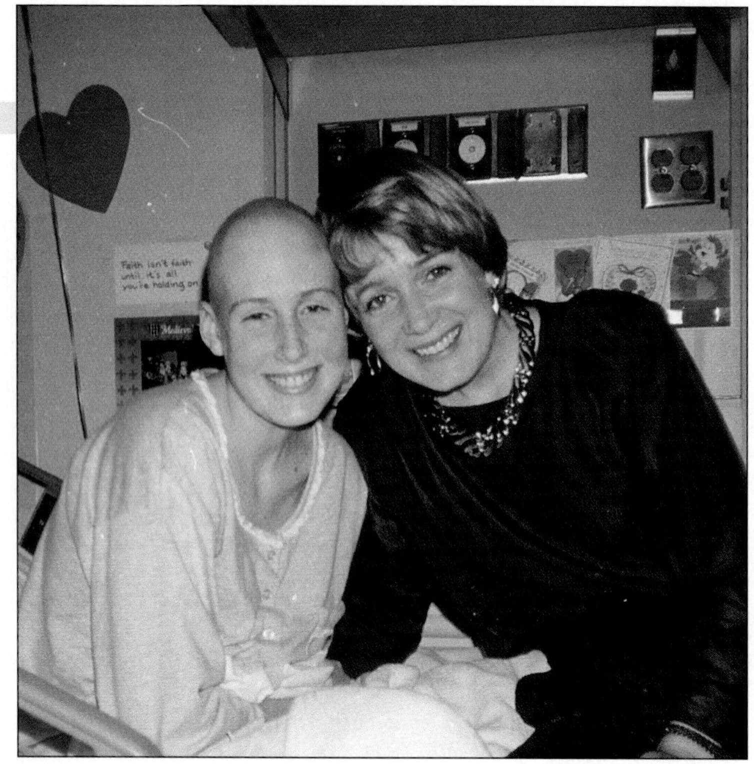

Courtesy of Cook Children's Medical Center, Fort Worth, Texas

CHAPTER OVERVIEW

LEARNING OBJECTIVES

After studying this chapter, you should be able to:

- List common clinical manifestations of childhood cancer.
- Discuss the therapies used in the treatment of cancer.
- Demonstrate an understanding of the nursing care associated with caring for a child with cancer.
- Discuss bone marrow transplantation in children.
- Describe the nursing care related to postoperative care of a child with a brain tumor.

KEY TERMS

blast cells: immature lymphocytes not normally present in peripheral blood

cellular immunity: immunologic response to an antigen that results in increased production of T-lymphocytes by the thymus

clean margins: evidence of normal, disease-free tissue in the outermost layer of cells of a surgical sample

hepatosplenomegaly: enlargement of the liver and spleen detected by palpation of the abdomen

humoral immunity: immunologic response to an antigen, resulting in production of B-lymphocytes

immunosuppression: a weakening or cessation of the body's normal immune response

intrathecal: within the spinal column

lymphadenopathy: swelling of the lymph nodes detected by palpation

neutropenia: decrease in the number of circulating neutrophils, which results in a decreased ability of the body to fight infection

protocol: a systematic plan of care outlining drug therapy and follow-up care based on research in cancer therapy

thrombocyte: platelet; necessary for blood clotting

Although childhood cancer is not common, it is the second leading cause of death in children. It is often difficult to diagnose, and health care providers must be aware of the clinical manifestations that provide an index of suspicion. The signs and symptoms the child shows depend on the child's age, the type of tumor, and the extent of the disease (Leonard, 1993). In a very short time, the child may have numerous tests, be diagnosed, and begin treatment. This can be devastating to both the child and the family. It may seem like a bad dream to the parents. The nurse becomes the lifeline for the child and the family as they go through the treatment process.

Pediatric oncology is an important subspecialty within nursing. Nurses who work with children who have cancer play an important role in the lives of those children. They support and educate the children and their families as they move through a process that is not only stressful, but also long-term. Nurses working in pediatric oncology are challenged to maintain a high level of technical competence and an ability to provide the psychological support required by the child and family. Working with children with cancer can be an emotional experience, and the nurse in this setting must have a support system and be aware of her limitations.

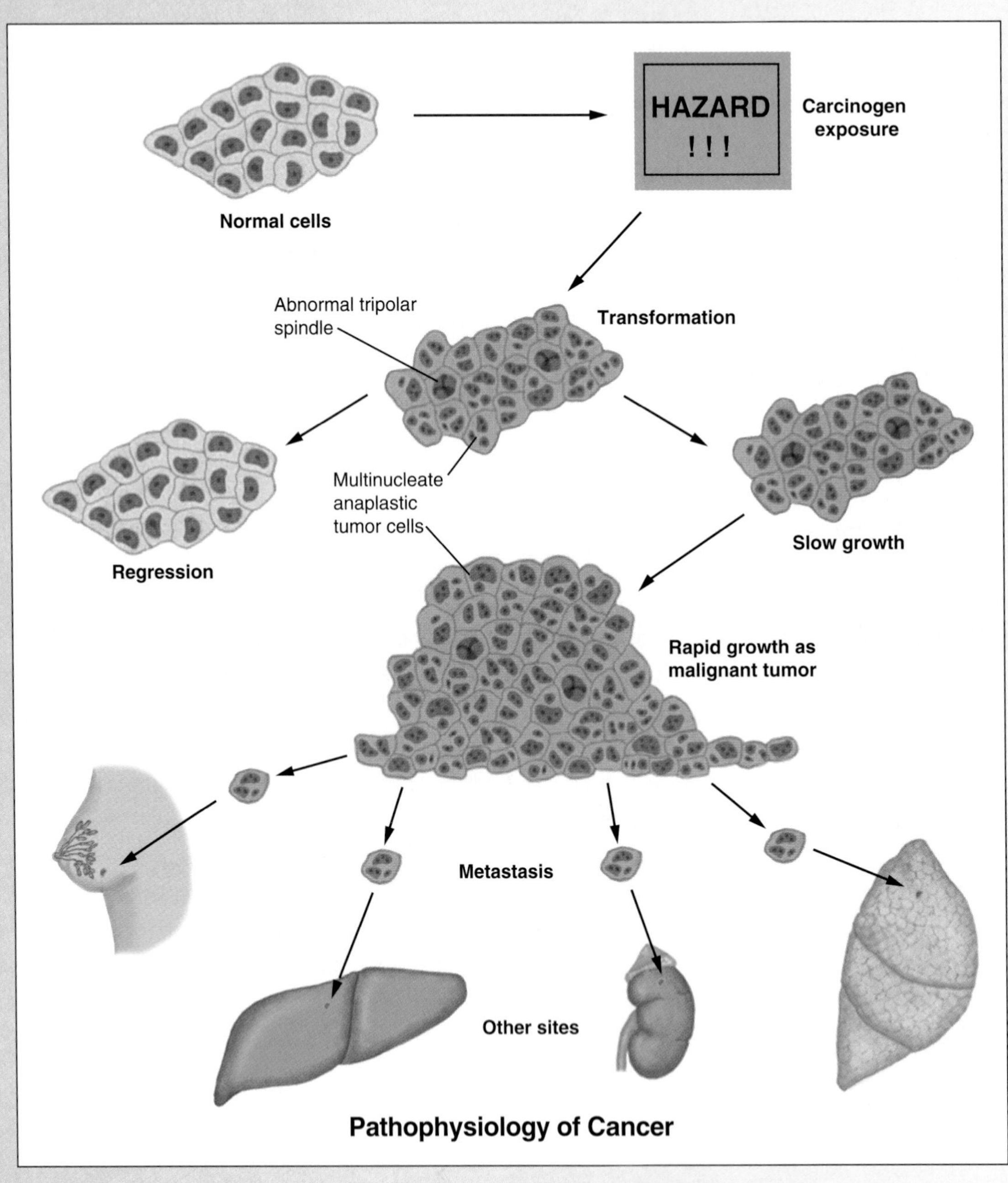

Pathophysiology of Cancer

REVIEW OF CANCER

A neoplasm is any tumor that arises from new, abnormal growth. Whereas a tumor may be either benign or malignant, a cancer is always malignant. The cancerous cells grow progressively; they have lost the ability to perform their intended functions because changes in the cell's DNA result in "wrong" information being transmitted. The cells therefore continue to proliferate.

It is currently believed that in cancer the immune system fails to provide the necessary cellular control; in a healthy immune system the aberrant cells will be identified and destroyed. There may be chemically induced cell suppression, as can occur with certain drugs, such as corticosteroids, or various viral diseases may underlie the cancer. Radiation, physical irritation, and heredity may contribute to the development of cancer. The malignant cells draw nourishment away from normal cells, eventually starving them out and replacing them.

Cancer cells spread in one of two ways: (1) by *invasion*, in which those cells grow in unrestricted disorderly fashion at the site of origin; and (2) by *metastasis*, in which the cells grow in sites other than the site of the primary cancer.

Based on the results of diagnostic studies and surgical examination, a tumor is staged. Staging describes the extent of disease locally, regionally, and systematically, and in most solid tumors guides the therapy (Leonard, 1993). Each tumor has its own specific system of staging, which assists in determination of treatment and prognosis.

Cardinal Signs and Symptoms of Cancer in Children

OVERT SIGNS AND SYMPTOMS

- A mass
- Purpura
- Pallor
- Weight loss
- Squint or change in the eye
- Vomiting in early morning
- Recurrent or persistent fever

SIGNS AND SYMPTOMS THAT MAY BE COVERT

- Bone pain
- Headache
- Persistent lymphadenopathy
- Change in balance, gait, or personality
- Fatigue, malaise

Staging of Cancer: TNM Classification

PRIMARY TUMOR (T)

TX: Primary tumor cannot be assessed
T0: No evidence of primary tumor
Tis: Carcinoma in situ
T1, T2, T3, T4: Increasing size and/or local extent of the primary tumor

REGIONAL LYMPH NODES (N)

NX: Regional lymph nodes cannot be assessed
N0: No regional lymph node metastasis
N1, N2, N3: Increasing involvement of regional lymph nodes

DISTANT METASTASIS (M)

MX: Presence of distant metastasis cannot be assessed
M0: No distant metastasis
M1: Distant metastasis

MEDICATIONS COMMONLY USED IN CHILDHOOD CANCER

	ROUTE	PRECAUTIONS AND SIDE EFFECTS	NURSING CONSIDERATIONS
Vincristine	IV	Little effect on bone marrow Lethal if given intrathecally Neurotoxicity (loss of deep tendon reflexes, footdrop, or neurotic pain of the jaw and abdomen)	May give if WBC is low Separate from intrathecal drugs Administer stool softener
Asparaginase	IM	Rare anaphylaxis Give deeply IM Rare hyperglycemia	Keep emergency drugs at hand Monitor patient for 1 hour after injection
Cyclophosphamide (Cytoxan)	PO IV	Toxic when in prolonged contact with bladder	Carefully note for development of hematuria Patient must void q 2 hr If not able to void, may need urinary catheter Provide adequate hydration 2–3 times maintenance
Methotrexate (MTX)	IV IT PO IM	Excreted through kidneys Nephrotoxic Not excreted in acidic urine	Do not infuse with a filter Blood levels of drug to be obtained throughout and after infusion Monitor urine pH and administer bicarbonate as ordered Compatible with bicarbonate Complete IV infusion on schedule; may obtain orders to increase infusion rate Administer leucovorin rescue *on schedule* as ordered
Cytarabine (Ara-C)	SQ IV IT	Occasional unexplained fevers in some patients Cell-cycle specific	Monitor temperature Do not interrupt infusion for more than 20 min
Daunorubicin (Daunomycin) or Doxorubicin (Adriamycin) *Ifosfamide*	IV IV	Late effect of cardiotoxicity Possible elevated temperature May cause urine to be red When given through a central venous access device, often causes bad taste Nephrotoxic	Give IVP over at least 20 min Monitor temperature Ensure IV is patent throughout Warn patient about red urine Offer chewing gum or strongly flavored candy Administer mesna rescue *on time* as ordered
Cisplatin	IV	Nephrotoxic Ototoxic	May give mannitol and furosemide to promote urine formation Notify doctor if urine output is <1ml/kg/hr BUN and creatinine must be measured before first dose Do not exceed l mg/min Audiogram may be done before and after therapy
Etoposide VP-16; (VePesid)	IV PO	May precipitate if not adequately diluted Hypotension	Should be diluted to 1 mg/ml Infuse over 45–60 min Establish baseline blood pressure
Mercaptopurine (6-MP)	IV PO	Hepatotoxic	Carefully note liver function studies
Mitoxantrone Hcl (Novantrone)	IV	Myocardiopathies Dark blue solution	Baseline electrocardiogram should be done Warn that sclera and urine may turn blue Patient should not wear contact lenses during therapy Infuse with D_5W or normal saline only Precipitates with heparin

MEDICATIONS COMMONLY USED IN CHILDHOOD CANCER *(continued)*

	ROUTE	PRECAUTIONS AND SIDE EFFECTS	NURSING CONSIDERATIONS
The Following Drugs Are Not Antineoplastic Agents, but Are Frequently Used in Children's Cancer Therapy			
Leucovorin	IV PO	Competes with MTX for transport into cells and promotes MTX excretion by the kidneys	Give as ordered with MTX therapy Usually begun within 36 hr of MTX therapy Give IVP over <1 min
Mesna	IV	Rescue for ifosfamide	Give as ordered and *on schedule*
Steroids	PO	Gastric upset Unpleasant taste Sodium and water retention Alters mood Appetite changes	Give with food Suggest crushing and mixing with chocolate syrup, juices, or cola drink for small children Warn parents of behavioral changes Expect odd food requests
Ondansetron (Zofran) or Granisetron (Kytril)	IV PO	Photosensitivity Antiemetic	Warn that sunburn may occur more easily Encourage low-sodium diet Give over 15–20 min

DIAGNOSTIC TESTS AND PROCEDURES FOR CANCER

TEST/DESCRIPTION	NORMAL VALUES	NURSING CONSIDERATIONS
Bone Marrow Aspiration Use of the anterior or posterior iliac crests to aspirate bone marrow. The tibia is sometimes used in infants.	The presence, absence, and ratio of cells that are specific and diagnostic to certain diseases. Some of the conditions used to diagnose include: leukemia, some specific vitamin deficiencies, neoplastic diseases in which the marrow is invaded by tumor cells, and agranulocytosis.	1. Describe the procedure to the child and parents. 2. Allow parents to stay with the child if they wish. 3. Depending on the protocol of the facility, the child may receive a wide range of sedation or anesthesia. Some centers use local anesthesia with no systemic sedation, while others use a combination of a sedative and an analgesic. Midazolam (Versed) is popular because of its rapid onset, short duration, and sedative and amnesiac effect. Topical anesthetics such as EMLA may also be used in some centers. 4. The child should be told that he or she will experience discomfort when the needle is inserted and when the marrow is aspirated, but that it will last only a few seconds. 5. Apply dressing to the area. If the child's platelet count is below 50,000/mm^3, use a pressure dressing.
Positron Emission Tomography (PET) Combines conventional nuclear medicine techniques with tomography and adds double photon imaging which images metabolic activity.	Used mainly to evaluate brain and cardiac function. Brain metabolism indicates tissue viability and PET can help identify the degree of malignancy present.	1. Be sure that the patient is not pregnant. 2. Younger children may require sedation. 3. Older children should be told about the scan and should be allowed to see the equipment.
Single Photon Emission Computed Tomography (SPECT) Nuclear medicine scan which combines the techniques of conventional nuclear medicine imaging with that of CT using gamma-emitting radioactive isotopes.	Normal organ. The organ is displayed in axial, parasagittal, and coronal sections.	Same as PET.

See Chapter 40 (CT scan, lumbar puncture, MRI) and Appendix I (CBC, serum chemistry, urinalysis) for other common tests used in the care of the child with cancer.

OVERVIEW OF CHILDHOOD CANCER AND ITS TREATMENT

Cancer is thought by most researchers to be a genetic disease. Either an acquired or inherited alteration in the DNA sequence perpetuates the mutation. The body's immune system, if it is working properly, will recognize those mutated cells as foreign and attempt to destroy them; therefore, each of us is probably making and destroying potentially cancerous cells every day. Unlucky occurrence may lead to mutated cell production, but the probability of mutations is increased by factors such as exposure to radiation, carcinogens, or physical irritants and heredity. The causes of cancer in children are not well defined. Children have limited exposure to carcinogens. Heredity may play a big part in the development of cancer in children due to the exposure of their parents to carcinogens.

Following accidents, cancer is the second leading cause of death in children. Fourteen childhood cancers per 100,000 children under age 15 years are diagnosed each year compared to 20 cancers per 100,000 between the ages 15 and 19 years (Foley, Fochtman, & Mooney, 1993). The aim of treatment is to cure the child with a minimum of long-term side effects. A challenge of treatment includes maintaining normal growth and development of the child, which can be affected by cancer treatments.

The cardinal signs of cancer in children are different from those seen in adults (see the box in the Clinical Reference Pages). Most adult cancers are carcinomas, and there are more screening tools available to assist with their early detection. The difficulty in diagnosing cancer in children is that most symptoms are attributable to common childhood illnesses and children often do not present until there are obvious signs and symptoms. Primary care providers are understandably reluctant to think about cancer as the cause of symptoms.

Much research has been done in past years searching for a cure to childhood cancers. Current success rates are attributed to cooperative, systematic research through the Pediatric Oncology Group (POG), Children's Cancer Study Group (CCSG), and the International Society for Pediatric Oncology (SIOP). Each group meets twice a year to develop new protocols and monitor the progress of current protocols; subgroups meet as needed throughout the year. Research shows that children have better outcomes if they are treated on a scientifically derived protocol that directs when drugs are to be given, how frequently, and in what dosages, as well as which diagnostic and follow-up studies are to be done and how often.

Only in recent years have successes in cancer treatment been so good that it has produced long-term survivors. Approximately 65% of children diagnosed with cancer will survive 5 years or longer. This represents a 40% increase in long-term survival from the 1960s (Baird et al., 1991). In that population, long-term side effects of treatment are being evidenced, challenging researchers to maximize effectiveness of treatment while minimizing side effects.

Therapeutic Management

Chemotherapy, radiation, bone marrow transplantation, and biologic response modifiers are the forms of treatment for children with cancer. Protocols for children call for longer treatment plans than for adults due to children's increased metabolic rate and thus increased rate of cell turnover. Recurrence of cancer in children who have been previously successfully treated can occur years after therapy. A second tumor may be of the original disease or of a new (or second) malignancy. For example, some children with acute lymphocytic leukemia (ALL) relapse with acute myelocytic leukemia (AML). Some children with ALL who were treated with prophylactic radiation to their central nervous system (CNS) relapse with brain tumors. Unfortunately, even more second malignancies may be found in future years as a result of the treatment used to cure the original malignancy.

Chemotherapy. Chemotherapy is the use of drugs (antineoplastic agents) to kill cancer cells. Different drugs affect different stages of cell development, so a combination of drugs known individually to be active against that specific disease is used. Because tumor cells do not go through the cell cycle at the same time, drugs are combined with others that are effective against tumor cells at different phases of division. Chemotherapy may be given orally, intravenously, intramuscularly, subcutaneously, or **intrathecally.** Rarely, it may be given directly into a body cavity (i.e., intra-arterial or intra-ommaya) for direct action. Depending on the protocol, a child may be hospitalized for chemotherapy, receive it on an outpatient basis, or be treated at home.

Chemotherapy does not differentiate between normal and cancer cells, so the most traumatic cytotoxic effects of the drugs are those produced to rapidly dividing healthy cells. The nadir—the time of the greatest bone marrow suppression—generally lasts 7 to 14 days, depending on the specific agent used. Even then, each child is individual and may be more or less sensitive to the side effects of the drugs and may need to have the subsequent dosages of a particular drug altered.

Side effects of chemotherapy (see box) represent challenges to caregivers and are due to the effect of chemotherapy on the more rapidly dividing cells of the gastrointestinal (GI) tract, hematopoeitic system, and integumentary system. The treatment of nausea and vomiting was revolutionized in 1992 with the release of the antiemetic ondansetron (Zofran) and in 1994 of granisetron (Kytril), which have been more effective in

Common Side Effects of Chemotherapy and Radiation Therapy

Chemotherapeutic drugs and radiation affect normal as well as abnormal cells, primarily cells that divide rapidly, such as cells of the GI tract, hair follicles, and bone marrow. As a result, children undergoing these therapies usually experience the following:

CHEMOTHERAPY SIDE EFFECTS

- Nausea
- Vomiting
- Alopecia
- Anorexia
- Malaise
- Bone marrow depression
- Stomatitis

RADIATION SIDE EFFECTS

- Fatigue
- Nausea
- Vomiting
- Anorexia
- Mucositis
- Bone marrow suppression
- Skin reactions

Photos courtesy of Cook Children's Medical Center, Fort Worth, Texas.

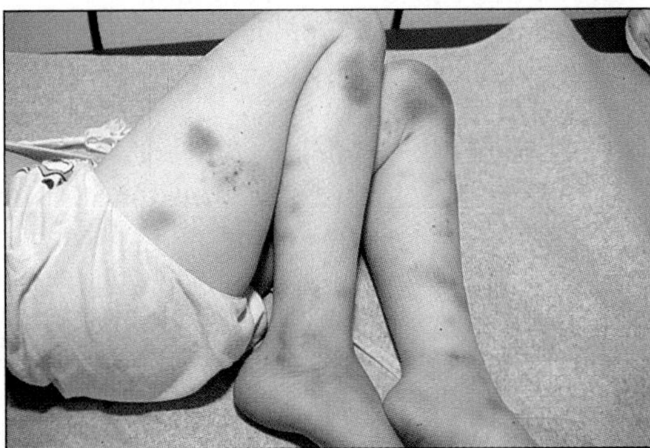

Suppression of the bone marrow in chemotherapy or radiation therapy reduces the cells produced by this organ. Low platelet levels lead to spontaneous bruising, as shown here. Nosebleeds and bleeding of the gums are other consequences. The nurse must make a special effort to observe for bruising in dark-skinned children because it will be more difficult to see.

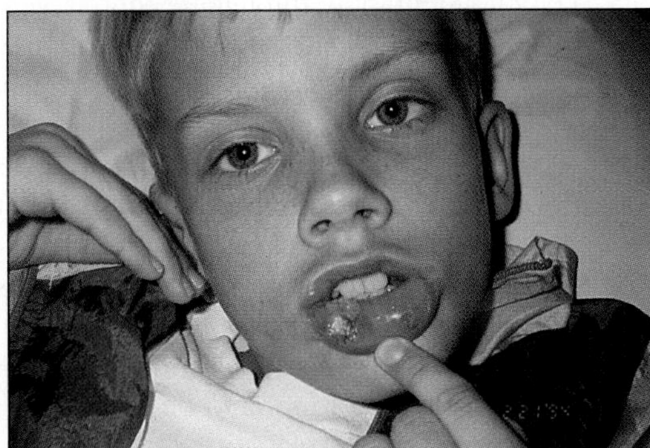

Mucositis (inflammation of the mucous membranes) and mouth ulcers are common side effects of chemotherapeutic drugs. Any mucous membrane can be affected.

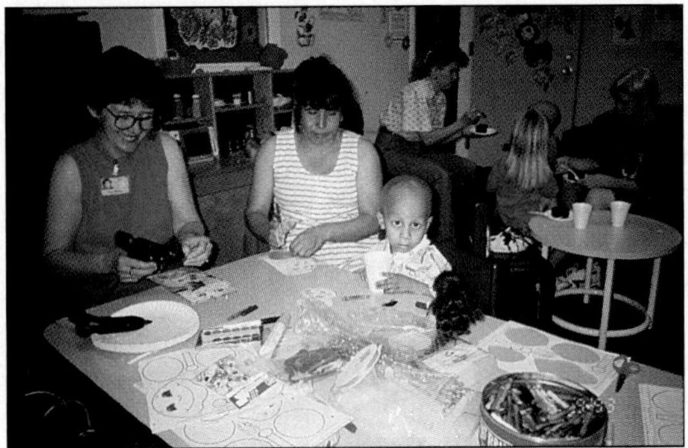

Hair loss is a distressing side effect of cancer treatment. School-age children and adolescents are most likely to feel this distress the most. Activities such as crafts or play groups help the children feel more normal and provide interaction with others.

combating chemotherapy-induced nausea and vomiting than earlier antiemetics. Adolescents commonly demonstrate anticipatory nausea and vomiting before receiving chemotherapy, based on their previous experience with chemotherapy; antianxiety drugs given before the patient comes to the hospital for chemotherapy sometimes helps alleviate this problem.

Hair loss has a tremendous psychologic effect, especially on the school-age and adolescent population. Some chemotherapeutic agents do not produce hair loss, but most do. Preparing the patient and family for this is one of the nurse's initial jobs on diagnosis. Purchase of a wig is advisable before the child actually loses his hair so that the natural color and texture can best be matched.

Anorexia is associated not only with nausea, but also with a change in taste experienced by some people in response to some chemotherapeutic agents. Small, frequent meals will help keep the child's weight from falling, but sometimes hospitalization for nutritional purposes is necessary. Hyperalimentation through a central venous catheter may be begun with the child as an inpatient and then continued on an outpatient basis by home health nurses.

Malaise is common in older children and adolescents and is often associated with depression. Normal activities are important to keep spirits and energy levels highest. Allow friends to visit the patient for prolonged periods as tolerated by the patient. Encourage video games, movies, and playroom or teen lounge activities with others of the same age. Allow the hospital routine to be as close to the child's home routine as possible.

Other side effects are specific to the agent being used as well as the dose.

The nurse's responsibility when giving chemotherapeutic agents is to know the following:

- length of infusion
- routes
- dosages
- OSHA guidelines for patient, family, and self.

Nursing responsibilities and precautions related to chemotherapy are detailed in the accompanying box.

Nursing Responsibilities and Precautions for Chemotherapy

- Body surface area (BSA in m^2) is used to calculate dosages.
- Accurate height and weight measurements are essential.
- Always double-check ordered dosage against BSA.
- Ensure informed consent has been signed if child is on a research protocol.
- A CBC should be done within 48 hours before chemotherapy is given.
- The WBC, hemoglobin, and platelet counts need to be at a predetermined level before chemotherapy is given.
- Ensure patency of IV site before giving drugs.
- If using an implantable infusion device, ensure needle placement and blood return.
- Vesicants (agents that produce blisters) should be given through a fresh IV site if site is older than 48 hours.
- The child may complain of vesicants burning through a peripheral IV, even if the IV is fresh and patent. Slowing down the administration may ease the discomfort. Apply a cool cloth just above the infusion site. Try speeding up the free-flowing IV fluid to help dilute the drug as it is infused.
- Have emergency drugs available.

Radiation. Radiation therapy is individually dosed for specific diseases and to the patient's size and age. Radiation may be given palliatively in low doses to prevent further growth of a tumor or curatively to eradicate disease. Total body irradiation is given before some bone marrow transplants in an attempt to irradicate microscopic disease and to cause bone marrow suppression. Radiation may be given in hyperfractionated doses; the daily dose is split into smaller, more frequently given doses in an attempt to minimize side effects.

Side effects of radiation are dose and location dependent and, as with chemotherapy, are a result of radiation's effect on healthy, rapidly dividing cells (see box). Manifested 7 to 10 days after the initiation of therapy, these side effects usually disappear within days or a few weeks of cessation of the radiation therapy.

Preparation of the child and family for radiation involves education about the process in addition to the side effects. Some institutions provide a pre-radiation tour so the child may experience the room and surroundings before therapy. During the tour, the child should be shown the window or monitor she will be observed through while undergoing radiation alone in the room. Some children will need to be sedated for their radiation therapy sessions. Others can be coached to lie still with the help of child life specialists and parents. Patients must lie still for prolonged periods because it is necessary for the radiation oncologist to very carefully control the depth and peripheral margins of the radiation.

The parents' first reaction to the erythematous skin that is evident after radiation therapy may be to apply lotion.

Some lotions and tape will worsen the skin's reaction to radiation. Remind parents not to use unapproved lotions or creams on the skin.

Loose clothing may be more comfortable. Sun protection is essential while undergoing radiation therapy. Fatigue associated with therapy may necessitate more frequent rest periods than parents are used to their child taking. Anorexia, nausea, and vomiting commonly occur; the parent will need to be creative in meal planning to prevent dehydration and weight loss. Radiation therapy will also cause bone marrow suppression, depending on the dose and site of therapy. Rarely is the anemia so bad as to necessitate transfusion, but it may add to the fatigue. The child's laboratory results should be monitored closely during radiation therapy for neutropenia, anemia, and thrombocytopenia.

Bone Marrow Transplantation. The use of bone marrow transplantation (BMT) has, in recent years, become accepted therapy for the treatment of several hematologic and oncologic disorders. BMT allows physicians to give doses of chemotherapy (with or without radiation) that are toxic to the patient and "rescue" the patient from total, irreversible bone marrow suppression by giving bone marrow unaffected by the chemotherapy or radiation. BMT is currently standard therapy for children in first remission with Philadelphia chromosome-positive ALL (a genetically determined ALL with >90% relapse rate), AML, and stage D neuroblastoma, as well as children with chronic aplastic anemia and severe combined immunodeficiency syndrome. BMT is also used for children with solid tumors, Hodgkin's disease, and non-Hodgkin's lymphoma resistant to conventional chemotherapy and radiation, as evidenced by their relapse while on therapy.

The doses of chemotherapy and radiation that can be used are limited by the toxic effects the therapies have on bone marrow.

There are three types of BMT—syngeneic, autologous, and allogeneic. The type used depends on the patient and on the disease's effect on the bone marrow. Rarely, a patient will have an identical twin and can receive a syngeneic BMT.

In autologous BMT, the patient undergoes general anesthesia for aspiration of the bone marrow, which is then processed in the laboratory and frozen until the time to infuse that marrow back into the patient. Then, the patient begins a regimen of chemotherapy and radiation (called conditioning) to try to irradicate any disease from the body. The white blood cell (WBC), red blood cell (RBC), and platelet counts begin to drop as the chemotherapy and radiation have their effects on the bone marrow. When this conditioning phase is over, the patient receives her own, now thawed marrow back into her body. The production by the bone marrow of normal cells, which can be seen on a complete blood count (CBC), is evidence that the infused marrow has "engrafted" or been accepted by the body.

In allogeneic BMT, a donor who matches the patient's tissue type is found. That bone marrow is then given to the patient. Only 35% of the population have a sibling who matches their tissue type (Foley, Fochtman, & Mooney, 1993), so a national or international search through the National Marrow Donor Program may be conducted to look for an unrelated matched donor.

The major problem associated with allogeneic transplants is graft-versus-host disease (GVHD) as the patient tries to reject the donor marrow. GVHD is the body's natural immunologic response to foreign tissue. Patients may exhibit a wide variety of symptoms associated with GVHD, such as mild to severely elevated liver enzyme levels, mild to copious diarrhea, and maculopapular skin reactions ranging from rashes to full skin desquamation. Antirejection drugs are given to help prevent this from occurring.

The process of extracting enough bone marrow for a transplant is considered a surgical procedure and is accomplished under general anesthesia because of the discomfort, but the process of giving bone marrow to a patient is not a surgical one. Processed bone marrow looks much like red fruit juice and is administered like a blood transfusion by infusing it into a central venous catheter.

Once the marrow is infused, nursing care focuses on preventing these **immunosuppressed** patients from developing a life-threatening infection until they engraft and produce their own WBCs with which to fight infection. The "waiting game" begins for parents and patients until the daily CBC begins to show signs of marrow recovery.

Common complications in the days and weeks after a BMT include mucositis, diarrhea, fevers, and nosebleeds. The patients receive intravenous (IV) nutritional support because most will not be able to take food and fluids orally due to severe mucositis and GI discomfort and diarrhea.

Initial post-transplant management includes strict isolation in either a hepafiltered room or a room equipped with laminar air flow. Both filter the air in the patient's room to eliminate many viruses, molds, and fungi that a person with a normal immune system would be able to handle. Regimented oral and skin care are required. All dressing changes are performed under sterile technique. Strict intake and output measurements are made. Vital signs are monitored frequently. Administration of blood products occurs several times a week. Many different medications are given to prevent infections, GVHD, peptic ulcers, and other complications of treatment.

Patients are not permitted to go home until their WBC count is sufficient to fight infections, and even then they must be considered immunosuppressed for months. Home care may include platelet transfusions, IV immune globulin, and antiviral medications. Patients must wear a mask when they venture out in public. Different institutions have different standards for how high the WBC count must be for discharge home. Home care varies as well. Follow-up visits are initially biweekly and continue for months.

Biologic Response Modifiers. The most recent additions to cancer therapy are the biologic response modifiers (BRMs). These are minute, naturally occurring substances found in the body that influence immune system functions. Examples are colony stimulating factors (CSFs), monoclonal antibodies, interleukins, tumor necrosis factor, and interferons (Foley, Fochtman, & Mooney, 1993).

Used to enhance cell recovery, different CSFs work on different types of cells to reduce the time and severity of bone marrow suppression. They may reduce the length of time a child must be hospitalized for fever and **neutropenia.** In individuals whose bone marrow is very susceptible to chemotherapy, requiring delaying chemotherapeutic cycles for bone marrow recovery, CSFs may reduce that recovery time, enabling the chemotherapeutic regimen to continue as scheduled for maximum effectiveness.

Monoclonal antibodies (MAbs) were developed by injecting mice with an antigen; the mice then produced an antibody to the antigen, and the antibody was recovered from their spleens. MAbs are produced for specific antigen expressed on the surface of a particular type of cancer cell. An antigen–antibody complex forms. MAbs are linked with chemotherapeutic agents and radioactive particles, enabling the removal of cancer cells with limited effect on surrounding tissue. MAbs were developed to recognize neuroblastoma cells and assist in purging of those cells from bone marrow in the laboratory in autologous BMT.

Interleukins are proteins that send messages between leukocytes (Foley, Fochtman, & Mooney, 1993). No specific action is exerted by them on cancer cells, but research is ongoing to determine how they can best be utilized to augment cancer therapy. Seven interleukins have been discovered (Foley, Fochtman, & Mooney, 1993), and their activity includes stimulation of platelet production, optimization of the graft-versus-host response in BMT patients, and enhancement of the activity of lymphocytes (Foley, Fochtman, & Mooney, 1993).

Tumor necrosis factor, when bound to cancer cells, actually causes hemorrhagic necrosis of tumors and stimulates macrophages and tumor-specific antibodies. Not all cancer cells are receptive to tumor necrosis factor, and clinical trials are ongoing to determine appropriate uses in pediatric cancers (Foley, Fochtman, & Mooney, 1993).

The mechanism of action of interferons is not known, but we know they are capable of inhibiting viral replication, modulating immune responses, and altering cellular proliferation (Foley, Fochtman, & Mooney, 1993). Studies are being conducted with alpha, beta, and gamma interferon to understand their application in pediatric cancer therapy.

LEUKEMIA

Leukemia is the disease that most often comes to mind when one discusses childhood cancer. A proliferation of immature WBCs, leukemia is the most common form of cancer in children under age 15 years. Considerable progress in its treatment has been achieved through years of research.

Etiology. Leukemia most likely arises from a fundamental alteration in the genetic makeup of the stem cell. All cells produced from this stem cell have a defect. These cells tend to replicate quickly, forming immature, or **blast,** cells in the bone marrow, which are released into peripheral circulation, crowding other cells produced. The blast cells do not properly respond to the body's feedback mechanism and continue to replicate in great numbers. Children with Down syndrome have a 10 to 20 times greater risk to develop leukemia than other children (Gaddy-Cohen, 1993). The twin of a child who has had leukemia also has a significant likelihood of developing the disease. Before age 5 years there is a 10% to 20% increased risk. At age 6 to 7 years the risk is similar to that for other siblings (Gaddy-Cohen, 1993).

Incidence. About 40 per million cases of leukemia in white children and 20 per million cases in black children are diagnosed each year (Gaddy-Cohen, 1993). ALL accounts for 80% of all cases of leukemia, AML for 15% to 20% (Gaddy-Cohen, 1993) and chronic myelocytic leukemia for 1% to 5% (Schultz, 1989). Peak incidence is age 3 to 5 years for ALL. Leukemia is more common in boys than girls after age 1 year.

Clinical Manifestations

- Pallor
- Excessive bruising
- Bone or joint pain (usually leg pain)
- Abdominal pain (often confused with a GI disorder)
- **Lymphadenopathy**
- Malaise
- Fever of unknown origin
- **Hepatosplenomegaly**
- Abnormal WBC counts (either lower or higher than normal for age)
- Mild to profound anemia and thrombocytopenia

Severity of the clinical manifestations varies with the cell type of leukemia and length of time before seeking medical attention.

Diagnostic Evaluation. The diagnosis will be strongly suspected from a history of the above clinical manifestations and an initial CBC. The confirmatory test for leukemia is microscopic examination of bone marrow obtained by bone marrow aspirate and biopsy. A lumbar puncture is also done to look for blast cells in the spinal fluid that are indicative of CNS disease. Serum electrolytes are obtained to ensure metabolic stability before chemotherapy is initiated. An elevated uric acid level, indicating rapid cell turnover, may be expected if the WBC count is very high. A bone scan or skeletal survey will check for bone involvement.

PATHOPHYSIOLOGY *of Leukemia*

In leukemia, normal bone marrow is replaced by malignant **blast cells.** As the blast cells take over the bone marrow, eventually RBC and platelet production is affected and the child becomes anemic and thrombocytopenic. The reticuloendothelial system is affected, thus disturbing the body's defense system and rendering these children unable to fight infections normally. The symptoms of the disease reflect bone marrow failure and organ infiltration.

In addition to being present in the blood and bone marrow, leukemia cells infiltrate extramedullary sites, most commonly, the CNS and the testicles. Although it is not common to see extramedullary leukemia at time of diagnosis, these are common sites of relapse.

Leukemias are classified by the type of WBC affected. Broadly, acute leukemias are classified as acute lymphocytic (ALL) and acute nonlymphocytic leukemia (ANLL). ALL originates from B-lymphocytes (B-cell ALL), T-lymphocytes (T-cell ALL), or is classified as "common ALL," which has B-cell lineage. ANLL is also known as acute myelocytic leukemia (AML) and can be further classified as acute promyelocytic leukemia (APL), acute myelomonocytic leukemia (AMMoL), and acute monocytic leukemia (AMoL). ANLL tends to be less responsive to therapy, more aggressive and difficult to treat, and more likely to result in relapse than ALL.

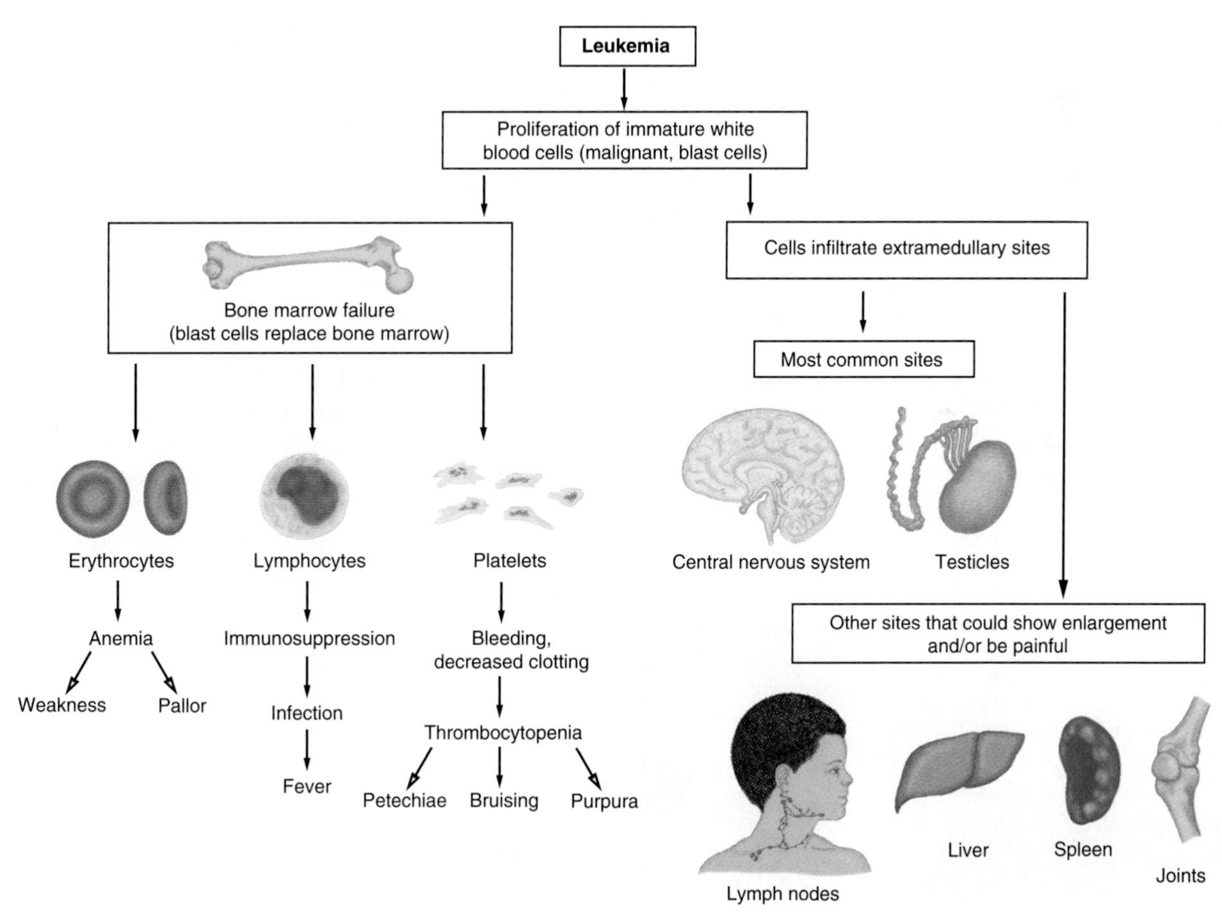

Therapeutic Management. Combination chemotherapy is the preferred treatment for leukemia. The length of treatment varies depending on the cell type, but is usually 2 to 3 years (ALL) and is divided into phases—remission induction, consolidation, and continuation or maintenance. Before induction, the child is treated for presenting symptoms, which may include sepsis, anemia, hemorrhage, and metabolic abnormalities.

Remission Induction. During induction, the hospitalized child receives his first doses of chemotherapy while his reaction to the drugs is assessed. Remission can be verified about 30 days after the initiation of chemotherapy by a bone marrow aspirate and lumbar puncture. If a significant number of blast cells are still present, a new and stronger drug regimen is given. This is an ominous sign indicative of a poorer prognosis. Less than 10% of children do not respond to standard induction therapy.

The particular drugs used, their dose, route, and scheduling depend on the **protocol** that will be used for that specific type of leukemia. Children are placed in prognostic categories with specifically tailored therapies. Before the child receives chemotherapy, allopurinol and IV fluids are given to decrease the serum uric acid and alkalinize the urine. This is especially important when the WBC count is very high, because as the WBCs break down in reaction to chemotherapy, they will release even more uric acid into the serum, which could compromise kidney function. Steroids are used in induction of ALL, as are vincristine, daunorubicin, and asparaginase. AML induction includes cytarabine (ara-C) and an anthracycline such as daunorubicin or doxorubicin. Intrathecal chemotherapy is given prophylactically to prevent relapse in the CNS.

Consolidation. Consolidation chemotherapy begins after remission is obtained and consists of cyclic doses of drugs that may require either inpatient or outpatient visits depending on the protocol. Continuation consists of outpatient therapy, the intensity of which is dependent on the cell type.

Maintenance. Maintenance therapy begins after the completion of remission induction and consolidation therapy. Combined drug therapies are used. CBCs are measured and periodic bone marrow aspirates are performed to be sure the child remains in remission. Children who relapse while on maintenance therapy have a poor prognosis. If relapse occurs, an attempt to reinduce a remission is made, usually with different chemotherapeutic agents.

Relapse. The gonads and the CNS are the most common sites of extramedullary relapse. Therapy includes a more aggressive regimen. The more relapses the child has, the poorer the prognosis.

NURSING CARE OF THE CHILD WITH LEUKEMIA

Assessment

Subjective data obtained almost always reveals an insidious onset of symptoms. The parents may state they realized their child was less active than normal. A persistent or recurrent fever of unknown cause is often in the history. The parents may have suddenly noticed their child had more bruises than usual. Sometimes the child will have complained of a stomachache off and on that the parent attributed to not wanting to go to school. Leg pain is often written off to laziness. Parents commonly express guilt because they did not recognize anything was wrong with their child sooner or, if they did notice, the symptoms were so vague they delayed in seeking treatment. Psychosocial assessment of the family is carried out throughout the care of the child.

The nurse is observing both the child's and the parents' reactions to the disease. The emotional maturity of the child and the family will affect how each copes with

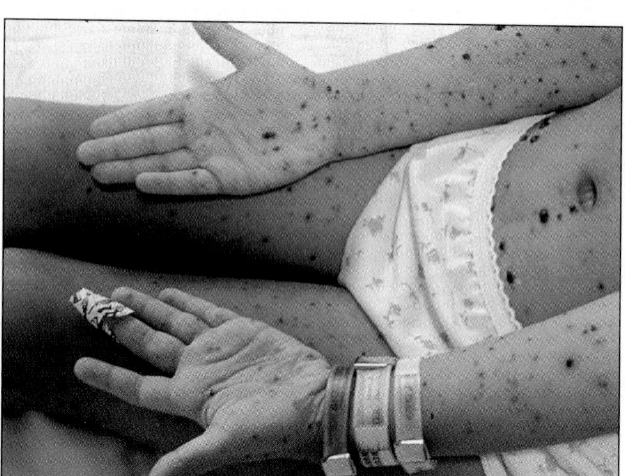

Figure 33–1
Varicella (chickenpox) can be deadly in the immunocompromised child. Thrombocytopenia (low platelet count) associated with chemotherapy can cause the varicella lesions to be hemorrhagic, as in those shown here. Secondary infections of the lesions are also common because of low white blood cell levels. (Courtesy of Cook Children's Medical Center, Hematology-Oncology Clinic, Fort Worth, Texas)

both the illness and the treatment. The child's chronological age and stage of development as well as previous experience in the health care system are critical factors in the assessment.

Parents who are unable to cope with the disease and who display a high level of anxiety will transfer this anxiety to their child. Children who have had previous negative experiences associated with hospitals, nurses, and doctors may exhibit increased anxiety. Children who have had a relative who had cancer and perhaps died, will naturally exhibit increased anxiety and need for support, even if the relative was an older person. The nurse's role is to identify and respond to these needs.

Objective data often shows some degree of fever. Fatigue, pallor, bruising on the extremities, petechiae in the mouth and sclera, and hepatosplenomegaly are all common symptoms. Children with very high WBC counts, AML, T-cell ALL, and B-cell ALL may present with more pronounced symptoms. The CNS is assessed because of the risk of infiltration into the CNS. The child's level of consciousness as well as signs of irritability, vomiting, and lethargy are assessed.

Nursing Diagnosis

- Risk for Infection related to immunosuppressed state (Fig. 33–1)
- Risk for Injury related to abnormal blood profile
- Altered Nutrition: Less Than Body Requirements related to nausea and vomiting or mucositis
- Knowledge Deficit related to disease process and treatment plan
- Body Image Disturbance related to hair loss
- Ineffective Family/Individual Coping related to chronic illness
- Pain related to disease process and procedures
- Impaired Skin Integrity related to radiotherapy
- Altered Mucous Membrane related to chemotherapy and radiation

Planning, Implementation, and Evaluation: The Child With Leukemia

NURSING DIAGNOSIS
- Risk for Infection related to immunosuppressed state

Expected Outcome:
- The child will be free of signs of infection, as evidenced by afebrile state, no redness of integument, no redness or swelling at site of central venous catheter, and negative cultures.

Intervention	Rationale
1. Monitor vital signs q 4 hr and p.r.n. if hospitalized. Have parents take temperature daily at home (oral, axillary, or tympanic temperatures only).	An elevated temperature may be the only visible sign of infection. Risk of injury to the fragile mucous membranes is so great that only oral or axillary temperatures should be taken. Rectal abscesses can easily occur to damaged rectal tissue. No rectal temperatures should be taken.
2. Practice proper handwashing, and teach this to the family.	Proper handwashing is the best way to prevent the spread of infection.
3. Inspect skin daily for breaks and redness.	Some neutropenic patients will not produce purulent drainage. Because pus is made of WBCs, drainage cannot be used as a sign of infection. Redness may be the only sign.
4. Inspect the mouth daily for oral ulcers. Inspect the perineum for fissures. Teach older children to do self-examination. No suppositories should be given.	The mucous membranes are fragile and easily affected by chemotherapy and radiation. Mouth ulcers and rectal abscesses are common side effects of chemotherapy and radiation and potential sites for bacteria entry due to the impaired mucosa.

Intervention	Rationale
5. Teach parents/child meticulous oral hygiene at diagnosis. a. Use soft bristled toothbrush. b. Perform oral hygiene four times a day. c. If platelet count is low, use cotton-tipped applicator instead of toothbrush.	Prevention of dental caries and ulcerations on fragile oral mucosa will help prevent infections.
6. At the first signs of mouth ulcers, begin a mouth care regimen three to four times daily, including an antifungal drug as ordered by the physician. Do not use over-the-counter mouthwashes.	Fungal infections originating from the mouth or GI tract can quickly become disseminated in immunosuppressed children. Over-the-counter mouthwashes may have a high alcohol content and may be drying to oral mucosa.
7. For the hospitalized neutropenic child, allow flowers or plants to be kept in the room only if institutional protocol allows. Do not use humidifiers.	Standing water and damp soil harbor *Aspergillus* and *Pseudomonas*, to which these children are very susceptible.
8. Place the hospitalized neutropenic child on a low bacteria diet.	Fruits and vegetables that are not peeled before being eaten harbor molds and should be avoided until the WBC count rises.
9. Change any dressings and IV lines using sterile technique.	Because the child with neutropenia is not able to normally fight infection, extra precautions must be taken.
10. Patient should not receive live-virus vaccines. Siblings should receive inactivated polio vaccine but may receive live MMR vaccine.	Shedding of live virus occurs in the stool after administration of the polio vaccine. The live MMR vaccine could produce infection in the severely immunocompromised patient, no virus shedding occurs to create a threat if given to the sibling.
11. Administer ordered Bactrim/Septra (trimethoprim/sulfamethoxazole).	Immunosuppressed patients are very susceptible to *Pneumocystis* infection and should be given prophylactic medicine.
12. Keep any child with chickenpox or any child who has been exposed to the virus away from the child with cancer. Inform the teacher of the importance of notifying parents immediately if a case of chickenpox occurs in another child at school.	Immunocompromised patients are unable to adequately fight varicella. Chickenpox can be deadly to the immunocompromised child (see Fig. 33–1). If a child who has not had chickenpox is exposed to someone with varicella, he should receive VZIG within 96 hours of exposure.
13. Obtain and monitor ordered cultures.	Physicians will order blood, urine, stool, and wound cultures as symptoms appear when the neutropenic child has fever.
13. Administer acetaminophen for fever.	Never give aspirin to a child who might already be thrombocytopenic because it can potentially cause spontaneous hemorrhage.
14. Administer antibiotics as ordered after cultures are obtained.	Cultures identify the specific organism in order to give the most effective antibiotic.

Evaluation:
- The child will receive appropriate treatment for infection and will demonstrate no long-term sequelae.
- The child/parents will promptly recognize warning signs of infection.

NURSING DIAGNOSIS • Risk for Injury related to abnormal blood profile

Expected Outcome: • The child will have no excessive, uncontrolled bleeding.

Intervention	Rationale
1. Apply firm pressure to any puncture sites. Apply pressure dressing to bone marrow aspirate sites.	Additional pressure may be required if platelet count is low.
2. If patient is severely thrombocytopenic (platelet count less than 20,000/mm^3), take the following steps: a. Limit any activity that could result in head injury; encourage patient to participate in quiet activities (i.e., reading books, watching videos, coloring). No contact sports. b. Provide soft-bristled toothbrush only or toothettes. c. Give stool softeners to prevent straining with constipation. d. Do not use suppositories. e. Check urine and stools for blood.	Decreased platelet count increases the risk for bleeding. There is a potential risk for intracranial hemorrhage.
3. Administer platelets as prescribed.	The life of platelets is about 72 hours.
4. Teach child how to control nosebleed and to blow nose gently.	One of the most common sites of bleeding is the nose. Gentle nose blowing can help prevent the vascular pressure that can cause bleeding.

Evaluation:
- The child will experience no excessive bleeding.
- The parents will demonstrate what to do for a nosebleed.

NURSING DIAGNOSIS • Altered Nutrition: Less Than Body Requirements related to nausea and vomiting or mucositis

Expected Outcome: • The child will maintain weight.

Intervention	Rationale
1. Administer antiemetics prophylactically and p.r.n. as ordered.	Antiemetics will decrease nausea.
2. When child is nauseated, offer cool, clear liquids. Be creative with liquids offered to make them more interesting and inviting.	Cool liquids are soothing and better tolerated than hot ones.
3. Offer small, frequent meals of high protein and high calorie content. Fortify foods with nutritional supplements. Allow the family to bring favorite foods to the hospital.	Small, frequent meals are better tolerated than large ones. Protein promotes tissue healing. High calories are needed for growth.
4. Do not offer favorite foods when child is nauseated.	Foods eaten within hours of nausea will be associated with being sick.

Intervention	Rationale
5. Administer ordered mouth analgesics before oral intake.	If mouth sores are present, analgesics will increase comfort and provide interest in eating.
6. Monitor daily weight. Keep strict intake and output. Weigh diapers.	Ensures adequate intake and provides objective assessment to alert nurse to further interventions.
7. Involve child in food selection.	Allowing the child control over as much as possible may increase his interest and participation in eating.

Evaluation: • The child will experience no more than 5% weight loss; growth will progress appropriate for age.

NURSING DIAGNOSIS • Knowledge Deficit related to disease process and treatment plan

Expected Outcome: • The child/parents will verbalize an understanding of the diagnosis and demonstrate compliance with treatment.

Intervention	Rationale
1. Assess child/parents' readiness for learning. Create an environment of learning.	Initially upon diagnosis, family may need time to adjust before they are ready for education. The appropriate setting for an educational session may be away from the child, unless he is an older school-age child or adolescent.
2. On initial diagnosis and with subsequent follow-up visits, spend time with family repeating and explaining diagnosis, sequelae, and treatment. Offer written literature or offer to tape educational sessions. (See Teaching Guidelines for the Child With Leukemia.)	Education is ongoing and will need reinforcing with stressed parents. Explaining rationale and sequelae will better ensure compliance with therapy. Written or taped information can be reviewed later for better absorption.
3. Keep explanations at family's level of understanding.	Nurse should vary explanations to meet the family's educational level.
4. Offer encouragement for parental recognition of danger signs and their appropriate use of medical care.	Praise will reinforce behavior. Parents want to know they are doing the right thing for their child.

Evaluation: The child/parents will:

- demonstrate understanding of treatment protocols by their compliance with therapy
- appropriately seek medical care for danger signs.

NURSING DIAGNOSIS • Body Image Disturbance related to hair loss

Expected Outcome: • The child will adapt to alopecia as evidenced by return to socialization with adaptive device (wig, hat, scarf).

Intervention	Rationale
1. Instruct child/parents on progression of hair loss and potential change in color and texture on regrowth. Suggest obtaining a wig before hair is lost.	Emphasize that hair loss is temporary (3 to 6 months). Some cranial radiation can result in patches of permanent hair loss. Matching a wig to original hair color, texture, and style is easier before hair is lost.

Intervention	Rationale
2. Encourage verbalization of feelings about hair loss. Enlist the help of the child life specialist to engage the child in play therapy.	Allowing the child to verbalize concerns about returning to social environment or school is an assessment tool for the nurse. Play therapy is a safe way for the child to express feelings and fears.
3. Discuss ways to minimize reaction to alopecia by promoting creative solutions, such as hats, wigs, or scarfs.	Allowing the child to create his own headpieces may minimize the negative impact of hair loss.
4. Make visits to the child's classroom.	Prepare classmates for the child's school reentry.
5. Encourage return to school as soon as possible.	The sooner the child returns to school, the less likely the child will begin a pattern of absenteeism.

Evaluation: The child will:
- demonstrate appropriate coping techniques related to hair loss
- continue in prediagnosis social life as soon as possible and as tolerated.

NURSING DIAGNOSIS
- Ineffective Individual/Family Coping related to chronic illness

Expected Outcome:
- The child will comply with the treatment plan.
- The parents will verbalize concerns about the impact of the illness on their family.
- The child/parents will utilize available support systems and community resources.

Intervention	Rationale
1. Teach family the necessity of adhering to the protocol. Teach the warning signs of problems to watch for and how to access after-hours emergency care.	Conscientious application of the treatment plan increases the chance of positive outcome.
2. Listen and encourage child/family to verbalize their feelings and express their concerns. Answer questions honestly and openly.	Identifying concerns and clarifying misconceptions helps families cope with the stress of chronic illness.
3. Introduce family to other families of children with cancer.	Families of other children with cancer can offer suggestions and support.
4. Consult social services and chaplains.	The financial and emotional burden of a child with cancer can be overwhelming.
5. Offer a list of local support groups appropriate to the child's age and family's individual needs.	Support groups of individuals with similar situations can provide much comfort and support to the child and the family.

Evaluation: The child/parents will:
- comply with the treatment plan
- verbalize appropriate concerns and questions
- utilize appropriate resources.

NURSING DIAGNOSIS • Pain related to disease process and procedures

Expected Outcome: • The child's pain will be kept to a tolerable level.

Intervention	Rationale
1. Explain procedures to child before performing them.	Honest explanations build rapport and reduce fear.
2. Assess p.r.n. for symptoms of pain, such as inactivity for age, increased heart rate or blood pressure, grimacing, verbalization of discomfort, irritability, and crying.	Younger children will not be able to verbalize pain. Stoic children may not express discomfort. Nurses must watch for physiologic signs of pain.
3. Administer comfort measures as needed, such as positioning, adjusting room temperature, and offering distractions appropriate to age.	Often comfort measures will decrease perception of pain and even decrease the amount of analgesic needed.
4. Administer analgesics promptly as ordered. Use topical anesthetics for procedural pain.	Analgesics reduce pain of procedures and of disease. Delays in pain administration can increase anxiety and, thus, increase pain.
5. Explain pain-control regimen to parents and to child as age-appropriate.	Parents know their child and can assist the nurse in assessing pain and reporting it promptly.
6. Notify physician if pain relief is not obtained with ordered dose of analgesic.	Pain tolerance varies greatly among children. Dosage increases may be needed, especially in the child suffering from chronic pain, or in the dying child.
7. Elicit the child life specialist's help before and during procedures.	Child life specialists are trained to use distraction techniques with children and represent a "safe" person to be with during repeated painful procedures.
8. Administer antianxiety drugs as ordered.	Especially in the adolescent patient, anticipation of a painful procedure may worsen the pain. Giving an antianxiety drug may help calm the patient so the procedure is better tolerated.

(See Chapter 20 for further discussion of pain reduction measures.)

Evaluation: The child will:

- express tolerable levels of discomfort
- be manageable for procedures.

NURSING DIAGNOSIS • Impaired Skin Integrity related to radiotherapy

Expected Outcome: • The child will have no signs of infection of integument.

Intervention	Rationale
1. Assess skin each shift.	Skin erythema is common with radiation, but should not progress to skin breakdown.
2. Use only approved lotions and creams on the skin, and instruct parents in the same.	Some commercial lotions can cause further irritation and redness to the skin.

Intervention	Rationale
3. Avoid excessive scrubbing of skin, hot water, and abrasive soaps.	Friction may increase breakdown. Hot water will be uncomfortable to irritated tissue.
4. Offer loose clothing of soft materials.	Tight clothing or abrasive fabrics may further irritate skin.
5. Notify physician if skin breakdown occurs.	Additional orders for therapeutic creams may be needed.
6. If child is immobile, turn and vary position at least every 2 hours.	Immobility may increase pressure on skin and promote breakdown.

Evaluation: The child will:
- develop no signs of skin infection
- heal without scarring of skin.

NURSING DIAGNOSIS
- Altered Oral Mucous Membrane related to chemotherapy and radiation

Expected Outcome:
- The child will be promptly treated for symptoms of mucous membrane breakdown.

Intervention	Rationale
1. Assess mouth and anus each shift for ulcers, erythema, or breakdown. Teach parent or child, if age-appropriate, the same. Report ulcerations to the physician.	Breakdown in mucous membranes usually begins with erythema and progresses to ulcerations. Home care should include this assessment for the duration of therapy. Additional medications, mouth rinses, or ointments will be ordered if ulcerations occur.
2. Do not take a rectal temperature in a patient undergoing chemotherapy or radiation. Do not take oral temperatures if mouth ulcers are present. Teach parents how to take accurate axillary temperatures.	Introduction of a thermometer into the rectum or mouth of a patient with fragile mucous membranes, no matter how carefully done, can tear tissue.
3. Begin meticulous mouth care, avoiding alcohol-based mouthwashes, several times a day with a soft-bristle toothbrush.	Frequent mouth care will help remove bacteria from the oral mucosa, decreasing the risk of infection to irritated tissue.
4. If rectum becomes irritated, begin sitz baths several times a day and after bowel movements.	Lukewarm sitz baths will keep perineum clean and be soothing to irritated tissue.
5. In diaper-wearing patients, use only diaper wipes that do not contain alcohol or perfumes. If perineum is very irritated, use only warm water wipes to the area.	Alcohol and perfumes will further irritate skin and can actually cause great discomfort. Very few commercial diaper wipes are appropriate for these patients.
6. If rectal prolapse occurs, place child in a warm water bath and notify physician.	Rectal prolapse is not uncommon. Usually warm water baths will relax the tissue and allow the rectum to ascend.
7. Offer bland, nonirritating foods and cool liquids.	Citrus products may be very painful to an ulcerated mouth, as may spicy foods. Cool liquids are soothing. Ice pops and slushes are usually well tolerated.

Evaluation: The child will:
- receive prompt intervention for mucosal breakdown
- exhibit no signs of infected mucosa.

TEACHING GUIDELINES *for the Child With Leukemia*

- Reinforce teaching concerning diagnosis, treatment, and side effects of chemotherapy.
- Encourage parents to participate actively in child's care.
- Provide written and verbal instructions concerning home care and provide ample opportunity for parents to return demonstrations of:
  - Central venous access dressing changes.
  - Oral medication administration.
  - Assessment of oral mucous membranes.
  - How to take axillary temperature.
- Teach signs and symptoms of infection and bleeding that require immediate treatment and how to access after-hours emergency treatment.
- Provide phone numbers needed for questions concerning diagnosis, treatment, and side effects of chemotherapy.
- Make appropriate referrals to social services, chaplain, and home health nursing agency.
- Encourage use of community resources.
- Stress importance of preventing infection and bleeding and need for follow-up visits, noting that many visits will involve blood draws to monitor WBC and platelet counts.
- If home hyperalimentation or dietary supplements have been ordered, provide appropriate instructions and referrals.

WILMS' TUMOR (NEPHROBLASTOMA)

Wilms' tumor, or nephroblastoma, is the most common renal tumor in children. Much research has been done on this disease and has produced changes in therapy that have resulted in favorable outcomes.

Pathophysiology. Arising from the renal parenchyma of the kidney, this tumor grows very rapidly. It may present unilaterally and localized or bilaterally, sometimes with metastases to other organs. As with other tumors, a staging system to direct treatment exists (refer to the Clinical Reference Pages).

Etiology. The cause of Wilms' tumor is unknown; however, a genetic predisposition exists. It is known to be associated with other congenital anomalies such as Beckwith-Wiedemann syndrome, genitourinary anomalies, hemihypertrophy, microcephaly, mental retardation, and sporadic aniridia (Green et al., 1991; Nathan & Oski, 1993). There are two histologic types of Wilms' tumor—favorable or nonmetastatic and unfavorable or metastatic (Drigan & Androkites, 1993).

Incidence. Annual incidence is 7.5 per million cases in white children and 7.8 per million cases in black children, with approximately 400 new cases diagnosed annually (Drigan & Androkites, 1993). About 65% of the tumors are seen in children between ages 2 and 6 years, with equal distribution between boys and girls (Exelby, 1991).

Clinical Manifestations

- Mobile abdominal mass
- Microscopic or gross hematuria
- Hypertension
- Abdominal pain
- Malaise
- Anemia
- Fever
- Lungs are primary site for distant metastasis

Diagnostic Evaluation. Diagnosis can be suspected from a good history. An abdominal ultrasound is the initial study done to detect a solid intrarenal mass. An abdominal computed tomography (CT) scan or magnetic resonance imaging (MRI) chest X-ray, and CT scan of the chest are done to confirm the diagnosis. A CBC as well as electrolytes, blood urea nitrogen and creatinine levels, and urinalysis are obtained. Definitive diagnosis is made at the time of surgery by pathology findings.

Therapeutic Management. After a thorough diagnostic workup, a nephrectomy of the involved kidney and lymph node sampling are done. In the few cases of bilateral disease, the patient may receive preoperative chemotherapy or radiation. The surgeon takes care to preserve as much of the renal parenchyma as possible as well as seeing that there is no spillage of the tumor in the surgical process, which would necessitate more aggressive treatment (Exelby, 1991). After pathologic review of the surgical specimen, staging of the tumor directs the therapeutic management of the child. Chemotherapy alone or in combination with radiation is used to treat these patients.

Survival rates for Wilms' tumor are much better than with many other forms of cancer. Favorable histology has a 90% long-term survival rate and unfavorable histology has an 80% long-term survival rate (Drigan & Androkites, 1993).

NURSING CARE OF THE CHILD WITH WILMS' TUMOR

Assessment

Parents often report that when bathing their child they noticed the child's stomach seemed swollen. Some parents will state the diaper no longer fit easily around the child's abdomen. More often than not, the child's activity level and appetite have not changed. Except for a palpable abdominal mass that usually does not cross midline, the exam of the child is normal.

> The tumor mass should not be palpated for the initial assessment by the practitioner. Excessive manipulation can cause seeding of the tumor and cause spread of the cancerous cells.

Nursing Diagnosis and Planning

The following nursing diagnoses and expected outcomes may be appropriate following assessment of the child with Wilms' tumor.

- Anxiety related to surgery with nephrectomy. ***Expected Outcome:*** *The child/parents will express decreased anxiety about outcomes of surgery.*
- Risk for Infection related to surgical interventions. ***Expected Outcome:*** *The child will exhibit no signs and symptoms of infection.*
- Knowledge Deficit related to disease process and treatment plan. ***Expected Outcome:*** *The child/parents will verbalize an understanding of the disease process and treatment plan.*

Implementation

Because the child usually feels good, nursing care is initially focused on preoperative teaching of the parents and the child. A sign should be placed on the bed warning against palpating the abdomen. A nephrectomy is a serious surgical procedure, and the family will have much anxiety about their child losing one of his kidneys. Nurses must offer support and reassurance.

Monitor the child for GI activity, bowel sounds, stool production, abdominal distension, signs and symptoms of infection, hemorrhage, and changes in blood pressure. Careful assessment of output by the remaining kidney is important. Strict intake and output measures are totaled at least every 4 hours. These children will probably come back from surgery with a nasogastric (NG) tube in place and with an order for replacement IV fluid for the NG drainage. Typically, NG tube output is totaled every 4 hours; that total is divided by 4, and either the resulting number is added to the current IV fluid rate or another IV solution is hung so that the amount lost by NG drainage is replaced over the next 4 hours. The process is repeated until the NG drainage has slowed enough that it does not affect overall fluid and electrolyte balance. The replacement fluid usually contains potassium because gastric contents are potassium-rich. Serum electrolyte levels will be checked every 8 to 12 hours during this process. Chapter 18 provides additional information regarding general postoperative care.

Once staging of the tumor is done, the child will be assigned to the appropriate therapeutic protocol. Teaching should center around the sequencing of tests and drugs on that protocol. Support for the family and assessment of their coping should continue throughout therapy. Therapy for Wilms' tumor is usually accomplished on an outpatient basis. See care plan for care of the child with leukemia for related nursing care.

Evaluation

- Is the family asking questions and sharing concerns and fears?
- Has the child remained free of infection and other complications of surgery?

HODGKIN'S DISEASE

Seen less commonly in children than non-Hodgkin's lymphoma, Hodgkin's disease is a neoplasm of lymphatic tissue. The presence of giant, multinucleated cells (Reed-Sternberg cells) is the hallmark of this disease.

Etiology. The cause is unknown; however, the possibility of an infectious agent is being investigated (Nathan & Oski, 1993). Infectious mononucleosis and the Epstein-Barr virus have both been associated with Hodgkin's disease, but the exact relationship is unknown.

Incidence. The incidence of Hodgkin's disease in the United States is about 7.3 per million cases in white children and 5.2 per million cases in black children (Liebhauser, 1993). Hodgkin's disease occurs more often in boys in children under age 15 years. Distribution evens after age 15 years to adulthood (Liebhauser, 1993). This disease is extremely uncommon under age 5 years. Diagnosis is usually in the teenage to adult years.

Clinical Manifestations

- Most commonly, anorexia, weight loss, malaise, and lethargy

- Painless, firm movable adenopathy in the cervical and supraclavicular regions
- Hepatosplenomegaly
- Mediastinal involvement with or without airway obstruction
- Fever

PATHOPHYSIOLOGY *of Hodgkin's Disease*

Hodgkin's disease originates in a single lymph node or a group of lymph nodes in the same anatomic region. Hodgkin's disease is characterized by giant, multinucleated cells called Reed-Sternberg cells, which are thought to represent activated B- and T-lymphocytes (see Chapter 23 Clinical Reference Pages). **Humoral immunity** remains normal in these patients, but they exhibit altered **cellular immunity.** Predictably, Hodgkin's disease will spread from lymph nodes to nonnodal sites such as the spleen, liver, bone, bone marrow, lungs, and mediastinum.

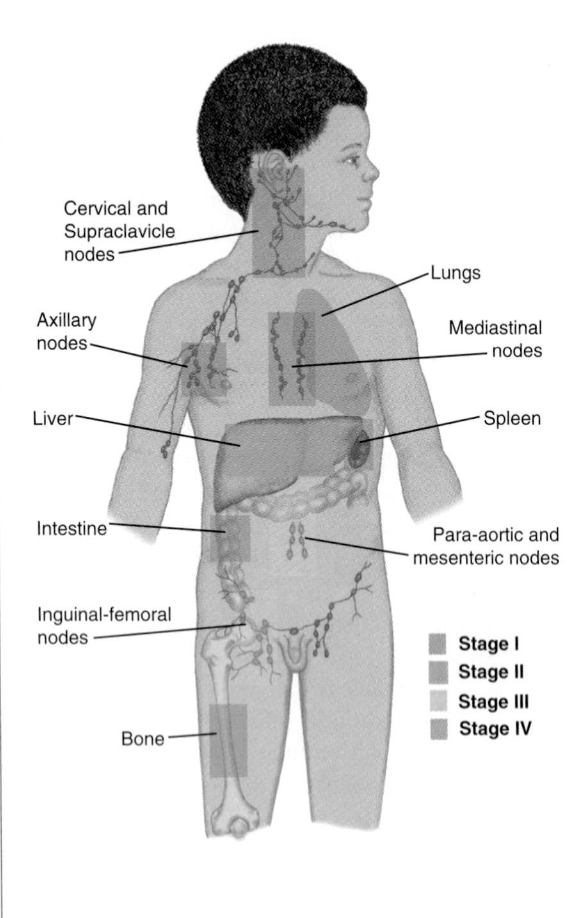

Diagnostic Evaluation. Diagnosis is determined by biopsy of cervical lymph nodes and histologic classification of that tissue. A bone marrow biopsy, CBC, sedimentation rate, serum copper and iron levels, serum ferritin and transferrin, renal and liver function tests, and baseline thyroid tests are done. Gallium scans are done to look for extent of disease. A lymphangiogram evaluates retroperitoneal involvement. A chest X-ray, as well as chest, abdominal, and pelvis CT scans, are done to examine extent of disease.

Some symptoms are of prognostic significance and so staging takes them into account. Unexplained weight loss of greater than 10% body weight in the past 6 months, unexplained fevers above 100.4°F (38°C), and night sweats increase with advancing disease. There are four stages, with Stage I having the most favorable prognosis and Stage IV the least favorable.

Therapeutic Management. Therapy depends on age at diagnosis, stage, and histologic type of disease. If the mediastinal disease is expansive, radiation may be used to shrink the tissue before having the patient undergo general anesthesia. In advanced disease, chemotherapy is the primary treatment.

Most patients are treated with both chemotherapy and radiation. If the disease is local only, radiation may be used alone. Greater than 90% survival can be expected from stage I and II disease. For stages III and IV, an 80% and 70% rate of long-term survival, respectively, is expected (Foley, Fochtman, & Mooney, 1993).

NURSING CARE OF THE CHILD WITH HODGKIN'S DISEASE

Assessment

When asked about activity level, these children may report not noticing any change until it was brought to their attention, because the onset is so insidious. Typically, the child noticed lumps around the neck while bathing. Initial assessment of these children includes a thorough lymph node examination. Depending on the severity of mediastinal disease, the respiratory system should be assessed for a change in status.

Preoperative teaching is done to prepare the patient for the biopsies. Assessment for future educational preparation is done.

Nursing Diagnosis and Planning

The following nursing diagnoses and expected outcomes may be appropriate following assessment of the child with Hodgkin's disease.

- Risk for Infection related to surgery, splenectomy, and immunosuppressed state. ***Expected Outcome:*** *The child will experience no signs or symptoms of infection.*

- Ineffective Breathing Pattern related to mediastinal disease (if present). ***Expected Outcome:*** *The child will experience no severe respiratory distress.*
- Knowledge Deficit related to disease process. ***Expected Outcome:*** *The parents will verbalize an understanding of the disease process.*

Implementation

Initially on diagnosis, the nurse will need to prepare the child for the diagnostic procedures and surgery, if indicated. A central venous catheter may be inserted during surgery. Postoperative care will include assessments for bleeding at dressing sites and administration of prophylactic antibiotics.

> The child who has had his spleen removed will need to receive oral, prophylactic antibiotics daily for the rest of his life.

The spleen removes organisms such as *Streptococcus pneumoniae* and *Haemophilus influenzae.* Without the spleen, these organisms can produce fulminating infections. Postoperative management of the airway is a concern if the child had any mediastinal disease.

Induction chemotherapy will be begun, unless disease is localized, within days after surgery after staging of disease is complete.

Education will include an explanation of the therapeutic protocol. Questions should be answered honestly. Realistic expectations of response to therapy will help parents deal rationally with their fears. The treatment of Hodgkin's disease during first remission is done in the outpatient setting at most centers.

See care plan for care of the child with leukemia for additional nursing care.

Evaluation

- Were any early signs of infection identified and treated early?
- Are the child and family verbalizing their fears?
- Is the child interacting with family and peers?

NON-HODGKIN'S LYMPHOMA

Non-Hodgkin's lymphoma, the third most common malignancy of childhood, refers to a group of neoplasms seen more commonly than Hodgkin's disease. They vary greatly from Hodgkin's disease in their clinical behavior, pathology, mode of metastasis, and responsiveness to therapy (McGowan-Quinlan, 1993). These diseases are rapid in onset and usually present with widespread involvement at diagnosis, but respond quickly to therapy.

Pathophysiology. Non-Hodgkin's lymphoma originates from a proliferation of either B- or T-lymphocytes. In children, T-cell lymphoblastic lymphoma, B-cell or Burkitt's lymphoma, non-Burkitt's lymphoma, or large cell lymphoma are the types usually seen.

Typically, diagnosis is made after the disease is widespread. Originally, the lymphocytes proliferate in lymph nodes, usually in the cervical or axillary areas. Spread of disease through the lymphatic system is rapid.

Etiology. Viral, immunologic, genetic, and environmental factors may contribute to the development of non-Hodgkin's lymphoma. Although the exact etiology is unknown, a linkage to the immune system is thought to exist. B-cell lymphoma has been associated with the Epstein-Barr virus. Patients with congenital immunodeficiency syndromes and AIDS and those who have undergone organ transplants have had their immune system chronically suppressed, and are at higher risk for developing non-Hodgkin's lymphoma.

Incidence. Non-Hodgkin's lymphoma is the third most common childhood malignancy. It has a peak incidence between ages 7 and 11 years (McGowan-Quinlan, 1993).

Clinical Manifestations

- Most commonly, symptoms of abdominal disease, including abdominal cramping, constipation, pain, anorexia, weight loss, ascites, obstruction, and vomiting as a late sign.
- Painless, enlarged lymph nodes are found in cervical or axillary region, less commonly in the inguinal area.
- If mediastinal disease is present, cough, respiratory distress, symptoms of bronchitis, and possibly significant tracheal deviation are seen.
- If bone marrow disease, the patient will exhibit general health decline and bone marrow suppression.

Diagnostic Evaluation. In addition to a physical exam looking for enlarged lymph nodes and hepatosplenomegaly, extensive laboratory work will include liver and renal function studies, electrolytes, magnesium, Epstein-Barr titers, and a urinalysis. The CBC may be normal unless the bone marrow is involved. Especially with Burkitt's lymphoma, the uric acid level will be high, indicating a rapid turnover of cells.

A chest X-ray will be done to look for mediastinal disease and tracheal deviation. A bone marrow aspirate and biopsy are done to assess involvement of disease in the marrow. Likewise, a lumbar puncture is performed to look for the presence of malignant lymphocytes in the spinal fluid. A bone scan is done to look for extent of disease in the bone. CT scans evaluate the extent of disease at diagnosis and are done throughout therapy to assess responsiveness. A biopsy of lymph nodes, the diagnostic test for non-Hodgkin's lymphoma, confirms the presence of malignant lymphoblasts in the nodes.

Therapeutic Management. Especially in Burkitt's lymphoma, children often present in metabolic disarray due to the rapidity with which the disease progresses. Before chemotherapy can be started, the metabolic state must be rectified because these children are prone to tumor lysis syndrome (TLS) due to the large tumor burden.

In TLS, the intracellular contents are dumped into the extracellular fluid as the tumor cells are lysed, or killed, with chemotherapy. Due to the large volume of these cells and because they are so quickly responsive to the chemotherapy, their intracellular electrolytes overload the kidneys and, if not monitored carefully, cause kidney failure.

In children prone to TLS, intensive hydration with an IV fluid containing bicarbonate alkalinizes the urine to help prevent the formation of uric acid crystals. Oral allopurinol is started to decrease the uric acid level. With the initiation of chemotherapy, serum electrolytes may be drawn several times a day to keep a close watch on the child's metabolic state. The urine may actually turn milky white as the tumor cells are filtered through the kidneys. If the child cannot be hemodynamically monitored on the general unit, she may be moved to the intensive care unit until metabolically stabilized.

Standard therapy for children with non-Hodgkin's lymphoma varies with the specific disease and stage, and involves multiagent chemotherapy. Therapy lasts for 6 months to $2\frac{1}{2}$ years, depending on the type of lymphoma, and requires frequent follow-up visits due to the likelihood of relapse right after therapy is stopped.

NURSING CARE OF THE CHILD WITH NON-HODGKIN'S LYMPHOMA

Assessment

With non-Hodgkin's lymphoma, parents will report an acute onset of symptoms that will vary with the type of organ involvement. Most parents will state their child has become very irritable and "just not herself." With metastatic disease, children often present appearing very toxic. Lymph nodes should be assessed. A very close check of the respiratory condition is warranted in a child with mediastinal disease, especially if the trachea is deviated. Assessment of a child prone to TLS includes subtle changes in behavior, such as restlessness and irritability and sensorium changes that are ominous signs of electrolyte imbalances (hyperuricemia, hyperkalemia, hyperphosphatemia, and hypocalcemia).

Nursing Diagnosis and Planning

The following nursing diagnoses and expected outcomes may be appropriate following assessment of the child with non-Hodgkin's lymphoma.

- Ineffective Breathing Pattern related to mediastinal disease. ***Expected Outcome:*** *The child will experience no severe respiratory distress.*
- Risk for Electrolyte Imbalances related to tumor lysis syndrome. ***Expected Outcome:*** *The child will maintain a stable metabolic state.*
- Risk for Infection related to immunosuppressed state. ***Expected Outcome:*** *The child will exhibit no signs and symptoms of infection.*
- Knowledge Deficit related to disease process. ***Expected Outcome:*** *The parents will verbalize an understanding of the disease process.*

Implementation

Initial nursing care is focused on following physician orders for maintaining a stable metabolic and electrolyte state before and during the induction phase of chemotherapy. Most children with Burkitt's lymphoma will need a urinary catheter inserted for measurement of output. However, urinary catheters are used very infrequently in immunocompromised patients because of the risk of introducing organisms into the urinary system. If a fever develops, urinalysis should be done to rule out an infection. All children undergoing induction should be placed under strict intake and output. These patients may be so sick that their nutritional status needs attention after induction, so the nurse should expect many of them to receive hyperalimentation.

Typically, a central venous catheter is in place or one may need to be placed to assist in nutritional support. These diseases are very responsive to chemotherapy. As a result, the blood counts may significantly drop after just 1 day of chemotherapy. Nurses must be prepared to initiate appropriate measures to prevent complications of bone marrow suppression such as infection, anemia, and bleeding.

Parents will need a lot of support because the chemotherapy may initially make the child sicker than when she presented. Questions should be answered directly and honestly. Time for extensive education on therapy may not exist for the parents until after their child has begun to recover from the initial round of chemotherapy.

Consults with chaplains and social workers may enhance nursing's psychosocial care of these families. Realistic expectations of therapy and response to therapy will help parents deal rationally with their fears.

See care plan for care of the child with leukemia for related nursing care.

Evaluation

- Has the child's respiratory status remained stable?
- Has electrolyte balance and an infection free state been maintained?
- Are the parents asking questions about the disease process and the case of their child?

BRAIN TUMORS

Brain tumors are the most common solid tumor and the second most common type of cancer in children after leukemia. In addition to the common side effects of cancer treatment, the sequelae of treatment for a brain tumor can be the most devastating to the child's cognition and overall developmental progress.

Etiology. The cause is unknown, but heredity and environment are both associated with brain tumors. Exposure to radiation seems to be a major environmental influence in the development of these tumors. Research is ongoing related to possible etiology. Alterations in chromosome 17 have been linked with medulloblastoma and astrocytoma, and loss on chromosome 10 with glioblastoma (Wisoff & Epstein, 1994).

PATHOPHYSIOLOGY *of Brain Tumors*

The histology of brain tumors ranges from benign to highly malignant. The impact these tumors has on the brain may have little to do with their relative malignancy and everything to do with the size of the tumor and the area of the brain being affected.

Most brain tumors arise in the posterior fossa. About 50% of tumors are astrocytomas, 25% are medulloblastomas, 11% are brainstem gliomas, and 9% are ependymomas (Foley, Fochtman, & Mooney, 1993). Prognostic percentages vary with the type of tumor, the amount resected, metastatic spread, age of the child and his physical status, and the individual response to therapy.

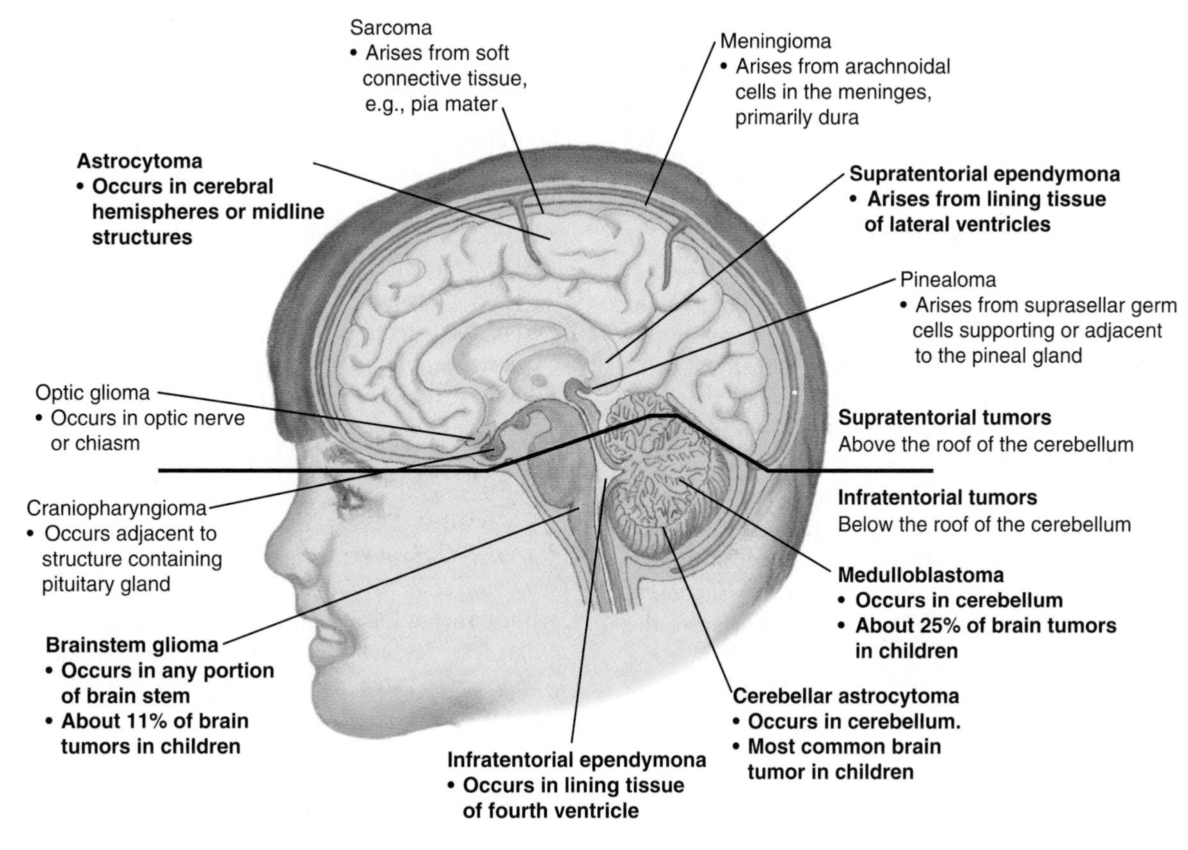

Location of brain tumors in children. Boldface labels indicate the most frequently occurring tumors in children.

Incidence. In the U.S., about 1500 children every year are diagnosed with a brain tumor (Friedman, Horowitz, & Oakes, 1991; Albright, 1993).

Clinical Manifestations

- Vomiting on arising, which becomes progressively more projectile
- Ataxia
- Visual changes (nystagmus, dyplopia, strabismus)
- Headaches that worsen on arising and improve during the day
- Nausea
- Seizures
- Lethargy
- Papilledema
- Positive Babinski's sign
- Cranial enlargement in infants
- Nuccal rigidity
- Bulging fontanel in infants
- Obscure behavioral changes, including irritability

Diagnostic Evaluation. Once a tumor is suspected, MRI, CT, single photon emission computed tomography (SPECT), or positron emission tomography (PET) scans are done. Adequate sedation is essential in order to diagnose a brain tumor. Chloral hydrate is the drug used most often to sedate young children. Usually a diagnosis is suspected from the symptoms the child exhibits and the location of the tumor. Pathologic examination then confirms the actual tissue type and tumor diagnosis. Depending on the type of tumor, a myelogram may be done to look for "drop mets," or metatastic disease in the spinal cord. A lumbar puncture examines the spinal fluid for the presence of tumor cells in the area.

Therapeutic Management. Initial intervention for a child with a brain tumor is "debulking," or operating to remove as much of the tumor as possible while minimally disturbing the surrounding brain tissue so that the child's neurologic functioning is preserved as much as possible. Children with the majority of the tumor removed have the best prognosis. In the case of a brain stem tumor, the risk to neurologic functioning outweighs the benefit of the debulking, so surgery may not be done. Depending on the location of the tumor and extent of surgical resection, a ventriculoperitoneal shunt may be inserted to relieve the hydrocephalus, thus relieving some of the symptoms. Dexamethasone is administered to reduce some of the brain tissue swelling that occurs from the manipulation of tissue during surgery.

Therapy depends on the type of tumor. More often than not, therapy will consist of surgery, radiation, and chemotherapy in a protocol form. Scanning performed at intervals will help determine progress with therapy.

NURSING CARE OF THE CHILD WITH A BRAIN TUMOR

Assessment

Because the majority of pediatric brain tumors arise in the posterior fossa, symptoms are related to increased intracranial pressure (ICP) and hydrocephalus.

> The hallmark symptoms of children with brain tumors are headache and morning vomiting related to the child getting out of bed.

The sudden increase in ICP with the change in position causes the vomiting. Parents may express much guilt for not paying attention to their child's complaint of headaches. These children are initially seen with neurologic symptoms. A thorough neurologic assessment should be performed (Chapter 11). Before allowing the child to get out of bed without help, the child's safety should be assessed. Children who have had insidious loss of visual function may have learned to compensate well, and excellent assessment skills will be required to determine that loss. Seizure precautions should be considered for any child with a brain tumor both preoperatively and postoperatively. Depending on the length of time the child has been feeling ill, weight loss and poor nutrition may be assessed.

Nursing Diagnosis and Planning

The following nursing diagnoses and expected outcomes may be appropriate following assessment of the child with a brain tumor.

- Pain related to increased intracranial pressure. ***Expected Outcome:*** *The child will verbalize a decrease in the severity of headache.*
- Risk for Infection related to surgery. ***Expected Outcome:*** *The child will exhibit no signs of infection.*
- Anxiety (child and parents) related to surgery and diagnosis. ***Expected Outcome:*** *The child/parents will exhibit decreased anxiety about outcomes of surgery and therapy.*
- Knowledge Deficit related to disease process. ***Expected Outcome:*** *The parents will verbalize an understanding of the disease process.*
- Body Image Disturbance related to a shaved head and hair loss. ***Expected Outcome:*** *The child will demonstrate appropriate coping techniques for hair loss and return to socializing.*

Implementation

When a child is suspected of having a brain tumor, the fear and anxiety is tremendous because of the potential neurologic impact of surgery and the fear of treatment failure and death.

Preoperative Care. Preoperative teaching should be done at the child's developmental level to prepare the child and family for the potential outcomes of surgery. The child should be educated about the anesthesia process and prepared to spend some time in the intensive care unit after surgery. Further discussion of preoperative care can be found in Chapter 18.

The child's head will be shaved before surgery. Although every effort is made to shave only as much hair as is necessary, it can still be traumatic for the child. The nurse should be aware of this and assist the child in verbalizing fears. Some children enjoy wearing a favorite cap or hat or making an outing of going to buy a hat. Prepare the child to wake up with a large dressing covering his head.

Postoperative Care. Postoperatively the child is at risk to develop increased ICP related to edema, hydrocephalus, or hemorrhage. Vital signs and mental and neurologic status are checked frequently. Special attention is paid to the child's temperature, which may be elevated because of hypothalamus or brainstem involvement during surgery. A cooling blanket should either be in place on the bed or readily available if the child becomes hyperthermic.

The child is assessed for signs of bleeding. Internal bleeding will manifest itself through changes in parameters associated with increasing ICP (i.e., pupil size, blood pressure, respiratory pattern). External bleeding is observed on the dressing. The back of the dressing is assessed for posterior pooling of blood. It is helpful to know the amount of expected drainage, especially if a drain has been placed in the wound. Areas of drainage are circled to monitor the amount of drainage and the dressing is reinforced. Colorless drainage indicates cerebrospinal fluid and should be reported immediately.

Postoperative positioning should be indicated by the surgeon. Location and size of the tumor are factors in determining positioning of the child. The child may have the head of the bed elevated to promote drainage of spinal fluid or, in the case of children who have tumors removed, they may lie flat. Care should be taken when turning the child to prevent tension on the suture line if it is in an area that movement will affect. The child is never placed in the Trendelenburg position because it increases ICP and the risk of bleeding. In the event of shock, the surgeon is notified immediately before changing the child's position.

From 30% to 40% of children with brain tumors will develop hydrocephalus, requiring placement of a permanent shunt catheter (Ryan & Shiminski-Maher, 1995). Chapter 40 addresses care of the child with a shunt.

The child may have a severe headache due to cerebral edema. A quiet environment, without bright lighting, should be provided together with comfortable positioning within the limits of the child's condition. Analgesia, according to the surgeon's protocol, should be provided. This will vary from morphine to Tylenol (acetaminophen). See Chapter 20 for discussion of pain management.

After the child is stabilized, he is assessed for functional deficits resulting from surgery (see box). These are somewhat predictable knowing the area of the brain involved and the function of that area. If these deficits are significant, the child may require rehabilitation to regain function.

Chemotherapy will begin after the child recovers from surgery, usually within a few weeks. Many of the current protocols use one or two courses of chemotherapy before radiation begins, depending on the age of the child. Additional nursing care related to the specific needs of the child with a brain tumor can be found in the care plan for a child with leukemia.

Functional Deficits Following Surgery for a Brain Tumor

After surgery, the child should be assessed for the following functional deficits:

- Ataxia, including head control and truncal stability
- Bilateral extremity strength and purposeful movement
- Speech
- Ability to swallow
- Vision and hearing
- Presurgical development task mastery
- Receptive and expressive language

If deficits are significant, the child may require rehabilitation to regain function.

Evaluation

- Are there both verbal and nonverbal indications of a positive comfort level?
- Is the family able to discuss the treatment plan and concerns related to the disease and treatment plan?
- Has the child remained free of infection?
- Is the child relating with peers in the same manner as prior to the disease?

NEUROBLASTOMA

Neuroblastoma is a solid tumor found only in children. Children younger than 12 months and those with a lower stage of disease have a favorable prognosis. Research is being done to improve outcomes for this disease.

Pathophysiology. The embryonal tumor arises from neural crest cells, which develop into the sympathetic nervous system and the adrenal medulla. Typically the tumor infringes on adjacent, normal tissue and organs. Discoveries in the cytogenetic makeup of this tumor have given researchers insight into prognostic indicators, which help them with treatment plans.

Etiology. The cause of neuroblastoma is unknown.

Incidence. Neuroblastoma occurs at a rate of 8.7 per million children, or 500–600 new cases annually in the United States (Santana, 1996) and is more common in boys than girls and more common in white children than black ones (Sullivan, 1993). About 70% of patients present with metastases (Sullivan, 1993).

Clinical Manifestations. These depend on the extent and involvement of the tumor.

- Abdominal mass
- Impaired range of motion and mobility, even pain and limping
- Decreased hemoglobin (rare)
- Large abdominal mass can produce disruption in bowel and bladder function.
- Chest tumors produce cough, decreased chest expansion with respiratory compromise.
- Compression of the superior vena cava results in facial and periorbital edema.
- "Dancing" eye movements
- Myoclonic jerks

Diagnostic Evaluation. Most children with neuroblastoma are diagnosed before age 2 years. A diagnostic workup includes chest X-ray, CT scan and bone scan to look for extent of disease. A bone marrow aspirate and biopsy, usually of both posterior iliac crests, evaluates marrow involvement.

Neuroblastoma cells may excrete catecholamines and their metabolites, vanillylmandelic acid (VMA) and homovanillic acid (HVA). Urine samples of children with neuroblastoma have elevated VMA and HVA 90% of the time (Nathan & Oski, 1993). Tumor samples will be sent to special reference laboratories to look at the genetic makeup of the tumor. Genetic information helps determine prognosis and treatment plan.

Therapeutic Management. Treatment depends on the presence and extent of metastasis. The *International Staging System for Neuroblastoma* is used to compare patients (see box). Staging criteria includes extent and location of metastasis, lymph node involvement, and whether the tumor is unilateral or crosses midline. Early-stage disease without metastasis may only require surgical excision of the tumor and follow-up evaluations. Children with later stage, poor prognosis disease may be taken to surgery for the purpose of obtaining tissue samples or for tumor debulking for pain control, not for resection of the tumor or tumors.

Age of diagnosis is also an important prognostic indicator. Cases diagnosed in children under age 1 year have a better prognosis. Some neuroblastoma that occurs in infants of less than 1 year has a high rate of spontaneous regression and may be only watched carefully or treated with low doses of chemotherapy (Foley, Fochtman, & Mooney, 1993).

After staging, treatment plans may include radiotherapy to tumor sites and systemic chemotherapy for several months. Another attempt at resection of the tumor may be carried out after combination chemotherapy and radiation have had an opportunity to reduce the tumor size. Bone marrow transplants are being done more routinely for later-stage neuroblastoma.

International Staging System for Neuroblastoma

Stage	Description
Stage 1	Localized tumor confined to the area of origin; complete gross excision, with or without microscopic residual disease, identifiable ipsilateral and contralateral lymph nodes negative microscopically.
Stage 2A	Unilateral tumor with incomplete gross excision; identifiable ipsilateral and contralateral lymph nodes negative microscopically.
Stage 2B	Unilateral tumor with complete or incomplete gross excision; with positive ipsilateral regional lymph nodes; identifiable contralateral lymph nodes negative microscopically.
Stage 3	Tumor infiltrating across the midline with or without regional lymph node involvement; or, unilateral tumor with contralateral regional lymph node involvement; or, midline tumor with bilateral regional lymph node involvement.
Stage 4	Dissemination of tumor to distant lymph nodes, bone, bone marrow, liver, and/or other organs (except as defined in stage 4S).
Stage 4S	Localized primary tumor as defined for stage 1 or 2 with dissemination limited to liver, skin, and/or bone marrow.

From Brodeur GM, Seeger RC, Barrett A, et al. (1988). International criteria for diagnosis, staging, and response to treatment in patients with neuroblastoma, *Journal of Clinical Oncology*, 6, 1874–1881.

NURSING CARE OF THE CHILD WITH NEUROBLASTOMA

Assessment

Parents may state their child has wanted to be held more often than usual. Activity level and appetite are usually reported as decreased. These children typically present as pale, very irritable, and uncomfortable appearing. Because of large abdominal tumors, many present with protuberant abdomens with masses palpated as hard and crossing midline. Range of motion and mobility are often impaired so much that the child will not bear weight.

Nursing Diagnosis and Planning

The following nursing diagnoses and expected outcomes may be appropriate following assessment of the infant with neuroblastoma.

- Pain related to tumor presence. ***Expected Outcome:*** *The infant will exhibit decreased crying and a relaxed body position.*
- Anxiety (parents) related to diagnosis of cancer, surgery, and treatment plan. ***Expected Outcome:*** *The parents will express decreased anxiety about the outcomes of therapy.*
- Knowledge Deficit related to disease process. ***Expected Outcome:*** *The parents will verbalize an understanding of the disease process.*

Implementation

Nursing care is focused initially on support of the family as they react and adjust to the diagnosis of cancer. Secondly the nurse should facilitate the educational process to allay fears based on unknowns. Initial care of the child will include pain management both preoperatively and postoperatively. Expect the child with an abdominal tumor to return from surgery with an NG tube in place. The wound should be carefully assessed for bleeding and signs of infection. Postoperative care of the child is discussed in Chapter 18.

Typically, later-stage disease will be treated immediately postoperatively with chemotherapy. With responsive tumors, improvements in the child's disposition will result very quickly. Refer to pages 996–999 for interventions for the child receiving chemotherapy and radiation. Additional nursing care may also be found in the care plan for the child with leukemia.

Evaluation

- Has the infant exhibited decreased crying and irritability?
- Is the infant resting quietly and comfortably in his mother's arms and having uninterrupted periods of rest?
- Are the parents asking questions related to the child's disease and treatment and seeking the support of family and friends?
- Are the parents verbalizing their fears and indicating the presence of coping skills?

OSTEOSARCOMA

Osteosarcoma, or osteogenic sarcoma, the most common bone malignancy in children, is a very aggressive tumor. The symptoms of this disease in its earliest stage are almost always attributed to extremity injury or normal "growing pains." Typically, trauma brings the tumor to the attention of medical personnel.

Pathophysiology. Osteosarcoma originates from bone-producing cells, which invade the medullary canal of the bone and quickly spread to surrounding soft tissue. The distal femur is the most common site followed by other lesions around the knee and shoulder. About 10% to 20% of patients have metastatic spread of disease at the time of diagnosis, usually first to the lungs (Betcher, 1993).

Etiology. The cause is unknown, although associations have been made between radiation for other diseases and osteosarcoma. Familial tendencies have been seen, suggesting that genetic factors are involved (Nathan & Oski, 1993).

Incidence. Because the peak incidence is in the teenage years, the rapid bone growth of the adolescent growth spurt is associated with the development of this tumor. Osteosarcoma occurs in girls at an earlier age than boys, which corresponds to their earlier maturation. Before adolescence, osteosarcoma is rare, but occurs with equal frequency in boys and girls (Betcher, 1993).

Clinical Manifestations

- Progressive, insidious, intermittent pain at tumor site
- Palpable mass
- Limping, if weight-bearing limb affected
- Progressive limited range of motion
- Eventually, pathologic fractures at tumor site

Diagnostic Evaluation. Initially X-rays of the primary site and chest are done, then a CT scan or MRI and bone scan. The CT scan will include the chest area to look for pulmonary metastases to help with staging of the disease. A biopsy must be done with great care so that there is no local contamination of tissue by tumor. Laboratory tests include a CBC, chemistries, serum alkaline phosphatase (ALP) and lactate dehydrogenase (LDH). Approximately 50% to 60% of patients will have elevated serum ALP (Nathan & Oski, 1993).

Therapeutic Management. Goals of therapy are to remove the tumor and prevent the spread of disease. Amputation has been the standard surgical intervention and is still necessary in some cases. However, some tumors are situated such that specially trained orthopedic surgeons are able to perform a limb-salvage operation. This is a complex procedure designed to remove the affected tissue with certainty of **clean margins** while preserving limb function by use of either bone grafts or surgically placed orthopedic devices. Many children with osteosarcoma are not candidates for limb salvage because of the location of their tumor.

Early research on this disease demonstrated that, even if a surgical resection of the tumor was accomplished, children had recurrent disease. This alerted physicians to the presence of microscopic disease. Therefore, after surgery, chemotherapy is begun even if the surgical procedure appears to have been successful. Chemotherapy is aimed at preventing the spread of disease by killing any microscopic tumor cells present anywhere in the body.

In children without overt metastasis, the cure rate is about 66% (Betcher, 1993). Extent of disease at diagnosis and elevation of LDH are the two most significant prognostic indicators. About 10% to 20% of patients with metastatic disease at diagnosis have a poor outcome. Elevated LDH at time of diagnosis decreases survival rate to 32% from 67% if the LDH is normal (Betcher, 1993).

NURSING CARE OF THE CHILD WITH OSTEOSARCOMA

Assessment

Subjective data to assess for includes history of injury to the affected limb and history of discomfort.

> Ask the child if any of his friends has noticed him limping or if he tires out more easily than his peers, making him unable to keep up in sports or play.

To prepare the child for outcomes of surgery, an assessment of his activity and sports involvement is essential to the psychosocial history. As in any child with cancer, body image changes, especially if the affected limb must be amputated, are of paramount importance. Preoperatively, the nurse should not only assess the child's values and fears, but also begin the process of preparing him for what he will look like after surgery.

By the time these patients come to medical attention, they may be in considerable pain from the tumor. Warmth, erythema, and tenderness at the site of tumor are not uncommon. If the swelling is great, the skin may appear shiny and taut with dilated blood vessels. Usually lung involvement is nonsymptomatic.

Nursing Diagnosis and Planning

The following nursing diagnoses and expected outcomes may be appropriate following assessment of the child with osteosarcoma.

- Pain related to tumor. ***Expected Outcome:*** *The child will verbalize decreased levels of pain using a pain assessment tool.*
- Fear and Anxiety related to loss of limb and diagnosis of cancer. ***Expected Outcome:*** *The child/parents will express decreased fears and anxiety related to surgery and diagnosis.*
- Risk for Infection related to surgical procedure. ***Expected Outcome:*** *The child will exhibit no signs and symptoms of infection.*
- Body Image Disturbance related to loss or impairment of limb. ***Expected Outcome:*** *The child will return to appropriate social situations.*
- Impaired Physical Mobility related to loss or impairment of limb. ***Expected Outcome:*** *The child will adapt to physical impairment with assistance with a return of mobility.*
- Knowledge Deficit related to disease process. ***Expected Outcome:*** *The child/parents will verbalize an understanding of the disease process.*

Implementation

Initial care is focused on making the patient comfortable. Preoperative teaching is extensive and must be specific to the procedure being done. If limb-salvaging is the procedure of choice, the surgeon and nurse should spend extensive time with the family explaining what is to be done. The nurse will be able to reinforce the preoperative and postoperative teaching. A central venous access device may be implanted while the child is undergoing anesthesia.

In addition to the usual postoperative care, pain, infection, and potential hemorrhage are concerns. The potential for postoperative pneumonia may be greater in the patient with pulmonary metastases.

If amputation occurs, phantom limb pain is a temporary condition some patients may experience. This sensation of burning, aching, or cramping in the missing limb is most distressing to the patient. He needs to be reassured that the condition is normal and only temporary.

Eventually, the child may be fitted with a permanent prosthesis once the surgical site has thoroughly healed. To begin to mold the stump for that, a temporary prosthesis may be used. This will more quickly enable the child to maintain use and strength of surrounding muscles in preparation for the permanent device. A prosthesis will address the issues of body image disturbance and enable the child to more quickly resume independence with activities of daily living. Prepare the child for much practice with physical therapists before he will achieve mo-

TEACHING GUIDELINES *for Home Care of the Child With Osteosarcoma*

- Provide written and verbal instructions concerning exercises to be done at home while surgical site is healing in preparation for fitting of prosthesis.
- Instruct on how to wrap stump for molding to adjust to prosthesis after surgical site has completely healed.
- Instruct to assess surgical site daily and wash with soap and water.
- Instruct on signs/symptoms of infection to report to physician.
- Make appropriate referrals as needed for financial, psychosocial, and physical support at home.
- Stress importance of follow-up care.

bility with the prosthesis. Teenagers, especially, may become discouraged if they expect the prosthesis to enable them to move "normally." Prepare them for a limp or for awkward movements with the prosthesis.

Assist the child to verbalize feelings about amputation. Involve the child in age-appropriate decision making concerning care. Encourage interaction with other children of the same age who have the same disease (support groups). Provide opportunities for the family to participate in care of the child and to provide support and encouragement. (See the Teaching Guidelines for Home Care of the Child With Osteosarcoma.)

Chemotherapy will begin several weeks after surgery to allow for proper healing of the surgical site. Radiation is used only for palliative pain control in advanced-stage disease because osteosarcoma is generally unresponsive to radiation.

Follow-up outpatient visits need to include a careful assessment of psychosocial adjustment. Questions should include the topics of social interactions, school attendance and performance, and behavioral changes. Additional related nursing care may be found in the care plan for the child with leukemia.

Evaluation

- Is the child experiencing minimal discomfort related to amputation?
- Are the family and child discussing fears related to disease and treatment?
- Is the child relating with peers?
- Has the child adapted to physical impairment with a return to mobility?

EWING'S SARCOMA

Ewing's sarcoma is the second most common bone tumor seen in children. Diagnosis is often challenging for physicians because this disease mimics infection and may be difficult to differentiate from other malignancies.

Pathophysiology. Ewing's sarcoma is a diagnosis made after all other small, round cell tumors have been excluded. Ewing's sarcoma has no defining characteristics. The disease is thought to arise from parasympathetic nerve tissue (Horowitz, Neff, & Kun, 1991). Like osteosarcoma, this tumor invades the soft tissue around the bone and is found most often in the midshaft of long bones, especially the femur, vertebrae, ribs, and pelvic bones. Gross metastasis is uncommon at diagnosis but does occur, most often in the lungs, bone, or bone marrow. Like osteosarcoma, microscopic disease is thought to be present early in the disease process.

Etiology. The cause is unknown and no genetic predispositions have been shown.

Incidence. Incidence is 1.7 per million per year in white children; the disease is very uncommon in black and Chinese children (Betcher, 1993). Ewing's sarcoma is rare in children under age 5 years and adults over age 30 years.

Clinical Manifestations

- Pain
- Soft tissue swelling around the affected bone
- If metastatic disease occurs, anorexia, fever, malaise, fatigue and weight loss are seen.
- If vertebral tumor is present, neurologic symptoms will be seen.
- If rib tumor is present, respiratory symptoms will be seen.

Diagnostic Evaluation. Diagnostic work-up is the same as osteosarcoma, and biopsy is necessary to differentiate between the two. Diagnostic work-up includes a plain chest X-ray, CT of the chest, CT or MRI of the primary site, bone scan, and a bone marrow aspirate and biopsy.

Therapeutic Management. Treatment begins with chemotherapy, followed by treatment directed at local control of the tumor. Clinicians debate whether to manage the primary tumor site with surgery or radiotherapy because this tumor is so sensitive to radiation (Horowitz, Neff, & Kun, 1991). Consideration is given to the expendability of the bone involved when surgery is considered as a treatment option. Bones such as a rib or a proximal fibula are considered expendable and may be removed to excise the tumor. Cure rates are over 70% in children with small extremity tumors and no metastasis (Meyer & Marina, 1996). With gross metastasis, the cure rate drops dramatically. Factors associated with a poor prognosis include an elevated LDH, a proximal rather than distal tumor, large tumor volume, and presence of metastatic disease, including bone marrow involvement.

NURSING CARE OF THE CHILD WITH EWING'S SARCOMA

Nursing care is similar to that described under osteosarcoma with the addition of care for the patient receiving radiotherapy. See previous sections for care of the child receiving chemotherapy and radiation and the care plan for the child with leukemia.

RHABDOMYOSARCOMA

Rhabdomyosarcoma is a malignancy of muscle, or striated, tissue that most often occurs periorbitally, in the head and neck in younger children, or in the trunk and extremities among older children. Long-term survival varies with the age of the patient, the histologic type of the tumor, and the location of the tumor.

Etiology. Although the exact etiology is unknown, rhabdomyosarcoma has been associated with familial cancer syndromes. There exists a higher incidence of maternal breast cancer in mothers of children with rhabdomyosarcoma.

Incidence. Rhabdomyosarcoma is the most common soft tissue malignancy in children and accounts for 5% to 10% of all malignant solid tumors in children (LaQuaglia, 1991). Annual incidence is estimated as 4.3 per million cases in white children and 3.3 per million cases in black children. Two age-groups predominate: age 2 to 6 years and age 15 to 19 years (Van Wezel-Bolen, 1993).

Clinical Manifestations

Dependent on tumor location:

- Soft to hard, nontender, relatively immobile mass may be mistaken for a traumatic hematoma.
- If periorbital, visual changes are present; the child may have ptosis, exophthalmos, or proptosis (bulging). Cranial nerve involvement may occur.
- In extremity tumors, limited range of motion is present.
- In pelvic tumors, disrupted organ function is seen around tumor.

PATHOPHYSIOLOGY *of Rhabdomyosarcoma*

Four histologic subtypes of rhabdomyosarcoma exist. Accounting for 50% to 60% of the tumors is the embryonic type, which carries the best prognosis. About 20% of cases are the alveolar type, which is most often found in the perineal area, trunk, and extremities and carries the worst prognosis. The pleomorphic type is very rare in children. Around 10% to 20% of tumors are considered undifferentiated (Holleb, Fink, & Murphy, 1991).

In addition to the histologic types described above, prognosis depends on several other factors. Children who have residual disease after attempted resection seem to have a poorer prognosis. If the tumor is in a location where symptoms appear early rather than deeply buried in a body cavity, the prognosis is better because the tumor is usually found before metastasis has occurred. Abnormalities in the DNA content of the tumor cells has prognostic significance. Staging of the tumor cells is based on whether the tumor was resected completely, resected with residual microscopic disease, incompletely resected, or presented with distant metastases (Rodary, Flaman, & Donaldson, 1989).

Diagnostic Evaluation. Diagnosis is made following a biopsy or attempted surgical resection of the tumor, a decision made depending on the location of the tumor. CT scans and ultrasounds are useful tools in determining extent of metastasis. Additional studies done depend on the location of the tumor and include lymphangiograms, a CBC, urinalysis, renal and liver function tests, skeletal surveys, bone scans, bone marrow aspirate and biopsy, and a lumbar puncture.

Therapeutic Management. The treatment of choice is a complete surgical resection of the tumor. However, a tumor attached to vital tissue may have to be left. When this occurs, the physician knows the child still has active tumor cells that need to be aggressively treated before they replicate and spread. Tumor cells not removed by surgery are referred to as residual disease. Radiotherapy is used for most patients except those with only local disease. Research is ongoing for the best regimen of chemotherapy to treat this disease. About 80% of children with metastatic disease at time of diagnosis relapse (Nathan & Oski, 1993).

NURSING CARE OF THE CHILD WITH RHABDOMYOSARCOMA

Assessment

Parents may relate that their first indication that something was wrong was the decreased activity level of the young child unable to verbalize pain. If the tumor is more superficially located, parents may have discovered a lump or swelling.

Findings of the physical exam will depend on the location of the tumor, but typically a soft to hard, nontender mass will be palpated. Surrounding lymph nodes should be palpated for enlargement that may indicate tumor involvement. The CBC is usually normal unless the tumor has extended into bone marrow causing a decrease in hemoglobin.

Nursing Diagnosis and Planning

The following nursing diagnoses and expected outcomes may be appropriate following assessment of the child with rhabdomyosarcoma.

- Anxiety (family/child) related to surgical procedure and outcome. ***Expected Outcome:*** *The child/parents will express decreased anxiety about surgery procedure and outcomes.*
- Risk for Infection related to surgery. ***Expected Outcome:*** *The child will exhibit no signs or symptoms of infection.*
- Knowledge Deficit related to disease process and treatment plan. ***Expected Outcome:*** *The child/parents will verbalize an understanding of the disease process and treatment.*

Implementation

Nursing care is focused initially on support of the family as they react and adjust to the diagnosis of cancer. Second, the nurse should facilitate the educational process to allay fears based on unknowns.

Postoperative care of the biopsy or surgical site will involve careful observations for signs of infection, hemorrhage, and edema. If surgery involves an abdominal or pelvic tumor excision, expect the child to return from surgery with an NG tube and possibly drains in place. Typically, a central venous catheter will be placed at the time of surgery.

Refer to the previous sections on interventions for the child receiving chemotherapy or radiation.

Follow-up care will involve periodic CT scans and/or MRIs to assess for response of the tumor to therapy or monitor any further disease progression. Most relapses will occur within 2 years of diagnosis and during therapy, although relapses have been reported as late as 6 years after diagnosis (Nathan & Oski, 1993). Additional related nursing care may be found in the care plan for the child with leukemia.

Evaluation

- Is anxiety decreased in the family and the child?
- Is the family supported by extended family members and friends, and are they asking questions related to their child's disease and care?
- Has the child remained free of infection?
- Does the child display a relaxed, comfortable body posture while relating with peers and family members?

RETINOBLASTOMA

Retinoblastoma is a rare, malignant tumor of the eye found only in children. Sometimes observant parents call this disease to the attention of the physician when they are looking at photographs and see a white reflection in one of the child's eyes instead of the normal red color when the camera flash is reflected off the retina.

Pathophysiology. The tumor develops in the posterior portion of the retina. It is possible for retinoblastoma to develop at a single site, but more commonly one sees multiple independent tumors of predominantly two types: familial and sporadic. Extension of the tumor down the optic nerve into the CNS occurs rarely. Metastasis is rarely seen before diagnosis (Pratt, 1996).

Like other forms of cancer, a staging system has been developed to standardize a method by which to communicate extent of disease and direct treatment regimens. Staging for retinoblastoma consists of Groups I through V, progressing from small single or multiple tumors to massive tumors with vitreous seeding.

Etiology. Retinoblastoma results from a genetic mutation. Research has isolated the mutation that causes familial disease to chromosome 13. Advances in genetic studies of this disease have led to genetic research of other forms of childhood cancer.

Incidence. Incidence is 1 in 20,000 live births, with equal distribution in boys and girls and among races (Foley, Fochtman, & Mooney, 1993).

Clinical Manifestations

- Leukokoria, or cat's eye reflex
- Vision loss
- Pain, redness, and inflammation of the eye
- Strabismus
- Squinting

Diagnostic Evaluation. Average age of diagnosis is 11 months for bilateral tumors and 23 months for unilateral tumors (Pratt, 1996). Diagnosis is usually made by visualization of leukokoria on routine examination. In children with a known family history of retinoblastoma, diagnosis usually follows routine fundoscopic examination under general anesthesia. CT scan and MRI of the orbits, as well as X-ray studies for extent of disease, should be done, as should a skeletal survey, bone scan, bone marrow aspirate, and lumbar puncture to look for metastasis.

Therapeutic Management. Typically in unilateral disease, there are multiple tumors present causing a loss of vision. Enucleation of the eye is standard therapy, but is becoming less frequent as nonsurgical therapies improve. With bilateral disease, treatment is aimed at preserving useful vision in one eye. Usually, the most involved eye is enucleated and the remaining eye receives radiotherapy. Chemotherapy is useful in achieving a response in metastatic disease, although not usually with long-term cure. Five-year survival is virtually 100% for Groups I through IV and approximately 85% for Group V patients (Nathan & Oski, 1993).

NURSING CARE OF THE CHILD WITH RETINOBLASTOMA

Assessment

Except for leukokoria (whitish reflex in pupillary area), the findings of physical examination of the child are usually normal.

Nursing Diagnoses and Planning

The following nursing diagnoses and expected outcomes may be appropriate following assessment of the child with retinoblastoma.

- Anxiety (child/family) related to enucleation and/or fear of blindness. ***Expected Outcome:*** *The child/family will express decreased anxiety about outcomes of therapy.*
- Risk for Infection related to enucleation. ***Expected Outcome:*** *The child will exhibit no signs or symptoms of infection.*
- Sensory/Perceptual Alterations (Visual) related to enucleation. ***Expected Outcome:*** *The child will develop compensatory mechanisms for vision.*
- Knowledge Deficit related to disease process. ***Expected Outcome:*** *The child/parents will verbalize an understanding of the disease process.*

Implementation

Nursing care is focused initially on support of the family as they react and adjust to the diagnosis of cancer. Secondly, the nurse should facilitate the educational process to allay fears based on unknowns.

Postoperative care of the enucleated orbit will involve careful observations for signs of infection, hemorrhage, and edema. The child will wear a patch over the socket for about 1 week postoperatively. To preserve the shape of the orbit for prosthesis fitting 5 to 6 weeks after surgery, a conformer is placed in the orbit. Nursing interventions include teaching the parents how to remove, clean, and reinsert first the conformer, then the prosthesis. Refer to the previous sections for the child receiving chemotherapy or radiation.

Whatever the extent of involvement of tumor or treatment modality involved, careful follow-up care by CT scans is indicated. Genetic counseling is recommended. If the retinoblastoma is found to be genetic, siblings should be periodically examined, as should any offspring produced by the patient.

Children with retinoblastoma have a high incidence of developing second malignancies later in life because of the genetic cause of the disease. Although no specific screening is recommended, symptomatology should be carefully evaluated with a high index of suspicion. Additional nursing care may be found in the care plan for a child with leukemia.

Evaluation

- Are the child and family verbalizing their understanding of the disease and treatment plan?
- Has the child remained free of infection?
- Is the child able to relate to peers and family?

KEY CONCEPTS

- The signs and symptoms of childhood cancer vary according to the child's age, the type of tumor, and the extent of the disease.
- One of the difficulties in diagnosing childhood cancer is that most symptoms are attributable to common childhood illnesses.
- Chemotherapy, radiation, bone marrow transplantation, and biologic response modifiers are the forms of treatment of children with cancer.
- Children typically have longer treatment plans than adults with cancer because of their increased metabolic rate, resulting in increased rate of cell turnover.

- When administering chemotherapy the nurse must be aware of the length of infusion, route, dosage, and OSHA guidelines for the patient, family, and self.
- Some lotions and tapes will increase the skin's reaction to radiation.
- Fatigue is a common side effect of radiation, and the child may need increased periods of rest.
- There are three types of bone marrow transplantation: syngeneic, autologous, and allogeneic.
- Nursing care of the child with a bone marrow transplant focuses on the prevention of infection until the child engrafts and produces his own white blood cells with which to fight infection.
- Biologic response modifiers are minute, naturally occurring substances found in the body that influence the immune system. They include colony-stimulating factors, monoclonal antibodies, interleukins, tumor necrosis factor, and interferons.
- Chemotherapy is the preferred treatment for leukemia and is divided into phases: remission induction, consolidation, and continuation or maintenance.
- Common nursing diagnoses associated with the child with cancer include: risk for infection, altered nutrition, less than body requirements, knowledge deficit, ineffective family/individual coping, pain, impaired skin integrity, body image disturbance, and altered oral mucous membranes.
- The mouth and anus are at increased risk for breakdown in the child receiving chemotherapy and/or radiation. Rectal temperatures should not be taken, and meticulous mouth and anal care should be given.
- The abdomen of a child with a Wilms' tumor should never be palpated.
- Postoperatively the child with a brain tumor is at risk to develop increased intracranial pressure related to edema, hydrocephalus, or hemorrhage. Vital signs and mental and neurologic status are checked frequently.
- A cooling blanket should be available postoperatively for the child who has had brain surgery because of the risk of hyperthermia resulting from hypothalamus or brainstem involvement.
- A quiet environment should be provided for the child who has had brain surgery. The position of the child is usually determined by the physician and depends on the location and size of the tumor.

REFERENCES

Albright, L. (1993). Pediatric brain tumors. *CA—Cancer Journal for Clinicians, 43,* 272–288.

Baird, S. B., Donehower, M. G., Stalsbroten, V. L., & Ader, T. B. (1991). *Cancer source book for nurses* (6th ed.). Atlanta: American Cancer Society.

Behrman, R. E., & Vaughn, V. C. (Eds.). (1992). *Nelson textbook of pediatrics* (14th ed.). Philadelphia: W. B. Saunders.

Betcher, D. (1993). Bone tumors. In G. V. Foley, D. Fochtman, & K. H. Mooney (Eds.), *Nursing care of the child with cancer* (2nd ed., pp. 300–309). Philadelphia: W. B. Saunders.

Drigan, R., & Androkites, A. (1993). Wilms' tumor. In G. V. Foley, D. Fochtman, & K. H. Mooney (Eds.), *Nursing care of the child with cancer* (2nd ed., pp. 272–277). Philadelphia: W. B. Saunders.

Exelby, P. R. (1991). Wilms' tumor 1991. *Urologic Clinics of North America, 18*(3), 589–597.

Foley, G. V., Fochtman, D., & Mooney, K. H. (Eds.). (1993). *Nursing care of the child with cancer* (2nd ed.). Philadelphia: W. B. Saunders.

Friedman, H. S., Horowitz, M., & Oakes, W. J. (1991). Tumors of the central nervous system. *Pediatric Clinics of North America, 38*(2), 381–391.

Gaddy-Cohen, D. (1993). Acute lymphocytic leukemia. In G. V. Foley, D. Fochtman, & K. H. Mooney (Eds.), *Nursing care of the child with cancer* (2nd ed., pp. 208–225). Philadelphia: W. B. Saunders.

Green, D. M., Finkelstein, J. Z., Breslow, N. E., & Beckwith, J. B. (1991). Problems in the treatment of patients with Wilms' tumor. *Pediatric Clinics of North America, 67*(3), 475–488.

Holleb, A. T., Fink, D. J., & Murphy, G. P. (1991). *Textbook of clinical oncology*. Atlanta: American Cancer Society.

Horowitz, M. E., Neff, J. R., & Kun, L. E. (1991). Ewing's sarcoma: Radiotherapy versus surgery for local control. *Pediatric Clinics of North America, 38*(2), 365–380.

LaQuaglia, M. (1991). Genitourinary rhabdomyosarcoma in children. *Urology Clinics of North America, 18*(3), 575–580.

Leonard, M. (1993). Nursing implications of diagnostic and staging procedures. In G. V. Foley, D. Fochtman, & K. H. Mooney (Eds.), *Nursing care of the child with cancer* (2nd ed., pp. 56–80). Philadelphia: W. B. Saunders.

McGowan-Quinlan, D. (1993). Non-Hodgkin's lymphoma. In G. V. Foley, D. Fochtman, & K. H. Mooney (Eds.), *Nursing care of the child with cancer* (2nd ed., pp. 264–271). Philadelphia: W. B. Saunders.

Meyer, W., & Marina, N. (1996). Ewing sarcoma/peripheral neuroepithelioma. In R. E. Behrman, R. M. Kliegman, & A. M. Arvin (Eds.), *Nelson textbook of pediatrics* (15th ed., pp. 1468–1470). Philadelphia: W. B. Saunders.

Nathan, D. G., & Oski, F. A. (Eds.). (1993). *Hematology of infancy and childhood* (4th ed.). Philadelphia: W. B. Saunders.

Pratt, C. (1996). Retinoblastoma. In R. E. Behrman, R. M. Kliegman, & A. M. Arvin (Eds.), *Nelson textbook of pediatrics* (15th ed., pp. 1470–1471). Philadelphia: W. B. Saunders.

Rodary, C., Flamant, F., & Donaldson, S. S. (1989). An attempt to use a common staging system in rhabdomyosarcoma: A report of an international workshop initiated by the International Society of Pediatric Oncology. *Medical Pediatric Oncology, 17*(3), 210–215.

Ryan, J. & Shiminski-Maher, T. (1995). Hydrocephalus and shunts in children with brain tumors. *Journal of Pediatric Oncology Nursing, 12*(4), 223–224.

Santana, V. (1996). Neuroblastoma. In R. E. Behrman, R. M. Kliegman, & A. M. Arvin (Eds.), *Nelson textbook of pediatrics* (15th ed., pp. 1460–1462). Philadelphia: W. B. Saunders.

Schultz, W. H. (1989). Recognizing cancer in children. *Journal of the American Academy of Physician Assistants, 2*(5), 338–352.

Sullivan, M. (1993). Neuroblastoma. In G. V. Foley, D. Fochtman, & K. H. Mooney (Eds.), *Nursing care of the child with cancer* (2nd ed., pp. 278–287). Philadelphia: W. B. Saunders.

Van Wezel-Bolen, G. (1993). Rhabdomyosarcoma. In G. V. Foley, D. Fochtman, & K. H. Mooney (Eds.), *Nursing care of the child with cancer* (2nd ed., pp. 288–299). Philadelphia: W. B. Saunders.

Wisoff, J., & Epstein, F. (1994). Management of pediatric brain tumors. In R. Morantz and J. Walsh (Eds.), *Brain tumors: A comprehensive text* (pp. 581–611). New York: Marcel Dekker.

BIBLIOGRAPHY

Abramson, D. H., Giovinazzo, V., Servodidio, C. A., & Weil, A. R. (1992). Visual fields in a successfully radiated retinoblastoma patient. *Journal of Ophthalmic Nursing and Technology, 11*(1), 17–19.

Abramovitz, L., & Senner, A. Pediatric bone marrow transplant update. *Oncology Nursing Forum, 22*(1), 107–115.

Betcher, D. L., & Burnham, N. (1991). Odansetron. *Journal of Pediatric Oncology Nursing, 8*(4), 183–185.

Birch, J. M. (1990). Epidemiology of childhood cancer. *Annales Nestle, 48*(3), 105–116.

Brandt, B. (1990). Nursing protocol for the patient with neutropenia. *Oncology Nursing Forum, 17*(1), 9–14.

Brown, R. B. (1991). Abdominal mass on a well child examination. *Journal of Pediatric Health Care, 5*(6), 333, 345–346.

Burke, M. B., Wilkes, G. M., & Ingwerson, K. (1992). *Chemotherapy careplans.* Boston: Jones and Bartlett.

Cheung, N. V. (1991). Immunotherapy: Neuroblastoma as a model. *Pediatric Clinics of North America, 38*(2), 425–441.

Dodet, B., & Lenoir, G. M. (1990). Aetiology of childhood cancers. *Annales Nestle, 48*(3), 117–124.

Donaldson, S. S., & Link, M. (1991). Hodgkin's disease: Treatment of the young child. *Pediatric Clinics of North America, 38*(2), 457–474.

Galbraith, L. K., et al. (1991). Treatment for alteration in oral mucosa related to chemotherapy. *Pediatric Nursing, 17*(3), 233–236.

Groenwald, S. K., Frogge, M. H., Goodman, M., & Yarbro, C. H. (1992). *The cancer problem.* Boston: Jones and Bartlett.

Heiney, S. P. (1989). Adolescents with cancer. *Cancer Nursing, 12*(2), 95–101.

Hockenberry, M. J., & Coody, D. K. (Eds.). (1989). *Pediatric oncology and hematology. Perspectives on care.* St. Louis: C. V. Mosby.

Hockenberry, M. J., Coody, D. K., & Bennett, B. S. (1990). Childhood cancers: Incidence, etiology, diagnosis, and treatment. *Pediatric Nursing, 16*(3), 239–246.

Houghton P. J., Shapiro, D. N., & Houghton, J. A. (1991). Rhabdomyosarcoma: From the laboratory to the clinic. *Pediatric Clinics of North America, 38*(2), 349–364.

Jonides, L., Rudy, C., & Walsh, S. (1991). Abdominal mass on a well child examination. *Journal of Pediatric Health Care, 5*(6), 333, 345–346.

Joy, S., & Grosfeld, J. L. (1991). Wilms' tumor. *AORN Journal, 53*(2), 437–448.

Kurtzberg, J., & Graham, M. L. (1991). Non-Hodgkin's lymphoma: Biologic classification and implication for therapy. *Pediatric Clinics of North America, 38*(2), 443–456.

Lilley, L. L. (1990). Side effects associated with pediatric chemotherapy: Management and patient education issues. *Pediatric Nursing, 16*(3), 252–255.

Lucarelli, G., et al. (1990). Bone marrow transplantation patients with thalassemia. *New England Journal of Medicine, 322*(7), 417–421.

Matthay, K. K. (1995). Neuroblastoma: A clinical challenge and biologic puzzle. *CA–A Cancer Journal for Clinicians, 45*(3), 179–192.

McGuire, P., & Moore, K. (1990). Recent advances in childhood cancer. *Nursing Clinics of North America, 25*(2), 447–460.

Meister, L. A., & Meadows, A. T. (1993). Late effects of childhood cancer therapy. *Current Problems in Pediatrics, 23*(3), 102–131.

Mulligan, C. M., & Wittman, B. K. (1990). Nursing care of the child with a brain stem glioma. *Journal of Pediatric Nursing, 5*(6), 375–386.

Nichols, M. L. (1995). Social support and coping in young adolescents with cancer. *Pediatric Nursing, 21*(3), 235–240.

Pediatric Oncology Group. (1992). Progress against childhood cancer: The Pediatric Oncology Group experience. *Pediatrics, 89*(4), 597–600.

Rahr, V. A., & Tucker, R. (1990). Non-Hodgkin's lymphoma: Understanding the disease. *Cancer Nursing, 13*(1), 56–61.

Servodidio, C. A., Abramson, D. H., & Romanella, A. (1991). Retinoblastoma. *Cancer Nursing, 14*(3), 117–123.

Shiminski-Maher, T. (1990). Brain tumors in childhood: Implications for nursing practice. *Journal of Pediatric Nursing, 4*(3), 122–130.

Shiminski-Maher, T., & Rosenberg, M. (1990). Late effects associated with treatment of craniopharyngiomas in childhood. *Journal of Neuroscience Nursing, 22*(4), 220–226.

Shiminski-Maher, T., & Shields, M. (1995). Pediatric brain tumors diagnosis and management. *Journal of Pediatric Oncology Nursing, 12*(4), 188–198.

Tucker, R., & Rahr, V. (1990). Nursing care of the patient with non-Hodgkin's lymphoma. *Cancer Nursing, 13*(4), 229–234.

Walters, P. (1990). Chemo: A nurse's guide to action, administration, and side effects. *RN, 53*(2), 52–67.

Young, J. A., Eslinger, P., & Galloway, M. (1989). Radiation treatment for the child with cancer. *Issues in Comprehensive Pediatric Nursing, 12*, 159–169.

34

The Child With Integumentary Alterations

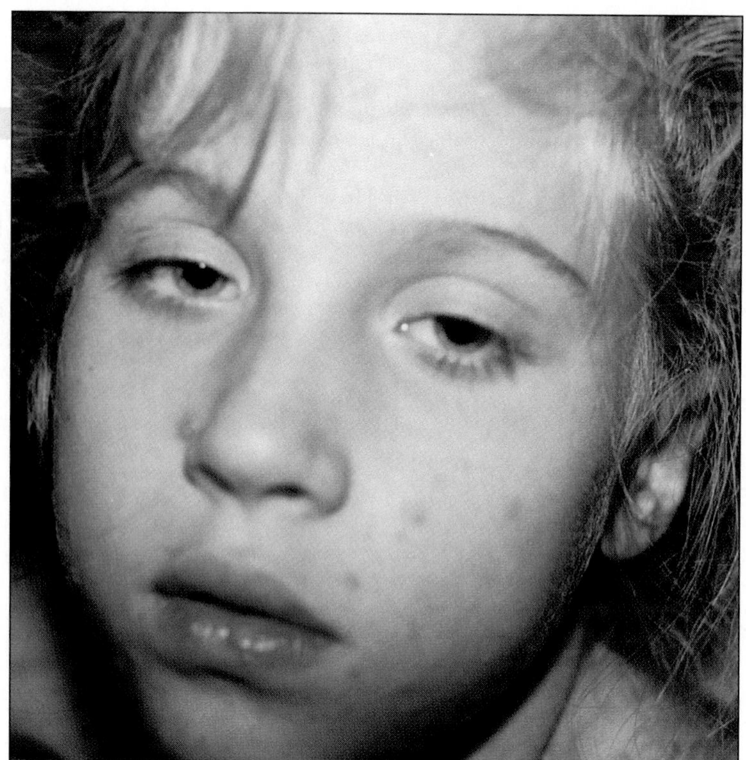

CHAPTER OVERVIEW

LEARNING OBJECTIVES

After studying this chapter, you should be able to:

- Describe the anatomy and physiology of normal skin.
- Describe the differences among the skin of the newborn, child, and adult.
- Identify common skin disorders of infants and children.
- Discuss manifestations of and treatment for common skin disorders, including bacterial, fungal, and viral infections; infestations; inflammatory disorders; acne vulgaris; and insect bites and stings.
- Discuss the nursing implications of common medications used in the treatment of skin disorders.
- Apply the nursing process in the care of infants and children with skin disorders.

KEY TERMS

alopecia: hair loss

apocrine sweat glands: secretory glands located in the axillae and genital regions; become active at puberty and respond to emotional and sexual stimulation

desquamation: sloughing of the skin in scales or sheets; can lead to loss of the deeper layers of the skin

ecchymoses: discoloration of the skin or mucous membranes caused by leakage of blood into the subcutaneous tissue

eccrine sweat glands: secretory glands distributed over the body that secrete sweat

erythema: redness of the skin

excoriation: scratch or abrasion of the skin

intertrigo: maceration of two skin surfaces in close opposition to each other

keratosis: overgrowth and thickening of the cornified epithelium

lichenification: thickening and hardening of the skin with accentuation of skin markings; often the result of chronic scratching

petechiae: tiny, flat purplish-red spots on the skin surface resulting from minute hemorrhages within the dermis

pruritus: itching

urticaria (hives): vascular reaction of the skin characterized by pruritic wheals, often caused by allergy or emotional stress

(See also key terms, Chapter 11.)

Skin is the largest organ of the body and is a sensitive indicator of a child's general health. Because skin disorders are among the most common health problems in children, they are seen frequently by nurses who work with pediatric patients. Skin disorders may cause pain, pruritus, or changes in local sensation. Because the skin is so visible and its disorders often disfiguring, dermatologic disorders can cause emotional and psychological stress for the child and family. Whether it is the discomfort and stress produced by an infant's eczema or the emotional upset caused by an adolescent's acne, skin disorders can influence the child's psychologic and social development.

Nurses caring for children are in a unique position to assess the condition of children's skin and to intervene to help children and families cope with these conditions. Nurses can play an important role by teaching parents and children strategies to maintain healthy skin and prevent future skin problems.

This chapter covers the various infectious and noninfectious skin disorders and infestations commonly seen in children. See also Chapter 11 for a discussion of skin assessment and illustrations of skin lesions.

CLINICAL REFERENCE PAGES

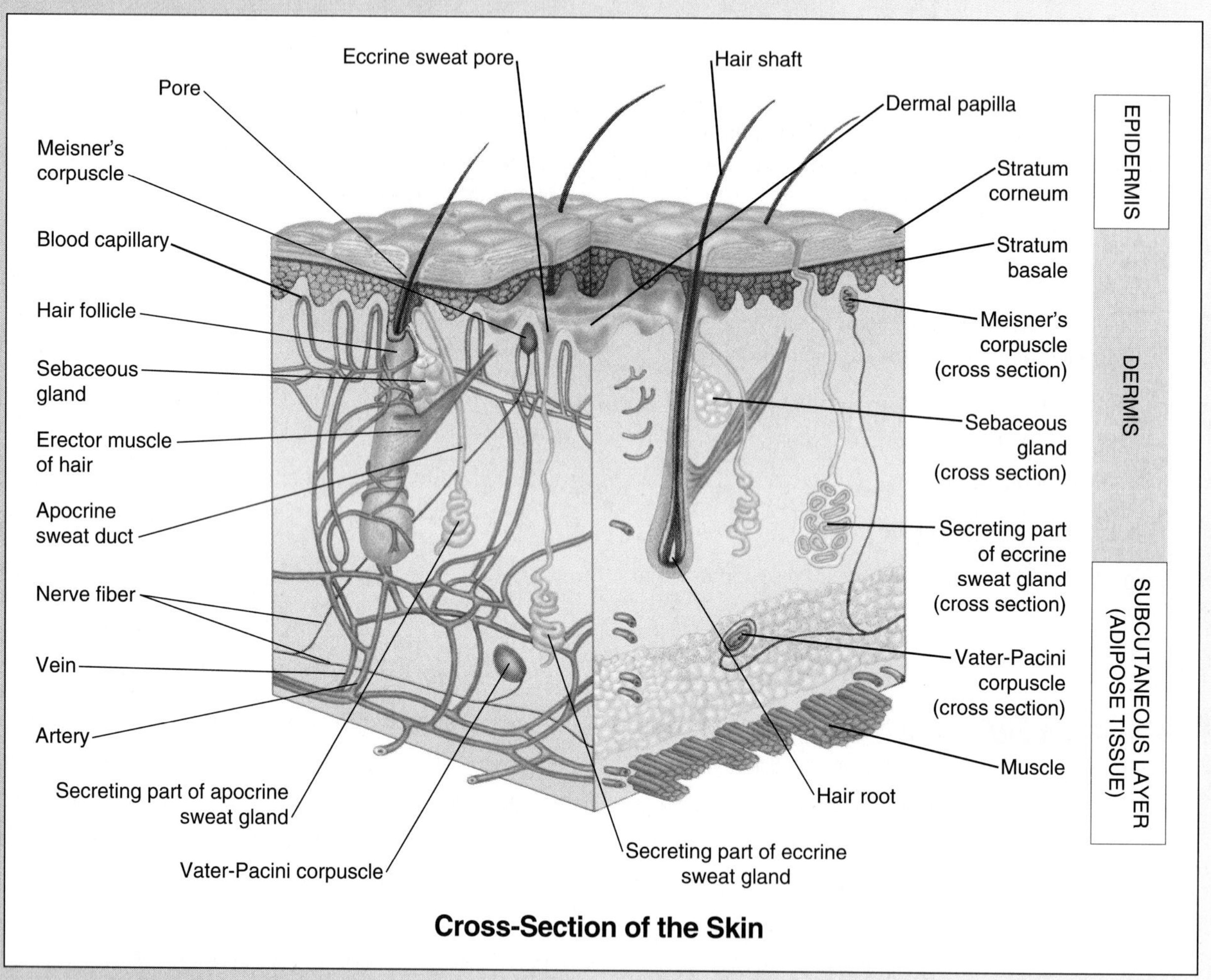

Cross-Section of the Skin

ANATOMY AND PHYSIOLOGY REVIEW

A knowledge of integumentary structure and function is necessary in order for the nurse to understand the changes that occur with disease. There are a number of important differences between the skin of infants and young children and that of adults (see box).

The skin is the body's largest organ. It has five major functions: (1) to protect the deeper tissues from injury, drying, and invasion by foreign matter; (2) to regulate temperature; (3) to aid in excretion of water; (4) to aid in production of vitamin D; and (5) to initiate the sensations of touch, pain, heat, and cold.

The skin is composed of two layers: the outer *epidermis* and the inner supportive *dermis*. Beneath these layers is the *subcutaneous layer*, which is composed largely of adipose tissue (see figure).

The *epidermis* is nonvascular stratified epithelium. It is divided into several layers, the two major layers being the *stratum corneum* and the *stratum basale*. The outermost stratum corneum is a tough, horny collection of dead keratinized cells that have migrated up from the underlying layers. Keratin, a fibrous protein, is also the principal component of the nails and hair. Skin cells are constantly being shed and replaced with new cells from the layers below. The epidermis is completely replaced every 4 weeks. The stratum basale, or basal cell layer, anchors the epidermis to the dermis. This innermost layer contains melanocytes, the source of melanin, the pigment that gives skin its color.

The *dermis*, composed of tough connective tissue, contains lymphatics and nerves. The highly vascular dermis nourishes the epidermis.

Appendages from the epidermis—sebaceous glands, sweat glands, and hair follicles—are embedded in the dermis. The sebaceous glands arise from the hair follicles and produce sebum, which lubricates the epidermis and is slightly bacteriostatic. Sebaceous glands are particularly abundant on the face and scalp. Their activity is influenced by hormones, testosterone increasing secretion and estrogen suppressing it. There are two types of sweat glands. The *eccrine sweat glands* open directly onto the skin surface and produce sweat, which evaporates to reduce body temperature. Eccrine sweat glands are widely distributed over the body and are mature in the 2-month-old infant. The *apocrine sweat glands* produce a thick, milky secretion and open onto hair follicles. They are located mainly in the axillary and genital areas and become active during puberty.

Each hair is composed of a shaft and a root, which lies in a deep cavity of dermal cells called the *hair follicle*. There are several types of hair. *Lanugo* is the first, fine hair that covers the body during fetal life, and generally disappears before or shortly after birth. It is replaced by fine, nonpigmented *vellus* hair. *Terminal* hair covers all the ordinarily hairy parts of the body and is coarse, long, and pigmented.

The *subcutaneous layer*, composed of fat cells, underlies the dermis. Adipose tissue helps to cushion and insulate underlying structures.

Pediatric Differences in the Skin

- The newborn's skin is thin and more susceptible to external irritants and to infection. Careful handling is required to avoid blistering the skin.
- Because of greater relative skin surface area to body volume ratio in infants and small children, there is a risk of greater absorption through the skin. Therefore, topical ointments and other skin preparations should not be used without a physician's order.
- The skin of infants and young children is more susceptible to bacterial infection.
- Immunoglobulin A (IgA) secreted by the epithelial cells of the mucous membranes does not reach adult levels until ages 2 to 5 years. This makes the infant less resistant to organisms, for example, on the hands or other objects the infant may put in his mouth.
- Eccrine glands do not reach mature function until age 2 or 3 years, making infants and young toddlers less able to regulate body temperature.

Data from Betz, C. L., Hunsberger, M. M., and Wright, S. [1994]. *Family-Centered Nursing Care of Children*, 2nd ed., p. 1652. Philadelphia: W. B. Saunders.

BACTERIAL INFECTIONS OF THE SKIN (PYODERMAS)

Skin infections are common during childhood. Bacterial flora are normally present on healthy skin. The susceptibility of the skin to infection from these organisms depends on several factors, including intactness of the skin, virulence of the organisms on the skin, and the immune status of the child.

Impetigo

Impetigo is the most common skin infection of childhood.

PATHOPHYSIOLOGY *of Impetigo*

Impetigo begins in an area of broken skin, such as an insect bite, scabies, or atopic dermatitis. Incubation period is 7 to 10 days. Impetigo is extremely contagious and may spread to other parts of the child's skin or to others who touch the child, use the same towel, or drink from the same glass. Spread of the infection is fostered by poor hygiene, crowded living conditions, and a hot, humid environment. Lesions resolve in 12 to 14 days with treatment.

Etiology. Impetigo may be caused by *Staphylococcus aureus*, group A beta-hemolytic streptococci, or a combination of these bacteria. *S. aureus* is the primary pathogen in most cases of impetigo.

Incidence. Impetigo is most common during hot, humid summer months. Toddlers and preschoolers are most frequently affected, often when recovering from an upper respiratory tract infection.

Clinical Manifestations

- Primary lesions are small red macules that quickly become vesicles or large bullae that rupture easily and release serous fluid.
- Secondary lesions are thick, honey-colored crusts that are lightly attached to the lesions. A superficial erosion that bleeds easily is present when crusts are removed.
- Lesions are pruritic. Scarring is not common, but may occur if the child picks or scratches the lesions.
- Lesions are usually located around the mouth and nose, but may be present on the extremities.

Figure 34–1 shows impetigo lesions. See also Chapter 11 for illustrations of common skin lesions.

Diagnostic Evaluation. Diagnosis is usually possible from the characteristic appearance of the lesions. Culture is not often performed unless the child fails to respond to treatment. If a culture is ordered, it should be obtained from beneath the crust or from the fluid inside the lesions.

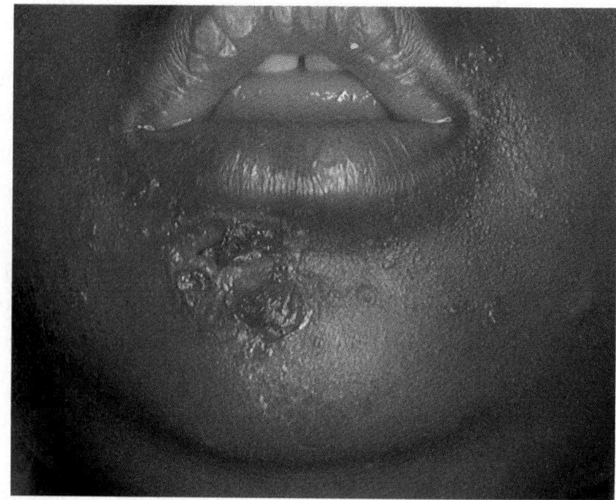

Figure 34–1
Impetigo lesions are usually located around the mouth and nose but may be located on the extremities. (From Hurwitz, S. [1993]. *Clinical pediatric dermatology: A textbook of skin disorders of childhood and adolescence* [2nd ed., p. 280]. Philadelphia: W. B. Saunders.)

Therapeutic Management. Impetigo is treated with topical and oral antibiotics. The lesions should be gently washed three times a day with a warm, soapy washcloth and crusts soaked and carefully removed. A topical ointment, such as bacitracin (Baciguent), mupirocin (Bactroban), or polymixin B sulfate-neomycin (Neosporin), is then applied to the lesions. Severe cases of impetigo are treated with oral antibiotics, usually erythromycin or dicloxacillin. Impetigo that is extensive or involves internal organs is treated with intravenous (IV) antibiotics. Antibiotic treatment of streptococcal impetigo does not prevent glomerulonephritis, but it does hasten healing of the lesions.

The necessity of good handwashing and careful hygiene to prevent spread of the infection should be emphasized. The child should not attend school for 24 to 48 hours after initiation of systemic antibiotics or 48 hours after using antibiotic ointment. The school should be notified of the diagnosis.

NURSING CARE OF THE CHILD WITH IMPETIGO

Assessment

The child's skin should be assessed for size, distribution, and spread of impetigo lesions. If the child is taking systemic antibiotics, signs of allergic reactions, such as rashes, should be monitored. If the impetigo is caused by beta-hemolytic streptococci, the child should be observed for periorbital edema or blood in the urine, which may signal the development of acute glomerulonephritis.

Nursing Diagnoses and Planning

The following nursing diagnoses and expected outcomes may be appropriate in the treatment of impetigo in the child.

- Impaired Skin Integrity related to destruction of skin layers secondary to bacterial infection. ***Expected Outcomes:*** *The child will maintain skin integrity as evidenced by the infection remaining confined to primary site; healing without evidence of scarring or secondary infection.*
- Knowledge Deficit related to prevention of spread of infection, care of impetigo lesions, and antibiotic administration. ***Expected Outcomes:*** *The child/family will comply with measures to prevent spread of infection; demonstrate knowledge of home care and administration of medications.*

Implementation

Parents should be taught to wash and soak off the crusts with a warm, soapy washcloth three times a day. The crusts should be gently removed after soaking, taking care not to spread the infection to other parts of the body with the contaminated washcloth. Antibiotic ointment should then be applied to the lesions and the affected areas left open to air. A small amount of bleeding after crust removal is common.

> The child can spread impetigo lesions merely by touching another part of the skin after scratching the infected areas. The child's fingernails should be kept short and hands washed often with antibacterial soap. The importance of good handwashing and careful hygiene by the entire household should be emphasized. Family members should not share towels, combs, or eating utensils with the infected child.

The child should sleep alone and should be bathed daily, alone, with antibacterial soap. The nurse should wear gloves when caring for a child with impetigo. The nurse should emphasize the importance of administering the full course of antibiotics as prescribed.

Evaluation

- Do child and family members practice handwashing and other techniques to prevent spread of infection?
- Do parents carry out home care measures, and are lesions healing?

Cellulitis

Cellulitis is a bacterial infection of the subcutaneous tissue and the dermis.

PATHOPHYSIOLOGY *of Cellulitis*

> Cellulitis may be caused by bacterial invasion through a break in the skin, but there may be no history of trauma near the affected area. Cellulitis of the head and neck may follow an upper respiratory infection, sinusitis, otitis media, or tooth abscess. Cellulitis may occur in any part of the body. The lower extremities, buccal (inside the cheek), and periorbital (surrounding the eye) regions are the areas most often affected. Complications of cellulitis include septic arthritis, meningitis, and brain abscess. Periorbital cellulitis may lead to decreased vision or blindness.

Etiology. Cellulitis is caused by Streptococcus, *Staphylococcus aureus*, or *Hemophilus influenzae.*

Incidence. Children age 2 years and younger are most often affected.

Clinical Manifestations

- Affected area is red, hot, swollen, and painful.
- Edema and purple discoloration of eyelids as well as decreased eye movement are present in periorbital cellulitis.
- Lymphangitis is seen, with red "streaking" of surrounding area.
- Regional lymph nodes are enlarged.
- Child demonstrates fever, malaise, and headache.

Diagnostic Evaluation. Complete blood count, blood cultures, and culture of the affected area are obtained. If no drainage is present, aspiration of the affected area may be performed. Orbital cellulitis may be diagnosed by computed tomography scan of the orbit.

Therapeutic Management. The child with cellulitis of an extremity is usually treated at home with oral antibiotics (penicillin or erythromycin) and warm compresses. Cellulitis involving a joint or the face requires hospitalization and IV antibiotics. Incision and drainage of the affected area may be necessary.

NURSING CARE OF THE CHILD WITH CELLULITIS

Assessment

A history should be taken, and the parents questioned regarding recent ear infections, dental caries, or trauma to the skin surrounding the affected area. Other pertinent data would include when the inflammation started and how rapidly it has progressed. The skin should be examined, noting temperature, swelling, and drainage. The child should be assessed for fever, pain, and irritability.

Nursing Diagnoses and Planning

The following nursing diagnoses and expected outcomes may be appropriate in the treatment of cellulitis in the child.

- Impaired Skin Integrity related to bacterial invasion. ***Expected Outcome:*** *The child will exhibit signs of healing, such as decreased redness, decreased swelling, and decreased fever.*
- Pain related to soft tissue swelling and inflammation. ***Expected Outcomes:*** *The child will be able to sleep; demonstrate decreased irritability.*
- Knowledge deficit related to illness and treatment. ***Expected Outcomes:*** *The family will state measures to prevent spread of infection; administer antibiotics as prescribed; demonstrate ability to carry out treatment measures.*

Implementation

The child should rest in bed and the affected extremity should be elevated and immobilized. Warm moist soaks applied every 4 hours increase circulation to the infected area, relieve pain, and promote healing. Acetaminophen may be given to control fever and pain. Frequent handwashing is essential to prevent spread of infection. Intravenous antibiotics should be administered accurately and on time to maintain a therapeutic blood level. If the child is being treated at home, the parents must understand the critical importance of administering the entire course of antibiotics as ordered. The child should be carefully monitored for signs of sepsis (increased fever, chills, confusion) or spread of infection.

Evaluation

- Does skin exhibit signs of healing?
- Do parents administer prescribed medications and carry out home care?

FUNGAL INFECTIONS OF THE SKIN

Thrush (Moniliasis)

Thrust (oral candidiasis, oral moniliasis) is a common infection of infants.

Etiology. A neonate may acquire candidiasis during delivery while passing through an infected vagina. An older infant may develop a fungal overgrowth during antibiotic therapy or from exposure to his mother's infected breasts or from inadequate cleaning of bottles and pacifiers.

PATHOPHYSIOLOGY *of Thrush*

Thrush (*monilia*) is a superficial fungal infection of the oral mucous membranes that occurs as a result of overgrowth of *Candida albicans.* Passage of *C. albicans* through the intestine can occur, causing a diaper dermatitis. Moisture in the diaper area creates an environment favorable to the development of *Candida* dermatitis.

Incidence. Thrush occurs most often in infants. Predisposing factors in all age groups include antibiotic therapy, diabetes, and altered immune status.

Clinical Manifestations

- White, curd-like plaques are noted on the tongue, gums, and buccal mucosa (Fig. 34–2). They may be distinguished from milk curds by difficulty in removal and bleeding of an erythematous base when plaques are removed.
- If infection is severe, child may have difficulty eating.

Diagnostic Evaluation. Diagnosis of oral candidiasis is made by the clinical appearance of the lesions.

Therapeutic Management. Nystatin oral suspension, swabbed onto the mucous membranes of the mouth, is effective in the treatment of thrush. Because *Candida* is present in the gastrointestinal tract, oral nystatin may be ordered as well to decreased the chance of recurrence.

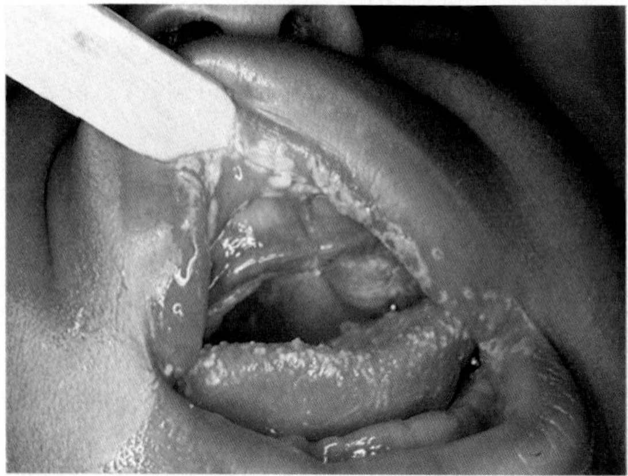

Figure 34–2
White, curd-like plaques of thrush (oral candidiasis, oral moniliasis), a common fungal infection in infants. (From Hurwitz, S. [1993]. *Clinical pediatric dermatology: A textbook of skin disorders of childhood and adolescence* [2nd ed., p. 36]. Philadelphia: W. B. Saunders.)

NURSING CARE OF THE CHILD WITH THRUSH

Assessment

Nursing assessment includes obtaining a history of maternal and infant monilial infections. The mother should be questioned regarding vaginal itching or discharge or any tenderness or redness of her nipples. Also, methods of cleaning bottles and pacifiers should be discussed. The infant's mouth and diaper area should be examined, and nutrition and hydration status should be assessed.

Nursing Diagnoses and Planning

The following nursing diagnoses and expected outcomes may be appropriate in the treatment of candidal infection in the infant.

- Impaired Skin Integrity related to increased susceptibility to infection. ***Expected Outcome:*** *The infant will exhibit signs of healing lesions, as evidenced by clear, intact mucous membranes.*
- Pain related to oral lesions. ***Expected Outcome:*** *The infant will have reduced discomfort, as evidenced by ability to take feedings without difficulty.*
- Knowledge Deficit related to cause of the infection and administration of medication. ***Expected Outcomes:*** *The family will demonstrate methods to prevent spread of infection; administer entire course of medication as prescribed.*

Implementation

Parents are taught to swab 1 ml of oral nystatin suspension onto the infant's gums and tongue every 6 hours for a week. Older children can receive up to 4 ml four times a day. Because cotton-tipped applicators tend to absorb the medication, a more effective method of administration is to rub the suspension onto the mucous membranes with a gloved finger. Another technique is to place a nystatin vaginal tablet in a nipple and allow the infant to suck on it four times a day. To increase the amount of time the medication is in contact with the mucous membranes, the nystatin should be given after feedings. Pacifiers, nipples, and bottles should be sterilized to decrease the chance of reinfection. Parents should also be taught the technique and importance of good handwashing. If the infant is breast-fed, the mother's breasts should also be treated with nystatin. If the infant also has a diaper rash, it is likely to be caused by *Monilia* as well. Parents should be told to request nystatin cream if the infant develops a diaper rash. Parents should be told to contact the health care provider if the infant refuses to eat, develops a fever over 100°F (37.8°C), or if the thrush does not clear with treatment.

Tinea Infection (Ringworm)

Tinea is a common superficial skin infection caused by a group of fungi known as dermatophytes. Tinea infections are designated by the word "tinea" followed by the Latin word for the affected part of the body. Figure 34–3 illustrates various types of tinea infections.

PATHOPHYSIOLOGY *of Tinea Infection*

Ringworm occurs when tinea fungus invades the hair, the stratum corneum of the skin, or the nails.

In tinea capitis, the fungus invades the hair shafts, causing the hairs to become brittle and to break off at the level of the scalp, leaving an area of stubbly, black-dotted alopecia. An immune reaction to the fungus may develop in the form of a kerion, a boggy, red, tender scalp mass that may contain *S. aureus* and is often accompanied by fever and lymphadenopathy. Children with allergies seem to be more susceptible to tinea capitis.

Tinea corporis, fungal infection of the face, trunk, or extremities, can be transmitted by humans or by dogs and cats. Most tinea corporis lesions clear without treatment in several months, but some may become chronic.

Tinea cruris (jock itch) causes an intense inflammatory reaction with severe pruritus. Tinea pedis (athlete's foot) may become chronic, particularly in adolescents who wear nonventilated athletic shoes. Tinea lesions may become secondarily infected with bacteria or *Candida*.

Etiology. Tinea infections are most commonly caused by two types of dermatophytes, *Trichophyton tonsurans* and *Microsporum. Trichophyton* affects all keratinized tissue, including skin, nails, and hair. *Microsporum* invades the hair. Tinea infections are transmitted from person to person, by animal contact, or by contact with contaminated fomites (combs, hats, head rests, pillows). Ninety percent of tinea capitis is caused by *T. tonsurans*, which is transmitted from person to person. Tinea cruris is not highly contagious. Poor hygiene, friction from tight clothing, and obesity are predisposing factors. Tinea pedis is not highly contagious and will not grow on healthy, dry skin.

Diagnostic Evaluation. Most tinea infections can be diagnosed by clinical appearance of the lesions. Confirmation of the diagnosis may by made by obtaining fungal cultures or by microscopic examination of skin scrapings prepared with potassium hydroxide (KOH). In the past, tinea infections were diagnosed when the lesions fluoresced under an ultraviolet Wood's light. However, the most common organism causing ringworm today, *Trichophyton tonsurans*,

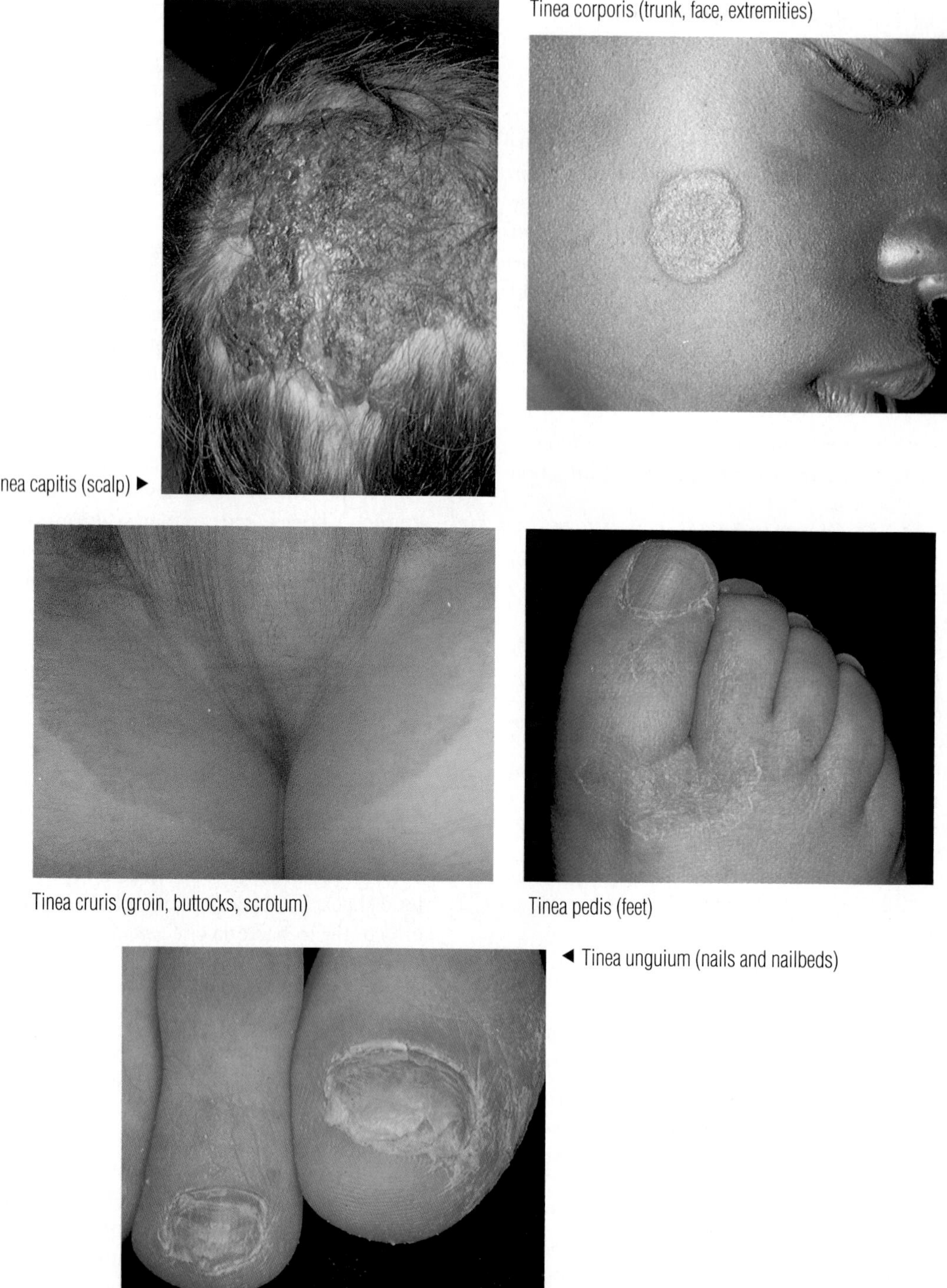
Tinea corporis (trunk, face, extremities)

Tinea capitis (scalp) ▶

Tinea cruris (groin, buttocks, scrotum)

Tinea pedis (feet)

◀ Tinea unguium (nails and nailbeds)

Figure 34–3

Tinea (ringworm) infections are caused by dermatophytes, a group of fungi. They are classified according to the part of the body affected. Five common types of tinea infections are shown here. (From Hurwitz, S. [1993]. *Clinical pediatric dermatology: A textbook of skin disorders of childhood and adolescence* [2nd ed., pp. 376, 380, 383, 385]. Philadelphia: W. B. Saunders.)

does not fluoresce. *Microsporum* lesions fluoresce a bright blue-green color.

Tinea Capitis

Affected Site: Scalp.

Incidence: Usually occurs in children ages 2 to 10 years.

Clinical Manifestations

- *Erythema* and scaling of the scalp are seen, as well as one or more round patches of *alopecia* that slowly increase in size.
- Begins as small papules at the base of hair follicles, which become crusting pustules and red scales.
- Thick, broken-off hairs close to the scalp surface result in patches of "black dot" alopecia.
- Scaling and flaking may resemble dandruff.
- Mild *pruritus* is present.
- A *kerion* may be present (allergic reaction to the fungus)—a swollen, boggy, pustular lesion surrounded by an area of alopecia.
- Surrounding lymph nodes may be enlarged.

Therapeutic Management. For treatment to be effective, medication must penetrate the hair follicles. Topical therapy alone is not effective for tinea capitis. Oral griseofulvin, 10 to 20 mg/kg/day for 6 to 8 weeks, is the treatment of choice. Because it is insoluble in water, absorption of this medication is increased if it is taken with a high-fat meal or with milk. Ketoconazole may be prescribed for children who cannot tolerate griseofulvin, or who fail to respond to it. Selenium sulfide shampoo (Selsun Blue, Exsel) should be used twice a week for 2 weeks to eliminate spores.

Tinea Corporis

Affected Sites: Trunk, face, extremities.

Incidence: Tinea corporis is not as common as tinea capitis, but has highest incidence in young boys and is most often seen in hot, humid climates. It also occurs in the diaper area of infants.

Clinical Manifestations

- Infection may appear anywhere on the body.
- Ringlike plaques with pale centers and scaly, red margins are seen.
- Lesions are usually ½ to 1 inch in diameter.
- Pruritus is present.

Therapeutic Management. Local treatment is usually effective for tinea corporis. Antifungal preparations such as clotrimazole (Lotrimin) or miconazole (Micatin) may be used three times daily until the lesions have been gone for 1 week. Infected pets should be treated as well. Micatin cream should be applied to visible ringworm patches on the pet's skin. If no patches are seen, but ringworm recurs in the child, Micatin powder should be applied to the pet's entire fur twice weekly for 3 weeks. The child should avoid close contact with the infected pet. Natural immunity develops in animals after 4 months (Schmitt, 1992).

Tinea Cruris

Affected Sites: Groin, buttocks, scrotum.

Incidence: Occurs most often in adolescent and adult males and is more common in obese individuals. Symptoms are usually worse in the summer.

Clinical Manifestations

- Pink papules and scales appear on the inner thighs, groin, and scrotum. The penis is not involved.
- Pruritus is present.

Therapeutic Management. Over-the-counter antifungal preparations such as Tinactin or Micatin should be applied twice daily to the lesions and at least 1 inch beyond the borders. Antifungal sprays and powders are not as effective as creams and lotions (McAnarney et al., 1992). Care should be taken to apply the medication to all creases.

Tinea Pedis

Affected Site: Nails and nail beds.

Incidence: Mainly occurs in adolescents and is more common in boys than in girls.

Clinical Manifestations

- Fine vesiculopustular or scaly lesions are seen on the soles of the feet and between the toes.
- Peeling, fissures, and maceration are present in severe cases.
- Pruritus and burning are present.

Therapeutic Management. A prescribed topical antifungal agent such as clotrimazole (Lotrimin) or miconazole (Monistat) is applied twice a day until the lesions have been cleared for 1 week. If the lesions do not respond to topical therapy, oral griseofulvin (Grifulvin, Fulvicin) may be given, 5 to 10 mg/kg/day for a month or longer, to promote healing. If the affected area is inflamed and oozing, soaking the feet in Burow's solution can promote healing.

NURSING CARE OF THE CHILD WITH A TINEA INFECTION

Assessment

A nursing history should be obtained, including description of the skin lesions and possible contacts. Animals the child has played with should be carefully inspected for ringworm. The child's siblings and playmates should also be examined, as children often share hairbrushes, hats, and barrettes, increasing the spread of infection.

Nursing Diagnoses and Planning

The following nursing diagnoses and expected outcomes may be appropriate in the treatment of tinea infection in the child or adolescent.

- Impaired Skin Integrity related to inflammation and scratching of lesions. ***Expected Outcomes:*** *The child will exhibit intact skin over impaired areas; demonstrate progressive healing of skin lesions.*
- Alteration in Comfort related to pruritic lesions. ***Expected Outcome:*** *The child will remain calm and exhibit no evidence of discomfort or pruritus.*
- Knowledge Deficit related to cause, treatment, and spread of the infection. ***Expected Outcomes:*** *The child/family will verbalize accurate information about the child's skin condition; demonstrate behaviors that prevent spread of the fungus; perform treatments correctly.*
- Body Image Disturbance related to visible skin lesions. ***Expected Outcome:*** *The child will verbalize feelings and concerns.*

Implementation

Adequate teaching is essential for successful treatment of tinea infection (see Teaching Guidelines for Fungal Skin Infections). Parents must understand that oral medication must be continued for 2 weeks beyond apparent clearing of lesions, sometimes for as long as 6 to 8 weeks. Discontinuing medication too soon may result in recurrence of lesions.

Fungus thrives in a warm, moist environment, so it is important to keep infected areas as dry as possible. Teaching regarding proper hygiene is essential for prevention and treatment of fungal infections. Children should be taught to avoid sharing personal items such as combs, hats, and hair ornaments. Children with tinea infections should sleep alone and should not share towels and washcloths with others. Feet should be washed daily and kept dry. Nonventilated athletic shoes should be allowed to dry thoroughly between wearings. Heavy cotton socks absorb sweat and keep the feet dry. If tinea pedis is present, the child should change socks at least twice a day and go barefoot or wear sandals as much as possible. Talcum powder or antifungal powder applied twice daily may help keep feet dry.

Tinea cruris heals much faster if the groin area is kept dry. Loose fitting cotton underwear should be worn, and athletic supporters and underwear should be washed frequently. The rash should be washed each day with plain water and carefully dried. Soap should be avoided. Scratching delays healing, so the child should be instructed to avoid scratching the area. The young man and his parents should be reassured that tinea cruris is not associated with venereal disease.

Parents should be instructed to call the physician if the infection has not cleared up in 4 weeks or if it continues to spread after a week of treatment. Parents should be reassured that fungal infection is not an indication of poor hygiene or neglect.

Evaluation

- Does the child have clean, intact skin?
- Do the child and parents perform treatments correctly and verbalize ways to prevent the spread of infection?

VIRAL INFECTIONS OF THE SKIN: HERPES SIMPLEX VIRUS, TYPE 1

Herpes simplex virus, type 1 (HSV-1) is responsible for a common, contagious, and often recurrent infection of the skin and mucous membranes. Herpes simplex virus infection can be asymptomatic or extremely painful. A wide spectrum of disease is caused by HSV-1: the common

TEACHING GUIDELINES *for Fungal Skin Infections*

- Keep infected areas as dry as possible.
- Do not share personal items such as towels, washcloths, combs, hats, or hair ornaments.
- *Athlete's foot:* Wash feet daily and keep them dry. Nonventilated athletic shoes should be allowed to dry thoroughly between wearings. Wear heavy cotton socks and change socks at least twice a day. Talcum powder or antifungal powder applied twice daily may help keep feet dry.
- *Tinea cruris:* Keep groin area dry. Wear loose-fitting cotton underwear. Wash athletic supporters and underwear frequently. Wash the rash each day with plain water and dry carefully. Do not use soap on the affected area. Avoid scratching the area.
- Continue to take oral medication as directed, even if condition has improved. Discontinuing medication too soon may result in recurrence of lesions.
- Call the physician if the infection has not cleared up in 4 weeks or if it continues to spread after a week of treatment.

fever blister or cold sore (herpes labialis), corneal lesions, and central nervous system infection.

PATHOPHYSIOLOGY *of Herpes Simplex Type 1*

There are four types of human herpesviruses: herpes simplex virus (HSV, types 1 and 2), cytomegalovirus (CMV), Epstein-Barr virus (infectious monoucleosis), and varicella-zoster virus. These viruses, with the exception of HSV-1, are discussed in Chapter 22. HSV-1 is the "oral" type of herpes and usually affects areas above the waist ("cold sores," "fever blisters," corneal lesions); HSV-2 affects areas below the waist (anal-genital area). However, either type can affect any region of the body. After an initial HSV infection the virus remains dormant within nerve cells innervating that portion of the skin originally infected. The virus can be reactivated by fever, stress, trauma, sun exposure, menstruation, or immunosuppression. When reactivated, the virus migrates to the skin area innervated by the ganglia that harbors it, near the site of the initial infection. The recurrent infection can be symptomatic or asymptomatic, but is just as contagious as the initial infection. Recurrent infections tend to be less severe than the initial infection. The immune status of the host determines the severity of HSV infection. HSV infection in the newborn or immunocompromised child can be fatal. HSV-1 is the most common cause of viral encephalitis in children. Mortality rate is over 75%.

Herpetic whitlow, a painful HSV infection of the fingers, can be transmitted to a nurse during oral or tracheal care of a child with herpes infection. Thumbsucking children may also develop this condition. Health care personnel with herpetic whitlow should not have patient contact until the infection has healed because the infection is highly contagious.

Etiology. Herpes simplex virus is transmitted by infected body fluids (such as saliva) coming in contact with breaks in the skin or mucous membranes. Newborns may become infected during delivery through an infected birth canal. HSV can be transmitted by nurses who fail to practice careful handwashing. Children with burns, eczema, or diaper rash or those who are immunosuppressed are particularly susceptible to HSV.

Incidence. The herpes simplex virus is widespread. Thirty-five percent of 5-year-olds carry HSV-1 antibodies. An initial HSV-1 infection commonly occurs by the time a child reaches age 5 (Gurevich, 1992). HSV infections in children are usually caused by HSV-1. Infection with HSV-2 is rare before age 14. These viral infections are more common in lower socioeconomic groups.

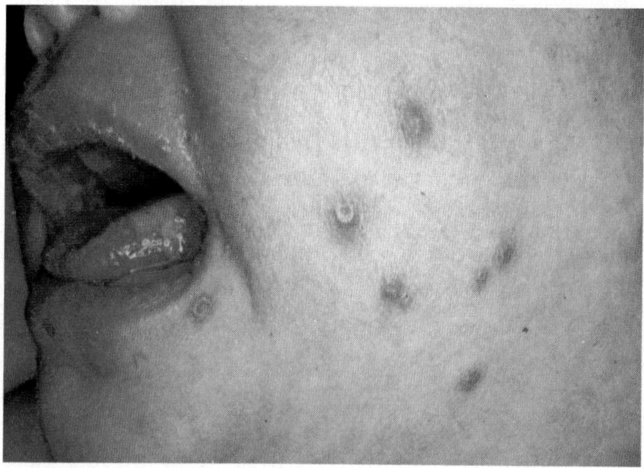

Figure 34–4
Herpes simplex infection in an infant. (From Feigin, R.D., & Cherry, J.D., Eds. [1992]. *Textbook of pediatric infectious diseases* [3rd ed., p. 773]. Philadelphia: W. B. Saunders.)

Clinical Manifestations (Fig. 34–4)

Herpes Labialis ("Cold Sore," "Fever Blister")

- Prodromal symptoms are burning, itching, or tingling. Symptoms appear 2 to 12 days after exposure.
- Clusters of fluid-filled vesicles ulcerate, dry, and crust.
- Lesions dry and crust within 7 to 10 days.
- Usually one or two lesions are present on the lips, tongue, gingiva, or buccal mucosa.
- Pruritus, pain are present.
- Approximately 85% of active HSV infections are asymptomatic.

Herpetic Gingivostomatitis

- Severe oral infection affects children under age 5 years.
- Vesicles and ulcerations, edematous throat, enlarged painful cervical lymph nodes are seen.
- Chills, fever, malaise, bad breath, drooling are present.

Herpetic Ocular Infection

- Irritation, inflammation of the conjunctiva or cornea are seen.
- Tearing, photophobia are present.
- Vesicles appear on eyelid and mucous membranes.

Herpetic Whitlow

- Symptoms appear 3 to 7 days after exposure.
- Vesicles, swelling, pruritus, and severe pain of the affected fingers are present.
- Discomfort may continue for weeks after the vesicles have healed.

Diagnostic Evaluation. Diagnosis may be made by clinical manifestations and history. A Tzanck or Papanicolau smear may be done. A positive smear cannot differentiate between varicella-zoster virus and HSV, and a negative smear does not rule out HSV infection. Tissue culture provides a more reliable method of diagnosis.

Therapeutic Management. Treatment is symptomatic. The child with oral HSV infection is usually cared for at home if he is able to take adequate fluids. If the child becomes dehydrated, IV fluids are needed. Although there is no cure for HSV, IV acyclovir (Zovirax) may used for immunocompromised children, neonates, and children with encephalitis or ocular HSV to decrease the severity of the infection.

Antibiotic ointment may be used to treat secondary bacterial infection of lesions. Corticosteroids are contraindicated, because they can worsen HSV infection. Oral or rectal acetaminophen with or without codeine may be prescribed, and topical anesthetics may be dabbed on lesions to help relieve pain. A prescribed anesthetic mouth rinse of equal parts of diphenhydramine (Benadryl) elixir, Kaopectate, and 2% viscous lidocaine may decrease pain and help the child to eat.

NURSING CARE OF THE CHILD WITH A HERPES SIMPLEX TYPE 1 INFECTION

Assessment

A nursing history should be taken and the parent or child should be asked about previous HSV infections. The skin should be carefully examined for lesions. The eye should be inspected for corneal ulcerations and edema, and the child's vision should be assessed for blurring and photophobia. Hydration status should be assessed.

Nursing Diagnoses and Planning

The following nursing diagnoses and expected outcomes may be appropriate in the treatment of HSV-1 infection in the child or adolescent.

- Impaired Skin Integrity related to inadequate secondary defenses. ***Expected Outcomes:*** *The child will demonstrate healing of lesions; have no signs of infection.*
- Pain related to inflammation and infection. ***Expected Outcome:*** *The child will have minimal pain, as evidenced by adequate fluid intake, decreased verbalization of pain, and decreased restlessness and irritability.*
- Risk for Infection related to changes in skin integrity. ***Expected Outcome:*** *The child will have no signs of secondary bacterial infection, as evidenced by healing lesions and normal body temperature.*
- Risk for Fluid Volume Deficit related to painful oral lesions. ***Expected Outcomes:*** *The child will maintain urine output of at least 1–2 ml/kg/hr; demonstrate moist mucous membranes and good skin turgor.*

Implementation

Children with oral HSV infection may be extremely uncomfortable. Swallowing can cause severe pain, and dehydration is a real danger. Parents should be told to contact the physician if the child develops signs of dehydration. Fluid intake is very important, and the child must be encouraged to drink. Frozen ice pops, noncitrus juices, milk, and flattened soft drinks are best. Frequent small feedings of bland, soft foods may be offered. Parents may need to be reassured that a few days without solid food will not harm the child as long as fluid intake is adequate. To prevent secondary infection, the mouth should be rinsed often with normal saline or $\frac{1}{4}$ strength hydrogen peroxide, especially after eating. Oral or rectal acetaminophen with codeine may be given as ordered for pain and fever. Topical anesthetics such as viscous lidocaine may be used with caution. Overuse of topical anesthetics in small children may depress the gag reflex and increase the risk of aspiration.

Hospitalized children infected with HSV should be placed under contact isolation or drainage and secretion precautions. The child is considered contagious until the scabs from visible lesions have fallen off. Because scabs do not form on mucous membranes, these lesions are considered contagious until they are completely healed. It is important to remember that active HSV infections may be asymptomatic.

> Health care personnel should always wear gloves when in contact with oral or genital secretions of a patient infected with HSV to prevent herpetic whitlow.

All personnel who have contact with the child should wear gloves when touching the patient near the lesions, during oral care or suctioning, and when handling bed linens or objects that might be contaminated with saliva or secretions from the lesions. Careful handwashing is essential. Children being cared for at home need the same precautions to prevent spread of infection. Bottles, nipples, toys, eating utensils, and towels should be washed in hot, soapy water. Family members should not share any of these items with the infected child. Because the infection can be spread to other parts of the body, the child should keep his fingers out of his mouth. Elbow restrains may be necessary. The child with HSV infection is usually miserable and needs generous cuddling and comfort in spite of his infectious condition. Careful handwashing and attention to hygiene decrease the risk of spread of infection.

Evaluation

- Are lesions healed, with no sign of spread of infection?

INFESTATIONS

Pediculosis

Pediculosis, infestation of lice in the scalp or body, is one of the largest and most exasperating problems in schools today. Although pediculosis is not a serious health problem, it causes much embarrassment and often elicits an emotional reaction among parents and school personnel.

PATHOPHYSIOLOGY *of Pediculosis*

Pediculosis may involve the scalp (pediculosis capitis), the body (pediculosis corporis), and the pubic area and eyelashes (pediculosis pubis). Each of these infestations is caused by a specific type of louse, each of which has a similar life cycle. All lice pierce the skin and suck blood. Head and pubic lice spend their life cycles on the skin of the human host; body lice live in clothing, coming to the skin only to feed. The female head louse lays eggs (nits) at the base of the hair shaft. The egg is covered with a gelatinous material, which hardens to semi-opaque, tiny pearly, whitish masses that are stuck tight to the hair shaft. Eggs incubate for about 1 week, and lice reach sexual maturity in about 2 weeks.

Pediculosis pubis is spread through sexual contact. Half of all patients with pediculosis pubis have another sexually transmitted disease, usually gonorrhea.

Lice may spread as long as the lice and nits remain alive on the infested person or belongings. Lice can live only 48 hours off the human host. Nits shed into the environment are capable of hatching for 10 days.

Etiology. Lice live only on humans and are transmitted by direct contact with infected persons and indirect contact with the infected person's belongings (brushes, hats). Lice cannot jump like fleas. Clean hair is no deterrent to head lice. It has been said that the healthiest lice live on the healthiest heads.

Incidence. It is estimated that 6–10 million school children are infested annually in the United States (Hurwitz, 1993). Incidence is as high as 40% among white school children in some areas. Pediculosis is rarely seen in blacks. Girls are affected twice as often as boys; all socioeconomic groups are affected. Peak incidence is in preschool and young school-age children. Pubic lice are usually seen in adolescents or young adults and are generally transmitted by sexual contact. Eyelid infestation in prepubertal children may be an indication of sexual abuse (Brimhall & Esterly, 1992).

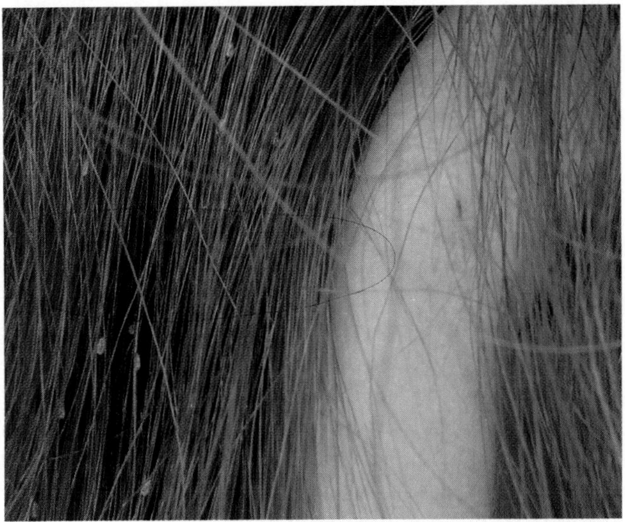

Figure 34–5
Head lice (pediculosis capitis). Note the nits attached to the hair shafts. (From Calen, J. P., Greer, K. E., Hood, A. F., Paller, A. S., and Swinyer, L. J. [1993]. *Color atlas of dermatology* [p. 373]. Philadelphia: W. B. Saunders.)

Clinical Manifestations

Pediculosis Capitis (Head Lice)

- Nits are visible, firmly attached to the hair shafts near the scalp, tiny silvery or grayish white specks resembling dandruff but more difficult to remove (Fig. 34–5). They are commonly found behind the ears and at the nape of the neck.
- Adult lice are difficult to see, and are small gray specks 1–4 mm. long that may crawl very fast.
- Pruritus of the scalp and/or back of the neck is seen. Secondary scalp infection may develop from scratching.

Pediculosis Corporis (Body Lice)

- Papular, rose-colored dermatitis appears in areas under tight clothing.
- Intense pruritus is present.
- Nits firmly attach to seams of clothing.

Pediculosis Pubis (Pubic Lice or Crab Lice)

- These lice may be found in pubic hair, facial hair, axillae, and body surface.
- Maculae cerulae (blue spots) may be found on thighs and trunk in cases of heavy infestation. Dark brown spots on underwear and sheets are insect waste materials.
- Intense pruritus is present.

Diagnostic Evaluation. Diagnosis of head lice is made by identification of nits and/or lice on the scalp. The hair should be parted with two tongue depressors, moving from side to side and front to back. The exposed scalp should be carefully examined under bright light or in a sunny area.

Therapeutic Management. A variety of antilice products are available. For many years treatment consisted of a single application of lindane shampoo (Kwell or Scabene) applied for 4 to 5 minutes and then rinsed out. Because lindane does not effectively kill nits, a second treatment 1 week later is recommended to ensure killing of newly hatched nymphs. Because of the danger of absorption through the skin and resulting neurotoxicity, lindane must be used with great caution. All family members should be treated to prevent reinfestation.

Because of the potential toxicity associated with lindane (Kwell), other products are frequently recommended. An over-the-counter antilice product, permethrin 1% (Nix), kills both lice and eggs with one application and has residual activity for 10 days. Nix is applied to the hair after shampooing and left for 10 minutes before rinsing out. The hair should not be shampooed for 24 hours after the treatment.

Over-the-counter products containing pyrethrins (RID, Triple X, R&C, Pronto) are safe and effective. Because they lack residual activity, they require a repeat treatment 1 to 2 weeks after the initial treatment if live nits are present.

Body lice are treated with a prescription drug or an over-the-counter medication (RID, Pyrinate–200, Triple X), following manufacturer's instructions. Clothing and bedding should be dusted with lindane or other recommended powder. Pubic lice are treated with an antilice shampoo, as for head lice. All sexual contacts should be treated.

NURSING CARE OF THE CHILD WITH PEDICULOSIS

Assessment

Examination for lice should be done unobtrusively and privately. All family members should be checked for the presence of nits and lice. Individuals with pubic lice should be assessed for signs of other sexually transmitted diseases and asked about sexual contacts, because they will need treatment as well.

Nursing Diagnoses and Planning

The following nursing diagnoses and expected outcomes may be appropriate in the treatment of pediculosis infestations in the child or adolescent.

- Pain related to inflammatory response and pruritus. ***Expected Outcome:*** *The child will rest comfortably and be free of scratching.*
- Risk for Infection related to scratching of scalp. ***Expected Outcome:*** *The child will have no signs of secondary bacterial infection, as evidenced by intact skin.*
- Knowledge Deficit related to treatment of lice infestation and prevention of recurrence. ***Expected Outcome:*** *The child/family will carry out prescribed treatment.*

Implementation

Because products containing lindane (Kwell) are potentially neurotoxic, they should never be used unless prescribed by a physician. A child with many open sores could absorb enough Kwell to cause seizures. Parents should carefully follow printed directions that come with the product. Nits should be removed by back-combing with a fine-toothed comb. Nits can be loosened with a mixture of half vinegar and half rubbing alcohol. Over-the-counter products such as Step 2 and Clear dissolve chitin, the substance that attaches nits to hair shafts. Many schools have a "no nit" policy, which requires children be free of all nits prior to reentry. Lice and nits may be removed from eyelashes by applying petrolatum to the eyelashes twice a day for 8 days. Bedding and linens should be washed with hot water and dried on a hot setting. Items that cannot be washed should be dry cleaned or sealed in plastic bags in a warm place for 3 weeks. Antilice sprays are unnecessary and should *never* be used on a child. Combs and brushes should be boiled or soaked in antilice shampoo or hot water (>140°F) for 15 minutes. Thorough home cleaning is necessary to remove any remaining lice or nits. Parents should vacuum floors, play areas, and furniture to remove any hairs that might carry live nits.

The child should be taught not to share hats, combs, or hair ornaments with other children. At school, individually assigned lockers or hooks for coats may help decrease spread of lice.

The child should be rechecked in 7 to 10 days for infestation. Parents should be told to call the physician if itching interferes with the child's sleep, if the condition does not clear up after 1 week, or if scalp lesions look infected. The National Pediculosis Association provides information about this disorder (see Appendix H).

Evaluation

- Is the child free of infestations?
- Do parents carry out the prescribed treatments?

Scabies

Scabies, or "itch mite," is a contagious condition that has been recognized for many centuries.

PATHOPHYSIOLOGY *of Scabies*

Scabies results from infestation with *Sarcoptes scabiei.* The female mite burrows into the epidermis, lays her eggs, and dies in the burrow after 4 to 5 weeks. The eggs hatch in 3 to 5 days, and larvae migrate to the skin surface to mature and complete the life cycle. The mites, eggs, and their excrement cause intense pruritus. One of the major complications of scabies is impetigo, the result of continued scratching.

Etiology. Scabies is transmitted by close personal contact with infected persons. Persons who share a bed or live in crowded conditions are likely to transmit scabies to each other. The scabies mite cannot survive for more than 3 days away from the human skin. For that reason, transmission of scabies by bedding or clothing is infrequent.

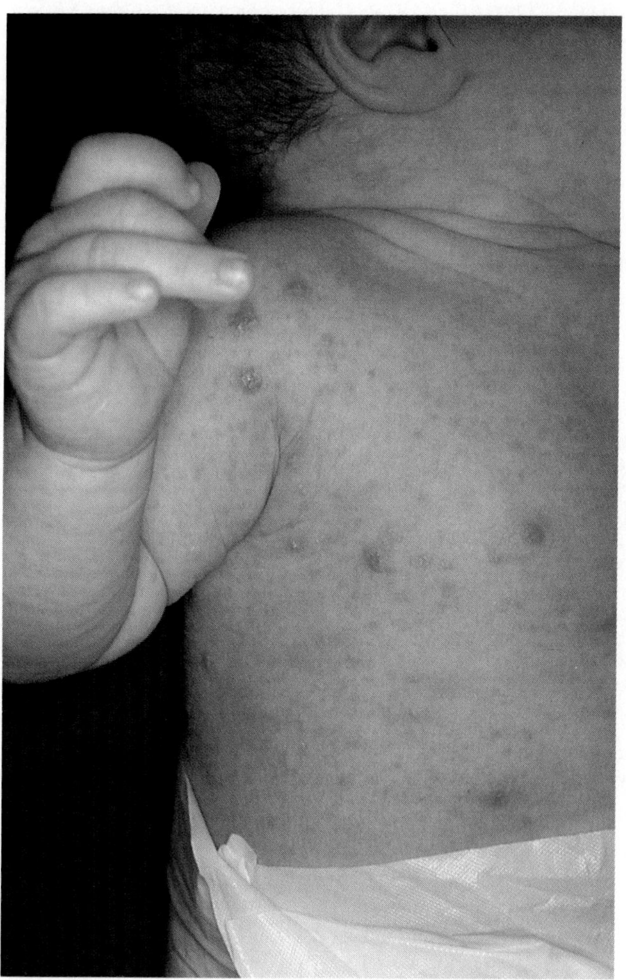

Figure 34–6
Scabies lesions on an infant. (From Calen, J. P., Greer, K. E., Hood, A. F., Paller, A. S., and Swinyer, L. J. [1993]. *Color atlas of dermatology* [p. 301]. Philadelphia: W. B. Saunders.)

Incidence. Scabies is widespread throughout the United States and is prevalent in many schools. All socioeconomic groups are affected.

Clinical Manifestations

- Intense pruritus is present, especially at night. Infants may be cranky, sleep fitfully, and rub their hands and feet together.
- Burrows (fine, grayish, threadlike lines) may be difficult to see. They are usually obscured by secondary changes of *excoriation* and inflammation.
- Papules, vesicles, and nodules are common (Fig. 34–6), and are most often found on the wrists, finger webs, elbows, umbilicus, axillae, groin, and buttocks. In infants the head, palms, and soles may be affected.
- Lesions are often secondarily infected from scratching.
- Scabies may be found on more than one family member.

Diagnostic Evaluation. Diagnosis is made by microscopic examination of scrapings of the lesions.

Therapeutic Management. Scabies can be treated with topical application of either lindane cream (Kwell, Scabene), crotamiton (Eurax), or permethrin 5% (Elimite). Because of the risk of neurotoxicity, lindane should not be used in children younger than age 2 years. Pruritus may last for several days after treatment and may be relieved by prescribed corticosteroid cream.

Family members and day care contacts (except for pregnant women) should also be treated. The child's bedding and clothing should be washed in hot water.

NURSING CARE OF THE CHILD WITH SCABIES

Assessment

Hands, elbows, umbilicus, groin, and buttocks should be inspected for burrows. Burrows may be difficult to see, however, and complaints of persistent itching may be the only symptom. Adolescents with scabies should be evaluated for sexually transmitted disease.

Nursing Diagnoses and Planning

The following nursing diagnoses and expected outcomes may be appropriate in the treatment of scabies infestations in the child or adolescent.

- Risk for Impaired Skin Integrity related to pruritus. ***Expected Outcome:*** *The child will demonstrate no increased redness, irritation, or abrasions.*
- Risk for Infection related to scratching of lesions. ***Expected Outcome:*** *The child will have no signs of secondary bacterial infection, as evidenced by normal body temperature and intact skin.*

Implementation

Parents should be instructed to use the scabicide according to manufacturer's instructions. The lotion is applied all over the body from the neck downward, making sure the soles of the feet, behind the ears, and under the toenails and fingernails are covered. The lotion should be kept on for the recommended period of time (4 to 8 hours for lindane and 8 to 14 hours for Elimite), and then the child should be given a bath. Infants should be clothed during treatment so they will not lick their skin. To minimize absorption and risk of toxicity from lindane, the lotion should not be applied for at least a half hour after bathing and should be applied only to cool, dry skin. Parents should be told that persistent itching following treatment is not a sign of reinfestation nor an indication for repeated application. Overuse of lindane may lead to neurotoxicity.

Scabies is usually cured with one treatment. Severe infestations may require a repeat application in 1 week. Clothing and bed linen should be dry-cleaned or washed in the washing machine and dried in the dryer on a hot setting.

Evaluation

- Is the child's skin intact and free of infestation?

NONINFECTIOUS SKIN CONDITIONS

Atopic Dermatitis

Atopic dermatitis, or eczema, is a common chronic inflammatory disease of the skin characterized by severe pruritus. Atopic dermatitis can have distressing psychosocial effects on the child and family.

Etiology. The cause of atopic dermatitis is unknown, but it is thought to be genetically determined and multifactorial, including an inherited tendency to dry, sensitive skin; allergy; and emotional stress. Seventy percent of children with atopic dermatitis have a family history of asthma, hay fever, or atopic dermatitis. Although the role of allergy in etiology of atopic dermatitis is controversial, food allergy has been shown to be an exacerbating factor in some children.

Incidence. Atopic dermatitis is a common disease, affecting 3% to 5% of U.S. children. The condition usually begins in infancy and clears by age 2 or 3 years. Atopic dermatitis affects all races and occurs more often in urban areas. Symptoms of this disease tend to be worse during winter months.

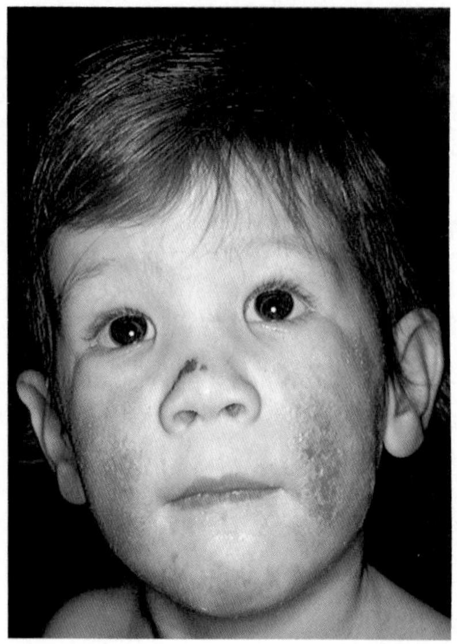

◀ Lesions on cheeks often spread to the forehead, scalp, and extensor surfaces of arms and legs.

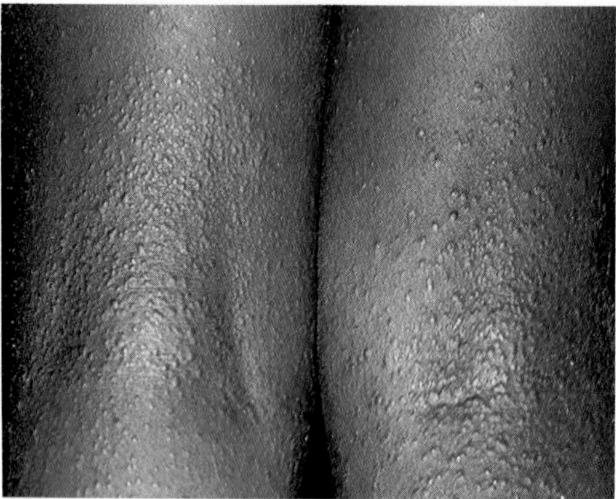

Flexor surfaces of wrists, ankles, knees, and elbows may be affected in the childhood form of the disease.

Figure 34–7

Atopic dermatitis, an allergic skin condition, affects 3% to 5% of children. It usually begins in infancy and clears by age 2 to 3 years. (From Hurwitz, S. [1993]. *Clinical pediatric dermatology: A textbook of skin disorders of childhood and adolescence* [2nd ed., pp. 49, 51]. Philadelphia: W. B. Saunders.)

PATHOPHYSIOLOGY *of Atopic Dermatitis*

Atopic dermatitis is an allergic skin condition. The skin of affected children releases twice as much histamine as that of normal children. The high levels of histamine trigger an inflammatory response, resulting in erythema, edema, and intense pruritus. Scratching increases itching, leading to an "itch-scratch-itch" cycle. Continual scratching and rubbing excoriates and damages the skin. Oozing, weeping, crusting, and cracking lesions develop. The skin of children with atopic dermatitis carries a higher than normal colonization of *Staphylococcus aureus* and secondary infection is common. Impetigo and viral infections (herpes, molluscum contagiosum) occur frequently in these children.

Exacerbations of atopic dermatitis can be triggered by many factors, including dry skin, emotional stress, irritants, allergens, infection, and sweating. The disease usually improves as the child gets older and in some cases completely remits. Approximately 50% of infants will experience remission by age 2 to 3 years. Seventy percent of children with atopic dermatitis develop asthma or allergic rhinitis later in life.

Clinical Manifestations (Fig. 34–7)

- Intense pruritus and dry, cracked, rough skin are present.
- Papulovesicular rash and scaly, red plaques become excoriated and lichenified.

Infantile Form (onset before age 2 years)

- Erythematous areas of oozing and crusting first appear on the cheeks, spreading to the forehead, scalp, and extensor surfaces of arms and legs.

Childhood Form (onset age 2 to 12 years)

- Skin appears scaly.
- Flexor surfaces of wrists, ankles, knees, and elbows, as well as neck creases, eyelids, and dorsum of hands and feet are affected.
- Chronic *lichenification* results from persistent scratching.
- Acute weeping areas may be seen with or without infection.

Adolescent/Adult Form (onset about age 12 years, continues into early adult years)

- Chronic skin changes (lichenified plaques) of face, sides of neck, flexural areas of extremities, and upper trunk are seen.

Diagnostic Evaluation. Diagnosis is made based on clinical features of intense pruritus, appearance of the lesions, pattern of remissions and exacerbations, and family history of allergy. Immunoglobulin E levels and eosinophils are often elevated.

Therapeutic Management. The main goals of treatment are to:

- control itching and scratching
- moisturize the skin
- prevent secondary infection
- remove irritants and allergens.

Control of pruritus includes avoiding trigger factors such as overheating, soaps, wool clothing, and other skin irritants. Proper hydration of the skin is essential. Bathing and use of wet compresses and occlusive creams and ointments are the mainstays of treatment. In humid climates, bathing should be as infrequent as possible, using only lukewarm water and mild, nonperfumed soap (Purpose, Dove, or Basis). The child who lives in a dry climate should bathe frequently (several times a day), using a hydrophilic agent such as Cetaphil instead of soap, and moisturize immediately after bathing. Application of moisturizer while the skin is still damp hydrates the skin. Corticosteroid creams (Aristocort, Kenalog) are prescribed for inflamed or lichenified areas. Oral antihistamines such as diphenhydramine (Benadryl) or hydroxyzine (Atarax) may be used to help break the "itch–scratch–itch" cycle. Because most children with atopic dermatitis itch more at night, antihistamines may be given before bedtime. Secondary infection is treated with antibiotic therapy.

Identification and elimination of allergens may be helpful. Allergy-proofing the home may be recommended (see Chapter 28). Allergy to certain foods is an exacerbating factor in some children. Eggs, soy, cow's milk, peanuts, and wheat are common offenders. If the child exhibits a sensitivity to particular foods, they should be eliminated from the diet. Infants at risk for allergy should be breast-fed for the first year, and solid foods should be delayed for the first 6 months of life.

NURSING CARE OF THE CHILD WITH ATOPIC DERMATITIS

Assessment

A thorough history should be obtained, including information about allergies in the family. The parents should be questioned about any environmental or dietary factors that seem to make the child's condition worse. Information on what treatments have been tried and their effectiveness should be obtained. Skin lesions should be examined for type, distribution, and evidence of secondary infection. The child's comfort level should be assessed. The family's feelings and coping methods should also be discussed.

Nursing Diagnoses and Planning

The following nursing diagnoses and expected outcomes may be appropriate in the treatment of atopic dermatitis in the child.

- Impaired Skin Integrity related to environmental and immunological factors. ***Expected Outcome:*** *The child's skin will have decreased evidence of excoriation.*
- Pain related to dry skin, secondary infection, and external irritants. ***Expected Outcomes:*** *The child will have reduced skin dryness and irritation; exhibit minimal pain and pruritus as evidenced by decreased irritability, absence of scratching, and uninterrupted periods of sleep.*
- High Risk for Infection related to skin excoriation. ***Expected Outcome:*** *The child will have no signs of secondary bacterial infection, as evidenced by normal body temperature and absence of purulent drainage.*
- Knowledge Deficit related to control of itching, prevention of secondary infection, and identification of aggravating factors. ***Expected Outcomes:*** *The child/family will identify and eliminate allergens and aggravating factors; carry out prescribed treatments correctly.*
- Altered Family Processes related to child's pruritus and involved treatment. ***Expected Outcome:*** *The child/family will discuss their feelings and concerns.*

Implementation

Care of the child with atopic dermatitis is demanding, and the entire family routine may center around the affected child. Parents need much support and reassurance as they care for an uncomfortable, often irritable child. (See Chapter 17.)

Keeping the skin hydrated helps relieve itching. Moisturizing creams such as Eucerin, Nivea, or Vaseline Dermatology Formula should be used several times a day and immediately after bathing. Parents need to be told that moisturizing creams contain no harmful drugs and should be applied whenever the child's skin looks dry. Soaks and cool wet compresses are soothing and may be applied to remove crusts, reduce inflammation, and dry weeping areas. Parents need explicit instructions on the use of soaks and topical medications. Strips of old cotton sheets moistened in lukewarm or cool tap water or Burow's solution work well for wet dressings. Wet compresses should not be used for more than 3 days.

Rough clothing may aggravate eczema, particularly wool or other fabrics that cause sweating. Soft cotton or cotton/polyester is tolerated best. Undergarments with irritating seams may be turned inside out so the soft seam is against the skin. Heat and sweating increase prutitus, so parents should be careful not to "bundle up" the child with heavy blankets or clothing. Because detergents and fabric softeners may also aggravate atopic dermatitis, clothes should be washed in mild detergent and rinsed twice.

Fingernails should be kept clean and short. Mittens and restraints may be needed to prevent scratching but should be used with caution, preferably only at night, because overuse may interfere with fine motor development and may eventually cause contractures. Long sleeves and one-piece outfits discourage scratching.

Skin must be kept clean to minimize secondary infection. The use of soap should be avoided. Bath oil or emulsifying ointment may be used as a soap substitute. Extra care must be taken when using bath oil because both child and tub tend to be very slippery. Tepid bath water helps prevent the child from becoming overheated and itchy. Parents should be instructed to contact the physician at the earliest signs of skin infection (weeping skin, pustules) and to administer topical and oral antibiotics as prescribed.

Sunlight can be helpful in controlling exacerbations but care should be taken to prevent sunburn. Children under age 2 years should not receive direct exposure to the sun (Blandthorn, 1990). Swimming may be beneficial if a moisturizer is applied before swimming and immediately upon exiting the pool. A humidifier in the child's room during winter months may decrease skin dryness. A resource for families of a child with atopic dermatitis is the Eczema Association for Science and Education.

Evaluation

- Is the child's skin intact with decreased pruritis?
- Do parents carry out prescribed treatments correctly?

Seborrheic Dermatitis

Seborrheic dermatitis is a common chronic inflammatory skin condition. "Cradle cap" in infants is the most common form of seborrhea. Seborrhea in older children may appear on the face, behind the ears, around the umbilicus, or in any other area with a large number of sebaceous glands.

PATHOPHYSIOLOGY ***of Seborrheic Dermatitis***

Seborrheic dermatitis is characterized by oily scales that block sweat and sebaceous glands, resulting in retained secretions and inflammation. Often there is overgrowth of normal skin bacteria and yeast, which increase inflammation and lead to secondary infection.

Etiology. The cause of seborrhea is unknown, but it appears to be related to dysfunction of the sebaceous glands. Unlike atopic dermatitis, seborrheic dermatitis is not associated with a family history of allergy.

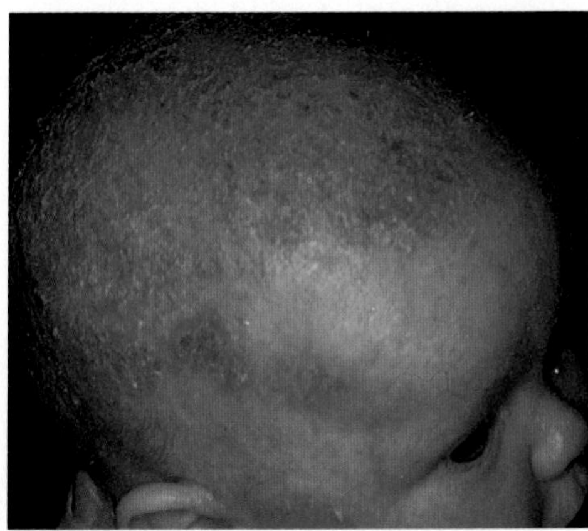

Figure 34–8

"Cradle cap," the most frequent form of seborrheic dermatitis in infants. The condition often begins in the first 2 to 3 weeks of life and usually disappears by age 12 months. (From Hurwitz, S. [1993]. *Clinical pediatric dermatology: A textbook of skin disorders of childhood and adolescence* [2nd ed., p. 17]. Philadelphia: W. B. Saunders.)

Incidence. Seborrhea is most common in infancy. The condition often begins in the first 2 to 3 weeks of life and usually disappears by age 12 months.

Clinical Manifestations (Fig. 34–8)

- Oily yellow scales are seen on the scalp, forehead, eyebrows, and behind the ears.
- Confluent erythema is present in the diaper and intertriginous areas and around the umbilicus.
- This dermatitis is nonpruritic.

Diagnostic Evalaution. Diagnosis is made based on the appearance of the lesions and absence of pruritus.

Therapeutic Management. Scales on the scalp should be scrubbed frequently with a mild baby shampoo or an over-the-counter antiseborrheic shampoo containing sulfur and salicylic acid (Fostex Medicated Cleansing, P&S, Sebulex) or tar (Neutrogena T/Gel, Polytar). Skin lesions that do not clear with frequent washing may be treated with 1% hydrocortisone cream applied twice daily. Seborrheic dermatitis of the diaper area is often secondarily infected with *Candida albicans* and requires appropriate treatment (Table 34–1). Lotions and creams tend to aggravate the condition and should not be used.

NURSING CARE OF THE CHILD WITH SEBORRHEIC DERMATITIS

Assessment

The infant's scalp or other affected areas should be inspected for lesions and inflammation. Parents should be questioned about frequency and technique of washing the infant's scalp.

Nursing Diagnoses and Planning

The following nursing diagnoses and expected outcomes may be appropriate in the treatment of seborrhea in the infant.

- Impaired Skin Integrity related to retained sebaceous secretions and inflammation. ***Expected Outcome:*** *The infant will maintain skin integrity as evidenced by healed lesions and no infection.*
- Knowledge Deficit related to cause and treatment of lesions. ***Expected Outcome:*** *The family will demonstrate understanding of proper skin care.*

Implementation

Scales are removed by daily shampooing. Massaging the scalp with warm mineral oil before shampooing helps loosen scales. Using a fine-toothed comb or clean, soft-bristled toothbrush during the shampoo helps loosen scales. Eyelid dermatitis (blepharitis) is treated with warm tap water compresses and cleansing with "no tears" baby shampoo. Care must be taken to keep topical medications out of the infant's eyes. Parents should be taught the importance of good hygiene of the infant's scalp and skin to prevent recurrence. They should be reassured that skin over the fontanel is not fragile and will not be damaged by gentle pressure and washing. Parents should be told to contact the physician if the sites become infected.

Diaper Dermatitis

Diaper dermatitis (diaper rash) is an inflammatory reaction to irritants in the diaper area.

PATHOPHYSIOLOGY *of Diaper Dermatitis*

Diaper dermatitis results from prolonged contact with irritants such as moisture, friction, and chemical substances. Urine ammonia, formed from breakdown of urea by fecal bacteria, is extremely irritating to sensitive infant skin. Ammonia by itself does not cause skin breakdown. Only skin damaged by infrequent diaper changes and constant urine and feces contact is prone to damage from ammonia in urine. Inadequate fluid intake, heat, and detergents in diapers aggravate the condition. Diaper rash begins with erythema in the perianal region. Left untreated, the area can quickly excoriate and progress to macules and papules, which form erosions and crusts. Diaper dermatitis may become secondarily infected with *Candida albicans*, streptococci, or staphylococci.

TABLE 34–1 *Diaper Rashes*

	DESCRIPTION	ETIOLOGY	TREATMENT	COMMENTS
Irritant Contact Dermatitis (Chafing Diaper Dermatitis)	Shiny, parchment-like erythema (similar to scald). Convex area of the buttocks, medial thighs, mons pubis, and scrotum, but not in the folds. Occurs at age 3 months or older.	Ammonia (urine) and putrefactive enzymes (feces) interact to create by-products. In older infants the contact dermatitis may be an allergic response to enzyme detergent or rubber.	Topical glucocorticoid cream (1% hydrocortisone or triamcinolone). Add Diaperene or 1 cup of vinegar to last diaper rinse and let soak $\frac{1}{2}$ hour before spinning (acidifies urine). Basic diaper and skin care.	Allergic contact dermatitis of diaper area is similar but does not usually occur in infancy.
Intertrigo	Red macerated area of sharp demarcation. Erythema, chafing, and fissuring develop. Area where skin surfaces are in opposition, particularly groin folds. Obese infants may develop intertrigo in gluteal and neck folds. Occurs at any age.	Heat, moisture, and sweat retention combine to irritate and macerate the skin.	Basic diaper and skin care. Teach appropriate wiping to child being potty trained.	Bacterial populations grow with maceration, increasing risk of secondary infections.
Seborrheic Dermatitis	Characteristic salmon-colored greasy lesion with yellowish scale, found primarily in intertriginous areas. Nonpruritic (differentiates it from eczema). Presence of intertrigo in groin and in other skin folds (neck or axilla) plus cradle cap indicates seborrheic dermatitis. Occurs at age 3 weeks to 4 months.	Inborn physiologic trait.	Same as for contact dermatitis.	May spread to entire diaper region after initial appearance in folds. Highly susceptible to secondary yeast or bacterial infection. Subsides spontaneously.

Miliaria	Small, sterile, clear vesicopustules. Anywhere that heat and moisture accumulate, especially diaper area. Occurs at any age.	Reaction to concentrated heat and humidity.	Basic diaper and skin care.	Also known as heat rash or prickly heat.
Primary Candidiasis	Small red papules with peripheral scaling. Sharply marginated area, usually involving the anterior thighs and abdomen, as well as the diaper area. Occurs at any age, usually after age 2 weeks.	*Candida albicans* from GI tract or an untreated infected caretaker.	Topical antimonilial (e.g., Vioform, Nilstat, Mycostatin, Micatin). Severe cases may benefit from wet soaks with tap water or Burow's solution. Oral Nilstat or Mycostatin is often indicated. Basic diaper and skin care.	Often secondary to seborrheic dermatitis, usually occurs following oral thrush. Do not use cornstarch on rash, as it may be metabolized by microorganisms, promoting infection.

Adapted from Betz, C. L., Hunsberger, M. M., & Wright, S. (1994). Family-centered nursing care of children (2nd ed., p. 1663). Philadelphia: W. B. Saunders. Irritant contact dermatitis and sebhorreic dermatitis photos: from Moschella, S. L. and Hurley, H. J. (1992). Dermatology (3rd ed., p. 239). Primary candidiasis photo: from Feigin, R. D., and Cherry, J. D., Eds. (1992). Textbook of pediatric infectious diseases (3rd ed., p. 776). Philadelphia: W. B. Saunders.

Incidence. Diaper rash occurs in about 10% of infants and is most common between ages 7 and 9 months. Some infants seem predisposed to diaper dermatitis.

Diagnostic Evaluation. Diagnosis is made by the characteristic appearance of the diaper area and the history of the onset and duration of the lesions.

Etiology, Clinical Manifestations, and Therapeutic Management. (See Table 34–1.)

NURSING CARE OF THE CHILD WITH DIAPER DERMATITIS

Assessment

The diaper area should be inspected carefully, noting the type and extent of lesions. The infant's hygiene should be evaluated, as well as the parents' knowledge of care related to the infant's skin integrity. Parents should be questioned about type of diapers used, laundering practices, and frequency and method used to clean the diaper area. Any recent changes in the infant's care such as foods, soaps, detergents, or lotions should be investigated. In case of candidal diaper dermatitis, the mother should be examined for signs of yeast infection.

Nursing Diagnoses and Planning

The following nursing diagnoses and expected outcomes may be appropriate in the treatment of diaper dermatitis in the infant.

- Impaired Skin Integrity related to irritation of the diaper area by ammonia and urea, feces, and detergents in cloth diapers. ***Expected Outcome:*** *The infant will maintain skin integrity as evidenced by clear, intact skin.*
- High Risk for Infection related to nonintact skin. ***Expected Outcome:*** *The child will have no signs of secondary bacterial infection, as evidenced by clean dry skin that is free of redness and excoriation.*
- Knowledge Deficit related to cause and prevention of rash. ***Expected Outcome:*** *The family will demonstrate correct methods of cleaning the infant and changing diapers.*

Implementation

Diaper dermatitis is much easier to prevent than to treat. Successful treatment and prevention of diaper rash, regardless of the cause, depends on thorough cleansing of the diaper area and on keeping the skin dry. Prompt, gentle cleansing after each voiding or defecation with water and mild soap (Dove, Neutrogena Baby Soap) rids the skin of ammonia and other irritants and decreases the chance of skin breakdown and infection. Careful attention should be given to skin folds and creases. Skin should be patted dry with a soft cloth towel after washing. Air drying the skin and frequently exposing the skin to air and light promotes healing of diaper rash. During bouts of diaper rash, the diaper may be left off during nap times.

Application of unmedicated powder when diapering can also reduce moisture and irritation. Parents should be taught to completely remove previous applications before applying new powder. Wet powder holds ammonia against the skin and forms tiny balls, which are extremely irritating. To decrease the risk of the infant's aspirating powder, parents should be taught to pour a small amount of powder onto a hand and not directly onto the infant's skin or near the infant's face. Application of a bland, protective ointment (A and D, Desitin, zinc oxide) to clean, dry, intact skin helps prevent diaper rash. Ointments should not be applied to inflamed areas, because they retain moisture. Steroid creams may be indicated for severe dermatitis but should be used for only 7 to 10 days, as prescribed.

Frequent diaper changes decrease irritation from urine and feces. The newborn's diaper should be checked every hour and the older infant's every 2 hours. The use of disposable diapers does not eliminate the need for frequent diaper changes. Although the "wicking" action of disposable diapers pulls moisture away from the skin toward the liner, ammonia and other by-products are left behind on the infant's skin, causing irritation. Rubber pants increase skin breakdown by holding in moisture and should be used infrequently.

If cloth diapers are laundered at home, they should be washed in hot water, using a mild soap and double rinsing. Soaking diapers before washing in a quaternary ammonium compound (Diaperene) decreases ammonia in the diapers.

The infant should have adequate fluid intake. Some diaper rashes clear with water supplementation alone (Gellis & Kagan, 1990). If a new food was introduced recently before the rash appeared, the food should be discontinued and gradually reintroduced after the rash has cleared.

Parents should be told to contact the physician if the rash does not improve in 3 days with treatment, if the rash becomes solid and bright red, if the rash becomes raw or bleeds, if blisters or boils develop, or if the infant develops a fever (over 100°F).

Contact Dermatitis

Etiology. Contact dermatitis may be caused by hundreds of substances. Among the most common causes of contact dermatitis are rubber, dyes in clothing, nickel (in jewelry, bra strap hooks, jean fasteners), and plants. Scented or strongly alkaline soaps, skin lotions, cosmetics, and wool clothing are also irritating to many children.

PATHOPHYSIOLOGY *of Contact Dermatitis*

Contact dermatitis is an inflammatory reaction of the skin caused by either direct exposure to an irritant (*irritant contact dermatitis*) or as a result of a delayed hypersensitivity response to an allergen (*allergic contact dermatitis*).

Irritant contact dermatitis may occur in any person who has repeated or prolonged contact with a primary irritant. Examples of primary irritants include citrus juices, detergents, bubble baths, and urine. Diaper dermatitis is an example of irritant dermatitis that results from prolonged exposure to urine (see Table 34–1). Teething infants may develop dermatitis on the face and neck folds from drooling.

Allergic contact dermatitis, a delayed hypersensitivity reaction, occurs in susceptible individuals who are sensitized to a substance by a previous exposure to the contact allergen. *Rhus dermatitis* (caused by poison ivy, oak, and sumac), the most common type of allergic contact dermatitis in children, is caused by oleoresins contained in all parts of the plant. Lesions appear several hours to several days after contact.

Incidence. Irritant contact dermatitis is more common in children than allergic contact dermatitis.

Clinical Manifestations

Irritant Contact Dermatitis

- Dry, inflamed, pruritic skin is seen.
- Distribution of lesions correlates with the skin surface in contact with the offending agent (e.g., watch band, clothing).

Allergic Contact Dermatitis

- Blistering, weeping lesions are seen over an area of inflamed skin.
- Intense pruritus is present.
- Lesions become crusted and scaly and heal in 10 to 14 days without treatment.
- Rhus dermatitis may cause severe systemic reactions.

Diagnostic Evaluation. Diagnosis is made by the characteristic appearance of the lesions and history of exposure to an irritating substance. Patch testing may be performed in children with persistent or recurrent dermatitis. (See Chapter 23 for a discussion of allergy testing.)

Therapeutic Management. Contact dermatitis is treated by discontinuing exposure to the offending agent. The skin should be washed thoroughly if any irritant remains on the skin. Cool compresses of tap water or Burow's solution soothe weeping, crusting lesions. Steroid cream (1%) may be applied several times daily after application of compresses. Oral steroids may be prescribed for severe contact dermatitis. Desensitization therapy is usually not effective in managing contact dermatitis.

NURSING CARE OF THE CHILD WITH CONTACT DERMATITIS

Assessment

A careful history should be obtained, including exposure to any potentially irritating substances. Assessment of skin lesions should include distribution, configuration, and evidence of pruritus.

Nursing Diagnoses and Planning

The following nursing diagnoses and expected outcomes may be appropriate in the treatment of contact dermatitis in the child.

- Pain related to skin inflammation. ***Expected Outcomes:*** *The child will have reduced skin irritation; demonstrate decreased evidence of excoriation; exhibit minimal pain and pruritus as evidenced by decreased irritability, absence of scratching, and uninterrupted periods of sleep.*
- Risk for Infection related to scratching of pruritic lesions. ***Expected Outcome:*** *The child will have no signs of secondary bacterial infection, as evidenced by clear intact skin.*
- Knowledge Deficit related to management and prevention of future skin inflammation. ***Expected Outcomes:*** *The child/family will identify and avoid irritating substances; carry out prescribed treatments correctly.*

Implementation

Nursing care of the child with contact dermatitis is aimed at relief of itching, prevention of infection, and identification and removal of offending substances. Cool compresses, antipruritic lotions (Calamine), and tepid Aveeno baths provide some relief from itching. Prescribed topical steroid creams should be applied in a thin layer following wet compresses to relieve inflammation. Antihistamines such as diphenhydramine (Benadryl) or hydroxyzine (Atarax) also help the child rest. Because overheating increases itching, the child should be occupied with quiet activities and room temperature kept at a comfortable level. Parents and child should be reassured that the lesions are not contagious and cannot be spread to others or to other parts of the body by scratching. Oils from *Rhus* plants that adhere to the skin, under the fingernails, and on clothing can cause new lesions if not removed with soap and water. Lesions may become secondarily infected, so the skin should be kept clean and every effort should be made to prevent scratching. Parents should contact the physician if the child develops fever or if the lesions become purulent.

Prevention of contact dermatitis depends on avoidance of offending substances. Children should be taught to recognize plants of the *Rhus* group (poison ivy, oak, and sumac). If the child is exposed to these plants, the skin should be rinsed with cool water immediately (within 15 minutes) and clothing washed in hot, soapy water. Oleoresins in the plants can be spread not only by direct contact with the plant, but also from smoke of burning leaves or by touching pets that have been playing in the plants. Other types of contact dermatitis may be prevented by avoiding known irritants such as cosmetics, jewelry, and canvas athletic shoes. Nickel-sensitive children can usually tolerate 14k gold or sterling silver jewelry. Pierced earrings should have hypoallergenic or surgical stainless steel posts.

Evaluation

- Is the child's skin intact, with healed lesions and no evidence of infection?
- Do the parents demonstrate an understanding of proper skin care?

PATHOPHYSIOLOGY ***of Acne Vulgaris***

Acne begins when sebaceous glands, stimulated by androgens at the onset of puberty, enlarge and secrete increased amounts of sebum. The sebaceous glands become plugged and dilated with sebum. When the enlarged gland is open to the skin surface, an open comedone, or blackhead, is formed. The characteristic black color is not a result of poor hygiene but is produced as fatty acids are oxidized on the skin. If the gland does not have an opening, a closed comedone, or whitehead, is formed. Closed comedones are small, nonerythematous papules just beneath the skin surface. Because a closed comedone has only a microscopic opening on the skin surface, pressure from excess sebum and keratin causes the comedone walls to rupture. Fatty acids produced by bacterial action on sebum are released into the surrounding tissues, causing inflammation. If the rupture occurs close to the surface, a pustule is formed. Ruptures deep in the dermis result in cysts and abcesses, which can lead to significant scarring.

Bacteria, particularly *Propionibacterium acnes,* play a role in the development of acne lesions by increasing inflammation and disrupting the integrity of the follicle walls.

Acne Vulgaris

Acne is a common inflammatory disease of the skin involving the sebaceous glands and hair follicles. Although acne is perceived by many as a minor disorder, it can cause significant anxiety and emotional pain for the affected adolescent. The disfiguring lesions of acne, although temporary, can lead to physical and emotional scarring.

Etiology. Although the exact cause is unknown, many variables seem to play a role in the development of acne lesions, including heredity, hormonal influences, and emotional stress. Foods do not appear to cause or increase the severity of acne.

Incidence. Acne affects approximately 85% of adolescents. Although acne may begin at any age, it usually develops during puberty and lasts into early adulthood. Acne is more common in males than in females. It seems to improve in the summer and flare during the winter months.

Clinical Manifestations (Fig. 34–9)

- Closed comedones (whiteheads), open comedones (blackheads), papules, pustules, and nodules are seen.
- Areas most often affected are the face, neck, back, shoulders, and upper chest.

Diagnostic Evaluation. Diagnosis is based on examination of the lesions and history.

Therapeutic Management. The aim of treatment is to prevent scarring and to promote a positive self-image in the adolescent. Treatment must be individualized, depending on the severity of the condition, types of lesions present, and sex of the individual. Improvement usually takes 4 to 6 weeks, so the adolescent needs support to keep from feeling discouraged.

Topical therapy such as tretinoin (Retin-A), a vitamin A derivative, reduces comedo formation and eliminates the lesions already present. The adolescent should be told that optimum results are achieved after 3 to 5 months of continuous therapy with this medication. Sunscreen should be used with tretinoin to reduce photosensitivity. Benzoyl peroxide applied daily reduces fatty acid production and is bactericidal for *P. acnes.* Benzoyl peroxide and tretinoin have reduced effectiveness and a potential additive irritant effect if applied together. The physician may prescribe the two medications to be applied on alternate days or may order benzoyl peroxide to be applied in the morning and tretinoin at bedtime. Other topical keratolytic agents containing sulfur, resorcinol, or salicylic acid may be prescribed for drying and peeling effects. Topical antibiotics, particularly tetracycline and erythromycin,

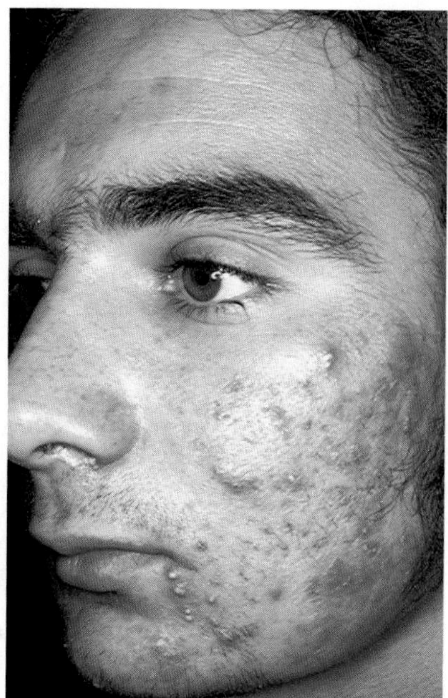

Figure 34–9
Acne affects 85% of adolescents, often causing anxiety and emotional pain related to self-consciousness about appearance. The sebaceous glands, stimulated by androgens at puberty, become plugged and dilated with the increased amounts of sebum produced. Comedones, papules, pustules, and nodules can result. Treatment is aimed at preventing scarring and promoting a positive self-image in the adolescent. (From Hurwitz, S. [1993]. *Clinical pediatric dermatology: A textbook of skin disorders of childhood and adolescence* [2nd ed., p. 137]. Philadelphia: W. B. Saunders.)

decrease the number of *P. acnes* organisms in hair follicles and are frequently used for inflammatory acne. Oral antibiotics (minocycline, erythromycin, clindamycin) may be prescribed for adolescents with severe inflammatory acne or those who are unresponsive to topical treatment. Exposure to sunlight should be avoided if tetracycline is used. Oral isotretinoin (Accutane) has dramatically improved the condition of patients with severe, nodulocystic acne. This drug suppresses sebum production and sebaceous gland activity. Because of the severity of side effects, isotretinoin is not indicated for all patients. Side effects include cataracts, cheilitis, dry skin, pruritus, conjunctivitis, and nosebleeds. Young women who anticipate becoming pregnant should not take isotretinoin because of its teratogenic effects. Sexually active female adolescents should use an effective form of contraception from the month before treatment until 1 month after discontinuing treatment. A negative pregnancy test must be obtained before initiating therapy. Informed consent is recommended for treatment with isotretinoin.

Estrogen may be prescribed for young women who are unresponsive to antibiotic therapy or who cannot take isotretinoin. The dermatologist may mechanically express comedones. The adolescent should be cautioned not to pick or squeeze lesions. Although scars cannot be completely removed, techniques such as dermabrasion, plastic repair, and collagen implants may improve appearance.

NURSING CARE OF THE CHILD WITH ACNE VULGARIS

Assessment

A detailed history should be obtained, including information such as how long acne lesions have been present and the effect of menses, clothing, and stress on severity and frequency of the lesions. Any acne treatments that have been tried and their effectiveness should be investigated. Hygiene measures should also be discussed, including frequency of washing skin and hair and type of cleansing agents used. Types of cosmetics used should also be ascertained. The adolescent's understanding of the development and treatment of acne should be assessed.

The face, chest, back, and neck should be carefully examined for the presence of lesions. Depth of tissue involvement and the presence of pustules, papules, cysts, and scars should be noted. The adolescent's feelings about herself and her appearance should be explored.

Nursing Diagnoses and Planning

The following nursing diagnoses and expected outcomes may be appropriate in the treatment of acne vulgaris in the adolescent.

- Impaired Skin Integrity related to increased sebaceous gland secretions, hormonal changes, and action of bacteria on the contents of clogged follicles. ***Expected Outcome:*** *Affected areas will exhibit signs of healing.*
- Risk for Infection related to inflammation of skin lesions. ***Expected Outcome:*** *The adolescent will have no signs of secondary bacterial infection, as evidenced by clear intact skin.*
- Body Image Disturbance related to appearance of skin lesions. ***Expected Outcome:*** *The adolescent will verbalize feelings and concerns.*
- Knowledge Deficit related to skin care and treatment regimen. ***Expected Outcome:*** *The adolescent will carry out prescribed treatment regimen to control excessive sebaceous gland activity.*

Implementation

Because acne is a long-term condition, the affected adolescent requires much support and encouragement if the treatment regimen is to be effective. Improvement may take as long as 12 weeks and exacerbations are common. Although there is no cure for acne, much can be done to control inflammation and reduce scarring.

TABLE 34–2 *Miscellaneous Skin Disorders*

DISORDER/ETIOLOGY	MANIFESTATIONS	MANAGEMENT	COMMENTS
Stevens-Johnson Syndrome, Erythema Multiforme			
Acute, sometimes recurrent autoimmune disease. May be triggered by infections or medications such as sulfonamides or anticonvulsants. New lesions continue to erupt for 1–4 weeks followed by healing during the next 6 weeks (Behrman, 1992).	Following a prodromal respiratory illness, bullae appear on the lips, mouth, eyes, and genitals. Fever, chills, malaise, neutropenia, anemia, weakness. Purulent conjunctivitis is common. Skin lesions rupture and may lead to significant fluid loss.	Treatment of skin lesions similar to extensive burns: reverse barrier isolation, IV fluids, air/fluid bedding, nutritional support, and pain management. Antibiotics for secondary infections. Ophthalmology consultation for eye lesions (Behrman, 1992).	Reassure child that the skin lesions will disappear. Inform parents about the possibility of recurrence and encourage them to avoid any implicated medications (Rathlev, 1994).
Neurofibromatosis Type 1 (von Recklinghausen Disease)			
Inherited (autosomal dominant) disorder. Manifestations begin in infancy or early childhood. Severity highly variable. Malignancy is a complication.	Neurofibromas (benign subcutaneous tumors arising from peripheral or CNS nerves in any part of the body). Café au lait spots, axillary or inguinal freckling, optic gliomas, headache, developmental delays, mental retardation, seizures, congenital malformations.	Symptomatic treatment; excision of painful or bothersome tumors.	Genetic counseling essential: 50% chance of transmitting disorder to offspring. National Neurofibromatosis Foundation* provides support to affected families.
Psoriasis			
Chronic, inflammatory rash caused by rapid proliferation of keratinocytes. Hereditary predisposition; onset in first two decades of life. Remissions and exacerbations; lasts throughout life. Arthritis is sometimes a complication.	Pruritus; erythematous, elevated plaques and silvery scales on the scalp, face, knees, elbows, and gluteal folds. Scales are attached at the center rather than edges and may bleed when removed.	Topical corticosteroids and tar preparations; keratolytic agents. Exposure to ultraviolet light and sunlight. Skin care to prevent secondary infection. Keratolytic agents enhance penetration of topical steroids. Sunlight may cause phototoxic reactions with tar preparations. To prevent tar folliculitis, tar should be applied down an extremity rather than up.	No cure for psoriasis. A resource for families of children with psoriasis is the National Psoriasis Foundation.†
Epidermolysis Bullosa (EB)			
Group of inherited disorders that vary in severity from occasional blisters (epidermolytic EB) to widespread and debilitating bullae formation with severe scarring and contractures (junctional EB).	Vesicles, bullae, and erosions develop spontaneously or as a result of friction or mechanical trauma. Dysphagia with esophageal involvement. Fusion or flexion deformities of hands and feet in severe forms.	Measures to prevent trauma and prevent pressure on skin are essential. Cool environment and lubrication of skin help prevent blister formation. No hot baths or tape on skin. Oral and topical antibiotics for secondary infection. Sterile aspiration of blister fluid may relieve pain. Large denuded areas treated as burns.	Genetic counseling should be offered. Dystrophic Epidermolysis Bullosa Research Association‡ provides support to patients with EB and their families.
Pityriasis Rosea			
Acute, inflammatory, self-limited skin disorder. Etiology unknown; may be viral.	Sudden eruption of salmon-pink, irregular patches on trunk and proximal portions of extremities. Symmetric distribution of lesions, "Christmas tree" appearance on back. "Herald patch" precedes rash by 7–10 days.	No treatment required for asymptomatic children. Pruritus can be treated with antipruritic lotions, ultraviolet light or sunlight.	Child generally feels well. Rash may last 6–12 weeks.

TABLE 34–2 *Miscellaneous Skin Disorders (continued)*

DISORDER/ETIOLOGY	MANIFESTATIONS	MANAGEMENT	COMMENTS
Warts Skin infection caused by human papilloma virus (HPV). Incubation period 1–6 months. Can persist from a few months to 5 or more years.	Painless, hyperkeratotic papule. Begins as a round, flesh-colored papule, later becomes brown or tan with a rough surface. Most common sites: dorsum of hands, fingers, feet, face, and genitalia.	Various methods of treatment: Daily application of lactic acid and salicylic acid (e.g., Compound W); freezing with liquid nitrogen; topical application of cantharidine for plantar or periungual warts.	Most warts disappear without treatment in 2–3 years. With treatment they usually resolve in 2–3 months. Picking at warts may cause them to spread to other areas of the body. Warts are not highly contagious to other people. Immunocompromised children are more susceptible to warts.
Molluscum Contagiosum Viral infection of the skin and mucous membranes. Transmitted by skin-to-skin and fomite-to-skin contact. May be transmitted by sexual contact.	Begin as pinpoint papules which increase in size to 2–3 mm or larger. Firm, solid, pink papules changing into soft, waxy, umbilicated papules. Curd-like core of the lesion can be expressed. Most common sites: face, trunk, extremities, oral mucous membranes, conjunctiva, and genitalia.	Lesions may be treated with cantharidin or liquid nitrogen. Treatment can be repeated once or twice a month, depending on the rate of appearance of new lesions. Usually respond well to treatment.	Lesions may be spread to other parts of the body and may be transmitted to others. Lesions disappear spontaneously over time. Children with eczema or impaired immunity are at risk for generalized spread of lesions.
Frostbite Freezing of tissue resulting from exposure to extreme cold. Exposed areas (fingers, toes, nose, cheeks, ears) are most often affected. Cold causes arteriolar vasoconstriction resulting in tissue anoxia and destruction.	*Early signs:* blanching of skin; stinging sensation followed by numbness and white, mottled appearance. Area feels cold, hard; may be without sensation. *First-degree:* redness and discomfort with return to normal in a few hours. *Second-degree:* redness; blisters and bullae 24–48 hours after rewarming. Pain during rewarming. *Third-degree:* cyanosis and mottling, followed by redness and swelling. Necrosis of epidermis, dermis, and subcutaneous tissue. Sensation is absent. Pain during rewarming. *Fourth-degree:* complete necrosis with gangrene, possible loss of body part.	Immediately cover affected areas with warm hands and warm clothing. Massaging areas causes further damage and should be avoided. Rapidly rewarm areas by immersion in a warm water bath (90–106°F) until all frozen tissues are thawed and the skin appears flushed. Pain during thawing can be severe and should be treated with analgesics and sedatives. Severely damaged areas are treated as burns. (See Chapter 35).	Children in cold climates should be taught to prevent frostbite by wearing adequate warm, layered clothing, hat, gloves, and two pairs of socks (one cotton, one wool). Children should be taught to warm themselves when hands or feet begin to sting. Young children should not be allowed to play outside in extremely cold temperatures.
Foreign Bodies Skin injury due to penetration of splinters, gravel, cactus spines, bee stingers, glass, or other foreign objects.	Pain, erythema, possible secondary infection. Foreign body may or may not be visible.	Area surrounding foreign body should be washed with soap and water before removal. Superficial splinters can be removed with a needle and tweezers disinfected with alcohol or flame.	Deeply imbedded foreign bodies, fishhooks, and other difficult-to-remove objects may require medical attention. Tetanus prophylaxis may be indicated.

*National Neurofibromatosis Foundation, 141 Fifth Ave., Suite 7–5, New York, NY 10010; (800) 323–7938.

†National Psoriasis Foundation, 6443 SW Beaverton Hwy, Suite 210, Portland, OR 97221.

‡D.E.B.R.A. of America, Inc., 141 Fifth Ave., Suite 75, New York, NY 10010.

TABLE 34–3 *Skin Lesions Caused by Insects and Arachnids*

AGENT/CHARACTERISTICS	MANIFESTATIONS	TREATMENT AND PREVENTION
Insects		
Mosquitoes, Fleas, Flies, Gnats		
Foreign protein in insect's saliva is injected as insect pierces skin to suck blood.	Itching, erythema, small wheal. Allergic reaction may occur.	Antipruritic lotions, cool compresses to relieve itching. Antihistamines if needed for sleep. *Prevention:* Wear insect repellent when contact anticipated. Treat potential breeding places (standing water for mosquitoes; pets, furniture, yard for fleas).
Hymenoptera (Bees, Wasps, Hornets, Yellow Jackets, Fire Ants)		
Venom is injected through a stinger.	Histamine and foreign proteins in venom cause local reaction of pain, swelling, redness, and itching. Systemic allergic reactions: nausea, generalized edema, respiratory distress, shock.	Carefully remove stinger by scraping it out horizontally. Avoid squeezing stinger, as more venom will be released. In honeybee stings, instant removal of the stinger and venom sac may prevent some symptoms since it takes 2–3 minutes for all of the venom in the sac to be injected (Adamski, 1990). Wash with soap and water. Paste made of powdered meat tenderizer and water is soothing. Ice and analgesics for discomfort. Antihistamines for itching. Systemic allergic reaction: epinephrine, corticosteroids immediately; transport to emergency facility. Children allergic to hymenoptera should wear medical identification.
Arachnids		
Brown Recluse ("Fiddle Back") Spider		
Yellowish to reddish brown with a violin-shaped mark on its back. Venom injected by fangs. Bites only when threatened. Lives in dark, protected areas (woodpiles, basements, closets, trash heaps).	Mild stinging at time of bite. Within 2–8 hours, area around bite becomes painful and develops erythema, followed by a blister. Venom is necrotoxic. Edema, redness, and purpura may involve entire limb. Central portion of lesion develops an indurated wheal that progresses to deep sloughing ulcer in 7–14 days. Ulcer often does not heal for several months. Usually results in a scar.	Immobilize and elevate affected extremity. Cool compresses, analgesics, tetanus prophylaxis. Observe for secondary infection. Skin graft may be necessary for large ulcers. No antivenin available. *Prevention:* Avoid areas inhabited by spiders.
Black Widow Spider		
Shiny black with a red hourglass-shaped mark on abdomen. Female's venom is very poisonous to humans. Males do not bite. Female builds irregular web in dark, sheltered spots and aggressively defends eggs.	Bite may be painless initially. Within 1 hour pain develops at site. Severe muscle pains and numbness spread from bite, and puncture site becomes red, swollen, and pruritic. Neurotoxic venom enters the bloodstream within an hour, causing dizziness, headache, nausea, vomiting, cramps, tremors, and rapid shallow respirations. Shock and renal failure may develop in young children.	Hospitalization for children. Antivenin if no allergy to horse serum. Supportive care, including morphine and muscle relaxants. Tetanus prophylaxis. *Prevention:* Avoid areas infested by spiders (woodpiles, outhouses).

TABLE 34–3 *Skin Lesions Caused by Insects and Arachnids (continued)*

AGENT/CHARACTERISTICS	MANIFESTATIONS	TREATMENT AND PREVENTION
Ticks		
Brown or gray. Live in fields, pastures, woods. Feed on blood of humans, dogs, livestock, or deer. Larvae feed on rodents. Tick buries head and mouthparts in the skin to suck blood.	Bites may cause local reactions or, rarely, systemic reactions (tick fever or tick paralysis). Ticks may transmit Lyme disease, Rocky Mountain spotted fever, Q fever, and tularemia.	*Methods to remove ticks:* Suffocate tick with nail polish, Vaseline, or oil; wait 30 minutes, then remove with tweezers, taking care to remove head. If mouthparts remain, remove with sterile needle. Wash site with soap and water. There is some evidence that prompt removal of ticks decreases chance of transmission of disease. *Prevention:* Wear long sleeves and pants and use insect repellent when walking in tick-infested areas. Inspect clothing and hair for ticks after walking through fields or woods.
Scorpion		
Most scorpions are not dangerous. They rarely attack humans unless accidentally disturbed or stepped on. If disturbed, they inflict a painful sting. One type, *C. sculpturatus,* is extremely poisonous and its sting can be fatal. It is found in Arizona. Scorpions are found mainly in the Southwestern U.S. Scorpions hide by day in basements, garages, closets, and crevices. Some varieties burrow and hide in gravel or children's sandboxes.	Sting is extremely painful. Local reaction of swelling at puncture site. Some species cause systemic reactions: tachycardia, hypertension, arrhythmias, irritability, seizures, pulmonary edema, coma. Fatal reactions most often occur in children under age 3 years.	Ice packs and tourniquet proximal to site slow spread of venom (Hurwitz, 1993). Wound should not be excised. Topical steroids and antihistamines for relief of symptoms. Severe reactions: supportive care for pain, shock, seizures. Narcotic analgesics act synergistically with scorpion venom and are contraindicated. Antivenin given for systemic reactions (available from the Antivenom Production Laboratory, Arizona State University). *Prevention:* Wear shoes to prevent stepping on scorpions. Inspect shoes and clothing before dressing. Apply creosote to garages, basements.
Chiggers (Harvest Mites)		
Live in tall grass and underbrush. Chiggers burrow into hair follicles and skin pores to feed.	Tend to concentrate in warm areas where clothing is snug (underwear elastic). Cause erythematous papules and intense itching.	Antipruritic agents. Prevention of secondary infection. *Prevention:* Insect repellent on clothing, ankles, and legs.

Explanations of the cause of acne and the rationale for treatment should be given at the outset so the adolescent can help plan her own treatment regimen. Written instructions and involvement in care improve compliance. Treatment must be individualized, but all treatment regimens include measures to reduce oil on the skin. Gently cleansing the face twice a day with soap (Purpose, Neutrogena) and shampooing the hair daily are important facets of care. The adolescent should be warned to avoid vigorous scrubbing and picking or squeezing of lesions, which can rupture pilosebaceous ducts and cause secondary infection. The adolescent should be taught how to apply topical medications and should be cautioned against overuse of these products to speed results. Because oily cosmetics and creams add to the plugging of follicles, only water-based cosmetics should be used.

A healthy lifestyle, including adequate rest, exercise, and a balanced diet, promotes healing of lesions. The adolescent's feelings about her appearance and coping mechanisms used should be explored. Positive self-image and self-esteem should be reinforced. Concerns and fears should be openly discussed and myths about acne dispelled.

Parents need information about acne to clear up misconceptions and to prevent needless nagging of the adolescent.

Evaluation

- Do acne lesions exhibit signs of healing?
- Does the adolescent carry out the treatment regimen to control acne and prevent scarring?

MISCELLANEOUS SKIN DISORDERS

There are a number of less common skin disorders with varied etiologies and manifestations. These disorders are listed in Table 34–2.

INSECT BITES AND STINGS

Insects are found almost everywhere, and children often come in contact with them during play. Bites of most insects are not serious, usually causing only itching and mild pain. Severe systemic reactions may occur in sensitized children, however. Approximately 2 million people in the United States are severely allergic to venomous stinging insects. The prevalence may be as high as 1% in children (Stafford et al., 1992). From 40 to 50 people die each year from allergic reactions to insect stings; of these, 1 or 2 are children (Graft, 1989). Children who are allergic to insect stings should wear identification describing the allergy and outlining appropriate treatment. An emergency kit containing antihistamine, epinephrine, and a syringe should be kept immediately available for such children. Parents should check the expiration date on the kit and replace it if it is outdated. (See Chapter 23 for a discussion of allergic reactions.)

Arachnids (scorpions, spiders, ticks, and mites) are found in areas where children play. Most arachnids are not dangerous or aggressive. In the United States only one type of scorpion and two types of spiders (black widow and brown recluse) cause life-threatening reactions.

Topical insect repellents are usually safe and effective in preventing insect bites. Repellents containing high concentrations of diethyltoluamide (DEET) should not be used on small children because of the risk of toxic encephalopathy. Such repellents should not be applied near the face, and children should be cautioned not to put their fingers in their mouths when wearing DEET.

Bites and stings of common insects and arachnids are discussed in Table 34–3, including manifestations, treatment, and prevention.

KEY CONCEPTS

- Functions of the skin include protection, thermoregulation, excretion, production of vitamin D, and sensation.
- The skin is composed of two layers—the outer epidermis and the inner supportive dermis, which contains blood vessels, nerves, and sweat glands. Beneath these layers is subcutaneous tissue, which attaches the dermis to the underlying structures.
- Developmental differences cause the skin of infants and children to be more susceptible to external irritants and infection than that of adults.
- Impetigo, the most common skin infection of childhood, is highly contagious. Nursing care includes administration of topical and/or oral antibiotics and education regarding good handwashing and careful hygiene to prevent spread of infection.
- Because tinea (fungus) thrives where it is moist and warm, infected areas should be kept as dry as possible. Proper hygiene should be taught to minimize spread of infection.
- Herpes simplex virus is transmitted by infected body fluids coming in contact with breaks in the skin or mucous membranes. Careful handwashing and attention to hygiene decrease the risk of spread of infection.
- Prevention of reinfestation is a primary goal in the treatment of pediculosis.
- Nursing care for the child with eczema includes frequent moisturizing of the child's skin and cautioning against clothing and soaps that might irritate the child's skin. Identification and elimination of allergens may be helpful.
- Diaper dermatitis is much easier to prevent than to treat. Successful treatment and prevention of diaper rash depends on thorough cleansing of the diaper area and keeping the skin dry.
- Nursing care of the child with acne includes teaching about regular, gentle cleansing of the skin; application of topical medications; and a healthy lifestyle with adequate rest, exercise, and a balanced diet. The nurse must be sensitive to the effect of acne on the adolescent's self-concept.
- Nursing care of the child with erythema multiforme is similar to that of a child who is burned.
- Insect bites and stings can cause severe systemic reactions in sensitized children.

REFERENCES

Adamski, D. B. (1990). Assessment and treatment of allergic response to stinging insects. *Journal of Emergency Nursing, 16*(2), 77–82.

Behrman, R. (1992). Vesicobullous disorders. In *Nelson's textbook of pediatrics* (14th ed., pp. 1639–1642). Philadelphia: W. B. Saunders.

Brimhall, C. L., & Esterly, N. B. (1992). Scabies, lice, and other unwelcome guests. Focus on Dermatology and Ophthalmology in *Contemporary Pediatrics, 2* (Special Edition), 10–19.

Gellis, S. S., & Kagan, B. M. (1990). *Current pediatric therapy* (13th ed.). Philadelphia: W. B. Saunders.

Graft, D. F. (1989). Stinging insect allergy: How management has changed. *Postgraduate Medicine, 85,* 173–178.

Gurevich, I. (1992). Varicella zoster and herpes simplex virus infections. *Heart and Lung, 21*(1), 85–91.

Hurwitz, S. (1993). *Clinical Pediatric Dermatology* (pp. 6–8). Philadelphia: W. B. Saunders.

McAnarney, E. R., Kreipe, R. E., Orr, D. P., & Comerci, G. D. (1992). *Textbook of adolescent medicine.* Philadelphia: W. B. Saunders.

Rathlev, M. (1994). Unpublished material.

Schmitt, B. D. (1992). *Instructions for pediatric patients.* Philadelphia: W. B. Saunders.

Stafford, C. T., Moffitt, J. E., & Yates, A. B. (1992). Insect sting anaphylaxis: Referral is imperative. *Emergency Medicine,* August 15, 1992, 230–232.

BIBLIOGRAPHY

Barker, N., Hadcraft, J., & Rutter, N. (1987). Skin permeability in the newborn. *Journal of Investigations in Dermatology, 88,* 409–411.

Barton, L., et al. (1988). Impetigo contagiosa: A comparison of erythromycin and dicloxacillin therapy. *Pediatric Dermatology, 5,* 88–91.

Blandthorn, J. (1990). Paediatric atopic dermatitis: Parameters of aetiology, diagnosis and management. *Australian Journal of Advanced Nursing,* 7(4), 18–28.

Brady, M. (1988). Common viral skin problems of childhood: Warts and molluscum. *Journal of Pediatric Health Care, 2*(4), 208–210.

Burks, A. W., et al. (1992). Atopic dermatitis and food hypersensitivity in children. *Allergy Proceedings, 13*(6), 285–289.

Ceilly, R. I., Goldberg, G. N., Prose, N. S. (1989). A guide to pediatric rashes. (K. B. Singer, Ed.), *Patient Care, 23,* 150–163.

Cobb, M. W. (1990). Human papilloma virus infection. *Journal of the American Academy of Dermatology, 22,* 547–566.

Eichfield, L. F., & Honig, P. J. (1991). Blistering disorders in childhood. *Pediatric Clinics of North America, 38*(4), 959–975.

Farber, E. M. (1992). Facial psoriasis. *Cutis, 50,* 25–28.

Gelmetti, C. (1992). Extracutaneous manifestations of atopic dermatitis. *Pediatric Dermatology, 9*(4), 380–382.

Goldberg, S. H., & Bronson, D. (1991). Blistering diseases. *Postgraduate Medicine, 89*(2), 159–162.

Grossman, L., & Rasmussen, J. E. (1991). Recent advances in pediatric infectious disease and their impact on dermatology. *Journal of the American Academy of Dermatology, 24*(3), 379–389.

Gurevich, I. (1990). Counseling the patient with herpes. *RN, 53*(2), 22–28.

Hanifen, J. M. (1991). Atopic dermatitis in infants and children. *Pediatric Clinics of North America, 38*(4), 763–787.

Hay, R. J. (1992). Fungal skin infections. *Archives of Disease in Childhood, 67*(9), 1065–1067.

Hogan, D. J., et al. (1991). Diagnosis and treatment of childhood scabies and pediculosis. *Pediatric Clinics of North America, 38*(4), 941–957.

Jablonska, S. (1991). Warts. In D. J. Demis (Ed.), *Clinical Dermatology* (pp. 1–22). Philadelphia: J. B. Lippincott.

Janniger, C. K. (1992). Childhood warts. *Cutis, 50*(1), 15–16.

Kohl, S. (1987). Postnatal herpes simplex infection. In R. D. Feign & J. D. Cherry (Eds.), *Textbook of pediatric infectious diseases* (2nd ed., pp. 1577–1601). Philadelphia: W. B. Saunders.

Levy, M. L. (1991). Disorders of the hair and scalp in children. *Pediatric Clinics of North America, 38*(4), 905–919.

Long, K. (1992). Oral acyclovir: Current recommendations for treatment. *Nurse Practitioner Forum, 3*(3), 126–128.

Mallory, S. B. (1991). Neonatal skin disorders. *Pediatric Clinics of North America, 38*(4), 745–761.

Milne, L. & Milne M. (1992). *The Audubon Society field guide to North American insects and spiders.* New York: Alfred A. Knopf.

Pochi, P. E. (1990). The pathogenesis and treatment of acne. *Annual Review of Medicine, 41,*187–198.

Shrand, H. (1961). Thrush in the newborn. *British Medical Journal, 2,* 1530–1533.

Tanz, R., et al. (1988). Treating tinea capitis: Should ketoconazole replace griseofulvin? *Journal of Pediatrics, 112*(June), 987–991.

U.S. Food and Drug Administration. (1991). Topical acne drug product for OTC use. *Federal Register, 5*(152), 37622–37635.

Ventura, A., et al. (1989). The effect of bacterial infection in the worsening of atopic dermatitis: Correlations with humoral immunologic patterns. *Annals of Allergy, 63*(August), 121–126.

Winston, M. H., & Shalita, A. R. (1991). Acne vulgaris. *Pediatric Clinics of North America, 38*(4), 889–903.

35

The Child With Burns

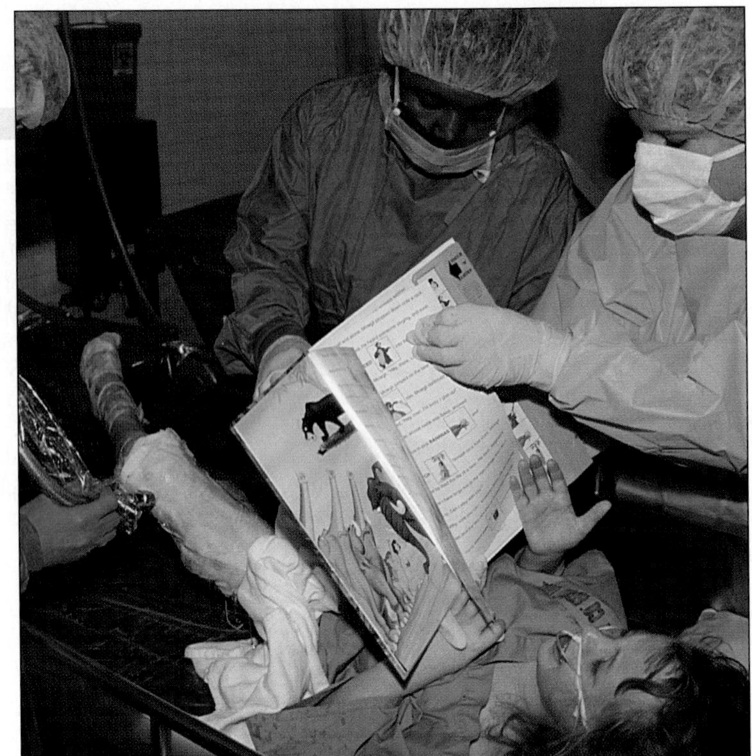

Courtesy of Parkland Memorial Hospital, Dallas, Texas

CHAPTER OVERVIEW

LEARNING OBJECTIVES

After studying this chapter, you should be able to:

- Discuss common causes of burns in children and the prevention of burn injuries.
- Describe the implications of a burn injury in a pediatric patient.
- Discuss the classifications of depth of a burn injury.
- List and describe complications of burn injuries.
- List common nursing diagnoses associated with the care of a child with burns.
- Formulate a plan of care for a child with minor burns.
- Formulate a plan of care for a child with moderate burns.
- Formulate a plan of care for a child with major burns.

KEY TERMS

allograft: a graft of tissue between the same species, but of a different genotype; a homograft

autograft: a graft of tissue taken from one part of one's own body and transferred to another part

debridement: removal of foreign material and devitalized or contaminated tissue from a traumatic or infected lesion until healthy tissue is exposed (Miller et al., 1994)

eschar: a slough produced by a thermal burn or corrosive application

heterograft: a graft of tissue transplanted between different species; a xenograft

hydrotherapy: washing of a portion of the body or the entire body

keloid: a sharply elevated, progressively enlarging scar due to excessive collagen formation during connective tissue repair

xenograft: a skin donation from another species of animal; heterograft

Burn injury may involve a small, painful area that hurts until healing occurs, or it may involve most of a child's body, with resulting severe trauma or death. Infants and toddlers are at greatest risk for sustaining burns because they are totally dependent upon their families for safety. Children may actually start a fire by playing with matches or flammable materials near open fires, they may be the victim of a house fire while they sleep, or they may be burned by an adult who is abusing them. Recovery from a major burn injury requires many months, and the child's appearance may be altered for life.

Caring for a child who is burned demands a multidisciplinary approach with a focus on the child and the family. Nursing care involves treatment of the physical injury and of the psychological effects of the injury on the child and family members. The challenges of burn nursing begin with acute burn care but continue through the rehabilitation phase until the child is restored to optimal function.

CLINICAL REFERENCE PAGES

REVIEW OF BURN INJURIES

Causes of burn injury may be thermal, chemical, electrical, or secondary to irradiation. With burn injury, the skin is unable to carry out its normal physiologic functions (see table on page 1065). The extent of the injury (depth and severity) determines whether the problem is local or systemic. Other factors, such as the location of the burned area; whether it is an electrical injury, concurrent inhalation injury, or trauma; and whether there is a pre-existing medical disease, contribute to morbidity and mortality.

Children who have been burned are at increased risk, compared to adults with burns, owing to the factors listed in the accompanying box.

Depth of Burn Injury. Depth of burn injury describes the local tissue damage and is largely a factor of the length of time of exposure, and the temperature or destructive potential of the agent causing the damage. Depth of injury is classified as superficial (first degree); partial thickness (second degree); and full thickness (third degree). (See the accompanying table on Depth of Burn Injury.)

Severity of Burn Injury. Severity of burn injury is determined by the degree to which the physiologic functions of the skin are disrupted beyond the body's normal ability to respond with compensatory mechanisms. Burn injuries are classified as minor, moderate uncomplicated, and major (see box, Classification of Severity of Burn Injury in Children). The severity of burn injury and its eventual morbidity and mortality are related to a combination of factors, including age, medical history, extent and depth of burn, special care of the body area involved (e.g., face or hands), and the presence of concomitant trauma, such as fractures or head injury, sustained at the time of the burn.

Pediatric Differences in the Effects of Burn Injury

- Very young children who have been severely burned have a higher mortality rate than do older children and adults with comparable burns.
- Because a child's skin is thinner than an adult's, lower burn temperatures and shorter exposure to heat or chemicals can cause a more severe burn.
- A larger body surface area as compared with adults places severely burned children at increased risk for fluid and heat loss. Children are also at increased risk for dehydration and metabolic acidosis secondary to diarrhea, evaporative water loss, and increased fluid requirements.
- The higher proportion of body fluid to mass in children increases the risk of cardiovascular problems owing to their less effective cardiovascular response to changing intravascular volume.
- Burns involving greater than 10% TBSA require a form of fluid resuscitation (Reeves et al., 1994).
- Infants and children are at increased risk for protein and calorie deficiency because they have smaller muscle mass and lower body fat than do adults. If they are not eating and their metabolism is increased, their protein and calorie needs will not be met.
- Hypertrophic scarring is more severe and scar maturation is prolonged (Reeves et al., 1994).
- An immature immune system means an increased risk of infection for infants and young children.
- A delay in growth may follow extensive burns.
- In children, Curling's ulcer occurs in the third or fourth week postburn, which is later than in adults.

Classification of Severity of Burn Injury in Children

MINOR BURN INJURY

- Partial-thickness burn of < 10% total body surface area (TBSA)
- Full-thickness burn of < 2% TBSA that does not involve special care areas (eyes, ears, face, hands, feet, perineum, joints)
- Excludes electrical injury, inhalation injury, concurrent trauma, all poor-risk patients (i.e., those of extremely young age or with intercurrent disease)

Clinical Manifestations

- Localized pain and blister formation in the area of injury
- No systemic effects
- No scarring

MODERATE, UNCOMPLICATED BURN INJURY

- Partial-thickness burns of 10% to 20% TBSA
- Full-thickness burns of < 10% TBSA that do not involve special care areas
- Excludes electrical injury, inhalation injury, concurrent trauma, all poor-risk patients (i.e., those of extremely young age or with intercurrent disease)

Clinical Manifestations

- Open wound that is a potential source of infection and a site for loss of fluids and electrolytes
- Pain that may interfere with routines of daily living
- Rate of wound healing influenced by nutritional status
- Possible scarring in areas of second- and third-degree injury

MAJOR BURN INJURY

- Partial-thickness burns of > 20% TBSA
- At full-thickness burns of 10% TBSA or greater
- All burns involving eyes, ears, face, hands, feet, perineum, or joints
- All inhalation injury, electrical injury, concurrent trauma, all poor-risk patients

Clinical Manifestations

- Life-threatening injuries with risk for severe complications and death
- Volatile hospital course characterized by periods of relative physiologic stability followed, within hours, by life-threatening emergencies, such as septic shock
- Repeated operative procedures for skin grafting which are always accompanied by major blood loss requiring multiple blood transfusions
- Potential risk for infection, either of the burn wound or related to pulmonary complications or systemic sepsis, until wound closure is achieved over 80% of the body surface area
- Much higher mortality associated with burn injury accompanied by inhalation injury than with burn injury alone

DEPTH OF BURN INJURY

	SUPERFICIAL (FIRST DEGREE)	PARTIAL-THICKNESS (SECOND DEGREE)		FULL-THICKNESS (THIRD DEGREE)
		Superficial	Deep	
Normal skin Epidermis Dermis Subcutaneous Muscle	Epidermis Dermis Subcutaneous Muscle	Epidermis Dermis Subcutaneous Muscle		Epidermis Dermis Subcutaneous Muscle
Morphology	Destruction of epidermis; physiologic functions remain intact	Destruction of epidermis and some dermis	Destruction of epidermis and dermis	Destruction of epidermis, dermis, and underlying tissue; may include fascia, muscle, tendon, and bone
Blister Formation	After 24 hours (e.g., from sunburn)	Within minutes; thin-walled, fluid-filled	May or may not appear as fluid-filled blisters; often, they are flat, dehydrated, and tissue paper–like. Body fluids lost through burn tissue must be replaced.	Rare; may appear as a tissue paper–like layer that is flat and dehydrated
Appearance	Peels after 24 to 48 hours	Red to pale ivory, moist surface	Mottled, waxy white, dry surface	White, cherry red, or black
Healing Time	3 to 7 days	7 to 21 days if no infection develops	30 days to several months if no infection; if infected, this type of burn may convert to full thickness	Will not heal; skin grafting required. Very small areas may heal from edges after a period of weeks.
Patient Reaction	Moderate discomfort, pain; chills; nausea; vomiting	May cause considerable pain	Severe pain upon exposure to air or water because nerve endings are intact	No pain in area of full-thickness burn because nerve endings are destroyed; surrounding areas of lesser depth are painful
Scarring	None	Minimal; influenced by genetic predisposition	Greatest because the slow healing of these burns increases scar tissue. Scar formation is influenced by genetic predisposition.	Autograft scarring is minimized by early excision and grafting. Scar formation is influenced by genetic predisposition.

FUNCTIONS OF SKIN ALTERED BY BURN INJURY

	STATUS AFTER BURN INJURY			
		PARTIAL THICKNESS (2ND DEGREE)		
NORMAL FUNCTION	**SUPERFICIAL (1ST DEGREE)**	**Superficial**	**Deep**	**FULL THICKNESS (3RD DEGREE)**
Protective barrier against infection and injury	Intact	Altered	Absent	Absent
Epidermis impermeable to most substances	Intact	Altered	Absent	Absent
Sensation from nerve endings	Intact	Intact	Absent	Absent
Vitamin D synthesis	Intact	Intact	Absent	Absent
Water vapor barrier to prevent water and electrolyte loss/absorption	Intact	Altered	Absent	Absent
Regulation of core body temperature	Intact	Altered	Absent	Absent
Immune components of skin present at dermal-epidermal junction	Intact	Altered	Absent	Absent
Local circulation	Intact	Altered	Absent	Absent
Elasticity of dermis	Intact	Intact	Altered	Absent
Ability to grow new skin	Intact	Intact	Altered	Absent

TOPICAL ANTIMICROBIAL AGENTS COMMONLY USED FOR BURNS

	ADVANTAGES	SIDE EFFECTS/DISADVANTAGES	NURSING CONSIDERATIONS
Silver Nitrate Solution	Effective against most gram-positive and some gram-negative organisms	Hyponatremia, hypokalemia, hypochloremia Decreased penetration of eschar Not effective against established infection Requires large, bulky dressings which limit mobility	0.5% solution in distilled water applied to wet dressing q 2 hr Dressing changes twice daily
Mafenide Acetate Cream (Sulfamylon)	Effective against a wide range of gram-positive and gram-negative organisms Rapidly diffuses through eschar (improved effectiveness in established infections) Permits open treatment of wound, thus increasing mobility	Painful on application May cause hypersensitivity reaction in 5%–7% of patients Associated with acid–base derangements	Applied to cleansed wound 1 to 2 times/day Treated area left open because wrapping causes maceration
Silver Sulfadiazine Cream (Silvadene)	Effective against a wide range of gram-positive and gram-negative organisms Soothing on application Softens eschar and increases joint mobility Absorbed slowly, reducing the possibility of nephrotoxicity	May cause hypersensitivity reaction in 5%–7% of patients Associated with initial decrease in leukocyte count	Applied to cleansed wound 1 to 3 times/day Wound may be left open or covered with light dressing

Adapted from Marvin, J. A. (1991). Burn injuries and skin trauma. In M. L. Patrick, S. L. Woods, R. F. Craven, J. S. Rokosky, & P. M. Bruno (Eds.), *Medical-surgical nursing: Pathophysiological concepts* (2nd ed., p. 1854). Philadelphia: J. B. Lippincott.

OVERVIEW OF BURN INJURIES IN CHILDREN

Burn injury to children may be accidental or nonaccidental. Nonaccidental injury involves child abuse by burning or neglect in supervision that results in harm to the child. In children younger than 5 years of age, burns are likely to occur as a result of environmental situations that are not controlled by caretakers. The natural curiosity and increasing mobility of the child this age contributes to the risk. Scald injury is the etiology of 72% of burn injuries in infants and toddlers (Finkelstein et al., 1992). Approximately 16% of burn injuries are related to child abuse (Herrin & Antoon, 1996).

Age-related risks for burn injury are listed in Table 35–1.

Incidence. Fire and burn injuries are a leading cause of accidental deaths in children ages 1 to 14 years. In the United States 30 to 40% of burn victims are children. Eighty-five percent of all burns are related to scalds; flame burns cause 13% of injuries; and the remainder of burns are electrical and chemical. The total number of reported burn injuries has decreased over the last 20 years. Of the approximately 50,000 children treated in hospitals for burns, about 45% are treated in one of the 120 burn centers in the United States. There are 15 pediatric burn centers. Triage criteria for referral to a burn center are presented in the accompanying box.

Extent of Burn Injury. The extent of injury refers to the percent of the total body surface area (TBSA) burned. The use of the standard rule of nines gives an inaccurate estimate because of the differences in body proportion between children and adults. When using the rule of nines in children, 9% is taken from the legs and added to the head for a child up to 1 year of age. Each subsequent year, 1% is returned to the legs until, at approximately age 9, the child's head is in proportion to that of an adult's (Miller et al., 1994). Many burn facilities use the Lund and Browder chart, which is a body surface chart corrected for age (see Fig. 35–1).

Prevention. Children can be taught to evacuate their house in the event of a fire using fire drills which identify two or more exits from each room and a location to meet outside the house. Other measures, such as the "stop, drop, and roll" program, can greatly decrease the severity of a burn injury by stopping the burning process and decreasing the amount of smoke inhalation and facial burns that occur (Powell, 1986). Public campaigns to educate adults to turn hot water heater thermostats down to 120°F can also reduce the number of accidental scald burns (Maley & Achauer, 1987). Many of these programs are taught in schools and youth groups, but nurses can implement these programs by contacting their local fire department or burn center. Public education regarding the presence of a working smoke detector can also significantly decrease the incidence of burns.

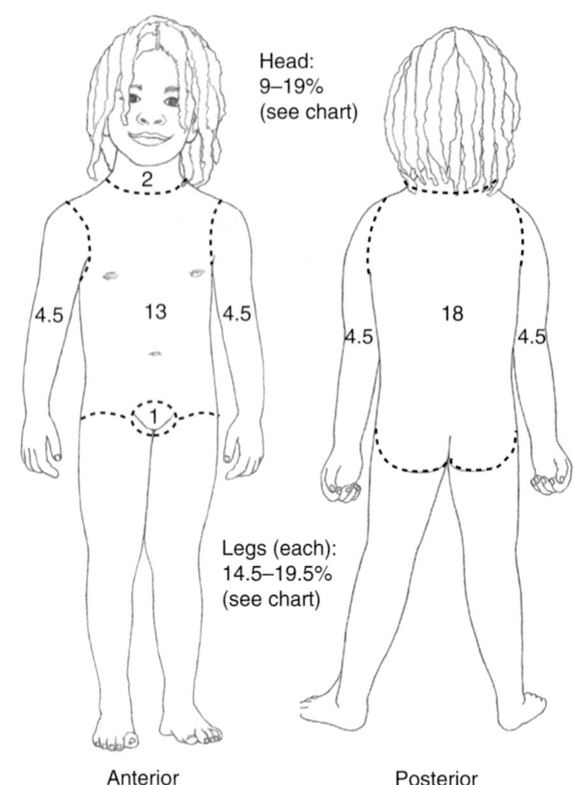

Child Burn Size Estimation Table
(percent total body surface area)

Burn area	Age (years) 1	1–4	5–9	10–14	15
Head	19	17	13	11	9
Neck	2	2	2	2	2
Anterior trunk	13	13	13	13	13
Posterior trunk	18	18	18	18	18
Genitalia	1	1	1	1	1
Upper extremity (each)	9	9	9	9	9
Lower extremity (each)	14.5	15.5	17.5	18.5	19.5

Figure 35–1
Calculating total body surface area (TBSA) burned in children. The standard "rule of nines" and standard body surface charts must be adapted because of the difference in body proportions between adults and children (see text). (Child Burn Size Estimation Table reprinted from Lund, C. C., & Browder, N. C. [1944]. Estimation of burn size. *Surgery, Gynecology, and Obstetrics, 79,* 352–358. By permission of *Surgery, Gynecology, and Obstetrics,* now known as the *Journal of the American College of Surgeons.*)

MINOR BURN INJURIES

In general, children with a minor burn injury are treated as outpatients in a physician's office, clinic, or hospital physical therapy department. Therapy is aimed at promoting wound healing, preventing infection, and providing pain relief.

The wound is cleansed with mild soap and tepid water. The area is debrided of loose debris and necrotic tissue. The debridement of blisters is controversial. Some

Burn Center Referral Criteria

The American Burn Association has identified the following injuries as those requiring referral to a burn center. Patients with these burns should be treated in a specialized burn facility after initial assessment and stabilization at an emergency department.

- Second and third degree burns of more than 10 percent BSA in patients under 10 or over 50 years old.
- Second and third degree burns of more than 20 percent BSA in all other age groups.
- Second and third degree burns with serious threat of functional or cosmetic impairment that involve face, hands, feet, genitalia, perineum, and major joints.
- Third degree burns of more than five percent BSA in any age group.
- Electric burns including lightning injury.
- Chemical burns with serious threat of functional or cosmetic impairment.
- Inhalation injury with burn injury.
- Circumferential burns of an extremity and/or the chest.
- Burned children should be transferred to a hospital with qualified personnel and equipment.
- Any burn patient with co-existing trauma, such as fractures, in which the burn injury poses the greatest risk of morbidity or mortality. However, if the trauma poses the greater immediate risk, the patient may initially be treated in a trauma center until stable, before being transferred to a burn center. Burn care may be provided simultaneously, or transfer may be accomplished after the burn patient has recovered from the immediate effects of the associated mechanical trauma. Should the burn injury present the dominant threat to mortality and the greatest risk of morbidity, then transfer to the burn center is appropriate. Physician judgement will be necessary in such situations and should be in concert with the regional medical control plan.

Pre-existing medical conditions frequently complicate burn management and prolonged recovery.

Patients at the extremes of age are subject to variable physiologic response to thermal injury. Infants and elderly patients are less tolerant of thermal, electric or chemical injuries. The burn team approach utilizing physicians, nurses, psychologists, dieticians, physical and occupational therapists has a significant influence on outcome for major burn and electric injuries.

Stabilization in Preparation for Transfer

Once the decision has been made to transfer a burn patient, it is essential that the patient be properly stabilized prior to the transfer process. The principles of stabilization are implemented during the primary and secondary assessment in the following manner.

Nebraska Burn Institute. (1994). ABLS (Advanced Burn Life Support) Course. Lincoln, NE: Author.

TABLE 35–1 *Age-Related Risks for Burn Injury*

AGE	INJURY TYPE	RISK FACTORS
< 5 Years	Flame	Playing with matches and cigarette lighters Playing with fires in fireplaces, barbecue pits, trash fires
	Scald	Kitchen injury from tipping scalding liquids Bathtub scalds associated with lack of supervision or child abuse ***Greatest number of pediatric burn patients are infants and toddlers younger than 3 years of age burned by scalding liquids***
5 to 10 Years	Flame	Male children are at increased risk Often associated with fire play and risk-taking behaviors
	Scald	Female children are at increased risk Likely to occur at home in the kitchen or bathroom
Adolescent	Flame	Injury associated with male peer-group activities involving gasoline or other flammable products Gasoline sniffing possibly involved Rarely occurs in female adolescents except in housefires or automobile accidents
	Electrical	Occurs most often in male adolescents involved in dare-type behaviors, such as climbing utility poles or antennas In rural areas, may be associated with moving irrigation pipes that touch an electrical source

researchers believe that all blisters should be opened and debrided because they can become a culture medium for bacteria (Saffle & Schnebly, 1994). Others contend that intact blisters should not be debrided because they form a moist, sterile, plasmatic environment that promotes wound healing and reepithelialization (Zuker, 1988). However, all agree that broken blisters should be debrided. The burned area is covered with an antimicrobial ointment (usually bacitracin or Silvadene) (see table in Clinical Reference Pages). A nonadherent dressing and light gauze is applied over the ointment. Dressings are usually changed twice daily.

The meticulous and regular performance of debridement is the cornerstone of successful burn wound management (Saffle & Schnebly, 1994).

Because anaerobic and aerobic bacteria can grow at the interface between burned and healthy tissue, tetanus toxoid is given to children whose immunizations are not up-to-date.

Nursing Care. The nurse should teach the parents to wash the area with mild soap and tepid water, apply the prescribed ointment and a light dressing; and promote use of the affected area. The parents should be instructed to soak the dressing in tepid water prior to its removal in order to loosen the dressing and decrease discomfort. Acetaminophen is usually effective as an analgesic. Burns of the face are usually left exposed, and antimicrobial ointment is applied twice daily. The parents should also be instructed about returning for follow-up visits.

If the parents are not able to provide needed care, home health assistance or even hospitalization may be indicated.

Treatment of minor burn injury is focused on promoting wound healing, pain management, and tetanus prophylaxis.

MAJOR BURN INJURIES AND ASSOCIATED CONDITIONS

The child with a severe burn undergoes multiple assessments when admitted to the hospital. The ABCs of airway, breathing, and circulation are assessed immediately, followed by other assessments and implementations.

Respiratory Compromise

Inhalation injury is a primary determinant of morbidity and mortality in burn patients. Pulmonary complications of burn injuries account for 60% to 70% of the patient deaths in burn centers (Carrougher, 1993). As with all trauma patients, the first priority in management of the pediatric burn patient is assessment of airway and breathing. There are three types of respiratory system injury that may occur with a burn: (1) upper respiratory tract injury, (2) pulmonary injury, and (3) carbon monoxide inhalation/hypoxia injury (Table 35–2).

Upper respiratory injury leads to swelling of the tissues in the throat and upper airway, resulting in mechanical obstruction of the airway. Swelling starts within a few minutes of the injury and the airway may occlude within a few minutes to a few hours. The edema remains in the tissues until it is slowly reabsorbed over a period of 2 to 5 days. Respiratory distress may be exhibited by abdominal breathing, head bobbing with respiratory efforts, nasal flaring, coughing, stridor, or wheezing. The young child may exhibit paradoxical inspiratory efforts, which draw the chest wall inward while thrusting out the abdomen. The small size of the pediatric airway may become occluded by mechanical obstruction related to tissue edema or to mucus plugs.

Burn Shock

Burn shock is a hypovolemic condition that develops following burn injury of greater than 15% to 20% of TBSA in children. Mechanisms of burn shock are not well understood, but the sequence of major burn injury, followed by massive capillary leakage of circulating fluid into the surrounding tissues, is well recognized.

Untreated burn shock leads to death from hypovolemia. The larger the total body surface burned, the greater the amount of fluid loss.

Within minutes of a major burn injury, all of the capillaries in the circulatory system—not just those in the area of the burn—lose their capillary seal, resulting in leakage of intravascular body fluid into the interstitial spaces. Erythrocytes and leukocytes remain in the circulation and produce an elevated hematocrit and leukocyte count. The process of burn shock continues for approximately 24 to 48 hours, at which time the capillary seal is restored.

As with any other trauma patient in hypovolemic shock, concurrent systemic changes also occur, including the following:

- Ileus, which persists for about 48 hours after the burn
- Decreased blood flow to the stomach and intestines, resulting in leakage from the gut into the peritoneum, with bacterial translocation
- Increased heart rate to compensate for hypotension
- Increased respiratory rate to meet the increased oxygen needs of the stressed body

TABLE 35–2 *Types of Respiratory Injury*

	CAUSE	AT RISK FOR:	TREATMENT
Upper Airway Obstruction	Edema of upper airway secondary to direct burn injury from inhaling superheated air, swallowing extremely hot liquids, or as an iatrogenic condition related to massive tissue swelling associated with extensive burns and burn shock therapy	Mechanical obstruction of upper airway	Intubation of airway; administration of warm, moist mist with oxygen as needed
Inhalation Injury	Inhalation of toxic products of combustion (smoke), resulting in chemical irritation and trauma to lung tissue	Impaired gas exchange related to interstitial respiratory distress syndrome 24–48 hours after burn injury	Early diagnosis of inhalation injury by bronchoscopy, or xenon-133 ventilation/perfusion scan, followed by intubation of airway and ventilatory support using a mechanical ventilator and oxygen as needed
Carbon Monoxide	Carbon monoxide released as a by-product of combustion, (especially common in structure fires) Carbon monoxide replaces oxygen on the hemoglobin molecule, leading to tissue hypoxia	Systemic hypoxia; brain damage; death	Administration of 100% oxygen by mask if the child is awake, alert, and able to protect the airway; otherwise, intubation and ventilatory support as required Continued monitoring of blood oxygen levels and oxygen administration until hypoxia resolves

Fluid and Electrolyte Deficits

In addition to fluids lost during burn shock, a healthy child has a relatively larger body surface area, in relation to weight, than an adult, thus increasing the degree of heat and evaporative water loss (Helvig, 1993). After the first 24 hours, even though the capillary seal is restored and circulating volume is maintained, major fluid and electrolyte losses continue to occur through the burn wound until wound closure is achieved. The fluid loss through the skin that follows a burn injury peaks at about the fourth day but continues to be a concern until the area heals. Fluid and electrolyte imbalances can occur rapidly. Whenever hypotension develops in burn patients, the body's ability to fight infection at the local level is compromised by low blood flow to the skin. Infection quickly develops and infected wounds lead to more tissue destruction. In the event of overwhelming infection, sepsis develops rapidly.

Metabolic Alterations

The major metabolic responses to burn injury are as follows:

Hypermetabolism. Hypermetabolism characterizes the metabolic response to burn injury, and is in proportion to the extent of burn. Energy expenditures may increase from 40% to 100% above basal levels in patients with burns of greater than 30% TBSA. Core body temperature for a child with major burn injury will reset at about 37.5°C or 99.5°F, and will remain at that level or higher until skin coverage is achieved. When exposed to cooler temperatures, the child will begin to shiver, increasing the oxygen and energy demands of the body tremendously.

Elevated Catecholamine Levels. Increased core temperature and metabolic rate are accompanied by an increase in catecholamine release. In addition, the stress associated with treatments, including the surface water evaporation that occurs with exposure of the patient to room temperature air, increase catecholamine release, metabolic stress, and energy demands.

Hyperglycemia. Glucose metabolism is also altered following burn injury. Hyperglycemia is a common occurrence, with the elevation of fasting blood glucose levels above normal being related to the severity of the injury or the presence of systemic infection. Young children may quickly deplete their glucose stores and become hypoglycemic unless they receive adequate nutritional support.

Nitrogen Imbalance. Nitrogen imbalance is associated with major burn injury related to increased nutritional needs that are not met.

Increased Nutritional Needs. The increased need for nutritional intake associated with major burn injury is related to increased energy demands associated with the hypermetabolic state and the need to heal a major wound. Major injury and infections can lead to weight loss and severe alterations in body composition, even when calories and protein are supplied in substantial amounts.

Growth Delay. Normal growth hormone levels are depressed following major burn injury. The child will not increase in height for many months while the body concentrates on survival by restoring and healing damaged tissue. About a year following the recovery phase, a growth spurt is usually noted.

Infection and Sepsis

Major burn wounds are an ideal location for bacterial growth because of the number of bacteria present and the warm, moist wound environment. If bacteria multiply to the extent that invasion into the underlying tissue occurs, infection results. The bacteria gain entrance into the systemic circulation and spread into other organs.

> Infection and the complications of infections remain a leading cause of death in burn patients. Survival depends on successfully controlling infection until the wound can be closed. This includes prevention of nosocomial infections. (Weber & Tompkins, 1993)

Wound Infection. Conditions that predispose the burn patient to the development of wound infection include:

- A source of organisms capable of producing disease
- A mode of transmission
- A susceptible host

Bacteria are found in the burn patient's own flora, especially those normally on the skin and in the gastrointestinal tract. Other bacteria can easily be spread to the patient by staff members caring for other patients (nosocomial infection). Because the local blood supply to the area of burn injury is destroyed with the burn, systemic antibiotics do not reach the burn wound.

Infection of partial-thickness burn wounds converts the area to a full-thickness injury, which then requires skin grafting.

Systemic Infection. In addition to the risk of wound infection, the burned child is also susceptible to infection from aspiration of gastrointestinal fluid into the lungs and pneumonia. The interface between the burn wound and healthy tissue is also a possible location for anaerobic bacteria to develop.

Pediatric diseases, such as chickenpox or measles, which happen at the same time the child is recovering from a major burn injury often prove lethal. This is especially true for chickenpox and its virus, herpes zoster.

The immune system is impaired following major burn injury and cannot protect the child from invasion by previously benign bacteria (Kravitz, 1993). Monocyte and macrophage components of the immune system are not functioning well, nor are the white blood cells, such as neutrophils, granulocytes, and basophils. Phagocytosis, the normal mechanism for removing debris from a wound, does not occur, allowing pockets of infection to develop.

Therapeutic Management of Associated Conditions

Respiratory Compromise. Children who are burned who do not have other injuries are awake, alert, and oriented. Initial treatment consists of establishing an airway and administering a high concentration (40%) of oxygen until an assessment and treatment plan are completed. Assessment of actual or potential pulmonary injury for patients with flame injury involves measurement of arterial blood gas and carbon monoxide levels.

> Patients with burn injuries who are unconscious are unconscious as a result of some factor other than the burn. The most common reason in flame injury is hypoxia associated with smoke inhalation.

Upper airway edema is managed by airway intubation and administration of humidified oxygen until the edema subsides, usually about 2 to 5 days later. When the assessment is made that airway edema is accumulating and will lead to airway compromise or occlusion, early planned intubation is preferred over emergency intubation. Inhalation injury is managed by airway intubation and ventilatory support at settings appropriate to the child's lung size. A full-thickness burn encircling the chest may limit full expansion of the lungs. In such cases, it may be necessary to perform an escharotomy of the chest tissue to allow for chest wall expansion.

Carbon monoxide inhalation and hypoxia are treated by administering high concentrations of oxygen by mask until the condition is resolved. Pure carbon monoxide intoxication resolves within about 30 minutes of 100% oxygen therapy. No further treatment is needed for the hypoxia, although there may be other related problems, such as neurologic damage secondary to hypoxia.

Burn Shock. Therapy for burn shock is aimed at supporting the patient through the period of hypovolemic shock until capillary integrity is restored. IV fluids are administered at a rate greater than the rate of fluid loss in order to maintain adequate circulating volume. Many formulas can be used to calculate the rate of fluid administration, the most common of which is the Parkland formula of fluid resuscitation (see the accompanying box). Because urine output reflects end-organ tissue perfusion, IV fluids are administered at a rate sufficient to keep the child's urine output at 1 ml/kg of body weight/hour. A Foley catheter is inserted into the bladder and output is measured hourly to determine the adequacy of fluid resuscitation. Ringer's lactate is the IV fluid of choice because it most closely approximates the composition of the extracellular fluid being lost.

If a child does not have adequate urine output during burn shock, the reason is insufficient administration of resuscitative fluids. Renal failure is not an expected component of burn shock if an adequate volume of IV fluids is being administered for burn shock resuscitation. It should be recognized that the Parkland formula and other burn shock fluid resuscitation formulas are guidelines; individual patients may require more than 4 ml/kg/% TBSA burn during the first 24 hours after the burn.

Sensorium is an important guide to the adequacy of fluid resuscitation. The burn injury itself does not affect the sensorium, so the child should be alert and oriented. Any alteration in sensorium should be evaluated further. When burn shock fluid resuscitation is delayed, cerebral hypoperfusion and hypoxia may occur, predisposing the child to development of cerebral edema upon initiation of massive fluid infusion. Children younger than 5 years of age handle free water poorly, making them susceptible to pulmonary and cerebral edema. Elevation of the head of the bed to decrease cerebral edematous fluid accumulation, along with monitoring for clinical signs of increased intracranial pressure, is essential.

Parkland Formula of Fluid Resuscitation for Burn Shock

4 ml Ringer's lactate solution
× kg of body weight
× % total body surface area (TBSA) burn

One-half of total is administered in the first 8 hours postburn
One-fourth of total is administered in the second 8 hours postburn
One-fourth of total is administered in the third 8 hours postburn

During the first 24 hours postburn, Ringer's lactate solution is administered IV using the formula as a guideline. The criterion for successful burn shock fluid resuscitation is based on an hourly urine output of 1 ml/kg/hr in children. Time is calculated from the time of injury, not from the time of admission.

Example: A 10-kg child with a 50% TBSA burn

4 ml × 10 kg × 50% TBSA burn = 2000 ml or 2 L of Ringer's lactate in 24 hours

Administer: 1000 ml in first 8 hours at 125 ml/h
500 ml in second 8 hours at 62 ml/hr
500 ml in third 8 hours at 62 ml/hr

In the event that fluid resuscitation is delayed, one-half of the amount is still administered in the remaining time. For example, if fluids are not started until 2 hours after the injury, one-half of the fluids are administered in the next 6 hours.

From Baxter, C. R. (1974). Fluid volume and electrolyte changes of the early postburn period. *Clinics in Plastic Surgery, 1,* 693–709.

Elevating the head of the bed or crib diminishes the amount of cerebral edema during burn shock resuscitation.

There are several reasons some patients may require fluid in excess of the calculated amount, among them an underestimation of burn size, pulmonary injury that sequesters fluid in the lungs, electrical injury with greater tissue destruction than is visible, extremely deep injury, and delayed initiation of fluid resuscitation.

Once burn shock has resolved, the child is given a colloid-containing solution, such as plasma or albumin, to replace the loss of plasma from the circulating volume.

Fluid and Electrolyte Deficits. When burn shock resuscitation is completed, a maintenance fluid plan is initiated using formulas based on normal basal fluid requirements plus calculated evaporative water loss from the burn wound. The fluid infused changes from Ringer's lactate to electrolyte-free solutions of 5% dextrose, with or without saline, depending on the patient's electrolyte status. A dextrose solution is used to meet some of the caloric needs of the hypermetabolic burn patient; 1 L of 5% dextrose solution contains 200 calories. Potassium may also be added to the IV infusion, if indicated, for hypokalemia.

Intake and output and serum electrolyte balance is monitored closely. Fluids are administered in amounts equally divided throughout each 24-hour period. IV fluids are administered until the child's bowel sounds return, usually within 48 hours after the burn. The child can then be started on oral fluids. The child must continue to maintain adequate fluid intake, either by IV infusion or orally, until wound closure is achieved.

At times during the clinical course, fluid losses may increase. This is especially true when the patient's core body temperature exceeds 39°C (102.2°F), when tracheal intubation is required, when a paralytic ileus necessitates prolonged nasogastric suction, when perioperative procedures are accompanied by massive blood loss, and when diarrhea occurs.

> Fluid and electrolyte imbalance lasting for only a few hours can lead to sepsis, seizures, and death in burned children.

Metabolic Alterations. The hypermetabolism of burn injury requires aggressive nutritional support. In addition, healing cannot occur in the presence of a negative nitrogen balance. Therefore, establishing and maintaining adequate nutritional intake to meet the caloric needs of the child is essential to survival. Caloric requirements are two to three times the normal basal requirements in the child with major burn injury.

A number of formulas have been proposed for estimating caloric requirements (see the accompanying box). Correct estimates are important, as too little nutritional intake causes protein mobilization from muscle and weight loss, whereas administration of excess calories can cause hyperglycemia, liver abnormalities, and increased carbon dioxide production. Weight, caloric and protein counts, and nitrogen balance are monitored daily, and when possible, indirect calorimetric measurements of resting energy expenditure are obtained.

> Healing of burn wounds cannot occur if the child is in negative nitrogen balance. Nutritional support is essential.

Most children with burns in excess of 25% of the TBS cannot consume an oral diet sufficient to meet their nutritional requirements. The child may refuse to eat because of the unfamiliarity of hospital food, because of pain, or in an effort to gain control over the environment. Many children require placement of enteral feeding tubes and tube feeding with supplemental liquid nutrition. In addition, vitamins (C, A, E, B, and B_5) and trace elements (iron, zinc, copper, manganese) are provided to promote wound healing. If the enteral route does not meet all of the child's nutritional needs, parenteral hyperalimentation can be used to supplement intake. This route is used only when necessary because of the risk of catheter-related infection and the desire to maintain intestinal integrity.

Estimating Caloric Requirements in Burned Children Using the Galveston Formula

Children younger than 12 years of age:
1800 kcal/m²/BSA plus 1300 kcal/m²/BSA burned

Adolescents:
1500 kcal/m²/BSA plus 1500 kcal/m²/BSA burned

From Hildreth, M.A., Herndon, D. N., Desai, M. H., & Broemeling, L. D. (1990). Current treatment reduces calories required to maintain weight in pediatric patients with burns. *Journal of Burn Care and Rehabilitation, 11*, 405–409.

ELECTRICAL INJURY AND ASSOCIATED CONDITIONS

Electrical injury is a major injury that often results in instant death, as the electrical current disrupts the electrical rhythm of the heart. The child who does not die instantly is at risk for four major complications during the acute phase:

- Cardiac arrest or arrhythmia
- Tissue damage
- Myoglobinuria (globulin from muscle serum)
- Metabolic acidosis

Cardiac Arrest/Arrhythmia. The immediate risk is cardiac arrest or arrhythmia secondary to damage to the heart's electrical conduction system. If cardiac arrest occurs, standard cardiac life support measures are initiated (see Chapter 14).

Tissue Damage. The electrical current follows the path of least resistance through the body. Entering through the skin, electricity causes heat damage to the skin layers, bone, nerves, tendons and blood vessels. The heat of the electrical current coagulates blood vessels and leaves the affected area without blood supply. Gangrene develops in necrotic tissue unless it is removed. Amputation is required in more than 90% of patients sustaining electrical injuries.

The location of the damage depends on the child's position and exposure. Electricity may enter one hand and exit from the other, for example, or it may travel through the body and exit from one or both legs. The greatest damage occurs at the entrance and exit sites.

Myoglobinuria. Myoglobinuria develops as a result of the release of products that are found in normal muscle, but that are released into the blood following electrical injury. Myoglobin is a large molecule that can mechanically obstruct the renal tubules and lead to acute tubular necrosis unless large amounts of IV fluid are administered to flush the myoglobin out of the kidney. Osmotic diuretics may be administered to promote increased urine volume. IV fluid is administered at a rate that maintains urine output at 2 ml/kg/hr until the myoglobinuria resolves.

Metabolic Acidosis. Metabolic acidosis follows electrical injury because of the associated cellular destruction and hypovolemic shock. Ringer's lactate, the fluid used for fluid resuscitation, contains sufficient bicarbonate to manage the acidosis that accompanies burn shock, but not enough to correct that associated with shock following electrical injury (i.e., pathophysiologic hypovolemic shock, not a "shock" from the electrical current).

Other Complications. The three complications just described usually resolve within 24 hours after injury. Other complications that follow electrical injury include loss of short-term memory and altered emotional states. The child can usually remember events up to the time of injury, including the names of family members, and his or her address, telephone number, and personal information, but is unable to recall more recent events. This loss of memory can be distressing to the child and frustrating to the family. For example, the child may be unable to remember visits by the family and thus feel abandoned by them. It is difficult for the child to follow instructions because of the inability to retain instructions, and this may lead to difficulty with planning care. Altered emotional states may include an absence of affect and blank stares or the opposite type of emotional response, such as manic behavior, hyperactivity, swearing, physical violence, and feelings of paranoia. Emotional responses usually become normal after about a week, but may persist longer in some patients. The electrical injury need not be to the head for these altered states to occur.

Long-term sequelae to electrical injury include gait-pattern instability and development of ocular cataracts. In addition to adaptation to any amputations, neurologic deficits may lead to gait-pattern instability and alterations in depth perception and other spatial orientation. Ocular cataracts may occur in one or both eyes at varying times from within 3 months to 18 months of injury. In the very young child, the patient may not notice changes in visual acuity; therefore, regular eye exams should be scheduled every 3 months for the first year.

CARE OF THE BURN WOUND

Burn wound closure and prevention of infection are the goals of burn wound management. Wound closure is accomplished either by supporting spontaneous healing or by initiating surgical repair. The method used is determined by the depth, extent, and location of the burn wounds. Burns to areas designated as special care areas are treated in specific ways (see the accompanying box).

Tetanus toxoid immunizations are administered as indicated to provide coverage appropriate for the child's age.

Application of Antimicrobial Agents and Dressings

Burn wounds receive daily care until closure is achieved. Wounds are cleansed using mild soaps and then are covered with topical antimicrobial agents. (See Photo Story, pp. 1075–1077. Topical Antimicrobial Agents are listed in a table in the Clinical Reference Pages at the beginning of this chapter.)

Topical antibacterial agents are placed on burn wounds to penetrate the eschar and to control bacterial growth in and around the burn wound. Systemic antibiotics are not used to control burn wound bacteria because there is no blood supply in the burn wound by which to deliver the drug. When sepsis is diagnosed, systemic antibiotics are administered and, if possible, the source of the sepsis eliminated. See Chapter 31 for a discussion of septic shock in children.

> If systemic sepsis occurs, patients will exhibit all the signs of hypovolemic shock, but the actual timing of the symptoms will depend on the volume status of the child at the time.

Silver sulfadiazine (Silvadene) is the topical agent that is most commonly used, but it is not typically used on the face or on electrical burns. Facial burns are covered with a light layer of antimicrobial ointment. Mafenide (Sulfamylon) is the topical agent of choice for burns to the ear or electrical burns because of its deep penetration into the eschar. Sulfamylon should not be applied to the face. In a small number of burn units, the established protocol calls for ointments to be placed on the wounds without a protective dressing. However, in most burn units, dressings are applied over the wound to keep the area moist and the topical agents in place.

Dressings are changed one to three times daily, depending on the agents used and specific wound care protocols. Dressing changes may occur in hydrotherapy tanks, bathtubs, showers, or, if the patient is too ill to be moved, at the beside. Placing the burned area in water facilitates cleansing of the area and softens the eschar, thereby promoting range of motion of the affected areas (see the section on Hydrotherapy that follows). Debris and previously applied topical agents are removed and the wounds re-dressed (see the section on Debridement that follows).

Treatment of Burns in Special Care Areas

Eyes: On admission, irrigate the eyes with sterile solution. Eyelids will swell shut for 3–5 days. Cleanse the area gently; do not attempt to force eyes open. After the edema resolves, wash the area every 8 hours and apply ointment and eye drops per physician's order. Inform the child that vision may be blurred owing to application of medications.

Ears: On admission, remove blisters and secure hair away from the burned area. Position the child without using a pillow to prevent further trauma to the ears, as wounds tend to adhere to pillows or linens. Apply Sulfamylon ointment every 12 hours as ordered by the physician.

Face: On admission, remove blisters and shave face,* except for eyebrows, as indicated. Apply bacitracin or other ointments per physician's order. Cleanse the area every 8 hours and reapply topical ointment. The area will heal quickly (7–10 days) if it is a superficial burn because of an abundant blood supply. Deeper burns are skin grafted early to decrease scarring. Pillows are not used with anterior neck burns so as to minimize scarring from chin to neck.

Hands: On admission, remove rings or other jewelry. Remove blisters and apply a topical antibiotic ointment (silver sulfadiazine), wrapping each finger individually and wrapping the entire hand in a manner that permits full range of motion. Cleanse the area every 8 hours and reapply ointment and dressings. Encourage full range of motion and use of hand. Elevate the patient's hand above the level of the heart to promote edema reabsorption. Administer pain medication to facilitate use of hand. The area will heal quickly (7–10 days) if it is a superficial burn because of abundant blood supply. Deeper burns should be skin grafted early to decrease scarring.

Feet: On admission, remove blisters. Apply topical antibiotic ointment (silver sulfadiazine) per physician's order. Wrap the toes individually, wrap the foot so that full range of motion is possible, and apply an elastic bandage, distal to proximal, over the dressing to promote comfort and reduce dependent edema. The patient should ambulate at least every 4 hours unless contraindicated; pain medication should be administered so as to be effective at ambulation times. Elevate the patient's lower extremities when at rest.

Joints: On admission, remove blisters and shave areas with hair. Apply topical ointment per physician's order. Wrap the area to permit full range of motion. Cleanse the area every 8 hours and reapply ointment and dressings. Shave areas of hair growth every 3–4 days. Encourage full range of motion. When at rest, joints should be kept in extension to prevent contracture formation.

Perineum: On admission, remove blisters and shave the area. Insert a bladder catheter before edema accumulates. Apply silver sulfadiazine, per physician's order, directly to the perineum or onto diapers before application. Maintain the bladder catheter until the edema subsides. Cleanse the area after each stool/voiding and reapply silver sulfadiazine. Scrotal edema can accumulate and may impair walking until resolved.

Circumferential burns: On admission, identify areas of full-thickness circumferential burn. Cleanse the area, remove blisters, and shave as needed. Monitor distal pulses every 15 minutes using a Doppler monitor. If distal pulses diminish or disappear, notify the physician immediately and prepare for escharotomy or fasciotomy. After the incision is made, check for pulses. Continue to monitor pulses every 15 minutes for 24 hours postburn. If pulses diminish or disappear again, notify the physician. Apply silver sulfadiazine and dressings to the area. Cleanse the area and change dressings every 8 hours.

*If age appropriate.

Aseptic technique is used during dressing changes. After dressings are applied to burn wounds, isolation is not necessary, and the child does not need to be restricted to a room or to an area of the hospital.

Pain medications are administered 20 to 30 minutes prior to dressing changes so that maximal effect can be achieved to control pain at the time of the procedure. In addition to pain control, measures to maintain the patient's core body temperature, minimize shivering, and conserve energy must be implemented as part of wound care activities. To the degree possible, the patient's capacity for self-care should be optimized.

Types of Dressings

Biologic, synthetic, or debriding dressings may be used for temporary closure of a wound during the acute phase of burn therapy.

Biologic Dressings. Biologic dressings are used to cover the burn wound temporarily during the acute phase of burn therapy. Biologic dressings have several functions: pain relief, reduction of evaporative fluid and heat loss, adherence, flexibility, protection from infection, reduction of bacterial colonization, and stimulation of local blood flow (Saffle & Schnebly, 1994). Common biologic dressings

Caring for Lauren, a Child With Burns

INTRODUCTION

Prevention of infection, removal of dead tissue, and wound healing are the primary objectives when caring for a child who has been burned. Dressing changes, of which hydrotherapy is an integral part, usually occur twice daily. The dressing changes are often quite painful. The child requires support by a multidisciplinary team both prior to and during the procedure.

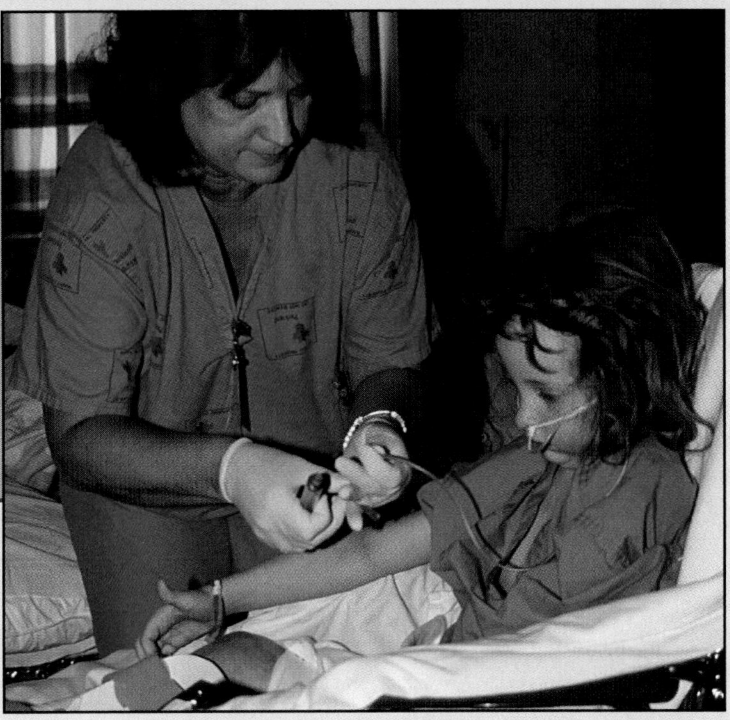

Thirty minutes before Lauren is scheduled to have her dressings changed, Linda, her nurse, administers 15 mg of morphine oral solution concentrated drops and 1 mg of Ativan to lessen Lauren's pain and anxiety during the procedure. Lauren's nasogastric tube provides an easy access site for medication administration, and Lauren doesn't have to taste or swallow the drugs, or feel the discomfort of an injection. The nasogastric tube was already in place to provide feedings for Lauren because she was refusing food. Assuring good nutrition is especially important for Lauren because as a burn patient she has increased caloric needs.

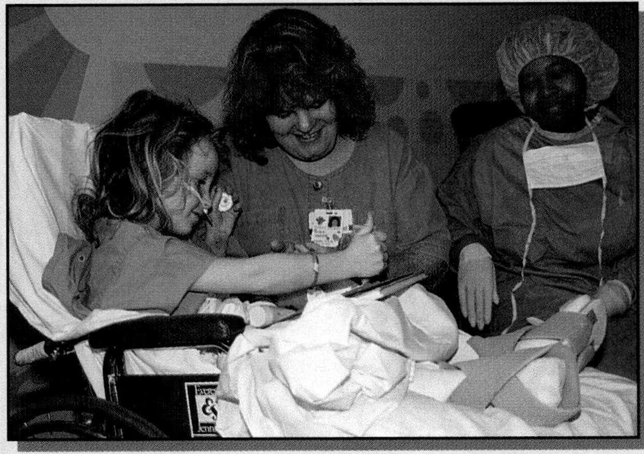

Lauren's mother cannot be with her today during the dressing change. The child life specialist joins Lauren and her nurse and explains that she will remain with them until the dressing change is completed. Child life specialists use play, art, and other forms of interaction to help children deal with their concerns and fears. The specialist gives Lauren the choice of remaining in her room or going to the playroom until it is time to begin the procedure. This gives Lauren a sense of control. Lauren chooses to go to the playroom and paint.

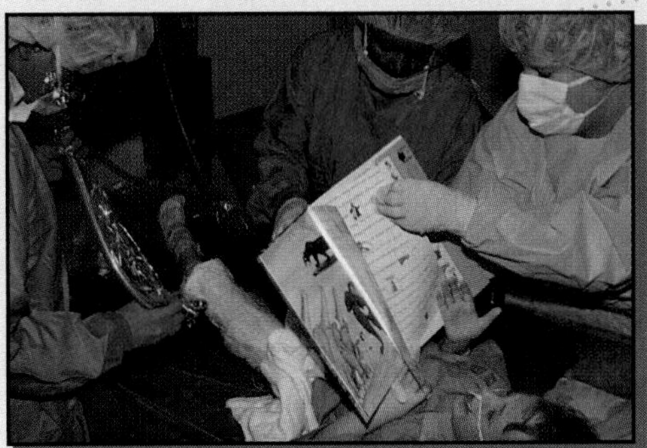

Once the medication has taken effect, Lauren is moved to the hydrotherapy room and the dressing change begins. The hydrotherapy room is kept warm because patients who have been burned have poor body temperature control. The therapist reads a book to Lauren as a means of distracting her from the discomfort associated with the procedure.

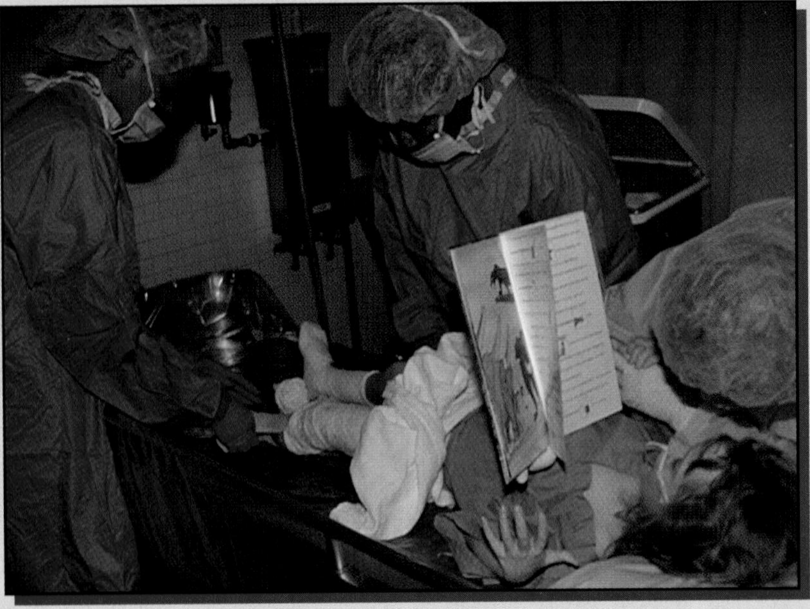

Bathing with water helps cleanse the area and softens the eschar. Natural debridement occurs with removal of dressings and hydrotherapy. The temperature of the water is adjusted for Lauren's comfort. The specialists who are changing Lauren's dressings wear impermeable gowns, gloves, masks, goggles, and hair covers to guard against contamination of the burn wounds. Gloves will be changed several times during the procedure: after removing soiled dressings, after cleansing the wound, and before applying new dressings.

The outer dressing is removed from Lauren's wounds, and the fine-mesh dressing touching the wound is loosened by spraying water on the area.

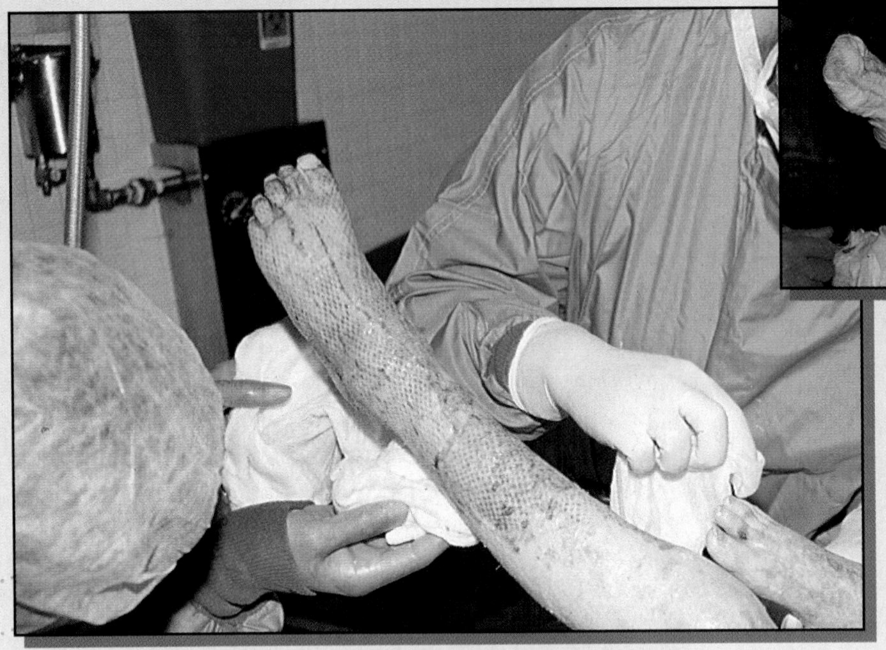

Lauren's wound is cleaned by spraying with water. Gauze pads are used to debride and remove exudate and the previously applied medication. Lauren is given the choice of assisting with removing the dressings, but she chooses not to help. Some children find that helping to remove the dressings is a way to have more control over the discomfort of the process.

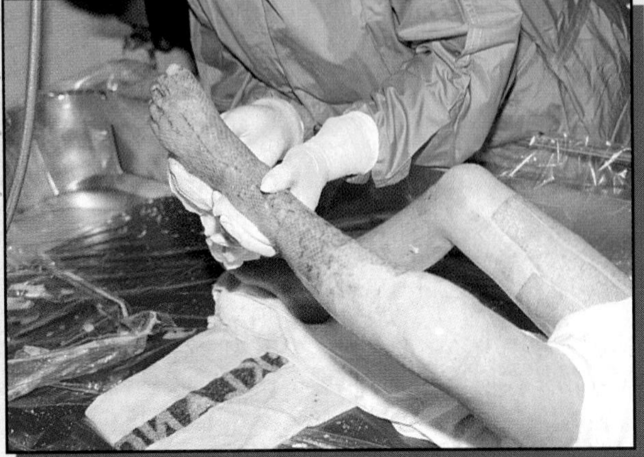

All of the previously applied medication must be removed before applying new medication, and the wound must be cleansed of any devitalized tissue or exudate. The debridement process is very painful; the nurse can minimize the length of the procedure by using firm pressure to clean the wound more quickly.

CONTINUED

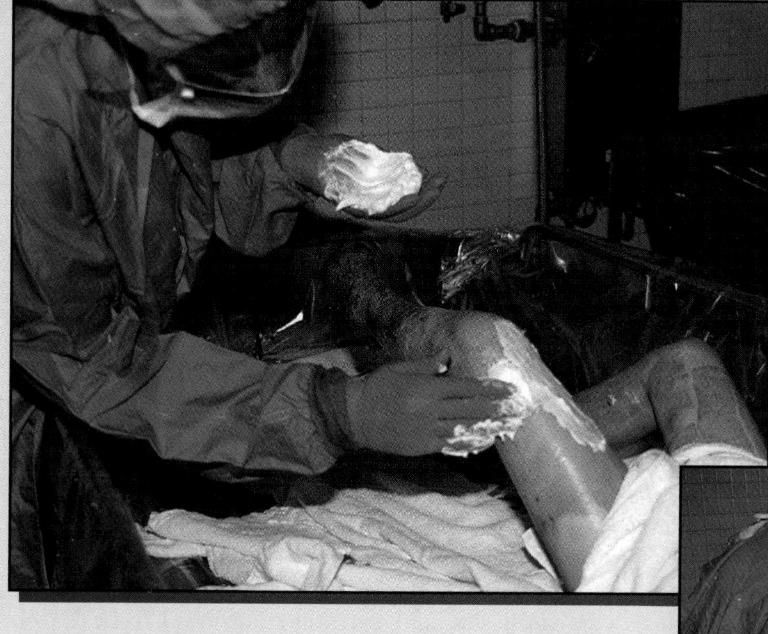

After the wound has been cleaned, a topical antimicrobial agent is applied. The most commonly used agent is silver sulfadiazene (Silvadene), which is applied directly to the wound. Care is taken to avoid getting the Silvadene on Lauren's unaffected skin or the grafted area, in order to avoid breaking down unburned tissue. The application of the Silvadene can best be compared to "icing a cake."

After the application of the Silvadene, a fine-mesh gauze is applied, and the area is secured by wrapping it with Kling.

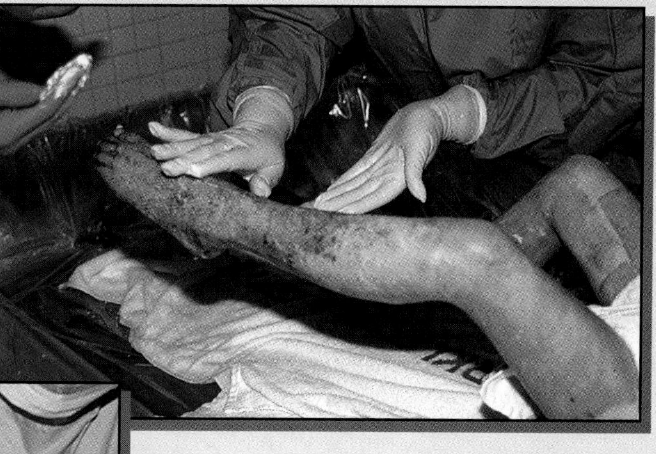

On the third day after Lauren's leg was grafted, the dressings were removed down to the fine-mesh gauze. On the fourth day the fine-mesh gauze was removed, and a new fine-mesh gauze impregnated with a topical ointment (Neomycin) was applied. When the wound is completely healed, it may be left exposed. The dark areas on the skin are grafted skin.

The donor site is covered with either a biosynthetic dressing (Biobrane), transparent film, or fine-mesh gauze. The dressing will begin to peel back like a scab and is trimmed when this happens. Dressings are not changed on donor sites to prevent tearing the delicate epithelium. The dressing is usually completely off the donor site in 10 to 14 days.

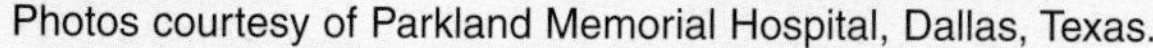

Photos courtesy of Parkland Memorial Hospital, Dallas, Texas.

include human skin **allograft** (cadaver), **xenograft** or **heterograft** (pig skin), and fresh human amniotic membrane (placenta). Fresh cadaveric allograft is used most often for temporary coverage of excised large burn areas.

Synthetic Dressings. Synthetic dressings protect the wound, provide a moist environment for epidermal growth, decrease pain, and allow for increased comfort with movement. They are used most frequently for fresh partial-thickness burns and donor sites. Examples include plastic films, hydrocolloids, hydrogels, and collagen-impregnated dressings. The major risk associated with these dressings is infection; thus, the wound must be clean and dry prior to application of the dressing.

Debriding Dressings. Although topical antibiotics loosen eschar, in some cases, a debridement dressing may be used. These dressings, which provide mechanical debridement, are applied after hydrotherapy and wound debridement. Gauze pads or rolls soaked in saline solution, Ringer's lactate, or antibiotic solution are wrung out, placed loosely on the wound, and covered with a dry gauze and elastic wrap. Removal of this type of dressing can be very painful and may cause excessive bleeding. The dressing may need to be moistened before removal. Use of debridement dressings should be discontinued once clean granulation tissue is present; otherwise, they will interfere with healing.

Debridement

In a burn injury, there is necrosis of skin and subcutaneous tissue. The burned tissue is called **eschar.** Eschar releases chemical mediators that stimulate leukocytes to digest debris, but this also damages capillaries and skin elements. Necrotic tissue within a wound prolongs inflammation and slows healing and epidermal coverage (Saffle & Schnebly, 1994).

Debridement is the removal of dead material within a wound in order to promote healing. Initial debridement may be performed in the emergency department or on the unit in the hydrotherapy treatment room. Burns are cleansed and debrided at least every 12 hours. Old creams and ointments must be removed as part of the debridement, and loose tissue is trimmed around the wound.

Hydrotherapy

Hydrotherapy is used to cleanse the wound and the patient. During this cleansing process, active range-of-motion exercises may also be performed. The hydrotherapy can take place in a tank, tub, or shower. Some facilities use disposable plastic liners to prevent contamination between patients. Hydrotherapy should last no longer than 20 minutes so as to prevent electrolyte loss (through skin into water secondary to osmosis). The room temperature should be kept warm, and the child should be covered and dried immediately following cleansing.

Skin Grafts and Donor Sites

Full-thickness burn injuries and most deep partial-thickness burn injuries are managed surgically. The procedure to remove the burn tissue is excision; wound coverage is achieved over healthy, unburned tissue. The skin used to cover the burn wound is harvested from an unburned area (donor site) of the patient's own skin (**autograft**). The skin that is surgically removed is a paper-thin section of the upper layers of the skin (split-thickness skin graft). In order to cover a greater area, autograft skin is usually prepared with a skin mesher. The mesher, which has variable settings, cuts small slits into the skin, allowing it to be stretched to cover a graft area one to nine times larger than the original size of the graft. The slit pattern disappears as the graft heals. If the patient does not have enough unburned skin to cover the wound, temporary coverage can be achieved by using a homograft (cadaver skin) or xenograft (pig skin) that has been specially prepared for that use.

In some burn units, the burn eschar is removed in a two-stage excision and grafting procedure. On the first day, the burn is surgically excised and the area is covered with antibiotic-soaked dressings, after which the patient is allowed to recover from anesthesia. On the second day, the patient is returned to surgery for a procedure that involves removing a paper-thin layer of unburned skin from the patient's body and applying that skin to the previously excised burn areas. In other burn units, excision and skin grafting is accomplished in one procedure, with an interval in between excision of the burn and application of the new skin to allow for control of blood loss. If blood collects between the excised area and the skin graft, the skin graft will not adhere. Infection can also cause loss of skin grafts.

Blood loss with excision of large burns is massive, and may require replacement of as much as one-half of the child's circulating blood volume. Burn patients receive many blood transfusions during their hospital course to replace blood lost during surgical wound management.

Scarring

Burn scars form in areas of healed burn, including those areas that received skin grafts. Scarring starts at the time healing starts and continues for about 8 to 12 months. Hypertrophic scarring results in an elevated, raised, reddened, and painful area that is very susceptible to traumatic injury from routine daily activities. Prevention of hypertrophic scarring is essential for optimal cosmetic and functional recovery. **Keloid** scars form in the area of the burn, and then expand onto unburned tissue.

Within a week or two after a wound is closed by either skin grafting or healing, scarring is minimized by application of pressure to the area using specially made anti-scarring compression garments. Garments, such as gloves, shirts, pants, or face masks, are individually measured and fitted to the burn area. They are worn 24 hours a day, except during bathing, for about 10 to 12 months after the burn (Kravitz, 1988). Some children wear them for shorter or longer periods of time, depending upon the rate of scar maturity. Although these garments have been available only in tan for many years, several manufacturers are now creating them in bright, interesting colors with attractive appliqued figures and designs. As donning and wearing these garments can be a difficult and painful process, compliance is often an issue, and the child's level of cooperation is almost totally dependent upon the attitude of the adult supervisor. Facial burns may be treated with masks of more rigid construction in order to restore a normal contour to the central face and chin.

Physical Therapy

Areas of burn become stiff, and range of motion is severely limited unless active range-of-motion therapy is initiated at the time of admission and continued for several months until the scars mature. Muscles tend to shorten, and skin contracts in burn areas involving the joints. Extension muscles are not as strong as flexor muscles, and injured areas over joints (especially the elbows, axilla, and knees) tend to become permanently fixed in the flexed position. Frequent physical therapy exercise is required to prevent flexion contractures, which severely limit mobility and may require surgical correction. If the child is able and willing to cooperate, active range of motion and use of the burned areas promote optimal functional recovery. If the child is unable or unwilling to cooperate, passive range of motion, performed by all staff, will help to maintain function. The parents and the child will be taught the physical therapy exercises prior to the child's discharge from the hospital, as therapy must continue for about 12 to 18 months after the burn, or until scar formation has peaked.

MANAGEMENT OF PAIN AND ITCHING

Pain and itching are both active components of recovery from a burn injury. With partial-thickness burns and in areas used for donor sites, nerve endings are exposed. Newly healed areas and those that have received skin grafts are highly sensitive to pressure pain, and the joints underneath develop an arthritic type of pain that is aggravated with movement. Burn patients awaken each day with chronic pain, stiffness, and aching in the burned areas for many months after the burn is healed.

Itching occurs in all healing areas and causes great distress unless it is relieved with medication. Itching persists for several months after burns heal, as new nerve endings and dermal elements reestablish themselves. Alterations in sweat glands after burning result in excessive sweat production, which leads to dry skin and itching, adding to the problem.

The perception of pain in the burned child varies widely but is usually related to procedural pain (from burn dressing changes or physical therapy) or background pain (from attempting to remain still to avoid the pain of movement). Chronically abused children learn not to verbalize pain, and often withdraw into a trance-like state when painful procedures occur. Other children in pain protest everything with every bit of volume and energy available to them. The amount of protest a child manifests in response to painful procedures should not be the criterion for pain management.

Procedural pain is real and can be minimized with a pain management program that involves the administration of adequate analgesia 20 to 30 minutes prior to initiation of the procedure, additional analgesia as the procedure continues, and analgesia at the completion of the procedure to allow rest and recovery time. For especially painful procedures, the use of short-acting, memory-altering medications may be indicated so that the child does not recall the procedure. One effective method of pain control is the patient-controlled analgesia pump (Chapters 19 and 20), a method which may be used by children as young as 6 years of age (Schumann, 1991).

> Pain medication should be administered in anticipation of painful procedures so that maximal effectiveness coincides with the timing of the procedure. When the child undergoes a procedure that is known to produce prolonged pain, such as a skin grafting, pain medication should be administered on a scheduled basis, rather than as needed once pain is reported.

Morphine is the drug of choice. It should be administered by the IV route rather than the intramuscular route because it will not be rapidly or evenly absorbed if it is injected into edematous tissue. To diminish pain between dressing changes, oral medications, such as acetaminophen with codeine, may be used (see Chapter 20).

In older children, anxiety and anticipatory stress may be factors that respond to anti-anxiety medications. Ensuring adequate sleep and uninterrupted quiet time is essential to allow the child to restore inner resources. Parental visiting should be unrestricted and individualized to the child's needs and those of the family. The child's pain is also a source of great distress to the family.

Itching can be controlled by medications, such as diphenhydramine hydrochloride (Benadryl), and the application of soothing lotions, such as Nivea or Eucerin, to healing skin.

PSYCHOSOCIAL ASPECTS OF BURN INJURY

The long-term effects of an accidental burn injury may be related to physical changes resulting from the healing/scarring process, or to the psychosocial alterations in the relationship between the child and family members (Molter, 1993).

The immediate psychosocial stresses for the burned child include separation from parents and from the home environment, as well as all of the known psychological traumas associated with hospitalization. Children who are intubated cannot speak or cry out, and often, their arms and legs are restrained to prevent pulling on IV lines and tubes. Physical restraint is terrifying to a young child who cannot understand the reason for restraint. Older children, who may be able to understand the rationale for restraint, may experience anger and a lack of trust.

Children must be allowed "safe time" during the day when no medical procedure, painful or not, is performed (Helvig, 1993). The period should be identified by the nurse as "safe" through a statement, such as "I am going to sit and read to you for the next 15 minutes, and nothing else will happen during that time."

Periods of uninterrupted sleep must be planned into the day so that the child has time to rest and regain strength, both mentally and physically.

Infants manage stress by sucking. If the child cannot take liquids by mouth, a pacifier should be provided so that the child can achieve stress reduction and comfort from sucking. Children who have recently given up bottles or pacifiers tend to regress, and these items should be made available to them if desired. The feelings of safety and comfort afforded by their use far exceed any problems associated with weaning after discharge from the hospital.

Recently mastered toileting skills will be lost with the stress of a major burn injury, so children should be placed in diapers until they are once again able to invest the emotional and physical work required to resume independent toileting. The child must be reassured that this behavior is acceptable during the burn injury, that punishment will not occur, and that diapering is not intended as a punishment. After discharge home, at a time the child and parents feel is appropriate, toilet-training can begin again.

After the acute crisis of burn injury is over and the child is nearing the time of discharge, short trips may be taken to nearby parks or shops to help the child and parents adjust to public reactions to the burn injury. The child may never look unburned, but the location of the burn and whether it can easily be covered with clothing during usual daily activities are factors that have a bearing on the child's and family's adjustment. Depending on the age of the child, peer pressure may also be a factor. Some severely burned children lose all facial features, including ears, and going out in public becomes an ordeal they and their family avoid. Other children lead well-adjusted lives despite major disfigurement. The inner strengths of the family and the value ascribed to the child by the family, both before and after the burn, appear to be deciding factors in the level of adjustment. More specifically, children appear to respond to the burn and give it meaning in a manner similar to their mother. Nevertheless, extensive, disfiguring burn scars have a tremendous long-term impact on the child and family. Occasionally, family members will not be able to accept the child, and will request foster placement.

Involving the family early in the care of the child facilitates acceptance. As soon as possible after discharge from the hospital, the child and family should resume normal daily activities. Most burn units have a formal program designed to facilitate the child's return to school. A staff member may accompany the child on the first day back to school in order to explain what has happened and to describe the purpose of pressure garments or other therapeutic interventions. Age-related issues of intimacy and sexuality will eventually arise, as will self-image and self-esteem issues. Social workers and psychologists monitor the patient's and family's adjustment during return clinic visits the first year after burn injury.

In the case of nonaccidental burn injuries, the child's placement after hospital discharge is determined by the legal system. Nurses should be prepared for the fact that the child may be returned to the home environment if it is believed that the child's safety can be assured. The younger child does not understand the concept of child abuse, and loves and depends on the parent(s) just as much as any other child. Separation of a child and parent carries significant psychosocial implications, and the goal of protective services is always to restore and maintain the family unit if the child's safety can be assured by close supervision by the agency.

NURSING CARE OF THE CHILD WITH BURNS

Assessment

In the first few seconds after the arrival of a child who has been burned, a determination is made as to the severity of the burn. If the burn is of minor or moderate severity, the care focus is on pain management and wound care. If a major burn injury has occurred, the initial assessment focuses on establishing and maintaining the child's airway, breathing, and circulation. After an airway and IV access have been established, a catheter is inserted into the bladder to begin hourly urine output measurements, and a nasogastric tube is inserted into the stomach to prevent aspiration. Vital signs are taken, with special attention to the child's body temperature. Without skin, the burned child, especially if very young, rapidly loses heat to the atmosphere and is at risk for hypothermia. Continuous monitoring of the child is required, with vital signs and urine output being measured and recorded at least hourly. Blood will be drawn for laboratory analysis every 6 to 8 hours during the first few days. To facilitate access for drawing blood samples and to allow continuous monitoring of blood pressure and pulse, arterial lines may be inserted. The child should be awake, alert, and oriented unless some condition other than an uncomplicated burn injury exists. Assessment for pain intensity takes place on a scheduled basis, and interventions to control pain occur as needed. Wound assessment is performed with each dressing change, taking note of any constriction of the distal circulation or signs of infection. The distal circulation of extremities with circumferential burns should be monitored hourly during burn shock.

Assessments will decrease in frequency after the first 2 to 3 days if the child is physiologically stable. Vital signs and urine measurements will be obtained and recorded every 4 hours, and then every 8 hours. Daily weights are also obtained. As the child begins oral intake, all fluids and foods are measured carefully for volume, calories, and protein, and bowel sounds are assessed to document continued peristalsis. Wound assessment continues with each dressing change.

Perioperative assessment of the child includes protection of the airway; administration of IV fluids, including blood products; and frequent monitoring of vital signs. Intake and output measurements, pain management, and protection of newly grafted areas by immobilizing the area for 24 to 48 hours are also integral parts of nursing care. An oral diet can be resumed as soon as the child is awake enough to protect the airway.

Assessment of the burn wound, and of the status of any donor sites following autografting, occurs several times each day. Assessment also includes range of motion abilities and frequency and effectiveness of physical therapy treatments. Daily assessment of the patient's independent activities is made with the goal of achieving as much independence as is age appropriate.

Nursing Diagnosis

The following nursing diagnoses and expected outcomes may be appropriate following assessment of the child with burns:

- Impaired Skin Integrity related to burn
- Pain related to thermal injury and related procedures
- Ineffective Airway Clearance/Impaired Gas Exchange related to upper airway edema, smoke inhalation injury, or carbon monoxide/hypoxia
- Altered Tissue Perfusion (peripheral) related to burn shock
- Risk for Fluid Volume Deficit related to loss of skin integrity in the area of the burn and shifting of plasma and plasma components from the circulatory system into the interstitial and intracellular spaces secondary to impaired capillary integrity
- Risk for Infection related to burn wound contamination or pulmonary complications
- Altered Nutrition Less Than Body Requirements, related to hypermetabolism and the increased energy requirements of wound healing
- Body Image Disturbance related to appearance
- Knowledge Deficit related to home care (see Teaching Guidelines following Care Plan)

Planning, Implementation, and Evaluation: The Child With Burn Injury

NURSING DIAGNOSIS • Impaired Skin Integrity related to burn

Expected Outcome: • The burn will heal without infection, as evidenced by restoration of the epithelial layer.

Intervention	Rationale
1. Cleanse and debride the wound daily and apply ointments/dressings as ordered. Assess the site and document.	Infection can be prevented by removing bacterial contamination, exudate, and previously applied medication.
2. Promote fluid and nutritional intake. Offer high-calorie, high-protein meals and snacks.	Healing occurs only in the presence of positive nitrogen balance. The child's protein and caloric needs are elevated owing to increased metabolism and catabolism.

Intervention	Rationale
3. Perform active and passive range of motion of the affected parts of the child's body.	Use of the burned area promotes edema reabsorption and prevents contracture deformity.
4. Make sure the child's tetanus toxoid immunizations are current.	Anaerobic bacteria can cause infection at the interface between the burn wound and healthy tissue.
5. Assess the child for signs and symptoms of infection: changes in sensorium, hypothermia, fever or wound appearance (drainage or odor).	Early detection of infection will ensure prompt treatment.
6. Administer vitamins and minerals (A, B, C, iron and zinc) as ordered.	Vitamin/mineral supplements facilitate wound healing and epithelialization.

Evaluation: • The burn wound shows signs of progressive healing.

NURSING DIAGNOSIS • Pain related to thermal injury and related procedures

Expected Outcome: • Pain relief will be achieved as evidenced by age-appropriate behaviors, adequate nutritional intake, and appropriate sleep patterns.

Intervention	Rationale
1. Determine the child's pain level using age-appropriate assessment tools (see Chapter 20).	The child's developmental stage affects response to pain.
2. Administer pain relief measures/medication on a scheduled basis, rather than p.r.n. Premedicate the child before painful procedures.	The fact that burns hurt is irrefutable, so there is no need to wait until pain is behaviorally indicated before administering medication.
3. Minimize the time spent on wound manipulation and exposure.	Exposure of the burned area to air or water hurts because the nerve endings are exposed. Dressing changes should be done as quickly as possible to minimize pain.
4. Use nonpharmacologic pain reduction measures (see Chapter 20).	The use of distraction, relaxation techniques, therapeutic touch, and other measures can help alleviate pain.
5. Perform passive and active range-of-motion exercises.	Exercise reduces the likelihood of contracture formation and increases functional ability.

Evaluation: • Except during times of direct wound care and physical therapy, the child is pain-free, as evidenced by normal sleep, play, and eating patterns.

NURSING DIAGNOSIS • Ineffective Airway Clearance/Impaired Gas Exchange related to upper airway edema, smoke inhalation injury, or carbon monoxide/hypoxia

Expected Outcome: • The child will maintain normal oxygen saturation levels, have unlabored respirations appropriate for age, and have clear bilateral breath sounds.

Intervention	Rationale
1. Assess the child's respiratory status hourly for the first 72 hours postburn, and then as indicated by the child's clinical condition.	Edema accumulates during the first 24 to 48 hours postburn, reaching maximum levels within about 24 hours after the burn injury. Acute respiratory distress syndrome (ARDS) is manifested within 48 to 72 hours postburn.
2. Monitor arterial blood gas levels and carboxyhemoglobin levels per physician's order.	The effectiveness of therapy will be reflected by systemic ventilation/perfusion.
3. Monitor oxygen levels continuously with pulse oximetry.	Changes in ventilatory status can rapidly be detected by pulse oximetry.
4. Administer humidified oxygen per physician's order.	Humidified oxygen administration helps to liquefy secretions and decrease mucous plug formation.
5. Encourage turning, coughing, and deep breathing every 1–2 hours while the child is awake as indicated by the child's clinical condition.	These interventions promote lung expansion and decrease the risk of atelectasis and dependent pulmonary edema.
6. Elevate the head of the bed 15° to 30°.	Head elevation facilitates lung expansion, especially in a child with a distended abdomen.
7. Suction the endotracheal or nasotracheal tube p.r.n.	Suctioning removes mucus accumulation and helps to maintain a patent airway.

Evaluation:

- The child is able to maintain ventilation/perfusion values that are within normal limits.
- Airway extubation is possible once the edema subsides.

NURSING DIAGNOSIS

- Altered Tissue Perfusion (peripheral) related to burn shock

Expected Outcome:

- The child will maintain a urine output of at least 1–2 ml/kg/hr for the first 24 hours postburn, and will remain alert and oriented.

Intervention	Rationale
1. Administer IV fluids per resuscitation formula.	Burn shock is a type of hypovolemic shock that requires administration of IV fluids to maintain circulating volume.
2. Monitor urine output hourly; report any output measure <1–2 ml/kg/hr.	Urine output reflects the adequacy of end organ tissue perfusion.
3. Monitor the child's electrolyte balance per physician's order.	Electrolyte imbalances may occur as fluids and electrolytes shift within the body.
4. Monitor the child's neurologic status hourly.	The child should be alert, awake, and oriented throughout burn shock unless complications arise.
5. Monitor blood flow distal to circumferential burns by monitoring distal pulses; notify the physician of any changes in distal pulses.	Accumulation of edema in areas of full-thickness circumferential burns may have a tourniquet effect, compromising distal blood flow. Escharotomy/fasciotomy is required if occlusion is evident.

Evaluation:
- The child maintains a urine output of 1–2 ml/kg/hr.
- The child's mental status is normal, and the child remains alert, awake, and oriented.
- The distal pulses in circumferential burn areas are not diminished.

NURSING DIAGNOSIS
- Risk for Fluid Volume Deficit related to loss of skin integrity in the area of the burn and shifting of plasma and plasma components from the circulatory system into interstitial and intracellular spaces secondary to impaired capillary integrity

Expected Outcome:
- The child will maintain normal fluid and electrolyte balance as evidenced by intake and output measurements and serum electrolyte values that are within normal limits.

Intervention	Rationale
1. Administer IV or oral fluids in the quantity ordered.	Fluids help to maintain capillary circulation to the viable skin appendages and general circulation to the vital organs. Fluid replacement continues until wound coverage is achieved.
2. Monitor the child's intake and output hourly until stable and every 4 hours thereafter.	Close monitoring is necessary to determine whether fluid resuscitation is adequate. Fluid intake that is sufficient to produce 1–2 ml/kg/hr of urine assures adequate tissue perfusion.
3. Weigh the child daily.	Weight is an accurate measurement of fluid hydration. Increasing weight indicates fluid overload.
4. Monitor the child's vital signs and sensorium hourly until burn shock resolves, then every 4 hours.	Alterations in electrolyte balance indicating a fluid excess/deficit can cause changes in sensorium and vital signs.
5. Monitor laboratory values for elevations in electrolyte or hemoglobin levels.	Early identification of abnormal laboratory values permits early treatment of fluid volume imbalances.

Evaluation:
- A normal fluid and electrolyte balance is maintained as evidenced by age-appropriate serum laboratory values, intake and output measurements, and weight.

NURSING DIAGNOSIS
- Risk for Infection related to burn wound contamination or pulmonary complications

Expected Outcome:
- The child will achieve wound closure without developing burn wound infection, systemic sepsis, or pneumonia.

Intervention	Rationale
1. Assess the burn wound during dressing changes for signs of infection, and assess the child for signs of sepsis: changes in sensorium, hypothermia, fever, or wound appearance (drainage or odor).	Infection and sepsis are related to the number of bacteria present in the burn wound; frequent cleansing removes bacteria and prevents overgrowth.
2. Use aseptic technique for wound care by wearing protective gear, practicing meticulous handwashing techniques, and changing protective gear between patients.	Cross-contamination of burn wounds from other patients or staff increases the risk and incidence of sepsis.

Intervention	Rationale
3. Provide nutritional support by individualizing meal plans.	Wound healing requires the positive nitrogen balance afforded by adequate nutritional and fluid intake.
4. Debride eschar, debris, and previously applied antimicrobials from the wound.	The wound can become a reservoir for infection if it is not kept clean.
5. Obtain wound cultures, as ordered, to document the bacteria present and to ascertain the development of any resistant strains.	Bacteria can become resistant to antibiotics; periodic wound cultures help to ensure the efficacy of antibiotic treatment.
6. Apply topical antimicrobials per physician's order. After removing all previously applied antimicrobial ointments, apply antimicrobial ointment at the depth recommended by the product manufacturer.	The time of action differs from one topical agent to another; correct timing and proper application of antimicrobials are necessary to ensure optimal effectiveness.
7. Recognize the indications for discontinuing airway intubation or nasogastric decompression and notify the physician as soon as possible.	The placement of tubes in the upper airway promotes aspiration of stomach contents into the lungs, which can lead to aspiration pneumonia and possible systemic sepsis.
8. Maintain elevation of the head of the bed at 15° to 30°.	Elevation of the patient's head decreases the incidence of aspiration of stomach contents into lungs.

Evaluation:

- Healing progresses without episodes of wound infection, pneumonia, or sepsis.
- Wound cultures exhibit minimal bacterial growth.

NURSING DIAGNOSIS

- Altered Nutrition: Less Than Body Requirements, related to hypermetabolism and the increased energy requirements of wound healing

Expected Outcomes:

- The child will maintain muscle mass and protein stores appropriate for age.
- Nitrogen balance and energy expenditure studies will consistently yield positive results.

Intervention	Rationale
1. Determine the child's daily nutrient requirements.	Caloric requirements are increased 2 to 3 times the normal basal requirements in a child with a major burn.
2. Provide high-caloric, high-protein feedings in small quantities throughout the day.	Children tolerate smaller, more frequent meals to meet daily requirements.
3. Encourage oral intake even if supplemented by tube feeding.	Infants can continue breastfeeding or bottle feedings supplemented by tube feedings.
4. Maintain a constant 24-hour infusion rate for tube feedings.	Diarrhea and cramping may occur if tube feedings are infused too rapidly or in large boluses.
5. Observe the child for gastrointestinal changes, such as diarrhea or constipation, and notify the physician.	Fluid overload, tube feeding excesses, bacterial infections, or oral antibiotics can cause diarrhea. Opioid pain medications, prolonged bedrest/immobility, or sepsis leading to paralytic ileus can cause constipation.

Intervention	Rationale
6. Arrange the timing of meals so that they do not immediately precede or follow painful or distressing events.	Vomiting occurs frequently when children cry excessively. In addition, severely injured children may use vomiting in an attempt to gain control over their environment.
7. Encourage the child's family to provide favorite, familiar foods.	Children tend to have limited food preferences. The availability of familiar or ethnic foods may be important in meeting the nutritional needs of individual children.
8. Arrange mealtimes so that they can be shared with family members or other patients. Turn off the television.	Mealtimes are social events, and should remain so during hospitalization, especially for a child.
9. Measure and record the child's weight on a weekly basis.	The child's ability to maintain or gain weight is an indicator of his/her nutritional status.
10. Measure and record the child's intake and output.	Objective evaluation of the child's intake and output helps determine the adequacy of nutritional intake.

Evaluation:

- The child maintains adequate nutrition as demonstrated by body weight, fluid and electrolyte balance, and restoration of serum protein levels.

NURSING DIAGNOSIS

- Body Image Disturbance related to appearance.

Expected Outcomes:

- The child will re-enter previous social settings and express a feeling of comfort in these areas.
- The family will provide emotional support for the child.
- The child will discuss feelings related to reactions of others to the child's change in appearance.

Intervention	Rationale
1. Encourage verbalization of feelings about appearance and about returning home and to school.	Identifies the child's concerns and anxieties and aids in working on coping strategies.
2. Provide honest answers to questions regarding appearance.	Builds trust and aids in developing realistic expectations.
3. Encourage family involvement in care.	Provides support for the child and decreases feelings of separation from significant others.
4. Encourage the child to provide for age-appropriate self-care.	Increases self-esteem.
5. Assess support systems and coping mechanisms used in previous times of stress or crisis.	Mobilizes previous strategies that were effective.
6. Engage the assistance of a child life specialist to work with the child to identify feelings about re-entry into home and school.	Children can often best express feelings through play and art.
7. Discuss ways in which the child can "cover up" disfigurement through clothing and make-up.	Provides a mechanism to decrease or minimize the disfigurement.

Intervention	Rationale
8. Visit the child's school prior to the child's return.	Prepares the child's classmates for the changes in the child's appearance and engages them in making the re-entry a positive experience through acceptance.

Evaluation:
- The child expresses a desire to return home and to school.
- The child expresses fears related to reactions of others to appearance.
- The family supports the child emotionally and encourages the child to express his feelings.

TEACHING GUIDELINES *for Home Care of the Child With Burns*

- Consult home health agency for nursing follow-up as ordered.
- Provide information regarding age-related risks for burn injuries and prevention actions.
- Provide instructions on nutritional needs, support, methods of increasing caloric and protein intake; if child still receiving tube feedings, instruct on procedures of tube feedings, checking residuals, recognizing and reporting complications.
- Provide instruction on importance of follow-up care with physician, physical therapy, consulting plastic surgeons.
- Assess parents understanding of growth and development and encourage of activities that best promote normal growth and development.
- Provide family with information concerning support groups for victims of burns and their families.
- Provide instruction on administration of medications as prescribed by physician.
- Provide instruction on signs/symptoms that should be reported to physician, home health nurse, clinic.
- Provide list of phone numbers for contacting physician, home health nurse, clinic.

KEY CONCEPTS

- Children are at increased risk for burn injuries because of their curiosity and their dependence upon their caretakers.
- The extent of a burn injury (depth and severity) determines whether there is a local or systemic reaction.
- The depth of a burn injury is classified as superficial (first degree), partial thickness (second degree), and full thickness (third degree).
- Pediatric differences in burn injuries include an increased risk for fluid and heat loss, hypertrophic scarring, cardiovascular problems, infection, and protein and caloric deficiency.
- When calculating the extent of TBSA burned, a body surface chart that is corrected for age should be used.
- A minor burn wound should be cleansed with mild soap and water, debrided of loose debris and tissue, and covered with an antimicrobial ointment and a sterile dressing.
- Complications associated with a major burn injury include respiratory compromise, burn shock, fluid and electrolyte imbalance, metabolic alterations, infection, and sepsis.
- Hydrotherapy is used to cleanse the wound as well as the patient. It can also be an ideal time for performing range-of-motion exercises.
- Wound debridement promotes healing and prevents infection.
- Morphine, administered IV, is the drug of choice for pain management in children with severe burn pain.
- The immediate focus of nursing care in a child with a minor or moderately severe burn wound is on wound care and pain management.
- The immediate focus of nursing care in a child with a major burn is on establishing and maintaining airway, breathing, and circulation.
- A child with a burn injury should always receive pain medication prior to hydrotherapy and wound debridement.
- Aseptic technique is used during dressing changes to prevent infection.
- The burned child requires a high-protein and high-calorie diet. Frequent, small meals and snacks of favorite foods should be offered.
- There may be long-term psychosocial effects associated with a burn injury. The child and family should receive psychological support.

REFERENCES

Carrougher, G. J. (1993). Inhalation injury. *AACN Clinical Issues in Critical Care Nursing, 4,* 367–377.

Finkelstein, J., Schwartz, S., Madden, M., Marano, M., & Goodwin, C. (1992). Pediatric burns. *Pediatric Clinics of North America, 39*(5), 1145–1163.

Helvig, E. (1993). Pediatric burn injuries. *AACN Clinical Issues in Critical Care Nursing, 4,* 433–442.

Herrin, J. T., & Antoon, A. Y. (1996). Burn injuries. In R. Behrman, R. Kliegman, & A. Arvin (Eds.), *Nelson textbook of pediatrics* (15th ed., pp. 270–277). Philadelphia: W. B. Saunders.

Kravitz, M. (1988). Thermal injuries. In *Trauma nursing: From resuscitation through rehabilitation* (pp. 707–745). Philadelphia: W. B. Saunders.

Kravitz, M. (1993). Immune consequences of burn injury. *AACN Clinical Issues in Critical Care Nursing, 4,* 399–413.

Maley, M. P., & Achauer, B. M. (1987). Prevention of tap water scald burns. *Journal of Burn Care & Rehabilitation, 8,* 62.

Miller, S., Richard, R., & Staley, M. (1994). Triage and resuscitation of the burn patient. In R. Richard & M. Staley (Eds.), *Burn care and rehabilitation: Principles and practice* (pp. 105–118). Philadelphia: F. A. Davis.

Molter, N. (1993). When is burn injury healed? Psychosocial implications of care. *AACN Clinical Issues in Critical Care Nursing, 4,* 424–432.

Powell, P. A. (1986). Learn Not to Burn Foundation. *Fire Journal, 80,* 12–16.

Reeves, S., Warden, G., & Staley, M. (1994). Management of the pediatric burn patient. In R. Richard & M. Staley (Eds.), *Burn care and rehabilitation: Principles and practice* (pp. 499–530). Philadelphia: F. A. Davis.

Saffle, J., & Schnebly, W. A. (1994). Burn wound care. In R. Richard & M. Staley (Eds.), *Burn care and rehabilitation: Principles and practice* (pp. 119–176). Philadelphia: F. A. Davis.

Schumann, L. L. (1991). Care of the patient with major burns. In R. B. Trofino (Ed.), *Nursing care of the burn injured patient* (pp. 135–181). Philadelphia: F. A. Davis.

Weber, J. M., & Tompkins, D. M. (1993). Improving survival: Infection control and burns. *AACN Clinical Issues in Critical Care Nursing, 4,* 414–423.

Zuker, R. M. (1988). Initial management of the burn wound. In H. Carvajal & D. Parks (Eds.), *Burns in children: Pediatric burn management* (pp. 99–105). Chicago: Year Book Medical Publishers.

BIBLIOGRAPHY

Abdullah, A., Blakeny, P., Hunt, R., Broemeling, L., Phillips, L., Herndon, D., Robson, M. (1994). Visible scars and self-esteem in pediatric patients with burns. *Journal of Burn Care and Rehabilitation, 15*(2),164–168.

Beard, S., Herndon, D., & Desai, M. (1989). Adaptation of self-image in burn-disfigured children. *Journal of Burn Care and Rehabilitation, 10,* 550–554.

Cioffi, W. G., & Rue, L. W. (1991). Diagnosis and treatment of inhalation injury. *Critical Care Clinics of North America, 3,* 191–198.

East, M. K., Jones, C. A., Feller, I., Saxon, M. I., & Wolfe, R. (1988). Epidemiology of burns in children. In H. F. Carvajal, D. H. Parks (Eds.), *Burns in children: Pediatric burn management* (pp. 3–10). Chicago: Year Book Publishers.

Engelhardt, V., & Clark, S. (1994). Early enteral feeding of a severely burned pediatric patient. *Journal of Burn Care and Rehabilitation, 15*(3), 293–297.

Faldmo, L., & Kravitz, M. (1993). Management of acute burns and burn shock resuscitation. *AACN Clinical Issues in Critical Care Nursing, 4,* 351–366.

Fallat, M. E., & Rengers, S. J. (1993). The effect of education and safety devices on scald burn prevention. *The Journal of Trauma, 34*(4), 560–563.

Hendricks, W. M. (1990). The classification of burns. *Journal of the American Academy of Dermatology, xx,* 838–839.

Herndon, D., Rutan, R., & Rutan, T. (1993). Management of the pediatric patient with burns. *Journal of Burn Care and Rehabilitation, 14*(1), 3–8.

Konop, D. J. General local treatment. In R. B. Trofino (Ed.), *Nursing care of the burn injured patient* (pp. 42–67). Philadelphia: F. A. Davis.

Kravitz, M. (Ed.) (1993). Burn care. *AACN Clinical Issues in Critical Care Nursing, 4,* 349–442.

Lund, C. C., Browder, N. C. (1944). Estimation of burn size. *Surgery, Gynecology, and Obstetrics, 79,* 352–358.

Martin, M. T., Seligman, R. (1991). Psychosocial care of the burn patient and significant others. In R. B. Trofino (Ed.), *Nursing care of the burn injured patient* (pp. 87–119). Philadelphia: F. A. Davis.

Martinez, S. (1992). Ambulatory management of burns in children. *Journal of Pediatric Health Care, 6*(1), 32–37.

Mayes, T., Gottschlich, M., Khoury, J., & Warden, G. (1996). Evaluation of predicted and measured energy requirements in burned children. *Journal of the American Dietetic Association, 96*(1), 24–29.

Meyer, W., Blakeney, P., Moore, P., Murphy, L., Robson, M., & Herndon, D. (1994). Parental well-being and behavioral adjustment of pediatric survivors of burns. *Journal of Burn Care and Rehabilitation, 15*(1), 62–68.

Nebraska Burn Institute. (1992). *Advanced burn life support course instructor's manual.* Lincoln, NE: Author.

Pollock, D., McGee, D., & Rodriguez, J. (1988). Deaths due to injury in the home among persons under 15 years of age, 1970–1984. Centers for Disease Control, CDC Surveillance Summaries. *MMWR, 37* (SS-1), 14.

Reynolds, E. M., Ryan, D. P., & Doody, D. P. (1993). Mortality and respiratory failure in a pediatric burn population. *Journal of Pediatric Surgery, 28*(10), 1326–1331.

Rieg, L. S. (1993). Metabolic alterations and nutritional management. *AACN Clinical Issues in Critical Care Nursing, 4,* 388–398.

Sampson, L. J. (1990). The development of a discharge planning index for use in a pediatric acute burn unit. *Journal of Burn Care and Rehabilitation, 11,* 365–371.

Showers, J., & Garrison, K. M. (1988). Burn abuse: A four-year study. *Journal of Trauma, 28,* 1581–1583.

Trofino, R. (1991). *Nursing care of the burn-injured patient.* Philadelphia: F. A. Davis.

Uitvlugt, N., & Ledbetter, D. (1995). Treatment of pediatric burns. In R. Arensman (Ed.), *Pediatric trauma* (pp. 173–199). New York: Raven Press.

36

The Child With Musculoskeletal Alterations

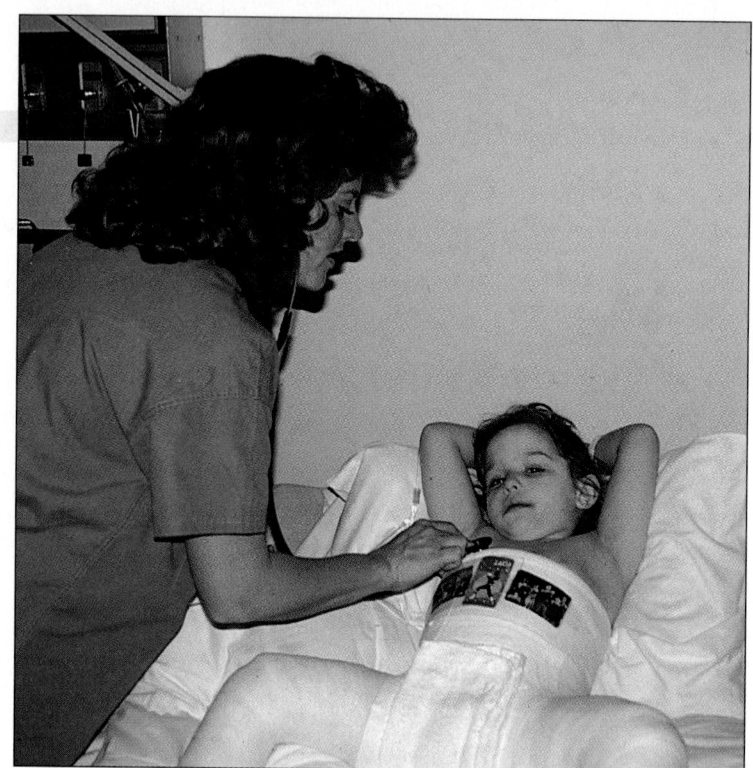

CHAPTER OVERVIEW

LEARNING OBJECTIVES

After studying this chapter, you should be able to:

- Demonstrate an understanding of the anatomy and physiology of the musculoskeletal system of the infant and young child.
- Describe the pathology, etiology, clinical manifestations, diagnostic evaluation, and therapeutic management of common pediatric musculoskeletal alterations.
- Select relevant assessment criteria that will be helpful in determining the etiology of common pediatric musculoskeletal alterations.
- State appropriate nursing diagnoses for alterations in musculoskeletal function.
- Identify characteristic behaviors that indicate alterations in musculoskeletal functioning.
- List significant diagnostic criteria used in diagnosing common pediatric musculoskeletal alterations.
- Summarize by treatment modalities the therapeutic management used to treat pediatric musculoskeletal alterations.
- Discuss teaching strategies associated with alterations in musculoskeletal function.
- Design and implement appropriate nursing interventions for the pediatric patient with altered musculoskeletal functioning.
- Evaluate and modify nursing interventions based on appropriate outcome criteria.
- Describe the pathophysiology, incidence, clinical manifestations, and nursing care of muscular dystrophy.

KEY TERMS

ankylosis: condition in which a joint is stiff or difficult to move

crepitus: a grating sensation at a fracture site that occurs when the ends of a broken bone move

ossification: formation of bone

osteoblastic: activity by osteoblasts that promotes bone formation

osteochondrosis: disorders of the epiphyses in which there is an interruption in the blood supply

osteoclastic: activity by osteoclasts that absorbs and removes old bony tissue

paresthesia: sensation of numbness and tingling

reduction: the repositioning of bone fragments into normal alignment

retention: the application of a device or mechanism that will maintain alignment of bone until healing occurs

This chapter is designed to prepare the nurse to care for children with commonly encountered musculoskeletal problems. Many of these problems occur because of vigorous motor activities that are part of a child's daily life, but the rapid growth of the skeletal system plays a significant role as well. Musculoskeletal problems involve muscles, bones, joints, and tendons, all of which are necessary for movement. Movement is critical to a child's development because it provides a forum in which the child can communicate and interact with the world. It even provides an outlet for anxiety.

Musculoskeletal disorders affect a child's ability to move and consequently have the potential to influence the successful resolution of various developmental stages. The majority of problems are short term, but there are a number of chronic musculoskeletal problems that require long-term treatment and nursing assistance in helping the child and family learn how to cope with the chronicity of the disorder.

This chapter discusses the structure and function of the musculoskeletal system, including developmental differences. Musculoskeletal disorders discussed include fractures, soft tissue injuries, infections of the bone, growth-related musculoskeletal disorders, and the more common joint and muscle diseases that affect children. Emphasis is placed on the child's adjustment to the stresses and demands of the disorders and the nurse's role in assisting the child and family to achieve their maximum level of functioning.

CLINICAL REFERENCE PAGES

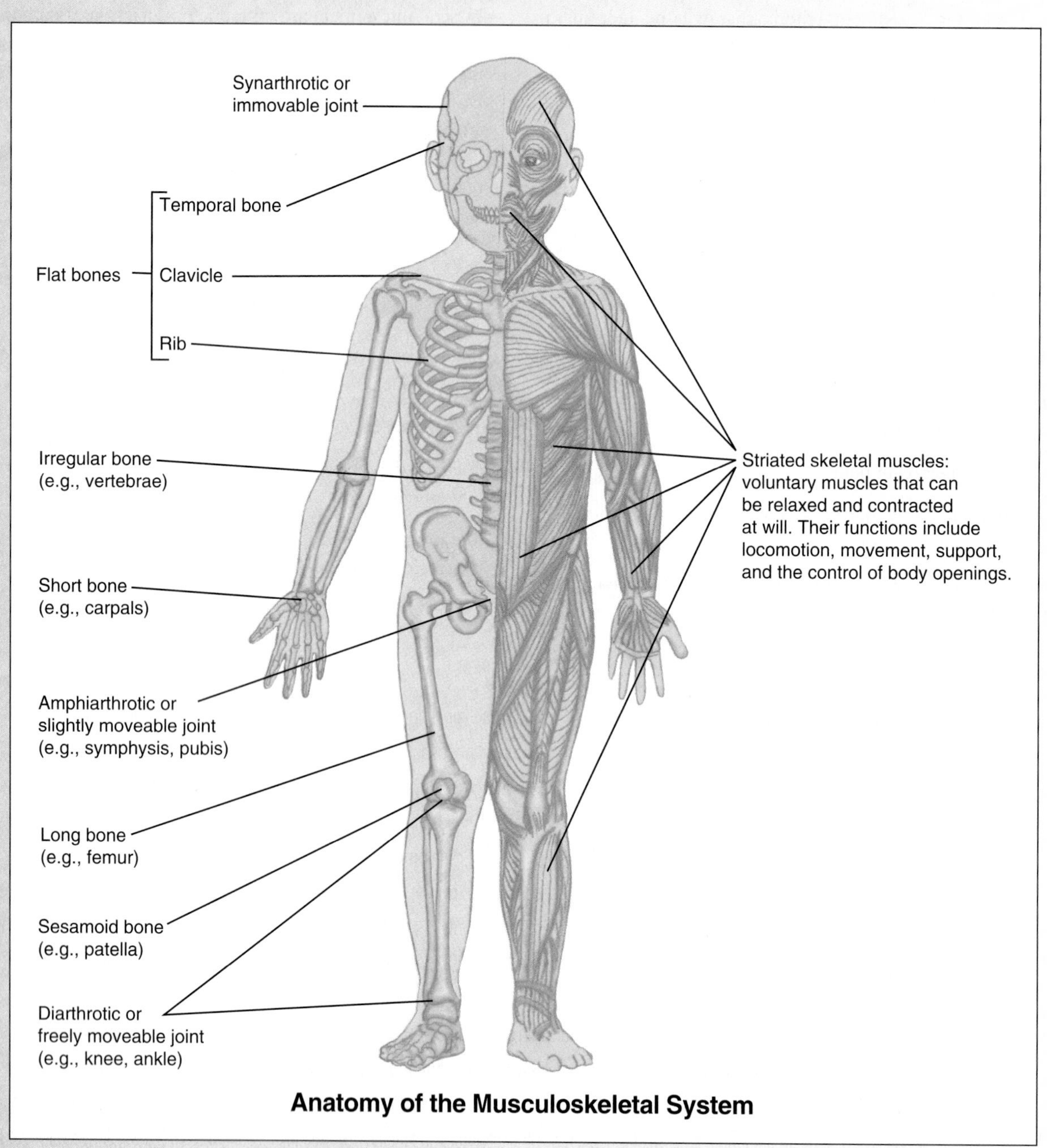

Anatomy of the Musculoskeletal System

Pediatric Differences in the Musculoskeletal System

- Muscle tissue is almost completely developed at birth. Growth occurs because of an increase in size, rather than number, of the muscle fibers.
- In the fetus, bony tissue begins to develop as closely packed connective tissue. Connective tissue is replaced by cartilage, and cartilage is replaced by mineral salts, which give rise to solid bone. The infant's bones are neither as firm nor as brittle as those of the older child. An infant's bones are only 65% ossified at eight months of age.
- New bony tissue is produced during periods of growth. The rate of growth varies at different ages. Skeletal growth is stimulated by pituitary growth hormone. Growth of long bones occurs at the epiphyses, which are located at the ends of the bones and separated from the main portion of the bone by cartilage during the period of growth. Injury at the epiphyses can cause growth disturbances.
- Growing bones produce callus and heal quickly, making internal fixation of fractures unnecessary in most children. Fractures in children younger than age 1 year are unusual because a large amount of force is necessary; abuse or underlying pathophysiology is often the cause of fractures in infants.
- The skull is not rigid during infancy, and the sutures of the cranium do not fuse until approximately 16 to 18 months of age. Increased intracranial pressure can separate the sutures, causing the infant's head to enlarge.
- Postural changes during infancy and childhood result from development of neurologic control, bone and muscle growth, and laying down of adipose tissue. Postural changes are a good indication of the level of development of the musculoskeletal and neurologic systems.
- Because soft tissues are resilient in children, dislocations and sprains are less common than in adults.

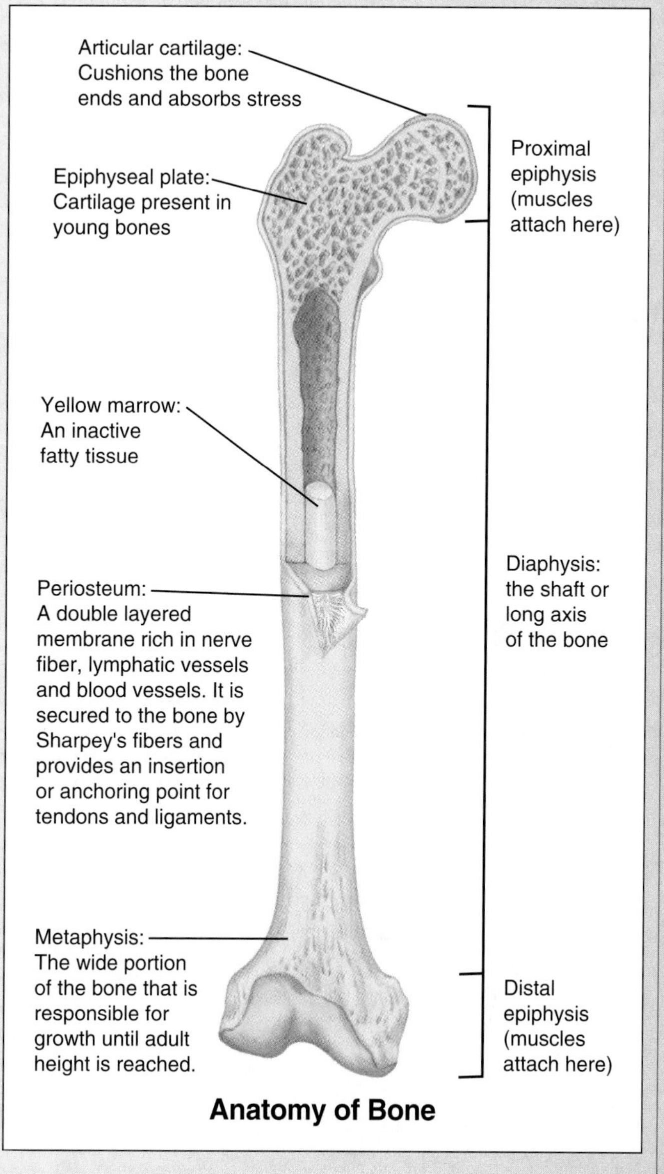
Articular cartilage: Cushions the bone ends and absorbs stress
Epiphyseal plate: Cartilage present in young bones
Yellow marrow: An inactive fatty tissue
Periosteum: A double layered membrane rich in nerve fiber, lymphatic vessels and blood vessels. It is secured to the bone by Sharpey's fibers and provides an insertion or anchoring point for tendons and ligaments.
Metaphysis: The wide portion of the bone that is responsible for growth until adult height is reached.
Proximal epiphysis (muscles attach here)
Diaphysis: the shaft or long axis of the bone
Distal epiphysis (muscles attach here)

Anatomy of Bone

REVIEW OF THE MUSCULOSKELETAL SYSTEM

The musculoskeletal system is composed of bones, joints, muscles, and cartilaginous tissue. To understand alterations in musculoskeletal function, it is necessary first to understand normal musculoskeletal structure and function, as well as growth and development patterns (see Pediatric Differences box).

Skeletal System. The skeleton furnishes surfaces for the attachment of muscles, tendons, and ligaments, which pull on individual bones. These actions make it possible for us to move about. The skeletal system consists of 206 bones, which are classified as long bones (e.g., humerus, radius), short bones (e.g., carpals, tarsals), flat bones (e.g., ribs), irregular bones (e.g., vertebrae), and sesamoid bones (e.g., kneecap).

Each long bone consists of a diaphysis (shaft) and an epiphysis (secondary ossification center) at each end. The muscles attach here and are responsible for joint stability. The metaphysis—the wide portion of the bone—is responsible for growth. The metaphysis consists of cartilage and actively produces bone. Periosteum, a vascular connective tissue, covers the bone. The medullary cavity is located in the center of the diaphysis.

COMMON DIAGNOSTIC AND LABORATORY TESTS AND PROCEDURES FOR MUSCULOSKELETAL DISORDERS IN CHILDREN

TEST	PURPOSE/DESCRIPTION	NURSING IMPLICATIONS
X-ray Films (Roentgenograms)	For detection of abnormalities or to determine bone age. X-rays (gamma radiation) pass through the body, reach the film on the other side of the body, and turn the film black. Areas filled with air appear dark on the film. Different densities of tissue absorb various amounts of radiation. The four densities of X-ray are: air: blackish fat: dark gray water: lighter gray bone: whitish	Food and fluids are not restricted. Clothing and jewelry should be removed, a paper or cloth gown is worn. Young children may require immobilization. Adequate preparation is essential to ensure cooperation.
Arthrography	To evaluate suspected joint damage such as tears of cartilage. Dye is injected into the joint, usually the knee, sometimes the shoulder or other joint.	Performed under local anesthesia. Check for allergies to iodine. May have mild to moderate discomfort after the procedure. Joint should rest for about 12 hours; compression dressing after procedure to reduce swelling.
Bone Scan	To detect tumors, infection, inflammation. Radioactive material given IV. In 2–4 hr the entire body is scanned, front and back.	Young children require sedation. Push fluids 2–4 hr before the test to ensure the client is well hydrated and to quickly eliminate radioactive material not absorbed by the bones. Child must void before scan to visualize pelvic bones.
Computed Tomography Scan	To visualize anatomic details. Narrow beam X-ray scans an area in successive layers. A computer processes readings and converts them to a picture shown on a screen, which is stored on disks. A three-dimensional cross section of body parts is shown.	Although procedure is painless, it may be frightening. Child must remain still during procedure, so young children require sedation. May or may not use contrast medium.
Magnetic Resonance Imaging (MRI)	Clearly defines organ structures, detects changes in tissue such as edema, blood flow patterns, or infarcts. Visualizes marrow, bone and soft tissue tumors, structure of muscles, ligaments, and bones. Huge magnet and radio waves create an energy field that can be transferred to a visual image. Child is placed on a moving stretcher which is pushed into the large cylinder that contains the magnet. A variety of noises will be heard during the procedure.	Food and fluids not restricted. Not used in patients with metal implants, pacemakers, or prostheses. Procedure may take an hour or more, so young children require sedation. Child should void before procedure. Adequate preparation, relaxation techniques, and parental presence decrease fear and feelings of claustrophobia.

Articular System. The joints provide for great freedom of movement, connecting bones to one another. The joints are composed of connective tissue and cartilage. They are classified by their degree of movement: synarthrosis or immovable (e.g., the skull), amphiarthrosis or slightly movable (e.g., the symphysis), and diarthrosis or freely movable (e.g., the knee). Muscles help stabilize joints and maintain contact between articular surfaces. The shape of the two ends of each bone and of the joint determine the extent of movement or articulation. Ligaments bind one bone firmly to another, and the joints are further strengthened by the overlying tendons and muscles.

Muscular System. Muscle, which is composed of elongated fibers, produces movement by contraction. There are three types of muscle: smooth muscle, found primarily in the internal organs; striated muscle or skeletal muscle, so called because of its striped appearance (seen under the microscope); and cardiac muscle, the heart muscle.

Cartilage. Cartilage is dense connective tissue that develops at the physis. Cartilage is capable of withstanding considerable tension. The skeleton of an embryo is mostly cartilage. In time it will largely convert to bone by **ossification.** Bone is necessary for longitudinal growth. Growth in the length of the long bones continues at the physis until adult height is reached. The epiphyseal plate absorbs shock, protecting the joint surfaces from serious fractures.

COMMON DIAGNOSTIC AND LABORATORY TESTS AND PROCEDURES FOR MUSCULOSKELETAL DISORDERS *(continued)*

TEST	PURPOSE/DESCRIPTION	NURSING IMPLICATIONS
Arthroscopy	To visualize the inside of a joint for diagnosis of injury and/or minor surgical repairs. Normally, arthrography is performed before arthroscopy. Fiberoptic endoscope is inserted to examine interior of joint.	Requires local or general anesthesia. NPO for 8 hr before test if general anesthesia. No restriction if local. Prepare patient for postoperative dressings, altered mobility, pain. Assess for infection. Prophylactic antibiotics may be ordered. Use ice bags postoperatively to reduce swelling.
Joint Aspiration	Fluid is withdrawn for analysis, usually for detection of infection or for relief of pain.	Local anesthesia. Prepare patient for some discomfort during and after procedure.
Ultrasound	To visualize body tissue structure or wave-form analysis of Doppler studies. Doppler probe is held over the skin surface or in a body cavity to produce an ultrasound beam in the tissues. Reflected echoes from the tissues are transformed by computer into visual image or audible sounds (Doppler).	Noninvasive; food and fluid are not restricted, except for small infants who may be NPO for 2–3 hr before the procedure so they can eat during the test.
Alkaline Phosphatase (ALP)	Enzyme found mainly in liver, bone, placenta, kidney. Elevated in bone disease, fractures, trauma, liver disease; may also be elevated during periods of rapid growth. Determinations may be ordered to differentiate between bone and liver problems.	2–10 yr: 100–320 U/L 11–18 yr: 100–390 U/L Nonfasting
Creatine Kinase (CK)	Enzyme found in heart and skeletal muscle; specific test for cardiac and muscle damage. Elevated in trauma, myocardial infarction, muscular dystrophy. Determinations may be ordered to differentiate between cardiac (MB) and skeletal (MM).	Male: 0–175 U/L Female: 10–55 U/L Nonfasting
Rheumatoid Factor (RA)	Macroglobulin antibody. May be responsible for destructive changes associated with RA. Positive RA factor supports possible diagnosis of JA.	< 20 IU/ml nonfasting
C-reactive Protein (CRP)	Appears in blood due to inflammatory process. Not seen in healthy people. Nonspecific, merely indicates presence of inflammation.	Negative nonfasting
Erythrocyte Sedimentation Rate (ESR)	Rate at which erythrocytes settle out of unclotted blood. Inflammation and necrotic problems cause an elevation.	Child 4–20 mm/hr, nonfasting

FRACTURES

Fractures, while not always considered a serious disorder, are important because they may lead to life-threatening complications. A fracture occurs when there is a break or disruption in the continuity of the bone. Generally, fractures occur when excessive or traumatic force exceeds the strength of the bone.

Etiology. Fractures in children usually result from increased mobility and inadequate or immature motor and cognitive skills. Fractures in children may result from trauma (falls, motor vehicle accidents, sports injuries, child abuse) or bone diseases that result in abnormally fragile bones (osteogenesis imperfecta).

An understanding of growth and development is helpful when assessing trauma in specific age-groups. For example, fractures in infancy are generally rare and, if they occur, are normally the result of trauma during birth or nonaccidental trauma. Therefore, fractures in infants warrant further investigation to rule out the possibility of child abuse.

Trauma is the leading cause of death in children of all ages (McCarthy & Surpure, 1990) (see Chapter 13). Trauma, probably the most ominous threat to children today, is a frequent cause of fractures. In fact, traffic-related injuries and falls are the leading causes of injuries and death among children (Allshouse, Rouse, & Eichelberger, 1993; Schaefermeyer, 1993). Children between ages 5 and 9 are most likely to experience fractures related to motor vehicle accidents. This is due in part to increased mobility as well as immature cognitive development. Fractures of the hip and femur would be seen with this type of injury. The child hit by an automobile often presents with Waddell's triad (see Fig. 14–3) (Rosenberg, Vranesich, & Bottenfield, 1982). This includes a fractured femur from contact with the car bumper, thoracic trauma from contact with the hood of the car, and a head injury from the subsequent fall.

Falls are a frequent occurrence in childhood. It is not surprising to find that the most frequently seen fracture in children is in the forearm (Mann & Raymaira, 1990). When a child begins to fall, he will attempt to cushion the fall by an outstretched arm, which in turn receives the full force of the fall (Fig. 36–2). This type of fall carries the potential of affecting every part of that outstretched arm (wrist, elbow, shoulder). Playground injuries are chiefly upper extremity fractures that result from falls on the arms (MacEwen, Kasser, & Heinrich, 1993).

PATHOPHYSIOLOGY *of Fractures*

When a fracture occurs, the break in the continuity of the bone results in fragments of bone and injury to the surrounding tissues. Torn blood vessels cause bleeding from the bone and tissues around the bone fragments. As blood clots at the site, fibrin strands provide a network for healing. Osteoblasts begin forming in immense numbers almost immediately after the injury. This increased **osteoblastic** activity results in formation of new bone matrix between the bone fragments. Calcium salts are deposited in the new bone matrix, forming a *callus.* The callus is responsible for stability and support of the fracture while healing occurs. Gradually the callus is formed into new bone. Remodeling, correction of an injury at the fracture site through the buildup of callus, occurs more rapidly in growing children.

Fractures are referred to as *simple* or *compound.* A fracture that is simple, or closed, is characterized as intact with no breaks in the skin. If there are wounds accompanying a simple fracture, they are usually superficial or unrelated to the fracture. The nurse should never assume that a simple fracture does not warrant close assessment. It is quite possible that other problems associated with the injury exist. For example, if hemorrhage occurs, it would be internal.

Fractures in which the skin, subcutaneous tissue, or muscle has been broken are called *compound,* or *open,* fractures. Infection is a risk with this type of fracture because organisms are able to enter the fracture site through the wound. Children with compound fractures are at risk for blood loss secondary to external hemorrhage.

Epiphyseal injuries occur when a break or fracture occurs between the shaft of the bone and the epiphyseal plate. In a growing bone, the region of least resistance to stress is the area between the metaphysis and the cartilaginous epiphyseal plate. An epiphyseal fracture is serious because it can interrupt and alter growth (Staheli, 1992). The amount of arrested growth is determined by the extent of the damage to the epiphyseal plate. If the germinal cells remain with the epiphysis and appear uninjured, healing is rapid and growth seldom affected. However, if the germinal layer is destroyed, growth disturbances will occur. The Salter-Harris classification system (Fig. 36–1) classifies epiphyseal growth plate injuries and their risk of growth disturbance.

Figure 36–1 illustrates fractures commonly seen in children, including the Salter-Harris classification of epiphyseal growth plate injuries.

Pediatric fractures are seldom complete breaks. Rather, children's bones tend to bend or buckle because of increased flexibility. This flexibility is due to a thicker periosteum and increased amounts of immature bone.

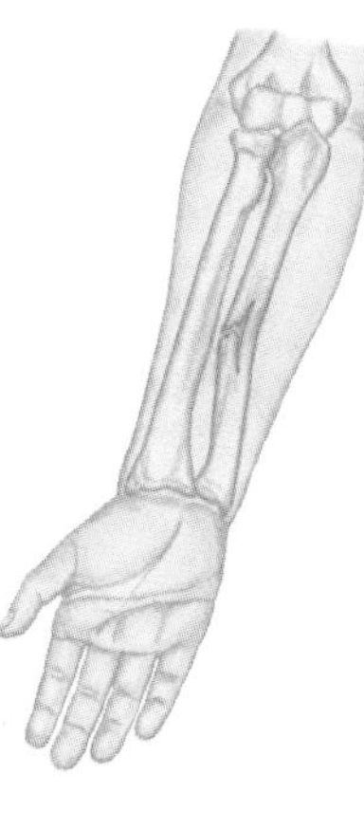
Greenstick
Break occurs through the periosteum on one side of the bone while only bowing or buckling on the other side. Seen most frequently in forearm.

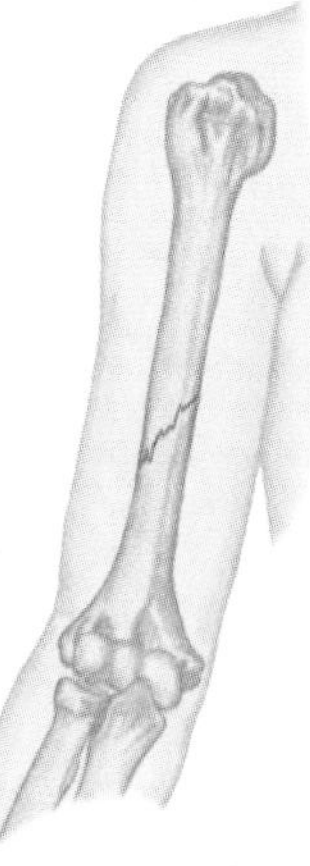
Spiral
Twisted or circular break that affects the length rather than the width. Seen frequently in child abuse.

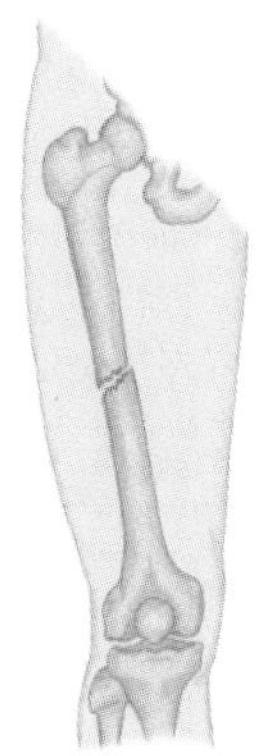
Oblique
Diagonal or slanting break that occurs between the horizontal and perpendicular planes of the bone.

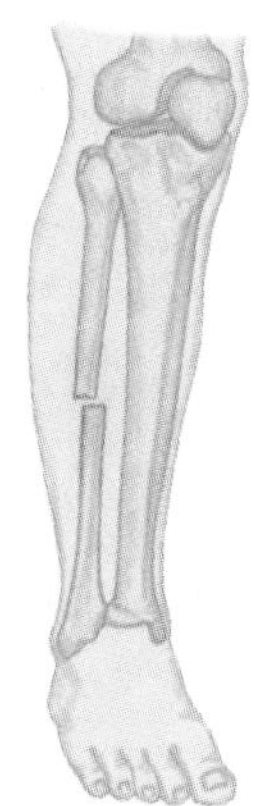
Transverse
Break or fracture line occurs at right angles to the long axis of the bone.

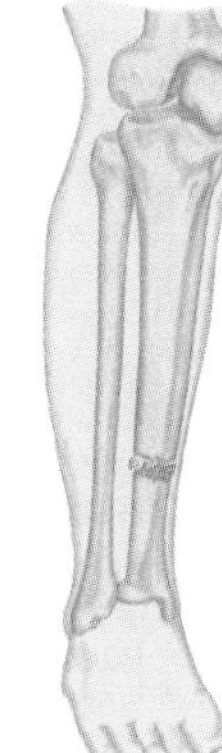
Comminuted
Bone is splintered into pieces. This is a rare occurrence in children.

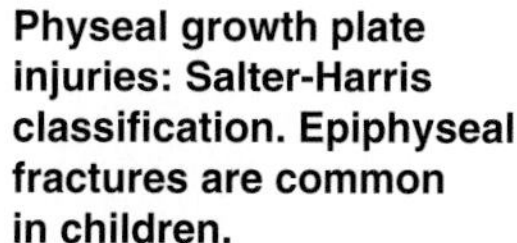
Physeal growth plate injuries: Salter-Harris classification. Epiphyseal fractures are common in children.

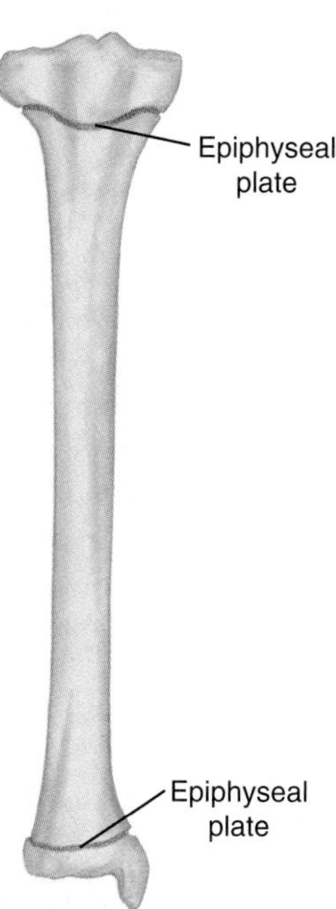
Epiphyseal plate
Epiphyseal plate

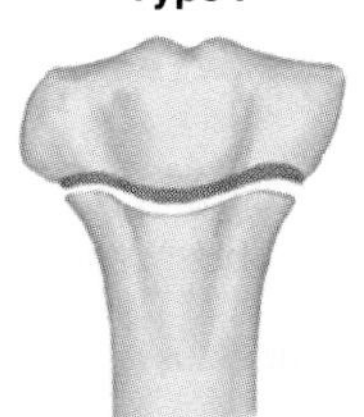
Type I
Epiphysis is completely separated from the metaphysis without fracture

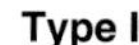
Type II

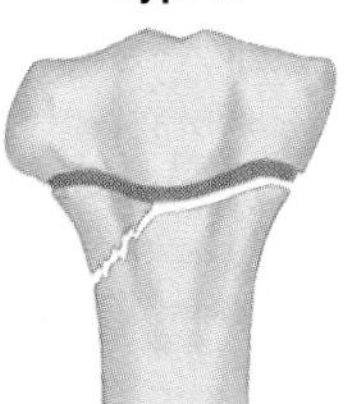
Transverse fracture extends through the separated epiphyseal plate producing triangular break

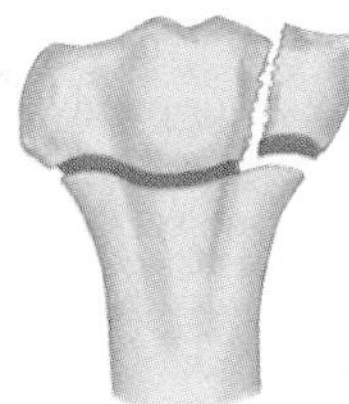
Type III
Fracture extends through part of the epiphyseal plate into the joint

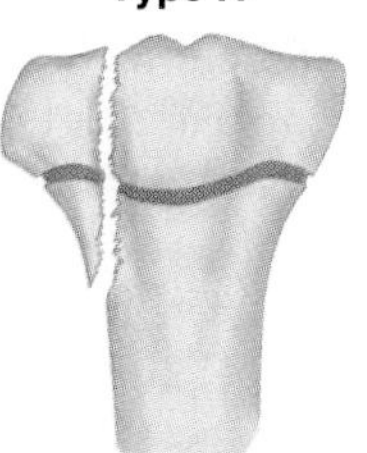
Type IV
Fracture extends through the epiphyseal plate and through the metaphysis

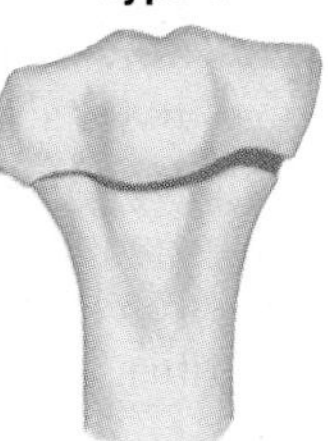
Type V
Epiphyseal plate is crushed, causing cell death in growth plate

Figure 36–1
Fractures commonly seen in children.

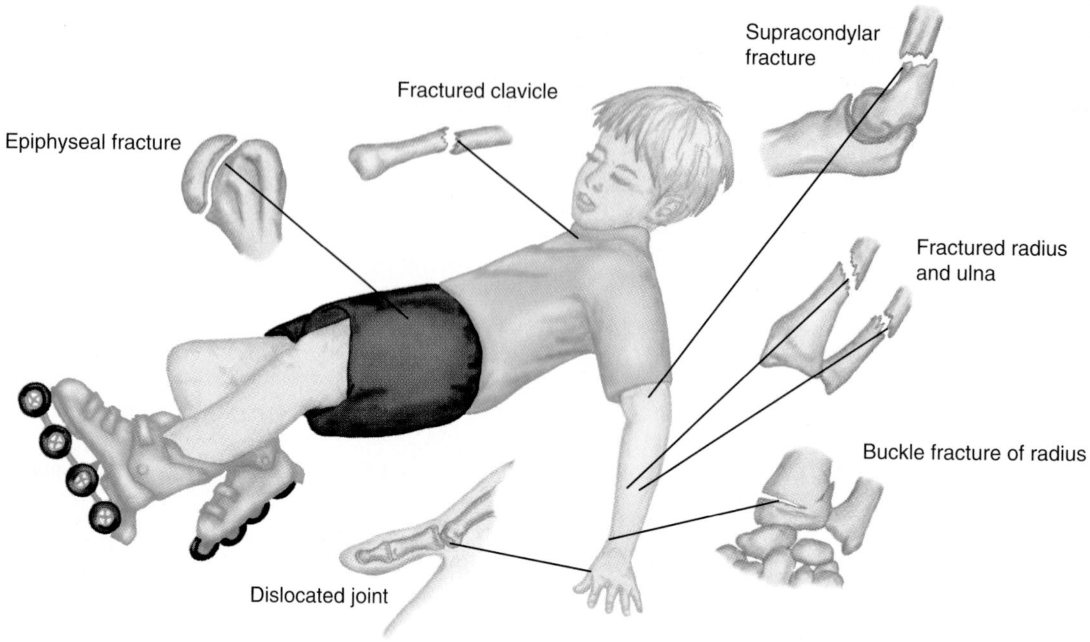

Figure 36–2

Upper extremity fracture in children often occurs when the child attempts to break a fall with an outstretched arm.

The upper arm is also a common site for fractures. A fractured clavicle may occur at any age. Lack of movement or a "pseudoparalysis" of the upper arm may be the only symptom in an infant. An older child will complain of pain (Staheli, 1992). A supracondylar humeral fracture is a serious injury because it may lead to circulatory impairment, cellular necrosis, and ischemic contracture (Volkmann's contracture).

Regardless of the cause of the fracture, it is important to remember that a child with an uncomplicated fracture should not present with signs of shock. If this occurs, more than likely there is a more serious problem and a thorough assessment should be conducted.

Incidence. Since the daily actions of children include numerous gross motor activities that place them at risk for injuries, fractures are a commonplace occurrence throughout childhood and adolescence.

The most common sites of fractures in children are the ulna, clavicle, tibia, and femur (Fig. 36–2). Epiphyseal fractures are also common in children (see Fig. 36–1).

Clinical Manifestations. Signs and symptoms of a fracture vary with location, type, and cause of the injury. General manifestations include:

- Pain or tenderness at the site
- Immobility or decreased range of motion
- Deformity of the extremity
- **Crepitus**
- Ecchymosis/erythema
- Edema
- Muscle spasm
- Inability to bear weight

Diagnostic Evaluation. Local signs and symptoms of a fracture are not always present, and assessment of a fracture can be difficult. Skeletal examination via radiography is the most effective tool for determining the type and location of a fracture. Often an X-ray of the unaffected extremity is taken for comparison purposes, especially when trying to determine if a line on the X-ray is a fracture or merely an epiphyseal line. Because the periosteum of children's bones is thicker and stronger, it is less likely to displace at the fracture site. Consequently, the fracture may not be visible on X-ray until healing begins. X-rays are also taken after reduction of the fracture and often during the healing process to assess progress.

Therapeutic Management of Fractures

The key to healing is the correct **reduction** and **retention** of the fracture. Reduction is the repositioning of the bone fragments into normal alignment. Retention is the application of a device or mechanism that will maintain alignment until healing occurs.

Reduction Methods

Fractures are treated by either closed or open reduction. Closed reduction is accomplished by manual alignment of the fragments followed by immobilization. Simple or closed fractures are treated by closed reduction. Hospitalization is seldom required for closed reduction, and the majority of these fractures heal without complications.

Open reduction requires the surgical insertion of internal fixation devices such as rods, wires, or pins that help maintain alignment while healing occurs. External fixation devices may also be used not only to stabilize fractures, but also to lengthen bones and correct angular deformities that involve bone and soft tissue. External fixators allow for periodic changes in alignment and length of the bone. In fact, external fixation devices are becoming so common in the treatment of fractures that the use of traction is not frequently seen. The Ilizarov external fixator is an external device frequently used in the treatment of fractures (Carlino, 1991).

When open reduction is employed, hospitalization is required and the child should be monitored for postoperative complications. Complications after open reduction include delayed healing and nonunion. Infections may also interfere with recovery. Close assessment by the health care team as well as strict adherence to sterile technique during dressing changes can decrease the risk of postoperative problems and promote healing.

Retention: Casting and Traction

Once correct alignment of the fracture is achieved, it is imperative to protect the fracture site as well as maintain position of the fragments. This is accomplished through the application of a cast or, in certain situations, traction, which effectively immobilizes the area while healing occurs.

Casts. A cast provides support and controls position while the fracture heals. Casts may also be used to correct deformities and to ensure compliance with treatment protocols. Materials most frequently used for casting are plaster of paris or synthetic material such as fiberglass. Plaster of paris is a heavier material that molds easily to the extremity and is less expensive than synthetic casts. It also takes approximately 24 hours to dry. Drying time could be longer depending on the size of the cast. Plaster of paris is not water resistant; when wet, a plaster of paris cast will begin to disintegrate.

Synthetic casts are more expensive but they tend to dry more quickly, are lighter, and are water resistant. If the synthetic cast becomes wet, parents need to be reminded to check the skin under the cast. Inadequate airflow prevents thorough drying of the skin, and damp skin is more susceptible to skin breakdown. Also synthetic casts do not mold well to the body and are not recommended for young children or those with serious fractures.

Most casts are applied on an outpatient basis and hospitalization is not required. The size of the cast is determined by the type of fracture and the amount of weight-bearing the extremity can tolerate. Short or long leg or arm casts are generally used for fractures of the upper and lower limbs. Fractures of the hip and knee require a body or spica cast (see Chapter 37, Caring for a Child in a Spica Cast, pp. 1154–1157).

Traction. Effective immobilization of a fracture may also be achieved through the use of traction. Traction is defined as a pull or force exerted on one part of the body and may be applied to the spine, pelvis, or long bones of the upper and lower extremities. The angle formed by the placement of the pulley on the bed frame and the angle of the involved joint determines the direction of the pull or force.

Once the direction of the pull or force has been determined, it is important to direct the traction along the long axis of the bone. Traction can be applied to the skin or the bone. Some traction, such as halo-femoral traction used for spinal problems, exerts a force without the use of weights.

An opposing pull or force must be provided at the same time if the traction is to be effective. This is called countertraction. The result is a two-way pull that maintains alignment of the affected extremity. The child's weight is usually sufficient to provide the countertraction. If body weight is not sufficient, additional weights may be used. Depending on the age of the child, restraining devices may be needed to maintain countertraction.

To assist with countertraction, the part of the bed that holds the traction apparatus is tilted or elevated. For example, if the leg was being placed in traction, the foot of the bed would be elevated. Otherwise the child would slide in the direction of the traction, disrupting the alignment of the extremity and reducing the effectiveness of treatment. Also, the mattress should be firm and a bed board or foot plate may be necessary to prevent flexion.

Traction is used to reduce and immobilize fractures by correcting and maintaining skeletal length and alignment. Without traction, muscle contraction would cause overriding and displacement of bone fragments. Effective traction prevents movement of the fracture site.

Disadvantages of traction include hospitalization and prolonged immobility. Currently, the use of traction is being replaced by early casting and percutaneous pinning of supracondylar fractures (MacEwen, Kasser, & Heinrich, 1993).

Traction may be described as either continuous or intermittent. Continuous traction exerts a constant pull and is used for fractures and dislocations. Intermittent traction provides a periodic pull or force and is used for contractures, low back pain, or muscle spasm. The nurse should always assume that traction is continuous unless the physician states otherwise. The removal of traction that was intended to be continuous could prove harmful to

Types of Skin Traction

BUCK EXTENSION

Purpose: Used to treat fractured hips, contractures, and muscle spasms.

Description: Continuous or intermittent boot or circular wrap is applied to the skin. Traction is applied to boot or wrap. Countertraction is provided by elevating foot of bed.

Nursing Interventions: Keep ropes and pulleys hanging free. Maintain heel off bed. Place rolled towels on external surface of knee to prevent external rotation of affected leg.

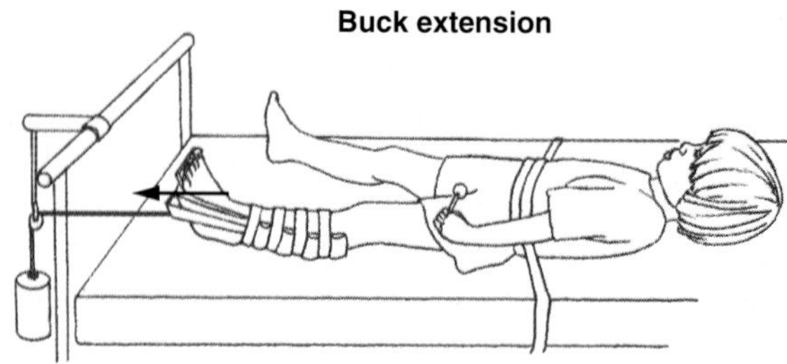

BRYANT TRACTION

Purpose: Used to treat congenital hip dysplasia and fractured femurs in children younger than 2–3 years of age.

Description: Intermittent traction. Child is supine with legs flexed slightly less than 90°, thus relaxing the hamstrings. Spreader bar or footplate is used to keep traction straps away from ankles. Sacrum should be off the mattress.

Nursing Interventions: Because the child's weight provides the countertraction, restraints are needed to maintain the child in the supine position. Remove the wraps at least once a shift and p.r.n. Assess for circulatory impairment and compartment syndrome.

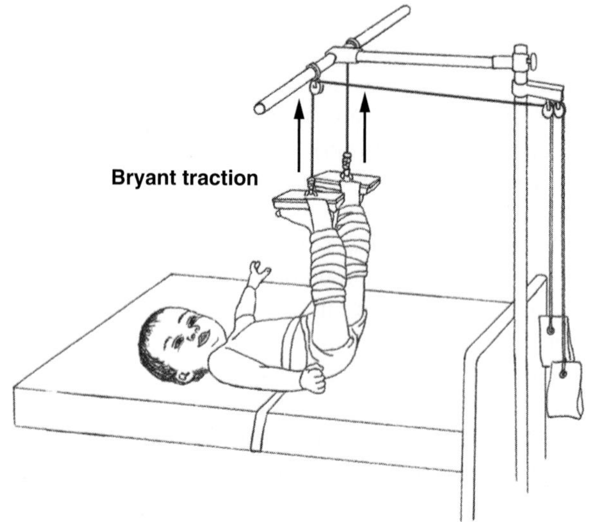

the patient and result in poor healing. The nursing care plan should always reflect the frequency and amount of time intermittent traction may be removed. While removing the traction, manual traction must be maintained by using one's hands to maintain pull on the body part.

Traction may also be described as running or balanced. Running, or straight, traction exerts a pull on the affected part without balanced support from a sling or splint. The child's weight provides the countertraction. Balanced, or suspension, traction also exerts a pull on the affected part but the extremity is supported by a sling or splint. Countertraction is provided through the use of weights and pulleys attached to the sling or splint. With balanced traction, even when the child moves, the pull remains constant because the countertraction offsets the movement. This type of traction allows more movement and results in fewer problems with immobility. Both balanced and running traction may be applied to either the skin or bone.

Skin Traction. Skin traction exerts force directly on the body surface. It is noninvasive, well tolerated, and does not require anesthesia. Skin traction is most effective with children who weigh less than 30 pounds or are younger than age 2 to 3 years. It can be applied to the pelvis, spine, or extremities (usually the long bones). The use of skin traction is preferred for conditions in which invasive procedures are contraindicated (such as hemarthrosis due to hemophilia). Foam rubber straps, adhesive moleskin, or cloth belts are applied to the skin and then attached to the weights and pulleys. Sometimes an elastic bandage will be wrapped around the skin to hold the traction apparatus in place. If skin traction to the lower leg is needed, a foam rubber boot may be used. The fit should be secure. Neurovascular status should be checked frequently to ensure adequate perfusion.

The effectiveness of skin traction is determined by the amount of pull that can be placed on the extremity. For this reason, skin traction is not appropriate if the child has a skin infection, open wound, or extensive tissue damage. Skin breakdown may also develop. Spraying the skin with tincture of benzoin before the application of the traction may offer some protection from skin irritation.

RUSSELL TRACTION

Purpose: Used to stabilize fractured femurs until callus forms.

Description: Continuous traction. Knee slightly flexed and supported with sling. Trapeze overhead may be used by child for repositioning and upper extremity muscle integrity.

Nursing Interventions: Check sling placement frequently to prevent peroneal nerve damage. Elevate foot of bed for countertraction; keep head of bed flat. Restraints may be needed to maintain correct alignment.

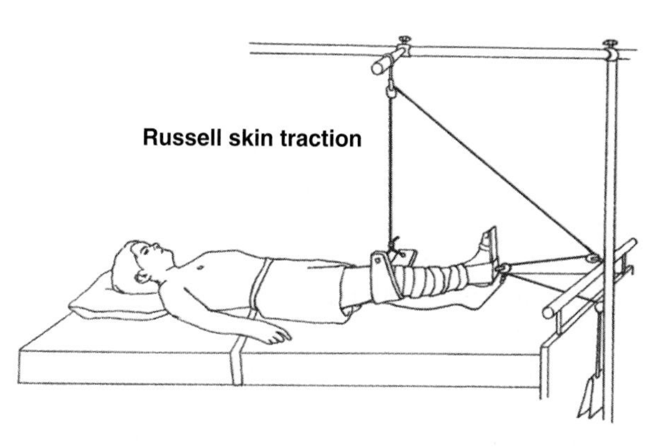

CERVICAL TRACTION

Purpose: Used to treat muscle or nerve irritation of shoulders and upper arms.

Description: May be continuous or intermittent. Maintains the head in extension via a halter: front straps fit under chin, rear straps at base rest at base of skull. Spreader bar equalizes force of pull.

Nursing Interventions: Elevate head of bed 20° to 30° for correct alignment. Maintain head in straight alignment. Notify physician if pain or discomfort occurs (not expected with cervical traction).

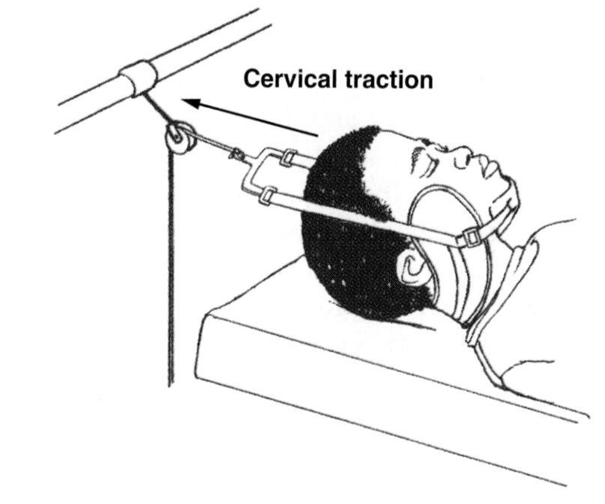

If the traction has not been set up correctly, neurovascular impairment may occur. The most common causes for this problem are hyperextension of the knee and elastic bandages that have been wrapped too tightly. To prevent this, a thorough assessment of the traction apparatus as well as the extremity itself should be conducted at least once a shift. (See the accompanying box for examples of skin traction.)

Skeletal Traction. Skeletal traction (Fig. 36–3) exerts greater force than skin traction and can be physiologically tolerated for longer periods of time. Traction is maintained via a metal device that is inserted into the bone. This is accomplished by introducing a Kirschner wire or Steinmann pin into the bone or Crutchfield tongs into the skull.

The insertion site of these stainless steel wires, pins, or tongs is determined by the fracture site. Common sites for skeletal traction include the skull, the proximal end of the ulna, and the distal end of the femur as well as the tibia and heel. Internal fixation, or the direct application of

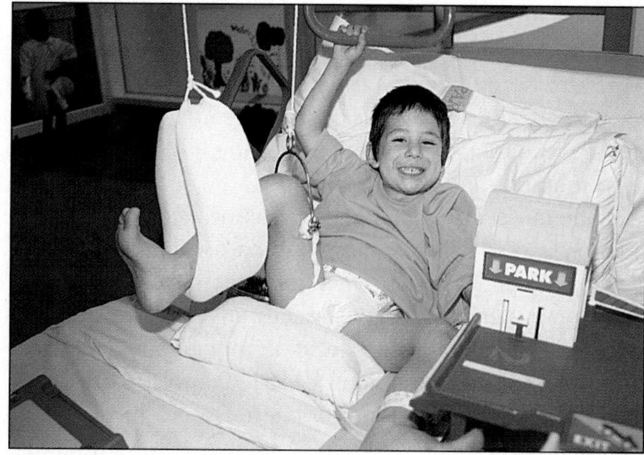

Figure 36–3

Skeletal traction is used to reduce and immobilize fractures and allows greater pull than would be possible with skin traction. Osteomyelitis is a serious complication because skeletal traction is invasive. (Courtesy of Parkland Memorial Hospital, Dallas, Texas)

Types of Skeletal Traction

CRUTCHFIELD TONGS

Purpose: To stabilize fractures or displaced vertebrae in cervical and thoracic areas.

Description: Tongs are inserted on either side of scalp through drill holes. Center of curved metal bar must extend along same planes as spinal cord. Traction pull is always along axis of spine.

Nursing Interventions: Check tongs q 8 hr and p.r.n. for displacement and looseness. Log roll or turn child as a unit when repositioning. Assess neurologic status frequently in first 24 hours because spinal cord injury frequently accompanies this type of injury. Do pin care every shift.

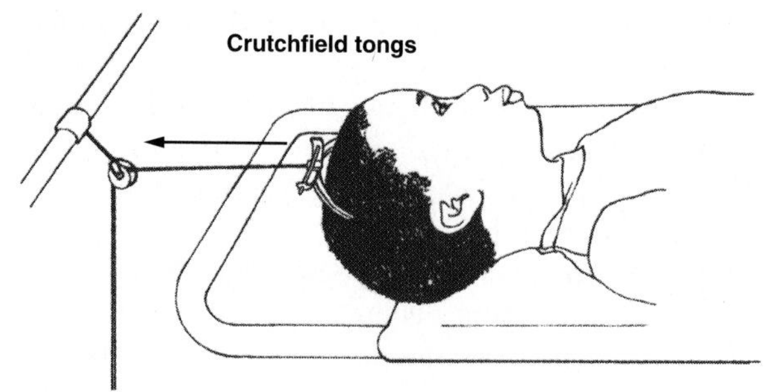

BALANCED SUSPENSION

Purpose: Suspends and immobilizes leg without applying traction to the body.

Description: May be applied to hip, tibia, fibula, or femur. Leg is supported by Pearson attachment and Thomas splint. Thomas splint is padded ring that fits around upper leg; Pearson attachment meets Thomas splint at knee and supports lower leg. Canvas sling may be used to further support lower leg.

Nursing Interventions: Attach footplate to prevent footdrop. Maintain bed in flat position to reduce flexion contracture of hip. If bed is in semi-Fowler position, at least once a shift make sure bed is in flat position for 20 minutes.

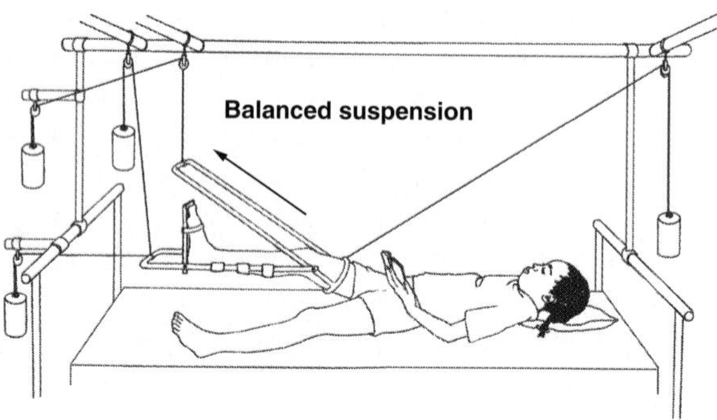

hardware to the bone, is a common occurrence in skeletal traction. It helps maintain correct alignment of the bony fragments and assists in proper healing. General anesthesia is required for internal fixation.

The most serious complication associated with skeletal traction is osteomyelitis, an infection involving the bone. Organisms gain access to the bone systemically or through the opening created by the metal pins or wires used for traction. Osteomyelitis may also occur with any open fracture. Clinical manifestations include complaints of localized pain, swelling, warmth, tenderness, or unusual odor. An elevated temperature may accompany the symptoms. (See pp. 1114–1117 for discussion of osteomyelitis.)

Skeletal traction is always continuous. If the force of the traction were altered, the muscles would contract and fracture alignment would be disrupted. The tissues around the fracture could also be injured. A good rule to follow is to assume all traction is continuous until adequate information regarding the traction apparatus can be obtained. (See the accompanying box for examples of skeletal traction.)

NURSING CARE OF THE CHILD WITH A FRACTURE

Assessment

Initial Trauma Assessment. Nursing assessment of the child with a fracture should begin with a thorough assessment of the patient's airway, breathing, and circulation. Because trauma is frequently the cause of fractures, determining physiologic stability is the number one priority. Once this is done, a history regarding the circumstances surrounding the fracture should be obtained.

Determining the cause of the fracture is important because non-accidental trauma may be involved. A complete history of how the fracture occurred as well as physical findings are important if child abuse is suspected.

90/90 FEMORAL TRACTION

Purpose: Most commonly used traction for complicated fractures of femur. Most effective in children over 6 years. Within 2 to 3 weeks, callus formation is sufficient to allow application of spica cast.

Description: Pin or wire is inserted through distal femur; low leg may be casted.

Nursing Interventions: Pin care every shift. Maintain correct alignment. Assess skin integrity every shift. Restraints may be needed to maintain correct position.

DUNLOP TRACTION

Purpose: Used to treat supracondylar fractures of humerus.

Description: Pin is inserted through distal humeral fragments. Elbow is flexed at 90° angle with forearm in neutral position.

Nursing Interventions: Maintain correct alignment to prevent contractures. Assess circulation q 2–4 hr to prevent vascular compromise. Pain, pallor, cyanosis, problems with movement, or absence of a pulse are indications of Volkmann's ischemia. Check for numbness, tingling, and decreased sensation by asking child to wiggle fingers.

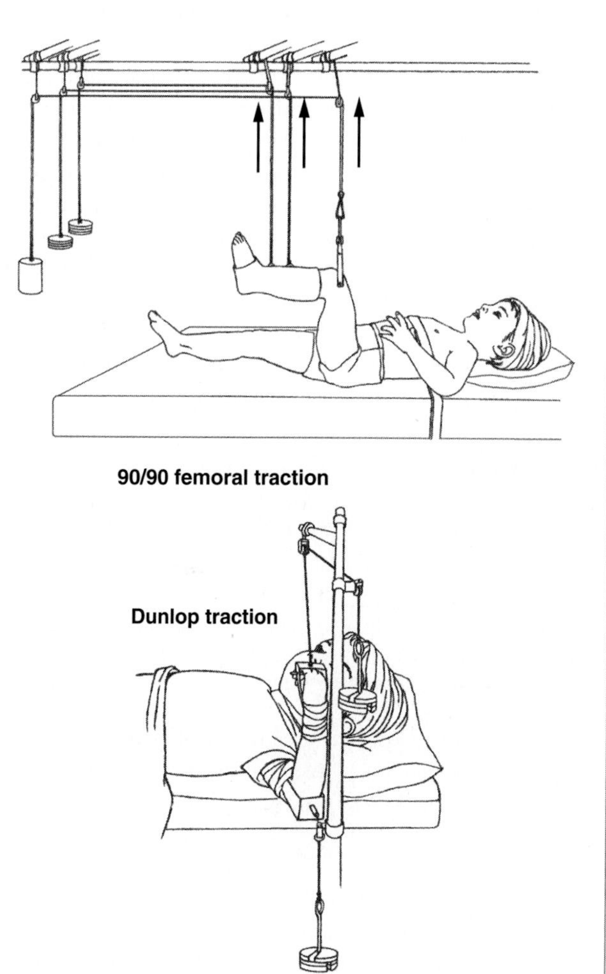

Tissue ischemia and nerve damage are serious complications that may accompany even a simple fracture. Neurovascular status (including skin color, temperature, movement and sensation of the extremity, quality of pulses and capillary refill of the extremity) should be assessed carefully because these problems must be handled quickly to prevent permanent disabilities.

The fracture site should be examined for bruising, skin lacerations, and swelling. Generally the child will favor the extremity, even to the point of cradling or supporting it. The area of the fracture is important to determine because growth plate injuries are not always evident on X-ray.

Assessing for Compartment Syndrome. Serious complications such as nerve compression, circulatory impairment, or compartment syndrome can result from swelling caused by trauma or an immobilizing device. Muscles and nerves of both upper and lower extremities are enclosed in compartments surrounded by tough, inelastic fascia. Compartment syndrome occurs when swelling causes pressure to rise within this closed space. The increased pressure compromises circulation to the muscles and nerves within the compartment and can result in paralysis and necrosis of tissues. Signs of compartment syndrome include severe pain often unrelieved by analgesics and signs of neurovascular impairment. Compartment syndrome is not uncommon in fracture of the forearm: therefore, the quality of the radial pulse and ability to extend the fingers should be assessed. If extension of the fingers produces pain, the physician should be notified.

Neurovascular Assessment. Neurovascular assessment should be performed every 1 to 2 hours during the first 48 hours after the injury. Quality of the pulse distal to the fracture site should be evaluated and compared with the pulse in the uninjured extremity. Sluggish capillary refill usually indicates neurovascular impairment.

General signs of circulatory impairment include coldness, pallor, blueness of the extremity, swelling, loss of motion, and numbness and tingling of the extremity. **Paresthesia,** or numbness and tingling, can be assessed by touching the fingers or toes and noting any decrease or loss in feeling. Paresthesia is of serious concern because paralysis can result if the problem is not corrected. A child's complaints of "pins and needles" or of the extremity "feeling asleep" should be reported. Since young children are not always able to describe a feeling or sensation, avoid questions such as "Do you feel this?" Asking a child to wiggle his fingers or toes is an appropriate way to determine motor impairment.

The five Ps of vascular impairment can be used as a guide when assessing neurovascular problems:

- Pain
- Pallor
- Pulselessness
- Paresthesia
- Paralysis

Pain unrelieved by analgesia or nursing interventions may be an indication of tissue ischemia. Prompt intervention is crucial if neurovascular impairment is to be prevented.

Motor function and sensation distal to the fracture should be assessed frequently. When assessing a complaint of pain, differentiation between pain related to the fracture and burning sensations distal to the fracture should be made.

A "burning" sensation is associated with tissue ischemia and can be an early indicator of serious neurovascular problems. This type of complaint must be reported to the physician.

Pain Assessment. Determining the level and source of pain with the preverbal child can be difficult. When the child is unable to clearly state the origin and type of pain, the nurse must frequently rely on assessment data to validate pain behaviors (see Chapter 20). It is important to remember that children in general are very adaptable to chronic or long-term pain. Expected behaviors in response to acute pain may be crying and increased restlessness, but with prolonged or chronic pain, young children learn very quickly the value of lying quietly and controlling their movements (Mills, 1989a, 1989b). When caring for preverbal children experiencing pain, the most effective tools available to the pediatric nurse are ongoing assessments of the child, which provide useful data regarding behaviors that recur as the child's pain threshold increases. Irritability, inability to move or wiggle the toes, odors or unusual smells from the cast, or color changes in a distal extremity should be noted.

When dealing with the preverbal child, it is important to use the parents as historians. Asking the parents how their child usually reacts to pain provides baseline information that can be used in determining the child's pain level (see Chapter 20).

Cast Application. It is the nurse's responsibility to assemble all necessary equipment as well as assist with the application of the cast. Before cast application, the nurse should assess the extremity for bruises or abrasions. Once it has been determined that casting is the appropriate treatment, the extremity should be covered with a protective tubular material (e.g., stockinette). Bony prominences should be covered with extra padding for comfort and protection.

Plaster of paris and materials for synthetic casts are packaged in the form of gauze strips or rolls that are soaked in water before application. The rolls are applied like an elastic bandage. As the last layer of material is applied, the stockinette should be pulled over the edges of the cast. This will provide a smooth edge around the cast and prevent skin irritation. If the nurse notices that the cast edges are rough or that a protective edge has not been provided, the nurse should "petal" the cast edges with adhesive moleskin or some other type of adhesive tape 1 to 2 inches wide, cut into strips approximately 3 to 4 inches long. One edge of the strip is rounded. Beginning with the straight end of the strip, place it on the inside of the cast edge; the rounded or "petaled" end is brought up and over the cast edge so it is on the outside of the cast. Each strip or "petal" overlaps the previous strip. The procedure is repeated until the cast edge is completely "petaled." When finished, the cast edge should be smooth.

Cast Care. A dry cast should sound hollow when tapped, have no unusual odors, and be cool to the touch. Any area of warmth or "hot spot" could be indicative of an early infection; the physician should be notified. It may be necessary to create a window in that area of the cast to monitor the site. Any drainage on the cast should be circled and the date and time marked on the cast. The area should be checked frequently. After open reduction, a certain amount of drainage may be expected but if it appears to be increasing, the physician should be notified.

The Nursing Care Plan that follows discusses care of the child in a cast or traction. Table 36–1 summarizes potential complications following the application of a cast.

Traction. Prior to the application of any type of traction, all procedures should be explained to the child and parents. The nurse should assess the condition of the extremity to be placed in traction. The skin should be inspected for abrasions, rashes, or vascular problems. Neurovascular

TABLE 36–1 *Potential Complications Following Cast Application*

COMPLICATION	ASSESSMENT	INTERVENTIONS
Ischemic tissue and nerve damage	Coldness Pallor Swelling Loss of motion Numbness and tingling Capillary refill >2 sec	Palpate distal pulse if possible. Neurovascular checks q 2 hr for the first 24 hr and then q 8 hr. Assess unaffected extremity for comparison purposes; document neurovascular assessment.
Pressure sores due to tight cast or poorly padded joint areas	Localized pain or burning sensation "Hot spot" over area of cast	Reposition frequently. Pad all joints before cast application. Keep small toys and objects away from cast. Neurovascular assessment q 1 hr and p.r.n. first 24hr, q 4 hr and p.r.n. after; trim cast as needed.
Compartment syndrome: accumulation of fluid within fascia that impedes venous flow and leads to ischemia	Deep, progressive pain; muscle will feel tense and full; pain upon passive stretching or when wiggling fingers and toes	Assist with fasciotomy. Pack wound and lightly wrap extremity, ROM by second day. Continue to assess neurovascular status.
Cast syndrome: portion of duodenum is compressed between superior mesenteric artery and aorta	Abdominal distention, vomiting, bowel obstruction	Frequent repositioning. Encourage fluids. Increase roughage in diet.

status should be evaluated. This includes skin color, temperature, and capillary refill. Peripheral pulses should also be evaluated. The unaffected extremity is always assessed as well. This will provide comparison data if problems arise in the future.

Nursing Diagnosis

- Risk for Injury related to neurovascular impairment
- Risk for Impaired Skin Integrity related to immobilization
- Impaired Physical Mobility related to cast or traction care
- Anxiety related to hospitalization and fracture
- Diversional Activity Deficit related to immobility, hospitalization, and limited interaction with peers
- Knowledge Deficit related to care and treatment of the fracture
- Altered Growth and Development related to immobilization and hospitalization

Planning, Implementation, and Evaluation: The Child in a Cast or Traction

NURSING DIAGNOSIS • Risk for Injury Related to neurovascular impairment

Expected Outcome: • The child's neurovascular integrity will be maintained or supported, as evidenced by normal skin color as compared to unaffected extremity, equal warmth and sensation in both extremities, no complaints of pain, equal and strong pulses in both extremities, and capillary refill less than 2 seconds.

Intervention	Rationale
1. Evaluate neurovascular status by assessing color, temperature, sensation, capillary refill (normal <2 seconds), and pulsation q 2 hr and p.r.n.; insert one finger between the cast and skin to check for cast tightness. Quality of the pulse distal to the fracture site should be evaluated and compared to the uninjured extremity.	Fractures and devices such as casts or traction may compress or restrict nerves or arteries, impeding healing and causing serious ischemic and circulatory problems. Swelling generally peaks 1 to 2 days after application of the cast.

Intervention	Rationale
2. Maintain correct body alignment. For child in traction, draw a line on the sheet and tell the parents to keep the child above that line and not to let him slip below it.	Proper alignment prevents pressure on the affected extremity and promotes healing.
3. Assess type and duration of pain. Ask parents how child normally reacts to pain. Be alert to preverbal children and their expressions of pain; irritability, inability to move or wiggle their toes, odors or unusual smells from the cast, or color changes in a distal extremity are typical behaviors the preverbal child might exhibit.	A complaint of burning pain or pain unrelieved by analgesia is an indicator of ischemia and nerve injury. Prompt intervention is crucial if neurovascular impairment is to be prevented. Odor from inside the cast can indicate infection.
4. Maintain cast integrity by supporting the drying cast with pillows. Reposition q 2–4 hr; turn the cast with the palms of the hands. If plaster of paris cast, keep it dry. Apply ice to reduce swelling.	An intact cast provides support and controls position while the fracture heals.
5. Elevate the casted extremity above level of heart; apply ice to cast p.r.n. If swelling persists after elevation, notify physician.	Elevating the extremity will reduce venous pooling; ice will reduce swelling and edema.
6. Maintain traction integrity by ensuring all weights and pulleys are hanging free and do not touch the floor or bed. Elevate the head or foot of the bed as indicated to maintain countertraction. Do not release the traction without a physician's order. Restrain child (if needed for safety) to maintain proper alignment. (Restraint should be used only if absolutely necessary for safety.) Assess that correct amount of weight is in use by checking with the physician's order.	Effective traction prevents movement of the fracture site and maintains skeletal alignment during healing.
7. Assess for complications of a fracture: nerve damage, epiphyseal injury, osteomyelitis (fever, pain, swelling), and compartment syndrome. Notify physician of signs of complications.	Occurrence of complications will interfere with healing and have long-term effects on the child's growth and development.
8. Circle any drainage on the cast and report any increase to the physician. Assess cast for areas of warmth or "hot spots."	Drainage on a cast or "hot spots" could be an early indication of infection or complications secondary to open reduction.

Evaluation: The child has appropriate neurovascular function, as evidenced by:

- Appropriate skin color as compared to unaffected extremity
- Equal warmth and sensation in both extremities
- No complaints of pain
- Equal and strong pulses in both extremities (if appropriate)
- Capillary refill less than 2 seconds.

NURSING DIAGNOSIS

- Risk for Impaired Skin Integrity related to immobilization

Expected Outcome:

- The child's skin will remain intact as evidenced by the absence of redness, irritation, and skin breakdown.
- The child will demonstrate intact skin over bony prominences; skin is smooth and without redness or irritation.

Intervention	Rationale
1. Assess skin integrity, especially over bony prominences, at least once a shift.	Regular assessment of the skin can identify problem areas early and prevent development of decubiti.
2. Reposition the child q 2 hr and p.r.n. Encourage use of trapeze to facilitate independent movement.	Frequent turning reduces pressure on sensitive skin.
3. Wash and dry the skin at least twice a day; massage the skin with circular movements; remove excess lotion with a towel. Do not use powder or talc because it tends to collect moisture and irritate the skin.	Skin that is clean and dry is less likely to develop decubiti. Frequent massage increases circulation to the skin and reduces the likelihood of skin breakdown.
4. Place an eggcrate or sheepskin mattress under the back and lower legs; use water-filled gloves under the heels to prevent skin breakdown.	These mattresses relieve pressure over bony prominences.
5. Petal the edges of the cast with adhesive tape or moleskin.	Infants' and children's skin is fragile and prone to injury from rough or jagged cast edges.
6. Protect the skin under the cast from moisture. Avoid getting the cast wet (no swimming, baths, or showers); cover the cast with plastic and waterproof tape if it is likely the child may get the cast wet (e.g., playing or due to bladder incontinence).	Damp or moist skin inside a cast is an excellent environment for bacterial growth.
7. Monitor the types of toys the child uses; do not allow a young child to play with small toys that could be hidden inside a cast or underneath the child. Supervise feeding because food may be hidden in the cast as well.	Objects or food hidden inside a cast place pressure on the skin and can lead to irritation and skin breakdown.

Evaluation:
- The child's skin integrity remains intact without evidence of redness, irritation, or tissue breakdown.

NURSING DIAGNOSIS
- Impaired Physical Mobility related to cast or traction care

Expected Outcome:
- The child will experience minimal immobilization problems, as evidenced by muscle and joint integrity, the absence of bone demineralization, clear breath sounds, intact skin, and age-appropriate elimination and nutritional habits.

Intervention	Rationale
1. Assess muscle strength and joint mobility every shift and p.r.n.	Baseline data is essential if an appropriate plan of care is to be developed for the child.
2. Maintain correct body alignment.	Inactive muscles lose tone and strength at a rate of 3%–5% a day, which may lead to loss of muscle mass and tissue breakdown.
3. Perform range of motion (ROM) and stretching exercises as appropriate. Consult with the physician regarding the need for occupational therapy and the use of splints and/or foot boards.	Joints become fibrotic from disuse, which leads to muscle shortening and joint contractures; exercise facilitates the movement of calcium into the bone.

Intervention	Rationale
4. Apply elastic stockings or TEDS.	Promotes venous return and decreases circulatory stasis.
5. Plan age-appropriate play activities that require the use of unaffected extremities. Provide colored markers to the child and his friends and let them decorate the child's cast.	Exercise will strengthen and enhance muscle and joint integrity while assisting with normal developmental needs.
6. Offer frequent small feedings of foods high in protein and calcium (milk, cheese, yogurt, green vegetables, puddings).	A diet high in calcium and protein will reduce problems associated with a negative nitrogen balance and increased bone catabolism.
7. Maintain hydration levels that are age-appropriate. Offer juices (cranberry, apple) and acid ash foods (cereal, meats) that will acidify the urine.	Encouraging fluids reduces problems associated with hypercalcemia, renal calculi, and stasis of respiratory secretions.
8. Maintain urine output at 1–2 ml/kg/hr; check urine for protein, blood, and specific gravity as ordered.	Ensuring adequate renal output aids in reducing the incidence of urinary tract infections secondary to urinary stasis and assists in reducing renal calculi.
9. Monitor bowel sounds and elimination pattern. Provide increased roughage in the diet and offer favorite foods. Determine child's usual bowel patterns; determine character of stool (amount, color, consistency and time). Position as upright as possible during defecation. Assess fluid intake and hydrate to meet fluid needs. Administer stool softeners and mild laxatives as needed; use familiar words for defecation.	Immobility decreases peristalsis and increases problems with constipation.
10. Assess respiratory status at least once a shift; encourage coughing and deep breathing through the use of such games as blowing bubbles, pin wheels, or magic tricks; older children may use the triflow or incentive spirometer as needed.	Immobility places the child at risk for stasis of secretions, which may lead to pneumonia and/or atelectasis.

Evaluation: The child experiences minimal problems of immobility, as evidenced by:

- Normal muscle and joint integrity
- The absence of cardiac or respiratory complications
- Age-appropriate nutritional, bowel, and bladder habits.

NURSING DIAGNOSIS

- Anxiety related to hospitalization and fracture (see Chapter 15)
- Diversional Activity Deficit related to immobility, hospitalization, and limited interaction with peers (see Chapter 15)
- Altered Growth and Development related to immobilization and hospitalization

Expected Outcome:

- The child will exhibit age-appropriate growth and developmental behaviors, as evidenced by decreased crying or acting-out, increased cooperation with self-care activities, and normal sleep habits.
- The parents will support and maintain appropriate developmental behavior for their child, as evidenced by increased involvement in the child's daily care and increased assistance in helping the child deal with the stress of hospitalization and immobility.

Intervention	Rationale
1. Assess the child's and parents' anxiety; acknowledge their anxiety and when possible model appropriate behaviors or teach activities that reduce anxiety.	Gathering assessment data is the first step in the nursing process and provides information regarding family strengths and nursing care needs.
2. Maintain a calm, consistent environment; organize nursing care to allow periods of developmentally appropriate activities. When possible assign the same nursing personnel.	Anxiety can be transferred to the child via parent or staff; a consistent care-giver will provide a sense of security to the child.
3. Recognize the child's need to regress in response to the injury or hospitalization; accept the behavior and assist the child to regain prior developmental stages when ready.	Schedules, routines, and rituals offer a sense of security to the young child; hospitalization and injuries such as fractures interrupt these routines and create stressful situations that impact on the child's ability to perform self-care activities such as toileting, sleeping, discipline, and feeding.
4. Encourage parents to stay with the child; if parents cannot stay, encourage them to leave an article of clothing or other personal item with the child. Audio tapes of parents reading favorite stories are also helpful.	The presence of a parent or significant family member can reduce the fear of separation and foster a sense of security.
5. Explain all routines and procedures to the child and parents; continue to offer explanations until understanding is verbalized by parents and/or child.	The unknown is a powerful influence on the child and increases anxiety; the presence of anxiety decreases the child's and parents' ability to process and analyze information.
6. Involve the parents in the care of the child when appropriate. Begin teaching the family about home care on the first day of hospitalization.	Encouraging the parents to participate in the child's care increases their sense of control and provides the child with a sense of security.
7. Provide age-appropriate play or diversional activities. When possible involve the parents in the child's play. Encourage expressive activities. (Throwing balls through a hoop or bean bags into a basket would be appropriate for a younger child; pounding boards are equally helpful in reducing stress and anxiety. Manipulating clay or play dough or expressing anger or frustration through painting would be appropriate activities for the older child.) Playing with remote control toys gives the child a feeling of mobility. Use therapeutic play: activities such as applying a cast to a doll, puppet play, storytelling utilizing pictures the child has drawn, or role playing.	Therapeutic play provides a safe and effective mechanism for reducing the stress of hospitalization and immobility. Therapeutic play puts the child in charge, provides a sense of control, and presents the child with opportunities to make choices. Play helps the child work through fears and anxieties.
8. When possible use age-appropriate dishes and cups for the young child. Let the child wear own clothing; jeans and shorts could still be used, slitting the sides of the pants and sewing Velcro closures on the legs. Allow the young child a transitional object in bed; use a night light and when possible follow night time rituals. Encourage therapeutic play with the preschool child; if possible place two preschoolers in the same room. Recognize the preschooler's use of magical thinking and encourage expressive play when dealing with the stress of immobility.	The use of familiar objects and maintaining routines provides the child with a sense of security and belonging; allowing contact with friends and family members reassures the child that he has not been forgotten and provides opportunities to enhance and support appropriate developmental behaviors.

Intervention	Rationale
9. Opportunities for keeping up with schoolwork should be provided for the school-age child and adolescent. Tutoring as well as Big Sister/Big Brother programs in the school can be very beneficial to the immobilized child. Tape recordings of classes can be very helpful in helping the child keep up with peers. If possible activities related to organizations like Boy Scouts or Girl Scouts should be maintained. Monitor time spent watching television or playing video games. Encourage involvement in hobbies and when possible select a roommate close in age.	Maintaining routines and helping the older child and adolescent maintain school activities provides opportunities for independence and productivity. Relating to the school-age child or adolescent on his level reinforces developmentally appropriate behavior as well as validating the importance of the child.

Evaluation: Normal growth and developmental behaviors are maintained, as evidenced by:

- The child/parents verbalize increased trust regarding health care providers.
- The child verbally or through play discloses feelings or concerns regarding the injury or hospitalization.
- The child demonstrates increased levels of control through increased self-care activities and age-appropriate sleep patterns.
- The parents accept the child's regressive behaviors and become more involved in the child's care.

NURSING DIAGNOSIS

- Knowledge Deficit Related to care and treatment of the fracture

Expected Outcome:

- The parents will verbalize accurate knowledge of fracture treatment, increased confidence with home care of the child, and an awareness of problems that may occur and the appropriate actions to take.

Intervention	Rationale
1. Assess parents' level of understanding regarding fractures, treatment method, cast care, and past experience with this type of injury.	Developing a teaching plan for the parents cannot begin until parents' knowledge level is determined.
2. Provide discharge instructions verbally as well as in writing; instruct parents to protect the cast from damage by keeping food and small objects away from the cast, to never allow the child to scratch under the cast, and to refrain from getting the cast wet. (See box, Discharge Instructions for Cast Care.)	Providing parents with information will increase their self-confidence and assist them in caring for their child in a safe and appropriate manner.
3. Discuss self-care activities with the parents and child (if age-appropriate) as well as modifications in home and school routines. Refer to appropriate resources for crutch walking as well as appropriateness of isotonic and isometric exercises. Referral to an occupational therapist may be needed to assist with adaptive devices for performance of activities of daily living and to increase independence.	The use of anticipatory guidance reduces parental anxiety and facilitates the transition from hospital to home.

Intervention	Rationale
4. Review neurovascular assessment and identify appropriate resources to contact if problems occur. Identify potential problems related to skin breakdown and infection. Follow-up all teaching with return demonstrations if appropriate.	Parents need to be instructed regarding potential complications and available resources.
5. Assist parents in understanding the impact of immobility on the child's growth and development.	It is important that parents realize that despite the cast, there are many ways they can enhance their child's development.

Evaluation: The parents will manage the transition from hospital to home smoothly and without problems, as evidenced by:

- Safe and effective home care
- Fracture heals without complications
- Age-appropriate developmental behaviors in child.

DISCHARGE INSTRUCTIONS *for Cast Care*

Check the edges of the cast:

- If they appear rough or are irritating the skin, "petal" the cast by overlapping moleskin or adhesive tape (1–2 inches in width; 3–4 inches in length) around the cast edges.

To assist with drying the cast:

- Place the child on a firm mattress.
- Support the cast and adjacent joints with pillows.
- Reposition every 2–4 hours to ensure thorough drying.
- Turn the cast using the palms of the hands.
- Fans directed toward the cast will facilitate drying.
- Once dry, the cast should sound hollow and be cool to the touch.
- DO NOT USE A HEAT LAMP TO DRY THE CAST.

Swelling generally peaks within 24–48 hours. To prevent problems:

- Apply ice to the casted area.
- Elevate the extremity with pillows.
- Apply pressure to the nailbed and count how long it takes for the color to return; it should take no longer than 2 seconds; do this every 2–3 hours for the first 24–48 hours.
- The casted extremity should be the same color and temperature as the other extremity.
- Check each finger or toe for sensation and movement several times a day for 2 days.

Protect the cast:

- When bathing or showering be sure and cover the cast with plastic to keep the cast dry.
- Do not put anything inside the cast; keep small toys and sharp objects away from the cast.
- Do not hit or strike the cast against anything.

Contact the physician if:

- The cast feels warm or "hot" or has an unusual smell or odor.
- Any drainage or blood suddenly appears on the cast.
- Your child begins complaining of pain, burning, numbness, or tingling or if the extremity changes color or temperature.

When it is time for the cast to be removed:

- Allow time for the child to adjust to the cast cutter; be sure and tell the child that the cutter works by vibrations.
- Use therapeutic play to help the young child deal with fears regarding the procedure.
- Once the cast is removed, the skin will be dry and flaky; wash the area with warm water and soap.
- The extremity will be stiff for awhile; it may need to be supported with a sling; normal movement will correct the stiffness.

Cast Removal

Cast removal can be very frightening for the child. The cast cutter operates by vibrations. These vibrations generate heat and create a "tickling" feeling on the skin. The noise generated by the cast cutter along with the debris of the disintegrating cast can be very frightening to a young child. It is important for the nurse to consider developmental needs as well as safety concerns when a cast is being removed. For example, the preschooler's magical thinking often arouses fears of body mutilation.

Therapeutic play can be effective in reducing the young child's fears of cast removal. Having the nurse demonstrate how the cast cutter works may help relieve some of the child's fears. Allowing the child to hold the cast cutter, even removing a cast from a doll (with supervision), can be very helpful in coping with the fears associated with this procedure. When possible, the parents or primary caregiver should be allowed to stay with the child during the procedure.

Once the cast has been removed, the skin under the cast will appear flaky and brown due to the accumulation of dead skin. Parents should be instructed to gently wash the extremity with mild soap and warm water. This will help remove the dead skin. The child may complain that the extremity looks smaller. If an extremity has been immobilized for a period of time, it is quite possible that muscle atrophy may have occurred. The extremity may also be stiff, and the child may want to protect it. Usually the stiffness diminishes in time, and with normal use and movement these problems should correct themselves.

Psychological Effects of Immobility

Mobility provides a forum in which the child may communicate and interact with the world. It even provides an outlet for anxiety. Children react to threatening situations by increasing their activity. Casts restrain a child's mobility. This restriction or lack of movement may be perceived by the child as punishment for becoming ill or being injured.

The immobilized child suffers from a lack of environmental stimuli and tactile perceptions that provide her with information about her world and how to interact in it. Regardless of age, the restrained child is constantly struggling between dependence and independence. For example, the casted infant will not be able to perform motor activities such as crawling and walking. This affects not only the infant's gross motor development, but also her cognitive growth because the infant is limited in her ability to explore and learn about her world.

In fact, immobility affects each age-group in unique ways. The immobilized toddler is limited in the development of autonomy. The preschooler's initiative is limited because of restricted physical activity, and magical thinking places her at risk for fears of body mutilation. The school-age child's development is centered around competition and physical activity that provides a sense of mastery. Immobility limits her interactions with her peers by preventing participation in school and sports activities. These activities are important because they assist the school-age child in developing a sense of industry. Without mobility the adolescent is limited in her interactions with peers as well as in developing a sense of identity apart from her parents.

Discharge planning should include information regarding ways parents can enhance their child's development. For example, the immobilized infant's position should be changed frequently—not only the infant's position in bed, but also the bed's position in the room—to increase the variety of stimuli available to the infant. Whenever possible and unless contraindicated, the infant should be taken outside. A wagon fitted with pillows and blankets would be a safe and easy way to transport the infant to the park or on a walk.

Fine motor activities should be emphasized as well. Age-appropriate activities for the young infant that would enhance fine motor development include the use of mirrors, mobiles with bright shiny objects, and toys that are of different textures. Being rocked to sleep or during a feeding (if not too awkward) provides great sensory stimulation. The older infant may enjoy stacking toys, cloth books with large pictures, building towers with oversized blocks, and playing with large balls. Large teething toys would also be appropriate because the older infant will begin teething. Parents should be encouraged to maintain eye contact at the infant's level as much as possible.

The nurse should also be aware that it is not uncommon to observe regressive behaviors in children who are immobilized. In fact, anxiety and depression may accompany the regression. Tasks easily accomplished by the child are now completed by others and there appears to be greater dependence on others. The classic example of regression is the toddler who is toilet trained and drinking from a cup who now wets the bed and demands a bottle. The older child may become more quiet or even revert to previous activities such as thumb sucking or demanding parental attention. Parents need to understand that regressive behavior is a healthy adaptation to the stress of immobility and that the regressive behavior should be accepted.

In time the child will begin to reclaim previous developmental stages (e.g., trust, autonomy) and it is at that point that parents or health care providers need to assist the child. For example, the toddler should be offered sips from a cup while drinking from a bottle and should wear training pants even though bed wetting is still occurring. The toddler should be offered choices whenever possible, such as clothing they would prefer to wear or type of cereal they would like for breakfast. Self-care activities should be encouraged as much as possible; the child should also be involved in planning care. Tutoring should be provided for the school-age child. Maintaining schoolwork encourages industry and helps the child remain involved in age-appropriate activities. Peer interactions should be encouraged through phone calls, letter writing, or visits. Even young children might like to speak with family members or friends on the phone. Providing assistance in dialing the phone would be a perfect opportunity for encouraging autonomy and individuality.

SOFT TISSUE INJURIES: SPRAINS, STRAINS, AND CONTUSIONS

Soft tissue injuries are common among children, usually due to accidents during play or from sports-related injuries. *Sprains* occur as a result of trauma to a joint in which ligaments are stretched or partially or completely torn. *Strains,* also known as pulls, tears, or ruptures, result from an excessive stretch of muscle. *Contusions* occur when soft tissue, muscle, or subcutaneous tissues are damaged. Sprains and contusions frequently accompany each other. Dislocations occur when a joint is disrupted in such a way that articulating surfaces are no longer in contact.

PATHOPHYSIOLOGY *of Soft Tissue Injuries*

When a sprain occurs, the twisting of the joint results in a process called inversion that disrupts the stability of the joint. If the inversion continues, surrounding structures may become involved. Damage to muscles and nerves may occur. Hemarthrosis and joint problems may also develop depending on the severity of the damage.

The joint most often involved in a sprain is the ankle. The ligament most often involved is the collateral ligament. When inversion begins secondary to force or trauma, damage to the ankle may be intensified by the involvement of other structures such as the malleolus. In severe sprains, a fracture may occur involving the fibula and malleolus. Sprains are classified as first-, second-, or third-degree.

Strains, very similar to sprains, are tearing injuries to a muscle or its tendon. The damage caused by the strains may not be immediately apparent; consequently, once the pain begins the child may have forgotten how the injury occurred (Hall, 1992). The presenting complaint is tenderness with or without swelling, redness, or limited ROM. When a contusion occurs, injury to the soft tissue, muscle, or surrounding structures is accompanied by bleeding into the tissues, swelling, and pain. The inflammatory response further exacerbates this phenomenon. This movement of blood into the surrounding tissues results in bruising, or ecchymosis.

Incidence. Sprains are not frequently seen in young children because of the poorly developed epiphyseal plate. A twisting or turning injury will more likely result in a fracture than a sprain because the epiphyseal plate is weaker and carries greater potential for injury. Sprains and strains are more commonly seen in the adolescent age-group and are frequently the result of athletic injuries. In general, sprains and contusions are more likely to occur with more physical or violent sports activities.

Clinical Manifestations

- Pain
- Swelling
- Localized tenderness
- Limited ROM
- Poor weight-bearing
- Pop or snapping sound (sprain)

Diagnostic Evaluation. Diagnosis is based on the clinical picture. However, an X-ray may be ordered to rule out fractures.

Therapeutic Management. The goal of treatment for sprains and contusions is to control the swelling and prevent further injury. Swelling can inhibit healing by keeping the ligament ends apart and increasing fibrous scarring. The earlier treatment is initiated, the less severe the swelling and immobility become.

The first 6 to 12 hours after soft tissue injury are the most important in controlling swelling and reducing muscle damage. Treatment of soft tissue injuries is summarized in the acronyms "RICE" or "ICES":

RICE	ICES
R = Rest	I = Ice
I = Ice	C = Compression
C = Compression	E = Elevation
E = Elevation	S = Support

The injured area should be wrapped immediately to support the joint and control the swelling. Ice is applied to reduce the swelling. Before the ice is applied, the joint should be wrapped with a thin layer of elastic bandage or elastic wrap to protect the skin. The ice is then applied to the injured area with additional wrap being used to secure the ice. Ice should be applied for no longer than 30 minutes (Dyment, 1988) every 4 to 6 hours even though the effects of the ice can last as long as 5 to 6 hours. Although the ice may be applied until the swelling has disappeared, conventional treatment recommends the application of ice for the first 24 to 48 hours. The joint should be immobilized and elevated.

Immobilizing the injured joint and cold therapy are generally very effective in the treatment of incomplete ligament tears. A complete rupture could require surgery to prevent excessive scar formation and long-term joint mobility problems. Application of a cast or splint for 4 to 5 weeks may also be necessary, especially for knee injuries.

NURSING CARE OF THE CHILD WITH A SOFT TISSUE INJURY

Assessment

One of the major functions of the nurse when assessing a sprain is to determine the severity of the injury as well as the presence of any fractures or other soft tissue injuries. The child should be assessed for neurovascular impairment as well as ROM. Generally the initial examination will reveal localized tenderness over the injured joint as well as limited joint mobility. The more difficulty a child has in weight-bearing, the more serious the injury (Nixon, 1989).

Nursing Diagnosis and Planning

The following nursing diagnoses and expected outcomes may be appropriate following assessment of the child with a sprain, strain, or contusion.

- Risk for Injury related to neurovascular impairment and complications secondary to the injury. ***Expected Outcomes:*** *The child will exhibit normal skin color as compared to unaffected extremity; have equal warmth and sensation in both extremities; have no complaints of pain; demonstrate equal and strong pulses in both extremities and capillary refill less than 2 seconds.*
- Pain related to swelling and soft tissue injury. ***Expected Outcome:*** *The child will have minimal pain, as evidenced by increased periods of rest, age-appropriate attention span, and physical indications of relaxation (decreased blood pressure and heart rate).*
- Impaired Physical Mobility related to swelling and soft tissue injury. ***Expected Outcome:*** *The child will tolerate activity restrictions, as evidenced by compliance with treatment protocol.*
- Knowledge Deficit related to home care of a child with a sprain. ***Expected Outcomes:*** *The parents will verbalize an understanding of the care of their child as evidenced by identifying their strengths and limitations; perform neurovascular assessments correctly; provide age-appropriate play activities for their child.*

Implementation

The child's neurovascular status should be monitored. This includes assessing skin color and temperature as well as sensation. Numbness and tingling should not be present. The quality of the pulse distal to the injured joint should be evaluated and compared with the uninjured extremity. Capillary refill should be brisk. It is helpful to use the unaffected extremity for comparison purposes when assessing neurovascular status.

Pain management is achieved through analgesics such as ibuprofen or acetaminophen. Distraction as well as age-appropriate play activities can be very effective in managing a child's pain.

It is important to keep the extremity elevated above the heart. This position enhances venous return and aids in reducing the swelling. Pillows placed beneath the extremity will provide support as well as comfort. When applying the elastic wrap, it is important to assess neurovascular status because it is possible to apply the wrap too tightly.

Stretching and strengthening exercises are helpful in maintaining joint and muscle integrity. These exercises are done passively at first. As healing progresses the child is taught active stretching and strengthening exercises. When instructing the parents regarding these exercises a return demonstration is most appropriate in evaluating the effectiveness of teaching. Physical therapy referrals may be helpful as well.

The amount of time needed for healing is determined by the severity of the injury. Weight-bearing is increased gradually as the pain subsides. More severe injuries may require partial weight-bearing exercises and full weight-bearing once the swelling has resolved. Sports activities may be restricted for anywhere from 3 to 8 weeks.

Home Care. Review principles of rest, support, and the application of ice with the parents and child. If wraps, splints, or casts are used, be sure the parents and child have been taught how to assess neurovascular status. If crutches are required, review principles of crutch walking with both parents and child. Make sure all family members understand activity and sports restrictions. Discuss follow-up appointments and the importance of adhering to activity restrictions until the injury has healed and the child has been cleared for sports.

Evaluation

After treatment/healing:

- Is the neurovascular function of the extremity intact?
- Can the child exhibit full range of motion and weight-bearing?
- Do the parents verbalize an understanding of home care?

OSTEOMYELITIS

Osteomyelitis is a bacterial infection of the bone involving the cortex and/or marrow cavity. It is classified as acute or chronic. Osteomyelitis is considered chronic if the infection persists longer than a month or does not respond to the initial antibiotic protocol. Regardless of advances in antibiotic treatment, osteomyelitis remains a serious problem that can be very difficult to diagnose and, if inadequately treated, results in high morbidity rates.

Incidence. Osteomyelitis may occur at any age, but its incidence is higher in children than in adults (Schwentker,

1992). Boys are affected two to four times as often as girls; although osteomyelitis is more likely to occur during growth spurts, age-groups generally affected are preschoolers and adolescents.

PATHOPHYSIOLOGY *of Osteomyelitis*

Osteomyelitis occurs most frequently in the metaphyseal region of the long bones, especially the femur or tibia. Bacteria enter the metaphysis via the osseous circulation, and the inflammatory process begins. Pus forms and spreads toward the medullary canal as well as the cortex of the bone. Because the periosteum of a child's bone is thick and easily displaced, pus quickly spreads along the shaft of the bone. Involucrum, or new bone, will develop in an attempt to isolate the infection. As a result the cortex of the bone becomes devascularized and the area of necrotic bone detaches to form a separate area called sequestrum (Herndon, 1993).

Large sections of sequestrum may eventually become honeycombed with cavities or sinuses that contain infective material. These cavities are so effectively walled off that antibiotic therapy may not be successful. Thus it is possible for osteomyelitis to recur in the chronic form.

Etiology. Bacteria infiltrate the bone via endogenous sources (skin or respiratory infections, abscessed teeth, acute otitis media) or exogenous sources (injury or surgical procedures). The infection is usually the result of vascular spread of the bacteria. However, osteomyelitis may also occur as a result of direct entry (open fracture) or injury to surrounding soft tissues (cellulitis). External fixation devices and skeletal traction can also lead to osteomyelitis. Although strict adherence to aseptic techniques and frequent assessments of pin sites have greatly controlled this problem, the development of osteomyelitis can be a serious deterrent to successful healing.

The most common causative organism in all ages is *Staphylococcus aureus. Streptococcus pneumoniae, Haemophilus influenzae* (in infants), and *Escherichia coli* and group B streptococci (in neonates) also are responsible for osteomyelitis. The most common causative organism for osteomyelitis in children with sickle cell anemia is *Salmonella.*

Clinical Manifestations

- Pain
- Favoring affected extremity
- Tenderness
- Warmth
- Erythema
- Limited ROM
- Systemic manifestations such as fever and lethargy

Diagnostic Evaluation. An elevated erythrocyte sedimentation rate (ESR) is the most consistent diagnostic finding in osteomyelitis. An elevated white blood cell count may or may not be present. Blood cultures will be drawn to determine the causative organism. Bone changes may not be apparent on X-ray until 7 to 14 days after the onset of symptoms (Herndon, 1993). Bone scans are helpful in localizing the area of increased vascularity.

Therapeutic Management. Once a culture has been obtained and the organism's sensitivity to antibiotics determined, antibiotic treatment is initiated. Controversy exists regarding the length of time required for antibiotic therapy, the need for intravenous versus oral antibiotics, and the role of bactericidal antibiotics and therapeutic blood levels. Nevertheless it is generally recommended that therapy for osteomyelitis requires 4 to 6 weeks of high-dose parenteral therapy. With acute osteomyelitis, it has been suggested that a 3-week course of therapy is adequate for most infections (Bamberger, 1990; Syrongiannopoulos & Nelson, 1988). In some cases, a short intensive course of intravenous therapy followed by oral therapy may be administered.

Because the antibiotics are administered over an extended period of time and high-dose therapy may be necessary to obtain the desired outcome, assessing the child's response to the antibiotics is an integral part of the treatment protocol. Peaks and troughs of serum antibiotic levels are monitored closely. Renal and hepatic function should be monitored as well as frequent blood counts to determine bone marrow activity. Children receiving aminoglycosides should be assessed periodically for side effects such as ototoxicity and nephrotoxicity.

To limit the spread of infection and to promote healing, the child is placed on complete bed rest. The extremity may be immobilized with a splint or bivalved cast. Surgical intervention may be necessary if an abscess is present or if the infection fails to respond to antibiotics. Invasive procedures include draining the abscess, debriding necrotic tissue, and performing a sequestrectomy. Osteomyelitis of the proximal femur generally requires some type of surgical decompression because septic arthritis of the hip may accompany this infection. Aseptic technique is critical after any type of orthopedic surgery because a secondary infection could inhibit the healing process.

NURSING CARE OF THE CHILD WITH OSTEOMYELITIS

Assessment

Although it may be difficult for parents to recall every injury their child has suffered, a thorough history of recent falls or traumas is helpful in determining the source of the infection. The nurse should carefully examine the affected area and note any pain, tenderness, erythema, or swelling. Usually the child will appear to protect the extremity, even tensing adjacent muscles and demonstrating reluctance to straighten or move the extremity.

In some cases the child will appear ill with a high fever, generalized lethargy, and even anorexia. If the infection has been present for a long time the symptomatology may not appear as clear and it may be more difficult to obtain a reliable history. In cases like this the nurse might want to assess the femur and tibia more carefully because osteomyelitis most frequently involves these bones.

Nursing Diagnoses and Planning

The following nursing diagnoses and expected outcomes may be appropriate following assessment of the child with osteomyelitis.

- Risk for Injury related to neurovascular impairment and complications related to antibiotic therapy. ***Expected Outcome:*** *The child will remain free from injury, as evidenced by age-appropriate neurovascular functioning and by absence of iatrogenic problems.*
- Pain related to the infectious process. ***Expected Outcome:*** *The child will experience a decrease in pain, as evidenced by increased rest periods, decreased restlessness and irritability, and increased attention span.*
- Impaired Physical Mobility related to the infectious process and activity restrictions. ***Expected Outcome:*** *The child will accept the activity restrictions, as evidenced by increased compliance with treatment plan.*
- Altered Growth and Development related to hospitalization and immobility. ***Expected Outcome:*** *The child will exhibit age appropriate growth and developmental behavior, increased self-care behavior and normal sleep patterns.*
- Knowledge Deficit related to long-term antibiotic therapy. ***Expected Outcomes:*** *The parents will identify the child's home care needs; identify concerns or issues regarding home care.*

Implementation

Assessment and documentation of the child's status should be carried out at least once a shift. The condition of the extremity should be assessed and any unusual change reported to the physician. Because any movement of the involved extremity will be accompanied by some degree of discomfort, the extremity should be immobilized and supported with pillows. When moving or turning is required, input should be obtained from the child since he will know the most comfortable ways to achieve position changes. When it is not age-appropriate to do this, the nurse should consult with the parents. During the acute phase, the pain may be quite severe and the child should be premedicated with an analgesic before any repositioning.

Intravenous Antibiotics. Because the antibiotics will be administered intravenously (IV), the nurse should frequently assess the IV site for signs of infiltration or phlebitis. If an infusion pump will be used, assess both the pump and IV site frequently during administration of the medication. Every effort should be made to protect the IV site; depending on the age of the child, restraints may be required.

Always remember to maintain sterile technique when performing a venipuncture, during any dressing change, and when accessing an existing IV line. If a peripheral line will be used, EMLA cream should be applied to the site 60 minutes before the venipuncture (see Chapter 15 for procedure). This will reduce the child's discomfort as well as help the child deal with fears of pain and powerlessness. For long-term antibiotic administration, a heparin lock or central line may be placed.

The nurse should have a thorough knowledge of the antibiotic being given. This includes calculating dosage based on body weight or surface area, reviewing side effects, and determining if therapeutic blood levels are required. If the patient's blood level exceeds the therapeutic range, the antibiotic should be withheld and the physician notified.

Since the child will probably be receiving multiple antibiotics, compatibility is important. History of allergies as well as any current problems the parents may have encountered with previous antibiotic administration should be noted. Periodically the nurse should review current laboratory data to ensure adequate liver and kidney function. A complete blood count and ESR should be measured on a regular basis to evaluate the child's response to treatment.

Standard Precautions and Wound Care. Standard precautions should be maintained at all times. Sterile technique and appropriate removal of soiled materials should be strictly enforced. Children with surgical wounds or drains require close monitoring. Drainage should be measured as accurately as possible and recorded at the end of the shift. The color and consistency of the drainage as well as any unusual odor should be noted in the nurses' notes. A description of the wound should also be included.

Neurovascular and Skin Assessment. Neurovascular assessment of the extremity should be obtained at least once a shift. If a cast or brace is being used to immobilize the extremity, neurovascular checks as well as periodic assessments of the skin are required. If a cast is used, the affected area will be left open by creating a window in the cast. The area should be checked for swelling, tenderness, and erythema at least once a shift and more frequently if needed.

Bed Rest and Immobility Interventions. Bed rest or non–weight-bearing is very important in preventing the spread of the infection. Returning the child to full weight-bearing and self-care activities is determined by the child's response to treatment and by the physician's assessment of the healing process.

Immobility can diminish the child's appetite. Meeting the child's nutritional needs is essential to facilitate growth and development and to assist with the healing process. The child should receive a diet high in calories and protein. Frequent small meals and food that has been brought from home are helpful in stimulating the child's appetite.

Nursing Care of the Parents. Parents may experience guilt regarding the diagnosis. They may believe that if they had been more attentive to the child this infection might not have happened. Allow the parents opportunities to discuss their concerns. It may be necessary to reinforce previous teaching by reviewing how the infection began and the specific therapeutic interventions. Listening to parents and acknowledging their concerns can be very helpful in reducing their anxiety and guilt.

Home Care. If the child is to receive IV antibiotic therapy at home, the parents need to be taught how to set up the medication as well as how to ensure the infusion is being administered safely. The teaching should be planned to fit the parents' schedule. Attention must be given to signs of frustration or anxiety. Repetitive questions, poor eye contact, and nervous gestures are indicators that anxiety may be interfering with the parents' ability to retain information. A return demonstration is the most effective way to evaluate teaching effectiveness. A referral to a home care agency should be made to assist the family with the IV infusions.

Frequently the child will go home on oral antibiotics if a short course of IV therapy has produced a favorable clinical response. At this point discharge planning must focus on the cost of the oral antibiotics, whether the parents are able financially to purchase the medications, what financial supports are available within the hospital that can assist the family in the purchase of the medications, and whether the parents will administer the medication in a timely fashion. Issues surrounding adherence to the treatment protocol and compliance must be addressed by the nurse. The importance of follow-up care must be emphasized. A referral to a home care agency would be appropriate.

Developmental issues need to be addressed by the nurse. If the child is to remain at home with restricted activity, the family must have a clear understanding of how the restrictions aid the healing process. The nurse should discuss age-appropriate activities that will maintain current developmental levels. If the child is exhibiting any residual fears or concerns related to hospitalization, therapeutic play activities may be needed. School-age children need to continue with their schoolwork as well as maintain contact with their friends. Tutoring should be implemented as soon as possible. Resources available to homebound children should be explored with the parents.

Evaluation

After treatment/healing:

- Is the neurovascular function of the extremity intact?
- Can the child exhibit full ROM and weight-bearing?
- Do the parents verbalize an understanding of home care?
- Do the parents provide developmentally appropriate activities for their child?

OSGOOD-SCHLATTER DISEASE

The classic picture of Osgood–Schlatter disease is that of a very active adolescent boy involved in sports activities complaining of bilateral knee pain that is exacerbated by running, jumping, or climbing stairs. The child will point to the tibial tubercle as the site of pain.

Etiology and Incidence. Although the etiology of Osgood-Schlatter is not completely understood, it is believed to be related to repetitive stress from sports-related activities combined with overuse of immature muscles and tendons over an extended period of time (National Youth Sports Foundation for the Prevention of Athletic Injuries, 1993). Osgood-Schlatter disease occurs in children between age 8 and 16 years and is three times more likely to occur in boys than girls. Usually both knees are involved.

Clinical Manifestations

- Knee pain and tenderness
- Swelling of the tibial tubercle
- Difficulty with weight-bearing

Diagnostic Evaluation. Diagnosis is based on the clinical picture presented by the child and X-ray examination.

Therapeutic Management. Treatment is conservative; because the disorder is usually self-limiting, avoiding activities such as kneeling, bicycling, and running provides adequate pain control. In some cases the physician may suggest wrapping the affected knee with elastic bandages. This limits knee flexion, reduces swelling, and provides time for healing.

In severe cases, ice, heat, and nonsteroidal anti-inflammatory medications are helpful. A knee immobilizer or casting with the knee in full extension may be necessary to decrease pain. Activity may be restricted for 6 weeks or more. Improvement is seen within 6 to 8 weeks and the problem disappears once growth stops.

PATHOPHYSIOLOGY *of Osgood-Schlatter Disease*

During the adolescent growth spurt "Sharpey fibres," which anchor the mature patellar tendon, are not yet formed and the tendon is attached by cartilage (Lloyd-Roberts & Fixsen, 1990). Repeated stress placed on the immature tendon insertion site results in tendinitis of the distal infrapatellar tendon. A fracture of the bony epiphysis of the upper tibia may also occur. Repetitive contractions of the quadricep muscles may elevate a small fragment of bone or cartilage from the distal portion of the tibia and contribute to the inflammatory process within the tendon (Weiner, 1993).

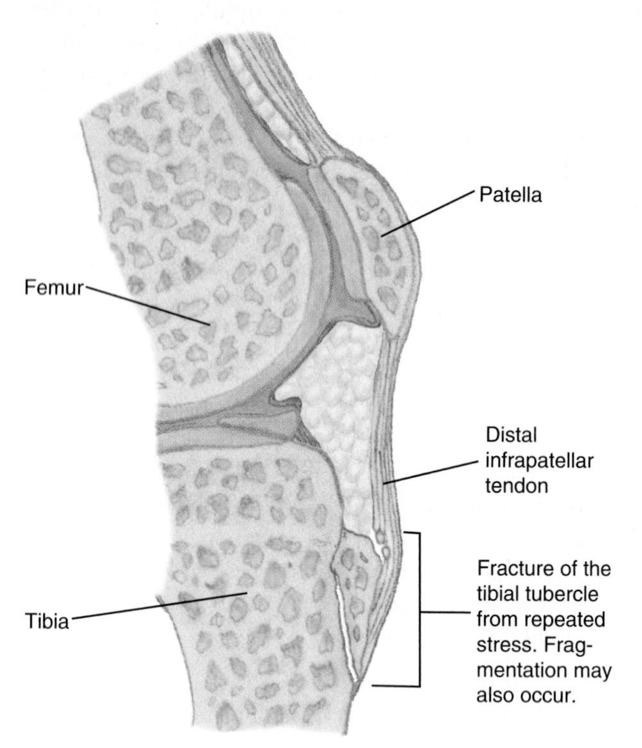
Patella
Femur
Distal infrapatellar tendon
Fracture of the tibial tubercle from repeated stress. Fragmentation may also occur.
Tibia

NURSING CARE OF THE CHILD WITH OSGOOD-SCHLATTER DISEASE

Assessment

Since Osgood-Schlatter disease develops in response to repetitive stress from sports-related activities, the nurse should obtain a thorough history of the child's activities. The knee should be examined for pain, tenderness, and swelling over the proximal tibia.

Pain that is aggravated by activities that require kneeling, running, or climbing stairs is an important feature of this disease. Inability to shift from a squatting to standing position without experiencing pain is highly significant. When asked to identify the area that hurts, the child will point to the tibial tubercle.

Nursing Diagnosis and Planning

The following nursing diagnoses and expected outcomes may be appropriate following assessment of the child with Osgood-Schlatter disease.

- Noncompliance related to age and activity restriction. ***Expected Outcome:*** *The child will accept the treatment plan, as evidenced by increased compliance with activity restriction.*
- Self-Esteem Disturbance related to decreased physical mobility and reduced involvement in age-appropriate activities. ***Expected Outcome:*** *The child will have an increased sense of self-worth, as evidenced by increased peer activities, involvement in school activities, and decreased periods of solitude.*
- Knowledge Deficit (parental) related to home care and therapeutic regimen. ***Expected Outcome:*** *The parents will demonstrate appropriate knowledge of the child's home care, as evidenced by verbalizing an understanding of the child's treatment plan and identifying concerns or issues regarding home care.*

Implementation

Nurses working with school-age children and adolescents should have a clear understanding of Osgood-Schlatter disease. A simple complaint of knee pain could easily be overlooked or incorrectly diagnosed. As a result, more serious problems could occur. Assessment of a child with Osgood-Schlatter disease includes inspection of the knee for swelling and tenderness. Range of motion and weight-bearing should also be evaluated. Inability to move from a squatting to standing position without experiencing pain is characteristic of Osgood-Schlatter disease and the physician should be notified.

The restrictions placed on the child's activity may interfere with the healthy development of peer relationships and self-esteem. Missing school or sports-related activities, limited interactions with peers, or even the need for special arrangements to participate in a peer-related activity contribute to the child's sense of isolation and alienation. Continued contact with peers is important to help the child achieve age-appropriate developmental tasks.

Parents need to be encouraged to express their fears and concerns. Since prevention of sports-related injuries should be the primary concern among all those involved in youth athletic participation, injury prevention education should be provided by the school nurse to all children involved in athletics (Ostrum, 1993).

Home Care. Parents may need reassurance that the child will indeed outgrow this problem. Although this disease is self-limiting, activity restrictions must be clearly understood by the parents. Before the child continues to engage in athletics, the parents and child should discuss the advisability of such activities with their physician. Hamstring stretching exercises may be helpful, but frequently physical therapy is required. This can prove to be expensive.

Evaluation

After treatment/healing:

- Does the child have full ROM and is he free of pain?
- Do the parents verbalize an understanding of the child's treatment regimen?
- Do the parents provide developmentally appropriate activities for their child?

LEGG-CALVE-PERTHES DISEASE

Legg-Calvé-Perthes disease (LCP), also known as **osteochondritis** deformans juvenilis or coxa plana, is a self-limiting disorder in which there is avascular necrosis of the femoral head. The child suffers from a painful limp that is exacerbated by activities such as walking or running.

Incidence. The incidence of LCP is approximately 15 per 100,000; it is five times more likely to occur in boys than girls (Rang, 1993). It occurs most frequently in boys between ages 4 and 8 years. Unilateral hip involvement is more common than bilateral. This disease is rare in African Americans and Asians.

Etiology. Although the cause of LCP is unknown, it is widely accepted that this is a disorder of growth. Weiner (1993) describes the child most susceptible to this disease as a blue-eyed male with very fine light-colored hair who is very alert, active, and shorter in stature than his peers.

Clinical Manifestations

- Complaints of hip/knee soreness or stiffness
- Painful limp
- Quadricep muscle atrophy

Diagnostic Evaluation. Diagnosis is made by radiographic examination. A bone scan or magnetic resonance imaging may reveal necrosis and irregularity of the femoral head. However, in the vast majority of cases plain X-rays of the femoral head easily diagnose the problem.

Therapeutic Management. The goal of treatment is to maintain the spherical shape of the femoral head as it regenerates and reduce the risk of permanent stiffness and degenerative arthritis. To accomplish this goal, the femoral head must be maintained in the acetabulum and protected from the stress of weight-bearing during the healing process. In addition, synovitis must be reduced if ROM is to improve. Some physicians do not believe weight-bearing is harmful as long as the femur remains in the acetabulum.

The femoral head is abducted and internally rotated in relation to the acetabulum through some type of "containment" that uses the acetabulum to maintain the spherical shape of the femoral head. Containment prevents the acetabulum from rubbing against the weakened portion of the femoral head and creating a flat shape. Methods of containment include traction, bracing, and surgical intervention.

Because LCP is first identified by the child's complaints of a painful, stiff hip joint, it is quite possible that the physician will hospitalize the child for non–weight-bearing ROM exercises and bed rest. If improvement is not seen within a week to 10 days and the child is still unable to abduct the hip, alternative methods of treatment are usually begun.

Surgical procedures include an osteotomy, which places the femur more securely into the acetabulum, or an innominate osteotomy, which rotates the acetabulum to completely cover the femoral head. Many physicians recommend surgical intervention because it reduces treatment time and eliminates problems with compliance.

Nonsurgical intervention involves bed rest and the use of traction, casts, or braces to position the femoral head in the acetabulum. This is accomplished by abducting the leg. The child may have to be hospitalized if traction is used. Following traction, the child will be fitted with a non–weight-bearing brace that prevents weight-bearing on the affected side. Remember for any brace to be effective the hip must move freely. Also, non–weight-bearing exercises are needed to maintain muscle integrity while the child wears the brace. Children may spend up to 1 to 3 years in non–weight-bearing braces.

PATHOPHYSIOLOGY *of Legg-Calvé-Perthes Disease*

A disturbance in the blood supply to the femoral epiphysis results in avascular necrosis of the femoral head. The most serious problem associated with LCP is the risk of permanent deformity. If the femoral head protrudes outside the acetabulum and the healing process within the femoral head is incomplete, over time the femoral head will flatten and take on a misshapen appearance. This could lead to problems with arthritis (Weiner, 1993).

The disease is considered self-limiting and is classified by the extent of the femoral head involvement and by the stage of the disease. The disease usually progresses through four stages. The disease generally lasts 1 to 2 years.

Stage 1, synovitis, lasts several weeks. During this stage the epiphysis begins to show the results of ischemia. The synovitis produces stiffness and pain. Stage 2 may last for 6 to 12 months and involves necrosis of bone cells. X-rays show a reduction in size and increased density of the femoral head. Once necrosis occurs, the bone weakens and dies, causing collapse of the femoral head. Stage 3 is the fragmentation stage in which avascular bone is reabsorbed. Healing occurs as new bone is formed. This process can last as long as 1 to 2 years. Stage 4 is called reconstitution, which results in final healing (Staheli, 1992).

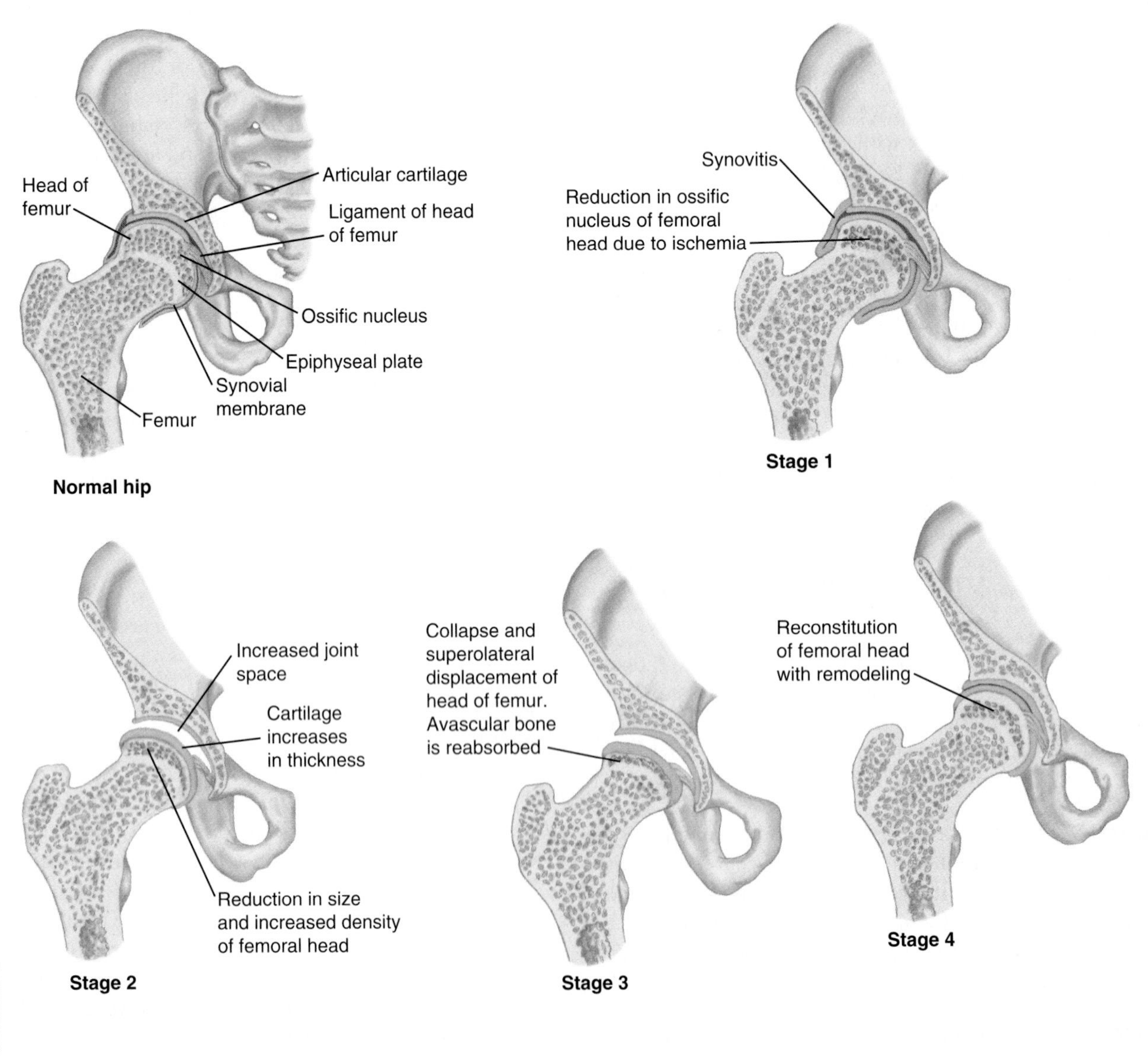

NURSING CARE OF THE CHILD WITH LEGG-CALVE-PERTHES DISEASE

Assessment

Assessment of a child with LCP reveals loss of internal hip rotation and limited abduction. The nurse should determine how long the child has been limping as well as the severity of the pain. The pain may be referred to the thigh or knee. The child will describe the pain as increasing with activity and decreasing with rest. A physical examination of the extremity may reveal muscle wasting of the thigh and buttock, which is a reflection of disuse. Shortening of the extremity on the affected side indicates collapse of the femoral head.

Nursing Diagnosis and Planning

The following nursing diagnoses and expected outcomes may be appropriate following assessment of the child with Legg-Calvé-Perthes disease.

- Risk for Injury related to necrosis and collapse of the femoral head. ***Expected Outcome:*** *The child will remain free of injury, as evidenced by age-appropriate neurovascular functioning and no evidence of permanent hip deformity.*
- Impaired Physical Mobility related to the disease process and activity restrictions. ***Expected Outcome:*** *The child will tolerate activity restrictions, as evidenced by increased compliance with braces or crutches.*
- Risk for Impaired Skin Integrity related to brace or traction. ***Expected Outcome:*** *The child will maintain skin integrity, as evidenced by smooth, clear, and unbroken skin.*
- Body Image Disturbance related to corrective brace or cast. ***Expected Outcome:*** *The child will have an increased sense of self-esteem and self-worth, as evidenced by increased peer activity and age-appropriate behaviors.*
- Knowledge Deficit related to disease process and home care needs. ***Expected Outcomes:*** *The parents will provide safe home care; demonstrate the correct use of the brace or crutches; perform neurovascular assessments; provide age-appropriate activities for their child.*

Implementation

Activity restrictions are perhaps one of the most problematic areas in the care of a child with LCP. The child may experience frustration and anger when unable to meet the physical and social demands of peers. Initially the child may appear to adjust to the lifestyle restrictions, but the nurse must be alert to subtle indicators of rebelliousness and uncooperativeness. Other children will adapt quickly to the appliance they wear and demonstrate incredible activity levels. Never confuse a child's refusal to comply with treatment regimens as an example of maladaptive behavior. The demands to keep up with their peers are sometimes so great that children are simply unable to make cognitively appropriate choices regarding their health.

Returning to school with a brace or cast poses unique problems as well. To facilitate the child's return to school, both the school nurse and the child's teacher should be involved in the discharge planning. It is important that the child participate in as many school-related activities as possible. Acknowledging the child's mobility limitations and working with school officials to identify appropriate alternatives will ensure a successful school re-entry. Emphasizing hobbies and other creative activities provides ways for the child to excel and feel a sense of accomplishment.

Home Care. Because the child will receive the majority of his or her care as an outpatient, nursing care should focus on home care and management of the appliance selected for therapy. Parents will need information concerning the purpose, application, and care of the appliance. The issue of compliance and the role it will play in the healing process must be clearly understood by the family. Parents will need to learn how to perform neurovascular assessments. Also, safety issues regarding the child's mobility when wearing the brace should be identified. The physical therapist and occupational therapist are important resources for the parents.

The purpose of any brace or cast used to treat LCP is to distribute the weight of the child to the ischial tuberosities. By design, the appliance will place additional stress on the child's skin. The condition of the skin should be assessed frequently and friction areas identified. Parents should be taught to check bony prominences; any reddened area on the skin that persists longer than 20 to 30 minutes demands immediate attention.

Mild soaps (Dove, Cetaphil) should be used during bathing. It is generally recommended that moisturizers not be applied to pressure areas. Instead rubbing alcohol (70%) is recommended to toughen the skin. If lotion or moisturizers are used on the skin it is important to wipe the excess off to prevent skin breakdown. Bony prominences should not be massaged. Place protective foam or transparent dressings over susceptible areas. If appropriate, protective clothing should be worn under the brace. Keep the clothing as free from wrinkles as possible.

Evaluation

After treatment/healing:

- Has the child regained full mobility?
- Does the child exhibit normal joint and muscular integrity?
- Has the hip healed without complications?
- Does the child participate in age-appropriate peer and school-related activities?
- Do the parents verbalize an understanding of the child's treatment regimen?
- Are the parents able to provide developmentally appropriate activities for their child?

OSTEOGENESIS IMPERFECTA

Osteogenesis imperfecta, also known as brittle bone disease, is an inherited disorder characterized by connective tissue and bone defects.

> **PATHOPHYSIOLOGY** *of Osteogenesis Imperfecta*
>
> In osteogenesis imperfecta, there is a biochemical defect in the synthesis of collagen. Because collagen is an essential component of connective tissue, the abnormal collagen results in the incomplete development of bones, ligaments, and sclera. Bones are brittle and extremely fragile and fracture easily.

Etiology and Classification. Osteogenesis imperfecta is an inherited disorder. The four types of osteogenesis imperfecta are described in the accompanying box.

Clinical Manifestations

- Blue sclera/cataracts
- Soft transparent skin
- Weak muscles
- Short stature
- Frequent fractures/pathologic fractures
- Hearing problems
- Bony deformities due to bending and bowing of softened bones
- Small brown deformed teeth
- Capillary fragility

Diagnostic Evaluation. The clinical picture is very helpful in diagnosing osteogenesis imperfecta. Genetic testing may be ordered to rule out hereditary problems as well as to advise the parents on the risk of the disease with other children.

> *Classification of Osteogenesis Imperfecta*
>
> **Type I: Autosomal Dominant.** Osteoporosis, excessive bone fragility, blue sclerae, normal teeth, deafness by age 20–30 years. (Most common type; 60% of cases.)
>
> **Type II: Autosomal Recessive.** Lethal. 50% stillborn. Multiple fractures at birth. (10% of cases.)
>
> **Type III: Autosomal Recessive.** Severe bone fragility, multiple fractures, short stature, progressive skeletal deformity, blue sclerae. Seldom survive to adulthood. (25% of cases.)
>
> **Type IV: Autosomal Dominant.** Mild to moderate bone fragility, normal sclerae, short stature. May experience spontaneous improvement at puberty. (6% of cases.)

Therapeutic Management. The goal of treatment is to maintain the integrity of the musculoskeletal system and prevent fractures. Until recently, this was chiefly accomplished through traction, casting, and, in severe cases, supporting the bone with an internal fixation device. Currently, cutting the bone into multiple segments subperiosteally and threading the segments over a stainless steel intramedullary nail has proven very successful. This technique provides stability to the bone while correcting the deformity which itself is the cause of future fractures. Union of the bone fragments is rapid and the surgery is well tolerated. As the child grows the nails may have to be replaced. This procedure appears to be most successful with the femur and tibia. Because of capillary fragility, blood loss must be monitored closely during any surgical procedure and replaced if necessary.

NURSING CARE OF THE CHILD WITH OSTEOGENESIS IMPERFECTA

Assessment

The child with osteogenesis imperfecta has a history of multiple fractures and delayed growth. The extremities may have an angular deformity secondary to old fractures. Upon examination, the nurse may note deformities of the leg and kyphoscoliosis. The child will appear short due to compression fractures of the spine, and joint mobility will be unusual due to relaxed ligaments. Teeth may appear discolored due to abnormal enamel. Too often, because of the child's appearance, people assume that the child is cognitively impaired. Children with osteogenesis imperfecta have normal or above normal intelligence.

Nursing Diagnosis and Planning

The following nursing diagnoses and expected outcomes may be appropriate following assessment of the child with osteogenesis imperfecta.

- Risk for Injury related to bone fragility and fractures. ***Expected Outcome:*** *The child will remain free from injury, as evidenced by age-appropriate neurovascular functioning, decreased fractures, and increased activity tolerance.*
- Ineffective Individual Coping/Ineffective Family Coping: Compromised, related to the chronic aspects of the disease. ***Expected Outcomes:*** *The child/family will cope effectively with the disease process, as evidenced by increased verbalization of fears and concerns; the child will demonstrate decreased regressive behaviors and increased involvement in age-appropriate activities.*

- Altered Growth and Development related to activity restrictions and decreased peer interaction. ***Expected Outcome:*** *The child will demonstrate appropriate developmental behaviors, as evidenced by increased self-care activities, age-appropriate behaviors, and increased peer involvement.*
- Knowledge Deficit related to the disease process and home care. ***Expected Outcomes:*** *The parents will verbalize an understanding of the disease process and rationale for treatment plan; increase participation in the child's care; anticipate the child's return home.*

Implementation

Because there is no effective treatment for this disease, providing care for a child with osteogenesis imperfecta requires attention to detail and the use of anticipatory guidance.

Identifying mobility issues that affect the child's functioning is important. The number one priority should always be prevention of fractures and maintenance of muscle and joint integrity. Gentle turning, passive ROM exercises, daily skin care, and thorough assessment of high-stress areas of the body are necessary to protect the child from fractures or related complications.

Diet. Excessive weight gain can place undue stress on the musculoskeletal system. Maintaining optimal physiologic functioning is critical if the complications of osteogenesis imperfecta are to be avoided. Attention should be directed toward assessing the nutritional status of the child. Information regarding current dietary habits would be helpful in determining the appropriateness of the child's diet and the need for additional foods.

Parents should be instructed regarding nutritional guidelines that support healthy growth and development. For example, carbohydrates should be the main source of calories. Complex carbohydrates found in fruits, vegetables, legumes, and whole grain cereals are preferable to the simple carbohydrates. High-fiber foods should be included, as should foods high in calcium, including milk, cheeses, and yogurt. If necessary, calcium, magnesium, and vitamin supplements may be added to the diet. From 2 to 3 servings a day of protein sources such as meats, poultry, fish, dry beans, eggs, and nuts should be eaten, depending on the child's age. Fats and sweets should be used sparingly. Fluid intake should be evaluated on an individual basis.

Home Care. Because each child is different, responses to the disease will vary. Coping with a chronic illness (see Chapter 17) that involves repeated hospitalizations and restricted mobility places incredible stress on the child and family. Learning how to accept the illness and how to adapt to the demands of the disease while meeting the needs of the family places stress on the parents' ability to cope. The nurse needs to develop an awareness of family dynamics, determine how the illness is affecting the family system, and assess the effectiveness of current coping strategies. Once this is done, appropriate interventions should be developed that address problematic areas.

Parents will need assistance with dressing and bathing the child. Clothing may have to be altered to allow for ease in dressing and undressing. If the child is to be discharged with a cast, the nurse should review principles of cast care and assessment of neurovascular status. Because of the risk of accidental fractures the nurse should review principles of safety during play as well as normal activities. A home referral may be appropriate to assist the family in the transition from hospital to home.

Evaluation

Following treatment,

- Is the child free from injury?
- Is neurovascular function normal?
- Is the child coping effectively with the disease process?
- Is the child involved in age-appropriate activities?
- Do the parents provide safe and effective home care?

JUVENILE RHEUMATOID ARTHRITIS

Juvenile rheumatoid arthritis (JRA) is an autoimmune inflammatory disease with no known cause. Although arthritis in children is most frequently called juvenile rheumatoid arthritis (JRA), the term is somewhat misleading in that it implies a positive rheumatoid factor (RF+), which is not always present in children with the disease. Because arthritis in children can manifest a number of different forms, each with a different treatment protocol and prognosis, a more accurate term is juvenile arthritis (JA).

Regardless of which term is used, there is overwhelming consensus that this is a systemic multisystem disorder that affects the body's connective tissue. It is characterized by joint swelling with limited ROM accompanied by pain, tenderness, and inflammation of one or more joints. For diagnostic purposes, the symptoms must be present 6 weeks or more.

Juvenile arthritis, one of the more common chronic diseases in children, is the leading cause of blindness and disability in children. JA is not a childhood version of rheumatoid arthritis. Rather the onset and course of the disease are very clearly defined. Prognosis is considered good but success is influenced by how well the child's growth and developmental needs are integrated into the treatment plan.

Etiology. In spite of extensive research, the cause of JA remains unknown. Infection, trauma, and emotional stress, frequently cited as factors that may trigger the autoimmune response, occur with such frequency in all children that it is difficult to demonstrate a relationship. More recently it is believed that genetic factors called human leukocyte antigens (HLA) may play a role in the development of JA (Hollister, 1995).

PATHOPHYSIOLOGY *of Juvenile Rheumatoid Arthritis*

The synovial joints are the primary structures involved in this rheumatic process. Normally synovial joints are moveable and contain synovium, a highly vascular tissue that produces a clear viscus synovial fluid that nourishes and lubricates cartilage. Cartilage is a firm resilient tissue that allows smooth articulation of bone ends. It also functions as a cushion to absorb the impact of movement.

In JA, immune complexes in blood and synovial tissue initiate the inflammatory response by activating the plasma protein complement. Kinin and prostaglandin are released, increasing the permeability of blood vessels in the synovial membranes and attracting leukocytes and lymphocytes to the synovial membrane. Phagocytic activity by neutrophils and macrophages ingest the immune complexes and as a result, enzymes are released and damage the articular surfaces of the joint (McCance & Huether, 1990).

As the synovium becomes inflamed, excessive fluid is produced. Unlike normal synovial fluid, this fluid is thin, watery, and lacks mucin. The synovium swells and thickened villi and nodules protrude into the joint cavity. Pannus formation occurs over the articular cartilage.

Periarticular structures outside the joint may also become involved. With further deterioration, the articular cartilage and contiguous bone become eroded and destroyed. The alignment, angle of tendon pull, ROM, and stability of the joint are affected. Restriction in the joint capsule and ligaments leads to limited joint movement and tendinitis. Adhesions between joint surfaces, **ankylosis** of the joints, and soft tissue contracture may occur if the process persists long enough.

Incidence. Juvenile arthritis affects approximately 250,000 children in the United States. It occurs before age 16; although the greatest number of cases occur between the toddler and adolescent years, prevalence is greatest between ages 1 and 3 years and ages 8 and 12 years (Page-Goertz, 1989). JA seldom occurs before age 6 months and is twice as likely to occur in girls than boys.

Clinical Manifestations

- Intermittent joint pain that lasts longer than 6 weeks.
- Joint may appear painful, stiff, swollen, warm to touch (no redness) with limited ROM.
- Morning stiffness.
- Child may protect the affected joint or refuse to walk.
- Systemic symptoms include malaise, fatigue, and lethargy.
- Anorexia, weight loss, and growth problems.
- History of late afternoon fever with temperature spiking up to 105°F.

Diagnostic Evaluation. The early diagnosis of JA is based on criteria established by the American Rheumatism Association (Emery & Miller, 1993) and focuses on the recognition of three distinct modes of onset: pauciarticular, polyarticular, and systemic onset (see Table 36–2). The character, frequency, and severity of the systemic and articular manifestations are also considered critical elements in the diagnostic process.

Therapeutic Management. The goals of therapeutic management are supportive and directed toward preserving joint function, controlling the inflammatory process, minimizing deformity, and reducing the impact the disease may have on the development of the child. These goals are accomplished through drug therapy, physical and occupational therapies, family education regarding home care, and developmental interventions.

It is important to remember that none of these treatment modalities are curative. However, when used appropriately, synovitis can be reduced, mobility increased, and the child's growth and developmental needs appropriately addressed.

Drug Therapy. The major groups of drugs used to suppress the inflammatory process and control pain are the nonsteroidal anti-inflammatory agents (NSAIDs) and the slower-acting or disease-modifying antirheumatic drugs (SAARDs) (see Table 36–3). These drugs may be given alone or in combination until the desired effect is achieved (Page, 1991).

Corticosteroid (e.g., prednisone) use is limited in the treatment of JA. Despite anti-inflammatory properties, their use neither cures JA nor prevents long-term joint damage. Moreover, the chronic side effects that frequently occur can be problematic for children. Indications for use are limited to life-threatening complications of JA such as pericarditis, profound anemia, and vasculitis.

The use of immunosuppressive and cytotoxic agents has been well established in the treatment of adults with rheumatoid arthritis. In the past 5 years, research has shown that the use of methotrexate provides symptomatic improvement in rheumatoid patients (Fife, 1993). Due to uncertainty regarding long-term effects on the immune and reproductive systems (Rosenberg, 1989), the use of immunosuppressive agents (e.g., cyclophospha-

TABLE 36–2 *Clinical Presentation of Juvenile Arthritis*

	INCIDENCE	JOINT INVOLVEMENT	CLINICAL MANIFESTATIONS	LABORATORY VALUES	COMPLICATIONS
Systemic "Still Disease"	15% of all JRA; more common in males	Any joint	Daily intermittent fever (up to 105°) Evanescent maculopapular rash Hepatosplenomegaly	Leukocytosis Anemia ↑ ESR ↑ CRP RF negative ANA negative	25–35% go on to severe crippling arthritis High mortality rate
Polyarticular	30–35% of all JRA Both types more common in females	5 or more joints Symmetrical involvement Any joint affected, but wrist, hands, feet most common	Mild systemic symptoms Low-grade temperature Fatigue Slowed growth	↑ ESR	Permanent deformities secondary to chronic arthritis
Subtype I (RF+)	10% more common 8–10 years of age				
Subtype II (RF−)	25% less crippling deformities than RF+				
Pauciarticular	50% of all JRA	4 or less joints Asymmetrical; knee most common	Infrequent systemic symptoms	May see mild leukocytosis ↑ ESR Maybe ANA + anemia	Iridocyclitis which leads to blindness
Early onset subtype 1	5–10% females below 6 years	Involves knees, ankles, elbows		HLA-DR5 antigen+	Leg length discrepancies Muscle atrophy Chronic iridocyclitis
Late onset subtype 2	5–10% boys over 8 years Family history of arthritis	Knees, ankles, toes		HLA-B27 antigen+	Spondyloarthritis Acute iridocyclitis
subtype 3	10–15%	3 or 4 joints involved	Begin as pauciarticular but evolve into polyarticular arthritis	ANA	Best prognosis

ESR = erythrocyte sedimentation rate, CRP = C-reactive protein, ANA = antinuclear antibodies.

Data from Gewanter, H. L. (1992). Juvenile arthritis. In R. A. Haekelman, S. B. Friedman, N. M. Nelson, & H. M. Seidel (Eds.), *Pediatric primary care* (2nd ed., pp. 1314–1320). St. Louis: C. V. Mosby.

TABLE 36-3 *Medications Commonly Used in the Treatment of Juvenile Arthritis*

TYPE	COMMENTS	SIDE EFFECTS	NURSING IMPLICATIONS
NSAIDs			
Acetylsalicylic acid (ASA) Naproxen sodium (Naprosyn) Tolmetin sodium (Tolectin) Ibuprofen (Advil)	Rapid-acting Inhibits synthesis of prostaglandins Increase dose stepwise over 4–6 week period	Epigastric distress GI upset Nausea/vomiting Bleeding problems Occult blood/GI Tinnitus (ASA)	Administer with food. Monitor therapeutic blood level (20–30 mg/dl) (ASA). Monitor CBC, platelet count, and prothrombin and bleeding times.
SAARDs			
Hydroxychloroquine Gold salts D-penicillamine Auranofin (oral preparation)	Used in children with progressive loss of joint function and poor response to NSAIDs May be administered in conjunction with NSAIDs	Gold salts IM: Auranofin PO: Skin rash Leukopenia Thrombocytopenia Hematuria Proteinuria Oral ulcers D-penicillamine PO: Similar to gold plus GI upset Hydroxychloroquine PO: Nausea/vomiting Anorexia Diarrhea Retinal deposits	Obtain baseline WBCs, platelets, and LFTs. Alternate injection sites. Monitor urine for blood and protein. Oral hygiene. Assess oral mucosa for irritation. Eye exam every month. Give with food or milk.

mides, methotrexate, and chlorambucil) is reserved for children with JA who are unresponsive to conventional treatment (NSAIDs). Side effects of these drugs include increased susceptibility to viral and fungal infections and bone marrow suppression.

Physical and Occupational Therapies. By controlling the synovitis of JA, drug therapy plays a role in preventing musculoskeletal problems. However, preserving muscle integrity and joint mobility is equally important. A joint not adequately supported by strong muscle is more prone to deformity. As muscle strength is lost, inactivity and further muscle wasting occurs. Range of motion is limited and general weakness of the extremity occurs. These musculoskeletal problems place the child at risk for impaired mobility, contractures, and altered growth and development.

The overall rehabilitation goals of JA are designed to prevent such problems from occurring. This is done by maintaining or restoring functional ROM in each joint and strengthening muscles surrounding the affected joints (Emery & Bowyer, 1991). This is best achieved through a program of rest, proper positioning, and exercises that have been developed by occupational and physical therapists. To ensure compliance when developing these aerobic exercise programs, the child's school and extracurricular activities should be considered.

To maximize the effectiveness of the exercise program, a thorough evaluation of the strengths and limitations of the child's joints must be obtained. With this information, an individualized exercise program can be developed. Swimming is an excellent way for the child to exercise. The warmth of the water coupled with the mild resistance it provides makes swimming the perfect medium for strengthening and ROM exercises while protecting the joint. When exercising, the child should focus on the joints that are most limited (Page-Goertz, 1989).

Children have a natural tendency to be active. All of this activity helps maintain normal muscle and joint integrity. Children with JA are no different. During remissions of the disease, their activity level assists in the maintenance of muscle strength. However during painful exacerbations of the disease, the child's natural reaction is to rest the painful joint. This inactivity could lead to muscle wasting and flexion deformity.

During painful episodes, hot or cold packs, splinting, and positioning the affected joint in a neutral position help reduce the pain. Although resting the extremity is appropriate, it is important to begin simple isometric or tensing exercises as soon as the child is able. These exercises are appropriate during exacerbations of the disease because they do not involve joint movement.

Besides physical and occupational therapy, several other treatment modalities have proven effective. The use of ultrasound, cold, and electrical stimulation assist in controlling the child's pain and increasing joint mobility. Heat also helps reduce joint stiffness and muscle spasm because the fibrous tissue found in joints and tendons yields better to stretching when it is heated. Examples of heat therapies include hot baths, whirlpools, hydrocollator packs, and paraffin baths.

Surgical Treatment. Surgical intervention is considered when the child or adolescent is having problems with joint contractures and unequal growth of extremities. This type of treatment can range from diagnostic procedures such as arthroscopic examination or open biopsy to soft tissue release (tenotomy) for contractures. Surgery to correct leg length discrepancies as well as arthroplasty and joint replacement may also be necessary.

Family Education. As part of the multidisciplinary approach, the nurse must take an active part in helping the parents and child learn how to cope with and adapt to the limitations of the disease. Because the majority of the child's care will occur in the home, the success of the therapeutic plan will be determined by the parents. Discharge planning is begun the moment the child is admitted. The parents should be involved in as many nursing activities as possible. This will reduce their anxiety and increase their sense of control over a very frightening situation.

NURSING CARE OF THE CHILD WITH JUVENILE RHEUMATOID ARTHRITIS

Assessment

Nursing assessment of the child with juvenile arthritis should begin with a thorough assessment of the child. Particular attention should be given to the status of the affected joints, the physical restrictions placed on the child, and the level and intensity of the pain as well as the child's and family's response to the disease process.

Any child with documented joint swelling or pain that has lasted longer than 6 weeks should be suspected of having JA. Because children may present with only one joint involved it is possible that JA will not even be considered. The joint should be examined for warmth, tenderness, pain, and limited ROM. Because children are not always able to clearly identify the problem, the nurse should be alert for increased irritability, guarding of the painful joint, or even refusal to bear weight. The child may limp or favor the extremity.

Because pain is a major component of this disease, the nurse should attempt to determine the intensity and severity of the pain. Activities that increase the pain should be determined as well as what the child does when the pain starts. The nurse should also explore with the child methods used to relieve the pain and if they were effective.

Joint stiffness should be assessed as well. With JA the stiffness is most noticeable in the morning and after long periods of inactivity. The duration of the stiffness and the child's description of how difficult it is to move around after periods of inactivity are important parts of the assessment. It is important to remember that the nonverbal child cannot complain about the pain. The parent may describe the child as very fussy and irritable in the morning. The young child may be reluctant to walk and want to be carried.

The presence of systemic involvement should be assessed as well. A history of temperature elevations, especially in the late afternoon or evening, is considered significant. The nurse should determine if a rash occurs with the fever. Anorexia, weight loss, and failure to grow may be the first indicators that something is wrong. The parent may complain the child is not sleeping at night or simply describe the child as irritable and fussy. Lethargy and malaise may also occur.

During the physical examination, the nurse should assess for lymphadenopathy, hepatosplenomegaly, and visual problems. Uveitis will only be apparent with a slit lamp examination. An accurate height and weight should be obtained and if possible, past growth parameters should be plotted on a growth chart to determine alterations in growth problems. Cardiac and respiratory assessment provides baseline information that will allow early detection of pericarditis and pleuritis.

Nursing Diagnosis

- Risk for Injury related to joint inflammation and synovitis
- Pain related to inflammatory process and painful joint and muscle weakness
- Impaired Physical Mobility related to inflammation of the joint and associated muscle weakness
- Altered Growth and Development related to activity intolerance
- Body Image Disturbance related to activity intolerance
- Altered Role Performance related to activity intolerance
- Knowledge Deficit related to care and treatment of JA

Planning, Implementation, and Evaluation: The Child With Juvenile Rheumatoid Arthritis

NURSING DIAGNOSIS • Risk for Injury related to joint inflammation and synovitis

Expected Outcome: • The child will remain free from injury, as evidenced by absence of joint inflammation, age-appropriate range of motion and muscle strength with no residual deformity.

Intervention	Rationale
1. Assess affected joints and muscles at least once a shift; note changes in pain, swelling, tenderness, or ROM.	Provides baseline information that will allow early detection and treatment of complications.
2. During periods of inflammation use splints, heat/cold, and positioning with support to protect the affected joint and reduce the occurrence of deformities.	Treatment modalities such as heat and splinting maintain position and function of the joint.
3. Administer NSAIDs as ordered. Assess child's response to the medications; monitor side effects and blood levels. Notify the physician of any untoward problems.	Anti-inflammatory medications reduce inflammation and control synovitis; joint function remains intact.
4. Assess complications related to inflammation and limited mobility, such as contractures and muscle wasting.	Early detection and treatment of JA-related complications reduces the long-term effects.
5. Chicken pox (varicella) and influenza vaccines should be administered; if child is receiving aspirin, be alert for manifestations of viral illness. If viral illness is suspected, aspirin should be stopped and another NSAID prescribed.	There is a strong link between Reye's syndrome, viral illnesses, and the use of aspirin.
6. If child receives immunosuppressant drugs, assess periodically for manifestations of infection. Keep child away from large crowds during peak flu season.	Immunosuppressant drugs reduce the child's ability to fight infection. Bone marrow depression is a serious problem with immunosuppressants.
7. Assess for visual complications of iridocyclitis. Stress importance of keeping scheduled appointments with ophthalmologist.	Ongoing assessment will prevent permanent visual impairment.

Evaluation: • The child will remain free from injury, as evidenced by appropriate joint mobility and muscle strength, and no residual complications.

NURSING DIAGNOSIS • Pain related to inflammatory process and painful joint and muscle weakness.

Expected Outcome: • The child will experience relief from the pain, as evidenced by increased sleep, decreased restlessness and irritability, and increased use of age-appropriate activities.

Intervention	Rationale
1. Assess child's verbal and nonverbal responses to pain. Assess for increased restlessness, withdrawal, decreased attention span, increased crying, and decreased sleep. (See also Chapter 20, The Child in Pain.)	Provides baseline information regarding child's coping ability. Regression behaviors are more easily identified from base-line information.
2. Administer NSAIDs as ordered; monitor side effects and therapeutic blood levels. Note child's response to medications.	Maintaining therapeutic blood level is the most effective way to control pain and ensure maximum comfort benefits.

Intervention	Rationale
3. Reposition affected joints in neutral position. Support joint with splints, pillows, or other devices. Apply heat or cold. Institute isometric exercises.	Reducing pressure on the affected joint and supporting the joint provides opportunity for healing and prevents the development of contractures.
4. Encourage parents to stay with the child. Assist with diversional activities.	Fear increases the child's perception of pain. The combination of pain medication and diversional activities enhances pain control.
5. Institute comfort measures used at home.	Familiar objects and routines provide a sense of security and aid in the reduction of anxiety.

Evaluation: • The child experiences relief from the pain, as evidenced by resting more comfortably, increased levels of self-care, and age-appropriate developmental activities.

NURSING DIAGNOSIS • Impaired Physical Mobility related to inflammation of the joint and associated muscle weakness

Expected Outcome: • The child will accept the activity restrictions, as evidenced by a decrease in pain, increased compliance with exercise program, and increased joint mobility and muscle strength.

Intervention	Rationale
1. Assist in the development of the exercise program. Incorporate developmental norms into the program. Coordinate referrals, daily routines, and family activities.	Compliance is increased when activity regimen is a normal part of the child's daily life.
2. Assess muscle strength and joint mobility every shift and p.r.n.	Baseline data is essential if an appropriate plan of care is to be developed for the child.
3. Maintain correct body alignment.	Inactive muscles lose tone and strength at a rate of 3%–5% a day, which may lead to loss of muscle mass and tissue breakdown.
4. Perform ROM and stretching exercises as appropriate. Consult with the physician regarding the need for occupational therapy, splints, and/or foot boards.	Joints become fibrotic from disuse, which leads to muscle shortening and joint contractures; exercise facilitates the movement of calcium into the bone.
5. Apply elastic stockings or TEDS.	Promotes venous return and decreases circulatory stasis.
6. Plan age-appropriate play activities that require the use of unaffected extremities.	Exercise will strengthen and enhance muscle and joint integrity; using unaffected extremity reduces problem of synovitis.
7. Offer frequent small feedings of foods high in protein and calcium.	A diet high in calcium and protein will reduce problems associated with a negative nitrogen balance and increased bone catabolism.
8. Maintain age-appropriate hydration levels. Offer fluids that will acidify the urine (e.g., cranberry juice).	Encouraging fluids reduces problems associated with hypercalcemia, renal calculi, and stasis of respiratory secretions.

Intervention	Rationale
9. Maintain urine output at 1–2 ml/kg/hr; check urine at least once a shift for protein, blood, and specific gravity.	Ensuring adequate renal output aids in reducing the incidence of urinary tract infections secondary to urinary stasis and assists in reducing renal calculi.
10. Monitor bowel sounds. Provide increased roughage in the diet and offer favorite foods.	Immobility decreases peristalsis and increases problems with constipation.
11. Assess respiratory status at least once a shift. Encourage coughing and deep breathing; incentive spirometer may be appropriate.	Immobility places the child at risk for stasis of secretions, which may lead to pneumonia and/or atelectasis.

Evaluation: The child has experienced no problems related to immobility, as evidenced by:

- Maintaining muscle and joint integrity
- Experiencing no cardiac or respiratory problems
- Maintaining age-appropriate weight and height
- Adhering to daily exercise program.

NURSING DIAGNOSIS

- Altered Growth and Development related to activity intolerance

Expected Outcome:

- The child will exhibit age-appropriate growth and development, as evidenced by increased cooperation with self-care activities, normal sleep habits, and age-appropriate behaviors.
- The parents will support and maintain appropriate developmental behavior for their child, as evidenced by increased involvement in the child's daily care and increased assistance in helping the child deal with her activity intolerance.

Intervention	Rationale
1. Assess the child's and parents' anxiety. Acknowledge their anxiety and when possible model appropriate behaviors or teach activities that reduce anxiety.	Gathering assessment data is the first step in the nursing process and provides information regarding family strengths and nursing care needs.
2. Maintain a calm, consistent environment. Organize nursing care to allow periods of developmentally appropriate activities. When possible assign the same nursing personnel.	Anxiety can be transferred to the child via parent or staff; a consistent caregiver will provide a sense of security to the child.
3. Recognize the child's need to regress in response to the hospitalization or illness. Accept the behavior and assist the child to regain prior developmental stages when ready.	Schedules, routines, and rituals offer a sense of security to the child. Hospitalization interrupts these routines and creates stressful situations that impact on the child's ability to perform self-care activities such as toileting, sleeping, discipline, and nutrition.
4. Encourage parents to stay with the child; if parents cannot stay, encourage them to leave an article of clothing or other personal item with the child.	The presence of a parent or significant family member can reduce the fear of separation and foster a sense of security.
5. Explain all routines and procedures to the child and parents. Continue to offer explanations until understanding is verbalized by parents and/or child.	The unknown is a powerful influence on the child and increases anxiety; the presence of anxiety decreases the child's and parents' ability to process and analyze information.

Intervention	Rationale
6. Involve the parents in the care of the child when appropriate.	Encouraging the parents to participate in the child's care increases their sense of control and provides the child with a sense of security.
7. Provide age-appropriate play or diversional activities. When possible involve the parents in the child's play. Encouraging expressive activities such as throwing balls through a hoop or bean bags into a basket would be appropriate for a younger child; pounding boards are equally helpful in reducing stress and anxiety; manipulating clay or play dough or expressing anger or frustration through painting would be appropriate activities for the older child.	Therapeutic play provides a safe and effective mechanism for reducing the stress of hospitalization and immobility.
8. Assess coping mechanisms used by the child. Recognize that age, gender, and self-concept play a role in a child's adjustment to a chronic illness. Use anticipatory guidance to assist the child in developing coping mechanisms that will foster the development of optimism and a sense of personal competence.	The use of healthy and appropriate coping mechanisms by the child increases the likelihood that the stressors associated with the chronic illness will not impact negatively on the child's growth and development.

Evaluation:

- The child/parents verbalize increased trust regarding health care providers.
- The child vocally or through play discloses feelings or concerns regarding the illness or hospitalization.
- The parents accept the child's regressive behaviors and become more involved in the child's care.
- The child demonstrates increased levels of control through increased self-care activities and age-appropriate sleep patterns.

NURSING DIAGNOSIS

- Body Image Disturbance and Altered Role Performance related to activity intolerance

Expected Outcome:

- The child will maintain optimal developmental level, as evidenced by age-appropriate behaviors, increased social interactions with friends or peers, and decreased school problems.

Intervention	Rationale
1. Assess child's perception regarding chronic illness. Ask child to draw a picture of perception of body.	Physical changes and failure to "keep up" with friends may cause feelings of being different.
2. Assist child in identifying strengths and areas of accomplishments. Identify creative hobbies or activities child may engage in that will enhance sense of worth.	Recognition of abilities and pride in the child's accomplishments increases self-esteem.
3. Encourage self-care activities. Discuss with parents importance of increasing child's sense of independence.	Autonomy and control are essential in any plan of care if the child is to be compliant and actively participate in her care; overprotection is a common parental reaction to chronic illness.
4. Use age-appropriate therapeutic play materials or support groups to assist the child in identifying areas of concern related to esteem and body image.	Developmental fears and anxieties are not always clear to the child. Play or support groups are safe avenues for the child to explore fears and concerns.

Intervention	Rationale
5. Involve school or related personnel regarding special needs. Assist with school reentry and focus on ways child may participate in age-appropriate activities.	Child's performance and acceptance by peers may be influenced by activity restrictions and frequent absenteeism.

Evaluation: • The child demonstrates age-appropriate behaviors, as evidenced by reentering school without problems and participating in peer-related activities.

NURSING DIAGNOSIS • Knowledge Deficit related to care and treatment of juvenile rheumatoid arthritis

Expected Outcome: • The parents will provide safe home care, as evidenced by accurate knowledge of juvenile arthritis, will be comfortable with the exercise program, and will verbalize an awareness of problems that require appropriate assistance.

Intervention	Rationale
1. Assess parents' level of understanding regarding the disease, treatment, and past experiences with a chronic illness.	Developing a plan of teaching for the parents cannot begin until the nurse has determined the parents' level of knowledge and understanding.
2. Assess risk factors present that might interfere with the child's home care.	Failure to recognize family system dynamics reduces success of home care.
3. Provide parents and child with verbal as well as written discharge instructions. Use return demonstrations to ensure parental understanding of procedures or exercises.	Providing parents with information will increase their self-confidence and assist them in caring for their child in a safe and effective manner.
4. Coordinate medical appointments, referrals, and physical therapy with the child's and parents' routines and schedules.	Organizing medical routines to fit the family's schedule provides a sense of normalcy for the family.
5. Review medications to be given by parents. Discuss side effects, importance of never missing a dose, and emergency situations that require a physician.	The use of anticipatory guidance reduces parental anxiety and facilitates the transition from hospital to home.
6. Use age-appropriate teaching strategies. Allow choices when planning care; provide time for child to discuss treatment regimen. Be alert for indications of anxiety or fatigue.	Compliance with the teaching plan depends on child's understanding of the illness and its management; increases child's coping ability.

Home Care: Children experiencing joint pain will limit their physical activity. They will need encouragement to resume pre-illness activities. If the child has consistently depended on her parents for assistance, the cycle of dependence will be difficult to break. Involving the child in the decision making process, if appropriate, is an excellent way to ensure her cooperation. To maintain developmental levels, a plan of care should be developed that aids the parents in providing age-appropriate activities and that fosters positive reinforcement for independent activities.

Throughout the course of the disease the child will need health and nutritional education and management, orthopedic evaluations to prevent deformities, and periodic eye examinations if iridocyclitis is a problem. Due to the chronic nature of this disease, attention should also be directed to the psychosocial adjustment of the child. Attention should be paid to peer involvement, school performance and the child's integration into the family system. (See Chapter 17.)

Evaluation: The parents provide safe and therapeutic home care, as evidenced by the following:

- Child experiences no untoward effects from treatment
- Exercise program becomes a routine part of child's day
- Parents demonstrate increased knowledge of JA.

MUSCULAR DYSTROPHIES*

Muscular dystrophies are a group of progressively degenerative inherited diseases that affect the muscle cells of specific muscle groups, causing weakness and atrophy. They vary in pattern of inheritance and age of onset, but most are identified in early childhood and are characterized by progressive muscle weakness. Duchenne muscular dystrophy is the most common of several forms of muscular dystrophy. Table 36–4 describes the types of muscular dystrophies of childhood.

Pathophysiology. Over time, muscle fibers degenerate and are replaced by fat and connective tissue. Progressive weakness and wasting of symmetric groups of skeletal muscles results in increasing disability and deformity.

Etiology. Muscular dystrophies are inherited by various genetic patterns. Duchenne muscular dystrophy is a sex-linked recessive disorder and therefore it affects only males. Females are carriers and pass the defect to their male children.

Incidence. Duchenne muscular dystrophy occurs in 1:3000 male children. Spontaneous mutations are responsible for 30% or more of those affected; therefore, many of these children have no family history of the disorder. Other forms of muscular dystrophy are less common, with varying patterns of inheritance (see Table 36–3). Females may be affected by some forms.

Clinical Manifestations

- Progressive symmetrical muscle wasting and weakness without loss of sensation.
- Symptoms first appear after walking is achieved (usually age 3 to 7 years).
- Child must use the Gower maneuver to rise from the floor (child puts hands on knees and walks hands up legs until standing erect).
- Gait is waddling and wide-based.
- Muscles of the pelvis and shoulders are most often affected in Duchenne muscular dystrophy.
- The calf muscles are characteristically weak but hypertrophied.
- Increasing disability and deformity include hip and knee contractures, foot deformities, scoliosis, and lordosis.
- Walking ability (Duchenne) is lost by age 9 to 12 years.
- Moderate obesity is common.
- IQ below 90 is common.
- In most forms, lifespan is shortened.
- Cardiopulmonary complications are the most common cause of death.

Diagnostic Evaluation. Children with a positive family history are especially at risk for muscular dystrophy and are monitored for clinical symptoms, which generally do not appear until the preschool years. Serum creatine kinase (CK) is elevated in the early stages of the disease and then will decrease as muscle bulk decreases. Electromyogram and muscle biopsy may also assist with diagnosis.

Therapeutic Management. Therapeutic management of the muscular dystrophies is aimed at maintaining ambulation and independence for as long as possible as muscle weakness progresses. Contractures further reduce mobility and therefore independence. Surgery, bracing, and physical therapy assist in keeping the child as mobile as possible. Later therapy is directed at maximizing sitting capabilities, respiratory function, and self-care. Prevention of obesity to facilitate mobility and care is a priority. Prompt attention to infection, especially in the respiratory tract, is essential.

Prognosis. Children with Duchenne muscular dystrophy rarely live beyond age 20. Death usually occurs as a result of respiratory complications, which may be compounded by spinal deformities.

NURSING CARE OF THE CHILD WITH MUSCULAR DYSTROPHY

Assessment

Where there is a family history of muscular dystrophy, infants and young children need to be monitored carefully for the possibility of muscular dystrophy. When a positive

*The Muscular Dystrophies section was written by Judith W. Gross, PhD, RN.

TABLE 36-4 *Muscular Dystrophies of Childhood*

TYPE	ONSET/PROGRESSION	INHERITANCE/INCIDENCE	CLINICAL MANIFESTATIONS
Duchenne	Onset: 1–4 yr Rapidly progressive; loss of walking by 9 to 10 yr; death in late teens from respiratory failure, heart failure, pneumonia.	X-linked recessive Most common hereditary neuromuscular disease. Affects all races. Incidence: 1:3000 male infants	Progressive generalized weakness and muscle wasting affecting limb and trunk muscles first; calves often enlarged; waddling gait; lordosis; cardiomyopathy; Gower maneuver; mental retardation common.
Myotonic (Steinert Disease)	Onset: In severe neonatal form: weakness at birth, may have paralysis of diaphragm. If child survives early weeks of life, steady improvement in motor function over the first decade, usually developing ability to walk. Often survive to late adulthood.	Autosomal dominant Incidence: 1:30,000	In the severe neonatal form, hypotonia and weakness at birth. Others may appear normal at birth. Mild weakness in first few years, with progressive muscle wasting of distal muscles. Myotonia worsened by cold, fatigue, stress. Mental retardation in about half of cases.
Becker	Onset: 5–10 yr Slowly progressive; maintain walking past early teens; life span into third decade.	X-linked recessive Incidence: 1:20,000 births	Almost identical to Duchenne but less severe; child is mobile until late teens; normal intelligence.
Congenital	Onset: Birth Typically slow but variable; many do not attain walking. Shortened life span.	Autosomal recessive Incidence: Rare	Generalized muscle weakness with possible joint deformities; hypotonia. Mental retardation and seizures common in types with CNS disease.
Facioscapulohumeral (FSH or Landouzy-Dejerine Disease)	Onset: First decade Slowly progressive loss of walking in later life; variable life expectancy; disease may span many decades.	Autosomal dominant or recessive Incidence: 3–10:million births	Earliest and most severe weakness occurs in facial and shoulder girdle muscles. May be unable to close eyes completely during sleep. Progressive disability, leading to inability to walk. May be mild, causing minimal disability.
Emery-Dreifus (Scapuloperoneal or Scapulolhumeral)	Onset: Middle childhood to early teens Progression is very slow; many survive to late adulthood.	X-linked recessive Incidence: Rare	Contractures of elbows and ankles develop early; shoulder muscles become wasted. Slowly progressive with eventual cardiac abnormality.

diagnosis is made, nursing intervention can become a major source of support for these children and their families. The family's ability to cope with chronic illness and the poor prognosis of muscular dystrophy need to be assessed. Over time, monitoring the child's mobility and self-care abilities to assure independence for as long as possible are essential. The potential for weight gain, respiratory infection, and the need for adequate support systems must be attended to regularly.

Nursing Diagnosis and Planning

The following nursing diagnoses and expected outcomes may be appropriate following assessment of the child with muscular dystrophy.

- Impaired Physical Mobility related to progressive muscle wasting, contractures, and deformity. ***Expected Outcome:*** *The child will remain as physically active as possible for as long as possible.*
- Ineffective Breathing Pattern related to progressively weakening respiratory muscles. ***Expected Outcome:*** *The child will maintain optimum respiratory function for as long as possible.*
- Self-Care Deficit related to weakness and inability to care for self. ***Expected Outcome:*** *The child will perform self-care for as long as possible.*
- Altered Nutrition: Potential for More Than Body Requirements related to reduced activity. ***Expected Outcome:*** *The child will maintain weight within the limits of normal.*

- Risk for Social Isolation related to inability to keep up with peers, frequent illness, hospitalization, and surgeries. ***Expected Outcome:*** *The child will modify activities to maintain peer relationships.*
- Ineffective Family Coping: Compromised, related to increasing demands of care, financial responsibilities, and needs and anxieties of other children. ***Expected Outcome:*** *The family will identify ways to cope effectively with the fears and frustrations of living with a progressive illness.*
- Anticipatory Grieving (family) related to child's poor prognosis. ***Expected Outcome:*** *The family will cope with the stressors of the child's illness and prognosis.*
- Knowledge Deficit related to complex care necessary for child with chronic disorder. ***Expected Outcome:*** *The parents will demonstrate the ability to care for the child without overprotection.*

Implementation

Nursing care for the child with muscular dystrophy is complex and long term, and involves the coordination of a variety of health care services. Anticipating the child's future needs requires a sensitive yet knowledgeable approach and the coordination of a variety of services. Maintenance of activity and self-care activities are important to the child and the family. Independence must be fostered within the limits of safety. Activities such as swimming, which promote ROM and mobility for as long as possible, are helpful. Later, activities that allow for reduced energy expenditure but keep the child involved with peers can be suggested.

Because the child in the later stages of Duchenne muscular dystrophy is unable to move himself, the nurse and family must assist with position changes every 2 hours to prevent injury to skin and other tissues from prolonged pressure. Adequate fluid intake must be encouraged to prevent urinary stasis. A bowel regimen, including stool softeners or laxatives, may be necessary.

Modifications of the home environment may be needed to allow for wheelchair mobility. Facilities for bathing and toileting may need modification. Creativity in clothing may be needed to allow for ease of dressing while meeting the needs of a child trying to fit in with peer norms.

Specific suggestions about dietary modification to control weight may be necessary. Families need specific ideas about how to make dietary changes for one child only, without creating unnecessary controversy surrounding food. The child needs to be protected from children with respiratory and contagious diseases to reduce the chance of life-threatening respiratory infections. As disability progresses, pulmonary hygiene and respiratory exercises are needed to maintain respiratory function as long as possible.

Regular monitoring by a multispecialty team is an ideal way to meet the varying needs of the child and family as the child's condition changes. Therapy is individualized to the specific needs of the child. Genetic screening and counseling is recommended for parents and siblings of children with muscular dystrophy.

Home Care. Parents must be taught how to perform basic nursing tasks and be referred to agencies that can assist with home care and equipment. Extended family and support groups such as the Muscular Dystrophy Association of America (see Appendix H) can provide needed emotional support and specific assistance as parenting energies are exhausted. Assistance is often needed to develop coping strategies to meet individual and family needs. As the disease progresses and energy wanes, the child is often a victim of social isolation. An electric wheelchair and portable telephone help some families to keep in contact with their child as he cruises in the neighborhood or help the child to maintain contact with his peer group.

In addition, attention to the needs of the grieving family need to be addressed. The student is referred to Chapter 16 (Family-Centered Nursing Care of the Child) and Chapter 17 (The Child With a Chronic Condition or Terminal Illness) for further study about the care of these children.

Evaluation

- Has child achieved maximum level of functioning?
- Do the family and child use adaptive equipment as necessary for positioning and mobility?
- Is the child as independent as possible?
- Does the child participate in family and peer activities?
- Can the family verbalize accurate knowledge about the condition and its management?

KEY CONCEPTS

- Because musculoskeletal problems are frequently caused by trauma, nursing assessment should always begin with a thorough assessment of the child's airway, breathing, and circulation.
- The cause of the musculoskeletal injury must be determined because nonaccidental trauma or child abuse may be involved.
- An open fracture, in which there is a wound or break in the skin, increases the possibility of infection.
- Immobilization of fractures involves the repositioning of the bone fragments (reduction) and the application of a cast or traction to maintain alignment (retention) until healing occurs.

- Tissue ischemia and nerve damage are serious complications that may occur following a fracture. Neurovascular assessment includes skin color, capillary refill, temperature, and sensation of the extremity. The quality of the pulse distal to the fracture site should also be evaluated and compared with the uninjured extremity.
- When evaluating neurovascular status after a musculoskeletal injury, always remember to assess for the five "Ps" of ischemia: pain, pallor, pulselessness, paresthesia, and paralysis.
- Nursing care of the child with osteomyelitis includes assessment and documentation of the child's status, support and immobilization of the extremity, administration of antibiotics without iatrogenic injury, and careful monitoring of the infusion equipment and IV site.
- Treatment for Osgood-Schlatter disease is conservative and involves limiting activities that require bending or kneeling. These restrictions may interfere with the achievement of developmental milestones and may result in isolation and alienation.
- Nursing care of the child with Osgood-Schlatter disease involves promoting compliance, reassuring the child that the problem is self-limiting, and assisting the child to achieve age-appropriate developmental tasks.
- The main goal of treatment for Legg-Calvé-Perthes disease is to maintain the femoral head in the acetabulum and protect the hip from the stress of weight-bearing during the healing process.
- Nursing outcomes for the child with Legg-Calvé-Perthes disease include compliance with activity restrictions, facilitating home care and management of the appliance selected for treatment, and promoting age-appropriate cognitive and emotional development.
- Osteogenesis imperfecta places the child at risk for pathologic fractures, bony deformities due to bending and bowing of softened bones, and kyphoscoliosis.
- Nursing outcomes for the child with osteogenesis imperfecta include keeping the child free from injury, the development of healthy coping behaviors, and the maintenance of developmental integrity.
- Therapeutic management of juvenile rheumatoid arthritis is supportive and directed toward preserving joint function, controlling the inflammatory process, minimizing deformity, and reducing the impact the disease may have on the development of the child.
- Nursing outcomes for a child with juvenile rheumatoid arthritis are keeping the child free from injury, pain control, enhanced physical mobility, and age-appropriate developmental behaviors.
- Nursing outcomes for a child with muscular dystrophy are maintaining physical activity, promoting respiratory function, weight management, and reducing the importance of the disease on the child's development.

REFERENCES

Allshouse, M., Rouse, T., & Eichelberger, M. (1993). Childhood injury: A current perspective. *Pediatric Emergency Care, 9,* 159–164.

Bamberger, D. (1990). Diagnosis and treatment of osteomyelitis. *Comprehensive Therapy, 16,* 48–53.

Carlino, H. (1991). The child with an Ilizarov external fixator. *Pediatric Nursing, 17,* 355–358.

Dyment, P. G. (1988). Initial management of minor acute soft tissue injuries. *Pediatric Annals, 17,* 99–106.

Emery, H. M., & Bowyer, S. L. (1991). Physical modalities of therapy in pediatric rheumatic diseases. *Rheumatic Disease Clinics of North America, 17,* 1001–1014.

Emery, H. M., & Miller, M. L. (1993). *Ambulatory pediatric care* (2nd ed.). Philadelphia: J. B. Lippincott.

Fife, R. Z. (1993). Methotrexate use in juvenile rheumatoid arthritis. *Orthopaedic Nursing, 12,* 32–36.

Hall, D. E. (1992). Sports injuries. In R. A. Hoekelman, S. B. Friedman, N. M. Nelson, & H. M. Seidel (Eds.), *Pediatric primary care* (pp. 1521–1527). St. Louis: C. V. Mosby.

Herndon, W. (1993). Acute osteomyelitis and septic arthritis. In J. Surpure (Ed.), *Synopsis of pediatric emergency care* (pp. 117–127). Boston: Andover Medical Publishers.

Hollister, J. R. (1995). Rheumatic diseases. In W. W. Hay, J. R. Groothuis, A. R. Hayward, & M. J. Levin (Eds.), *Current pediatric diagnosis and treatment* (12th ed., pp. 807–814). East Norwalk, CT: Appleton and Lange.

Levy, J., & Ward, W. T. (1993). Pediatric femur fractures: An overview of treatment. *Orthopaedics, 16,* 183–190.

Lloyd-Roberts, G. C., & Fixsen, J. (1990). *Orthopedics in infancy and childhood.* Boston: Butterworth-Heinemann.

MacEwen, D., Kasser, J., & Heinrich, S. (1993). *Pediatric fractures: A practical approach to assessment and treatment.* Baltimore: Williams & Wilkins.

McCance, K., & Huether, S. (1990). *Pathophysiology: The biologic basis for disease in adults and children.* St. Louis: C. V. Mosby.

McCarthy, D. L., & Surpure, J. S. (1990). Pediatric trauma: Initial evaluation and stabilization. *Pediatric Annals, 19,* 584–596.

Mann, D. C., & Raymaira, S. (1990). Dislocation of physeal and non-physeal fractures in 1650 bone fractures in children 0–16 years. *Journal of Pediatric Orthopedics, 10,* 713–716.

Mills, N. (1989a). Acute pain behavior in infants and toddlers. In S. G. Funk, E. M. Tornquist, M. T. Champagne, L. A. Copp, & R. A. Wiese (Eds.), *Key aspects of comfort, management of pain, fatigue, and nausea* (pp. 52–59). New York: Springer.

Mills, N. (1989b). Pain behaviors in infants and toddlers. *Journal of Pain and Symptom Management, 4,* 184–190.

National Youth Sports Foundation For the Prevention of Athletic Injuries, Inc. (1993). *Fact sheet—Youth sports injuries.* Needham, MA: Author.

Nixon, J. E. (1989). The lower leg, ankle and foot. In S. Gates & P. Mooar (Eds.), *Orthopaedics and sports medicine for nurses* (pp. 209–237). Baltimore: Williams & Wilkins.

Ostrum, G. (1993). Sports-related injuries in youth: Prevention is the key and nurses can help. *Pediatric Nursing, 19,* 333–342.

Page, G. G. (1991). Chronic pain and the child with juvenile rheumatoid arthritis. *Journal of Pediatric Health Care, 5,* 18–23.

Page-Goertz, S. (1989). Even children have arthritis. *Pediatric Nursing, 15,* 11–16.

Rang, M. (1993). Perthes disease. In D. Wenger & M. Rang (Eds.), *The art and practice of children's orthopaedics* (pp. 297–330). New York: Raven Press.

Rosenberg, A. (1989). Advanced drug therapy for juvenile rheumatoid arthritis. *The Journal of Pediatrics, 114,* 171–178.

Rosenberg, N. M., Vranesich, P., & Bottenfield, G. (1982). Fractured femurs in pediatric patients. *Annals of Emergency Medicine, 11,* 84–85.

Schaefermeyer, R. (1993). Pediatric trauma. *Emergency Medicine Clinics of North America, 11,* 187–205.

Schwentker, E. P. (1992). Osteomyelitis. In R. A. Hoekelman, S. B. Friedman, N. M. Nelson, & H. M. Seidel (Eds.), *Pediatric primary care* (pp. 1413–1416). St. Louis: C. V. Mosby.

Staheli, L. (1992). *Fundamentals of pediatric orthopedics.* New York: Raven Press.

Syrongiannopoulos, G., & Nelson, J. D. (1988). Duration of antimicrobial therapy for acute suppurative osteoarticular infections. *Lancet, 1,* 37–40.

Weiner, D. (1993). *Pediatric orthopedics.* New York: Churchill Livingstone.

BIBLIOGRAPHY

Behrman, R. E., & Vaughan, V. C. (1992). *Nelson textbook of pediatrics* (14th ed.). Philadelphia: W. B. Saunders.

Bubulka, G. M., & Cipolla, F. (1991). Preparing for pediatric emergencies. *Journal of Emergency Nursing, 17,* 236–240.

Campbell, L. S., & Campbell, J. D. (1991). Musculoskeletal trauma in children. *Critical Care Nursing Clinics of North America, 3,* 445–456.

Canale, S. T., & Beaty, J. H. (1991). *Operative pediatric orthopaedics.* St. Louis: Mosby–Year Book.

Carpenito, L. J. (1989). *Nursing diagnosis: Application to clinical practice.* Philadelphia: J. B. Lippincott.

Dyment, P. G. (1991). How to make the sports physical exciting. *Contemporary Pediatrics, 10,* 93–106.

Einhorn, T. (1991). Mechanisms of fracture healing. *Hospital Practice, 26,* 41–45.

Faden, H., & Grossi, M. (1991). Acute osteomyelitis in children. *American Journal of Diseases of Children, 145,* 65–69.

Fantini, F. (1992). Future trends in pediatric rheumatology. *Journal of Rheumatology (Supplement), 37,* 49–53.

Fink, C. W., & Nelson, J. D. (1986). Septic arthritis and osteomyelitis in children. *Clinical Rheumatic Diseases, 12,* 423–435.

Gagliardi, B. A. (1991). The impact of Duchenne muscular dystrophy on families. *Orthopaedic Nursing, 10*(5), 41–48.

Hart, K. (1994). Using the Ilizarov external fixator in bone transport. *Orthopaedic Nursing, 13,* 35–40.

Herndon, W. A., Alexieva, B. T., & Schwindt, M. I. (1985). Nuclear imaging for musculoskeletal infections in children. *Journal of Pediatric Orthopedics, 5,* 343–347.

Hughes, R. B., & D'Ambrosia, K. (1993). Nursing management of a child with juvenile rheumatoid arthritis. *Orthopaedic Nursing, 12,* 17–22.

Jones-Walton, P. (1991). Clinical standards in skeletal pin site care. *Orthopaedic Nursing, 10,* 12–17.

Ledwith, C. A., & Fleisher, G. R. (1992). Slipped capital femoral epiphysis without hip pain leads to missed diagnosis. *Pediatrics, 89,* 660–662.

Mansfield, M. J., & Emans, S. J. (1993). Growth in female gymnasts: Should training decrease during puberty? *Journal of Pediatrics, 122,* 237–240.

Martinez, A. G., Weinstein, S. L., & Dietz, F. R. (1992). The weight-bearing abduction brace for the treatment of Legg-Perthes disease. *The Journal of Bone and Joint Surgery, 74A,* 12–21.

Mason, K. J. (1989). Pediatric orthopaedics: Developmental norms. *Orthopaedic Nursing, 8,* 45–50.

Meehan, P. L., Angel, D., & Nelson, J. M. (1992). The Scottish-Rite abduction orthosis for the treatment of Legg-Perthes disease. *The Journal of Bone and Joint Surgery, 74A,* 2–11.

Morrissy, R. T. (Ed.). (1990). *Lovell & Winter's pediatric orthopaedics* (3rd ed.). Philadelphia: J. B. Lippincott.

Nance, D. K., & Mardjetko, S. M. (1994). Technical aspects and nursing considerations of limb lengthening. *Orthopaedic Nursing, 13,* 21–33.

Nypaver, M., & Treloar, D. (1994). Neutral cervical spine positioning in children. *Annals of Emergency Medicine, 23,* 208–211.

Reed, J. L., & Keegan, M. J. (1993). Fat embolism syndrome: A complication of trauma. *Critical Care Nursing, 13,* 33–37.

Renshaw, T. S. (1986). *Pediatric orthopedics.* Philadelphia: W. B. Saunders.

Rockwood, C. A., Wilkins, K. F., & King, R. E. (Eds.). (1991). *Fractures in children* (3rd ed.). Philadelphia: J. B. Lippincott.

Scoles, P. V. (1988). *Pediatric orthopedics in clinical practice.* (2nd ed.). Chicago: Year Book Medical Publishers.

Sipos, D. A. (1993). M. P. implants for rheumatoid arthritis of the hand. *Orthopaedic Nursing, 12,* 7–14.

Sonzogni, J. J., & Gross, M. (1993). Hip and pelvic injuries in the young: Fractures and special disorders, part 2. *Emergency Medicine, 25,* 18–20+.

Tachdjian, M. O. (1990). *Pediatric orthopaedics* (2nd ed.). Philadelphia: W. B. Saunders.

Unkila-Kallio, L. (1994). Serum C-reactive protein, erythrocyte sedimentation rate, and white blood cell count in acute hematogenous osteomyelitis of children. *Pediatrics, 93,* 59–62.

White, P. H., & Ansell, B. M. (1992). Methotrexate for juvenile rheumatoid arthritis. *New England Journal of Medicine, 326,* 1077–1078.

Williams, P. F., & Cole, W. G. (Eds.). (1991). *Orthopaedic management in childhood* (2nd ed.). London: Chapman and Hall.

37

The Child With Structural Disorders of the Bones and Joints

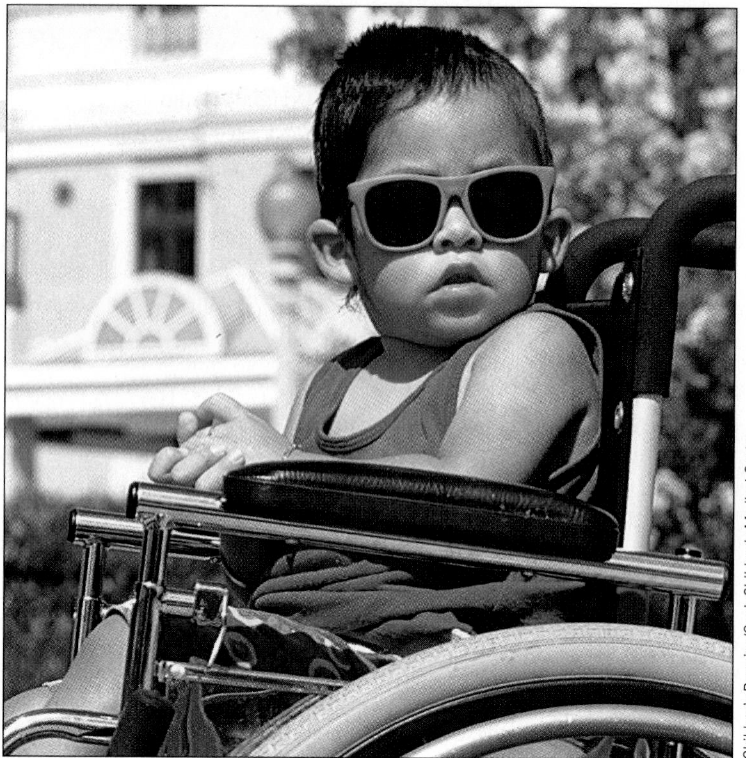

Children's Promise/Cook Children's Medical Center

CHAPTER OVERVIEW

LEARNING OBJECTIVES

After studying this chapter, you should be able to:

- Provide a rationale to substantiate the need for routine well child assessment.
- Describe the pathophysiology, incidence, and clinical manifestations of children exhibiting specific disorders of the bones and joints.
- Describe common diagnostic measures associated with structural disorders of the bones and joints in children.
- Provide a rationale to substantiate the need for periodic follow-up of children with identified structural disorders of bones and joints.
- Describe the role of the nurse in the care and treatment of the child exhibiting structural disorders of bones and joints.

KEY TERMS

abduction: movement away from the midline

acetabulum: the hip socket in the pelvis

adduction: movement toward the midline

anomaly: abnormality

autologous blood transfusion: transfusion of one's own blood which has been harvested previously

avascular necrosis: tissue damage secondary to inadequate blood supply

dislocation: displacement of a bone from its normal articulation within a joint

dysplasia: abnormal development

external fixation: pins, screws and bars placed through bone and soft tissue to immobilize, or to correct a deformity

internal instrumentation: instruments placed inside the body to immobilize parts

inversion: a turning toward the midline

myelomeningocele: a birth anomaly involving the vertebrae and spinal canal that causes paralysis

orthoses: braces, external supports, artificial limbs made by a specialist to meet individual needs

ossification: formation of bone from osseous tissue or cartilage

osteotomy: surgical cutting of bone

Pavlik harness: a device that holds an infant's hips in flexion and external rotation

plantar flexion: to bend toward the sole of the foot

polydactyly: extra fingers or toes

pseudarthrosis: failure of the bones to fuse

spica cast: a cast used to immobilize the hips that extends from above the waist to the knees or ankles

subluxation: partial dislocation of a joint

superior mesenteric artery syndrome: a condition resembling intestinal obstruction caused by reduced blood supply to a segment of the mesentery

syndactyly: fusion or webbing of two or more fingers or toes

valgum: abnormal position of a limb that involves bending away from the midline of the body. Genu valgum results in knock knees.

varum: abnormal position of the limb that involves bending toward the midline of the body. Genu varum results in bowlegs.

Musculoskeletal disorders are common among children. They may vary from mild alterations of normal to severe malformations. They may be congenital or inherited, or acquired through injury or infection. The nurse plays an important role in caring for children with musculoskeletal conditions, providing screening and treatment, reassuring parents, and educating families about home care.

Because children have a natural tendency to be active, impaired physical mobility or mobility restrictions imposed by treatment present a challenge to the child, health care staff, and parents. Immobility can interfere with the child's normal growth and development in every area. Nurses maximize normal development by teaching families strategies that promote independence and mobility. Another important nursing role is providing psychosocial support to help children and families cope with the impact of musculoskeletal disorders.

Often, musculoskeletal disorders of children change with growth. For this reason, they usually require long-term monitoring. Patient compliance is critical to a successful outcome, and helping the child and family comply with the treatment plan is often challenging. By educating parents and encouraging them to take an active role in the child's care, nurses facilitate the treatment plan.

Families and children with musculoskeletal disorders need education, reassurance, and support. This chapter discusses how to provide effective care to children with musculoskeletal disorders.

For a review of the anatomy and physiology of the musculoskeletal system and for information about related laboratory and diagnostic tests, see the Clinical Reference Pages at the beginning of Chapter 36.

SCOLIOSIS

Although scoliosis is defined as lateral curvature of the spine, it is, in fact, a three-dimensional deformity involving rotation of the vertebral bodies. The forces of a curved spine on the structure of the body cause the rib cage to become misshapen. The body develops a compensatory curve in order to maintain posture and balance. Scoliotic curves are measured in degrees. Curves of less than 20 degrees are slight curves. Curves of greater than 40 degrees usually require surgery, and curves of greater than 80 degrees are severe and compromise respiratory function.

PATHOPHYSIOLOGY AND ETIOLOGY *of Scoliosis*

The causes of scoliosis are numerous. Most cases of scoliosis can be classified into three major categories, which offer some insight into the causes of the disorder. *Idiopathic scoliosis* is the predominant form of scoliosis. Although there is no recognizable cause for idiopathic scoliosis, there is a genetic component to its incidence. Most idiopathic scoliosis occurs in adolescent girls and tends to progress more rapidly during growth spurts, such as the period immediately preceding menarche. Idiopathic scoliosis can also occur in other age groups. *Congenital scoliosis* is another major category of scoliosis. It is the result of vertebral abnormalities, such as hemivertebra or vertebral bars, and is associated with other congenital anomalies. A third major category of scoliosis is *paralytic scoliosis.* This type of scoliosis is relatively common in individuals with certain neuromuscular diseases, such as cerebral palsy, muscular dystrophy, paraplegia, or quadriplegia. Scoliosis may also develop in children with certain other disorders, such as osteogenesis imperfecta, juvenile rheumatoid arthritis, and spinal cord tumors, and it may also occur secondary to radiation therapy.

Incidence. The incidence of scoliosis varies with its cause. Idiopathic scoliosis is a common disorder, affecting approximately 10% of the population. Most idiopathic scoliosis is so slight that it goes undetected and is of no clinical significance. Idiopathic scoliosis is most common in female patients and in families in which another member is affected. The incidence of congenital scoliosis is variable. It is believed to be caused by a variety of factors and is also associated with certain other congenital anomalies. Scoliosis is a relatively common occurrence in children with neuromuscular disorders.

Clinical Manifestations. The clinical manifestations of scoliosis include the following:

- Visible curve of the spine
- Rib hump when the child is bending forward
- Asymmetric rib cage
- Uneven shoulder and/or pelvic heights
- Prominence of the hip or scapula
- Difference in the space between the arms and the trunk when standing
- Apparent leg-length discrepancy
- In severe cases, reduced vital capacity
- Disproportionately short thorax and long arms

(See Fig. 37–1 and the box opposite, Screening Procedure for Scoliosis.)

Diagnostic Evaluation. Scoliosis may be detected at any time during childhood or adolescence and is often first discovered during routine scoliosis screening sessions. Evidence of clinical manifestations should lead to more thorough assessment of the spine. Radiographic examination of the thorax will confirm the diagnosis and assist with the treatment regimen. In addition, children with disorders commonly associated with scoliosis should be monitored routinely for the development of spinal deformity.

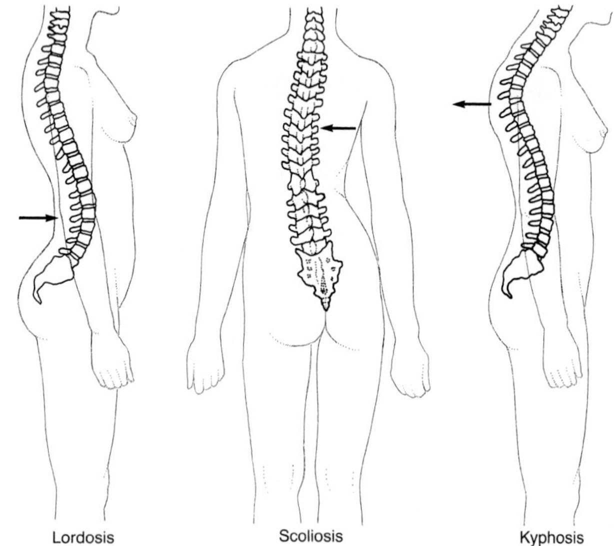

Figure 37–1
Most spinal abnormalities in children are abnormal curvatures. In *scoliosis,* the spine curves laterally and the vertebrae rotate, pulling the ribs along. *Kyphosis* is a front-to-back rounding, usually of the thoracic spine; it is often accompanied by scoliosis. *Lordosis* is an exaggerated concave curvature of the spine, usually in the lumbar area. (From Ignatavicius, D. D., Workman, M. L., & Mishler, M. A. [1995]. *Medical surgical nursing: A nursing process approach* [2nd ed., p. 1399]. Philadelphia: W. B. Saunders.)

Screening Procedure for Scoliosis

Children ages 9 through 15 should be screened for scoliosis to ensure early detection and treatment. At greatest risk are girls from age 10 through adolescence.

The child should be unclothed or wearing underpants only so that the chest, back, and hips can be clearly seen. Have the child stand with weight equally on both feet, legs straight, and arms hanging loosely at the sides. Observe for the following signs of scoliosis:

- Nonpainful lateral curvature of the spine.
- The curve can have one turn ("C curve") or may include two compensating curves ("S curve").
- Lateral deviation and rotation of each vertebra is accentuated by looking at the ribs as well as the spinal column itself.
- Unequal shoulder heights.
- Congenital scoliosis may be visible in the infant lying prone; is sometimes more prominent if the infant is suspended prone.
- Unequal scapula prominences and heights. (Note that the muscle masses may be somewhat unequal, especially if the child uses one shoulder more than the other as in carrying books. Look for bony, not muscular prominence.)
- Unequal waist angles.
- Unequal rib prominences and chest asymmetry.
- Unequal rib heights when the child stands in Adam's position (see photo).

The physical examination should also include:

- Observation for equal leg lengths.
- Examination of the skin for hairy patches, nevi, café au lait spots, lipomas, dimples.
- Neurological examination.
- Cardiac examination for Marfan syndrome.

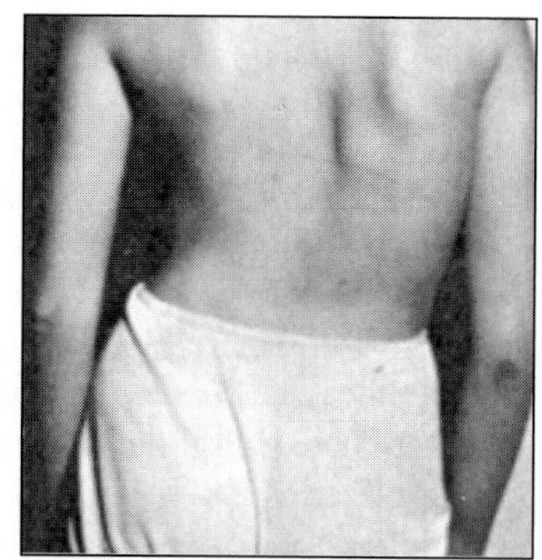

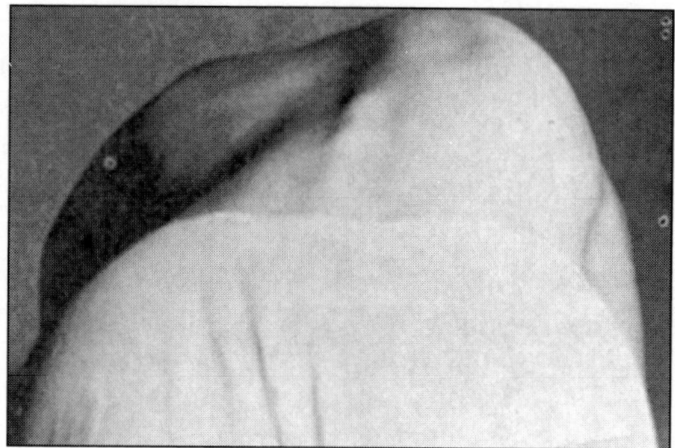

Adam's position with rib hump of structural scoliosis. Lateral curvature of thoracic and lumbar segments of the spine, usually with some rotation of involved vertebral bodies.

Functional scoliosis is flexible; it is apparent with standing and disappears with forward bending. It may be compensatory for other abnormalities such as leg-length discrepancy.

Structural scoliosis is fixed; the curvature shows both on standing and on bending forward. Note rib hump with forward flexion. When the person is standing, note unequal shoulder elevation, unequal scapulae, obvious curvature, unequal elbow level, and unequal hip level.

Data from Burns, C. E. (1996). Musculoskeletal disorders. In C. E. Burns, N. Barber, M. A. Brady, & A. M. Dunn (Eds.). *Pediatric primary care: A handbook for nurse practitioners* (p. 778). Philadelphia: W. B. Saunders. Photos from Delp, M. H., & Manning, R. T. (1981). *Major's physical diagnosis: An introduction to the clinical process* (9th ed., p. 450). Philadelphia: W. B. Saunders.

Therapeutic Management. Treatment of scoliosis is a major and complex undertaking. Surgical and nonsurgical interventions are employed in the treatment of scoliosis. Treatment options include regular and periodic observation with radiographic evaluation, bracing, or spinal fusion surgery. The type of treatment depends on the degree of the curvature as well as the age of the child and the amount of growth that is anticipated. Children who are diagnosed as having scoliosis need careful and long-term monitoring of their condition. Although mild curvatures may never progress to the point that treatment is warranted, the curvature can become increasingly pronounced and require further treatment.

Children with curvature of the spine should undergo long-term interval monitoring to detect any progression of the curve.

In the past, bracing was used extensively in the treatment of scoliosis and is used today to stabilize some mild curves. Although bracing does not correct a curve, it may slow its progress until the child's skeletal maturity allows for an optimal treatment option (Winter, 1994).

Surgical treatment by means of spinal fusion is a common means of treatment for scoliosis today. Because fusion results in cessation of spinal growth, it is delayed for as long as possible to allow for maximum skeletal growth. Recently many new techniques for surgical intervention have been developed which improve outcomes while decreasing the length of hospitalization. Sometimes spinal fusion is preceded by traction. Most surgical techniques rely on some form of **internal instrumentation** rods that assist with correction of the deformity (curve) and hold the spine immobile for the long healing period. These operative procedures are usually accomplished through incisions in the back, but some complex fusions of the spine are approached through anterior thoracic and/or retroperitoneal incisions. Iliac bone graft may be used for the spinal fusion (Puno et al., 1994).

Significant blood loss may be expected during the spinal fusion, and replacement of blood is frequently necessary. Because spinal fusion for scoliosis is a planned procedure, children are often able to donate their own blood in the weeks preceding the surgery for use at the time of surgery. Such **autologous blood transfusions** have become commonplace since the advent of the human immunodeficiency virus (HIV) epidemic.

Prognosis. With close monitoring and follow-up, the treatment outcomes for idiopathic scoliosis are excellent. The older the child is at the time of appearance of manifestations of scoliosis and treatment, the more successful the ultimate result is likely to be. The prognosis for congenital scoliosis is variable and depends on the underlying defect. Treatment of scoliosis in children with neuromuscular disorders is a challenge and can be very complex; outcomes are variable. These children must be monitored for an indefinite period for the possibility of progression of the curve.

Complications. A variety of complications can occur during treatment for scoliosis. The use of casts and braces can result in skin irritation and even pressure sores. Neurologic damage can result from mechanical injury during surgery or from stretching of the spinal column during correction. Although electronic monitoring (somatosensory evoked potentials) during surgery helps to reduce the possibility of spinal cord damage intraoperatively, postoperative sensation and motor function are the only definitive indicators of neurologic function. Another complication in the surgical treatment of scoliosis is **superior mesenteric artery syndrome.** This disorder is caused by mechanical changes in the position of the patient's abdominal contents, resulting from lengthening of the body. It results in a syndrome of emesis and abdominal distension similar to that which occurs with intestinal obstruction or paralytic ileus. Postoperative vomiting in children with body casts or those who have undergone spinal fusion warrants attention because of the possibility of superior mesenteric artery syndrome. Fluid/electrolyte imbalances can also result in the postoperative period, as can atelectasis and sluggish bowel function. Superficial or deep wound infection is also possible (Therss et al., 1996). The major long-term complication of spinal fusion is **pseudarthrosis,** or failure of one or more segments of the spine to fuse. Spinal fusion retards longitudinal growth of the spine (Husu & Upadhygy, 1994).

NURSING CARE OF THE CHILD WITH SCOLIOSIS

Assessment

Nursing assessment strategies are an important part of the care of children with scoliosis. Nurses are involved in routine screening of children and adolescents for scoliosis in acute care settings, in outpatient settings, and in schools (see box). School nurses screen children for scoliosis, usually beginning in the fifth grade. For children who have been diagnosed but are not undergoing treatment, periodic evaluation is necessary to monitor possible progression of the curve. For those undergoing treatment, assessment focuses on determining the child's and parents' level of knowledge about scoliosis and learning capacity. It also involves evaluation for body image concerns, anxiety about the various treatment modalities, compliance with prescribed treatments, including bracing, and an understanding of the many issues surrounding spinal fusions. Patient education is essential to promote compliance with treatment.

Children undergoing non-surgical treatment and their families must understand and correctly apply treatment measures and be committed to compliance. For example, patients in bracing need to be monitored closely to ensure that the curve does not progress and that treatment goals are being met. The drawbacks of braces include discomfort in warm weather and skin irritation. Adolescent girls may find braces to be cosmetically offensive, and patient cooperation is often a problem. Clothing modifications are necessary if compliance is to be expected.

Children undergoing spinal fusion have special needs in the perioperative period. Preoperatively, explanations about the procedures and the care anticipated are aimed at reducing the anxiety and fear surrounding surgery. Coordination of autologous blood donation may be the nurse's responsibility.

In the immediate postoperative period, patients are monitored to determine the neurologic status of the lower extremities, as well as to assess pain, fluid status (by monitoring IV fluid intake, urinary output, edema, and vital signs), bleeding (by monitoring hemoglobin and hematocrit values, wound and chest drainage, and blood loss on dressings), and return of bowel function (by auscultating for bowel sounds). Pulmonary hygiene, including various incentive measures and log rolling the patient from side to side every 2 hours, is also an essential nursing task in the immediate postoperative period.

As the patient stabilizes postoperatively, mobility is quickly increased, and the diet can be progressed with monitoring of gastrointestinal status. Orthoplast jackets may be used postoperatively with some patients. Patients must understand their function and use. A cotton T-shirt between the plastic and the skin reduces discomfort and irritation.

It is not unusual for these patients to be discharged from the hospital by the fifth postoperative day. Because the treatment of scoliosis is a long-term process and can affect a child for most of the growing-up years, close monitoring is important to ensure positive outcomes.

Nursing Diagnosis

- Risk for Impaired Skin Integrity related to wearing of a brace
- Knowledge Deficit related to lack of information about the natural history of scoliosis and available treatment modalities
- Body Image Disturbance related to a postural deformity, to bracing, or to a surgical scar on the back
- Anxiety related to impending surgery
- Risk for Injury related to neurovascular deficit secondary to instrumentation
- Pain related to the operative procedure
- Ineffective Airway Clearance related to long-term anesthesia and intubation, immobility, and pain associated with spinal fusion
- Knowledge Deficit related to home care following spinal fusion

Planning, Implementation, and Evaluation: The Child With Scoliosis

NURSING DIAGNOSIS • Risk for Impaired Skin Integrity related to wearing of a brace

Expected Outcome: • The child will maintain intact skin.

Intervention	Rationale
1. Teach the child that the brace must be worn according to the prescribed schedule. Either full-time or part-time bracing may be prescribed. Full-time bracing is usually 18–23 hours/day with 30 minutes to several hours off for exercises and bathing.	Compliance with treatment is necessary to prevent progression of the curvature (Allington & Bowen, 1996).
2. Check the brace for proper fit. Inspect the skin for signs of redness or breakdown every 8 hours.	An improperly fitting brace may rub against the skin, causing breakdown.
3. Instruct the child/family to keep the skin clean and dry, bathe daily, and dry the skin thoroughly. Use of lotions or powders should be avoided, as they can become sticky or cake under the brace, causing irritation.	Cleanliness minimizes the risk of skin irritation.
Advise the child to wear soft, nonirritating fabrics (cotton T-shirts) under the brace.	Soft fabrics decrease irritation and absorb perspiration.
4. Encourage child to perform prescribed exercises.	Exercises increase flexibility and strengthen muscles.

Evaluation:
- The child's skin has no lesions, redness, or signs or infection.
- The brace is properly fitted.
- The child attends follow-up appointments.

NURSING DIAGNOSIS • Knowledge Deficit related to lack of information about the natural history of scoliosis and the treatment modalities available

Expected Outcomes: The child and family will:

- Express an understanding of what has been taught about scoliosis, including the reasons for therapy.
- Demonstrate the skills taught (such as performance of prescribed exercise).
- Ask appropriate questions which indicate a knowledge of scoliosis and treatment (e.g., "Will I be able to play basketball?").
- Follow through with needed therapy.

Intervention	Rationale
1. Determine the child's and family's knowledge level about scoliosis and treatment modalities.	Teaching needs to begin at the client's level of understanding.
2. Teach the child and family about scoliosis, its signs and symptoms, progression, and its treatment.	Knowledge and understanding increase motivation and compliance with treatment while reducing anxiety.
3. Identify the child's and family's areas of concern (e.g., activity restriction, operative concerns, outcomes of therapy).	Teaching will be most effective if it is directed at the individual's needs.
4. Select instructional methods that are appropriate to the child's developmental level (puppets, audiovisuals).	Learning styles vary with the individual and his abilities.
5. Communicate in a clear and honest manner.	This approach establishes trust between the staff and family and, by extension, promotes confidence in the effectiveness of treatment.
6. Explain the reason for the various interventions (such as coughing in the postoperative period).	It is likely that the patient will be more cooperative in the postoperative period if she knows the reason for the intervention.
7. Have the child (or parents) demonstrate specific skills (such as coughing or recumbent logrolling).	This allows the nurse to evaluate learning and allows the patient to gain confidence in her own ability to perform the maneuver.
8. Encourage the child to ask questions and discuss concerns. Correct any inaccurate information. Allow the child to handle equipment.	Children use their senses to learn.
9. Include the parents in teaching.	Their comfort level will be reflected in the child.

Evaluation: The child and family will:

- Express an understanding of scoliosis and its treatment, ask appropriate questions, demonstrate the skills taught, and follow through with required therapy.

NURSING DIAGNOSIS

- Body Image Disturbance related to a postural deformity, to bracing, or to a surgical scar on the back

Expected Outcomes: The child will:

- Talk about how she feels about her body and the effect of the scoliosis, and the brace or surgical scar, on her self-image.
- Demonsrate confidence in herself and in her abilities (academic, extracurricular activities, or other qualities).

Intervention	Rationale
1. Encourage the child or teen to talk about the diagnosis, treatment, and feelings about the experience.	This allows assessment of the patient's perceptions and provides opportunities to clarify misconceptions and to vent feelings.
2. Encourage conversation that focuses on how the child feels about herself and her body.	This allows the nurse to provide emotional support, and may ease anxiety.
3. Encourage the child to discuss experiences with friends.	Friends are likely to be very supportive and helpful if they share in a knowledge of the disorder.
4. Provide information about the disorder and the treatment. Encourage the child to consider an activity which she can master and feel a sense of accomplishment (soccer, science club).	This helps the child gain a sense of control over the experience.
5. During hospitalization, provide privacy to the greatest degree possible.	Children and teens are very modest.

Evaluation: • The child demonstrates acceptance of her body and expresses confidence in her abilities.

NURSING DIAGNOSIS • Anxiety related to impending surgery

Expected Outcome: • The child will discuss her anxiety and identify effective coping mechanisms to address it.

Intervention*	Rationale
1. Determine whether the child is anxious about surgery.	The child may not be anxious or may be hiding her anxiety.
2. Initiate a conversation with the child about how anxiety makes one feel and how anxiety is a normal response to anticipated surgery. For example, "Many girls facing surgery are nervous about what it will be like to have this operation. Perhaps you would like to know more about what it will be like."	The child may need permission to discuss her anxiety and may require assistance verbalizing her feelings. She needs to be assured that she is normal.
3. Assist the child in identifying positive and effective means for resolving anxiety (e.g., talking with a friend, exercising or engaging in other activities, practicing relaxation techniques).	In role modeling for the child and discussing various possibilities for coping, the nurse allows the child to find a comfortable means for expressing feelings.
4. Identify and discourage negative behaviors associated with anxiety (e.g., verbal outbursts, physical aggression, withdrawal). Try telling the child, "It's OK and normal to be anxious about surgery. This is hard for your parents, too. Let's talk about ways you might let your parents know how you are feeling."	The child needs to understand that there are acceptable and unacceptable ways to express one's feelings.

*Also refer to Chapter 15.

Intervention	Rationale
5. Reassure the child about specific fears ("Can my mom be with me?" "Will I get a shot?").	Reassurance and conversation may help to resolve some fears.
6. Assess the child's need for specific information and teach accordingly.	Fears about the unknown may be reduced by increasing knowledge.

Evaluation: • The child will identify the source of anxiety and demonstrate ways of coping effectively with the anxiety.

NURSING DIAGNOSIS • Risk for Injury related to neurovascular deficit secondary to instrumentation

Expected Outcome: • The child will maintain neurovascular integrity as evidenced by adequate circulation, strong pulses, movement, and sensation of extremities.

Intervention	Rationale
1. Assess all extremities for color, circulation, capillary refill, warmth, sensation, and motion. Perform neurovascular checks q 2 hr for the first 24 hours and then q 4 hr for the next 48 hours. Check and record the quality of pedal pulses every hour for 48 hours.	The risks of instrumentation during surgery include complications such as altered neurovascular status, paralysis, and thrombus formation. Frequent monitoring of the child's condition postoperatively is crucial.
2. Monitor the child for signs of urinary retention or bowel incontinence.	Bowel or bladder incontinence may indicate spinal cord trauma.
3. Strictly maintain flat bedrest postoperatively as ordered. Logroll q 2 hr. Place a pillow behind the child's back and between the legs. Place a thin, small pillow under the child's head. Have the child roll from a side-lying position to a sitting position.	Maintaining alignment promotes healing and prevents injury to the spine.
4. Assist the child to ambulate when ordered.	Because of possible hypotension, narcotics, postoperative weakness, pain, or anxiety, patient needs assistance with early ambulation.

Evaluation: • The child ambulates without difficulty and exhibits no evidence of neurologic deficit.

NURSING DIAGNOSIS • Pain related to the operative procedure

Expected Outcome: • The child will indicate decreasing amounts of pain as measured on a pain scale; she will appear calm and relaxed; and she will turn, cough, and deep breathe effectively with assistance.

Intervention	Rationale
1. Assess the child's pain level frequently in the postoperative period. (Statements of pain, anxiety, an inability to cough, hyperalertness, reluctance or refusal to move, and/or sweating may indicate pain.)	Children and adolescents may be unable or unwilling to verbalize their pain. The child may not ask for pain medication because of a fear of injections.

Intervention	Rationale
2. Provide prescribed analgesics in a timely manner.	Appropriate and timely use of analgesics provides optimal control of pain.
3. Assist family members in understanding the patient's experience and interventions.	When parents understand and can participate in the child's care, they can provide support to the child.
4. Explore alternative means for relieving pain (using anxiety-reducing techniques, dimming the room lights, reducing stimuli, playing music, therapeutic touching).	Alternative therapy may be very effective.
5. Assess the patient's response to pain relief measures and communicate with the physician about possible adjustments, if needed. (Also refer to Chapter 20 for a thorough discussion of the nursing care of pain in children and teenagers.)	Adjustments may be necessary to achieve optimal pain relief.

Evaluation:
- Using a pain scale, the child rates her pain on the low end; she appears calm and relaxed; she turns, coughs, and deep breathes effectively with assistance.

NURSING DIAGNOSIS
- Ineffective Airway Clearance related to long-term anesthesia and intubation, immobility, and pain associated with spinal fusion

Expected Outcome:
- The child will demonstrate effective coughing and adequate air exchange.

Intervention	Rationale
1. Teach deep breathing and coughing exercises preoperatively.	In the postoperative period, the child will be familiar and skilled at exercise even though well medicated.
2. Assist the patient to cough and deep breathe q 2 hr during the first 2 postoperative days.	The patient needs frequent prompting and assistance during the immediate postoperative period.
3. Ensure that the patient rolls from side to side q 2 hr. Nursing assistance is needed in the early postoperative period.	With frequent position changes, secretions do not pool in the airways.
4. Ensure adequate pain control.	Turning and optimal coughing are difficult without adequate analgesia.
5. Use an incentive spirometer, "blow bubbles," or a balloon as an incentive for deep breathing.	The challenge provided by a "toy" promotes effective breathing exercises.

Evaulation:
- The child demonstrates adequate air exchange and coughs effectively.
- The patient's core temperature remains at or below 38.5°C.
- The child's lungs are free of adventitious sounds.

NURSING DIAGNOSIS
- Knowledge Deficit related to home care following spinal fusion

Expected Outcome:
- The family and child will successfully manage treatment at home.

Intervention	Rationale
1. Teach the family and child the correct technique for wound care. Discuss the importance of a well-balanced diet.	Proper wound care and good nutrition decrease the chance of infection.
2. Discuss activity restrictions. (Usually, these patients cannot ride a bike, use roller blades, ski, mow lawn, or lift more than 10 lb.) Activity restrictions are usually maintained for 6 to 9 months, depending on the type of surgery and the physician. Show the child how to perform activities without twisting or bending at the waist.	Home care instructions for activity are important to reduce the possibility of complications.
3. Instruct the family and child to be alert for unfavorable signs, such as skin breakdown, pain, or difficulty breathing, and inform them about problems that can be anticipated.	Home care instructions reduce the possibility of complications.
4. Provide the name and phone number of an easily accessible health care provider in case questions arise at home. Inform the family about community resources available.	Accessibility to a health care provider and/or community resources decreases anxiety and improves compliance with treatment.
5. Schedule a follow-up appointment prior to discharge. Emphasize the importance of keeping appointments.	Periodic evaluation is important to recovery.

Home Care: Home care of the nonsurgical patient includes physical therapy regimens and bracing if required. Long-term monitoring of the spinal curvature is essential. Patients and their parents should know that periodic evaluation is important, and convenient appointments should be made and kept.

For postoperative patients, home care instructions should be provided for wound care and activity restrictions to reduce the possibility of complications. The child should be shown how to perform activities of daily living without twisting or bending at the waist. Instructions will vary with the physician's desires. Restrictions usually apply to such activities as bicycle riding, roller blading, horseback riding, skiing, mowing the lawn, or lifting more than 10 pounds. Activity restrictions are usually maintained for 6 to 9 months, depending on the type of surgery and the physician.

Evaluation:

- The family demonstrates the procedures necessary to care for the child at home.
- The family is aware of sources of help, if needed.
- The family keeps follow-up appointments.

KYPHOSIS

Kyphosis is defined as a front to back rounding of the thoracic spine. Mild kyphosis occurs normally and in varying amounts in the thoracic spine. It may be a postural deviation related to self-consciousness that is manifested by round shoulders. Although kyphosis usually occurs in the thoracic area, it can occur in other areas of the spine, and it becomes especially problematic when it progresses uncontrollably and results in neurologic damage or reduced respiratory function. Kyphosis is often accompanied by scoliosis, although the reverse is not necessarily true.

Pathophysiology. Kyphosis can occur as a postural defect (idiopathic), as a result of structural abnormalities of the vertebral bodies of the spine, or secondary to certain neuromuscular disorders, such as myelomeningocele, or to other factors, such as tumors, surgery, or radiation therapy.

Incidence. Postural kyphosis is found in about 4% of otherwise healthy adolescents. The incidence of kyphosis that occurs secondary to other conditions and disorders and that is severe enough to treat is variable.

Clinical Manifestations. The clinical manifestations of kyphosis include the following:

- Visually appreciable humpback or convex deformity
- Predominantly affects the thoracic area, but may involve a lower portion of the spine (see Fig. 37–1)

Diagnostic Evaluation. The diagnosis of kyphosis is relatively easy to establish based on visual examination of the spine. It is often associated with other conditions, necessitating a comprehensive analysis of its cause.

Therapeutic Management. Exercises may be recommended for mild postural curves. The treatment for severe kyphosis is similar to the treatment for scoliosis. Because the two conditions are often found in the same patient, treatment is directed at both conditions. In patients who have not yet reached skeletal maturity and whose curves are flexible, casting or bracing may be attempted first. For complex progressive curves, spinal fusion frequently becomes necessary.

Nursing Care

Nursing care of the patient with kyphosis, including home care, is based on the same principles as outlined for scoliosis management.

LORDOSIS

Lordosis is an exaggerated concave curvature of the spine, usually in the lumbar area, where a mild concave curve is normal. Occasionally, it occurs in other areas of the spine, in which case it is not considered to be normal as it can compress vital organs, such as the heart and lungs, and may require immediate intervention.

Pathophysiology. Lumbar lordosis, by itself, is usually not severe enough to cause concern. It may, however, occur secondary to other defects, such as hip flexion contracture, muscular dystrophy (Fig. 37–2), obesity, or developmental dysplastic hip (DDH). Lordosis is a frequent complication of myelomeningocele and several other neuromuscular disorders.

Incidence. The incidence of lordosis is variable and depends on the presence of associated conditions.

Clincial Manifestations. The clinical manifestations of lordosis include the following:

- An exaggerated concave curve in the lumbar area
- Pain in the lower back
- An accompanying defect, such as DDH, hip flexion contracture, or obesity

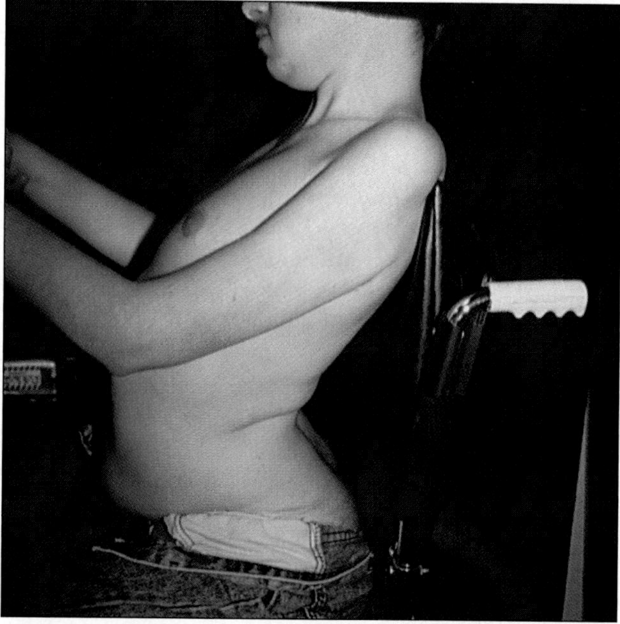

Figure 37–2
Lordosis may occur secondary to other defects, as in this boy with muscular dystrophy. Care of the child with lumbar lordosis is similar to that outlined for scoliosis, with concurrent management of any accompanying disorders.

Diagnostic Evaluation. The diagnosis is confirmed by physical examination and by x-ray studies.

Therapeutic Management. Treatment for lordosis depends on its cause, but treatment modalities are grounded in the principles outlined for scoliosis management.

Nursing Care

The nursing care for children with lordosis, including home care, is similar to that outlined for the care of children with scoliosis. In addition, accompanying disorders must be monitored and treated concurrently.

DEVELOPMENTAL DYSPLASIA OF THE HIP

Developmental dysplasia of the hip (DDH) has traditionally been known as congenital dislocation of the hip (CDH). DDH is a condition in which the head of the femur (ball) is improperly seated in the acetabulum or hip socket of the pelvis. The term **dysplasia** implies an alteration in normal development. There is a wide range of severity of hip dysplasia, ranging from very mild to severely dislocated. It is believed that DDH can be present at birth (in which case it is congenital), but in some children, it develops after birth, hence the term developmental.

PATHOPHYSIOLOGY *of DDH*

Hip **dislocation** denotes a condition in which the ball of the femur is outside the hip socket. It can occur as a late stage of DDH, or it can occur in children with certain neuromuscular disorders, such as cerebral palsy or **myelomeningocele.** Dislocation secondary to neuromuscular disorders varies in a number of ways from DDH, and so will be covered as a separate entity. In either type of hip disease, one or both hips may be affected.

In the normal infant hip, the head of the femur is well seated in the **acetabulum** (hip socket) and is stable. Developmental dysplasia of the hip occurs in varying degrees ranging from instability of the hip joint to frank dislocation, as defined below:

- Instability of the hip is the appropriate term when the head of the femur is located in the acetabulum but may be subluxated (partially dislocated) or even dislocated with manual manipulation.
- **Subluxation** of the hip occurs when the head of the femur is positioned under the edge of the acetabulum. It is not well seated in the acetabulum, yet it is not completely dislocated.
- Dislocation of the hip occurs when the head of the femur lies outside of the acetabulum.

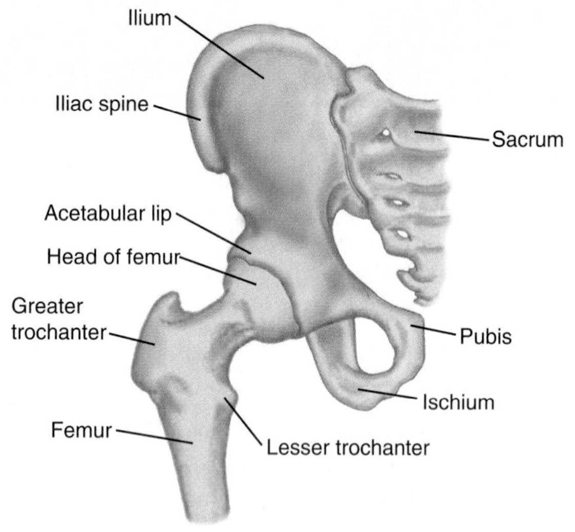

Normal hip joint

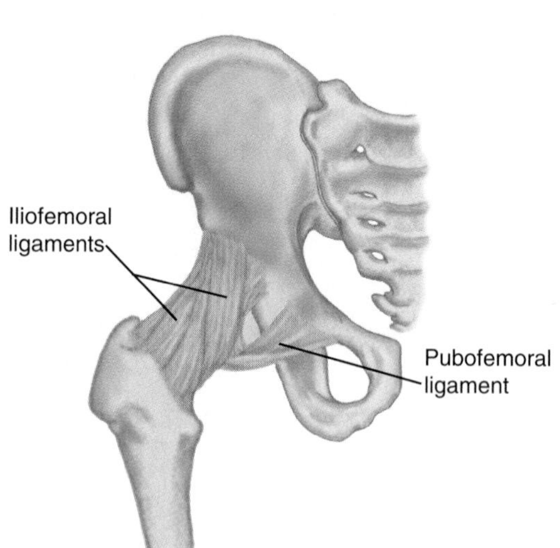

Ligaments of normal hip joint

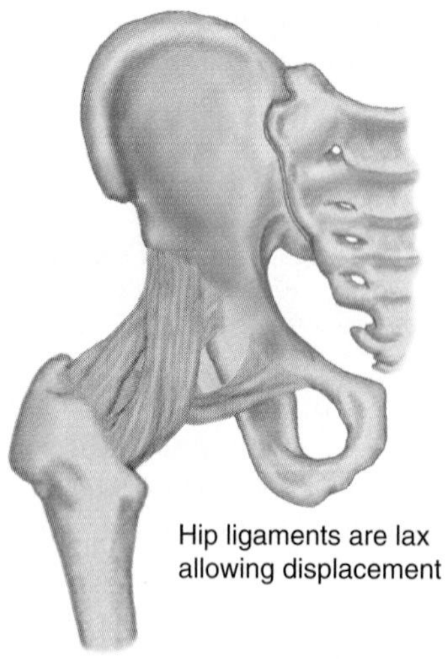

Unstable hip

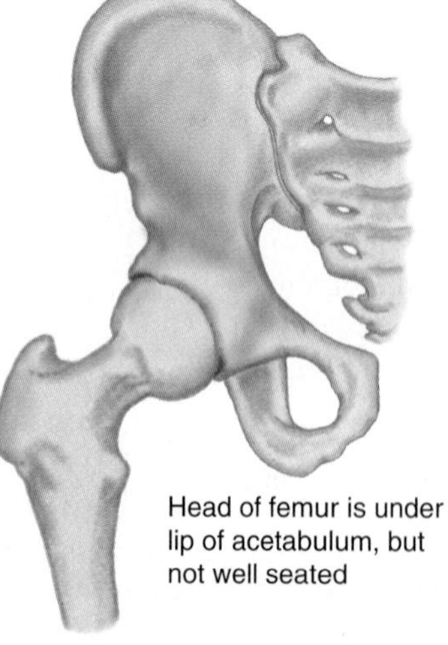

Subluxated hip

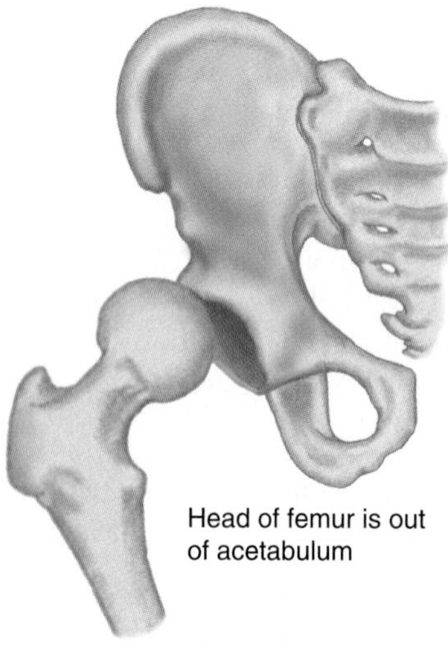

Dislocated hip

Incidence. The incidence of DDH varies greatly among the races. It is less common in African-American and Chinese infants and more common in American Indians. It is most common in Caucasians, in females, and in first born infants. It is associated with breech deliveries, and it carries a familial tendency.

Etiology. The cause of DDH is not known but appears to be multifactorial in origin. Genetic factors and pre- and post-natal positioning seem to be related.

Clinical Manifestations. The clinical manifestations of DDH, according to age, are as follows:

Neonates

- Laxity of the ligaments around the hip, which allows the femoral head to be displaced from the acetabulum upon manipulation

Infants Beyond the Newborn Period (Unilateral) (Fig. 37–3)

- Asymmetry of the gluteal skin folds when the infant is placed prone and the legs are extended against the examining table (or infant may be held upright with legs dangling)
- Limited range of motion in the affect hip
- Asymmetric **abduction** of the affected hip when placed supine with the knees and hips flexed
- Apparent short femur on the affected side

The Walking Child

- Minimal to pronounced variations in gait, with lurching toward the affected side

Diagnostic Evaluation. DDH is best diagnosed during routine screening assessments. Because of the complexities of diagnosis, screening for DDH should be done at birth and during each routine infant well-child visit by a well-trained nurse or physician.

Diagnosis of DDH in the neonate can be very difficult because the signs and symptoms may be very subtle. In general, symptoms result from laxity of the ligaments surrounding the hip joint. In newborn infants with DDH, the hip joints appear lax, rather than completely dislocated. Subluxation, or laxity with the tendency of the hip to dislocate, can often be assessed by the Ortolani and Barlow maneuvers. In the Barlow maneuver, the examiner gently pushes the unstable femoral head out of the acetabulum. In the Ortolani maneuver, the examiner reduces the dislocated femoral head back into the acetabulum. A positive finding is a palpable clink upon entry or exit of the femoral head over the acetabular ring. These techniques should be performed only by a well-trained nurse or physician. Unilateral DDH is easier to diagnose than bilateral disease because of the asymmetry of physical findings. Radiography is not useful in the neonate because bony **ossification** is not complete. Ultrasonography is now used to assist with the diagnosis of DDH (Rosendahl et al., 1995). Computerized axial tomography (CAT) and magnetic resonance imaging (MRI) may also be helpful, but their use is limited.

In the infant who is no longer a neonate, the physical signs of DDH are different. The symptoms change from lax ligaments to contractures and stiffness in the affected hip joint(s). Abduction is limited on the affected side(s).

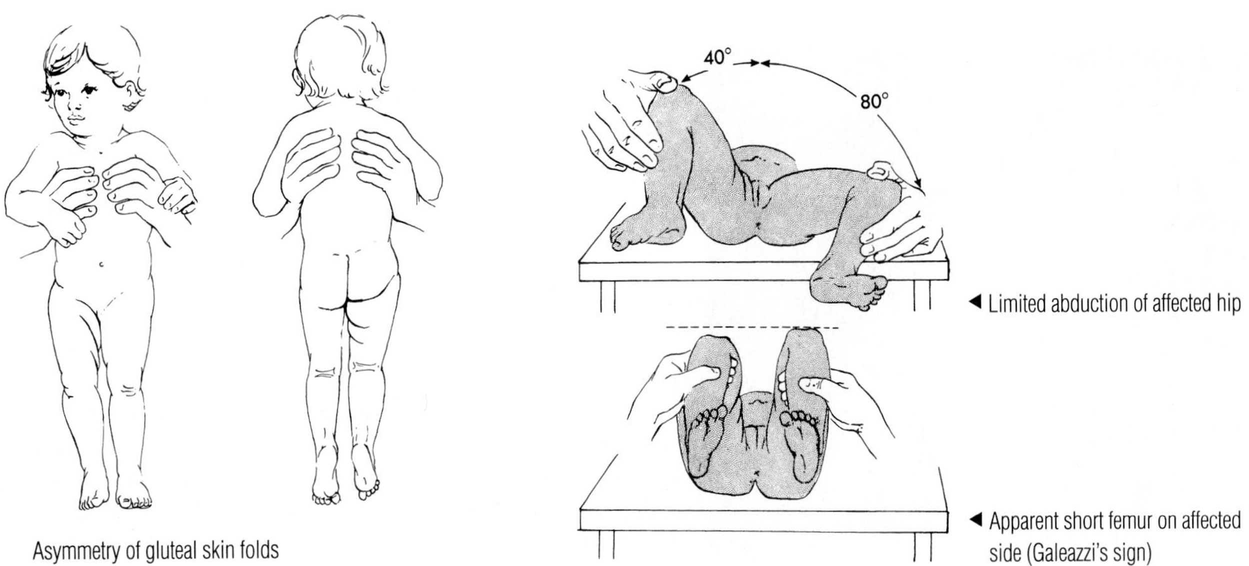

Figure 37–3
Physical findings in unilateral congenital dislocation of the hip. (From Tachdjian, M. O. [1990]. *Pediatric orthopedics* [2nd ed., p. 326]. Philadelphia: W. B. Saunders.)

The femur on the affected side (in unilateral disease) appears to be shortened.

Children with DDH who are walking may exhibit a "waddling" gait, with the child leaning toward the affected side (unilateral) or lurching from one side to the other (bilateral). Any abnormalities in gait need to be carefully evaluated as possible signs of DDH. Radiography is useful in diagnosing older infants and children.

Bilateral DDH is always more difficult than unilateral DDH to identify because there is no normal hip that can be used for comparison. Interestingly, many unstable hips resolve spontaneously. If left untreated, only about 20% will settle into a dislocated position.

> Because of the diagnostic complexities of DDH, routine well-child screening at birth and during infancy is necessary to ensure identification of this disorder.

Therapeutic Management. Early diagnosis and treatment of DDH are important to maximize a successful outcome. Treatment depends on the age of the child at the time of diagnosis and on the severity of the dysplasia. Because the musculoskeletal development of the neonate is immature, early diagnosis and successful treatment of DDH in the neonate can result in normal or near-normal hip(s).

In the neonatal period, treatment involves splinting of the hips with a **Pavlik harness** to maintain flexion and abduction and external rotation. The Pavlik harness consists of chest and shoulder straps and foot stirrups (Fig. 37–4). Initially, the harness is worn continuously. Positioning in the harness promotes development of a functional hip socket and a well-formed femoral head. This splinting may be the only treatment necessary to allow the hip to mold and grow normally. Hips that remain unstable become progressively deformed as bone maturity takes place, resulting in functional disability. Parents must be taught the proper use of the harness, as improper positioning of the infant's hip can cause interruption of the blood supply to the head of the femur, resulting in **avascular necrosis** (tissue damage secondary to inadequate blood supply). In addition, skin care, techniques for holding and feeding, and the importance of vigilant follow-up must be stressed.

Treatment is more complicated in those children whose diagnosis is made after the newborn period. Traction and/or surgery to release muscles and tendons is usually necessary to allow for adequate control of the hip joint. The procedure is followed by positioning and immobilization in a **spica cast** (see Chapter 36). For many of these profoundly affected children, traction is often followed by **osteotomy** (surgical cutting of the bone) and repositioning of the femur. Following surgery, long-term immobilization in a spica cast is required until healing is achieved.

The child's progress is followed closely. Radiographs document the progress achieved with treatment. Follow-up monitoring is essential, as the treatment may need to be modified.

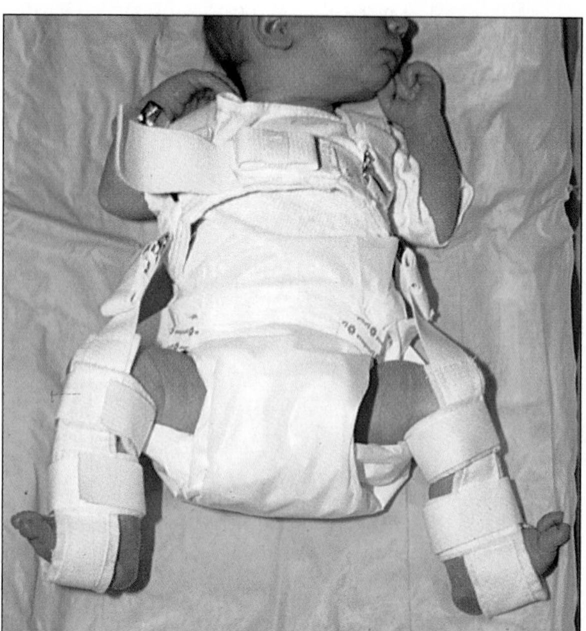

Figure 37–4
The Pavlik harness is used to treat neonates with hip displacement. By maintaining the infant's hips in flexion, abduction, and external rotation, the device promotes development of a functional hip socket and a well-formed femoral head. Because the family will be using the Pavlik harness with their infant at home, the nurse must make sure that the parents understand its purpose, as well as how to apply the device properly to avoid avascular necrosis. The nurse should also provide instructions on skin care and techniques for holding and feeding the infant. The importance of follow-up must also be stressed.

NURSING CARE OF THE CHILD WITH DEVELOPMENTAL DYSPLASIA OF THE HIP

Assessment

Assessment of all infants for the possibility of DDH during routine neonatal and well-child visits is necessary to ensure prompt diagnosis and treatment. Assessment procedures are complex and change with the age of the child. Bilateral disease is particularly difficult to identify. Assessment should be performed by well-trained nurses or nurse practitioners, or by trained physicians. Parents should be advised of the importance of routine well-child care throughout infancy and childhood.

> Because the needs of children with disorders of the musculoskeletal system are often long-term, parents usually have a good understanding of their child's progress. Questions such as, "What concerns do you have about your child's progress today?" or "How you are doing at home?" acknowledge that their feelings and ideas are valued and important. Information generated by such questions can become the focus for assessment and further intervention.

Once the diagnosis of DDH is established, nursing assessment is directed at determining the parents' learning needs and ensuring that the treatment regimen is followed. The skin of the infant in a Pavlik harness or cast must be monitored, and the anxiety levels and coping abilities of the parents need to be assessed.

When surgery becomes necessary, nursing priorities shift to an assessment of circulation to the lower extremities and pain.

Nursing Diagnoses

- Knowledge Deficit related to the diagnosis of DDH and its treatment, the use and care of a Pavlik harness, and/or to care of a child in a spica cast
- Anxiety (Parental) related to having a less-than-perfect child and to the need to provide complex care for an extended period of time
- Risk for Impaired Skin Integrity related to chafing of the skin by the Pavlik harness or to cast and dampness
- Altered Tissue Perfusion (Lower Extremities) related to impaired circulation secondary to surgery and/or casting
- Risk for Injury related to difficult positioning of a child in infant carrying devices (infant seats, strollers, car seats)
- Knowledge Deficit related to home care

Planning, Implementation, and Evaluation: The Child With Developmental Dysplasia of the Hip

NURSING DIAGNOSIS

- Knowledge Deficit related to the diagnosis of DDH and its treatment, the use and care of a Pavlik harness, and/or to care of a child in a spica cast

Expected Outcomes:

- The parents will demonstrate the therapeutic and safe use of a Pavlik harness, as evidenced by the child returning for follow-up appointments properly positioned in a harness and by the worn appearance of the harness.
- The parents will verbalize care of the spica cast and, at the time of follow-up visits, the cast will be reasonably clean and dry, and the child's skin will be clear and intact, without abrasions or sores.
- The parents will demonstrate proper technique for diapering and dressing of the child in the spica cast. (See Photo Story, pp. 1154–1157.)

Intervention	Rationale
1. Demonstrate and teach the parents the proper care and/or application of a Pavlik harness or spica cast. Ask the parents to demonstrate this skill when they are comfortable. Provide parents with a phone contact if questions arise. Harness straps should be secure enough to keep the child's hips flexed without being tight. The harness should be worn 23 hours/day and should be removed only to check the skin and for bathing. Hips and buttocks should be supported carefully when the infant is out of the harness.	Requirements of harness use may change during therapy, making teaching, demonstration, and return demonstration at every visit essential. Parents need to be confident and comfortable in performing these skills accurately. The Pavlik harness must ensure proper femur and acetabular placement.

Text continued on page 1158

Caring for Nicole, a Child in a Spica Cast

INTRODUCTION

Four-year-old Nicole is immobilized in a spica cast after hip surgery and receives IV morphine for pain. The therapies imposed by surgery and casting can lead to complications of respiration, elimination, skin breakdown, nutrition, and boredom. These potential complications, along with Nicole's growth and development needs, present challenges to her parents and the nurses caring for her.

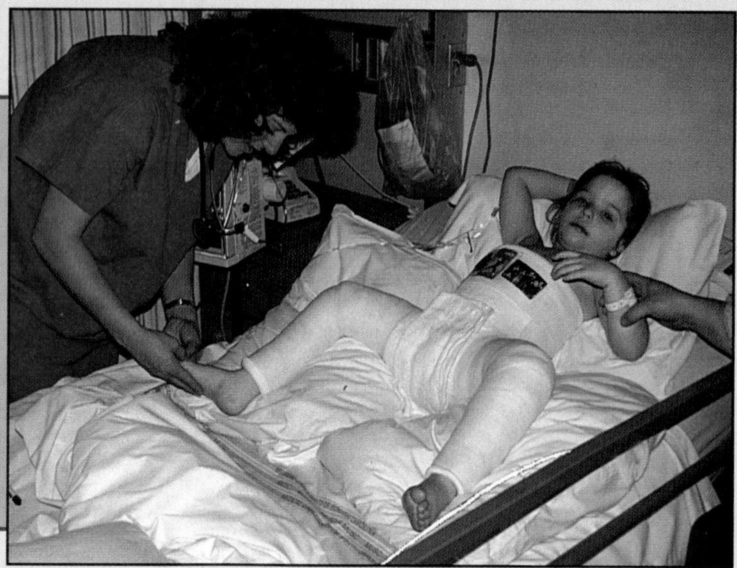

Nicole is positioned to her level of comfort with pillows at her back. A folded pillow under each leg keeps her heels from pressing against the mattress, thereby preventing pressure points. If Nicole were a few years younger, she would not be able to tell her caregivers where to place pillows for comfort, or if her heels or toes were hurting or bent. Particular attention to potential pressure points is necessary with pre-verbal children.

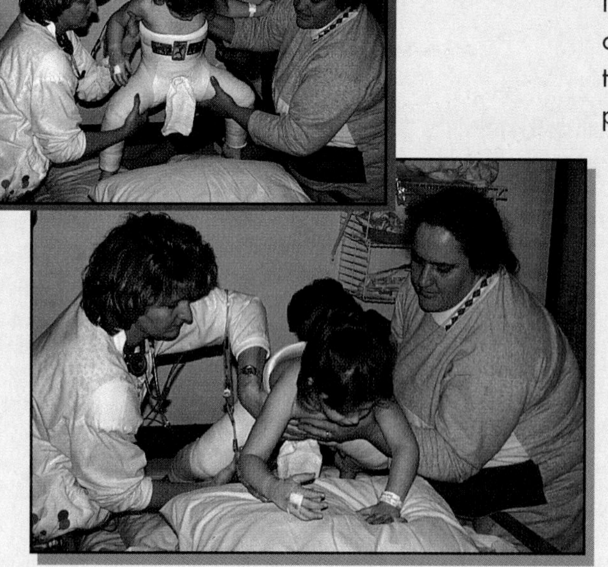

Three people are needed to turn Nicole: two to lift and turn her and a third to reposition pillows. Nicole is repositioned every 2 hours to prevent respiratory stasis. The crossbar between the legs of a spica cast (not present on this cast) should not be used as a handle when lifting the child. Once the child is feeling better and develops trust that she will not be dropped, repositioning is less frightening.

When prone, Nicole has a pillow under her chest to keep her face off the mattress and to allow her head mobility. A pillow under each leg keeps her feet and toes free. The prone position provides independence and increases Nicole's perception of control.

To prevent aspiration, Nicole eats in a prone position. Because independence and autonomy are important to children, every opportunity to enhance the child's independence should be encouraged. Food should be served in bite-sized pieces; finger foods may be preferred. Straws are used for liquids. The child should not be left unattended while eating.

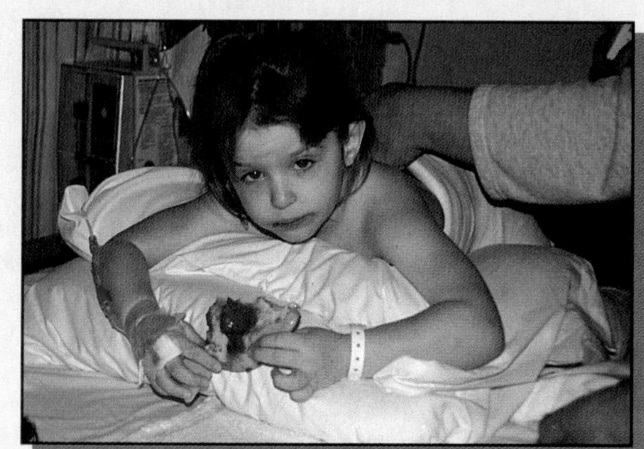

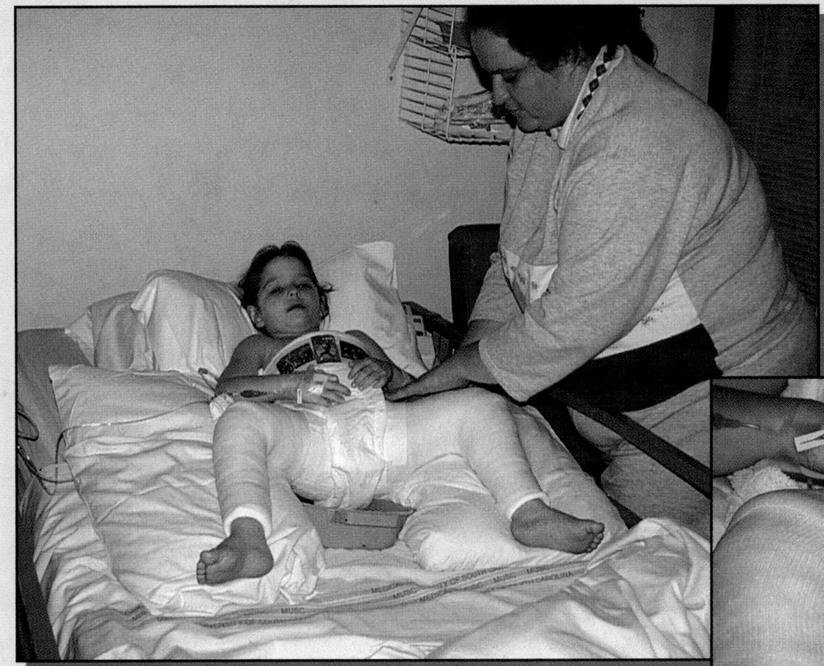

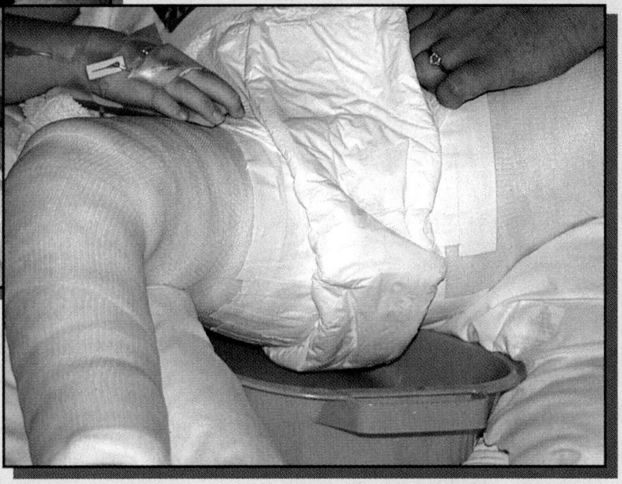

Nicole's mother is assisting her to void without soiling the webril and stockinette inside the cast. An infant-sized disposable diaper is tucked snugly into the posterior edge of the perineal opening of the cast. The edges of the diaper are folded along each side to prevent leakage of urine onto the cast. A fracture bedpan is used to keep Nicole's buttocks off the mattress. Defecation may be performed in a similar manner.

For a child not yet toilet trained, protecting the cast from urine and feces becomes a major concern. Disposable diapers tucked snugly under the edges of the perineal opening are usually successful in keeping excrement from running under the cast and onto the webril and stockinette. For any method, keeping the head higher than the buttocks reduces seepage into the sacral area. Meticulous attention to elimination is important as only one episode of leakage creates a permanently odorous cast.

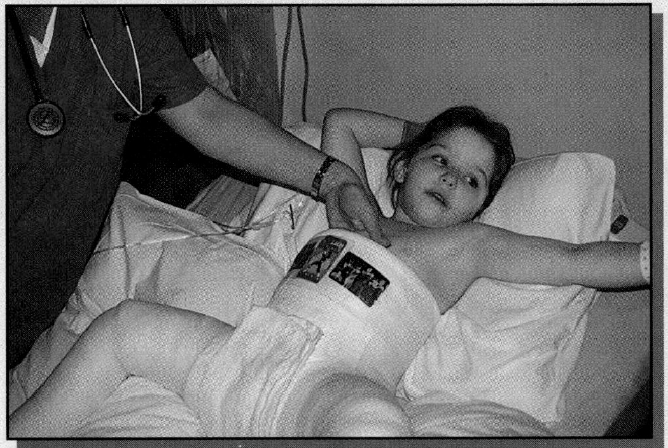

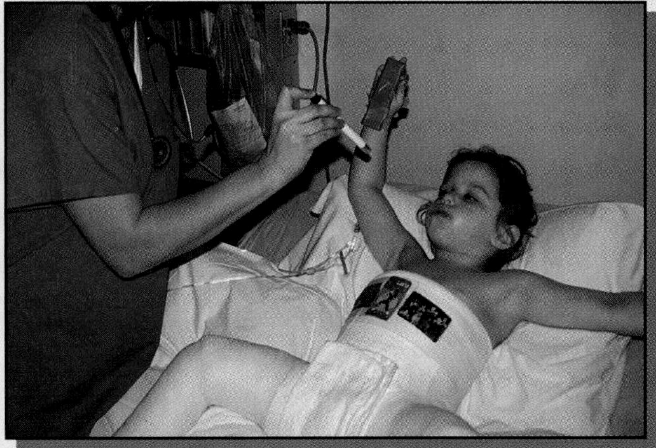

Nicole's nurse assesses her respiratory status. The cast must allow adequate room for respiratory excursion. Note how the nurse is able to fit several fingers under the edge of the cast around Nicole's chest. Respiratory assessment is performed at least every 8 hours. Deep breathing should be accomplished every 2 to 4 hours in the immediate post-operative period. Here the nurse asks Nicole to "blow out the light." Pinwheels, soap bubbles, and other tricks may be used to encourage deep breathing. In young children, crying provides the exercise of deep breathing.

CONTINUED

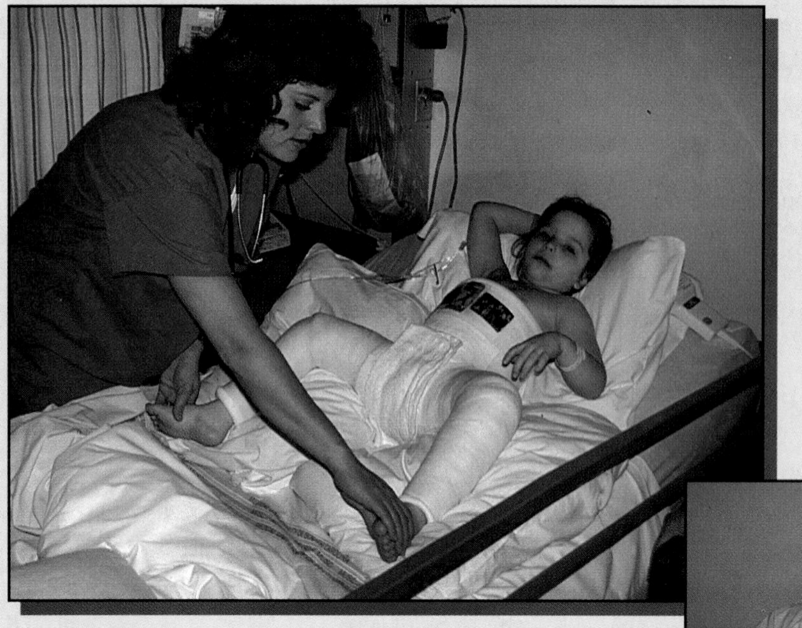

The nurse performs neurological checks to ensure the adequacy of circulation and sensation in Nicole's feet. She assesses bilaterally for color, temperature, sensation, swelling, and pulses.

Nicole's mother lightly applies a skin lubricant to Nicole's skin to prevent dryness and reduce itching and chafing. Itching under the cast causes considerable discomfort for Nicole. At times, Benadryl is necessary to reduce severe itching.

After Nicole is discharged from the hospital, her safety on the trip home is ensured by a special car-seat restraint available for children in spica casts. Whenever she travels in the car, Nicole is secured safely with this restraint..

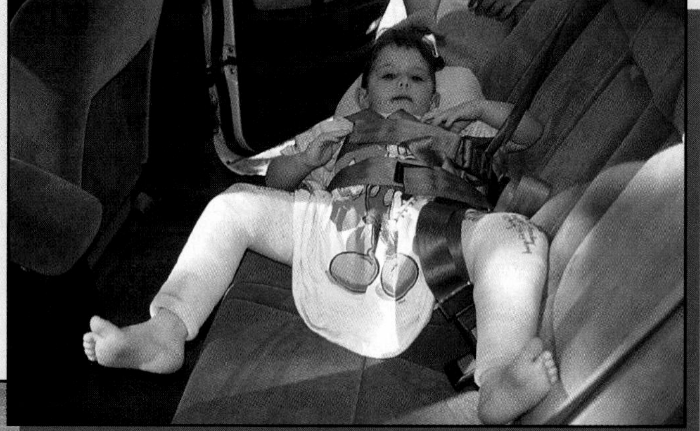

Before Nicole's discharge, her parents were instructed in body mechanics to prevent injury when lifting and turning Nicole in her heavy cast. At home, Nicole's mother washes her hair at the kitchen sink. Towels are used for comfort and to prevent water from running under the cast. Nicole is never left unattended on the kitchen counter or in other high places. Nicole's mother is careful to check the water temperature to prevent burning Nicole.

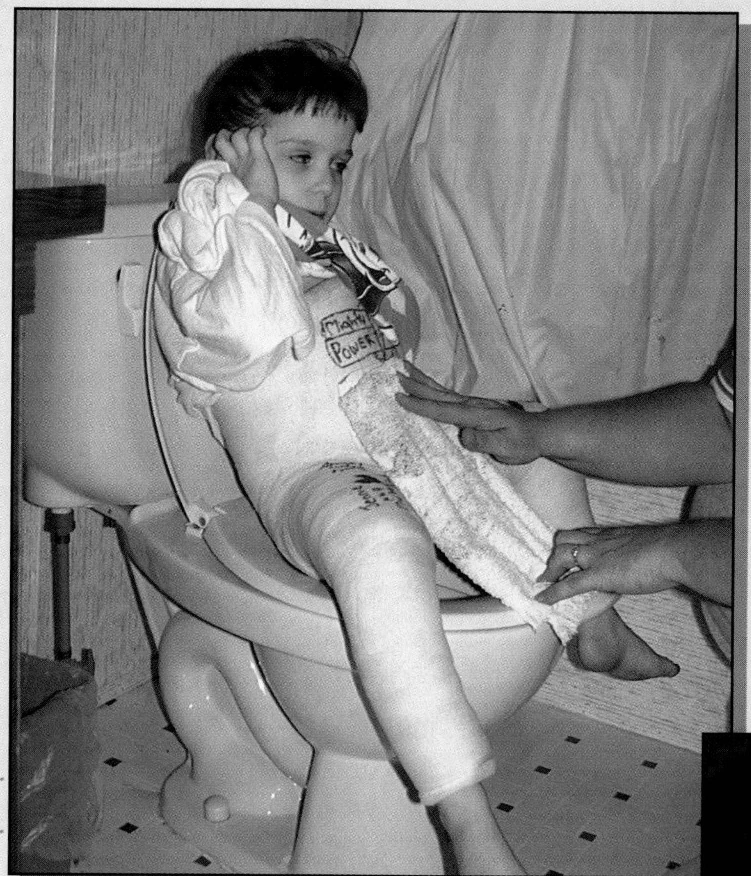

Nicole's mother has devised a system for toileting at home. Keeping Nicole in an upright position prevents soiling of the cast. Attention to bowel function is important as constipation is a potential problem. Increased dietary fiber and fluid intake, including prune juice, are usually adequate to promote regularity.

With pillows for positioning and comfort, Nicole uses a wheelchair for mobility. A younger child in a spica cast may be placed in a wagon padded with pillows. Children in wheelchairs and wagons should be strapped in to prevent falls. A child in a spica cast may also be placed on a blanket on the floor in an area of activity. This decreases the child's sense of isolation by increasing interactions with family members and friends.

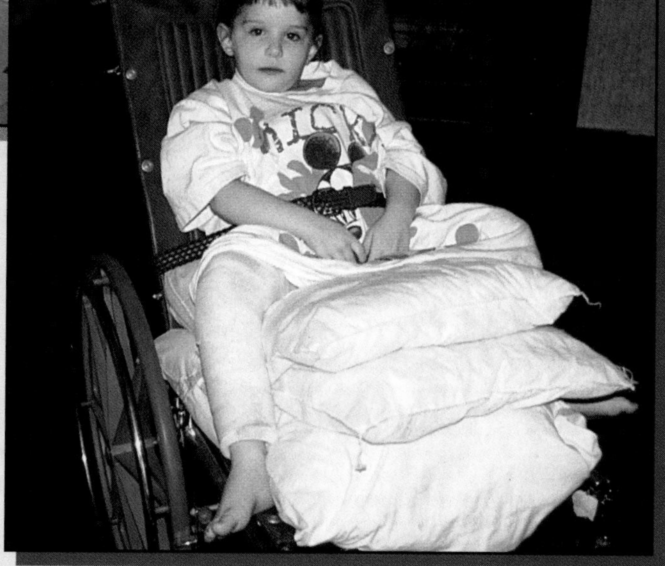

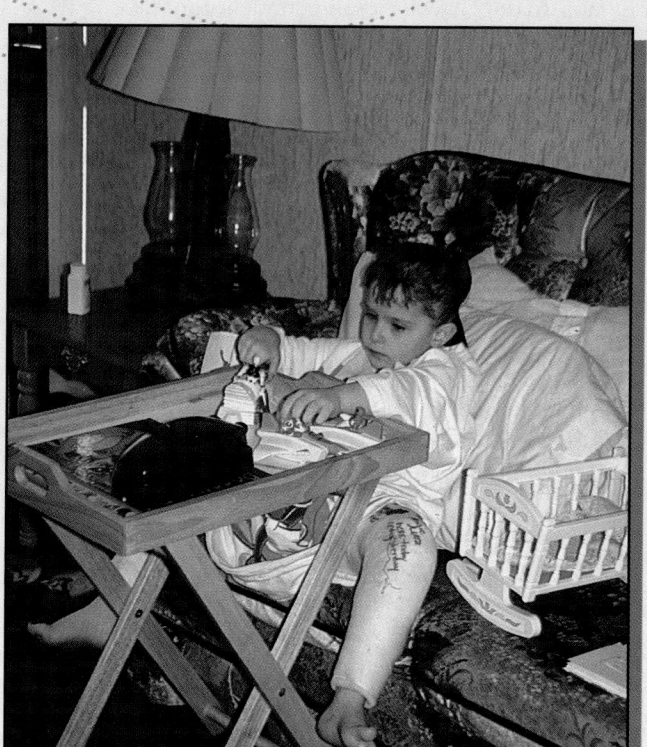

Photos courtesy of Judy Gross and Children's Hospital, Orthopediatric Unit, Medical University of South Carolina, Charleston, South Carolina.

Nicole is usually dressed in large tee shirts, which are soft, absorbent, and easy to put on and take off. Although Nicole is continent, a disposable diaper is taped under her perineal area in place of underpants. Clothing may be adapted using Velcro closures. Socks are used when needed to keep Nicole's feet warm.

Age-appropriate activities help to pass the time for the immobilized child and can challenge and enhance development. Dolls, books, and coloring interest Nicole. At home, Nicole prefers to sit on the edge of the couch. She is never left alone and is old enough to request assistance if she feels herself sliding.

Intervention	Rationale
2. Demonstrate the proper use of the Pavlik harness, including feeding and bathing, and ask the parents for a return demonstration.	Improper use of harness straps can cause skin irritation. During some periods of therapy, the harness may not be removed for several weeks.
3. Teach skin care (as outlined later in this chapter), emphasizing the reasons for each intervention and the risks posed by a wet cast or skin breakdown.	The skin of infants requires special care and attention. Caregivers are more likely to carry out instructions if they understand the reasons for each of the instructions.
4. Instruct parents about ways to dress their child to accommodate climate, style, and other needs (e.g., fitting of socks over toes of cast, use of Velcro closures, and relative ease of knit clothes).	Clothing must be suited to the environmental conditions to ensure the infant's comfort. The parents want the child to look as much like other infants as possible.

Evaluation:

- Parents use the Pavlik harness or spica cast in a safe and therapeutic manner.

NURSING DIAGNOSIS

- Anxiety (Parental) related to having a less-than-perfect child, and to the need to provide complex care for an extended period of time

Expected Outcomes:

The parents will:

- Describe DDH and its treatment in lay terms to other family members.
- Carry out treatment regimens, demonstrating increased self-confidence in the care of the child in the Pavlik harness or spica cast.
- Treat the child as a normal infant to the greatest extent possible.
- Interact with health care providers and others in a calm and friendly manner.

Intervention	Rationale
1. Communicate information to parents in a clear, kind, and straightforward manner.	Complex or ambiguous messages raise anxiety.
2. Adjust teaching to accommodate parents' need for information and support.	This helps parents gain a sense of control.
3. Teach methods to hold, nurse, and cuddle the infant while he/she is confined to the harness or spica cast.	Parent/infant bonding is important for both child and parents. Fear of harming child may prevent parents from cuddling the child.
4. Provide reliable, respectful, and empathetic care. Reduce waiting time during follow-up visits. Express an interest in the child and the parents.	Demonstrating respect for clients builds trust and reduces stress. The subtleties and complexities of this disorder often create confusion and uncertainty for parents.

Evaluation:

- The parents will describe DDH and its treatment in lay terms to other family members, carry out the prescribed therapy to the greatest extent possible, and treat the child as a normal (not handicapped) child.
- The parents will seek recommended health care, expressing concerns, questions, and frustrations in a calm and straightforward manner.

NURSING DIAGNOSIS • Risk for Impaired Skin Integrity related to chafing of the skin by the Pavlik harness or cast and to dampness

Expected Outcome: • The child's skin will remain clear and free of lesions.

Intervention	Rationale
1. Teach parents to protect the child's skin and legs under the harness by reducing rubbing of the harness. Use of long socks and Webril around the shoulder straps is helpful. Lotion may also be helpful in protecting delicate skin. Teach the parents to inspect the child's skin for reddened or irritated areas and to reposition the child frequently.	Protective layers reduce skin irritation. During some periods of therapy, the harness may not be removed. Cleanliness and skin care can be a particular challenge during these times.
2. Teach the family how to place disposable diapers snugly under the edges of the perineal hole in a spica cast, using sanitary napkins to absorb excess urine, or to use another method for containing urine and stool (see photo story). Teach the parents how to change diapers without removing the harness. (Refer to Chapter 36 for a discussion of cast care.)	Excess urine can trickle under the cast, irritating and macerating the skin, resisting drying, and becoming malodorous.

Evaluation: • The child's skin will remain clear and free of lesions.

NURSING DIAGNOSIS • Altered Tissue Perfusion (lower extremities) related to impaired circulation secondary to surgery and/or casting

Expected Outcome: • Circulation to the child's feet and toes will remain adequate, as evidenced by warm, well-perfused feet and toes, and absence of severe pain in the legs.

Intervention	Rationale
1. Assess the warmth and color of the child's feet and toes, and evaluate the child for excessive pain after hip surgery or after cast application according to the prescribed schedule (every 30 minutes for 4 hours; then every hour for 8 hours; then every 4 hours).	Snug casting and/or surgery can cause tissue swelling, resulting in circulatory compromise to the extremity. Swelling may increase in the hours after surgery and ecchymoses develop on the buttocks postoperatively.
2. If circulation distal to the operative site or cast is compromised, notify the physician promptly so that constricting forces can be relieved as soon as possible.	Without oxygen, metabolism is compromised and tissues will necrose, causing permanent tissue damage to the muscles and nerves.

Evaluation: • The child's toes and feet remain warm and pink throughout the treatment period.

NURSING DIAGNOSIS • Risk for Injury related to difficult positioning of child in infant-carrying devices (infant seats, strollers, car seats)

Expected Outcome: • The child will be safe from falls and will be adequately restrained when traveling in an automobile.

Intervention	Rationale
1. Assume a proactive role in discussing safety issues with parents.	In initiating a discussion about safety issues related to spica casts, the nurse advises the parents of the potential for injury and the importance of taking safety precautions.
2. Assist parents in identifying strategies for transporting their infant in a safe and comfortable manner, including use of a car seat that can accommodate the wide spread of legs of a child in a Pavlik harness or spica cast.	Most infant-carrying devices are not suitable or safe for infants in spica casts. Alternatives need to be safe, yet roomy enough to prevent discomfort and pressure points.
3. Suggest using an open area of the floor covered with a blanket to place the infant during waking hours as an alternative to traditional placement (e.g., in an infant seat).	On the floor, the child is safe from falls. The floor provides unrestricted play space.
4. Remind parents that the child must not be left unattended.	Infants often develop a surprising ability to move, despite the restrictions imposed by a cast.

Evaluation: • The child does not sustain injury.

NURSING DIAGNOSIS • Knowledge Deficit related to home care

Expected Outcome: • The family will successfully manage treatment at home.

Intervention	Rationale
1. Teach parents the correct use of the Pavlik harness or care of the child in a spica cast. Emphasize the importance of wearing the harness as prescribed.	Use of these devices requires skill to prevent complications and to achieve desired results.
2. Emphasize the importance of excellent hygiene and skin care.	Meticulous skin care and early detection and prompt treatment of irritation prevent skin breakdown.
3. Teach the parents the signs of infection (fever, wound drainage, indications of discomfort). Teach the parents the signs of neurovascular impairment (coolness or paleness of the feet, decreased motion of the legs or feet, swelling).	Parents must be alert for early signs of infection and altered tissue perfusion, and should be instructed to report complications promptly.
4. Teach the parents ways to provide environmental and development stimulation (e.g., moving the child to different areas of the home during the day, placing the child's bed near a window, placing toys within the child's reach, providing age-appropriate activities).	Providing stimulation decreases the boredom associated with immobility. Providing age-appropriate activities helps to promote normal development.
5. Explain the importance of feeding the child a diet that is high in calories, calcium, protein, and fiber fluids.	Such a diet promotes healing and bone development. Fiber helps prevent constipation.

Intervention	Rationale
6. Provide the parents with the name and phone number of an easily accessible health care provider in case questions arise at home. Inform the family of community resources available.	Accessibility of a health care provider or community resource decreases anxiety and improves compliance with treatment.
7. Schedule follow-up appoints prior to hospital discharge. Emphasize the importance of keeping these appointments.	Periodic evaluation is important to recovery.

Evaluation: • The parents verbalize an understanding of home care instructions.

HIP DISLOCATION IN THE CHILD WITH NEUROMUSCULAR IMPAIRMENT

Hip dislocation is a common occurrence in children with neuromuscular disorders, such as cerebral palsy and myelomeningocele. Although this disorder shares some similarities with DDH, the two disorders are separate entities. In some children with neuromuscular conditions, hip dislocation may be noted at birth. Usually, however, the child's hips are normal at birth, but become dislocated later.

Pathophysiology. Hip dislocation in children with associated neuromuscular disorders results from contractures and other imbalances of the muscles and tendons. In these children, the hip joint is often stable at birth. Over time, the unequal pull of muscles and tendons causes the hip(s) to become dislocated.

Incidence. Hip dislocation is a common occurrence in children with neuromuscular disorders, such as cerebral palsy and myelomeningocele. The incidence of dislocation increases with the severity of the neuromuscular impairment. Dislocation often occurs in the nonambulatory child with cerebral palsy in whom muscle imbalance is severe.

Clinical Manifestations. The clinical manifestations of hip dislocation are as follows:

- Severe contracture of the hip(s) in **adduction,** causing difficulty in diapering and seating
- Painful hip(s)
- Posterior displacement of the head of the femur, as evidenced by a bulge in the gluteal area

Diagnostic Evaluation. Diagnosis of dislocated hip and other disorders of the hip in the neuromuscularly impaired child may be made at any time during infancy and childhood. Although not all of these children appear to be uncomfortable, some may cry or otherwise complain of hip pain as dysplasia develops. Because many of these children are profoundly retarded, their complaints may go unrecognized. Seating and hygiene of children with cerebral palsy may become difficult as hip disease develops and abduction becomes difficult. In extreme cases, pressure points secondary to the dislocations can lead to decubitus ulcers. Because hip disorders are so common in these children, routine radiographic hip screening is done throughout childhood. Assessment varies depending on the underlying neuromuscular disease.

Therapeutic Management. Often, dislocation of the hip can be prevented or delayed in neuromuscularly impaired children by surgical release of muscle and tendons. When dislocation does occur, treatment can be very difficult. Traction, surgical release of muscles and tendons, and/or osteotomy of the femur or pelvis may be necessary. These procedures are followed by positioning and long-term immobilization in a spica cast to allow for healing.

Therapy is aimed at maximizing functional ability (including seating), eliminating pain, and facilitating diapering and other hygiene-related activities. Treatment progress is closely monitored by clinical examination and radiographs. Close follow-up is essential, as hip displacement in these children can recur, and treatment may need to be reinstituted or modified.

Nursing Care

Nursing care, teaching needs, and home care of the neuromuscularly impaired child with a dislocated hip centers around care of the child in a spica cast (see the previous section on DDH) and is adjusted to the functional abilities and needs of the individual child. The reader is referred to Chapter 40 for further discussion of the nursing care of the child with neurological/developmental alterations.

LIMB DEFECTS

Defects of the limbs are common in children and are a concern of parents. Most alterations of arms and legs are mild variations of normal posturing, but some are severe anomalies or abnormalities.

Etiology and Incidence. A wide range in the type and severity of malformations of the limbs exists. Limb defects result from birth anomalies and sometimes from trauma. These defects take many forms, including webbing (syndactyly) or extra (polydactyly) fingers or toes; congenital absence of all or part of an extremity; and club foot (covered below) and club hand. The structure and function of congenital limb malformations can be improved with therapy but the affected limbs are never normal.

Trauma or infection to an extremity may result in a variety of difficulties. Leg-length discrepancy can result after trauma, infection, or radiation as a result of the child's continued growth.

Pathophysiology. Mild limb defects most frequently occur secondary to the forces of extrinsic pressure such as in utero positioning, or to the sitting and sleeping postures of young children. Heredity may also play a part in mild alterations of the limbs. These disorders are usually cosmetic in nature, although occasionally they alter functional ability. They tend to correct with the growth of the child. Common mild developmental alterations of the limbs include knock-knees (genu valgum) and bowlegs (genu varum), metatarsus adductus, toeing-in, toeing-out, and flat feet.

Severe limb defects are often congenital; they include club foot and absence of limbs.

Diagnostic Evaluation. Severe congenital defects are readily apparent at birth. Mild defects and deformations that develop over time are usually identified by parents or school nurses and are evaluated by specialized clinicians. X-rays may be necessary to fully evaluate limb defects and to assist with developing a treatment plan.

Therapeutic Management. Mild limb deformities often resolve without treatment. Sometimes, exercises, splints, special shoes, or casts are prescribed. For severe deformities, surgical intervention may be required to release tendons, reposition bones, reconstruct parts, retard growth of an extremity, or exacerbate growth of a limb. In some situations, long-term immobility of an extremity is necessary using casts or **external fixation. Orthoses** may be prescribed for specific needs, and physical therapy may be necessary.

Nursing Care

Nursing care varies with the defect and with the treatment. Parents may need a great deal of reassurance about the outcomes of their child's therapy. The nurse must reinforce the principles of therapy and teach parents to carry out treatments at home. For example, exercises, special appliances, or braces may require daily use. For children in casts, parents must be taught how to provide care at home (see Chapter 36 and the previous section in this chapter on DDH). Parents may need referral to an orthotist for construction of a device to assist with the child's function or mobility. The nurse must reinforce correct use of these appliances. Special emphasis on protection of skin is another task of the nurse. Periodic follow-up is often necessary for children with limb defects.

Clubfoot

Clubfoot is congenital malformation of the lower extremity.

Etiology. Although the cause of clubfoot deformity is unknown, there is a genetic predisposition. In addition, children with certain neuromuscular disorders, such as myelomeningocele, are especially prone to having clubfoot.

Incidence. Clubfoot occurs in 1:1000 births. There is a 2:1 ratio of males to females.

Clinical Manifestations. The clinical manifestations of clubfoot are as follows:

- The foot is plantar-flexed, with an inverted heel and adducted forefoot.
- The defect may be unilateral or bilateral.
- Defects are rigid and cannot be manipulated into a neutral position.

Diagnostic Evaluation. Clubfoot is readily apparent on clinical examination at birth.

Therapeutic Management. Treatment for clubfoot is started as soon after birth as possible. Serial manipulation and casting are performed at least weekly. If sufficient correction is not achieved in 3 to 6 months, surgery is usually indicated. Some malformations respond readily to treatment, whereas other more severe forms respond less well to even vigorous and prolonged therapy. Although early treatment may result in a foot that appears normal, recurrence is common. For this reason, long-term follow-up of the child with clubfoot is essential, as further treatment may be indicated. Even with aggressive treatment, the foot is seldom completely normal. Lifelong atrophy of the calf is common (Handlesman & Badalamente, 1981; Hyam et al., 1977; Irani & Sherman, 1963), and is often accompanied by structural deformity of the ankle and foot.

PATHOPHYSIOLOGY *of Clubfoot*

In clubfoot, the foot is **plantar-flexed,** the heel is inverted, and the forefoot is adducted. The foot is rigid and is resistant to manipulation. The malformation involves the foot, ankle, and lower leg, and must be differentiated from a flexible **inversion** of the foot found commonly in neonates.

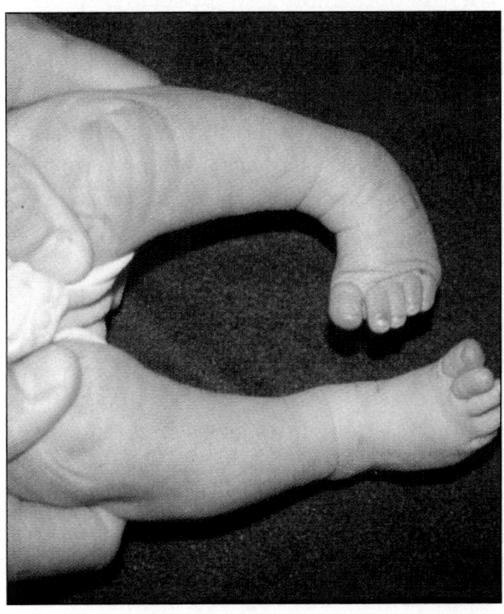

NURSING CARE OF THE CHILD WITH CLUBFOOT

Assessment

Initially the nurse must assess and explore the parents' feelings about not having a completely normal newborn infant. As treatment is initiated, parents' knowledge about the disorder of clubfoot, the treatment, and the need for long-term follow-up must also be assessed. Long-term casting with frequent cast changes place great responsibility on the parents (Fig. 37–5). Their ability to adequately monitor the child for complications must be assessed. In addition, when the child must undergo surgical correction of the defect, pain monitoring and treatment interventions are necessary and require particular nursing skill.

Nursing Diagnosis and Planning

The following nursing diagnoses and expected outcomes may be appropriate following assessment of the child with clubfoot.

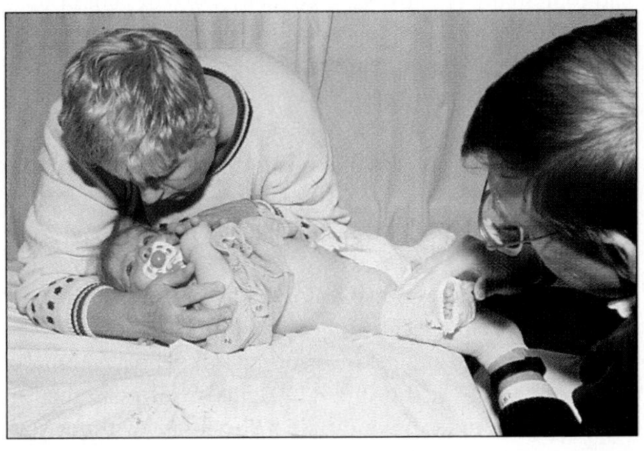

Figure 37–5
In the infant with clubfoot, serial manipulation and casting are started as soon after birth as possible to take advantage of the natural pliability of the neonate's bones. Long-term casting with frequent cast changes places great responsibility on the parents. The nurse is responsible for teaching the parents cast care and monitoring the child for complications. Recurrence is common, making long-term follow-up essential. (Courtesy of Cook Children's Medical Center, Fort Worth, Texas)

- Dysfunctional Grieving (Parental): related to actual loss of anticipated perfect neonate and to missing the experience of parenting a perfect newborn infant. ***Expected Outcome:*** *The parents will discuss their feelings about their child's deformity and about not being able to parent a perfect child.*
- Knowledge Deficit related to treatment, home management in a cast, and need for long-term follow-up. ***Expected Outcome:*** *The parents will explain and demonstrate the care of their child in a clubfoot cast and what to do when difficulties arise.*
- Risk for Impaired Skin Integrity related to irritation from casts or splints. ***Expected Outcome:*** *The child will maintain intact skin on the legs and feet.*
- Altered Tissue Perfusion (Peripheral) related to surgery and/or casting of the lower extremities. ***Expected Outcome:*** *The child will exhibit adequate tissue perfusion in the toes of the affected foot at all times.*
- Pain related to surgery on the foot or feet. ***Expected Outcome:*** *The child will exhibit comfort as evidenced by normal patterns of sleeping and feeding.*
- Altered Growth and Development related to immobility. ***Expected Outcome:*** *The child will achieve optimal growth and development.*

Implementation

Nursing care is related to the stage of treatment. Initially, parents need help understanding the defect and the possibilities for treatment and outcome. They also may need help acknowledging the defect as a source of disappointment. The nurse can encourage parents to discuss the defect with each other and to recognize each other's unique strategies for coping with the defect.

Pain management in the immediate postoperative period is the role of the nurse. Initially intravenous analgesia is used, with progression to oral analgesia such as codeine, and then to non-aspirin, non-narcotic analgesics. The feet should be elevated in the postoperative period and ice bags should be applied to reduce swelling and pain and to help ensure adequate circulation to the foot or feet. The neurovascular status of the toes needs to be assessed at least every 2 hours in the immediate postoperative period. Parents will need help positioning the child for comfortable feeding. Usually, the infant's feet are elevated above the level of his heart to reduce swelling and pain. The reader is referred to Chapter 20 (The Child in Pain) for additional strategies for managing pain in children.

The nurse is responsible for teaching the parents how to keep the cast(s) clean and dry at home. Cast edges must be petalled with moleskin or other soft fabric to protect the tender skin of the infant. Parents need assistance in learning how to bathe and diaper the infant without soiling or wetting the cast(s). When cast changes are done on an outpatient basis, parents need instructions about how to assess the child's neurovascular status and who to notify if assistance is needed. See Chapter 36 (The Child With Musculoskeletal Alterations) for further discussion about the care of a child in a cast.

The nurse must decide whether referral of the family to the local visiting nurse agency is necessary. Because clubfoot can recur, all children with this condition require interval follow-up until they reach skeletal maturity. Parents must understand that this periodic follow-up assessment is essential.

> Because the condition of clubfoot can recur, all children with clubfoot require long-term interval follow-up until they reach skeletal maturity to ensure an optimal outcome.

Home Care. Nonsurgical home care for the infant undergoing treatment for clubfoot centers around care of the cast(s). Hygiene and skin care should be emphasized.

Postoperatively, the child's foot will be casted for several months. Not only must parents care for the cast, but they must be taught to monitor the child for signs of neurovascular compromise (coolness or paleness of foot, weak or absent pulses).

Parents caring for a child at home need to be provided with the name and phone number of an easily accessible health care provider in the event that they have concerns. Follow-up monitoring is necessary for all patients with clubfoot, even those who have undergone surgical correction, because of the potential for recurrence.

Evaluation

- Are the child's feet warm, with normal color and intact skin?
- Can the parents verbalize those symptoms that must be reported immediately to the primary care practitioner?
- Do the parents attend follow-up appointments?
- Do the parents describe activities that promote the child's growth and development?
- Does the child demonstrate age-appropriate tasks and skills?
- Do parents discuss their feelings and experiences about the child's feet with friends and family members?
- Does the child exhibit usual sleep and feeding patterns?

Genu Valgum (Knock Knees) and Genu Varum (Bowlegs)

Genu varum (bowlegs) and genu valgum (knock knees) are usually variations of normal growth and development or are familial (physiologic), but they may have a pathologic origin. Bowlegs are common in infants and toddlers, and it is estimated that 20% of all 3-year-olds have knock knees. In most of these cases, the condition resolves spontaneously without treatment. The pathologic form of genu valgum and genu varum usually occurs secondary to another condition and may require treatment. In addition, asymmetric deformity may require treatment.

Pathophysiology. Almost always, knock knees and bowlegs are normal variations in the growth of children. However, both may occur as a result of trauma to the tibia or femur, or may be secondary to other disorders, such as profound obesity, osteomyelitis, rickets, juvenile rheumatoid arthritis, neurofibromatosis, Blount's disease, or osteogensis imperfecta.

Incidence. Bowlegs are common in sturdily built infants and toddlers. This condition is also associated with tibial torsion, which is a normal variation in toddlers. Knock knees are common in the preschool age group (ages 3 to 7 years). The incidence of either condition varies with the child's age and the presence of other disorders or conditions.

Clinical Manifestations. The clinical manifestations of genu varum and genu valgum include the following:

- Angulation of the legs causing the knees to touch or to bow
- Awkward appearance, with occasional stumbling
- Pain (infrequent)
- Only a mild deformity in most cases
- No effect on function usually
- May be associated with a specific age (e.g., bowlegs in toddlers)
- Decreasingly severe deformity (or vanishing entirely) with age

Diagnostic Evaluation. The diagnosis is established on the basis of a visual examination (Fig. 37–6). Assessment by a skilled practitioner yields information that will determine the need for treatment. An asymmetric deformity or a cosmetically unacceptable and progressing deformity, requires further evaluation.

Therapeutic Management. In most children, knock knees and bowlegs have little clinical significance. Until the age of $2\frac{1}{2}$ years, bowlegs are a common variation in the normal child. Knock knees are common in children ages 2 to 7 years. A severe or asymmetric deformity is cause for further investigation. Both conditions tend to self-correct as the child ambulates and grows. Night splints may be prescribed to encourage a postural or positional change. Manual manipulation to encourage flexibility, or casting, may be indicated. Clothing may disguise a mild deformity. For some children, weight reduction may be the only treatment necessary to correct the deformity. In children in whom the deformity does not resolve spontaneously or in whom underlying pathology exists, stapling of the growth

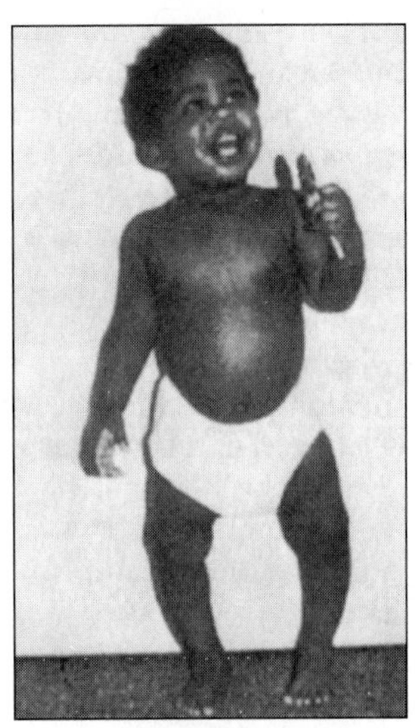

Bowlegs

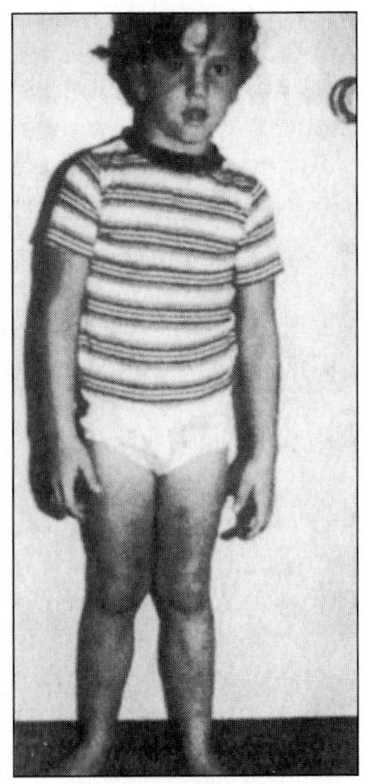

Knock Knees

Figure 37–6

In the child with genu varum, or bowlegs, there is a persistent space measuring more than 2.5 cm between the knees when the ankles are together. Genu varum is a normal finding for 1 year after the child begins walking. In the child with genu valgum, or knock knees, there is a space of more than 2.5 cm between the ankles when the knees are together. Genu varum occurs as a normal variation in children 2 to $3\frac{1}{2}$ years of age. To remember the terminology, link the r's and g's: genu varum—knees apart; genu valgum—knees together. (From McDade, W. [1977, November]. Bowlegs and knock knees. *Pediatric Clinics of North America, 24*(4), 831, 833.)

plates on the lateral or medial side may allow correction of the deformity as further growth takes place. For severe deformity, osteotomy may be indicated.

Nursing Care

Nursing care focuses on assisting the child's parents to understand the treatment program so they will comply with it. They may need to be discouraged from purchasing expensive corrective shoes, which are not necessary. For children who must wear night splints or braces, parents may need assistance adhering to the regimen in the face of loud protestations from the child. Sleeping may be interrupted as the child adjusts to new sleeping positions. For children with severe obesity, the goal may be to change the eating behaviors for the entire family to allow the child every opportunity for significant and successful weight reduction.

Reinforcement of the explanations offered by the physician increases the parents' understanding of these disorders and helps to reduce concern about normal variations of growth and development. Home care focuses on ensuring compliance with the prescribed treatment regimen and recommended follow-up evaluation.

KEY CONCEPTS

- All children should undergo routine interval well-child evaluation to assess for normal growth and development.
- Children with identified structural disorders of the bones and joints require periodic follow-up evaluations until they reach skeletal maturity to assess the efficacy of treatment and to ensure positive outcomes.
- Children and families require empathetic care to deal with the anxieties and altered body image caused by deformity.
- Attention must be directed toward preventing skin irritation and breakdown under casts and braces.
- To the greatest degree possible, children with structural deformities should be treated as normal children.
- Children in casts and braces need special monitoring to ensure safety.
- The nurse plays a pivotal role in teaching and in ensuring routine follow-up care for children with structural deformities.

REFERENCES

Allington, N. J. & Bowen, J. R. (1996). Adolescent idiopathic scoliosis: Treatment with the Wilmington brace. A comparison of full-time and part-time use. *Journal of Bone and Joint Surgery (Am), 78*(7), 1056–1062.

Handlesman, J. E., & Badalamente, M. A. (1981). Neuromuscular studies in clubfoot. *Journal of Pediatric Orthopaedics, 1*(1), 23–32.

Hsu, L. C. & Upadhyay, S. S. (1994). Effect of spinal fusion on growth of the spine and lower limbs in girls with adolescent idiopathic scoliosis. *Journal of Pediatric Orthopaedics, 14*(5), 564–568.

Hyam, I., Handlesman, J. E., Badenhorst, M., & Pickering, A. (1977). The muscles in the club foot—A histological, histochemical and electron microscope study. *The Journal of Bone and Joint Surgery, 59B*(4), 465–72.

Irani, R. N., & Sherman, M. S. (1963). The pathological anatomy of the club foot. *The Journal of Bone and Joint Surgery, 45A*, 45–52.

Puno, R. M., Mehta, S., & Byrd, J. A. (1994). Surgical treatment of idiopathic thoracolumbar and lumbar scoliosis in adolescent patients. *Orthopaedic Clinics of North America, 25*(2), 275–286.

Rosendahl, K., Aslaksen, A., Lie, R. T., & Markestad, T. (1995). Reliability of ultrasound in the early diagnosis of developmental dysplasia of the hip. *Pediatric Radiology, 25*(3), 219–224.

Theiss, S. M., Lonstein, J. E., & Winter, R. B. (1996). Wound infections in reconstructive spine surgery. *Orthopaedic Clinics of North America, 27*(1), 105–110.

Winter, R. B. (1994). The pendulum has swung too far. Bracing for adolescent idiopathic scoliosis in the 1990s. *Orthopaedic Clinics of North America, 25*(2), 195–204.

BIBLIOGRAPHY

Abramson, S. J. (1992). Real ultrasonographic evaluation of the infant hip. *Orthopaedic Nursing, 11*(1), 72–3.

Barlow, T. G. (1962). Early diagnosis and treatment of congenital dislocation of the hip. *Journal of Bone and Joint Surgery, 44B*(2), 292–301.

Behrman, R. E., & Vaughan, V. C. (1992). *Nelson's textbook of pediatrics* (14th ed.). Philadelphia: W. B. Saunders.

Brosnan, H. (1991). Nursing management of the adolescent with idiopathic scoliosis. *The Nursing Clinics of North America, 26*, 17–31.

Canale, S. T., & Beaty, J. H. (1991). *Operative pediatric orthopaedics*. St. Louis: Mosby–Year Book.

Carpenito, L. J. (1989). *Nursing diagnosis: Application to clinical practice*. Philadelphia: J. B. Lippincott.

Cassella, M. C., & Hall, J. E. (1991). Current treatment approaches in the operative and nonoperative management of adolescent idiopathic scoliosis. *Phyiscal Therapy, 71*(12), 897–909.

Corbett, D. (1988). Information needs of parents of a child in a Pavlik harness. *Orthopaedic Nursing, 7*(2), 20–3.

Cotton, L. A. (1991). Unit rod segmental spinal instrumentation for the treatment of neuromuscular scoliosis. *Orthopaedic Nursing, 10*(5), 17–23.

Gross, R. H. (1985). Common angular and rotational problems of early childhood. *Orthopaedic Surgery Update Series, 3*(39). Princeton, NJ: Continuing Professional Education Center.

Killam, P. E. (1989). Orthopedic assessment of young children: Developmental variations. *Nurse Practitioner, 14*(7), 27–36.

Kyzer, S. P. (1991). Congenital idiopathic clubfoot. *Orthopaedic Nursing, 10*(4), 11–18.

Mason, K. J. (1989). Pediatric orthopaedics: Developmental norms. *Orthopaedic Nursing, 8*(4), 45–50.

Mason, K. J. (1991). Congenital orthopedic anomalies and their impact on the family. *The Nursing Clinics of North America, 26*, 1–16.

McDade, W. (1977). Bowlegs and knock-knees. *Pediatric Clinics of North America, 24*(4), 825–839.

Renshaw, T. S. (1986). *Pediatric orthopedics*. Philadelphia: W. B. Saunders.

Schaming, D., Gorry, M., Soroka, K., & Catullo, M. E. (1990). When babies are born with orthopaedic problems. *RN, 53*(4), 62–7.

Scoles, P. V. (1988). *Pediatric orthopedics in clinical practice*. (2nd ed.). Chicago: Year Book Medical Publishers.

Shoppee, K. (1992). Developmental dysplasia of the hip. *Orthopaedic Nursing, 11*(5), 30–36.

Sparks, S. M., & Taylor, C. M. (1993). *Nursing diagnosis and reference manual*. Springhouse, PA: Springhouse.

Speers, A. T., & Speers, M. (1992). Care of the infant in a Pavlik harness. *Pediatric Nursing, 18*(3), 229–32.

Stout, J. D., Bandy, P., Feller, N., Stroup, K. B., & Bull, M. J. (1992). Transportating resources for pediatric orthopaedic clients. *Orthopaedic Nursing, 11*(4), 26–30.

Waters, L. (1992). Pharmacologic strategies for managing pain in children. *Orthopaedic Nursing, 11*(1), 34–40.

Williams, P. F., & Cole, W. G. (Eds.). (1991). *Orthopaedic management in childhood* (2nd ed.). London: Chapman and Hall.

38

The Child With Endocrine Alterations

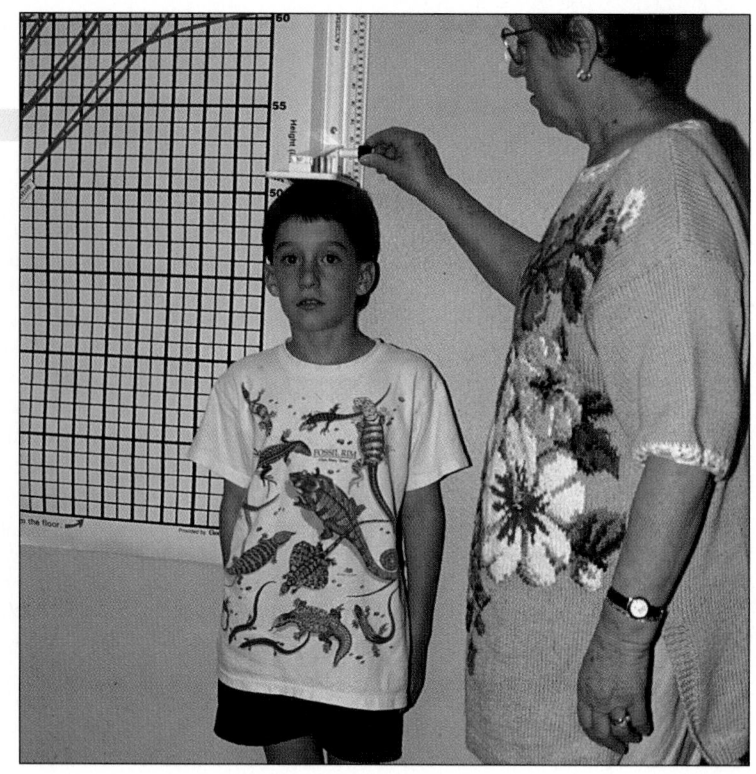

CHAPTER OVERVIEW

LEARNING OBJECTIVES

After studying this chapter, you should be able to:

- List the six major hormones of the endocrine system.
- Describe the negative feedback system.
- Discuss nursing strategies to improve compliance with medications.
- Describe the difference between hypothyroidism and hyperthyroidism.
- Compare and contrast the relationship between diabetes insipidus and syndrome of inappropriate antidiuretic hormone as they relate to water metabolism.
- Describe the psychosocial issues concerning children with precocious puberty.
- Describe two tests that assess for hypocalcemia.

KEY TERMS

euthyroid: having normal thyroid function

gland: an organ or structure that secretes a substance or hormones to be used in some other part of the body

hormone: a chemical substance produced by one gland or tissue and carried by the blood to other tissues or organs, where it causes a specific effect

hypothalamus: portion of the brain that secretes releasing factors to the pituitary gland for the maintenance of endocrine/metabolic activities

idiopathic: for unknown reasons

pituitary: an endocrine gland attached to the base of the brain that secretes numerous hormones; often referred to as "the master gland"

This chapter looks at the main endocrine glands and how alterations in the hormones they secrete affect infants and children. Some of the disorders discussed, such as precocious puberty and growth hormone deficiency, are most often seen in an outpatient setting. Because several of the disorders require long-term management, the nurse's priority is teaching and advocacy. In those disorders that may affect the child's appearance, the child's psychologic needs must be a priority. Diabetes mellitus, a common disorder of the endocrine system, is discussed in Chapter 39.

CLINICAL REFERENCE PAGES

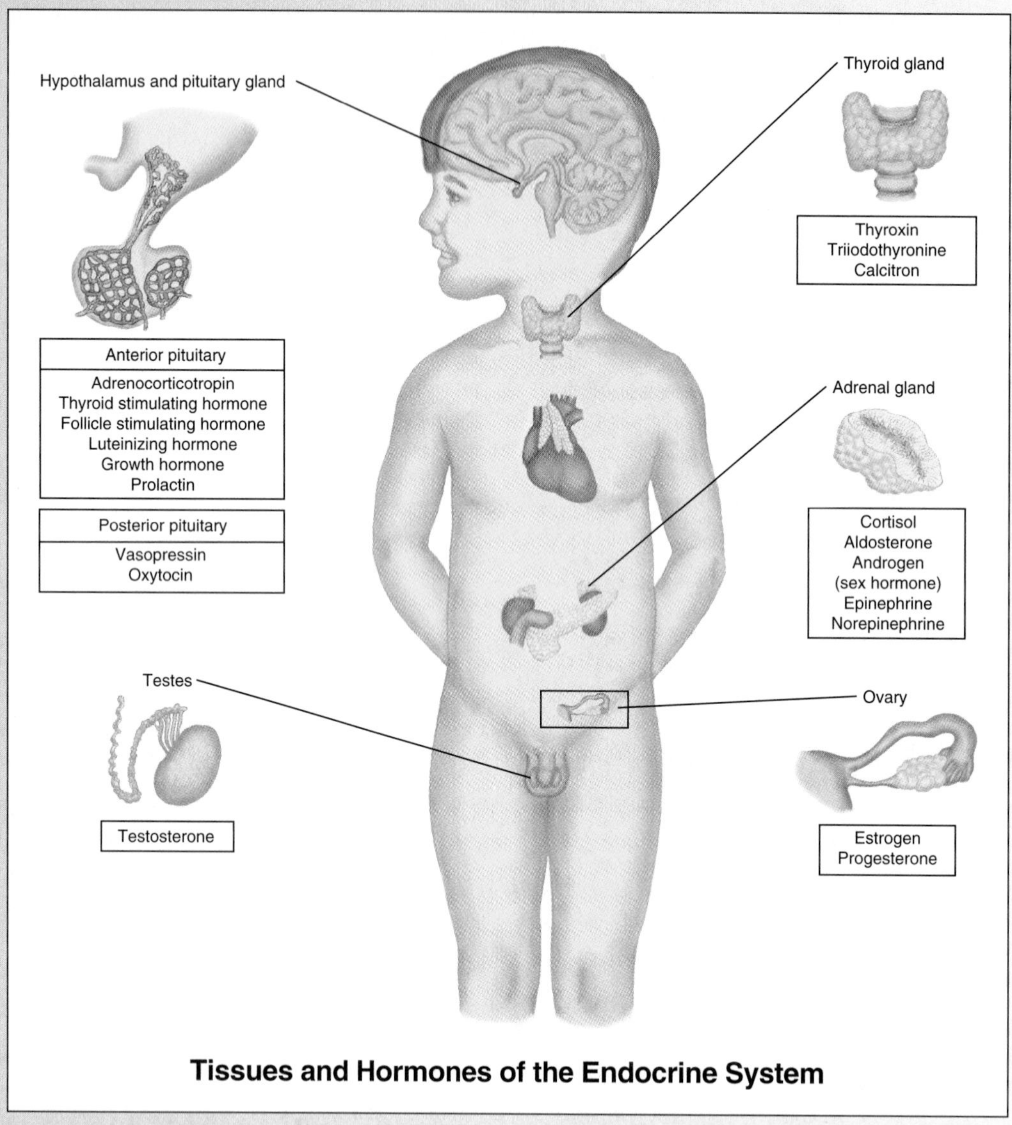

Tissues and Hormones of the Endocrine System

REVIEW OF THE ENDOCRINE SYSTEM

The endocrine system comprises various tissues that produce and secrete chemicals called **hormones.** The hormones stimulate and regulate the actions of other tissues, the target tissues. The endocrine system and the autonomic nervous system function together to regulate growth, metabolism, and reproduction. The hypothalamic-pituitary axis controls their activities. The autonomic nervous system reacts to stimuli, transmitting its message to the hypothalamus. In turn, the **hypothalamus** manufactures and secretes the appropriate factors. These are transmitted to the anterior pituitary gland, which then stimulates or inhibits the release of the involved hormones.

The principle of feedback control is involved in hormone production and secretion (see figure). Negative feedback is involved when the concentration of a particular hormone increases, inhibiting the system responsible for releasing that hormone; thus, as the hormonal secretion rises, there is a corresponding decrease in secretion of the stimulating hormone. When there is too little circulating hormone, the target gland is stimulated to secrete additional hormone.

The **pituitary gland** is composed of an anterior lobe and a posterior lobe. The anterior pituitary lobe produces six hormones: adrenocorticotropic hormone (ACTH), thyroid-stimulating hormone (TSH), follicle-stimulating hormone (FSH), luteinizing hormone (LH), growth hormone (GH), and prolactin. Four of these hormones—ACTH, TSH, LH, and FSH—in turn stimulate their target glands to secrete the appropriate specific hormones. The posterior pituitary lobe produces antidiuretic hormone (ADH) and oxytocin.

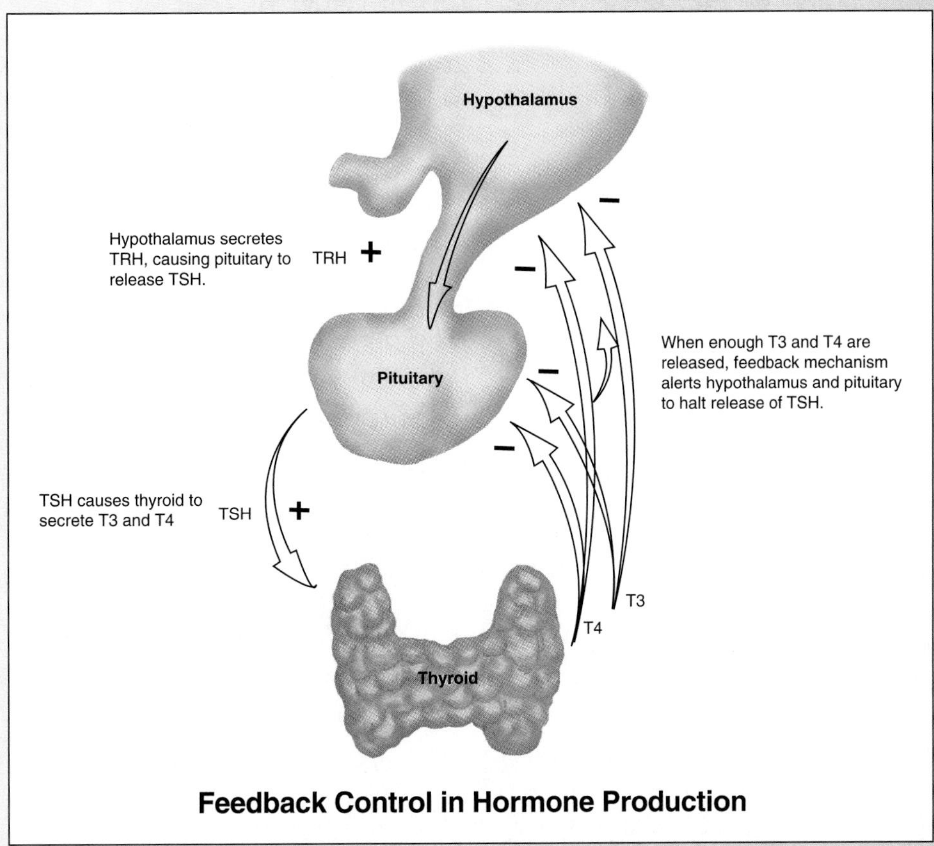

Feedback Control in Hormone Production

Disruption in the neurologic or chemical control of hormone secretion will cause an endocrine disorder. Possible underlying causes include malfunction of the nervous system, the hypothalamus, the pituitary gland, or the target gland. Congenital, infectious, neoplastic, autoimmune, or **idiopathic** factors may play a role. Abnormal activity of the pituitary gland can result in genetic alterations, developmental and degenerative problems, tumor formation, and other manifestations of abnormality.

DIAGNOSTIC TESTS AND PROCEDURES

Diagnosing endocrine dysfunction most commonly involves laboratory testing. Serum samples of hormones are measured to determine if the levels are adequate, deficient, or excessive. Laboratory screening is useful for diagnosis of disease, as well as for monitoring children on hormone therapy.

Normal hormone levels for children are related to age and stage of puberty. Hormones are secreted at various times during the day or on a circadian rhythm. Therefore, random blood samples may be difficult to interpret. In order to avoid this, stimulation testing is frequently used to obtain more accurate and definitive test results. This usually requires the child to be admitted for a limited morning stay in the hospital.

With stimulation testing, a releasing factor or other agent is given to trigger the release of a specific hormone. The peak level of the hormone can then be measured and more accurately interpreted.

Other diagnostic tests include bone age X-rays for bone maturation and growth potential. Computed tomography (CT) scans and magnetic resonance imaging (MRI) scans are used to determine the presence of tumors and/or cysts that may be affecting either the hypothalamus, pituitary, or target glands.

Accurate measurement of height and weight is important when assessing the child for endocrine dysfunction. Evaluation of sexual development according to Tanner stages is also a part of the diagnostic workup (see Table 8–2 in Chapter 8). Developmental milestones and school performance should also be monitored, because delays may be associated with endocrine disorders.

Pediatric Differences in the Endocrine System

- The endocrine system is less developed at birth than any other body system.
- Hormonal control of many body functions is lacking until age 12 to 18 months. As a result, infants may manifest imbalances in concentration of fluids, electrolytes, amino acids, glucose, and trace substances.

COMMON LABORATORY AND DIAGNOSTIC TESTS FOR ENDOCRINE SYSTEM DYSFUNCTION

TEST	DESCRIPTION	NORMAL FINDINGS	INDICATIONS	PREPARATION AND NURSING CONSIDERATIONS
Blood				
Growth hormone test	An agent such as insulin, arginine, or clonidine is given to stimulate release or production of GH	One or more peak GH levels greater than 7 ng/ml	Evaluate GH deficiency	Time specific; specimens must be drawn accurately NPO after midnight before test Notify physician if severe or prolonged hypoglycemia develops when insulin is given as stimulating agent
Cosyntropin test (Cortrosyn)	IV cosyntropin (ACTH) is given to test ability of adrenal gland to respond to ACTH	A rise of cortisol level 7 mEq/dl or more above baseline	Evaluate adrenal insufficiency (may be associated with GH deficiency or hypopituitarism)	NPO after midnight Blood samples must be drawn before and after cosyntropin is given
Diagnostic				
Water deprivation study	Child is deprived of water and other fluids for 7 hr	Decreased urine output Increased urine specific gravity Normal serum sodium	Confirm diagnosis of diabetes insipidus	Strictly monitor serum sodium and urine osmolality Stop test if significant weight loss, or change in vital signs or neurologic status develop Weigh child before, during, and after test
Radiologic				
Bone age X-ray film	X-ray study of wrist to determine bone maturation	Bone age consistent with chronologic age	Delayed bone age may indicate GH deficiency or hypothyroidism; advanced bone age may be associated with precocious puberty	None
CT/MRI of brain	Noninvasive imaging techniques to identify structures/abnormalities of the brain	Normal structures	Determine presence of tumors or cysts, or structural abnormalities that may be affecting either hypothalamus or pituitary gland	May require sedation
Pelvic ultrasound study	Noninvasive sound waves identify anatomy of pelvic structures/abnormalities	Normal structures	Identify tumors/cysts within ovaries or adrenal glands in disorders associated with puberty	May require full bladder

MEDICATIONS COMMONLY USED IN TREATING ENDOCRINE DISORDERS

DRUG	ACTION	DOSAGE AND ADMINISTRATION	SIDE EFFECTS	NURSING CONSIDERATIONS
Levothyroxine (Synthroid, Levothroid)	Replacement therapy for hypothyroidism	*PO* <1 yr: 25–50 μg/day >1 yr and adolescents: 3–6 μg/kg/day Initial dose is one-fourth maintenance dose *IV* 75% of oral dose	Hyperthyroidism, palpitations, increased sweating, heat intolerance	Administer at same time each day Use pill dispenser to increase compliance
Methimazole (Tapazole)	Blocks thyroid production; treatment of hyperthyroidism	Initial dose: 0.05–0.7 mg/kg/day, divided into 3 doses q 8 hr Maintenance therapy: half of initial dose q 8 hr	Skin rash, pruritus, arthralgia, neutropenia, hepatotoxicity, hypothyroidism	Inform patient or parent to notify physician if skin rash or sore throat occurs
Propylthiouracil (PTU)	Inhibits thyroid hormone synthesis. Diverts iodine from thyroid hormone synthesis	Children 6–10 yr 50–150 mg/day divided into 3 doses q 8 hr	Urticaria, rash, pruritus, nausea, skin pigmentation, hair loss, headache, hepatotoxicity	Obtain baseline weight/pulse Check for skin eruptions, itching, and swollen lymph glands Space evenly around clock Notify physician of sudden or continuous weight increase
Desmopressin acetate (DDAVP)	Controls increased urination caused by insufficient ADH Regulates thirst and serum sodium	*Intranasal* Concentration: 100 mcg/ml Dose: 0.05–0.2 ml bid; titrated to regulate urine output *Subcutaneous* Concentration: 4 μg/ml Dose: 1/10 intranasal dose	Too much DDAVP may cause decreased urine output, decreased serum sodium, headache, water retention Not enough DDAVP may cause increased urine output and thirst, decreased serum sodium, dehydration	Monitor urine output Follow sodium levels Explain signs and symptoms of hyponatremia (refer to Table 36–5)
Gonadotropin releasing factor agonist (Depo-Lupron)	Suppresses puberty by inhibiting binding of GnRH to pituitary gland, which causes decrease in production of LH, FSH, estrogen, and testosterone	*IM* 7.5 mg q 4 wk Dose range: 140–300 μg/kg/month	Local irritation at injection site	Instruct parent or older child in proper IM injection technique
Growth hormone (Protropin, somatrem)	Replacement therapy for GH deficiency Increases rate of growth Protects against hypoglycemia	*Subcutaneous* 0.15–0.30 mg/kg/wk divided into 6 or 7 doses 7 times/wk supplied Powder form; must be diluted	Local irritation at injection site	Teach parent proper subcutaneous injection technique Observe for local irritation Teach correct dilution and administration of medication Refrigerate after diluting
Hydrocortisone (Cortef)	Replacement therapy for adrenal insufficiency/hypopituitarism	*PO or IV* Maintenance: 10–20 mg/m²/day divided into 2–3 doses Stress: 150 mg/m² divided into 3–4 doses	Edema, weight gain, glucosuria, greater risk of infection, ulcers, acne, hirsutism	Give with food or milk Increase dose for illness/fever per physician's instructions

CONGENITAL HYPOTHYROIDISM

Congenital hypothyroidism is a condition present from birth in which the thyroid gland does not produce enough thyroid hormone to meet the metabolic needs of the body.

Untreated hypothyroidism leads to mental retardation.

Incidence. Congenital hypothyroidism occurs in 1:4000 births as detected by newborn screening. Because untreated hypothyroidism causes mental retardation, most states have mandatory newborn screening programs to diagnose hypothyroidism before symptoms occur. Early detection and treatment favors increased intellectual function. Approximately 90% of cases are sporadic; the other 10% are hereditary, caused by inborn errors of thyroid metabolism (LaFranchi, 1986).

Clinical Manifestations (Fig. 38–1)

- Prolonged jaundice
- Lethargy
- Constipation
- Feeding problems
- Cold to touch
- Skin mottling
- Umbilical hernia
- Hypotonia/slow reflexes
- Large tongue
- Large fontanel
- Distended abdomen
- Hoarse cry
- Excessive sleeping

Diagnostic Evaluation. Congenital hypothyroidism is usually diagnosed by newborn screening. Ideally, testing should be done between ages 3 to 6 days. Tests done 24 to 48 hours after delivery may be falsely interpreted due to the rise in TSH immediately after birth.

Any infant with a low T_4 and TSH value greater than 40 μU/ml is considered to have primary hypothyroidism until proven otherwise (American Academy of Pediatrics, 1987).

Table 38–1 lists the normal T_4 and TSH values for age. Thyroid scans may be useful in identifying any functioning thyroid tissue. However, treatment should never be delayed while waiting for scan results.

Therapeutic Management. Treatment of congenital hypothyroidism consists of lifelong thyroid hormone replace-

PATHOPHYSIOLOGY AND ETIOLOGY *of Congenital Hypothyroidism*

The thyroid gland is a butterfly-shaped gland located in front of the neck. Thyroid-stimulating hormone (TSH), secreted by the pituitary, induces the thyroid to produce thyroxine (T_4) and triiodothyronine (T_3). The thyroid traps iodine and produces T_4, which is essential for normal growth and development, especially brain development, in the first 2 years of life. Immediately after delivery, there is a dramatic increase in TSH most likely related to the stress of the birth process. Within the first week of life, the TSH level gradually falls (LaFranchi, 1986).

Congenital hypothyroidism is caused by an absent (aplastic) or underdeveloped (lingual) thyroid gland. For unknown reasons, the fetal thyroid gland fails to develop or does not fully develop. Other causes may be hypothalamic or hypopituitary disorders in which there is insufficient TSH to stimulate the thyroid gland. Maternal intake of medications during pregnancy or exposure to radiation may cause transient or permanent hypothyroidism in the infant.

An infant with congenital hypothyroidism will have an elevated TSH and a low T_4.

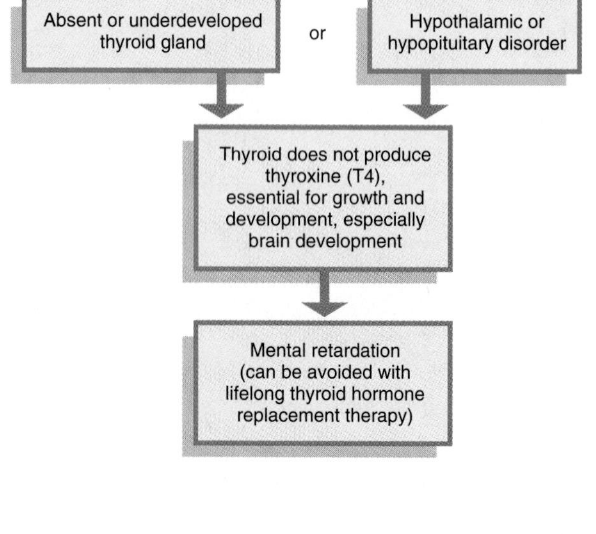

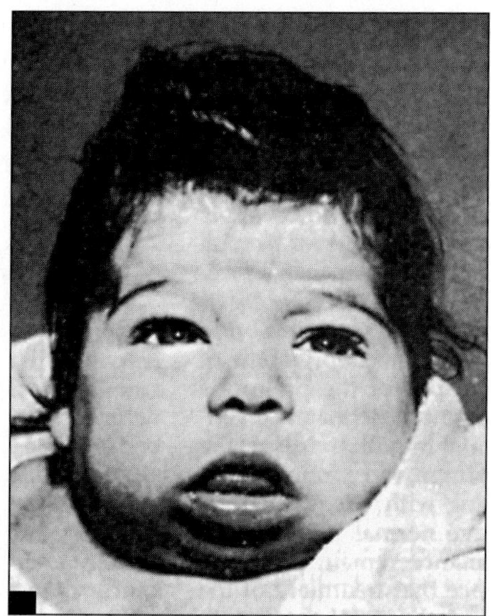

◀ Untreated congenital hypothyroidism in a 6-month-old infant.

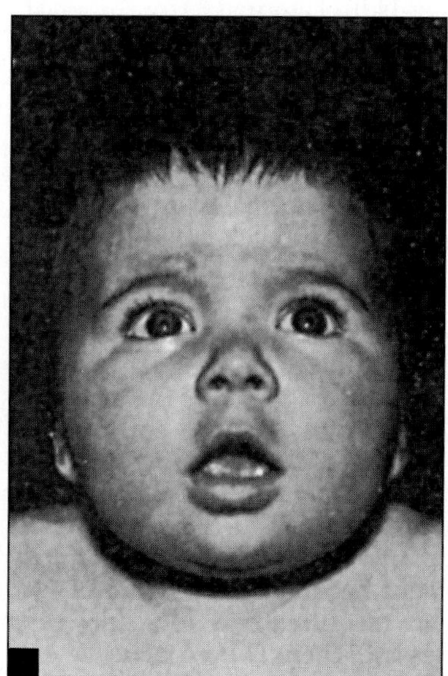

Four months after treatment. ▶

Figure 38–1

This infant with congenital hypothyroidism fed poorly and was constipated. She was very lethargic and had no social smile and no head control. In the pretreatment photo, notice her puffy face, large tongue, dull expression, and hirsute forehead. The post-treatment photo shows decreased facial puffiness, decreased hirsutism of the forehead, and an alert appearance. Newborn screening for hypothyroidism is important because treatment should begin in the first weeks of life to prevent mental retardation and other problems. Treatment consists of lifelong thyroid hormone replacement. (From Behrman, R. E., Kliegman, R. M., & Arvin, A. M. [1996]. *Nelson textbook of pediatrics* [15th ed.]. Philadelphia: W. B. Saunders, p. 1592.)

TABLE 38–1 *Normal T_4 and TSH Values*

	TOTAL T_4 (μg/dl)		TSH (μU/ml)	
AGE	MEAN	RANGE	MEAN	RANGE
Cord blood	10.2	7.4–13.0	9.0	<2.5–17.4
1–3 days	17.2	11.8–22.6	8.0	<2.5–13.3
1–2 weeks	13.2	9.8–16.6	—	—
2–4 weeks	11.0	7.0–15.0	4.0	0.6–10.0
1–4 months	10.3	7.2–14.4	<2.5	<2.5
4–12 months	11.0	7.8–16.5	2.1	0.6–6.3
1–5 years	10.5	7.3–15.0	2.0	0.6–6.3
5–10 years	9.3	6.4–13.3	2.0	0.6–6.3
10–15 years	8.1	5.6–11.7	1.9	0.6–6.3
Adult	8.4	4.3–12.5	1.8	0.2–7.6

LaFranchi, S. (1986). Newborn thyroid disorders and screening. In N. Lavin (Ed.), *Manual of endocrinology and metabolism* (p. 401). Boston: Little, Brown.

ment, usually in the form of levothyroxine. It is given as a single daily oral dose. Dose is between 3 and 6 mcg/kg/day. The dosage is titrated to suppress the TSH and keep the T_4 in the upper half of normal (Aronson et al., 1990).

NURSING CARE OF THE INFANT WITH CONGENITAL HYPOTHYROIDISM

Assessment

Nursing care of the infant with congenital hypothyroidism involves assessing growth and development and ensuring compliance with medication. Nurses have a major role in recognizing the infant with hypothyroidism. Mental retardation caused by untreated hypothyroidism cannot be reversed, but it can be prevented through early identification and proper treatment. Generally, infants are followed every month for the first year of life, and then every 3 to 6 months thereafter. Accurate measurements of height, weight, and head circumference should be obtained at each visit. Screening for developmental milestones is also essential.

Nursing Diagnosis and Planning

The following nursing diagnoses and expected outcomes may be appropriate in the treatment of congenital hypothyroidism in the infant.

- Knowledge Deficit related to congenital disorder. ***Expected Outcomes:*** *The parents will demonstrate the ability to monitor their infant for signs and symptoms of hypothyroidism and hyperthyroidism; verbalize an understanding of normal growth and development milestones; give thyroid medication properly; verbalize understanding of lifelong needs and routines of the child.*
- Altered Growth and Development related to disease process. ***Expected Outcome:*** *The infant will demonstrate growth and developmental milestones appropriate for age.*
- Ineffective Thermoregulation related to decreased basal metabolic rate. ***Expected Outcome:*** *The infant will maintain normal body temperature.*

Implementation

Education is directed toward the parents. They should have an understanding of the importance of compliance with therapy.

Parents should be aware of the correct dose and timing of the medication their infant is to receive. Levothyroxine is given orally as a single daily dose. The medication may be dissolved in a small amount of water and given by syringe. It may also be dissolved and put into the nipple of a baby bottle with a small amount of formula. The medication should not be given in a whole bottle, because if the infant does not finish it, she will not receive the full dose. When the infant is older, the medication may be given in a spoonful of cereal or baby food. If the infant or child vomits within 1 hour of taking medication, the dose should be given again.

> Frequently missed doses may lead to developmental delays and poor growth.

Parents should also be instructed on the signs and symptoms of both hypothyroidism and hyperthyroidism (see box) and when to notify the physician if symptoms occur. Infants receiving too much medication may become hyperthyroid. Parents can be taught to count their child's pulse and instructed to withhold the dose and contact their practitioner if the pulse rate is above the value set by the practitioner.

Because this is a lifelong condition, school-age children and teenagers should be made aware of the importance of taking their medication and of keeping regular follow-up visits with the physician.

Evaluation

- Has the infant exhibited any signs or symptoms of hypothyroidism or hyperthyroidism?
- Is the child developing appropriately for age according to growth charts and Denver Development scores?
- Does the child have normal results on thyroid function tests?
- Have the parents verbalized an understanding of the lifelong needs and routines of their child?

Hypothyroidism Versus Hyperthyroidism

SIGNS AND SYMPTOMS OF HYPOTHYROIDISM

- Tiredness/fatigue
- Constipation
- Cold intolerance
- Weight gain
- Dry, thick skin
- Edema of face, eyes, hands
- Decreased growth

SIGNS AND SYMPTOMS OF HYPERTHYROIDISM

- Nervousness/anxiety
- Diarrhea
- Heat intolerance
- Weight loss
- Smooth, velvety skin
- Exophthalmos
- Increased appetite

ACQUIRED HYPOTHYROIDISM

Hypothyroidism is a condition in which there is inadequate thyroid hormone to meet the metabolic needs of the body.

Pathophysiology. Refer to pathophysiology for congenital hypothyroidism. In contrast to congenital hypothyroidism, adverse effects from hypothyroidism acquired after age 2 to 3 years are often reversible. A goiter, an enlarged thyroid gland $1\frac{1}{2}$ to 2 times normal size, occurs in response to TSH secretions.

Etiology. Primary causes of acquired hypothyroidism include the following: Hashimoto's thyroiditis, which is usually associated with a goiter; surgical thyroidectomy; radioactive iodine therapy for hyperthyroidism; and radiation therapy for malignancies. Excessive iodine ingestion may also cause hypothyroidism.

Decreased TSH secretion by the pituitary is a secondary cause. A tertiary cause is decreased thyrotropin releasing hormone (TRH) secretion by the hypothalamus. This accounts for less than 5% of hypothyroidism in pediatric patients (Lavin, 1986).

> Thyroiditis is the most common cause of acquired hypothyroidism in children and adolescents. It often occurs in families with a history of thyroid hormone disease. Other family members may have positive thyroid antibodies. Thyroiditis is more common in females.

Clinical Manifestations

- Goiter (one lobe usually larger than the other)
- Dry, thick skin and coarse hair
- Tiredness/fatigue
- Cold intolerance
- Constipation
- Weight gain
- Decreased growth
- Edema of face, eyes, and hands
- Irregular menses

Diagnostic Evaluation. Hypothyroidism is diagnosed by having an elevated TSH and a low T_4. An elevated TSH is the most sensitive indicator of primary hypothyroidism.

Thyroiditis is diagnosed when there are circulating thyroid antibodies and is usually associated with a firm goiter. Initially the TSH is elevated with a normal T_4, although, over time, the T_4 will decrease.

With secondary or tertiary hypothyroidism, the TSH is not elevated; therefore, TRH stimulation testing is usually required for diagnosis.

Therapeutic Management. Management of hypothyroidism consists of thyroid hormone replacement, usually with levothyroxine. Dosage is 3 to 6 mcg/kg/day, depending on the age and weight of the child. Levothyroxine is given as a single daily dose. The dose is titrated to maintain T_4 in the upper half of normal and to suppress TSH.

NURSING CARE OF THE CHILD WITH ACQUIRED HYPOTHYROIDISM

Assessment

Care of the child with acquired hypothyroidism consists of monitoring response to treatment and compliance with medication. With proper treatment, the goiter should decrease in size. Signs and symptoms of hypothyroidism should also resolve with adequate thyroid hormone replacement. Growth and development should be closely followed by monitoring height, weight, and performance on the Denver Development at each visit as well as school performance.

Nursing Diagnosis and Planning

The following nursing diagnoses and expected outcomes may be appropriate in the treatment of acquired hypothyroidism in the child.

- Constipation related to decreased basal metabolic rate secondary to hypothyroidism. ***Expected Outcome:*** *The child will maintain normal bowel movements.*
- Activity Intolerance related to fatigue. ***Expected Outcome:*** *The child will be able to exercise at the same level as her peers.*
- Altered Nutrition: More Than Body Requirements related to weight gain/obesity. ***Expected Outcome:*** *The child will grow and gain weight at an age-appropriate rate.*
- Ineffective Thermoregulation related to decreased basal metabolic rate secondary to hypothyroidism. ***Expected Outcome:*** *The child will maintain normal body temperature.*

Implementation

Parents and school-age and older children should be instructed on the correct dose and timing of thyroid medication. Thyroid hormone levels are usually checked every 3 to 6 months and normal thyroid function indicates good response to therapy. Parents need to be instructed on the signs and symptoms of hypothyroidism and hyperthyroidism and when to notify the physician if symptoms occur (see box Hypothyroidism versus Hyperthyroidism).

Evaluation

- Does the child have normal results on thyroid function tests?

- Has the child maintained normal bowel movements?
- Can the child tolerate exercise at the same level as peers?
- Has the child maintained age-appropriate height and weight?
- Has the child maintained normal body temperature?

GRAVES' DISEASE (HYPERTHYROIDISM)

Graves' disease is the production of excessive thyroid hormones by an enlarged thyroid gland. It is the most common cause of hyperthyroidism in children.

Pathophysiology. Refer to the previous discussion on the pathophysiology of the thyroid gland under Congenital Hypothyroidism. An enlarged gland is usually associated with Graves' disease.

Etiology. Circulating autoantibodies known as thyroid stimulating immunoglobulin (TSI) stimulate the thyroid gland to make T_3 and T_4. These antibodies attach themselves to the TSH receptor sites on the thyroid gland. Therefore, it is not the TSH that stimulates the thyroid gland but the antibodies. Therefore, in Graves' disease, the production of excessive thyroid hormones is not under pituitary control. The cause of antibody production is unknown at this time.

Incidence. Graves' disease accounts for 10% to 15% of thyroid disorders in children (Levy, Schumacher, & Gupta, 1988). The female to male ratio is approximately 4:1. There may also be a familial tendency toward Graves' disease. Children with autoimmune disease are at risk for other autoimmune disorders.

Clinical Manifestations

- Goiter
- Weight loss
- Increased appetite
- Nervousness
- Diarrhea
- Increased perspiration
- Heat intolerance
- Increased heart rate
- Palpitations
- Tremors
- Exophthalmos
- Poor attention span; behavior/school problems

Diagnostic Evaluation. Graves' disease is diagnosed by an elevated T_4 level and a suppressed TSH, associated with symptoms of hyperthyroidism. Autoantibodies are generally positive. Thyroid uptake of radioactive iodine is increased.

Therapeutic Management. The three approaches to the management of Graves' disease include antithyroid drug therapy, radioactive iodine, and surgery. Antithyroid drug therapy with propylthiouracil or methimazole has been the major form of medical management for childhood hyperthyroidism (Sills, Horlick, & Rapaport, 1992). These drugs act by blocking thyroid hormone production by the thyroid gland. The medications are generally given three times a day and will lower thyroid hormone levels in approximately 6 weeks. Minor adverse effects include arthralgia, skin rash, pruritus, and gastric intolerance. Major adverse effects of antithyroid drugs may include neutropenia, hepatotoxicity, and hypothyroidism.

A second approach to management is oral radioiodine treatment. With this therapy the thyroid gland takes up the radioactive iodine, which destroys the thyroid tissue. Repeat uptake scan and thyroid function studies should be done approximately 2 months after the initial radioiodine therapy (Levy, Schumacher, & Gupta, 1988). Hypothyroidism is common once the thyroid gland is radiated; therefore, lifelong thyroid replacement may be necessary.

Subtotal or partial thyroidectomy is the surgical removal of thyroid gland tissue and the third form of management. With surgery there is the possibility of injury to the parathyroid glands, which are located near the thyroid gland. Damage to the parathyroids could result in hypocalcemia; therefore, calcium levels should be monitored postsurgery. There is also a 60% to 80% chance of developing hypothyroidism, which can be treated with thyroxine.

Once the child is successfully treated and no longer demonstrates hyperthyroidism, follow-up visits with the endocrinologist should be scheduled one to two times a year to evaluate thyroid function.

NURSING CARE OF THE CHILD WITH GRAVES' DISEASE

Assessment

The goal of treatment consists of normalizing thyroid hormone levels, alleviating symptoms of hyperthyroidism, and decreasing the goiter. The nurse should assess for compliance with therapy, because most medications are given three times a day.

If a child is being treated with propylthiouracil, there is an increased risk of neutropenia and hepatotoxicity.

> A child receiving propylthiouracil who develops a fever or sore throat should be evaluated by a physician; a complete blood count should be obtained.

Contact sports should be limited while the child is being treated to decrease the possibility of damage to the liver.

Nursing Diagnosis and Planning

The following nursing diagnoses and expected outcomes may be appropriate in the treatment of Graves' disease in the child.

- Ineffective Management of Therapeutic Regimen (Individual) related to noncompliance with medication. ***Expected Outcome:*** *The child will comply with the medication regimen.*
- Altered Nutrition: Less than Body Requirements related to increased metabolic rate. ***Expected Outcome:*** *The child will maintain weight appropriate for age and height.*
- Diarrhea related to increased basal metabolic rate secondary to hyperthyroidism. ***Expected Outcomes:*** *The child will be euthyroid as evidenced by normal results on thyroid function tests; have normal bowel movements.*
- Risk for Activity Intolerance related to increased basal metabolic rate secondary to hyperthyroidism. ***Expected Outcome:*** *The child will be able to exercise at the same level as her peers.*
- Sleep Pattern Disturbance related to increased basal metabolic rate secondary to hyperthyroidism. ***Expected Outcome:*** *The child will sleep through the night without waking.*
- Risk for Altered Body Temperature related to increased basal metabolic rate secondary to hyperthyroidism. ***Expected Outcome:*** *The child will maintain normal body temperature.*

Implementation

The antithyroid drugs propylthiouracil and methimazole are generally given two to three times per day. This regimen may be difficult for some children to follow. Pill dispensers and watches with alarms may be utilized for reminders to take the medication at specific times. Children should be seen by the endocrinologist and have thyroid function tests every 2 to 3 months while undergoing treatment. Normal thyroid function tests and alleviation of symptoms indicate good response to therapy. Once the child is euthyroid and asymptomatic he should be seen one to two times a year because hyperthyroidism may recur.

Evaluation

- Does the child have normal results on thyroid function tests?
- Is the child free of symptoms of hyperthyroidism?
- Is the child growing at an age-appropriate rate?
- Does the child demonstrate normal bowel movements?
- Is the child able to exercise at an age-appropriate level?
- Does the child sleep throughout the night?
- Has the child maintained a normal body temperature?

DIABETES INSIPIDUS

Diabetes insipidus is an inability to concentrate urine due to a deficiency of vasopressin, also known as antidiuretic hormone (ADH).

Etiology. Diabetes insipidus is frequently the result of head trauma, tumors, or infection in the area of the hypothalamus. The most common type of tumor involving the hypothalamus and causing diabetes insipidus is craniopharyngioma.

Cranial radiation for treatment of tumors may also lead to ADH deficiency. Other causes include infections of the central nervous system such as meningitis or encephalitis, or congenital malformations such as septic optic dysplasia or hypopituitarism.

Incidence. Head trauma and surgical resection of suprasellar tumors account for most cases of diabetes insipidus. Approximately 50% to 75% of children with these types of tumors will develop permanent diabetes insipidus; the remainder will experience transient diabetes insipidus postoperatively (Shiminski-Maher, 1991).

Clinical Manifestations

- Increased urination (polyuria)
- Increased thirst (preferring water), polydipsia
- Nocturia
- Dehydration
- Increased serum sodium (greater than 150 mEq/L
- Decreased urine specific gravity (less than 1.005)

Diagnostic Evaluation. Diagnostic criteria include polyuria with associated hypernatremia and low urine specific gravity in the absence of hyperglycemia (Seckl et al., 1990). Urine should be checked for glucose to rule out hyperglycemia as a cause for increased urine output.

A water deprivation test may also be necessary to confirm the diagnosis. This is a 7-hour procedure during which the child is deprived of water. A normal response is decreased urine output with a high urine specific gravity and no change in serum sodium. In diabetes insipidus, when fluid is restricted the child continues to have large amounts of dilute urine, evidenced by a low specific gravity. The serum sodium will also increase.

To ensure the child's safety, this test is done in a hospital setting with frequent monitoring of serum sodium, hematocrit, and osmolality. The urine osmolality and output are also measured. The child should be weighed at the beginning of the test, midway, and at the conclusion.

> Water deprivation should be stopped if the child loses 3% to 5% of baseline body weight, becomes dehydrated, or demonstrates a significant change in vital signs or neurologic status.

PATHOPHYSIOLOGY *of Diabetes Insipidus*

ADH is produced within the **hypothalamus** and then is transported through the pituitary stalk and stored in the posterior pituitary. It is carried through the blood to the kidneys, where it acts on the distal tubules and collecting ducts to increase reabsorption of free water, thereby concentrating urine and decreasing output.

ADH is under the control of osmoreceptors in the anterior pituitary. These osmoreceptors operate on a negative feedback system based on the serum osmolality, particularly the sodium concentration. When the osmolality is low there is decreased production of ADH. This causes increased urine output and normalizes osmolality; conversely, when the osmolality is increased, there is increased ADH production, which causes water retention and decreases urine output. In diabetes insipidus, there is a deficiency of ADH, and therefore the body is unable to conserve water, which results in large volumes of dilute urine. With this loss of free water, there is an increase in serum sodium concentration. If the child has an intact thirst center, he may be able to compensate for the large fluid loss by increasing his oral intake. If the thirst drive is not intact or the child is unable to drink enough, the child may become dehydrated and have a high serum sodium level.

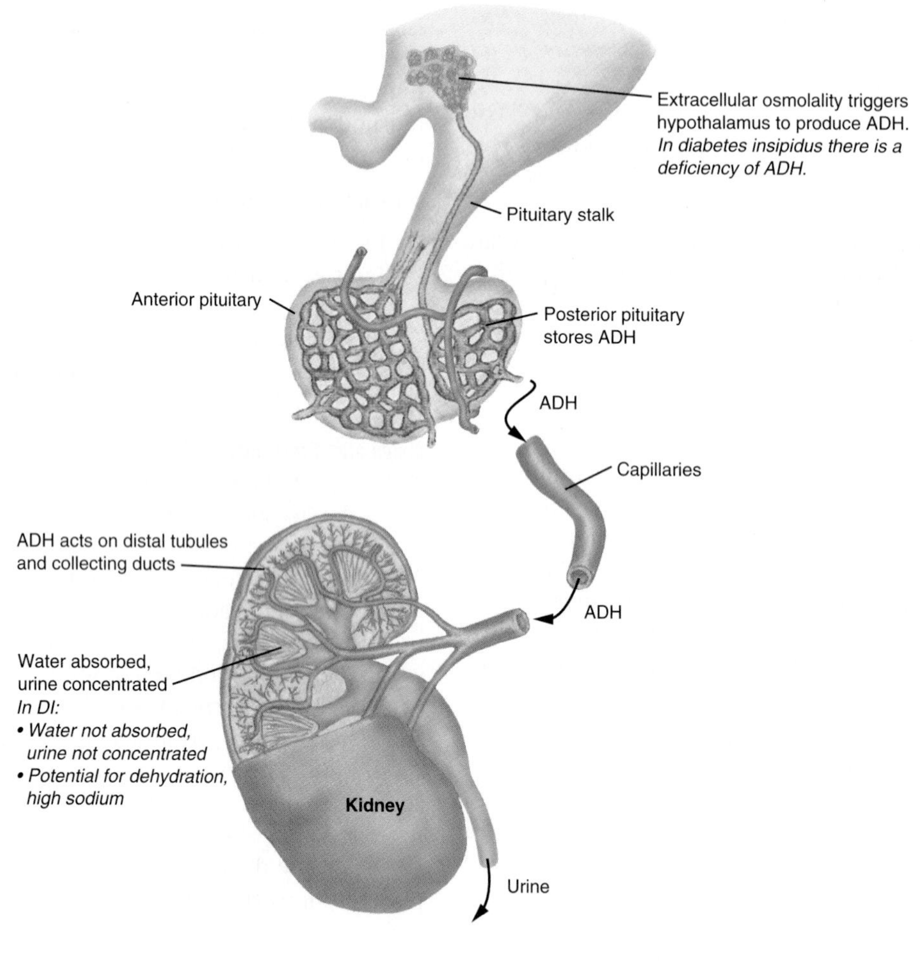
Extracellular osmolality triggers hypothalamus to produce ADH.
In diabetes insipidus there is a deficiency of ADH.
Pituitary stalk
Anterior pituitary
Posterior pituitary stores ADH
ADH
Capillaries
ADH acts on distal tubules and collecting ducts
ADH
Water absorbed, urine concentrated
In DI:
• Water not absorbed, urine not concentrated
• Potential for dehydration, high sodium
Kidney
Urine

Therapeutic Management. Treatment consists of maintaining fluid balance and administering synthetic vasopressin (DDAVP). The dose of DDAVP ranges from 0.05 to 0.2 ml and is usually given twice a day. It is administered either intranasally or by subcutaneous injection. The concentration of intranasal DDAVP is 100 μg/ml; the concentration of subcutaneous DDAVP is 4 μg/ml.

Intranasal DDAVP is given through a soft flexible tube that has premarked doses. It may also be given by a metered spray, which delivers the medication in 0.1-ml increments. The subcutaneous dose is one-tenth of the intranasal dose.

Dosage is individualized and based on the child's age, size, urine output, and specific gravity. The accompanying

Symptoms of Excessive or Insufficient DDAVP

TOO MUCH DDAVP

- Decreased urine output
- Decreased serum sodium
- Headaches
- Water retention

TOO LITTLE DDAVP

- Increased urine output
- Increased thirst
- Increased serum sodium
- Dehydration

box lists the symptoms of too much or too little DDAVP. The duration of action varies from 12 to 24 hours. Doses will be timed so that before the next dose the child will be allowed to have mild increased urination. This will help prevent overtreatment and water retention. Parents are often taught to measure urine specific gravity at home to monitor effectiveness of treatment.

A child with an intact thirst center will be able to regulate his fluid needs and intake. If the child is not able to recognize thirst due to head trauma/surgery, the physician may prescribe a 24-hour fluid requirement.

NURSING CARE OF THE CHILD WITH DIABETES INSIPIDUS

Assessment

Nursing care involves assessing the parents' and child's understanding of diabetes insipidus. They should be instructed in the symptoms indicating the need for DDAVP, as well as symptoms of too much DDAVP. The family should also be instructed in the proper administration of DDAVP.

Nursing Diagnosis and Planning

The following nursing diagnoses and expected outcomes may be appropriate in the treatment of diabetes insipidus in the child.

- Fluid Volume Deficit related to abnormal fluid loss from polyuria. ***Expected Outcome:*** *The child will avoid dehydration as evidenced by increasing fluid intake and taking DDAVP in response to excessive urine output.*
- Risk for Fluid Volume Excess related to excessive DDAVP. ***Expected Outcome:*** *The child will maintain normal skin turgor, specific gravity, and electrolytes.*
- Knowledge Deficit related to diabetes insipidus. ***Expected Outcomes:*** *The parents will describe the symptoms of excessive DDAVP; describe the symptoms and treatment of diabetes insipidus.*

Signs and Symptoms of Hyponatremia

Review the following signs and symptoms of hyponatremia with the child's parents:

EARLY

Anorexia
Headache
Nausea
Vomiting

MODERATE

Confusion
Irritability
Lethargy
Altered level of consciousness

SEVERE

Seizures
Coma

Implementation

The nurse should educate the family on the basic pathophysiology of water metabolism and the cause of diabetes insipidus. They should be instructed on the symptoms of diabetes insipidus. Parents and school-age and older children should be taught how to administer DDAVP by the route prescribed by the physician. They should be able to demonstrate proper administration of the medication. The family also needs to be instructed in how to measure urine specific gravity and how to recognize increased urination or low specific gravity that would necessitate the need for DDAVP. Signs and symptoms of hypernatremia and hyponatremia must also be reviewed with the parents (see box). The child should wear a Medic Alert bracelet noting the diagnosis of diabetes insipidus. The child's teachers need to be aware of the diagnosis and must allow the child free access to water.

Evaluation

- Has the child avoided episodes of dehydration requiring hospitalization?
- Has the child maintained urine specific gravity between 1.010 and 1.020?
- Can the child/parents describe the symptoms of too much DDAVP?
- Can the child/parents describe the symptoms and treatment of diabetes insipidus?

SYNDROME OF INAPPROPRIATE ANTIDIURETIC HORMONE

Syndrome of inappropriate antidiuretic hormone (SIADH) results from the excessive production or release of ADH, or vasopressin.

PATHOPHYSIOLOGY *of SIADH*

Refer to the discussion of the pathophysiology of water metabolism under diabetes insipidus. Table 38–2 lists the differences between diabetes insipidus and SIADH. Excessive ADH results in the kidneys reabsorbing too much free water. This causes decreased output of concentrated urine, evidenced by a high urine specific gravity (greater than 1.030). The excess water also causes an expanded fluid volume and a low serum sodium level. Normal sodium level is between 135 and 145 mEq/L. Once the sodium level falls below 125 mEq/L, the child may become symptomatic and experience anorexia, nausea, weakness, weight gain, confusion, and irritability.

Etiology. Childhood SIADH generally is caused by disorders affecting the central nervous system, including infections such as meningitis, head trauma, and brain tumors. After surgery for brain tumors, children may experience transient SIADH. Often there is a triple response after surgery: Initially, the child will have diabetes insipidus, then experience temporary SIADH, and then return to diabetes insipidus (Seckl et al., 1990).

Incidence. SIADH is rare in children and is usually related to an underlying cause. It is generally transient and resolves when the underlying condition is corrected.

Clinical Manifestations

- Decreased urine output
- Increased urine specific gravity
- Fluid retention
- Weight gain
- Hyponatremia
- Increased urine osmolality

Diagnostic Evaluation. SIADH should be suspected in children with central nervous system involvement, such as infections or head trauma, who have decreased urine output in spite of adequate intake. Laboratory diagnosis includes evidence of hyponatremia, hypochloremia, and low serum osmolality. Urine osmolality is generally greater than serum osmolality (Bacon et al., 1990). Urine specific gravity will be increased, greater than 1.030. It is also important to obtain laboratory studies for adrenal, thyroid, and renal function to rule out other causes for hyponatremia (Lindamin, 1992).

TABLE 38–2 *Diabetes Insipidus Versus Syndrome of Inappropriate Antidiuretic Hormone*

DIABETES INSIPIDUS	SIADH
Increased urination	Decreased urination
Increased thirst	Increased urine osmolality
Nocturia	Weight gain
Dehydration	Fluid retention
Hypernatremia	Hyponatremia
Urine specific gravity < 1.005	Urine specific gravity > 1.030

Therapeutic Management. The first line of treatment is fluid restriction to correct hyponatremia. The physician will order fluid limitations. The underlying cause of SIADH must also be corrected. If hyponatremia is severe, the child may require intravenous infusion of sodium chloride. Drug therapy may also be used, although it usually is not indicated for transient SIADH. Medications such as lithium and demeclocycline block the action of ADH at the renal collecting tubules, and have been used in the management of chronic SIADH (Bacon et al., 1990).

NURSING CARE OF THE CHILD WITH SIADH

Assessment

The child with SIADH should be assessed for signs and symptoms of fluid overload, which include edema, weight gain, urine specific gravity less than 1.010, and dilutional hyponatremia. Neurologic status should also be monitored if the child is hyponatremic by assessing mental status for level of consciousness, headache, irritability, or seizures.

Severe hyponatremia may cause seizures.

Nursing Diagnosis and Planning

The following nursing diagnoses and expected outcomes may be appropriate in the treatment of SIADH in the child.

- Fluid Volume Excess related to decreased urine output. ***Expected Outcome:*** *The child will maintain a balanced intake and output, as evidenced by maintenance of weight.*
- Risk for Injury related to seizures caused by hyponatremia. ***Expected Outcome:*** *The child will be protected from possible injury due to seizures.*

Implementation

The child should be assessed every 2 to 4 hours for hydration and neurologic status. Strict intake and output must be recorded. The child should be weighed daily.

It may be difficult for a child to comply with the fluid restrictions. Explain to the child and parents the need for limited fluids and that it is temporary. Hard sugarless candies or wet washcloths may be used to help keep mucous membranes moist.

Diet should include foods with high sodium content, because extra sodium may help correct hyponatremia, although salty foods such as chips may also make the child thirsty.

Electrolytes should be closely monitored as ordered by the physician.

Because there is the potential for seizures with severe hyponatremia, seizure precautions must be initiated if the serum sodium is less than 125 mEq/L.

Alert the physician immediately to any change in neurologic status. Evaluation of the child with SIADH should include maintaining a balanced intake and output, maintaining weight, and having a normal serum sodium and urine specific gravity between 1.010 and 1.020.

Evaluation

- Has the child had a balanced intake and output?
- Has the child maintained his weight?
- Has the child avoided seizures related to hyponatremia?

PRECOCIOUS PUBERTY

Precocious puberty is early onset of puberty, occurring before age 8 in girls and before age 9 in boys. It is defined as the premature appearance of secondary sexual characteristics and an advanced growth rate and bone maturation.

The major concern of precocious puberty is rapid bone growth, which causes early fusion and ultimate short stature as an adult.

Incidence. Precocious puberty is more common in females; approximately 70% of cases are idiopathic. Males have a higher incidence of CNS lesions. Both males and females may have hypothalamic hamartomas. Approximately 50% of true precocious puberty occurs in children under age 6 years (Kaplan & Grumbach, 1990).

Clinical Manifestations

Females

- Breast development
- Pubic hair
- Axillary hair
- Enlargement of vagina, uterus, and ovaries
- Acne
- Adult body odor
- Onset of menstrual periods

Males

- Testicular enlargement
- Increase in penis size
- Pubic hair
- Axillary/chest hair
- Facial hair
- Acne
- Adult body odor
- Deepening of voice

PATHOPHYSIOLOGY AND ETIOLOGY *of Precocious Puberty*

Puberty occurs when the hypothalamus releases gonadotropin releasing hormone (GnRH). This stimulates the pituitary gland to release LH and FSH (Fig. 38–2). In females, FSH stimulates formation of ovarian follicles to produce estrogen. Estrogen is necessary for the development of secondary sexual characteristics such as breast development and maturation of the vagina and labia. Luteinizing hormone is involved in the process of ovulation. In males, FSH triggers the testes to support the development of sperm. Luteinizing hormone stimulates the production of testosterone, which is necessary for the development of sexual characteristics and sperm production. Puberty development is classified according to Tanner stages I through V (see Table 8–2). The adrenal glands produce the hormone dehydroepiandrosterone (DHEA), which causes pubic and axillary hair growth. During puberty, there is also an increase in growth rate, or a "growth spurt," in which a child grows an average of 4 to 6 inches per year.

In precocious puberty, the sex hormones that accelerate growth also cause the bone plates to close early. Bone generally fuses at age 14 for girls and age 15 for boys. With true precocious puberty, children have hormonal changes that mimic the onset of normal puberty (Kaplan & Grumbach, 1990). These hormonal changes may be central, arising from the hypothalamus, or peripheral, arising from the ovaries, testes, or adrenal glands.

Central or true precocious puberty may be idiopathic or may be caused by central nervous system (CNS) tumors (most commonly hamartomas), head trauma, or cranial radiation.

Peripheral causes may include abnormalities or tumors of the adrenal glands, ovaries, or testes. Congenital adrenal hyperplasia, a genetic disorder of the adrenal pathway, is the most common cause of peripheral precocious puberty. The McCune-Albright syndrome may cause early puberty in females; the genetic disorder familial testotoxicosis causes early puberty in males.

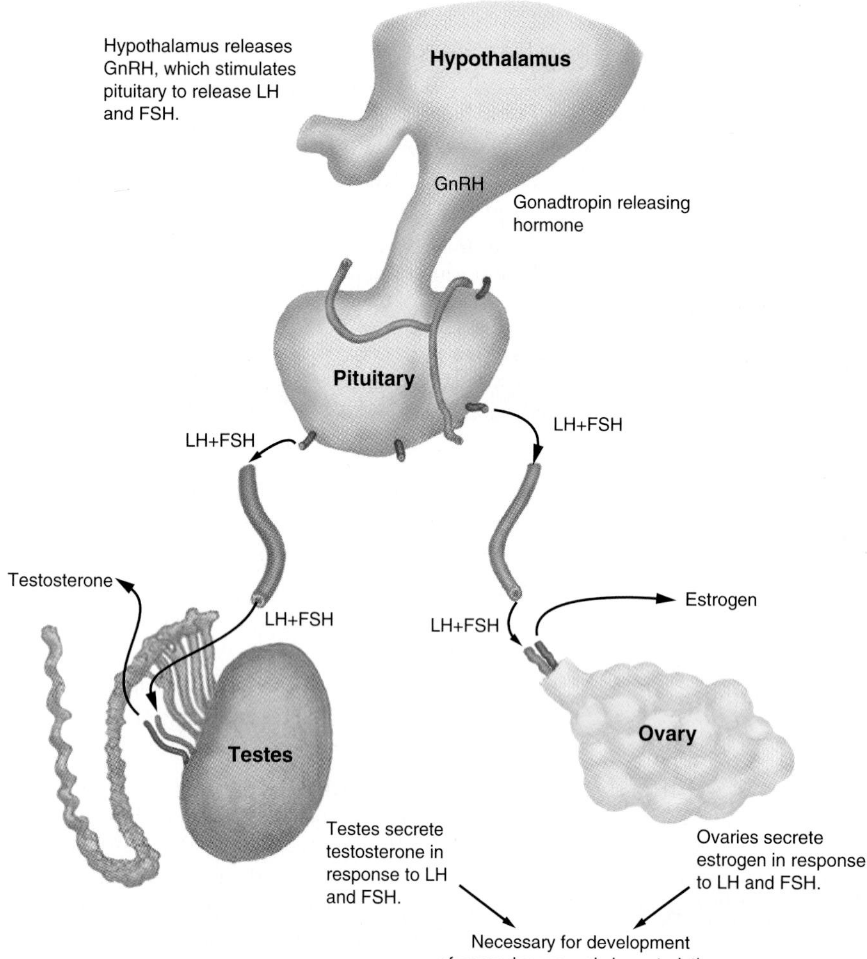
Hypothalamus releases GnRH, which stimulates pituitary to release LH and FSH.
Hypothalamus
GnRH
Gonadtropin releasing hormone
Pituitary
LH+FSH
LH+FSH
Testosterone
LH+FSH
LH+FSH
Estrogen
Testes
Ovary
Testes secrete testosterone in response to LH and FSH.
Ovaries secrete estrogen in response to LH and FSH.
Necessary for development of secondary sexual characteristics.

Figure 38–2
Endocrine changes in puberty.

Diagnostic Evaluation. Diagnosis of precocious puberty begins with a thorough history, including onset of sexual characteristics, and a physical examination. Blood tests are then necessary to evaluate for elevated levels of LH, FSH, testosterone, and estrogen. Unfortunately, these hormones are released in small bursts during the day. Therefore, random samples may not be adequate.

The GnRH stimulation test is a more accurate and definitive test to determine early puberty. Synthetic GnRH is administered intravenously to stimulate the release of LH and FSH from the pituitary gland. Serial samples of LH and FSH are then obtained over a 2-hour period.

Before puberty, the FSH peak is higher than the LH peak, whereas with the onset of puberty, the LH peak is higher than the FSH peak.

Radiographic studies are also essential for the diagnosis. Bone age X-rays of the wrist determine bone maturation and can assist in predicting final adult height. Skull X-rays may be useful in screening for CNS lesions, although CT scans and MRIs are more accurate in visualizing tumors.

Abdominal and pelvic ultrasound are beneficial in diagnosing adrenal and ovarian tumors or cysts. Pelvic ultrasound also provides evidence of pubertal changes in the uterus and ovaries.

Finally, if there is isolated pubic hair development, DHEA levels may be elevated; this suggests an adrenal origin for premature sexual hair growth.

Therapeutic Management. The goal of treatment is to stop or reverse the development of secondary sexual characteristics and to slow down the rapid growth rate and bone age advancement.

Current therapy for true precocious puberty is to administer a GnRH agonist or blocker. GnRH blockers inhibit the binding of GnRH to the pituitary gland, which will cause a decrease in the production of LH, FSH, estrogen, and testosterone. This in turn will stop sexual development from progressing and will stop or slow down bone age advancement, thus preserving adult height.

Several GnRH agonists are commercially available and can be administered either intranasally or by subcutaneous injection. Until recently, these drugs had to be administered on a daily basis, which led to problems with compliance. Currently, a depot form is available that can be given as a monthly injection.

Once therapy is initiated, GnRH secretion is suppressed within 2 to 4 weeks. The increased growth rate and bone maturation as well as the sexual characteristics regress within the first year of treatment. There is no current evidence that GnRH agonist therapy will interfere with the child's reproduction in the future. Studies have shown that once therapy is discontinued, GnRH function returns within 1 year (Jay et al., 1992).

For patients with peripheral precocious puberty, treatment is aimed at correcting the underlying cause.

NURSING CARE OF THE CHILD WITH PRECOCIOUS PUBERTY

Assessment

Nursing care of the child with precocious puberty should address the physical and behavioral changes associated with puberty. Nurses who work with these children may notice that they feel more comfortable around older children rather than peers of their own age. They often experience teasing about their bodies and may limit social activities such as swimming. Boys will often exhibit aggressive behavior. Children who go through early puberty appear older than their chronological age and are often treated accordingly by adults.

> Children with precocious puberty are at greater risk for sexual abuse.

Nursing Diagnosis and Planning

The following nursing diagnoses and expected outcomes may be appropriate in the treatment of precocious puberty in the child.

- Altered Sexuality Patterns related to early puberty. ***Expected Outcome:*** *The child will discuss feelings related to sexual development.*
- Body Image Disturbance related to early sexual development. ***Expected Outcome:*** *The child will voice an acceptance of body appearance.*
- Impaired Social Interaction related to appearing older than chronologic age. ***Expected Outcome:*** *The child will exhibit age-appropriate behaviors and social interactions.*
- Altered Family Processes related to having a child with precocious puberty. ***Expected Outcomes:*** *The child/parents will understand the physical and emotional changes that occur with early puberty; verbalize concerns about the child's sexual development and its effect on the family.*

Implementation

Many parents may not be comfortable with their child's early development. The nurse may assist with explaining the stages of puberty and the associated behavioral changes. Parents need to know that even though the child is experiencing puberty early, these are normal changes that the body goes through. Explanations given to the child should be geared to his chronological age and kept brief and simple. Psychological counseling may be necessary to help the family deal with the sensitive issues of sexuality.

> If a child appears embarrassed or uncomfortable when being interviewed about sexual development, the nurse should explain to the child: "Everyone goes through changes in his body; it's just that these changes are happening to you sooner than most children. Can you tell me in your own words how you feel about your body?"

Evaluation

- Has the child verbalized an understanding of the changes occurring in his body?
- Is the child free of sexually precocious behavior?
- Have the parents verbalized their concerns about their child's early sexual development?

HYPOPARATHYROIDISM

Hypoparathyroidism is a condition in which the body does not produce adequate parathyroid hormone (PTH), which is necessary to maintain normal calcium levels.

PATHOPHYSIOLOGY *of Hypoparathyroidism*

There are four parathyroid glands (two on the right and two on the left) located in the neck behind the thyroid gland. These glands secrete parathyroid hormone (PTH), which is essential for calcium conservation and excretion of phosphorus.

The primary action of PTH is to increase calcium absorption from the gastrointestinal tract. It also facilitates reabsorption of calcium from the bones. PTH acts on the kidneys to increase urinary excretion of phosphorus and to decrease excretion of calcium.

Normally, PTH is released in response to calcium levels in the blood. When calcium is low, PTH is increased; when calcium is high, PTH production is decreased. In hypoparathyroidism, PTH levels remain low or absent in the presence of hypocalcemia.

Etiology. The primary cause of hypoparathyroidism is the manipulation or removal of the parathyroid glands during neck or thyroid surgery. Radiation to the neck may also cause hypoparathyroidism.

Autoimmune destruction of the parathyroid glands is another cause and is often associated with Addison's disease and chronic *Candida* infections. Familial hypoparathyroidism is inherited as an autosomal dominant trait.

In the neonatal period, infants may experience transient hypocalcemia with low PTH levels. Predisposing factors include prematurity and intrauterine growth retardation. Maternal factors include diabetes, toxemia, hyperparathyroidism, and poor dietary intake of calcium.

DiGeorge's syndrome is a congenital syndrome associated with absent thymus and parathyroid glands resulting in hypoparathyroidism.

Incidence. Hypoparathyroidism is a very rare condition in children. Approximately 80% to 90% of hypoparathyroidism results from removal/manipulation of the parathyroid glands during thyroid or neck surgery (Lavin, 1986). Idiopathic hypoparathyroidism occurs most frequently in children aged 5 to 15 years (Bacon et al., 1990).

Clinical Manifestations

- Dry, scaly skin
- *Candida* infections
- Transversed ridged nails
- Alopecia
- Poor dental enamel
- Late teeth eruption
- Cataracts
- Diarrhea
- Increased intracranial pressure
- Hyperreflexia
- Papilledema

Diagnostic Evaluation. Primary hypoparathyroidism is diagnosed by low or absent PTH levels associated with hypocalcemia and elevated phosphorus. Alkaline phosphatase may be normal or low. Hypocalcemia is a classic feature of hypoparathyroidism. (The accompanying box lists the signs and symptoms of hypocalcemia).

Signs and Symptoms of Hypocalcemia

Paresthesia
Irritability
Abdominal cramping
Confusion
Carpopedal spasm (positive Trousseau's sign)*
Laryngospasm*
Seizure*

*Medical emergencies.

Electrocardiography may show prolonged Q-T intervals and nonspecific T-wave changes.

Therapeutic Management. The goal of treatment is to maintain normal calcium levels. For long-term therapy, oral replacement is generally provided by calcium gluconate. The dose is 115 mg elemental calcium/kg/day. This is approximately 800 mg a day for prepubertal children and 1000 to 1500 mg a day for adolescents. Children may also require vitamin D or a metabolite in conjunction with calcium replacement.

It is imperative to closely monitor serum and urinary calcium levels as well as phosphorus. Overtreatment may cause hypercalcemia and/or kidney stones. (See the box on the next page for the signs and symptoms of hypercalcemia.)

For emergency treatment of severe hypocalcemia resulting in seizures or tetany, intravenous calcium is required. This is given as 100 mg/kg over a 30-minute period.

Intravenous calcium may cause bradycardia and cardiac arrest if given too rapidly.

NURSING CARE OF THE CHILD WITH HYPOPARATHYROIDISM

Assessment

Nursing care consists of assessing the child for signs and symptoms of hypocalcemia. Chvostek's sign is elicited by tapping the facial nerve anterior to the ear. A positive sign is unilateral contraction of the facial muscle. A positive Trousseau's sign occurs when a blood pressure cuff elevated above the systolic blood pressure produces carpopedal spasm of the hand.

The nurse should also assess the parents' understanding of the medical condition and compliance with therapy.

Nursing Diagnosis and Planning

The following nursing diagnoses and expected outcomes may be appropriate in the treatment of hypoparathyroidism in the child.

- Knowledge deficit related to hypoparathyroidism. ***Expected Outcomes:*** *The child/parents will have a basic understanding of hypoparathyroidism; verbalize the signs and symptoms of both hypercalcemia and hypocalcemia; describe medical emergencies related to hypocalcemia.*
- Risk for Injury related to hypocalcemic seizures. ***Expected Outcome:*** *The child will maintain normal calcium levels and will be free of seizures.*

Implementation

The parents need instruction in the basic pathophysiology of hypoparathyroidism. They must be educated on the signs and symptoms of hypocalcemia and when to notify the physician of emergency situations.

The child will need to take daily calcium and may also need vitamin D. Follow-up visits with the endocrinologist are every 2 to 3 months. At this time, serum and urinary calcium levels will be monitored and dosages adjusted as needed.

Evaluation

- Have the parents verbalized a basic understanding of hypoparathyroidism?
- Can the parents verbalize the signs and symptoms of hypocalcemia and hypercalcemia?
- Can the parents describe medical emergencies related to hypocalcemia?
- Does the child have normal calcium levels?
- Is the child free of seizures related to hypocalcemia?

HYPERPARATHYROIDISM

Hyperparathyroidism is an overproduction of the parathyroid hormone (PTH), which leads to hypercalcemia.

Pathophysiology. Refer to the section on hypoparathyroidism for a discussion of the pathophysiology of the parathyroid glands and calcium metabolism.

The exact mechanism of hyperparathyroidism is unknown at this time, although PTH levels remain elevated in the presence of hypercalcemia. Severe hypercalcemia may be life-threatening.

Etiology. The primary cause of primary hyperparathyroidism in children is parathyroid adenoma. Infants may have hyperplasia or enlargement of the parathyroid glands.

Incidence. Hyperparathyroidism is a rare condition in children.

Clinical Manifestations

- Abdominal pain
- Pancreatitis
- Kidney stones
- Rib cage deformities/fractures
- Hypotonia (infants)
- Poor feeding (infants)
- Failure to thrive (infants)

Diagnostic Evaluation. Hypercalcemia associated with elevated PTH level is diagnostic for hyperparathyroidism. Phosphorus is usually decreased, and alkaline phosphatase is increased.

Therapeutic Management. Acute treatment for hypercalcemia is performed with the infusion of a saline solution (Jansson et al., 1991) often followed with the diuretic furosemide. Other forms of medical therapy include the use of medications including calcitonin and disodium pamidronate.

Total or partial surgical removal of the parathyroid glands is the standard treatment. Often part of one of the glands is transplanted to the forearm (Bacon et al., 1990). Hypoparathyroidism and/or hypocalcemia may occur after surgery.

NURSING CARE OF THE CHILD WITH HYPERPARATHYROIDISM

Assessment

Nursing care involves assessing the child for hypercalcemia (see box). If the child undergoes surgery, hypocalcemia may be present postoperatively. Therefore, laboratory results must be closely followed and the nurse should notify the physician immediately of any abnormal values.

Nursing Diagnosis and Planning

The following nursing diagnoses and expected outcomes may be appropriate in the treatment of hyperparathyroidism in the child.

- Knowledge Deficit related to hyperparathyroidism and/or hypercalcemia. ***Expected Outcomes:*** *The child will maintain normal calcium levels; The parents will have a basic understanding of hyperparathyroidism and be able to describe the signs and symptoms of hypercalcemia.*

Implementation

The family should be educated about the signs and symptoms of hypercalcemia. Follow-up visits with the endocrinologist to monitor calcium levels will be necessary.

Evaluation

- Has the child maintained normal calcium levels after intervention?

Signs and Symptoms of Hypercalcemia

Irritability	Headaches
Weakness	Anorexia
Confusion	Constipation
Increased thirst	Hematuria
Increased urination	Seizure*

*Medical emergency.

- Do the parents verbalize a basic understanding of hypercalcemia?
- Can the parents describe the signs and symptoms of hypercalcemia?

GROWTH HORMONE DEFICIENCY

Growth hormone deficiency results from inadequate production or secretion of growth hormone (GH), which results in poor growth and short stature.

PATHOPHYSIOLOGY *of Growth Hormone Deficiency*

Hormones such as growth hormone, thyroxine, cortisol, and sex hormones influence growth. The hypothalamus secretes growth hormone releasing factor, which stimulates the pituitary to release GH. This hormone is secreted in pulses throughout the day, with increased secretion during the night. In the presence of hypoglycemia, GH is secreted to counteract insulin and raise the blood glucose level. Many children with GH deficiency may present with hypoglycemia.

The majority of children with short stature have constitutional growth delay. Children with short stature or poor growth rates may also be deficient in other hormones. Normal thyroid function is essential for growth; therefore, hypothyroidism may also present with short stature. Sex hormones are required for the growth spurt and sexual maturation that occurs with puberty. Children lacking more than one hormone produced by the pituitary gland are referred to as having hypopituitarism. Rate of growth and final adult height are dependent on factors such as family heights and nutrition. Any child growing less than 5 centimeters a year should be referred to an endocrinologist for further evaluation.

Etiology. Growth hormone deficiency may be isolated or may be associated with an underlying cause. Such causes include hypopituitarism, brain tumors (most commonly craniopharyngioma), and cranial irradiation. Other disorders associated with short stature that may respond to GH therapy include Turner's syndrome and chronic illnesses, such as renal disease.

Incidence. The incidence of GH deficiency is approximately 1 in 10,000 to 20,000 children. In the United States, about 30,000 children are being treated with GH replacement.

Clinical Manifestations

- Height less than 5% for age and sex
- Immature/cherubic facies
- High-pitched voice
- Delayed puberty
- Hypoglycemia
- Micropenis (associated with hypopituitarism)

Diagnostic Evaluation. Diagnosis of GH deficiency begins with thorough measurements of growth over an extended period of time (usually 6 to 12 months). Height should be measured on a consistent scale, preferably with a calibrated stadiometer.

If a child demonstrates consistently poor growth (less than 5 cm/yr), is more than two standard deviations from the mean for height, or deviates from the previous growth curve, further diagnostic testing is warranted.

Initial screening involves thyroid function tests, complete blood count (CBC), somatomedin-C, and a bone age X-ray. Normal thyroid function is essential for adequate growth and should always be checked when evaluating for short stature. CBC and other specific blood screening for any systemic/chronic illness should be done. Somatomedin-C is an indirect measurement of GH level. A bone age X-ray demonstrates skeletal maturation and growth potential. Bone age is usually more retarded with hypothyroidism than with isolated GH deficiency or hypopituitarism (Bacon et al., 1990).

Because GH is normally secreted in pulses throughout the day and night, stimulation testing is necessary to confirm the diagnosis of GH deficiency. Agents used in provocative testing to stimulate the production of GH include insulin, arginine, clonidine, glucagon, and L-dopa. Once the stimulating agent is given, serial GH levels are drawn. Although criteria vary from agency to agency, a GH level lower than 7 ng/mL is usually indicative of GH deficiency (Grunt & Schwartz, 1992). Two positive tests are required for diagnosis.

Therapeutic Management. If a child demonstrates GH deficiency, replacement therapy is indicated. From the early 1960s until 1984, patients were treated with GH derived from human pituitaries. In 1984, there were reports of patients who had been treated with human growth hormone developing Creutzfeldt-Jakob disease, a progressive and fatal neurologic disease. Use of human growth hormone was therefore discontinued. In 1985, synthetic GH produced by recombinant DNA technology became available (Shulman, Miller, & Rose, 1990). Currently, GH therapy is very expensive.

Growth hormone is supplied in a powdered form that must be diluted for administration. Once diluted, it must be refrigerated. It is given as a subcutaneous injection six to seven times per week, usually in the evening. Dose ranges from 0.15 to 0.30 mg/kg/week (Moshang, 1996) depending on the child's age and his response to therapy.

Treatment is usually considered effective if there is an increase of 2 cm/yr over the pretreatment growth rate (Shulman, Miller, & Rose, 1990). The earlier treatment is initiated, the greater the height potential. Treatment is continued until the bone plates close or the patient reaches predicted final height.

NURSING CARE OF THE CHILD WITH GROWTH HORMONE DEFICIENCY

Assessment

Nursing care of the child with GH deficiency includes assessment of the whole family. The parents' attitudes regarding the child's size may influence the child's self-esteem. If the parents are overly concerned or place too much emphasis on the child's height, the child may be more self-conscious or have low self-esteem. It is also important to address psychosocial adjustment such as school performance and involvement in extracurricular activities. Many times, short children appear younger and are often treated as such by adults or may be teased by their peers.

> When assessing a child with short stature, the nurse should ask the child if height causes any problems at school. For example, the nurse may ask, "Have you ever been teased or been in any fights at school because of your height?"

The nurse should also assess compliance with the medication regimen, because many patients have difficulty receiving daily injections. Nurses need to make sure the medication is being diluted correctly and the proper dose is given.

Nursing Diagnosis and Planning

The following nursing diagnoses and expected outcomes may be appropriate in the treatment of growth hormone deficiency in the child.

- Altered Growth and Development related to growth hormone deficiency. ***Expected Outcome:*** *The child will show an increase in growth rate.*
- Body Image Disturbance related to short stature. ***Expected Outcome:*** *The child will demonstrate acceptance of body image.*
- Self-Esteem Disturbance related to short stature. ***Expected Outcome:*** *The child will demonstrate appropriate feelings of self-esteem.*
- Ineffective Management of Therapeutic Regimen: Families, related to noncompliance with daily injection. ***Expected Outcome:*** *The child/parents will comply with the injection schedule.*

Implementation

The nurse should offer reassurance to the child and parents that compliance with the injections will improve growth rate. It is also helpful to remind the patients that the injections are temporary and are helping them to grow. Keeping a growth chart at home and needing larger clothes are physical signs the child can use to monitor growth. These indicators also assist with compliance.

There are injection aids available to assist with giving medication. Many children are able to give their own injections.

The nurse also has an important role in educating patients on the proper dilution and administration of the medication. Patients also need to be taught proper subcutaneous injection technique and be able to demonstrate giving an injection.

Effectiveness of therapy is evaluated by growth rate. Children are seen approximately every 3 months by the endocrinologist. Nurses need to perform accurate measurements of height and record them on the growth chart. Generally, the child is measured at least three times; then the average height is recorded. Therapy is continued until the child reaches predicted adult height or the bone plates fuse.

Evaluation

- Has the child shown an increase in growth rate?
- Does the child verbalize feelings regarding body image/self-esteem?
- Is the child compliant with injection schedule?

KEY CONCEPTS

- The six major hormones of the endocrine system are adrenocorticotropic hormone (ACTH), thyroid-stimulating hormone (TSH), follicle-stimulating hormone (FSH), luteinizing hormone (LH), growth hormone (GH), and prolactin.
- The pituitary gland stimulates target organs to produce specific hormones. When enough hormone is produced, the gland signals the pituitary to stop stimulation. This is referred to as a negative feedback system.

- To improve compliance with daily medications, nurses may suggest the use of pill dispensers or watches with alarms as reminders to take medication at specific times.
- Signs and symptoms of hypothyroidism include tiredness/fatigue, constipation, cold intolerance, weight gain, dry thick skin, edema, and poor growth. The signs and symptoms of hyperthyroidism include nervousness, diarrhea, heat intolerance, weight loss, smooth velvety skin, exophthalmos, and increased appetite.
- Diabetes insipidus is an inability to concentrate urine due to a deficiency of antidiuretic hormone. Diabetes insipidus is characterized by polyuria, dehydration, increased serum sodium, and a low urine specific gravity. In comparison, the syndrome of inappropriate antidiuretic hormone (SIADH) results from excessive production of antidiuretic hormone. This is evidenced by decreased urine output, increased urine specific gravity, and decreased serum sodium.
- Puberty occurs in five stages according to Tanner. These stages are related to breast development and pubic hair growth for females; and testicular enlargement and pubic hair growth for males.
- Psychosocial issues concerning children with precocious puberty include self-consciousness about their bodies, being treated as older than their chronologic age, and aggressive behavior by boys.
- Two ways to assess for hypocalcemia are by eliciting Chvostek's sign and Trousseau's sign. Chvostek's sign is elicited by tapping the facial nerve anterior to the ear. A positive sign is unilateral contraction of the facial nerve. Positive Trousseau's sign is present when a blood pressure cuff elevated above the systolic blood pressure produces carpopedal spasm of the hand.

REFERENCES

American Academy of Pediatrics. (1987). Newborn screening for congenital hypothyroidism: Recommended guidelines. *Pediatrics, 80*(5), 745–749.

Aronson, R., Ehrlich, R., Bailey, J., & Rovet, J. (1990). Growth in children with congenital hypothyroidism detected by neonatal screening. *The Journal of Pediatrics, 116*(1), 33–37.

Bacon, G., Spencer, M., Hopwood, N., & Kelch, R. (1990). *A practical approach to pediatric endocrinology* (3rd ed). Chicago: Yearbook Publishers.

Grunt, J., & Schwartz, D. (1992). Growth, short stature, and the use of growth hormone: Considerations for the practicing pediatrician. *Current Problems in Pediatrics,* Oct., 390–409.

Jansson, S., Tisell, L., Lindstedt, G., & Lundberg, P. (1991). Disodium pamidronate in the preoperative treatment of hypercalcemia in patients with primary hyperparathyroidism. *Surgery, 110*(3), 480–486.

Jay, N., Mansfield, J., Blizzard, R., et al. (1992). Ovulation and menstrual function of adolescent girls with central precocious puberty after therapy with gonadotropin-releasing hormone agonist. *Journal of Clinical Endocrinology and Metabolism, 75*(3), 890–894.

Kaplan, S., & Grumbach, M. (1990). Clinical review 14: Pathophysiology and treatment of sexual precocity. *Journal of Clinical Endocrinology and Metabolism, 71*(4), 785–789.

LaFranchi, S. (1986). Newborn thyroid disorders and screening. In N. Lavin (Ed.), *Manual of endocrinology and metabolism* (pp. 389–412). Boston: Little, Brown and Co.

Lavin, N. (1986). Thyroid disorders in children. In N. Lavin (Ed.), *Manual of endocrinology and metabolism* (pp. 412–440). Boston: Little, Brown.

Levy, W., Schumacher, P., & Gupta, M. (1988). Treatment of childhood Graves' disease. *Cleveland Clinic Journal of Medicine, 55*(4), 373–382.

Lindamin, C. (1992). SIADH: Is your patient at risk? *Nursing92, 22*(6): 60–63.

Moshang, T. (1996). Short Stature. In F. Burg et al. (Eds.) *Gillis and Kagans Current Pediatric Therapy* (pp. 329–331). Philadelphia: W. B. Saunders.

Seckl, J., Dunger, D., Bevan, J., et al. (1990). Vasopressin antagonist in early postoperative diabetes insipidus. *Lancet, 335,* 1353–1356.

Shiminski-Maher, T. (1991). Diabetes insipidus and syndrome of inappropriate secretion of antidiuretic hormone in children with midline suprasellar brain tumors. *Journal of Pediatric Oncology Nursing, 8*(3), 106–111.

Shulman, L., Miller, J., & Rose, L. (1990). Growth hormone therapy. *American Family Physician, 41*(5), 1541–1546.

Sills, I., Horlick, M., & Rapaport, R. (1992). Inappropriate suppression of thyrotropin during medical treatment of Graves' disease in childhood. *The Journal of Pediatrics, 121*(2), 206–209.

BIBLIOGRAPHY

Doherty, G., et al. (1992). Results of a multidisciplinary strategy for management of mediastinal parathyroid adenoma as a cause of persistent primary hyperthyroidism. *Annals of Surgery, 215*(2), 101–106.

Fisher, D. (1991). Clinical Review 19: Management of congenital hypothyroidism. *Journal of Clinical Endocrinology and Metabolism, 72*(3), 523–529.

Frasier, D., & Lippe, B. (1990). Clinical Review 11: The rational use of growth hormone during childhood. *Journal of Clinical Endocrinology and Metabolism, 71*(2), 269–273.

Henry, J. (1992). Routine growth monitoring and assessment of growth disorders. *Journal of Pediatric Health Care, 6*(5), 291–301.

Rieser, P. (1992). Educational, psychologic, and social aspects of short stature. *Journal of Pediatric Health Care, 6*(5), 325–332.

39

The Child With Diabetes Mellitus

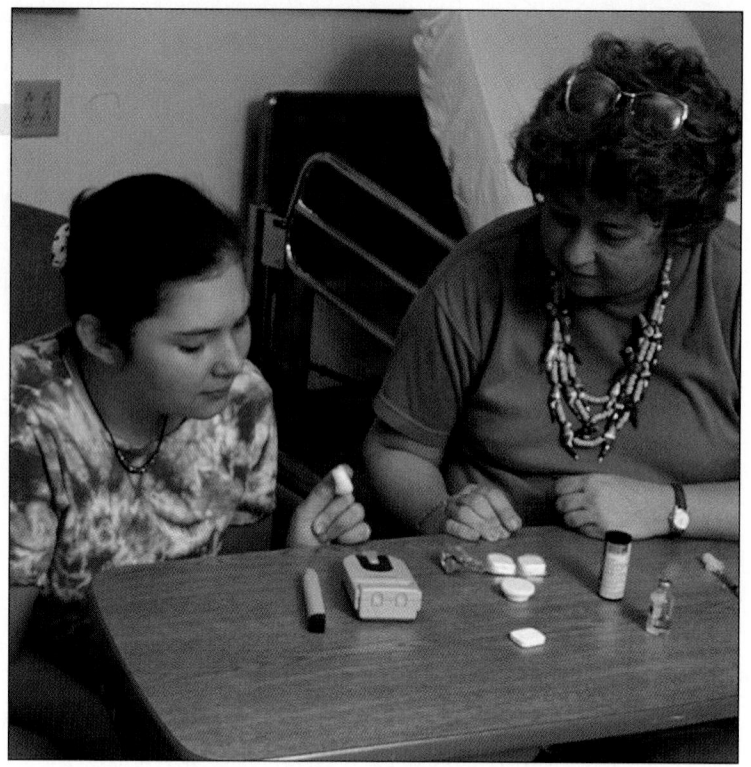

CHAPTER OVERVIEW

LEARNING OBJECTIVES

After studying this chapter, you should be able to:

- Identify the role of insulin in the metabolism of carbohydrates, fats, and proteins in both the fasting and postprandial state.
- Compare and contrast insulin-dependent diabetes mellitus (IDDM; Type 1 diabetes) and non-insulin-dependent diabetes mellitus (NIDDM; Type 2 diabetes).
- Identify management goals for the child with IDDM.
- List the nursing diagnoses associated with IDDM.
- Identify the patient/family teaching needs associated with home management of IDDM.
- Identify the role and nursing implications of insulin therapy, diet therapy, exercise, self-monitoring of blood glucose, and urine ketone monitoring in the management of diabetes.
- Describe the signs, symptoms, causes, and treatment of hypoglycemia and hyperglycemia.
- Identify the pathophysiology of diabetic ketoacidosis, treatment, and nursing care of the child in diabetic ketoacidosis.

KEY TERMS

beta cells: specialized cells within the pancreas that manufacture and secrete insulin; thought to be the target of the autoimmune destructive process of IDDM

diabetic ketoacidosis (DKA): metabolic consequence of severe insulin deficit; marked by hyperglycemia, acidosis, and ketosis

glucagon: a hormone produced by the alpha cells of the pancreas; counteracts the action of insulin by converting liver stores of glycogen to blood glucose, resulting in an elevation of the blood glucose level

glucose: the substrate of choice for cellular energy; the breakdown product of carbohydrate

glycosuria: glucose in urine; occurs when the blood glucose level exceeds the renal threshold and glucose "spills" into the urine

glycosylated hemoglobin: a laboratory test used to evaluate glycemic control by measuring glycosylation (or sugar coating) on the hemoglobin portion of the red blood cell; offers a 3-month average of blood sugar control

honeymoon phase: an early stage of diabetes characterized by relatively small exogenous insulin requirements to maintain normal blood sugar

hyperglycemia: blood glucose levels above 120 mg/dl (fasting) and/or 200 mg/dl (random)

hypoglycemia: blood glucose levels below 70 mg/dl

ketone/ketoacid: an acid manufactured by the liver in response to starvation (in diabetic child, a result of insulin deficit); produced from fat stores, can be used for energy when glucose is unavailable

Kussmaul's Respiration: deep, rapid respiration seen with DKA, in which CO_2 is expelled in a respiratory compensation for acidosis; also described as "air hunger"

neuroglycopenic signs: signs due to decreased cerebral glucose utilization (headache, personality, behavior changes, etc.)

Insulin-dependent diabetes mellitus (IDDM), the most common childhood endocrine disorder, presents challenges in the areas of teaching, compliance, maintenance, and prevention. Because of recent changes in the health care delivery system, meeting the needs associated with management of IDDM has become more complicated. Unless the newly diagnosed child with diabetes is in diabetic ketoacidosis (DKA), the child most likely will not be hospitalized. This creates a major challenge for the nurse, who must have a plan of care that will involve teaching either in a clinic or the home. An awareness of normal growth and development assists the nurse in providing the support the child will need to comply with the treatment plan and hopefully control or limit the complications associated with the disease. Inclusion of the family in the care and support of the child must be part of planning and implementation of nursing care of the child with IDDM. Because IDDM is a chronic disease, see Chapter 17 for a discussion of that aspect of care.

CLINICAL REFERENCE PAGE

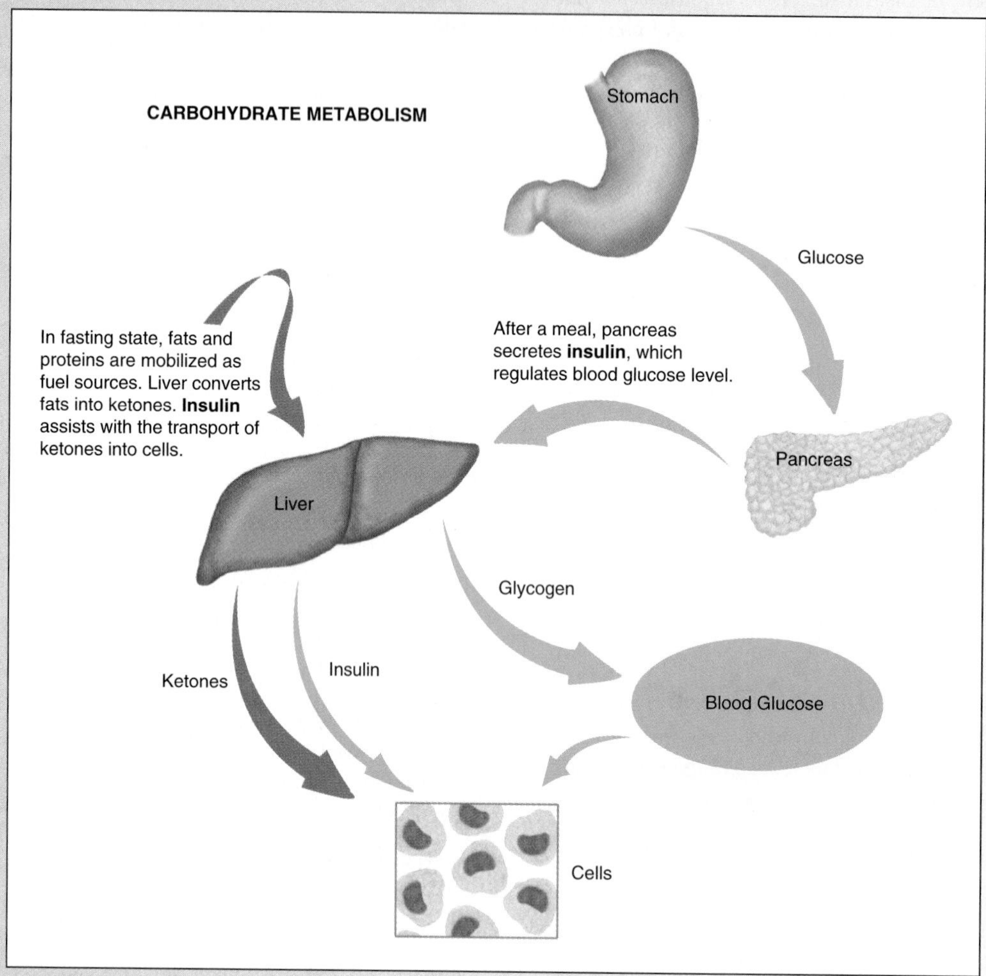
CARBOHYDRATE METABOLISM
Stomach
Glucose
After a meal, pancreas secretes **insulin**, which regulates blood glucose level.
In fasting state, fats and proteins are mobilized as fuel sources. Liver converts fats into ketones. **Insulin** assists with the transport of ketones into cells.
Pancreas
Liver
Glycogen
Ketones
Insulin
Blood Glucose
Cells

REVIEW: PHYSIOLOGY OF CARBOHYDRATE METABOLISM

Glucose is the primary source of energy for body cells. Small amounts of glucose can be stored in the fat tissues and in the form of glycogen in muscle or liver cells. Because the glucose can be stored in only small quantities, a minimum blood glucose level must be maintained by the body.

Insulin, a hormone, is secreted by the **beta cells** of the pancreas. Its main function is to regulate the blood glucose level. It does this by controlling the rate of glucose uptake by the cells. Little or no insulin is secreted by the beta cells when a person is in the fasting state; greater quantities are secreted after the person has eaten a meal. In the fasting state, with relatively small quantities of available insulin, the body's fats and proteins are mobilized to be used as fuel sources. The liver then converts the fats into **ketoacids,** or **ketones.** With the assistance of insulin, the ketones are transported into the cells, and can then be used as an alternative source of fuel for the body functions. This process assures an energy source during periods of fasting.

ACTIONS OF INSULIN

ANABOLIC ACTIONS OF INSULIN	CATABOLIC CONSEQUENCES OF INSULIN DEFICIT
Promotes glucose as a fuel source	Promotes fats and proteins as fuel sources
Promotes storage of glucose as glycogen	Allows glycogen stores to be broken down
Prevents breakdown of fat stores	Allows fat stores to be depleted
Increases protein synthesis	Allows protein breakdown into amino acids

INSULIN-DEPENDENT DIABETES MELLITUS (IDDM)

Insulin-dependent diabetes mellitus results when the pancreas is unable to produce and secrete insulin.

PATHOPHYSIOLOGY *of IDDM*

In the absence of insulin, the metabolism of fats, proteins, and carbohydrates is impaired. Glucose is unable to move into the intracellular space, resulting in **hyperglycemia.** As blood glucose levels exceed the renal threshold, glucose is "spilled" into the urine via osmotic diuresis, resulting in polyuria. Excessive thirst follows in response to fluid loss. Fatigue, hunger, and weight loss also accompany the onset of IDDM, as cellular starvation continues in the absence of insulin.

Ketones (ketoacids), manufactured by the liver from adipose tissue, are produced in response to cellular starvation. In the absence of insulin, ketones are also unavailable to the cell for nourishment. Increasing blood levels of ketones (ketonemia) will result in ketoacidosis.

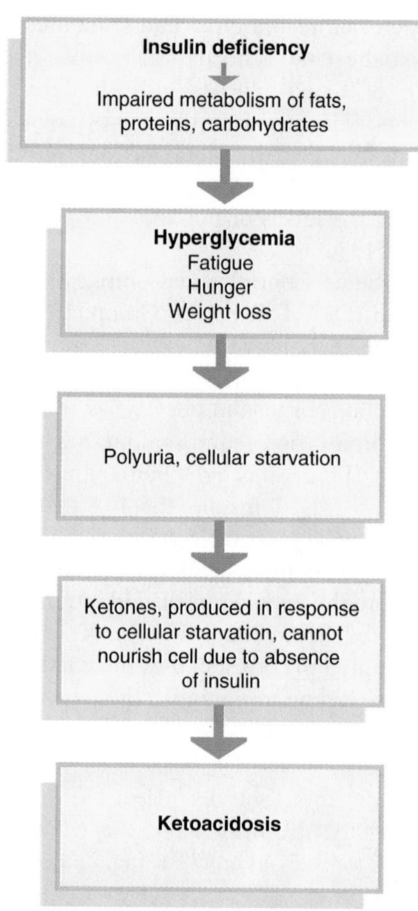

Etiology. IDDM is an autoimmune process that results in the destruction of the insulin-secreting cells of the pancreas. A genetic predisposition plus an environmental or viral trigger are thought to initiate the onset of the autoimmune destructive process. Current research focuses on identifying specific genes that may affect an individual's susceptibility to IDDM, as well as exploring methods of interrupting or preventing the autoimmune response in susceptible individuals (first-degree relatives of a diabetic individual). The NIH is presently conducting a multicenter Diabetes Prevention Trial (DPT), which explores possible intervention strategies for high-risk individuals, including the use of low dosages of long-acting insulin. No prevention or cure is presently available for IDDM.

Incidence. The incidence of IDDM is 15 per 100,000 people in the North American population younger than age 20 years (or a risk of 1 in 600), and decreases to 5 per 100,000 for the population over age 20. The risk of diabetes increases to 1 in 20 if the individual has a first-degree relative (parent or sibling) with IDDM, and increases to 1 in 3 if an identical twin has the disease. The average age of onset of IDDM is the early pubertal years, although onset can occur as early as the neonatal period and throughout adulthood (Wetterhaul et al., 1992).

IDDM Compared With NIDDM. The term diabetes mellitus encompasses a variety of diseases, the most prevalent of which is non-insulin dependent diabetes (NIDDM). NIDDM is related to either insufficient production of insulin, or excessive insulin production combined with insulin resistance in the peripheral tissues. NIDDM is treated with diet and exercise alone, or in combination with oral hypoglycemic agents, and/or in combination with insulin. Oral hypoglycemic agents are not insulin, but are medications that prompt the pancreas to produce insulin and work to decrease insulin resistance in the peripheral tissues. Both IDDM and NIDDM involve abnormal carbohydrate metabolism. NIDDM is contrasted with IDDM in Table 39–1.

Clinical Manifestations

Hyperglycemia

The first three symptoms are known as the three Ps.

- Polyuria, or enuresis in a toilet-trained child
- Polydipsia
- Polyphagia
- Fatigue
- Weight loss
- Blurred vision

Hypoglycemia

Early symptoms are caused by adrenaline release.

- Trembling
- Tachycardia
- Sweating
- Anxiety

TABLE 39–1 *IDDM Versus NIDDM*

	IDDM	NIDDM
Incidence	2/1000	25/1000 (Wetterhaul et al., 1992)
Average age at onset	Prepubertal, < 20 years	>40 years
Body size	Lean	Obese
Sex	Males and females equally affected	Females affected > males
Ethnic targets	None, although less common in nonwhite populations	Native American, Black, Hispanic
Treatment	Insulin therapy, diet, exercise	Varies: diet, exercise, may require oral agents or insulin therapy
Ketosis prone	Yes	No

- Hunger
- Pallor
- Headache

Later symptoms are caused by cerebral glucose deficit.

- Loss of coordination
- Personality/mood/behavior change (especially in the young child)
- Slurred speech
- Sleepiness
- Nightmares
- Decreasing level of consciousness or loss of consciousness
- Seizure activity

Table 39–2 provides an overview of hypoglycemia, hyperglycemia, and ketoacidosis.

Diagnostic Evaluation. Diagnosis of IDDM is based on a clinical picture of hyperglycemia (and acidosis, if present) combined with the laboratory data of a fasting serum glucose of greater than 120 mg/dl and a random serum glucose greater than 200 mg/dl. Ketonuria, although not diagnostic for IDDM, will be a frequent finding, as will **glycosuria.** Glucose tolerance testing is rarely used in diagnosing IDDM. The **glycosylated hemoglobin** value will be elevated in response to prolonged elevations of blood glucose.

Therapeutic Management

The goals of diabetes management are

- appropriate growth (height and weight)
- age-appropriate lifestyle
- near normal glycosylated hemoglobin
- absence of acute complications (hypoglycemia, hyperglycemia)

Insulin Therapy. The child with IDDM loses the ability to make insulin via an autoimmune destruction of the insulin-producing cells: the beta cells. Symptoms of hyperglycemia begin to be evident when the majority of beta cells are destroyed. After initiation of insulin therapy, the child may experience the **honeymoon phase.** This stage is characterized by a decreasing need for insulin and **hypoglycemia.** It may last from a few weeks to a year or longer. It is important to prepare the child and family for this possibility of a honeymoon phase both to avoid the misconception that the diabetes is "going away," as well as to provide instruction on recognition and treatment of hypoglycemia.

The goal of insulin therapy is to replace the insulin the child is no longer able to make. Synthetic human insulin, made by recombinant DNA technology, is free of animal impurities and is recommended for children. Oral hypoglycemic agents, while useful in the treatment of NIDDM (Type 2 diabetes), are not effective in the treatment of IDDM.

The choice of insulin types and schedule of injections is based on the child's needs (Table 39–3). Daily self-monitoring of blood glucose aids in defining insulin requirements. The child in the honeymoon phase will need less insulin than the child making no endogenous insulin. The pubertal child requires larger insulin dosages due to increasing levels of pubertal and growth hormone (Amiel et al., 1986).

The Diabetes Control and Complications Trial Research Group (DCCT Research Group, 1993) concluded that long-term diabetic complications can be minimized by intensive treatment. This treatment, defined as three or more injections of insulin per day (or the use of a continuous insulin infusion pump), mimics physiologic delivery of insulin. Three injections per day have become the most frequently used insulin therapy for the pediatric patient: intermediate-acting combined with rapid-acting insulin injected before breakfast, rapid-acting insulin injected before the evening meal, and intermediate-acting insulin injected before bed. The peak actions of these insulins are timed to correspond to the child's usual mealtimes and snack time to minimize the possibility of hypoglycemia (see Fig. 39–1).

Store insulin in a cool, dry place. Do not freeze nor expose to excessive heat or agitation. Check the expiration date on the vial before using. Once opened, the vial should be dated and discarded as recommended by the health care professional.

TABLE 39–2 *Comparison of Hypoglycemia, Hyperglycemia, and Ketoacidosis*

DESCRIPTOR	HYPOGLYCEMIA	HYPERGLYCEMIA	KETOACIDOSIS
Onset	Rapid	Slow	Slow
Signs and Symptoms	*Adrenergic signs:* Trembling Sweating Tachycardia Pallor Clammy skin Hunger	Increased urination Increased thirst Fatigue Weight loss (gradual, over several weeks) Blurred vision	*Hyperglycemia signs plus:* Abdominal pain Chest pain Kussmaul's respirations Nausea and vomiting Acetone (fruity) odor to the breath *Signs and symptoms of dehydration:* Dry lips and mucous membranes Sunken eyes Sudden weight loss Decreased urination
Sensorium	*Neuroglycopenic symptoms:* Personality change Irritability Drunken behavior Decreasing level of consciousness, to loss of consciousness Seizure activity	Normal sensorium	Increasing lethargy Decreasing level of consciousness Coma
Laboratory Data	Blood glucose below 70 mg/dl Urine ketones negative or trace	Serum glucose over 200 mg/dl	Serum glucose over 300 mg/dl Urinary ketones positive Serum pH below 7.25 Serum ketones positive
Causes	Too much insulin Excessive activity without eating extra carbohydrate Missed or delayed meal	Excessive intake of carbohydrate Little or no exercise Inadequate amount of insulin Increased stress, either emotional or physical	Inadequate amount of insulin Excessive stress
Treatment	15 grams oral carbohydrate *For loss of consciousness or seizure activity:* Glucagon SQ or IM IV glucose	Insulin Exercise	IV fluids IV insulin Electrolyte replacement

TABLE 39–3 *Insulin Action by Type (Humulin)*

	ONSET	PEAK	DURATION
Lispro	≤15 minutes	30–90 minutes	≤5 hours
Regular Insulin*	30 minutes	2–4 hours	4–6 hours
NPH or Lente Insulin	1–2 hours	6–8 hours	12–24 hours
Ultralente Insulin	Slow; >2 hours	Peakless	24–36 hours

*Data from Galloway, et al. (1981). Factors influencing the absorption, serum insulin concentration, and blood glucose responses after injections of regular insulin and various insulin mixtures. *Diabetes Care, 4*(3), 366–376.

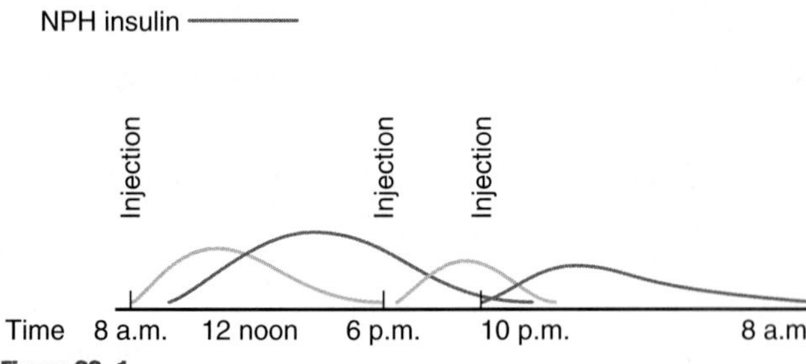

Figure 39–1

For the pediatric IDDM patient, three injections of insulin per day is the usual therapeutic regimen. Peak action of these injections is timed to correspond with the child's usual meal and snack time to minimize the chance of hypoglycemia.

Nutrition Therapy. The goal of nutrition therapy is to promote normal growth, encourage good nutrition, and maintain blood glucose goals. Because the insulin dosage is balanced with food intake, the diet should stress a consistent intake, particularly of carbohydrate food products. The diet therapy chosen should be easy to understand and should help the child and family learn to make healthy food choices. One diet therapy is based on the *ADA Exchange Lists for Meal Planning (1995),* a system in which foods are grouped into six categories according to carbohydrate content. Using these categories, the nutritionist can generate a meal plan, or a guideline for daily food intake. The meal plan is based on the child's diet history. As the child grows, the meal plan is tailored to meet increasing dietary needs.

> Meals and snacks are balanced with insulin action. Both the amount of food and the timing of the meal and snack are important in avoiding hypoglycemia and hyperglycemia. Encourage families to adhere to a daily schedule that maintains *consistency of food intake, of injection times, and of mealtimes.*

Exercise. Exercise is an important aspect of diabetes management. Exercise aids insulin in lowering blood glucose levels. The child with diabetes should be encouraged to participate in age-appropriate sports. Early enjoyment of a sport or activity can promote a lifelong active lifestyle. Because exercise lowers glucose levels, the child must be taught how to prevent hypoglycemia. The child should try to schedule activities to avoid exercising when an insulin dose is peaking. Teach the family to add extra snacks of 15 to 30 grams carbohydrate for each 45 to 60 minutes of exercise. With experience, the child and parent will be able to tailor the snack guidelines to meet the child's specific needs. Coaches and teammates should be taught how to recognize and treat hypoglycemia. Delayed or nocturnal hypoglycemia can occur after strenuous activity. Additional carbohydrate may be required after exercise to maintain blood glucose levels. The child should always wear a medical identification emblem.

Blood Glucose Monitoring. Self-monitoring of blood glucose provides an objective tool to assist with diabetes control. Monitoring is recommended before meals and before the bedtime snack. More frequent monitoring may be useful during prolonged exercise, during an illness, or if nighttime hypoglycemia is suspected.

Blood glucose goals must be tailored to the abilities of the family and the age of the child. Goals for the infant or toddler are usually liberalized to aid in preventing severe hypoglycemia.

Preprandial Blood Glucose Goals

Non-diabetic:	70–110 mg/dl
Children with IDDM:	80–150 mg/dl
Infants/toddlers:	100–200 mg/dl

The identified goals are a target range: not *all* glucose levels will fall in this range, even in the child with excellent diabetes control.

Glucose test results should be recorded in a glucose diary or record book. Patterns or trends in blood glucose levels indicate a need to adjust the insulin dose. Three to four days of a consistent pattern of glucose values (for example, 200 mg/dl before the evening meal for three consecutive days) indicates a need to increase the appropriate insulin (the morning intermediate-acting insulin in this example). The healthcare team may provide the family with a guideline for increasing insulin based on glucose patterns.

Blood glucose meters are accurate only if used according to manufacturers' recommendations. Regardless of the brand selected, quality control procedures must be performed as recommended. Test supplies must be stored according to manufacturers' specifications and discarded when outdated.

Glucose meters available as of this writing require a drop of blood to perform glucose determinations. (Fig. 18–10 in Chapter 18 shows the finger stick method for obtaining a small blood sample.) Methods of blood glucose determination that do not require a drop of blood may be available in the future. Transdermal glucose sensors or implantable glucose sensors are future possibilities for glucose monitoring.

NURSING CARE OF THE CHILD WITH IDDM

Developmental Issues

The Infant and Toddler

The infant or toddler with diabetes poses special challenges for diabetes management. The burden of management falls on the parent(s) or other caregivers. Achieving consistency in dietary intake with the infant can be quite difficult. Inconsistent intake, particularly of carbohydrates, will contribute to blood glucose variability. Food control issues can easily become a battleground between the child and the parent. A diet strategy that stresses carbohydrate consistency rather than specific food groups offers more flexibility than a structured meal plan. Allow the toddler to participate in making food choices (from perhaps two or three options) to offer the child a sense of control.

Diluted insulin may be required for some infants. U-20 insulin rather than the standard U-100 (that is, 20 units of insulin per ml rather than 100 units of insulin per ml) may be necessary to provide small enough dosages to avoid hypoglycemia. This diluted insulin solution should be clearly labeled to avoid dosage errors. The signs and symptoms of hypoglycemia are difficult to recognize in the infant or might be mistaken for the toddler's temper tantrum. The glucose goals for this age-group are liberalized to avoid episodes of severe hypoglycemia.

Establishing rituals and routines will help the toddler feel more in control. Encourage the parent to have a specific place to perform the blood test and a special place to keep supplies. The toddler will feel more in control if able to predict and participate in diabetes activities (see Table 39–4).

The Preschooler

The preschool years are characterized by increasing motor maturity, a widening social circle, and magical thinking. The preschooler can understand simple explanations regarding diabetes. Such explanations help to allay fears that the diabetes was caused by the child's being "bad." Play therapy using dolls and diabetes equipment will help the preschooler express concerns regarding injections and finger sticks.

The preschooler has a more predictable appetite than the toddler and is frequently willing to try new foods. Still, supervision is necessary to ensure that meals and snacks are eaten, especially if the child is in a daycare setting with many distractions.

The preschooler may be able to identify the feelings associated with hypoglycemia. Use the child's description as a code word for the onset of hypoglycemia symptoms. The preschooler's preference for high energy activities makes him a candidate for hypoglycemia. The caregiver should be prepared with readily available carbohydrate foods as well as emergency medications.

The School-Age Child

The school-age child and family face the challenge of incorporating diabetes care within a busy school day. In order to avoid singling the child out, the diabetes care should be as unobtrusive as possible while still maintaining a safe environment for the child. The family should communicate with school personnel about the child's diabetes. A school nurse or health aide should be identified to supervise pre-lunch blood glucose monitoring, to assist with insulin injections, and to educate other school personnel in recognizing and treating hypoglycemia. Schools vary on the availability of nursing services. Parents may have to work with school personnel to identify appropriate staff to supervise their child's diabetes care.

Planning ahead for field trips, school parties, and athletic events will allow the child with diabetes to safely participate in age-appropriate activities. For example, the child who has soccer practice three afternoons per week will need to plan how to prevent hypoglycemia during practice. An extra snack of 15 to 30 grams carbohydrate before practice will avert hypoglycemia.

The Adolescent

The developmental milestones of the adolescent are often in conflict with the recommendations for achieving diabetes control. The early adolescent is concerned with body image and peer group acceptance, and is moving away from the family for support and identity. Clothing, diet, lifestyle, and speech are areas in which the early adolescent strives to conform with peers. The mid-adolescent is open to risk-taking behaviors and is more openly challenging of parental authority. By late adolescence, the individual becomes more future oriented, with behaviors based more on abstract morals and less on peer group demands. (Refer to Chapter 8 for further discussion on developmental issues affecting the adolescent.) These normally recognized milestones become dilemmas when diabetes control is affected. Missed injections, omitted blood tests, irregular meals, and dietary splurges are frequent complaints of parents of diabetic adolescents.

The parents and their adolescent must accept that diabetes responsibility will increasingly shift to the adolescent. Encourage parents to work as partners with the adolescent to achieve diabetes control. Identify what is important to the adolescent, and use that information as a tool to motivate compliance. The adolescent is not motivated by predictions of complications in the distant future. Rather, motivation should focus on issues important to the adolescent: personal appearance, athletic ability, strength/muscle mass, endurance, and/or ideal weight.

Delegating Diabetes Responsibilities

The child with diabetes is functionally able to perform diabetes skills far sooner than he is cognitively able to understand the implications of the activity or consequences of omitting the activity. When queried as to the appropriate age to delegate specific responsibilities, parents tended to delegate responsibility at a younger age than the professionals who responded (Follansbee, 1989).

Transfer of responsibility should be on a step-by-step basis, as demonstrated in Table 39–4. Diabetes responsibilities shift from full parent responsibility to a partnership between parent and child, and on to the acceptance of responsibility by the young adult.

Delegation of diabetes responsibility at an *inappropriate* age results in poor diabetes control and frequent bouts of DKA. The importance of ongoing parental support and supervision cannot be overemphasized.

Administration of Insulin

Because insulin is a protein, and would be digested if taken orally, it is given parenterally. Insulin is administered by subcutaneous injection into the adipose tissue over large muscle masses: the back of the arms, the top and outer portion of the thighs, the abdomen, and the hip (Fig. 39–2). To avoid injecting into the muscle or vascular space, an injection angle of 45 degrees and aspiration before injection may be used on thin children or infants. Rotation of injection sites helps prevent adipose hypertrophy (fatty lumps), which absorb insulin poorly. Lipodystrophy (pitting of the adipose tissue at the injection site) is seen with animal-derived insulin, but rarely with human insulin. Various injection sites absorb insulin at slightly different rates, as described in Figure 39–2. Absorption is also affected by the amount of exercise the underlying muscle engages in and by the body temperature. To help decrease variations in absorption from day to day, the child should use one location within a major site for the morning injection, rotating to another site for the evening injection, and a third site for the bedtime injection for a period of 2 to 3 weeks before changing major sites.

Insulin may be administered by an insulin syringe, air injector, or insulin pump. Disposable syringes are to be used one time and safely discarded (dispose of syringe in coffee can or bleach bottle before placing in trash). Studies have indicated a low incidence of infection with syringe reuse (Poteet, Reinert, & Ptak, 1987), but the instructions of the diabetes team should be adhered to regarding reuse of syringes.

The air injector uses compressed air to deposit the insulin within the fatty tissue, without the use of a needle. The child/family must learn to use the device correctly; to load insulin, adjust pressure settings to avoid intramuscular delivery, and clean properly.

TABLE 39–4 *Examples of Delegation of Diabetes Tasks (With Supervision)*

DEVELOPMENTAL CHARACTERISTICS	DIABETES TASK	DIET TASK
Toddler/Preschooler		
Likes rituals Finicky eater Not yet able to understand need for insulin	Chooses and cleans finger for puncture Helps by holding still for injection Identifies a word or phrase to describe feeling of hypoglycemia	Helps by choosing foods
School-Age Child		
Thinking is present oriented Spending large amounts of time away from parents Begins to develop self-concept	Performs finger puncture and blood glucose test Chooses injection site according to rotation schedule Pushes plunger on insulin syringe after the needle is inserted by parent or gives own injection Performs ketone test	Recognizes need to eat on time to avoid hypoglycemia Knows treatment for hypoglycemia
Early Adolescent		
Looks to peer group for identity Needs to conform to peer group norms Increased risk-taking behaviors	Records blood glucose values in diary Performs insulin injection	Knows meal plan Can choose correct foods for snack Adds extra snack for increased activity
Middle/Late Adolescent		
Future oriented Wants to take charge of life Able to recognize consequences of behaviors and choices Emotional separation from parents	Draws up and injects insulin Looks for patterns in blood glucose values Recognizes when to test for ketones Initiates treatment for ketones (fluids)	Can plan meals and snacks based on meal plan Can choose appropriate foods at a party

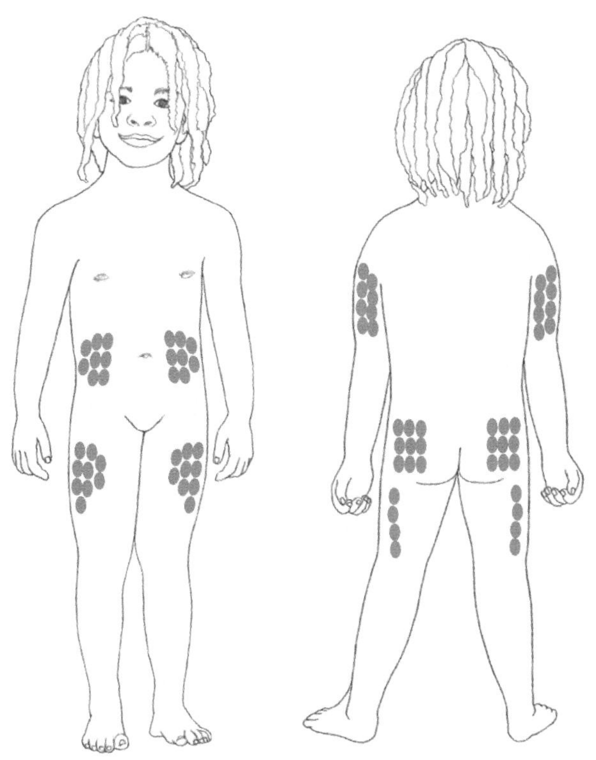

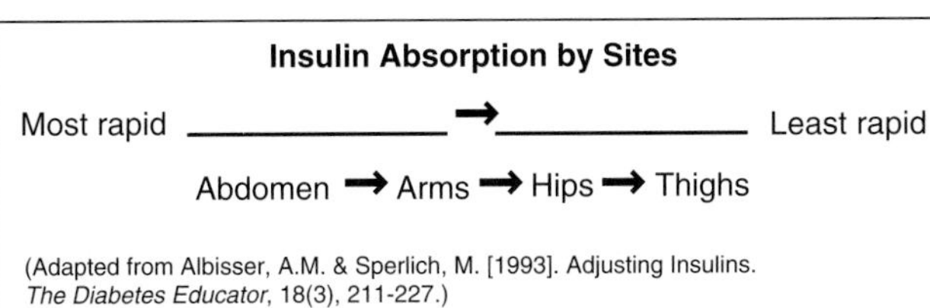

Insulin Absorption by Sites
Most rapid → Least rapid
Abdomen → Arms → Hips → Thighs
(Adapted from Albisser, A.M. & Sperlich, M. [1993]. Adjusting Insulins. *The Diabetes Educator*, 18(3), 211-227.)

Figure 39–2
Subcutaneous insulin injection sites most commonly used are illustrated here, although almost any area on the body may be used. Sites are rotated on a daily basis to help prevent the formation of fatty lumps, which absorb insulin poorly. However, since the rate of absorption varies by site (see chart), the child is advised to rotate sites within the same general area (e.g., arm, thigh) for a period of 2 to 3 weeks before changing to another area. This will help decrease variations in absorption from day to day.

The insulin pump is a device that provides a continuous infusion of regular insulin. The pump consists of a computer, a reservoir of regular insulin, and thin tubing through which the insulin is delivered via a small needle inserted into the abdomen. A continuous basal, or background, rate of insulin infusion is programmed into the device, and bolus dosages are administered as determined by blood glucose testing. The pump most closely mimics physiologic delivery of insulin. The candidate for insulin pump therapy must be willing to meticulously measure blood glucose throughout the day (and often night) to avoid hypoglycemia and to respond to hyperglycemia.

THE NURSING PROCESS IN IDDM MANAGEMENT

Assessment

Nursing assessment of the child diagnosed with IDDM begins with a careful history. Identify signs and symptoms of hyperglycemia: polyuria (increased urination), polydipsia (increased thirst), and polyphagia (excessive eating)—the three Ps. Daytime polydipsia and polyuria may not worry a parent, but enuresis or accidents in the previously toilet-trained child and nighttime requests for water will spark concern. New onset diabetes is frequently overlooked in light of specific symptoms. A urinary tract infection might be suspected based on urinary frequency. An infective process frequently accompanies the onset of diabetes, but is not the cause of the diabetes. The stress associated with an infection can compromise the function of the remaining insulin-secreting cells. A history of weight loss or fatigue is also a common parental observation. Nausea and vomiting will be present in the child who is acidotic.

Ask about other medications used. Glucocorticoids and some chemotheraputic agents can cause hyperglycemia.

Physical assessment should include signs and symptoms of dehydration: dry mucous membranes, flushed skin, acute weight change, absence of tearing, or poor skin turgor. Identify the time of most recent voiding. Oliguria is a significant finding in the assessment of dehydration.

Assess for signs and symptoms of acidosis: abdominal pain, nausea and vomiting (which also contribute to dehydration), **Kussmaul's respirations** coupled with a fruity odor to the breath, and/or decreasing LOC. Ongoing assessment of the child in acidosis should include vital signs, LOC, and intake and output. Vital signs and LOC should be monitored frequently until stable.

Assess the family's present knowledge of diabetes. For the newly diagnosed child, prepare the family to participate in a diabetes education program to learn home care skills. Encourage parents to arrange for time away from work and school to participate. Assess the family's ability to cope with the diagnosis of a chronic disease. Identify usual methods of coping with stress and usual support systems. Explore the availability of financial resources to meet the child's health care needs.

Nursing Diagnosis

- Knowledge Deficit related to the home care needs of the child with IDDM
- Altered Family Processes related to the chronic health care needs of a child with IDDM
- Altered Nutrition: Less Than Body Requirements related to insulin deficit
- Risk for Injury related to hypoglycemia or hyperglycemia

Planning, Implementation, and Evaluation: The Child With IDDM

NURSING DIAGNOSIS • Knowledge Deficit related to home care needs of the child with IDDM

Expected Outcome: • The child and family will be able to successfully manage diabetes, as evidenced by demonstration of skills and verbalization of concepts necessary for home care.

Intervention	Rationale
1. Identify barriers to learning that might hinder the ability of the family to learn home care information. Barriers could include issues such as language fluency, literacy, employment pressures, and child care. These issues should be addressed before initiating education.	Identifying and addressing these issues will optimize the learning ability of the family. For example, provide appropriate written materials for the individual with low literacy skills.
2. Identify learning objectives with the family (see Teaching Guidelines).	A written list of specific objectives will help the family prioritize education, as well as provide a sense of accomplishment as learning objectives are met.
3. Present information at a developmentally appropriate level for the child (see box: Therapeutic Communication With the Child Who Has IDDM)	The child must understand diabetes within his cognitive ability. More advanced information can be presented as the child matures.

Evaluation: The child and family can successfully manage home care, as evidenced by demonstrations of skill mastery and verbalization of home care concepts.

NURSING DIAGNOSIS • Altered Family Processes related to the chronic health care needs of a child with IDDM

Expected Outcome: • The family will recognize/identify stresses and identify strategies for dealing with the stress of a chronic disease.

Intervention	Rationale
1. Assist family to identify age-appropriate diabetes skills for the child and the responsibilities of the parent.	Delegation of responsibilities should occur as the child is both able to perform the skill and to understand the implications of the skill. Parental support and supervision is essential for all age children for successful home management of diabetes.
2. Assist the child and family to identify behaviors that the child recognizes as supportive. Supportive family behaviors might include the following: all family members follow the child's meal plan, avoid having sweets in the home, offer to record blood glucose levels in the diary for the child, or recognize and praise the child's attempts at adherence.	Discussions of family support will help to involve all family members in the child's care, as well as give the child the opportunity to identify behaviors he considers supportive (McKelvey et al., 1993). Adaptation is enhanced by focusing on the strengths of the child and family.
3. Identify community support systems available for the family. For the child with diabetes, summer diabetes camp and age-specific support groups are invaluable for motivation and building self-esteem. A parent support group or participation in fund-raising activities in a local diabetes community group can provide support for other family members.	Community resources offer a variety of opportunities for support, as well as an alternative to relying solely on family coping skills.

Intervention	Rationale
4. Identify a "vacation" plan in which the major caregiver can take a break from diabetes responsibilities. The ongoing, day-to-day responsibility of diabetes management can be shared, between parents, siblings, and others. Although total responsibility might not be delegated, perhaps the child (or parent) can take a break from one aspect of responsibility as another family member takes on the responsibility.	Taking responsibility for diabetes control is very stressful and demanding. Sharing responsibilities among family members will help to prevent burnout, discouragement, and frustration.

Evaluation: The child and family are able to verbalize a plan for sharing diabetes responsibility.

NURSING DIAGNOSIS • Altered Nutrition: Less Than Body Requirements related to insulin deficit

Expected Outcome: • The family will demonstrate ability to utilize insulin therapy, diet therapy, and self-monitoring of glucose to maximize nutritional status.

Intervention	Rationale
1. Teach family the action of food (carbohydrates, fats, and proteins) on blood glucose level: carbohydrates raise blood glucose levels, fats and proteins have minimal effects on glucose levels.	Understanding the relationship of food to blood glucose levels will help the family recognize the rationale for adhering to the diabetic diet.
2. Based on the child's usual schedule, generate a daily schedule that includes times for blood glucose test, medication, meals, and snacks.	Consistency in timing of meals and snacks in relationship to insulin injections is essential. Encouraging child and family input into this aspect of planning will impart a sense of control, as well as promote compliance.
3. Ask the child to identify favorite foods and demonstrate how to incorporate these into the meal plan.	Most foods can be incorporated into the meal plan, even if only in small amounts. Allowing small amounts of favorite "treats" can encourage compliance.
4. Assess the child's satiety on the prescribed diet. Instruct the child/parent to notify the nutritionist if the meal plan forces the child to overeat, or if the child is persistently hungry. Utilize appropriate growth chart to track the child's height and weight with respect to age.	The meal plan is tailored to the child and his activity level. Nutrition needs will vary with age, as well as with variations in activity level. For example, a morning gym class may require that the child add a mid-morning snack.
5. Discuss the relationship between insulin, food (carbohydrate), and exercise. Identify ideal blood glucose goals for the child. Present an example situation in which the blood glucose is out of the ideal range, and encourage the family to identify possible options using diet, insulin, and/or exercise to more closely attain the blood glucose goal.	Diet, exercise, and insulin therapy are the tools of diabetes management. This exercise will develop problem-solving skills within the family and provide a sense of competency.
6. Instruct the family to plan 3 to 4 days of menus based on the meal plan. Both the *type* of food as well as *amount* of food should be included.	This exercise will help the family operationalize the diet instructions.

Evaluation:
- The child's height and weight are appropriate for age as compared to growth chart percentiles.
- The child is free of episodes of severe hypoglycemia or hyperglycemia.

TEACHING GUIDELINES *for the Family of the Child With IDDM*

Family education is an essential component of caring for the child with IDDM. The family and child will understandably be overwhelmed with questions and fears about the diagnosis. Prepare the family by emphasizing the importance of education, and encourage all family members to participate.

Choose a comfortable location which will have few interruptions. The learning objectives listed on the facing page can be used as a checklist for reviewing the family members' knowledge about the disease process and therapy.

Provide appropriate literature and materials for family members. Videotapes, booklets, and pamphlets should be developmentally appropriate. Educational materials for the parent should also be matched to the parent's literacy skills. Choose materials wisely; too much information may be less helpful than too little information.

Practice Sessions. Encourage all family members to get involved: let each person test his or her own blood glucose, as well as give a self-injection of sterile saline. Practicing these procedures will help allay family fears, as well as allow the child to supervise as a family member performs the procedure.

To develop problem-solving skills, present scenarios in which the child and/or parent must make management decisions. Include a situation in which hypoglycemia must be identified and responded to, a situation requiring a urine ketone test, and an example of missing an insulin dose. Help the family to decide what responses to make with insulin, diet, or exercise.

Follow-up Care. Many questions will arise as a family leaves the hospital or clinic and begins to live with diabetes. A contact person should be available for ongoing discussion, education, and motivation. Education of the child and family is an ongoing process.

When other parts of the treatment regimen have become familiar, the injections can be taught. Initially, self-injecting insulin will be scary for the school-age child. It is usually advisable to start with the parent inserting the needle and the child pushing the plunger. The child can then progress to performing self-injection.

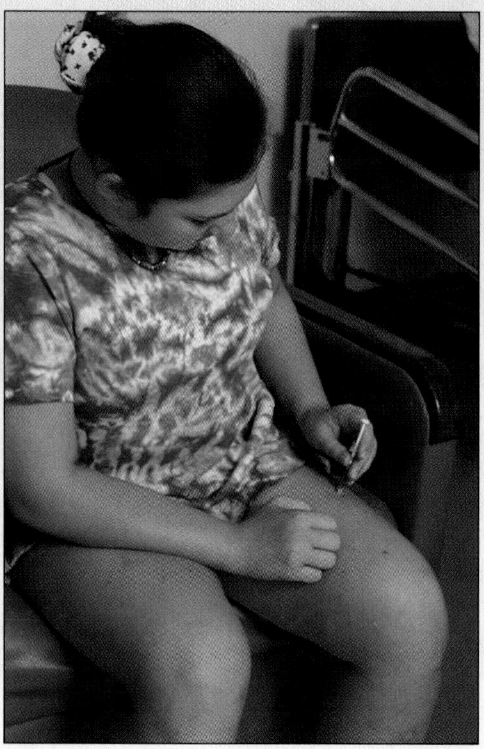

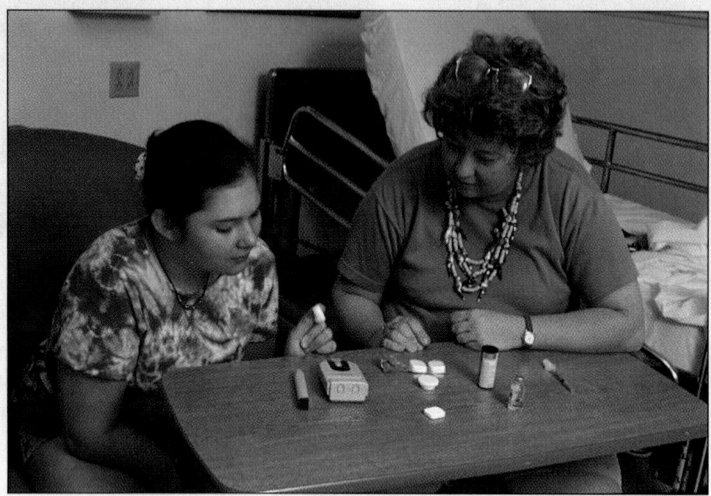

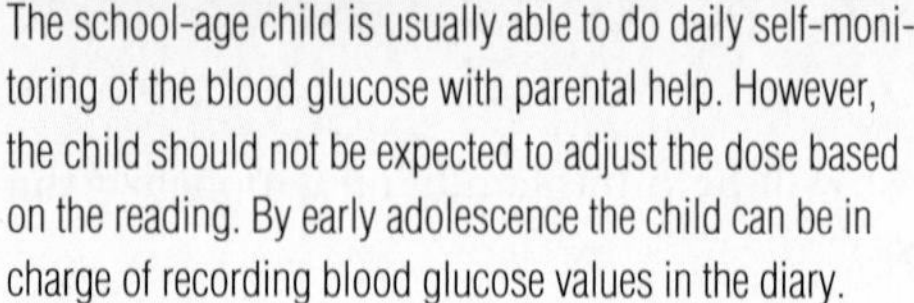

The school-age child is usually able to do daily self-monitoring of the blood glucose with parental help. However, the child should not be expected to adjust the dose based on the reading. By early adolescence the child can be in charge of recording blood glucose values in the diary.

LEARNING OBJECTIVES

A. *General Information*
The child and family will be able to:
1. Describe the action of insulin in the body.
2. Describe the characteristics of Type 1 vs Type 2 diabetes.
3. Identify three factors that can be used to control blood glucose levels.

B. *Medication Therapy*
The child and family will be able to:
1. Name the child's insulin and identify the onset, peak, and duration of action.
2. State the storage recommendations for insulin.
3. State the recommended expiration date of the insulin.
4. Demonstrate accurate syringe preparation for a single type of insulin.
5. Demonstrate syringe preparation using two types of insulin.
6. Demonstrate subcutaneous insulin injection technique.
7. Identify insulin injection sites and describe a pattern of rotation.
8. Identify a plan for safe syringe disposal.
9. Identify recommended insulin dosages and injection times.

C. *Home Glucose Monitoring*
The child and family will be able to:
1. Identify nondiabetic blood glucose levels and target goals for good glucose control.
2. Demonstrate the use, calibration, control testing, and cleaning of the blood glucose monitor.
3. Identify a plan for recording blood glucose values.

D. *Hypoglycemia*
The child and family will be able to:
1. Identify the signs and symptoms of a hypoglycemic reaction.
2. Describe appropriate treatment for both a mild and severe hypoglycemia reaction.
3. Identify three potential causes of a hypoglycemia reaction.
4. Identify the importance of medical emergency identification.
5. Describe typical blood glucose trends during the honeymoon phase.

E. *Hyperglycemia/Sick Day*
The child and family will be able to:
1. Identify the signs and symptoms of hyperglycemia.
2. Identify strategies to control hyperglycemia.
3. Describe the possible effects of stress or illness on diabetes control.
4. Demonstrate the procedure for urinary ketone testing.
5. State when to test for urinary ketones.
6. State basic treatment for urinary ketones.
7. Describe the signs and symptoms requiring physician/health care team contact.

F. *Exercise*
The child and family will be able to:
1. State the effect of exercise on blood glucose levels.
2. State the benefits of and precautions for exercise.
3. Identify the relationship of diet, exercise, and insulin on blood glucose control.
4. Generate a home schedule that identifies mealtimes, blood test times, and insulin injection times.

G. *Complications*
The child and family will be able to:
1. Identify the role of glucose control in the prevention or delay of diabetes-related complications.
2. Identify appropriate health care follow-up for the child with diabetes.

H. *Psychological Adjustment/Family Involvement*
The child and family will be able to:
1. Create a plan for the entire family to participate in diabetes care and management.

I. *Community Resources*
The child and family will be able to:
1. Identify available community resources for ongoing diabetes education and support.

Therapeutic Communication With the Child Who Has IDDM

EXAMPLE 1: CHRISTINA

Christina is 10 years old and newly diagnosed with diabetes. The conversation covers a discussion of what causes her diabetes (and what did not cause her diabetes), as well as offering an everyday analogy to help Christina understand a chronic disease.

Nurse: Christina, I've been talking with you and your mother about your diabetes. Do you have any questions for me?

Christina: No. Yes, Grandma told me that I ate too much candy, and that gave me diabetes.

Nurse: That is incorrect. Let me tell you why. The nickname for blood glucose is blood sugar. Many people think that eating too much sugar or candy will result in diabetes, or high blood sugar. Blood sugar is *not* the same thing as the white sugar that you put on cereal. You have diabetes because your body is not able to make insulin. What is the name of the medicine that you and your mother have learned to give you?

Christina: Insulin.

Nurse: That's right. We help your body by giving you insulin. Your body needs *help* to work correctly. Just like my eyes. My eyesight is poor, so I wear glasses *to help me see better*. My eyes are not sick, they just need some help. Your body needs help, too. That's why your doctor has asked you and your mom to learn about insulin.

EXAMPLE 2: AARON

Aaron is 13 with diabetes. Because he is beginning to spend more time with friends and less time with his parents, Aaron's nurse wants to emphasize the need to tell his friends about diabetes, especially hypoglycemia. He uses role play to involve Aaron in learning.

Nurse: Aaron, I want you to think about how you will explain low blood sugars to your friends. Since low blood sugars are an emergency, I want your friends to know how to help you. Let's pretend that I am your best friend, Bob. You are over at my house, and I am asking you some questions. Now remember, I'm Bob, and I don't know anything about diabetes. (Speaking as Bob): Aaron, I heard that you have diabetes, but sometimes you have low blood sugars. That's strange because I thought your problem was high blood sugar. Why do you have low blood sugars?

Aaron: I could have a low blood sugar if I don't eat enough food, or if I exercise a lot, or if I take too much insulin.

Nurse (as Bob): What happens when you have a low blood sugar? Do you feel any different?

Aaron: Well, I might get shaky, and dizzy. Or get a headache. Or get sweaty.

Nurse (as Bob): What do you do about a low blood sugar? Lay down?

Aaron: Well, I need to test my blood to see if it is low. If it's low, I should eat something.

Nurse (as Bob): Like what?

Aaron: A half a glass of juice, or 6 Life Savers, or a half of a can of soda.

Nurse (as Bob): Oh, I could help by getting you a diet soda. Since you are diabetic, I know you can't have regular sodas. Is that right?

Aaron: No, I need a regular soda.

Nurse (as Bob): But you have diabetes!

Aaron: But when I'm low, I can have regular soda because it *has* sugar.

Nurse (as himself): Good job, you explained that well!

NURSING DIAGNOSIS • Risk for Injury related to hypoglycemia or hyperglycemia

Expected Outcome: • Family members will demonstrate knowledge of the signs, symptoms, and treatment of hypoglycemia and hyperglycemia, as evidenced by initiating appropriate treatment for hypoglycemia and hyperglycemia.

Intervention	Rationale
Hypoglycemia: Blood Glucose below 70 mg/dl	
1. Teach the child and family to recognize the signs and symptoms of hypoglycemia (refer to Table 39–2). School personnel should also be involved in teaching.	Signs and symptoms of hypoglycemia should prompt the child or parent to test the blood glucose level. Some children do not display adrenergic signs of hypoglycemia.

Intervention	Rationale
The school nurse, if available, can play a key role in the care of a child with diabetes.	**Neuroglycopenic** signs may be the only clues to hypoglycemia in these children. These signs are very hard for the *child* to recognize, but can be observed by a parent or teacher. Blood glucose goals for this child may need to be modified to prevent hypoglycemia unawareness.
2. Treat hypoglycemia promptly with 15 grams of easily digested carbohydrate. If symptoms are not relieved (or blood glucose level is not above 80 mg/dl) in 15 minutes, repeat the treatment. If the hypoglycemia occurs during the night, treat with 30 grams carbohydrate: 15 grams simple carbohydrate, and 15 grams complex carbohydrate with protein. Examples of 15 grams of carbohydrate include 4 ounces of fruit juice, 6 ounces of regular cola, 6 Life Savers, or a commercial glucose product.	Prompt treatment reduces the possibility of a severe reaction. Candy bars, donuts, and cookies are poor treatment choices due to the high fat content, which can delay carbohydrate digestion. The child could also interpret these treats as a reward for hypoglycemia.
3. Help the child and family identify strategies to prevent hypoglycemia based on common causes of hypoglycemia: missed or delayed meal, too much insulin, or unusual amount of exercise without increasing carbohydrate intake. Help the family identify a plan to teach hypoglycemia signs, symptoms, and necessary treatment to school personnel and daycare workers. Help the child prepare to explain hypoglycemia to his friends (see Therapeutic Communication box, Example 2). Compile a diabetes box for school and daycare. The box should contain carbohydrates for treating hypoglycemia as well as written information. Instruct the child to wear a medical emergency identification emblem at all times.	Many episodes of hypoglycemia can be avoided by careful planning and anticipating potential situations that could result in hypoglycemia. Instruction on the signs, symptoms, and treatment of hypoglycemia is essential information to be shared with individuals caring for the child. Hypoglycemia is a potential emergency. Prompt treatment includes recognition of symptoms, testing of blood glucose, and treatment with 15 grams of carbohydrate. If hypoglycemia occurs during the night, increase the carbohydrate to 30 grams.
4. Teach the parents how to treat severe hypoglycemia. For the unconscious child or the child having a seizure a small amount of glucose gel (cake frosting or honey will also work) can be rubbed on the inner cheek and gums. Avoid placing a large amount of gel in the mouth because the child could choke. **Glucagon** (available by prescription as Glucagon Emergency Kit from Eli Lilly Co.) can be injected subcutaneously or intramuscularly. Inject 1 mg for the child weighing greater than 50 lb or 0.5 mg for the child weighing less than 50 lb. The onset of action is 10 to 15 minutes. Position the unconscious child on her side. Once conscious, the child will need a large snack to replace lost glycogen stores.	The unconscious child or the child having a seizure requires prompt treatment. Severe hypoglycemia has been associated with developmental delay and should be avoided (Daneman et al., 1989). Glucagon is a pancreatic hormone that opposes the action of insulin and promotes the conversion of liver glycogen to blood glucose. The child is positioned on her side to prevent aspiration. Both severe hypoglycemia and glucagon administration can result in nausea with vomiting.
Hyperglycemia: Blood Glucose Levels Higher Than Target Range	
1. Teach family to recognize potential causes of hyperglycemia: inadequate amount of insulin, increased dietary intake, decreased amount of exercise, and stress response (either emotional or physical stress such as illness).	Anticipating situations that might result in hyperglycemia can help the family plan for such events. The signs and symptoms of hypoglycemia and hyperglycemia may be difficult to distinguish from one another for both the child and the parent. Test blood glucose before treating to verify glucose level. If testing is impossible, treat for hypoglycemia.

Intervention	Rationale
2. Instruct family on sick day diabetes management, including when and how to test for urinary ketones. (See box Sick Day Rules for the Child with IDDM.) Identify a home treatment plan for ketones, and identify precautions for vomiting.	Testing for ketones when ill and/or when blood glucose is 250 mg/dl or higher will aid in detecting insulin deficit. Ketones are treated with (calorie-free) fluids, and additional regular insulin per physician order. Nausea with vomiting will lead to dehydration, and cannot be treated with oral fluids. Physician contact is essential if the child is vomiting.
3. Identify strategies to prevent or treat hyperglycemia.	Consistency in diet, exercise, and insulin injection times will aid in preventing hyperglycemia. Persistent hyperglycemia may indicate a need for an insulin dosage adjustment. The growing child will need periodic increases in baseline insulin dosages.

Evalution: The child and family are able to correctly recognize and promptly treat hypoglycemia and hyperglycemia.

Sick Day Rules for the Child With IDDM

1. Always give the insulin injection, even if the child does not have an appetite. If you feel that the child will become hypoglycemic with the usual dose, contact the physician or nurse educator for specific instructions. If ordered, use sliding scale regular insulin for hyperglycemia, every 3 to 4 hours.
2. Test blood glucose level at least every 4 hours, more often for persistent hypoglycemia or hyperglycemia.
3. Test for urinary ketones with each voiding. Notify the physician or nurse educator if moderate or large amounts of urinary ketones are present. Additional regular insulin may be ordered.
4. Encourage calorie-free liquids. If ketones are present, liquids are essential to aid in clearing.
5. Follow the child's usual meal plan. If the child has a poor appetite, a sick day diet consisting of simple carbohydrates can be substituted. Try to replace the usual grams of carbohydrate with simple carbohydrate foods.
6. Encourage rest—especially if urinary ketones are present. Exercising while ketones are present will result in increased ketone formation.
7. Notify the physician or nurse educator for:
   - nausea and vomiting
   - fruity odor to the breath
   - deep, rapid respirations
   - decreasing level of consciousness
   - moderate or high urinary ketones
   - persistent hyperglycemia

DIABETIC KETOACIDOSIS (DKA)

Diabetic ketoacidosis (DKA) is the metabolic consequence of a severe insulin deficit. Refer to Table 39–2 for the sequence of events leading to acidosis, as well as the signs and symptoms that accompany the diagnosis.

Etiology. DKA results from an absolute or relative insulin lack. In the younger diabetic child, the most common cause is insulin resistance, such as a stress response initiated by an infection. In the adolescent, the most common cause is missed insulin injection(s).

Clinical Manifestations

- Abdominal pain
- Chest pain
- Nausea/vomiting
- Fruity (ketone) odor to the breath
- Kussmaul's respirations
- Decreasing level of consciousness
- Increased urination, followed by decreased urine output
- Dehydration, as evidenced by weight loss, dry mucous membranes, poor skin turgor, and decreased urine output

Diagnostic Evaluation. Diabetic ketoacidosis is confirmed by the following test results:

Blood glucose: Elevated
Arterial or venous pH: Low
Urinary ketones: Large
Serum ketones (beta-hydroxybutyric acid): Elevated
Serum potassium: Elevated, normal, or low
Serum phosphorus: Low
White blood cell count: Elevated, especially with infection
Serum CO_2: Low

NURSING CARE OF THE CHILD IN DIABETIC KETOACIDOSIS

Assessment

Assessment of the child in DKA includes assessing the following:

- level of consciousness
- hydration status
- respiratory status
- weight

Assessment of the child with a known history of IDDM should include:

- most recent blood glucose values
- history of urinary ketones, and the steps taken to manage ketones at home
- usual insulin dosages, and the time and amount of the most recent injection
- time of last meal and amount of food eaten
- identification of the family member usually given the responsibility for injections and blood tests
- the family's understanding of the daily management of diabetes
- usual sick day management plan

Nursing Diagnosis

- Fluid Volume Deficit related to abnormal fluid losses through diuresis and emesis
- Risk for Injury related to alteration in acid-base balance from lack of insulin, leading to ketoacid production
- Risk for Injury related to electrolyte imbalance from emesis and acidosis
- Risk for Injury related to cerebral edema due to resolving DKA
- Knowledge Deficit related to diabetes home management during sick days

Planning, Implementation, and Evaluation: The Child in DKA

NURSING DIAGNOSIS • Fluid Volume Deficit related to abnormal fluid losses through diuresis and emesis

Expected Outcome: • The child will be safely rehydrated, as evidenced by normal for age, weight, skin turgor, mucous membranes and urine output.

Intervention	Rationale
1. Assess the child for hydration status, evaluating weight, skin turgor, mucous membranes, and urine output.	Identify baseline hydration status. A comparison of the child's usual weight with the admission weight provides an estimation of percent of total body fluid loss.
2. Encourage calorie-free fluids if the child is not nauseated. Initiate intravenous (IV) fluids as ordered. Normal saline is the initial fluid used, followed by half normal saline.	Rehydration is the initial step in resolving DKA. If acidosis has resulted in nausea and vomiting, IV fluids are required. Fluid losses occur primarily from the osmotic diuresis occurring with hyperglycemia. Emesis can also contribute to fluid loss. Normal saline is the initial IV rehydration fluid. Although normally a hypertonic solution in comparison to blood, it is isotonic in states of dehydration.
3. Maintain strict intake and output monitoring.	Accurate intake and output records are essential in calculating rehydration status.
4. Observe for edema and/or pulmonary congestion during rehydration.	Overhydration may be manifested by these signs.
5. Weigh on arrival and frequently during rehydration (every 8 hours may be appropriate).	A comparison of the admission weight to the child's usual weight provides an indication of hydration status. Follow-up weights will provide ongoing assessment.

Evaluation: Child is safely rehydrated as ketosis is resolved, as evidenced by normal for age weight, urine output, skin turgor, and mucous membranes.

NURSING DIAGNOSIS

- Risk for Injury related to alteration in acid-base balance from lack of insulin, leading to ketone production and acidosis

Expected Outcome:

- The child will experience a resolution of ketosis and acidosis, as evidenced by laboratory results and clinical assessment.

Intervention	Rationale
1. Test all urine samples for the presence of ketones. Assess the child's breath for acetone. Observe respirations to identify Kussmaul's respirations.	The presence of urinary ketones indicates possible acidosis. Serum ketone analysis, or beta-hydroxybutyric acid, is a direct measurement of ketone activity. The liver produces three ketoacids: betahydroxybutyric acid, acetoacetate, and acetone. Acetone, the weakest of the acids, is expelled via the lungs and can be assessed as a fruity smell to the child's breath. High acid levels trigger a rapid and deep respiration (Kussmaul's respiration) in an effort to remove excessive acetone.
2. Encourage calorie-free fluids, if the child is able to drink. If ordered, begin IV fluids.	Fluids are essential in flushing ketones as well as in maintaining hydration. In severe dehydration, the osmotic pull of the blood glucose helps to hold fluid in the bloodstream, thus preventing circulatory shock. Insulin is not given until rehydration has begun to avoid circulatory shock.
3. Initiate insulin therapy as ordered.	Insulin therapy is initiated *after* rehydration has begun. A continuous IV infusion of *regular* insulin is titrated to keep blood glucose in a safe range while avoiding hypoglycemia. Insulin therapy inhibits the production of ketones. Subcutaneous insulin is not an appropriate therapy for the dehydrated child. With dehydration, peripheral vessels constrict, resulting in poor absorption and distribution of the insulin. Insulin adheres to the plastic of the IV bag and tubing, and it is not known whether this affects therapy. Some clinicians recommend priming the IV tubing with the insulin solution and flushing with a fresh solution before patient delivery. This technique saturates the binding sites of the plastic and provides nonfluctuating insulin delivery.
4. Monitor blood glucose frequently.	IV insulin has a rapid onset. A continuous infusion of insulin could quickly result in hypoglycemia.
5. Provide glucose-containing IV fluids as ordered.	Insulin is needed to inhibit ketone formation. Even though blood glucose values may be in an acceptable range, the insulin infusion must continue until the serum ketones are cleared. To prevent hypoglycemia, glucose is added to the saline hydration solutions.

Evaluation: Within 24 hours of admission, the child displays no evidence of ketosis, as evidenced by negative serum or urinary ketones.

NURSING DIAGNOSIS • Risk for Injury related to electrolyte imbalance from emesis and acidosis

Expected Outcome: • The child will not experience adverse consequences of electrolyte abnormalities, as evidenced by normal serum potassium values.

Intervention	Rationale
1. Monitor potassium levels closely. Assess for signs and symptoms of hyperkalemia, including bradycardia, muscle weakness, hyperreflexia, and respiratory arrest. Also assess for signs and symptoms of hypokalemia, including muscle weakness, fatigue, hypotension, and hyporeflexia.	During acidosis, potassium moves out of the cell and into the intravascular spaces. Intravascular potassium is lost via diuresis. Initially, serum potassium levels may appear in an acceptable range, but this does not reflect the lost intracellular potassium. As rehydration and correction of acidosis begins, potassium will move back into the cells, resulting in lower serum levels. Serum potassium levels are obtained frequently (every 1–2 hours initially) during treatment of DKA to adequately assess potassium needs. See Chapter 24 for further discussion.
2. Utilize cardiac monitor to assess electrocardiogram resulting from altered potassium levels. Hypokalemia produces prolonged ST segment; notched, flat, or inverted T waves; and arrhythmias. Hyperkalemia produces flattened P wave, and/or peaked T wave and ventricular fibrillation.	Hypokalemia or hyperkalemia can result in a medical emergency, requiring rapid response.
3. Assess urine output before initiating potassium therapy. If anuric, notify the physician. Initiate potassium therapy as ordered.	Renal failure can result from severe dehydration. If anuric, potassium will not be lost via urinary excretion. Replacement therapy must be made cautiously.

Evaluation: The child experiences no signs or symptoms of electrolyte imbalance.

NURSING DIAGNOSIS • Risk for Injury related to cerebral edema due to resolving DKA

Expected Outcome: • The child will not experience adverse consequences of cerebral edema, as evidenced by appropriate level of consciousness.

Intervention	Rationale
1. Observe child frequently for signs of cerebral edema: complaints of headache, decreasing level of consciousness, or unequal, fixed, or dilated pupils. Notify physician of any changes from the baseline assessment.	Cerebral edema is a complication of resolving DKA and can result in brain damage or death. The causes are unclear, but may be related to overhydration; rapid fluid shifts, particularly into the cerebral intracellular space; and electrolyte imbalance. Frequent neurologic checks will aid in prompt recognition and prevention of neurologic deficits.
2. Monitor blood glucose values frequently (hourly) when IV insulin is being infused.	Blood glucose values should not drop more than 50–100 mg/dl/hr to aid in preventing rapid osmotic shifts. As the serum glucose approaches the mid-200s, glucose will be added to the IV fluids. Blood glucose levels are maintained in the mid-200s for the duration of the IV insulin therapy.

Evaluation: The child experiences no adverse consequences of cerebral edema, as evidenced by appropriate neurologic evaluation.

NURSING DIAGNOSIS • Knowledge Deficit related to home management during sick days

Expected Outcome: • The family will promptly recognize and respond to situations requiring sick day management.

Intervention	Rationale
1. Teach the family how and when to test for urinary ketones: a. Test for urinary ketones when the blood glucose is over 250 mg/dl. b. Test for urinary ketones when the child is ill.	Ketones are formed in response to an insulin deficit. Either high glucose values or an illness could be associated with an insulin deficit.
2. Instruct family on sick day management. (See Sick Day Rules box.)	Stress, either from an infection or the environment, can result in hyperglycemia and uncontrolled diabetes. Early recognition and treatment of ketones can prevent acute complications.
3. Identify situations requiring the family to contact the diabetes health care team, including nausea with vomiting, high levels of urinary ketones, procedures requiring NPO status, and signs of acidosis.	Early intervention is essential in preventing acidosis and its sequelae. Outpatient management of ketones can be initiated by the family with direction from the diabetes team.
4. Provide the patient and family with phone numbers of appropriate health care professionals for questions on sick day management.	The child and family should know who to call and how to reach the appropriate health care professional for guidance during sick days. The pediatrician/primary health care provider should respond to usual childhood complaints, and issues related to diabetes control should be addressed by the diabetes team.
5. Frequent bouts of DKA require evaluation of home care knowledge, compliance with recommended regimen, home supervision, and coping skills.	Frequent episodes of DKA may reflect poor compliance, poor understanding of home care needs, inappropriate or absent parental supervision, and/or depression. A team approach (including nurse educator, nutritionist, social worker, psychologist, physician) can address many of these issues.

Evaluation: The child and family promptly recognize and respond appropriately to situations requiring sick day management, as evidenced by no occurrences of DKA.

LONG-TERM HEALTH CARE NEEDS OF THE CHILD WITH IDDM

Serious complications are associated with long-term diabetes: retinopathy, nephropathy, neuropathy, and cardiovascular disease. Studies have demonstrated that intensive control of diabetes may decrease the onset or severity of complications by 35% to 70% (DCCT Research Group, 1993). Intensive control is defined as three or more insulin injections per day, as well as frequent blood glucose monitoring. Intensive control of diabetes is most effectively provided by a multidisciplinary team, including the dietitian, nurse educator, endocrinologist, social worker, and psychologist. Regular visits with the team aid in addressing issues that affect diabetes control: growth, anticipatory guidance, motivation, new products, and relevant research updates. Telephone contact with the nurse educator provides an essential link to the health care team between regular visits. Specific issues such as ketone management, sick days, birthday parties, or schedule changes can be addressed and managed by telephone contact.

Routine health care for the child with diabetes should include yearly dental and ophthalmologic evaluations, as well as prophylactic interventions such as influenza vaccinations. Other referral sources should be utilized as specific needs are identified.

FUTURE THERAPIES

Diabetes research may one day make current therapies obsolete. Current research is aimed at both preventing diabetes (as mentioned in the Epidemiology section) and finding a cure after diagnosis. Transplantation of islet cells is a significant area of research that might one day offer such a cure. Several issues must be addressed before this therapy is a possibility: what is the best site for transplantation, from what source will the islet cells be obtained, and how can the transplanted islet cells avoid destruction by the immune response? As these issues are resolved, transplantation may become the first-line treatment for IDDM.

KEY CONCEPTS

- In the absence of insulin, the metabolism of fats, proteins, and carbohydrates is impaired and glucose is unable to move into the intracellular space, resulting in hyperglycemia.
- Both IDDM and NIDDM involve abnormal carbohydrate metabolism, but risk related to age of onset, body size, gender, and ethnic background, and treatment are different for the two types of diabetes.
- The goals of diabetes management are to maintain appropriate height and weight, maintain age-appropriate lifestyle, maintain near-normal glycosylated hemoglobin, and prevent acute complications of hypoglycemia and hyperglycemia.
- Common nursing diagnoses associated with IDDM include Knowledge Deficit, Alteration in Family Process, Alteration in Nutrition, and Potential for Injury related to Hypoglycemia and Hyperglycemia.
- Teaching needs associated with home management of IDDM are related to the disease process, medication, home glucose monitoring, hypoglycemia, hyperglycemia, exercise, complications, and support services.
- There are adrenergic and neuroglycopenic clinical manifestations of hypoglycemia. Hypoglycemia should be treated with 15 grams of easily digested carbohydrate.
- Hyperglycemia is caused by an inadequate amount of insulin, increased dietary intake, decreased amount of exercise, and a response to emotional or physical stress. Persistent hyperglycemia may indicate a need for an insulin dosage adjustment.
- Nursing diagnoses related to care of the child in DKA include Fluid Volume Deficit, Risk for Injury related to Alteration in Acid-Base Balance, Risk for Injury related to Electrolyte Imbalance, Risk for Injury related to Cerebral Edema, and Knowledge Deficit.

REFERENCES

Albisser, A. M., & Sperlich, M. (1993). Adjusting insulins. *Diabetes Educator, 18*(3), 211–227.

Amiel, S. A., Sherwin, R. S., Simonson, D. C., Lauriano, A. A., & Tamborlane, W. V. (1986). Impaired action in puberty: A contributing factor to poor glycemic control in adolescents with diabetes. *New England Journal of Medicine, 315*(4), 215–219.

Daneman, D., Frank, M., Perlman, K., Tamm, J., & Ehrlich, R. (1989). Severe hypoglycemia in children with insulin dependent diabetes: Frequency and predisposing factors. *Journal of Pediatrics, 115*(11), 681–685.

DCCT Research Group (1993). The effect of intensive treatment of diabetes on the development and progression of long-term complications in insulin-dependent diabetes mellitus. *New England Journal of Medicine, 329*(14), 977–986.

Exchange lists for meal planning. (1995). The American Diabetes Association, Inc., Alexandria, VA, and the American Dietetic Association, Chicago, IL.

Follansbee, D. S. (1989). Assuming responsibility for diabetes management: What age? What price? *Diabetes Educator, 15*(4), 347–351.

Galloway, J. A., Spradlin, C. T., Nelson, R. L., Wentworth, S. M., Davidson, J. A., & Swarner, J. L. (1981). Factors influencing the absorption, serum insulin concentration, and blood glucose responses after injections of regular insulin and various insulin mixtures. *Diabetes Care, 4*(3), 366–376.

McKelvey, J., Waller, D., Schreiner, B., North, A. J., Marks, J. F., Murphy, J. N., & Travis, L. B. (1993). Reliability and validity of the diabetes family behavior scale. *Diabetes Educator, 19*(2), 125–132.

Poteet, G., Reinert, B., & Ptak, H. (1987). Outcome of multiple usage of disposable syringes in the insulin-requiring diabetic. *Nursing Research, 36*(6), 350–352.

Wetterhaul, S. F., Olson, D. R., DeStefano, F., Stevenson, J. M., Ford, E. S., German, R. R., Will, F. C., Newman, J. M., Sepe, S. J., & Vinicor, F. (1992). Trends in diabetes and diabetes complications 1980–1987. *Diabetes Care, 15*(8), 960–967.

BIBLIOGRAPHY

Armentrout, D. (1995). Neonatal diabetes mellitus. *Journal of Pediatric Health Care, 9*, 75–78.

Balik, B., Haig, B., & Moynihan, P. M. (1986). Diabetes and the school age child. *American Journal of Maternal Child Nursing, 11*(5), 324–330.

Denne, J. R., Andrews, K. L., Lees, D. V., & Mook, W. (1992). A survey of patient preference for insulin jet injectors versus needle and syringe. *Diabetes Educator, 18*(3), 223–227.

Hodges, L. C., & Parker, J. (1987). Concerns of parents with diabetic children. *Pediatric Nursing, 13*(1), 22–24, 68.

Holler, H. J. (1991). Understanding the use of the exchange lists for meal planning in diabetes management. *Diabetes Educator, 17*(6), 474–484.

Holtzmeister, L. A. (1992). Nutrition update: Baby food exchanges and meal planning for the infant with diabetes. *Diabetes Educator, 18*(5), 375–385.

Howey, D. C., Bowsher, R. R., Brunelle, R. L., & Woodworth, J. R. (1994). [Lys (B28) Pro (B29)] human insulin: A rapidly absorbed analogue of human insulin. *Diabetes, 43*, 395–402.

Jacobson, A. M., Hausser, S. T., Lavori, P., Willett, J. B., Cole, C. F., Wolfsdorf, J. I., Dumont, R. H., & Wertlieb, D. (1994). Family environment and glycemic control: A four-year prospective study of children and adolescents with insulin-dependent diabetes mellitus. *Psychosomatic Medicine, 56*, 401–409.

Jarrett, L., Hilliam, K., Bartsch, C., & Lindsay, R. (1993). The effectiveness of parents teaching elementary school teachers about diabetes mellitus. *Diabetes Educator, 19*(3), 193–197.

Jawadi, M. H., & Ho, L. S. (1986). Stability and reproducability of the biological activity of premixed short-acting and intermediate-acting insulins. *American Journal of Medicine, 81*(3), 467–471.

Kushion, W., Salisbury, P. J., Seitz, K. W., & Wilson, B. E. (1991). Issues in the care of infants and toddlers with insulin-dependent diabetes mellitus. *Diabetes Educator, 17*(2), 107–110.

LaGreca, A. M., Swales, T., Klemps, S., Madigan, S., & Skyler, J. (1995). Adolescents with diabetes: Gender differences in psychosocial functioning and glycemic control. *Child Health Care, 24*, 61–78.

Lipman, T. H., DiFazio, D. A., Meers, R. A., & Thompson, R. L. (1989a). A developmental approach to diabetes in children: Birth through preschool, part 1. *American Journal of Maternal Child Nursing, 14*(4), 255–259.

Lipman, T. H., DiFazio, D. A., Meers, R. A., & Thompson, R. L. (1989b). A developmental approach to diabetes in children: School age—adolescents, part 2. *American Journal of Maternal Child Nursing, 14*(5), 330–332.

Martin, R., Kupsis, B., Novak, P., & Kushion, W. (1994). The infant with diabetes mellitus: A case study. *Pediatric Nursing, 20*(1), 27–32.

Nuttall, S. Q. (1993). Carbohydrate and dietary management of individuals with insulin-requiring diabetes. *Diabetes Care, 16*, 1039–1042.

Pansey, P. W. (1987). Hyperglycemia at dawn. *American Journal of Nursing, 87*, 1424–1426.

Peters, A. L., & Davidson, M. B. (1987). Effect of storage on action of NPH and regular insulin mixtures. *Diabetes Care, 10*(6), 799–800.

Puczynski, S., Puczynski, M. S., & Ryan, C. M. (1992). Hypoglycemia in children with insulin-dependent diabetes mellitus. *Diabetes Educator, 18*(2), 151–153.

Rodine, G., Craven, J., & Daneman, D. (1989). Eating disorders and insulin manipulation in adolescent females with insulin dependent diabetes. *Psychosomatic Medicine, 51*, 244–266.

Rodriguez, J. R., Gefkan, G. R., Clark, J. E., Hunt, F., & Fishel, P. (1994). Parenting satisfaction and efficacy among caregivers of children with diabetes. *Child Health Care, 23*, 181–191.

Rossini, A. A., Mordes, J. P., & Handlewr, E. S. (1991). A tumbler hypothesis: The autoimmunity of insulin dependent diabetes. *Diabetes Spectrum, 2*(3), 195–201.

Rubovits, D. S., & Siegel, A. W. (1994). Developing conception of chronic disease: A comparison of disease experience. *Child Health Care, 23*, 267–285.

Savinetti-Rose, B. (1994). Developmental issues in managing children with diabetes. *Pediatric Nursing, 20*(1), 11–15.

Sperling, M. A. (1894). Diabetic ketoacidosis. *Pediatric Clinics of North America, 31*(3), 591–610.

Strowig, S., & Raskin, P. (1992). Glycemic control and diabetic complications. *Diabetes Care, 15*(9), 1126–1131.

Tomky, D. (1995). Advances in monitoring. *RN, 58*(3), 38–45.

Travis, L. B., Brouhard, B. H., & Schriener, B. (1987). *Diabetes mellitus in children*. Philadelphia: W. B. Saunders.

Van-Ginkle, J. (1992). Diet education for children with IDDM. *Diabetes Educator, 18*(3), 201–204.

Weissburg-Benchell, J., Glascgow, A. M., Tynan, W. D., Wirtz, P., Turek, J., & Ward, J. (1995). Adolescent diabetes management and mismanagement. *Diabetes Care, 18*, 177–182.

Wise, J. E., Kolb, E. L., & Saunder, S. E. (1992). Effect of glycemic control on growth velocity in children with IDDM. *Diabetes Care, 15*(7), 826–830.

Wysocki, T., Meinhold, P. A., Abrams, K. C., Barnard, M. U., Clarke, W. L., Bellando, B. J., & Bourgeois, M. J. (1992). Parental and professional estimates of self-care independence of children and adolescents with IDDM. *Diabetes Care, 15*(1), 43–52.

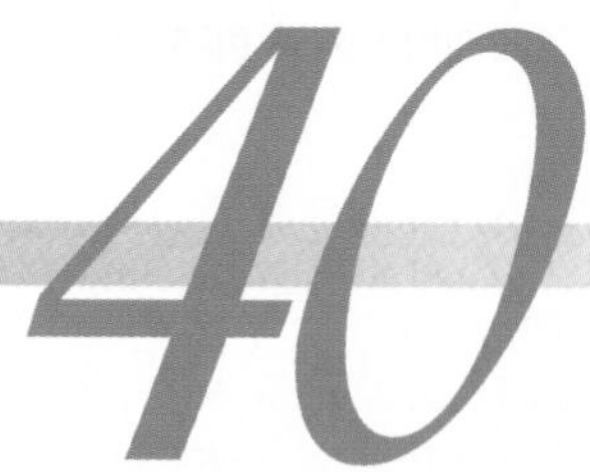

40

The Child With Neurologic Alterations

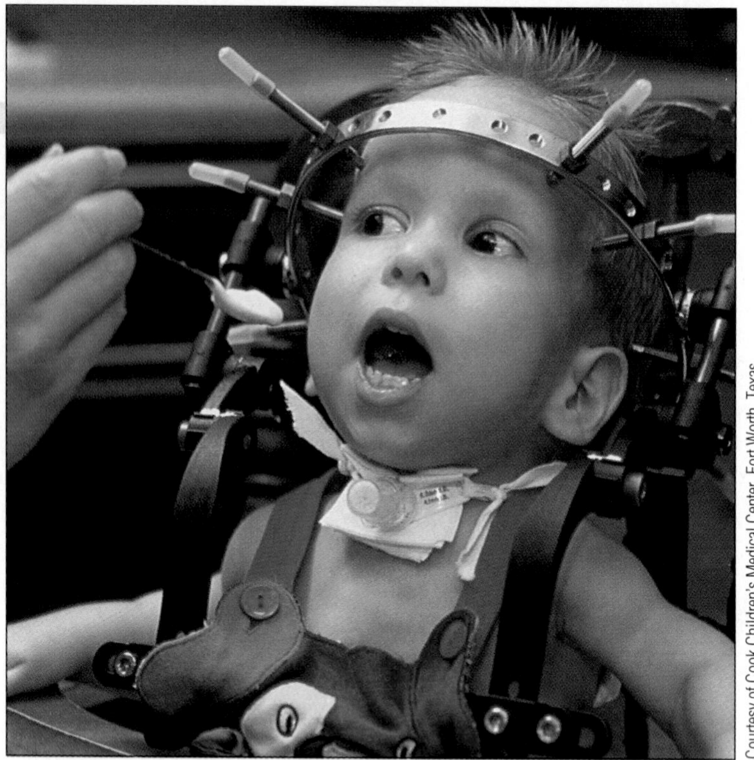

Courtesy of Cook Children's Medical Center, Fort Worth, Texas

CHAPTER OVERVIEW

LEARNING OBJECTIVES

After studying this chapter, you should be able to:

- Describe the embryologic development of the nervous system.
- Describe the anatomy and physiology of the nervous system.
- Describe the normal compensatory mechanisms that keep intracranial pressure within a constant range.
- Identify the neurologic differences among the infant, child, and adult.
- Be able to perform and document a neurologic assessment of a child.
- Describe the steps and procedures in a neurologic assessment.
- Discuss the nursing implications of common medications used in the management of neurologic disorders.
- List the measures used to prevent or treat cerebral edema.
- Differentiate between abnormal flexion and extension, and discuss the significance of each.
- List the compensatory mechanisms that affect intracranial blood flow and extravascular fluid volume if hydrocephalus develops.
- Describe teaching strategies that can be used with the child experiencing neurologic problems and with the child's family.

KEY TERMS

autoregulation: the unique ability of the cerebral arteries to change their diameter in response to alterations in cerebral perfusion pressure, to maintain a steady blood flow during changes in blood pressure and perfusion

basal ganglia: serves as a major communication and sorting area for messages to and from the cerebral hemispheres; composed of masses of gray matter; controls movement, and participates in emotion and cognition

blood–brain barrier: separates brain tissue and blood; very selective and normally permeable only to glucose, water, carbon dioxide, and some chemicals and drugs

brain stem: connected to the cerebral hemispheres by thick bunches of nerve fibers; all nerve fibers traverse through the brain stem from the hemispheres to the cerebellum and spinal cord

cerebral cortex: gray matter of the cerebrum, where the higher functions of thinking occur

cerebral herniation: shift of brain tissue sideways under the falx cerebri or downward, causing severe neurologic dysfunction

cerebral perfusion pressure (CPP): difference between mean arterial blood pressure and intracranial pressure

Cushing's response: late sign of increased intracranial pressure; includes increased blood pressure, widened pulse pressure, decreased heart rate, and decreased or irregular respiratory rate

decerebrate posture: abnormal extension of the upper extremities with internal rotation of the upper arms and wrists; lower extremities will extend with some internal rotation

decorticate posture: abnormal flexion of the upper extremities and extension of the lower extremities

extrapyramidal tract: descending pathway of the motor neurons concerned with involuntary or unconscious skeletal muscle coordination and reflex control of coordination

glia cells: make up support tissue that nourishes and protects the neurons

Monroe-Kellie doctrine: theory describing the compensatory mechanism of the cranial contents that maintains a steady volume and pressure

myelinization: formation of the proteolipid coating of the nerves that facilitates conduction of impulses

pyramidal tract: descending pathway of the upper motor neuron concerned with voluntary movement

Care of the child with neurologic problems requires knowledge of neuroanatomy, neurophysiology, and normal growth and development. The nurse plays an important role in the early recognition of pediatric neurologic problems, some of which may have the potential for devastating long-term outcomes. The nurse assesses the child's condition by comparing the normal behavior of that child to the current behavior. The family is an invaluable source of information about their child's normal behavior and how the current behavior deviates from that norm. The child and the family are in need of support and understanding because the child's illness represents a crisis in the lives of all the family members. Nursing support of the family is important because the family's ability to respond and influence the child's coping mechanisms directly influence the recovery and adaptation process.

CLINICAL REFERENCE PAGES

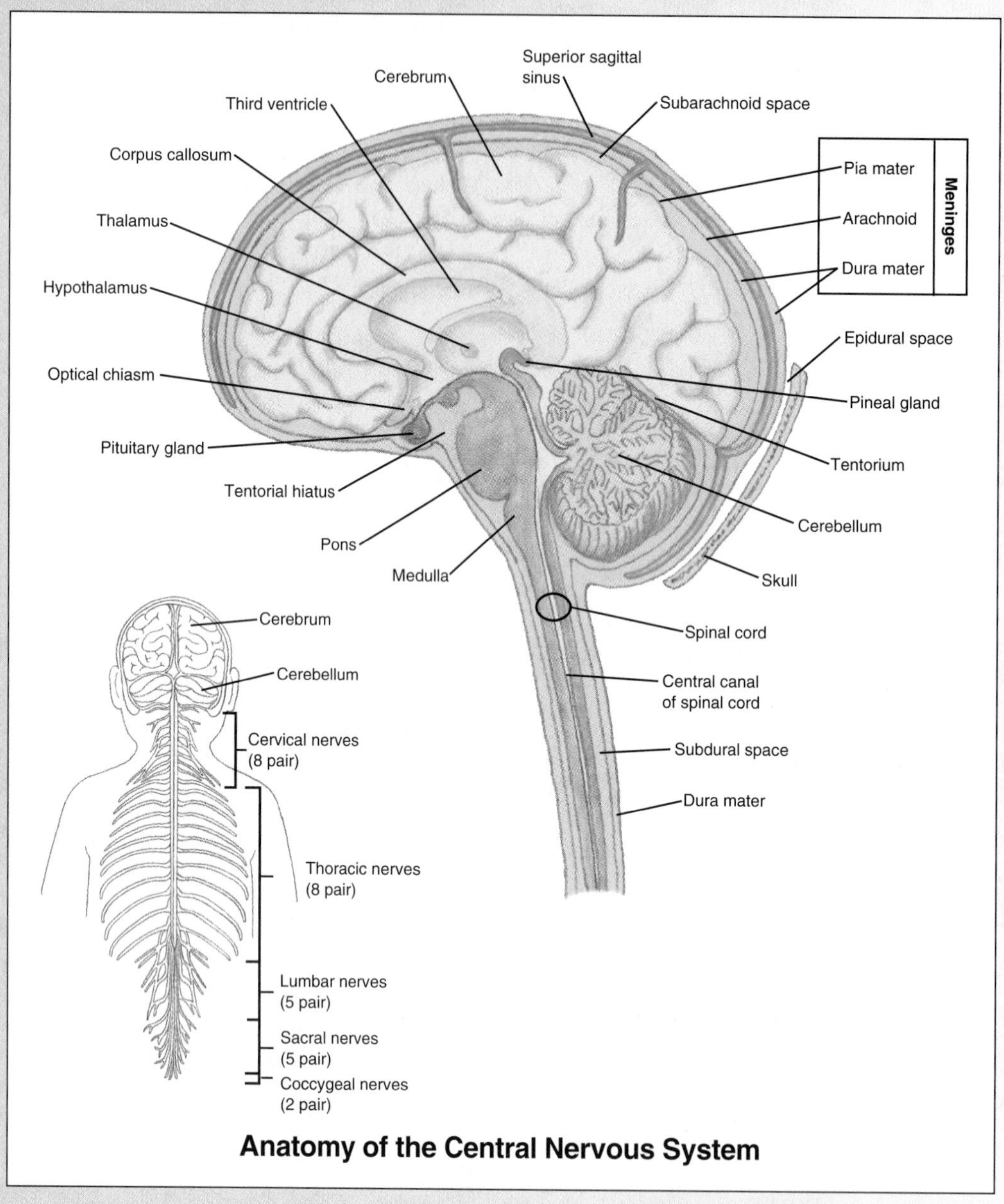

Anatomy of the Central Nervous System

Pediatric Differences in the Central Nervous System

- The brain of a term infant is two-thirds the weight of an adult's brain. By age 1 it weighs 80% as much as an adult's brain, and by age 6, approximately 90% as much as an adult's brain.
- An infant has about 50 ml of cerebrospinal fluid, as compared with 150 ml in an adult.
- The peripheral nerves are not completely myelinated by birth. As myelinization progresses, so does the child's coordination and fine muscle movements.
- The head circumference in a term infant is 34 to 35 cm. By age 6 months the head circumference is 44 cm, and by age 1, 47 cm.
- Papilledema rarely occurs in infancy because of the open fontanels and sutures that can expand with increased intracranial pressure. (See Fig. 11–5.)
- The primitive reflexes of Moro, grasp, and rooting—present at birth—disappear by about age 12 months. These primitive reflexes may reappear with neurologic disease.

REVIEW OF THE CENTRAL NERVOUS SYSTEM

Embryologic Development. The nervous system is one of the first systems formed in utero. By the fourth week of gestation the neural tube closes at the anterior end to form the brain and at the posterior end to form the spinal cord.

During the second month of gestation the brain becomes the prominent body structure. It grows rapidly and continues to grow until around the fifth year of life. There appear to be two periods of rapid brain cell growth during gestation. Between the fifteenth and twentieth weeks of gestation the number of neurons increases significantly. At 30 weeks the number of neurons increases again.

It is thought that brain cells arise only during the first 100 days of gestation and that the brain then grows through continued cell division and multiplication. It is further believed that no new nerve cells appear after the sixth month of fetal life; brain growth depends on the development and multiplication of existing neurons. Therefore, it is critical to have early prenatal care to prevent or minimize the potential for birth defects.

The Myelin Sheath. Myelin, the fatty substance that surrounds the nerves of both the central and the peripheral nervous systems, begins to form at about the sixteenth week of gestation. Myelin insulates the nerves and conducts electrical impulses. Coordination of fine and gross motor skills progresses with the deposition of the myelin sheath. Nerve fibers can conduct impulses in the absence of myelin; however, the impulses travel more slowly. Gross motor skills obviously precede fine motor skills, as coordination and control advance throughout childhood. The myelin sheath can be destroyed by certain viruses, drugs, or the aging process itself.

The Neural System. The neural system develops multiple connections between the areas of the brain that control specific functions, including vision, hearing, motor function, sensation, coordination, and speech. Each function is under the control of a specific area of the brain. The right half, or hemisphere, of the brain controls the left side of the body, and is concerned with the social aspects of perception, intuition, and experience; the left hemisphere controls the right side of the body, and is largely concerned with language acquisition and use and logical, verbal reasoning.

The neonate's neurologic system functions at a subcortical level. Spinal cord reflexes such as sucking and cardiorespiratory functions are present; cortical functions such as memory and coordination are only partially developed.

Axial Skeleton. The axial skeleton protects the underlying structures of the central nervous system (CNS). For convenience of study the bones of the skull and the vertebral column are divided into regions that form the wall of the cranial cavity and the spinal column. The frontal, occipital, temporal, and parietal bones form the cranial vault. The floor of the cranial vault is composed of three compartments, or fossae—the anterior, middle, and posterior fossae. The anterior fossea houses the frontal lobes of the brain; the middle fossae contains the upper **brain stem** and the pituitary gland; and the posterior fossae contains the lower brain stem. Blood vessels and cranial nerves enter and leave the skull through the foramina.

At birth the skull plates are not fused, but are separated by nonossified spaces called fontanels. The posterior fontanel is usually fused by age 2 months and the anterior fontanel is fused by age 16 to 18 months. The fontanels allow the cranium to expand in response to rapid brain growth. Before fusion of the fontanels and sutures, an increase in intracranial pressure (ICP) will produce an increase in head circumference.

The neonate's brain is 25% of its mature adult weight; at age $2\frac{1}{2}$ years, it is 75% of its adult size, and by age 6 years, the brain is 90% of its adult weight. It is consequently difficult to predict the long-term sequelae of neurologic insults that occur in infancy. Brain growth can be assessed through head circumference measurements. These measurements are an important part of the child's routine physical examination and should be plotted on a growth chart to determine whether insufficient or excessive head and brain growth might point to a potential neurologic problem. Premature closing of the fontanels or sutures can cause massive neurologic damage and continued evaluation by the physician will be needed.

The Meninges. Three membranes surround the brain and spinal column. The first layer is the dura mater, a fibrous connective tissue structure containing many blood vessels and fibroblast-like cells that secrete collagen to produce a tough protective membrane (Martin, 1996). It comprises two layers having outer and inner meningeal components. Between the periosteum of the bone and the dura mater lies the epidural space. Sheets of dura also extend downward and inward to form partitions within the cranium. The falx cerebri separates the cerebral hemispheres, and the falx cerebelli separates the cerebellar hemispheres.

The tentorium is a tentlike structure separating the cerebellum from the occipital lobe of the cerebrum. The large gap through which the brain stem passes is the tentorial hiatus.

The next layer is the arachnoid, a delicate, avascular, weblike, serous membrane loosely covering the brain. Between the arachnoid and the dura lies the subdural space, which contains a small amount of fluid, just sufficient to prevent adhesion of the two membranes.

Between the pia mater and the arachnoid is the subarachnoid space, which is filled with cerebrospinal fluid (CSF). The CSF acts as a cushion to reduce the force of trauma felt by the brain.

The third layer is the pia mater. It is a delicate, transparent membrane that adheres closely to the outer surface of the brain. The pia mater is a vascular membrane, consisting of arteries and veins.

The Brain. The three sections of the brain are the cerebrum, the cerebellum, and the brain stem. The cerebrum is the largest component, filling the upper portion of the skull. It is divided into two hemispheres, right and left, separated by a longitudinal fissure. The cerebral hemispheres are further divided into lobes in relation to the cranial bones: frontal, parietal, temporal, and occipital. The cerebrum also includes part of the thalamus, hypothalamus, **basal ganglia,** and the olfactory and optic nerves.

The cerebellum is composed of white and gray matter. It is attached to the brain stem by paired bundles of fibers.

The brain stem consists of the midbrain, the pons, the medulla, the thalamus, and the third ventricle.

The Cranial Nerves. Twelve pairs of cranial nerves arise from the brain and brain stem, each with a specific function. Testing these nerves can indicate the location and degree of CNS injury. (See Chapter 11 for discussion of assessment of cranial nerve function.)

The Spinal Cord. For purposes of study the spinal cord is segmented into the cervical, thoracic, lumbar, and sacral regions. The spinal nerves are named for their corresponding vertebral segments.

The spinal cord transmits signals to and from the brain and responds to local sensory information through its automatic motor responses called reflexes. The simplest type of spinal cord response is the reflex arc. Sensation is transmitted to the spinal cord from a sensory nerve fiber. It synapses with a motor neuron in the same cord segment, causing a muscle or tendon contraction in the corresponding motor nerve. Deep tendon reflexes are examples of the reflex arc.

Sensory innervation occurs as sensory nerves carrying body sensations enter the spinal cord on the dorsal surface. Most sensory fibers for pain and temperature ascend to the brain by way of lateral spinal tracts. Sensory fibers for touch and pressure ascend through anterior tracts. Almost all sensory fibers pass through the thalamus, where perception of touch, pressure, and temperature is interpreted. Perceptions of texture, size, and weight are interpreted in the cortex.

Motor nerves are stimulated to respond after the brain receives a signal from a sensory nerve. The motor nerves cross over to the contralateral (opposite) side of the spinal cord from which they originate, then exit on the ventral surface of the spinal cord.

> The side contralateral to the injured side will be the side affected by the injury.

Functional differences exist between the upper and lower motor neurons; thus the outcome of a spinal cord injury is affected by the site of the injury. An injury between the brain and the dendrites (the nerve fibers that carry impulses toward the cell body) will render the brain incapable of signaling the muscle cells to cease responding reflexively, and the muscle will become contracted, or spastic. If the injury is to a section of the nerve between the muscle and axons (the nerve fibers that carry impulses away from the cell body), the muscles will become incapable of responding reflexively, causing them to become flaccid.

Cerebrospinal Fluid. CSF is a clear liquid produced in the choroid plexus of the ventricles. The CSF aids in protecting the brain, spinal cord, and meninges by acting as a watery cushion surrounding them, to absorb the shocks to which they are exposed. It is reabsorbed through the arachnoid villi into the venous sinuses.

Cerebral Blood Flow. The internal carotid arteries supply blood to all parts of the brain. Approximately 17% of cardiac output, and 20% of body oxygen, is transported to the brain. The brain has the largest requirement for oxygen—about 10 times that of all the rest of the body.

Cerebral blood flow (CBF) is controlled by **cerebral perfusion pressure** (CPP), which is the difference between the mean arterial blood pressure and the intracranial pressure.

Autoregulation or self-regulation is the unique ability of the cerebral arteries to change in diameter in response to changes in the CPP. The cerebral vessels can maintain a steady blood flow to the brain during alterations in blood pressure and perfusion; however, autoregulation fails when the limits of cerebrovascular dilation are reached.

Autoregulation may be impaired as a result of trauma and/or ischemia. It is influenced significantly by changes in $Pa{O_2}$ and $Pa{CO_2}$. An increase in $Pa{CO_2}$ (above 40 mm Hg) produces cerebral vasodilation and an increase in CBF. A decrease in $Pa{CO_2}$ (25 to 30 mm Hg) causes cerebral vasoconstriction and thus reduces blood flow to the brain. Alterations in $Pa{O_2}$ between 80 and 100 mm Hg have little effect on CBF, though hypoxia will dramatically increase CBF.

CEREBROSPINAL FLUID ANALYSIS IN CHILDREN: NORMAL FINDINGS

	NEONATE		CHILD OVER 6 MONTHS
	PRETERM	FULL TERM	
WBC/mm³	9	8	0
Protein			
mg/100 ml:	115	90	Less than 40
Range:	65–150	20–170	
Glucose			
mg/100 ml:	50	52	Greater than 40
Range:	24–63	34–119	
CSF/Blood			
Glucose:	74%	81%	50%
Range:	55–150%	44–248%	40–60%

COMMON DIAGNOSTIC TESTS AND PROCEDURES FOR NEUROLOGIC DISORDERS IN CHILDREN

	DESCRIPTION	PURPOSE	NURSING CONSIDERATIONS
Computed Tomography (CT Scan)	Computerized image of horizontal and vertical cross-sections of brain at any axis	Identifies abnormal tissue and structures, as in brain tumor, bleeding, hydrocephalus	May need an IV if contrast medium is used. Notify radiologist if child is allergic to iodine. May be sedated if necessary.
Digital Subtraction Angiography	IV contrast dye injected; clear image of vessels obtained as computer eliminates all tissue that has not received the contrast dye	Visualizes vascular abnormalities	May be NPO. Notify radiologist if child is allergic to iodine. Permit signed. No restrictions on activity after the test.
Echo-encephalography	Echoes from ultrasonic waves are recorded as they reflect off various surfaces of the skull	Identifies abnormal structure, position, function	Painless procedure No preparation
Electro-encephalography	Electric potential of the brain is measured and recorded as electrodes placed on the scalp conduct and amplify electrical activity	Identifies abnormal electrical brain discharges, as in seizures	May have regular diet or fluids. No caffeine or stimulants. Hair should be clean. Tell child procedure is painless.
Lumbar Puncture	CSF pressure is measured and specimen obtained as needle is inserted into subarachnoid space between L3 and L4	Measures pressure; CSF analysis identifies infections; used for administration of medications	Permit signed. Have the infant or child lay in a lateral position with knees up to chest. After procedure, lay flat.
Magnetic Resonance Imaging (MRI)	Computerized images of brain produced by radiofrequency emissions from certain elements	Visualizes morphologic features of tissue and structures at a level of detail not possible by other methods	No pain to the procedure but may be sedated if necessary. Loud noises from clicking. Patient's head will be restrained.
Nuclear Brain Scan	Radioactive substance injected IV; amount of substance measured and recorded; abnormal uptake indicates abnormal tissue or structure	Identifies focal brain lesions; visualizes CSF pathways	Patient needs to remain still during test. Will need an IV.

CEREBROSPINAL FLUID ANALYSIS FINDINGS IN PATHOLOGIC CONDITIONS

	APPEARANCE	PRESSURE	CELLS	PROTEIN	GLUCOSE/OTHER
Normal Lumbar CSF	Clear and colorless	70–200 mm H_2O	0–5/μl	15–45 mg/dl	50–75 mg/dl
Traumatic Tap	Bloody; supernatant fluid clear	Normal	Red blood cells	4 mg/dl rise per 5000 red cells	NA
Acute Purulent Meningitis	Cloudy-milky or xanthochromatic	100–300 mm H_2O	Polymorphonuclear cells over 1000	Increased	Decreased early
Viral Meningitis	Clear	Normal or increased	0 to a few hundred, mostly leukocytes	50–200 mg/dl	Normal
Encephalitis	Clear and colorless	Normal or slightly elevated	Normal or increased	50–200 mg/dl	<40 mg/dl
Subdural Hematoma	Yellow/clear and colorless	Increased	Normal	Normal or increased	Normal
Lead Encephalopathy	Clear or slightly cloudy	Increased	Leukocytes	Normal or slightly increased	NA; lead in spinal fluid
Multiple Sclerosis	Clear and colorless	Normal or low	Normal or increased	Normal or increased (increased gamma globulin)	NA; negative serology
Diabetic Coma	Clear and colorless	Decreased	Normal	Normal or slightly increased	May be 200–300 mg/dl

MEDICATIONS COMMONLY USED IN PEDIATRIC NEUROLOGIC DISORDERS

	DOSE AND ROUTE	THERAPEUTIC SERUM DRUG CONCENTRATIONS	ACTION/USES	SIDE EFFECTS AND NURSING CONSIDERATIONS
		Anticonvulsants		
Lorazepam (Ativan)	0.05 mg/kg over 2 min IV		Benzodiazepine, acts on subcortical levels of the CNS	Sedation, respiratory suppression
Clonazepam (Klonopin)	0.01–0.02 mg/kg/d PO, in divided doses	20–80 ng/ml	Benzodiazepine, anticonvulsant	Ataxia, drowsiness, weight gain, irritability, increases salivation, changes appetite
Phenytoin (Dilantin)	10–15 mg/kg IV/PO per day, in divided doses. Children older than age 6 yr may require 300 mg/d.	10–20 μg/ml	Anticonvulsant	Depression of myocardial function; heart block; bradycardia. Incompatible with many IV drugs and glucose. Tubing must be flushed to prevent precipitation. Rash, anemial behavioral and cognitive problems.
Phenobarbital	4–6 mg/kg/day PO or 10–15 mg/kg/day IV or IM	15–40 μg/ml	Barbiturate, sedative, hypnotic, anticonvulsant	Hyperactivity, drowsiness, ataxia, GI upset, allergic rash
Primidone (Mysoline)	10–25 mg/kg/day PO	5–12 μg/ml	Used for generalized and complex partial seizures	Vertigo, sedation, nausea, vomiting, ataxia, nystagmus
Valproic acid (Depakene)	15–30 mg/kg/day PO	40–50 μg/ml	Inhibits the neurotransmitter GABA. Used for absence and multiple seizure types	Nausea, vomiting, sedation, hair loss, hepatic dysfunction. Use with caution in children <2 yr old
Diazepam (Valium)	0.1–0.5 mg/kg/dose IV		Benzodiazepine, used for status epilepticus, generalized seizures	Slurred speech, ataxia, drowsiness, respiratory failure
Carbamazepine (Tegretol)	5–20 mg/kg/day PO	4–12 μg/ml	Used for partial, generalized, and mixed seizures	Dizziness, nausea, vomiting, ataxia, visual disturbances, hematologic disorders
Ethosuximide (Zarontin)	20–40 mg/kg PO	40–100 μg/ml	Used for absence seizures	Abdominal pain, irritability, anorexia
		Medications Used to Decrease ICP		
Mannitol	0.25 g/kg to 1 g/kg/dose over 30–60 min		Osmotic diuretic	Dizziness, headache, nausea, dry mouth, hypotension, pulmonary congestion, fluid and electrolyte imbalances
Furosemide (Lasix)	1–2 mg/kg q 6–8 hr. May be increased to a maximum of 6 mg/kg.		Produces a quick diuresis as well as decreasing venous tone and production of CSF	Dizziness, vertigo, weakness, nausea, vomiting, orthostatic hypotension, rash, muscle cramps
Pancuronium	0.1 mg/kg with morphine 0.1 mg/kg q 2–4 hr		Neuromuscular blocker (use with sedation) to prevent agitation and resistance to mechanical ventilation	

Data from Burns, C. E., Barber, N., Brady, M. A., & Dunn, A. M. (1996). *Pediatric primary care: A handbook for nurse practitioners*. Philadelphia: W. B. Saunders.

GENERAL NURSING CARE OF THE CHILD WITH A NERVOUS SYSTEM DISORDER

Assessment

The child with a neurologic injury or illness needs a complete neurologic assessment (see Chapter 11 for assessment of the cranial nerves). Test the child's level of consciousness, cerebral function, cerebellar function, and orientation. Note the child's mood and behavior. Knowledge of normal developmental milestones, as measured by the Denver Developmental Screening Test II (DDST-II) is essential (see Chapter 2 and Appendix D). The child's level of consciousness may be assessed using the Glasgow Coma Scale Modified for Children (Chapter 14, Table 14–2). The child's interaction with his family and the environment will also yield information about level of consciousness. Note lethargy or drowsiness, hyperactivity, tremors, or jitteriness.

Balance, coordination, and motor skills are assessed by observing the child dressing or undressing, buttoning, or playing. Other tests for coordination are rapid alternating movements, the finger-to-nose test, throwing a ball, or handling a pencil. Observe the child's walking gait for hemiplegia, scissors gait, or an abnormally wide-spaced gait. Observe and record the child's muscle development, strength, and tone. Test range of motion of all joints as well as deep tendon reflexes. Check sensory function of the face, trunk, arms, and legs. Test both sides of the child for vibration, superficial tactile sensation, and superficial pain and temperature.

Nursing Diagnosis

Many diseases or disorders of the brain and spinal column share problems in common, as reflected in the following nursing diagnoses:

- Altered Tissue Perfusion (Cerebral) related to alteration of arterial or venous blood flow, cerebral infarction, hemorrhage, hematoma, increased ICP, cerebral edema, seizures, hypoventilation, or increased cerebral metabolism
- Altered Nutrition: Less Than Body Requirements related to restricted intake; neurologic impairment; swallowing and/or chewing difficulty; or risk for aspiration, nausea, or vomiting
- Risk for Impaired Skin Integrity related to neuromuscular impairment, decreased level of consciousness, inadequate physical activity, immobility, or improper fluid or nutritional intake
- Anxiety related to change in health status, threat to self-concept, behavior changes, possible injury, social isolation, seizures, neurologic impairment, or lack of privacy during skin inspection and hygiene care
- Knowledge Deficit related to infectious process, disease process, medication regimen, dietary or fluid needs, measures for prevention, or chronic illness of a child or infant

Planning, Implementation, and Evaluation: The Child With a Neurologic Disorder

NURSING DIAGNOSIS

- Altered Tissue Perfusion (Cerebral) related to alteration of arterial or venous blood flow, cerebral infarction, hemorrhage, hematoma, increased ICP, cerebral edema, seizures, hypoventilation, or increased cerebral metabolism

Expected Outcome:

- The child will have improved cerebral perfusion, no cranial nerve deficits, improved or normal level of consciousness, vital signs in baseline normal, Glascow Coma Scale within normal limits, and appropriate behavior or thought patterns.

Intervention	Rationale
1. Assess age and developmental level of child.	Document a baseline age-appropriate level to gauge changes in neurologic status.
2. Establish neurologic baseline assessment and vital signs on admission.	Changes in neurologic signs can indicate deterioration or improvement in status.
3. Monitor factors that may further increase cerebral edema and ICP (hypoxia, fever, seizures, hypotension, hypercapnia).	Allows for correction of conditions that increase ICP and keep cerebral metabolic needs to a minimum.

Intervention	Rationale
4. Maintain head of bed at 30° to 45° angle.	Venous outflow drainage of the brain is facilitated by gravity.
5. Avoid prone position, neck flexion, or hip flexion.	All these positions tend to increase ICP. Lying flat in bed increases ICP. Neck flexion kinks the jugular vein where venous drainage occurs. Hip flexion may increase intra-abdominal or intrathoracic pressure, thus increasing ICP.
6. Organize nursing care around periods of low ICP.	Nursing care such as suctioning, bathing, and repositioning has been shown to increase ICP.
7. Monitor pupil size and reactivity every hour, p.r.n., or as ordered.	An increase in pupil size may indicate an increase in CSF accumulation.
8. Measure head circumference daily or p.r.n. and document on growth chart if age-appropriate.	Cranial expansion takes place when the CSF is under pressure, if fontanelles are open.
9. Palpate the anterior fontanel every shift if age-appropriate.	An increase in size may indicate an increase in CSF accumulation.
10. Palpate the cranial suture lines every shift if age-appropriate.	The cranial sutures may separate with an increase in CSF volume or pressure.
11. Assess the infant for irritability, lethargy, and feeding intolerance.	All are signs of increasing ICP and deteriorating neurologic status.
12. Place emergency equipment (oxygen, suction, bag-valve-mask) near the child's room or at the bedside.	Increased ICP can cause apnea and may lead to cardiopulmonary arrest.
13. Monitor intake and output hourly.	Indicates fluid volume imbalance.
14. Check urine specific gravity every 4–6 hours or p.r.n. Notify physician if urine specific gravity is above 1.030 or less than 1.010, or if output is below 1 ml/kg/hr or above 2 ml/kg/hr.	Urine specific gravity normally is 1.010 to 1.030, and normal urine output is 1–2 ml/kg/hr. With increasing ICP diabetes insipidus (DI) or syndrome of inappropriate antidiuretic hormone (SIADH) may occur (Behrman, Kliegman, & Arvin, 1996).

Evaluation: The child:

- demonstrates a normal respiratory rate and pattern and vital signs
- demonstrates a stable level of consciousness
- has normal urine output, normal urine specific gravity
- shows no decrease in cranial nerve function, an optimum level on the Glascow coma-scale, and appropriate behavior and thought patterns for age

---

NURSING DIAGNOSIS

- Altered Nutrition: Less Than Body Requirements related to restricted intake; neurologic impairment; swallowing and/or chewing difficulty; risk for aspiration; nausea, or vomiting

Expected Outcome:

- The child's weight is stable or normal for age and height.
- The child has normal serum proteins, moist mucous membranes, and adequate urine output.
- Nausea and vomiting are controlled.

Intervention	Rationale
1. Weigh the child daily on the same scale, at the same time of day, and in the same clothes. Record on a growth chart.	Changes in weight indicate fluid balance and nutritional status. Weigh only if the procedure does not increase ICP.
2. Monitor skin turgor, mucous membranes, eye orbits, urine output, urine specific gravity and serum and urine electrolytes.	These are indicators of fluid and electrolyte status.
3. Position the child or infant upright after feedings. If the child is old enough and the ICP is not elevated, his head should be slightly flexed and facing forward. Arms should be positioned forward with feet placed on a firm surface.	Decreases the risk of aspiration. Proper positioning will enhance comfort, prevent contractures, and provide for safety while feeding.
4. Provide a flexible feeding schedule with small feedings of favorite foods.	These techniques facilitate digestion and the ability to maintain adequate caloric intake.
5. Minimize handling around feeding times.	Decreases likelihood of vomiting and aspiration.
6. Stroke the child's throat upward while he is swallowing. Assist the child with chewing with the child's chin and jaw in the nurse's hand, if swallowing is impaired.	Swallowing may be facilitated by this method.
7. Assess level of consciousness prior to giving liquids.	Decreased LOC may cause aspiration with swallowing.
8. Consult dietician.	The dietician will advise how best to meet metabolic demands and plan the most efficient way to get calories.
9. Verify placement of oral or nasogastric (NG) tube before tube feedings are initiated.	Incorrect placement of NG tube will result in placing feedings into the lungs.
10. Obtain order to medicate for nausea and vomiting if necessary.	With nausea controlled the child will be more likely to tolerate feedings.

Evaluation: The child:

- shows normal growth for age, with no weight loss
- has nausea and vomiting controlled
- has age-appropriate caloric intake daily
- has proper hydration with moist mucous membranes

NURSING DIAGNOSIS

- Risk for Impaired Skin Integrity related to neuromuscular impairment, decreased level of consciousness, inadequate physical activity, immobility, or improper fluid or nutritional intake

Expected Outcome:

- The child will demonstrate a progressive increase in or adequate physical activity, optimal range of motion, and no skin breakdown.
- The parents will participate in their child's care.

Intervention	Rationale
1. Use eggcrate mattress or special flotation mattress to protect bony prominences. Reposition q 2 hr and p.r.n. Check for redness and pressure areas.	The child with a lower level of consciousness may not be active, and the immobility can cause skin breakdown.
2. Assess skin q 2 hr with the repositioning of the child or infant.	Prolonged pressure on the skin will quickly lead to breakdown.
3. If the child has had a shunt placed postoperatively, avoid putting temperature probes, cardiac monitor leads, or excessive tape over the shunt site.	Irritation from adhesives will contribute to skin breakdown and possible infection.
4. Encourage parents to participate in passive range of motion (PROM) exercises for the child, if appropriate.	Participating in the child's care enhances the child's sense of well-being and provides emotional and physical support for the child and increases the child's activity.
5. If braces or splints are used, assess the skin before and after the splints or assistive devices are put on and taken off.	Correct application of braces will minimize pressure points and reduce skin breakdown.
6. Implement a daily skin care regimen. Teach parents or family to check skin frequently.	Bathing, moisturizing, and inspecting the skin will facilitate skin integrity.

Evaluation: The child:

- has intact, clean, and dry skin with no pressure areas or sores
- participates in own care as tolerated.

The parents:

- participate in the child's skin care regimen
- assists in ROM activities for the child as possible

NURSING DIAGNOSIS

- Anxiety related to change in health status, threat to self-concept, behavior changes, possible injury, social isolation, seizures, neurologic impairment, or lack of privacy during skin inspection and hygiene care

Expected Outcome:

- The parents demonstrate management of anxiety; maintain social and personal relationships; verbalize relaxation; verbalize feelings about neurologic impairment; and demonstrate coping skills.

Intervention	Rationale
1. Keep the parents informed of the child's progress, prognosis, and plan of care. Encourage parents to talk about concerns and ask questions. Allow parents to make decisions where possible.	Control over any event of the child's care helps the parents to feel a part of the caregiving team and will lessen anxiety.
2. Encourage parents to participate actively in ADLs (oral hygiene, bathing, feeding, etc).	Touching the child and active participation in the child's care lowers parental anxiety.
3. Orient the parents to hospital routine and refer to clergy, social worker, and other team members.	A familiar environment is less threatening and will enable the parents to better deal with the child's condition and prognosis.

Intervention	Rationale
4. Encourage rooming-in when possible.	This will involve the parents more in the child's care, and make them part of the health team, and decrease anxiety in the child.
5. Aid in anxiety reduction techniques such as relaxation techniques, music, and guided imagery.	Facilitates coping and stress reduction.

Evaluation: The parents:

- participate in caregiving for their child when possible
- meet with the health care team periodically
- discuss concerns and fears
- plan with the team for the child's future and participate in decision making
- state reduced feelings of loneliness
- demonstrate coping and problem-solving skills

NURSING DIAGNOSIS

- Knowledge Deficit related to infectious process, disease process, medication regimen, dietary or fluid needs, measures for prevention, or chronic illness of a child or infant

Expected Outcome: The child/parents will

- state age-appropriate, realistic factors about the child's condition
- list factors to decrease neurologic deficits and measures to prevent further occurrences of illness
- demonstrate that the grieving process has begun

Intervention	Rationale
1. Allow time for teaching. If the child will be having an operation, do preoperative teaching for the parents as well.	Answers questions and reinforces information given to the parents by the physician. This will include the parents in learning.
2. Assess the parents' understanding of the child's disability. Assess the parents' understanding of the child's need for physical, speech, or occupational therapies.	Parents need to understand the intellectual and physical abilities and disabilities of their child to give informed consent or reinforce need for therapies.
3. Put parents in touch with community support groups.	Support may be gained by seeing or hearing how others coped with similar situations.
4. Supply the parents with phone numbers to call for needed information once they are home.	Health care workers can help parents feel in touch and educate them at the same time by talking over the child's condition on the telephone.
5. Teach the parents important signs and symptoms in the child's illness, side effects to medications, and when to call the physician or nurse. Provide written instructions.	The parents need to state important signs and symptoms that indicate a change in the child's condition and be aware of when to seek medical attention. Anxiety reduces learning and attention span. A written copy of signs and symptoms will stay with them longer than verbal instructions.
6. Review the signs of symptoms of a wound infection.	Until the surgical incision is healed the risk of infection is present.
7. Review with the parents the signs and symptoms of urinary tract retention or infection.	Due to retention and reflux the child will be at risk for urinary tract infections.

Evaluation: The parents:
- discuss the child's care appropriately
- list situations in which the child needs to be seen by the physician or nurse
- contact community support

INCREASED INTRACRANIAL PRESSURE

Intracranial pressure reflects the pressure exerted by the blood, brain, CSF, and any other space-occupying fluid or mass. Increased ICP occurs when a disturbance in autoregulation occurs so that the ICP is increased and sustained at 20 mm Hg or higher.

Etiology. Alterations in the brain can result from a space-occupying lesion such as a brain tumor or hematoma. The brain can swell as a result of head trauma, hematoma, or an hypoxic episode. The inflammatory response associated with an infectious process can alter ICP as well, although to a lesser degree. CSF dynamics can be disrupted as a result of the overproduction of fluid, the malabsorption of fluid, or a communication problem within the system.

Clinical Manifestations

Infants

- Poor feeding/vomiting
- Irritability/restlessness
- Lethargy
- Bulging fontanel
- High-pitched cry
- Increased head circumference

PATHOPHYSIOLOGY *of Increased ICP*

The major pathophysiologic changes associated with increased ICP result from alterations in the brain, CSF dynamics, and CBF. To maintain cerebral pressure and volume within normal range, changes in one or more of the contents of the cranium must be compensated for by changes in the others; this is referred to as the **Monroe-Kellie doctrine.**

Compensatory mechanisms include reduction in CSF production, increase in CSF absorption, and reduction in cerebral mass as a result of fluid displacement. Once the limits of compensation are reached, any further increase in volume or pressure will cause a sudden increase in ICP and an associated decline in the clinical status of the child. Ultimately, increased ICP will compromise cerebral perfusion and produce shifting of brain tissue, causing herniation. The consequences of herniation depend on its severity and location.

There are four types of herniation. *Transtentorial herniation* occurs when part of the brain herniates downward and around the tentorium cerebelli. It may be unilateral or bilateral, and may involve anterior or posterior portions of the brain. If a large amount of tissue is involved it may cause death because vital brain structures are compressed and become unable to perform their vital functions.

Temporal lobe herniation, or uncal herniation, refers to a shifting of the temporal lobe laterally across the tentorial notch. This produces compression of the third cranial nerve and ipsilateral pupil dilation. If pressure continues to rise, flaccid paralysis, pupil dilation, pupil fixation, and death will result. *Tonsillar herniation* occurs when the cerebellar tonsils herniate through the foramen magnum. The child will develop nuchal rigidity, shoulder or arm numbness, and changes in heart and respiratory rate and pattern. *Brain stem herniation* through the foramen magnum results in death as a result of compression of vital cardiorespiratory centers.

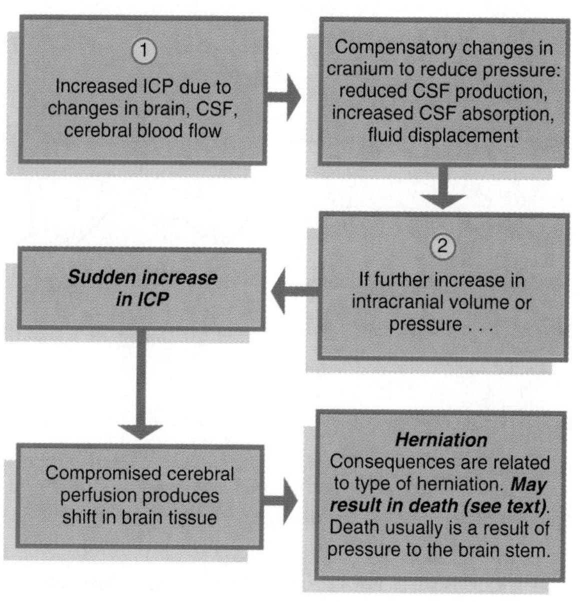

- Separation of cranial sutures
- Distended scalp veins
- Eyes deviated downward (sunset sign or setting sun sign)
- Increased or decreased response to pain

Children

- Headache
- Diplopia
- Mood swings
- Slurred speech
- Papilledema (after 48 hours)
- Altered level of consciousness
- Nausea and vomiting

Late Signs

- Tachycardia leading to bradycardia
- Apnea
- Systolic hypertension
- Widening pulse pressure
- **Decorticate/decerebrate posturing** (Fig. 40–1)

Diagnostic Evaluation. Diagnostic tests for increased ICP include computed tomography scan (CT), magnetic resonance imaging (MRI), lumbar puncture (LP), electrolyte levels, arterial blood gases (ABGs), complete blood count (CBC), electroencephalogram (EEG), and X-rays.

> Normal blood gas levels are PaO_2 of greater than 80 mm Hg and $PaCO_2$ less than 45 mm Hg in a child with normal ICP. The goal of hyperventilation is $PaCO_2$ between 30 and 35 mm Hg (Geraci & Geraci, 1996).

Therapeutic Managment. The management of increased ICP is directed toward reduction of the volume of the CSF, preservation of cerebral metabolic function, and avoidance of those situations which increase ICP.

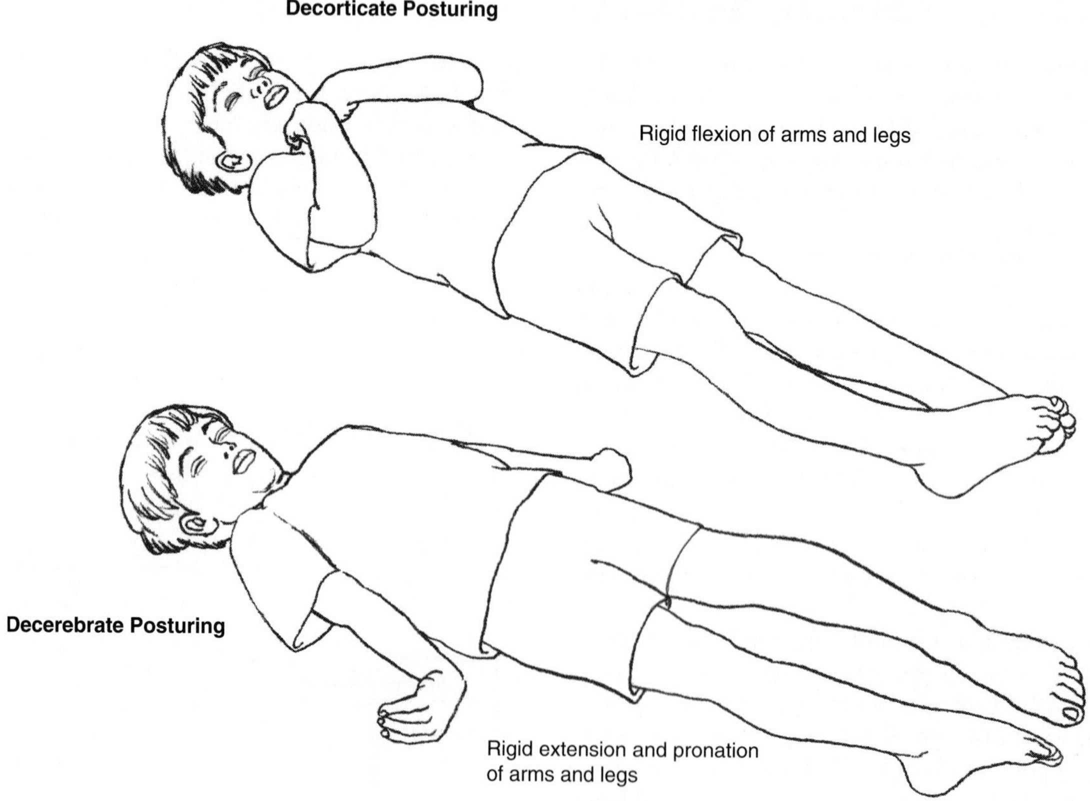

Figure 40–1
Decorticate posturing is an abnormal flexion of the upper extremities and extension of the lower extremities with possible plantar flexion of the feet. It indicates a lesion in the cerebral hemisphere or disruption of the corticospinal tracts. *Decerebrate posturing* is an abnormal extension of the upper extremities with internal rotation of the upper arm and wrist and extension of the lower extremities with some internal rotation. It usually indicates damage in the diencephalon, midbrain, or pons.

NURSING CARE OF THE CHILD WITH INCREASED INTRACRANIAL PRESSURE

Assessment

Assessment of the child with increased ICP requires astute clinical observation. Common signs and symptoms may not occur until the ICP is significantly elevated and the child is deteriorating rapidly.

Nursing care depends on the progression of CNS involvement. The assessment parameters are those common to all children with an underlying neurologic problem. Special attention needs to be focused on level of consciousness, behavior, pupil status, cranial nerve function, motor function, reflexes, and vital signs.

Level of Consciousness. The baseline level of conciousness is assessed and documented. Information about the child's normal behavior is obtained from the parents or primary caregivers. Serial observations are made to assess changes in the child's condition.

STANDARD TERMS FOR LEVEL OF CONSCIOUSNESS

Level of consciousness should be described by the nurse using standard terminology:

Full consciousness: awake, alert, oriented, interacts with environment

Confused: the ability to think clearly and rapidly is lost

Disoriented: the ability to recognize place or person is lost

Lethargic: awakens easily but exhibits limited responsiveness

Obtunded: sleeps unless aroused and once aroused has limited interaction with the environment

Stupor: requires considerable stimulation to arouse

Coma: vigorous stimulation produces no motor or verbal response

Behavior. Changes in the child's normal behavior pattern may be an important early sign of increased ICP. Parents often are the first to notice a change in the child's behavior. A parent's comment such as "he isn't acting like himself" should be taken seriously. The child who no longer recognizes his parents, who cannot follow commands, or who has minimal response to pain is deteriorating.

> Decreased responsiveness to painful stimuli is a significant sign of alteration in level of consciousness.

Pupil Evaluation. Pupil evaluation is done to detect increasing ICP. As ICP rises, compression of the third cranial nerve occurs, resulting in pupil dilation with sluggish or absent constriction to light.

Motor Function. The child with increased ICP will exhibit changes in motor function. Purposeful movement will decrease and abnormal posturing may be observed (see Fig. 40–1). **Decorticate posturing** refers to flexion of the upper extremities (elbows, wrists) and extension of the lower extremities. Plantar flexion of the feet may also be observed. This type of posturing implies an injury to the cerebral hemispheres. **Decerebrate posturing** involves extension of the upper extremities with internal rotation of the upper arm and wrist. The lower extremities will extend with some internal rotation noted at the knees and feet. This type of posturing is indicative of damage to more areas of the brain, such as the diencephalon, midbrain, or pons.

> The progression from decorticate to decerebrate posturing usually indicates deteriorating neurologic function and warrants physician notification. Flaccid paralysis indicates further deterioration in the child's condition.

Vital Signs. Vital sign measurement, with particular attention to blood pressure, pulse, and respiratory rate, is important. Cushing's response is usually apparent just before or when the brain stem herniates. This usually indicates an alteration in brain stem perfusion, with the body attempting to improve CBF by increasing blood pressure.

> Cushing's response is a late sign of increased ICP. Cushing's response consists of an increased systolic blood pressure with widening pulse pressure, bradycardia, and change in respiratory rate and pattern.

As ICP rises, the child may present with a change from the baseline respiratory pattern, such as Cheyne-Stokes respiration, central neurogenic hyperventilation, or apneustic breathing. Cheyne-Stokes respiration refers to a pattern of breathing characterized by increasing rate and depth, then decreasing rate and depth with a pause of variable length. The cycle will be repeated again and again. Central neurogenic hyperventilation is identified by a rapid rate despite normal ABGs. This type of breathing pattern usually indicates midbrain or pontine involvement. Apneustic breathing occurs when the child demonstrates prolonged inspiration and expiration. As Cushing's response occurs, the child will develop apnea.

> CPP is the mean arterial blood pressure minus ICP (Hickey, 1992).

Nursing Diagnosis

Nursing diagnoses that may apply to increased ICP include those common to other neurologic disorders:

- Altered Tissue Perfusion (Cerebral) related to increased ICP, cerebral edema, or decreased CPP

- Altered Nutrition: Less Than Body Requirements related to nausea, vomiting, inability to swallow, or impaired level of consciousness
- Anxiety related to change in health status or life crisis
- Knowledge Deficit related to medication regimen

Care for children with these nursing diagnoses is detailed in the general care plan at the beginning of the chapter.

Other nursing diagnoses that apply to the child with ICP are as follows:

- Ineffective Breathing Pattern related to neuromuscular impairment
- Altered Tissue Perfusion (Skin) related to immobility
- Risk for Infection related to invasive lines
- Fluid Volume Deficit related to restricted intake, inability to swallow, and change in mental status

Planning, Implementation, and Evaluation: The Child With Increased Intracranial Pressure

NURSING DIAGNOSIS • Risk for Infection related to invasive lines

Expected Outcome: • The child will be afebrile, have normal white blood cell (WBC) count, no evidence of meningitis or pneumonia, no CSF or purulent drainage, and no urinary tract infection.

Intervention	Rationale
1. Maintain strict asepsis when manipulating ventriculostomy drainage system.	Helps prevent an infection of the catheter site and CSF
2. Assess invasive sites for redness or drainage.	Report signs of infection to the physician.
3. Monitor temperature, WBC count, chest X-rays, and urinalysis for signs of infection.	Steroids may mask infection and decrease immunity to infectious organisms.
4. Use aseptic techniques with foley catheter.	With bedrest/immobility, these children are prone to urinary tract infection

Evaluation: • The child has no temperature elevation and demonstrates no signs of infection.

NURSING DIAGNOSIS • Fluid Volume Deficit related to restricted intake, inability to swallow, and change in mental status.

Expected Outcome: • The child will have moist mucous membranes, serum osmolality and electrolytes within normal limits for age, and intake and output normal for age.

Intervention	Rationale
1. Monitor intake and output and urine specific gravity. Notify physician of urine output <1 ml/kg/hr or >2ml/kg/hr.	SIADH or DI can occur with stress, surgery, brain disorders, or some medications. (See box for clinical manifestations of DI and SIADH.)
2. Administer fluids within fluid restriction.	Fluid restriction aids in decreasing extracellular fluid and in turn decreasing ICP.
3. Administer medications as ordered. (See Common Medications table in Clinical Reference Pages.)	Osmotic and loop diuretics will decrease cerebral edema and cause fluid loss.
4. Monitor serum sodium, electrolytes, and serum osmolality.	These indicate fluid status and what measures to take to keep electrolytes in balance. Hyponatremia will cause cerebral edema.

Evaluation: • The child will demonstrate appropriate fluid balance and normal electrolyte levels.

Monitoring for DI and SIADH in the Child With Increased ICP

Diabetes insipidus (DI) or syndrome of inappropriate antidiuretic hormone (SIADH) can occur in the child with increased ICP. The nurse must monitor intake and output in the child with increased ICP and be alert for the following clinical manifestations:

DI (HIGH AND DRY)	SIADH (LOW AND WET)
High urine output	Low urine output
Specific gravity below 1.005	Specific gravity above 1.020
High serum sodium	Low serum sodium
Osmolality above 295 mOsm/L	Osmolality below 275 mOsm/L
Low volume (vascular fluid)	High volume (vascular fluid)
Weight loss	Weight gain
Hypotension	Hypertension
Tachycardia	Lethargy
Thirst	Coma
Anxiety	Seizures
Depression	Nausea
Apathy	Vomiting
Constipation	

CONGENITAL DISORDERS

Spina Bifida

Spina bifida, a congenital disorder, is a neural tube defect in which there is incomplete closure of the vertebrae and neural tube. Spina bifida is classified as spina bifida occulta and spina bifida cystica (Fig. 40–2). Spina bifida occulta usually occurs between L5 and S1, with failure of the vertebrae to completely fuse. The child may have no sensory or motor defects. The only clinical manifestation that may appear is a dimple, small tuft of hair, hemangioma, or lipoma in the lower lumbar or sacral area. These defects may be detected accidentally on a routine X-ray. Spina bifida cystica results in incomplete closure of the vertebrae and neural tube, resulting in a saclike protrusion in the lumbar or sacral area with varying degrees of nervous tissue involvement. Spina bifida cystica is further divided into meningocele, myelomeningocele, lipomeningocele, and lipomeningomyelocele. Meningocele is a saclike protrusion filled with spinal fluid and meninges. The most severe form of meningocele is myelomeningocele, in which the sac is filled with spinal fluid, meninges, nerve roots, and spinal cord.

Etiology. The etiology of spina bifida is unknown in most cases. There is evidence that there may be a genetic predisposition. Folic acid deficiency of the mother has been linked to neural tube defects. There is also evidence that

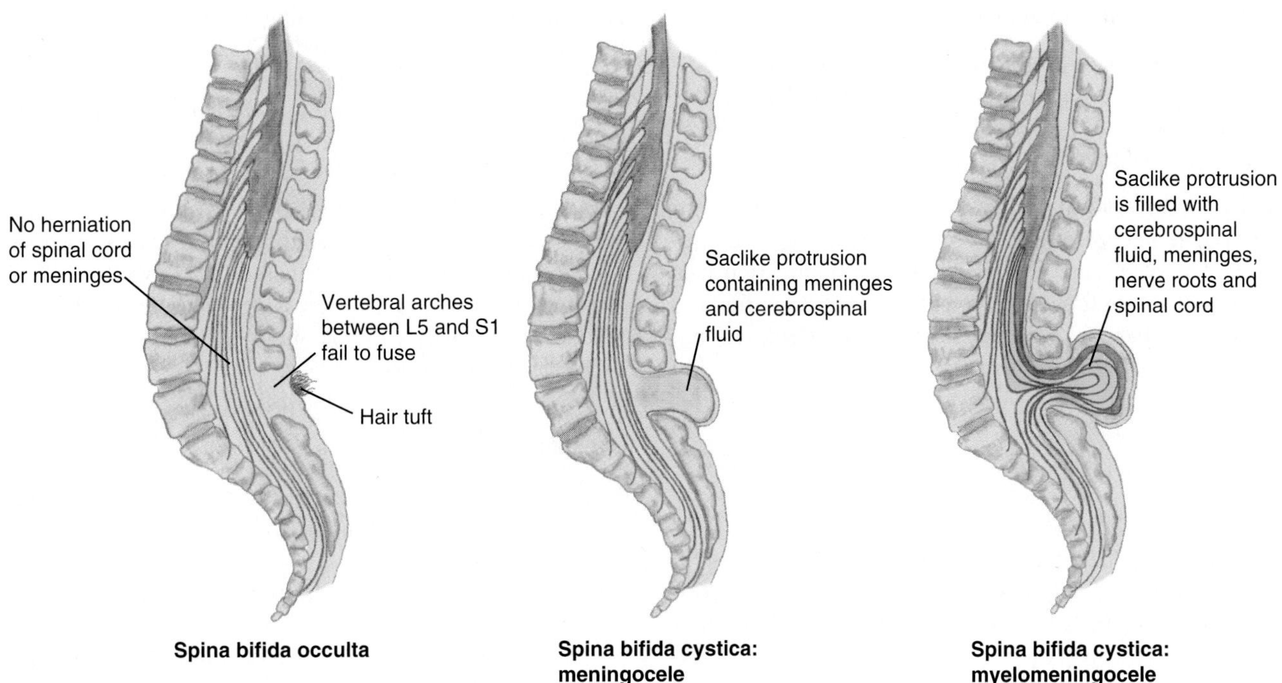

Figure 40–2
Three forms of spina bifida.

it may be viral in origin; however, research has yet to determine the actual cause and preventive measures that may be taken.

PATHOPHYSIOLOGY *of Spina Bifida*

During the fourth week of gestation (days 24 to 28) ventral induction of the neural tube fails to occur. The degree of impairment is related to the level of the defect on the spinal cord and on the size of the defect. Ninety percent of spinal cord lesions are at L2 and below. The lesion results in paralysis, partial paralysis, or varying sensory defects. Club feet, scoliosis, contracture, and dislocation of the hips may also be associated with the defect. Associated malformations may include hydrocephalus and Arnold-Chiari malformation.

Incidence. The incidence is 1 to 5 per 1000 live births. There is variability in geographic locations within the United States and worldwide (Hobdell, 1996).

Clinical Manifestations. The degree of deficit is from the level of the lesion or below.

Location of Lesion and Deficit

- **T12:** Flaccid lower extremities, decreased sensation and lack of bowel control, incontinence and dribbling of urine
- **L1–L3:** Hip flexion, flail feet
- **L2–L4:** Hip adduction
- **L3–S2:** Hip adduction, hip extension, knee flexion
- **S3 and below:** No motor impairment
- **Sacral roots:** Plantar flexion

Diagnostic Evaluation. Diagnostic tests include alpha-fetoprotein levels in amniotic fluid at 16 to 18 weeks of gestation, ultrasound of the fetus, and CT after delivery. Myelogram may be done.

Therapeutic Management. Immediate surgical closure is the most common choice (Fig. 40–3). The rationale for immediate surgical closure is decreased risk of infection and decreased morbidity and morality. Other benefits are improved prognosis without further cord deterioration, and earlier and easier physical handling and bonding.

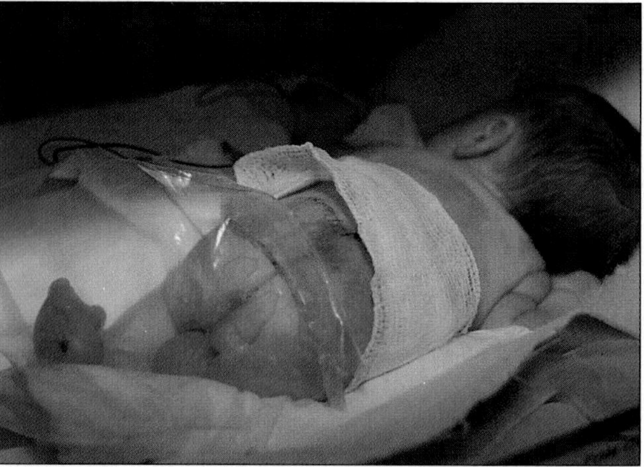

Figure 40–3
This infant has a repaired myelomeningocele. Note the left club foot. This deformity often accompanies the defect because normal intrauterine movement does not occur in the fetus with spina bifida, interfering with the development of the extremities. The legs are flaccid, and normal neonatal flexion is absent. The infant is also incontinent, dribbling stool and urine constantly. Hydrocephalus also commonly accompanies these neural tube defects. (Courtesy of Parkland Memorial Hospital, Dallas, Texas)

NURSING CARE OF THE CHILD WITH SPINA BIFIDA

The sac is evaluated and the lesion is measured. The infant's head circumference is measured. The anterior fontanel is palpated for fullness. The infant is placed in a prone position to avoid stress or pressure on the sac. A roll is placed under the infant's ankles to maintain foot alignment, and a roll is placed between the knees with the hips slightly flexed to maintain hip alignment and decrease tension on the sac.

Assessment

The infant's overall tone is assessed with special note of spontaneous movement of the extremities. The motor examination is done at rest. Using painful stimuli from the torso downward, observations are made regarding voluntary movement below the level of the lesion.

The infant is at risk for infection before closure of the sac. Therefore, the infant's temperature must be monitored every 1 to 2 hours. Signs of infection should be noted along with irritability, lethargy, or nuchal rigidity. A sterile saline dressing is placed over the sac to maintain the moisture of the sac and its contents. However, there is a risk of infection and the dressing needs to be changed whenever soiled, or with documentation of the appearance of the sac and contents.

Nursing Diagnosis

Nursing diagnoses that may apply to infants with spina bifida include those common to other neurologic disorders:

- Altered Tissue Perfusion (Cerebral) related to increased ICP
- Altered Nutrition: Less Than Body Requirements related to NPO status for surgery
- Knowledge Deficit related to home care

Care for these nursing diagnoses is detailed in the general care plan at the beginning of the chapter. Other nursing diagnoses that apply to the child with spina bifida are:

- Risk for Impaired Skin Integrity related to presence of sac
- Risk for Infection related to the open sac
- Impaired Physical Mobility related to neuromuscular impairment
- Altered Urinary Elimination related to neuromuscular impairment
- Constipation related to sensory deficit and neurologic impairment

Planning, Implementation, and Evaluation: The Child With Spina Bifida

NURSING DIAGNOSIS • Risk for Impaired Skin Integrity related to presence of sac

Expected Outcome: The child will:
- have no postoperative infection
- have no signs of pressure sores

Intervention	Rationale
1. Use special mattress or pad for infant's bed.	Prone position may cause pressure points.
2. Assess the infant's skin and reposition frequently. Change the diaper and clean the area frequently.	Keeping the infant's diaper open will enable frequent cleaning of the perineal area because oozing of stool and dribbling of urine may occur.
3. Use stoma adhesive on each side of the lesion; consult the stoma therapist if needed.	Frequent dressing changes may irritate the skin and the potential for irritation will be less if the tape is stuck to the stoma adhesive. The stoma therapist may make special recommendations for neonatal skin needs.

Evaluation: • The infant has no skin breakdown, and maintains clean dry buttocks and perineal area.

NURSING DIAGNOSIS • Risk for Infection related to the open sac

Expected Outcome: The child will:
- have no drainage from the sac and no areas of redness
- remain afebrile
- maintain WBC count within normal limits

Intervention	Rationale
1. Monitor vital signs. Assess the sac for redness, and clear or purulent drainage.	These are signs of infection that need to be documented and reported to the physician.
2. Begin feedings when bowel sounds are present.	Adequate nutrition is needed for healing.
3. Maintain sterile dressings over the sac or incision site.	Sterile dressings will facilitate healing and decrease the risk of infection.

Evaluation: • The infant has good skin integrity with good healing of the incision line.

NURSING DIAGNOSIS • Impaired Physical Mobility related to neuromuscular impairment

Expected Outcome: The child will:
- learn to use whatever devices he or she can to become mobile
- maximize abilities to be mobile

Intervention	Rationale
1. Assess and document physical impairments and abilities. Note the activities the child is able to participate in and encourage as much activity as is tolerated.	Notes advances or regression in activities or abilities of the child.
2. Maintain splints, braces, and casts. Use wheelchairs, walkers, and other assistive devices as needed.	These may be used for proper alignment and to decrease contractures. Other devices may increase independence and mobility.
3. Ensure the child attends therapy classes and participates to his or her fullest. Encourage self-care.	This will help prevent contractures and encourage independence and increased self-esteem.

Evaluation:
- The child enjoys as much mobility as he or she desires, keeping in mind his or her impairments.
- The parents handle the child gently, but encourage occupational and physical therapy.

NURSING DIAGNOSIS • Altered Urinary Elimination related to the neuromuscular impairment

Expected Outcome: • The child will have no urinary infections; urine will be clear and odor free.

Intervention	Rationale
1. Assess urinary stream.	Urinary dribbling indicates interrupted innervation to the bladder.
2. Maintain moist mucous membranes. Offer adequate fluids.	Good hydration will help prevent UTIs.
3. Teach and maintain regular toilet habits. Use intermittent clean catheterization to keep bladder empty if necessary.	Facilitates complete and regular emptying of the bladder; helps prevent retention and UTIs.
4. Check urinary frequency, output, and specific gravity.	May be initial indicators of urinary pattern alteration.

Evaluation: • The child establishes regular voiding patterns and has normal urinalysis.

NURISNG DIAGNOSIS • Constipation related to sensory deficit and neurologic impairment

Expected Outcome: • The child will have regular bowel movements.

Intervention	Rationale
1. Observe and document the infant's or child's anal opening and pattern of bowel movements.	Absence of rectal sphincter tone indicates abnormal bowel function, noting the pattern will alert caregivers to implement a bowel program.

Intervention	Rationale
2. Assess for abdominal distension, vomiting, and poor feeding.	Signs of constipation
3. Develop bowel program: suppository before breakfast, sit on toilet after breakfast, may need to stimulate anal spincter.	Bowel program will ensure elimination needs are met.
4. Consult dietician to assure diet provides adequate fluid and fiber.	Facilitates softer stools and easier passage.

Evaluation: The child:

- is free of constipation or impaction
- has regular bowel movements

Hydrocephalus

Hydrocephalus develops as a result of an imbalance between production and absorption of CSF. As excess CSF accumulates in the ventricular system, the ventricles become dilated and the brain is compressed against the skull. This results in enlargement of the skull if the sutures are open, or signs and symptoms of increased ICP if the sutures are fused.

Etiology. Hydrocephalus may be congenital, acquired, or of unknown etiology. In infancy hydrocephalus is most often congenital or related to prematurity. Congenital hydrocephalus results from developmental defects such as Arnold-Chiari malformations, congenital arachnoid cysts, congenital tumors, or aqueduct stenosis. In premature infants neonatal meningitis or subarachnoid hemorrhage may result in hydrocephalus. Hydrocephalus is often associated with myelomeningocele. Intrauterine infection and perinatal hemorrhage cause hydrocephalus in some infants. In older children hydrocephalus is usually acquired as a complication of meningitis, tumor, or hemorrhage.

Incidence. The incidence of hydrocephalus in infancy is 5.8 per 10,000 births. Incidence of hydrocephalus with spina bifida is considered to be 3 to 4 per 1000 births. Obstructive, or noncommunicating, hydrocephalus accounts for 99% of all cases of hydrocephalus in children.

Clinical Manifestations

Infant: Early Signs

- Rapid growth—increase in head circumference above the normal growth curve
- Full, bulging anterior fontanel
- Irritability
- Poor feeding
- Distended, prominent scalp veins
- Widely separated cranial sutures
- Thinning of skull bones

Infant: Late Signs

- "Setting sun" sign—sclera are visible above the iris
- Frontal bone enlargement or bossing
- Vomiting, difficulty swallowing or feeding
- Increased blood pressure, decreased heart rate
- Altered respiratory pattern
- Shrill high-pitched cry
- Sluggish or unequal pupillary response to light

Child: Early Signs

- Strabismus
- Frontal headache that occurs in the morning and is relieved by emesis or sitting upright
- Nausea and vomiting that may be projectile
- Diplopia
- Restlessness
- Personality changes
- Ataxia
- Papilledema
- Irritability
- Sluggish and unequal pupillary response to light
- Confusion

Disorders Associated With Hydrocephalus

Arnold-Chiari malformation is deformity of the cerebellar tonsils into the cervical canal. Arnold-Chiari malformations may or may not be associated with hydrocephalus and a myelomeningocele.

Craniosynostosis is premature closure of the cranial sutures. This abnormal skull development causes an abnormally shaped skull. In some cases craniectomy is needed for management of increased ICP. Hydrocephalus is an associated disorder in many cases of craniosynostosis.

PATHOPHYSIOLOGY *of Hydrocephalus*

Cerebrospinal fluid is produced primarily by the choroid plexus, which lines the lateral ventricles. CSF circulates through the ventricular system and flows into the subarachnoid space around the brain and the spinal cord. The CSF is then reabsorbed within the subarachnoid spaces.

Hydrocephalus results when there is either (1) impaired absorption of CSF within the subarachnoid space (communicating hydrocephalus); or (2) obstruction of flow of CSF within the ventricles that prevents CSF from circulating around the spinal cord and the subarachnoid space (noncommunicating hydrocephalus). Hydrocephalus rarely may be caused by overproduction of CSF by a tumor of the choroid plexus.

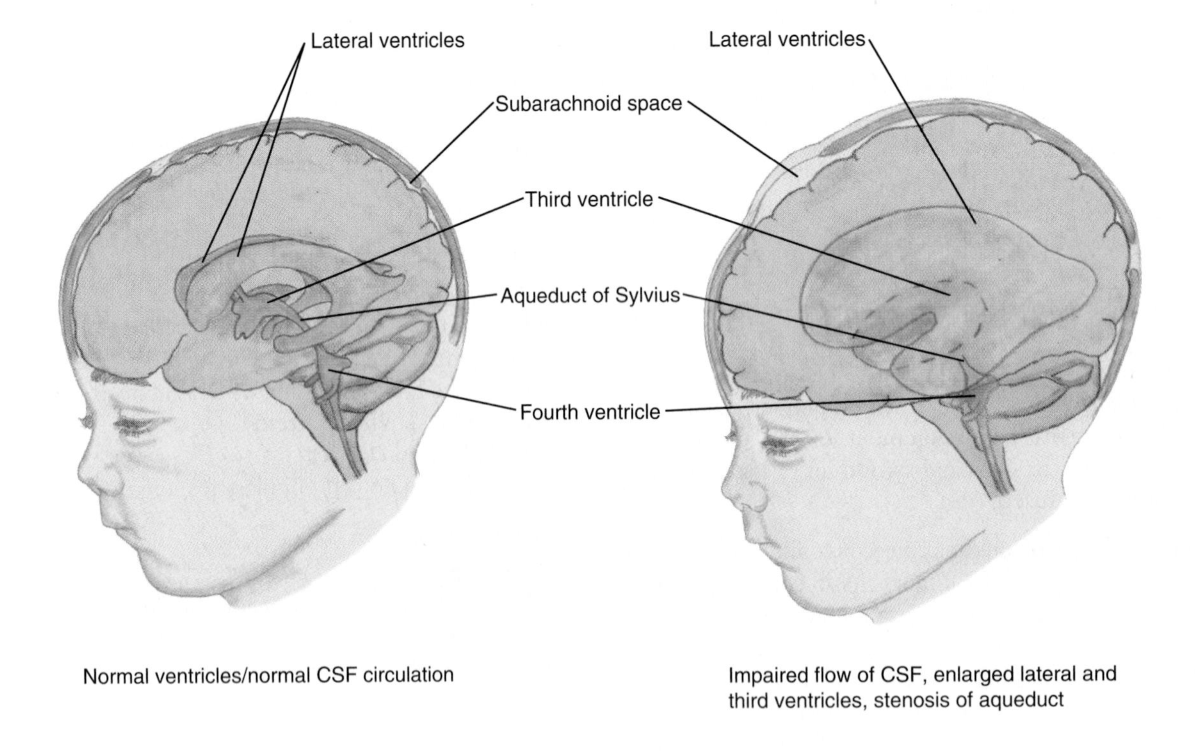

Normal ventricles/normal CSF circulation

Impaired flow of CSF, enlarged lateral and third ventricles, stenosis of aqueduct

Child: Late Signs

- Increased blood pressure
- Decreased heart rate
- Alteration in respiratory pattern
- Seizures
- Lethargy
- Blindness from herniation of the optic disk
- Decerebrate rigidity
- Vomiting

Diagnostic Evaluation. Diagnostic tests include serial measurements of head circumference, CT, MRI, and LP.

Therapeutic Management. The objectives of therapy are to prevent further CSF accumulation and reduce disability and death. The aim is to bypass the blockage and drain the fluid from the ventricles to an area where it may be reabsorbed. Tubes leading from the ventricles out of the skull and passing under the skin to the peritoneal cavity accomplish this (ventriculoperitoneal shunt; Fig. 40–4).

NURSING CARE OF THE CHILD WITH HYDROCEPHALUS

The care of the child with hydrocephalus includes giving medications to decrease the CSF production. However, because the majority of cases of hydrocephalus require shunting to drain the excess CSF, most of the nursing care will be postsurgical.

Assessment

When an infant is born with hydrocephalus he may have apparent signs at birth or signs of an obstruction may

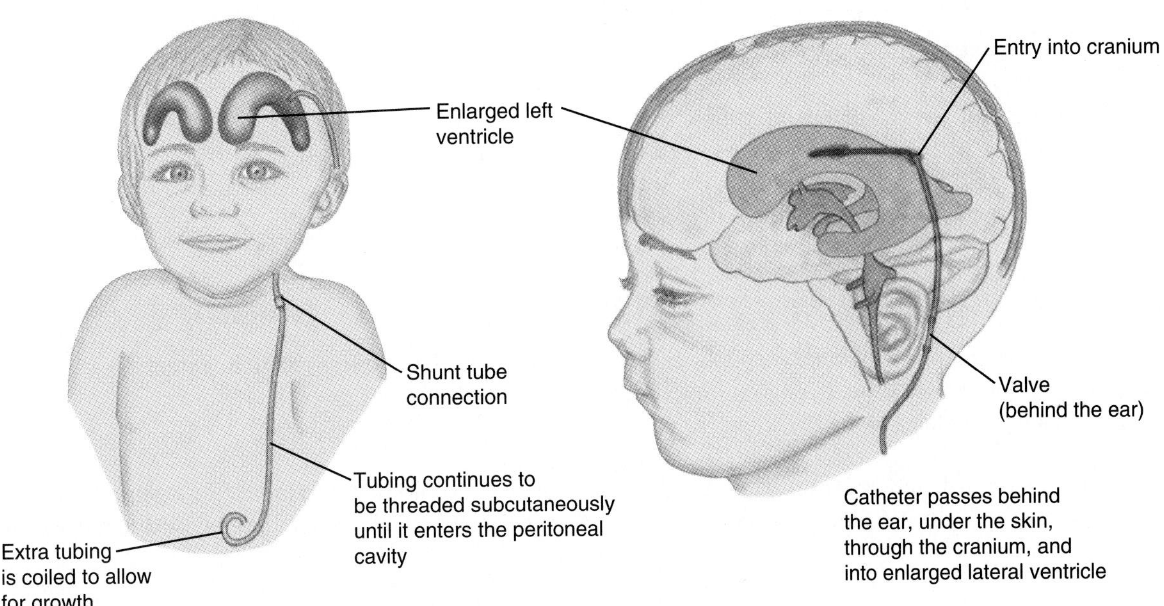

Figure 40–4

A ventriculoperitoneal shunt is implanted in the child with hydrocephalus to prevent excess accumulation of CSF in the ventricles. The tubing diverts the CSF from the ventricles into the peritoneal cavity, where it is reabsorbed. Nursing care of the child with a ventricular shunt includes monitoring for infection and pain, administering antibiotics and pain medications as ordered, and teaching the family how to change dressings and how to recognize shunt problems.

appear over the next few months. The first symptom may be an abnormal head circumference. Head circumference should be measured daily or more frequently depending on the child's condition, and should be recorded and plotted on a graph. To facilitate accuracy when different personnel take the measurement, a pen mark should be made on the scalp where the tape measure is being placed. The tape measure is usually placed just above the top of the ears and around the head, around the mid-forehead and the most prominent portion of the occiput. The infant's anterior fontanel should be palpated for size, bulging, tenseness, and cranial suture separation. Assessment of the fontanel is made when the baby is sitting in an upright position and is quiet. It may bulge or pulsate if the infant is crying.

Attention is paid to the infant's behavior when the fontanel is full or tense. The parent is asked if the baby is irritable, lethargic, or if any change in feeding behavior has been noticed. Ask if the infant has had any seizures. Vital signs are assessed to identify any changes from the infant's baseline.

If the child is older, any change in level of consciousness, personality, interaction with the environment, sleep patterns, or delays in developmental milestones needs to be explored with the parents. Attention must be given to complaints of headache that may be relieved with sitting upright and vomiting with no other explanation. If the child has a history of vomiting, the hydrational status should also be assessed.

Nursing Diagnosis

Nursing diagnoses that may apply to the infant or child with hydrocephalus include those common to other neurologic disorders:

- Altered Tissue Perfusion (Cerebral) related to increased ICP
- Altered Nutrition: Less Than Body Requirements related to nausea, vomiting, or decreased level of consciousness
- Anxiety related to change in the child's health status or the child's need for surgery
- Risk for Injury related to seizures
- Risk for Impaired Skin Integrity related to surgical placement of shunt and tubing tunneled under skin

Care related to these nursing diagnoses is detailed in the general care plan at the beginning of the chapter. Other nursing diagnoses that apply to the infant or child with hydrocephalus are:

- Risk for Infection related to shunt placement
- Pain related to operative procedure
- Knowledge Deficit related to home care and signs and symptoms of shunt malfunction or complications

Planning, Implementation, and Evaluation: The Child With Hydrocephalus

NURSING DIAGNOSIS

- Risk for Infection related to shunt placement

Expected Outcome: The child will:

- demonstrate no elevated temperature
- have a clean, dry suture line
- tolerate feedings well
- exhibit no signs of increased ICP

Intervention	Rationale
1. Monitor temperature q 1–2 hr and p.r.n. Assess for decreased level of consciousness, or vomiting. Also assess for swelling or redness along the shunt tract.	These are the first signs of an infection.
2. Assess head, abdominal, and chest dressings for drainage. Test drainage for glucose on a Dextrostix or check for a halo sign on gauze.	Drainage could be CSF, indicating a route for infection to reach the brain. CSF contains glucose and makes a halo on gauze.
3. Position the child off the shunt site so that no weight is placed on the valve for the first 2 days.	Prevents skin breakdown and reduces risk of infection
4. Administer intravenous antibiotics as ordered and monitor serum levels to prevent subtherapeutic or toxic levels.	*Staphylococcus epidermis* infection is the major complication of shunts.
5. Teach the parents the dressing change technique, and show them how to recognize shunt infection or malfunction.	Parents need to know how to care for their child at home and when to seek medical attention for him.

Evaluation: The child:

- is infection free
- has a clean, dry suture site

The parents will:

- demonstrate dressing changes with aseptic technique
- state the signs of infection

NURSING DIAGNOSIS

- Pain related to operative procedure

Expected Outcome:

- The child will have pain relief, as evidenced by sleeping restfully, playing whenever possible, and verbalizing pain relief.

Intervention	Rationale
1. Assess child's pain level, activity, and irritability, and give pain medications p.r.n. Administer analgesics (e.g. codeine) as ordered if needed.	Pain relief will help decrease crying and decreases ICP and metabolic demands. Codeine does not interfere with the child's level of consciousness.
2. Hold, cuddle, and distract the child. Teach therapeutic play to family/caregivers.	Nonpharmacologic methods of pain management also decrease ICP.

Evaluation: The child will:

- smile and react with the caregivers
- have vital signs that are normal for age

NURSING DIAGNOSIS

- Knowledge Deficit related to home care and signs and symptoms of shunt malfunction or complications

Expected Outcome: The parents will:

- demonstrate assessment of the child's level of consciousness
- discuss the shunt's purpose and function
- discuss signs of infection

Intervention	Rationale
1. Assess parents' knowledge of changes in the child's level of consciousness. Begin teaching on their level of understanding.	Parents need to understand that shunt malfunction will cause increased ICP.
2. Teach the parents to observe the child for abdominal distension or discomfort (Williams, Hays & McCool, 1996).	Shunt placement may cause an ileus or peritonitis.
3. Teach the parents to observe for poor feeding, nausea or vomiting, elevated temperature, and skin redness or tenderness.	All signs of an infection should be reported to the physician.
4. Teach parents safety measures about home care, playing, and car seats with padding.	It is important to provide anticipatory guidance for the growing child.
5. Stress the importance of neurosurgical follow-up care.	The shunt may need revision as the child grows.

Evaluation: The parents:

- discuss care of child with a shunt
- describe signs of shunt malfunction

Cerebral Palsy

Cerebral palsy is a chronic, nonprogressive major cause of pediatric disability. It is characterized by a difficulty in controlling the muscles due to an abnormality in the extrapyramidal or pyramidal motor system (motor cortex, **basal ganglia,** cerebellum).

Etiology. The damage to the motor system can occur during the prenatal, perinatal, or postnatal periods and is classified as such.

Prenatal

Maternal diabetes
Rh or ABO incompatibility
Rubella in the first trimester
Genetic
Intrauterine ischemic event
Toxoplasmosis
Cytomegalovirus
Congenital brain abnormality

Perinatal

Asphyxia from umbilical cord around the neck
Low birth weight
Premature
Precipitous delivery
Pregnancy-induced hypertension
Birth trauma
Anoxia
Prolonged labor
Perinatal metabolic condition (diabetes)
Intracranial hemorrhage

Postnatal

Infections
Trauma
Stroke
Poisoning

Incidence. Approximately 1.5 to 5 per 1000 live births in the United States results in a child with cerebral palsy.

PATHOPHYSIOLOGY *of Cerebral Palsy*

A number of neuromuscular disabilities are associated with cerebral palsy. The alteration in voluntary muscular control is related to a cerebral insult. The type of neuromuscular disability is related to the area of the brain that has been injured.

There are five classifications of cerebral palsy: atheoid, spastic, ataxic, rigid, and mixed. *Atheoid (dyskinetic) palsy* refers to an injury in the basal ganglia. This is characterized by slow, writhing movements that are uncontrolled and involuntary, involving all extremities.

Spastic cerebral palsy is the most common type; the affected area of the brain is the cortex. It is characterized by increased deep tendon reflexes, hypertonia, flexion, and sometimes contractures. The child's muscles are very tense, and any stimulus may cause a sudden jerking movement. The child needs to make a conscious effort to relax. There may be a scissor gait, hip flexion with adduction and internal rotation, or toe walking due to tight heel cords.

In *ataxic cerebral palsy* the affected area of the brain is the cerebellum. There is a loss of coordination, equilibrium, and kinesthetic sense. The overall appearance of the child is clumsy.

The child with *rigid/tremor/atonic cerebral palsy* is relatively rare. This child has rigidity of both flexor and extensor muscles. The child with tremors demonstrates them both at rest and on movement. There is a poor prognosis for the child with this type of cerebral palsy because of associated deformities and lack of active movement.

Approximately half the children with cerebral palsy will have some degree of mental retardation and other handicaps. Other than epilepsy and mental retardation, there may be problems with learning, poor attention span, hyperactivity, hearing or visual loss, and emotional problems. Gastroesophageal reflux may be a problem (see Chapter 25). There is a high expenditure of calories with the intense movements, and difficulty feeding leads to a calorie deficit.

Clinical Manifestations

The manifestations of cerebral palsy may vary, and one or more of the following may be observed in any one child.

- Persistence of primitive reflexes
- Delayed gross motor development
- Lack of progression through the developmental milestones
- Abnormal posturing, inability to maintain normal posture and balance
- Spasticity or uncontrollable movements in the extremities
- Disturbances of gait, particularly ataxia and toe walking
- Seizures
- Attention deficit disorder
- Sensory impairment
- Failure of automatic reactions (equilibrium)
- Speech and swallowing impairments

Diagnostic Evaluation. Diagnostic tests include EEG, CT, electrolyte levels, and a thorough neurologic examination. Persistent primitive reflexes are seen, as well as abnormal muscle tone and posture, and abnormal motor development.

Therapeutic Management. The goal of managing the child with cerebral palsy is early recognition and intervention to maximize the child's abilities. It is often not diagnosed before age 2 years. The child will learn through repetition to develop patterns through alternative receptor sites in the brain to gain new pathways for proper motor function. The child may be intellectually intact, but this may be overlooked because of the child's physical limitations.

The multidisciplinary health care team approach is necessary to meet the many needs of the child with cerebral palsy. The team includes the child and family, a pediatrician, neurologist, orthopedic surgeon, nurse, speech and hearing therapist, social worker, occupational physical therapist, and educators.

NURSING CARE OF THE CHILD WITH CEREBRAL PALSY

The nursing care of the child with cerebral palsy includes the multidisciplinary approach. Family teaching includes techniques for feeding, carrying, dressing, bathing, playing, and use of adaptive equipment.

Assessment

The most important component of assessment is identification. Identifying and tracking the infant at risk is imperative. The infant identified at risk is then monitored for irritability, feeding difficulties, delayed development, poor motor development, abnormal posturing, persistence of infant reflexes, ataxic gait, and poor muscle tone. Assessing the child's response to therapy is important. Monitoring and documenting progress or lack of progress is just as important as identifying problems.

> The nurse needs to be aware of normal growth and development with special attention to developmental milestones. Delay in reaching these milestones is one of the key indicators of cerebral palsy (Burns et al., 1996).

Nursing Diagnosis

Nursing diagnoses that may apply to the child with cerebral palsy include those common to other neurologic disorders:

- Altered Nutrition: Less Than Body Requirements related to difficulty chewing or swallowing and increased activity
- Risk for Impaired Skin Integrity related to use of splints and braces
- Anxiety (Parental) related to uncertainty of child's condition
- Knowledge Deficit (Parental) related to home care and needed therapies

Care related to these nursing diagnoses is detailed in the general care plan at the beginning of the chapter. Other nursing diagnoses that apply to the infant or child with cerebral palsy are:

- Impaired Physical Mobility related to spasticity and muscle weakness
- Altered Growth and Development related to neuromuscular impairment
- Impaired Verbal Communication related to neuromuscular impairment and difficulty with articulation
- Risk for Injury related to spasticity, uncontrolled muscle movements, or seizures

Planning, Implementation, and Evaluation: The Child With Cerebral Palsy

NURSING DIAGNOSIS • Impaired Physical Mobility related to spasticity and muscle weakness

Expected Outcome: The child will:
- maximize ability for movement
- be free of contractures or injuries
- be free of complications from immobility

Intervention	Rationale
1. Reinforce physical therapy exercises to strengthen and help coordination of muscles.	Early intervention and consistent therapy will facilitate proper posture and avoid contractures.
2. Encourage parents to be active in the child's daily physical and occupational therapy.	Parents will integrate therapy skills into the child's ADLs.
3. Assess and document the child's response to physical therapy.	Alterations in therapies may be made in a timely fashion for a higher degree of success.
4. Evaluate the need for special equipment for reading, writing, eating, and mobility.	Use of special equipment will enhance chances of success in self-care.

Evaluation:
- The child demonstrates improved mobility and self-care.
- The parents demonstrate physical therapy techniques used for their child.

NURSING DIAGNOSIS • Altered Growth and Development related to neuromuscular impairment

Expected Outcome: The child will:
- explore ways to learn
- participate with other children in some activities

Intervention	Rationale
1. Assess child's developmental level and intelligence.	The child with cerebral palsy should be given opportunities to learn and be exposed to new experiences.
2. Encourage early intervention and participation in school programs.	Interventions with multidisciplinary groups will maximize the child's potential for learning.
3. Communicate and interact with the child on his functional level, not his chronological age.	A child with normal intelligence should be spoken to on his level, but a child with decreased intelligence needs to be spoken to at his developmental level.

Evaluation:
- The child attends public school and plays with peers whenever possible.
- The child receives physical, speech, and occupational therapies at school.
- The parents maximize the child's potential.

NURSING DIAGNOSIS
- Risk for Injury related to spasticity, uncontrolled muscle movements, or seizures

Expected Outcome:
- The child will have a safe environment and not be injured.

Intervention	Rationale
1. Provide a safe environment; remove sharp objects.	Providing a safe environment will reduce the risk of injury.
2. Use protective helmet if the child falls frequently.	Protects from sustaining a head injury.
3. Implement bedside seizure precautions. (Do not pad the rails with pillows.)	Keeping suction, oxygen, and airway equipment at the bedside, and padding the side rails are all measures to prevent injury, and provide for resuscitation of the child if necessary. Pillows may cause suffocation.
4. Provide safe, appropriate toys for age and developmental level.	No sharp, very small, or easily shattered toys should be allowed for the child who may fall while having a seizure.
5. Position upright after meals.	Prevents aspiration secondary to gastroesophageal reflux.

Evaluation:
- The child is not injured.
- The child does not aspirate.
- The parents demonstrate safety measures for the child.

NURSING DIAGNOSIS
- Impaired Verbal Communication related to neuromuscular impairment and difficulty with articulation

Expected Outcome: The child will:
- express needs
- develop methods for communication with others

Intervention	Rationale
1. Use flash cards and talking boards to facilitate communication.	Helps reinforce language and speech development, and increases self-esteem.

Intervention	Rationale
2. Refer the child to a speech therapist.	Early intervention will maximize speech capabilities.
3. Encourage and reinforce speech therapy techniques, nonverbal methods to communicate, proper feeding techniques, and jaw control.	Facilitates communication and decreases the child's frustration with not being understood. Facilitates goals of speech therapy.

Evaluation: The child:

- participates with groups with appropriate communication
- uses various methods to communicate

The parents:

- allow time for the child to respond to questions and conversations
- learn the communication method that the child learns

INFECTIOUS DISORDERS

Meningitis

Meningitis is an infectious process of the CNS that may occur as a primary disease or as the result of complications of neurosurgery, trauma, systemic infection, or sinus/ear infections. A wide variety of bacteria and viruses can be responsible for the primary infection. Earlier diagnosis and improved antibiotic therapy have reduced the mortality and incidence of complications from bacterial meningitis.

Etiology. The primary bacterial organisms responsible for causing bacterial meningitis vary according to age. However, among children aged 2 months to 12 years, three pathogens seem to be the most prevalent. *Haemophilus influenzae* (type B), *Neisseria meningitidis,* and *Streptococcus pneumoniae* cause 95% of the cases of purulent meningitis in this age-group. These types of meningitis usually result from an extension of a localized infection such as otitis media, sinusitis, pharyngitis, or pneumonia into the CSF. The organisms primarily responsible for neonatal meningitis are group B streptococci and *Escherichia coli.*

Organisms may also be introduced directly after an injury in which the skin is broken and communication between skin, sinuses, and CSF occurs. Entry may occur in association with a lumbar puncture, skull fracture, or surgery.

Meningococcal meningitis caused by *Neisseria* usually occurs in older children and adolescents. Because it is transmitted primarily by droplet infection, the risk increases as the number of contacts increases.

Viral meningitis is associated with such viruses as mumps, paramyxovirus, herpes, and enterovirus. In rare

PATHOPHYSIOLOGY *of Meningitis*

Meningitis causes an inflammation of the meninges of the brain. This inflammatory process is the result of a pathogen entering the CNS and causing a toxic response. As the process continues, increased ICP develops along with subdural empyema. If the infection spreads to the ventricles, edema and tissue scarring around the ventricle results in obstruction of the CSF, resulting in hydrocephalus.

This process can happen very rapidly because the CSF is an excellent growth medium for bacteria, containing nutrient substances such as protein and glucose. Leukocytes are unable to function as a defense mechanism in the fluid environment of the CSF. Leukocytes require a tissue surface to destroy bacteria, so there is little defense to stop the growth of bacteria and it can multiply quickly.

As the infection spreads further into brain tissue, changes occur in the permeability of capillaries and blood vessels in the dura mater. These changes lead to increased passage of albumin and water into the subdural space with a subsequent accumulation of protein and fluid. This results in further increased ICP.

The most common neurologic sequelae of meningitis are hearing loss, mental retardation, seizures, visual impairment, and behavioral problems (Behrman, Kliegman, & Arvin, 1996). Other complications include cranial nerve dysfunction, brain abscess, and syndrome of secretion of inappropriate antidiuretic hormone (SIADH).

cases, protozoa or fungi are the infecting organisms. These are seen most frequently in children with AIDS.

Incidence. Meningitis most commonly affects children between ages 1 month and 5 years. Boys are affected more frequently than girls, and risk factors increase where individuals are in close contact with one another (day-care centers or large families in small dwellings). There is a higher incidence in African American children than in Caucasian children. The incidence of *H. influenzae* type B related to meningitis is rapidly declining since the immunization of infants was begun.

Clinical Manifestations. Signs and symptoms of meningitis vary depending on the age of the child and the duration of the preceding illness. There is no one hallmark sign or symptom.

Clinical Signs in the Neonate

- Poor feeding
- Poor sucking
- Vomiting
- Diarrhea
- Poor muscle tone
- Poor cry
- Hypothermia and/or hyperthermia
- Apnea
- Seizures
- Sepsis
- Disseminated intravascular coagulation

Clinical Signs in the Infant and Child

- Fever
- Poor feeding
- Vomiting
- Irritability
- Seizures
- High-pitched cry
- Bulging anterior fontanel

In the neonate, infant, and young child the symptoms of meningitis are frequently vague and nonspecific.

Early Clinical Signs in Children and Adolescents

- Severe headache
- Photophobia
- Nuchal rigidity
- Fever
- Altered level of consciousness (lethargy, irritability)
- Poor feeding
- Vomiting
- Diarrhea
- Muscle or joint pain
- Purpura or joint pain
- Kernig's sign: pain with extension of leg and knee (Fig. 40–5)
- Brudzinski's sign: flexion of head causes flexion of hips and knees (Fig. 40–5)

Late Clinical Signs in Children and Adolescents

- Changes in the level of consciousness
- Seizures

Diagnostic Evaluation. Diagnosis is made by testing CSF obtained by lumbar puncture. Findings usually include increased pressure, cloudy CSF (in the case of bacterial meningitis), high protein, and low glucose (see chart of CSF findings in Clinical Reference Pages). Blood cultures may be done, and nose and throat cultures may occasionally be helpful if the CSF is negative.

Therapeutic Management

Acute bacterial meningitis is a medical emergency requiring early recognition and prompt, aggressive management.

Isolation is begun and maintained for at least 24 hours after antibiotics are given. Prompt initiation and uninterrupted administration of appropriate intravenous antibiotics is essential with a suspected diagnosis of bacterial meningitis. Treatment is started before the causative organism is identified because cultures may take up to 3 days to yield results. It is vital to start antibiotics early because delay could be fatal. Antibiotic therapy is based on the age of the child, the most frequently encountered pathogen for that age-group, and the initial appearance of the CSF. If intravenous access is difficult, the first dose of antibiotics should be administered intramuscularly.

Treatment for neonatal bacterial meningitis consists of ampicillin and an aminoglycoside or a third-generation cephalosporin. For older children and adolescents, the treatment of choice is ampicillin and penicillin G. The initial choice of antibiotics must be a broad-spectrum one so that most of the suspected pathogens will be covered. After the culture and sensitivity reports are available, initial treatment regimens may have to be changed. The treatment for viral meningitis is symptomatic and supportive, usually with complete recovery.

NURSING CARE OF THE CHILD WITH MENINGITIS

Assessment

The information from the history and physical will provide baseline data and a complete neurologic assessment, including presence or absence of headaches, photophobia, hearing loss, seizure activity, changes in the level of consciousness, changes in pupil reactions and size, nuchal rigidity, or muscle flaccidity, should be performed. Personality changes and irritability may be noted. Also important to note are any food and fluid intake, nausea, vomiting, or loss of appetite. Other important points to note from the history are recent immunizations or any recent

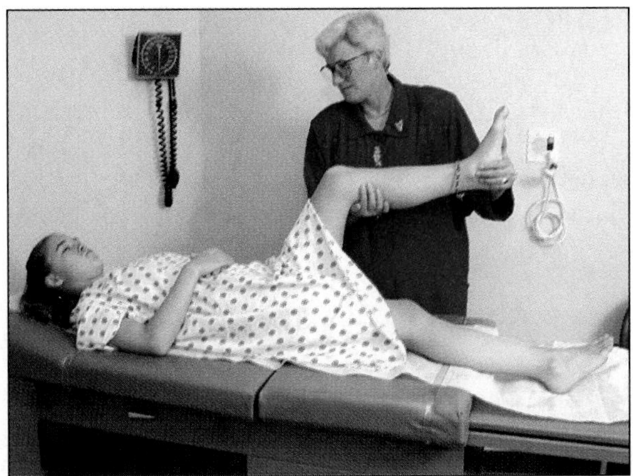

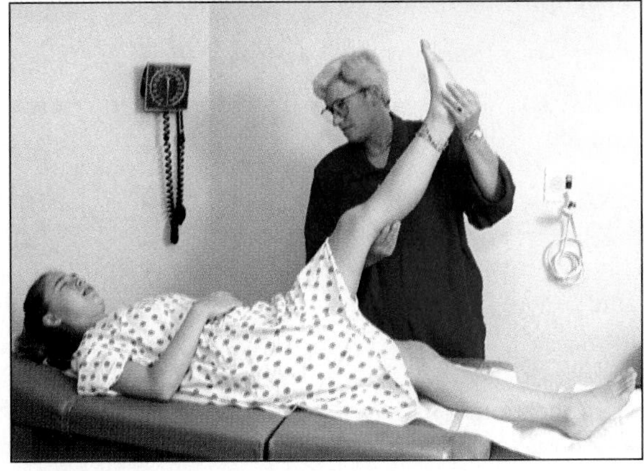

Kernig's Sign
The child can easily extend the leg when in the supine position. However, when the thigh is flexed toward the abdomen, pain prevents complete extension of the leg.

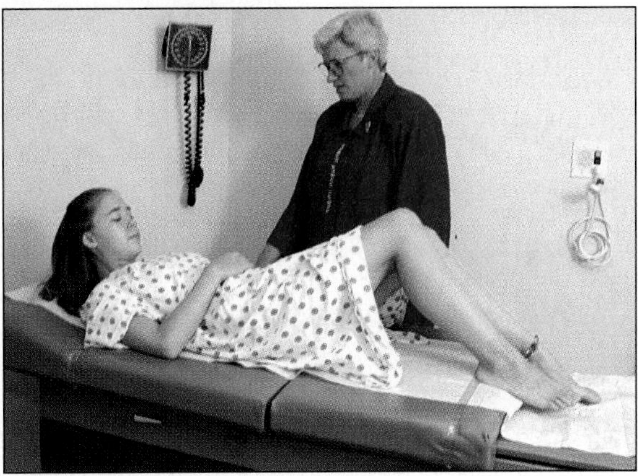

Brudzinski's Sign
In the supine position, the child bends her head toward her chest. (In a younger child, the nurse can bend the child's head.) This action usually produces involuntary hip and knee flexion in the child with meningitis.

Figure 40–5
As part of the assessment for meningitis, the nurse can attempt to elicit Kernig's sign and Brudzinski's sign. Both are early signs of meningitis in children and adolescents. (Courtesy of Parkland Memorial Hospital, Dallas, Texas)

illnesses, such as upper respiratory infections, otitis media, surgery, skull fracture, or previous lumbar puncture.

Early recognition and treatment of complications is essential and can substantially reduce morbidity and mortality. Thorough knowledge of the disease process is vital, and assessments must be complete and frequent to note any changes in the child's condition.

Nursing Diagnosis

Nursing diagnoses that may apply to the child with meningitis include those common to other neurologic disorders:

- Altered Tissue Perfusion (Cerebral) related to increased ICP
- Altered Nutrition: Less Than Body Requirements related to decreased level of consciousness, nausea, and vomiting
- Anxiety related to seriousness of meningitis and possible residual neurologic deficits
- Pain related to meningeal irritation (headache)
- Risk for Fluid Volume Deficit related to vomiting
- Risk for Injury related to seizures, increased ICP
- Risk for Altered Body Temperature related to acute infectious process
- Altered Family Processes related to child with an acute illness
- Anticipatory Grieving related to possible neurologic deficits

Care related to these nursing diagnoses is detailed in the general care plan at the beginning of the chapter as well as in other care plans throughout this chapter. Nursing care related to the following diagnosis is detailed in the care plan below:

- Knowledge Deficit related to seriousness of meningitis and possible residual neurologic deficits

TEACHING GUIDELINES *for the Child With Meningitis*

- The close contacts of the child with *H. influenzae* need prophylactic treatment with rifampin.
- Anyone spending at least 4 hours out of the 5–7 days previous to the child's hospitalization with *H. influenzae* need prophylactic treatment if they are not already immunized.
- All close contacts of children with *Neisseria meningitidis* need prophylactic treatment regardless of age or immunization status.
- Rifampin colors the urine and sweat red-orange, and will stain contact lenses.

Planning, Implementation, and Evaluation: The Child With Meningitis

NURSING DIAGNOSIS • Knowledge Deficit related to seriousness of meningitis and possible residual neurologic deficits

Expected Outcome: • The parents will discuss the disease process and possible sequelae, treatment, and possible implications for spread of the disease.

Intervention	Rationale
1. Discuss the disease process and prognosis with the parents. Assess their knowledge of the disease process.	The parents will learn what the disease is, how it is spread, and how to follow up on treatment (see Teaching Guidelines).
2. Teach the family the possible complications and sequelae of meningitis. Discuss the importance of follow-up care.	Complications of meningitis may include hydrocephalus, vision and hearing loss, delayed growth and development, seizures, subdural effusions, and cranial nerve palsy.
3. Have parents identify others exposed to meningitis and refer for treatment.	Close contacts should not wait for signs of meningitis to develop. They should seek medical attention because they could be incubating the infection.
4. Instruct parents on prescribed medications and treatments. Document instructions and return demonstration by parents or caregiver.	Parents will be anxious and grieving about the child's illness and outcome; learning will be difficult. To be sure the parents have learned, watch them perform the necessary procedures.

Evaluation: The parents:

- demonstrate that they can administer the child's care and medication
- discuss the disease and treatments
- refer close contacts for treatment

Encephalitis

Encephalitis is an inflammation of the brain as a result of a viral illness or CNS infection. The signs and symptoms of encephalitis are a change in the level of consciousness, irritability, motor or sensory deficits, and seizure activity. It may follow measles, chickenpox, rubella, or immunizations.

Pathophysiology. A toxin or infectious pathogen enters the brain, producing an inflammatory response. This inflammation causes cerebral edema, cellular damage, and neurologic dysfunction. Invasion of the CNS occurs via the blood and peripheral nerve pathways.

Etiology. Encephalitis is usually associated with an antecedent illness. Viral illnesses such as herpes simplex, rabies, measles, chickenpox, mumps, and rubella have all been implicated. Equine encephalitis, a virus carried by mosquitoes associated with horses, has also been implicated. Herpes simplex I is the most common cause of encephalitis in the neonatal period. Other infections such as meningitis have been associated with encephalitis as well. Toxic encephalitis can follow hyperbilirubinemia or exposure to toxins such as with lead poisoning.

Incidence. Encephalitis occurs in all age-groups. The peak incidence is between ages 5 and 14 years. It affects more than 12,000 children each year in the United States.

Clinical Manifestations

- Headache
- Irritability
- Lethargy
- Altered level of consciousness
- Nuchal rigidity
- Seizures
- Visual, auditory, and speech disturbances

The signs and symptoms of encephalitis depend on the causative agent and the location of the infection within the brain.

Diagnostic Evaluation. Lumbar puncture to culture CSF is performed. Brain biopsy or serum antibody test may be done if cultures are negative. CT or MRI to rule out a focal tumor or lesion may be performed. EEG may be helpful in diagnosis, as generalized slowing of variable degrees is common.

Therapeutic Management. Treatment of encephalitis is supportive. Acyclovir or a third-generation cephalosporin may be ordered until the cause of the encephalitis is determined. The child is hospitalized, monitored, and treated for increased ICP. Anticonvulsant drugs are administered.

NURSING CARE OF THE CHILD WITH ENCEPHALITIS

Assessment

Assessment data includes a thorough history. The nurse should be alert for any history of recent illness, rash, immunizations, or exposure to infectious diseases. Any recent travel, animal bite, or ingestion of poison, drugs, or toxic material should be noted.

A comprehensive neurologic assessment will follow with a focus on neurologic symptoms such as onset, frequency, duration, progression, and specific descriptions.

Nursing Diagnosis and Planning

The following nursing diagnoses and expected outcomes may be appropriate following assessment of the child with encephalitis:

- Altered Tissue Perfusion (Cerebral) related to increased ICP. ***Expected Outcome:*** *The child will maintain normal ICP, as evidenced by having the usual or improved level of consciousness; return to normal motor and sensory function; and stable vital signs.*
- Risk for Injury related to seizures. ***Expected Outcome:*** *The child will sustain no injury during a seizure.*
- Pain related to meningeal irritation. ***Expected Outcome:*** *The child will have diminished severity of headaches.*
- Ineffective Breathing Pattern related to increased ICP and decreased level of consciousness. ***Expected Outcome:*** *The child will have a patent airway with good gas exchange, as evidenced by normal or improved ABGs, no cyanosis, and normal pulse oxygen level.*
- Altered Nutrition: Less Than Body Requirements related to decreased level of consciousness. ***Expected Outcome:*** *The child will maintain a stable body weight.*
- Anxiety (Parental) related to having a child with an acute (critical) illness. ***Expected Outcome:*** *Family members will discuss their fears and begin to prioritize their needs.*
- Knowledge Deficit (Parental) related to the inflammatory process and the child's condition. ***Expected Outcome:*** *The family will verbalize an understanding of the child's condition and participate in the child's care.*
- Anticipatory Grieving (Parental) related to possible neurologic complications. ***Expected Outcome:*** *The parents will discuss the possible outcomes of the illness.*
- Altered Family Process related to having a critically ill child. ***Expected Outcome:*** *The family will discuss possible support mechanisms and begin to plan for discharge.*

Implementation

Encephalitis is caused by a viral infection that produces an inflammatory process in the brain. The response to this process can result in altered neurologic function. Accurate, ongoing assessment of the CNS status of the child is essential to detect changes and institute appropriate clinical management. The nurse must anticipate increasing ICP, minimize the factors that influence a rise in ICP, and be prepared to treat it. The child should be continually assessed for changes in level of consciousness or behavior, headache, nuchal rigidity, alterations in pulse and respirations, pupillary responses, and seizure activity.

The child's temperature should be maintained within a normal range. Fever increases cerebral metabolism and metabolic demands. Antipyretics, cool compresses, or a tepid bath may be indicated. In certain situations a hypothermia blanket may be appropriate. If a hypothermia blanket is used, the nurse must monitor the child's body temperature every hour because it can be reduced rapidly with a hypothermia blanket. The child's skin condition must be assessed often because peripheral circulation is decreased with the use of cooling devices, which could easily lead to skin breakdown.

Fluid and electrolyte balance is another important nursing consideration. Careful attention must be paid to the child's intake and output, as well as other common indicators of hydrational status. Watch the child for signs of fluid overload, such as increasing weight, abnormal electrolytes and hematocrit, edema, and changes in level of consciousness.

The child with encephalitis may have headaches that range in intensity from mild to severe. Pain management is an important issue. Once the presence of headache has been determined and the intensity ascertained, the nurse will administer appropriate pharmacologic agents as prescribed by the physician. The nurse can institute nonpharmacologic pain management strategies as well, including distraction, rhythmic breathing, and cutaneous stimulation. Reducing environmental stimuli such as light and noise will help.

The seriousness of encephalitis combined with a long recovery period and possible subsequent neurologic deficit are major stressors for the child and her family. The nurse must be alert to their behavioral responses and anticipate reactions such as fear, anxiety, and ineffective coping. The nurse should be calm, supportive, and understanding with an ability to listen and encourage verbalization. Parent participation is an effective coping mechanism and should be encouraged by the health care team.

Encephalitis may present with mild to severe symptoms. The child may progress rapidly to recovery or to neurologic deterioration and coma or death. The prognosis depends on a number of factors: causative agent, patient health status, prompt recognition of the child's declining condition, and effective early intervention by the health care team. The nurse at the bedside plays a key role in maximizing a positive outcome by being alert to subtle changes in the child's condition.

Evaluation

- Has the child's neurologic status improved?
- Have the vital signs returned to baseline for the child?
- Do the parents/caregivers verbalize a realistic understanding of the disease process and the follow-up care that is needed?

Reye Syndrome

Reye syndrome is an acute encephalopathy characterized by a viral infection followed by hepatic, metabolic, neurologic failure.

Pathophysiology. Liver cell damage interrupts the normal waste removal process. The urea cycle is disrupted, resulting in an accumulation of ammonia in the serum (0–80 μg/dl is normal). As the disease progresses, serum ammonia level continues to rise to toxic levels, resulting in cerebral dysfunction. Further liver dysfunction results in fluid and electrolyte imbalance, metabolic acidosis, hypoglycemia, dehydration, and coagulopathies. The development of encephalopathy, cerebral edema, and increased ICP results in neurologic complications.

Etiology. The exact cause of Reye syndrome is not clear. Many theories of susceptibility exist; some point to exposure to viral agents or toxins; others suggest that such exposure merely precipitates the disease in infants or children already at risk. The role of salicylates is also unknown. It may be a synergistic co-factor, with an unknown host factor in combination with a viral illness, such as varicella or influenza.

> The American Academy of Pediatrics recommends that aspirin not be administered to children with varicella or influenza because of its association with Reye syndrome. Acetaminophen is considered the drug of choice for pediatric patients (Behrman, Kliegman, & Arvin, 1996).

Incidence. Reye syndrome occurs in children from infancy through adolescence, with the average age being 6 to 7 years. It is rare in adults. Males and females are affected equally. Because pediatricians now recommend that aspirin not be administered to pediatric patients, the incidence of Reye syndrome has dramatically decreased in recent years.

Clinical Manifestations

- History of systemic viral illness 4 to 7 days before the onset of symptoms
- Malaise
- Nausea
- Vomiting
- Progressive neurologic deterioration

A proposed staging system for Reye syndrome is presented in Table 40–1.

TABLE 40–1 *Clinical Staging of Reye Syndrome*

GRADE	SYMPTOMS AT TIME OF ADMISSION
I	Usually quiet, **lethargic** and sleepy, vomiting, laboratory evidence of liver dysfunction
II	Deep lethargy, **confusion,** delirium, combative, hyperventilation, hyperreflexic
III	Obtunded, **light coma** ± seizures, decorticate rigidity, intact pupillary light reaction
IV	Seizures, deepening coma, **decerebrate rigidity,** loss of oculocephalic reflexes, fixed pupils
V	Coma, loss of deep tendon reflexes, respiratory arrest, fixed dilated pupils, **flaccidity/decerebrate** (intermittent); isoelectric electroencephalogram

From Behrman, R. E., Kliegman, R. M., & Arvin, A. M. (1996). *Nelson textbook of pediatrics* (15th ed., p. 1144). Philadelphia: W. B. Saunders.

Diagnostic Evaluation. Elevated serum ammonia levels are noted. Liver biopsy reveals liver dysfunction. Respiratory dysfunction and increased ICP are noted. Blood glucose levels reveal hypoglycemia. Coagulation times may be altered due to liver dysfunction.

Therapeutic Management. The major elements of medical and nursing care are to maintain effective cerebral perfusion and control increasing ICP. On admission, a rapid but thorough neurologic assessment is performed to establish a baseline. Further assessment in the form of diagnostic testing may be undertaken at a later time. A complete set of vital signs is obtained with special emphasis on cardiovascular and respiratory function. These evaluations are important because increasing ICP will alter the function of these systems first. Assessment of hydration is also important. Reye syndrome begins with severe vomiting that may quickly lead to dehydration. However, overreplacement of fluids may led to cerebral edema, so maintenance of fluid and electrolyte balance is very important.

NURSING CARE OF THE CHILD WITH REYE SYNDROME

Assessment

The key to nursing care for a child with Reye syndrome is assessment because the child is at high risk for sudden deterioration. The child is cared for in the intensive care unit, where frequent neurologic assessments and frequent vital sign checks can be made. Increased ICP should be monitored and interventions to lower increased ICP initiated to prevent neurologic sequelae. The progression of Reye syndrome may be gradual or fulminant so the value of rapid recognition and swift effective management cannot be overemphasized.

Nursing Diagnosis and Planning

The following nursing diagnoses and expected outcomes may be appropriate following assessment of the child with Reye syndrome:

- Altered Tissue Perfusion (Cerebral) related to increased ICP. ***Expected Outcomes:*** *The child will have a high level of consciousness, remain alert and oriented, obey commands, and interact with the environment and caregivers.*
- Ineffective Breathing Pattern related to decreased level of consciousness or increased ICP or to cerebral edema. ***Expected Outcomes:*** *The child will have normal ABGs, clear breath sounds, and normal rate and depth of respiration.*
- Decreased Cardiac Output related to decreased circulatory volume. ***Expected Outcomes:*** *The child will have a normal blood pressure, pulse, and urine output of 1 to 2 ml/kg/hr.*
- Risk for Injury related to hypoglycemia. ***Expected Outcome:*** *The child will maintain blood glucose levels as follows:*

  Infant: 50–90 mg/dl
  Child: 60–100 mg/dl
  Adolescent: 70–105 mg/dl
- Knowledge Deficit related to disease process. ***Expected Outcome:*** *The parents will discuss the disease process and possible outcomes for the child, and begin to plan discharge to home or rehabilitation facility.*

Implementation

The nurse must assess the child's neurologic status, including level of consciousness, reflexes, posturing, and seizure activity. The child may be in the intensive care unit so direct ICP monitoring may be used. The child may need to be intubated and hyperventilated.

The child's cardiovascular and respiratory status is monitored hourly. Observations should include the rate, depth, and symmetry of respirations. Pulse oximetry is valuable. Other important hourly assessments are heart rate, blood pressure, and peripheral perfusion. Hypovolemia or poor systemic perfusion is treated with aggressive fluid administration if signs of increased ICP are not present. Hypertonic intravenous solutions (10% to 15% glucose), blood products, or colloids may be used to maintain the serum osmolality between 275 and 295 mOsm/L.

As liver functions are altered, the nurse should be alert to signs of bleeding. Overt as well as covert bleeding is possible. This may be treated with vitamin K, fresh frozen plasma, or platelet transfusions.

The level of the parents' anxiety may be profound. Any child with an altered level of consciousness generates tremendous anxiety and concern in his parents. The inability to predict the outcome adds to the anxiety. Verbalization and expression of feelings needs to be encouraged, and accurate information about the child's condition needs to be provided with referrals to appropriate resources. The nurse can support the role of the parent as the primary caregiver by encouraging participation in the care of the child when possible. Frequent visitation and interaction should be supported by the nurse if possible, and the environment and treatment modalities explained.

Evaluation

- Is the child's level of consciousness improved?
- Do the ABGs show good oxygenation?
- Are the results of neurologic checks normal?
- Does the child have any signs of liver dysfunction?
- Do the parents verbalize an understanding of the disease process and uncertain outcome of their child?
- Do the parents participate in some of the child's care?

Guillain-Barré Syndrome (Postinfectious Polyneuritis)

Guillian-Barré syndrome (GBS) is a progressive motor weakness in association with an infection. The infection may have been upper respiratory, possibly viral in nature, such as rubella, enterovirus, or varicella. The syndrome may also occur as a toxic response to immunizations. The cause is unknown but may be related to an autoimmune or inflammatory response, which produces demyelination of the motor and sometimes sensory nerves.

Pathophysiology. The most prominent feature of GBS is the infiltration of lymphocytes in peripheral nerves, causing inflammation. Initially, the myelin sheath becomes edematous; as further inflammation takes place, segmental demyelinization occurs. This process takes place along the membrane surrounding the Schwann cells. As the inflammatory process continues, myelin loss increases and results in axonal degeneration.

Incidence. GBS affects approximately 1 to 1.5 people per 100,000 per year worldwide. It affects all ages. It occurs moderately more often in males.

Clinical Manifestations

- *Limb paresthesias and/or pain,* including numbness, tingling, and weakness of the lower extremities with an ascending loss of deep tendon reflexes leading to a flaccid paralysis.
- *Autonomic instability,* including blood pressure fluctuations, cardiac arrhythmias, postural hypotension, and urinary and bowel incontinence, may occur.
- *Cranial nerve dysfunction* may occur, such as facial nerve paralysis, dysphagia, and poor cough, gag, and swallow reflexes. If this occurs respiratory function will be impaired.
- *Respiratory failure* results from the progressive motor paralysis of the intercostal and phrenic nerves.

> Respiratory failure is the greatest threat and the primary cause of death in Guillain-Barré syndrome.

- *Neuromuscular impairment* (bilateral ascending weakness or paralysis) usually progresses upward from the feet to the head and is reversed as healing takes place.

Diagnostic Evaluation. Bilateral ascending weakness or paralysis following an upper respiratory infection by a week or two is a diagnostic indication. The CSF may demonstrate high protein levels.

Therapeutic Management. Medical management of the child with GBS is supportive, with attention given to the neurologic, respiratory, and cardiovascular systems. Special attention to respiratory support is needed, as most deaths are attributed to respiratory failure. Plasmapheresis may be beneficial.

NURSING CARE OF THE CHILD WITH GUILLAIN-BARRÉ SYNDROME

Assessment

A complete history and physical examination is important to determine the presence of an antecedent viral illness and to establish baseline clinical status. Special attention is given to the respiratory and neurologic systems. Respiratory assessment should take place frequently because of the risk of respiratory compromise and the need for prompt action should the child's respiratory status deteriorate. Major assessment parameters include respiratory rate, chest excursion, work of breathing, and breath sounds. Pulse oximetry is helpful. Daily pulmonary function testing is necessary. The frequency of neurologic assessment depends on the clinical condition of the child. Neurologic parameters include cranial nerve function, motor capabilities, sensory perception, and deep tendon reflexes.

Nursing Diagnosis and Planning

The following nursing diagnoses and expected outcomes may be appropriate following assessment of the child with Guillain-Barré syndrome.

- Ineffective Breathing Pattern related to neuromuscular impairment. ***Expected Outcomes:*** *The child will have clear bilateral breath sounds, good chest expansion, and normal tidal volume.*
- Sensory/Perceptual Alterations (Visual, Auditory, Kinesthetic, and Tactile) related to neuromuscular impairment. ***Expected Outcomes:*** *The child will communicate with caregivers by use of eye blinks or direction of eye movements to express answers to questions about positioning, comfort, movements, and need for touch.*
- Decreased Cardiac Output related to autonomic instability. ***Expected Outcomes:*** *The child will have brisk capillary refill, normal urine output, good pulses in all extremities, and no arrhythmias.*
- Risk for Impaired Skin Integrity related to immobility with paralysis. ***Expected Outcome:*** *The child will have no skin breakdown and no pressure sores.*
- Impaired Verbal Communication related to neuromuscular impairment. ***Expected Outcome:*** *The child will demonstrate new ways to communicate using available muscles.*
- Altered Urinary Elimination related to paralysis. ***Expected Outcomes:*** *The child will have an empty bladder and no urinary tract infection or distension of the abdomen. Urine output will be 1 to 2 ml/kg/hr.*
- Anxiety related to increasing ascending paralysis. ***Expected Outcome:*** *The child will calmly interact with caregivers, with decreased fretful periods and increased restful periods.*
- Knowledge Deficit related to disease progression and home care. ***Expected Outcomes:*** *The child and parents*

will make plans about discharge care. The parents will discuss the child's illness and possible complications.

- Altered Family Processes related to having a child with a prolonged illness. ***Expected Outcome:*** *The parents will discuss support systems and changes in the family.*

Implementation

The goal of nursing care for the child with GBS is to achieve optimal neurologic functioning with an emphasis on maintaining independence in activities of daily living, and facilitate a recovery without complication.

Treatment is largely supportive with a focus on assessing and monitoring the clinical status of the child, and preventing or minimizing complications. The nurse must be able to recognize changes in the child's condition and intervene in a timely and effective manner. Initially, the nurse must provide respiratory support if the respiratory system becomes compromised and muscles weaken and become flaccid. Resuscitation and ventilatory support may be needed, the appropriate emergency equipment and personnel should be at hand.

> Anticipate a deterioration in respiratory status. Emergency equipment such as a bag-valve-mask device, oxygen, suction, endotracheal tubes, laryngoscope, blade, and stylet should be at the bedside.

Interruption in the autonomic nervous system reflexes can cause circulatory changes, resulting in arrhythmias, hypotension, dizziness, and night sweats. Early detection of neurologic changes are made by serial assessments and prompt action should be taken to correct problems and prevent complication.

The child with GBS is at an increased risk for developing complications associated with immobility. Maintaining skin integrity is a priority. Frequent turning and repositioning, attention to pressure points, and use of special mattresses are all important steps to take to prevent skin breakdown. Managing incontinence also will help prevent skin breakdown.

To prevent contractures, physical and occupational therapy must be initiated as part of the child's daily routine. Range of motion, self-help exercises, correct alignment, and application of splints and braces are part of the child's daily care.

> Anticipate loss of motor function and initiate preventive nursing measures, such as passive range of motion, turning, and repositioning at least every 2 hours. Chest physiotherapy should be done every 2 to 4 hours.

The risk of pulmonary embolus as a result of deep vein thrombosis is always a threat; frequent turning and positioning with special attention to positioning of the child's legs to alleviate pressure on the dorsal aspect of the knees is essential. Anticoagulant therapy may be initiated; if so, the nurse should monitor clotting times and watch for any signs of bleeding.

As cranial nerve function is altered and interference with gag and swallow occurs, nutrition becomes an important issue. Adequate caloric intake is essential to prevent catabolism. Alternative methods of providing nutrition must be employed. The physician may consider nasogastric (NG), nasojejunostomy, or gastrostomy feedings. The nurse monitors the type and amount of feeding, tube placement and patency, tolerance of feedings as evidenced by residuals, abdominal distension, stools, and weight gain. Total parenteral nutrition is also an option. This is usually reserved for the acute or critical phase of the illness, or if the child does not tolerate alternative methods of nutritional support.

The progression of the disease is unpredictable, the loss of functioning frightening, and the recovery time variable—from months to years. The long-term implications for nursing care are easily identified. The child and family will require a great deal of emotional support. Full recovery from GBS is possible.

The uncertainty of the progression of the disease can contribute to the anxiety of the child and family. Keep them well informed and answer their questions. If there are questions that cannot be answered by the nurse, refer those to the appropriate health care member. Encourage verbalization of feelings concerning the illness and hospitalization and support and validate the feelings of the family and child.

Foster the child's positive development during the illness by normalizing the situation as much as possible. As the child's clinical condition worsens and he becomes more dependent on the parents, encourage control by offering choices and encouraging decision making when appropriate. Contact the child's teacher for continuation of studies and communication with school friends. Support the role of parent as the primary caregiver by facilitating parent participation. Help the parent support the child. If the child's clinical condition deteriorates enough to warrant transfer to a critical care unit, prepare the family for the move. Initiate telephone contact with the receiving nurse to establish a relationship before transfer to lessen the family's anxiety. If possible, a physician or nurse orientation to the critical care unit will help the family deal with the stress of the transfer. Compassionate and competent health care team members can optimize the child's recovery.

Evaluation

- Does the child demonstrate normal respiratory function?
- Has the child's neurologic status returned to normal?
- Do the parents participate in and discuss the child's care?

SEIZURE DISORDERS

A seizure is an occasional excessive disorderly discharge of neuron activity. Epilepsy is recurrent seizure activity, which can be classified as partial (focal) or generalized (without focal onset). Partial seizures do not necessarily alter consciousness. Generalized seizures are recurrent attacks of altered consciousness usually accompanied by tonic or clonic muscle spasms.

Pathophysiology. During a seizure there is excessive, self-limiting neuronal discharge. The result of this discharge is activation of associated motor or sensory organs. The extent of the seizure depends on the location and extent of the abnormal neuronal discharges. The brain consists of millions of nerve cells. Electrical impulses are sent through many of these cells by means of neurotransmitters. When many of these nerve cells fire abnormally at the same time, a seizure may result.

Etiology. There are many reasons why seizures occur. Seizures are categorized as cerebral, biochemical, post-traumatic, and idiopathic. Cerebral lesions account for a large category of factors that may cause increased neuronal activity. In many children the cause of a cerebral lesion is a static or nonprogressive encephalopathy secondary to hypoxia, hemorrhage, CNS infections, head trauma, or developmental defects of the brain. Biochemical causes of seizures include metabolic and toxic disorders. Any form of head injury can be traumatic enough to cause seizures. About 50% of childhood seizures are idiopathic.

Febrile seizures occur in 3% to 4% of children. The most common age for febrile seizures is 3 months to 5 years. Only about a third of these children ever have another seizure, and about 3% of this group of children develop epilepsy. The height and rapidity of temperature elevation seems to be a factor in precipitating febrile seizures. Temperature is usually elevated above 101.8°F (38.8°C). The seizure activity occurs during the temperature rise rather than after prolonged elevation. Ninety percent of febrile seizures occur as a result of fever caused by otitis media, pharyngitis, and adenitis. The family of a child who experiences a febrile seizure should be given information about these seizures and instructed what to do if another seizure occurs (see Teaching Guidelines).

Incidence. An estimated 3% to 5% of children have seizures during their early years (after age 6 months and before age 3 years). Seizures are unusual after age 5.

Clinical Manifestations. There are many types of seizures. The International Classification of Seizures is used to divide the seizures into two groups: generalized and partial (see the accompanying box).

Because of the lack of **myelinization** of fiber tracts, neonates do not experience the same type of tonic-clonic seizure an older child experiences. Neonatal seizures may be subtle with eyes deviating; clonic, with random and irregular movements; focal; tonic; and/or myoclonic with jerking movements of the extremities. (See Neonatal Seizures, Chapter 21.)

Diagnostic Evaluation. The child's health history and any family history of seizures is important to ascertain. A thorough description of the child's behavior during the seizure activity is important to delineate the type of seizure. Video recording and EEG monitoring will help identify the seizure. Serum electrolyes, CBC, blood glucose, and blood urea nitrogen (BUN) help indicate metabolic causes. Lumbar puncture will help to identify a CNS infection. CT and MRI will indicate trauma or tumor.

Therapeutic Management. The basic tenet of treatment for seizures is to treat the whole child. The goals are to identify and correct the cause of the seizure, eliminate the seizure, prevent further episodes of seizure activity with a minimum of side effects, and normalize the child's and family's lives.

TEACHING GUIDELINES *for the Child With Febrile Seizures*

During the seizure:

1. Turn the child on his side. Do not try to restrain the child.
2. Do not put anything in the child's mouth. Allow the child to drool. You may use a suction bulb to remove saliva or fluids.
3. Call the physician or nurse if any of the following occurs:
   - The seizure lasts more that 2–3 minutes.
   - Another seizure occurs.
   - The child's neck is stiff.
   - The child is delirious or difficult to awaken after the seizure.

Of children who have a febrile seizure, 60% have only one seizure. The other 40% have two to three seizures over the years, usually stopping by age 5 or 6. The average body temperature at which a febrile seizure occurs is 104°F (40°C).

(See Chapter 18 for discussion of care of the child with fever.)

International Classification of Seizures

GENERALIZED SEIZURES

Onset at any age. Clinical features indicate involvement of both cerebral hemispheres. Consciousness is impaired.

Tonic-Clonic Seizures

Tonic-clonic seizures cause an abrupt arrest of activity and loss of consciousness.

The *tonic phase* consists of a sustained, generalized contraction of muscles, including the diaphragm, lasting a few seconds.

The *clonic phase* is symmetrical and rhythmic, consisting of alternating contraction and relaxation of major muscle groups. This phase usually ends spontaneously in less than 5 minutes. Respirations are irregular and may be stridorous. Sphincter incontinence may or may not be present.

The tonic-clonic seizure is followed by a variable period of confusion, lethargy, and sleep.

Atonic Seizures

Atonic seizures cause an abrupt loss of postural tone, loss of consciousness, confusion, lethargy, and sleep.

Myoclonic Seizures

Myoclonic seizures are brief, random contractions of a muscle group. They can occur on one or both sides of the body, and they may occur singularly or in clusters. Consciousness is not lost during myoclonic seizures. The onset may be as early as age 2 years, but they are more frequently seen in school-age children or adolescents.

Absence Seizures

Formerly called petit mal seizures, absence seizures are very brief episodes of altered awareness. There is no muscle activity, except eyelid fluttering or twitching. The child has a blank facial expression. Absence seizures last only 5 to 10 seconds, but they may occur one after the other several times a day. The onset of absence seizures does not usually occur before age 5 (Behrman, 1996).

PARTIAL SEIZURES

Onset at any age. Clinical features suggest that only a limited functional area on one hemisphere of the brain is involved. Partial seizures begin focally, but they may become generalized.

Partial seizures are further divided into those with simple and those with complex symptomatolgy.

Simple Partial Seizures

Simple partial seizures consist of twitching of an extremity, face, or neck, or the sensation of twitching or numbness in an extremity or face or neck. This seizure may last 10 to 20 seconds.

Complex Partial Seizures

Complex partial seizures may begin with or without an aura. Symptoms include impaired consciousness, transient staring, altered mental status, and feelings of unreality, detachment, and disrupted memory. There may be unexplained feelings of fear or dread, distortions of perception or hallucinations, teeth grinding, lip smacking, chewing, swallowing, scratching, or pulling at shirt buttons. The average duration of a complex partial seizure is 1 to 2 minutes.

From Behrman, R. E., Kliegman, R. M., & Arvin, A. M. (1996). *Nelson textbook of pediatrics* (15th ed.). Philadelphia: W. B. Saunders.

NURSING CARE OF THE CHILD WITH SEIZURES

Assessment

A detailed history including the prenatal, perinatal, and neonatal periods is important in determining precipitating factors related to the seizure activity. Pathologic precipitating factors include a history of hypoxia, cerebral trauma, high fever, lead poisoning, metabolic disorders, brain tumors, birth trauma, and/or CNS infections. Nonpathologic factors include overhydration, oversedation, drug abuse, sleep deprivation, antihistamine drug use, and alcohol intoxication.

Seizure activity is often not witnessed by the health care professional. The parents should be asked about the age of onset, time of onset, precipitating events, and behavior prior to and after the seizure. A detailed description of the seizure itself is essential, including what the child does during the seizure, how the seizure progresses, and how long it lasts.

The child is given a comprehensive physical examination with special emphasis on the neurologic system. Parameters include evaluation of behavior, motor skills, and developmental level. Evaluation of the child and family's emotional response to the seizure disorder is done at this time. Identification of emotional and educational needs, planning, and interventions are based on this information.

The nursing care of the child with seizures is either acute or long term. Acute management includes identification of the type of seizure and factors that precipitate the event. Long-term management focuses on medication administration and education.

Nursing Diagnosis

Nursing diagnoses that may apply to the child with seizures include:

- Ineffective Breathing Pattern related to tonic-clonic seizure
- Altered Tissue Perfusion (Cerebral) related to prolonged seizure activity
- Knowledge Deficit related to management of a seizure disorder or medication regimen
- Altered Family Processes related to having a child with a chronic illness (see Chapter 17)
- Risk for Injury related to seizure activity

Planning, Implementation, and Evaluation: The Child With Seizures

NURSING DIAGNOSIS

- Risk for Injury related to seizure activity

Expected Outcome: The child will:

- remain uninjured after a seizure
- have good control of the seizure disorder
- demonstrate knowledge of seizures and seizure first aid

The parents will:

- demonstrate correct anticonvulsant medication administration; discuss prevention of seizures
- demonstrate seizure first aid

Intervention	Rationale
1. Pad side rails with blankets, keep bed in low position. Place child on a soft surface if not in bed. Remove sharp objects and furniture out of the way.	These actions modify the environment to make it safer for the seizing child.
2. Do not put anything into the child's mouth.	Forcing something into the child's mouth may cause injury to the child's mouth, gums, or teeth.
3. Place the child on his side in a lateral position. Do not restrain the child.	Positioning the child on the side will prevent aspiration as the saliva drains out of the corner of the child's mouth. Restraints could cause injury to the child. The nurse or family may gently guide or protect the child's movements.
4. Document time of seizures, precipitating factors, type of movements or seizure, incontinence, or frequency of seizure and notify the physician.	These observations help pinpoint the focus of the seizure and will help the physician treat the seizure correctly.
5. Check for breathing during and after the seizure. Loosen clothing around the child's neck.	If breathing does not spontaneously start after the seizure is over, suction the child and administer rescue breathing. Call for help. If these measures do not start breathing again, continue rescue breathing. Respiratory depression is a side effect of valium and antivan.
6. Stay with the child.	Reduces the risk of injury and allows for observation and documentation of the seizure.
7. If the seizure lasts longer than 2–3 minutes, notify physician.	May need to administer medication to stop prolonged seizures.

Evaluation:

- The child remains injury-free.
- Seizures are monitored and documented.
- The parents demonstrate seizure first aid.

NURSING DIAGNOSIS • Knowledge Deficit related to having a seizure disorder

Expected Outcome: • The child/parents will discuss seizures and educational needs.

Intervention	Rationale
1. Assess educational needs of the child and parents.	Provides baseline information in order to develop a teaching plan
2. Provide an individual teaching plan for the child and parents on handling seizures.	With an individualized teaching plan, what is needed by the child and parents will be taught.
3. Explore actual and potential problems that may arise and interfere with treatment.	Facilitates adjustment and normalizes life; provides anticipatory guidance
4. Measure outcomes of education to assure that learning has taken place and is facilitating acceptance.	Evaluation of teaching is an ongoing process to assure continued learning
5. Refer to an epilepsy support group. (See Appendix H for list of resource organizations.)	Social support is helpful for some families and may promote adjustment to lifestyle changes.
6. Educate the child and parents about the medication regimen. Emphasize the importance of complying with medical treatment (see Teaching Guidelines).	The goal of pharmacologic management is to raise the seizure threshold, thus preventing seizures.
7. Identify the side effects of the medication and when medical attention should be sought.	Knowledge of what is expected and normal will facilitate proper use and compliance with medication.
8. Identify hazards of noncompliance with medications. Encourage parents/child not to discontinue medications even if the child is seizure-free.	Noncompliance will affect the serum levels of anticonvulsants and may cause a seizure to occur.
9. Stress to the child and parents the importance of regular medical evaluation and follow-up, including obtaining blood levels of the medication and teaching signs of toxicity.	Facilitates appropriate therapeutic blood levels of anticonvulsants.

TEACHING GUIDELINES *for the Child Taking Seizure Medication*

THE CHILD TAKING PHENYTOIN (DILANTIN)

- Gums may become swollen and tender.
- Oral care is very important. The child should brush and floss after every meal, using a soft brush.
- The child should see the dentist every 3–6 months for a checkup and cleaning of the teeth.
- Therapeutic blood levels should be monitored. After the therapeutic level is attained, blood levels should be monitored periodically if a seizure occurs or if side effects are noticed.

THE ADOLESCENT TAKING ANTIEPILEPTIC MEDICATIONS

- Some states require a driver to be seizure-free for 1 year to obtain a driver's license.
- Birth control pills may be less effective while taking antiepileptic medications. The patient should consult a nurse or physician for additional forms of birth control.
- Acne or oily skin may be a problem. The patient should consult a dematologist for skin problems.
- Alcohol, marijuana, and street drugs will lower the seizure threshold. It is best to avoid or limit these drugs.
- The adolescent should not stop taking antiepileptic medications suddenly or without discussing it with a doctor or nurse. Suddenly stopping medications may cause the patient to have a seizure or status epilepticus.

Intervention	Rationale
10. Inform the parents about the need for an identification band for the child.	If the child has a seizure in a public place the identification will inform passers-by of what to do for the child.
11. Encourage the family to find alternative activities besides contact sports for the child. The child should avoid swimming or climbing alone. Identify the child's strengths, not what he cannot do.	Appropriate activities will reduce the risk of injury while promoting a positive self-image.
12. Encourage verbalization of fears and concerns about having seizures.	This therapeutic communication may identify issues that need to be addressed.
13. Teach the child and parents to educate other family members, friends, and teachers about seizures.	Accurate information reduces the stigma associated with epilepsy.

Evaluation:

- The child discusses having seizures; discusses fears and concerns about seizures and life with them; participates in medication regimen; discusses medication side effects and dosage; and demonstrates a positive self-image.
- The family demonstrates safety with the child having seizures; administers anticonvulsants safely and appropriately; and discusses when to call the physician (Austin, 1996).

Status Epilepticus

Status epilepticus is a pediatric emergency. It is prolonged seizure activity, which may be either a single seizure of 10 minutes or more or recurrent seizures that last more than 30 minutes with no return to consciousness between seizures. The most common form of status epilepticus is generalized tonic-clonic status, which has the highest potential for complications and possible death.

Pathophysiology. Status epilepticus is caused by random discharge of large numbers of neurons firing abnormally. The discharges cause abnormal repetitive motor activity. In the CNS there is an increased metabolic rate, depletion of glucose stores, and an increase in oxygen consumption. If cerebral metabolic demands are not met, these changes cause neuronal injury. Prolonged seizures cause lactic acidosis, an altered blood–brain barrier, and increased ICP.

Etiology. The causes of status epilepticus are many. Acute CNS injury caused by head trauma, meningitis, and electrolyte imbalance frequently precipitate status epilepticus. The condition can also be caused by toxins and specific medications. Other causes are chronic CNS injury and sudden withdrawal from anticonvulsants.

Incidence. Status epilepticus occurs in 5 to 10% of children with epilepsy. The most common cause in children under age 3 years is febrile status epilepticus.

Clinical Manifestations. See International Classification of Seizures in previous section.

Diagnostic Evaluation. Laboratory work to be done includes: blood glucose, ABGs, electrolytes, anticonvulsant drug levels, toxicology screen, and possibly a lumbar puncture. The child may have many of the same problems as the child with increased ICP.

Therapeutic Management. Generalized tonic-clonic status epilepticus is a medical emergency, and treatment consists of maintaining optimal respiratory and hemodynamic function, and identification and treatment of the causes of the seizure activity. Diazepam (Valium) or lorazepam (Ativan) are given intravenously, or rectally if intravenous access cannot be obtained. The intramuscular route is not used as it is unpredictable.

Intravenous diazepam must be given directly into the vein (not the tubing, because it interacts with the plastic), at a rate no greater than 1 mg/min. It should not be mixed with other drugs or solutions, and can be diluted only with normal saline. Resuscitative equipment should be at the bedside and respirations monitored closely during IV administration.

NURSING CARE OF THE CHILD WITH STATUS EPILEPTICUS

Assessment

On arrival at the hospital, the child is often in a coma and has unstable vital signs. Along with general seizure precautions, this child requires rapid assessment and vigorous supportive therapy. Supportive measures include assessing and maintaining a patent airway, and administration of oxygen. Intravenous hydration and drug therapy are initiated to arrest the seizure activity. A variety of drugs are used in the treatment of status epilepticus. (See the medications table in the Clinical Reference Pages at the beginning of this chapter.)

Nursing Diagnoses and Planning

- Impaired Gas Exchange related to seizures. ***Expected Outcome:*** *The child's ABGs will be within normal limits.*
- Ineffective Breathing Pattern related to seizures. ***Expected Outcome:*** *The child's pulse oxygen saturation remains > 95%.*
- Ineffective Airway Clearance related to possible aspiration during seizure. ***Expected Outcome:*** *The child will have clear breath sounds.*
- Altered Tissue Perfusion (Cerebral) related to lactic acidosis with prolonged seizing. ***Expected Outcome:*** The child's level of consciousness will return to normal.

Implementation and Evaluation

See the nursing care plan for epilepsy.

TRAUMA

Head Injury

Head injury refers to the pathologic result of any mechanical force to the scalp, skull, meninges, or brain.

Incidence. Multiple trauma is the leading cause of death in children beyond infancy. Approximately 200,000 children are hospitalized yearly in the United States for evaluation and treatment of a head injury.

Clinical Manifestations. The clinical manifestations depend on the type of injury and the subsequent amount of increased ICP.

Skull and Scalp Injuries

- Lacerations
- Abrasions
- Bleeding
- Subgaleal hematoma

Skull Fractures

- *Linear:* Straight line fracture, dura is not involved
- *Depressed:* Bone is pressing downward, indented
- *Basilar:* Fracture of the base of the skull: symptoms are Battle's sign, raccoon's eyes, rhinorrhea, otorrhea, hemotympanum

Concussion

- Transient loss of consciousness
- Headache
- Nausea
- Vomiting
- Dizziness

Contusion

- Transient loss of consciousness
- Transient memory loss
- Headache
- Vomiting
- Seizures

Vascular Injuries (Fig. 40–6)

- *Epidural:* Possible loss of consciousness followed by a lucid period and then deterioration into coma. Other manifestations include decreased responsiveness, headache, abnormal anisocoria, and contralateral hemiparesis.
- *Subdural:* Headache, confusion, deterioration in the level of consciousness.
- *Subarachnoid:* Headache, deterioration in the level of consciousness.

Diagnostic Evaluation. A complete history of the event is important to determine the mechanism of injury and if the child lost consciousness or not. A complete neurologic examination is done after X-rays to assure there is no cervical spinal cord injury. Any indication of increased ICP is quickly reported to the physician. A CT or MRI is the most precise test to diagnose the specific kind of head injury sustained.

Therapeutic Management. Initial management of the child with a head injury includes assessment of ventilatory function, neurologic impairment, and the presence of other injuries (see the section on Pediatric Trauma in Chapter 14). Interventions to maintain vital functions are provided until all injuries are determined. The child with a head injury may develop increased intracranial pressure and/or seizures. See earlier discussion of these disorders.

NURSING CARE OF THE CHILD WITH A HEAD INJURY

Assessment

Initial assessment of the child with a head injury includes the ABCs—airway, breathing, circulation (see Chapter

PATHOPHYSIOLOGY AND ETIOLOGY *of Head Injury*

The cranium is a rigid structure that contains blood, brain tissue, and CSF. The pressure exerted by these components on the cranium is between 4 and 15 mm Hg. According to the Monroe-Kellie doctrine, an increase in one of these components must be accompanied by a decrease in one of the others to maintain the ICP within normal range. Cerebral function is dependent on adequate delivery of nutrients such as oxygen, glucose, and other substrates; an abnormal increase in ICP will interfere with the balance and delivery of these nutrients.

Head injuries are either primary or secondary. Primary head injuries are the damage to the head at the time of the injury; secondary head injuries refer to the consequences of the primary injury, particularly increased ICP. The severity of the injury depends on the amount of stress to the cranium and brain. These injuries may be concussions, contusions, lacerations, fractures, and/or hematomas.

Most head injuries in children are the result of motor vehicle collisions, falls, sports injuries, child abuse, and neglect. Acceleration-deceleration is the term used to describe the mechanism of injury. The shearing force of the initial impact moves the brain forward followed by a counter movement of the brain in the skull. The shearing force produces bruising, tearing, and bleeding (see figure below).

Shaken baby syndrome results in epidural hematomas and retinal hemorrhages (see Fig. 40–6 and Chapter 41).

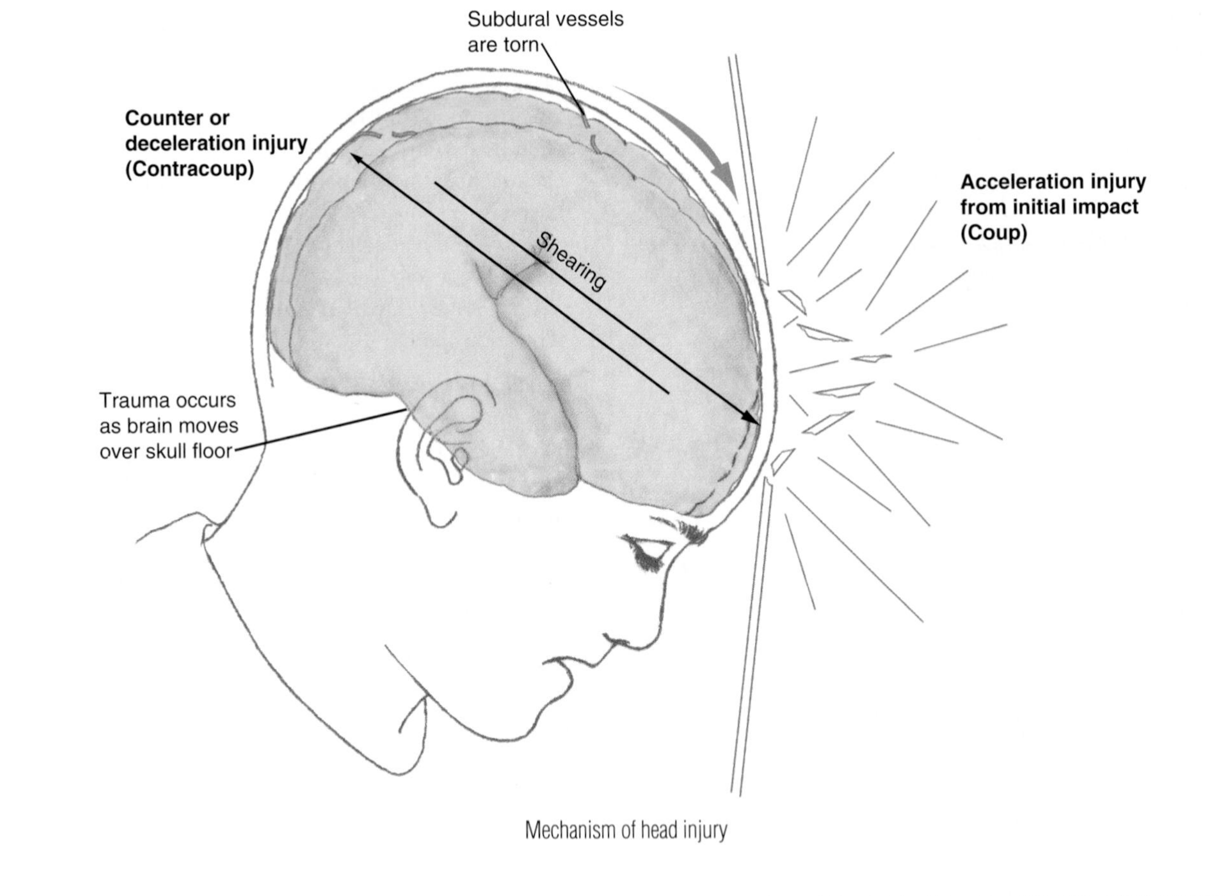

Mechanism of head injury

14). The child's neck is immobilized as special attention is given to the cervical spine. Baseline vital signs are obtained and documented, and further signs are obtained as indicated by the child's clinical condition. A complete history and comprehensive neurologic examination are completed. Assessment includes level of consciousness, pupillary size and reactivity to light, and motor and verbal response, using the Glasgow Coma Scale or other assessment tool (see Chapter 14, Table 14–2).

The cranial nerves are evaluated to identify deficits as a result of the injury or to monitor for increased ICP. The clinical signs and symptoms of increased ICP with or with-

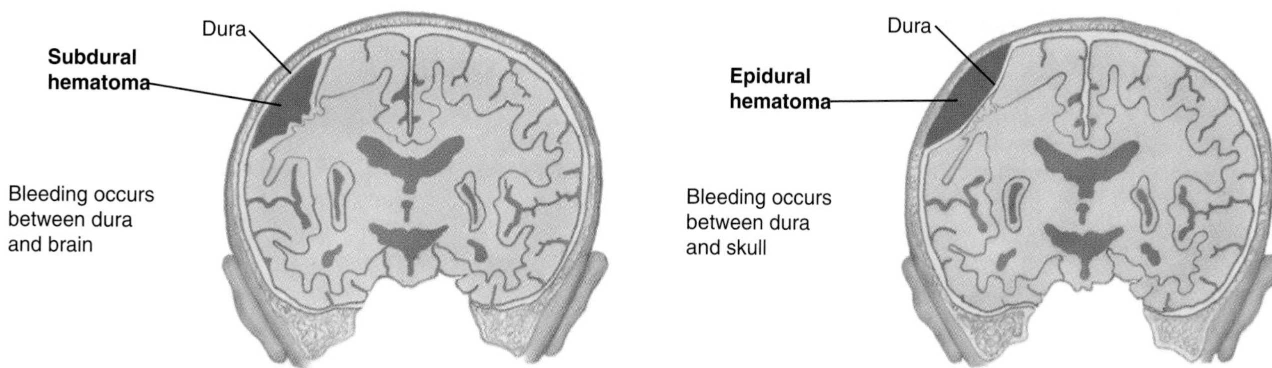

Figure 40–6

Subdural and epidural hematomas are the two most common cranial hematomas, occurring in 6% to 7% of head injuries in children. A *subdural hematoma* is often caused when the head strikes an immovable object. However, in an infant a subdural hematoma may result from aggressive shaking (a form of child abuse); retinal hemorrhage is also a classic sign of shaking injury in infants. With *epidural hematoma*, rapid decline in neurologic function may occur 4 to 8 hours after a brief period of lucidity. If untreated, the increased cranial pressure can cause death in a short period of time.

out actual measurement of the ICP will determine both the clinical status of the child and the medical and nursing interventions.

> Nasotracheal suctioning is contraindicated in a child with a basilar skull fracture. Because of the nature of the injury the suction catheter may be introduced into the brain.

Nursing Diagnosis

Nursing diagnoses that may apply to the child with a head injury include the following:

- Altered Tissue Perfusion (Cerebral) related to increased ICP or cerebral edema
- Risk for Fluid Volume Deficit related to diabetes insipidus
- Fluid Volume Excess related to SIADH
- Ineffective Airway Clearance related to possible decreased level of consciousness or facial trauma
- Risk for Injury related to lacerations or possible hematoma
- Risk for Altered Nutrition: Less Then Body Requirements related to nausea, vomiting, NPO status, dysphagia, or facial trauma
- Knowledge Deficit (Family) related to head injury
- Anxiety (Family) related to having a child with a critical illness or uncertain outcome
- Altered Family Processes related to having a child with a sudden critical illness
- Altered Growth and Development related to head injury causing learning disabilities

Planning, Implementation, and Evaluation: The Child With a Head Injury

NURSING DIAGNOSIS • Risk for Fluid Volume Deficit related to diabetes insipidus

Expected Outcome: • The child will have urine output of 1–2 ml/kg/hr and keep serum sodium levels between 135 and 145 mEq/L.

Intervention	Rationale
1. Carefully monitor IV fluid intake.	The child with head injury is at risk for cerebral edema, SIADH, and diabetes insipidus.
2. Obtain accurate intake and output. Child may need an indwelling urinary catheter or diapers may be weighed before and after use.	Monitoring intake and output documents fluid loss.

Intervention	Rationale
3. Monitor for other fluid losses, diarrhea, or vomiting. Notify physician and replace fluids as prescribed.	Prevents dehydration and hypovolemic shock.

Evaluation:
- The child has minimal weight loss (less than 3% of total preinjury body weight), maintains moist mucous membranes, and has urine specific gravity > 1.006.

NURSING DIAGNOSIS
- Fluid Volume Excess related to SIADH

Expected Outcome:
- The child will have urine specific gravity between 1.002 and 1.030, serum sodium 135 to 145 mEq/L, and serum osmolality between 275 and 295 mOsm/kg.

Intervention	Rationale
1. Restrict fluid intake as prescribed.	Prevents fluid overload and complications of hyponatremia such as cerebral edema and increased ICP.
2. Monitor electrolytes and serum osmolality. Monitor intake and output, daily weights, urine specific gravity.	Allows the nurse to modify the fluid intake or types of fluids given; reduces complications of fluid overload if treated early.
3. Keep an IV line patent. Change IV fluids as prescribed.	Manipulate IV fluids to maintain homeostasis.
4. Teach parents about signs and symptoms of DI and SIADH.	Parents may assist the health care team by monitoring of signs and symptoms of DI and SIADH once discharged from the hospital or rehabilitation hospital.

Evaluation:
- The child maintains normal electrolytes and urine specific gravity, and appropriate hydration.
- The parents discuss observations to be made once they are at home to monitor for DI or SIADH (see Teaching Guidelines).

TEACHING GUIDELINES *for the Child With a Head Injury*

Call the doctor immediately if the child:
- has bleeding that does not stop after 10 minutes of holding pressure
- needs sutures
- is less than 1 year old
- had a seizure after the head injury
- was unconscious or confused
- has a severe headache or vomiting
- has slurred speech or blurred vision
- has blood or watery fluid coming from the ear or nose
- has unequal pupils or crossed eyes
- has difficulty walking, crawling, or the arms are weak
- has other symptoms that concern you

Post-concussion Syndrome

Your child may be upset easily and may be irritable if tired or stressed. Memory problems are common, as are learning difficulties, double vision, vertigo, headaches, fatigue, photophobia, and hyperacoutism. These symptoms may last many months.

Data from Schmitt, B. D. (1992). *Instructions for pediatric patients* (p. 127). Philadelphia: W. B. Saunders.

Spinal Cord Injury

Spinal cord injury can be sustained by any trauma or injury to the spinal cord or to its vascular supply or venous drainage.

PATHOPHYSIOLOGY *of Spinal Cord Injury*

Spinal cord injuries occur in children when vertebral bodies are fractured, or when subluxation of the vertebra occurs. Subluxation results in malalignment of contiguous vertebra, so that the spinal cord is compressed. The cord may be crushed, overstretched, or completely divided. All neurons carrying sensations from those parts of the body below the lesion are unable to pass their message on to the brain. A severe cord injury will cause complete paralysis and complete loss of sensation below the severed level.

Flaccid paralysis of the affected limbs immediately follows a spinal cord injury. This is due to spinal shock, which may last 3 weeks or more. The flaccidity changes to spasticity when the spinal shock resolves.

Etiology. In the pediatric patient, spinal cord injury is usually caused by motor vehicle accidents, falls, diving accidents, sports injuries, gunshot or knife wounds, or attempted suicide. In the infant, a common cause of spinal cord injury is intentional aggressive shaking.

Incidence. Although spinal cord injuries are less frequent in children than adults, 75% of spinal cord injuries in children occur in the cervical spine, between the occiput and C3. As the child grows older the site of the spinal cord injury moves distally.

Clinical Manifestations

- Loss of some or all movement or sensation below the level of injury
- Respiratory depression or apnea
- Hypotension and bradycardia
- Hypothermia
- Neck pain

Diagnostic Evaluation. After taking the history of the injury and complete neurologic exam, X-rays, CT, or MRI determine the extent of the spinal cord injury. The extent of motor or sensory deficit may resolve somewhat as spinal shock resolves.

Therapeutic Management. Treatment includes steroid therapy, which may be administered within 8 hours of the injury as a bolus of 30 mg/kg followed by a continuous infusion of 5.4 mg/kg/hr for 23 hours. Other treatments include halo traction (Fig. 40–7) or Gardner-Wells tongs for unstable injuries or for subluxation, or until surgical stabilization can be performed.

NURSING CARE OF THE CHILD WITH A SPINAL CORD INJURY

Assessment

Spine immobilization must occur before any attempt is made to move the child. Airway assessment is made immediately, and if intubation is necessary it is done without hyperextension of the neck. Next, circulation should be assessed, keeping in mind that hypotension may be a result of either hypovolemia or neurologic shock. Bradycardia and hypothermia may ensue. Attempts should be made to maintain the body temperature and keep the child well oxygenated.

Neurologic assessment includes mobility, sensation, and reflexes. The injury may be referred to as complete or incomplete. With a complete spinal cord injury the cord is completely severed and there is no spinal innervation below the injury. With an incomplete spinal cord injury the cord has some function remaining. Such an assessment is ongoing and carefully documented so changes can be dealt with in a timely fashion. The patient is then assessed for other systems trauma.

Nursing Diagnosis and Planning

The following nursing diagnoses and expected outcomes may be appropriate following assessment of the child with spinal cord injury:

- Ineffective Breathing Pattern related to spinal cord injury. ***Expected Outcome:*** *The child will have ABGs within normal limits, stable vital signs, and motor and sensory function.*
- Risk for Impaired Skin Integrity related to immobility. ***Expected Outcome:*** *The child will have no evidence of skin breakdown.*
- Anxiety related to having an acute illness, or having a child with an acute illness. ***Expected Outcome:*** *The child/parents will verbalize what the spinal cord injury means to them.*
- Altered Family Processes related to having a child with an acute and chronic injury. ***Expected Outcome:*** *The parents will participate in the child's care.*

Implementation

The goal of nursing care is to minimize the potential for further injury, prevent sequelae of immobility, and promote maximal spinal cord recovery. The spinal cord is

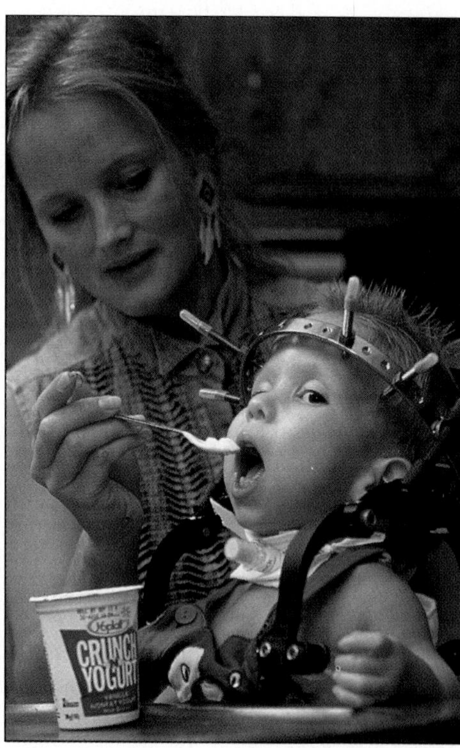

Figure 40–7
Children who have injuries or birth defects that involve the upper spine may require halo traction to stabilize the spine and prevent added nerve damage. Spinal cord injury is a catastrophic event for the child and family, who will need intense nursing support and education, as well as referral to support groups. (Courtesy of Cook Children's Medical Center, Forth Worth, Texas)

immobilized by use of tongs or halo traction. The child will remain in traction for several weeks. The nurse is responsible for maintaining proper alignment by monitoring the status of the traction every 1 to 2 hours. Towels and rolls may be useful to help position the child. The nurse should perform a motor and sensory assessment after each change of position.

If the child's situation becomes unstable, surgical stabilization may become necessary. Progressive neurologic deterioration is the major indicator for surgery.

The immobilized and neurologically impaired child is at risk for respiratory complications. Respiratory status and pulse oximetry are assessed and documented every 1 to 2 hours. Supplemental oxygen may be indicated. Nebulizer, incentive spirometry, and intermittent positive pressure breathing (IPPB) may be ordered. Some children may require tracheostomy and mechanical ventilation if the respiratory muscles are involved or if weaning from the ventilator is slow and difficult to accomplish.

The nurse assesses perfusion by monitoring vital signs, color, skin temperature, urine output, and mentation. An indwelling urinary catheter will be inserted to facilitate bladder emptying and accurate measurement of intake and output, which is monitored hourly. If alterations in perfusion occur the child will receive crystalloids by bolus infusion. Vasopressors such as dopamine and dobutamine may also be used.

The spinal cord injured child may have a problem with body temperature control, and so should be warmed or cooled as appropriate. If there is an elevated temperature, wound and blood cultures are taken. Sputum cultures may be necessary. Antipyretic and broad-spectrum antibiotic therapy is initiated after the cultures are sent.

The child may have an NG tube in place. The nurse will maintain tube patency and monitor and document drainage. The pH of the gastric fluid may be tested and the child treated with antacids, sucralfate (carafate), or histamine blockers. The child is at risk for stress ulcers and a gastrointestinal bleed. A bowel regimen will be initiated and maintained to prevent impaction. Bowel training includes a high fiber diet, stool softeners, and increased water intake. While the indwelling catheter is in place, care will be taken to prevent infection. The child will eventually be progressed to intermittent catheterization if necessary.

The skin should be inspected frequently and skin care administered each time the child is repositioned. Pressure on the bony prominences is minimized by use of special mattresses and padding.

Adequate nutrition is essential to the healing process. Caloric intake is monitored and the child may receive nutrition via oral intake, tube feeding, or total parenteral nutrition. A good indicator of a favorable response to the nutrition is timely healing of wounds.

Spinal cord injury is a catastrophic event. The life of the child and his family has been suddenly and permanently altered. They will need intense assistance and support. These goals can be attained through therapeutic play, promotion of independent functioning, referral to support groups, and thorough discharge planning and home care teaching.

Evaluation

- Has the child's neurologic function improved?
- Are bodily functions maintained as normally as possible?
- Do the child/parents verbalize feelings and emotions about the injury and the prognosis?
- Do the parents demonstrate abilities to provide physical and emotional support for the child?

DISORDERS CAUSED BY TOXINS

Botulism

Botulism is a form of food poisoning caused by a toxin produced by the anerobic bacillus *Clostridium botulinum*. The source is usually honey or improperly sterilized canned foods.

Clinical manifestations include constipation, CNS symptoms 12 to 36 hours after ingestion, weakness or dizziness, headache, double vision, vomiting, difficulty talking, respiratory paralysis, decreased deep tendon reflexes, and impaired gag reflex.

Therapeutic Management and Nursing Care. Management includes respiratory support and the administration of antitoxoid. The infant or child will usually recover after the diagnosis is made and treatment started. **Hospital stay for infant botulism averages one month.**

To prevent botulism, educate parents not to give infants honey or syrup in their milk or water.

Tetanus (Lockjaw)

Tetanus is caused by an endotoxin produced by the anaerobic spore-forming gram-positive bacillus *Clostridium tetani*. The disorder incubates in 3 days to 3 weeks. Puncture wounds, burns, lacerations, and compound fractures are examples of entry sites.

Clinical manifestations include painful muscular rigidity of the masseter and neck muscles, facial spasms, dysphagia, and laryngospasm. There may be respiratory arrest. Pain is severe.

Therapeutic Management and Nursing Care. Ventilation and respiratory support are vital. Fluids and electrolytes must be monitored. Tube feedings or total parenteral nutrition may be necessary. Valium is given for seizures, and antibiotics may be given for the initial wound. A quiet environment should be provided for the child.

Prevention is accomplished with tetanus toxoid. Tetanus immune globulin may be given for quick immunity.

KEY CONCEPTS

- By the fourth week of gestation the nervous system has begun to develop. The neural tube closes first at the anterior end to form the brain and then at the posterior end to form the spinal cord. The brain continues to grow until about the fifth year of life.
- The CNS is composed of the brain and spinal cord, which are protected by bony coverings, the skull and vertebral column. The skull has several bones that are not fused at birth and do not fuse until 12 to 18 months of life. The brain and spinal cord are also covered by the meninges, a fibrous connective tissue structure that contains many blood vessels. Cerebrospinal fluid surrounds the brain and spinal cord. The brain consists of the cerebrum, cerebellum, and brain stem. The peripheral nervous system consists of 12 pairs of cranial nerves and 31 pairs of spinal nerves. The autonomic nervous system consists of the sympathetic and parasympathetic systems, which are in control of the body's automatic functions.
- Autoregulation is the body's ability to change vascular diameter in response to changes in cerebral perfusion pressure. When autoregulation fails cerebrovascular dilatation is impaired and cerebral blood flow decreases. Hypercapnia and/or hypoxia lead to cerebral dilation and increased ICP. Hypocapnia leads to cerebral arterial constriction and decreased ICP.
- The brain of an infant is two-thirds the size of an adult's. The brain grows to 80% of adult size by age 1 year. CSF production is about 24 ml/day whereas the adult produces about 400 to 600 ml/day. Head circumference can change in the infant and young child, but the head of the adolescent and adult is unyielding. This has implications for head circumference measurement for growth and development in the infant and young child. The spinal cord, cranial nerves, and peripheral nerves get longer during childhood; the spinal cord terminates at L3 in the newborn and L1–L2 in the adult. Myelinization of nerves begins in the third month of gestation and is completed in adolescence, as demonstrated by progressive development and coordination. Neurologic changes may be more subtle in the infant or child, and may be indicated by irritability or poor feeding behaviors.
- The neurologic examination includes level of consciousness and Glasgow Coma Scale, pupil size and reaction to light, cranial nerve testing, motor and sensory functions, respiratory status and function, vital signs, and measurement of head circumference.

- Anticonvulsants have many side effects; if given IV, respiratory depression is the most serious. Other anticonvulsants may cause blood dyscrasias or liver damage; complete blood counts and liver enzymes should be measured routinely. Mannitol and furosemide (Lasix) are diuretics that are used to help decrease ICP. Monitor serum electrolytes and serum osmolality with diuretics. Paralyzing agents may be used to decrease agitation and ICP; with these drugs the child needs total care and respiratory support. Codeine is useful for pain and will not interfere with a neurologic assessment.
- Measures to prevent cerebral edema range from prevention of trauma, wearing seat belts and helmets, teaching bicycle safety, and discouraging risk taking and driving while under the influence of alcohol or drugs. Cerebral edema is decreased by hyperoxygenating and hyperventilating the child, administering diuretics, elevating the head of the bed 30° to 45°, keeping the child in good alignment so venous drainage is not impaired, and reducing agitation and noxious stimuli.
- Abnormal posturing is an ominous neurologic sign. Flexion (decorticate) posturing refers to flexion of the upper extremities, arms, hands, and wrists. The child's legs are extended. Flexion indicates cortical damage. Extension (decerebrate) posturing refers to extended arms that are inwardly rotated and the extended legs. Extension indicates damage to more of the brain, theoretically extending to the brain stem.
- Fibrosis or scarring of the meninges may occur with a hemorrhage or infection and prevent CSF from being absorbed in the arachnoid villi; this is referred to as communicating hydrocephalus. The blockage of the flow of CSF through the ventricular system is referred to as noncommunicating hydrocephalus. The changes in the brain are enlarged ventricles. If the cranial sutures are not ossified the head circumference will be abnormally large.
- Teaching strategies are begun after an assessment of the family's and child's needs is made. The family's grieving may be verbalized; their emotions and fears should be expressed and validated. Reinforce information that has been supplied by the other members of the health care team. Encourage parents in their caregiving efforts when appropriate. Assist the family in setting realistic goals for the child. Identify support systems and refer to community agencies. Have family members demonstrate skills necessary for home care. Encourage therapeutic play. Promote peer contact when possible and appropriate. Provide incentives for accomplishments. Point out positive aspects of the child. Identify positive coping mechanisms.

REFERENCES

Austin, J. K. (1996). A model of family adaptation to new onset childhood epilepsy. *Journal of Neuroscience Nursing, 28*(2), 82–92.

Behrman, R. E., Kliegman, R. M., & Arvin, A. M. (1996). *Nelson textbook of pediatrics* (15th ed.) Philadelphia: W. B. Saunders.

Burns, C. E., Barber, N., Brady, M. A., & Dunn, A. M. (1996). *Pediatric primary care: A handbook for nurse practitioners.* Philadelphia: W. B. Saunders.

Geraci, E., & Geraci, R. (1996). A look at recent hyperventilation studies: Outcomes and recommendations for early use in the head-injured patient. *Journal of Neuroscience Nursing, 28*(4), 222–233.

Hickey, J. V. (1992). *The clinical practice of neurological and neurosurgical nursing* (3rd ed.). Philadelphia: J. B. Lippincott.

Hobdell, E. F. (1996). Perceptual accuracy and gender-related differences in parents of children with myeolmenigocele. *Journal of Neuroscience, 27*(4), 240–244.

Martin, J. H. (1996). *Neuroanatomy: Text and atlas* (2nd ed.). Stamford, CT: Appleton & Lange.

Wildrick, D., Parker-Fisher, S., & Morales, A. (1996). Quality of life in children with well-controlled epilepsy. *Journal of Neuroscience Nursing, 28*(3), 192–198.

Williams, D. G., Hayes, J., & McCool, S. (1996). Shunt infections in children: Presentation and management. *Journal of Neuroscience Nursing, 28*(3), 155–162.

BIBLIOGRAPHY

Barker, E. (1994). *Neuroscience nursing.* St. Louis: C. V. Mosby.

Baron, M. C. (1991). Advances in the care of children with brain tumors. *Journal of Neuroscience Nursing, 23*, 39.

Behrman, R. E., Kliegman, R. M., & Arvin, A. M. (1996). *Nelson textbook of pediatrics* (15th ed.). Philadelphia: W. B. Saunders.

Bysshi, J. (1993). Bacterial meningitis: Why vigilance must continue. *Professional Care of Mother & Child, 3*, 222.

Carno, M. (1994). Meningococcemia: Recognizing and reducing complications in pediatric patients. *AACN: Clinical Issues in Critical Care Nursing, 5*, 276.

DeRogetes, H. (1993). A different reflection . . . growing up with cerebral palsy. *Nursing Outlook, 41*, 235.

Dormans, J. P. (1993). Orthopedic management of children with cerebral palsy. *Pediatric Clinics of North America, 40*, 645.

Fecht-Gramley, M. E. (1995). Emergency pediatric head trauma. *American Journal of Nursing, 95*, 54.

Harper, J. (1988). Use of steroids in cerebral edema: Therapeutic implications. *Heart and Lung, 17*, 70.

Hazinski, M. F. (1991). *Nursing care of the critically ill child.* St. Louis: Mosby–Year Book.

Kurtz, M. J. (1993). Case study of an adolescent spinal cord injury patient. *Rehabilitation Nursing, 18*, 237.

Lee, S. (1989). Intracranial pressure changes during positioning of patients with severe head trauma. *Heart and Lung, 18*, 411.

Moore, P. C. (1988). When you have to think small for a neurologic exam. *RN, 6*, 38.

Morrison, C. (1987). Brain herniation syndromes. *Critical Care Nurse, 5*, 34.

Morrow, J. D. (1995). Treatment of the infant with myelomeningocele. *Journal of Pediatric Nursing, 10*, 99.

Paratz, J., et al. (1993). Intracranial dynamics in preterm infants and neonates. *Australian Journal of Physiotherapy, 39*, 171.

Peterson, P. M., et al. (1994). Spina bifida: The transition into adulthood begins in infancy. *Rehabilitation Nursing, 19*, 229.

Pieper, P. (1994). Pediatric trauma: An overview. *Nursing Clinics of North America, 29*, 563.

Reimer, M. (1989). Head injured patients: How to detect early signs of trouble. *Nursing89, 19*, 34.

Rising, C. J. (1993). The relationship of certain nursing activities to intracranial pressure. *Journal of Neuroscience Nursing, 25*, 302.

Rolak, L. A. (1993). *Neurology secrets.* St. Louis: C. V. Mosby.

Rosman, N. (1986). Pediatric emergencies: Managing acute head trauma. *Contemporary Pediatrics, 11*, 24.

Schmitt, B. D. (1992). *Instructions for pediatric patients.* Philadelphia: W. B. Saunders.

Shiminski-Maher, E., et al. (1994). Current trends in the diagnosis and management of hydrocephalus in children. *Journal of Pediatric Nursing, 9*, 74.

Shpritz, D. W. (1994). Practical points in understanding ICP. *Journal of Post Anesthesia Nursing, 9*, 357.

Stewart-Amedei, C. (1988). What to do until the neurosurgeon arrives. *Journal of Emergency Nursing, 14*, 296.

Swoboda, C. J., et al. (1994). Seizure disorders: Syndromes, diagnosis and management. *Contemporary Therapy, 20*, 67.

Vos, H. (1993). Making headway with intracranial hypertension. *American Journal of Nursing, 2*, 28.

Walsh, E., et al. (1994). Childhood near drowning: Nursing care and primary prevention. *Pediatric Nursing, 20*, 265.

Werdman, M. J. (1994). Pediatric drowning. *Emergency, 26*, 28.

Whiting, S. (1994). A child's first seizure: Should you treat it? *Medical Clinics of North America, 17*, 55.

Wolman, C., et al. (1994). Factors influencing self-esteem and self-consciousness in the adolescent with spina bifida. *Journal of Adolescent Health, 15*, 543.

Zickler, C. F., & Dodge, N. N. (1994). Office management of the young child with cerebral palsy and difficulty growing. *Journal of Pediatric Health Care, 8*, 111.

Ziemba, S. K. (1995). Clinical snapshot: Seizures. *American Journal of Nursing, 95*, 32.

Zimmerman, S., & Gildea, J. (1985). *Critical care pediatrics.* Philadelphia: W. B. Saunders.

41

The Child With a Psychosocial Disorder

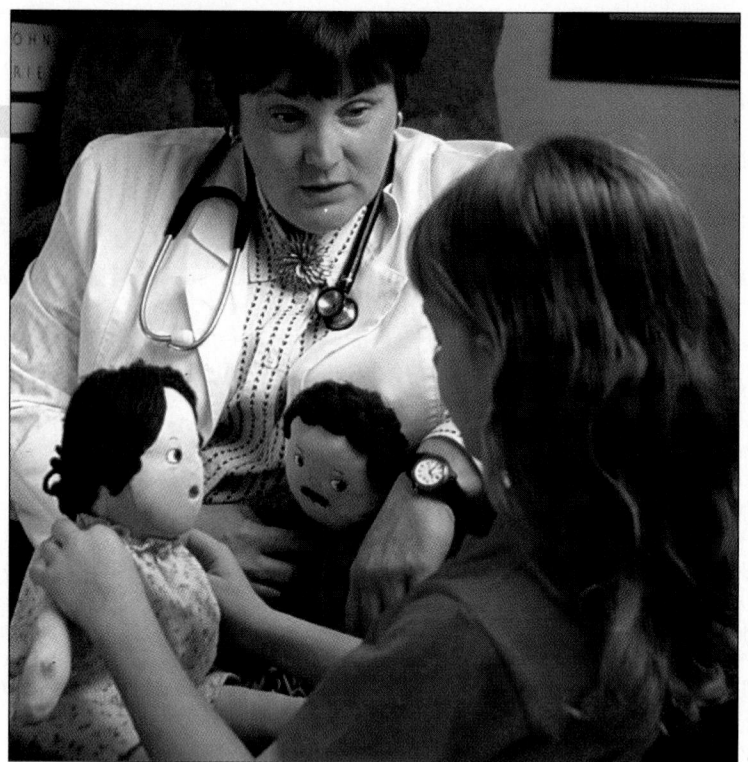

Courtesy of Cook Children's Medical Center, Fort Worth, Texas

CHAPTER OVERVIEW

LEARNING OBJECTIVES

After studying this chapter, you should be able to:

- Identify common characteristics of anxiety and depressive symptoms.
- Identify the factors and behaviors that correlate with childhood depression, suicide, or suicide attempts.
- Develop a nursing care plan for a potential suicide patient or for support of the family of a child who has committed suicide.
- Explore the symptomatology, etiology, risk factors, and psychologic dynamics associated with eating disorders.

- Use the nursing process to develop a nursing care plan for a patient with an eating disorder.
- Identify the primary symptoms and manifestations of attention-deficit hyperactivity disorder (ADHD).
- Use the nursing process to develop a nursing care plan for children and families with ADHD.
- Identify signs and symptoms of various types of substance abuse.
- Describe the family characteristics and social factors that contribute to physical, emotional, and sexual abuse of children.
- Identify the nurse's responsibilities for the safety and welfare of children relative to emotional, physical, and sexual abuse.
- Develop a nursing care plan for a child who has been abused.
- Develop a care plan for a family with a child who is described as having failure to thrive.

KEY TERMS

abuse: a general term that includes nonaccidental physical injury, or the nonaccidental act of omission by a parent or person responsible for the care of a child. This term includes physical injury, sexual molestation, neglect, and emotional injury

comorbidity: the presence of two different but interactive conditions existing simultaneously within a single individual

double message: a verbal message that is contradictory to the underlying tone or meaning of the message

substance abuse: excessive or inappropriate use of medication in order to modify mood or behavior or in a manner that results in social, occupational, psychological, or physical problems, or in a situation that creates a physical hazard

substance addiction: a physical or psychological dependence on a substance, with continued use even when it is known to impair cognitive or social functioning

substance dependence: a physical or psychological craving for a chemical substance, the cessation of which causes withdrawal symptoms

suicide: a voluntary and intentional cessation of one's life

suicide attempt: any actions taken by an individual toward self that will result in death if not interrupted

suicide gesture: a suicide attempt that is undertaken primarily to get attention rather than to actually take one's life; nonetheless, it is still considered a serious behavior

suicide threat: a statement or behavior that usually occurs prior to overt suicidal activity

violence: the use of extreme force or a destructive action that results in injury, discordance, or outrage, and/or engaging in sudden intense activity to the point of loss of control

Pediatric nursing includes a number of disorders and conditions that are best viewed as psychosocial disorders, as they primarily involve the way in which the child or adolescent relates to others and copes with stress. For most psychosocial disorders, there is a familial or biologic predisposition that is triggered if the environment is demanding or unsupportive. Psychosocial disorders may be produced by physical stressors, such as birth defects, physical injuries, and chronic illness. They may also be produced by emotional stressors, such as inconsistent or contradictory child-rearing practices, marital conflict, or neglect. Some psychosocial disorders, such as autism or mental retardation, are inheritable disorders. Other disorders are primarily related to an inaccurate or inappropriate relationship between the child and significant others in the social environment. Research consistently shows that psychosocial disorders are caused by a combination of predisposing or inherent factors and environmental or interactional factors.

This chapter discusses several common psychosocial issues in children and adolescents: depression and anxiety, suicide, eating disorders, abuse (including failure to thrive), attention-deficit hyperactivity disorder, and substance abuse. Related disorders, including mental retardation and pervasive developmental disorders, are presented in Chapter 42. Encopresis is discussed with constipation in Chapter 26, and enuresis is covered in Chapter 27.

CLINICAL REFERENCE PAGES

OVERVIEW OF CHILDHOOD PSYCHOPATHOLOGY

Neurobiologic factors, family factors, and sociocultural factors can contribute to the development of psychosocial disorders in children. Neurobiologic factors are briefly reviewed in the section that follows; family, social, and cultural factors are discussed in conjunction with the various disorders presented within this chapter.

Neurobiologic Factors. For disorders with a psychological basis, the primary organ involved is the brain, together with chemicals produced and used by the brain to initiate specific actions. These actions include memory, learning, attention and concentration, mood, and cognition. Because the brain develops throughout childhood, significant changes in the anatomy and physiology of the brain also occur. The most significant changes affecting psychosocial development include myelinization, growth of new tissue, and extension of the neural system throughout the brain. (See the Clinical Reference Pages in Chapter 40 for a review of brain anatomy and physiology.)

The brain increases in tissue mass and size throughout childhood and adolescence. The increase in the size of the brain results in an increased potential for memory and complex cognitive reasoning, as well as the capacity to learn new skills and acquire new information. Cognitive development proceeds from the simple to the complex, and from the concrete to the abstract. (For a more complete description of cognitive development, refer to Chapter 42.)

The effect of damage to the brain is dependent upon several factors. One of the most significant factors is the maturational stage of the brain at the time the damage occurs. Early damage spares more language functions, but may cause changes in all subsequent areas of development related to the specific area of the brain that is injured. Another factor is the length of time the brain tissue is impaired (as a result of swelling, hemorrhage, or tissue destruction). Finally, the specific area of the brain that is damaged may determine the specific areas of deficit. One factor, which is not directly related to actual tissue damage but is clearly related to effects on behavior, is the individual's perception of an experience, which is encoded into the brain's memory system and used as a basis for later behaviors.

Manifestations of Psychopathology. Psychosocial disorders are responses to stress and may be manifested as disturbances in feeling (e.g., depression, anxiety), in body functions (e.g., encopresis, enuresis), in behavior (e.g., conduct disturbance, school avoidance, or passive-aggressive behaviors), or in performance (learning problems). The manner in which an individual responds to stress is dependent on multiple factors.

FACTORS DETERMINING INDIVIDUAL RESPONSES TO STRESS

- Temperament
- Developmental level
- Nature and duration of the stress
- Past experiences
- Coping and adaptive abilities of the family

Disorders that are typically first evident in childhood are listed in the accompanying box.

Psychosocial Disorders Typically Manifested in Childhood

Mental retardation (see Chapter 42)

Pervasive developmental disorders/autistic disorder

Learning disorders: reading, arithmetic, etc.

Disruptive behavior disorders: Attention-deficit hyperactivity disorder, conduct disorder, oppositional defiant disorder

Anxiety disorders: separation anxiety disorder, overanxious disorder, post-traumatic stress disorder, reactive attachment disorder; dissociative disorders

Mood disorders: depression; bipolar disorder

Eating disorders: anorexia nervosa, bulimia nervosa, pica, obesity, rumination disorder of infancy

Tic disorders: Tourette's disorder, chronic motor or vocal tics, transient tics

Elimination disorders: functional encopresis, functional enuresis (see Chapters 26 and 27)

Speech disorders: receptive or expressive language disorders, cluttering, stuttering, elective mutism

Data from American Psychiatric Association. (1994). *Diagnostic and Statistical Manual of Mental Disorders* (4th ed.). Washington, DC: Author; Johnson, B. S., et al. (1995).

Diagnostic Evaluation. Diagnosing psychosocial disturbance in a child is difficult for several reasons. First, there is a wide range of normal emotional and social behaviors for young children. Even through adolescence, the individual is maturing and developing in terms of coping skills, attitudinal responses, and perspective. During childhood, there is marked inconsistency and unpredictability in behavioral responses to various situations. Also, during examinations, both the child and adolescent are markedly affected by their relationship and level of comfort with the examiner, as well as the setting. Finally, children and adolescents are affected and shaped by their relationships with parents and other social figures. For a thorough assessment of psychosocial disorders, a structured mental status examination of the child must be completed (see the accompanying box). Various laboratory and diagnostic tests may also be appropriate (see pertinent box). The results of these tests will help to determine whether pharmacologic intervention may be effective. Medications commonly used to treat psychosocial disorders in children and adolescents are presented in the accompanying table.

Mental Status Examination of Children

Appearance—dress, gestures, posture, tics or other repetitive movements; physical presentation, such as age, stature, race, age-appropriate behaviors

Ability to attend to task

Mood or affect—predominant feelings, mood fluctuations, mood congruence with verbalizations

Manner of relating to the examiner—exploration of their understanding of the purpose of the interview, approach or avoidance behaviors, use of play materials available, verbalizations

Intellectual skills—problem-solving abilities, conceptualization of causality, body image, memory, judgment, general fund of knowledge, insight (as compared to developmental norms)

Capacity for imaginative thinking and play

Sensorimotor development—fine and gross motor skills, symmetry and coordination of movement, hand and eye dominance, right-left discrimination

Presence/absence of suicidal-homicidal ideation, intent, plan; delusions or illusions; hallucinations

Speech—fluency, tone, volume, age-appropriateness

Common Laboratory and Diagnostic Tests for Psychosocial Disorders in Children and Adolescents

- **Urine Tests:** Used to assess for specific drugs excreted by the kidneys
- **Blood and Serum Tests:** Used to assess the long-term effects of malnutrition, evidence of specific drugs or ingested chemicals, and potency of selected pharmacotherapeutic agents prescribed for symptom reduction
- **X-ray Studies of the Skull and Long Bones:** Frequently used to identify current and previous fractures, as these are common signs of physical abuse
- **Genital and Anal Examinations:** Performed by a physician and used, together with slides of secretions, to help determine whether sexual abuse has occurred
- **Measurement of Subcutaneous Tissue:** May be ordered if physical neglect associated with malnutrition is suspected

MEDICATIONS COMMONLY USED TO TREAT PSYCHOSOCIAL DISORDERS IN CHILDREN AND ADOLESCENTS

DRUG, DOSAGE, ADMINISTRATION ROUTE	ACTION	SIDE EFFECTS	NURSING CONSIDERATIONS
Stimulants			
Dextroamphetamine (Dexedrine): 0.3–1.5 mg/kg daily PO	Increased concentration, decreased impulsivity	Insomnia, decreased appetite, nausea, weight loss, depression, increased heart rate and blood pressure, tics	Instruct the parents to administer the medication following meals, rather than before. Avoid caffeine, which potentiates the actions of stimulants. Do not administer the final dose after 4 to 5 p.m. Monitor weight and growth changes. Offer rest opportunities. Monitor heart rate changes as the child matures. The child may require more medication with age.
Methylphenidate (Ritalin): 0.3–2.0 mg/kg daily PO	Same as above		
Pemoline (Cylert): 1–3 mg/kg/day PO	Same as above	Abnormal liver function	
Neuroleptics			
Chlorpromazine (Thorazine): 3–6 mg/kg/day PO or IM	To reduce agitation, aggressive behaviors, thought disturbance	Sedation; extrapyramidal symptoms, including lowered blood pressure, sun sensitivity, alterations in appetite and weight, anticholinergic effects (dry mouth, dilated pupils, increased heart rate, delayed urination)	Instruct the child/parents to avoid direct and intense sunlight and to use sunscreen. Monitor the child's intake and output, and blood pressure. Avoid skin contact with medication. Suck hard candy or sugarless gum. Do not withdraw medication abruptly.
Thioridazine (Mellaril): 0.5–3 mg/kg/day PO			
Fluphenazine (Prolixin): 0.1–0.5 mg/kg/day IM			
Thiothixene (Navane): 1–3 mg/kg/day PO			
Haloperidol (Haldol): 0.1–0.5 mg/kg/day PO or IM			
Antianxiety Medications			
Paroxetine (Paxil): 0.25–0.70 mg/kg AM PO	Similar to other selective serotonin reuptake inhibitors (SSRIs)	Irritability, insomnia, gastrointestinal symptoms, headaches	Similar to other SSRIs
Tricyclic Antidepressants			
Imipramine (Tofranil): 1.5 mg/kg/day PO. May increase by 1 mg/kg, not to exceed 5 mg/kg/day.	Elevates mood	Sedation, anticholinergic effects, lightheadedness, tachycardia	Provide a minimum supply to decrease suicide risk. Monitor the child's intake and output. Taper medication. Avoid activities that require alertness and psychomotor coordination until the child's CNS response to the drug is determined. Expect a lag time of 10–14 days before noticeable effects.
Nortriptyline (Pamelor): 10–50 mg/day PO (adolescent patients)			
Selective Serotonin Reuptake Inhibitors			
Fluoxetine hydrochloride (Prozac): 0.5–1.0 mg/kg/day PO	Inhibits serotonin uptake in CNS, enhancing serotoninergic function For treatment of major depression Suppresses appetite, elevates mood, decreases gastric secretions	Nausea, headache, nervousness, insomnia, anxiety, dry mouth	Give in a.m. to decrease insomnia side effect. Administer with food or milk if gastrointestinal distress occurs. Observe the patient for suicidal risk as depression lowers and energy level rises.
Sertraline hydrochloride (Zoloft): 1.5–3.0 mg/kg/day PO	Similar to fluoxetine; selective blocking of serotonin uptake with enhancement of synaptic activity	Headache, tremor, insomnia, agitation, nervousness, nausea, diarrhea, dry mouth	Same as for fluoxetine hydrochloride
Paroxetine (Paxil): 0.25–0.70 mg/kg/day PO	Same as for sertraline hydrochloride	Nausea, headache, dry mouth, weakness, sweating, tremor, fatigue, weight gain, insomnia	Same as for fluoxetine hydrochloride. Caution the patient to avoid tasks that require alertness.
Fluvoxamine (Luvox): 1.5–4.5 mg/kg/day PO	Selectively inhibits serotonin uptake in CNS, enhancing serotoninergic function For treatment of depression, obsessive-compulsive disorders	Nausea, somnolence, asthenia, headache, dry mouth, insomnia	Side effects are minimized by giving the entire daily dose at bedtime.

Abbreviations: PO, per os; IM, intramuscularly; CNS, central nervous system

ANXIETY AND DEPRESSION

Mood or affective disturbances in children and adolescents are generally of two types: anxiety and/or depression. It is difficult to differentiate between anxiety and depressive disorders in children for several reasons. In children and adolescents, the behavioral presentation of both disorders may be similar. For example, the child who is anxious may be withdrawn, tearful, unwilling to engage in play, or prone to acting aggressively toward others. These same symptoms typically present in children who are depressed. Moreover, it is often difficult to differentiate between normal mood changes secondary to normal developmental maturation and adaptation, and abnormal, persistent mood disturbances. Generally, however, mood disturbance is more intense and persistent, and interferes with social relations and daily functioning. Finally, the child or adolescent may have evidence of both anxiety and depression.

Classification

Anxiety Disorders. Anxiety is the most common mood disturbance in childhood and may present as one of several specific disorders. Separation anxiety is normal for children ages 6 months to 24 months, but it is considered a *separation anxiety disorder* if it occurs past 24 months of age, persists for more than 4 weeks, and creates functional difficulties (e.g., refusal to leave the house to play with friends). This disorder occurs in about 40% of children and young adolescents (American Psychiatric Association, 1994). One form of separation anxiety is *school phobia.* In this disorder, the child is so fearful of separation from the parent or other major attachment figure that they are afraid to attend school. Another common anxiety disorder is *social phobia,* whereby individuals avoid social or performance situations to such a degree that their daily routine is affected (e.g., by refusing to participate in physical education exercises, or failing to raise their hands to ask a question in class). The anxiety may be so intense that the child experiences a sense of panic, in which case the disorder may be termed *panic disorder.* One type of panic disorder that follows a specific and terrifying event is *post-traumatic stress disorder.* Symptoms of this disorder include intense fear, helplessness, or horror, along with physiologic symptoms of increased arousal. The individual demonstrates persistent avoidance of stimuli associated with the traumatic event. This disorder is frequently seen in children who have been sexually or physically abused.

Depressive Disorders. Depressive disorders are also varied and are specified by the intensity or duration of depressive symptoms or the particular behaviors displayed by the individual. Children or adolescents who exhibit a depressed or irritable mood for at least 1 year meet the criteria for *dysthymic disorder.* If the child experiences chronic, fluctuating mood disturbances for 1 year, *cyclothymic disorder* or *bipolar mood disorder* may be diagnosed. If the clinical presentation includes a 2-week (or longer) episode of depressed or irritable mood, in addition to disturbances in appetite, sleep, psychomotor activity, energy, or self-esteem, the child meets the criteria for *major depressive disorder.* A psychiatric nursing text should be reviewed for more detailed information about these specific disorders.

Psychophysiology. Research supports the view that both anxiety and depression have a biologic basis. Among the biochemical agents that appear to modulate mood are monoamines, including catecholamines and indolamines, and neurotransmitters, such as noradrenaline, serotonin, and acetylcholine. The limbic region in the brain is considered to be the "seat of emotions," and chemical or physical alterations in this region have been found to impact mood, as well as some other characteristics, such as energy, self-valuation, and sleep patterns.

Etiology. Affective disorders are believed to have a genetic basis, as first-degree relatives with an anxiety or depressive disorder may predict an increased risk of the disorder in offsprings. Monozygotic twins have been shown to have as high a concordance rate as 65% for affective disorders when compared to dizygotic twins, who have only a 14% concordance rate (Bernstein & Borchardt, 1991).

Psychosocial theories emphasize the importance of the interaction within the family system, behavioral patterns of the individual, and interpersonal factors in the development of depression. There is evidence that individuals in dysfunctional families, those with behavioral disorders, and individuals with limited social interactions are at increased risk for both anxiety and depressive disorders. For example, children who come from families with overprotective, hostile, overly controlling, or unaffectionate parents are more likely than their peers with healthy family patterns to develop anxiety symptoms or depression (Messer & Beidel, 1994). The likelihood that anxiety or depressive symptoms are inherent in most psychosocial disorders is without dispute. So, in addition to meeting criteria for an anxiety or depressive disorder, it is likely for the affected individual to also suffer from substance abuse, attention-deficit disorder, sleep disorders, encopresis, conduct disorder, or a host of other difficulties.

Incidence. Current epidemiologic information about anxiety disorders in children indicate that, by 11 years of age, 8.9% meet the criteria for some form of anxiety disorder, and by age 17, 17.3% meet the same criteria (Costello, 1989; Bernstein & Borchardt, 1991).

It is estimated that the incidence of depressive disorders for adolescents in the general population is in the range of 0.4% to 6.4%. Depression before puberty is uncommon. The rate for depressive symptoms for children and adolescents is higher than for actual depressive disorders, ranging from 1.8% to 59% depending on the population surveyed.

Clinical Manifestations. The clinical manifestations of anxiety/depressive disorders include the following:

- Sad or irritable mood
- Diminished interest in daily activities
- Significant weight loss or gain
- Insomnia or hypersomnia
- Psychomotor agitation or retardation
- Fatigue or loss of energy
- Feelings of worthlessness, hopelessness, or excessive guilt
- Diminished ability to think or concentrate
- Recurrent thoughts of death or suicide
- Somatic complaints, such as recurrent abdominal pain or headaches, with no physical cause

Therapeutic Management. Although medications are frequently prescribed for anxiety and depressive disorders, there is wide variation in response. Typically, even if medication is prescribed, the most effective treatment includes an opportunity for the child and family to explore situations and environmental factors that are related to the child's symptoms. Individual and family therapy are essential for patients with suicidal ideation or persistent mood disturbances. Social skills training or group therapy may be most helpful for social anxiety. School phobia is usually treated by insisting that the child attend school, offering interventions during school time to reduce anxiety symptoms, and refusing to pick up the child from school, even if the child insists. This form of intervention is a type of desensitization therapy. Other strategies for decreasing anxiety and/or depressive symptoms include relaxation therapy, distraction strategies, self-talk, or cognitive strategies, as well as support from adults or friends who are safe and reassuring.

NURSING CARE OF THE CHILD WITH ANXIETY OR DEPRESSION

Assessment

A thorough history should be obtained from the perspective of both the child and the family. Initially, it may be necessary to interview the child in front of the parent(s), but once the child becomes more comfortable with the nurse, time alone with the child should be offered. The interview should cover both the child's mood and the events that are related to those moods, physiologic symptoms, patterns of daily activities, identification of stressors, and information about the duration, frequency, and intensity of symptoms. Suicidal ideation or plan should be assessed by asking both direct and indirect questions (see the box entitled Questions to Assess Suicidal Potential in the subsequent section on suicide).

Questions about the family environment should seek to identify those with whom the child relates most easily, recent stressors (e.g., changes in residence or schools), and family interaction patterns. It is important to explore any family history of mood disturbance, as well as other emotional problems or substance abuse problems.

Several self-reporting instruments and interview schedules are available for the specific assessment of anxiety and depression. The Schedule for Affective Disorders and Schizophrenia for School-Aged Children (K-SADS) is often used in psychiatric settings (Puig-Antich & Chambers, 1978). The Children's Depression Rating Scale (CDRS) (Pozanski et al., 1979) and the Children's Depression Inventory (CDI) (Kovacs, 1981) are often used in outpatient settings to assess depression symptoms (Spielberger, 1975). The State-Trait Anxiety Inventory for Children (STAIC) and the Revised Children's Manifest Anxiety Scale (REMAS) are frequently used to assess anxiety symptoms (Reynolds & Richmond, 1979).

NURSING DIAGNOSIS AND PLANNING

The following nursing diagnoses and expected outcomes may be appropriate following assessment of the child with anxiety or depression:

Nursing Diagnoses

- Ineffective Individual Coping related to loss of energy, sleep disturbance, biochemical imbalance, loss of control
- Self-Esteem Disturbance related to cognitive distortions, inability to manage daily events, sense of hopelessness or guilt
- Risk for Violence: Self-Directed, related to suicidal ideation, guilt, or hopelessness
- Sleep Pattern Disturbance related to anxiety, depression, and inactivity

Expected Outcomes

The child will:

- display adaptive ability to attend to activities of daily living
- relate an increase in self-confidence and an increase in positive feelings about self
- identify and interact in a socially positive manner with significant others
- report a decrease in frequency and/or severity of depressed or anxious mood
- express feelings of being well rested and show no signs of sleep deprivation (irritability, lethargy, restlessness)

Implementation

The nurse is part of a team who will offer support for the entire family while exploring the contributing factors for the emotional distress in the child. The nurse should participate in identifying specific changes in the environment and interaction patterns that would support a sense of control and positive regard for the child. Setting up a schedule for activities of daily living with frequent rest periods (or "recovery periods") are generally helpful for anxious or depressed patients. Privacy and space for the child and/or family members to discuss their feelings as treatment progresses should be made available on a regular basis.

If the child requires hospitalization, admission will generally be to a psychiatric unit, where specialized nursing is available. However, it is common for children who are cared for on pediatric units, in outpatient clinics, or in school systems to be identified with mood disturbance. Education of parents and teachers about depression and anxiety in childhood is an important service for nurses to provide to the community.

Evaluation

In assessing the effectiveness of therapeutic interventions, the nurse should ask:

- Does the child report feeling happier, less sad, or less "upset"?
- Does the child exhibit normal patterns of eating and sleeping?
- Does the child exhibit an energy level that allows for interactions, play, and work?
- Does the child seem interested in people and events?

SUICIDE

Suicide is a leading cause of death in adolescents. It may also be the underlying cause of some accidents in adolescents. Children most at risk are those who are vulnerable to depression, including youngsters who are HIV-positive and those who have family members who have attempted suicide (Kelly, 1991). As in other psychosocial disorders, there appear to be sociologic, genetic, and psychological components that contribute to an understanding of suicide in children and adolescents.

Psychopathology. There are several theories about the dynamics of suicide. The first is a psychological perspective that examines intrapsychic willingness to identify with a deceased or unavailable love object, an internalization of anger, and use of interpersonal goals to gain love or to inflict punishment. The sociological perspective focuses on the life situation or position in society that is unacceptable to the individual, and the view that suicide is the only logical escape from an intolerable situation. The psychiatric perspective emphasizes the distortions of perceptions and judgment that characterize a disturbance in the mental state of the individual (Pallikkathayil & Flood, 1991).

Development of a concept of mortality and death follows the general laws of the development of cognitive and affective abilities, from the concrete to the abstract. Up to the age of 6 years, it is unlikely that a child has any realistic concept of death or that the child looks for death in an active way. However, there are children as young as 3 years of age who have tried to commit suicide and seemed to understand what they were doing. Between the ages of 6 and 8 years, the child abandons an egocentric view and discovers that death is one of many events out of an individual's control. From the age of 9 years on, the child most likely views death as inevitable and universal. As the child's understanding of the concept of death increases, so does the risk for suicide within that population (Vaz-Leal, 1989).

Etiology. Underlying depression and poor self-concept appear to be the most significant contributing factors for suicide, regardless of age or gender. Long-standing family dysfunction is generally present, with emotional detachment and isolation between family members. Typically, the suicide victim is a vulnerable individual who, under stress, seeks and finds a way to die. The individual is, for some reason, unable to elicit adequate adult support to stop the suicide process.

Incidence. Estimates of prevalence for moderate to severe suicidal ideation are 4.5% for male individuals and 8.7% for female individuals. The prevalence of **suicide attempts** is 1.9% in males and 1.5% in females. For completed suicides, the ratio is 2 to 3 males for every female (Pallikkathayil & Flood, 1991). Statistics for suicide attempts in children younger than 10 years of age are generally not collected. However, there is evidence that the incidence of suicide ideation and attempt is increasing among children younger than 10 years of age.

Clinical Manifestations and Risk Factors

The risk of suicide should be considered if the following are present:

- Suicidal clues, such as cryptic verbal messages, giving away of personal items, and changes in expected patterns of behaviors (i.e., sudden calmness in a normally anxious teenager)
- Specific statements about suicide or self-harm
- Preoccupation with death, often manifested by interest in death themes in literature and art
- Frequent risk-taking or self-abusive behaviors
- Overwhelming sense of guilt or shame
- Obsessional self-doubt
- Open signs of mental illness manifested as delusions or hallucinations
- Significant change in a major life event that is internally disruptive
- History of physical or sexual abuse

Therapeutic Management. Suicide prevention is viewed as the most significant mental health contribution and is promoted at the local, state, and federal level. Prevention is offered through multimedia educational presentations in schools, support groups at local mental health centers, emphasis in communities on stress reduction, social affiliations, and networking within support systems.

One of the most significant prevention strategies is screening for depression, both within the school system and the health care system. Most individuals who commit suicide have been in contact with one of these systems and have offered at least veiled information about their suicidal ideation or feelings of despair prior to the event. Federal funds are provided for education, research, and treatment in order to reduce the incidence of suicide.

Following a child's suicide, services must be provided to family members and immediate friends of the child. It is important for these services to be offered quickly, preferably within the first 24 hours after the suicide, and to remain available for the first year following the event. Grief and emotional adjustment often takes several months and may peak around the anniversary date of the suicide event.

It is common for suicides to occur in a cluster within a community.

Persistent suicidal ideation is a significant clue to a potential suicide attempt. Children with these thoughts should undergo a thorough psychiatric evaluation by a mental health professional. The child may require pharmacotherapeutic agents, such as antidepressants or antipsychotic medications.

The use of medications in children at risk for suicide requires close monitoring and allocations in small dosages, as they may be used in a suicide attempt or act.

NURSING CARE OF THE CHILD AT RISK FOR SUICIDE

Assessment

The risk of suicide is best assessed using a systematic approach to behaviors, attitudes, and risk factors. Several instruments have been developed to assess lethality and potentiality, which have lessened the likelihood of overlooking contributing factors. Each of the instruments is similar in that they explore risk factors, such as age and gender, stressors, lethality of the proposed method of suicide, coping mechanisms, and support systems to arrive at an overall score measuring suicide potential. When assessing an individual for suicide ideation or potential (see accompanying box), it is important not to overlook subtle symptoms of depression and/or anxiety, such as decreased energy or persistent restlessness. It is also important to explore thought content and organization, awareness and expression of feelings, perceived level and types of stress, perceived availability of support resources, prior suicidal behaviors, and medical status.

Questions to Assess Suicide Potential

1. Have you ever thought of trying to hurt yourself? How might you do this?
2. Have you ever thought of killing yourself? How might you do this?
3. Have you known anyone who has committed suicide/killed themselves? When did this occur? What was it like for you?
4. Do you have access to firearms? Knives?
5. Do you ever do things to deliberately place yourself in danger, such as driving when you are drunk or playing Russian roulette with a gun?
6. Have you ever told anyone about wanting to kill yourself?
7. Have you ever been hospitalized for suicidal behavior?
8. How do you feel right now?

A **suicide gesture** or threat should NEVER be ignored. The child should be encouraged to discuss the thought specifically, and help should be obtained from qualified health professionals.

Nursing Diagnosis and Planning

The following nursing diagnoses and expected outcomes may be appropriate following assessment of the child at risk for suicide.

Nursing Diagnoses

- Risk for Violence: Self-Directed, related to a desire to cease emotional pain, to solicit attention of others, or to avoid responsibility
- Self-Esteem Disturbance related to a sense of failure and hopelessness about the ability to change self or circumstances
- Anxiety related to current or anticipated events
- Altered Family Processes related to relational disturbance or possible abuse or neglect
- Ineffective Individual Coping related to a sense of despair or limited availability of support

Expected Outcomes

The child/adolescent and family will:

- regain a sense of internal balance and control, lessening the likelihood of a repeated suicide attempt
- elicit the necessary support from others to meet needs of attention, belonging, and worth
- assume responsibility for personal actions and decisions
- mobilize support systems in an effective manner to reduce the likelihood of another suicide decision
- develop a "Suicide Prevention Plan"

Implementation

The nurse's therapeutic approach should be empathetic and nonjudgmental in order to decrease the child's sense of isolation and rejection. This can be conveyed by adopting a voice and demeanor that are clear, direct, and supportive. Protecting the youth from inflicting harm to self can be accomplished by being emotionally and physically available, offering opportunities to discuss feelings and the suicidal event, and removing potentially harmful objects.

The nurse should suggest alternative coping strategies, such as choosing alternative activities when impulses arise, and remaining near other people. The nurse can help the child identify specific feelings and effective ways to manage those feelings. It is important for the nurse to assess how closely a child needs to be monitored throughout the day, realizing that the potential for self-harm fluctuates.

Anticipatory guidance/grieving for families of suicidal or potentially suicidal individuals is best provided on both an individual and group basis in order to allow a balance between the need to explore personal issues and the need for social support. It is important to be aware that grieving will occur even if the suicide attempt was unsuccessful. Individual and family therapy will also provide an opportunity to explore contributory factors that can be altered to reduce the suicide potential. Working with the parents in a collaborative approach, with other therapeutic team members, will help the parents regain their ability to assist their child and manage the home environment. It is important to increase the adult-child interactions, thereby decreasing the risk of another suicide attempt.

Evaluation

In assessing the effectiveness of therapeutic intervention, the nurse should ask:

- Is the child able to identify times when suicidal potential is greatest and to seek help during these times?
- Does the child participate in activities that reduce feelings of despair and hopelessness?
- Does the child display evidence of positive self-esteem?

EATING DISORDERS: ANOREXIA NERVOSA AND BULIMIA NERVOSA

Eating disorder is a general term that encompasses anorexia nervosa, bulimia nervosa, pica, obesity, and rumination disorders. Anorexia nervosa and bulimia nervosa are discussed here, as they are two of the most common eating disorders among children. (Obesity is discussed in Chapter 12.) Although they have distinguishing features, both anorexia and bulimia have overlapping features and similar etiology, and there is support for viewing these disorders as a continuum, rather than as separate entities.

Anorexia nervosa is characterized by a deliberate refusal to maintain adequate body weight, a distorted body image, and amenorrhea (in females). The term anorexia is a misnomer, as the individual rarely experiences loss of appetite. *Bulimia nervosa* is characterized by recurrent episodes of binge eating; a sense of lack of control over eating binges; self-induced vomiting or excessive use of laxatives, diuretics, and/or emetics to prevent weight gain; and a persistent overconcern with body image. Shame and guilt about many life experiences, but especially eating, is typically reported by children and adolescents with eating disorders.

Individuals with severe eating disorders have a mortality rate of 6% to 10% from complications of the disorder or from suicide (Love & Seaton, 1991). Treatment resistance is very high in individuals with anorexia and bulimia, because their entire psychological and sociologic experiences are framed by their body image and self-esteem, and because of secondary gains such as attention, admiration, envy, and control over others through eating patterns. Unfortunately, in addition to the eating disorder, about 50% of the patients with eating disorders meet criteria for other serious psychiatric disorders, such as major depression or a personality disorder.

Ritualistic behaviors are common in these children and adolescents, particularly around issues of food. For example, the patient may eat only at a particular time of day, eat foods only in a certain order, or insist on washing all foods before eating. The rituals are often an attempt to control the portions, fat content, or nutrients ingested. The rituals also serve to enhance the individual's sense of control over food and/or dietary intake. Frequently, the individual will spend hours preparing foods, but will refuse to eat any of the food prepared.

PATHOPHYSIOLOGY ***of Eating Disorders***

Frequently, an impaired carbohydrate metabolism in the hypothalamic-pituitary axis is noted in individuals with an eating disorder. The conversion of thyroxine (T_4) to triiodothyronine (T_3) is inadequate. Phosphate concentrations are inadequate, especially in patients with severe anorexia complicated by bulimic episodes. Patients with eating disorders commonly experience hypokalemia, hypochloremia, hyponatremia, alkalosis, dental enamel erosion, parotid and salivary gland enlargement, decreased transferrin levels, and malabsorption complications.

The child or adolescent will go to extreme measures to prevent others from becoming aware of their weight loss or lack of food intake. The patient may ingest large amounts of water or insert heavy objects in the vaginal cavity prior to weighing in order to give the impression of weight gain. The patient may eat in front of people and then go to the bathroom to "purge" themselves following the meal.

Etiology. Disordered eating emerges from multiple risk factors. One of the most salient factors appears to be "enmeshed" family relationships, in which the individual is considered to be an extension of the parent or is viewed as a means of meeting the parents' needs rather than being allowed to develop as an autonomous individual. The family system typically includes a mother who is overprotective, lacks empathy, and is overly invested in daily activities with the child. The father is often emotionally distant from the mother and the child. This type of family structure results in a suppression of the child's growth as an individual. The disorder is more common among sisters and mothers of those with the disorder than among the general population, suggesting some familial predisposition.

The development and severity of the individual's risk for eating disorders appear to be related to the child's response to biologic maturity, and to the psychological and social demands of sexual development. Also, if life events disrupt developmental progress or make premature demands on the child, there is an increased risk of an eating disorder. Thirty-three percent to 70% of women with eating disorders report early sexual abuse and trauma, which provides further evidence that the child assumes a role in meeting the needs of adults, rather than benefiting from adult protection and support (Calam & Slade, 1989; Palmer et al., 1990). There are significant psychological and social factors that have been found to be relevant in the pathogenesis of eating disorders. These include such factors as depressive tendencies, alterations in brain neurotransmitters, cultural expectations to be thin, and the individual's pervasive sense of ineffectiveness.

Individuals with eating disorders usually have a family history of affective disorders. The family dynamics for male anorexics are reported to include poor father-son relationships, with the father typifying the strong, cultural image; and mothers that are overinvolved, overprotective, and overdependent on the mother-son relationship. In at least 50% of the males with eating disorders, there is a homosexual conflict, sexual isolation, anxiety about sexual behaviors with either sex, attempts to suppress sexual drives, and the presence of a gender identity disorder (Hamlett & Curry, 1990).

Incidence. Bulimia nervosa appears to be more prevalent than anorexia nervosa, with as many as 2% to 8% of the female adolescent population reporting symptoms. For girls between the ages of 12 and 18 years, the reported incidence for eating disorders of some type ranges from 1 in 800 to 1 in 1000. Eating disorders are more rare in boys, and clear information about their incidence in this population is not available.

Clinical Manifestations. The clinical manifestations of anorexia nervosa and bulimia nervosa include the following:

Anorexia Nervosa

- Refusal to maintain a body weight that exceeds the minimal weight recommended for height and weight (15% below expected weight)
- Intense preoccupation with and unrelenting fear of obesity
- Disturbance in body image (weight, size, or shape) that is obviously contrary to observable information (Fig. 41–1)
- In females, at least three missed menstrual periods (primary or secondary amenorrhea)
- Misperception of internal and external stimuli, particularly food-related cues, such as hunger
- Overwhelming feelings of ineffectiveness and inadequacy
- Lanugo
- Fatigue
- Dry, flaky skin
- Dull, brittle hair
- Muscle wasting

Boys with eating disorders demonstrate many behavior patterns similar to girls, including weight loss through excessive dieting, compulsive activities, and purging "to get strong" or to develop an athletic build (rather than "to be thin" as reported by females). Male individuals typically demonstrate obsessive and affective disturbances predominantly evidenced by irritability, anxiety, and depression (Hamlett & Curry, 1990).

Bulimia Nervosa

- Recurrent episodes of binge eating
- A sense of uncontrol over eating behaviors during binges
- Strategies employed to prevent weight gain (self-induced vomiting; use of laxatives, diuretics, or emetics; fasting; or vigorous exercise)
- A minimum of two binge eating episodes per week for at least 3 months
- Persistent overconcern with body shape and weight

Diagnostic Evaluation. An electrocardiogram and chest radiograph are typically performed if symptoms of bradycardia, hypotension, or hypothermia are noted. Complete liver and renal function tests and serum electrolyte studies are usually included in the medical work-up.

Therapeutic Management. The treatment of eating disorders is initially focused on the secondary effects of self-induced vomiting, excessive use of diuretics and laxatives, and the lack of nutrients to sustain function of body systems. Efforts to stabilize electrolyte levels and body chemistry values are crucial in order to prevent sustained damage to body systems, especially the cardiac, respiratory, and elimination systems. Adequate caloric intake is the next major

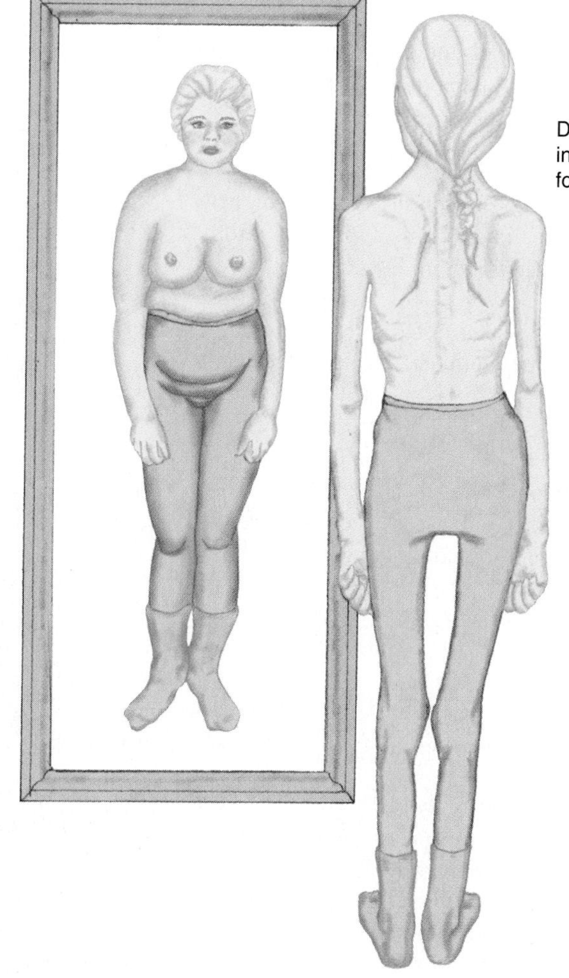

Figure 41–1
In anorexia nervosa, the adolescent refuses to maintain adequate body weight, partly because of a distorted body image: she perceives herself as overweight when, in fact, she is below minimum weight. The causes of eating disorders are complex, and can include troubled family relationships, as well as difficulty dealing with the demands of biologic maturity and sexual development. Cultural expectations to be thin, as well as an individual's pervasive sense of ineffectiveness, can also be contributing factors in eating disorders. About 50% of patients with eating disorders also have other serious psychiatric disorders, such as depression or personality disorder.

goal of treatment and often requires strict monitoring of the patient in order to prevent sabotage of medical treatment. Ongoing individual therapy is needed for the patient to cope with complex issues. Therapy must be intensive and highly individualized for the patient to begin adequate nutritional intake. Finally, alteration of misperceptions about body image and a reorientation to issues of control and self-management are necessary. Follow-up therapy for the individual and family is indicated for a period of several months, often up to 3 years.

NURSING CARE OF THE CHILD OR ADOLESCENT WITH AN EATING DISORDER

Assessment

Children and adolescents with eating disorders typically have varying degrees of mistrust, ambivalence, and denial. It is generally better if the assessment is conducted in a structured and concrete manner (rather than as an open-ended exploration), with emphasis placed on alliance building and periodic review of the assessment process for the child or adolescent. Determining the motivation for changing behaviors is crucial, and should be assessed for each specific behavior (i.e., weight gain, induced vomiting, altered self-perception of body). A mental status examination should also be included, as the side effects of restrictive dieting can impair cognitive functioning and perpetuate affective disturbances. Any history of self-injury should be noted. The nurse should assist the child or adolescent in gaining an understanding of impulse control problems and ritualistic and compulsive behaviors.

The medical history and physical assessment should be comprehensive, focusing on any medically based illness that mimics an eating disorder or that exists concomitantly. Psychological assessment of body image and identification of problems, substance abuse, and social support systems utilized by the patient are important components of the assessment. A family history of eating disorders or other psychiatric illnesses should be explored. Family dynamics, including level and/or quality of interaction, support, discipline, and differentiation of members, should be explored in depth. Previous treatment attempts and coping strategies should also be identified.

Nursing Diagnosis and Planning

The following nursing diagnoses and expected outcomes may be appropriate following assessment of the child or adolescent with an eating disorder.

Nursing Diagnoses

- Altered Nutrition: Less than Body Requirements, related to inadequate intake, malabsorption from extended periods of starvation, and/or distorted body image
- Anxiety/Fear or Powerlessness related to weight gain, sense of self-inadequacy, and fear of lack of control over body and self
- Activity Intolerance/Sleep Pattern Disturbance related to fatigue, depression, and an excessive drive to exercise and expend energy
- Fluid Volume Deficit related to excessive use of diuretics or laxatives and/or inadequate fiber and fluid intake

Expected Outcomes

The child/adolescent will:

- Gain sufficient weight and/or maintain an adequate weight to sustain systemic homeostasis and physiological health
- Demonstrate the ability to seek help with anxiety management and will demonstrate improved coping strategies, including open expression of feelings
- Establish improved sleeping and activity patterns with a corresponding improvement noted in affect, energy, and sense of well-being
- Have electrolyte levels that are within normal limits, normal skin turgor, and moist mucous membranes

Implementation

Children and adolescents with severe eating disorders may require hospitalization in order to support physiologic stability. These patients are then generally transferred to a day treatment program. The focus of care is to restructure cognitive perceptions, reduce opportunities to engage in ritualistic and self-injurious behaviors, and reestablish physiologic homeostasis. The programs typically include interventions that enlist the patient's cooperation in a refeeding program. Nutritional consultation is provided to facilitate gradual weight gain. Monitoring of intake and output, vital signs, laboratory values, electrolyte status, and cardiac status is essential. The adolescent will need to be supported in exploring refeeding sensations of fullness, bloating, and delayed gastric emptying and will need help tolerating these feelings and body sensations. The nurse and the adolescent jointly participate in monitoring affect, mood, and potential for suicide. The nurse and the adolescent agree to a contract specifying necessary interventions to ensure safety, as well as to monitor daily food intake and feelings. These interventions may take the form of interacting with the staff at regular intervals or agreeing to approach the staff if suicidal ideation is present. The nurse will need to validate the patient's feelings of ambivalence, fear, and powerlessness. If hyperalimentation or nasogastric tube feedings are needed for adequate nutritional intake, the nurse should provide support to the patient and monitor feedings. Finally, the nurse should provide educational information about the short- and long-term effects of starvation.

> During the early phase of treatment, it may be necessary to observe the adolescent following meals to prevent episodes of purging.

The nurse is likely to participate in providing or supporting psychological treatments, such as individual, group, and family therapy sessions. Especially in the early phase of treatment, the adolescent may be very resistant to efforts to increase nutritional intake and may resort to denial, trickery, or manipulation in order to prevent weight increase or thwart adherence to dietary regimens. For example, the patient may drink large amounts of water prior to weighing, to convey that weight is being gained. Or, the patient may deny deliberately vomiting after meals.

Keeping the family informed and involved about the treatment goals and progress is essential. Participation of the family in family therapy is generally a required part of the treatment plan, as the etiology of the disorder is generally directly related to family interaction patterns. It is important for the nurse to support the family in voicing their concerns about the patient while encouraging the family to view the adolescent as having an identity and sense of control that is independent of the family.

Evaluation

Has the child or adolescent:

- demonstrated an increase in food consumption adequate to sustain growth and developmental needs?
- reduced binging/purging activities?
- demonstrated a positive alteration in self-perceptions and body image, as evidenced by an increased sense of self-control and decreased anxiety about the present and the future?
- demonstrated a decrease in ambivalence and mistrust about self and significant others?

ATTENTION-DEFICIT HYPERACTIVITY DISORDER

Attention-deficit hyperactivity disorder (ADHD) is a diagnostic label for children presenting with significant problems in three specific areas: (1) attention and concentration, (2) impulse control, and (3) overactivity. Over the years, it has variously been called postencephalitic behavior disorder, restlessness syndrome, hyperkinetic impulse disorder, minimal brain dysfunction, and hyperactive child syndrome. At present, the term for this disorder is attention-deficit hyperactivity disorder (ADHD). The most comprehensive definition has been provided by Barkley (1990):

> *ADHD is a developmental disorder characterized by developmentally inappropriate degrees of inattention, overactivity, and impulsivity. These often arise in early childhood, are relatively chronic in nature, and are not readily accounted for on the basis of gross neurological, sensory, language, or motor impairment; mental retardation; or severe emotional disturbance. These difficulties are typically associated with deficits in rule-governed behavior and in maintaining a consistent pattern of work performance over time.*

There is increasing evidence that impulsivity and hyperactivity, or poor response regulation and inhibition, are the underlying foundations for this condition.

ADHD is one of the most common reasons for referral of children to mental health services. These referrals are made by either parents or teachers. Adults are often not only concerned about the primary symptoms, which often result in frequent injuries, poor scholastic performance, and low performance motivation, but also because of associated symptoms, which may include affective distress (anxiety or depression), aggressiveness toward peers, and antisocial or oppositional defiance toward authority figures (see accompanying box).

Childhood Problems Associated With ADHD

Lowered intellectual development:
- Lowered academic performance
- Learning difficulties
- Impaired complex problem-solving skills

Impaired organizational skills

Minor physical abnormalities:
- Curved fifth finger
- Adherent ear lobes
- Furrowed tongue
- Greater skin on nasal side of the eyelid

Increased incidence of sleeping problems

Comorbidity with other behavioral or emotional disorders:
- Oppositional and defiant behaviors
- Aggressive behaviors
- Conduct disorder behaviors
- Antisocial behaviors

Significant difficulty in social relationships

Within a single individual affected with ADHD, there may be wide variations in response to the environment. For example, if the complexity of the task is high, the child with ADHD is likely to perform poorly. If the structure is rigid and the restrictions on behavior are high, the child with ADHD becomes increasingly distinguishable from unaffected children. If instructions are repeated frequently or if the task is novel or unfamiliar, the child's performance tends to improve. One of the most significant environmental variables that affects the behavior of children with ADHD is the rate of immediate reinforcement. These children require much higher rates of reinforcement than their same-age peers. Fatigue may also affect the degree to which ADHD symptoms are exhibited.

PATHOPHYSIOLOGY *of ADHD*

The research is inconclusive, but there is some consistent evidence that the basis of this disorder is a sluggish or underreactive neurologic, electrophysiologic response to stimulation. Prefrontal and limbic system connections in the brain are viewed as the most likely locations for neurologic functional abnormalities. The most likely neurochemical transmitter associated with ADHD appears to be decreased dopamine levels in the brain.

Etiology. ADHD occurs more commonly in first-degree biologic relatives of people with the disorder than in the general population, providing some evidence for a genetic predisposition for the disorder. Other central nervous system abnormalities, such as the presence of neurotoxins and epilepsy, or other neurologic disorders, are thought to be predisposing factors, although less than 5% of children with ADHD have definitive neurologic findings. Environments that are chaotic or abusive may be predisposing factors.

Incidence. Estimates of the incidence of ADHD range from 1% to 20%, but the general consensus is that 3% to 5% of the childhood population are accurately diagnosed with ADHD. Sex ratios also vary, but 6 boys affected for every 1 girl affected is the ratio that is most often cited for clinic-referred samples. Epidemiologic studies find the proportion to be approximately 3:1 among nonreferred children displaying these symptoms. Aggressive and antisocial behaviors are thought to explain the increased rate of referrals of boys.

Clinical Manifestations. The child with ADHD:
- often fidgets with hands or feet or squirms in seat
- is easily distracted by internal or external stimuli
- has difficulty awaiting turns in games or group situations

- often blurts out answers to questions before the questions have been completed
- has difficulty following through on instructions from others, even when instructions are clearly understood
- has difficulty sustaining attention in tasks or play activities
- often shifts from one uncompleted activity to another
- has difficulty playing quietly
- often talks excessively
- often interrupts or intrudes on others
- often does not seem to listen to what is being said
- often loses things necessary for tasks or activities at school or at home (pencils, books, clothes, assignments)
- often engages in physically dangerous activities without considering the possible consequences, but not for the express purpose of thrill-seeking

(Adapted in part from American Psychiatric Association [1994]. *Diagnostic and Statistical Manual of Mental Disorders* [4th ed., pp. 83–85], Washington, DC: Author.)

Diagnostic Evaluation. Although high-resolution magnetic resonance imaging (MRI) and blood and urine studies of metabolites of brain neurotransmitters have been performed in individuals with ADHD, none of these has provided consistent information. The diagnosis of ADHD is currently established on the basis of self-reports, parent reports, and teacher reports. These reports are coupled with psychological assessments conducted by psychologists while the child is completing tasks requiring vigilance, attention, and concentration, as well as those involving delayed gratification. Clinical interviews may be coupled with clinical trials of psychopharmocologic agents, such as methylphenidate (Ritalin) or dextroamphetamine (Dexedrine), to determine the child's behavioral response.

Therapeutic Management. The most significant goal of therapeutic management is to reduce the frequency and intensity of unsocialized behaviors. This requires achievement of a balance between the child's temperament and environmental demands, expectancies, and supports. Therefore, treatment goals and interventions must be targeted at enhancing the child's capabilities and self-esteem. The interventions often require altering the environmental demands. Expectations that may be appropriate for a child without ADHD—"he should be able to sit still in school for 40 minutes" or "she should be able to handle 1 hour of homework"—may need to be modified for the child with ADHD. In every case, the nurse and other members of the health care team must work with the parents, both to modify the environment and to develop strategies for fostering competencies in the child. Most clinicians working with these children propose a combination of psychopharmacotherapy and behavior-oriented family therapy to achieve the necessary alterations in the child's internal functioning and external environment. Research indicates that methylphenidate works equally well for attention-deficit disorder with or without hyperactivity, but ADHD, primarily nonhyperactive type, requires lower doses of medication for effectiveness (Barkley et al., 1991). Medication is typically administered during the school day, but recently, there has been an increased awareness on the part of pediatricians that attention/concentration and alertness are needed for any learning task, such as baseball or learning to drive a car. The side effects and potency of the medications often make parents and physicians hesitate to administer the medication other than during critical learning periods.

> Support groups for parents are vital in assisting families to cope with and modify their interactions with and expectations of the child with ADHD.

NURSING CARE OF THE CHILD WITH ADHD

Assessment

The nurse should discuss with the parents the child's typical behavior while playing alone as well as with other children, during mealtimes, and while the parent is on the telephone or occupied with chores or other activities. Explore the length of time it takes the child to bathe or dress and the frequency with which the child becomes distracted during these tasks. This behavior is then compared to behaviors exhibited when the child is engaged in highly stimulating activities and those with frequent feedback, such as Nintendo games. Also, the child's behavior is compared when engaged in novel versus routine activities. The child's developmental and family history is explored in detail, noting the age at which the child began to exhibit independent behaviors, such as walking, getting out of bed alone, and searching out the environment. It is not uncommon for children with ADHD to explore the environment at an early age, with only limited need to return to the caregiver for support or approval. Also among the factors noted are any family members who have been diagnosed as having ADHD or who exhibit similar behaviors. Provide parents with self-report inventories, such as the Child Behavior Checklist, Conners Teacher Rating Scale–Revised, or the School Situations Questionnaire, to be completed and returned to the appropriate professional.

Observation within the home or school setting is likely to generate the most valid information, as the clinic environment may constitute a novel experience and, by the nature of the disorder, may inhibit the child's natural tendency to explore, become distracted, or display limited motivation in task completion.

Nursing Diagnosis and Planning

The following nursing diagnoses and expected outcomes may be appropriate following assessment of the child with ADHD.

Nursing Diagnoses

- Impaired Social Interaction related to impulsivity, poor self-management skills, and aggressive behaviors
- Risk for Injury related to impulsivity, limited judgment skills, and/or excessive need for mobility and stimulation
- Ineffective Family Coping: Compromised or Disabling, related to the need for consistent and close supervision of the child, hyperactivity of the child, and/or social stigma for a child with impulsive or aggressive behaviors
- Knowledge Deficit related to parents' or others' perceptions that the child is willfully defiant or disobedient in following directions or in limit-testing

Expected Outcomes

The child with ADHD will:

- improve impulse control and ability to sustain attention on tasks
- remain safe from injury as a result of adequate supervision and provision of safe ways to meet the child's need for increased activity and movement

The family will:

- discuss the child's needs and a plan to provide the needed support
- discuss the child's disease and display an understanding of the disease process and treatment

Implementation

One of the primary nursing interventions in caring for the child with ADHD is to teach the family about the disorder. Emphasis is placed on reducing the parents' blame and guilt about the problems exhibited by the child. Also, efforts are made to alter the parents' perceptions of the child as intentionally misbehaving or lacking motivation to learn or to achieve. Teaching also includes instructing the family about ways to provide frequent positive reinforcement. Instruction about medications is important for both parents and child, as is instruction about the adaptations of the family environment that are needed to allow the child to practice new skills while taking the medication.

It may be necessary to facilitate communication between the family and the school about ways to accommodate the child's shortened attention span and increased need for mobility and frequent breaks. Often, cognitive-behavioral therapy, provided by a specially trained professional, is helpful in identifying specific exercises that can reduce bothersome traits.

Ordinarily, positive effects of medication are seen within 1 to 2 weeks if the medication is taken as prescribed. It is common for the family to observe a rapid change in the child's behavior, and to experience much relief as symptoms subside. However, because this disorder is lifelong, and progress in self-control and behavioral patterns is usually slow, these families require ongoing support. Parents may need to be actively involved in dispensing medication, even through adolescence, as the child may fluctuate in his willingness to take the medication. Affected children may also experience difficulty in remembering to take the medication because of the attentional deficits characteristic of the disorder.

Evaluation

Does the child:

- comply with the cognitive strategies designed to increase self-control, as evidenced by a decrease in impulsivity?
- comply with the pharmacologic regimen, which is aimed at increasing the child's ability to attend and concentrate at school or in attention-demanding situations?
- complete school assignments in a shorter amount of time, with less distractibility?
- demonstrate increased skill in peer relations, as evidenced by fewer conflicts and more frequent positive statements to and about peers?

Does the family:

- demonstrate acceptance of the child and the special needs of the child?
- demonstrate an increased acceptance of the child's condition as a medical problem, rather than a social or behavioral problem?
- provide a safe and supportive environment within the home, as evidenced by adequate supervision and opportunities for meeting mobility needs in a safe manner?
- comply with the medication regimen?

SUBSTANCE ABUSE

Chemical agents that are typically abused by children and adolescents include alcohol, hallucinogens, sedatives, analgesics, anxiolytics, steroids, and stimulants. The substance abused depends on its availability and cost, as well as social influences and parental behaviors or tolerance for drug use. (For example, parents may consider tobacco use to be more acceptable than use of marijuana or cocaine.) Most professionals differentiate between **substance abuse** and **substance addiction.** However, the basic treatment concerns are similar. Substance abuse is generally considered to increase over time. The phases of substance abuse are outlined in the accompanying box.

PATHOPHYSIOLOGY *of Substance Abuse*

The primary effect of substance abuse is on the brain, which acts to control the rest of the body. The actual action on the brain is largely dependent on the type of substance used, as substances act in accordance with their specific chemical composition. For example, alcohol decreases the responsiveness of the brain to stimuli and affects the entire brain. Table 41–1 lists specific drugs and describes their effects on the body.

Etiology. Rather than considering causes of substance abuse, it is more productive to think in terms of risk factors, which include social, personal, and familial factors. Substance abuse and **substance dependence** tend to

Phases of Substance Abuse

Four phases of abuse have been identified:

Phase 1: Experimentation. The drug is taken to see what it does, or to appease peers.
Phase 2: Early drug use. A specific drug or various drugs are used with some regularity for their pleasurable effects or to reduce anxiety. Social use of drugs typically falls into this category.
Phase 3: True drug addiction. Drugs are used regularly, and physical dependence begins if it is characteristic of the drug. Social functioning revolves around a drug focus.
Phase 4: Severe drug addiction. The physical condition of the addict deteriorates. All activities are related to obtaining or using the drug, with isolation from nondrug culture.

TABLE 41–1 *Commonly Abused Drugs and Their Effects*

	EXPECTED BEHAVIORS/EFFECTS	SPECIAL CONSIDERATIONS
Tobacco	Chronic cough, wheezing, increased phlegm production, atherosclerosis.	Considered a "gateway" drug; initial use usually begins in elementary school
Alcohol	Amount-related effects include euphoria followed by depression and/or hostility, decreased inhibitions, impaired judgment, incoordination, and slurred speech	Considered a "gateway" drug; easily accessible/available drug
Marijuana	Relaxation, mild euphoria, loss of inhibition, decreased motivation, red eyes, dry mouth	Considered a "gateway" drug
Opiates	Euphoria, elation, pain relief, detachment and apathy, drowsiness, constricted pupils, constipation, slurred speech, impaired judgment	Long-term apathy about self often leads to physical malnutrition and dehydration Criminal behaviors associated with obtaining drugs are likely to occur. Infections at injection sites are common
Barbiturates	Similar to those associated with alcohol	Often used in conjunction with stimulants; may have a paradoxical effect of hyperactivity in children
Amphetamines	Euphoria, hyperactivity, agitation, irritability, insomnia, weight loss, tachycardia, hypertension	May have a paradoxical effect of depression in children
Cocaine	Euphoria, elation, agitation, hyperactivity, irritability, pressured speech, grandiosity, tachycardia, hypertension diaphoresis, anorexia, weight loss, insomnia	Psychotic behavior may occur if the dose is large; can be fatal if combined with other drugs
Hallucinogens	Distorted perceptions, heightened awareness, hallucinations, illusions, depersonalization, dilated pupils, hypertension, increased salivation	Psychotic behaviors, panic flashbacks long after drug use ceases, self-destructive behaviors
Phencyclidine Hydrochloride (PCP)	Euphoria, distorted perceptions, agitation, violence, antisocial behaviors, hypertension, increased salivation, increased pain response	Panic, irrational behaviors, psychosis

cluster in families, and there is evidence that there is a genetic influence. For alcohol, as well as for most other drugs, there is some evidence that substance abuse often represents the individual's attempt to cope with anxiety generated by impaired social skills, poor interpersonal relationships, or lack of adaptive behaviors. With some psychosocial disorders, such as ADHD, depression, and conduct disorder, there is an increased association with substance abuse. Other factors that seem to coincide with increased substance abuse include aggressiveness, delinquent behavior, low self-esteem, and poor scholastic performance (Garfinkel et al., 1990; Lowinson et al., 1992).

> Family systems that are closed to outsiders; have a history of psychiatric disturbance, including substance abuse; and have poor communication skills are at risk for creating an environment in which substance abuse in youth is perpetrated.

Incidence. There is much variation in the types of substances abused across gender and age. Typically, boys are heavier consumers of alcohol than girls. Female junior-high students are increasing their use of tobacco, whereas tobacco use by their male counterparts has remained consistent. In 1994, the National Institute on Drug Abuse reported a continued sharp increase in the use of marijuana, LSD, inhalants, and cigarette smoking among high school students. This is a reversal of a downward trend in drug use since the 1980s (Chatlos, 1996).

The 1994 rates for drug use among youth ranged from 26% use of alcohol and 17% use of tobacco among eighth graders to 50% use of alcohol and 30% use of tobacco for high school seniors. Marijuana use was 8% for eighth graders and 19% for high school seniors. Research consistently supports the hypothesis that drug use progresses from beer or wine to cigarettes or hard liquor and then marijuana followed by other illicit drugs (Chatlos, 1996).

Nearly one-third of the high school seniors questioned in 1993 believed there was no significant risk associated with regular smoking (Johnson, O'Malley, & Bachman, 1995). Public awareness and emphasis on treatment and prevention have had very limited impact on teenagers in the 1990s.

An awareness of the possibility of substance abuse is the responsibility of the parent, teacher, and health professional. Knowing the clinical behavioral manifestations of substance abuse is essential, and much information is readily available to adults interested in prevention and early identification.

Clinical Manifestations. The clinical manifestations of substance abuse include the following:

- Low grades or poor school performance
- Irregular school attendance
- Aggressive or rebellious behavior
- Excessive influence by peers
- Deterioration of relationships with family members or former friends
- History of a lack of parental support and supervision
- Rapid or extreme changes in behavior or mood
- Loss of interest in hobbies, sports, or other favorite activities
- Changes in eating or sleeping patterns that increase as manipulative behaviors increase, especially those that are related to the need to acquire desired substances
- Increased antisocial behavior as the desire for social conformity and acceptance decreases and the need for the substance(s) increases

Therapeutic Management. The treatment for substance abuse includes individual, group, and family therapy. Treatment in a center specifically designed for substance abuse is recommended. Participation in Alcoholics Anonymous or Narcotics Anonymous is recommended. These organizations also offer support groups geared toward helping family members. The programs are designed to provide support and to promote needed alterations in the family system so as to decrease the likelihood of relapse.

> The rate of refusal on the part of the substance abuser to adhere to therapeutic recommendations, resulting in relapses, is quite high; more than 50% of those completing a course of treatment continue to abuse substances throughout their lifetime.

NURSING CARE OF THE CHILD OR ADOLESCENT WITH A SUBSTANCE ABUSE PROBLEM

Assessment

Physical assessment should include evaluation of the patient's respiration rate, heart rate, blood pressure, activity level (hyperactive or hypoactive), mood, affect, judgment, speech, sensory responses, and memory. A thorough history of current and past drug use should be obtained. A family and social history; a medical history, including any prior treatment for substance abuse; and a legal history (e.g., past and current charges related to substance abuse) should be obtained.

Nursing Diagnosis and Planning

The following nursing diagnoses and expected outcomes may be appropriate following assessment of the child or adolescent with a substance abuse problem.

Nursing Diagnoses

- Altered Thought Processes related to the specific effects of the particular substance involved

- Sensory/Perceptual Alterations related to the specific effects of the particular substance involved
- Anxiety related to a decrease in sense of control over self and/or the environment
- Ineffective Individual Coping related to limited development of effective social interactions and problem solving skills
- Impaired Social Interaction related to anxiety or limited social skills
- Self-Esteem Disturbance related to limited social skills, ineffective coping skills, and a poor sense of self-management.

Expected Outcomes

The child/adolescent will:

- maintain orientation to time, place, and person.
- not experience falls or other injuries related to sensory/perceptual changes.
- express increased feelings of self-worth and the ability to change behavior.
- identify current stressors leading to substance use/abuse.
- identify alternative activities, people, and social situations that promote nonuse of abuse substance.
- replace substance abuse with more appropriate social skills and develop meaningful relationships with nonabusing peers and family members.

Implementation

The nurse's responsibilities in caring for children or adolescents with substance abuse problems depend on the severity of the abuse and the treatment goals. If the nurse is the first to encounter the abuse, it is his or her responsibility to notify the family and make referrals for treatment. If the youth has been identified and referred to a substance abuse treatment facility, the nurse's primary responsibility will be to stabilize the physiologic status of the youth and to consistently support the recommendations for treatment. Explaining the expectations and the types of services offered is important for both the youth and the family, as most treatment programs offer programs that increase patient and family responsibilities over time.

Initially, maintaining safety and an optimal level of physical comfort will be necessary, especially if detoxification is required. These tasks are accomplished by keeping the youth under close observation, removing from the area any items that could be potentially dangerous, and monitoring vital signs. Being readily available to discuss thoughts, concerns, and perceptions is important to create an emotional sense of safety for the youth. Primary interventions include educating the patient and family members about necessary laboratory tests and providing ongoing information about the nature of substance abuse.

One of the most significant nursing interventions is to assist the patient and family in developing social support systems, and to refer them to appropriate resources that can offer additional support as they make long-term changes in their social and emotional patterns of relating. It is also essential to help the youth assume responsibility for the substance abuse problem, rather than passing the blame on to others. The nurse also has a responsibility to provide emotional support for the youth and family as they develop insight into their behaviors and the need for behavioral changes, as these changes are often difficult to effect.

The relapse rate among youthful substance abusers is extremely high, and success with a short-term treatment program is not necessarily an indicator of successful, long-term control of the problem. The incidence of relapse is generally reduced if the child and family maintain active, long-term involvement in support groups. These groups include Alcoholics Anonymous, Ala-Teen, Ala-Tot, Narcotics Anonymous, and the like. Tough Love support groups for parents may also be beneficial in providing counsel and support. All of these programs are self-help organizations aimed at providing information and support derived from others who have been in similar situations.

Evaluation

Does the child:

- remain substance-free?
- demonstrate an increased sense of self-confidence?
- take ownership of the responsibility to change behaviors related to the substance abuse?
- show improvement in peer and family relationships?

CHILD ABUSE

Child abuse includes emotional or physical abuse or neglect, as well as sexual exploitation or molestation by caretakers or other individuals.

Physical Abuse, Neglect, and Emotional Abuse

Etiology. Family dysfunction is the problem underlying most forms of child abuse. The specific profile of the family varies depending on the type of **abuse,** although it is not uncommon for multiple types of abuse to exist in a single family system (see the accompanying box, Characteristics of the Abusive Family). Generally, the dysfunctional family dynamics are multigenerational, involving both parents.

> It is common for the abuser, the noninvolved parent, and/or the child to deny the abuse, either by denying the event or awareness of the event, denying the impact of the event, or denying any responsibility for the event.

Characteristics of the Abusive Family

Isolation from community and social groups
Intense competition for emotional resources within the family, such as affection, attention, and nurturance
Low levels of differentiation among family members
Low trust for outsiders and family members
Unpredictable and unstable family environment
Conflict resolution generally achieved through aggression and a power struggle between family members
Present focus and crisis-oriented actions for immediate gratification
Communication often characterized by mixed or **double messages,** threats, or a focus on nonverbal communication, rather than direct verbalization
Family roles that are typically fixed and traditional, with rigid rules
Frequent domination by a single family member who maintains control through manipulation, intimidation, deceit, and aggression

Sociologic and economic factors also appear to influence the incidence and etiology of child abuse, with an increase in child abuse being observed during periods of economic hardship or external stress. The typical perpetrator is a direct relative of the child, usually the parent or primary caretaker. Often, this individual exhibits limited coping skills and has been abused as a child or teenager. The typical profile of an abused child is more difficult to determine. However, some research has indicated that the typical abused child is younger than five years of age, often has mild physical abnormalities, is developmentally or physically delayed, displays a difficult temperament, and/or reminds the abuser of someone else. Overall, the child does not meet the expectations of the parent(s), or may remind the parent of someone else with whom a negative association has been made.

Incidence. The most frequent and severe physical abuse occurs in children younger than 2 years of age. Estimates indicate that 2.9 million children are reported for suspected abuse annually, and that more than 1000 deaths occur as a result of abuse in this population.

Clinical Manifestations of Physical Abuse

Physical Indicators (Fig. 41–2)

- Unexplained bruises or welts that appear in various stages of healing, often in clustered patterns that reflect the shapes of the articles used to inflict injury
- Unexplained burns, especially on the soles, palms, back, or buttocks; immersion burns (sock-like, glove-like, or doughnut-shaped [on buttocks or genitals])
- Infected burns, indicating a delay in seeking treatment
- Unexplained fractures to the skull, nose, or facial structures; multiple or spiral fractures; or dislocations and numerous fractures in various stages of healing
- Bald patches on the scalp

Behavioral Indicators

- Wariness in response to adult contact
- Apprehension when others cry
- Extreme aggressiveness or withdrawal
- Fear of parents or fear of going home
- Vacant or frozen stares
- Lying very still when surveying surroundings
- Lack of crying when approached by a stranger or examiner
- Monosyllablic responses to questions
- Manipulative behaviors to get attention
- Inappropriate or precocious maturity
- Capacity for superficial relationships only
- Indiscriminate seeking of attention

Clinical Manifestations of Physical Neglect

Physical Indicators

- Inadequate weight gain for age, poor growth pattern, failure to thrive
- Consistent hunger
- Poor hygiene
- Dressing in clothes that are not seasonally suitable (i.e., no coat or shoes in winter)
- Reports of lack of supervision for long periods of time, or permission to engage in unsafe activities
- Wasting of subcutaneous tissue
- Unattended physical problems or medical needs
- Abandonment
- Bald patches on the scalp

Behavioral Indicators

- Begging; stealing of food
- Extended stays at school (comes very early or stays very late)
- Inconsistent school attendance
- Constant fatigue, listlessness, or falling asleep in class
- Assumption of adult responsibilities or roles
- Alcohol or substance abuse
- Delinquency
- Reports of there being no caretaker or evidence of lack of adult supervision

Clinical Manifestations of Emotional Abuse

Physical Indicators

- Speech disorders
- Lags in physical development
- Failure to thrive
- Hyperactive/disruptive behavior

Behavioral Indicators

- Habit disorders (sucking, biting, rocking, etc.)
- Conduct/learning disorders

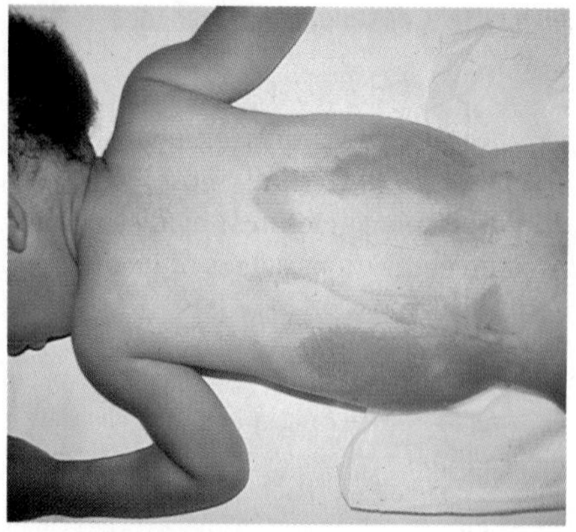

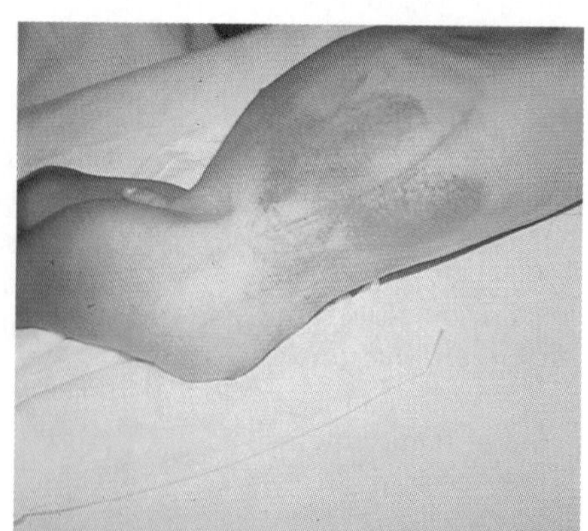

Nonaccidental distribution of bruises—All four surfaces of the mid-body are involved, but there are no bruises on arms and legs.

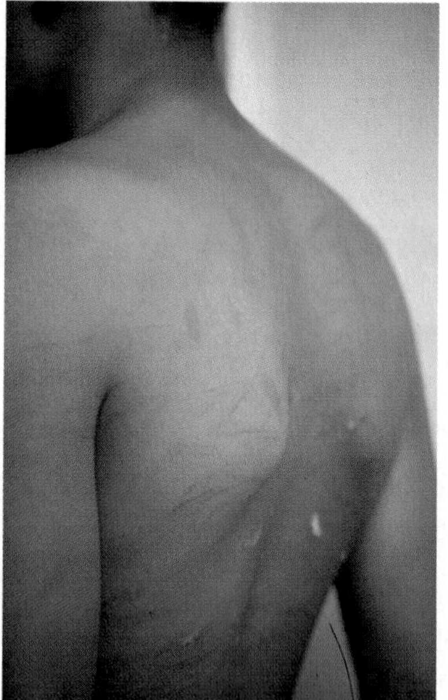

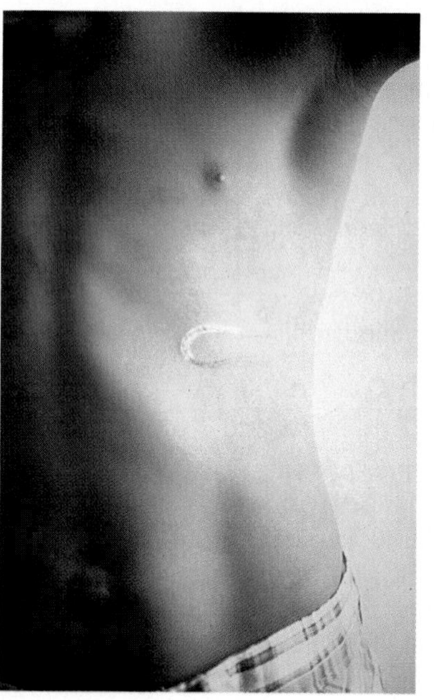

Pattern of injury—Linear scars of various ages indicate repeated abuse using a switch or whip. The loop pattern on the boy's anterior torso is consistent with a looped electrical cord used as a whip.

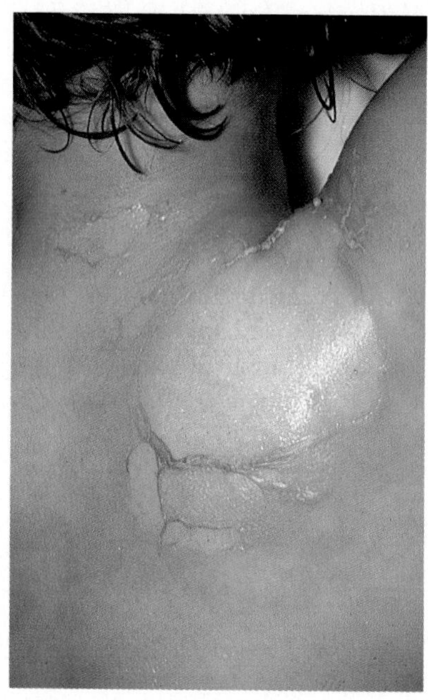

Scald burn of shoulder and neck—The typical distribution of a scald burn in a toddler is shown. This type of injury occurs when a toddler pulls a cup of coffee or pan of water off a stove.

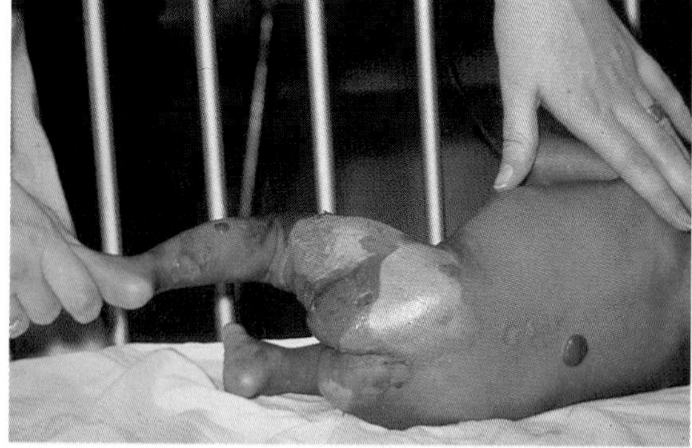

Nonaccidental immersion scald—Involvement of virtually the entire posterior surface of the legs indicates that the legs were held under scalding water; even an infant this young would flex the knees to avoid the hot water.

Figure 41–2

Physical signs of child abuse. The nurse should be alert for the typical behavioral indicators of abuse (see text). The nurse or other professional who performs an abuse assessment must write down the child's comments verbatim, without coaching the child, because these statements may later be used in legal proceedings. (Courtesy of Barbara Tenney, M.D. From Henry, M. C., & Stapleton, E. R. [1992]. *EMT: Prehospital care* [p. 675]. Philadelphia: W. B. Saunders)

- Neurotic traits (sleep disorders, inhibition of play, unusual fearfulness)
- Psychoneurotic reactions (hysteria, obsessions, compulsions, phobias, hypochondriasis)
- Extremes in behaviors (withdrawal, aggression, etc.)
- Overly adaptive/compliant behaviors
- Suicide attempts

Shaken Baby Syndrome. Shaken baby syndrome is a widely recognized form of child abuse that is caused by vigorous shaking while the infant is held by the extremities or shoulders. This type of physical abuse leads to whiplash-induced intracranial and intraocular bleeding. There is generally no external signs of head trauma, which makes this syndrome difficult to detect. Shaken baby syndrome should be considered in infants who present with failure to thrive, seizures, apnea, respiratory irregularities, coma, or vomiting associated with drowsiness or lethargy (Coody et al., 1994; Chiocca, 1995).

Munchausen Syndrome by Proxy. Munchausen syndrome by proxy is a form of physical abuse, most often inflicted by the mother or primary caretaker. The caretaker falsifies illness in the child through simulation and/or production of illness and then takes the child for medical care, claiming no knowledge of how the child became ill. The most common reasons these caretakers give for seeking medical treatment are bleeding, seizures, central nervous system depression, apnea, diarrhea, vomiting, fever, and rash. Long-term morbidity in these cases is as high as 8%. In one study, failure to thrive was associated with Munchausen syndrome in 14% of cases. Often, while under the supervision of other adults, the child exhibits no symptoms reported by the primary caretaker, and may, in fact, appear to be normal and healthy. This behavior reflects a serious disturbance in the parent and requires specialized psychiatric treatment for the parent and removal of the child from the parents' care. The long-term effects on the child range from conduct and emotional disturbance; problems in school, such as difficulties with attention and concentration; and poor school attendance (Bools et al., 1993; Rosenberg, 1987).

Sexual Abuse

Incidence. Sexual abuse victims are usually between 6 and 9 years of age at the onset of the abuse, and the ratio of females:males is 3:1. However, this ratio is considered to represent less than the actual incidence for boys.

The youth often copes with sexual victimization in what has been termed the "child sexual abuse accommodation syndrome." The coping mechanisms are the child's normal behaviors in response to an abnormal event, as there is little or nothing the child can do to prevent the abuse. The initial strategy involves *secrecy*. It is normal for the child to keep the abuse secret, as the lack of social acceptance of the situation is sensed by the child. This awareness dominates the child's sense of self. Because the sexual abuse generally occurs in a private setting rather than in a public one, the child experiences a great deal of guilt. This guilt may be intensified by the child's ambivalence about the pleasure that might have been experienced by the event. The secrecy is typically reinforced by threats that the child, the perpetrator, or another loved one will "get into trouble." The second behavioral response observed in child abuse victims arises from a sense of *helplessness*. The child feels responsible for holding the family system together and feels isolated from peers because of a deep sense of shame and guilt. The normal strategy for accommodating this sense of helplessness is to "play possum," pretending to be asleep or unaffected by the sexual abuse. This is an attempt by the child to manage the intrusion experienced. Next, the child often employs strategies to cope with an enduring sense of *entrapment* because as long as the child is accessible and the relationship exists, the molestation continues. This strategy involves minimizing the pain and taking responsibility for the abuse. Almost universally, sexually abused children believe that their own personal "badness" is the reason the abuse is continuing, rather than placing the responsibility on the perpetrator. Often, these children develop strategies for dissociating during the abuse to avoid feelings or physical pain. Frequently, the child will make *veiled attempts at disclosure or will delay disclosure* in order to keep the abuse secret and to avoid the risk alienating significant others. Often, the child fears that revealing the abuse will prove to be worse than keeping the secret. In fact, most sexually abused children keep the abuse secret throughout their lives, unless there is some intervention from outside the system that prompts them to reveal the abuse. Finally, the typical behavior of the sexually abused child is to *retract* the revelation of abuse once it is made. Consistent advocacy by and permission of an "outsider" are often required before a child will reveal the full story of the abuse (Summit, 1983).

Clinical Manifestations of Sexual Abuse

Physical Indicators

- Difficulty walking or sitting
- Torn, stained, or bloody underclothing
- Pain, swelling, or itching of genitals
- Pain on urination
- Bruises, bleeding, or lacerations involving the external genitalia, vagina, or anal area
- Vaginal/penile discharge
- Sexually transmitted disease
- Poor sphincter tone
- Excessive masturbation

Behavioral Indicators

- An unwillingness to change clothes or participate in gym activities
- Withdrawal, fantasy, or infantile behavior
- Bizarre, sophisticated, or unusual sexual behavior or knowledge

- Promiscuity
- Poor peer relations
- Delinquency or running away
- Depression or suicidal ideation/gestures/attempts
- Aggressive behavior
- Change in school performance
- Sleep disturbances/nightmares
- Eating disturbances (obesity, anorexia/bulimia)
- Self-destructive behaviors (substance abuse, self-mutilation)
- Sexual acting out toward a younger child

NURSING CARE OF THE ABUSED CHILD

Assessment

The nurse's assessment should include a thorough evaluation for skin integrity, including examination of the scalp, bottoms of the hands and feet, front and back of the trunk, and genitals. A baseline measurement of height and weight should be obtained, along with documentation of the birth weight for infants. An assessment of the patient's level of anxiety, ability to relate to the examiner, and emotional tone is also crucial. Finally, a thorough assessment of the family support system, including patterns of interaction, belief systems, and social support systems, should be conducted.

During the physical assessment of the child's entire body, information about bruises and injuries, and information directly relating to sexual abuse should be requested in a nonemotional, matter-of-fact manner with particular attention to the child's need for privacy and dignity. Comments made by the child should be written down verbatim, as disclosure of abuse is often subtle, and this information may be able to be used in legal proceedings at a later time. Assessment should include an account of written or verbal contact with teachers, relatives (including both parents, siblings, and grandparents), and others who have been involved with the child over an extended period of time.

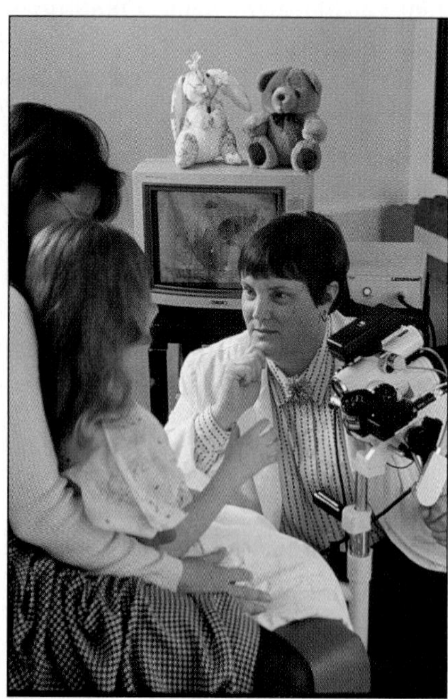

◀ Note the communication techniques illustrated in this photo which are designed to reassure the child and give the child some power. The little girl is not immediately positioned for a genital examination. The physician first sits to talk with the child at her eye level and makes eye contact with her.

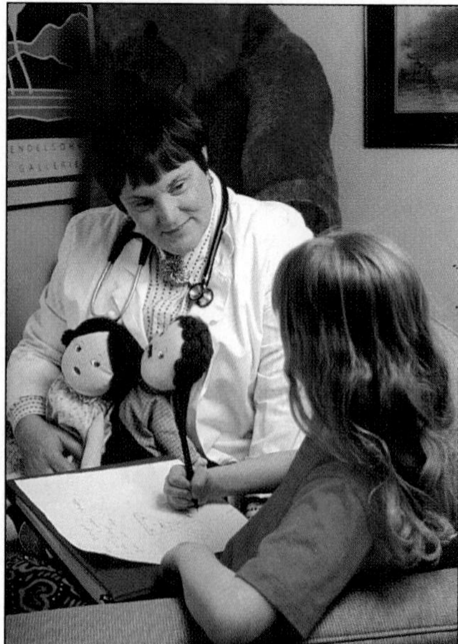

Drawings may help to identify the abused child, and ▶ may assist in therapy. As with the dolls, art can help the child express what cannot be expressed in words.

Figure 41–3

Disclosure of abuse may be slow because the child often has difficulty trusting any adult. Identification of sexual abuse requires particular sensitivity, as physical examination of the child's genitals to identify signs of injury or sexually transmitted disease can be frightening for the child, who associates handling of the genitals with pain or shame. Anatomically correct dolls are often used in the assessment of abuse within a family. These dolls help children express what they cannot express in words; young children, in particular, have a limited vocabulary to use when describing the events that have occurred. (Courtesy of Cook Children's Medical Center, Fort Worth, Texas)

Child Sexual Behavior Inventory, Version 1

Please circle the number that tells how often your child has shown the following behaviors *recently or in the last 6 months*:

Never	Less than 1/month	1–3 times/month	At least 1/week
0	1	2	3

1. 0 1 2 3 Dresses like the opposite sex
2. 0 1 2 3 Talks about wanting to be the opposite sex
3. 0 1 2 3 Touches sex (private) parts when in public places
4. 0 1 2 3 Masturbates with hand
5. 0 1 2 3 Scratches anal or crotch area, or both
6. 0 1 2 3 Touches or tries to touch mother's or other women's breasts
7. 0 1 2 3 Masturbates with object
8. 0 1 2 3 Touches other people's sex (private) parts
9. 0 1 2 3 Imitates the act of sexual intercourse
10. 0 1 2 3 Puts mouth on another child's or adult's sex parts
11. 0 1 2 3 Touches sex (private) parts when at home
12. 0 1 2 3 Uses words that describe sex acts
13. 0 1 2 3 Pretends to be the opposite sex when playing
14. 0 1 2 3 Makes sexual sounds (sighing, moaning, heavy breathing, etc.)
15. 0 1 2 3 Asks others to engage in sexual acts with him or her
16. 0 1 2 3 Rubs body against people or furniture
17. 0 1 2 3 Inserts or tries to insert objects in vagina or anus
18. 0 1 2 3 Tries to look at people when they are nude or undressing
19. 0 1 2 3 Imitates sexual behavior with dolls or stuffed animals
20. 0 1 2 3 Shows sex (private) parts to adults
21. 0 1 2 3 Tries to view pictures of nude or partially dressed people (may include catalogs)
22. 0 1 2 3 Talks about sexual acts
23. 0 1 2 3 Kisses adults not in the family
24. 0 1 2 3 Undresses self in front of others
25. 0 1 2 3 Sits with crotch or underwear exposed
26. 0 1 2 3 Kisses other children not in the family
27. 0 1 2 3 Talks in a flirtatious manner
28. 0 1 2 3 Tries to undress other children or adults against their will (opening pants, shirts, etc.)
29. 0 1 2 3 Asks to view nude or sexually explicit TV shows (may include video movies or HBO-type shows)
30. 0 1 2 3 When kissing, tries to put tongue in other person's mouth
31. 0 1 2 3 Hugs adults he or she does not know well
32. 0 1 2 3 Shows sex (private) parts to children
33. 0 1 2 3 If a girl, overly aggressive; if a boy, overly passive
34. 0 1 2 3 Seems very interested in the opposite sex
35. 0 1 2 3 If a boy, plays with girls' toys; if a girl, plays with boys' toys
36. 0 1 2 3 Other sexual behaviors (please describe)

A. ____________________

B. ____________________

Figure 41–4

This inventory, by Friedrich, can be used in assessing children for sexual abuse. (From Friedrich, W. [1990]. *Psychotherapy of sexually abused children and their families.* New York: W. W. Norton. Copyright 1990 by W. W. Norton.)

> Generally, information about abuse is veiled or denied initially, with disclosure occurring as a process, over time, in the presence of trusted people within the child's social system.

Trust between the health care system and the family system can be enhanced by answering questions directly and specifically, by assuming a nonjudgmental and supportive stance throughout all interactions, and by acting as an advocate for the holistic care of the child as well as of the family. Recognition of the child's low self-esteem, feelings of inadequacy, and fear will enable the nurse to relate in a manner that is supportive. The child will need encouragement to make self-care decisions and to discuss thoughts and feelings, which will have been repressed in order to survive the trauma (Fig. 41–3). Often, sexually abused children will identify with the abuser, believing that they are responsible for what the abuser did, or that they deserved the "punishment" received. The child may also have a sense of affection for the perpetrator, believing that the abuse is a necessary part of the relationship.

When there is suspected sexual abuse, the child and parent are interviewed in the same manner as described for physical abuse. Observe for clinical manifestations of sexual abuse in a manner that provides dignity and respect for both the child and the parent. Friedrich (1990) offers an inventory that describes typical behaviors (Fig. 41–4.)

Nursing Diagnosis

The following nursing diagnoses may be appropriate following assessment of the child/adolescent and family thought to be affected by abuse:

- Altered Parenting related to immaturity, lack of knowledge, empathy on the part of parental caregivers, or limited or negative past parenting experience
- Fear or Powerlessness (Child's) related to the possible outcomes of disclosure, sense of shame, and possible loss of control within the family system
- Knowledge Deficit (Parental) related to the developmental abilities of the child, external support resources, or ways to manage internal and external stressors
- Risk for Injury related to a family with a history of physical abuse, physical neglect, emotional abuse, and/or sexual abuse

Planning, Implementation, and Evaluation: The Abused Child

NURSING DIAGNOSIS

- Altered Parenting related to immaturity, lack of knowledge, empathy on the part of parental caregivers, or limited or negative past parenting experience

Expected Outcomes:

- The family will express an understanding of positive parenting models.
- The family will respond to the child's needs in a timely and appropriate manner.

Intervention	Rationale
1. Assess parents' strengths and weaknesses, normal coping mechanisms, and the presence or absence of support systems. Special attention should be paid to the following characteristics of the parents: a. expectations with regard to the child b. comforting behaviors c. response to the child d. general knowledge about the child	In order to provide optimal care for the child, involvement of the family is crucial. By understanding the needs of the family, a plan of care can be developed, including referral to appropriate supportive agencies.
2. Discuss with the parents the parenting they received as children.	Parenting is a learned behavior.
3. Observe the parents' interactions with the child.	Although parents may verbalize a positive relationship with their child, observation of actual interactions provides a more realistic view of the parent-child relationship.
4. Provide an accepting environment.	Communication is encouraged through the demonstration of acceptance.
5. Provide information regarding normal growth and development for parents.	Parents who are abusers often have unrealistic expectations of their children which, in part, may be related to their lack of knowledge regarding growth and development.
6. Include role modeling as a method of teaching parenting.	By observing the way the nurse touches and talks to the child in an affirming manner, the parents can observe firsthand the child's response to positive parenting type skills.
7. Devote part of the time spent with the child and family to focusing on the child's positive attributes (e.g., "You are such a pretty little girl," or "Look at that wonderful smile.").	Parents' negative perceptions of the child, which may be based on their own life experiences, can be altered by viewing the child through another's eyes.
8. Encourage the parents to participate in the care of the child. Reinforce positive behaviors.	These strategies build self-esteem and confidence in parenting skills.

Evaluation: The parents:

- interact appropriately with the child through verbal, physical, and visual contact.
- verbalize an understanding of normal growth and development.
- verbalize positive statements regarding the child.
- bring the child for follow-up visits.

NURSING DIAGNOSIS

- Fear and/or Powerlessness (Child's) related to the possible outcomes of disclosure, sense of shame and possible loss of control within the family system

Expected Outcomes:

- The child will verbalize the source of his or her fear.
- The child will explore aspects of life in which there is a feeling of control and power.

Intervention	Rationale
1. Reassure the child about his or her personal safety.	Verbal reassurance can provide a sense of security.
2. Identify specific strategies the child can use to maintain a sense of stability (i.e., stay with a trusted adult, refuse to answer intrusive questions, limit exposure to adults who are not trusted).	By providing some viable options, the child can begin to gain a sense of control over the experience.
3. Acknowledge the child's fear.	This helps the child to identify feelings and opens new areas of communication.
4. Spend time with the child. Use both verbal and nonverbal forms of communication.	These actions provide comfort and encourage verbalization of feelings.
5. Offer choices, when available, regarding activities of daily living, recreation time, and time with other children and adults.	Being offered choices gives the child a sense of control and diminishes feelings of powerlessness.

Evaluation: The child:

- participates in play activities.
- verbalizes specific fears related to abuse and disclosure.

NURSING DIAGNOSIS

- Knowledge Deficit (Parental) related to the developmental abilities of the child, external support resources, or ways to manage internal and external stressors

Expected Outcomes:

- The family will gain an understanding of the child's developmental and emotional needs in a framework that is oriented to the child's welfare.
- The family will identify support systems.

Intervention	Rationale
1. Assess the parents' knowledge of child growth and development.	A baseline assessment must be done in order to develop a plan of care.
2. Serve as a role model for positive parenting skills.	Learning can be enhanced through observing the application of parenting skills, which is more effective than listening to a lecture.

Intervention	Rationale
3. Assist the family in identifying stressors and the support systems and resources that may help to decrease the parents' stress level.	By decreasing the level of stress on the parents, the risk of abuse is decreased.
4. Refer the family to pertinent support groups, such as Parents Anonymous.	A lack of support and isolation are common among abusive families. A support group may decrease isolation.
5. Involve the parents in the care of the child.	Participation in care will provide opportunities for positive reinforcement, teaching, and increased emotional attachment to the child.
6. Provide education in the areas of: a. growth and development b. nutrition c. care related to activities of daily living d. routine well-child care e. manifestations of illness f. need for care and loving	Education in parenting skills may decrease unrealistic expectations, increase awareness of the needs of children, and increase the chances of positive parenting. Parents may not have had positive parenting role models as children.
7. Provide a consistent caregiver from among the nursing staff.	Consistency of care increases the child's feelings of trust and security and provides increased opportunities for the child to verbalize feelings.

Evaluation:
- The parents verbalize an understanding of child growth and development.
- The child does not experience intentional harm.
- The parents join a support group.

NURSING DIAGNOSIS
- Risk for Injury related to a family with a history of physical abuse, physical neglect, emotional abuse, and/or sexual abuse

Expected Outcomes:
- The child will remain free from physical or psychological injury and neglect.
- The family will seek psychological support to overcome the problem of abuse.

Intervention	Rationale
1. Assess the child's physical and mental status.	All children should undergo a thorough physical assessment upon presentation to the health care setting, and should be assessed for bruises, burns, scars, and other signs of abuse. Children may enter the health care system for reasons other than injury.
2. Observe the interactions between child and family.	Subtle signs of abuse may be detected in the way the child interacts with the abuser and other adults.
3. Obtain a thorough history.	Frequent presentation of the child for injuries and/or signs of healed injuries may indicate a pattern of abuse.
4. Use a nonthreatening, nonjudgmental manner when interacting with the child's parents.	By building a trusting relationship with the parents, the child can be helped. If the parents become suspicious or alienated, they may deny the child access to health care. They will become defensive, and will not be open to teaching.

Intervention	Rationale
5. Report all cases in which abuse is suspected.	All 50 states require health care professionals to report all cases of suspected abuse.
6. Assist in removing children from an unsafe environment.	Suspected abuse should be evaluated immediately in order to remove the child to an environment that is safe, thereby preventing further injury.
7. Document the following: a. results of the child's physical assessment b. obsevations of interactions between the child and family and between the child and other adults, as well as the child's reaction to hospitalization or the health care setting c. direct comments made by the child and the family that pertain to the child or the child's injury d. child's developmental level	Objective documentation is essential in all cases of suspected abuse.
8. If the child is removed from the home, provide the child and family with support and opportunities to verbalize feelings. Play therapy may be used effectively with children.	Children who are removed from the custody of their parents will grieve their loss. Parents will need support in dealing with guilt and loss.

Evaluation:

- The child remains free of inflicted injury.
- The child is placed in a safe environment.
- The child verbalizes feelings regarding placement outside the home.
- The family seeks psychological counseling.

The care plan will change dramatically depending on the specific nature of the abuse, the likelihood of repeated abuse, and the point in time at which the child enters the health care system. The child may initially be removed from the home, which often limits the nurse's ability to assess parents for teaching or motivation for change.

FAILURE TO THRIVE

Most clinicians agree that "failure to thrive" is not an actual diagnosis, but rather a term that describes a cluster of concurrent symptoms. In practice, if a child's weight falls below the fifth percentile, if the child's weight drops more than two major percentile groups, or if the average daily growth gain in grams is less than the normal values (Table 41–2), the child is considered to be at risk for failure to thrive, and a more thorough evaluation is warranted.

Etiology. Typically, studies of nonorganic failure to thrive have shown a relationship to poverty, maternal depression, and poor social support systems, all of which ultimately affect the mother-infant relationship (Benoit et al., 1989; Gorman et al., 1993). In addition, mothers of these infants frequently report significant caregiver instability and crises during their own childhood, increased negative life stress at the time of the infant's birth, and a negative perception of their infant (Gorman et al., 1993).

The most commonly used model for understanding nonorganic failure to thrive and mixed failure to thrive is an interactive-transactional model. This model is based on neurobehavioral phenomena and identifies multiple factors in the genesis of failure to thrive (see accompanying

TABLE 41–2 *Normal Growth for Infants and Children*

AGE	MEDIAN DAILY GAIN (g)	RECOMMENDED DAILY ALLOWANCE (Kcal/kg/day)
0–3 months	26–31	108
3–6 months	17–18	108
6–9 months	12–13	98
9–12 months	9	98
1–3 years	7–9	102
4–6 years	~6	90

Reproduced from the National Research Council, Food and Nutrition Board. (1989). Recommended daily allowances. Washington, DC: National Academy of Sciences.

PATHOPHYSIOLOGY *of Failure to Thrive*

Three types of failure to thrive are typically described: organic failure to thrive, nonorganic failure to thrive, and mixed failure to thrive.

Organic failure to thrive is failure to gain weight secondary to physical factors. These physical factors may be a specific physiologic impairment, such as a congenital heart defect, gastrointestional disorder, or endocrine disorder. Alternatively, the physical factor may be a chronic infection, a central nervous system abnormality, a chromosomal disorder, or a metabolic disorder.

Nonorganic failure to thrive is a term used in the absence of a history contributing to, or physical or laboratory findings suggestive of, an organic disease capable of causing failure to gain weight. Generally, environmental factors are the strongest influence on the child's intake or use of calories. This form of the disorder is commonly believed to result from a complex interactive pattern between the infant and the primary caregivers.

Mixed failure to thrive is caused by a combination of organic and inorganic factors. The initial problem may be physical, such as respiratory distress, which limits effective suckling. This difficulty, in turn, interferes with the caregiver's sense of adequacy and ability to provide nurturing care to the infant. The infant becomes more irritable and difficult to manage, further increasing the caregiver's sense of inadequacy.

Persistent failure to gain weight is considered to originate with malnutrition. Table 41–3 presents a staging system for malnutrition in infants, which can be used as the criteria for hospitalization and the types of intervention selected. The long-term effects of undernutrition, regardless of the cause, may include secondary immune dysfunction, micronutritional deficiencies, and developmental delays in all major areas. Associated immune dysfunctions include diminished complement, secretory immunoglobulin A (IgA), and T-cell function. Affected children may develop repeated gastrointestinal or respiratory infections, with each episode raising the child's caloric needs and lowering intake, resulting in even greater vulnerability. Micronutrient deficiencies often complicate undernutrition by causing anemia and rickets. Iron and calcium deficiencies tend to increase lead absorption, which can then lead to constipation, abdominal pain, or anorexia. Zinc deficiency impairs growth directly and can also interfere with taste bud function. Chronic undernutrition in the first 2 years of life can result in limited brain size, a reduction in neuronal number, and decreased synaptic complexity. Acquired microcephaly may persist even when somatic growth recovers.

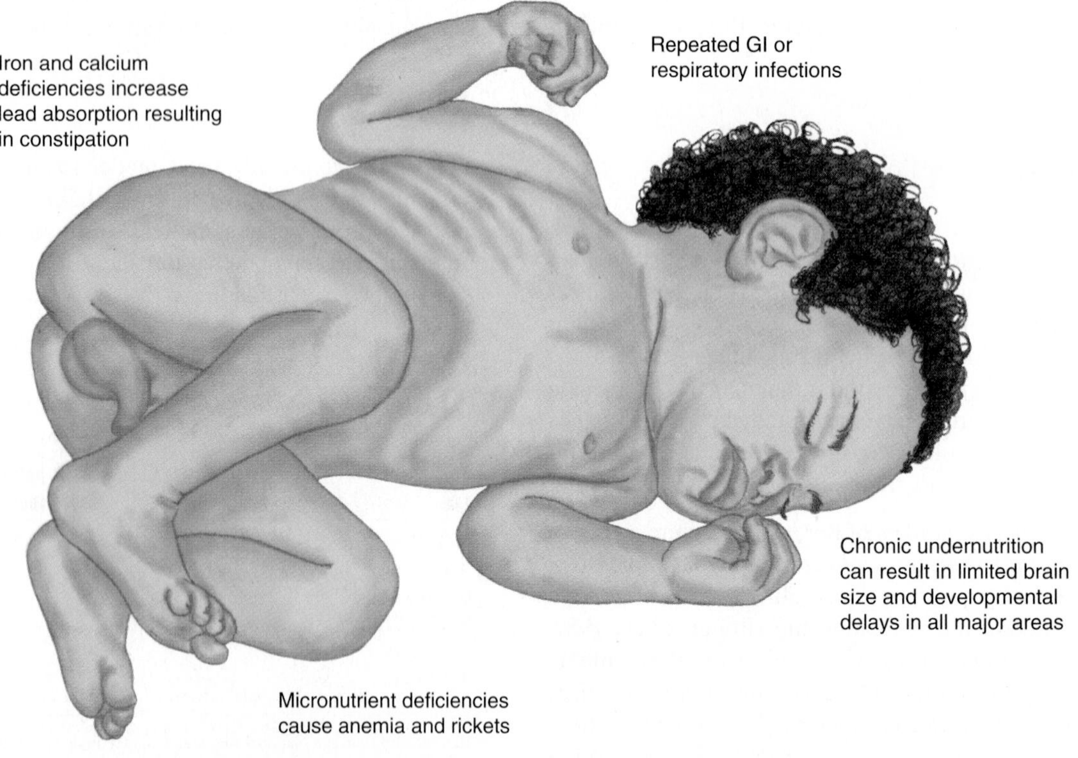
Iron and calcium deficiencies increase lead absorption resulting in constipation
Repeated GI or respiratory infections
Chronic undernutrition can result in limited brain size and developmental delays in all major areas
Micronutrient deficiencies cause anemia and rickets

TABLE 41–3 *Staging System for Malnutrition in Infants*

	WEIGHT FOR AGE (% of Median)	HEIGHT FOR AGE (Stunting) (% of Median)	WEIGHT FOR HEIGHT (Wasting) (% of Median)
Normal	>90	>95	>90
Mild	75–90	90–95	81–90
Moderate	60–74	85–89	70–80
Severe	<60	<85	<70

Reprinted with permission from Frank, D. A., Silva, M., & Needlman, R. (1993, February). Failure to thrive: Mystery, myth, and method. *Contemporary Pediatrics, 10*, 118.

box, Possible Causes of Failure to Thrive). The interactions involved are all mediated through a maladaptive parent-infant relationship. The parent displays impaired skills in "reading" or responding to the infant's cues appropriately. The infant then has difficulty eliciting attention and appropriate care, often becoming irritable or stiff, or exhibiting feeding difficulties. These symptoms are difficult for the new parent(s) to manage, resulting in parental anxiety and difficulty in bonding emotionally with the infant.

Incidence. Generally, 2% to 3% of hospitalized infants are listed as being admitted for failure to thrive, but some reports indicate that as many as 9.6% of the total number of infant hospital admissions may be related to this cluster of symptoms and weak interactional parent-child pattern (Drotar, 1991). Although failure to thrive occurs in children of all social classes, a disproportionate number of these children are from low-income families.

Clinical Manifestations and Risk Factors for Failure to Thrive

Physical Indicators

- Weight below the 5th percentile
- Sudden or rapid deceleration in the growth curve
- Delay in reaching developmental milestones
- Decreased muscle mass
- Muscular hypotonia
- Abdominal distension
- Generalized weakness and cachexia (general ill health and malnutrition)

See also Chapter 12, Table 12–5, for the physical signs and symptoms of malnutrition.

Behavioral Indicators

- Avoidance of eye contact
- Avoidance of physical touch
- Intense watchfulness
- Sleep disturbances
- Lack of age-appropriate stranger anxiety
- Inappropriate lack of preference for parent(s)
- Disturbed affect, such as apathy, extreme irritability, extreme compliance
- Repetitive self-stimulating behaviors, such as rocking, head-banging, intense sucking, intense chewing on fingers or hands, and head-rolling

Diagnostic Evaluation. A differential diagnosis is generally made by a multidisciplinary team whose initial task is to search for an organic cause of the growth failure. If no known cause is found, then the approach is to focus on "diagnosis by response." This approach includes provision of nutrition and nurturing in a consistent manner. If the infant gains the expected weight, the term nonorganic failure to thrive is considered to be the appropriate diagnosis.

The initial screening may include the following:

- Physical examination to rule out congenital defects and obtain baseline data
- Developmental screening to determine current level of attainment of developmental milestones
- Tuberculin test to rule out tuberculosis
- Bone survey radiographs of long bones, joints, and skull to rule out fractures, determine bone age, and check epiphyseal development
- Anteroposterior and lateral chest films to rule out pulmonary disease
- Urinalysis to rule out urinary tract infections and diabetes, as well as certain metabolic defects
- Complete blood count (CBC) and differential studies to rule out anemia and chronic or systemic infections

Possible Causes of Failure to Thrive

PERINATAL

Intrauterine infection
Chromosomal abnormalities
Poor prenatal care
Poor intrauterine environment

POSTNATAL

Insufficient nutrition
Susceptibility to teratogen exposure
Infection
Immune insufficiency
Susceptibility to lead intoxication
Impaired emotional attachment
Chronic illness

- Sweat test to rule out cystic fibrosis
- Stool test to rule out monosaccharide and disaccharide deficiency, milk intolerance, internal bleeding, parasitic infestation, and malabsorption
- T-4 tests to rule out hypothyroidism
- Electrocardiogram to rule out cardiac abnormalities or circulatory defects
- IV pyelogram to rule out urinary tract abnormalities or internal injuries
- Bowel and muscle biopsies to rule out Hirschsprung's disease, congenital muscular dystrophy, or celiac disease
- Upper and lower gastrointestinal radiographic studies to rule out dysphagia, gastrointestinal anatomic abnormalities, or internal injuries
- Serum studies to rule out lead toxicity and zinc or iron deficiencies

Therapeutic Management of Nonorganic Failure to Thrive. The first goal of treatment is to provide nutritional therapy to increase the child's caloric intake. The goal for growth is two to three times the average rate for age (see Table 41–2). Daily multivitamins with minerals are often prescribed to ensure that specific nutritional deficiencies do not occur in the course of rapid growth. Caloric enrichment of food is essential, and formula may be concentrated in titrated amounts up to 24 calories/oz. Greater concentrations can lead to diarrhea and dehydration.

Common Reasons for Inadequate Nutritional Intake in Infants and Children

- Overdilution of formula
- Large quantities of cereal or baby food in bottles
- Excessive fluid intake other than formula or milk
- Selection of foods with inappropriate texture for infant's stage of development
- Infrequent feedings, especially in children who are temperamentally quiet or undemanding
- No set feeding times
- No high chair
- Frequent small sips from a bottle (grazing)
- Distractions during feedings (television or social interactions)
- Struggles over feeding between caregiver(s) and child
- Poor breastfeeding skills of mother and/or infant

NURSING CARE OF THE CHILD WITH FAILURE TO THRIVE

Assessment

The initial assessment should include a complete history of the presenting problem, with emphasis on age of onset, recent changes in the child's routines (i.e., travel out of the country), and attendance at large day-care centers or in a shelter-type living environment. The nurse should also obtain information about any chronic nasal obstruction, episodes of bronchitis or wheezing, or other respiratory difficulties. Information about stool frequency, consistency, and any discomfort associated with excretion should be obtained. A thorough dietary history should include all drinks, meals, and snacks consumed by the child, as well as where, when, how, and by whom the child is typically fed. The nurse should explore possible reasons for low intake, such as recurrent infections or medical complications of earlier episodes of malnutrition. The accompanying box presents common dietary patterns that may be overlooked if the dietary history is not carefully investigated.

The physical examination should focus especially on the skin, hair, nails, and mucous membranes of the child to identify signs of malnutrition. Also, the nurse should look for lesions that could interfere with eating, such as dental caries, tongue enlargement, mandibular hypoplasia, unrecognized submucosal cleft palate, or tonsillar hypertrophy.

The nurse should complete a thorough psychosocial history that focuses on income, family (dis)organization, social isolation, stress factors, support systems, and family psychopathology, such as maternal depression, family violence, or alcoholism. It is important to ask about the availability of food, especially around the time of arrival of a paycheck, Aid for Dependent Children (AFDC) check, or food stamps. Finally, the psychosocial history should include questions about facilities for storing and preparing food.

Assessment of infant-parent interactions should focus on the ways in which the child is held and fed, how eye contact is initiated and maintained, and the facial expressions of both the child and the caregiver during interactions. Observations of various kinds of interactions are important, too, and should include play, talk, and touch by both the child and caregiver, as well as the other's reaction to these attempts to engage in interaction. The nurse should note the responses of the caregiver to the child's cues, such as when the child cries, reaches out, or looks toward the caregiver. A sense of synchrony or harmony should be sensed in the interaction.

Nursing Diagnosis

The following nursing diagnoses may be appropriate following assessment of the infant or child with failure to thrive:

- Altered Nutrition: Less Than Body Requirements, related to insufficient intake of calories, incomplete absorption of nutrients, impaired interactions with caregivers, or inadequate care by caregivers
- Knowledge Deficit related to lack of experience and of positive parenting training

Planning, Implementation, and Evaluation: The Child With Failure to Thrive

NURSING DIAGNOSIS • Altered Nutrition: Less Than Body Requirements, related to insufficient intake of calories, incomplete absorption of nutrients, impaired interactions with caregivers, or inadequate care by caregivers

Expected Outcome: • The child will experience normal growth and development for age and sex.

Intervention	Rationale
1. Monitor the child's nutritional status.	
a. Document physical alterations, especially changes in physical status during or following feedings.	Fatigue, colic, or respiratory distress may indicate an underlying cause of the disorder.
b. Document the child's feeding patterns.	Subtle deficits may have a significant bearing on nutritional intake.
c. Document the nature of parent-child interactions, especially before, during, and after feedings.	Psychological components revealed in the context of interactions may be the most significant indicators of the cause for undernutrition.
2. Encourage the caregiver to discuss both positive and negative feelings about care, procedures, and interactions with the child.	The caregiver may be unaware of some of the underlying feelings that may be affecting the infant-caregiver relationship.
3. Increase the child's caloric intake by feeding the child on demand or increasing intake as tolerated; offering high-protein snacks between meals; offering small portions of a wide variety of food at mealtimes; teaching the child healthy mealtime behaviors (decrease distractions; make mealtime pleasurable); planning naps/rest periods and intervening in the event of fretfulness or crying.	The child's intake must be greater than his/her caloric expenditure.
4. Monitor the child's intake and output.	Fluid loss may affect daily weight patterns.
5. Daily weight measurements should be obtained at the same time, with the same scales, and with the child dressed in the same amount of clothing each time.	This approach decreases the variability of internal factors that impact weight.
6. Provide a consistent caregiver from the nursing staff.	This strategy increases trust and provides the child with an adult who anticipates needs, thus decreasing the child's level of frustration.

Evaluation:
- The child gains weight.
- The child eats the food offered.
- The parents participate in feeding the child.

NURSING DIAGNOSIS • Knowledge Deficit related to lack of experience and of positive parenting training

Expected Outcome: • The child and caregiver will experience positive responses in their relationship with each other.

Intervention	Rationale
1. Provide instruction in child care, being sure to model appropriate adult/child interactions. Include techniques for holding, touching, and feeding the child.	Instruction, coupled with modeling and practice, will facilitate integration of information.
2. Exhibit a positive attitude toward the parents.	Acceptance increases trust and fosters an openness to learning.
3. Provide information regarding normal growth and development.	Parents may lack an understanding of normal growth and development and may have unrealistic expectations of the child.
4. Provide for rooming-in with the child.	This arrangement allows the nurse to observe parent-child interactions and to provide further teaching if necessary.
5. Teach the parents ways to increase the child's caloric intake and to minimize the control issues associated with mealtimes. (See box, Teaching Guidelines for Effective Feeding.)	Lack of previous experience and knowledge may result in ineffective parenting skills.

Evaluation:
- The parents are observed interacting appropriately with the child during meals.
- The parents verbalize an openness to learning new techniques of feeding.

TEACHING GUIDELINES *for Effective Feeding Practices*

Almost all children, at one time or another, do not eat as well as parents would like. If you are concerned about your child's eating, these guidelines may help:

- Children do well with schedules. Try to maintain consistent mealtimes and snack times each day.
- Children need to eat often, not constantly. Offer something every 2 to 3 hours, allowing three meals and two to three snacks per day.
- Make sure your child can easily reach the food served. Use a high chair, phone books, or small table.
- Allow your child to feed himself/herself. Try very small amounts at first. Offer seconds later. Expect messiness, and prepare in advance for easy clean-up (use of bibs, newspapers under the high chair, or whatever works for you). If you are worried about what little food actually gets into the child's mouth, use two spoons: one for the baby to control, and one for you to use for feeding.
- No force feeding, bribing, or cajoling! These approaches will backfire.
- Don't worry if your child wants to eat the same food every day; many children are like that. Variety is not important to a toddler's nutrition; what matters are total calories and protein.
- At mealtimes, offer solids first. Liquids are filling and provide fewer calories.
- Limit the amount of juice, water, and carbonated drinks consumed. Offer milk or formula instead.
- Offer foods that are easy for your child to handle. "Finger foods" are ideal, such as Cheerios, French fries, slices of banana, and peas. Make sure pieces are small so as to avoid choking.
- For more calories per bite, add margarine, mayonnaise, gravies, and grated cheese to foods. For snacks, use peanut butter, cheese, pudding, bananas, or dried fruit.
- Limit "junk foods," such as soda, donuts, and candy. They have little protein and fewer calories than some other foods, and take up valuable space in the stomach without promoting growth.
- Eat with your child or allow your child to eat with others, so meals and snacks can be fun.

Adapted with permission from Frank, D. A., Silva, M., & Needlman, R. (1993, February). Failure to thrive: Mystery, myth, and method. *Contemporary Pediatrics, 10,* 121.

KEY CONCEPTS

- In children and adolescents, the behavioral manifestations of anxiety and depression may be similar. Both may be withdrawn, tearful, unwilling to engage in play, and/or aggressive toward others.
- It is difficult to differentiate between normal mood changes secondary to developmental maturation and abnormal, persistent mood disturbances.
- A suicide gesture or statement should never be ignored.
- Protecting a youth from inflicting harm to self involves being emotionally and physically available to him, offering opportunities to discuss feelings and the suicidal event, and removing potentially harmful objects.
- Support for grieving families of suicidal or potentially suicidal individuals is best provided on both an individual and group basis in order to allow exploration of personal issues and social support.
- Anorexia nervosa is characterized by a deliberate refusal to maintain adequate body weight, a distorted body image, and amenorrhea (in female patients).
- One common factor among children with an eating disorder is a family system in which the individual is considered to be an extension of the parent, or serves as a means of meeting the parents' needs, rather than being allowed to develop as an autonomous individual. The mother tends to be overprotective, lacking in empathy, and overly invested in the daily activities of the child. The father is often emotionally distant from the mother and the child.
- The focus of care for a youth with an eating disorder involves restructuring cognitive perceptions, reducing opportunities for engaging in ritualistic and self-injurious behaviors, and reestablishing physiologic homeostasis.
- During the early treatment phase of eating disorders, it may be necessary to observe the youth following meals to prevent episodes of purging.
- ADHD is a developmental disorder characterized by developmentally inappropriate degrees of inattention, overactivity, and impulsivity.
- Support groups are vital in assisting families to cope with and modify expectations and interactions involving the child with ADHD.
- Education of the family about ADHD is a crucial component of caring for the child with this disorder.
- Low grades, irregular school attendance, aggressive or rebellious behavior, deteriorating relationships with family members or former friends, rapid or extreme changes in behaviors or mood, and loss of interest in hobbies, sports, or other activities are some common signs of substance abuse.
- The youth with a substance abuse problem, together with the family, should receive help in developing social support systems, with referral to appropriate resources that can offer additional support as they attempt to make long-term changes in their social and emotional patterns of relating.
- Child abuse tends to increase during times of economic hardship or external stress. Abusive families tend to be isolated, lack a support system, have low levels of trust, resolve conflict through aggression, assume fixed and traditional roles within the family, and establish rigid rules.
- All suspected child abuse must be reported to the appropriate authorities.
- Abusive parents often have unrealistic expectations of their children, which may relate to a lack of knowledge of normal growth and development.
- Role modeling positive parenting skills is an effective intervention in the care of the child who has been abused.
- The assessment of infant-parent interactions in cases of nonorganic failure to thrive should include observation of the ways in which the child is held and fed, how eye contact is initiated and maintained, and the facial expressions of both the child and the caregiver during interactions.

REFERENCES

American Psychiatric Association. (1994). *Diagnostic and Statistical Manual of Mental Disorders* (4th ed.). Washington, DC: Author.

Barkley, R. A. (1990). *Attention-deficit hyperactivity disorder*. New York: Guilford Press.

Barkley, R. A., DuPaul, G. J., & McMurray, M. B. (1991). Attention deficit disorder with and without hyperactivity: Clinical response to three dose levels of methylphenidate. *Pediatrics, 87*(4), 519–531.

Benoit, D., Zeanah, C. H., & Barton, M. (1989). Maternal attachment disturbances and failure to thrive. *Infant Mental Health Journal, 10*, 185–202.

Bernstein, G. A., & Borchardt, C. M. (1991). Anxiety disorders of childhood and adolescence: A critical review. *Journal of the American Academy of Child and Adolescent Psychiatry, 30*(4), 519–532.

Bools, C. N., Neale, B. S., & Meadow, S. R. (1993). Follow-up of victims of fabricated illness (Munchausen syndrome by proxy). *Archives of Diseases in Childhood, 69*, 625–630.

Calam, R. M., & Slade, P. D. (1989). Sexual experiences and eating problems in female undergraduates. *International Journal of Eating Disorders, 8,* 391–397.

Chatlos, J. C. (1996). Recent trends and a developmental approach to substance abuse in adolescents. In *Child and Adolescent Psychiatric Clinics of North America, 5*(1), 1–27.

Chiocca, E. (1995). Shaken baby syndrome: A nursing perspective. *Pediatric Nursing, 21*(1), 33–37.

Coody, D., Brown, M., Montgomery, D., Flann, A., & Yetman, R. (1994). Shaken baby syndrome: Identification and prevention for nurse practitioners. *Journal of Pediatric Health Care, 8,* 50–56.

Costello, E. J. (1989). Child psychiatric disorders and their correlates: A primary care pediatric sample. *Journal of the American Academy of Child and Adolescent Psychiatry, 28,* 851–855.

Drotar, D. (1991). The family context of nonorganic failure to thrive. *American Journal of Orthopsychiatry, 61,* 23–34.

Frank, D. A., Silva, M., & Needlman, R. (1993, February). Failure to thrive: Mystery, myth, and method. *Contemporary Pediatrics, 10,* 114–133.

Friedrich, W. (1990). *Psychotherapy of sexually abused children and their families.* New York: W. W. Norton.

Garfinkel, B. D., Carlson, G. A., & Weller, E. B. (1990). *Psychiatric disorders in children and adolescents.* Philadelphia: W. B. Saunders.

Gorman, J., Leifer, M., & Grossman, G. (1993). Nonorganic failure to thrive: Maternal history and current maternal functioning. *Journal of Clinical Child Psychology, 22*(3), 327–336.

Hamlett, K. W., & Curry, J. F. (1990). Anorexia nervosa in adolescent males: A review and case study. *Child Psychiatry & Human Development, 21*(2), 79–94.

Johnson, L., O'Malley, P., & Bachman, J. (1995). *National survey results on drug use from the monitoring the future study, 1975–1994.* Washington, DC: National Institute on Drug Abuse.

Kaysar, N., Kronenberg, J., Polliack, M., & Gaoni, B. (1991). Severe hypophosphataemia during binge eating in anorexia nervosa. *Archives of Diseases in Childhood, 66*(1), 138–139.

Kelly, G. (1991). Childhood depression and suicide. *Nursing Clinics of North America, 26*(3), 545–558.

Kovacs, M. (1981). Rating scales to assess depression in school-aged children. *Acta Paedopsychiatrica, 46,* 305–315.

Love, C. C., & Seaton, H. (1991). Eating disorders: Highlights of nursing assessment and therapeutics. *Nursing Clinics of North America, 26*(3), 677–697.

Messer, S. C., & Beidel, D. C. (1994). Psychosocial correlates of childhood anxiety disorders. *Journal of the American Academy of Child and Adolescent Psychiatry, 33*(7), 975–983.

National Research Council, Food and Nutrition Board. (1989). Recommended daily allowances. Washington, DC: National Academy of Sciences.

Pallikkathayil, L., & Flood, M. (1991). Adolescent suicide: Prevention, intervention, and postvention. *Nursing Clinics of North America, 26*(3), 623–634.

Palmer, R. L., Oppenheimer, R., Dignon, A., Chaloner, D. A., & Howell, K. (1990). Childhood sexual experiences with adults reported by women with eating disorders: An extended series. *British Journal of Psychiatry, 156,* 699–703.

Pozanski, E. O., Cook, S. C., & Carroll, B. J. (1979). Children's Depression Rating Scale. *Pediatrics, 64*(4), 442–450.

Puig-Antich, J., & Chambers, W. (1978). *The schedule for affective disorders and schizophrenia for school-aged children.* Pittsburgh: Western Psychiatric Institute and Clinic.

Reynolds, C. R., & Richmond, B. O. (1979). Factor structure and content validity of "What I think and Feel": The Revised Children's Manifest Anxiety Scale. *Journal of Personality Assessment, 43,* 281–283.

Rosenberg, D. A. (1987). Web of deceit: A literature review of Munchausen syndrome by proxy. *Child Abuse & Neglect, 11,* 547–563.

Spielberger, C. (1973). *State-Trait Anxiety Scale for Children.* Palo Alto, CA: Consulting Psychologists Press.

Summit, R. C. (1983). The child sexual abuse accommodation syndrome. *Child Abuse and Neglect, 7,* 177–193.

BIBLIOGRAPHY

Ambrosini, P. J., Bianchi, M. D., Rabinovish, H., & Elia, J. (1993). Antidepressant treatments in children and adolescents: Anxiety, physical and behavioral disorders. *Journal of the American Academy of Child and Adolescent Psychiatry, 32*(3), 483–493.

American Medical Association Diagnostic and Treatment Guidelines on Child Sexual Abuse. (1993). *Archives of Family Medicine, 2*(1), 19–27.

August, G. J., & Garfinkel, B. D. (1993). The nosology of attention-deficit hyperactivity disorder. *Journal of the American Academy of Child and Adolescent Psychiatry, 32*(1), 155–165.

Baren, M. (1994). Managing ADHD. *Contemporary Pediatrics, 11*(12), 29–48.

Behrman, R. E., Kliegman, R. M., Nelson, W. E., & Vaughan, V. C. III. (1992). *Nelson's textbook of pediatrics* (14th ed.). Philadelphia: W. B. Saunders.

Berthier, M., Oriot, D., Bonneau, D., Chevrel, J., Magnin, G., & Garnier, P. (1993). Failure to prevent physical child abuse despite detection of risk factors at birth and social work follow-up. *Child Abuse and Neglect, 17*(5), 691–692.

Biederman, J., Newcorn, J., & Sprich, S. (1991). Comorbidity of attention deficit hyperactivity disorder with conduct, depressive, anxiety, and other disorders. *American Journal of Psychiatry, 148*(5), 564–77.

Bithoney, W. G., McJunkin, J., Michalek, J., Snyder, J., Egan, H., & Epstein, D. (1991). The effect of a multidisciplinary team approach on weight gain in nonorganic failure-to-thrive children. *Journal of Developmental and Behavioral Pediatrics, 12,* 254–258.

Borst, S. R., & Noam, G. G. (1993). Developmental psychopathology in suicidal and nonsuicidal adolescent girls. *Journal of the American Academy of Child and Adolescent Psychiatry, 32*(3), 501–508.

Brent, D. A., Perper, J. A., Morita, G., Baugher, M., & Allman, C. (1993). Psychiatric risk factors for adolescent suicide: A case-control study. *Journal of the American Academy of Child and Adolescent Psychiatry, 32*(3), 521–529.

Brent, D. A., Perper, J. A., Morita, G., Baugher, M., & Allman, C. (1993). Suicide in adolescents with no apparent psychopathology. *Journal of the American Academy of Child and Adolescent Psychiatry, 32*(3), 494–500.

Broddy, J. M., & Skuse, D. H. (1994). Annotation: The process of parenting in failure to thrive. *Journal of Child Psychology and Psychiatry, 35*(3), 401–424.

Cicchetti, O., & Toth, S. (1995). A developmental psychopathology perspective on child abuse and neglect. *Journal of the American Academy of Child and Adolescent Psychiatry, 34*(5), 541–562.

Dashiff, C. (1995). Understanding separation anxiety. *Journal of Child and Adolescent Psychiatric Nursing, 8*(2), 27–38.

Davis, H. W., & Zitelli, B. J. (1995). Childhood injuries: Accidental or inflicted? *Contemporary Pediatrics, 12*(1), 94–112.

Devlin, B. K., & Reynolds, E. (1994, March). Child abuse. *American Journal of Nursing, 3*, 26–32.

DeWilde, E. J., Kienhort, I., Dieskstra, R., & Wolter, W. (1993). The specificity of psychological characteristics of adolescent suicide attempters. *Journal of the American Academy of Child and Adolescent Psychiatry, 32*(1), 51–59.

DiNicola, V. F., Roberts, N., & Oke, L. (1989). Eating and mood disorders in young children, *Nursing Clinics of North America, 12*(4), 873–893.

Dusenbury, L., Khuri, E., & Millman, R. B. (1992). Adolescent substance abuse: A sociodevelopmental perspective. In J. H. Lowinson, P. Ruiz, & R. B. Millman (Eds.), *Substance abuse: A comprehensive textbook* (2nd ed.). Baltimore: Williams & Wilkins.

Finkelhor, D. (1979). *Sexually victimized children*. New York: Free Press.

Finkelhor, D., & Berliner, L. (1995). Research on the treatment of sexually abused children: A review and recommendations. *Journal of the American Academy of Child and Adolescent Psychiatry, 34*(11), 1408–1422.

Fischer, M., Barkley, R. A., Fletcher, K. E., & Smallish, L. (1993). The adolescent outcome of hyperactive children: Predictors of psychiatric, academic, social, and emotional adjustment. *Journal of the American Academy of Child and Adolescent Psychiatry, 32*(2), 324–332.

Fleming, J. E., & Offord, D. R. (1990). Epidemiology of childhood depressive disorders: A critical review. *Journal of the American Academy of Child and Adolescent Psychiatry, 29*(4), 571–580.

Frank, E. S. (1991). Shame and guilt in eating disorders. *American Journal of Orthopsychiatry, 61*(2), 303–306.

Johnson, B. (1993). *Psychiatric-mental health nursing*. Philadelphia: J. B. Lippincott.

Kelleher, K. J., Casey, P. H., Bradley, R. H., Pope, S. K., Whiteside, L., Barrett, K. W., Swanson, M. E., and Kirby, R. S. (1993). Risk factors and outcomes for failure to thrive in low birth weight preterm infants. *Pediatrics, 91*(5), 941–948.

Kiser, L. J., Heston, J., Millsap, P. A., & Pruitt, D. B. (1991). Physical and sexual abuse in childhood: Relationship with post-traumatic stress disorder. *Journal of the American Academy of Child and Adolescent Psychiatry, 30*(5), 776–783.

Kovacs, M., Goldston, D., & Gatsonis, C. (1993). Suicidal behaviors and childhood-onset depressive disorders: A longitudinal investigation. *Journal of the American Academy of Child and Adolescent Psychiatry, 32*(1), 8–20.

Kutcher, S. P., Reiter, S., Gardner, D. M., & Klein, R. G. (1992). The pharmacotherapy of anxiety disorders in children and adolescents. *Pediatric psychopharmacology, 15*(1), 41–65.

Levine, M. D., Carey, W. B., & Crocker, A. C. (1992). *Developmental-behavioral pediatrics* (2nd ed.). Philadelphia: W. B. Saunders.

Lewinsohn, P. M., Clarke, G. N., Seeley, J. R., & Rohde, P. (1994). Major depression in community adolescents: Age at onset, episode duration, and time to recurrence. *Journal of the American Academy of Child and Adolescent Psychiatry, 33*(6), 809–818.

Lobo, M. L., Barnard, K. E., Coombs, J. B. (1992). Failure to thrive: A parent-infant interaction perspective. *Journal of Pediatric Nursing, 7*(4), 251–261.

Los Angeles Suicide Prevention Center. (1991). Assessment of suicidal potentiality. Los Angeles: Author.

Martin, F. E. (1990). The relevance of a systematic model for the study and treatment of anorexia nervosa in adolescents. *Canadian Journal of Psychiatry, 35*(6), 495–500.

McLeer, S. V., Deblinger, E., Henry, D., & Orvaschel, H. (1992). Sexually abused children at high risk for post-traumatic stress disorder. *Journal of the American Academy of Child and Adolescent Psychiatry, 31*(5), 875–879.

Moreau, D., Mufson, L., Weissman, M. M., & Klerman, G. L. (1991). Interpersonal psychotherapy for adolescent depression: Description of modification and preliminary application. *Journal of the American Academy of Child and Adolescent Psychiatry, 30*(4), 642–651.

Niven, R. G. (1986, June). Adolescent drug abuse. *Hospital & Community Psychiatry, 37*, 596.

Nowinski, J. (1990). *Substance abuse in adolescents and young adults: A guide to treatment.* New York: W. W. Norton.

Pheffer, C. R., Klerman, G. L., Hurt, S. W., Kakuma, T., Peskin, J. R., & Siefker, C. A. (1993). Suicidal children grow up: Rates and psychosocial risk factors for suicide attempts during follow-up. *Journal of the American Academy of Child and Adolescent Psychiatry, 32*(1), 106–113.

Rao, U., Weissman, M. M., Martin, J. A., & Hammond, R. W. (1993). Childhood depression and risk of suicide: A preliminary report of a longitudinal study. *Journal of the American Academy of Child and Adolescent Psychiatry, 32*(1), 21–27.

Robins, L. N. (1991). Conduct disorder. *Journal of Child Psychology and Psychiatry and Allied Disciplines, 32*(1), 193–212.

Rogers, S. J., & DiLalla, D. L. (1990). Age of symptom onset in young children with pervasive developmental disorders. *Journal of American Academy of Child and Adolescent Psychiatry, 29*(6), 863–872.

Schachar, R., & Wachsmuth, R. (1990). Oppositional disorders in children: A validation study comparing conduct disorder, oppositional disorder and normal control children. *Journal of Child Psychology and Psychiatry and Allied Disciplines, 31*(7), 1089–1102.

Schetky, D., & Green, A. H. (1988). *Child sexual abuse: A handbook for health care and legal professionals.* New York: Brunner/Mazel (Classic book).

Smith, C., & Steiner, H. (1992). Psychopathology in anorexia nervosa and depression. *Journal of the American Academy of Child and Adolescent Psychiatry, 31*(5), 841–843.

Sullivan, B. (1991). Growth-enhancing interventions for nonorganic failure to thrive. *Journal of Pediatric Nursing, 6*(4), 236–242.

42

The Child With a Cognitive Deficit

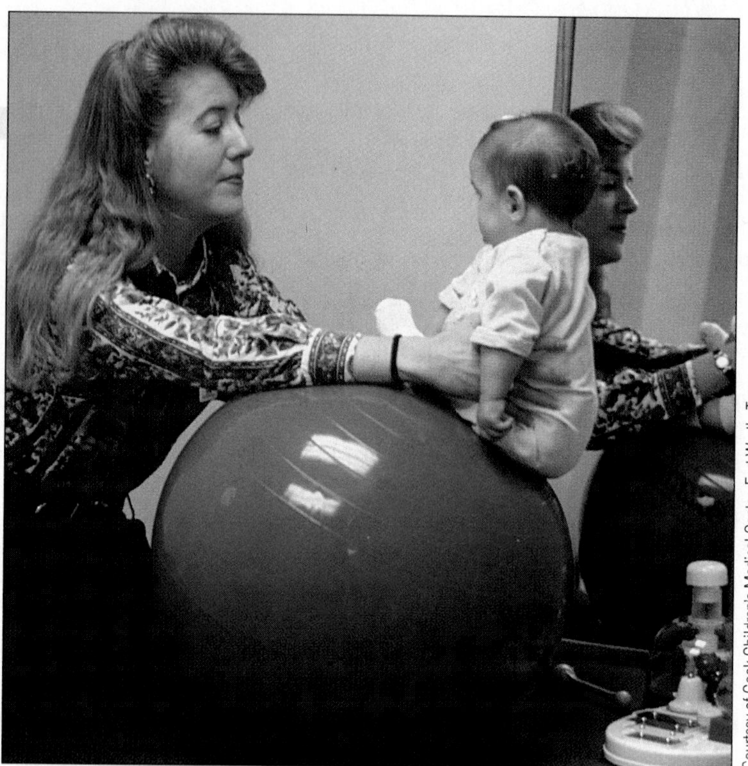

Courtesy of Cook Children's Medical Center, Fort Worth, Texas

CHAPTER OVERVIEW

LEARNING OBJECTIVES

After studying this chapter, you should be able to:

- Identify the various causes for mental retardation.
- Identify specific tools used in assessing the presence and degree of mental retardation.
- Identify educational and support resources for families with a child who is mentally retarded or developmentally delayed.
- Develop appropriate nursing strategies for supporting the family and child who is mentally retarded or developmentally delayed.
- Develop nursing strategies for families caring for a child with Down syndrome.

- Identify behavioral characteristics and appropriate nursing actions when working with a child with fragile X syndrome.
- Identify the basic diagnostic criteria for autism and how it differs from other types of pervasive developmental disorders.
- Identify the major aspects to be considered in working with the family of an autistic child.
- Develop home care interventions for a child with a cognitive deficit that are appropriate to the family system's ability and the child's developmental needs.

KEY TERMS

comorbidity: the presence of two different disorders occurring in the same individual. It is common for children with cognitive impairments to have coexisting psychiatric disorders

functional age: the age equivalent at which the child is actually able to perform specific self-care or relational tasks. For example, the child may be 6 years old chronologically, but may only be able to perform skills representative of children 4 years of age. The child's functional age, then, would be 4 years

intelligence: intelligence has different meanings. The three most common definitions are: (1) the innate capacity of the individual; (2) what individuals can do relative to learning, thinking, and problem-solving; and (3) results obtained on intelligence tests that measure specific skills, such as verbal, nonverbal, or mechanical abilities

pervasive developmental disorders (PDD): infant and childhood disorders characterized by severe and pervasive impairment in several areas of development in a manner that is distinctly deviant from the individual's developmental level or mental age (American Psychiatric Association, 1994)

Children with cognitive deficits have significant impairments in measured intelligence and adaptive behavior. Cognitive impairments can be a result of malformations of the brain and central nervous system, injury, infections, anoxia, or poisoning, or the cause may be unknown. Specific disabilities are differentiated based on an assessment of language, cognition, academic ability, self-help skills, social behaviors, and motor performance.

A cognitive impairment may be classified as a general delay, as in mental retardation, or as a part of a larger constellation of failures in skill acquisition, as in pervasive developmental disorders (PDDs). There is considerable overlap within several cognitive-related disorders. For example, children with autism, a specific disorder classified as a PDD, are often moderately or severely mentally retarded.

The family of a child with a cognitive deficit must cope with frequent and exceptionally high demands. The family is confronted with serious medical and environmental issues that seem rarely to be solved, only managed. Independence and self-management should be emphasized throughout childhood and adolescence so that, as the individual reaches adulthood, the possibility for independent living and gainful employment can be maximized.

The nurse is an integral part of the multidisciplinary team that manages the care of a child with a cognitive deficit. The nurse is involved in early assessment of the child, support of the family, assisting with self-care training, referral to support services, behavior training, and providing the necessary nursing care for other disabilities the child may have. School and community nurses require a broad range of knowledge to support children in the public school system who often have multiple cognitive and physical deficits.

COMMON DIAGNOSTIC TESTS FOR COGNITIVE DISORDERS

	DESCRIPTION	NORMAL FINDINGS	INDICATIONS	NURSING IMPLICATIONS
Vision Test	Assessment of vision, ocular pressure, and structural defects	Normal vision Normal structures	40%–45% of children with Down syndrome have refractive errors, cataracts, or other visual problems (Pueschel & Pueschel, 1992).	Explain pupil dilation. Provide protective eyewear following the examinations.
Hearing Test	Assessment of perception of sound frequency and volume	Normal hearing range	70%–80% of children with Down syndrome have hearing defects. Children with autism and PDD often appear to have defective hearing, despite normal hearing function. Hearing tests should be conducted.	Explain the test in simple terms. The test may require that the child wear a headphone, which may be difficult to tolerate.
Thyroid Studies	Blood serum tests to determine thyroid levels	Ages 1–3 years: 5.4–12.5 Ages 3–10 years: 5.7–12.8 Puberty-adulthood: 4.2–13.0	Slowed growth rates in children with Down syndrome are common.	These studies should not be performed within 7 days of a radionuclide scan.
Adaptive Behavior Scales (AAMR, MCDI, DDST, Vineland)	Assessment of language, motor, social, and self-care skills	Age-expected skills with 1 standard deviation from the mean	Children with suspected developmental delays	
IQ tests: Bayley Scales (Birth–3 Years); Stanford-Binet (2 Years of Age and Up); WPPSI (3–6 Years); WISC-III (6–16 Years); WAIS-R (16 Years of Age and Up)	Assessment of cognitive abilities	Age-normal skills within $1\frac{1}{2}$ standard deviations from the mean	Children with suspected developmental delays	

Bone Roentgenograms	Assessment of bone plates and joint spaces	Age-expected bone age	A decreased growth rate is common in children with Down syndrome.	This test requires that the patient be motionless during the radiographic study.
Brain Sonogram	Ultrasonogram of cranium	Normal position of brain's midline structures and normal blood flow velocity; no hemorrhages	Microcephaly or macrocephaly; misshapen cranium; family history of hydrocephaly	The patient must be supine. Any jewelry or metal objects should be removed from the child's head. The child may need sedation or may need to be restrained as this procedure takes 1 hour to complete. Explain to the parents that the test is noninvasive. Keep the patient warm during the procedure.
Genetic Analysis	Cytogenic bonding; culture media analysis		Suspected genetic or neoplastic disorders	Allow parents an opportunity to ask questions and express concerns about the possible results and implications of the testing.
Computed Tomography (CT)	Special noninvasive radiographic technique that allows visualization of cross-sections of brain tissue.	No blood clots, tumors, or infections	Impaired development, such as microcephaly; family history of central nervous system malformations; possible tumors or subdural hematomas	The child may need to be sedated or restrained, and will need to assume supine position. CT scans require the use of contrast medium and so require informed consent.
Magnetic Resonance Imaging (MRI)	Noninvasive method used to create images corresponding to density of tissue	Normal anatomy and physiology of the brain and/or spinal column	Same as for CT	The test requires informed consent. Remove metal or ferromagnetic objects before MRI. Sedation of the child is usually required.
Positron Emission Tomography (PET)	Noninvasive means of comparing cerebral brain flow and metabolic changes; used to localize seizure foci, visualize brain hemodynamics, and study brain pharmacology using radioisotopes	Normal metabolism of glucose in brain; normal blood flow and electrical activity	Seizures; hydrocephaly; evidence of cerebral dysfunction	The test requires informed consent. The child will need to be sedated. Liquids may be limited prior to the procedure. The child will need to void before the procedure if not in diapers. Parents may be able to remain with the child during the procedure.

AAMR, American Association on Mental Retardation; MCDI, Minnesota Child Development Inventory Profile; DDST, Denver Developmental Screening Test; WPPSI, Wechsler Preschool and Primary Scale of Intelligence; WISC-III, Wechsler Intelligence Scale for Children; WAIS-R, Wechsler Adult Intelligence Scale—Revised

MENTAL RETARDATION

Mental retardation is most commonly defined as "significantly subaverage general intellectual functioning existing concurrently with deficits in adaptive behavior and manifested during the developmental period" (American Psychiatric Association, 1994). When using standardized tests of intelligence, subaverage general intellectual functioning refers to a score that is at least two standard deviations below the mean. Mental retardation continues to be the most common term used by the medical profession, but other descriptive labels are more commonly used within the educational system. These labels include mentally handicapped, mentally impaired, or mentally deficient (American Psychiatric Association, 1994). Adaptive behavior refers to effective coping with common life demands, as well as the ability to maintain acceptable community standards of personal independence expected of individuals in the same age group, sociocultural background, and community setting. "Manifested during the developmental period" specifically means acquired or determined prior to the age of 18 years. The American Association on Mental Retardation (AAMR) has proposed that this definition be modified to include individuals with an intellectual functioning score of 70 to 75, and to reduce the number of levels to two—mild and severe—rather than four (mild, moderate, severe, and profound). Finally, the AAMR proposes that the individual must demonstrate limitations in at least two of the following 10 areas of adaptive behaviors: "communication, self-care, home living, social skills, community use, self-direction, health and safety, functional academics, leisure, and work." (Luckasson, 1992).

Relationship Between Developmental Disabilities and Child Abuse. There appears to be a significant relationship between developmental disabilities and child abuse. Experts believe that as many as 40% of children requiring child protective services have some type of developmental disability (West et al., 1992). The reasons given for this strong relationship include the intense stress in these families, parental isolation, and unrealistic expectations for the child's performance owing to a lack of knowledge about normal growth and development. There is also evidence that abuse can result in developmental disabilities or handicapping conditions. The identification of disabilities and health problems among children reported to child protective services is poor, as the primary focus of these services has been on substantiation of abuse or determination of risk for abuse. In addition, there is evidence that medical and other service providers spend little time with families during a typical week, and provide no increase in services despite increased funding availability (Herman & Hazel, 1991; West et al., 1992). The limited contact with families often serves to isolate them from supportive services and limits the professionals' understanding of the needs of the child, further perpetuating the sense of helplessness and lack of control in these family systems.

Defining Cognitive Impairment. Cognitive impairment is a general term that denotes limitations of intellectual and functional abilities. **Intelligence** is a difficult concept and is one that has been defined in a number of ways. It is important to determine the meaning of the word when used both by the professional and by the parent. Often, the intelligence quotient (IQ) of the child has little meaning for the parent, so the nurse must provide an explanation of its meaning and purpose. Mental age or **functional age** are terms that are often used to define a child's mental ability compared to the expected abilities of other children of the same chronological age. This score also gives some information about the level of cognitive understanding. For example, if an individual has a mental age of 5 years, the nurse's explanations need to be simple and specific, requiring no inferences on the part of the patient. However, if the individual has a mental age of 12 years, the nurse's explanations can provide more description and detail, or require some degree of inductive reasoning. Some psychologists suggest that intellectual functioning peaks around 16 years of age. Testing at this age period would be a functional estimate of the individual's ability level throughout adulthood.

Since the 1960s, cognitive disabilities, and especially mental retardation, have been approached from a developmental perspective. Hypothetically, mentally retarded children are believed to follow universal sequences of development and to perform identically with nonretarded children of the same mental age on cognitive-linguistic tasks. However, these notions have been challenged. It appears that those processes that are biologically mediated, such as motor functioning and cognition, do tend to begin early in life and follow a sequential pattern of development. However, moral, social, and cultural behaviors appear to be predominantly influenced by environmental determinants, as well as the cause of the mental retardation (Cicchetti & Mans-Wagener, 1987; Miller, 1986; Wetherby, 1986).

Safety Challenges. Cognitively impaired children are, by definition, less capable of managing environmental challenges than their peers. Injuries are generally more common in these children, when compared to same-age peers, probably as a result of their impaired function. However, among preschool-age children, injuries in children with cognitive impairment are less common, as the parents of these children are very protective and the children experience a decreased exposure to risk. There appear to be no gender differences in the risk for injury among this population (Dunne et al., 1993). Because of the prevalence of

TABLE 42–1 *Safety Concerns for Developmentally Delayed or Impaired Children*

	POSSIBLE INJURY	EDUCATION/TRAINING ISSUES
		Home
Kitchen	Burns Poisoning	*Preschool age:* Preventive education (i.e., instruct not to touch hot stove, not to ingest, etc.) *Elementary age:* Safe use of equipment; basic safety *High school age:* Cooking safety, emergency precautions
Bathroom	Falls Burns Cuts	*Elementary age:* Tub safety, precautions on wet floors *High school age:* Safe use of hair care equipment, shaving utensils, etc.
General		*Preschool & elementary age:* Avoidance of electrical outlets, safe passage around objects
		Outdoors
Yard or Playground	Animal bites Poisoning Abduction	*Preschool age:* Staying within boundaries; appropriate response to strange animals; safe use of equipment; avoidance of ingestion of berries, etc. *Elementary age:* Stranger safety, bicycle safety, traffic safety, water safety
Vehicles	Cuts Falls Serious injury	*Preschool & elementary age:* Seat belt use, keeping hands in car *High school age:* Traffic safety

safety concerns and the increased national focus on increasing self-reliance and independence in disabled individuals, safety in several domains needs to be emphasized across the lifespan of these individuals. Table 42–1 presents typical concerns for teaching in the home and in the community. Although it is clear from the table that the learning needs of these individuals are similar to those of children without disabilities, there may be a need for prolonged teaching, a greater degree of demonstration during teaching, frequent verbal and visual reminders, and more practice (Collins et al., 1991).

> Safety is a persistent concern of parents, teachers, and health professionals. This is particularly true for cognitively impaired children, as maturation in anticipating danger, problem solving, and judgment are generally impaired across the lifespan of these individuals. Additionally, those with motor disabilities are often unable to perform skills in a fashion that fosters safety.

Legal and Educational Considerations. Mental retardation has been more a consideration in legal, administrative, and educational spheres than in terms of medical diagnosis and treatment. Indeed, under many insurance plans, the single diagnosis of mental retardation does not qualify as a medical condition, and funds are not available for treatment. In some states, another psychiatric diagnosis must accompany the Axis II diagnosis of mental retardation in order for psychotropic medications to be prescribed (Vitiello & Behar, 1992).

The medical criteria, as well as the terminology used, are often somewhat different from the educational criteria for identifying mentally retarded students. In addition, the educational system uses slightly different criteria for placement purposes in the classroom, based on intellectual testing. The IQ score is an important measure in education, as this score often either limits or makes accessible various resources to the child. Public laws define and limit the placement of students in the school system, emphasizing the least restrictive environment for learning and the greatest inclusion possible with nonimpaired children (PL 94-142, PL 99-457). Also, recent revisions to laws for ensuring educational services for children with mental or physical disabilities make provisions for services from birth through the age of 21 years. When working with these children and families, the nurse may need to serve as a resource for helping families locate advocate services for their child.

Comorbidity With Psychiatric Conditions. Psychiatric disorders are likely to coexist with mental retardation, as the brain malfunctions that cause cognitive deficits also frequently affect those areas of the brain that monitor emotional states. The most frequent accompanying diagnoses include disruptive behavioral disorders, depression, and atypical psychosis (Vitiello & Behar, 1992).

Etiology. Mental retardation may be the result of congenital or early environmental factors. However, mental retardation may also occur secondary to head injury, anoxia, intracranial hemorrhage, infections, or poisoning, or from the presence or treatment of a brain tumor. As medical

Causes of Mental Retardation

HEREDITARY ORIGIN (5%)

Inborn errors of metabolism: aminoacidopathies, galactosemia, Tay-Sachs disease, phenylketonuria
Hereditary syndromes: muscular dystrophy, tuberous sclerosis, neurofibromatosis
Chromosomal aberrations: Down syndrome, fragile X syndrome
Familial retardation of probable polygenic origin

EARLY EMBRYONIC ALTERATIONS (30%–35%)

Sporadic chromosomal changes: Down syndrome
Multiple congenital anomalies: congenital rubella, toxoplasmosis, herpes, congenital hypothyroidism

EARLY INTRAUTERINE OR NEONATAL ALTERATIONS (10%–15%)

Fetal malnutrition: placental insufficiency, toxemia, drug addiction, maternal uterine cancer, multiple pregnancy
Neonatal conditions: prematurity, neonatal asphyxia, hyperbilirubinemia, hypoglycemia, central nervous system hemorrhage; ABO incompatibilities

ACQUIRED CHILDHOOD CONDITIONS OR DISEASES (3%–5%)

Complications of infections: meningitis, encephalitis, pertussis, varicella
Lead poisoning
Cranial trauma
Cerebral tumors
Cardiac arrest
Asphyxiation

ENVIRONMENTAL PROBLEMS AND BEHAVIORAL SYNDROMES (20%)

Psychosocial deprivation
Parental neurosis, psychosis, character disorder
Childhood psychosis, autism, other pervasive developmental disorders

UNKNOWN CAUSES (30%–35%)

Data from Reber, M. (1992). Mental retardation. *Psychiatric Clinics of North America, 15*(2), 511–522; American Psychiatric Association. (1994). *Diagnostic and Statistical Manual of Mental Disorders* (4th ed.). Washington, DC: Author.

technology advances, an increasing proportion of mentally retarded children are found to have a medical basis for their cognitive and adaptive impairments. Often the cause is a subtle, but nonetheless significant, biologic factor, such as minor chromosomal abnormalities, rare genetic syndromes, subclinical lead intoxication, nutritional deficiencies, or exposure to numerous prenatal risks and/or trauma. There is evidence that early neurodevelopmental functioning and later neurologic integrity and intellectual ability are strongly associated. Factors associated with low socioeconomic status have also been consistently reported as influences on cognitive function.

The accompanying box presents examples of the factors that can result in mental retardation.

Incidence. Mental retardation occurs in at least 1% of the population and may affect up to 3% of the total population in the United States (Vitiello & Behar, 1992). Among those diagnosed with mental retardation, 85% display only mild cognitive impairment. Ten percent of mentally retarded individuals are classified as moderately mentally retarded, 3% to 4% are severely mentally retarded, and only 1% to 2% are profoundly mentally retarded. This has clinical significance in that most families are able to care for mild to moderately impaired children and adolescents at home. As adults, most mildly impaired individuals are able to marry (often to individuals with normal intellectual function), maintain employment, and have relationships that are satisfying to them.

Clinical Manifestations. Specific congenital malformations often result in specific clinical manifestations. In addition, the severity of the mental retardation also affects the types and frequency of problem behaviors.

Mildly Mentally Retarded

- Presence or absence of physical features largely determined by the cause of the cognitive disability
- Social isolation and loneliness
- Depression

Severely Mentally Retarded

- Self-injury
- Fecal smearing
- Tearing of personal clothes and objects
- Severe temper tantrums
- Disrobing

In addition to general clinical manifestations based on the degree of the impairment, many syndromes present particular features that are helpful in determining the cause of the cognitive impairment. The two most common genetic disorders having mental retardation as a central feature are Down syndrome and fragile X syndrome. These will be presented as separate diagnostic syndromes later in this chapter.

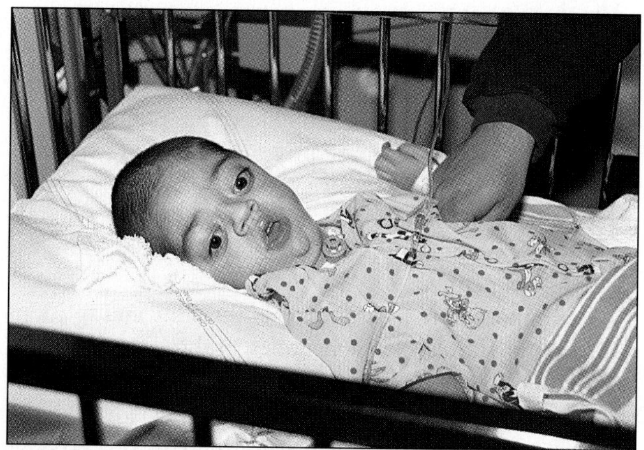

Figure 42–1

Children with cognitive deficits may have other dysfunctions as well. The family of a cognitively impaired child often experiences grieving that is ongoing because the child does not meet their expectations. This child has Marshall-Smith syndrome, which does not appear to be hereditary. His bones ossified unusually early, necessitating a craniotomy to allow greater brain development. He has a tracheostomy because of respiratory difficulties associated with an abnormally developed larynx. A gastrostomy button facilitates his nutrition. (Courtesy of Children's Medical Center, Dallas, Texas)

There are many disabilities associated with mental retardation that can further limit a child's adaptive skills. These deficits include cerebral palsy, visual deficits, seizure disorders, communication deficits, feeding problems, PDDs, failure to thrive, or attention-deficit hyperactivity disorder. It is common for speech and language deficits to be profoundly affected. Seizure disorders frequently develop as the child matures.

Although mentally retarded children can be generally healthy, the presence of associated deficits may place them at increased risk for illness (Fig. 42–1). For example, if a mentally retarded child also has cerebral palsy, the risk for gastroesophageal reflux and aspiration pneumonia is high. Motor or swallowing problems may result in inadequate oral intake or insufficient weight gain.

Diagnostic Evaluation. Diagnostic evaluations may be performed in utero, during the neonatal period, or when the child fails to achieve expected developmental milestones. Tests may be general, as well as specific to the neurologic or cognitive area in question. Several neuropsychologic tests are used to assess the individual's current level of functioning, as well as to anticipate persistent cognitive deficits that will remain following surgical repair and healing. These tests, which may involve administration of pencil-and-paper tasks, motor tasks, sensory tasks, or problems whose solutions require various degrees of cognitive processing, help to determine both the severity and type of cognitive impairment. Learning disabilities are often identified using some of these same instruments, and many are often available through the school system. Nurses can also be educated to administer developmental screening tools, such as the Denver Developmental Screening Test II (DDST-II; see Chapter 2 and Appendix D). It is important to note that the DDST-II has low reliability in diagnosing mental retardation for children ages 1 to 3 years (Batshaw, 1993).

Often, the diagnosis of mental retardation is not made until the child enters school and experiences significant academic failure, prompting formal psychological testing. However, routine assessment of development during pediatric visits is the best method of early detection. The accompanying box offers a description of IQ-specific developmental skills for motor, language, and social adaptive behaviors (Batshaw, 1991).

Expected Skills According to IQ Scores

NORMAL (IQ: 85–115)

Normal age skills across all domains
Borderline (IQ: 68–84)
Early milestones achieved
Likely to be noticed when school performance is monitored
Vocational skills adequate for competitive employment

MILD MENTAL RETARDATION (IQ: 52–67)

Slight delay in achieving developmental milestones
No alteration in sequence of skill acquisition
Likely to require special education services with an emphasis on vocational and self-maintenance skills
Able to form and maintain adult relationships

MODERATE MENTAL RETARDATION (IQ: 36–51)

Noticeable delay in motor and speech development
Early and persistent training in self-care required
Supervision required for complex activities or problem-solving

SEVERE MENTAL RETARDATION (IQ: 20–35)

Marked delay in all motor skills
Limited expressive speech, even though some receptive language skills may be present
Constant supervision required

PROFOUND MENTAL RETARDATION (IQ: 0–19)

May be able to walk
May have primitive speech
Constant supervision required

Therapeutic Management. Medical strategies are directed at preventing and treating infections, correcting structural deformities, and treating associated behaviors, such as aggressiveness. Corrective measures might include congenital heart surgery for malformations, the insertion of tympanostomy tubes, or splints for joints that are hypotonic and hyperextended. Frequently, prophylactic antibiotics are used to reduce the likelihood of infections. The treatment of behavioral difficulties and psychosocial disturbances may involve administration of medications, such as those described in Chapter 41, Psychosocial Deficits. However, because of marked differences in metabolic rates among developmentally delayed children, the doses may be more varied than for other children of the same height and weight.

Therapeutic management is largely dependent on community and educational resources. However, as already noted, obtaining services for these children requires multidisciplinary efforts and strong advocacy on the part of both parents and professionals.

NURSING CARE OF THE CHILD WITH MENTAL RETARDATION

Assessment

Assessing the Child. When assessing cognitive skills and level of adaptive functioning, it is necessary to become familiar with age-expected abilities that can be used as a standard for comparison (see growth and development chapters, Unit II). Life experiences also affect a child's abilities. Children who have had limited exposure to social rules and opportunities for thinking about their experiences will talk and act differently than children who have had more practice in these areas. Alternating between question-type information and demonstration-type information may be helpful in maintaining the child's interest in the assessment.

It is important to look directly at the child and speak in a direct and simple, yet noncondescending, manner. Ask the child as much of the necessary information as possible rather than relying solely on the parents to provide the information. As the child speaks, attend to the level of communication, the skill in using words to communicate, and the ability to follow one-step commands or more complicated requests.

Assessing Family Functioning. It is crucial to assess the family's level of functioning, the specific coping skills available and typically used, and the ability of the family to demonstrate awareness of and involvement in addressing the needs of the child. The child may come from a home where the parents have below-average intellectual functioning. Or, the parents may be young and may lack an understanding of developmental information, making them less aware of their child's abilities and functional deficits. Social and financial resources need to be explored in a manner that is informative but does not invade privacy. A matter-of-fact approach is helpful in assessing how

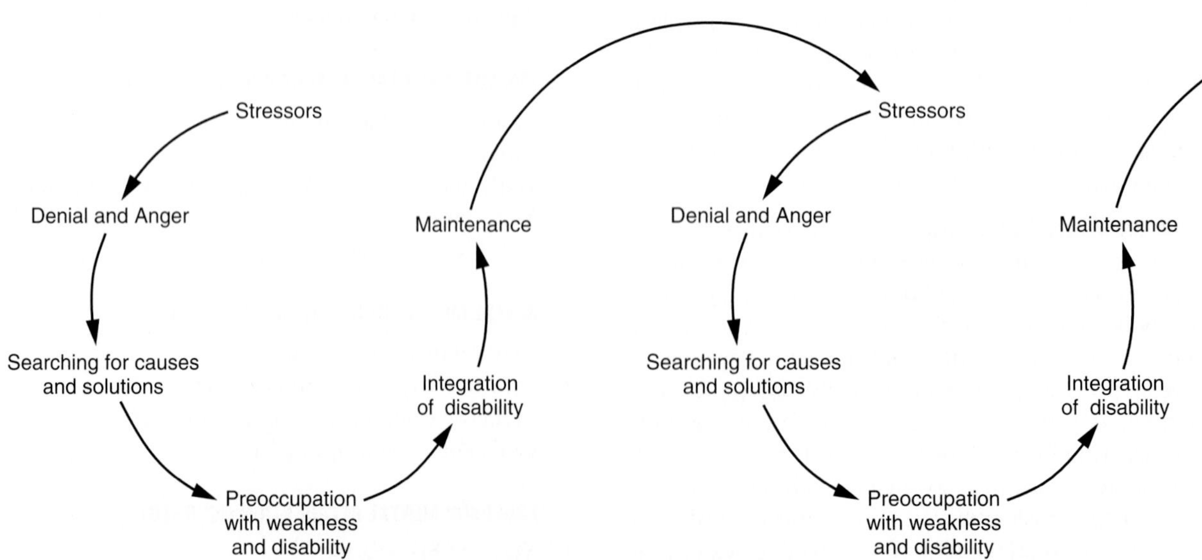

Figure 42–2

Typical coping style of the family of a child with a cognitive deficit. (Reprinted with permission from Finke, L. [1995]. Mental retardation. In B. S. Johnson [Ed.]. *Child, adolescent, and family psychiatric nursing.* Philadelphia: J. B. Lippincott, p. 176.)

the family meets the basic needs of each family member and manages the exceptional needs of the cognitively impaired child. This part of the assessment may be lengthy, as it may be necessary to assist the family in seeking long-term assistance for meeting the medical, psychological, and social needs of the child.

The family's interactional patterns should be assessed on an ongoing basis. Family patterns may trigger unacceptable behaviors in the child, and the child's behaviors may initiate particular responses in family members. These patterns may be outside the awareness of the family but be observable to others. In addition, the family's level of coping with the diagnosis or current situation should be assessed. Families with mentally retarded children experience grief in a manner similar to families of children with other chronic illnesses (see Chapter 17). This grief cycle begins with a stage of disbelief and denial, then progresses to anger. A process of searching for answers generally follows, a process that is particularly difficult when no specific etiology can be identified. The family then moves to a stage of preoccupation with the child's disabilities and symptoms. Finally, the family begins to identify the child's strengths and resources, moving toward a sense of integration and homeostasis. This process is repeated with each new developmental stage or situational setback, such as surgery or illness (Fig. 42–2). The goal is for the child to be accommodated into the family system and to receive safe, nurturing care and the opportunity to develop skills to the maximum degree possible.

Multidisciplinary Assessment. An interdisciplinary approach is critical for the effective management of these children. The team generally includes physicians, nurses, psychologists, speech and language pathologists, educational and recreational professionals, and, possibly, physical therapists and occupational therapists. In addition to nursing care, the family may be referred for genetic counseling and supportive psychotherapy. The assessment should include components that identify the need for other team members or auxiliary services. Long-term services may include respite care, in-home services, parent training, and support groups.

Nursing Diagnosis

- Risk for Injury related to an inability to anticipate danger or to level of self-care skills
- Knowledge Deficit (family members) related to the cause and likely outcomes of the child's cognitive disabilities, available support systems, or information about sexuality, vocational options, leisure skills, and so on.
- Impaired Social Interaction related to an inability to initiate and maintain social relationships
- Ineffective Family Coping: Compromised or Disabling, related to excessive emotional and financial strain on family members caring for a cognitively impaired individual, lack of acceptance by society, or an extended grieving process associated with a chronic disability

Planning, Implementation, and Evaluation: The Child With Mental Retardation

NURSING DIAGNOSIS • Risk for Injury related to an inability to anticipate danger or to level of self-care skills

Expected Outcome: • Self-injury or accidental injury will be avoided.

Intervention	Rationale
1. Provide anticipatory guidance relative to the child's developmental abilities to perform or understand.	Parents may not be able to accurately anticipate the child's cognitive or functional level. This is particularly true if the parents are inexperienced or have limited cognitive skills themselves.
2. Keep safety rails up on hospital beds and on the bed at home if the child is predisposed to falling or roaming at night. Provide child-sized furniture, and select age- and skill-related play equipment.	These strategies help to prevent accidental falls, as these children are accident-prone and have a limited ability to assess the environment for safety.
3. Give simple explanations about unsafe areas in the environment. Use the child's cognitive level as a key to what the child can understand or the degree of unsupervised freedom that can safely be allowed.	Concrete explanations can be understood by young or cognitively delayed individuals.

Evaluation: • The child does not sustain injury.

NURSING DIAGNOSIS

- Knowledge Deficit (family members) related to the cause and likely outcomes of the child's cognitive disabilities, available support systems, or information about sexuality, vocational options, leisure skills, and so on.

Expected Outcome:

- The child and family will utilize personal and community resources to increase the child's ability to develop personal skills for appropriate social, leisure, and vocational abilities.

Intervention	Rationale
1. During hospitalization, provide information that is simple, concrete, and solution-focused.	Hospitalization is stressful and may impair the family's adaptive coping skills.
2. Explain medical terms without assuming that the family knows the terminology. Give explanations to both the child and parents. Use demonstrations and therapeutic play.	The child may have a limited capacity to understand words, but may be able to understand a demonstration.
3. Select skills that enhance self-care and socially appropriate behaviors. As the child reaches puberty, provide simple information about sexuality and physical changes. Support training in leisure skills.	Education that is practical and functional to the child's mental and chronological age fosters self-esteem, compliance, and cooperation.
4. Provide parents with local and national resources for home care, education, and training facilities for mentally retarded individuals.	Additional services will be needed as the child grows or requires more specialized training. Often, families have to find out-of-home placement if the child's disability is severe or destructive to the family.
5. Provide parents with anticipatory guidance about developmental milestones and anticipated skills, including safety, sexuality, skills that can be expected, and behavioral changes throughout the developmental process.	Parents may have unrealistic expectations or expect too little from the child.

Evaluation:

- The family uses the resources available in the community to maximize the abilities of the child.

NURSING DIAGNOSIS

- Impaired Social Interaction related to an inability to initiate and maintain social relationships

Expected Outcome:

- The child will have some relationships that are satisfying and meaningful, as well as some solitary leisure skills.

Intervention	Rationale
1. Encourage the parents to support the child in participating in group activities that promote peer interactions (Special Olympics, special camps, etc.; Fig. 42–3).	Children who are mentally retarded need to be exposed to nonimpaired children, as well as to children with similar handicaps, to accommodate to social expectations and demands.
2. Encourage the parents to participate in interactive activities, such as reading books and playing, on a regular basis.	Families are likely to limit their interactions, as the child offers reduced reinforcements in social situations.

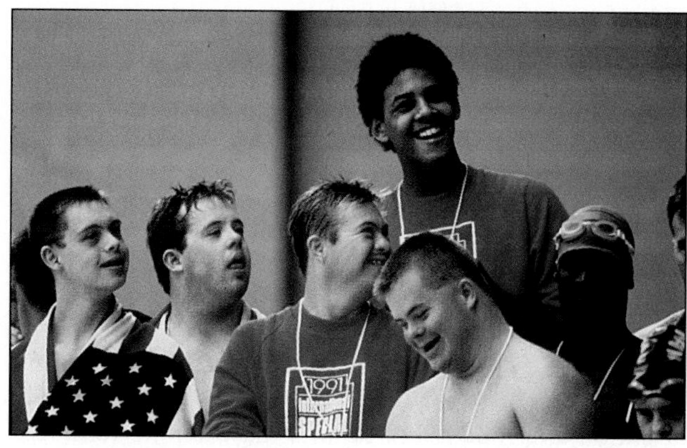

Figure 42–3
Programs such as the Special Olympics offer opportunities for social interaction with peers and assist mentally retarded children in reaching their maximum potential. (© Special Olympics International.)

Evaluation:

- Both the family and the child demonstrate a sense of pleasure in social interactions with family members and with other individuals within their social sphere.

NURSING DIAGNOSIS

- Ineffective Family Coping: Compromised or Disabling, related to excessive emotional and financial strain on family members caring for a cognitively impaired individual, lack of acceptance by society, or an extended grieving process associated with a chronic disability

Expected Outcome:

- The child and family will experience a sense of mastery and self-satisfaction in their family management and a sense of social acceptance within the community.

Intervention	Rationale
1. Provide anticipatory and ongoing support for the grieving process. Parents should be told the diagnosis and needed information as quickly as possible; this information should be given when both parents or supportive family members are available. Information may need to be explained in different ways (verbal, written materials, videos, etc.) to help parents grasp the meaning of the diagnosis.	Families typically experience a cycle of grieving that is repeated when milestones are not reached or when the child experiences an illness or a change in behavior (see Fig. 42–1).
2. Assist in identifying appropriate resources for social interactions and social training (early intervention programs; special education programs; recreational programs for mentally retarded children, etc.).	Mildly and moderately retarded individuals often experience loneliness and depression as a result of insufficient stimulation and social contact. Such programs can assist the child in reaching his or her maximum potential.
3. Identify and refer to appropriate community resources for both emotional support and family/child education. The nurse may need to act as an advocate and referral center (support groups; education consultants; home health agencies).	The grieving process and the need to accommodate to the child's skill level are ongoing; families often feel isolated and helpless in locating necessary resources.
4. Assist family members in identifying realistic short- and long-term goals for the child and themselves. Encourage the family to express feelings and concerns; provide hope when appropriate.	Stress, grieving, and limited knowledge may impair the family's ability to set reasonable goals themselves.
5. Provide parent education for monitoring the child for alterations in health status. Help the family recognize nonverbal signs of discomfort.	The child may be unable to verbalize pain typically associated with ear infections, colds, or major illnesses.

Intervention	Rationale
6. Assist the family in exploring their choices in terms of home care, group home, or residential facility.	Families may be hesitant to discuss care options for fear of being perceived as uncaring or unable to provide home care.

Evaluation:
- The child and family are able to manage the anxiety and grieving experience as they understand the diagnosis and the severity of the disorder.
- The family accommodates the child in the family system in a manner that facilitates growth and maturity to the maximum level possible.
- Family members are able to act as primary care providers and provide a safe environment.
- The family seeks medical attention as needed, and utilizes the multiple resources available to meet the child's social, emotional, educational, and medical needs.

DOWN SYNDROME

Down syndrome is a congenital condition that results in moderate to severe mental retardation. A high percentage of cases are linked to an extra group G chromosome, chromosome 21 (trisomy 21). The assessment and nursing interventions described for mentally retarded individuals are also applicable to these individuals. However, there are additional considerations for those identified as having Down syndrome.

Depending on the severity of the symptoms, the most common experience is for parents to rear the child at home until early adulthood. Following late adolescence or early adulthood, group home placement is typical. Supported employment is encouraged, and parents are typically advised to initiate vocational training in elementary school. The partnership of parents and professionals is vital in managing the symptoms and in providing the comprehensive services that are needed. The network of professionals includes educators, prevocational trainers, mental health workers, psychologists, social workers, physical therapists, occupational therapists, and speech and language pathologists, in addition to physicians and nurses (Fig. 42–4). Services required throughout the lifespan include education and vocational training, transitional services, respite care, social services, financial supplements, psychotherapy, and preventive and/or corrective medical care. It is easy to see how this array of needed services might be overwhelming to the family, and the potential for frustration on the part of both the parents and the professional team is high. Communication and coordination of services is considered to be a primary task for each team member.

Etiology. Although the specific cause is unknown, late maternal age has been consistently identified as one of the most significant factors associated with Down syndrome. The risk of a 35- to 39-year-old woman having a child with trisomy 21 is 6.5 times greater than that of a 20- to 24-year-old woman; at 40 to 44 years of age, the risk is 20.5 times greater (Hayes & Batshaw, 1993). As a result of preventive approaches for women who are at high risk for having a child with Down syndrome, recent studies indicate that most of these children are now born to women younger than 35 years of age. Recent molecular genetic studies reveal that in 5% of these, chromosome 21 translocation is identified as a paternal genetic contribution (Pueschel & Pueschel, 1992).

Several chromosomal alterations that result in Down syndrome have been identified. Most of these children (92% to 95%) have trisomy 21. In the remainder of these children, chromosome 21 translocates to chromosome 14 or 22. Mosaicism, a condition where two or more cells contain different numbers of chromosomes, occurs in 2% to 3% of children with Down syndrome (Pueschel & Pueschel, 1992).

Incidence. In the United States, there are more than 300,000 individuals with Down syndrome, with up to 10,000 new cases each year. This syndrome accounts for

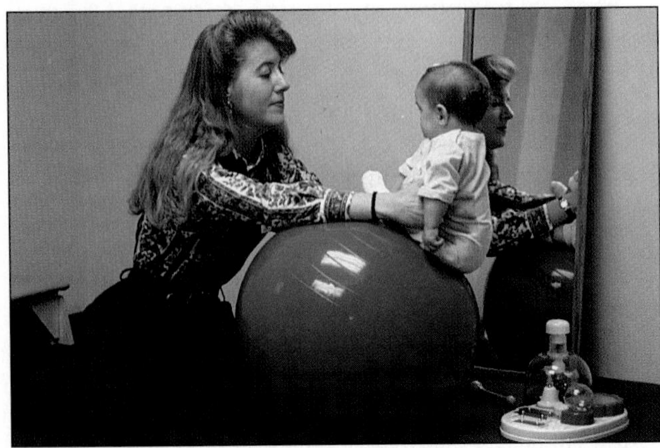

Figure 42–4
Children with delayed motor or cognitive function, whether temporary or pervasive, benefit from early and vigorous therapy to help them reach their maximum development. (Courtesy of Cook Children's Medical Center, Fort Worth, Texas)

PATHOPHYSIOLOGY *of Down Syndrome*

Although the pathogenesis of Down syndrome is not clear, it is presumed that the additional gene products of the triplicated chromosome 21 cause changes in the normal processes regulating embryogenesis. There is some evidence that a particular region of the chromosome 21 is responsible for facial features, heart defects, mental retardation, and dermatologic changes (Hayes & Batshaw, 1993). Second, it appears that many of the malformations in this disorder result from "incomplete" rather than "abnormal" embryogenesis. Examples include malformations of the atrioventricular canal, tracheoesophageal fistula, and imperforate anus. Finally, it appears that alterations in neurotransmitters, particularly in the cholinergic system, are responsible for the premature aging and Alzheimer's type dementia that are common in individuals with Down syndrome.

A number of medical problems in the newborn period can seriously compromise health and survival. If the child survives these complications, there are a number of less serious difficulties that are generally encountered in childhood. See the accompanying list of medical conditions typically associated with Down syndrome.

Medical Conditions Associated With Down Syndrome

CONDITIONS FREQUENTLY IDENTIFIED DURING THE NEONATAL PERIOD

- Cardiac conditions
  - Endocardial cushion defect
  - Tetralogy of Fallot
  - Atrial septal defects
  - Patent ductus arteriosus
  - Ventricular septal defects
- Gastrointestinal conditions
  - Tracheoesophageal fistula
  - Pyloric stenosis
  - Imperforate anus
  - Duodenal atresia
  - Aganglionic megacolon (Hirschsprung's disease)
- Congenital cataracts
- Hypothyroidism
- Dysplastic hips
- Leukemia-like conditions

CONDITIONS FREQUENTLY IDENTIFIED DURING THE CHILDHOOD PERIOD

- Endocrine disorders
  - Decreased growth
  - Obesity secondary to overeating, underexercise, or undetected hypothyroidism
  - Thyroid dysfunction
  - Infertility
  - Alopecia
  - Thin hair
- Sensitive skin and propensity for rashes
- Ophthalmic problems, such as myopia, strabismus, nystagmus, cataracts, blepharitis, and keratoconus
- Chronic serous otitis media
- Hematologic abnormalities
  - Subtle immune deficiencies
  - Acute nonlymphoblastic leukemia
  - Acute lymphoblastic leukemia
- Craniofacial defects
  - Malocclusions
  - Delayed teeth eruption
  - Periodontal disease and gingivitis
  - Bruxism
  - Sinusitis and rhinitis
  - Sleep apnea secondary to cranial malformations
- Musculoskeletal abnormalities
  - Hypotonia
  - Joint laxity and dislocations
  - Atlantoaxial subluxation or dislocation
- Sensory deficits
- Seizure disorders
- Psychiatric disorders, particularly adjustment reaction disorders, anxiety disorders, depression, behavior disorders, dementia
- Pervasive developmental disorders

one-third of all cases of moderate to severe mental retardation. Worldwide, the prevalence of Down syndrome is 1 in 700 births; in the United States, it is reported to be 1 in 500 births. Boys who are affected outnumber girls 1.3 to 1.0. As a result of increased prenatal diagnosis, approximately 40% of fetuses with Down syndrome in women aged 35 years or older are now terminated voluntarily. This has resulted in a recent decrease in the birthrate of children with Down syndrome.

Clinical Manifestations

Facial Features

- Brachycephaly (disproportionate shortness of the head)
- Flat occiput
- Oblique palpebral fissures
- Inner epicanthal folds
- Narrow, high-arched palate
- Protruding tongue
- Small, short ears which may be low set
- Delayed teeth eruption and frequent poor alignment

Body Features

- Short, broad hands
- Simian line (transverse palmar crease)
- In-curved little finger (clinodactyly)
- Broad, stubby feet with plantar crease
- Short, broad neck
- Prone to diastasis recti abdominis and umbilical hernia
- Small penis in males; bulbous vulva in females
- Dry skin with tendency for cracking and fissuring
- Hyperextensibility of joints and hypotonicity of muscles

Intellectual/Language/Social Function

- Generally moderate to severe mental retardation with intellectual abilities that continue to decline with age
- Onset of Alzheimer's type dementia with increasing age
- Language development characterized by particular difficulty with grammar but general strength in pragmatic language (social usage). (Pragmatic language includes such skills as maintaining the conversation on a specific topic and taking turns during conversation.)
- Social skills that surpass expected skills based on intellectual capacity.
- Social skills and adaptive self-care skills that decline with age.
- A limited ability to use the environmental cues available (i.e., infrequent scanning and use of only a few referential cues, such as eye contact with the primary caregiver, which often results in their inability to extract the information needed to draw conclusions).
- Blunted affect
- Fewer disruptive behaviors than other chromosomal disorders (Cicchetti & Beeghly, 1990; Evenhuis, 1990; Cullen et al., 1981).

Diagnostic Evaluation. Frequently, the diagnosis of Down syndrome is made at birth as a result of the characteristic prominent features. However, if there is some question, chromosomal analysis is conducted. Other diagnostic tests are conducted on the basis of the associated features, such as nasopharyngeal abnormalities or cardiac defects.

In order to rule out associated disorders and to detect frequently encountered difficulties, it is recommended that these children be monitored frequently throughout the first 12 months of life, with an emphasis on gastrointestinal and cardiac symptoms. This often requires a full cardiac work-up initially, and an electrocardiogram (ECG) at the end of the first year. In the second to fourth years of life, the medical emphasis is on sleep and behavioral difficulties, along with annual thyroid screening and ophthalmologic assessment. Generally, these children are referred for dental assessments at 24 months and followed at least annually throughout childhood.

Therapeutic Management. The management of Down syndrome is symptom-specific, as there is no cure for the disorder. Surgery to correct cardiac abnormalities, gastrointestinal malformations, and craniofacial deviations have been used to prolong life, alleviate discomfort, and decrease the likelihood of further medical complications. (For nursing responsibilities during these procedures, please refer to the appropriate chapters.)

Plastic surgery to correct some of the appearance characteristics of Down syndrome is controversial. Proponents believe that the surgery helps to reduce the stigma of mental retardation, as well as to improve speech, eating, breathing, and general health and acceptance by family and society. Others are opposed to the surgery on the basis of the child's inability to understand and give consent, and the degree of discomfort typically experienced as a result of the procedure. The surgery generally consists of tongue reduction; implants to the bridge of the nose, chin, cheeks, and jawbone; and Z-plasty of the eyelids to reduce the epicanthal folds (May & Turnbull, 1992).

NURSING CARE OF THE CHILD WITH DOWN SYNDROME

Assessment

The neonatal assessment described in Chapter 3 is crucial in diagnosing Down syndrome on the basis of physiologic characteristics. The reader is also referred to the assessment of mentally retarded children included in the nursing care plan presented earlier in this chapter. In addition to these processes, the assessment for Down syndrome is also based on family history, especially the mother's age. If Down syndrome is suspected or already confirmed on the basis of earlier genetic testing, serum alpha-fetoprotein levels, or amniotic fluid samples, an assessment is conducted to determine the severity of symptoms and the family's ability to cope with and accommodate the needs of the infant.

A thorough physical examination should be conducted, including hearing and vision examinations.

> As many as 80% of children with Down syndrome have hearing deficits. These children are also more likely to have refractive errors or cataracts.

If the child with Down syndrome is hospitalized for surgical repair, infections, or injury, it is important to assess the child's typical coping patterns in order to support those strategies already in place. These children prefer routine and consistency, so an assessment of their daily routine is important, including times and habits related to mealtimes, bathing, and order of dressing.

Assessing the child's ability to communicate and understand language is important in order to provide information that is geared to an appropriate level of comprehension. Knowing the child's words for specific body functions, such as voiding, defecating, or sleeping, will allow for greater comfort for the child while in the hospital. Assessment of their learning abilities will be important prior to initiating any education or procedure-related play.

An assessment of motor skills is performed to determine the procedures necessary to ensure safety. Frequently, these children are awkward and somewhat uncoordinated, increasing the likelihood for falls. The presence of self-stimulating behaviors needs to be assessed, as these are often used as coping strategies, but may also be self-injurious. The presence of sensory deficits, such as vision or hearing difficulties, should be determined as part of the routine assessment. Such deficits can be detected through close observation of the child while reaching for objects, by listening to conversation, or by announcing the child's name. However, the child with Down syndrome may respond to a lesser degree, or with blunted affect, to sensory stimuli, even if hearing or vision deficits are not present.

An assessment of the environment will help to determine whether it is conducive to safety and provides sufficient stimulation. Affected children frequently do not seek out stimulation, and may need encouragement through colors, sound, and motion. An assessment of social behaviors is also important, and should include play, social judgment skills, and social interest in the environment. The child may demonstrate inappropriate behaviors, such as those listed under severe mental retardation. Moreover, their natural curiosity may be diminished as a result of fear or frustration.

Nursing Diagnoses

- Altered Parenting related to delayed development, physical appearance, and medical complications
- Self-Care Deficits related to cognitive immaturity
- Altered Growth and Development related to poor sucking abilities or mouth deformities, flaccid facial muscles, and other abnormalities

Planning, Implementation, and Evaluation: The Child With Down Syndrome

See also the care plan for children with mental retardation for related nursing care.

NURSING DIAGNOSIS

- Altered Parenting related to delayed development, physical appearance, and medical complications

Expected Outcome:

- The family will be able to develop satisfying and supportive relationships that meet the physical and emotional needs of each family member.

Intervention	Rationale
1. Offer assistance and support to parents by giving clear explanations and by relating to the child as a unique and significant individual. Give clear statements about what you observe about the child's behaviors and skills. Assist in identifying positive features and behaviors in the child.	Parents are often fearful of how others will respond to their child and may need encouragement to identify positive characteristics of their child.

Evaluation:

- Parent-child interactions are positive and mutually satisfying.

NURSING DIAGNOSIS • Self-Care Deficit related to cognitive immaturity

Expected Outcome: • The child is able to meet his/her needs related to toileting, feeding, bathing, and dressing.

Intervention	Rationale
1. Keep the environment as routine as possible. Obtain information about the child's home routines and record it in the care plan so that the information can easily be accessed.	A change in routine often results in excessive frustration and decreased coping abilities.
2. The plan of care is based on the child's cognitive and motor abilities, rather than on chronological age. Observe the child for signs of readiness to learn a new task (reaching for cup, attempting to dress self, etc.).	The child's skills in some areas may be age-appropriate, but may be markedly delayed in others. Self-care should be encouraged.
3. Adaptive tools for dressing, bathing, and eating may be necessary (see Fig. 42–4).	The child's level of coordination, muscle strength, and dexterity may not allow the child to zip, button, or feed self in the usual way.

Evaluation: The evaluation of the effectiveness of nursing care will depend on the reasons the child is being treated. A general evaluation includes the following:

- The child demonstrates continued development and use of self-care skills already present, satisfying interactions with others, and a sense of mastery and competency with the learning of new skills.
- The parents demonstrate acceptance of the child's disabilities, with a tolerance for delayed skill development, as well as an interest and willingness in helping the child learn new skills through demonstration, repetition, and much positive feedback.

NURSING DIAGNOSIS • Altered Growth and Development related to poor sucking abilities or mouth deformities, flaccid facial muscles, or other abnormalities

Expected Outcome: • The child will maintain a steady growth velocity pattern throughout childhood.

Intervention	Rationale
1. Explore options for fluid and calorie intake; care may require special bottles or adaptive utensils as the child develops.	Breastfeeding may not be possible if the child's muscle tone or sucking reflex is immature. The child may not have the strength or ability to use ordinary eating or drinking tools owing to facial, mouth, or trunk abnormalities.
2. Parents may require nutritional consultation or the child may need behavioral training to encourage intake of new foods or acquisition of new skills.	These children like to maintain routines and are often resistant to food or environmental changes.

Evaluation: • The child exhibits a normal growth pattern appropriate for age and abilities.

FRAGILE X SYNDROME

Fragile X syndrome is one of the more common chromosomal defects that result in significant cognitive deficits. It has only recently been recognized as a distinct condition. The disorder does not usually manifest itself as mental retardation in female individuals, but the fragile X chromosome is normally passed to the offspring by a female carrier. This syndrome has a unique profile of behavioral and cognitive patterns.

PATHOPHYSIOLOGY *of Fragile X Syndrome*

Fragile X syndrome is an X-linked disorder characterized by an abnormal gene at the Xq27.3 location. The responsible gene has been identified as FMR-1, which has a cytosine, guanine, guanine (CGG) nucleotide repeat.

Etiology. The gene that causes fragile X syndrome is transmitted by the mother, who is the carrier. Interestingly, these mothers have specific strengths in verbal memory and specific deficits in skills thought to be monitored by the frontal lobes, and there is some evidence to suggest global right hemisphere deficits (Mazzocco et al., 1993).

Incidence. Fragile X syndrome affects approximately 1 in every 1000 male children and 1 in every 2000 female children (Reber, 1992; Laxova, 1994). As many as 1 in 625 individuals may carry the fragile X gene (Wilson & Mazzocco, 1993). Approximately 20% of males with the phenotype and 75% of the heterozygous females exhibit no discernible clinical features of the syndrome, yet remain capable of transmitting the genetic abnormality to their children (Bregman & Hodapp, 1991). In general, male individuals are the only ones who exhibit the full effects of the X-linked recessive disorder because their only X chromosome has the abnormal gene. If female individuals show signs of the disorder, those signs are usually less severe.

Clinical Manifestations

Physical Features

- Facial dysmorphism, with large or prominent ears and a long, narrow face; a head circumference that may be disproportionate to height and weight; lowered epicanthic folds; and prominent nasal alae (cartilaginous flap on outer side of each nostrile)
- Postpubertal macro-orchidism
- Flat feet
- Lax ankles
- Hyperextensible fingers
- Extremely soft and smooth skin
- Mitral valve prolapse (common)

Intellectual/Language/Social Function

- Autistic-like behaviors, such as gaze avoidance, hand flapping, echolalia, and abnormal speech patterns
- Hyperkinetic behaviors, including restlessness, agitation, and attention deficits
- Hand-biting
- Sensory motor integration deficits, such as poor coordination, motor planning deficits, and tactile defensiveness
- *In boys:* cognitive deficits in the moderate to severe range; strengths in visual memory, but weakness in auditory processing abilities and abstract reasoning; improved performance with simultaneous rather than sequential processing; language delays, perseveration, tangential speech, and other communicative disorders. *In girls:* generally only mild cognitive deficits, but with many variations
- High degree of disruptive behaviors, including temper tantrums, self-injurious behaviors, extreme agitation
- Progressive dementia

(Data from Smith, 1993; Vitiello & Behar, 1992; and Warren Holroyd, & Folstein, 1989.)

Diagnostic Evaluation. Prenatal diagnosis is now available through DNA analysis (Brown et al., 1993; Coplan, 1993). "All mentally retarded males with a matrilineal family history of learning problems or physical stigmata associated with the disorder should be tested for fragile X chromosome. Treatable conditions, such as hypothyroidism, plumbism, phenylketonuria, and Wilson's disease, must be clearly ruled out" (Reber, 1992).

Therapeutic Management. Treatment with folic acid is often initiated in infancy, although the effectiveness of this treatment as a supportive medication for behavioral management has not been well studied. Medications used in the behavior management of other disorders, such as attention-deficit hyperactivity disorder (ADHD) and autism, may also be prescribed.

Speech and language evaluation/therapy is generally prescribed during the first year of life and is made available on an ongoing basis. Sensorimotor integration therapy may be offered to enhance motor planning, joint stability, coordination, and integration of visual, auditory, and tactile information, and is considered to be the therapy of choice for learning disabilities. The accompanying box presents one family's experience with a child with fragile X syndrome.

NURSING CARE OF THE CHILD WITH FRAGILE X SYNDROME

The nursing care of individuals with fragile X syndrome is similar to the care outlined for mentally retarded children earlier in this chapter, with specific attention to the behav-

*A Child With Fragile X Syndrome: One Family's Experience**

When our son Eric was born, we anticipated his arrival with great excitement. We were unaware of any problems until he had a diphtheria-pertussis-tetanus (DPT) shot at 2 months of age, which was followed by encephalitis. His father is a physician and I am a nurse, and we began to observe developmental delays about this time. By 9 months of age, he was still unable to roll over and could not sit unsupported. At 15 months of age, we began to work with a physical therapist but noted little improvement. We were then referred to an Adaptive Learning Center, where he received supportive treatment for 5 years. He was unable to walk until his third birthday. When he was 4 years old, we were referred to a geneticist, but there was no firm diagnosis. My husband read some information about fragile X syndrome and requested specific testing for this disorder.

Our son has the typical behavior of avoiding eye gaze. When people insist that he look them in the eye when listening or speaking, he becomes very anxious. Eric also displays a tendency to repeat questions and seems unable to stop even when he has the answer. His play is also atypical, more like that of a 5-year-old than a child of his chronological age of 12 years. This makes it difficult for him to make or keep friends. We continue to take Eric to a therapeutic play group to work on this skill and to give him time with others who are more accepting of his differences.

Eric's difficulties have been painful for our family. My husband and I have had little time to talk or be alone, as he has required so much of our attention. His older sister believed he was favored and resented the changes we had to make in the family schedule to accommodate his behaviors and needs.

We have had varied responses from both the medical and educational systems. Some people have been willing to listen instead of merely doing things in the typical way. For example, Eric tolerates some medical procedures better if he is held at an angle rather than lying supine or sitting upright. He needs time to hear an explanation of what is going to happen, and more time to process the information. He needs to be able to ask questions and see a demonstration. Once a nurse tried to hide a needle from him before administering an injection; he needed her to show him the needle and tell him what she was going to do. We tried to tell her what would work best for him, but she would not listen. After a while we lost some of our confidence in the medical profession.

Often, I feel like I have to repeat myself over and over because few people in education know about this disorder. Some are very willing to learn and adapt, but others insist on their own way of teaching. For example, our son learns words globally first, called logo-reading, and is only later able to break down the word into phonetic sounds. He learns incidentally rather than by direct instruction. The teacher is most effective when working with another student and letting Eric just "listen in" rather than speaking to him directly. Eric is afraid of loud noises, so events, such as a fire drill, are very difficult for him. One teacher changed the fire drill evacuation route to avoid passing by the fire alarm, and this was very helpful.

*As related by Karen Greenhood, a master's-prepared nurse and the mother of two children.

ioral and cognitive difficulties presented by the individual child. The plan should include a multidisciplinary team approach to assessment. Special education services will be necessary to address the child's specific cognitive and academic difficulties, as well as to foster continued skill development and to reduce the stress created within the typical educational setting. Remediation services should include behavioral interventions specific to the child's needs, speech and language assistance, and possible occupational and physical therapy to address visuomotor, and motor skill deficits. Family members of individuals with fragile X should receive genetic counseling and testing.

Precautions for apnea may be prescribed, as sudden infant deaths occur with increased frequency in these children (Laxova, 1994). Assessment for other related abnormalities, such as cleft palate, foot deformations, hip dislocations and other conditions involving joint hyperextensibility, hernias, and hypertonia, should also be performed. Seizures occur in 17% to 50% of these children, so medications and education of the family about seizure disorders may be warranted.

AUTISM

Autism is the most severe condition classified as a **pervasive developmental disorder** (PDD) by the American Psychiatric Association (1994). PDDs are those disorders characterized by "severe and pervasive impairment in several areas of development: reciprocal social interaction skills, communication skills, or the presence of stereotyped behavior, interests, and activities" (American Psychiatric Association, 1994). Typically, these conditions are evident in the first 12 months of life, but may be overlooked if gross motor skills are progressing normally. Frequently, these conditions are observed with a diverse group of other medical conditions. Other conditions included in this category are Rett syndrome and childhood thought disorders, formerly known as childhood schizophrenia, symbiotic psychosis, and childhood psychosis. Autism will be discussed because it is the most severe of these disorders, but it is clearly not the most frequently encountered disorder among PDDs.

There is no evidence that autism can be cured, so treatment is generally lifelong and is characterized by varying degrees of success. Children with IQs of less than 50 generally remain cognitively stable. In those with IQs greater than 50, the outcome varies depending on education and early treatment. Research indicates that language functions, rather than social behaviors, can be used most successfully to predict short-term outcomes. The early onset of social symptoms does not necessarily indicate increased severity of symptoms, lower intelligence, or insecure attachments.

Etiology. The cause of autism is unknown; however, it is believed that the disorder can be caused by a wide range of prenatal, perinatal, and postnatal conditions, including maternal rubella, untreated phenylketonuria, tuberous sclerosis, anoxia during birth, encephalitis, and fragile X syndrome. It was once believed that family child-rearing practices and parental personality characteristics influenced the development of autism, but there are no controlled studies that confirm this view. Because siblings are more likely to develop the disorder than children in the general population, genetic factors are believed to play a role.

Incidence. Autism is three to four times more common in boys than in girls, occurring with a frequency of 10 to 15 children in every 10,000. No differences in incidence have been noted to correlate with race, socioeconomic level, or culture.

Clinical Manifestations. Autism is a severely incapacitating, lifelong developmental disability that is characterized by a qualitative impairment in four developmental areas: (1) disturbance in the rate and appearance of physical, social, and language skills; (2) abnormal responses of the body sensations; (3) thinking capacity, but with absent or delayed speech and language; (4) abnormal ways of relating to people, objects, and events. The child may have a vast vocabulary, yet have no comprehension of the meaning of the words; likewise, he or she may be able to solve intricate mathematical problems, but not be able to make change from a dollar. The child may seem oblivious to the sound of his own name but may come running into the room at the sound of a truck. Generally, there is a fixed, unchanging response to a particular stimulus. Self-stimulation is common and generally involves repetition of a particularly pleasing sensory stimulus, such as twirling a toy or rubbing the top of the head. The autistic child typically repeats an act, such as fingering an object or continuously spinning around, rather than responding to new stimulus. It appears that interest is limited by nature, rather than by choice, to an extremely narrow range. These children generally overreact to any change within the environment. Often, autistic children do not have a typical sense of personal space, and so may touch others on the face or stand face to face, with noses touching, even when encountering a total stranger.

Autism is usually apparent to parents before the age of 3 years, although there may be a period of apparently normal development followed by rapid deterioration. There is a wide range in the degree of impairment produced. Autism shares some similarities with the characteristic presentation of what has been called childhood schizophrenia and mental retardation, but there are definitive differences. These differences are outlined in Table 42–2. Eighty percent of autistic individuals are mentally retarded (Reber, 1992). A few individuals with autism also demonstrate an extremely developed skill in a particular

TABLE 42–2 *Differential Diagnosis of Autism, Mental Retardation, and Schizophrenia*

Autism	*Mental Retardation*
Peaked skill profile	Flat skill profile
Lack of imitative skills	Imitation skills and gesturing; social behavior; initiation of social contact
Nonsocial behaviors with little initiation	
Abnormal communication and language	Limited language ability, but sufficient for communication
Development seizures possible during adolescence	Usually no seizures; Alzheimer's type dementia in adulthood
Autism	***Schizophrenia***
Onset before 30 months of age	Onset during pubescence or adolescence
No remissions	Remissions and relapses
Rare hallucinations/delusions	Hallucinations/delusions common
Absence of thought disorder	Thought disorder
No family history of schizophrenia	Family history of schizophrenia
Self-stimulating behaviors	Odd behavior, but no self-stimulating behaviors
Medications of limited use	Medications often helpful in reducing symptoms

area, such as music or mathematics. These individuals are sometimes known as idiot-savants because of their demonstration of both a severe cognitive deficit and an extraordinary cognitive skill or expertise.

Social Behaviors

- Marked lack of awareness of the existence or feelings of others (i.e., ignores emotions of others)
- Lack of or abnormal amount of comfort-seeking at times of distress (i.e., does not show pain when hurt)
- Lack of or abnormal imitation of others' actions
- Lack of or abnormal social play (generally plays alone or involves others only as mere objects)
- Gross impairment in social peer relationships (appears not to want or need friends)

Language

- Lack of or impaired verbal communication and abnormalities in the production of speech (inappropriate volume, pitch, rate, rhythm, and/or intonation, such as a monotone voice or echolalia)
- Markedly abnormal nonverbal communication (i.e., uses no gestures or behavioral cues)
- Absence of imaginative play (no imitative or dramatic role playing)
- Impaired interactive speech/communication (does not allow for the normal give and take of conversation; becomes preoccupied with a given subject or word and is out of context with the conversation)

Restrictive Repertoire

- Stereotyped body movements (e.g., spinning around, head-banging, "flapping," or rocking)
- Persistent preoccupation with characteristics of objects (smell, taste, texture) or an abnormal attachment to objects (e.g., piece of string, a picture of a whale, etc.)
- Marked distress over a minor change in the environment (e.g., exhibiting tantrums when a light is turned on, refusing to look at teacher wearing a new dress)
- Unreasonable insistence on routine (following a schedule to the very minute or second; refusal to attend an assembly during a scheduled mathematics class)
- Self-injurious behaviors, such as biting, picking at skin, or scratching of eyes
- Marked restriction in range of interests (e.g., may repeatedly align objects and cannot be diverted from doing so)

(Data from American Psychiatric Association 1994 and Larsson et al., 1992).

Diagnostic Evaluation. A diagnosis of autism is usually established on the basis of symptoms. Often, the family is interviewed initially, followed by observation of the child alone, with the parent, and interacting with the examiner or others in the environment. Interviews are coupled with observations and clinician rating scales. Advanced practitioners may participate in the observations and rating scales used to diagnose this disorder. Two assessment instruments that may be useful include the Childhood Autism Rating Scale (CARS) (Schopler et al., 1988) and the Psychoeducational Profile-Revised (PEP-R) (Schopler, Reichler, & Renner, 1990). Both offer opportunities for evaluating skills in gross and fine motor development, affect, language, sensory modes, social relations, and ability to interact with play materials. Many of the instruments used to categorize autism require formalized training and are beyond the scope of this text.

Therapeutic Management. Early identification of autism is essential, and treatment generally involves placement in an environment that facilitates interaction and promotes replacement of stereotypical behaviors with more normalized behaviors using behavioral methods. Autistic people have a normal lifespan; consequently, they require significant financial resources for treatment and supervision. Because of the severity of the social impairment and the ineffectiveness of normal environmental interventions, affected children are usually referred to special programs designed to offer stimulation, modify stereotypical behaviors, or establish routines for teaching as soon as identification of the disorder has been made. Programs usually focus on safety precautions for self-injurious behaviors, such as head-banging, and the promotion of communication. Facilitative communication through the use of picture boards or keyboards is controversial, but has been used in many educational settings to assist these children to interact with their environment.

NURSING CARE OF THE CHILD WITH AUTISM

Assessment

Prior to diagnosis, the nurse must assess the child with possible autism as if there were no physical conditions present, as no classical physical features exist to highlight this disorder. The primary characteristic of autism is lack of social interaction and awareness. For this reason, if the child is very young, the nurse who interacts only with the child's parents is not likely to be aware of the child's degree of social disengagement. If the child has already been diagnosed as having autism and the assessment is to determine the severity of the disorder or is part of a preprocedural or prehospitalization assessment, assessment is performed in the same manner as with any normal child. However, the nurse will quickly become aware of the child's social detachment or lack of language as the assessment continues. A systematic exploration of the child's skills compared to developmental norms is essential. For the staff nurse, this may include evaluating the child's ability to feed, dress, and toilet. The assessment should include the child's interactive patterns and verbalization skills. The child's motor skills will be important to note, too, as these have major implications for safety and self-care. For initial, generalized screening, the Denver Developmental Screening Inventory may be helpful (see Chapter 2). A family history of autism or other mental disorders, family coping skills, and available social support systems also should be assessed.

Nursing Diagnosis and Planning

The following nursing diagnoses and expected outcomes may be appropriate following assessment of the child with autism.

Nursing Diagnoses

- Risk for Injury related to an inability to anticipate danger, a tendency for self-mutilation, and sensory perceptual deficits
- Impaired Social Interaction related to an inability to initiate and maintain social relationships and to limited verbal skills
- Altered Thought Processes related to an inability to perceive self or others accurately and to cognitive and perceptual dysfunction

Expected Outcome

The child will:

- maintain integrity of skin and avoid self- or accidental injury
- develop understandable and socially acceptable ways to communicate needs and wants
- show interest in surroundings and have the ability to acknowledge others in the environment
- demonstrate orientation to person, place, and time and perform activities of daily living that are appropriate to this orientation

Implementation

When working with autistic children, it is essential for the nurse to work closely with the family to determine the child's routines, habits, and preferences. Children with autism are often unable to tolerate even the slightest change in routine and may become withdrawn, self-abusive, or violent if their routines are altered. The nurse should write down any specific cues that will help the child remain oriented to the environment and will facilitate tolerance to change. For example, the nursing staff should be limited to as few individuals as possible. The child may need to perform toileting and self-care activities in a particular order. The child may require an environmental cue, such as stroking a favorite blanket, before being able to move from one activity to the next. The nurse can generally evaluate the child's tolerance to the situation by monitoring signs of anxiety or emotional comfort, as evidenced by behaviors, such as attending or observing the nurse when she is in the room or demonstrating a willngness to participate in self-care.

The nurse must work closely with the family to determine the specific ways in which the child communicates. The child may use sign language or pictures to specify needs if no verbal skills are developed. These children are often reluctant to initiate or sustain direct eye contact, so the nurse may interpret this as meaning that the child is not listening or is unaware of what is being said. In addition, the child may answer questions after several minutes' delay. The nurse should identify these behaviors, allowing extra time and being alert to differences in communication styles. These children generally have the ability to understand much more language than they are able to express.

The child may require a helmet or side rolls if a tendency for head-banging is demonstrated. Wrist restraints may be necessary if the child is unable to remain in the bed at night. It is important for the nurse to help the parents understand, and to explain to their child, any safety precautions that are unfamiliar to the child. The presence of a parent or older sibling is almost always required when an autistic child is hospitalized. Evaluating the child for safety is an ongoing nursing function. Reducing the adjustment demands for the child may be necessary if the nurse recognized behaviors indicating stress or anxiety.

Evaluation

Has the child:

- remained free of injury?
- developed a way to communicate needs?
- demonstrated an interest in surroundings?
- acknowledged the presence of others in his environment?
- developed the ability to perform activities of daily living?
- accommodated to the hospital setting by adjusting to the change in environment and schedule?

SUMMARY

Children with a cognitive deficit experience limitations in social interactions, use of language for self-expression, and self-care abilities. If these limitations are severe, the individual will require involvement with mature, caring adults throughout their lives. These individuals have many normal needs, including the need for positive attention and opportunities for self-discovery and growth. The nurse needs to work closely with the family to identify the child's specific patterns of interacting with the environment. This will require asking relevant and clear questions about how the child communicates and perceives experiences in the environment. Another nursing consideration relates to the fact that families with a cognitively impaired child experience repeated stress and grief as the child continues to fail to reach developmental expectations. The nurse can be most helpful in this process by offering family members an opportunity to discuss feelings and by identifying resources to help meet the child's needs. This may require acting as an advocate for the parents within the school system and the community.

KEY CONCEPTS

- Mental retardation may be the result of congenital or early environmental factors, or it may occur secondary to head injury, anoxia, intracranial hemorrhage, infections, poisoning, or the presence or treatment of a brain tumor.
- Several neuropsychologic tests are available to assess levels of mental retardation. The best method of early detection is through assessment of development during routine pediatric preventive care visits.
- Parents of children with cognitive deficits should be provided with anticipatory guidance relative to their child's developmental abilities.
- The family of a child with a cognitive deficit experiences repeated stress and grief as the child continues to fail to reach developmental expectations.
- Nurses must work closely with the family of a child with a cognitive deficit to identify the specific patterns the child uses to interact with the environment. This is accomplished by asking relevant and clear questions about how the child communicates and perceives experiences in the environment.
- The nurse acts as an advocate for the parents within the school system and the community.
- Changes in routine can cause frustration for the child with Down syndrome.
- The family of a child with Down syndrome may require assistance in identifying and obtaining adaptive tools for dressing, bathing, and eating.
- The family of a child with Down syndrome should be encouraged and assisted in helping the child learn new skills through demonstration, repetition, and positive feedback.
- Children with fragile X syndrome exhibit autistic-like behaviors, such as gaze avoidance, hand flapping, echolalia, and abnormal speech patterns. In addition, affected children have poor coordination, hyperkinetic behaviors, and cognitive deficits that are moderate to severe.
- Autism is characterized by an impairment in the rate and appearance of physical, social, and language skills; abnormal responses of the body sensations; thinking capacity, but with absent or delayed speech and language, and abnormal ways of relating to people, objects, and events.
- Autism shares similarities with childhood schizophrenia and mental retardation, but there are definitive differences.
- When working with children with autism it is important to work with the family to determine the child's routines, habits, and preferences.

REFERENCES

American Psychiatric Association. (1994). *Diagnostic and Statistical Manual of Mental Disorders (4th ed.).* Washington, DC: Author.

Batshaw, M. L. (1993). Mental retardation. *Pediatric Clinics of North America, 40*(3), 507–521.

Batshaw, M. L. (1991). *Your child has a disability. A complete sourcebook of daily and medical care* (pp. 53–54). Boston: Little, Brown.

Bregman, J. D., & Hodapp, R. M. (1991). Current developments in the understanding of mental retardation. Part I: Biological and phenomenological perspectives. *Journal of the American Academy of Child and Adolescent Psychiatry, 30*(5), 707–719.

Brown, W. T., Houck, G. E., Jeziorowska, A., Levinson, F. N., Ding, X., Dobkin, C., Zhong, N., Henderson, J., Brooks, S. S., & Jenkins, E. D. (1993). Rapid fragile X carrier screening and prenatal diagnosis using a nonradioactive PCR test. *Journal of the American Medical Association, 270*(13), 1569–1575.

Cicchetti, D., & Beeghly, M. (1990). *Children with Down syndrome: A developmental perspective.* New York: Cambridge University Press.

Cicchetti, D., & Mans-Wagener, L. (1987). Sequences, stages, and structures in the organization of cognitive development in infants with Down syndrome. In I. Uzgiris & J. McV. Hunt (Eds.), *Infant performance and experience: New findings with the ordinal scales.* Urbana: University of Illinois Press.

Collins, B. C., Wolery, M., & Gast, D. L. (1991, September). A survey of safety concerns for students with special needs. *Education and Training in Mental Retardation,* pp. 305–317.

Coplan, J. (1993, February). Child development. *Current Problems in Pediatrics,* pp. 44–49.

Cullen, S., Cronk, C., Pueschel, S., Schnell, R., & Reed, R. (1981). Social development and feeding milestones of young Down syndrome children. *American Journal of Mental Deficiencies, 85,* 410–415.

Dunne, R. G., Asher, K. N., & Rivara, F. P. (1993). Injuries in young people with developmental disabilities: Comparative investigation from the 1988 national health interview survey. *Mental Retardation, 31*(2), 83–88.

Evenhuis, H. M. (1990). The natural history of dementia in Down's syndrome. *Archives of Neurology, 47,* 263–267.

Fink, L. (1995). Mental retardation. In B. S. Johnson (Ed.), *Child, adolescent and family psychiatric nursing.* Philadelphia: J. B. Lippincott.

Hayes, A., & Batshaw, M. L. (1993). Down syndrome. *Pediatric Clinics of North America, 40*(3), 523–535.

Herman, S. E., & Hazel, K. L. (1991). Evaluation of family support services: Changes in availability and accessibility. *Mental Retardation, 29*(6), 351–357.

Larsson, E. V., Luce, S. C., Anderson, S. R., & Christian, W. P. (1992). Autism. In M. D. Levine, W. B. Carey, & A. C.

Crocker (Eds.), *Developmental-behavioral pediatrics* (2nd ed.) (pp. 534–542). Philadelphia: W. B. Saunders.

Laxova, R. (1994). Fragile X syndrome. *Advances in Pediatrics, 41,* 305–341.

Luckasson, R. (Ed.). (1992). *Mental retardation: Definition, classification and systems of support* (9th ed.). Washington, DC: American Association on Mental Retardation.

May, D. C., & Turnbull, N. (1992). Plastic surgeons' opinions of facial surgery for individuals with Down syndrome. *Mental Retardation, 30*(1), 29–33.

Mazzocco, M. M. M., Pennington, B. F., & Hagerman, R. J. (1993). The neurocognitive phenotype of female carriers of fragile X: Additional evidence for specificity. *Developmental and Behavioral Pediatrics, 14*(5), 328–335.

Miller, J. (1986). Early cross-cultural commonalities in social explanation. *Developmental Psychology, 22,* 514–520.

Pueschel, S. M., & Pueschel, J. K. (1992). *Biomedical concerns in persons with Down syndrome.* Baltimore: Paul H. Brookes.

Reber, M. (1992). Mental retardation. *Psychiatric Clinics of North America, 15*(2), 511–522.

Schopler, E., Reichler, R. J., Bashford, A., Lansing, M. D., & Marcus, L. M. (1990). *Individualized assessment and treatment for autistic and developmentally disabled children. Volume 1: Psychoeducational Profile-Revised (PEP-R).* Austin, TX: Pro-Ed.

Schopler, E., Reichler, R. J., & Renner, B. R. (1988). *Childhood Autism Rating Scale (CARS).* Los Angeles: Western Psychological Services.

Smith, S. E. (1993). Cognitive deficits associated with fragile X syndrome. *Mental Retardation, 31*(5), 279–283.

Vitiello, B., & Behar D. (1992). Mental retardation and psychiatric illness. *Hospital and Community Psychiatry, 43*(5), 494–499.

Warren, A. C., Holroyd, S., & Folstein, M. F. (1989). Major depression in Down's syndrome. *British Journal of Psychiatry, 155, 202–205.*

West, M. A., Richardson, M., LeConte, J., Crimi, C., & Stuart, S. (1992). Identification of developmental disabilities and health problems among individuals under child protective services, *Mental Retardation, 39*(4), 221–225.

Wetherby, A. (1986). Ontogeny of communicative functions in autism. *Journal of Autism and Developmental Disorders, 16,* 295–316.

Wilson, P. G., & Mazzocco, M. M. M. (1993). Awareness and knowledge of fragile X syndrome among special educators. *Mental Retardation, 31*(4), 221–227.

BIBLIOGRAPHY

Bauer, S. (1995). Autism and the pervasive developmental disorders: Part 1. *Pediatrics in Review, 16*(4), 130–136.

Bauer, S. (1995). Autism and the pervasive developmental disorders: Part 2. *Pediatrics in Review, 16*(5), 168–176.

Bruininks, R., Thurlow, M. L., & Ysseldyke, J. E. (1992, June). Assessing the right outcomes: Prospects for improving education for youth with disabilities. *Education and Training in Mental Retardation,* pp. 93–100.

Chernecky, C. L., Krech, R. L., & Berger, B. J. (1993). *Laboratory tests and diagnostic procedures.* Philadelphia: W. B. Saunders.

Coplan, J. (1993). Child development. *Current Problems in Pediatrics, 23*(2), 44–49.

Coplan, J. (1995). Normal speech and language development: An overview. *Pediatrics in Review, 16*(3), 91–100.

Hagerman, R. J. (1988). Fragile X syndrome. *Current Problems in Pediatrics, 17*(11), 621–674.

Levine, M. D., Carey, W. B., & Crocker, A. C. *Developmental-behavioral pediatrics* (2nd ed.). Philadelphia: W. B. Saunders.

Mahoney, G., & O'Sullivan, P. (1990). Early intervention practices with families of children with handicaps. *Mental Retardation, 28*(3), 169–176.

Smith, B., Chung, M. C., & Vostanis, P. (1994). The path to care in autism: Is it better now? *Journal of Autism and Developmental Disorders, 24*(5), 551–563.

Wehman, P. (1992, June). Transition for young people with disabilities: Challenges for the 1990's. *Education and Training in Mental Retardation,* pp. 112–118.

43

The Child With Sensory Alterations

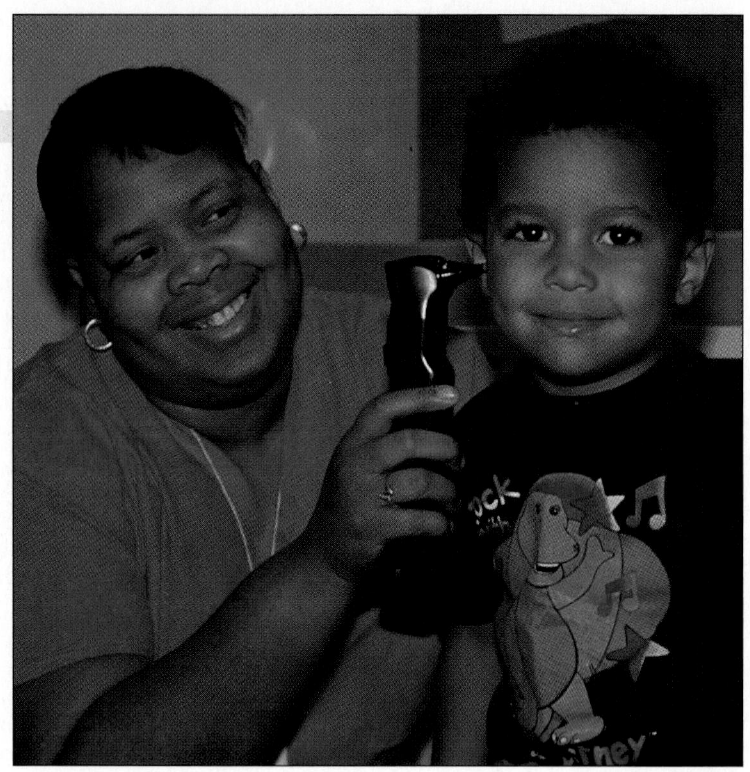

CHAPTER OVERVIEW

LEARNING OBJECTIVES

After studying this chapter, you should be able to:

- Describe the specific information required for a health history in a child with potential sensory deficits.
- Describe the structure and function of the eye and ear.
- Define the nurse's role in assessing for sensory deficits.
- Describe specific nursing care for children with health problems affecting the eye and ear.
- Describe how alterations in the sensory organs affect the child's ability to communicate.
- Identify potential growth and development interruptions that may occur with problems affecting the sensory organs.

KEY TERMS

amblyopia: reduced visual acuity not correctable by refractive means and not attributable to structural or pathologic ocular anomalies

astigmatism: abnormal curvature of the cornea or the lens

cataract: a loss of transparency of the crystalline lens or its capsula

central hearing loss: result of damage to the conduction system between the brain stem and cerebral cortex

concomitant strabismus: not of paralytic origin; remains constant for all directions of gaze

conductive hearing loss: reversible loss caused by damage, inflammation, or obstruction to outer or middle ear; sound is prevented from progressing across middle ear

congenital (infantile) glaucoma: increased intraocular fluid pressure that occurs during first 3 years of life; due to a defect in the drainage network of the eye

diplopia: double vision

esotropia (convergent) strabismus: eye turns inward; most common type of strabismus in infants

exotropia (divergent) strabismus: eyes turn away from the midline; occurs most often when the child attempts to focus on a distant object; may be present at birth

hyphema: a hemorrhage or sanguineous exudate in the anterior chamber of the eye

mixed hearing loss: combination of conductive and sensorineural loss

nonconcomitant strabismus: angle of deviation varies with direction of gaze due to paralysis or paresis of one or more extraocular muscles

nonparalytic strabismus: most common type of strabismus in children; all extraocular muscles function, but are not coordinated; child often squints

nystagmus: involuntary eye movements that make the eyes appear to be darting back and forth

ophthalmia neonatorum: conjunctivitis noted in the first few weeks of life, usually gonococcal or chlamydial

paralytic strabismus: caused by a weakness or paralysis of one or more of the extraocular muscles

pseudostrabismus: not a true strabismus; the eyes appear to deviate inward, but are actually in alignment; the appearance of misalignment is caused by facial features such as epicanthal folds and a broad, flat nasal bridge

secondary glaucoma: increased intraocular fluid pressure that occurs after age 3 and may be the result of disease or surgery

sensorineural hearing loss: result of damage or malformation of the middle ear and/or auditory nerve; hearing loss is usually permanent

strabismus: "squint" or "lazy eye"; a condition in which the eyes are not straight due to lack of coordination of the extraocular muscles; most often due to muscle imbalance or paralysis of the extraocular muscles, but may also result from conditions such as a brain tumor, myasthenia gravis, or infection

subconjunctival hemorrhages: bleeding situated beneath the conjunctiva. In children, most frequent cause is trauma or following severe coughing or sneezing episodes (valsalva maneuvers). Also caused by *S. pneumoniae* and *haemophilus*

visual accommodation: ability to focus on distant and near objects

Because a child learns so much through the senses, deficits in hearing and vision can have profound effects on development. Appropriate screening and early intervention are crucial. Early identification of vision and hearing deficits allows for early intervention, either correction or the provision of adaptive measures, so that "normal" growth and development may be preserved for the child. Because a child cannot report sensory deficits, nurses must assess carefully for alterations in vision or hearing.

The health history of a child with a potential sensory deficit is essentially the same as for any child (see Chapter 11), but should also include some additional pieces of information. These include a thorough prenatal history, growth and developmental history, past history of any infections (including treatment, because many medications can cause sensory deficits), previous trauma to the eye or ear, any changes noted in behavior (such as rubbing the eyes, turning up the volume on the television, decreased attention span), any changes in appearance (red, inflamed eyes; drainage from the eye or ear), and any physical complaints (complaints of ear or eye pain, headache, nausea and vomiting). After carefully reviewing the health history, a thorough physical examination should be carried out utilizing age-appropriate measures of visual and hearing acuity (see Chapter 11).

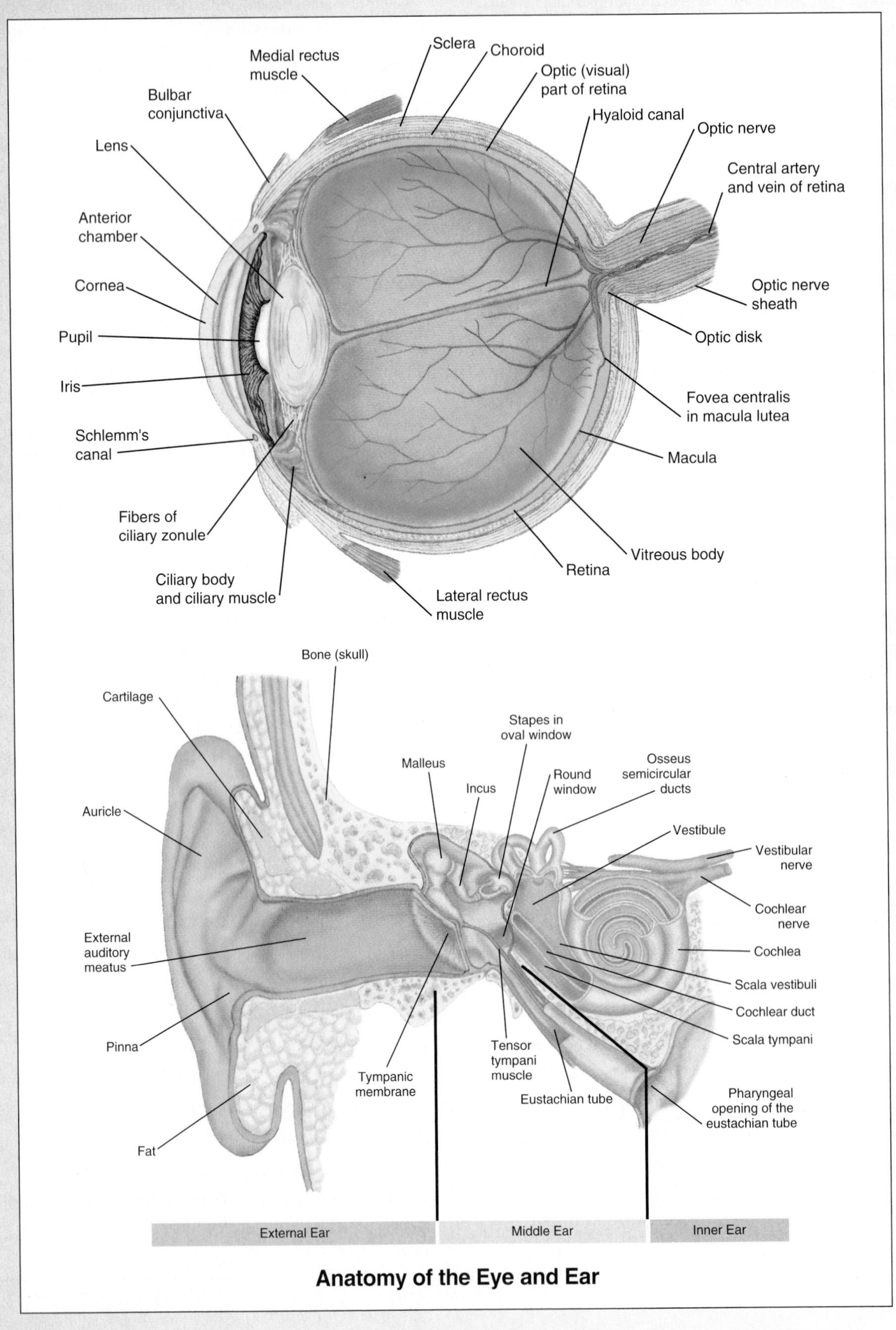

Anatomy of the Eye and Ear

REVIEW OF THE EYE

The eye is attached to the skull by six accessory muscles. These are used to move the eye to achieve vision. Ciliary muscles function to alter the shape of the eye to provide focus and accommodation at various distances. Cranial nerves II, III, IV, V, and VI all affect the eye.

The "orb" or eye is made up of several parts. The cornea is the clear area located in the front of the eye. This is where light enters the eye. The cornea and sclera (white outer covering) make up the eye's outer layer. The middle layer is composed of the choroid (vascular lining), the lens (a clear structure that changes shape to allow accommodation of light on the retina), and the iris (the colored muscular ring located behind the cornea that expands or contracts to control the amount of light entering the eye). The inner layer of the eye is known as the retina. This area contains the rods and cones. These receive light impulses and transmit them via the optic nerve (cranial nerve II) to the brain. The macula contains the greatest concentration of nerve endings. Light is focused here by the cornea and the lens. The optic disk is the area where the optic nerve enters the eye.

Neonatal Development. The eyes begin to develop at about 22 days' gestation. The "critical period" for development is considered to be 22 to 50 days. Congenital abnormalities appear to be caused by either genetic or environmental factors or a combination of the two. The eye is especially sensitive to teratogens, in particular infections such as cytomegalovirus and rubella.

REVIEW OF THE EAR

The ear is divided into three parts: the outer, middle, and inner ear. The outer ear includes the auricle and external ear canal. It is separated from the middle ear by the tympanic membrane (eardrum). The tympanic membrane vibrates to conduct sound waves to the middle ear. The middle ear contains the "bones of hearing"—the malleus (hammer), incus (anvil), and stapes (stirrup). These bones conduct sound waves from the tympanic membrane to the inner ear. The inner ear contains the nerve endings that conduct sound impulses to the brain. These are located in a snail-shaped chamber (the cochlea) that is filled with fluid. The inner ear also controls balance. The eustachian tube connects the middle ear with the nasopharynx. It functions to allow fluids to drain into the nasopharynx and to assist in equalizing pressure between the outer and middle ear.

Neonatal Development. The ear begins to develop during the third week of gestation. The critical period for the development of the ear is between 4 and 6 weeks' gestation. Like the eye, the ear is very sensitive to teratogens. It is innervated by the acoustic nerve (cranial nerve VIII). (Congenital deafness appears to be largely due to genetic factors.)

Pediatric Differences in the Sensory Organs

- The eyes begin to develop at about 22 days gestation. The "critical period" for development is considered to be 22–50 days. The developing eye is especially sensitive to teratogens, particularly infections such as cytomegalovirus (CMV) and rubella.
- Development of the eye is not complete at birth, but the newborn is able to fix his gaze, follow an object to midline, and react to a change in intensity of light.
- By 3 months of age, the infant can follow moving objects with her eye. By 4 months of age, she can recognize familiar objects.
- Binocularity, the ability to fixate on one visual field with both eyes, is not present at birth but is established by 6 months of age. Frequent eye-crossing after 6 months of age is abnormal and indicates strabismus.
- Visual acuity changes with age:

4 months:	20/50 to 20/80
1 year:	20/40 to 20/70
4 years:	20/30 to 20/40
5 years:	20/20 to 20/30

- Lacrimal glands are not fully developed at birth. Tears are not often present with crying until after 1–3 months. Temporary obstruction of lacrimal ducts may cause overflow of tears.
- The size of the orbits doubles by the time the child is 1 year of age and doubles again by 6 years of age. Eye growth is completed at 10–12 years of age.
- Development of the ear begins during the third week of gestation and is complete by the third month of embryonic life. Infection or other insult to the fetus during this time can cause irreparable damage to the ear. Ear development occurs at the same time as kidney development, so malformation in one system may indicate problems in the other.
- An infant as young as 3 days old is able to distinguish between familiar and unfamiliar sounds and can recognize his mother's voice.
- The infant can distinguish between frequently heard words and other words ("nonsense" language) by 1 year. Basic auditory skills are in place by 3 years of age. Hearing can be evaluated by audiometry testing by this age.
- Infants can imitate sounds heard by 3–5 months of age. Verbal "dialogue" that is similar to that of an adult is noted by about 6 months of age.
- Infants and young children have shorter, more horizontal, and more flaccid eustachian tubes, predisposing them to otitis media.

DISORDERS OF THE EYE

The nurse holds a very important role in the prevention and early detection of eye problems. All children should have vision screening done at birth, age 6 months, at the preschool examination, and then periodically throughout the school years (Gerali, 1991). Careful attention to behavioral and appearance changes as well as physical complaints assist in the early detection and treatment of eye disorders. These signs and symptoms of potential problems are summarized in the accompanying box. Children who have these symptoms should be referred for further evaluation.

Refractive Errors

Refractive errors cause alterations in the path of light rays through the eye that result in visual disturbances. In these disorders, the orb may be flattened or elongated. They are defined in Table 43–1. Refractive errors are often discovered when a child is noted to squint or frown or move objects so that they are more easily seen. Parents may also be alerted by a teacher or by complaints from the child. *Legal blindness* is defined as a correction of 20/200 or less in the better eye or a visual field of 20° or less.

Corrective lenses are used to improve the child's vision. Glasses should be impact resistant and have "spring loaded" frames that are less likely to be bent or

Signs and Symptoms of Potential Eye Problems

Behavioral:
- Rubbing eyes excessively
- Shutting or covering one eye when reading or concentrating
- Tilting head or thrusting head forward to see
- Difficulty in reading or doing "close-up" tasks
- Increased incidence of blinking, especially when doing "close-up" tasks
- Cannot see distant objects clearly
- Squinting or frowning to see

Appearance:
- Crossed eyes
- Redness or swelling
- Drainage
- Excessive tearing
- Recurring infections

Physical complaints:
- Can't see
- Headaches, dizziness, nausea/vomiting with "close-up" tasks
- Double vision
- Blurred vision

Adapted from Gerali, P.S. (1991). Childsight: Helping children grow up with good vision. *Journal of Ophthalmic Nursing and Technology, 10*(5), 222–223.

TABLE 43–1 *Types of Refractive Disorders*

REFRACTIVE ERROR	DESCRIPTION	CLINICAL MANIFESTATIONS	TREATMENT
Myopia	Near-sightedness Ability to see near objects more clearly than those at a distance Caused by the image focusing in front of the retina	Difficulty seeing the blackboard or TV clearly, decreased interest in activities requiring distance vision. Squinting, head tilting, holding book close to eyes. Decreased attention span, poor school performance.	Treated with biconcave lenses. New lenses may be required every year or two as the child grows.
Hyperopia	Far-sightedness Ability to see distant objects more clearly than those close up Caused by the image focusing beyond the retina	Most children are normally hyperopic until about age 7 years but are able to accommodate to see clearly. May develop strabismus or amblyopia from prolonged hyperopia.	Most young children with hyperopia need no correction. If correction is required, convex lenses are used.
Astigmatism	Unequal curvature of the cornea or the lens, causing light rays to bend in different directions May coexist with myopia or hyperopia	Mild astigmatism may be asymptomatic. Manifestations may be similar to myopia.	Treated with special lenses to compensate for the unequal curvature of the cornea.

TEACHING GUIDELINES *Caring for Glasses*

- Always remove glasses with both hands to prevent warping of the frame.
- To prevent scratches, never lay glasses face down.
- Use only the recommended method for cleaning lenses; paper towels and other dry cloths may scratch lenses.
- If a harness is used to hold a young infant's glasses in place, care should be taken to avoid getting the elastic bands too tight.
- Never replace missing screws with paper clips or wires, since these may come loose and cause eye trauma.
- Glasses have been outgrown when the bend of the temple is in front of the ear.

From Catalano, R. A., & Nelson, L. B. (1990). *Pediatric ophthalmology: A test atlas.* East Norwalk, CT: Appleton and Lange.

warped. Because the bridge of the nose is flat, cable temples (ear pieces that wrap around the ear) are recommended in children under 4 years of age (Catalano & Nelson, 1994). Straps may also be used in helping to hold the glasses in place.

The accompanying Teaching Guidelines present tips for instructing parents and children about caring for glasses.

Contact lenses should not be prescribed for a child until he is old enough to independently care for them in a responsible manner.

Strabismus

Strabismus (squint, lazy eye) is a condition in which the eyes are not aligned due to lack of coordination of the extraocular muscles. It is present in up to 4% of children under age 6 (Lavrich & Nelson, 1993). Strabismus is most often due to muscle imbalance or paralysis of the extraocular muscles, but may also result from conditions such as a brain tumor, myasthenia gravis, or infection. About 50% of children with strabismus have a family history of the condition. Strabismus is defined by the type of deviation noted (see box).

Strabismus is normal in the young infant but should not be present after about age 4 months.

When both eyes are unable to focus simultaneously, the brain suppresses the image from the deviating eye to avoid double vision (diplopia). Amblyopia, or decreased vision in the deviated eye, can develop if strabismus is not treated early. If untreated amblyopia occurs in a child younger than age 4 years (the critical period for development of the visual cortex), permanent loss of vision in the deviated eye may result. Because the child loses binocular vision, depth perception may also be impaired (Lavrich & Nelson, 1993). Early detection and treatment of strabismus are essential to prevent loss of vision.

The Hirschberg test, cover-uncover test, and the alternate-cover tests are used in the diagnosis of strabismus (Castiglia, 1994; Lavrich & Nelson, 1993). See Chapter 11 for an explanation of the use of these tests. The nurse may suspect strabismus when the child complains of frequent headaches, squints, or tilts the head to see. Children with family members with strabismus should be regularly assessed for development of the condition.

Treatment of strabismus may include special glasses, vision therapy, patching, surgery, or pharmacologic treatment. If the deviation is caused by hyperopia, corrective lenses are indicated to correct vision. Glasses with specially ground prism power may also be indicated. These glasses correct vision in the affected eye so that the brain receives the same image from both eyes.

Patching may also used to strengthen the weak eye. In this treatment, the "good" eye is patched. This encourages the child to use the weaker eye. It is most successful when done during the preschool years (American Academy of Ophthalmology, 1994). The schedule for patching is individualized (e.g., one week for every year of the child's age, wearing the patch every other day, and is prescribed by the ophthalmologist. See the accompanying Teaching Guidelines for educating parents about eye patching.

Surgery may be indicated to realign the weakened muscles. It is most often indicated when amblyopia is present (Castiglia, 1994) and should be performed before the child is 2 years old. The stronger eye may be patched before surgery to treat any existing amblyopia. Surgery may be required only on the weakened eye or on both eyes. More than one surgery may be necessary. During the surgery, small incisions are made and the weakened muscles are tightened. Glasses may still be required after surgery to maintain the alignment (Kaye, 1990).

Finally, botulinum toxin (Botox) was approved in 1989 by the U.S. Food and Drug Administration as an alternative to surgery. The toxin is injected into the eye muscle

Types of Strabismus

nonparalytic (nonconcomitant) strabismus: Most common type of strabismus in children. Constant deviation in all fields of gaze; not associated with eye muscle paralysis. All extraocular muscles function, but are not coordinated. Child has difficulty seeing at close range; often squints. Accommodative nonparalytic strabismus may develop between ages 2 and 4 years as a result of a large refractive error.

paralytic (concomitant) strabismus: Caused by a weakness or paralysis of one or more of the extraocular muscles. The eye appears crossed when turned in the direction of the affected muscle. May cause headache, incoordination. Diplopia may cause child to close one eye or tilt head.

esotropia (convergent): The eye turns inward; most common type of strabismus in infants. May occur with hyperopia as the eyes compensate for the refractive error by overconvergence.

exotropia (divergent): The eyes turn away from the midline; occurs most often when the child attempts to focus on a distant object. May be present at birth.

pseudostrabismus: Not a true strabismus. The eyes appear to deviate inward, but are actually in alignment. The appearance of misalignment is caused by facial features such as epicanthal folds and a broad, flat nasal bridge.

phoria: A tendency for the eye to deviate. More evident during times of stress, fatigue, or illness.

tropia: A continuous misalignment of the eye.

Photos from Albert, D. M., & Jakobiec, F. A. (Eds.). (1994). *Principles and practice of ophthalmology* (pp. 2731, 2733). Philadelphia: W.B. Saunders.

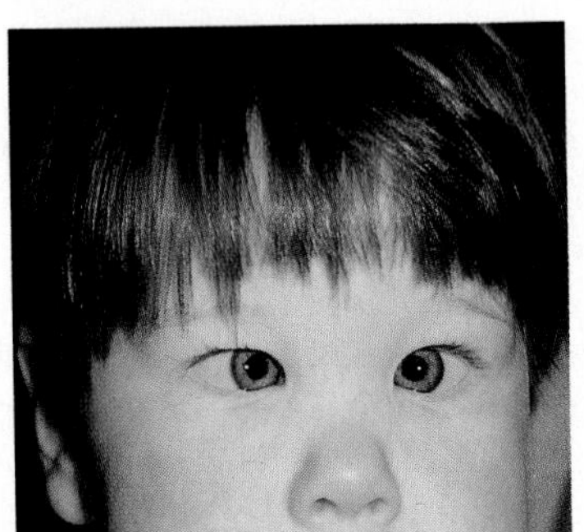

Infant with early onset esotropia. The deviation may not be apparent until age 3 or 4 months.

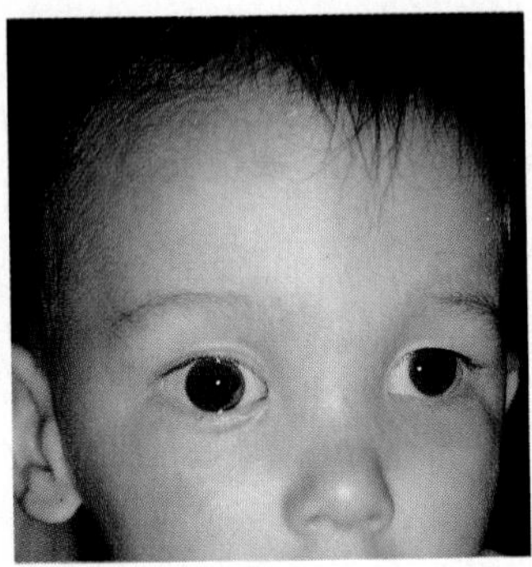

Child with left exotropia. Most exodeviations in childhood are intermittent in nature.

and produces temporary paralysis. This allows the muscles opposite the paralyzed muscle to straighten the eye. With successful treatment, once the medication wears off (in about 2 months), the correction will remain. The success rate is about 50% (Day, Eggers, Gammon, & Spivey, 1990). The most common side effect is a drooping eyelid (ptosis), which resolves spontaneously (Castiglia, 1994).

Nursing Care of the Child With Strabismus

As previously stated, early identification of the child with strabismus is crucial in preventing visual loss. Parent education is essential for prescribed treatment to be successful. Teaching should include why patching or corrective lenses are necessary, the expected results of wearing the patch or lens, how to correctly place the patch, how many hours per day the patch or lens is to be worn, and the expected length of treatment. The child needs to understand that wearing the patch or lens is not negotiable. It is often essential to teach parents strategies for dealing with resistant behaviors. If the child is to have a surgical correction, the nurse should *preoperatively* prepare the child and parents for what to expect after surgery and provide information about dressing changes, eyedrops, corrective

TEACHING GUIDELINES *Educating Parents About Eye Patching*

Parent teaching is imperative when patching is prescribed. Parents should be taught that prescribed patching will not harm the stronger eye, that patching alone will not straighten the eye, and that the patch should be applied directly to the face (not to glasses) (Kaye, 1990). The importance of complying with the prescribed regimen and returning for follow-up visits should also be stressed.

lenses, and any other postoperative treatments that may be required. See the nursing care plan for the child having eye surgery for further information.

Color Blindness

Color "blindness" or color deficiency occurs in 8% of the population and affects primarily males. It affects the ability to distinguish between colors within certain groups such as red, blue, and green.

Testing should be done if there is suspicion of a problem (i.e., a suspected optic nerve or retinal dysfunction), when there is a family history of color blindness, and routinely in preschool boys (Catalano & Nelson, 1994). The most common detection test is the pseudoisochromatic (color confusion) test. In this test, color plates are designed to have patterns that will be hidden to the color deficit (Bensinger, 1992). Pseudoisochromatic plates are also available for children who cannot yet read. If a problem is detected, more sophisticated testing may be necessary to determine the exact type of color blindness. Although there is no cure for color blindness, certain types of tints may be used in contact lenses and glasses to help the child discriminate color differences.

Nursing Care of the Child With Color Blindness

Because color blindness cannot be cured, nursing care focuses on adaptive and supportive measures. Parents should be encouraged to have children tested if there is a family history of color blindness, or if they suspect the child is having trouble distinguishing colors.

Parent/patient education is very important for the child with color blindness. Teaching should focus on alternative ways to discriminate colors that are in deficit. For the older child who can dress himself, clothes may be labeled or organized within the closet and bureau in a set manner so that he can "match" items without assistance.

Safety is a major concern for the color-blind child. For example, the child who cannot distinguish red and green must learn another way to distinguish traffic signals and other warning lights. Finally, anticipatory guidance must also be given in the areas of appropriate career choices. For example, color blindness may prohibit an adult from certain career choices such as pilot, police officer, or fire fighter.

Glaucoma

Glaucoma is a disease in which the intraocular fluid pressure of the eye is increased. This pressure increase, if left untreated, will lead to atrophy of the optic disk and, ultimately, blindness.

Glaucoma in children is one of two types. Congenital or infantile glaucoma occurs during the first 3 years of life and is due to a defect in the drainage network of the eye. Greater than 50% of all infantile glaucoma is of this type (Catalano & Nelson, 1994). Juvenile glaucoma refers to disease that occurs after age 3 and may be the result of inherited disease, or may occur after disease (such as congenital rubella), trauma, or cataract removal (Wagner, 1994).

Clinical signs of glaucoma include excessive tearing, light sensitivity, blepharospasm (muscle spasm causing involuntary closing of the eyelid), and enlargement of the globe and cornea (Wagner, 1994). Parents often note excessive tearing, or corneal haziness due to edema, and bring the child in for clinical evaluation. The child may also be brought to the practitioner for what appears to be conjunctivitis, or "pinkeye."

Physical examination includes an assessment of visual acuity, measurement of intraocular pressure (tonometry), assessment of corneal diameter and clarity, and an examination of the retina to assess for optic nerve cupping. Any infant with a visible iris diameter greater than 10.5 mm should be evaluated. If retinal edema is present, the light reflex will be diffuse. Because young children may not be able to cooperate during an examination, they are often sedated. Intraocular pressure should be measured only under light sedation, however, because deeper sedation may alter readings (either high or low, depending on the agent used).

The preferred treatment for pediatric glaucoma is surgery. Medications to clear the cornea may be used before surgery to allow better visualization. This should occur as soon as possible after diagnosis to prevent loss (or further loss) of vision. The goal of surgery is to increase the outflow of the aqueous humor from the anterior chamber. Medications such as cholinergic agents, beta-adrenergic blocking agents, or adrenergic agents may be indicated after surgery to maintain a low intraocular pressure.

Prognosis varies from child to child. The earlier the onset of glaucoma, the poorer the prognosis (Wagner, 1994). Over half of children who have glaucoma present at birth and 20% of those with later onset will be legally blind in the affected eye(s) (Wagner, 1994). About one third of those children who undergo successful surgery will have vision better than 20/50 (Wagner, 1994). Decreased vision may result from damage to the optic nerve, opacity of the cornea or cataract, or amblyopia resulting from refractive errors.

Nursing Care of the Child After Surgery for Glaucoma

Postoperative nursing care includes monitoring for signs and symptoms of increased intraocular pressure (pain, nausea and vomiting, increased inflammation) and administering of any ordered medications such as miotic eyedrops (used to constrict the pupils) and antibiotic oint-

Working With a Visually Impaired Child

- Orient the child to her environment on admission. This may be done by assisting her in walking around the room and identifying objects such as the bed, bathroom, doorways, windows, and chairs.
- Never touch the child without identifying yourself and telling her why you will be touching her.
- When describing objects or the environment to a blind child, use familiar terms. For example, if the child is an older child who is recently blinded, you may be able to use color when describing objects. If the child has been blind since birth, color has no meaning. It is also useful to describe how many steps away something is. Remember, parents are often your best source for communication.
- Identify noises for the child, because blind children often have difficulty in establishing the source of a noise.
- Keep all items in the room in the same location and order. Changing the order or spacing of objects may cause confusion or lead to injury.
- Provide detailed explanations and allow the child to progress through care "in steps" to allow her to learn the order.
- As with any child, allow as much control over the situation as possible.
- Supervise the child and counsel parents to supervise the child as needed.

ments or eyedrops. If the child's eyes are patched, special attention should be paid to the resulting sensory deficits. (See box, Working With a Visually Impaired Child.)

Patient/parent education is essential to maintain the appropriate intraocular pressure and prevent complications (including blindness). This includes the use of any prescribed medications, patching, and any other measures designed to correct refractive errors. The importance of returning for follow-up care should be stressed. The child and caregivers should also be taught signs and symptoms of increasing intraocular pressure. Any signs of increasing intraocular pressure or infection should be reported immediately to the ophthalmologist.

Cataract

A cataract is an opacity or loss of transparency of the lens. Causes include heredity (usually an autosomal dominant trait), infection (such as rubella), trauma, or a metabolic imbalance. Cloudiness of the lens may be noted during examination in the newborn nursery (as indicated by a white instead of red reflex) or by parents. Ophthalmoscopy may reveal a dark spot in the lens. Parents may note that the infant exhibits visual inattentiveness and come in for an evaluation. Other clinical signs include nystagmus (involuntary eye movements in which the eyes appear to be darting back and forth) and strabismus.

The cataract alters vision because it does not allow a sharp, clear image to be formed on the retina. Early intervention (before age 17 weeks) for the infant born with cataracts is crucial to allow vision to develop normally (Cheng et al., 1991).

Treatment for cataracts is the surgical removal of the opaque lens. The resultant hyperopia is then dealt with using a contact lens or an intraocular lens implant. Glasses may also be used to correct the resultant vision problem.

Amblyopia may also be present. In this case, the normal eye may be patched after surgery to develop the weakened eye.

Nursing Care of the Child With a Cataract

Care should be taken postoperatively to avoid increasing intraocular pressure (see Care Plan, The Child Having Eye Surgery). This includes prevention of coughing, straining, vomiting, and touching of the operative site. A patch and "hard shield" are usually in place after surgery to prevent injury to the operative site. To prevent edema and pressure on the site, the nurse should avoid placing the child with the affected eye in a dependent position (Symanski, Newman, & Bachynski, 1994). The child should be monitored for signs and symptoms of infection (fever, drainage, redness). Medications including antibiotics, mydriatics, and steroids may be used after surgery.

Postoperative teaching includes how to insert, remove, and care for the child's contact lens. Parents must be taught the signs and symptoms of infection and increasing intraocular pressure. To provide visual stimulation to the affected eye and prevent further loss of vision, the importance of complying with the patching regimen should also be stressed. Finally, the importance of returning for follow-up visits should be stressed. This is important to ensure that the lens fits correctly, that vision correction is appropriate, and that there are no signs and symptoms of complications.

Inflammatory Disorders

Conjunctivitis

Conjunctivitis (or "pinkeye") is an inflammation of the conjunctiva (the clear, membranous lining of the lid and sclera). Signs and symptoms of conjunctivitis may include itching, burning, light sensitivity (photophobia), "scratchy" eyelids, redness, edema, and discharge. It is usually caused by either allergy or infection. Accurate diagnosis before treatment is important, because inappropriate treatment may lead to complications.

Conjunctivitis noted in the first few weeks of life is called "ophthalmia neonatorum." In infants, conjunctivitis occurring in the first 24 hours of life is usually due to chemical irritation from infection prophylaxis administered soon after birth. (See Chapter 3, The Newborn). Conjunctivitis occurring after the first 24 hours may be caused by either infection or a blocked lacrimal (tear) duct. Infection may be acquired during birth (from passing through the birth canal) or after birth. Chlamydia is responsible for most (about 80%) of eye infections noted in infants (Trobe, 1993). Medical treatment should be directed at the cause of the infection. Antibiotic or antiviral eyedrops or ointments are most often used to treat infectious conjunctivitis. If chlamydia is the cause, however, systemic antibiotics are also used to prevent pneumonia.

Conjunctivitis in older children may have a variety of etiologies. Among them are allergy, infection, and trauma. As with the infant, treatment depends on the cause. A detailed history should be obtained to help determine the cause. Infection should be suspected if the child has recently been exposed to another individual with conjunctivitis or an upper respiratory infection (Catalano & Nelson, 1994). Itching often identifies the cause as an allergic response. Chlamydial conjunctivitis is rare in older children. It may be suspected, however, in a sexually active adolescent with chronic infection that is unresponsive to other treatment (King, 1993).

A diagnosis of chlamydial conjunctivitis in a nonsexually active child should signal the health care provider to assess the child for possible sexual abuse (Catalano & Nelson, 1994).

Nursing Care of the Child With Conjunctivitis

Medical management depends on the cause of the conjunctivitis. If the cause is infection, antibiotic or antiviral eyedrops or ointment may be prescribed. If allergies are suspected, antihistamines, either oral or in the form of eyedrops, may be indicated. In severe cases of allergic conjunctivitis, steroid eyedrops and cromolyn sodium eyedrops may be indicated. The steroid eyedrops will be tapered over about 7 days. Because steroids can worsen the severity of many infections, they are used with caution and only for a short time. Long-term use of steroids has been associated with an increased risk of cataract and glaucoma (Catalano & Nelson, 1994).

Parents must be taught to keep the eye clean and to administer any prescribed medications (see Chapter 19). Because bacterial and viral conjunctivitis is extremely contagious, infection control measures should also be taught. These include good handwashing and not sharing towels and washcloths. Bottles of eye medication should never be shared with another person. The tip of the dropper or ointment tube should not touch the child's eye or eyelid during administration. The child should also be kept home from school or day care until he has received antibiotic eyedrops for 24 hours.

Preventing injury from rubbing the eye is also important. Mittens may be used for infants. These may be fashioned from "booty" type socks or be commercially made mittens. Distraction and constant reminding are recommended for toddlers and older children. If the child wears contact lenses, he should be instructed to discontinue wearing them until the infection has completely cleared. Securing new contact lenses will eliminate the chance of reinfection from contaminated contact lenses and will also lessen the risk of a corneal ulceration. Eye make-up should also be discarded and replaced, because the chance of reinfecting eyes from contaminated make-up is high (King, 1993). Mascara should be replaced at least every 3 months.

Finally, if the conjunctivitis is allergic in origin, cool compresses and dark glasses may also help to lessen the irritation and photophobia. If cromolyn sodium eyedrops are prescribed, parents should be taught to begin using them *before* the "allergy season," because they have little effect on an active inflammatory process (King, 1993). Ophthalmic nonsteroidal anti-inflammatory preparations (NSAIDs) may also be helpful.

Blocked Lacrimal Duct

A blocked lacrimal (tear) duct is characterized by excessive tearing (epiphora) and crusting, or "mattering," of the eyelids on awaking. Parents may also notice a small mass just below the inner aspect of the eye. Treatment usually consists of massaging the duct. If the duct remains blocked despite massaging or after age 1 year, surgical opening of the duct is indicated.

Nursing Care of the Child With a Blocked Lacrimal Duct

Care should be taken to assess the nature of the mucoid drainage. In a noninfected duct, the drainage is usually white or clear. If the duct has become infected, however, the drainage may be green or yellow. If the drainage appears infected, antibiotic eyedrops or ointment are indicated.

Parent education includes teaching the proper technique for lacrimal massage. This involves washing hands thoroughly and placing the index finger over the lacrimal duct (at the inner aspect of the eye by the bridge of the nose) and "milking," or gently massaging the duct, in an upward motion. Parents should be taught that massaging down the nasal bone has very little effect on the duct, because the lacrimal system is intraosseous and not affected by massage. Other teaching includes monitoring for signs and symptoms of infection.

Periorbital Cellulitis

Orbital cellulitis is caused by an infection of the soft tissues of the orbit. It may be the result of trauma or an infection of the ethmoid sinus. Clinical signs and symptoms include severe eyelid edema and an anteriorly displaced eye. The child will also be febrile and have an elevated white blood cell count.

Treatment includes intravenous antibiotics and decongestants. If the area is painful, analgesics may also be prescribed.

Left untreated, the infection causing the orbital cellulitis can spread to the optic nerve directly to the brain, causing meningitis.

Nursing Care of the Child With Orbital Cellulitis

Nursing care involves administration of prescribed medications and monitoring of the child receiving intravenous therapy. The child should also be carefully monitored for signs and symptoms that the infection is spreading. This includes a thorough neurologic assessment. Finally, the child's pain status should be assessed frequently (see Chapter 20). Pain may be relieved by the use of prescribed analgesics or hot packs up to four times a day.

Corneal Ulcers

Corneal ulcers are usually caused by ocular infection. Signs and symptoms include pain, tearing, purulent discharge, and blurred vision. Risk factors for corneal ulceration include trauma, extended soft contact lens wear, surgical procedures, and viral infection in the eye. Immunosuppression and prolonged use of topical antibiotics in the eye also increase the risk of corneal ulceration (Catalano & Nelson, 1994).

Treatment includes aggressive topical antibiotic therapy. Cultures are often done and treatment started with a potent new generation of fluoroguinolones: ciprofloxacin, oflaxacin, and norfloxacin.

Nursing Care of the Child With a Corneal Ulcer

Parental teaching includes the administration of any prescribed medications and the cause and prevention of future ulcerations. Parents should also be taught to prevent rubbing of the eyes (which can worsen the injury). If the child wears contact lenses, they should not be worn until the ulceration and infection are completely healed. Any lenses worn during the episode should be discarded.

Eye Trauma

Corneal Abrasion

Corneal abrasions usually result from a scraping of the cornea by foreign bodies, contact lenses, fingernails, and exposure to sunlamps (Hiatt, 1991). The child may present with light sensitivity, pain, excessive tearing, and decreased vision. The abrasion is diagnosed by instilling a fluorescein dye in the eye and examining the eye under a blue filtered light (Wood's lamp) to highlight the injury. If foreign bodies remain in the eye, they should be removed.

If the abrasion is a small one, treatment may consist only of the instillation of antibiotic ointment four times a day. Larger abrasions require patching for 24 hours followed by the instillation of an antibiotic ointment (Catalano, 1993). Cycloplegia for pain control may be used. Many authorities now recommend no patching unless the wound is very large. If patched, the eye should be examined in 24 hours.

Failure to treat an abrasion may result in loss of visual acuity and/or permanent scarring and opacity of the cornea.

Nursing Care of the Child With a Corneal Abrasion

Parent education is very important in caring for the child with a corneal abrasion. Because an abrasion increases the risk of infection, parents should be taught the importance of administering antibiotics as prescribed. The child should not rub the eye, because rubbing can worsen an abrasion. If the eye is patched, parents should be taught not to remove the patch for 24 hours, even to instill ointment. This prevents further damage to the eye from blinking. Finally, injury prevention should be reinforced. This includes the wearing of safety goggles during sports and other activities, such as wood working.

Hemorrhages

Subconjunctival Hemorrhage. Subconjunctival hemorrhages present as red areas beneath the conjunctiva. They are often the result of valsalva maneuvers such as coughing, vomiting, or straining. Subconjunctival hemorrhages resolve on their own within 2 to 3 weeks and require no treatment. Although they often appear worse than they are, they may be associated with other ocular or physical problems and should be evaluated.

Nursing Care. Because these hemorrhages resolve on their own, care is aimed at reassurance. Parents should be told that the hemorrhage will appear to "grow larger" in the first few days. This is due to the weight of the eyelid and the effects of gravity (Catalano & Nelson, 1994).

Hyphema. A hyphema is a hemorrhage resulting from a blow to the eye. Symptoms include a recent history of injury, pain, light sensitivity, decreased vision, and excessive tearing. If there is no known history of injury, the child should be assessed for a bleeding disorder, anticoagulant therapy, renal or hepatic disease, retinoblastoma, or child abuse. An examination of the eye reveals blood in the anterior chamber of the eye. Traumatic hyphema will usually fill less than one-third of the anterior chamber.

Recommendations for management vary. Treatment usually includes hospitalization, bed rest, sedation, and patching. Because of the risk of a "rebleed" between the second and fifth days, bed rest and patching are often recommended (Hiatt, 1991; Catalano, 1993). Medications such as steroid eyedrops, antifibrinolytic eyedrops (tranexamic acid is best for pediatric use [cyklokapron], antiglaucoma medications, and cycloplegic eyedrops (atropine) may also be used.

Nursing Care. Careful assessment is required for the child with a hyphema. The eye should be assessed frequently for a secondary hemorrhage, or "rebleed." This is characterized by an increase in size of the hyphema with bright red "new" blood noted over the existing clot. The child should also be monitored for signs and symptoms of increasing intraocular pressure (pain, nausea and vomiting, increased inflammation). The child should also be closely monitored for side effects of medications. These include nausea and vomiting, orthostatic hypotension, tinnitus, and hematuria (Catalano & Nelson, 1994).

The child is usually restricted to bed rest with bathroom privileges. Elevating the head of the bed 30°–40° helps settle the hyphema in the inferior anterior chamber angle. Television viewing may or may not be allowed, and reading and other "near" activities are usually forbidden. Therefore, boredom is a problem for most children. Diversionary activities that don't involve reading or straining the eyes should be offered. These include music and books on tape. If both of the child's eyes are patched, care should be taken to orient him to his environment and provide for his safety. (See Chapter 13, Safety, and Chapter 10, Communicating With Children.)

Discharge teaching includes use of prescribed home medications, patching regimen (the eye is usually patched at night for 2 weeks after discharge), and prevention of further injury (see Teaching Guidelines). The child's eye should be protected with a shield if an eye patch is worn at night. The child can usually return to all normal activities 1 month after the injury, but eye protection should be worn for the rest of the child's life (Catalano & Nelson, 1994). The importance of follow-up should also be stressed, because the child is at risk for complications such as glaucoma and cataracts.

Chemical Burns

Chemical burns are an ocular emergency. Burns may occur from any of a number of common household items such as bleach, ammonia, drain opener, and oven cleaner.

They are managed by immediate irrigation of the affected eye(s) with water or saline. If the chemical is alkaline, the irrigation may continue for several hours, because the damaging action of alkaloids may be prolonged (Hiatt, 1991). Irrigation should continue for at least 30 minutes with at least 2 liters of irrigant if the burn is mild and for 2 to 4 hours or with at least 10 liters of irrigant if the burn is severe (Catalano, 1993). The cornea may appear cloudy after an alkali burn.

Further treatment may include topical steroids, medications to dilate the pupils (and decrease the risk of adhesions), antibiotic ointment, and patching. Oral antibiotics and analgesics may also be indicated. Follow-up care includes monitoring visual acuity and monitoring for side effects such as increased intraocular pressure and cataracts.

Nursing Care of the Child With a Chemical Burn

Initial care of the child with a chemical burn to the eyes is focused on irrigation to prevent further injury. Irrigation of

TEACHING GUIDELINES *Prevention of Eye Injuries During Sports*

- High-risk sports include those in which no eye protection is worn, such as boxing and martial arts, or those in which there is a rapidly moving ball, bat, or puck.
- The highest percentage of injuries are seen in basketball and baseball.
- Protective eyewear such as goggles and face shields should be worn when at all possible.
- Goggles should be worn under helmets and with hockey masks.
- Orthodontic headgear should always be removed when playing sports.

Adapted from Catalano, R. A. (1993). Eye injuries and prevention. *Pediatric Clinics of North America, 40*(4), 827–839.

a frightened, hurting child's eyes can be very difficult. Helping the child lean over a water fountain that is spraying upward makes the task easier. After the initial period of irrigation is completed, nursing care focuses on prescribed medical treatments, comfort measures, and injury prevention (particularly if both of the child's eyes are patched). Discharge teaching focuses not only on the prescribed medical treatments, but also on the importance of compliance with long-term follow-up and injury prevention.

The Child Having Eye Surgery

Any surgical procedure is stressful for the child and family. Eye surgery is particularly stressful, as the child's visual fields or acuity may be greatly reduced or absent for a period of time. If both eyes are affected, the child's ability to maneuver and care for herself is also affected.

Special attention should be paid to education. If the child is going home with patches, drops, or any other procedure that must be performed, it is imperative that the family know how to perform this care. Education regarding safety must also be done. This includes wearing patches, eye glasses, avoiding blows to the head, etc.

Assessment

The child and family should have a thorough assessment that begins with their understanding of what surgical procedure is planned and why this is necessary. Discharge planning should begin at admission, with the family being educated on the care that will be necessary following discharge, as well as any other changes that may be necessary. These might include such changes as home schooling if both eyes are affected. Safety should also be addressed at admission and should be reinforced during the child's hospitalization. Finally, any special adaptations for procedures should be assessed for and implemented at admission.

Nursing Diagnoses

- Sensory/Perceptual Alterations: Visual impairment related to eye patching or surgical procedure
- Risk for Injury related to increased intraocular pressure resulting from bleeding edema or hematoma
- Risk for Infection related to surgical incision
- Pain related to surgical procedure
- Fear related to bandaged eyes following surgery
- Knowledge Deficit related to care of eyes following surgery

Planning, Implementation, and Evaluation: The Child Having Eye Surgery

NURSING DIAGNOSIS

- Sensory/Perceptual Alterations: Visual impairment related to eye patching or surgical procedure

Expected Outcome:

- The child and family will be prepared for any anticipated visual changes.
- The child and parents will be oriented to the surroundings and will be prepared for unfamiliar sights and sounds.
- The child will remain alert and oriented to time and self.

Intervention	Rationale
1. Prepare the child and family preoperatively for any changes expected in vision, including blurred vision or patched eyes.	Preoperative preparation allows the family to know what to expect, thus lessening anxiety.
2. Preoperatively, orient the child and family to the surroundings, including the recovery room and hospital room.	Preoperative orientation to surroundings allows the child to have a feeling of familiarity during the postoperative period.
3. Provide reality orientation for the child during the postoperative period, especially if his vision is impaired or his eyes are patched.	Providing a sense of time passage, and orienting to day and night prevents the child from becoming disoriented and confused.
4. Provide emotional support and allow expression of feelings of anger and frustration. This may be done through use of play therapy and therapeutic communication.	Allowing the child and family to express their fears and frustrations in a "healthy" manner provides an appropriate outlet and encourages the use of other senses.

Evaluation:
- The child and family express understanding of visual changes.
- The child and parents are oriented to surroundings.
- The child remains alert and is oriented to time and self.

NURSING DIAGNOSIS
- Risk for Injury related to increased intraocular pressure resulting from bleeding, edema, hematoma

Expected Outcome:
- The child will not experience a physical injury.
- The child will wear eye patches and/or shields as ordered.
- Restraints will be used according to institutional policy and physician order. The child will not receive an injury from the restraints.

Intervention	Rationale
1. Fully orient the child to his surroundings and ensure that unsafe objects are removed from the environment.	Orienting the child to the environment and ensuring that the environment is safe will prevent falls and other injuries when the child is out of bed.
2. Ensure that the child wears eye patches and/or shields as ordered.	Eye patches and shields are often prescribed to prevent any further injury to the eye.
3. Restrain arms as necessary and as ordered.	Restraints may be necessary to prevent the child from rubbing his eye and, thus, damaging the eye.
4. Monitor for signs and symptoms of increased intraocular pressure.	The child should be monitored closely for signs and symptoms of increasing intraocular pressure, which can damage the eye and seriously impair vision.

Evaluation:
- The child does not experience a physical injury.
- Eye patches and/or shields are worn as ordered.
- Restraints are used according to institutional policy and physician order. The child does not receive an injury from the restraints.

NURSING DIAGNOSIS
- Risk for Infection related to surgical incision

Expected Outcome:
- Any signs and symptoms of infection are reported and treated immediately.

Intervention	Rationale
1. Monitor the child for signs and symptoms of infection, including redness, drainage, fever, and excessive tearing or edema.	These are physical signs that the eye is developing a postoperative infection.
2. Administer antibiotic therapy as ordered.	Antibiotics may be used as a prophylaxis against infection

Evaluation:
- Any signs and symptoms of infection are reported and treated immediately.

NURSING DIAGNOSIS • Pain related to surgical procedure

Expected Outcome: • The child will experience minimal discomfort during the postoperative period.

Intervention	Rationale
1. Assess the child frequently (q 4 hr while awake) for pain using an age-appropriate pain scale.	Providing pain control decreases the child's need to rub or touch the eyes, which can cause trauma to the surgical site.
2. Administer pain medications as ordered.	
3. Provide nonpharmacologic pain relief measures such as ice pack, moist heat, etc., as indicated.	

Evaluation: • The child evidences minimal discomfort as measured using an age-appropriate pain scale.

DISORDERS OF THE EAR: HEARING LOSS

Hearing loss may be caused by damage to or impairment of any part of the ear. Four types of hearing loss have been identified: conductive, sensorineural, mixed, and central (see box). Each has a different treatment regimen and response to intervention.

Assessment for hearing loss should be done on any infant or child who is at high risk for hearing loss due to heredity, birth factors, exposure to ototoxic medications or infections, trauma, or medical conditions that may result in hearing loss. Factors associated with hearing loss based on age are listed in the accompanying box.

Testing should be done by an audiologist and may be done using auditory brain stem response or otacoustic emissions. Visual reinforcement audiometry is used to measure behavioral testing of a child's hearing ability in children older than age 6 months (Kramer & Williams, 1993).

Audiometry measures the sounds that the human ear can hear, with "0" being the softest sound that can be heard. Sound is measured in a scale from 0 to 110 decibels (dB). Sounds above 140 dB cause pain. Hearing loss is divided into four categories (Aram, 1987):

Mild: Failure to hear 26 to 40 dB
Moderate: Failure to hear 41 to 65 dB
Severe: Failure to hear 66 to 95 dB
Profound: Failure to hear above 96 dB

Treatment of hearing loss depends on the type of loss. For example, nonconductive hearing loss is often associated with craniofacial abnormalities that block the ear canal. It may also be associated with a canal blocked with cerumen. Most hearing loss of this type can be treated either medically or surgically (Northern & Downs, 1991).

Sensorineural hearing loss, on the other hand, is almost always irreversible (Northern & Downs, 1991) and requires a different approach. Hearing aids are often recommended for these children. The type of aid chosen depends on the specific needs of the child. It should provide the best acoustics and be appropriate in a cosmetic

Types and Causes of Hearing Loss

Conductive: Outer or middle ear affected by damage, inflammation, or obstruction; sound prevented from progressing across the middle ear; may be the result of excessive cerumen (wax), foreign bodies, perforated tympanic membrane, or otitis media (Webster & Wood, 1989; Bevan, 1988); hearing loss is often reversible

Sensorineural: Result of damage or malformation of the middle ear and/or auditory nerve; may be result of infection (meningitis or intrauterine), heredity, exposure to loud noise, ototoxic medications, or prematurity (Kravitz & Selekman, 1992); hearing loss is usually permanent

Mixed: Combination of conductive and sensorineural loss; conductive loss is often reversible, whereas sensorineural loss is not

Central: Result of damage to the conduction system between the brain stem and cerebral cortex; may be result of trauma, neurovascular changes, or brain tumors; may cause difficulty in differentiation of sounds, auditory memory

Factors Indicating the Need for Hearing Screening

NEONATES (BIRTH TO 28 DAYS)

- Family history of inherited sensorineural hearing loss
- Intrauterine infections such as rubella, cytomegalovirus, and toxoplasmosis
- Craniofacial abnormalities
- Birth weight < 1.5 kg (3.3 lb)
- Hyperbilirubinemia requiring exchange transfusion
- Ototoxic medications given in multiple courses or with loop diuretics
- Bacterial meningitis
- Apgar scores of 0 to 4 at 1 minute or 0 to 6 at 5 minutes
- Mechanical ventilation for 5 or more days
- Any findings associated with a syndrome that includes hearing loss

INFANTS DEVELOPING CERTAIN CONDITIONS ASSOCIATED WITH HEARING LOSS (29 DAYS TO 2 YEARS)

- Caregiver concerns about hearing, speech, language, or developmental delay
- Infections associated with sensorineural hearing loss
- Head trauma resulting in loss of consciousness or skull fracture
- Any findings associated with a syndrome that includes hearing loss
- Hyperbilirubinemia requiring exchange transfusion
- Ototoxic medications given in multiple courses or with loop diuretics
- Recurrent otitis media with effusion lasting at least 3 months

INFANTS (29 DAYS TO 3 YEARS) NEEDING PERIODIC HEARING SCREENING

Sensorineural:

- Family history of inherited sensorineural hearing loss
- Intrauterine infections such as rubella, cytomegalovirus, and toxoplasmosis
- Neurofibromatosis Type II or other neurodegenerative disorder

Conductive:

- Recurrent otitis media with effusion lasting at least 3 months
- Anything that affects eustachian tube function
- Neurodegenerative disorders

Adapted from Joint Committee on Infant Hearing (1994). 1994 Position Statement. *ASHA, 36*(12), 38–41.

sense. For example, an adolescent will seldom choose a body type hearing aid if an "ear level" aid (one inserted into the ear canal) will suffice. The four types of hearing aids most commonly used for pediatric patients are the "behind the ear," the "ear level" (in the ear), eyeglass (aids attached to the temples of eyeglass frames), and body.

Finally, cochlear implants offer new options for children suffering from sensorineural hearing loss. The implant is a small device that is surgically implanted. It delivers electrical stimulation to the inner ear, and stimulates cranial nerve VIII. The nerve impulses travel to the brain, where they are "interpreted" as normal sound (Northern & Downs, 1991). Minimum selection criteria are as follows (adapted from Northern, 1986, p. 342):

- At least 2 years of age
- Bilateral sensorineural deafness (either profound or total)
- Pre-evaluation to determine sensorineural deafness
- Normal IQ
- No other handicaps such as autism or learning disabilities
- Strong family support
- Team decision that hearing aids and training are not providing satisfactory progress

The Nurse's Role in Assessing for Hearing Deficits

Hearing should be assessed at each well child visit and whenever there is a complaint specific to ears (including otitis media—see Chapter 28). This may be done by noting the child's response to bells, rattles, clapping of hands, or horns held about 12 inches from the ear. Older children may be asked to repeat whispered words or phrases or listen for a ticking watch. Language skills should also be assessed. Deaf infants will babble the same as hearing infants until about age 5 to 6 months, when babbling is noted to cease in deaf children. Parents should also be questioned about the child's attention span, disruptive behavior, and other behaviors such as increasing the volume on the television. If the child appears to have hearing loss or is noted to be lagging behind in developmental milestones, he should be referred for further evaluation by an audiologist and ENT physician.

Caring for the Hearing-Impaired Child

- If the child has a hearing aid, encourage him to use it. Make sure it is in place before you begin speaking to him.
- Look directly in the child's face. You should have his complete attention before beginning to speak.
- Speak clearly. You should also slow your speech slightly.
- Eliminate background noise.
- Use visual aids to assist your communication. These include pictures, your hands, and written messages for older children.

LANGUAGE DEVELOPMENT AND LANGUAGE DISORDERS

Until age 10 months to 1 year, a child is considered to be "prelingual." The sounds the child makes have no direct meaning or connection to future language. They are, instead, practice of a learned skill. Before about age 6 months, infants make few sounds other than crying. At about 6 months, however, they enter the "babbling phase." These are the cooing, happy sounds that an infant makes when she is content. The first words appear at about age 10 months to 1 year. First sentences appear at about age 18 months. By age 2 years, most children have at least a 50-word vocabulary.

Girls have more rapid language development until about age 3 years, when the difference disappears. However, by adolescence, girls again show superior verbal skills. Although there is a relationship between developmental delay and verbal skills, the relationship between language development and intelligence is unclear. There seems to be no scientific evidence that a child who "talks early" is brighter than one who does not. Children who talk very early do appear, however, to usually be "bright," whereas those who talk "extremely late" appear to have some developmental delay.

Language disorders in the pediatric patient are usually one of two types. The first is the inability to comprehend (receptive disorder). The second is a disorder in which the child cannot express thoughts through speech (expressive

TEACHING GUIDELINES *for Improving Parent–Child Interaction and Communication*

THE IMPORTANCE OF TALKING

Talking to your child is necessary for his language development. Because children usually imitate what they hear, how much you talk to your child, what you say, and how you say it will affect how much and how well your child talks.

LOOK

Look directly at your child's face and wait until you have his attention before you begin talking.

CONTROL DISTANCE

Be sure that you are close to your child when you talk (no farther than 5 feet). The younger the child, the more important it is to be close.

LOUDNESS

Talk slightly louder than you normally do. Turn off the radio, TV, dishwasher, to remove background noise.

BE A GOOD SPEECH MODEL

- Describe to your child daily activities as they occur.
- Expand what your child says. For example, if your child points and says "car," you say, "Oh, you want the car."
- Add new information. You might add, "That car is little."
- Build vocabulary. Make teaching new words and concepts a natural part of every day's activities. Use new words while shopping, taking a walk, or washing dishes, for example.
- Repeat your child's words using adult pronunciation.

PLAY AND TALK

Set aside some times throughout each day for "play time" for just you and your child. Play can be looking at books, exploring toys, singing songs, coloring, and so on. Talk to your child during these activities, keeping the conversation at his level.

READ

Begin reading to your child at a young age (under 12 months). Ask a librarian for books that are right for your child's age. Reading can be a calming-down activity that promotes closeness between you and your child. Reading provides another opportunity to teach and review words and ideas. Some children enjoy looking at pictures in magazines and catalogs.

DON'T WAIT

Your child should have the following skills by the ages listed below:

- 18 months: 3-word vocabulary
- 2 years: 25- to 30-word vocabulary and several 2-word sentences
- $2\frac{1}{2}$ years: At least a 50-word vocabulary and 2-word sentences consistently

IF YOUR CHILD DOESN'T HAVE THESE SKILLS, TELL YOUR DOCTOR

A referral to an audiologist and speech pathologist may be indicated. Hearing and language testing may lead to a better understanding of your child's language development.

From Northern, J. L., & Downs, M. P. (1991). *Hearing in children* (4th ed., pp. 26–27). Baltimore: Williams & Wilkins. Adapted from "Suggestions for Parents," Dr. Noel Matkin, PhD.

disorder). Receptive disorders result from some type of central nervous system failure. This may be the result of trauma, a congenital malformation, or other failure of language development. This child cannot express symbols and abstract ideas in spoken words or in a logical manner.

Expressive disorders are most often of three types. The first is a disorder of the voice. This is an alteration in the pitch and intonation that may result from a medical condition such as a cleft palate. The second is a defect of articulation, or the way in which words are pronounced. This is the most common type of speech defect and may be related to neuromuscular disease or to structural abnormalities of the nose, throat, and mouth, or may be idiopathic. Finally, fluency disorders interrupt the flow of normal speech. Included in this category is lisping. If stuttering persists after age 5 years, the child should receive appropriate referrals for speech evaluation (Fig. 43–1).

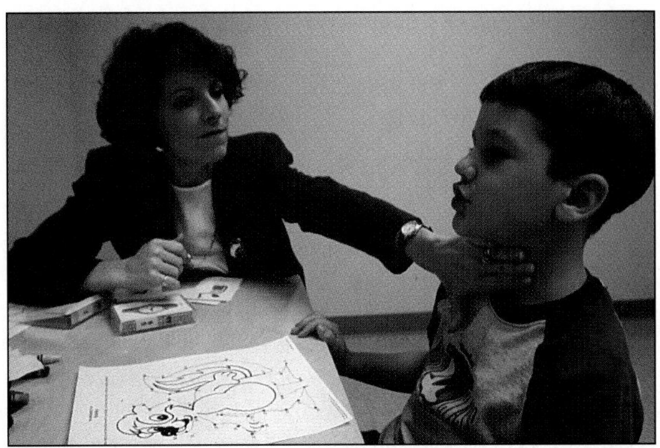

Figure 43–1
Expressive speech disorders include disorders of voice, articulation, and fluency. A speech therapist works with the child to help him speak more clearly and be better understood. Early intervention is very important to correct speech disorders; for that reason, the nurse should assess speech patterns during each health screening visit. Referrals should be made for any problems that are noted. (Courtesy of Cook Children's Medical Center, Fort Worth, Texas)

Nursing Care of the Child With a Language Disorder

As with screens for hearing loss, the nurse should assess the child's communication patterns with each well child visit. Any problems should be noted and referrals should be made to provide appropriate intervention as soon as possible. The accompanying Teaching Guidelines list measures that parents can take to encourage speech and prevent speech problems.

KEY CONCEPTS

- Anything that alters a child's sensory perception can affect growth and development.
- Sense organs develop very early and are sensitive to teratogens. Any interference with development can result in later sensory alteration.
- Special care should be taken when caring for the child with sensory alterations. Orientation to a new environment is critical in preventing stress and possible injury.
- Most screenings for sensory alterations are noninvasive and relatively painless.
- Parent education and support are critical in assisting the child with sensory alteration to develop as normally as possible.
- Early intervention for the child with sensory alterations allows for more normal growth and development.
- Health teaching should include injury prevention.

REFERENCES

American Academy of Ophthalmology. (1994). Strabismus: Etiology, diagnosis, and treatment. *Journal of Ophthalmic Nursing and Technology, 13*(3), 121–123.

Aram, D. (1987). Disorders of speech and language. In R. E. Behrman & V. C. Vaughn (Eds.), *Nelson textbook of pediatrics* (13th ed.). Philadelphia: W. B. Saunders.

Bevan, R. (1988). *Hearing impaired children.* Springfield, IL: Charles C. Thomas.

Besinger, R. (1992). Color vision testing. *Journal of Ophthalmic Nursing and Technology, 11*(4), 161–163.

Castiglia, P. T. (1994). Strabismus. *Journal of Pediatric Health Care, 8*(5), 236–238.

Catalano, R. A. (1993). Eye injuries and prevention. *Pediatric Clinics of North America, 40*(4), 827–839.

Catalano, R. A., & Nelson, L. B. (1994). *Pediatric ophthalmology: A text atlas.* Norwalk, CT: Appleton & Lange.

Cheng, K. P., et al. (1991). Visual results after early surgical treatment of unilateral congenital cataracts. *Ophthalmology, 98*(6), 903–910.

Day, S., Eggers, H., Gammon, J. A., & Spivey, B. E. (1990). Early strabismus/amblyopia screening. *Patient Care, 24,* 83–94.

Gerali, P. S. (1991). Childsight: Helping children grow up with good vision. *Journal of Ophthalmic Nursing and Technology, 10*(5), 222–223.

Hiatt, R. L. (1991). Eye trauma in children. *Southern Medical Journal, 84*(6), 747–750.

Joint Committee on Infant Hearing. (1994). 1994 Position Statement. *ASHA, 36*(12), 38–41.

Kaye, B. (1990). The cure for lazy eye. *Journal of Ophthalmic Nursing and Technology, 9*(3), 90–93.

King, R. A. (1993). Common ocular signs and symptoms in childhood. *Pediatric Clinics of North America, 40*(4), 753–766.

Kramer, S. J., & Williams, D. R. (1993). The hearing-impaired infant and toddler: Identification, assessment, and intervention. *Infants & Young Children, 6*(1), 35–49.

Kravitz, L., & Selekman, J. (1992). Understanding hearing loss in children. *Pediatric Nursing, 18*(6), 591–594.

Lavrich, J. B., & Nelson, L. B. (1993). Diagnosis and treatment of strabismus disorders. *Pediatric Clinics of North America, 40*(4), 737–752.

Northern, J. L. (1986). Selection of children for cochlear implantation. *Seminars in Hearing, 7,* 341–347.

Northern, J. L., & Downs, M. P. (1991). *Hearing in children* (4th ed.). Baltimore: Williams & Wilkins.

Symanski, M. E., Newman, C. O., & Bachynski, B. N. (1994). Treating congenital cataracts. *MCN, 19*(6), 335–338.

Trobe, J. D. (1993). *The physician's guide to eye care.* San Francisco: American Academy of Ophthalmology.

Wagner, R. S. (1994). Glaucoma in children. *Pediatric Clinics of North America, 40*(4), 855–867.

Webster, A., & Wood, D. (1989). *Children with hearing difficulties.* London: Cassell Educational Limited.

GLOSSARY

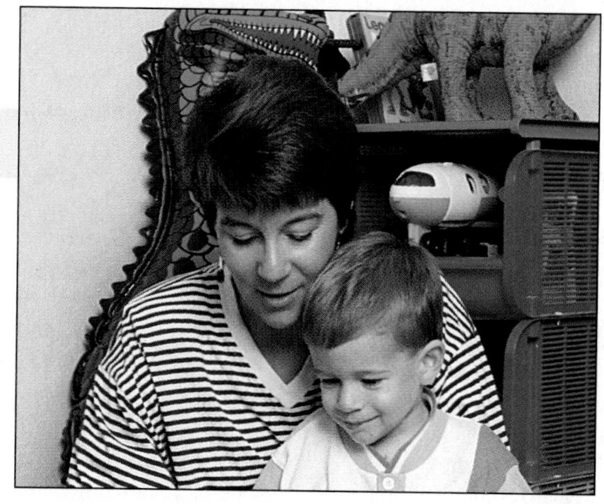

ABCDEs: Airway, Breathing, Circulation, Disability, and Exposure. When assessing children, it is important to remember to assess each one of these areas.
abduction: movement away from the midline
abuse: a general term that includes nonaccidental physical injury, or the nonaccidental act of omission by a parent or person responsible for the care of the child. This term includes physical injury, sexual molestation, neglect, and emotional injury.
acetabulum: the hip socket in the pelvis
achalasia: failure of smooth muscle fibers of the GI tract to relax, resulting in a functional obstruction and difficulty in passage of food and chyme along the GI tract
acholic: free from bile
acidosis: abnormal accumulation of acid or loss of base from the body, with pH equal to or less than 7.35
active immunity: the protection, which can last months, years, or even a lifetime, that forms in response to exposure to antigens in nature or vaccines
active listening: the ability to empathetically listen in order to gain better understanding of the actual as well as implied message
adaptive immune system: a defense system that recognizes foreign invaders, synthesizes and delivers immune products to infection sites, directs action against invaders, and has deactivation mechanisms
adduction: movement toward the midline
adolescence: the biological and psychosocial transition from childhood to adulthood
advocacy: speaking or arguing in support of a policy or a person's rights
afterload: the amount of resistance against which the heart pumps
AHCPR: Agency for Health Care Policy and Research; a federal agency established in 1989
airway management: correct positioning of airway, and appropriate interventions used to ensure patency of the airway and adequate oxygenation and ventilation
alkalosis: abnormal accumulation of bicarbonate or loss of acid in the body, with pH equal to or greater than 7.45
allergy: the immune system's response to an allergen that causes a hypersensitivity reaction in various body systems
allograft: a graft of tissue between the same species, but of a different genotype; a homograft
alopecia: hair loss
amblyopia: reduced visual acuity not correctable by refractive means and not attributable to obvious structural ocular anomalies
anergy: impaired or absent ability to react to specific antigens
angioplasty: vessel dilation
animism: attributing lifelike characteristics to inanimate objects
ankylosis: condition in which a joint is stiff or difficult to move
anomaly: abnormality
anthropometric measurements: measurement of height, weight, head circumference, skinfold thickness, and arm circumference
antibody: a protein that the immune system produces to bind to specific antigens and eliminate them from the body
anticipatory grief: the processes of mourning, coping, interacting, planning, and psychosocial reorganizing that are begun in part as a response to the impending loss of a loved one
antigen: a substance that possesses unique configurations enabling the immune system to recognize it as foreign
antipyretic: an agent that reduces or relieves fever
antitoxin: a particular kind of antibody produced by the body in response to the presence of a toxin
anuria: severe diminution of urine formation, less than 0.5 ml/kg/hr, usually indicative of kidney failure; may be secondary to severe dehydration
Apgar: scoring system that evaluates the newborn's heart rate, respiratory rate, muscle tone, irritability, and color and is indicative of adaptation to extrauterine life
apical pulse rate: heart rate determined by placing the stethoscope over the point of maximum intensity (PMI) and counting for 1 minute
apocrine sweat glands: secretory glands located in the axillae and genital regions; become active at puberty and respond to emotional and sexual stimulation
arrhythmia: an abnormal rhythm of the heart

arteriovenous fistula: a connection between an artery and vein, usually for the purpose of hemodialysis
arteriovenous graft: a U-shaped plastic tube inserted between an artery and a vein, usually for the purpose of hemodialysis
artery: a vessel that carries blood away from the heart
asphyxiation: a state of suffocation that severely compromises oxygen delivery to the body
aspiration: accidentally drawing foreign objects into the nose, throat, or lungs on inspiration
astigmatism: abnormal curvature of the cornea or the lens
atelectasis: collapsed or airless state of the lung (may involve all or part of the lung)
atresia: congenital absence or closure of a body orifice; obliteration of a tubular organ
attenuated vaccines: vaccines derived from microorganisms or viruses whose virulence has been weakened owing to passage through another host
auscultate: to listen to body sounds (e.g., heart sounds, breath sounds)
auscultation: the art of listening to sounds produced by the body; frequently using a stethoscope to magnify body sounds
autograft: a graft of tissue taken from one part of one's own body and transferred to another part
autoimmune disease: disease that occurs when the immune system produces antibodies—called autoantibodies—against cells of the body
autoimmune disorder: a disorder in which the body launches an immunologic response against itself
autologous blood transfusion: transfusion of one's own blood which has been harvested previously
autonomy: ability to function independently without the control of others
autoregulation: the unique ability of the cerebral arteries to change their diameter in response to alterations in cerebral perfusion pressure, to maintain a steady blood flow during changes in blood pressure and perfusion
autosomal recessive: a genetic trait carried on 1 of the 22 pairs of chromosomes not concerned with determination of sex. An autosomal recessive trait is evident in the infant only when it is transmitted by both parents.
avascular necrosis: tissue damage secondary to inadequate blood supply
basal ganglia: serves as a major communication and sorting area for messages to and from the cerebral hemispheres; composed of masses of gray matter; controls movement; and participates in emotion and cognition
bereavement: the objective condition or state of loss
beta cells: specialized cells within the pancreas that manufacture and secrete insulin; thought to be the target of the autoimmune destructive process of IDDM
blast cells: immature lymphocytes not normally present in peripheral blood
blood–brain barrier: selective anatomic or physiologic capillary feature that prevents passage of potentially harmful substances, such as certain medications, radioactive ions, and viruses, from the blood into the central nervous system
body mass index (BMI): body weight (kg) divided by height squared used as an index of relative weight and obesity
bradycardia: slow heart rate for age
brain stem: connected to the cerebral hemispheres by thick branches of nerve fibers; all nerve fibers traverse through the brain stem from the hemispheres to the cerebellum and spinal cord
calcitonin: a hormone, secreted by cells within the thyroid gland, that inhibits bone resorption or breakdown. Under normal circumstances, its production is increased when serum calcium concentrations are elevated.
caput succedaneum: edema of the soft tissues of the scalp and head caused by squeezing during the delivery process; usually disappears in 2 to 3 days
cardiac catheterization: the process of examining the heart by introducing a catheter into a vein or artery and passing it into the heart to sample oxygen, measure pressure, and X-ray the area
cardiac output: the volume of blood in liters pumped from the heart each minute
cardiomegaly: an enlarged heart on chest X-ray
cardiopulmonary resuscitation (CPR): performed when a patient's respiratory and cardiovascular systems require support, as in the pulseless, nonbreathing patient. Airway management, ventilation, and chest compressions are provided to improve tissue perfusion until the patient can receive definitive care.
caries: decay of the teeth
case management: a practice model that uses a systematic approach to identify specific patient needs and to manage patient care to ensure optimal outcomes
cataract: a loss of transparency of the crystalline lens or its capsule
cellular immunity: immunologic response to an antigen that results in increased production of T lymphocytes by the thymus
central hearing loss: result of damage to the conduction system between the brain stem and cerebral cortex
central venous access device: venous access device in which the catheter is centrally placed, usually in the superior vena cava or jugular vein; used for long-term intravenous therapy
central venous pressure: pressure measured in the right atrium; helpful in determining the amount of circulating blood volume
centration: tendency to focus on only one aspect of an event or object rather than all aspects
cephalhematoma: unilateral swelling caused by bleeding below the periosteum of the cranium; swelling does not cross suture lines
cephalocaudal: growth and development that proceed from head to toe
cerebral cortex: gray matter of the cerebrum, where the higher functions of thinking occur
cerebral herniation: shift of brain tissue sideways under the flax cerebri or downward, causing severe neurologic dysfunction
cerebral perfusion pressure (CPP): difference between mean arterial blood pressure and intracranial pressure
chelation: binding of a metallic ion with a structure so that the ion is inactivated
chromosomes: packages of genetic material that occur in pairs within the nucleus of cells; contain genes
chronic illness/condition: a condition or illness that is long-term and either without cure or with residual characteristics that result in limitations upon activities of daily living
chronic sorrow: recurrent feelings of grief, loss, and fear related to the child's condition and the loss of the ideal, healthy child

chronological age: age in years
clean margins: evidence of normal, disease-free tissue in the outermost layer of cells of a surgical sample
communication: the act of transmitting and receiving information
comorbidity: the presence of two different disorders occurring in the same individual. It is common for children with cognitive impairments to have coexisting psychiatric disorders.
compensation: maintenance of an adequate blood flow without distressing symptoms, accomplished by cardiac and circulatory adjustments such as tachycardia, cardiac hypertrophy, and increased blood volume from sodium and water retention
complement: an accessory system to a humoral response which is composed of serum proteins that facilitate enzyme action and antigen death
complex carbohydrates: classed as complex because they are large molecules with many bonds that must be broken so that monosaccharides can be released and absorbed; include starch, glycogen, and cellulose
concomitant strabismus: not of paralytic origin; deviation remains constant for all directions of gaze
conductive hearing loss: reversible loss caused by damage, inflammation, or obstruction to the outer or middle ear; sound is prevented from progressing across middle ear
congenital (infantile) glaucoma: increased intraocular fluid pressure that occurs during first 3 years of life and is due to a defect in the drainage network of the eye
conscious sedation: "light sedation" during which the patient retains airway reflexes and responds to verbal stimuli
conservation: ability to understand that certain properties of objects do not change simply because their order, form, or appearance has changed
coping: efforts directed toward managing and solving various problems, events, and stressors
crackle: abnormal discontinuous nonmusical breath sound heard on auscultation, primarily during inhalation; also called rale
crepitus: a grating sensation at a fracture site that occurs when the ends of a broken bone move
culture: shared values, beliefs, and practices of a particular group of people
Cushing's response: late sign of increased intracranial pressure; includes increased blood pressure, widened pulse pressure, decreased heart rate, and decreased or irregular respiratory rate
cytotoxicity: the degree to which an agent possesses a specific destructive action on certain cells, or the possession of such action
dead space: space in the hub of the syringe and needle; medication remains in the dead space after a medication has been injected (usually 0.2 ml)
debridement: removal of foreign material and devitalized or contaminated tissue from traumatic or infected lesion until healthy tissue is exposed
decerebrate posture: abnormal extension of the upper extremities with internal rotation of the upper arms and wrists; lower extremities will extend with some internal rotation
decompensation: inability of the heart to maintain adequate circulation, marked by dyspnea, venous engorgement, cyanosis, and edema
decorticate posture: abnormal flexion of the upper extremities and extension of the lower extremities
denial: a defense mechanism in which unpleasant realities are denied and kept out of conscious awareness
dental emergency: injury or infection of a tooth or teeth, when the length of time to definitive care is critical for the care of the tooth or to alleviate pain
desquamation: sloughing of the skin in scales or sheets; can lead to loss of the deeper layers of the skin
development: changes that occur over time in function, psychosocial, and cognitive behavior
developmental age: age based on functional behavior and ability to adapt to the environment; does not necessarily correspond to chronological age
diabetic ketoacidosis (DKA): metabolic consequence of severe insulin deficit, marked by hyperglycemia, acidosis, and ketosis
diarrhea: an increase in the volume of stool output and/or a change in the consistency of stool compared to the individual's normal stool pattern
dilatation: to make larger using artificial means (such as a balloon catheter)
diplopia: double vision
discipline: the structure an adult sets for a child's life designed to allow him to happily and effectively fit into the real world
dislocation: displacement of a bone from its normal articulation within a joint
double message: a verbal message that is contradictory to the underlying tone or meaning of the message
dramatic play: allows children to act out roles and experiences that may have happened to them, that they are fearful will happen to them, or that they observed happening to someone else
Dubowitz: scale developed in 1970 to assess gestational age according to 10 neurologic and 11 physical criteria
dysphagia: inability or difficulty in swallowing
dysplasia: abnormal development
dyspnea: difficulty breathing
dysuria: pain on urination
ecchymoses: discoloration of the skin or mucous membrane caused by leakage of blood into the subcutaneous tissue
eccrine sweat glands: secretory glands distributed over the body that secrete sweat
echocardiogram: a graphic record of the walls, valves, and vessels of the heart that is produced by reflective sound (ultrasound), of which there are several different types
edema: presence of abnormally large amounts of fluid in the intercellular tissue spaces of the body
egocentric: preoccupied with one's own interests and needs
egocentrism: complete absorption with self; an inability to understand that others have a different point of view
emergency: a psychological, medical, or traumatic condition that requires immediate care or care within an hour to prevent further deterioration
empathy: the ability to remain objective while seeing from another's perspective
empowerment: providing the family with the appropriate tools (education, information, support) that enable them to fully participate in decision making and care of the child
encopresis: fecal incontinence after age 4 years
enteral: by way of the alimentary canal (e.g., enteral feeding)

envenomation: injection of venom by an animal (usually snakes, lizards, spiders, scorpions, etc.) into a human body
epidural: situated within the spinal canal, on or outside the dura mater; synonyms are *extradural* and *peridural*
epidural medication: medication administered directly into the epidural space in the spine; administered either as a bolus injection or on a continuous basis through an infusion pump
epiglottitis: inflammation of the epiglottis
erythema: redness of the skin
erythropoiesis: production of erythrocytes
eschar: a slough produced by a thermal burn or corrosive application
estropia (convergent) strabismus: eye turns inward; most common type of strabismus in infants
eutectic mixture of local anesthetics (EMLA): cream used to numb the skin at a depth of 0.5 mm; used before needlesticks
euthyroid: having normal thyroid function
exanthem: an eruption or rash on the skin
excoriation: scratch or abrasion
expressive play: provides children opportunities to express feelings and energy in appropriate and active ways
external fixation: pins, screws, and bars placed through bone and soft tissue to immobilize, or to correct a deformity
extracellular fluid (ECF): found outside the cell, comprising approximately one third of the body's fluid in older children and about half of the fluid in infants
extramedullary: outside the bone marrow
extrapyramidal tract: descending pathway of the motor neurons concerned with involuntary or unconscious skeletal muscle coordination and reflex control of coordination
exotropia (divergent) strabismus: eyes turn away from the midline; occurs most often when the child attempts to focus on a distant object; may be present at birth
familiarization play: the providing of materials that are commonly associated with health care situations and using them in creative and playful activities
family: two or more emotionally involved people living in close proximity and having reciprocal obligations with a sense of commonness, caring, and commitment
family-centered nursing care: a philosophy of care that recognizes the family as the constant in a child's life, as well as the need for personnel and service systems to encourage, respect, and support family competencies
fistula: abnormal communication between two organs or from one organ to the outside of the body
food jags: the refusal of previously liked foods or the requesting of a particular food at every meal
frequency: urination at short time intervals
functional age: the age equivalent at which the child is actually able to perform specific self-care or relational tasks. For example, the child may be 6 years old chronologically, but may only be able to perform skills representative of children 4 years of age. The child's functional age, then, would be 4 years.
fundoplication: a 270° to 360° wrap of the stomach fundus around the distal esophagus to tighten the lower esophageal sphincter and prevent gastric reflux
ganglion: a cluster of nerve cells outside the central nervous system; responsible for intestinal peristalsis
genes: units of heredity that control formation and function of proteins throughout the body and transmit inherited information
genetics: the study of heredity
gestation: length of pregnancy
gestational age: age of a fetus or newborn stated in terms of the number of weeks dating from the first day of the mother's last menstrual period.
gland: an organ or structure that secretes a substance or hormones to be used in some other part of the body
glia cells: make up support tissue that nourishes and protects the neurons
glucagon: a hormone produced by the alpha cells of the pancreas; counteracts the action of insulin by converting liver stores of glycogen to blood glucose, resulting in an elevation of the blood glucose level
glucose: the substrate of choice for cellular energy; the breakdown product of carbohydrate
glycosuria: glucose in urine; occurs when the blood glucose level exceeds the renal threshold and glucose "spills" into the urine
glycosylated hemoglobin: a laboratory test used to evaluate glycemic control by measuring glycosylation (or sugar coating) on the hemoglobin portion of the red blood cell; offers a 3-month average of blood sugar control
gradient: a pressure difference
granulocytes: polymorphonuclear leukocytes (neutrophils, eosinophils, or basophils)
grief: a psychophysiologic process that occurs in response to a specific loss
growth: measurable physical and physiologic changes that occur over time
growth spurts: brief periods of rapid increase in growth rate
grunting: sound similar to "grunting" noise that can be heard with or without a stethoscope
hematemesis: vomiting of bright red blood or of denatured blood that looks like "coffee grounds"; usually represents a bleeding source proximal to the jejunum
hematopoiesis: production of blood cells; normally occurs in the bone marrow, but may occur in extramedullary sites
hemolysis: breakdown of red blood cells
hemosiderosis: focal or general increase in tissue iron stores without associated tissue damage
heparin lock (intermittent infusion port): IV catheter placed and used to administer intravenous medications intermittently
hepatosplenomegaly: enlargement of the liver and spleen detected by palpation of the abdomen
heredity: the transmission of genetic characteristics from parent to offspring
heterograft: a graft of tissue transplanted between different species; a xenograft
history: the collection of subjective data to describe past and present health status
homozygote: an individual who inherited two identical genes for a certain trait
honeymoon phase: an early stage of diabetes characterized by relatively small exogenous insulin requirements to maintain normal blood sugar
hormone: a chemical substance produced by one gland or tissue and carried by the blood to other tissues or organs, where it causes a specific effect
hospice care: a system of specialized and comprehensive care that provides support and assistance to patients (and their

families) affected by terminal illness. The purpose of the care is to rehumanize the dying experience while providing the means for the patient and family to live as comfortably and as fully as possible. This is accomplished through the provision of respectful, noninvasive care, pain and symptom control, and emotional, physical, psychological, and spiritual support services.

humoral immunity: immunologic response to an antigen, resulting in production of B lymphocytes

hydrotherapy: washing of a portion of the body or the entire body

hypercalciuria: excessive calcium in the urine

hypercapnia: increased levels of carbon dioxide in the blood, as indicated by an elevated P_{CO_2} determined by blood gas analysis

hyperglycemia: blood glucose levels about 120 mg/dl (fasting) and/or 200 mg/dl (random)

hyperlipidemia: high cholesterol and triglyceride levels in the blood

hypertonic (hypernatremic) dehydration: state in which the solute concentration is above that of normal body fluids (i.e., sodium > 145 Eq/L)

hypertrophy: thickening of the wall

hyphema: a hemorrhage or sanguineous exudate in the anterior chamber of the eye

hypoalbuminemia: low albumin levels in the blood

hypocapnia: decreased levels of carbon dioxide in the blood

hypoglycemia: blood glucose levels below 70 mg/dl

hypothalamus: portion of the brain that secretes releasing factors to the pituitary gland for the maintenance of endocrine/metabolic activities

hypothermia: cooling of body temperature to subnormal levels; temperature levels considered to be dangerous to infants and children are core body temperatures below 96°F

hypotonic (hyponatremic) dehydration: state in which the solute concentration is below that of normal body fluids (i.e., sodium < 135 mEq/L)

hypoxemia: decreased oxygen level in the blood

hypoxia: decreased oxygenation of cells and tissues

identity formation: the acquisition of psychosocial, sexual, and vocational identity

idiopathic: for unknown reasons

ileocecal valve: the ringlike mucous membrane at the junction of the terminal ileum and cecum

illness trajectory: the impact of a disease or condition upon all family members, the physiologic progression of the disease, and the work organization done by the family as part of the coping process

immune (lymphoreticular) system: the body's internal defense against foreign substances, such as bacteria, viruses, parasites, and fungi

immunity: resistance of the body to the effects of a harmful organism or its toxin

immunodeficiency: a defect in the immune system leading to increased susceptibility to multiple infections, including repeat infections

immunosuppression: a weakening or cessation of the body's normal immune response

implanted venous access device (IVAD, infusaport): implanted port reservoir that is surgically implanted with the catheter tip placed in the superior vena cava; used for long-term intravenous therapy

inactivated vaccines: vaccines that contain killed microorganisms

inborn error of metabolism: a genetically determined biochemical disorder in which specific congenital defects in the structure or function of a protein molecule produce a metabolic block that may result in pathologic consequences at birth or later

inertial forces: the external forces of motion that are exerted on the body during impact with blunt energies

infarction: the formation of an infarct, which is a localized area of ischemic necrosis produced by occlusion of the arterial supply or the venous drainage of the part

infection: invasion of an organism by a pathogenic or nonpathogenic organism, such as bacteria, viruses, protozoa, helminths, or fungi

inflammation: a tissue response to injury or destruction of cells

informed consent: a requirement, both legal and ethical, that the patient and the parent/guardian completely understand proposed procedures and/or treatments, including their benefits and risks

ingestion: swallowing of a potentially toxic substance, such as a large amount of medication, petroleum products, or toxic plants

injury control: interventions that reduce the incidence or severity of injury events

injury prevention: activities or educational efforts to promote or increase an individual's awareness of safety issues

innate immune system: a host defense system that consists of barriers (skin), phagocytosis, and circulating soluble factors

inspection: the art of careful observations to identify physical findings

intelligence: the innate capacity of the individual; what individuals can do relative to learning, thinking, and problem-solving; and results obtained on intelligence tests that measure specific skills, such as verbal, nonverbal, or mechanical abilities

internal instrumentation: instruments placed inside the body to immobilize parts

interstitial fluid: fluid surrounding the cell, including lymph fluid

intertrigo: maceration of two skin surfaces in close opposition to each other

intracellular fluid (ICF): fluid found within the cells

intrathecal: within the spinal column

intravascular fluid: fluid contained within the blood vessel (e.g., plasma)

inversion: a turning toward the midline

irreversibility: inability to understand a process in reverse or to mentally undo an action that has been performed

ischemia: deficiency of blood supply to an organ

isotonic (isonatremic) dehydration: state in which the solute concentration is practically identical to that of body fluids (i.e., sodium between 135 and 145 mEq/L)

keloid: a sharply elevated progressively enlarging scar due to excessive collagen formation during connective tissue repair

keratosis: overgrowth and thickening of the cornified epithelium

ketone/ketoacid: an acid manufactured by the liver in response to starvation (in diabetic child, a result of insulin deficit); produced from fat stores, can be used for energy when glucose is unavailable

Kussmaul's Respiration: deep, rapid respiration seen with DKA, in which CO_2 is expelled in a respiratory compensation or acidosis; also described as "air hunger"
latchkey children: children who care for themselves at home after school
learning: behavior changes that occur as a result of both maturation and experience with the environment
leukocytes: white blood cells, whose chief function is to protect the body against foreign substances. There are five types: lymphocytes, monocytes, neutrophils, eosinophils, and basophils.
levator ani muscle: part of pelvic diaphragm, responsible for elevating anus into correct area in embryologic development
LGA: large for gestational age infant; most often associated with maternal diabetes, but may also be caused by genetics
lichenification: thickening and hardening of the skin with accentuation of skin markings; often the result of chronic scratching
lymphadenopathy: swelling of the lymph nodes detected by palpation
lymphocytes: the primary white blood cells of the immune sytem (e.g., B lymphocytes or B cells and T lymphocytes or T cells)
maceration of skin: degenerative changes resulting in discoloration and softening of the skin
malocclusion: misalignment of the teeth or dental arches; teeth may be crowded, crooked, or out of alignment
McBurney's point: one-half to 2 inches from the right anterior superior iliac spine, a point of special tenderness in appendicitis
meconium: first stool passed by neonate; greenish-black, sticky substance that results from bile, epithelial cells, and amniotic fluid in the GI tract
Medicaid: a state-operated program providing medical care to certain eligible persons
melena: rectal passage of black, tarry stools, indicating denatured blood from the upper GI tract
menarche: onset of menstruation
metered dose inhaler: handheld device that delivers "puffs" of medication for inhalation
microphthalmia: a developmental defect causing moderate or severe reduction in the size of the eye
mild hearing loss: failure to hear 26 to 40 dB
mistrust: the negative resolution of the first developmental task according to Erikson's theory, resulting in acute emotional tension and behavioral signs of unmet needs
mixed hearing loss: combination of conductive and sensorineural loss
moderate hearing loss: failure to hear 41 to 65 dB
Monroe-Kellie doctrine: theory describing the compensatory mechanism of the cranial contents that maintains a steady volume and pressure
morbidity: ratio of sick to well persons in a defined population
mortality: ratio of the number of deaths to the total number of persons in a given population
murmur: a sound in the cardiac cycle caused by turbulent blood flow
myelinization: the process by which myelin, a fatty, insulating covering, is formed around the axons of nerve fibers; this process begins during the latter part of fetal life and continues during the first postnatal year
myelomeningocele: a birth anomaly involving the vertebrae and spinal canal that causes paralysis
myocardial contractility: the property by which myocardial cells and tissues shorten in response to an appropriate stimulus; force of contraction of the myocardium
nasal flaring: serious sign of air hunger; widening of nares to enable infant to take in more oxygen
negativism: attitude of opposing or resisting the directions of others
neonatal mortality: infant deaths that occur during the first 27 days of life
neuroglycopenic signs: signs due to decreased cerebral glucose utilization (headaches, personality behavior changes, etc.)
neutral thermal environment: an environmental temperature range within which the infant can maintain normal body temperature with the least amount of metabolic expenditure and oxygen consumption
neutropenia: decrease in the number of circulating neutrophils, which results in decreased ability of the body to fight infection
nonconcomitant strabismus: angle of deviation varies with direction of gaze due to paralysis or paresis of one or more extraocular muscles
nonparalytic strabismus: most common type of strabismus in children; all extraocular muscles function, but are not coordinated; child often squints
nonspecific immune functions: protective barriers, such as chemicals, interferon, inflammation, and phagocytosis, which are activated in the presence of an antigen, but are not specific to that antigen
nonsteroidal anti-inflammatory drug (NSAID): an aspirin-like drug that reduces pain and inflammation arising from injured tissue
normalization: responses of the family of a child with a chronic illness that are used to negate the illness and/or abnormal behaviors in order to maintain valued social roles
nursing diagnosis: a clinical judgment about individual, fammily, or community responses to actual or potential health problems/life processes. Nursing diagnoses provide the basis for selection of nursing interventions to achieve outcomes for which the nurse is accountable.
nutrients: foods that supply the body with elements necessary for metabolism
nystagmus: involuntary eye movements that make the eyes appear to be darting back and forth
object permanence: the realization that objects continue to exist even though they are out of sight
occult bleeding: bleeding in such minute quantity that it can only be recognized by microscopic or chemical means
oliguria: diminished amounts of urine output
ophthalmia neonatorum: conjunctivitis noted in the first few weeks of life, usually gonococcal or chlamydial
orthopnea: difficulty breathing except in an upright position
orthoses: braces, external supports, artificial limbs made by a specialist to meet individual needs
ossification: formation of bone from osseous tissue or cartilage
osteoblastic: activity by osteoblasts that promoted bone formation
osteochondrosis: disorders of the epiphyses in which there is an interruption in the blood supply

osteoclastic: activity by osteoclasts that absorbs and removes old bony tissue
osteotomy: surgical cutting of bone
oxygen saturation: a measure of the degree to which oxygen is bound to hemoglobin
pain: an unpleasant sensory and emotional experience associated with actual or potential tissue damage or described in terms of such damage
pain threshold level: the level of intensity at which pain becomes appreciable or perceptible
palliative treatment: medical treatments or procedures that aim to promote patient comfort and quality of life, not to cure the underlying disease
palpation: the art of touching to determine such factors as texture, temperature, moisture, and organ location
palpitations: sensation of rapid or irregular heart beat
pancytopenia: a reduction in all types of blood cells
parallel play: playing alongside, but not with, other children
paralytic strabismus: caused by a weakness or paralysis of one or more of the extraocular muscles
parathyroid hormone: a hormone produced by the parathyroid glands in response to low serum calcium levels; it increases the breakdown of bone, releasing calcium and phosphorous; increases absorption of calcium from the gastrointestinal tract; and increases reabsorption of calcium in the kidneys
parent/infant attachment: a sense of belonging to or connection with a parent and infant
paresthesia: sensation of numbness and tingling
passive immunity: antibody transfer from a person with active immunity to a person who does not have that antibody
pathogen: a disease-producing microorganism
patient-controlled analgesia (PCA): pain medication administered through an infusion pump, either as a continuous (background) infusion, with or without bolus doses, or as a bolus only; allows the patient to retain some control over how often and how much pain medication is administered
Pavlik harness: a device that holds an infant's hips in flexion and external rotation
percussion: the art of tapping the body to determine density, location, and size of organs
peripherally inserted central line: central line that is inserted peripherally (usually through an antecubital vein) into the superior vena cava
peristalsis: progressive, wavelike movements caused by contraction and relaxation of the longitudinal and circular muscles of the GI tract; propels a bolus of food or fluid forward
pervasive developmental disorders (PDD): infant and childhood disorders characterized by severe and pervasive impairment in several areas of development in a manner that is distinctly deviant from the individual's developmental level or mental age
petechiae: tiny, flat purplish red spots on the skin surface resulting from minute hemorrhages within the dermis
pharmacokinetics: study of the properties of medications
-phoria: tendency for one eye to deviate when fusion is prevented
photophobia: light sensitivity
physiologic anorexia: decreased appetite because of relatively decreased caloric need
pincer grasp: use of index finger and thumb to grip objects
pituitary: an endocrine gland attached to the base of the brain that secretes numerous hormones; often referred to as "the master gland"
plantar flexion: to bend toward the sole of the foot
polydactyly: extra fingers or toes
portoenterostomy: a connection created from the portal system to the GI system, specifically diverting bile from liver tracts to jejunum
postmature infant: infant born after 42 weeks of gestation
postneonatal mortality: infant deaths occurring between the ages of 28 days and 1 year
preload: amount of stretch of the myocardial fibers before contraction; most easily measured by determining central venous pressure (CVP)
preparation: providing the child with information in advance of procedures, treatments, and/or events in order to facilitate coping
preterm infant: infant born before 38 weeks of gestation
primary sexual characteristics: internal and external reproductive organs in males and females (i.e., uterus, fallopian tubes, testes, spermatic cord)
prodrome: the initial stage of a disease; symptoms indicative of an approaching disease
professional boundaries: self-awareness that allows an individual to recognize the differences between professional and personal relationships and maintain these in work settings
profound hearing loss: failure to hear above 96 dB
projectile vomiting: vomiting that is projected with force, perhaps 2 to 4 feet away from the mouth; may be preceded by deep gastric left to right peristaltic waves; characteristic of pyloric stenosis
proteinuria: protein in the urine
protocol: a systematic plan of care outlining drug therapy and follow-up based on research in cancer therapy
pruritus: itching
pseudarthrosis: failure of the bones to fuse
pseudostrabismus: not a true strabismus; the eyes appear to deviate inward, but are actually in alignment; the appearance of misalignment is caused by facial features such as epicanthal folds and a broad, flat nasal bridge
puberty: the period of time during which adolescents experience a growth spurt, develop secondary sex characteristics, and achieve reproductive maturity
pubescence: the period of time prior to sexual maturity characterized by the development of breast tissue and pubic hair in females and genital growth and pubic hair in males
pulmonary edema: collection of excessive fluid in the alveoli of the lungs
pulmonary hypertension: increased pressure in the pulmonary arteries and arterioles
pulmonary vascular resistance: the amount of resistance in the pulmonary arteries against which the right heart must pump
pulmonary venous congestion: increased pulmonary pressure leading to the accumulation of excessive fluid and blood in the pulmonary veins
pylorus: the distal opening of the stomach where the stomach contents pass into the duodenum; surrounded by muscle bands
pyramidal tract: descending pathway of the upper motor neuron concerned with voluntary movement

recommended dietary allowance (RDA): recommendations for the average amounts of nutrients that should be consumed daily by healthy people in the United States

reduction: the repositioning of bone fragments into normal alignment

regression: use of behavior that is more appropriate to an earlier stage of development; often used to cope with stress or anxiety

regurgitation: an abnormal backward flow (i.e., blood through a heart valve)

renal scarring: area of nonfunction in the kidney

reproductive maturity: the establishment of menstruation/ovulation in females and the development of spermatogenesis in males

retention: the application of a device or mechanism that will maintain alignment of bone until healing occurs

reticulocyte: immature red blood cells; normal value for children is 1%

reticuloendothelial system: the collection of cells, throughout the body, which are capable of phagocytosis

retractions: abnormal movement of the chest walls during inspiration; may occur intercostally and substernally

rhonchi: adventitious breath sounds caused by the passage of air through an airway obstructed by thick secretions; do not clear with coughing

risk-taking behaviors: behaviors that predispose the adolescent to physical or psychosocial harm

ritualism: the need to maintain sameness and reliability

secondary glaucoma: increased intraocular fluid that occurs after age 3 and may be the result of disease or surgery

secondary sexual characteristics: physical characteristics of males and females influenced by reproduction hormones, but having no direct role in reproduction (i.e., voice, body shape, pubic hair distribution)

self-esteem: the personal value that an individual places on himself or herself

sensorimotor stage: Piaget's first stage of cognitive development in which the infant and young toddler use mainly senses and movement to begin to understand and control their environment

sensorineural hearing loss: result of damage or malformation of the middle ear and/or auditory nerve; hearing loss is usually permanent

sensory information: sharing concepts with children using techniques that incorporate sight, taste, touch, smell, and hearing

separation anxiety: distress and apprehension caused by being removed from parents, home, or familiar surroundings

severe hearing loss: failure to hear 66 to 95 dB

sexual maturity rating (SMR): stages of sexual maturation based on pubic hair and breast development in girls and pubic hair and genital development in boys

shock: inadequate tissue perfusion, usually caused by illness or injury, that causes respiratory or cardiovascular compromise

shunt: abnormal blood flow from one side of the heart to the other

situational crisis: unanticipated event that poses a threat to an individual's psychosocial or psychologic well-being

small for gestational age infant (SGA): may be two types: (1) symmetrical, in which the whole body, including the head, is involved; and (2) asymmetrical (most common), in which the body is starved in appearance, but the head of normal size

specific immune functions: a humoral (B cell and antibody production) and cell-mediated (T cell) response that is activated in a highly discriminatory way to antigens that survive in the body

spica cast: a cast used to immobilize the hips that extends from above the waist to the knees or ankles

Standard Precautions: infection control guidelines developed by the National Center for Infectious Disease (NCID) and the Hospital Control Practices Advisory Committee (HICPAC) to prevent the spread of infectious organisms from blood, body fluids, secretions and excretions, mucous membranes, and nonintact skin

stenosis: the narrowing or constriction of an opening (such as a heart valve)

strabismus: squint or lazy eye: a condition in which the eyes are not straight due to lack of coordination of the extraocular muscles; most often due to muscle imbalance or paralysis of the extraocular muscles, but may also result from conditions such as a brain tumor, myasthenia gravis, or infection

stranger anxiety: the ability of an infant to distinguish between caregivers and others, to prefer parents over other caregivers, and to become distressed when separation occurs

stress: any situation or condition, positive or negative, requiring adjustment on the part of the individual, family, or group

stridor: a shrill, harsh sound that can be heard during inspiration or expiration, or both; produced by the flow of air through a narrowed segment of the respiratory tract

subconjunctival hemorrhage: bleeding situated beneath the conjunctiva. In children the most frequent cause is trauma, or after severe coughing or sneezing episodes (Valsalva maneuvers). Also caused by *S. pneumoniae* and *haemophilus*.

subluxation: partial dislocation of a joint

submersion injury: injury resulting from a near-drowning incident. Such an injury may be immediately apparent or may appear up to 48 hours after the submersion incident.

substance abuse: excessive or inappropriate use of medication in order to modify mood or behavior or in a manner that results in social, occupational, psychological, or physical problems, or in a situation that creates a physical hazard

substance addiction: a physical or psychological dependence on a substance, with continued use even when it is known to impair cognitive or social functioning

substance dependence: a physical or psychological craving for a chemical stubstance, the cessation of which causes withdrawal symptoms

suicide: a voluntary and intentional cessation of one's life

suicide attempt: any actions taken by an individual toward self that will result in death if not interrupted

suicide gesture: a suicide attempt that is undertaken primarily to get attention rather than to actually take one's life; nonetheless, it is still considered serious behavior

suicide threat: a statement or behavior that usually occurs prior to overt suicidal activity

superior mesenteric artery syndrome: a condition resembling intestinal obstruction caused by reduced blood supply to a segment of the mesentery

surrogate play: offering to play for a child who is too ill or immobilized or who lacks physical stamina to sustain play interactions on his or her own

sustained-release medication: medication designed to be taken in its complete form; it slowly dissolves and releases medication into the bloodstream over a specified length of time (usually 12–24 hours)
symbolic play: uses games and interactions that represent an issue or concern to be addressed
symbolic thought: ability to allow a mental image (word or object) to represent something else that is not present
syndactyly: fusion or webbing of two or more fingers or toes
systematic assessment: following an organized method to collect data
systemic vascular resistance: the amount of resistance in the systemic arteries against which the left heart must pump
systemic venous congestion: increased systemic venous pressure leading to the accumulation of excessive fluid in the systemic veins
tachycardia: increased heart rate compared to norms for age
tachypnea: increased respiratory rate
tenesmus: ineffective, painful, or continuous urge to defecate
term newborn: infant born between 38 and 42 weeks of gestation
terminal care: a philosophy of care for the dying child in a hospital setting that is based on the tenet that the remaining time is precious for both the patient and the family. During terminal care, procedures and treatments deemed necessary for comfort and pain relief are arranged so as not to disrupt the family. Such care is provided on a 24-hour basis and reflects the needs and desires of the family.
therapeutic play: guided play that promotes the psychophysiologic well-being of a child
thrombocyte: platelet; necessary for blood clotting
tissue perfusion: the amount of blood flow distributed to an area
toddler: child between the ages of 12 and 36 months
toxin: a poison produced by pathogenic microorganisms
transcutaneous electrical nerve stimulation (TENS): a method of producing electroanalgesia through electrodes applied to the skin
transductive reasoning: reasoning from the particular to the particular rather than from the general to the particular
transmural: through all layers of the wall of a cavity
trauma: injury from an external cause, such as a motor vehicle accident, gunshot wound, or stabbing. Trauma may be self-inflicted, may be deliberately inflicted or accidental, and may be physical or psychological.
trauma score: a numeric score assessed by health care providers to determine the condition of patients. The score usually results from adding, subtracting, dividing, or multiplying numbers representing physiologic parameters or specific types of injuries. These scores are used for field triage and are assessed serially to determine whether a patient's condition is improving or deteriorating.
triage: a sorting process used to decide the urgency of a patient's illness or injury and allocate appropriate resources effectively. The purpose of triage is to assure that the most seriously ill or injured patients receive the highest level of care possible.
-tropia: continuous misalignment of the eye
trust: the basic emotion established during infancy as a result of satisfying interactions between child and caregiver that provides the foundation upon which a healthy personality is built
tunneled central line: surgically placed central line held in place by a Dacron cuff located in a subcutaneous tunnel; most commonly placed in the external jugular vein
urgency: sudden urge to urinate
urticaria (hives): vascular reaction of the skin characterized by pruritic wheals, often caused by allergy or emotional stress
valgum: abnormal position of a limb that involves bending away from the midline of the body. Genu valgum results in knock-knees.
valve: an opening, covered by membranous flaps; when closed, normally no blood passes through
valvuloplasty: opening of a valve using mechanical means
varum: abnormal position of the limb that involves bending toward the midline of the body. Genu varum results in bowlegs.
vector: a carrier that transfers an ineffective agent from one host to another
vernix caseosa: cheesy, white substance composed of epitrichium (outer layer of embryonic skin) cells and secretions from the sebaceous glands; appears at about 20 weeks of fetal life and is present until about 42 weeks of gestational age
villi: finger-like projections in the mucosa of the intestine; responsible for absorption
violence: the use of extreme force or destructive action that results in injury, discordance, or outrage, and/or engaging in sudden intense activity to the point of loss of control
virulence: the ability of an organism to produce its effect
visual accommodation: ability to focus on distant and near objects
wheezing: high-pitched, musical whistles, heard with or without a stethoscope, which may be inspiratory or expiratory and which are caused by bronchial constriction or obstruction of the airway; commonly occurs in asthma
WIC: the special supplemental food program for women, infants, and children that provides nutritious food and nutrition education to low-income pregnant and postpartum women and their children.
win/win solution: establishment of a common goal, as resolution to a conflict, that both parties can support
xenograft: a skin donation from another species of animal; heterograft

APPENDICES

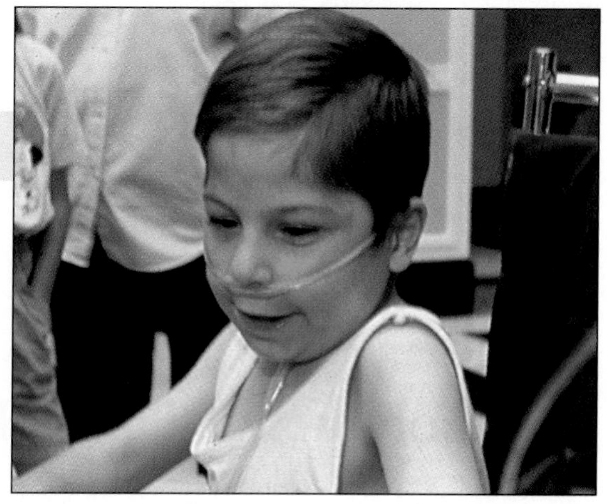

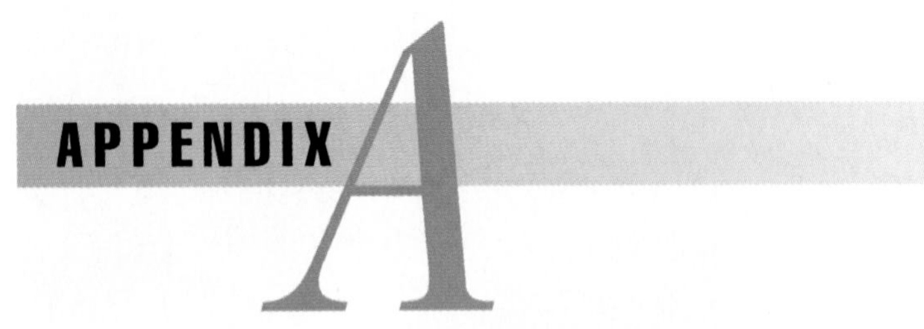

Recommended Childhood Immunization Schedule

United States, July–December 1996

Vaccines are listed under the routinely recommended ages. Shaded bars indicate range of acceptable ages for vaccination. Red shaded bars indicate *catch-up vaccination:* at 11–12 years of age, hepatitis B vaccine should be administered to children not previously vaccinated, and Varicella Zoster Virus vaccine should be administered to children not previously vaccinated who lack a reliable history of chickenpox.

Age ▶ / Vaccine ▼	Birth	1 mo	2 mo	4 mo	6 mo	12 mo	15 mo	18 mo	4–6 yrs	11–12 yrs	14–16 yrs
Hepatitis B[1,2]	Hep B-1										
			Hep B-2		Hep B-3					Hep B[2]	
Diptheria, Tetanus, Pertussis[3]			DTP	DTP	DTP	DTP[3] (DTaP at 15+ m)			DTP or DTaP	Td	
H. influenzae type b[4]			Hib	Hib	Hib[4]	Hib[4]					
Polio[5]			OPV[5]	OPV	OPV				OPV		
Measles, Mumps, Rubella[6]						MMR			MMR[6] or	MMR[6]	
Varicella Zoster Virus Vaccine[7]						Var				Var[7]	

[1]*Infants born to HBsAg-negative mothers* should receive 2.5 μg of Merck vaccine (Recombivax HB) or 10 μg of SmithKline Beecham (SB) vaccine (Engerix-B). The 2nd dose should be administered ≥1 mo after the 1st dose. *Infants born to HBsAg-positive mothers* should receive 0.5 mL hepatitis B immune globulin (HBIG) within 12 hrs of birth, and either 5 μg of Merck vaccine (Recombivax HB) or 10 μg of SB vaccine (Engerix-B) at a separate site. The 2nd dose is recommended at 1–2 mos of age and the 3rd dose at 6 mos of age. *Infants born to mothers whose HBsAg status is unknown* should receive either 5 μg of Merck vaccine (Recombivax HB) or 10 μg of SB vaccine (Engerix-B) within 12 hrs of birth. The 2nd dose of vaccine is recommended at 1 mo of age and the 3rd dose at 6 mos of age.

[2]Adolescents who have not previously received 3 doses of hepatitis B vaccine should initiate or complete the series at the 11–12-year-old visit. The 2nd dose should be administered at least 1 mo after the 1st dose, and the 3rd dose should be administered at least 4 mos after the 1st dose and at least 2 mos after the 2nd dose.

[3]DTP4 may be administered at 12 mos of age, if at least 6 mos have elapsed since DTP3. DTaP (diphtheria and tetanus toxoids and acellular pertussis vaccine) is licensed for the 4th and/or 5th vaccine dose(s) for children aged ≥15 mos and may be preferred for these doses in this age group. Td (tetanus and diphtheria toxoids, adsorbed, for adult use) is recommended at 11–12 years of age if at least 5 years have elapsed since the last dose of DTP, DTaP, or DT.

[4]Three *H. influenzae* type b (Hib) conjugate vaccines are licensed for infant use. If PRP-OMP (PedvaxHIB [Merck]) is administered at 2 and 4 mos of age, a dose at 6 mos is not required. After completing the primary series, any Hib conjugate vaccine may be used as a booster.

[5]Oral poliovirus vaccine (OPV) is recommended for routine infant vaccination. Inactivated poliovirus vaccine (IPV) is recommended for persons with a congenital or acquired immune deficiency disease or an altered immune status as a result of disease or immunosuppressive therapy, as well as their household contacts, and is an acceptable alternative for other persons. The primary 3-dose series for IPV should be given with a minimum interval of 4 wks between the 1st and 2nd doses and 6 mos between the 2nd and 3rd doses.

[6]The 2nd dose of MMR is routinely recommended at 4–6 yrs of age or at 11–12 yrs of age, but may be administered at any visit, provided at least 1 mo has elapsed since receipt of the 1st dose.

[7]Varicella zoster virus vaccine (Var) can be administered to susceptible children any time after 12 months of age. Unvaccinated children who lack a reliable history of chickenpox should be vaccinated at the 11–12-year-old visit.

Approved by the Advisory Committee on Immunization Practices (ACIP), the American Academy of Pediatrics (AAP), and the American Academy of Family Physicians (AAFP). From American Academy of Pediatrics, Committee on Infectious Diseases. Recommended childhood immunization schedule, United States, July–December 1996. *Pediatrics* 1996;97:158–160.

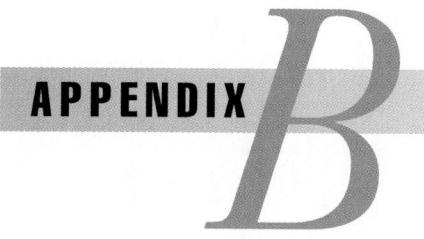

Recommendations for Preventive Pediatric Health Care

Committee on Practice and Ambulatory Medicine

Each child and family is unique; therefore, these **Recommendations for Preventive Pediatric Health Care** are designed for the care of children who are receiving competent parenting, have no manifestations of any important health problems, and are growing and developing in satisfactory fashion. **Additional visits may become necessary** if circumstances suggest variations from normal.

These guidelines represent a consensus by the Committee on Practice and Ambulatory Medicine in consultation with national committees and sections of the American Academy of Pediatrics. The Committee emphasizes the great importance of **continuity of care** in comprehensive health supervision and the need to avoid **fragmentation of care.**

A **prenatal visit** is recommended for parents who are at high risk, for first-time parents, and for those who request a conference. The prenatal visit should include anticipatory guidance and pertinent medical history. Every infant should have a newborn evaluation after birth.

	INFANCY[3]								EARLY CHILDHOOD[3]					MIDDLE CHILDHOOD[3]				ADOLESCENCE[3]										
AGE[4]	NEWBORN[1]	2-4d[2]	By 1mo	2mo	4mo	6mo	9mo	12mo	15mo	18mo	24mo	3y	4y	5y	6y	8y	10y	11y	12y	13y	14y	15y	16y	17y	18y	19y	20y	21y
HISTORY																												
Initial/Interval	•	•	•	•	•	•	•	•	•	•	•	•	•	•	•	•	•	•	•	•	•	•	•	•	•	•	•	•
MEASUREMENTS																												
Height and Weight	•	•	•	•	•	•	•	•	•	•	•	•	•	•	•	•	•	•	•	•	•	•	•	•	•	•	•	•
Head Circumference	•	•	•	•	•	•	•	•	•	•	•																	
Blood Pressure												•	•	•	•	•	•	•	•	•	•	•	•	•	•	•	•	•
SENSORY SCREENING																												
Vision	S	S	S	S	S	S	S	S	S	S	S	O[5]	O	O	S	S	O	S	O	S	S	O	S	S	O	S	S	S
Hearing[6]	S/O	S	S	S	S	S	S	S	S	S	S	O	O	O	S	S	O	S	O	S	S	O	S	S	O	S	S	S
DEVELOPMENTAL/ BEHAVIORAL ASSESSMENT[7]	•	•	•	•	•	•	•	•	•	•	•	•	•	•	•	•	•	•	•	•	•	•	•	•	•	•	•	•
PHYSICAL EXAMINATION[8]	•	•	•	•	•	•	•	•	•	•	•	•	•	•	•	•	•	•	•	•	•	•	•	•	•	•	•	•
PROCEDURES – GENERAL[9]																												
Hereditary/Metabolic Screening[10]	←	—	•																									
Immunization[11]	•—	—	→	•	•	•		←	•	→			←	•	→			•—	—	—	—	—	→					
Lead Screening[12]							•—	→			•																	
Hematocrit or Hemoglobin			←	—	—	—	•											←	—	—	—	•[13]	—	—	—	—	—	→
Urinalysis														•				←	—	—	—	•[14]	—	—	—	—	—	→
PROCEDURES – PATIENTS AT RISK																												
Tuberculin Test[15]								*	*	*	*	*	*	*	*	*	*	*	*	*	*	*	*	*	*	*	*	*
Cholesterol Screening[16]											*	*	*	*	*	*	*	*	*	*	*	*	*	*	*	*	*	*
STD Screening[17]																		*	*	*	*	*	*	*	*	*	*	*
Pelvic Exam[18]																		*	*	*	*	*	*	←*	*	*[18]	*	*→
ANTICIPATORY GUIDANCE[19]	•	•	•	•	•	•	•	•	•	•	•	•	•	•	•	•	•	•	•	•	•	•	•	•	•	•	•	•
Injury Prevention[20]	•	•	•	•	•	•	•	•	•	•	•	•	•	•	•	•	•	•	•	•	•	•	•	•	•	•	•	•
INITIAL DENTAL REFERRAL[21]								←	—	—	—	•																

1. Breastfeeding encouraged and instruction and support offered.
2. For newborns discharged in less than 48 hours after delivery.
3. Developmental, psychosocial, and chronic disease issues for children and adolescents may require frequent counseling and treatment visits separate from preventive care visits.
4. If a child comes under care for the first time at any point on the schedule, or if any items are not accomplished at the suggested age, the schedule should be brought up to date at the earliest possible time.
5. If the patient is uncooperative, rescreen within six months.
6. Some experts recommend objective appraisal of hearing in the newborn period. The Joint Committee on Infant Hearing has identified patients at significant risk for hearing loss. All children meeting these criteria should be objectively screened. See the Joint Committee on Infant Hearing 1994 Position Statement.
7. By history and appropriate physical examination: if suspicious, by specific objective developmental testing.
8. At each visit, a complete physical examination is essential, with infant totally unclothed, older child undressed and suitably draped.
9. These may be modified, depending upon entry point into schedule and individual need.
10. Metabolic screening (eg, thyroid, hemoglobinopathies, PKU, galactosemia) should be done according to state law.
11. Schedule(s) per the Committee on Infectious Diseases, published periodically in *Pediatrics*. Every visit should be an opportunity to update and complete a child's immunizations.
12. Blood lead screen per AAP statement "Lead Poisoning: From Screening to Primary Prevention" (1993).
13. All menstruating adolescents should be screened.
14. Conduct dipstick urinalysis for leukocytes for male and female adolescents.
15. TB testing per AAP statement "Screening for Tuberculosis in Infants and Children" (1994). Testing should be done upon recognition of high risk factors. If results are negative but high risk situation continues, testing should be repeated on an annual basis.
16. Cholesterol screening for high risk patients per AAP "Statement on Cholesterol" (1992). If family history cannot be ascertained and other risk factors are present, screening should be at the discretion of the physician.
17. All sexually active patients should be screened for sexually transmitted diseases (STDs).
18. All sexually active females should have a pelvic examination. A pelvic examination and routine pap smear should be offered as part of preventive health maintenance between the ages of 18 and 21 years.
19. Appropriate discussion and counseling should be an integral part of each visit for care.
20. From birth to age 12, refer to AAP's injury prevention program (TIPP®) as described in "A Guide to Safety Counseling in Office Practice" (1994).
21. Earlier initial dental evaluations may be appropriate for some children. Subsequent examinations as prescribed by dentist.

Key: • = to be performed   * = to be performed for patients at risk   S = subjective, by history   O = objective, by a standard testing method   ←•→ = the range during which a service may be provided, with the dot indicating the preferred age.

NB: Special chemical, immunologic, and endocrine testing is usually carried out upon specific indications. Testing other than newborn (eg, inborn errors of metabolism, sickle disease, etc.) is discretionary with the physician.

The recommendations in this publication do not indicate an exclusive course of treatment or serve as a standard of medical care. Variations, taking into account individual circumstances, may be appropriate.

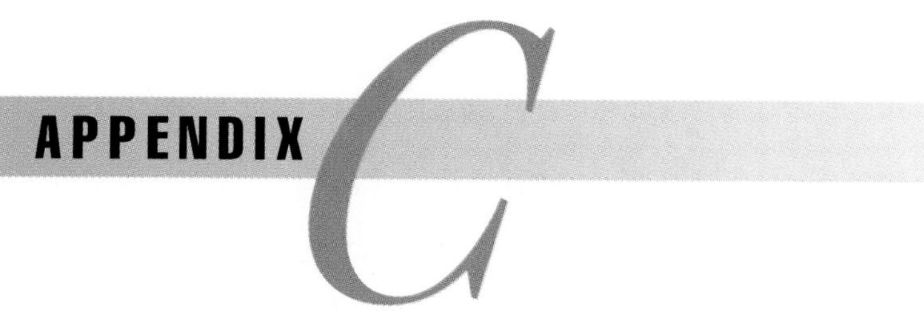

Growth Charts

Ross
Growth &
Development
Program

GROWTH RECORD FOR INFANTS*
BIRTH TO 1 YEAR,
SEXES COMBINED

NAME: ______________

DATE OF BIRTH: ______________

I.D. NO.: ______________

HEAD CIRC (cm): 22 24 26 28 30 32 34 36 38 40 42 44 46

LENGTH (cm): 44 48 52 56 60 64 68 72 76 80

WEIGHT (kg): 1.0 1.5 2.0 2.5 3.0 3.5 4.0 4.5 5.0 6.0 7.0 8.0 9.0 10 11

Length (left scale): 32 36 40

Head circ (right scale): 42 44 46

26 28 30 32 34 36 40 (Weeks)

1 2 3 6 9 12 (Months)

▬ Mean
± 1 SD
------ ± 2 SD

DATE	AGE	LENGTH	WEIGHT	HEAD CIRC

DATE	AGE	LENGTH	WEIGHT	HEAD CIRC

*Adapted with permission: Babson SG, Benda GI: Growth graphs for the clinical assessment of infants of varying gestational age. *J Pediatr* 89:814-820, 1976.

Provided as a service of The Ross Hospital Formula System

ROSS LABORATORIES
COLUMBUS, OHIO 43216
Division of Abbott Laboratories, USA

G413(0.05)/DECEMBER 1987 LITHO IN USA

GIRLS: BIRTH TO 36 MONTHS
PHYSICAL GROWTH
NCHS PERCENTILES*

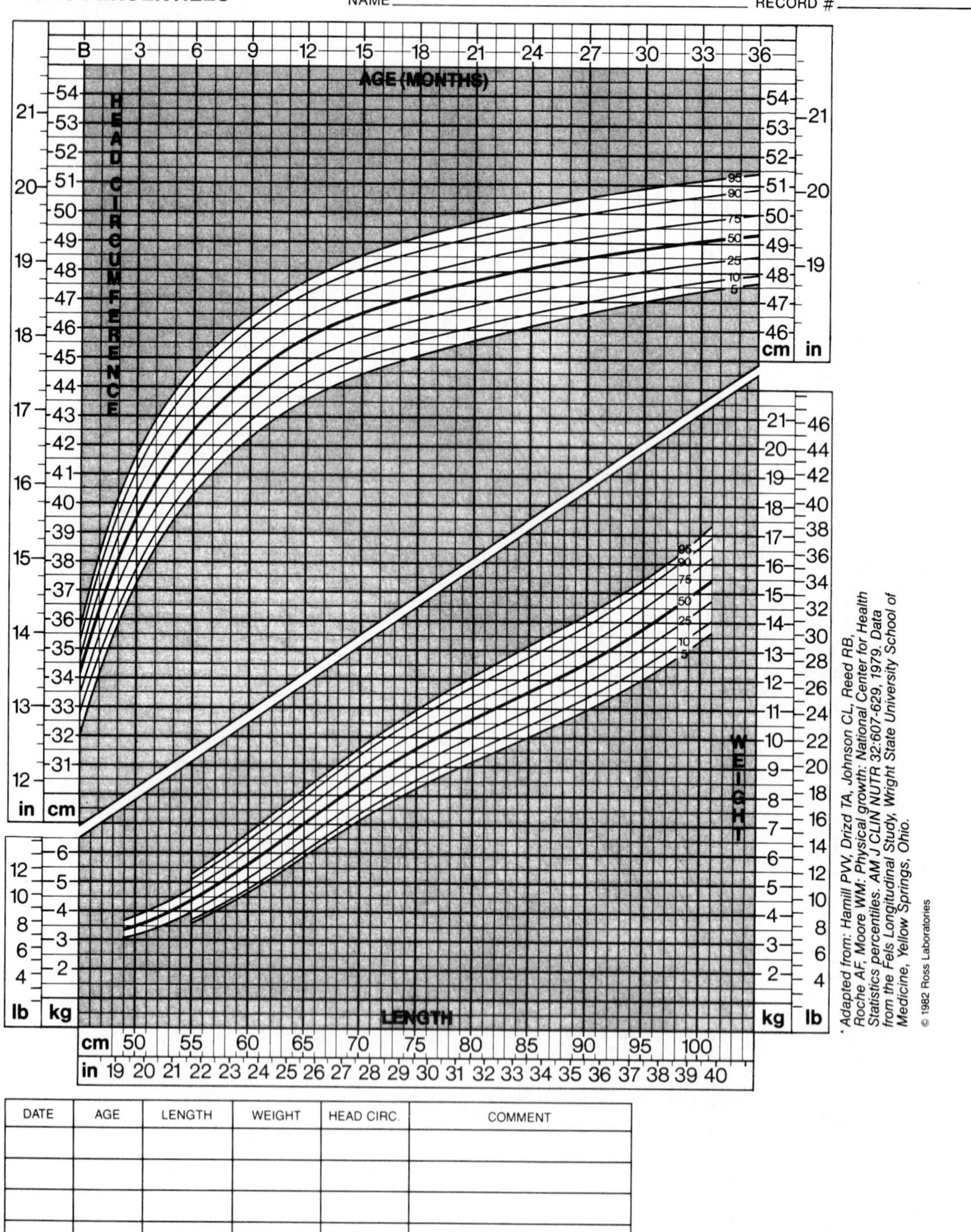

DATE	AGE	LENGTH	WEIGHT	HEAD CIRC.	COMMENT

GIRLS: BIRTH TO 36 MONTHS
PHYSICAL GROWTH
NCHS PERCENTILES*

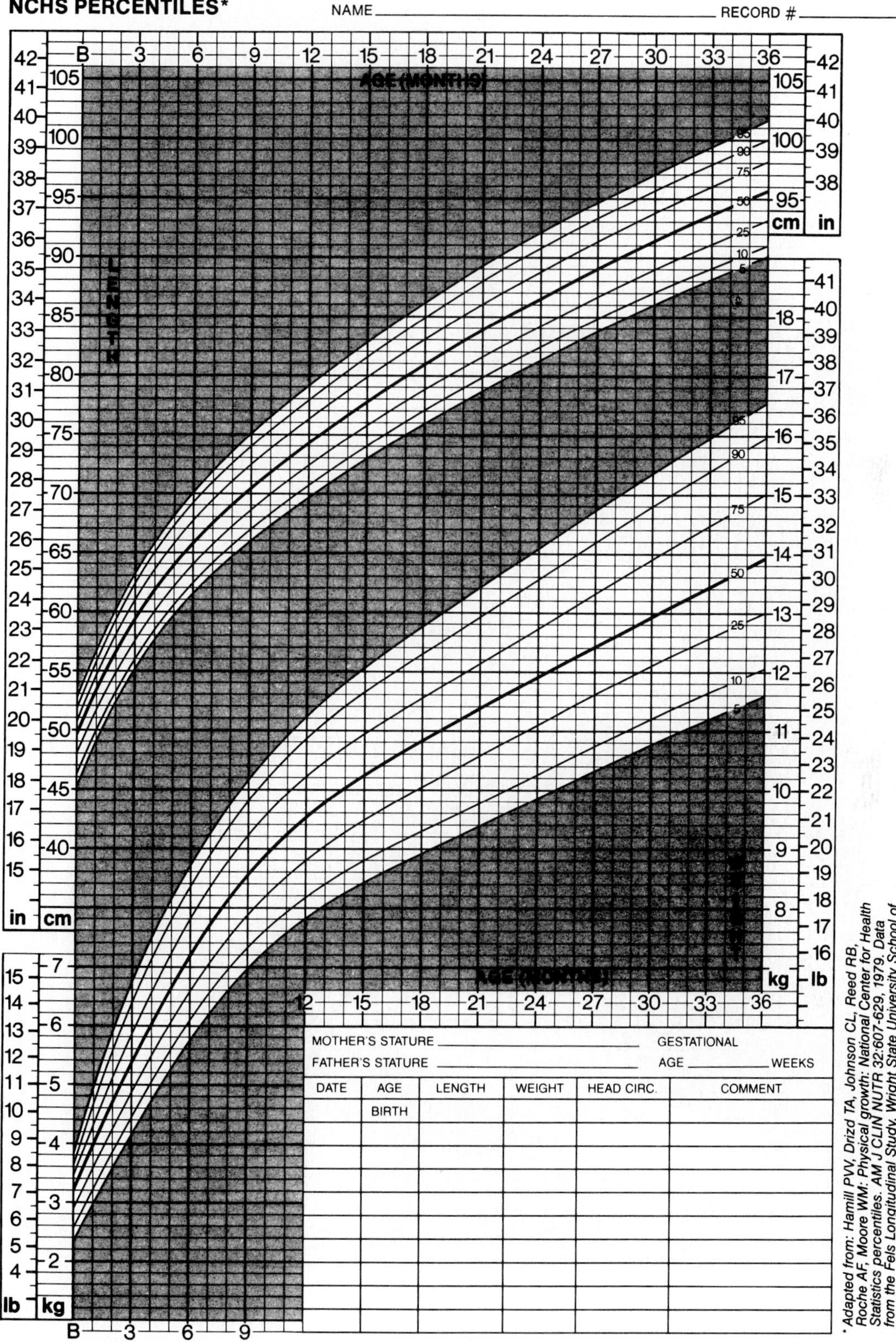

* Adapted from: Hamill PVV, Drizd TA, Johnson CL, Reed RB, Roche AF, Moore WM: Physical growth: National Center for Health Statistics percentiles. AM J CLIN NUTR 32:607-629, 1979. Data from the Fels Longitudinal Study, Wright State University School of Medicine, Yellow Springs, Ohio.

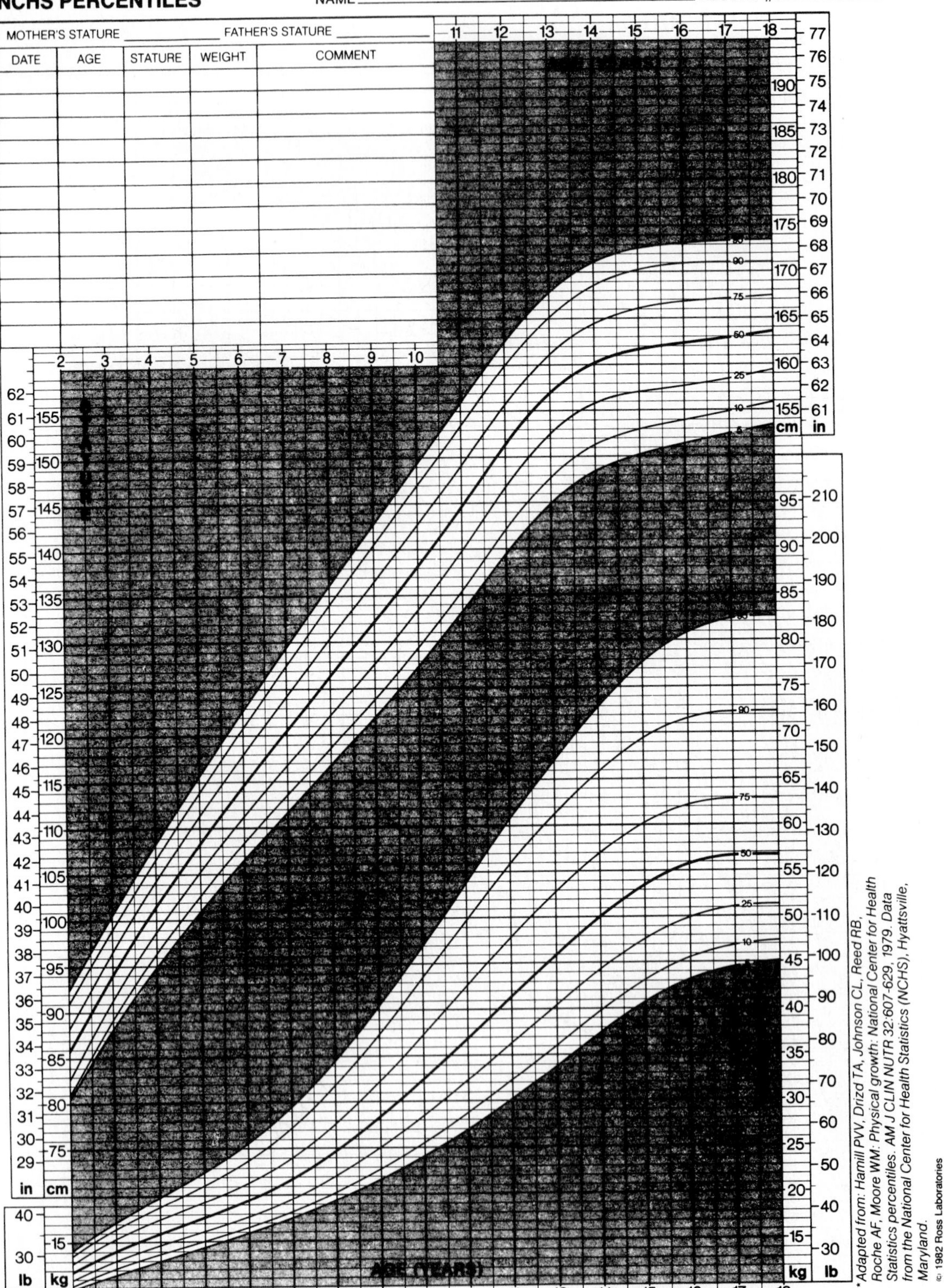

Adapted from Behrman, R. E., Kliegman, R. M., & Arvin, A. M. (1996). *Nelson textbook of pediatrics* (15th ed.). Philadelphia: W. B. Saunders, pp. 2033–2058.

GIRLS: PREPUBESCENT PHYSICAL GROWTH NCHS PERCENTILES*

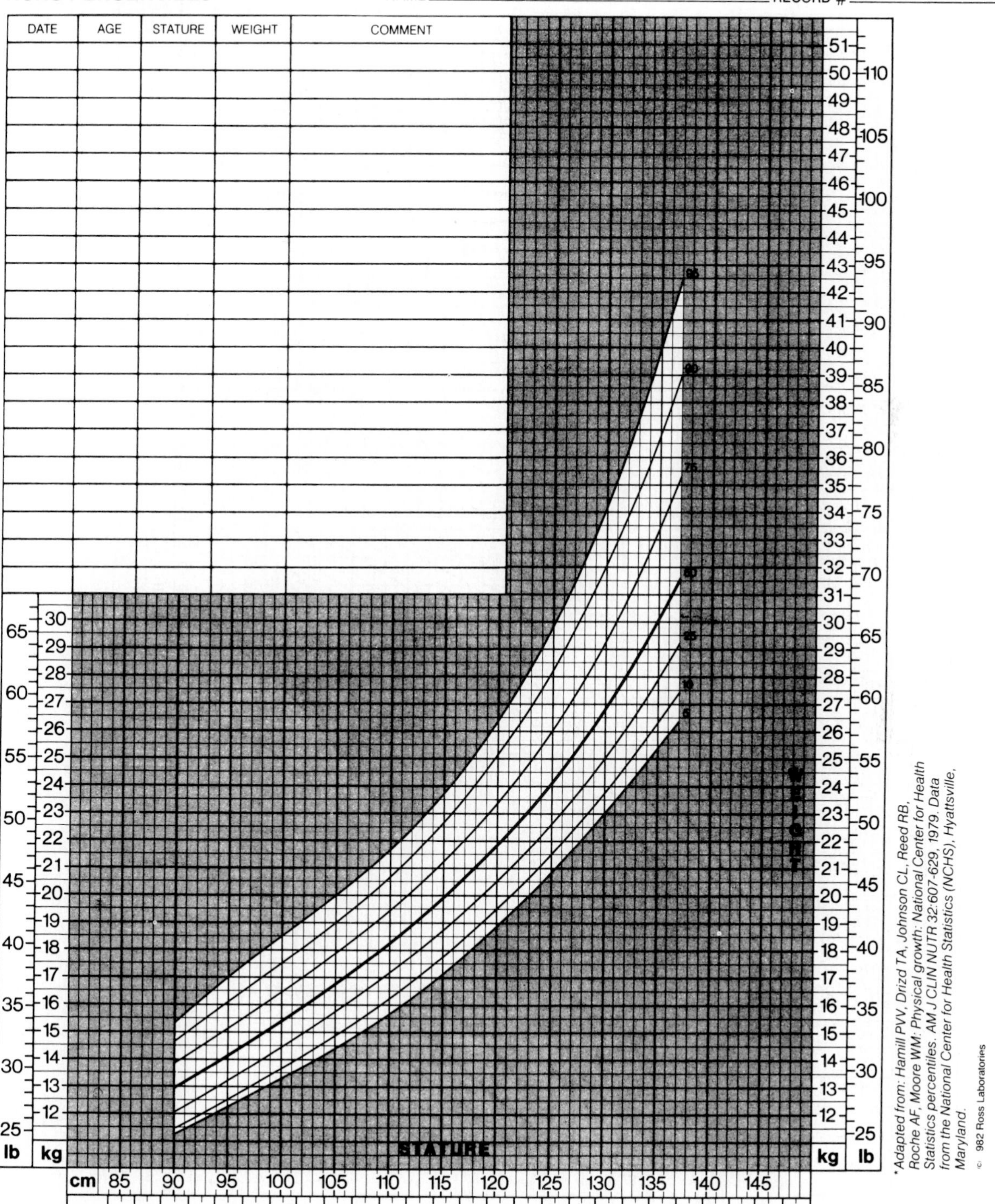

*Adapted from: Hamill PVV, Drizd TA, Johnson CL, Reed RB, Roche AF, Moore WM: Physical growth: National Center for Health Statistics percentiles. AM J CLIN NUTR 32:607-629, 1979. Data from the National Center for Health Statistics (NCHS), Hyattsville, Maryland.

BOYS: BIRTH TO 36 MONTHS PHYSICAL GROWTH NCHS PERCENTILES*

NAME ______________________ RECORD # ______________

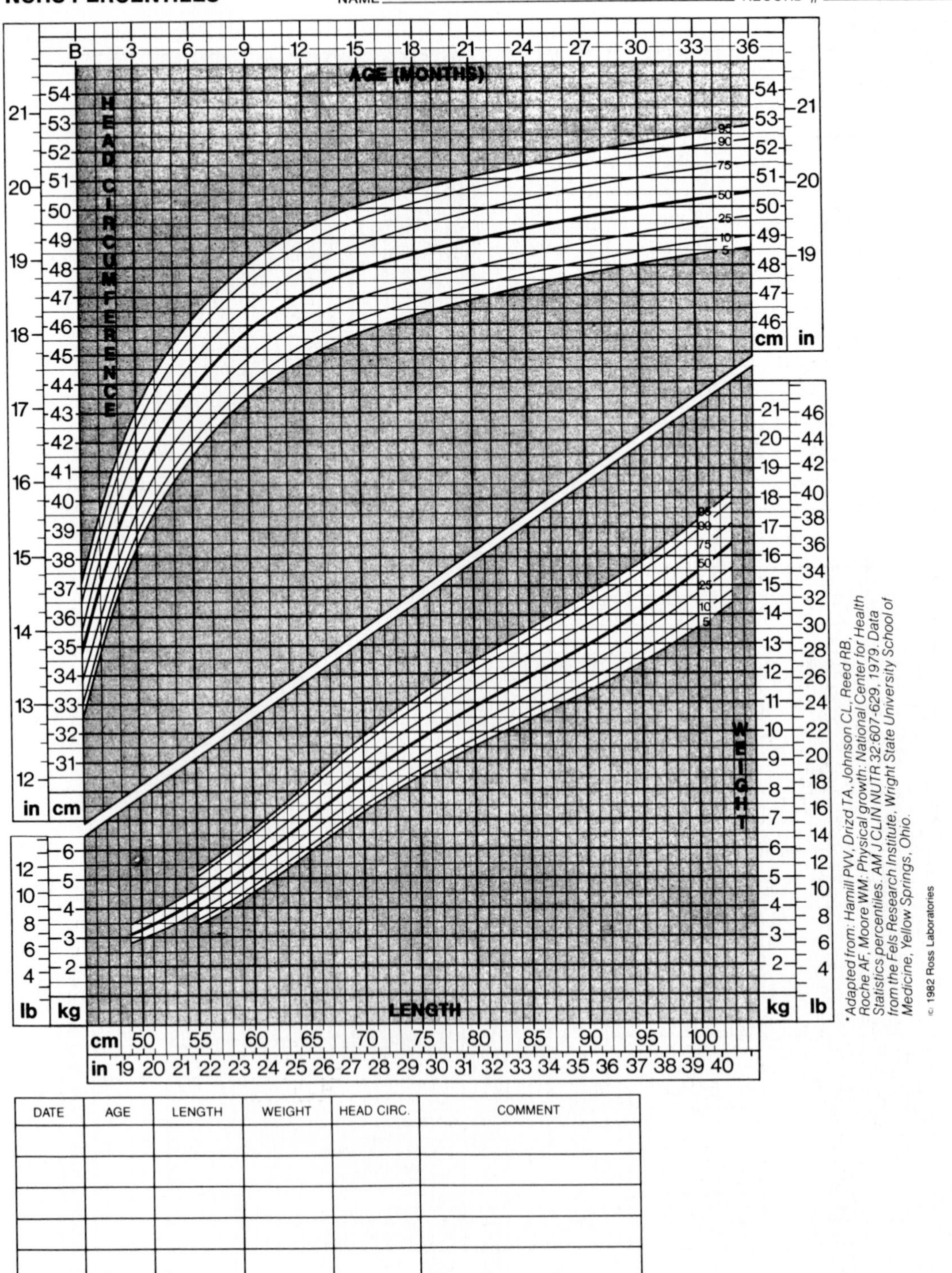

*Adapted from: Hamill PVV, Drizd TA, Johnson CL, Reed RB, Roche AF, Moore WM: Physical growth: National Center for Health Statistics percentiles. AM J CLIN NUTR 32:607-629, 1979. Data from the Fels Research Institute, Wright State University School of Medicine, Yellow Springs, Ohio.

DATE	AGE	LENGTH	WEIGHT	HEAD CIRC.	COMMENT

BOYS: BIRTH TO 36 MONTHS
PHYSICAL GROWTH
NCHS PERCENTILES*

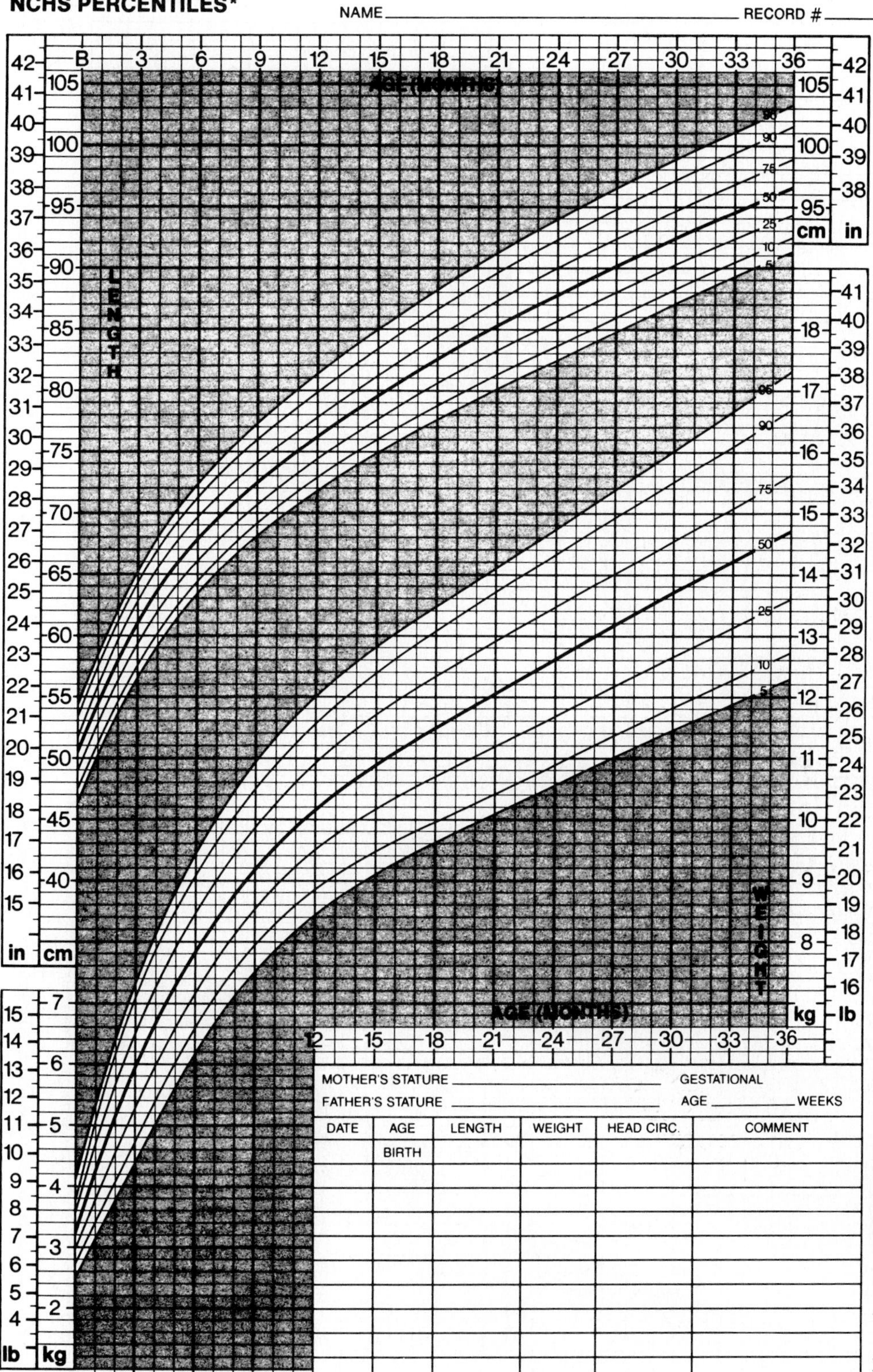

*Adapted from: Hamill PVV, Drizd TA, Johnson CL, Reed RB, Roche AF, Moore WM: Physical growth: National Center for Health Statistics percentiles. AM J CLIN NUTR 32:607-629, 1979. Data from the Fels Research Institute, Wright State University School of Medicine, Yellow Springs, Ohio.

BOYS: 2 TO 18 YEARS PHYSICAL GROWTH NCHS PERCENTILES*

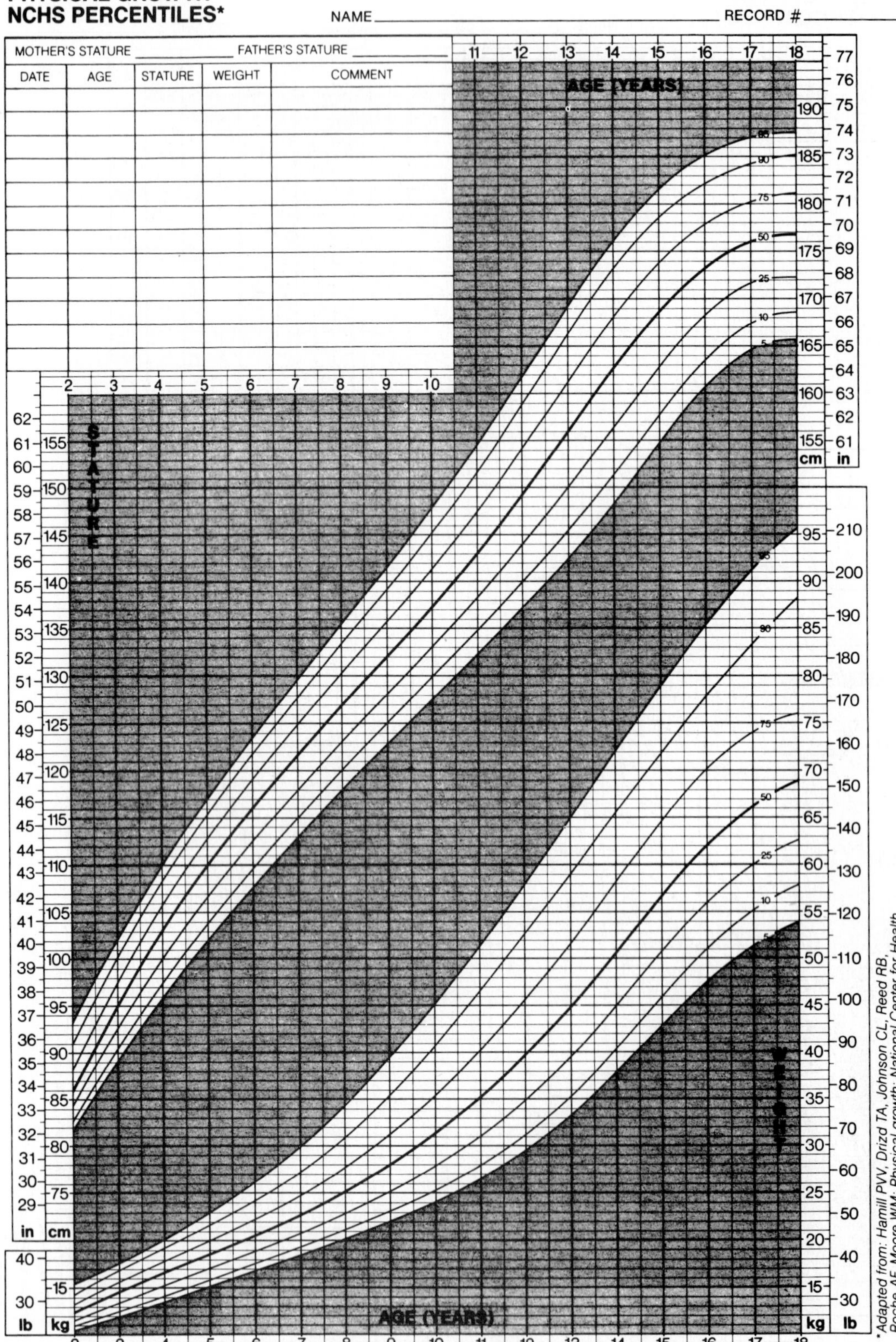

*Adapted from: Hamill PVV, Drizd TA, Johnson CL, Reed RB, Roche AF, Moore WM: Physical growth: National Center for Health Statistics percentiles. AM J CLIN NUTR 32:607-629, 1979. Data from the National Center for Health Statistics (NCHS), Hyattsville, Maryland.

BOYS: PREPUBESCENT PHYSICAL GROWTH NCHS PERCENTILES*

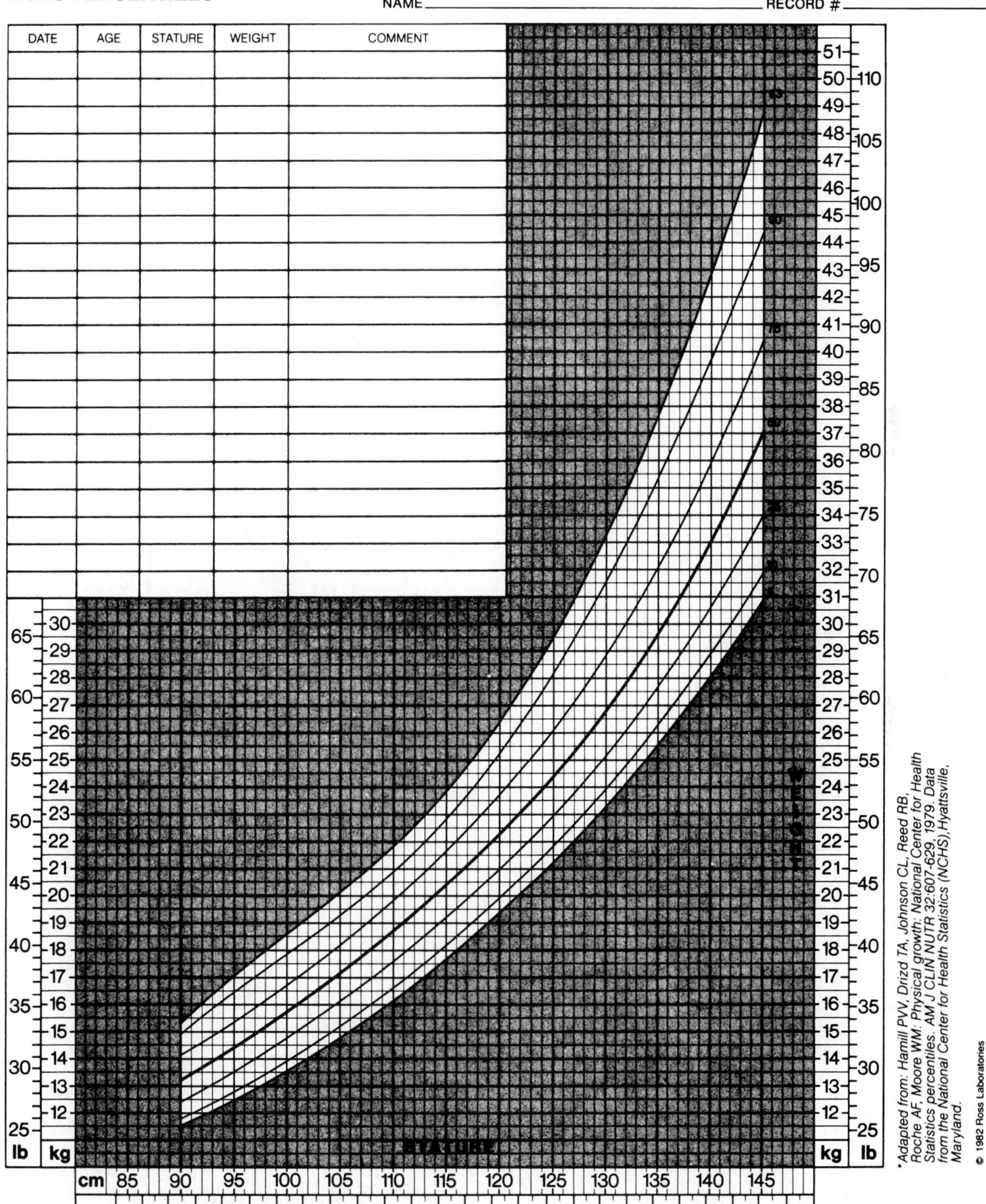

*Adapted from: Hamill PVV, Drizd TA, Johnson CL, Reed RB, Roche AF, Moore WM: Physical growth: National Center for Health Statistics percentiles. AM J CLIN NUTR 32:607-629, 1979. Data from the National Center for Health Statistics (NCHS), Hyattsville, Maryland.

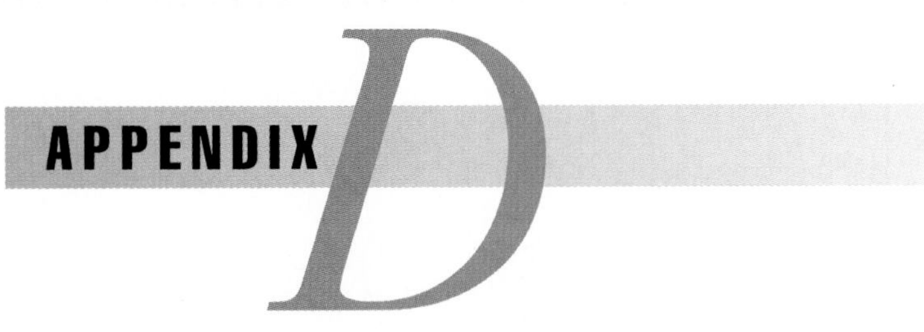

Denver Developmental Screening Test II*

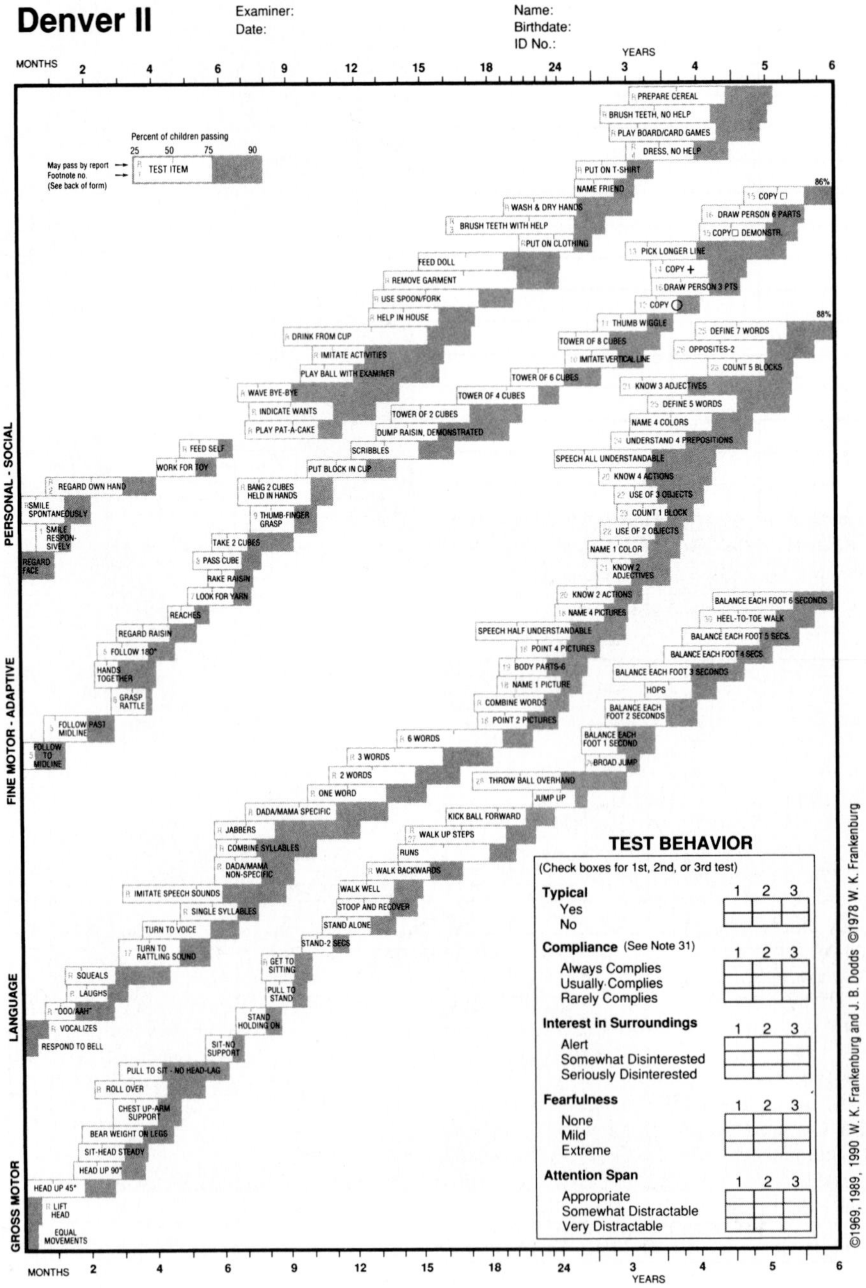

Denver II

Examiner:
Date:

Name:
Birthdate:
ID No.:

MONTHS 2 4 6 9 12 15 18 24 — YEARS 3 4 5 6

Percent of children passing: 25 50 75 90
May pass by report →
Footnote no. →
(See back of form)
TEST ITEM

PERSONAL - SOCIAL

PREPARE CEREAL
BRUSH TEETH, NO HELP
PLAY BOARD/CARD GAMES
DRESS, NO HELP
PUT ON T-SHIRT
NAME FRIEND
WASH & DRY HANDS
BRUSH TEETH WITH HELP
PUT ON CLOTHING
FEED DOLL
REMOVE GARMENT
USE SPOON/FORK
HELP IN HOUSE
DRINK FROM CUP
IMITATE ACTIVITIES
PLAY BALL WITH EXAMINER
WAVE BYE-BYE
INDICATE WANTS
PLAY PAT-A-CAKE
FEED SELF
WORK FOR TOY
REGARD OWN HAND
SMILE SPONTANEOUSLY
SMILE RESPONSIVELY
REGARD FACE

FINE MOTOR - ADAPTIVE

86%
COPY □
DRAW PERSON 6 PARTS
COPY □ DEMONSTR.
PICK LONGER LINE
COPY +
DRAW PERSON 3 PTS
COPY ○
THUMB WIGGLE
TOWER OF 8 CUBES
IMITATE VERTICAL LINE
TOWER OF 6 CUBES
TOWER OF 4 CUBES
TOWER OF 2 CUBES
DUMP RAISIN, DEMONSTRATED
SCRIBBLES
PUT BLOCK IN CUP
BANG 2 CUBES HELD IN HANDS
THUMB-FINGER GRASP
TAKE 2 CUBES
PASS CUBE
RAKE RAISIN
LOOK FOR YARN
REACHES
REGARD RAISIN
FOLLOW 180°
HANDS TOGETHER
GRASP RATTLE
FOLLOW PAST MIDLINE
FOLLOW TO MIDLINE

LANGUAGE

88%
DEFINE 7 WORDS
OPPOSITES-2
COUNT 5 BLOCKS
KNOW 3 ADJECTIVES
DEFINE 5 WORDS
NAME 4 COLORS
UNDERSTAND 4 PREPOSITIONS
SPEECH ALL UNDERSTANDABLE
KNOW 4 ACTIONS
USE OF 3 OBJECTS
COUNT 1 BLOCK
USE OF 2 OBJECTS
NAME 1 COLOR
KNOW 2 ADJECTIVES
KNOW 2 ACTIONS
NAME 4 PICTURES
SPEECH HALF UNDERSTANDABLE
POINT 4 PICTURES
BODY PARTS-6
NAME 1 PICTURE
COMBINE WORDS
POINT 2 PICTURES
6 WORDS
3 WORDS
2 WORDS
ONE WORD
DADA/MAMA SPECIFIC
JABBERS
COMBINE SYLLABLES
DADA/MAMA NON-SPECIFIC
IMITATE SPEECH SOUNDS
SINGLE SYLLABLES
TURN TO VOICE
TURN TO RATTLING SOUND
SQUEALS
LAUGHS
"OOO/AAH"
VOCALIZES
RESPOND TO BELL

GROSS MOTOR

BALANCE EACH FOOT 6 SECONDS
HEEL-TO-TOE WALK
BALANCE EACH FOOT 5 SECS.
BALANCE EACH FOOT 4 SECS.
BALANCE EACH FOOT 3 SECONDS
HOPS
BALANCE EACH FOOT 2 SECONDS
BALANCE EACH FOOT 1 SECOND
BROAD JUMP
THROW BALL OVERHAND
JUMP UP
KICK BALL FORWARD
WALK UP STEPS
RUNS
WALK BACKWARDS
WALK WELL
STOOP AND RECOVER
STAND ALONE
STAND-2 SECS
GET TO SITTING
PULL TO STAND
STAND HOLDING ON
SIT-NO SUPPORT
PULL TO SIT - NO HEAD-LAG
ROLL OVER
CHEST UP-ARM SUPPORT
BEAR WEIGHT ON LEGS
SIT-HEAD STEADY
HEAD UP 90°
HEAD UP 45°
LIFT HEAD
EQUAL MOVEMENTS

TEST BEHAVIOR

(Check boxes for 1st, 2nd, or 3rd test)

Typical	1	2	3
Yes			
No			
Compliance (See Note 31)	1	2	3
Always Complies			
Usually Complies			
Rarely Complies			
Interest in Surroundings	1	2	3
Alert			
Somewhat Disinterested			
Seriously Disinterested			
Fearfulness	1	2	3
None			
Mild			
Extreme			
Attention Span	1	2	3
Appropriate			
Somewhat Distractable			
Very Distractable			

*The Denver II Training Manual is required to administer the test. The Manual and other Denver II materials (kits, forms, training videotapes) can be obtained from Denver Developmental Materials, P.O. Box 6919, Denver, Colorado 80206-0910. Telephone: 303-355-4729 or 800-419-4729.

DIRECTIONS FOR ADMINISTRATION

1. Try to get child to smile by smiling, talking or waving. Do not touch him/her.
2. Child must stare at hand several seconds.
3. Parent may help guide toothbrush and put toothpaste on brush.
4. Child does not have to be able to tie shoes or button/zip in the back.
5. Move yarn slowly in an arc from one side to the other, about 8" above child's face.
6. Pass if child grasps rattle when it is touched to the backs or tips of fingers.
7. Pass if child tries to see where yarn went. Yarn should be dropped quickly from sight from tester's hand without arm movement.
8. Child must transfer cube from hand to hand without help of body, mouth, or table.
9. Pass if child picks up raisin with any part of thumb and finger.
10. Line can vary only 30 degrees or less from tester's line.
11. Make a fist with thumb pointing upward and wiggle only the thumb. Pass if child imitates and does not move any fingers other than the thumb.

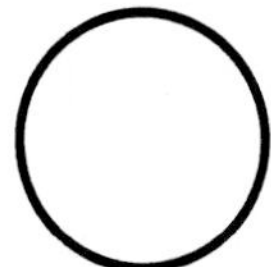

12. Pass any enclosed form. Fail continuous round motions.

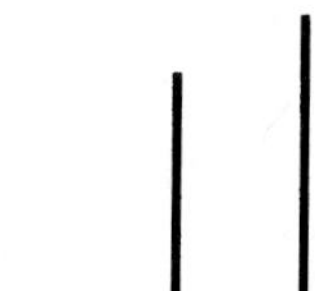

13. Which line is longer? (Not bigger.) Turn paper upside down and repeat. (pass 3 of 3 or 5 of 6)

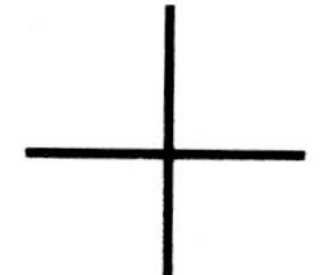

14. Pass any lines crossing near midpoint.

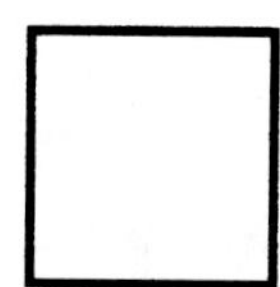

15. Have child copy first. If failed, demonstrate.

When giving items 12, 14, and 15, do not name the forms. Do not demonstrate 12 and 14.

16. When scoring, each pair (2 arms, 2 legs, etc.) counts as one part.
17. Place one cube in cup and shake gently near child's ear, but out of sight. Repeat for other ear.
18. Point to picture and have child name it. (No credit is given for sounds only.) If less than 4 pictures are named correctly, have child point to picture as each is named by tester.

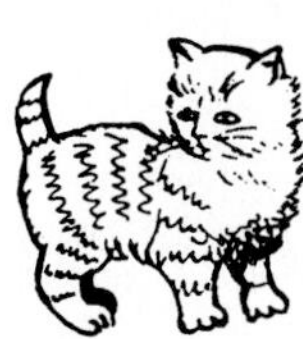
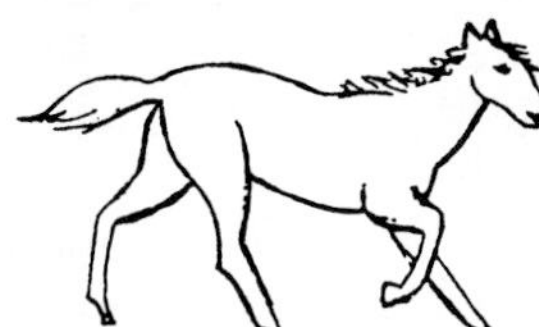
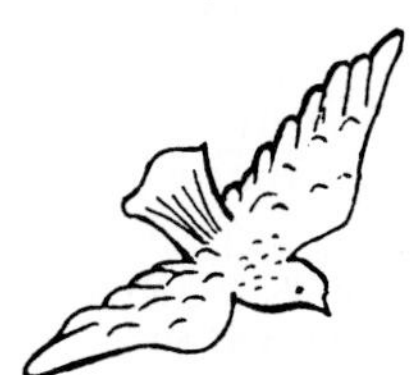
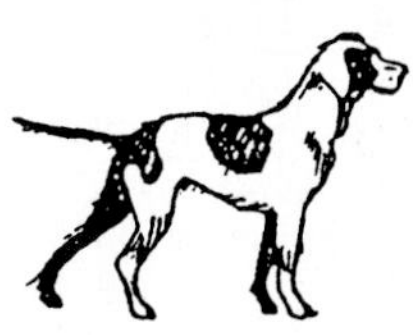
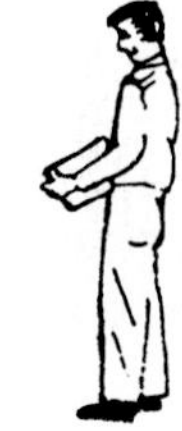

19. Using doll, tell child: Show me the nose, eyes, ears, mouth, hands, feet, tummy, hair. Pass 6 of 8.
20. Using pictures, ask child: Which one flies?... says meow?... talks?... barks?... gallops? Pass 2 of 5, 4 of 5.
21. Ask child: What do you do when you are cold?... tired?... hungry? Pass 2 of 3, 3 of 3.
22. Ask child: What do you do with a cup? What is a chair used for? What is a pencil used for? Action words must be included in answers.
23. Pass if child correctly places and says how many blocks are on paper. (1, 5).
24. Tell child: Put block **on** table; **under** table; **in front of** me, **behind** me. Pass 4 of 4. (Do not help child by pointing, moving head or eyes.)
25. Ask child: What is a ball?... lake?... desk?... house?... banana?... curtain?... fence?... ceiling? Pass if defined in terms of use, shape, what it is made of, or general category (such as banana is fruit, not just yellow). Pass 5 of 8, 7 of 8.
26. Ask child: If a horse is big, a mouse is __? If fire is hot, ice is __? If the sun shines during the day, the moon shines during the __? Pass 2 of 3.
27. Child may use wall or rail only, not person. May not crawl.
28. Child must throw ball overhand 3 feet to within arm's reach of tester.
29. Child must perform standing broad jump over width of test sheet (8 1/2 inches).
30. Tell child to walk forward, ⊂⊃⊂⊃⊂⊃⊂⊃→ heel within 1 inch of toe. Tester may demonstrate. Child must walk 4 consecutive steps.
31. In the second year, half of normal children are non-compliant.

OBSERVATIONS:

DENVER ARTICULATION SCREENING EXAM ▼

DENVER ARTICULATION SCREENING EXAM
for children 2 1/2 to 6 years of age

Instructions: Have child repeat each word after you. Circle the underlined sounds that he pronounces correctly. Total correct sounds is the Raw Score. Use charts on reverse side to score results.

NAME

HOSP. NO.

ADDRESS ______________________

Date: __________ Child's Age: ________ Examiner: ____________________ Raw Score: __________
Percentile: ________ Intelligibility: ______________ Result: ______________________

1. table	6. zipper	11. sock	16. wagon	21. leaf
2. shirt	7. grapes	12. vacuum	17. gum	22. carrot
3. door	8. flag	13. yarn	18. house	
4. trunk	9. thumb	14. mother	19. pencil	
5. jumping	10. toothbrush	15. twinkle	20. fish	

Intelligibility: (circle one)
1. Easy to understand
2. Understandable 1/2 the time.
3. Nct understandable
4. Can't evaluate

Comments:

Date: __________ Child's Age: __________ Examiner: ____________________ Raw Score ________
Percentile: __________ Intelligibility: ______________ Result: ______________________

1. table	6. zipper	11. sock	16. wagon	21. leaf
2. shirt	7. grapes	12. vacuum	17. gum	22. carrot
3. door	8. flag	13. yarn	18. house	
4. trunk	9. thumb	14. mother	19. pencil	
5. jumping	10. toothbrush	15. twinkle	20. fish	

Intelligibility: (circle one)
1. Easy to understand
2. Understandable 1/2 the time.
3. Not understandable
4. Can't evaluate

Comments:

Date: ____________ Child's Age: ________ Examiner: __________________ Raw Score___________
Percentile: ___________ Intelligibility: ______________ Result: ______________________

1. table	6. zipper	11. sock	16. wagon	21. leaf
2. shirt	7. grapes	12. vacuum	17. gum	22. carrot
3. door	8. flag	13. yarn	18. house	
4. trunk	9. thumb	14. mother	19. pencil	
5. jumping	10. toothbrush	15. twinkle	20. fish	

Intelligibility: (circle one)
1. Easy to understand
2. Understandable 1/2 the time.
3. Not understandable
4. Can't evaluate

Appendix continued on following page

DENVER ARTICULATION SCREENING EXAM *Continued* ▼

To score DASE words: Note raw score for child's performance. Match raw score line (extreme left of chart) with column representing child's age (to the closest *previous* age group). Where raw score line and age column meet denotes percentile rank of child's performance when compared with other children that age. Percentiles above heavy line are *abnormal,* below heavy line are *normal.*

PERCENTILE RANK

Raw Score	2.5 yr	3.0 yr	3.5 yr	4.0 yr	4.5 yr	5.0 yr	5.5 yr	6 yr
2	1							
3	2							
4	5							
5	9							
6	16							
7	23							
8	31	2						
9	37	4	1					
10	42	6	2					
11	48	7	4					
12	54	9	6	1	1			
13	58	12	9	2	3	1	1	
14	62	17	11	5	4	2	2	
15	68	23	15	9	5	3	2	
16	75	31	19	12	5	4	3	
17	79	38	25	15	6	6	4	
18	83	46	31	19	8	7	4	
19	86	51	38	24	10	9	5	1
20	89	58	45	30	12	11	7	3
21	92	65	52	36	15	15	9	4
22	94	72	58	43	18	19	12	5
23	96	77	63	50	22	24	15	7
24	97	82	70	58	29	29	20	15
25	99	87	78	66	36	34	26	17
26	99	91	84	75	46	43	34	24
27		94	89	82	57	54	44	34
28		96	94	88	70	68	59	47
29		98	98	94	84	84	77	68
30		100	100	100	100	100	100	100

To score intelligibility:

	NORMAL	ABNORMAL
2.5 years	Understandable half of the time or easy to understand	Not understandable
3 years and older	Easy to understand	Understandable half of the time or not understandable

Test result: 1. Normal on DASE and intelligibility = *normal*
2. Abnormal on DASE or intelligibility = *abnormal**

* If abnormal on initial screening, rescreen within 2 weeks. If abnormal again, child should be referred for complete speech evaluation.

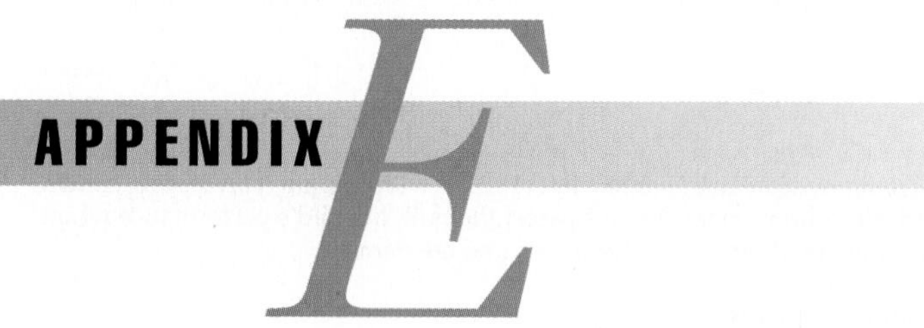

Normal Blood Pressure Readings for Children

Normal Blood Pressure Readings for Girls

AGE	SYSTOLIC BLOOD PRESSURE PERCENTILE 5TH	10TH	50TH	90TH	95TH	AGE	DIASTOLIC BLOOD PRESSURE* PERCENTILE 5TH	10TH	50TH	90TH	95TH
1 day	46	50	65	80	84	1 day	38	42	55	68	72
3 days	53	57	72	86	90	3 days	38	42	55	68	71
7 days	60	64	78	93	97	7 days	38	41	54	67	71
1 mo	65	69	84	98	102	1 mo	35	39	52	65	69
2 mo	68	72	87	101	106	2 mo	34	38	51	64	68
3 mo	70	74	89	104	108	3 mo	35	38	51	64	68
4 mo	71	75	90	105	109	4 mo	35	39	52	65	68
5 mo	72	76	91	106	110	5 mo	36	39	52	65	69
6 mo	72	76	91	106	110	6 mo	36	40	53	66	69
7 mo	72	76	91	106	110	7 mo	36	40	53	66	70
8 mo	72	76	91	106	110	8 mo	37	40	53	66	70
9 mo	72	76	91	106	110	9 mo	37	41	54	67	70
10 mo	72	76	91	106	110	10 mo	37	41	54	67	71
11 mo	72	76	91	105	110	11 mo	38	41	54	67	71
1 yr	72	76	91	105	110	1 yr	38	41	54	67	71
2 yr	71	76	90	105	109	2 yr	40	43	56	69	73
3 yr	72	76	91	106	110	3 yr	40	43	56	69	73
4 yr	73	78	92	107	111	4 yr	40	43	56	69	73
5 yr	75	79	94	109	113	5 yr	40	43	56	69	73
6 yr	77	81	96	111	115	6 yr	40	44	57	70	74
7 yr	78	83	97	112	116	7 yr	41	45	58	71	75
8 yr	80	84	99	114	118	8 yr	43	46	59	72	76
9 yr	81	86	100	115	119	9 yr	44	48	61	74	77
10 yr	83	87	102	117	121	10 yr	46	49	62	75	79
11 yr	86	90	105	119	123	11 yr	47	51	64	77	81
12 yr	88	92	107	122	126	12 yr	49	53	66	78	82
13 yr	90	94	109	124	128	13 yr	46	50	64	78	82
14 yr	92	96	110	125	129	14 yr	49	53	67	81	85
15 yr	93	97	111	126	130	15 yr	49	53	67	82	86
16 yr	93	97	112	127	131	16 yr	49	53	67	81	85
17 yr	93	98	112	127	131	17 yr	48	52	66	80	84
18 yr	94	98	112	127	131	18 yr	48	52	66	80	84

Reprinted with permission from the Second Task Force on Blood Pressure Control in Children, National Heart, Lung and Blood Institute, Bethesda, MD. Tabular data prepared by Dr. B. Rosner, 1987.

*K4 was used for ages less than 13; K5 was used for ages 13 and over.

Normal Blood Pressure Readings for Boys

	SYSTOLIC BLOOD PRESSURE PERCENTILE						DIASTOLIC BLOOD PRESSURE* PERCENTILE				
AGE	5TH	10TH	50TH	90TH	95TH	AGE	5TH	10TH	50TH	90TH	95TH
1 day	54	58	73	87	92	1 day	38	42	55	68	72
3 days	55	59	74	89	93	3 days	38	42	55	68	71
7 days	57	62	76	91	95	7 days	37	41	54	67	71
1 mo	67	71	86	101	105	1 mo	35	39	52	64	68
2 mo	72	76	91	106	110	2 mo	33	37	50	63	66
3 mo	72	76	91	106	110	3 mo	33	37	50	63	66
4 mo	72	76	91	106	110	4 mo	34	37	50	63	67
5 mo	72	76	91	105	110	5 mo	35	39	52	65	68
6 mo	72	76	90	105	109	6 mo	36	40	53	66	70
7 mo	71	76	90	105	109	7 mo	37	41	54	67	71
8 mo	71	75	90	105	109	8 mo	38	42	55	68	72
9 mo	71	75	90	105	109	9 mo	39	43	55	68	72
10 mo	71	75	90	105	109	10 mo	39	43	56	69	73
11 mo	71	76	90	105	109	11 mo	39	43	56	69	73
1 yr	71	76	90	105	109	1 yr	39	43	56	69	73
2 yr	72	76	91	106	110	2 yr	39	43	56	68	72
3 yr	73	77	92	107	111	3 yr	39	42	55	68	72
4 yr	74	79	93	108	112	4 yr	39	43	56	69	72
5 yr	76	80	95	109	113	5 yr	40	43	56	69	73
6 yr	77	81	96	111	115	6 yr	41	44	57	70	74
7 yr	78	83	97	112	116	7 yr	42	45	58	71	75
8 yr	80	84	99	114	118	8 yr	43	47	60	73	76
9 yr	82	86	101	115	120	9 yr	44	48	61	74	78
10 yr	84	88	102	117	121	10 yr	45	49	62	75	79
11 yr	86	90	105	119	123	11 yr	47	50	63	76	80
12 yr	88	92	107	121	126	12 yr	48	51	64	77	81
13 yr	90	94	109	124	128	13 yr	45	49	63	77	81
14 yr	93	97	112	126	131	14 yr	46	50	64	78	82
15 yr	95	99	114	129	133	15 yr	47	51	65	79	83
16 yr	98	102	117	131	136	16 yr	49	53	67	81	85
17 yr	100	104	119	134	138	17 yr	51	55	69	83	87
18 yr	102	106	121	136	140	18 yr	52	56	70	84	88

Reprinted with permission from the Second Task Force on Blood Pressure Control in Children, National Heart, Lung and Blood Institute, Bethesda, MD. Tabular data prepared by Dr. B. Rosner, 1987.

*K4 was used for ages less than 13; K5 was used for ages 13 and over.

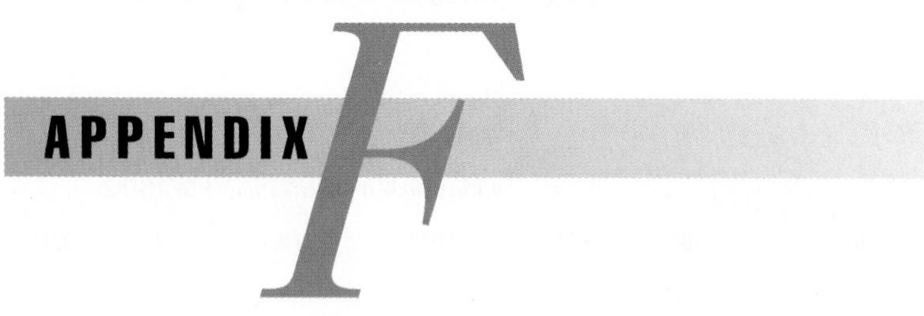

Skinfold Thickness by Age and Sex

50th Percentiles

Skinfold thickness by age and sex, as measured by Harpenden skinfold calipers over triceps and under scapula. Scale is in millimeters on the left side and logarithmic transformation units on the right side. The lines shown are the 50th percentiles for British children.

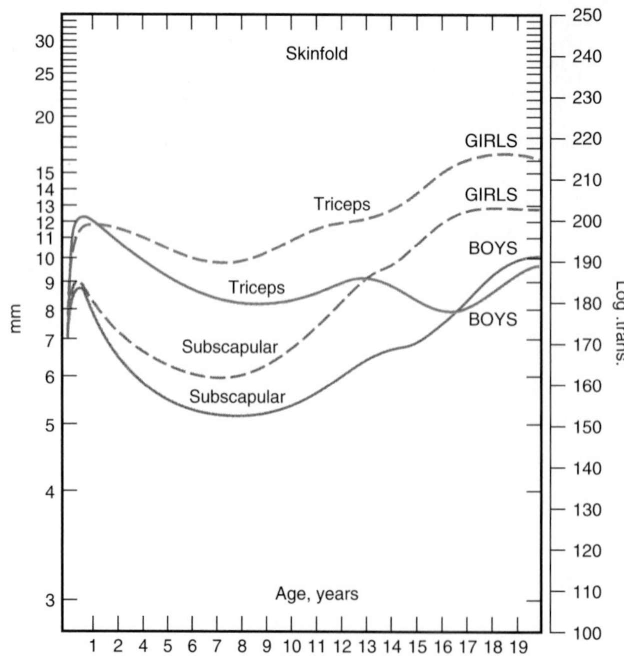

Reprinted by permission from Tanner, J. M. (1978). *Fetus into man: Physical growth from conception to maturity.* Cambridge, MA: Harvard University Press.

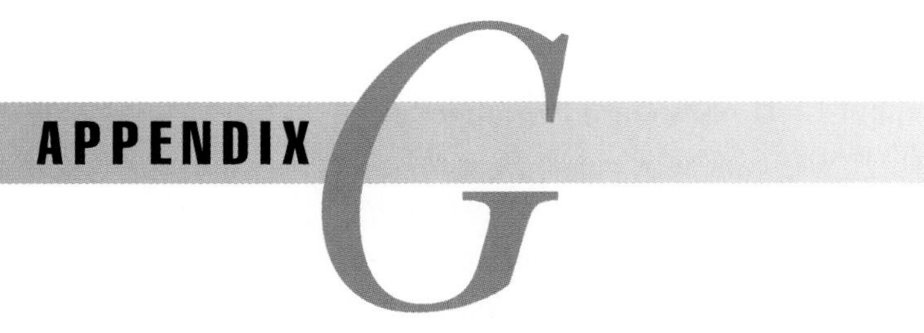

Guidelines for Isolation Precautions in Hospitals

To assist hospitals in maintaining up-to-date isolation practices, the Centers for Disease Control and Prevention (CDC) and the Hospital Infection Control Practices Advisory Committee (HICPAC) have revised the "CDC Guideline for Isolation Precautions in Hospitals."

The revised guideline contains two parts. Part I, "Evolution of Isolation Practices," reviews the evolution of isolation practices in U.S. hospitals, including their advantages, disadvantages, and controversial aspects, and provides the background for the HICPAC-consensus recommendations contained in Part II, "Recommendations for Isolation Precautions in Hospitals." The guideline supersedes previous CDC recommendations for isolation precautions in hospitals.

The guideline recommendations are based on the latest epidemiologic information on transmission of infection in hospitals. The recommendations are intended primarily for use in the care of patients in acute-care hospitals, although some of the recommendations may be applicable for some patients receiving care in subacute-care or extended-care facilities. The recommendations are not intended for use in daycare, well-care, or domiciliary care programs. Because there have been few studies to test the efficacy of isolation precautions, and because gaps still exist in the knowledge of the epidemiology and modes of transmission of some diseases, disagreement with some of the recommendations is expected. A working draft of the guideline was reviewed by experts in infection control and published in the *Federal Register* for public comment. However, all recommendations in the guideline may not reflect the opinions of all reviewers.

Adapted from Garner, J. S., and the Hospital Infection Control Practices Advisory Committee. (1996). Guideline for isolation precautions in hospitals—Public Health Service, U.S. Department of Health and Human Services, Centers for Disease Control and Prevention, Atlanta, Georgia. *Infection Control and Hospital Epidemiology 17*, 53–80. For a reprint of the entire report, address requests to Mailstop E-69, Hospital Infections Program, National Center for Infectious Diseases, Centers for Disease Control and Prevention, Atlanta, GA 30333.

SUMMARY

The "Guideline for Isolation Precautions in Hospitals" was revised to meet the following objectives: (1) to be epidemiologically sound; (2) to recognize the importance of all body fluids, secretions, and excretions in the transmission of nosocomial pathogens; (3) to contain adequate precautions for infections transmitted by the airborne, droplet, and contact routes of transmission; (4) to be as simple and user-friendly as possible; and, (5) to use new terms to avoid confusion with existing infection control and isolation systems.

The revised guideline contains two tiers of precautions. In the first, and most important, tier are those precautions designed for the care of all patients in hospitals regardless of their diagnosis or presumed infection status. Implementation of these "Standard Precautions" is the primary strategy for successful nosocomial infection control. In the second tier are precautions designed only for the care of specified patients. These additional "Transmission-Based Precautions" are used for patients known or suspected to be infected or colonized with epidemiologically important pathogens that can be transmitted by airborne or droplet transmission or by contact with dry skin or contaminated surfaces.

Standard Precautions synthesize the major features of Universal (Blood and Body Fluid) Precautions (designed to reduce the risk of transmission of blood-borne pathogens) and Body Substance Isolation (designed to reduce the risk of transmission of pathogens from moist body substances). Standard Precautions apply to (1) blood; (2) all body fluids, secretions, and excretions *except sweat*, regardless of whether or not they contain visible blood; (3) nonintact skin; and, (4) mucous membranes. Standard Precautions are designed to reduce the risk of transmission of microorganisms from both recognized and unrecognized sources of infection in hospitals.

Transmission-Based Precautions are designed for patients documented or suspected to be infected or colonized with highly transmissible or epidemiologically important pathogens for which additional precautions beyond Standard Precautions are needed to interrupt transmission in hospitals. There are three types of Transmission-Based Precautions: Airborne Precautions, Droplet Precautions, and Contact Precautions. They may be combined for diseases that have multiple routes of transmission. When used either singularly or in combination, they are to be used in addition to Standard Precautions.

The revised guideline also lists specific clinical syndromes or conditions in both adult and pediatric patients that are highly suspicious for infection and identifies appropriate Transmission-Based Precautions to use on an empiric, temporary basis until a diagnosis can be made; these empiric, temporary precautions are also to be used in addition to Standard Precautions.

A synopsis of the types of precautions and the patients requiring the precautions is listed in Table 1, page 1381.

RECOMMENDATIONS

The recommendations presented below are categorized as follows:

Category IA. Strongly recommended for all hospitals and strongly supported by well-designed experimental or epidemiologic studies.

Category IB. Strongly recommended for all hospitals and reviewed as effective by experts in the field and a consensus of HICPAC based on strong rationale and suggestive evidence, even though definitive scientific studies have not been done.

Category II. Suggested for implementation in many hospitals. Recommendations may be supported by suggestive clinical or epidemiologic studies, a strong theoretical rationale, or definitive studies applicable to some, but not all, hospitals.

No recommendation; unresolved issue. Practices for which insufficient evidence or consensus regarding efficacy exists.

The recommendations are limited to the topic of isolation precautions. Therefore, they must be supplemented by hospital policies and procedures for other aspects of infection and environmental control, occupational health, administrative and legal issues, and other issues beyond the scope of this guideline.

I. Administrative Controls

A. Education

Develop a system to ensure that hospital patients, personnel, and visitors are educated about use of precautions and their responsibility for adherence to them. *Category IB*

B. Adherence to Precautions

Periodically evaluate adherence to precautions, and use findings to direct improvements. *Category IB*

II. Standard Precautions

Use Standard Precautions, or the equivalent, for the care of all patients. *Category IB*

A. Handwashing

(1) Wash hands after touching blood, body fluids, secretions, excretions, and contaminated items, whether or not gloves are worn. Wash hands immediately after gloves are removed, between patient contacts, and when otherwise indicated to avoid transfer of microorganisms to other patients or environments. It may be necessary to wash hands between tasks and procedures on the same patient to prevent cross-contamination of different body sites. *Category IB*

(2) Use a plain (nonantimicrobial) soap for routine handwashing. *Category IB*

(3) Use an antimicrobial agent or a waterless antiseptic agent for specific circumstances (e.g., control of outbreaks or hyperendemic infections), as defined by the infection control program. *Category IB* (See Contact Precautions for additional recommendations on using antimicrobial and antiseptic agents.)

B. Gloves

Wear gloves (clean, nonsterile gloves are adequate) when touching blood, body fluids, secretions, excretions, and contaminated items. Put on clean gloves just before touching mucous membranes and nonintact skin. Change gloves between tasks and procedures on the same patient after contact with material that may contain a high concentration of microorganisms. Remove gloves promptly after use, before touching noncontaminated items and environmental surfaces, and before going to another patient, and wash hands immediately to avoid transfer of microorganisms to other patients or environments. *Category IB*

C. Mask, Eye Protection, Face Shield

Wear a mask and eye protection or a face shield to protect mucous membranes of the eyes, nose, and mouth during procedures and patient-care activities that are likely to generate splashes or sprays of blood, body fluids, secretions, and excretions. *Category IB*

D. Gown

Wear a gown (a clean, nonsterile gown is adequate) to protect skin and to prevent soiling of clothing during procedures and patient-care activities that are likely to generate splashes or sprays of blood, body fluids, secretions, or excretions. Select a gown that is appropriate for the activity and the amount of fluid likely to be encountered. Remove a soiled gown as promptly as possible, and wash hands to avoid transfer of microorganisms to other patients or environments. *Category IB*

E. Patient-Care Equipment

Handle used patient-care equipment soiled with blood, body fluids, secretions, and excretions in a manner that prevents skin and mucous membrane exposures, contamination of clothing, and transfer of microorganisms to other patients and environments. Ensure that reusable equipment is not used for the care of another patient until it has been cleaned and reprocessed appropriately. Ensure that single-use items are discarded properly. *Category IB*

F. Environmental Control

Ensure that the hospital has adequate procedures for the routine care, cleaning, and disinfection of environmental surfaces, beds, bedrails, bedside equipment, and other frequently touched surfaces, and ensure that these procedures are being followed. *Category IB*

G. Linen

Handle, transport, and process used linen soiled with blood, body fluids, secretions, and excretions in a manner that prevents skin and mucous membrane exposures and contamination of clothing, and that avoids transfer of microorganisms to other patients and environments. *Category IB*

H. Occupational Health and Blood-borne Pathogens

(1) Take care to prevent injuries when using needles, scalpels, and other sharp instruments or devices; when handling sharp instruments after procedures; when cleaning used instruments; and when disposing of used needles. Never recap used needles, or otherwise manipulate them using both hands, or use any other technique that involves directing the point of a needle toward any part of the body; rather, use either a one-handed "scoop" technique or a mechanical device designed for holding the needle sheath. Do not remove used needles from disposable syringes by hand, and do not bend, break, or otherwise manipulate used needles by hand. Place used disposable syringes and needles, scalpel blades, and other sharp items in appropriate puncture-resistant containers, which are located as close as practical to the area in which the items were used, and place reusable syringes and needles in a puncture-resistant container for transport to the reprocessing area. *Category IB*

(2) Use mouthpieces, resuscitation bags, or other ventilation devices as an alternative to mouth-to-mouth resuscitation methods in areas where the need for resuscitation is predictable. *Category IB*

I. Patient Placement

Place a patient who contaminates the environment or who does not (or cannot be expected to) assist in maintaining appropriate hygiene or environmental control in a private room. If a private room is not available, consult with infection control professionals regarding patient placement or other alternatives. *Category IB*

III. Airborne Precautions

In addition to Standard Precautions, use Airborne Precautions, or the equivalent, for patients known or suspected to be infected with microorganisms transmitted by airborne droplet nuclei (small-particle residue [5 μm or smaller in size] of evaporated droplets containing microorganisms that remain suspended in the air and that can be dispersed widely by air currents within a room or over a long distance). *Category IB*

A. Patient Placement

Place the patient in a private room that has (1) monitored negative air pressure in relation to the surrounding areas, (2) 6 to 12 air changes per hour, and (3) appropriate discharge of air outdoors or monitored high-efficiency filtration of room air before the air is circulated to other areas in the hospital. Keep the room door closed and the patient in the room. When a private room is not available, place the patient in a room with a patient who has active infection with the same microorganism, unless otherwise recommended, but with no other infection. When a private room is not available and cohorting is not desirable, consultation with infection control professionals is advised before patient placement. *Category IB*

B. Respiratory Protection

Wear respiratory protection when entering the room of a patient with known or suspected infectious pulmonary tuberculosis. Susceptible persons should not enter the room of patients known or suspected to have measles (rubeola) or varicella (chickenpox) if other immune caregivers are available. If susceptible persons must enter the room of a patient known or suspected to have measles (rubeola) or varicella, they should wear respiratory protection. Persons immune to measles (rubeola) or varicella need not wear respiratory protection. *Category IB*

C. Patient Transport

Limit the movement and transport of the patient from the room to essential purposes only. If transport or movement is necessary, minimize patient dispersal of droplet nuclei by placing a surgical mask on the patient, if possible. *Category IB*

D. Additional Precautions for Preventing Transmission of Tuberculosis

Consult CDC "Guidelines for Preventing the Transmission of Tuberculosis in Heath-Care Facilities" for additional prevention strategies.

IV. Droplet Precautions

In addition to Standard Precautions, use Droplet Precautions, or the equivalent, for a patient known or suspected to be infected with microorganisms transmitted by droplets (large-particle droplets [larger than 5 µm in size] that can be generated by the patient during coughing, sneezing, talking, or the performance of procedures). *Category IB*

A. Patient Placement

Place the patient in a private room. When a private room is not available, place the patient in a room with a patient(s) who has active infection with the same microorganism but with no other infection (cohorting). When a private room is not available and cohorting is not achievable, maintain spatial separation of at least 3 ft between the infected patient and other patients and visitors. Special air handling and ventilation are not necessary, and the door may remain open. *Category IB*

B. Mask

In addition to standard precautions, wear a mask when working within 3 ft of the patient. (Logistically, some hospitals may want to implement the wearing of a mask to enter the room.) *Category IB*

C. Patient Transport

Limit the movement and transport of the patient from the room to essential purposes only. If transport or movement is necessary, minimize patient dispersal of droplets by masking the patient, if possible. *Category IB*

V. Contact Precautions

In addition to Standard Precautions, use Contact Precautions, or the equivalent, for specified patients known or suspected to be infected or colonized with epidemiologically important microorganisms that can be transmitted by direct contact with the patient (hand or skin-to-skin contact that occurs when performing patient-care activities that require touching the patient's dry skin) or indirect contact (touching) with environmental surfaces or patient-care items in the patient's environment. *Category IB*

A. Patient Placement

Place the patient in a private room. When a private room is not available, place the patient in a room with a patient(s) who has active infection with the same microorganism but with no other infection (cohorting). When a private room is not available and cohorting is not achievable, consider the epidemiology of the microorganism and the patient population when determining patient placement. Consultation with infection control professionals is advised before patient placement. *Category IB*

B. Gloves and Handwashing

In addition to wearing gloves as outlined under Standard Precautions, wear gloves (clean, nonsterile gloves are adequate) when entering the room. During the course of providing care for a patient, change gloves after having contact with infective material that may contain high concentrations of microorganisms (fecal material and wound drainage). Remove gloves before leaving the patient's environment and wash hands immediately with an antimicrobial agent or a waterless antiseptic agent. After glove removal and handwashing, ensure that hands do not touch potentially contaminated environmental surfaces or items in the patient's room to avoid transfer of microorganisms to other patients or environments. *Category IB*

C. Gown

In addition to wearing a gown as outlined under Standard Precautions, wear a gown (a clean, nonsterile gown is adequate) when entering the room if you anticipate that your clothing will have substantial contact with the patient, environmental surfaces, or items in the patient's room, or if the patient is incontinent or has diarrhea, an ileostomy, a colostomy, or wound drainage not contained by a dressing. Remove the gown before leaving the patient's environment. After gown removal, ensure that clothing does not contact potentially contaminated environmental surfaces to avoid transfer of microorganisms to other patients or environments. *Category IB*

D. Patient Transport

Limit the movement and transport of the patient from the room to essential purposes only. If the patient is transported out of the room, ensure that precautions are maintained to minimize the risk of transmission of microorganisms to other patients and contamination of environmental surfaces or equipment. *Category IB*

E. Patient-Care Equipment

When possible, dedicate the use of noncritical patient-care equipment to a single patient (or cohort of patients infected or colonized with the pathogen requiring precautions) to avoid sharing between patients. If use of common equipment or items is unavoidable, then adequately clean and disinfect them before use for another patient. *Category IB*

F. Additional Precautions for Preventing the Spread of Vancomycin Resistance

Consult the HICPAC report on preventing the spread of vanomycin resistance for additional prevention strategies.

TABLE 1 *Synopsis of Types of Precautions and Patients Requiring the Precautions**

Standard Precautions

Use Standard Precautions for the care of all patients.

Airborne Precautions

In addition to Standard Precautions, use Airborne Precautions for patients known or suspected to have serious illnesses transmitted by airborne droplet nuclei. Examples of such illnesses include:

- Measles
- Varicella (including disseminated zoster)*
- Tuberculosis†

Droplet Precautions

In addition to Standard Precautions, use Droplet Precautions for patients known or suspected to have serious illnesses transmitted by large particle droplets. Examples of such illnesses include:

- Invasive *Haemophilus influenzae* type b disease, including meningitis, pneumonia, epiglottitis, and sepsis
- Invasive *Neisseria meningitidis* disease, including meningitis, pneumonia, and sepsis
- Other serious bacterial respiratory infections spread by droplet transmission, including:
  - Diphtheria (pharyngeal)
  - Mycoplasma pneumonia
  - Pertussis
  - Pneumonic plague
  - Streptococcal pharyngitis, pneumonia, or scarlet fever in infants and young children
- Serious viral infections spread by droplet transmission, including:
  - Adenovirus*
  - Influenza
  - Mumps
  - Parvovirus B19
  - Rubella

Contact Precautions

In addition to Standard Precautions, use Contact Precautions for patients known or suspected to have serious illnesses easily transmitted by direct patient contact or by contact with items in the patient's environment. Examples of such illnesses include:

- Gastrointestinal, respiratory, skin, or wound infections, or colonization with multidrug-resistant bacteria judged by the infection control program, based on current state, regional, or national recommendations, to be of special clinical and epidemiologic significance
- Enteric infections with a low infectious dose or prolonged environmental survival, including:
  - *Clostridium difficile*
  - For diapered or incontinent patients: enterohemorrhagic *Escherichia coli* O157:H7, *Shigella*, hepatitis A, or rotavirus
- Respiratory syncytial virus, parainfluenza virus, or enteroviral infections in infants and young children
- Skin infections that are highly contagious or that may occur on dry skin, including:
  - Diphtheria (cutaneous)
  - Herpes simplex virus (neonatal or mucocutaneous)
  - Impetigo
  - Major (noncontained) abscesses, cellulitis, or decubiti
  - Pediculosis
  - Scabies
  - Staphylococcal furunculosis in infants and young children
  - Zoster (disseminated or in the immunocompromised host)*
- Viral/hemorrhagic conjunctivitis
- Viral hemorrhagic infections (Ebola, Lassa, or Marburg)

*Certain infections require more than one type of precaution.

†See CDC "Guidelines for Preventing the Transmission of Tuberculosis in Health-Care Facilities.

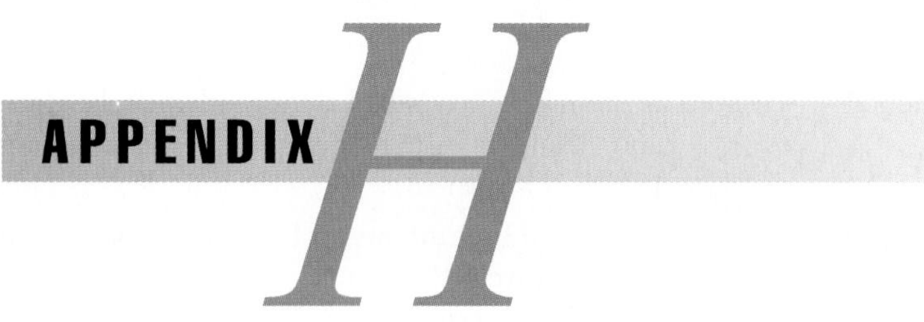

Resources for Health Care Providers and Families

UNIT II (CHAPTERS 2–8) GROWTH AND DEVELOPMENT: THE CHILD AND THE FAMILY

DENTAL CARE RESOURCES

AMERICAN DENTAL ASSOCIATION
Bureau of Health Education and Audiovisual Services
211 East Chicago Avenue
Chicago, IL 60611

AMERICAN SOCIETY OF DENTISTRY FOR CHILDREN
211 East Chicago Avenue, Suite 920
Chicago, IL 69611

ACADEMY OF DENTISTRY FOR THE HANDICAPPED
Educational Materials Clearinghouse
1726 Champa Road, Suite 422
Denver, CO 80202

LATCHKEY CHILDREN

Books

American Home Economics Association. *Beyond the latchkey: Expanding community options for school-age care.* AHEA Publications, 1555 King Street, Alexandria, VA 22314. (703) 706-4600. (The manual for Project Home Safe's community training program. It includes complete instructions and materials for the trainer plus 400 pages of resources for program participants.)

Bergstrom, Joan. (1984). *School's out—Now what? Creative choices for your child.* Berkeley, CA: Ten Speed Press.

Dana, Trudy. (1988). *Safe and sound: A parents guide to the care of children home alone.* New York: McGraw-Hill.

Kyte, Kathy. (1983). *In charge: A complete handbook for kids with working parents.* New York: Knopf.

Leiner, Katherine. (1986). *Both my parents work.* New York: Franklin Watts. Photographs by Steve Sax.

Long, Lynette. (1984). *On my own: A kids' self-care book.* Washington, DC: Acropolis Books.

Long, Lynette, & Long, Thomas. (1983). *The handbook for latchkey children and their parents.* New York: Arbor House.

Project Home Safe. *Developmentally appropriate practice in school-age child care programs* (2nd ed.). Kendall/Hunt Publishing. (800) 228-0810. (Project Home Safe's resource for school-age child care providers and educators who teach child care and child development courses.)

Swan, Helen, & Houston, Victoria. (1985). *Alone after school: A self-care guide for latchkey children and their parents.* Englewood Cliffs, NJ: Prentice Hall.

Toinson, Bryan, Rowland, Bobbie, & Coleman, Mark. (1989). *Home alone kids: The working parents guide to providing the best care for your child.* Lexington, MA: D.C. Heath and Co.

Other Resources

Materials are available from the following Phone Line programs for those who wish to establish similar programs in their communities:

PHONE FRIEND
P.O. Box 735
State College, PA 16804

GRANDMA, PLEASE
4520 N. Beacon
Chicago, IL 60640

DENVER DEVELOPMENTAL SCREENING TEST

DENVER DEVELOPMENTAL MATERIALS, INC.
P.O. Box 6919
Denver, CO 80206-0919

CHAPTER 10
COMMUNICATING WITH CHILDREN

ASSOCIATION FOR THE CARE OF CHILDREN'S HEALTH
7910 Woodmont Avenue, Suite 300
Bethesda, MD 20814
(800) 808-2224

CHILD LIFE COUNCIL
7910 Woodmont Avenue, Suite 310
Bethesda, MD 20814
(301) 654-1343

INSTITUTE FOR FAMILY-CENTERED CARE
7900 Wisconsin Avenue
Bethesda, MD 20814
(301) 652-0281

NATIONAL ASSOCIATION FOR THE EDUCATION OF YOUNG CHILDREN
1509 16th Street, NW
Washington, DC 20036-1426
(800) 424-2460

ZERO TO THREE
National Center for Clinical Infant Programs
2000 14th Street, North
Suite 380
Arlington, VA 22201-2500
(703) 528-4300
(800) 899-4301

CHAPTER 12
NUTRITION

AMERICAN DIETETIC ASSOCIATION
216 West Jackson Boulevard
Suite 800
Chicago, IL 60606-6995
(800) 877-1600

BEST START (BREASTFEEDING)
3500 East Fletcher Avenue
Suite 308
Tampa, FL 33613
(800) 277-4975

CENTER FOR CHILD AND ADOLESCENT OBESITY
Department of Family and Community Medicine
University of California, San Francisco
MU3 East, Box 0900
San Francisco, CA 94143-0900
(415) 476-2502

CLEARINGHOUSE ON INFANT FEEDING AND MATERNAL NUTRITION
American Public Health Association
1015 15th Street, N.W.
Washington, DC 20005
(202) 789-5600

FOOD RESEARCH AND ACTION CENTER
1875 Connecticut Avenue, N.W., Suite 540
Washington, DC 20009
(202) 986-2200

INTERNATIONAL LACTATION CONSULTANT ASSOCIATION
201 Brown Avenue
Evanston, IL 60202
(708) 260-8874

LA LECHE LEAGUE INTERNATIONAL
1400 North Meacham Road
Schaumburg, IL 60173-4840
(800) 525-3243

NATIONAL CENTER FOR NUTRITION AND DIETETICS
American Dietetic Association
216 West Jackson Boulevard
Chicago, IL 60606-6995
(800) 366-1655

NATIONAL DAIRY COUNCIL
O'Hare International Center
10255 West Higgins Road, Suite 900
Rosemont, IL 60018
(800) 426-8271

CHAPTER 13
SAFETY

AMERICAN ACADEMY OF PEDIATRICS
The Injury Prevention Program (TIPP)
141 Northwest Point Blvd.
P.O. Box 927
Elk Grove Village, IL 60057
(800) 433-9016

AMERICAN SPINAL INJURY ASSOCIATION
250 E. Superior Street, Room 619
Chicago, IL 60611
(312) 908-3425

AMERICAN TRAUMA SOCIETY
8703 Presidential Parkway
Suite 512
Upper Marlboro, MD 20772-2656
(800) 556-7890

NATIONAL HEAD INJURY FOUNDATION
333 Turnpike Road
Southborough, MA 01772
(617) 485-9950

NATIONAL HEAD & SPINAL CORD INJURY PREVENTION PROGRAM
"Think First" Program
American Association of Neurological Surgeons & Congress of Neurosurgical Surgeons
22 South Washington Street
Park Ridge, IL 60068
(708) 692-9500

NATIONAL HIGHWAY TRAFFIC SAFETY ADMINISTRATION
400 7th Street SW
Washington, DC 20590

NATIONAL SAFEKIDS CAMPAIGN
111 Michigan Avenue NW
Washington, DC 20010-2970

NATIONAL SAFETY COUNCIL
P.O. Box 1171
Chicago, IL 60611

PHYSICIANS FOR AUTOMOTIVE SAFETY
P.O. Box 208
Rye, NY 10580

HARBORVIEW INJURY PREVENTION AND RESEARCH CENTER
University of Washington
325 Ninth Avenue ZX-10
Seattle, WA 98104
(206) 223-8388

THE CHILDREN'S SAFETY NETWORK
National Center for Education in Maternal and Child Health
38th & R Streets NW
Washington, DC 20057
(202) 625-8400

U.S. CONSUMER PRODUCT SAFETY COMMISSION
Washington, DC 20207
(800) 638-CPSC

NATIONAL RIFLE ASSOCIATION OF AMERICA
Safety and Education Department
1600 Rhode Island Ave., NW
Washington, DC 20036

Safe Home. A tested program for creating safe homes for children by reducing common hazards. The Safe Home kit includes a Leader's Guide, Inspector's Notes, filmstrip, checklists, and a demonstration supply board. To order, write or call:

SCIPP/STATEWIDE COMPREHENSIVE INJURY PREVENTION PROGRAM
Massachusetts Department of Public Health
Division of Family Health Services
150 Tremont Street
Boston, MA 02111
(617) 727-1246

Safe Day Care. A teacher's guide for creating safe environments for preschool children. Program serves as a guide to creating and maintaining a safe daycare environment, reinforcing habits of preschoolers, preparing for an emergency, and advocating child safety to parents. To order, write or call: SCIPP/Statewide Comprehensive Injury Prevention Program (address and telephone as listed earlier).

TIPP: The Injury Prevention Program: A Guide to Safety Counseling in Office Practice. A 24-page guide that includes safety counseling schedules, safety surveys, counseling guidelines, safety sheets, and safety slips. Catalog code HE0042; cost $5.00 per copy. To order, write or call:

AMERICAN ACADEMY OF PEDIATRICS
Department of Publications
141 Northwest Point Blvd.
P.O. Box 927
Elk Grove Village, IL 60009-0927
(800) 433-9016

Further Reading

Bass, J. L., et al. (1985). Educating parents about injury prevention. *Pediatric Clinics of North America, 32*:233–242.
Gallagher, S. S., et al. (1985). A home injury prevention program for children. *Pediatric Clinics of North America, 32*:95–112.

FIRE AND BURN INJURY

Protect Your Home Against Fire . . . Planning Saves Lives. Child safety slip that describes steps for prevention. Catalog Code HE0039; cost $5.00 per 100 copies. To order, write or call: American Academy of Pediatrics (address and phone as listed earlier).

Further Reading

Dershewitz, R. A., & Williamson, J. W. (1977). Prevention of childhood household injuries: A controlled clinical trial. *American Journal of Public Health, 67*, 1148–1153.
Gorman, R. L., et al. (1985). A successful city-wide smoke detector giveaway program. *Pediatrics, 75*, 14–18.
Katcher, M. L. (1981). Scald burns from hot tap water. *Journal of the American Medical Association, 246*, 1219–1222.
Katcher, M. L. (1987). Prevention of tap water scald burns: Evaluation of a multimedia injury control program. *American Journal of Public Health, 77*, 1195–1197.
McLoughlin, E., et al. (1982). Project burn prevention: Outcome and implications. *American Journal of Public Health, 72*, 241–247.
Miller, R. E., et al. (1982). Pediatric counseling and subsequent use of smoke detectors. *American Journal of Public Health, 72*, 392–393.

SUFFOCATION

Choking Prevention and First Aid for Infants and Children Brochure. Catalog code HE0066; cost $15.00 per 100 copies. To order, write or call: American Academy of Pediatrics (address and telephone as listed earlier).

Safety News. Free publication of the Consumer Product Safety Commission (CPSC) that lists CPSC and manufacturers' warnings and recalls; information on crib, nursery, toy, and playground safety. To order, write or call:

CPSC
5401 Westbard Avenue
Washington, DC 20207
(800) 638-CPSC or (301) 492-6424

Infant Furniture: Cribs. Child safety slip that describes buying recommendations and safety tips. Catalog Code HE0030; cost $6.00 per 100 copies. To order, write or call: American Academy of Pediatrics (address and telephone as listed earlier).

CHAPTER 17
THE CHILD WITH A CHRONIC OR TERMINAL ILLNESS

AIDS/HIV

THE NAMES PROJECT FOUNDATION
2362 Market Street
San Francisco, CA 94114
(415) 863-5511
Sponsor of the international AIDS memorial quilt, fundraiser for people with AIDS and their loved ones

ARTHRITIS

ARTHRITIS FOUNDATION
1314 Spring Street, NW
Atlanta, GA 30309
(404) 872-7100

CARDIAC DISORDERS

AMERICAN HEART ASSOCIATION
7272 Greenville Ave.
Dallas, TX 75231
(214) 373-6300

CANCER

AMERICAN CANCER SOCIETY
1599 Clifton, NE
Atlanta, GA 30329
(404) 320-3333 or (800) ACS-2345

THE ALPHA BOOK ON CANCER AND LIVING
(800) 866-4111
Listing of many resources relating to children and cancer

CANDLELIGHTERS CHILDHOOD CANCER FOUNDATION
7910 Woodmont Avenue
Suite 460
Bethesda, MD 20814
(800) 366-2223
Resources and support for children with cancer and their families

CHILDREN'S ONCOLOGY CAMPS OF AMERICA
2309 West Whiteoaks Drive, Suite B
Springfield, IL 62704
(217) 793-3949
Annual directory of summer camps for children with cancer

CORPORATE ANGEL NETWORK
Westchester County Airport
Building One
White Plains, NY 10604
(914) 328-1313
Nonprofit organization that coordinates free air transportation for ambulatory cancer patients traveling to and from treatment, check-ups, and consultations

THE NATIONAL LEUKEMIA ASSOCIATION, INC.
585 Stewart Avenue, Suite 536
Garden City, NY 11530
(516) 222-1944
Provides information and financial aid to patients with leukemia

THE LEUKEMIA SOCIETY OF AMERICA
600 Third Avenue
New York, NY 10016
(800) 955-4572
Offers information, financial aid, and support to patients with leukemia, Hodgkin's disease, and lymphoma

SUNSHINE KIDS FOUNDATION
2902 Ferndale Place
Houston, TX 77098
(800) 594-5756

GENERAL SUPPORT, GRIEF AND BEREAVEMENT

THE CENTER FOR ATTITUDINAL HEALING
19 Main Street
Tiburon, CA 94920
(415) 435-5022
Provides services, including support and bereavement services, to children with cancer and other terminal illnesses

CHILDREN'S HOSPICE INTERNATIONAL
700 Princess St.
Suite 22314, Lower Level
Alexandria, VA 22301
(800) 242-4453

THE COMPASSIONATE FRIENDS
P.O. Box 3696
Oak Brook, IL 60522-3696
(708) 990-0010
Support group for parents whose children have died

THE DOUGY CENTER FOR GRIEVING CHILDREN
3909 SE 52nd Ave.
P.O. Box 86852
Portland, OR 97286
(503) 775-5683
A resource for helping children impacted by loss through grief

HOSPICELINK
Hospice Education Institute
190 Westbrook Road
Essex, CT 06426
(800) 331-1620
Hospice information

THE HARMONY PROJECT
Ted Menten
Box 28K
300 East 40th Street
New York, NY 10016

MAKE-A-WISH FOUNDATION OF AMERICA
1624 East Meadowbrook
Phoenix, AZ
(602) 248-9474
Grants wishes to children with life-threatening illnesses. Contact the national office for information on the nearest local chapter.

RONALD MCDONALD HOUSE
McDonald's Campus Office Building
Croc Drive
Oak Brook, IL 60521
(708) 575-7418
Provides housing near treatment centers for children with cancer and other life-threatening diseases and their families

STARLIGHT FOUNDATION
12424 Wiltshire Blvd.
Suite 1050
Los Angeles, CA 90025
(800) 274-STAR
FAX: (310) 207-2554
Grants wishes to children with life-threatening illnesses

THE WARM PLACE
1510 Cooper Street
Fort Worth, TX 76108
(817) 877-2272
Grief support for children who have experienced the loss of a significant relationship through death

Grief Periodicals: Adults and Children

Bereavement: A Magazine of Hope and Healing
Andrea Gambell, ed.
350 Gradle Drive
Carmel, IN 46032

Fernside Inside
Newsletter of the Fernside Center for Grieving Children
P.O. Box 8944
Cincinnati, OH 45208
(513) 321-0282

The Forum Newsletter
Albert L. Strickland, ed.
Association for Death Education and Counseling
533 Stagg Lane
Santa Cruz, CA 95062
(408) 475-6527

Just For Us: A Bereavement Newsletter for Children and Teens
Saint Mary's Hospital for Children
29-01 216th Street
Bayside, NY 11360
(718) 281-8500

Professional Journals

Death Studies
Hannelore Wass, ed.
Hemisphere Publishing
1010 Vermont Ave.
Washington, DC 20005

Loss, Grief, and Care: A Journal of Professional Practice
Haworth Press
28 West 22nd Street
New York, NY 10010-6194

Professional Associations for Death Education and Counseling

ASSOCIATION RESOURCES
638 Prospect Ave.
Hartford, CT 06105

THE CENTER FOR DEATH EDUCATION AND RESEARCH
1167 Social Science Building
University of Minnesota
Minneapolis, MN 55455

Resource Information and Distributors

CENTERING CORPORATION
1531 N. Saddle Creek Road
Omaha, NE 68104-5064
(402) 553-1200

COMPASSION BOOK SERVICE
479 Hannah Branch Road
Burnsville, NC 28714
(704) 675-9670

THE GOOD GRIEF PROGRAM
Judge Baker Children's Center
295 Longwood Ave.
Boston, MA 02115
(617) 232-8390

MEDIC PUBLISHING COMPANY
P.O. Box 89
Redmond, WA 98073
(206) 881-2883

MOUNT IDA COLLEGE OF DEATH EDUCATION
777 Dedham Street
Newton Center, MA 02159
(617) 969-7000, ext. 249

THE RAINBOW CONNECTION
477 Hannah Branch Road
Burnsville, NC 28714
(704) 675-5909

NATIONAL HEMOPHILIA FOUNDATION
110 Greene St., Suite 303
New York, NY 10012
(212) 219-8180, ext. 3027

CHAPTER 20
THE CHILD IN PAIN

Quick Reference Guide for Clinicians

CENTER FOR RESEARCH DISSEMINATION AND LIAISON
AHCPR Publications Clearinghouse
P.O. Box 8547
Silver Spring, MD 20907
(800) 325-9295 or (301) 495-3453

Oucher

JUDITH E. BEYER, R.N., PH.D
University of Colorado Health Science Center
School of Nursing
Campus Box C-288
4200 East Ninth Avenue
Denver, CO 80262

Poker Chip Tool

NANCY HESTER, R.N., PH.D, F.A.A.N.
Associate Professor, School of Nursing
Campus Box 288
University of Colorado Health Science Center
4200 East Ninth Avenue
Denver, CO 80262

Adolescent Pediatric Pain Tool

MARILYN SAVEDRA, D.N.S., R.N.
University of California, San Francisco School of Nursing
Box 0606
San Francisco, CA 94143

CHAPTER 25
THE CHILD WITH UPPER GASTROINTESTINAL ALTERATIONS

CLEFT PALATE FOUNDATION
1218 Grandview Ave.
Pittsburgh, PA 15211
(800) 24-CLEFT

MARCH OF DIMES BIRTH DEFECTS FOUNDATION
1275 Mamaroneck Ave.
White Plains, NY 10605
(914) 428-7100

CHAPTER 26
THE CHILD WITH LOWER GASTROINTESTINAL ALTERATIONS

AMERICAN CELIAC SOCIETY/DIETARY SUPPORT COALITION
58 Musano Court
West Orange, NJ 07052
(201) 325-8837

CELIAC/SPRUE ASSOCIATION/UNITED STATES OF AMERICA
P.O. Box 31700
Omaha, NE 68131-070
(402) 558-0600

GLUTEN INTOLERANCE GROUP OF NORTH AMERICA
P.O. Box 23053
Seattle, WA 98102-0353
(206) 325-6980; FAX: (206) 850-2394

PULL-THRU NETWORK
62 Edgewood Avenue
Wyckoff, NJ 07481
(201) 891-5932

AMERICAN PSEUDO-OBSTRUCTION AND HIRSCHSPRUNG DISEASE SOCIETY
P.O. Box 772
Medford, MA 02155
(617) 395-4255; FAX: (617) 396-6868

CROHN'S DISEASE FOUNDATION OF AMERICA
368 Park Avenue S.
New York, NY 10015
(800) 932-2423

CHAPTER 28
THE CHILD WITH AN ACUTE RESPIRATORY DISORDER

THE AMERICAN LUNG ASSOCIATION
1740 Broadway
New York, NY 10019
(212) 315-8700

AMERICAN ACADEMY OF ALLERGY AND IMMUNOLOGY
611 East Wells Street
Milwaukee, WI 53202
(414) 272-6071

AMERICAN ALLERGY ASSOCIATION
P.O. Box 7273
Menlo Park, CA 94026
(415) 322-1663

INFANT DEATH SYNDROME CLEARINGHOUSE
8201 Greensboro Drive, Suite 600
McLean, VA 22102
(703) 821-8955

AMERICAN SUDDEN INFANT DEATH SYNDROME INSTITUTE
275 Carpenter Dr., Suite 100
Atlanta, GA 30328
(800) 847-SIDS

NATIONAL SUDDEN INFANT DEATH SYNDROME FOUNDATION
10500 Little Patuxent Parkway, Suite 420
Columbia, MD 21044
(800) 221-5105

NATIONAL CENTER FOR THE PREVENTION OF SUDDEN INFANT DEATH SYNDROME
330 N. Charles St.
Baltimore, MD 21201
(714) 968-7623

NATIONAL SUDDEN INFANT DEATH SYNDROME FOUNDATION
2 Metro Plaza, Suite 104
8200 Professional Place
Landover, MD 20785
(800) 221-7437

CHAPTER 29
THE CHILD WITH CHRONIC RESPIRATORY ALTERATIONS

ORGANIZATIONS

NATIONAL HEART, LUNG, AND BLOOD INSTITUTE, NATIONAL ASTHMA EDUCATION PROGRAM
7200 Wisconsin Ave.
P.O. Box 329
Bethesda, MD 20814-4820
(301) 951-3260

ASTHMA AND ALLERGY FOUNDATION OF AMERICA
1125 15th St., NW, Suite 502
Washington, DC 20005
(202) 466-7643 or (800) 7-ASTHMA

NATIONAL ALLERGY AND ASTHMA NETWORK/MOTHERS OF ASTHMATICS
3554 Chain Bridge Rd., Suite 200
Fairfax, VA 22030-2709
(703) 385-4403; (800) 878-4403

AMERICAN LUNG ASSOCIATION
1740 Broadway
New York, NY 10019
(212) 315-8700

NATIONAL JEWISH CENTER FOR IMMUNOLOGY AND RESPIRATORY MEDICINE
Lung Line
(800) 222-LUNG

Programs/Resources on Self-Management of Asthma

ASTHMA CARE TRAINING FOR KIDS (ACT)
Asthma and Allergy Foundation of America
1125 15th Street, NW, Suite 502
Washington, DC 20005
(800) 7-ASTHMA

CALM: CHILDHOOD ASTHMA, LEARNING TO MANAGE
Asthma and Allergy Foundation of America
(see earlier listing for address)
(202) 466-7643

SUPERSTUFF
American Lung Association
1740 Broadway
New York, NY 10019

TEACHING MY PARENTS/MYSELF ABOUT ASTHMA
Health Education Associates
14 North Lake Road
Columbia, SC 29223

NATIONAL JEWISH CENTER OF IMMUNOLOGY AND RESPIRATORY MEDICINE
1400 Jackson Street
Denver, CO 80206
(800) 222-LUNG

NATIONAL ASTHMA EDUCATION PROGRAM
Information Center
4733 Bethesda Ave., Suite 530
Bethesda, MD 20814
(301) 951-3260

CHILDREN WITH ASTHMA: A MANUAL FOR PARENTS
Pedipress, Inc.
125 Redgate Lane
Amherst, MA 01002

WINNING OVER WHEEZING
Rhone-Poulenc-Rorer, Inc.
500 Virginia Drive
Fort Washington, PA 19304

CHAPTER 30
THE CHILD WITH CONGENITAL CARDIAC DEFECTS

AMERICAN HEART ASSOCIATION
Council on Cardiovascular Disease in the Young
7272 Greenville Ave.
Dallas, TX 75231
(214) 373-6300

AMERICAN SOCIETY OF HYPERTENSION
515 Madison Avenue, Suite 1212
New York, NY 10022
(212) 644-0650

CHAPTER 31
THE CHILD WITH CARDIOVASCULAR ALTERATIONS

AMERICAN HEART ASSOCIATION
Council on Cardiovascular Disease in the Young
7272 Greenville Ave.
Dallas, TX 75231
(214) 373-6300

AMERICAN SOCIETY OF HYPERTENSION
515 Madison Avenue, Suite 1212
New York, NY 10022
(212) 644-0650

CHAPTER 32
THE CHILD WITH HEMATOLOGIC ALTERATIONS

AHEPA COOLEY'S ANEMIA ORGANIZATION
1909 Q Street, NW, Suite 500
Washington, DC 20009
(202) 232-6300

APLASTIC ANEMIA FOUNDATION OF AMERICA
P.O. Box 22689
Baltimore, MD 21203
(800) 747-2820

COOLEY'S ANEMIA FOUNDATION
105 E. 22nd Street, Suite 911
New York, NY 10010
(800) 221-3571

THALASSEMIA ACTION GROUP
105 E. 22nd Street, Suite 911
New York, NY 10010
(800) 221-3571

NATIONAL HEMOPHILIA FOUNDATION
110 Greene St., Suite 303
New York, NY 10012
(212) 219-8180

AMERICAN SICKLE CELL ANEMIA ASSOCIATION
10300 Carnegie Avenue
Cleveland, OH 44106
(216) 229-8600

NATIONAL ASSOCIATION FOR SICKLE CELL DISEASE
3345 Wilshire Blvd., Suite 1106
Los Angeles, CA 90010-1800
(800) 421-8453

HEMOPHILIA AND AIDS/HIV NETWORK
FOR THE DISSEMINATION OF INFORMATION
110 Greene St., Suite 303
New York, NY 10012
(212) 431-8541

CHAPTER 33
THE CHILD WITH CANCER

Refer to the resources listed for Chapter 17 under "Cancer" and "General Support, Grief and Bereavement" for addresses of organizations.

THE ALPHA BOOK ON CANCER AND LIVING
(800) 866-4111
Lists resources relating to children and cancer

THE AMERICAN CANCER SOCIETY
(800) ACS-2345
Offers many resources for children with cancer

THE ASSOCIATION OF PEDIATRIC ONCOLOGY NURSES
(804) 379-9150
Offers membership for nurses interested in pediatric oncology

CANDLELIGHTERS CHILDHOOD CANCER FOUNDATION
(800) 366-2223
Offers resources and support for families of children with cancer

CENTER FOR ATTITUDINAL HEALING
(415) 435-5022
Offers support and bereavement services for children and families with terminal illnesses

CHILDREN'S ONCOLOGY CAMPS OF AMERICA
(217) 793-3949
Offers an annual directory of camps for children with cancer

CORPORATE ANGEL NETWORK
(914) 328-1313
Coordinates free air transportation for ambulatory cancer patients traveling to and from treatment centers

THE LEUKEMIA SOCIETY OF AMERICA
(800) 955-4572
Offers information, financial aid, and support to patients with leukemia, lymphoma, and Hodgkin's disease

THE NATIONAL LEUKEMIA ASSOCIATION, INC.
(516) 222-1944
Provides information and financial aid to patients with leukemia

MAKE-A-WISH FOUNDATION OF AMERICA
(602) 248-9474
Grants wishes to children with life-threatening illnesses

RONALD MCDONALD HOUSES
(708) 575-7418
Provides lodging for families of hospitalized children

SUNSHINE KIDS FOUNDATION
(800) 594-5756
Provides activities for children with cancer

CHAPTER 35
THE CHILD WITH BURNS

NATIONAL INSTITUTE FOR BURN MEDICINE
909 East Ann Street
Ann Arbor, MI 48104
(313) 769-9000

AMERICAN BURN ASSOCIATION
New York-Cornell Medical Center
525 E. 68th St.
Room L-706
New York, NY 10021
(800) 548-BURN

INTERNATIONAL SHRINERS HEADQUARTERS
2900 Rocky Point Drive
Tampa, FL 33607
(800) 237-5055; in Florida: (800) 282-9161

CHAPTER 36
THE CHILD WITH MUSCULOSKELETAL ALTERATIONS

OSTEOGENESIS IMPERFECTA FOUNDATION, INC.
P.O. Box 14807
Tampa, FL 34629-4807
(813) 855-7077

ARTHRITIS FOUNDATION
1314 Spring St. NW
Atlanta, GA 30309
(404) 872-7100

ARTHRITIS SOCIETY OF CANADA
250 Bloor St., E., Suite 401
Toronto, Ontario, Canada M4W 3P2
(416) 967-5679

MUSCULAR DYSTROPHY ASSOCIATION OF AMERICA, INC.
3300 East Sunrise Drive
Tucson, AZ 85718
(520) 529-2000

MUSCULAR DYSTROPHY ASSOCIATION OF CANADA
150 Eglinton Ave., E., Suite 400
Toronto, Ontario, Canada M4P 1E8
(416) 488-0030

CHAPTER 37
THE CHILD WITH STRUCTURAL DISORDERS OF THE BONES AND JOINTS

NATIONAL SCOLIOSIS FOUNDATION, INC.
72 Mount Auburn St.
Watertown, MA 02172
(617) 926-0397
FAX: (617) 926-0398

SCOLIOSIS ASSOCIATION, INC.
P.O. Box 811705
Boca Raton, FL 33481-1705
(800) 800-0669

CHAPTER 39
THE CHILD WITH DIABETES MELLITUS

AMERICAN DIABETES ASSOCIATION
1660 Duke Street
Alexandria, VA 22314
(703) 549-1500

HUMAN BIOLOGICAL DATA INTERCHANGE
1880 John F. Kennedy Blvd., 6th Floor
Philadelphia, PA 19103
(800) 345-HBDI, ext. 4234

INTERNATIONAL DIABETES CENTER
5000 West 39th Street
Minneapolis, MN 55416
(612) 927-3393

JUVENILE DIABETES FOUNDATION INTERNATIONAL
432 Park Avenue S., 16th Floor
New York, NY 10016
(212) 889-7575

AMERICAN ASSOCIATION OF DIABETES EDUCATORS
444 North Michigan Ave., Suite 1240
Chicago, IL 60611-3901
(800) 338-DMED

CHAPTER 41
THE CHILD WITH A PSYCHOSOCIAL DISORDER

PHYSICAL OR SEXUAL ABUSE

PARENTS ANONYMOUS (P.A.)—NATIONAL HEADQUARTERS
22330 Hawthorne Blvd., Suite 208
Torrence, CA 90505
(800) 421-0353

PARENTS UNITED, INC.
P.O. Box 952
San Jose, CA 95108
(408) 280-5055

NATIONAL COMMITTEE FOR THE PREVENTION OF CHILD ABUSE
332 S. Michigan Ave., Suite 1250
Chicago, IL 60604-4357

Books

Matsakis, A. (1991). *When the bough breaks: A helping guide for parents of sexually abused children.* New Harbinger Publications, Inc.

I can't talk about it: A child's book about sexual abuse. (1986). Portland, OR: Mulnomah Press.

Hindman, J. (1992). *A touching book.* Ontario, OR: Alexandria Associates.

ATTENTION-DEFICIT HYPERACTIVITY DISORDER

CHILDREN WITH ATTENTION DEFICIT DISORDERS (CHADD)
National Headquarters
499 NW 70th Ave.
Plantation, FL 33322
(305) 587-3700

ATTENTION DEFICIT DISORDERS ASSOCIATION (ADDA)
4300 West Park Blvd.
Plano, TX 75093

NATIONAL ATTENTION DEFICIT DISORDER ASSOCIATION
P.O. Box 972
Mentor, OH 44061
(800) 487-2282 or (313) 769-6690
ADAFAX BACK: (313) 769-6729
Website: http://www.92starnet.con~sled

CHALLENGE (ADHD NEWSLETTER)
P.O. Box 488
West Newbury, MA 01985
(508) 462-0495

CHAPTER 42
THE CHILD WITH A COGNITIVE DEFICIT

FRAGILE X SYNDROME

FRAGIX X ASSOCIATION OF AMERICA
P.O. Box 39
Parkridge, IL 60068
(708) 724-8626

NATIONAL FRAGILE X FOUNDATION
1441 York Street, Suite 215
Denver, CO 80206
(800) 688-8765 or (303) 333-6155

AUTISM

ADRIANA FOUNDATION
1911 11th Street, Suite 301
Boulder, CO 80302
(303) 786-9530

AUTISM SOCIETY OF AMERICA
7910 Woodmont Avenue, Suite 650
Bethesda, MD 20814-3015
(301) 657-0881

NATIONAL INSTITUTE OF MENTAL HEALTH
5600 Fisher's Lane
Rockville, MD 20857
(301) 443-4513

DIVISION TEACH
Department of Psychiatry
University of North Carolina
Chapel Hill, NC 27514

MENTAL RETARDATION

AMERICAN ASSOCIATION ON MENTAL RETARDATION
1719 Kalorama Road, NW
Washington, DC 20009-2683
(800) 424-3688

MENTAL RETARDATION ASSOCIATION OF AMERICA
211 East 300 South St., Suite 212
Salt Lake City, UT 84111
(801) 328-1575

THE ARC
500 East Border St., Suite 300
Arlington, TX 76010
(817) 261-6003

AMERICAN ASSOCIATION OF MENTAL DEFICIENCY
5201 Connecticut Avenue, NW
Washington, DC 20015

NATIONAL ASSOCIATION FOR RETARDED CITIZENS (NARC)
2709 Avenue E. East
Arlington, TX 76010

CHAPTER 43
THE CHILD WITH SENSORY ALTERATIONS

ALEXANDER GRAHAM BELL ASSOCIATION FOR THE DEAF
3417 Volta Place, NW
Washington, DC 20007
(202) 337-5220

AMERICAN COUNCIL FOR THE BLIND
1010 Vermont Avenue, NW, Suite 1100
Washington, DC 20005
(202) 393-3666 or (800) 424-8666

AMERICAN COUNCIL OF PARENTS OF BLIND CHILDREN
Route A, Box 78
Franklin, LA 70538

AMERICAN DEAFNESS ASSOCIATION
P.O. Box 55369
Little Rock, AR 72225
(501) 663-4617

AMERICAN FOUNDATION FOR THE BLIND
15 West 16th Street
New York, NY 10011
(212) 620-2000

AMERICAN SOCIETY FOR DEAF CHILDREN
814 Thayer Avenue
Silver Spring, MD 20910
(301) 585-5400

THE BLIND CHILDREN'S CENTER
4120 Marathon Street
P.O. Box 29159
Los Angeles, CA 90029
(213) 664-2153

CENTER FOR SPEECH, LANGUAGE AND HEARING ASSOCIATION
10801 Rockville Pike
Rockville, MD 20852
(800) 638-8255

HELEN KELLER NATIONAL CENTER FOR DEAF-BLIND YOUTH AND ADULTS
111 Middleneck Road
Sands Point, NY 11050
(516) 944-8900

NATIONAL ASSOCIATION FOR PARENTS OF THE VISUALLY HANDICAPPED
2011 Hardy Circle
Austin, TX 78757
(800) 562-6265

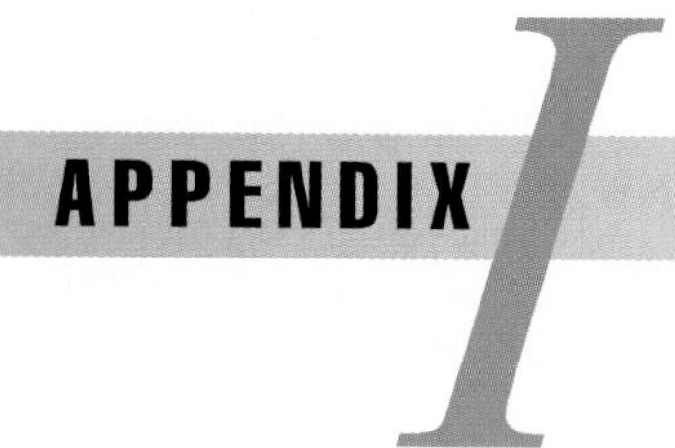

Common Laboratory Tests and Normal Values

To conserve space, the following common abbreviations are used.

ABBREVIATIONS ▼

Ab	absorbance
AU	arbitrary unit
CKBB	brain isoenzyme of creatine kinase
CKMB	heart isoenzyme of creatine kinase
d	diem, day, days
F	female
g	gram
hr	hour, hours
Hb	hemoglobin
HbCO	carboxyhemoglobin
IU	International Unit of hormone activity
L	liter
M	male
MCV	mean corpuscular volume
mEq/L	milliequivalents per liter
min	minute, minutes
mm^3	cubic millimeter; equivalent to microliter (µl)
mm Hg	millimeters of mercury
mo	month, months
mol	mole
mOsm	milliosmole
MW	relative molecular weight
N	nitrogen
Pa	pascal
pc	postprandial
RBC	red blood cell(s); erythrocyte(s)
RT	room temperature
s	second, seconds
U	International Unit of enzyme activity
vol	volume
WBC	white blood cell(s)
wk	week, weeks
yr	year, years

SYMBOLS ▼

>	greater than
≥	greater than or equal to
<	less than
≤	less than or equal to
±	plus/minus
≅	approximately equal to

Adapted from Behrman, R. E., Kliegman, R. M., & Arvin, A. M. (1996). *Nelson textbook of pediatrics* (15th ed.). Philadelphia: W. B. Saunders, pp. 2033–2058.

ABBREVIATIONS FOR SPECIMENS ▼

S	serum
P	plasma
(H)	heparin
(LiH)	lithium heparin
(E)	EDTA
(C)	citrate
(O)	oxalate
W	whole blood
U	urine
F	feces
CSF	cerebrospinal fluid
AF	amniotic fluid
(NaC)	sodium citrate
(NH_4H)	ammonium heparinate

KEY TO COMMENTS ▼

30°, 37°	temperature of enzymatic analysis (Celsius)
a	colorimetry
b	Ektachem, proprietary analytic system of Johnson & Johnson Clinical Diagnostics, Inc.
c	enzyme-amplified immunoassay
d	values obtained are significantly method dependent
e	nephelometry
f	cation-exchange chromatography
g	values in older males higher than those in older females
h	ion-selective electrode
i	fluorescence polarization
j	enzymatic assay

Prefixes Denoting Decimal Factors

PREFIX	SYMBOL	FACTOR
mega	M	10^6
kilo	k	10^3
hecto	h	10^2
deka	da	10^1
deci	d	10^{-1}
centi	c	10^{-2}
milli	m	10^{-3}
micro	µ	10^{-6}
nano	n	10^{-9}
pico	p	10^{-12}
femto	f	10^{-15}

Common Laboratory Tests and Normal Values

TEST	SPECIMEN	REFERENCE RANGE (CONVENTIONAL UNITS)		FACTOR	REFERENCE RANGE, INTERNATIONAL UNITS (SI)	COMMENTS
Acetaminophen	S, P(H,E)	Therapeutic concentration	10–30 μg/ml	× 6.62	66–200 μmol/L	i z
		Toxic concentration	>200 μg/ml		>1,300 μmol/L	
Activated partial thromboplastin time (APTT)	P(C)	25–35 s			25–35 s	
		Infant: <90 s			Infant: <90 s	
Adrenocorticotropic hormone (ACTH)	P(H)	Cord blood	130–160 pg/ml	× 1	130–160 μg/L	
		1–7 d postnatal	100–140 pg/ml		100–140 μg/L	
		Adult				
		0800 hr	25–100 pg/ml		25–100 μg/L	
		1800 hr	<50 pg/ml		<50 μg/L	
Alanine aminotransferase (ALT, SGPT)	S	0–5 d	6–50 U/L	× 1	6–50 U/L	37° s b
		1–19 yr	5–45 U/L		5–45 U/L	
Albumin	P	Premature 1 d	1.8–3.0 g/dl	× 10	18–30 g/L	
		Full-term <6 d	2.5–3.4 g/dl		25–34 g/L	
		<5 yr	3.9–5.0 g/dl		39–50 g/L	
		5–19 yr	4.0–5.3 g/dl		40–53 g/L	
	U	4–16 yr	3.35–15.3 mg/24 hr/1.73 m^2			c
	CSF	10–30 mg/dl			100–300 mg/L	
Ammonia nitrogen	S, P(LiH)	Neonate	90–150 μg N/dl	× 0.714	64–107 μmol/L	j f
		0–2 wk	79–129 μg N/dl		56–92 μmol/L	
		>1 mo	29–70 μg N/dl		21–50 μmol/L	
		Thereafter	15–45 μg N/dl		11–32 μmol/L	
		1–90 d	59–202 μg N/dl	× 0.714	42–144 μmol/L	
		3 mo–3 yr	48–195 μg N/dl		34–139 μmol/L	
	U		500–1,200 mg N/24 hr	× 0.0714	36–86 mmol/d	
Amphetamine	S, P(H,E)	Therapeutic concentration	20–30 ng/ml	× 7.396	150–220 nmol/l	
		Toxic concentration	>200 ng/ml		>1,500 nmol/l	
Antistreptolysin-O titer (ASO titer)	S	≤166 Todd units				
		170–330 Todd units in school-age children				
Base excess	W(H)	Neonate	(−10)–(−2) mmol/L		(−10)–(−2) mmol/L	
		Infant	(−7)–(−1) mmol/L		(−7)–(−1) mmol/L	
		Child	(−4)–(+2) mmol/L		(−4)–(+2) mmol/L	
		Thereafter	(−3)–(+3) mmol/L		(−3)–(+3) mmol/L	
Bicarbonate	S, P	Arterial	21–28 mmol/L		21–28 mmol/L	
		Venous	22–29 mmol/L		22–29 mmol/L	
Bilirubin	S, P					

TEST	SPECIMEN	Premature		Full-Term	FACTOR	Premature	Full-Term	COMMENTS
Total	S	Cord blood	<2.0 mg/dl	<2.0 mg/dl	× 17.10	<34 μmol/L	<34 μmol/L	
		0–1 d	<8.0 mg/dl	<6.0 mg/dl		<137 μmol/L	<103 μmol/L	
		1–2 d	<12.0 mg/dl	<8.0 mg/dl		<205 μmol/L	<137 μmol/L	
		2–5 d	<16.0 mg/dl	<12.0 mg/dl		<274 μmol/L	<205 μmol/L	
		>5 d	<2.0 mg/dl	0.2–1.0 mg/dl		<34 μmol/L	3.4–17.1 μmol/L	

(continued)

Common Laboratory Tests and Normal Values (continued)

TEST	SPECIMEN	REFERENCE RANGE (CONVENTIONAL UNITS)		FACTOR	REFERENCE RANGE, INTERNATIONAL UNITS (SI)	COMMENTS
	U	Negative			Negative	
	AF	28 wk <0.075 mg/dl		× 17.10	<1.3 µmol/L	
		(or Ab450 <0.048)			(or Ab450 <0.048)	
		40 wk <0.025 mg/dl			<0.43 µmol/L	
		(or Ab450 <0.02)			(or Ab450 <0.02)	
Conjugated	S	0–0.2 mg/dl		× 17.10	0–3.4 µmol/L	
Bleeding time (BBT)						
Ivy		Normal 2–7 min			Normal 2–7 min	
		Borderline 7–11 min			Borderline 7–11 min	
Simplate (G–D)		2.75–8 min			2.75–8 min	
Blood volume	W(H)	M 52–83 ml/kg		× 0.001	M 0.052–0.083 L/kg	
		F 50–75 ml/kg			F 0.050–0.075 L/kg	
C-reactive protein	S	Cord blood	52–1,330 ng/ml	×1	52–1,330 µg/L	c
		2–12 yr	67–1,800 ng/ml		67–1,800 µg/L	
Calcium, ionized (Ca)	S, P(H), W(H)	Cord blood	5.0–6.0 mg/dl	× 0.25	1.25–1.50 mmol/L	
		Neonate				
		3–24 hr	4.3–5.1 mg/dl		1.07–1.27 mmol/L	
		24–48 hr	4.0–4.7 mg/dl		1.00–1.17 mmol/L	
		Thereafter	4.8–4.92 mg/dl, or		1.12–1.23 mmol/L	
			2.24–2.46 mEq/L	× 0.5	1.12–1.23 mmol/L	
Calcium, total	S	Cord blood	9.0–11.5 mg/dl	× 0.25	2.25–2.88 mmol/L	
		Neonate				
		3–24 hr	9.0–10.6 mg/dl		2.3–2.65 mmol/L	
		24–48 hr	7.0–12.0 mg/dl		1.75–3.0 mmol/L	
		4–7 d	9.0–10.9 mg/dl		2.25–2.73 mmol/L	
		Child	8.8–10.8 mg/dl		2.2–2.70 mmol/L	
		Thereafter	8.4–10.2 mg/dl		2.1–2.55 mmol/L	
	U	Ca in diet				
		Ca-free	5–40 mg/24 hr	× 0.025	0.13–1.0 mmol/24 hr	
		Low to average	50–150 mg/24 hr		1.25–3.8 mmol/24 hr	
Carbon dioxide	W(H)	Neonate	27–40 mm Hg	× 0.1333	3.6–5.3 kPa	
		Infant	27–41 mm Hg		3.6–5.5 kPa	
Partial pressure (Pco_2)		Thereafter				
		M	35–48 mm Hg		4.7–6.4 kPa	
		F	32–45 mm Hg		4.3–6.0 kPa	
Total (tco_2)	S, P(H)	Cord blood	14–22 mmol/L	× 1	14–22 mmol/L	
		Premature	14–27 mmol/L		14–27 mmol/L	
		Neonate	13–22 mmol/L		13–22 mmol/L	
		Infant	20–28 mmol/L		20–28 mmol/L	
		Child	20–28 mmol/L		20–28 mmol/L	
		Thereafter	23–30 mmol/L		23–30 mmol/L	
Carbon monoxide	W(E)	Nonsmokers	<2% HbCO	× 0.01	HbCO fraction <0.02	
		Smokers	<10%		<0.10	
		Lethal	>50%		>0.5	

Cerebrospinal fluid							
Pressure	CSF	70–180 mm H_2O			70–180 mm H_2O		
Volume	CSF	Child	60–100 ml	× 0.001	0.06–0.10 L		
		Adult	100–160 ml		0.1–0.16 L		
Chloral hydrate	S	As trichloroethanol					
		Therapeutic concentration	2–12 μg/ml	× 6.694	13–80 μmol/L		
		Toxic concentration	>20 μg/ml		>134 μmol/L		
Chloride	S, P(H)	Cord blood	96–104 mmol/L	× 1	96–104 mmol/L		
		Neonate	97–110 mmol/L		97–110 mmol/L		
		Thereafter	98–106 mmol/L		98–106 mmol/L		
	CSF		118–132 mmol/L	× 1	118–132 mmol/L		
	U	Infant	2–10 mmol/24 hr	× 1	2–10 mmol/24 hr		
		Child	15–40 mmol/24 hr		15–40 mmol/24 hr		
		Thereafter	110–250 mmol/24 hr (varies greatly with Cl intake)		110–250 mmol/24 hr		
	Sweat	Normal	<40 mmol/L	× 1	<40 mmol/L		
		Borderline	45–60 mmol/L		45–60 mmol/L		
		Cystic fibrosis	>60 mmol/L		>60 mmol/L		
Cholesterol, total	S	1–3 yr	45–182 mg/dl	× 0.0259	1.15–4.70 mmol/L		j
		4–6 yr	109–189 mg/dl		2.80–4.80 mmol/L		
	S			× 0.0259			
Clotting time, Lee-White, 37°C	W	Glass tubes	5–8 min (5–15 min at RT)		Glass tubes	5–8 min (5–15 min at RT)	
		Silicone tubes	About 30 min prolonged		Silicone tubes	About 30 min prolonged	
Creatine kinase	S	Cord blood	70–380 U/L	× 1	70–380 U/L		30° g
		5–8 hr	214–1,175 U/L		214–1,175 U/L		
		24–33 hr	130–1,200 U/L		130–1,200 U/L		
		72–100 hr	87–725 U/L		87–725 U/L		
		Adult	5–130 U/L		5–130 U/L		
Creatine kinase isoenzymes	S		***CKMB***	***CKBB***			
		Cord blood	0.3–3.1%	0.3–10.5%			
		5–8 hr	1.7–7.9%	3.6–13.4%			
		24–33 hr	1.8–5.0%	2.3–8.6%			
		72–100 hr	1.4–5.4%	5.1–13.3%			
		Adult	0–2%	0			
Creatinine, plasma							
Jaffe, kinetic, or enzymatic	S, P	Cord blood	0.6–1.2 mg/dl	× 88.4	53–106 μmol/L		
		Neonate	0.3–1.0 mg/dl		27–88 μmol/L		
		Infant	0.2–0.4 mg/dl		18–35 μmol/L		
		Child	0.3–0.7 mg/dl		27–62 μmol/L		
		Adolescent	0.5–1.0 mg/dl		44–88 μmol/L		
		Adult					
		M	0.6–1.2 mg/dl		53–106 μmol/L		
		F	0.5–1.1 mg/dl		44–97 μmol/L		

(continued)

Common Laboratory Tests and Normal Values (continued)

TEST	SPECIMEN	REFERENCE RANGE (CONVENTIONAL UNITS)		FACTOR	REFERENCE RANGE, INTERNATIONAL UNITS (SI)	COMMENTS
Jaffe, manual	S, P		0.8–1.5 mg/dl	× 88.4	70–133 μmol/L	
	AF	After 37-wk gestation	>2.0 mg/dl	× 88.4	>180 μmol/L	
Creatinine, urinary	U	Premature	8.1–15.0 mg/kg/24 hr	× 8.84	72–133 μmol/kg/24 hr	d b
		Full-term	10.4–19.7 mg/kg/24 hr		92–174 μmol/kg/24 hr	
		1.5–7 yr	10–15 mg/kg/24 hr		88–133 μmol/kg/24 hr	
		7–15 yr	5.2–41 mg/kg/24 hr		46–362 μmol/kg/24 hr	
Creatinine clearance (endogenous)	S, P, U	Neonate	40–65 ml/min/1.73 m^2			
		<40 yr				
		M	97–137 ml/min/1.73 m^2			
		F	88–128 ml/min/1.73 m^2			
		Decreases	~6.5 ml/min/decade			
Diazepam	S, P(H,E) at trough	Therapeutic concentration	100–1,000 ng/ml	× 3.512	350–3,500 nmol/L	
		Toxic concentration	>5,000 ng/ml		>17,500 nmol/L	
Digoxin	S, P(H,E) (12-hr post)	Therapeutic concentration				
		CHF	0.8–1.5 ng/ml	× 1.281	1.0–1.9 nmol/L	i c
		Arrhythmias	1.5–2.0 ng/ml		1.9–2.6 nmol/L	
		Toxic concentration				
		Child	>2.5 ng/ml		>3.2 nmol/L	
		Adult	>3.0 ng/ml		>3.8 nmol/L	
Eosinophil count	W(E,H) capillary	50–350 cells/mm^3 (μl)		× 10^6	50–350 × 10^6 cells/L	
Erythrocyte count (RBC count)	W(E)		***Millions of cells/mm^3 (μl)***		***× 10^{12} cells/L***	
		Cord blood	3.9–5.5	× 1	3.9–5.5	
		1–3 d (capillary)	4.0–6.6		4.0–6.6	
		1 wk	3.9–6.3		3.9–6.3	
		2 wk	3.6–6.2		3.6–6.2	
		1 mo	3.0–5.4		3.0–5.4	
		2 mo	2.7–4.9		2.7–4.9	
		3–6 mo	3.1–4.5		3.1–4.5	
		0.5–2 yr	3.7–5.3		3.7–5.3	
		2–6 yr	3.9–5.3		3.9–5.3	
		6–12 yr	4.0–5.2		4.0–5.2	
		12–18 yr				
		M	4.5–5.3		4.5–5.3	
		F	4.1–5.1		4.1–5.1	
		18–49 yr				
		M	4.5–5.9		4.5–5.9	
		F	4.0–5.2		4.0–5.2	

Test	Specimen		Conventional	Factor	SI	
Erythrocyte sedimentation rate (ESR)	W(E)					
Westergren, modified		Child	0–10 mm/hr		0–10 mm/hr	
		Adult				
		M < 50 yr	0–15 mm/hr		0–15 mm/hr	
		F < 50 yr	0–20 mm/hr		0–20 mm/hr	
Wintrobe		Child	0–13 mm/hr		0–13 mm/hr	
		Adult				
		M	0–9 mm/hr		0–9 mm/hr	
		F	0–20 mm/hr		0–20 mm/hr	
			41–54%		41–54 AU	
Fat, fecal	F (72 hr)	Infant, breast-fed	<1 g/24 hr	× 1	<1 g/24 hr	
		0–6 yr	<2 g/24 hr		<2 g/24 hr	
		Adult				
		Normal diet	<7 g/24 hr		<7 g/24 hr	
		Fat-free diet	<4 g/24 hr		<4 g/24 hr	
		Coefficient of Fat Absorption (%)			***Absorbed Fraction***	
		Infant		× 0.01		
		Breast-fed	>93		>0.93	
		Formula-fed	>83		>0.83	
		>1 yr	≥95		≥0.95	
α-Fetoprotein (AFP)	S maternal	***Pregnancy (wk)***	***Median***		***Median***	
		15	34 ng/ml	× 1	34 μg/L	
		16	38 ng/ml		38 μg/L	
		17	44 ng/ml		44 μg/L	
		18	49 ng/ml		49 μg/L	
		19	56.5 ng/ml		56.5 μg/L	
		20	66 ng/ml		66 μg/L	
	AF		***Mean***			
		15	13.5 ± 3.42 μg/ml			
		16	11.7 ± 3.38 μg/ml			
		17	10.3 ± 3.03 μg/ml			
		18	9.5 ± 3.22 μg/ml			
		19	7.1 ± 2.86 μg/ml			
		20	5.0 ± 2.45 μg/ml			
Fibrinogen	P(NaCl)	Neonate	125–300 mg/dl	× 0.01	1.25–3.00 g/L	
		Adult	200–400 mg/dl		2.00–4.00 g/L	
Galactose	S	Neonate	0–20 mg/dl	× 0.0555	0–1.11 mmol/L	
	P	5 mo–17 yr	0.0–0.5 mg/dl		0.0–0.03 mmol/L	j
	U	Neonate	≤60 mg/dl	× 0.0555	≤3.33 mmol/L	
		Thereafter	14 mg/24 hr	× 0.00555	<0.08 mmol/24 hr	

(continued)

Common Laboratory Tests and Normal Values (continued)

TEST	SPECIMEN	REFERENCE RANGE (CONVENTIONAL UNITS)			FACTOR	REFERENCE RANGE, INTERNATIONAL UNITS (SI)		COMMENTS
Glucose	S	Cord blood	45–96 mg/dl		× 0.0555	2.5–5.3 mmol/L		
		Neonate						
		1 d	40–60 mg/dl			2.2–3.3 mmol/L		
		>1 d	50–90 mg/dl			2.8–5.0 mmol/L		
		Child	60–100 mg/dl			3.3–5.5 mmol/L		
		Adult	70–105 mg/dl			3.9–5.8 mmol/L		
	W (H)	Adult	65–95 mg/dl			3.6–5.3 mmol/L		
	CSF	Adult	40–70 mg/dl			2.2–3.9 mmol/L		
Quantitative, enzymatic	U	<0.5 g/24 hr			× 5.55	<2.8 mmol/24 hr		
Qualitative	U	Negative				Negative		
Glucose, 2 hr pc	S	<120 mg/dl (For diabetes, see Glucose tolerance test, oral)			× 0.0555	<6.7 mmol/L		
Glucose tolerance test (GTT), oral	S		*Normal*	*Diabetic*		*Normal*	*Diabetic*	
Adult dose: 75 g		Fasting	70–105 mg/dl	>115 mg/dl	× 0.0555	3.9–5.8 mmol/L	>6.4 mmol/L	
Child dose: 1.75 g/kg of ideal weight up to maximum of 75 g		60 min	120–170 mg/dl	≥200 mg/dl		6.7–9.4 mmol/L	≥11 mmol/L	
		90 min	100–140 mg/dl	≥200 mg/dl		5.6–7.8 mmol/L	≥11 mmol/L	
		120 min	70–120 mg/dl	≥140 mg/dl		3.9–6.7 mmol/L	≥7.8 mmol/L	
Growth hormone (hGH, so matotropin)	S, P(E,H)	Neonate						
		1 d	5–23 ng/ml		× 1	5–53 μg/L		
		1 wk	5–27 ng/ml			5–27 μg/L		
		1–12 mo	2–10 ng/ml			2–10 μg/L		
	Fasting, at rest	Child	<0.7–6 ng/ml			<0.7–6 μg/L		
		Adult	<0.7–6 ng/ml			<0.7–6 μg/L		
Hematocrit (HCT, Hct)	W(E)		***Percent Packed Red Cells (Vol Red Cells/Vol Whole Blood Cells × 100)***			***Volume Fraction (Vol Red Cells/Vol Whole Blood)***		
Calculated from MCV and RBC (electronic displacement or laser)		1 d (capillary)	48–69%		× 0.01	0.48–0.69		
		2 d	48–75%			0.48–0.75		
		3 d	44–72%			0.44–0.72		
		2 mo	28–42%			0.28–0.42		
		6–12 yr	35–45%			0.35–0.45		
		12–18 yr						
		M	37–49%			0.37–0.49		
		F	36–46%			0.36–0.46		
		18–49 yr						
		M	41–53%			0.41–0.53		
		F	36–46%			0.36–0.46		

Hemoglobin (Hb)	W(E)	1–3 d (capillary)	14.5–22.5 g/dl	× 0.155	2.25–3.49 mmol/L	MW Hb = 64,500
		2 mo	9.0–14.0 g/dl		1.40–2.17 mmol/L	
		6–12 yr	11.5–15.5 g/dl		1.78–2.40 mmol/L	
		12–18 yr				
		M	13.0–16.0 g/dl		2.02–2.48 mmol/L	
		F	12.0–16.0 g/dl		1.86–2.48 mmol/L	
		18–49 yr				
		M	13.5–17.5 g/dl		2.09–2.27 mmol/L	
		F	12.0–16.0 g/dl		1.86–2.48 mmol/L	
	P(H)	<10 mg/dl		× 0.155	<1.55 μmol/L	
		<3 mg/dl with butterfly set-up and 18G needle			<0.47 μmol/L with butterfly set-up and 18G needle	
	U	Negative			Negative	
Hemoglobin A	W(E,C,H)		>95%	× 0.01	Fraction of hemoglobin >0.95	
Hemoglobin F	W(E)					
Alkali denaturation		1 d	63–92 %HbF	× 0.01	0.62–0.92 mass fraction	
		5 d	65–88 %HbF		0.65–0.88 mass fraction	
		3 wk	55–85 %HbF		0.55–0.85 mass fraction	
		6–9 wk	31–75 %HbF		0.31–0.75 mass fraction	
		3–4 mo	<2–59 %HbF		<0.02–0.59 mass fraction	
		6 mo	<2–9 %HbF		<0.02–0.09 mass fraction	
		Adult	<2 %HbF		<0.02 mass fraction	
Immunoglobulin A (IgA)	S	Cord blood	1.4–3.6 mg/dl	× 10	14–36 mg/L	e
		1–3 mo	1.3–53 mg/dl		13–530 mg/L	
		4–6 mo	4.4–84 mg/dl		44–840 mg/L	
		7 mo–1 yr	11–106 mg/dl		110–1,060 mg/L	
		2–5 yr	14–159 mg/dl		140–1,590 mg/L	
		6–10 yr	33–236 mg/dl		330–2,360 mg/L	
		Adult	70–312 mg/dl		700–3,120 mg/L	
Immunoglobulin D (IgD)	S	Neonate	None detected	× 10	None detected	
		Thereafter	0–8 mg/dl		0–80 mg/L	
Immunoglobulin E (IgE)	S	M	0–230 IU/ml	× 1	0–230 kIU/L	
		F	0–170 IU/ml		0–170 kIU/L	
Immunoglobulin G (IgG)	S	Cord blood	636–1,606 mg/dl	× 0.01	6.36–16.06 g/L	e
		1 mo	251–906 mg/dl		2.51–9.06 g/L	
		2–4 mo	176–601 mg/dl		1.76–6.01 g/L	
		5–12 mo	172–1,069 mg/dl		1.72–10.69 g/L	
		1–5 yr	345–1,236 mg/dl		3.45–12.36 g/L	
		6–10 yr	608–1,572 mg/dl		6.08–15.72 g/L	
		Adult	639–1,349 mg/dl		6.39–13.49 g/L	
Immunoglobulin M (IgM)	S	Cord blood	6.3–25 mg/dl	× 10	63–250 mg/L	e
		1–4 mo	17–105 mg/dl		170–1,050 mg/L	
		5–9 mo	33–126 mg/dl		300–1,260 mg/L	
		10 mo–1 yr	41–173 mg/dl		410–1,730 mg/L	
		2–8 yr	43–207 mg/dl		430–2,070 mg/L	
		9–10 yr	52–242 mg/dl		520–2,420 mg/L	
		Adult	56–352 mg/dl		560–3,520 mg/L	

(continued)

Common Laboratory Tests and Normal Values (continued)

TEST	SPECIMEN	REFERENCE RANGE (CONVENTIONAL UNITS)		FACTOR	REFERENCE RANGE, INTERNATIONAL UNITS (SI)	COMMENTS
Iron	S	Neonate	100–250 µg/dl	× 0.179	17.90–44.75 µmol/L	
		Infant	40–100 µg/dl		7.16–17.90 µmol/L	
		Child	50–120 µg/dl		8.95–21.48 µmol/L	
		Thereafter				
		M	50–160 µg/dl		8.95–28.64 µmol/L	
		F	40–150 µg/dl		7.16–26.85 µmol/L	
		Intoxicated child	280–2,550 µg/dl		50.12–456.5 µmol/L	
		Fatally poisoned child	>1,800 µ/dl		>322.2 µmol/L	
Iron-binding capacity, total (TIBC)	S	Infant	100–400 µg/dl	× 0.179	17.90–71.60 µmol/L	
		Thereafter	250–400 µg/dl		44.75–71.60 µmol/L	
17-Ketogenic steroids (17-KGS)	U	0–1 yr	<1.0 mg/24 hr	× 3.467	<3.5 µmol/24 hr	Conversion based on dehydroepiandrosterone, MW 288
		1–10 yr	<5 mg/24 hr		<17 µmol/24 hr	
		11–14 yr	<12 mg/24 hr		<42 µmol/24 hr	
		Thereafter				
		M	5–23 mg/24 hr		17–80 µmol/24 hr	
		F	3–15 mg/24 hr		10–52 µmol/24 hr	
Ketone bodies						
Qualitative	S	Negative			Negative	
	U	Negative			Negative	
Quantitative	S	0.5–3.0 mg/dl		× 10	5–30 mg/L	
LDL-cholesterol (LDLC)	S, P(E)					
			M (mg/dl) / ***F (mg/dl)***		***M (mmol/L)*** / ***F (mmol/L)***	
		Cord blood	10–50 / 10–50	× 0.0259	0.26–1.30 / 0.26–1.30	
		1–9 yr	60–140 / 60–150		1.55–3.63 / 1.55–3.89	
		10–19 yr	50–170 / 50–170		1.30–4.40 / 1.30–4.40	
		20–29 yr	60–175 / 60–160		1.55–4.53 / 1.55–4.14	
		30–39 yr	80–190 / 70–170		2.07–4.92 / 1.81–4.40	
		40–49 yr	90–205 / 80–190		2.33–5.31 / 2.07–4.92	
		Recommended (desirable) range for adults	<130 mg/dl		1.68–4.53 mmol/L	
Lead	W(H)	Child	<10 µg/dl	× 0.0483	<0.48 µmol/L	
		Adult	<40 µg/dl		<1.93 µmol/L	
		Acceptable for industrial exposure	<60 µg/dl		<2.90 µmol/L	
		Toxic	≥100 µg/dl		≥4.83 µmol/L	
	U (24-hr)	<80 µg/dl		× 0.00483	<0.39 µmol/L	
Leukocyte count (WBC)	W(E)		***× 1,000 cells/mm^3 (µl)***		***× 10^9 cells/L***	
		Birth	9.0–30.0		9.0–30.0	
		24 hr	9.4–34.0		9.4–34.0	
		1 mo	5.0–19.5		5.0–19.5	
		1–3 yr	6.0–17.5		6.0–17.5	
		4–7 yr	5.5–15.5		5.5–15.5	
		8–13 yr	4.5–13.5		4.5–13.5	
		Adult	4.5–11.0		4.5–11.0	

Test	Specimen	Age	Reference range	Conversion factor	SI units
Leukocyte differential	W(E)				
Myelocytes		0		× 0.01	0
Neutrophils—"bands"		3–5%			0.03–0.05 no. fraction
Neutrophils—"segs"		54–62%			0.54–0.62 no. fraction
Lymphocytes		25–33%			0.25–0.33 no. fraction
Monocytes		3–7%			0.03–0.07 no. fraction
Eosinophils		1–3%			0.01–0.03 no. fraction
Basophils		0–0.75%			0–0.0075 no. fraction
Mean corpuscular hemoglobin concentration (MCHC)	W(E)	Birth	31–37 pg/cell	× 0.0155	0.48–0.57 fmol/cell
		1–3 d (capillary)	31–37 pg/cell		0.48–0.57 fmol/cell
		1 wk–1 mo	28–40 pg/cell		0.43–0.62 fmol/cell
		2 mo	26–34 pg/cell		0.40–0.53 fmol/cell
		3–6 mo	25–35 pg/cell		0.39–0.54 fmol/cell
		0.5–2 yr	23–31 pg/cell		0.36–0.48 fmol/cell
		2–6 yr	24–30 pg/cell		0.37–0.47 fmol/cell
		6–12 yr	25–33 pg/cell		0.39–0.51 fmol/cell
		12–18 yr	25–35 pg/cell		0.39–0.54 fmol/cell
		18–49 yr	26–34 pg/cell		0.40–0.53 fmol/cell
Mean corpuscular hemoglobin	W(E)		***Percentage Hb/cell or g Hb/dl RBC***		***mmol Hb/L RBC***
		Birth	30–36	× 0.155	4.65–5.58
		1–3 d (capillary)	29–37		4.50–5.74
		1–2 wk	28–38		4.34–5.89
		1–2 mo	29–37		4.50–5.74
		3 mo–2 yr	30–36		4.65–5.58
		2–18 yr	31–37		4.81–5.74
		>18 yr	31–37		4.81–5.74
Mean corpuscular volume (MCV)	W(E)	1–3 d (capillary)	95–121 μm^3	× 1	95–121 fl
		0.5–2 yr	70–86 μm^3		70–86 fl
		6–12 yr	77–95 μm^3		77–95 fl
		12–18 yr			
		M	78–98 μm^3		78–98 fl
		F	78–102 μm^3		78–102 fl
		18–49 yr			
		M	80–100 μm^3		80–100 fl
		F	80–100 μm^3		80–100 fl
Occult blood	F	Negative (>2 ml blood/24 hr in ~ 100–200 g stool)			Negative
	U	Negative			Negative
Osmolality	S	Child and adult	275–295 mOsm/kg H_2O		
	U	50–1,400 mOsm/kg H_2O, depending on fluid intake. After 12 hr of fluid restriction, normal range is >850 mOsm/kg H_2O			
	U (24-hr)	300–900 mOsm/kg H_2O			
Oxygen, partial pressure of (PO_2)	W(H), arterial	Birth	8–24 mm Hg	× 0.133	1.1–3.2 kPa
		5–10 min	33–75 mm Hg		4.4–10.0 kPa
		30 min	31–85 mm Hg		4.1–11.3 kPa
		>1 hr	55–80 mm Hg		7.3–10.6 kPa
		1 d	54–95 mm Hg		7.2–12.6 kPa
		Thereafter (decreases with age)	83–108 mm Hg		11–14.4 kPa

(continued)

Common Laboratory Tests and Normal Values (continued)

TEST	SPECIMEN	REFERENCE RANGE (CONVENTIONAL UNITS)		FACTOR	REFERENCE RANGE, INTERNATIONAL UNITS (SI)	COMMENTS
Oxygen saturation	W(H), arterial	Neonate	85–90%	× 0.01	0.85–0.90 Saturated fraction	
		Thereafter	95–99%		0.95–0.99 Saturated fraction	
Partial thromboplastin time (PTT)	W(NaCl)					
Nonactivated		60–85 s (Platelin)			60–85 s	
Activated		25–35 s (differs with method)			25–35 s	
Phenobarbital	S, P(H,E) at trough	Therapeutic concentration	15–40 μg/ml	× 4.306	65–170 μmol/L	i c
		Toxic concentration				
		Slowness, ataxia, nystagmus	35–80 μg/ml		150–345 μmol/L	
		Coma				
		With reflexes	65–117 μg/ml		280–504 μmol/L	
		Without reflexes	>100 μg/ml		>430 μmol/L	
Phenylalanine	S	Premature	2.0–7.5 mg/dl	× 60.54	120–450 μmol/L	
		Neonate	1.2–3.4 mg/dl		70–210 μmol/L	
		Thereafter	0.8–1.8 mg/dl		50–110 μmol/L	
	U	10 d–2 wk	1–2 mg/24 hr	× 6.054	6–12 μmol/24 hr	
		3–12 yr	4–18 mg/24 hr		24–110 μmol/24 hr	
		Thereafter	Trace–17 mg/24 hr		Trace–103 μmol/24 hr	
Plasma volume	P(H)	M	25–43 ml/kg	× 0.001	M 0.025–0.043 L/kg	
		F	28–45 ml/kg		F 0.028–0.045 L/kg	
Platelet count (thrombocyte count)	W(E)	Neonate 84–478 × 10^3/mm^3 (μl) (after 1 wk same as adult)		× 10^6	84–478 × 10^9/L	
		Adult 150–400 × 10^3/mm^3 (μl)			150–400 × 10^9/L	
Potassium	S	<2 mo	3.0–7.0 mmol/L	× 1	3.0–7.0 mmol/L	h
		2–12 mo	3.5–6.0 mmol/L		3.5–6.0 mmol/L	Increased by hemolysis
		>12 mo	3.5–5.0 mmol/L		3.5–5.0 mmol/L	
	P(H)				3.5–4.5 mmol/L	Serum values systematically higher than plasma values
	U (24-hr)	2.5–125 mmol/L (varies with diet)			2.5–125 mmol/L (varies with diet)	
Protein						
Total	S	Premature	4.3–7.6 g/dl	× 10	43–76 g/L	
		Neonate	4.6–7.4 g/dl		46–74 g/L	
		1–7 yr	6.1–7.9 g/dl	× 10	61–79 g/L	
		8–12 yr	6.4–8.1 g/dl		64–81 g/L	
		13–19 yr	6.6–8.2 g/dl		66–82 g/L	
Total urinary	U (24-hr)	1–14 mg/dl			10–140 mg/L	
		50–80 mg/24 hr (at rest)			50–80 mg/24 hr (at rest)	
		<250 mg/24 hr after intense exercise			<250 mg/24 hr after intense exercise	
Total protein (column)	CSF	Lumbar	8–32 mg/dl	× 10	80–320 mg/L	

Prothrombin time (PT)						
One-stage (quick)	W(NaC)	In general, 11–15 s (varies with type of thromboplastin)			11–15 s	
		Neonate: prolonged by 2–3 s			Neonate: prolonged by 2–3 s	
Two-stage modified (Ware and Seegers)	W(NaC)	18–22 s			18–22 s	
RBC count. See Erythrocyte count						
Red cell volume	W(H)	M	20–36 ml/kg	× 0.001	0.020–0.036 L/kg	
		F	19–31 ml/kg		0.019–0.031 L/kg	
Reticulocyte count	W (E,H,O)	Adults 0.5–1.5% of erythrocytes, or		× 0.01	0.005–0.015 number fraction	
		25,000–75,000/mm^3 (µl)		× 10^6	25,000–75,000 × 10^6/L	
	W (capillary)	1 d	0.4–6.0%	× 0.01	0.004–0.060 number fraction	
		7 d	<0.1–1.3%		<0.001–0.013 number fraction	
		1–4 wk	<1.0–1.2%		<0.001–0.012 number fraction	
		5–6 wk	<0.1–2.4%		<0.001–0.024 number fraction	
		7–8 wk	0.1–2.9%		0.001–0.029 number fraction	
		9–10 wk	<0.1–2.6%		<0.001–0.026 number fraction	
		11–12 wk	0.1–1.3%		0.001–0.013 number fraction	
Salicylate	S, P(H,E) at trough	Therapeutic concentration	15–30 mg/dl	× 0.0724	1.1–2.2 mmol/L	
		Toxic concentration	>30 mg/dl		>2.2 mmol/L	
Sedimentation rate. See Erythrocyte sedimentation rate						
Sickle cell tests						
Sodium metabisulfite	W(E,H,O)	Negative				
Dithionite test	W(E,H,O)	Negative				
Sodium	S,P(LiH, NH_4H)	Neonate	134–146 mmol/L	× 1	134–146 mmol/L	
		Infant	139–146 mmol/L		139–146 mmol/L	
		Child	138–145 mmol/L		138–146 mmol/L	
		Thereafter	136–146 mmol/L		136–148 mmol/L	
	U (24-hr)	(depending on diet)	40–220 mmol		40–220 mmol	
	Sweat	Normal	<40 mmol/L	× 1	<40 mmol/L	
		Indeterminate	45–60 mmol/L		45–60 mmol/L	
		Cystic fibrosis	>60 mmol/L		>60 mmol/L	
Specific gravity	U	Adult	1.002–1.030		1.002–1.030	
		After 12-hr fluid restriction	>1.025		>1.025	
	U (24-hr)		1.015–1.025			
Theophylline	S, P(H,E)	Therapeutic concentration, bronchodilator	10–20 µg/ml	× 5.550	56–110 µmol/L	i j
		Premature apnea	5–10 µg/ml		28–56 µmol/L	
		Toxic concentration	>20 µg/ml		>110 µmol/L	
Thrombin time	W(NaC)	Control time ± 2 s when control is 9–13 s			Control time ± 2 s when control is 9–13 s	

(continued)

Common Laboratory Tests and Normal Values (continued)

TEST	SPECIMEN	REFERENCE RANGE (CONVENTIONAL UNITS)			FACTOR	REFERENCE RANGE, INTERNATIONAL UNITS (SI)		COMMENTS
Thyroxine								
Total	S	Full-term infant			× 12.8700			
		1–3 d	8.2–19.9 μg/dl			106–256 nmol/L		
		1 wk	6.0–15.9 μg/dl			77–205 nmol/L		
		1–12 mo	6.1–14.9 μg/dl			79–192 nmol/L		
		Prepubertal child						
		1–3 yr	6.8–13.5 μg/dl			88–174 nmol/L		
		3–10 yr	5.5–12.8 μg/dl			71–165 nmol/L		
		Pubertal children and adults	4.2–13.0 μg/dl			54–167 nmol/L		
Free	S	Neonate			× 12.87			
		3 d	2.0–4.9 ng/dl			26–631 pmol/L		
		Infant						
		1–12 mo	0.9–2.6 ng/dl			12–33 pmol/L		
		Prepubertal child	0.8–2.2 ng/dl			10–28 pmol/L		
		Pubertal children and adults	0.8–2.3 ng/dl			10–30 pmol/L		
Thyroxine, total	W	Neonatal screen (filter paper)	6.2–2.2 μg/dl					
Tourniquet test		<5–10 petechiae in 2.5-cm circle on forearm (halfway between systolic and diastolic); pressure maintained for 5 min				<5–10 petechiae in 2.5-cm circle on forearm (halfway between systolic and diastolic); pressure maintained for 5 min		
		0–8 petechiae in 6-cm circle (50 mm Hg for 15 min)				0–8 petechiae in 6-cm circle (50 mm Hg for 15 min)		
		10–20 petechiae in 5-cm circle (80 mm Hg)				10–20 petechiae in 5-cm circle (80 mm Hg)		
Triglycerides	S after ≥ 12-hr fast		***M (mg/dl)***	***F (mg/dl)***		***M (g/L)***	***F (g/L)***	
		Cord blood	10–98	10–98	× 0.01	0.10–0.98	0.10–0.98	
		0–5 yr	30–86	32–99		0.30–0.86	0.32–0.99	
		6–11 yr	31–108	35–114		0.31–1.08	0.35–1.14	
		12–15 yr	36–138	41–138		0.36–1.38	0.41–1.38	
		16–19 yr	40–163	40–128		0.40–1.63	0.40–1.28	
		20–29 yr	44–185	40–128		0.44–1.85	0.40–1.28	
		Adults: Recommended (desirable) levels				Adults: Recommended (desirable) levels		
		M	40–160 mg/dl			M	0.40–1.60 g/L	
		F	35–135 mg/dl			F	0.35–1.35 g/L	

Urea nitrogen	S, P	Cord blood	21–40 mg/dl	× 0.357	7.5–14.3 mmol urea/L
		Premature (1 wk)	3–25 mg/dl		1.1–9 mmol urea/L
		Neonate	3–12 mg/dl		1.1–4.3 mmol urea/L
		Infant/child	5–18 mg/dl		1.8–6.4 mmol urea/L
		Thereafter	7–18 mg/dl		2.5–6.4 mmol urea/L
Urine, volume	U (24-hr)	Neonate	50–300 ml/24 hr	× 0.001	0.050–0.300 L/24 hr
		Infant	350–550 ml/24 hr		0.350–0.550 L/24 hr
		Child	500–1,000 ml/24 hr		0.500–1.000 L/24 hr
		Adolescent	700–1,400 ml/24 hr		0.700–1.400 L/24 hr
		Thereafter			
		M	800–1,800 ml/24 hr		0.800–1.800 L/24 hr
		F	600–1,600 ml/24 hr (varies with intake and other factors)		0.600–1.600 L/24 hr
WBC. See Leukocytes.					

		REFERENCE RANGE					REFERENCE RANGE (SI)				
		Peak		Trough			SI Peak		SI Trough		
DRUGS	**SPECIMEN**	*Therapeutic (μg/ml)*	*Toxic (μg/ml)*	*Therapeutic (μg/ml)*	*Toxic (μg/ml)*	**FACTOR**	*Therapeutic (μmol/ml)*	*Toxic (μmol/ml)*	*Therapeutic (μmol/ml)*	*Toxic (μmol/ml)*	**COMMENTS**
Antibiotics											
Amikacin	S	20–25	>30	1–4	>8	× 1.708	34–43	>51	1.7–6.8	>14	i c
Chloramphenicol	S	10–20	>25			× 3.095	31–62	>77			c
Gentamicin	S	6–10	>12	0.5–2.0	>2.0	× 2.064	12–21	>25	1.0–4.1	>4.1	c i
Netilmicin	S	6–10	>12	0.5–2.0	>2	× 2.103	13–21	>25	1.1–4.2	>4.2	c i
Tobramycin	S	6–10	>12	0.5–2.0	>2	× 2.139	13–21	>26	1.1–4.3	>4.3	c i
Vancomycin	S	30–40	>60	5–10	>20	× 0.303	9.1–12.1	>18.2	1.5–3.0	>6.1	c i

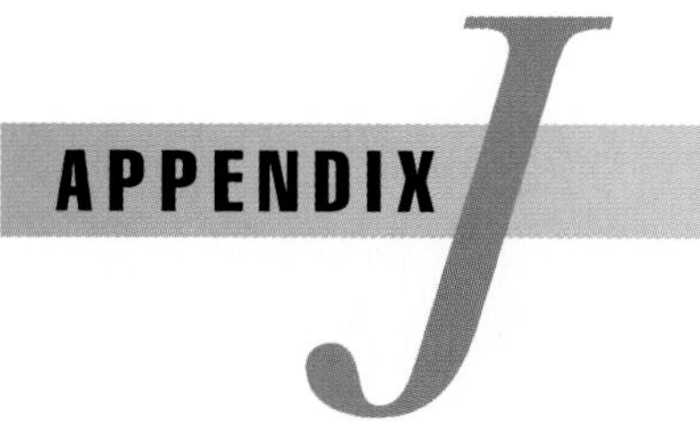

NANDA-Approved Nursing Diagnoses

Activity Intolerance
Activity Intolerance, Risk for
Adaptive Capacity: Intracranial, Decreased
Adjustment, Impaired
Airway Clearance, Ineffective
* Anticipatory Grieving
Anxiety
Aspiration, Risk for
Body Image Disturbance
Body Temperature, Risk for Altered
* Bowel Incontinence
Breastfeeding, Effective
Breastfeeding, Ineffective
Breastfeeding, Interrupted
Breathing Pattern, Ineffective
Caregiver Role Strain
Caregiver Role Strain, Risk for
* Chronic Low Self Esteem
* Chronic Pain
* Colonic Constipation
Communication, Impaired Verbal
Community Coping, Ineffective
Community Coping, Potential for Enhanced
Confusion, Acute
Confusion, Chronic
Constipation
* Constipation, Colonic
* Constipation, Perceived
Decisional Conflict (Specify)
Decreased Cardiac Output
Defensive Coping
Denial, Ineffective
Diarrhea
Disorganized Infant Behavior
Disorganized Infant Behavior, Risk for
Disuse Syndrome, Risk for
Diversional Activity Deficit
Dysfunctional Grieving
Dysfunctional Ventilatory Weaning Response
Dysreflexia
Energy Field Disturbance
Environmental Interpretation Syndrome, Impaired
Family Coping: Compromised, Ineffective
Family Coping: Disabling, Ineffective
Family Coping: Potential for Growth
Family Process: Alcoholism, Altered
Family Processes, Altered
Fatigue
Fear
Fluid Volume Deficit
Fluid Volume Deficit, Risk for
Fluid Volume Excess
Functional Incontinence
Gas Exchange, Impaired
Grieving, Anticipatory
Grieving, Dysfunctional
Growth and Development, Altered
Health Maintenance, Altered
Health Seeking Behaviors (Specify)
Home Maintenance Management, Impaired
Hopelessness
Hyperthermia
Hypothermia
Incontinence, Bowel
Incontinence, Functional
* Incontinence, Reflex
* Incontinence, Stress
* Incontinence, Total
* Incontinence, Urge
Individual Coping, Ineffective
Infant Feeding Pattern, Ineffective
Infection, Risk for

*These are duo-referenced for ease and speed in locating the correct diagnosis.

From North American Nursing Diagnosis Association (1994). *NANDA nursing diagnoses: Definitions and Classifications 1995–1996.* Philadelphia: Author.

Injury, Risk for
Knowledge Deficit (Specify)
Loneliness, Risk for
Management of Therapeutic Regimen: Community, Ineffective
Management of Therapeutic Regimen: Families, Ineffective
Management of Therapeutic Regimen: Individual, Effective
Management of Therapeutic Regimen (Individuals), Ineffective Noncompliance (Specify)
Memory, Impaired
Nutrition: Less than Body Requirements, Altered
Nutrition: More than Body Requirements, Altered
Nutrition: Potential for more than Body Requirements, Altered
Oral Mucous Membrane, Altered
Organized Infant Behavior, Potential for Enhanced
Pain
* Pain, Chronic
Parent/Infant/Child Attachment, Risk for Altered
Parental Role Conflict
Parenting, Altered
Parenting, Risk for Altered
* Perceived Constipation
Perioperative Positioning Injury, Risk for
Peripheral Neurovascular Dysfunction, Risk for
Personal Identity Disturbance
Physical Mobility, Impaired
Poisoning, Risk for
Post-Trauma Response
Powerlessness
Protection, Altered
Rape-Trauma Syndrome
Rape-Trauma Syndrome: Compound Reaction
Rape-Trauma Syndrome: Silent Reaction
* Reflex Incontinence
Relocation Stress Syndrome
Role Performance, Altered
Self Care Deficit
  Bathing/Hygiene
  Feeding
  Dressing/Grooming
  Toileting
* Self Esteem, Chronic Low
* Self Esteem, Situational Low
Self Esteem Disturbance
Self-Mutilation, Risk for
Sensory/Perceptual Alterations (Specify)
  (visual, auditory, kinesthetic, gustatory, tactile, olfactory)
Sexual Dysfunction
Sexuality Patterns, Altered
* Situational Low Self-Esteem
Skin Integrity, Impaired
Skin Integrity, Risk for Impaired
Sleep Pattern Disturbance
Social Interaction, Impaired
Social Isolation
Spiritual Distress
Spiritual Well-Being, Potential for Enhanced
* Stress Incontinence
Suffocation, Risk for
Sustain Spontaneous Ventilation, Inability to
Swallowing, Impaired
Thermoregulation, Ineffective
Thought Processes, Altered
Tissue Integrity, Impaired
Tissue Perfusion, Altered (Specify Type)
  (Renal, cerebral, cardiopulmonary, gastrointestinal, peripheral)
* Total Incontinence
Trauma, Risk for
Unilateral Neglect
* Urge Incontinence
Urinary Elimination, Altered
Urinary Retention
Violence, Risk for: Self-directed or directed at others

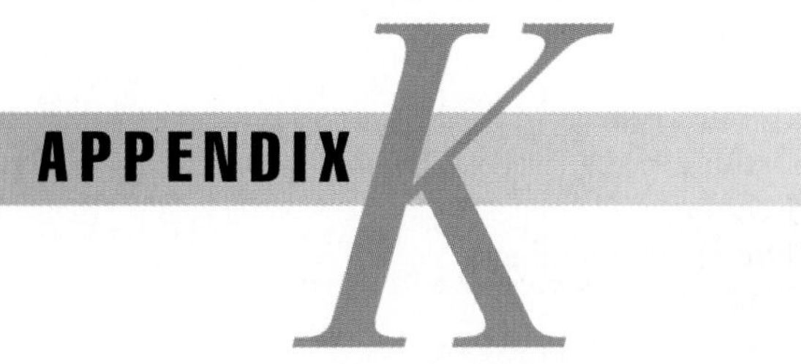

APPENDIX K

Sample Pediatric Clinical Pathways

APPENDECTOMY-PERFORATED
(Uncomplicated -without multi-system problems)
ICD-9 Codes 540.0 and 540.1

Expected LOS- 7 Days
D#.# = Key interventions for this study.

Examples of appropriate Co-morbidities
Otitis Media
Acute Sinusitis
Pharyngitis
chronic illness not in active stage

Examples of Co-morbidities that are not appropriate:
HIV
Pneumonia
Sickle Cell
Hemophilia
Immuno-compromised patients
cardiac patients
reflux
oncology diagnoses

Refer to Variance Sheet for Recording

	Admission Day	Day 2	Day 3	Day 4	Day 5	Day 6	Day 7
Aspect of Care	Date___Unit___ ED/OR_______	Date___Unit____	Date___Unit____	Date___Unit____	Date___Unit____	Date___Unit____	Date___Unit____
DAILY OUTCOME			Ambulating	NG tube out	Afebrile	Eating	Discharge *(D 7.1 If not d/c by Day 7, record on tracking sheet)*
TESTS	CBC Electrolytes (+ / -) Sonogram (if ind)	Electrolytes (+ / -) Gent level (if ind)		CBC (+ / -)	CBC (+ / -)	CBC (+ / -)	
CONSULTS	Surgeon		Consider Home Health				
FLUID/ELECTROLYTE MANAGEMENT	I&O	I&O	I&O	I&O	I&O	I&O	I&O
TREATMENTS/ PROCEDURES	Appendectomy NG Irrigation Wound Care	NG Irrigation Wound Care	NG Irrigation Wound Care	Wound Care	Wound Care	Wound Care	
MEDICATIONS	IV (pump, site check) ***D1.1 Gentamicin w/ Clindamycin q 8 hrs. Ampicillin q 6 hrs. Methadone or morphine for pain***	IV (pump, site check) ***D2.1 Gentamicin w/ Clindamycin q 8 hrs. Ampicillin q 6 hrs. Methadone or morphine for pain***	IV (pump, site check) ***D3.1 Gentamicin w/ Clindamycin q 8 hrs. Ampicillin q 6 hrs. Methadone or morphine for pain.***	IV (pump, site check) ***D4.1 Gentamicin w/ Clindamycin q 8 hrs. Ampicillin q 6 hrs. Methadone or morphine for pain.***	Hep lock ***D5.1 Gentamicin w/ Clindamycin q 8 hrs. Ampicillin q 6 hrs. Methadone or morphine for pain.***	Hep lock ***D6.1 Gentamicin w/ Clindamycin q 8 hrs. Ampicillin q 6 hrs. Analgesics p.o.***	Hep lock ***D7.2 Gentamicin w/ Clindamycin q 8 hrs. Ampicillin q 6 hrs. Analgesia p.o.***
CLINICAL SUPPORT	NPO Pain Management Parent Support Bed/Chair Extra Patient Checks Reposition q 4	NPO Pain Management Parent Support Chair Routine Safety Reposition prn	NPO Pain Management Parent Support Ambulate Routine Safety	NPO/Cl liq (+ / -) Pain Management Parent Support Ambulate Routine Safety	Cl liquid/Full liq Pain Management Parent Support Ambulate Routine Safety	Regular Pain Management Ambulate Routine Safety	Regular Pain Management Ambulate Routine Safety Pain Control Wound Care Activity Follow-up Visit
Original 7/22/1994	Revised 11/2/1995						

Disclaimer: This clinical pathway is provided as a general guideline for use by physicians and staff in planning the care and treatment of patients and their families. **It is not intended to be and and does not establish a standard of care.** Each patient's care is individualized according to specific needs.

QI TRACKING
-Ultrasound for R/O appendicitis
-Use of abdominal films
-Pt seen in ER within 7 days prior to admission
-Antibiotics
-Pain control

Cook Children's Medical Center
N:\WPFILES\COMM-MS\SURG\APPYPERF.FRM

This pathway is not a permanent part of the patient's medical record.

APPENDECTOMY-NON/PERFORATED
(Uncomplicated -without multi-system problems)
ICD-9 Codes 540.9 and 542

Expected LOS- 2 Days
D#.# = Key interventions for this study.

Examples of appropriate Co-morbidities
Otitis Media
Acute Sinusitis
Pharyngitis
chronic illness not in active stage

Examples of Co-morbidities that are not appropriate:
HIV
Pneumonia
Sickle Cell
Hemophilia
Immuno-compromised patients
reflux
cardiac patients
oncology diagnoses

Refer to Variance Sheet for Recording

	Admission Day	Day 2	Day 3	Day 4
Aspect of Care	Date___Unit___ ED/OR	Date____Unit____	Date____Unit____	Date____Unit____
DAILY OUTCOME	Ambulating	Afebrile Eating ***D2.1 If not d/c by Day 2, record on tracking sheet.***		
TESTS	CBC UA (if ind) Sonogram (if ind)			
CONSULTS	Surgeon			
FLUID/ELECTROLYTE MANAGEMENT	I&O	I&O		
TREATMENTS/ PROCEDURES	Appendectomy			
MEDICATIONS	***D1.1 Mefoxin 1 dose prior to surgery.*** ***D1.2 Analgesics***	***D2.2 Analgesics p.o.***		
CLINICAL SUPPORT	Bed/Chair/Ambulate Routine Safety Pain Management Parent Support Discharge Date NPO/Clear liq	Ambulate Activity Routine Safety Pain Management Parent Support Follow-up Visit Full liq/Reg. Pain Control Wound Care		
Original 7/24/1994	Revised 11/2/1995			

Disclaimer: This clinical pathway is provided as a general guideline for use by physicians and staff in planning care and treatment of patients and their families. **It is not intended to be and does not establish a standard of care.** Each patient's care is individualized according to specific needs.

QI TRACKING
-Ultrasound for R/O appendicitis
-Use of abdominal films
-Pt seen in ER within 7 days prior to admission
-Antibiotics
-Pain control

Cook Children's Medical Center
n:\WPFILES\COMM-MS\SURG\APPYNONP.FR4

This pathway is not a permanent part of the patient's medical record.

BRONCHIOLITIS & BRONCHIOLITIS (+) RSV
(Uncomplicated-without multi-system problems)
ICD-9 Codes 466.1& 466.1 with 07989

Expected LOS- 3.7 Days
D#.# = Key interventions for this study.

Examples of appropriate Co-morbidities
Acute Pharyngitis
Acute Sinusitis NOS
Cellulitis
Other Specific Viral Infection
Otitis Media NOS

Examples of Co-morbidities that are not appropriate
Asthma
Bronchopneumonia
Bronchopulmonary Dysplasia
Cardiac Conditions that extend the LOS
Cerebral Palsy
Cystic Fibrosis
Esophageal Reflux
HIV
Pneumonia
Pulmonary Collapse
Respiratory Failure
RSV pneumonia
Sickle Cell Anemia

Refer to Tracking Sheet for Recording

Clinical Pathway	Admission Day	Day 2	Day 3	Day 4
Aspect of Care	Date____Unit____ ED	Date____Unit____	Date____Unit____	Date____Unit____
DAILY OUTCOME		↓ nebs if tolerated ↓ O2 if tolerated	*nebs if tolerated* *↓ O2 if tolerated*	Discharge
TESTS	CBC ***D1.1 RSV prep if hi-risk**** CXR CBG if resp distress or ↑ O2 requirements Possible: Pertussis preps Chlamydia preps Viral panel	CBG if distress (↓ oxygenation) Lytes if indicated		
CONSULTS	Discharge Planner: Discharge needs & possible home nebulizer Specialist: Pulmonary or Inf Disease consult if hi-risk*		Specialist if not improved	Specialist if not improved
FLUID/LYTES MANAGEMENT	Possible IV pump I/O	Hep lock if tolerating p.o.		
TREATMENTS/ PROCEDURES	***D1.2 Albuterol Nebs q 2-4 hrs*** R.T. to wear mask Monitor O2 O2 as needed Consider epi nebs CA monitor Possible CPT	***D2.5 Albuterol Nebs q 3-8 hrs*** Wean O2 if tolerated	Albuterol nebs q 3-8 hrs ***D3.7 Wean O2***	
MEDICATIONS	***D1.3 Possible steroids (if no response in 24-36 hrs then stop)*** ***D1.4 Consider ribavirin if hi-risk. ****		Review all IV meds & antibiotics	
CLINICAL SUPPORT	Diet p.o. if RR < 60 Contact Isolation during season, even if RSV prep is (-), gown & gloves when touching patient. Emotional support for family Education: Activity Exposure (smoke) & follow-up	***D2.6 Diet p.o. if RR < 60***	Diet p.o. if RR < 60	
Original 10/10/95	Rev. Date 11/9/95			

*** AAP guideline- CHD, parenchymal lung disease, infants less than 6 weeks old, prematurity, immunodeficiency, severely ill (impaired gas exchange)**

Disclaimer: This clinical pathway document is provided as a general guideline for use by physicians and staff in planning the care and treatment of patients and their families. It is not intended to be and does not establish a standard of care. Each patient's care is individualized according to their specific needs.

Cook Children's Medical Center
N:\WPFILES\COMM-MS\CCAR\BRONCHCP.FRM

Privileged and Confidential Committee Document
TEX.REV.CIV.STAT.ANN. art. 4995b § 5.0

This pathway is not a permanent part of the patient's medical record.

SICKLE CELL DISEASE WITH VASO-OCCLUSIVE PAIN

(Uncomplicated-without multi-system problems)
ICD-9 Codes 282.62 (Sickle Cell with Crisis)

D#.# = Key interventions for this study.

Examples of appropriate Co-morbidities

Anemia
Otitis Media
Hypoxemia
Pyrexia
Respiratory Abnormality
Thrush

Examples of Co-morbidities that are not appropriate

Asthma w/Status Asthmaticus
Nephrotic Syndrome
Pleural Effusion
Pneumonia
Septicemia
Chest Syndrome

Clinical Pathway	Pre-Admission	
Aspect of Care	Date____Unit____ ED	Comments
DAILY OUTCOME	* Pain Scale	* Pain Scale Requirements to activate Pathways Faces scale >= 3 Numerical >=6
TESTS	CBC + Diff Reticulocyte Count Blood Bank Clot ***P1.1 Blood culture if T> 38.5 C*** CXR if respiratory symptoms or if supplemental O_2 is needed to keep sats >92%	
CONSULTS		
FLUID/ELECTROLYTE MANAGEMENT	***** P1.2 D5W + 1/2 NS (no KCL) at maintenance*** NS Bolus 10-20cc/kg	***<u>Maintenance fluid formula:</u>* *4cc/kg/hr for 1st 10kg* *2cc/kg/hr for 2nd 10kg* *1cc/kg/hr for each additional kg*
TREATMENTS/ PROCEDURES		
MEDICATIONS	***P1.3 Morphine sulfate 0.1 mg/kg q 2 hr PRN pain*** ***P1.4 Ketorolac: 1 mg/kg (max 60 mg) initial dose*** ***P1. 5 Ceftriaxone 50 mg/kg, for fever > 38.5° C (max dose 2 gm)*** Oxygen: ***P1.6 Pts in no respiratory distress w/ pulse ox ≥ 92% require no O_2 therapy; record variation if on O_2.*** Patients with respiratory distress and/or pulse ox of <92 %: administer O_2 2L/min by nasal cannula, increase or change to face mask as needed to SATS > 92% Wean O_2 if possible to keep SATS > 92%	
CLINICAL SUPPORT	H & P Vital signs with BP Pulse Oximetry Weight Activity as tolerated Diet as tolerated Introduction to carepath	
Original 10/03/1995	Revised 11/2/1995 Rev. 11/9/95 Rev. 11/21/1995 Rev. 12/6/95 Rev 3/6/96	

Disclaimer: This clinical pathway is provided as a general guideline for use by physicians and staff in planning care and treatment of patients and families. **It is not intended to be and does not establish a standard of care.** Each patient's care is individualized according to specific needs.

Cook Children's Medical Center
N:\WPFILES\COMM-MS\SUBS\SICKLECP.FR3

Privileged and Confidential Committee Document
TEX.REV.CIV.STAT.ANN. art. 4995b § 5.06

This pathway is not a permanent part of the patient's medical record.

SICKLE CELL DISEASE WITH VASO-OCCLUSIVE PAIN
(Uncomplicated-without multi-system problems)
ICD-9 Codes 282.62 (Sickle Cell with Crisis)

Expected LOS- 4 Days

D#.# = Key interventions for this study.

Examples of appropriate Co-morbidities

Anemia	Pyrexia
Otitis Media	Respiratory Abnormality
Hypoxemia	

Examples of Co-morbidities that are not appropriate

Asthma w/Status Asthmaticus	Pneumonia
Nephrotic Syndrome	Septicemia
Pleural Effusion	Chest Syndrome

Refer to Tracking Sheet for Recording

Clinical Pathway	**Admission Day (Incl. first 30 hrs)**	**Day 2**	**Day 3**	**Day 4**
Aspect of Care	Date____Unit____	Date____Unit____	Date____Unit____	Date____Unit____
DAILY OUTCOME				(D4.1 If not d/c by Day 4, record on tracking sheet)
TESTS	***D1.1 H/H Repeat daily until stable or baseline.*** Retic count (initially) CXR if O_2 requirement has increased or clinically worsened.	Electrolytes w/o pH. Consider LFTs if on Ketolorac		
CONSULTS	Notify of Admit By Day 1: Sickle Cell Nurse, Child Life and Social Services			
FLUID/ELECTROLYTE MANAGEMENT	**D1.2 D5W + ½ NS (no KCl). Total fluids @ 1 to 1 ½ maintenance***	D5W + 1/2 NS (no KCL) at maintenance	D5W + 1/2 NS 1/2 maintenance	*D4.2 Discontinue IV fluids by Day 4*
TREATMENTS/ PROCEDURES	Local Heat PRN	Local Heat PRN	Local Heat PRN	Local Heat PRN
MEDICATIONS	***D1.3 Continue established morphine dose 0.1-0.15mg/kg IV q 2 hrs.*** If no decrease in pain score after dose and subjective/objective assessment shows no improvement morphine infusion may be instituted. Continuous monitor while on drip. If substantial decrease in pain score after dose and subjective/objective assessment shows significant improvement, ↓ morphine to .05 to .075 mg/kg IV q 2 hrs. PRN If pain relief continues, skip to day 3 of pathway. ***Maintenance fluid formula:** 4cc/kg/hr for 1st 10kg 2cc/kg/hr for 2nd 10kg 1cc/kg/hr for each additional kg	*D2.1 Decrease morphine by 25% of established dose (IV q 2 hrs PRN)* If no decrease in pain score after dose and subjective/objective assessment shows no improvement, morphine infusion may be instituted. If substantial decrease in pain score after dose and subjective/objective assessment shows significant improvement, ↓ morphine to .05 mg/kg IV q 2 hrs. PRN If substantial decrease in pain score and subjective/objective assessment shows significant improvement, skip to Day 3 of carepath.	*D3.1 Decrease morphine by 25% of Day 2 dose (50% of original dose) IV q 2 hrs PRN)* *D3.2 Begin Tylenol #3 q 4 hrs po (dose by codeine 1-2 mg/kg) (No PRN)*	*D4.3 Discontinue morphine by Day 4* *D4.4 Time between last morphine dose and discharge.* *D4.5 Tylenol #3 po q 4 hrs (dose by codeine 1-2 mg/kg) PRN*

Clinical Pathway	Admission Day (Incl. first 30 hrs)	Day 2	Day 3	Day 4
MEDICATIONS (CONTINUED)	***D1.4 IV Ketorolac*** 1 mg/kg (max 60mg) initial dose, then 0.5mg/kg q 6 hrs x 8 doses. ***D1.5 Continue cefuroxime if febrile 50 mg/kg, for fever > 38.5° C (max dose 2 gm)*** If blood/urine cultures are +, change to appropriate antibiotic. Vistaril 1mg/kg IV q 4 hrs prn pruritus. May consider Benadryl. ***D1.6 Methylprednisolone (15 mg/kg, max 1000 mg) IV over 1 hr for severe pain, @ M.D. discretion.*** **May give x twice, 24 hours apart.** Oxygen: ***D1.7 Pts in no respiratory distress w/ pulse ox ≥ 92% require no O_2 therapy; record variation if on O_2.*** Pts w/ respiratory distress and/or pulse ox of <92 %. Administer O_2 2 L/min by nasal cannula, increase or change to face mask as needed to sats > 92% Wean O_2 if possible to keep sats > 92%	***D2.2 D/C Ketorolac.*** ***D2.3 Start Ibuprofen 10 mg/kg po q 6 hrs.*** Continue cefuroxime if febrile If blood/urine cultures are +, change to appropriate antibiotic. Vistaril 1mg/kg IV q 4 hrs prn pruritus. May consider Benadryl. ***D2.4 Methylprednisolone 5mg/kg IV if given on Day 0 and Day 1*** Oxygen: ***D2.5 Pts in no respiratory distress w/ pulse ox ≥ 92% require no O_2 therapy; record variation if on O_2.*** Pts w/ respiratory distress and/or pulse ox of <92 %. Administer O_2 2 L/min by nasal cannula, increase or change to face mask as needed to sats > 92% Wean O_2 if possible to keep sats > 92%	Continue ibuprofen If blood/urine cultures are +, change to appropriate antibiotic. If blood/urine cultures (-) discontinue cefuroxime, restart penicillin. Vistaril 1mg/kg IV q 4 hrs prn pruritus. May consider Benadryl. ***D3.3 Methylprednisolone 3mg/kg IV if given on Day 0 and Day 1*** Oxygen: ***D3.4 Pts in no respiratory distress w/ pulse ox ≥ 92% require no O_2 therapy; record variation if on O_2.*** Pts w/ respiratory distress and/or pulse ox of <92 %. Administer O_2 2 L/min by nasal cannula, increase or change to face mask as needed to sats > 92% Wean O_2 if possible to keep sats > 92%	Continue Ibuprofen Vistaril 1mg/kg IV q 4 hrs prn pruritus May consider Benadryl. Oxygen: ***D4.6 Pts in no respiratory distress w/ pulse ox ≥ 92% require no O_2 therapy; record variation if on O_2.*** Pt w/ respiratory distress and/or pulse ox of <92 %. Administer O_2 2 L/min by nasal cannula, increase or change to face mask as needed to sats > 92% Wean O_2 if possible to keep sats > 92%
CLINICAL SUPPORT	Activity as tolerated Pain Flowsheet Pain Scale q 8 hrs H & P LOC, VS with BP q 4 hrs I & O Pulse Oximetry TID if not continuous Diet as tolerated Encourage PO fluids Review of carepath with family Review of pain scale	OOB at least BID & ad lib Pain Flowsheet Pain Scale q 8 hrs H & P LOC, VS with BP q 4 hrs I & O Continue pulse ox TID if not continuous Diet as tolerated Encourage PO fluids Education regarding pain management at home: 1. Medication & nonpharmacologic interventions 2. Nutrition: Encourage fluids	OOB at least BID & ad lib Pain Flowsheet Pain Scale q 8 hrs H & P LOC, VS with BP q 4 hrs I & O Continue pulse ox TID if not continuous (if on O_2) Diet as tolerated Encourage PO fluids Education regarding pain management at home: 1. Medication & nonpharmacologic interventions 2. Nutrition: Encourage fluids	OOB at least BID & ad lib Pain Flowsheet Pain Scale q 8 hrs H & P Change VS to q shift I & O Continue pulse ox TID if not continuous (if on O_2 Diet as tolerated Encourage PO fluids Education regarding pain management at home: 1. Medication & nonpharmacologic interventions 2. Nutrition: Encourage fluids and high fiber diet
Original 10/3/1995	Revised 11/2/1995 Rev. 11/12/95 Rev. 1/15/96 Rev. 3/6/96			

Disclaimer: This clinical pathway is provided as a general guideline for use by physicians and staff in planning care and treatment of patients and their families. **It is not intended to be and does not establish a standard of care.** Each patient's care is individualized according to specific needs.

Cook Children's Medical Center
N:\WPFILES\COMM-MS\SUBS\SICKLECP.FR3

Privileged and Confidential Committee Document
TEX.REV.CIV.STAT.ANN. art. 4995b § 5.06

This pathway is not a permanent part of the patient's medical record.

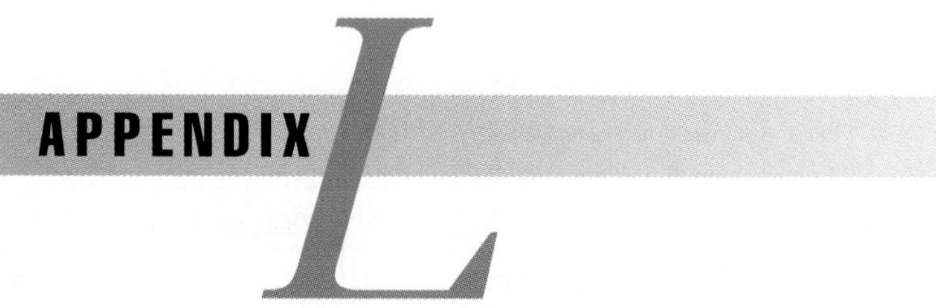

Nutrient Charts

National Research Council Recommended Dietary Allowances[a], Revised 1989: Designed for the Maintenance of Good Nutrition of Practically All Healthy People in the United States

CATEGORY	AGE (YEARS) OR CONDITION	WEIGHT[b] (kg)	WEIGHT[b] (lb)	HEIGHT (cm)	HEIGHT (in)	PROTEIN (g)	FAT-SOLUBLE VITAMINS: VITAMIN A (μg RE)[c]	VITAMIN D (μg)[d]	VITAMIN E (mg α-TE)[e]	VITAMIN K (μg)
Infants	0.0–0.5	6	13	60	24	13	375	7.5	3	5
	0.5–1.0	9	20	71	28	14	375	10	4	10
Children	1–3	13	29	90	35	16	400	10	6	15
	4–6	20	44	112	44	24	500	10	7	20
	7–10	28	62	132	52	28	700	10	7	30
Males	11–14	45	99	157	62	45	1,000	10	10	45
	15–18	66	145	176	69	59	1,000	10	10	65
	19–24	72	160	177	70	58	1,000	10	10	70
	25–50	79	174	176	70	63	1,000	5	10	80
	51+	77	170	173	68	63	1,000	5	10	80
Females	11–14	46	101	157	62	46	800	10	8	45
	15–18	55	120	163	64	44	800	10	8	55
	19–24	58	128	164	65	46	800	10	8	60
	25–50	63	138	163	64	50	800	5	8	65
	51+	65	143	160	63	50	800	5	8	65
Pregnant						60	800	10	10	65
Lactating	1st 6 Months					65	1,300	10	12	65
	2nd 6 Months					62	1,200	10	11	65

[a]The allowances, expressed as average daily intakes over time, are intended to provide for individual variations among most normal persons as they live in the United States under usual environmental stresses. Diets should be based on a variety of common foods in order to provide other nutrients for which human requirements have been less well defined. See the RDA publication for detailed discussion of allowances and of nutrients not tabulated.

[b]Weights and heights of Reference Adults are actual medians for the U.S. population of the designated age, as reported by NHANES II. The use of these figures does not imply that the height to weight ratios are ideal.

[c]RE = retinol equivalents; 1 retinol equivalent – 1 μg retinol or 6 μg β carotene.

[d]As cholecalciferol; 10 μg of cholecalciferol = 400 IU of vitamin D.

[e]α-Tocopherol equivalents; 1 mg d-α-tocopherol = 1 α-TE.

[f]1 NE (niacin equivalent) is equal to 1 mg of niacin or 60 mg of dietary tryptophan.

From Food and Nutrition Board, National Academy of Sciences, in Williams, S. R. (1994). *Essentials of nutrition and diet therapy* (6th ed.). St. Louis: C. V. Mosby.

WATER-SOLUBLE VITAMINS							MINERALS									
VITAMIN C (mg)	THIAMIN (mg)	RIBOFLAVIN (mg)	NIACIN (mg NE)[f]	VITAMIN B_2 (mg)	FOLATE (μg)	VITAMIN B_{12} (μg)	CALCIUM (mg)	PHOSPHORUS (mg)	MAGNESIUM (mg)	IRON (mg)	ZINC (mg)	IODINE (μg)	SELENIUM (μg)
30	0.3	0.4	5	0.3	25	0.3	400	300	40	6	5	40	10
35	0.4	0.5	6	0.6	35	0.5	600	500	60	10	5	50	15
40	0.7	0.8	9	1.0	50	0.7	800	800	80	10	10	70	20
45	0.9	1.1	12	1.1	75	1.0	800	800	120	10	10	90	20
45	1.0	1.2	13	1.4	100	1.4	800	800	170	10	10	120	30
50	1.3	1.5	17	1.7	150	2.0	1,200	1,200	270	12	15	150	40
60	1.5	1.8	20	2.0	200	2.0	1,200	1,200	400	12	15	150	50
60	1.5	1.7	19	2.0	200	2.0	1,200	1,200	350	10	15	150	70
60	1.5	1.7	19	2.0	200	2.0	800	800	350	10	15	150	70
60	1.2	1.4	15	2.0	200	2.0	800	800	350	10	15	150	70
50	1.1	1.3	15	1.4	150	2.0	1,200	1,200	280	15	12	150	45
60	1.1	1.3	15	1.5	180	2.0	1,200	1,200	300	15	12	150	50
60	1.1	1.3	15	1.6	180	2.0	1,200	1,200	280	15	12	150	55
60	1.1	1.3	15	1.6	180	2.0	800	800	280	15	12	150	55
60	1.0	1.2	13	1.6	180	2.0	800	800	280	10	12	150	55
70	1.5	1.6	17	2.2	400	2.2	1,200	1,200	320	30	15	175	65
95	1.6	1.8	20	2.1	280	2.6	1,200	1,200	355	15	19	200	75
90	1.6	1.7	20	2.1	260	2.6	1,200	1,200	340	15	16	200	75

Estimated Sodium, Chloride, and Potassium Minimum Requirements of Healthy Persons[a]

AGE	WEIGHT (kg)[a]	SODIUM (mg)[a,b]	CHLORIDE (mg)[a,b]	POTASSIUM (mg)[c]
Months				
0–5	4.5	120	180	500
6–11	8.9	200	300	700
Years				
1	11.0	225	350	1,000
2–5	16.0	300	500	1,400
6–9	25.0	400	600	1,600
10–18	50.0	500	750	2,000
>18[d]	70.0	500	750	2,000

[a]No allowance has been included for large, prolonged losses from the skin through sweat.

[b]There is no evidence that higher intakes confer any health benefit.

[c]Desirable intakes of potassium may considerably exceed these values (>3.500 mg for adults).

[d]No allowance included for growth. Values for those below 18 years assume a growth rate at 50th percentile reported by the National Center for Health Statistics and averaged for males and females.

Data from National Research Council, Food and Nutrition Board, National Academy of Sciences, 1989. Williams, S. R. (1994). *Essentials of nutrition and diet therapy* (6th ed.). St. Louis: C. V. Mosby.

Estimated Safe and Adequate Daily Dietary Intakes of Selected Vitamins and Minerals[a]

CATEGORY	AGE (YEARS)	VITAMINS: Biotin (μg)	VITAMINS: Pantothenic Acid (mg)
Infants	0–0.5	10	2
	0.5–1	15	3
Children and adolescents	1–3	20	3
	4–6	25	3–1
	7–10	30	4–5
	11 +	30–100	4–7
Adults		30–100	4–7

CATEGORY	AGE (YEARS)	TRACE ELEMENTS[b]: Copper (mg)	Manganese (mg)	Fluoride (μg)	Chromium (μg)	Molybdenum (mg)
Infants	0–0.5	0.4–0.6	0.3–0.6	0.1–0.5	10–40	15–30
	0.5–1	0.6–0.7	0.6–1.0	0.2–1.0	20–60	20–40
Children and adolescents	1–3	0.7–1.0	1.0–1.5	0.5–1.5	20–80	25–50
	4–6	1.0–1.5	1.5–2.0	1.0–2.5	30–120	30–75
	7–10	1.0–2.0	2.0–3.0	1.5–2.5	50–200	50–150
	11 +	1.5–2.5	2.0–5.0	1.5–2.5	50–200	75–250
Adults		1.5–3.0	2.0–5.0	1.5–4.0	50–200	75–250

[a]Because there is less information on which to base allowances, these figures are not given in the main table of RDA and are provided here in the form of ranges of recommended intakes.

[b]Since the toxic levels for many trace elements may be only several times usual intakes, the upper levels for the trace elements given in this table should not be habitually exceeded.

Data from National Research Council, Food and Nutrition Board, National Academy of Sciences, 1989. Williams, S. R. (1994). *Essentials of nutrition and diet therapy* (6th ed.). St. Louis: C. V. Mosby.

INDEX

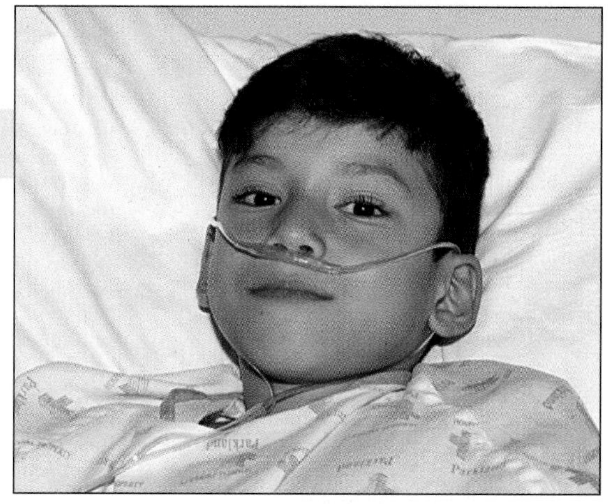

Page numbers in *italics* refer to figures; page numbers followed by t refer to tables; page numbers followed by c refer to charts.

NORMAL VITAL SIGNS BY AGE

AGE	TEMPERATURE* FAHRENHEIT	TEMPERATURE* CELSIUS	PULSE RATE (bpm)	RESPIRATORY RATE (breaths/min)	BLOOD PRESSURE (mmHg)
Newborn	96.8–99 (axillary)	36–37.2 (axillary)	120–160	30–60	Systolic: 46–92 Diastolic: 38–71
3 Years	97.5–98.6 (axillary)	36.4–37 (axillary)	80–125	20–30	Systolic: 72–110 Diastolic: 40–73
10 Years	97.5–98.6 (oral)	36.4–37 (oral)	70–110†	16–22	Systolic: 83–121 Diastolic: 45–79
16 Years	97.5–98.6 (oral)	36.4–37 (oral)	55–90	15–90	Systolic: 93–131‡ Diastolic: 49–85

*The normal range of the child's temperature will depend on the method used. Temperatures are subject to circadian rhythms in all ages.

†After age 12 years, a boy's pulse is 5 bpm slower than a girl's.

‡After age 14 years, blood pressure in boys is higher than in girls.

TEMPERATURE EQUIVALENTS *Celsius and Fahrenheit*

CELSIUS	FAHRENHEIT	CELSIUS	FAHRENHEIT
34.0	93.2	38.4	101.1
34.2	93.6	38.6	101.4
34.4	93.9	38.8	101.8
34.6	94.3	39.0	102.2
34.8	94.6	39.2	102.5
35.0	95.0	39.4	102.9
35.2	95.4	39.6	103.2
35.4	95.7	39.8	103.6
35.6	96.1	40.0	104.0
35.8	96.4	40.2	104.3
36.0	96.8	40.4	104.7
36.2	97.1	40.6	105.1
36.4	97.5	40.8	105.4
36.6	97.8	41.0	105.8
36.8	98.2	41.2	106.1
37.0	98.6	41.4	106.5
		41.6	106.8
37.2	98.9	41.8	107.2
37.4	99.3	42.0	107.6
37.6	99.6	42.2	108.0
37.8	100.0	42.4	108.3
38.0	100.4	42.6	108.7
38.2	100.7	42.8	109.0

Conversion formulas:

Fahrenheit to Celsius (°F −32) × (5/9) = °C

Celsius to Fahrenheit (°C) × (9/5) + 32 = °F